Schmidek & Sweet

Operative Neurosurgical Techniques

Schmidek & Sweet

Operative Neurosurgical Techniques

INDICATIONS, METHODS, AND RESULTS

Henry H. Schmidek, MD, FACS

David W. Roberts, MD

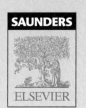

SAUNDERS

ELSEVIER

FIFTH EDITION

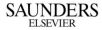

1600 John F. Kennedy Blvd.
Suite 1800
Philadelphia, PA 19103-2899

SCHMIDEK & SWEET OPERATIVE
NEUROSURGICAL TECHNIQUES:
INDICATIONS, METHODS, AND RESULTS

Part number 9997627121 (vol.1)
Part number 999762713x (vol.2)
ISBN-13: 978-0-7216-0340-7
ISBN-10: 0-7216-0340-8

NOTICE

Knowledge and best practice in this field are constantly changing. As new research and experience broaden
our knowledge, changes in practice, treatment, and drug therapy may become necessary or appropriate.
Readers are advised to check the most current information provided (i) on procedures featured or (ii) by
the manufacturer of each product to be administered, to verify the recommended dose or formula, the
method and duration of administration, and contraindications. It is the responsibility of the practitioner,
relying on their own experience and knowledge of the patient, to make diagnoses, to determine dosages
and the best treatment for each individual patient, and to take all appropriate safety precautions. To the
fullest extent of the law, neither the Publisher nor the Editors assume any liability for any injury and/or
damage to persons or property arising out or related to any use of the material contained in this book.

Previous editions copyrighted 2000, 1995, 1988, 1982 by W. B. Saunders.

Library of Congress Cataloging-in-Publication Data

Schmidek & Sweet operative neurosurgical techniques : indications, methods, and results /
  [edited by] Henry H. Schmidek, David W. Roberts.—5th ed.
     p. ; cm.
  Includes bibliographical references and index.
  ISBN 0-7216-0340-8 (set)
    1. Nervous system—Surgery. I. Title: Schmidek and Sweet operative neurosurgical techniques.
  II. Title: Operative neurosurgical techniques. III. Schmidek, Henry H. IV. Roberts, David W.
  [DNLM: 1. Neurosurgical Procedures—methods. 2. Craniocerebral Trauma—surgery. 3. Nervous System
Diseases—surgery. WL 368 S348 2006]
  RD593.O63 2006
  617.4'8—dc22

                                                              2005043215

Acquisitions Editor: Rebecca Schmidt Gaertner
Developmental Editor: Agnes Hunt Byrne
Editorial Assistant: Suzanne Flint

Printed in the United States of America.

Last digit is the print number: 9 8 7 6 5 4 3 2 1

To William Herbert Sweet, MD, DSc, FACS

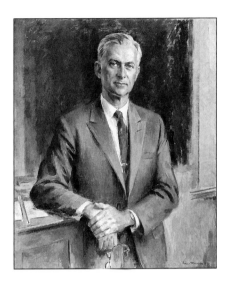

Dr. William Sweet died in his home in Brookline, Massachusetts, on January 22, 2001, after a long siege with Parkinson's disease complicated by dementia. It was as if a meteor that had traveled a lifetime of luminous miles was suddenly gone.

Dr. Sweet was passionate about astronomy, radio-astronomy, particle physics, classical music, history, and medicine, but especially those disciplines with the prefix "neuro." Life was a continual intellectual feast. It took an enormous amount of energy to feed this voracious intellect. He subscribed to, and read, each issue of over 60 journals. His private library contained at least 5000 books reflecting his interests in the basic neurosciences, neurosurgery, neurology, psychiatry, neuropathology, and surgery.

In his funeral oration, Pericles intoned, "the whole world is a sepulchre of the illustrious man." Sweet did indeed travel the world seeking knowledge at its premier clinical and research facilities. From a multitude of disciplines he translated observations into solutions of problems encountered in the nervous system.

Dr. Sweet was an intensely private person: he could be warm and charming when relaxed but he would never be confused with the touchy, feely, sensitive man now in vogue. He was a man of his own times and traditions. Like the majority of academic neurosurgeons of his generation, he grew up in rural America, was the son of a doctor, excelled scholastically, went to the local land grant university, and then migrated to one of the major east coast research universities to further his career. As a youth in Washington state his precocious intelligence and curiosity were already apparent. In high school he could easily have been made the principal and run the institution but his teachers preferred to graduate him at the age of 14. At age 18 he graduated from the University of Washington first in a class of 1000. He loved the classical piano: it was mathematical, ordered, controlled, yet creative. He also loved aviation: it was full of risks, challenge, and exhilaration. He debated being a concert pianist and considered being a naval aviator. He decided against the piano because he felt he would never attain world-class stature in this area.

In the late 1920s the major powers were all at peace so being a military officer and fighter pilot did not seem a fruitful endeavor. So when the time came for him to choose a career, he decided to follow in his father's footsteps: he became a doctor and then a surgeon. In 1930 he enrolled in the Harvard Medical School.

Dr. Cushing was at the time the senior professor of surgery at Harvard and was at the height of his fame. Between 1930 and 1932 Sweet had the opportunity to take Cushing's measure. Here was the personification of the focused, single-minded individual trying to understand and deal with pathology within the most complex system known to man—the human brain. To Sweet this was a challenge worth emulating. After his sophomore year in medical school, and with a Rhodes scholarship to Magdalen College, Oxford, he spent the next two years in Sherrington's laboratory, as had Cushing and as had Penfield.

Although he was the world's leading neurophysiologist, Sherrington stopped working and was never to return to his laboratory following the sudden and unexpected death of Lady Sherrington. As a result, Sweet found himself in England with an empty closet-sized laboratory, without guidance, and without a project. Fortunately, John Fulton and John Eccles were also in the laboratory at that time, and with their help Sweet obtained a bachelor's degree in neurophysiology rather than the doctorate he had planned to work toward. Still not sure of his path, he returned to the Harvard Medical School and at night and on weekends worked at the Boston Psychopathic Hospital so that he could gain some insight into psychiatry. After a year and a half at this endeavor he said he found this field "far too nebulous" and—with typical Sweetian syntax—"a complete morass of ignorance." Still in medical school, he did an elective rotation in neurosurgery at the Massachusetts General Hospital with Drs. Jason Mixter and J. C. White. Because one of the residents, Henry Heyl (subsequently Chief of Neurosurgery at Dartmouth and editor of the *Journal of Neurosurgery*), had left the service and the lab was short-staffed, Sweet was given a great deal of responsibility, and he thrived in this environment. This experience crystallized his decision to make neurosurgery his life's work. After graduating from medical school, six years after enrolling, he went to the University of Chicago to train with Percival Bailey, Earl Walker, and Paul Bucy. Bailey was to become his intellectual role model. Bailey was Cushing-trained in neurosurgery, he was trained in psychiatry, he was trained in neurology, and he had a doctorate in neurophysiology. Sweet was to immerse himself in these same disciplines.

After the University of Chicago Sweet returned to England to train in neurology just as England was going to war. Sweet described how within a 24-hour period after World War II was declared the National Hospital at Queen's Square removed its patients to outlying hospitals and made ready to receive the wounded. With the British neurosurgeons going into the military, Sweet volunteered to take over as *the* consultant neurosurgeon to the Queen Elizabeth Hospital in Birmingham—serving a community of 4.5 million inhabitants in the British midlands. For the next four years he enjoyed a surgical bonanza, and when needing advice with a difficult case, turned to another neurosurgeon who was to have a brilliant career, Sir Geoffrey Jefferson, the neurosurgeon in Manchester. Sweet and Jefferson shared many of the same attributes, and they were to remain lifelong friends.

As medicine had fed his mind, England nurtured his soul. He had great respect for the stoicism of the English people, and he loved England, with its beautiful Gothic architecture and its verdant and manicured gardens. He loved the controlled, understated, ever-articulate British with their droll humor. He remained a committed Anglophile and over the subsequent years made innumerable trips back to England.

In 1945 Dr. Sweet, 35 years old, returned home to the Massachusetts General Hospital ready to continue his academic career. He was to be tremendously productive and prolific. In 1961 he was named Chief of the Neurosurgical Service at the MGH and Professor of Surgery at the Harvard Medical School. I am reminded here of Winston Churchill's characterization of T. E. Lawrence: "Here was a man in whom existed an immense capacity for service. He reigned over those with whom he came in contact, and they felt themselves in the presence of an extraordinary being. They felt that the latent reserves of force and willpower were beyond measurement. When he roused himself to action, who could say what crisis he could not surmount or quell" (or, in Dr. Sweet's case, sometimes precipitate). As a chief, every day there were crises to surmount, committees to cajol, residents to be reined in, aneurysms to be clipped, research to be directed, funds to be procured, journals to be devoured, and more planes to be boarded. It just kept going and going. To this maelstrom of 110–120 hour work weeks, Sweet brought a penetrating unemotional intellect. He was also supremely confident of his surgical abilities. He raised more money for research than any other MGH surgical service. He established laboratories staffed with full-time

scientists working within neurosurgery in electron microscopy, neurophysiology, immunology, neurochemistry, experimental neuropathology, and biophysics. He transformed the MGH Neurosurgical Service from what Dr. Churchill, then Chief of Surgery, characterized as an "intellectual backwater" to a service of international renown. This did not always endear him to those around him, especially if one did not reach his standards or if someone was competing with him for resources and influence within the hospital—for he was a tough and tenacious competitor.

Sweet's qualities enabled him to attract an extraordinary group of men to train. During his 16 years as chief he trained 13 residents who became full professors and chiefs of neurosurgical services in the United States alone. He also was instrumental in the training of dozens of others who went on to distinguished careers both in neurosurgery and in the basic sciences. He provided advice to study sections of the NIH, to NASA, to the Neurosciences Research Program at MIT, and to the Brookhaven National Laboratory. He was routinely asked for advice on the careers of neurosurgeons worldwide. It was largely because of the discussions between Sweet and his friend Hugo Krayenbuhl, then Chief of Neurosurgery in Zurich, that Gazi Yasargil found himself in Burlington, Vermont, working with Pete Donaghy, and there laying the foundation of microvascular neurosurgery.

Dr. Sweet's interests are reflected in his 538 publications and 15 books. A major effort was devoted to investigating the uses of various forms of radiation to study (for example) CSF production, brain tumor localization, and treatment of glioblastomas, and to produce focal intracranial lesions. He published widely on stereotactic and functional neurosurgery in epilepsy, and in movement and behavioral disorders. He and J. C. White produced two classic monographs on the neurosurgical management of pain. To him is owed the concept of the production of focal lesions in the nervous system with the radiofrequency current. He made a major advance in the treatment of trigeminal neuralgia with the technique of differential thermal rhizotomy. He also made contributions in vascular neurosurgery: it was under his direction that the service performed the first operations on the brain at body temperatures of 24°C to 27°C. In 1954 he carried out one of the first carotid endarterectomies ever performed. He was the first to report the routine use of intracarotid pressure measurements with carotid occlusion for treatment of aneurysms. He published a remarkable series on the radical removal of craniopharyngiomas in adults. In addition, he was on the committee that defined the Harvard Brain Death criteria and devoted considerable effort to helping a large number of neurosurgeons with their medicolegal problems.

Anecdotes about Dr. Sweet abound, and everyone who spent time with him had a war story. I will share with you two of my stories. Presented with an annoying situation, Dr. Sweet could be surprisingly creative in how he dealt with it or avoided dealing with it. Consider this example, when he was called to participate in a gripe-session in which the pediatricians were to vent their dissatisfaction about the management of a case. This meeting was scheduled for a Monday morning at 8 AM in the Vincent Burnham Building of the MGH. As Dr. Sweet's resident, I arrived at 7:50 AM to meet with him in his office in the

White Building. I reminded him of the meeting—he invited me to have a cup of coffee. At 8:15 AM I again reminded him of the meeting—he suggested some more coffee. It was dawning on me that something was afoot. At about 8:20 AM we made our way down one elevator and up another and ten minutes later entered a room full of disgruntled pediatricians.

Dr. Sweet strode to the front of the room and began a monologue that had something of the following flavor: "I have just returned from the desert in New Mexico, where at an altitude of 2124 meters, a latitude of 30.4 degrees north, longitude of 107.37 degrees west, sits the world's premier radioastronomical observatory. This observatory consists of an array of 27 antennas, each antenna is 81 feet in diameter and sits on railroad tracks so the position can be changed. When dispersed this array is spread over 36 kilometers and when these antennae are combined electronically at a frequency of 43 gigaherz they give a resolution of 0.04 seconds—sufficient to see a golf ball 100 miles away." He continued this tutorial on radioastronomy. Promptly at 9:00 AM he glanced at his wristwatch, thanked the dumbstruck and silent audience for their attention, said that he had to be in the Operating Room forthwith and that he was delighted to have had an opportunity to join them at their conference. He walked out of the room. At the elevator he smiled and one could almost hear him say "check-mate."

Another anecdote involved a famous vascular surgeon who came to the MGH to present his successes with carotid endarterectomy at Surgical Grand Rounds. Sweet was in the audience along with the other MGH surgical "greats." The visitor held forth. During the discussion following the presentation this high-pitched voice emanated from the front row and it began: "Sir, could I please see slide __ again." After the mandatory fumbling at the projector, a lateral projection of a carotid angiogram with a high grade extracranial internal carotid stenosis was shown. "Well, how did this patient do?" "Oh, very well, Dr. Sweet." "Really!" There was a pause, "Tell me, do you find it a useful tactic to revascularize glioblastomas?" On the angiogram one could see a part of the head and there was the tumor blush—unnoticed by anyone else in the room.

Churchill also said of T. E. Lawrence that he was "one of those men whose pace of life was faster and more intense than what is normal, such as an airplane only flies by its speed and pressure against the air, so he flew best and easiest in the hurricane." Through this hurricane of activity, this intense pressure of life, Elizabeth assisted with the focus, structured the chaos, and found humor in the pathos. She ran the service on a day-to-day basis during his chiefship, and when Dr. Sweet left the chiefship in 1977, she traveled the rest of the miles with him. He never retired but slowed as the infirmities accumulated. His last papers were published in 1997. In describing his parents' relationship in the last years of Sweet's life, I paraphrase their son David: As his giant mind and indomitable world broke apart and ebbed away into eternity, all those around him who knew him found this terribly painful to watch. One person, Elizabeth, had the love and the strength to take care of him—at home—for every one of those difficult days. She did this so well, she knew him so well, she guarded and shielded him so well that he never fully recognized the degree of his impairment, for she could always fill in the blanks for him.

Sweet was proud of the honorary fellowships, memberships, prizes, and decorations from the world's medical, scientific, and general learned societies, and also from national governments. As he looked back over his life, he felt he had accomplished his goal: as Cushing was the dominant neurosurgeon of his era and Penfield was of his, Sweet was the leading intellect of the third generation of neurosurgeons; he was once again first in his class.

He was an extraordinary person, and it was a privilege to have known him as teacher, mentor, colleague, and friend.

Henry H. Schmidek, MD, FACS
Dartmouth Medical School
Lebanon, New Hampshire

CONTRIBUTORS

KHALID M. ABBED, MD
Chief Resident, Neurosurgery, Academic Fellow,
Department of Neurosurgery, Harvard Medical School,
Massachusetts General Hospital, Boston, Massachusetts
Surgical Management of Cerebellar Astrocytomas in Adults

DIANA L. ABSON KRAEMER, MD
Clinical Associate Professor, University of Washington,
Swedish Medical Center, Seattle, Washington
*Diagnostic Techniques in Surgical Management of Epilepsy:
Strip Electrodes, Grids, and Depth Electrodes*

CHRIS B. T. ADAMS, MChir, FRCS
Radcliffe Infirmary, Department of Neurological Surgery,
Oxford, England
Transcranial Surgery for Pituitary Macroadenomas

JOHN R. ADLER, JR., MD
Professor, Department of Neurosurgery; Director,
Radiosurgery and Stereotactic Surgery, Stanford University
School of Medicine, Stanford, California
CyberKnife Radiosurgery for Spinal Lesions

MANISH AGHI, MD, PhD
Resident in Neurosurgery, Harvard Medical School,
Massachusetts General Hospital, Boston, Massachusetts
Surgical Management of Intracerebral Hemorrhage

ARUN P. AMAR, MD
Assistant Professor and Director of Endovascular
Neurosurgery, Yale University School of Medicine,
New Haven, Connecticut
*Surgical Management of Growth Hormone–Secreting and
Prolactin-Secreting Pituitary Adenomas*

SEPIDEH AMIN-HANJANI, MD
Assistant Professor, Department of Neurosurgery,
University of Illinois at Chicago, Chicago, Illinois
*Surgical Management of Cavernous Malformations of the
Nervous System*

JOSHUA M. AMMERMAN, MD
Resident, Department of Neurosurgery, The George
Washington University Medical Center, Washington, DC
Video-Assisted Thoracoscopic Discectomy

JULIO ANTICO, MD
Professor, University of Buenos Aires; Chairman,
Department of Radiosurgery, University Hospital,
Buenos Aires, Argentina
Sphenoid Ridge Meningiomas

TOOMAS ANTON, MD
Resident, Department of Neurosurgery, Henry Ford
Hospital, Detroit, Michigan
Posterior Fossa Meningiomas

RONALD I. APFELBAUM, MD
Professor, Department of Neurosurgery, University of Utah
Health Sciences Center, Salt Lake City, Utah
*Neurovascular Decompression in Surgical Disorders of
Cranial Nerves V, VII, IX, and X*

JEFFREY E. ARLE, MD, PhD
Assistant Professor, Department of Neurosurgery,
Tufts University School of Medicine, Boston,
Massachusetts; Director, Functional Neurosurgery,
Lahey Clinic, Burlington, Massachusetts
Current Management of Cervical Dystonia

TAKAO ASANO, MD, DMSc
Professor, Department of Neurosurgery, Saitama Medical
School, Saitama, Japan
*Surgical Management of Ossification of the Posterior
Longitudinal Ligament*

ERIK-OLOF BACKLUND, MD, PhD
Professor Emeritus, Department of Neurosurgery,
Linköping University Hopsital, Linköping,
Sweden
*Stereotactic Radiosurgery for Pituitary Adenomas and
Craniopharyngiomas*

JOACHIM BAEHRING, MD
Assistant Professor of Neurology and Neurosurgery,
Yale University School of Medicine; Attending
Neurologist, Yale New Haven Hospital, New Haven,
Connecticut
Approaches to Lateral and Third Ventricular Tumors

PERRY A. BALL, MD
Associate Professor, Departments of Surgery and
Anesthesiology, Dartmouth Medical School; Staff
Neurosurgeon, Dartmouth-Hitchcock Medical Center,
Lebanon, New Hampshire
*Spinal Cord Stimulation and Intraspinal
Infusions for Pain*

JONATHAN J. BASKIN, MD
Atlantic NeuroSurgical Specialists, Morristown,
New Jersey
*Surgical Techniques for Stabilization of the Subaxial
Cervical Spine (C3–C7)*

ARMANDO BASSO, MD, PhD
Professor Emeritus, University of Buenos Aires School of
Medicine; Director, Neurosciences Institute, University
Hospital, Buenos Aires, Argentina
*Transcranial Approach to Lesions of the Orbit; Sphenoid
Ridge Meningiomas*

ULRICH BATZDORF, MD
Professor of Neurosurgery, Division of Neurosurgery,
UCLA Medical Center, Los Angeles, California
*Microsurgery of Syringomyelia and Syringomyelia Cord
Syndrome*

DONALD P. BECKER, MD
Professor of Surgery, Division of Neurosurgery, David
Geffen School of Medicine at UCLA; Director of UCLA
Neurosurgery Brain Tumor Program, UCLA Medical
Center, Los Angeles, California
Surgical Management of Severe Closed Head Injury in Adults

JOSHUA BEDERSON, MD
Professor, Department of Neurosurgery, Mount Sinai
School of Medicine, New York, New York
*Surgical Management of Spinal Cord Tumors and
Arteriovenous Malformations*

RUDOLF BEISSE, MD
Adjunct Professor, Department of Neurosurgery,
University of Utah, Salt Lake City, Utah; Head Trauma
Surgeon and Vice Chairman, Berufsgenossenchaftliche
Unfallklinik Muranau, Muranau, Germany
*Endoscopically Assisted Surgical Management of Thoracic
and Lumbar Fractures*

ALIM LOUIS BENABID, MD, PhD
Professor of Biophysics; Director, Laboratory of Neuro-
biophysics; Director, INSERM Preclinical Neurobiology,
Joseph Fourier University Medical School, Grenoble, France
Multilobar Resections in Epilepsy Surgery

LUDWIG BENES, MD
Neurosurgeon, Department of Neurosurgery, Philipps
University Marburg, Marburg, Germany
*Surgical Management of Aneurysms of the Vertebral and
Posterior Inferior Cerebellar Artery Complex*

VALLO BENJAMIN, MD
Professor, Department of Neurosurgery, New York
University School of Medicine; Attending Physician,
New York University Tisch Hospital, Bellevue Hospital,
New York, New York
*Surgical Management of Tuberculum Sellae and Medial
Sphenoid Ridge Meningiomas*

EDWARD C. BENZEL, MD
Chairman, Cleveland Clinic Spine Institute, Cleveland, Ohio
Surgical Management of Cervical Spondylotic Myelopathy

HELMUT BERTALANFFY, MD
Neurosurgeon, Professor, and Chairman, Department of
Neurosurgery, Philipps University Marburg, Marburg,
Germany
*Surgical Management of Aneurysms of the Vertebral and
Posterior Inferior Cerebellar Artery Complex*

SANAT N. BHAGWATI, MBBS, MS
Professor, Department of Neurosurgery, University of
Bombay; Senior Consultant Neurosurgeon,
Bombay Hospital and Medical Research Centre,
Mumbai, India
*Surgical Management of Fungal Infections of the Central
Nervous System*

RAVI BHATIA, MS, MCh
Professor of Neurosurgery, Department of Neurosurgery,
Indraprastha Apollo Hospital, New Delhi, India
*Surgical Management of Tuberculous Infections of the
Nervous System*

MARK H. BILSKY, MD
Attending Neurosurgeon, Memorial Sloan-Kettering
Cancer Center, New York, New York
Superior Sulcus Tumors

KEITH L. BLACK, MD
Director, Division of Neurosurgery; Director, Maxine
Dunitz Neurosurgical Institute, Ruth and Lawrence
Harvey Chair in Neurosciences, Cedars-Sinai Medical
Center, Los Angeles, California
Current Surgical Management of High-Grade Gliomas

LEWIS S. BLEVINS, JR., MD
Associate Professor of Medicine and Neurological
Surgery, Department of Neurological Surgery,
Vanderbilt University School of Medicine,
Nashville, Tennessee
*Endocrinologic Approach to the Evaluation and
Management of the Patient Undergoing Surgery for a
Pituitary Tumor*

NIKOLAS BLEVINS, MD
Assistant Professor, Department of Otolaryngology–Head
and Neck Surgery, Stanford University;
Attending Surgeon, Stanford Hospital and Clinics,
Lucile Packard Children's Hospital, Stanford,
California
Surgical Management of Glomus Jugulare Tumors

GEORGE T. BLIKE, MD
Associate Professor, Department of Anesthesia, Dartmouth
Medical School, Dartmouth-Hitchcock Medical Center,
Lebanon, New Hampshire
*Ensuring Patient Safety in Surgery—
"First Do No Harm"*

GÖRAN C. BLOMSTEDT, MD, PhD
Associate Professor, Docent of Neurosurgery, Helsinki
University; Vice Chairman, Helsinki University Hospital,
Helsinki, Finland
Considerations of Infections after Craniotomy

MAXWELL BOAKYE, MD
Assistant Professor, Department of Neurosurgery,
Stanford University Medical Center, Stanford,
California
Treatment of Odontoid Fractures

JAMES M. BORTHWICK, BSc, MB, ChB, FRCA
Honorary Clinical Senior Lecturer, University of Glasgow;
Consultant Anaesthetist, Department of
Neuroanaesthesia, Institute of Neurological Sciences,
Southern General Hospital, Glasgow, Scotland
  Surgical Management of the Rheumatoid Cervical Spine

ANNE BOULIN, MD
Department of Neuroradiology, Hôpital Foch,
Suresnes, France
  *Transbasal Approach to Tumors Invading the Skull Base;
  Surgical Management of Endocrinologically Silent Pituitary
  Tumors*

CHRISTOPHER M. BOXELL, MD
Clinical Assistant Professor, The University of Oklahoma
College of Medicine; Attending Physician, St. John
Medical Center, Tulsa Spine and Specialty Hospital, Tulsa,
Oklahoma
  Cervical Laminoplasty

ALBINO BRICOLO, MD
Professor and Chairman, Department of Neurosurgery,
University of Verona Medical School, University Hospital
of Verona, Verona, Italy
  Petroclival Meningiomas

RONALD BRISMAN, MD
Associate Professor of Clinical Neurosurgery, Columbia
University; Neurosurgeon, New York Presbyterian
Hospital, New York, New York
  Gamma Knife Radiosurgery for Trigeminal Neuralgia

GAVIN W. BRITZ, MD, MPH
Assistant Professor, Department of Neurological Surgery,
University of Washington School of Medicine;
Harborview Medical Center, Seattle, Washington
  *Craniofacial Resection for Anterior Skull Base
  Tumors; Surgical Management of Moyamoya Disease
  in Adults*

JASON A. BRODKEY, MD
Neurosurgeon, Michigan Brain and Spine Institute,
Ypsilanti, Michigan
  *Transtemporal Approaches to the Posterior
  Cranial Fossa*

JACQUES BROTCHI, MD, PhD
Professor of Neurosurgery, Faculty of Medicine, Université
Libre de Bruxelles; Chairman and Head, Department of
Neurosurgery, Erasme Hopsital, Brussels, Belgium
  *Surgical Management of Intramedullary Spinal Cord
  Tumors in Adults*

JEFFREY N. BRUCE, MD
Professor of Neurological Surgery, Columbia University
College of Physicians and Surgeons; Attending Physician
in Neurological Surgery, New York Presbyterian Hospital,
New York, New York
  *Surgical Management of Intraorbital Tumors;
  Pineal Region Masses: Clinical Features and
  Management; Supracerebellar Approach for Pineal
  Region Neoplasms*

FRANZ XAVER BRUNNER, MD
Professor, Zentralklinikum Augsburg, Augsburg,
Germany
  *Surgical Management of Trauma Involving the Skull Base
  and Paranasal Sinuses*

JOHN C. M. BRUST, MD
Professor, Department of Neurology, Columbia University
School of Medicine; Director, Harlem Hospital Neurology
Service, Harlem Hospital Center, New York, New York
  *Surgical Management of Intracranial Aneurysms Caused by
  Infection*

KIM J. BURCHIEL, MD, FACS
Professor and Chair, Department of Neurological Surgery;
Professor, Department of Anesthesiology and Perioperative
Medicine, Oregon Health and Science University School
of Medicine, Portland, Oregon
  *Deep Brain Stimulation in the Management of Parkinson's
  Disease and Disabling Tremor*

JAMES A. BURNS, MD
Assistant Professor, Division of Laryngology,
Department of Otolaryngology-Head and Neck
Surgery, University of Virginia, Charlottesville,
Virginia
  Transnasal Endoscopic Repair of Cranionasal Fistulas

RICHARD W. BYRNE, MD
Associate Professor, Rush University Medical School;
Associate Attending Physician, Rush University Medical
Center, Chicago, Illinois
  Multiple Subpial Transection for Epilepsy

PAOLO CAPPABIANCA, MD
Professor and Chairman of Neurological Surgery,
Department of Neurological Sciences, Federico II
University School of Medicine, Naples, Italy
  *Repair of the Sella Turcica after Transsphenoidal
  Surgery*

ANTHONY J. CAPUTY, MD, FACS
Professor and Chairman, Department of Neurosurgery,
The George Washington University, Washington, DC
  Video-Assisted Thoracoscopic Discectomy

FRANCESCO CARDINALE, MD
"Claudio Munari" Epilepsy Surgery Center, Niguarda
Hospital, Milan, Italy
  Multilobar Resections in Epilepsy Surgery

THOMAS P. CARLSTEDT, MD
Professor of Neurosurgery, University College London,
Consultant Orthopaedic Surgeon, The Royal National
Orthopaedic Hospital, Stanmore, England
  Surgical Management of Spinal Nerve Root Injuries

ANTONIO G. CARRIZO, MD, PhD
Professor, University of Buenos Aires School of Medicine;
Chairman, Department of Neurosurgery, University
Hospital, Buenos Aires, Argentina
  *Transcranial Approach to Lesions of the Orbit; Sphenoid
  Ridge Meningiomas*

BOB S. CARTER, MD, PhD
Assistant Professor of Surgery, Department of Cerebrovascular Surgery, Harvard Medical School; Attending Neurosurgeon, Massachusetts General Hospital, Boston, Massachusetts
Decompressive Craniectomy: Physiologic Rationale, Clinical Indications, and Surgical Considerations; Management of Dissections of the Carotid and Vertebral Arteries; Surgical Management of Intracerebral Hemorrhage

ADRIAN CASEY, MD
Consultant Neurosurgeon, National Hospital for Neurology and Neurosurgery, London, England
Innovations in Anterior Cervical Spine Surgery

LAURA CASTANA, MD
"Claudio Munari" Epilepsy Surgery Center, Niguarda Hospital, Milan, Italy
Multilobar Resections in Epilepsy Surgery

STEVEN D. CHANG, MD
Assistant Professor, Department of Neurosurgery; Director, CyberKnife Radiosurgery, Stanford University School of Medicine, Stanford, California
CyberKnife Radiosurgery for Spinal Lesions

E. THOMAS CHAPPELL, MD
Associate Clinical Professor, University of California, Irvine, University of California, Irvine Medical Center, Orange, California
Neurosurgical Management of HIV-Related Focal Brain Lesions

CLARK CHEN, MD, PhD
Post-Doctoral Fellow, Radiation Oncology, Dana-Farber Cancer Institute, Harvard Medical School; Resident, Department of Neurosurgery, Massachusetts General Hospital, Boston, Massachusetts
Decompressive Craniectomy: Physiologic Rationale, Clinical Indications, and Surgical Considerations

P. ROC CHEN, MD
Fellow in Endovascular Neurosurgery and Interventional Neuroradiology, Department of Neurosurgery, Brigham and Women's Hospital, Harvard Medical School, Boston, Massachusetts
Management of Unruptured Cerebral Aneurysms

SAMUEL H. CHESHIER, MD, PhD
Resident, Department of Neurosurgery, Stanford University School of Medicine, Stanford, California
CyberKnife Radiosurgery for Spinal Lesions

E. ANTONIO CHIOCCA, MD, PhD
Dardinger Family Endowed Chair in Oncological Neurosurgery, Professor and Chairman, Department of Neurosurgery, The Ohio State University Medical Center/James Cancer Hospital, Columbus, Ohio
Surgical Management of Cerebellar Astrocytomas in Adults

RAY M. CHU, MD
Attending Neurosurgeon, Maxine Dunitz Neurosurgical Institute, Cedars-Sinai Medical Center, Los Angeles, California
Current Surgical Management of High-Grade Gliomas

IVAN S. CIRIC, MD
Professor, Department of Neurological Surgery, Northwestern University Feinberg School of Medicine, Chicago, Illinois; Division of Neurosurgery, Evanston Hospital, Evanston, Illinois
Complications of Transsphenoidal Microsurgery

ALAN R. COHEN, MD
Professor, Departments of Neurological Surgery and Pediatrics, Reinberger Chair in Pediatric Neurological Surgery, Case Western Reserve University School of Medicine; Surgeon-in-Chief and Chief of Pediatric Neurosurgery, Rainbow Babies and Children's Hospital, University Hospitals of Cleveland, Cleveland, Ohio
Surgical Management of Tumors of the Fourth Ventricle

G. REES COSGROVE, MD, FRCS(C)
Professor, Department of Neurosurgery, Tufts University School of Medicine, Boston, Massachusetts; Chairman, Department of Neurosurgery, Lahey Clinic, Burlington, Massachusetts
Cingulotomy for Intractable Psychiatric Illness

MASSIMO COSSU, MD
"Claudio Munari" Epilepsy Surgery Center, Niguarda Hospital, Milan, Italy
Multilobar Resections in Epilepsy Surgery

PAUL R. COSYNS, MD
Professor and Chairman, Department of Psychiatry, University of Antwerp, Wilrijk, Belgium, University Hospital Antwerp, Edegem, Belgium
Neurosurgery for Psychiatric Disorders

WILLIAM T. COULDWELL, MD, PhD
Professor and Chairman, Department of Neurosurgery, University of Utah Medical Center, Salt Lake City, Utah
Surgical Management of Growth Hormone–Secreting and Prolactin-Secreting Pituitary Adenomas

SEAN P. CULLEN, MD
Instructor, Department of Radiology, Brigham and Women's Hospital, Boston, Massachusetts
Surgical and Endovascular Management of Aneurysms and Fistulas Involving the Cavernous Sinus

T. FORCHT DAGI, MD, MPH, MTS, FACS, FCCM
Department of Health Sciences and Technology, Harvard-MIT Health Science and Technology Program, Boston, Massachusetts
Management of Cerebrospinal Fluid Leaks

RONAN M. DARDIS, MD
Consultant Neurosurgeon, University Hospital Coventry and Warwickshire, Warwickshire, England
Innovations in Anterior Cervical Spine Surgery

ARTHUR L. DAY, MD
Professor of Surgery, Department of Neurosurgery, Harvard
Medical School; Program Director and Vice Chairman,
Department of Neurosurgery, Brigham and Women's
Hospital, Boston, Massachusetts
*Perioperative Management of Severe Traumatic Brain
Injury in Adults; Surgical and Endovascular Management
of Aneurysms and Fistulas Involving the Cavernous Sinus;
Management of Unruptured Cerebral Aneurysms*

J. DIAZ DAY, MD
Clinical Assistant Professor, Department of Neurological
Surgery, University of Southern California; Director,
Neurological Surgery, Hoase Ear Clinic, Los Angeles,
California
*Surgical Management of Tumors Involving the Cavernous
Sinus*

ENRICO DE DIVITIIS, MD
Professor and Chairman of Neurological Surgery;
Chief, Department of Neurological Sciences, Frederico II
University School of Medicine, Naples, Italy
Repair of the Sella Turcica after Transsphenoidal Surgery

JACQUEZ CHARL DE VILLIERS, MD
Emeritus Professor, Department of Neurosurgery,
University of Cape Town, Cape Town, South Africa
*Surgical Management of Arteriovenous Malformations of
the Scalp*

VEDRAN DELETIS, MD, PhD
Associate Professor, Albert Einstein College of Medicine
of Yeshiva University, Bronx, New York; Director of
Intraoperative Neurophysiology, St. Luke's Roosevelt
Medical Center, New York, New York
*Intraoperative Neurophysiology: A Tool to Prevent and/or
Document Intraoperative Injury to the Nervous System*

ROBERT DERUTY, MD
Professor, Department of Neurosurgery, Laennec
University, Neurological Hospital, Lyon, France
*Surgical Management of Cerebral Arteriovenous
Malformations*

HAREL DEUTSCH, MD
Assistant Professor, Department of Neurosurgery, Rush
University, Chicago, Illinois
Endoscopic and Minimally Invasive Surgery of the Spine

JESSICA KOCH DEVIN, MD
Clinical Fellow in Endocrinology, Vanderbilt University
School of Medicine, Vanderbilt University Medical
Center, Nashville, Tennessee
*Endocrinologic Approach to the Evaluation and Management
of the Patient Undergoing Surgery for a Pituitary Tumor*

HARGOVIND DEWAL, MD
Fellow, Spine Surgery, Cleveland Clinic Foundation,
Cleveland, Ohio
*Surgical Management of Degenerative Lumbar Stenosis and
Spondylolisthesis*

P. C. TAYLOR DICKINSON, MD
Good Samaritan Hospital, New York, New York
*Surgical Management of Intracranial Aneurysms
Caused by Infection*

CURTIS A. DICKMAN, MD
Associate Chief, Spine Section; Director, Spinal Research,
Division of Neurological Surgery, Barrow Neurological
Institute, Phoenix, Arizona
*Surgical Techniques for Stabilization of the Subaxial
Cervical Spine (C3–C7)*

**ZAYNE DOMINGO, MBChB(Natal), FCS(SA), MMed(UCT),
DPhil(OXON)**
Specialist Neurosurgeon, Constantiaberg Mediclinic,
Wynberg, South Africa
*Surgical Management of Arteriovenous Malformations of
the Scalp*

CHARLES G. DRAKE, MD, FACD, FRCS[†]
*Surgical Techniques of Terminal Basilar and Posterior
Cerebral Artery Aneurysms*

JAMES M. DRAKE, BSE, MBBCh, MSc, FRCSC, FACS
Professor of Surgery, University of Toronto;
Neurosurgeon-in-Chief, Hospital for Sick Children,
Toronto, Ontario, Canada
*Cerebrospinal Fluid Shunting and Management of Pediatric
Hydrocephalus*

THOMAS B. DUCKER, MD
Professor of Neurosurgery, Johns Hopkins University
School of Medicine and Hospital, Baltimore, Maryland
Circumferential Spinal Fusion (Cervical)

ANNE-CHRISTINE DUHAIME, MD
Professor of Neurosurgery, Dartmouth Medical School;
Director, Pediatric Neurosurgery, Children's Hospital At
Dartmouth (CHAD), Dartmouth-Hitchcock Medical
Center, Lebanon, New Hampshire
Craniopharyngiomas: A Summary of Data—Commentary

IAN F. DUNN, MD
Resident in Neurosurgery, Department of Neurosurgery,
Harvard Medical School, Bringham and Women's
Hospital and Children's Hospital, Boston,
Massachusetts
*Perioperative Management of Severe Traumatic Brain
Injury in Adults; Surgical and Endovascular
Management of Aneurysms and Fistulas Involving the
Cavernous Sinus*

SUSAN R. DURHAM, MD
Assistant Professor, Department of Neurosurgery,
Dartmouth Medical School, Dartmouth-Hitchcock
Medical Center, Lebanon, New Hampshire
Surgical Management of Sciatic Nerve Lesions

[†]Deceased.

JOSHUA R. DUSICK, MD
Resident and Research Fellow, Division of Neurosurgery, David Geffen School of Medicine, University of California, Los Angeles, Los Angeles, California; Department of Physical Therapy, Mount St. Mary's College, Newburgh, New York
Surgical Management of Severe Closed Head Injury in Adults

KURT M. EICHHOLZ, MD
Resident, University of Iowa College of Medicine, Iowa City, Iowa
Management Options in Thoracolumbar Fractures

ALAA EL-NAGGAR, MD
Lecturer, Neurosurgery Department, Faculty of Medicine, University of Alexandria, Egypt
Orbitozygomatic Infratemporal Approach to Parasellar Meningiomas

DILANTHA B. ELLEGALA, MD
Clinical Fellow in Surgery, Department of Neurosurgery, Brigham and Women's Hospital, Boston, Massachusetts, Department of Neurological Surgery, Oregon Health and Sciences University, Portland, Oregon
Surgical and Endovascular Management of Aneurysms and Fistulas Involving the Cavernous Sinus

PAMELA ELY, MD, PhD
Associate Professor of Medicine, Director, Lymphoma Clinical Oncology Group, Dartmouth-Hitchcock Medical Center, Lebanon, New Hampshire
Management of Primary Central Nervous System Lymphomas

JOSEPH A. EPSTEIN, MD
Clinical Professor Emeritus of Neurological Surgery, The Albert Einstein College of Medicine, Bronx, New York; The North Shore–Long Island Jewish Health System, Manhasset and New Hyde Park; Long Island Neurological Associates, P.C., New Hyde Park, New York
Far Lateral Lumbar Disc Herniations: Diagnosis and Surgical Management

NANCY E. EPSTEIN, MD, FACS
Clinical Professor of Neurosurgery, The Albert Einstein College of Medicine, Bronx, New York; Chief, Division of Spinal Neurosurgery, Winthrop University Hospital, Mineola, New York
Far Lateral Lumbar Disc Herniations: Diagnosis and Surgical Management

THOMAS J. ERRICO, MD
Associate Professor, Departments of Orthopaedic Surgery and Neurosurgery, New York University School of Medicine; Chief, Spine Service; Director, Spine Fellowship Program; Attending Physician, NYU Hospital for Joint Diseases; Attending Physician, Tisch Hospital, New York, New York
Surgical Management of Degenerative Lumbar Stenosis and Spondylolisthesis

R. FRANCISCO ESCOBEDO, MD†
Neurosurgical Aspects of Neurocysticercosis

CLIFFORD J. ESKEY, MD, PhD
Asssistant Professor, Department of Radiology, Dartmouth Medical School; Director, Interventional Neuroradiology, Dartmouth-Hitchcock Medical Center, Lebanon, New Hampshire
Vertebroplasty and Kyphoplasty

CAMILO E. FADUL, MD
Associate Professor of Medicine, Dartmouth Medical School, Dartmouth-Hitchcock Medical Center, Lebanon, New Hampshire
Management of Primary Central Nervous System Lymphomas

RUDOLF FAHLBUSCH, MD
Chairman and Professor, Department of Neurosurgery, University of Erlangen-Nuremberg, Erlangen, Germany
Surgical Management of Convexity, Parasagittal, and Falx Meningiomas

GILBERT J. FANCIULLO, MD, MS
Associate Professor, Dartmouth Medical School; Director, Section of Pain Medicine, Dartmouth-Hitchcock Medical Center, Lebanon, New Hampshire
Spinal Cord Stimulation and Intraspinal Infusions for Pain

RICHARD G. FESSLER, MD, PhD
Professor and Chief, Section of Neurosurgery, The University of Chicago, Chicago, Illinois
Primary Reconstruction for Spinal Infections; Surgical Approaches to the Cervicothoracic Junction

GEORGES FISCHER, MD, PhD
Professor of Neurosurgery, Faculty of Medicine R. T. H. Leannec; National Expert in Neurosurgery, Domaine Scientifique de la Doua, Université Claude Bernard Lyon 1, Lyon, France
Surgical Management of Intramedullary Spinal Cord Tumors in Adults

NORMAN D. FISHER-JEFFES, MD
Department of Orthopedic Surgery, University of Natal, Durban, South Africa
Surgical Management of Arteriovenous Malformations of the Scalp

IAN G. FLEETWOOD, MD, FRCS(C)
Assistant Professor of Neurosurgery, Dalhousie University; Director of Cerebrovascular Surgery, Co-Director of Stereotactic Radiosurgery, Queen Elizabeth II Health Sciences Centre, Halifax, Nova Scotia, Canada
Surgical Management of Midbasilar and Lower Basilar Aneurysms

---

†Deceased.

JOHN C. FLICKINGER, MD, FACR
Professor, Department of Radiation Oncology,
University of Pittsburgh School of Medicine; Radiation
Oncologist, UPMC-Presbyterian Hospital, Pittsburgh,
Pennsylvania
Radiosurgery of Vestibular Schwannomas

KEVIN T. FOLEY, MD
Professor, Department of Neurosurgery, University of
Tennessee School of Medicine, Semmes-Murphey Clinic,
Memphis, Tennessee
Image-Guided Spine Surgery

DARYL R. FOURNEY, MD, FRCSC
Assistant Professor, Division of Neurosurgery,
University of Saskatchewan, Royal University Hospital,
Saskatoon, Saskatchewan, Canada
Sacral Resection and Stabilization

STEFANO FRANCIONE, MD
"Claudio Munari" Epilepsy Surgery Center, Niguarda
Hospital, Milan, Italy
Multilobar Resections in Epilepsy Surgery

STEPHEN R. FREIDBERG, MD
Chair Emeritus, Division of Surgery; Chairman Emeritus,
Department of Neurosurgery, Lahey Clinic, Burlington,
Massachusetts
*Surgical Management of Cerebrospinal Fluid Leakage after
Spinal Surgery*

KAI FRERICHS, MD, PhD
Assistant Professor of Surgery, Department of
Neurosurgery, Harvard Medical School; Endovascular
Neurosurgery, Brigham and Women's Hospital, Boston,
Massachusetts
*Perioperative Management of Severe Traumatic Brain Injury
in Adults; Management of Unruptured Cerebral Aneurysms*

JONATHAN A. FRIEDMAN, MD
Assistant Professor, Dartmouth Medical School; Staff
Neurosurgeon, Dartmouth-Hitchcock Medical Center,
Lebanon, New Hampshire
*Surgical Management of Posterior Communicating,
Anterior Choroidal, and Carotid Bifurcation Aneurysms*

GERHARD M. FRIEHS, MD
Associate Professor of Neurosurgery, Department of Clinical
Neurosciences Program in Neurosurgery, Brown Medical
School; Director, Trauma and Functional Neurosurgery,
Rhode Island Hospital, Providence, Rhode Island
*Surgical Management of Injuries of the Cervical Spine and
Spinal Cord; Surgical Management of Segmental Spinal
Instability*

DAVID M. FRIM, MD, PhD
Associate Professor of Surgery and Pediatrics,
Biological Sciences Division, The University of Chicago;
Chief, Pediatric Neurosurgery, The University of Chicago
Children's Hospital, Chicago, Illinois
*Surgical Management of Adult Hydrocephalus; Surgical
Treatment of Neurofibromatosis*

AARON M. FROM, MD
Resident, Department of Internal Medicine, Mayo Clinic,
Rochester, Minnesota
*Ankylosing Spondylitis and Management of Spinal
Complications; Management Options in Thoracolumbar
Fractures*

TAKANORI FUKUSHIMA, MD, DMSc
Professor of Neurosurgery, Duke University Medical
Center, Durham, North Carolina; West Virginia
University Medical Center, Morgantown, West Virginia
*Surgical Management of Tumors Involving the
Cavernous Sinus*

MICHAEL R. GAAB, MD, PhD
Professor of Neurosurgery, Hannover Medical School;
Head, Department of Neurosurgery, Hannover Nordstadt
Hospital, Hannover, Germany
Neuroendoscopic Approach to Intraventricular Tumors

STEPHAN GAILLARD, MD
Department of Neurosurgery, Hôpital Foch, Suresnes, France
*Transbasal Approach to Tumors Invading the Skull Base;
Surgical Management of Endocrinologically Silent Pituitary
Tumors*

GALE GARDNER, MD
Clinical Professor, Department of Otolaryngology,
University of Tennessee College of Medicine, Memphis,
Tennessee
*Transtemporal Approaches to the Posterior Cranial Fossa;
Surgical Management of Glomus Jugulare Tumors*

BERNARD GEORGE, MD
Professor, Department of Neurosurgery, University of Paris;
Head, Department of Neurosurgery, Lariboisiere Hospital,
Paris, France
Meningiomas of the Foramen Magnum

VENELIN GERGANOV, MD
Department of Neurosurgery, Sofia Medical University,
Sofia, Bulgaria
Surgical Management of Craniopharyngiomas

CARL A. GEYER, MD
Assistant Professor of Radiology, Tufts University Medical
School; Clinical Lecturer, Harvard Medical School,
Boston; Neuroradiologist, Lahey Clinic, Burlington,
Massachusetts
Intraspinal Cerebrospinal Fluid Cysts

RENATO GIUFFRÈ, MD†
Surgical Management of Low-Grade Gliomas

ZIYA L. GOKASLAN, MD, FACS
Professor of Neurosurgery, Oncology, and Orthopedic
Surgery; Vice Chairman, Department of Neurosurgery;
Director, Neruosurgical Spine Program, Johns Hopkins
University, Baltimore, Maryland
Sacral Resection and Stabilization

---

†Deceased.

ALFREDO GOMEZ-AVINA, MD
Instituto Nacional de Neurología y Neurocirugía,
Mexico City, Mexico
Neurosurgical Aspects of Neurocysticercosis

SERGEY K. GORELYSHEV, MD
Professor and Chief, Department of Pediatric
Neurosurgery, Burdenko Neurosurgical Institute, Moscow,
Russia
*Surgical Management of Brain Stem, Thalamic,
and Hypothalamic Tumors*

TAKEO GOTO, MD
Lecturer, Department of Neurosurgery, Osaka City
University Graduate School of Medicine, Osaka, Japan
*Orbitozygomatic Infratemporal Approach to Parasellar
Meningiomas*

CHARLES W. GROSS, MD
Professor Emeritus, Rhinology, Departments of
Otolaryngology-Head and Neck Surgery and Pediatrics,
University of Virginia, Charlottesville, Virginia
Transnasal Endoscopic Repair of Cranionasal Fistulas

ROBERT G. GROSSMAN, MD
Chairman, Department of Neurosurgery; Director,
The Neurological Institute, The Methodist Hospital,
Houston, Texas
Temporal Lobe Operations for Drug-Resistant Epilepsy

DANIEL J. GUILLAUME, MD
Chief Resident, Neurosurgery, Roy J. and
Lucille A. Carver College of Medicine, University of
Iowa Hospitals and Clinics, Iowa City, Iowa
*Diagnosis and Management of Traumatic Intracranial
Aneurysms*

RICHARD W. GULLAN, MD
Senior Neurosurgeon, King's College Hospital, London,
England
Innovations in Anterior Cervical Spine Surgery

NIHAL T. GURUSINGHE, MBBS, FRCSE
Clinical Lecturer, Department of Neurosurgery, University
of Lancashire, Preston, Lancashire; Senior Consultant
Neurosurgeon, Preston Acute Hospitals, Preston, England
*Surgical Management of Fungal Infections of the Central
Nervous System*

BARTON L. GUTHRIE, MD
Associate Professor, University of Alabama, Birmingham
Medical Center, Birmingham, Alabama
*Neurosurgical Management of HIV-Related Focal Brain
Lesions*

JAN M. GYBELS, MD, PhD
Professor Emeritus of Neurology and Neurosurgery,
Laboratory of Experimental Neurosurgery and
Neuroanatomy, Katholieke Universiteit Leuven; Member,
Royal Academy of Medicine of Belgium, Leuven,
Belgium
Neurosurgery for Psychiatric Disorders

FUAD S. HADDAD, MD
Professor of Neurosurgery, American University of Beirut,
Beirut, Lebanon
*Diagnosis and Management of Traumatic Intracranial
Aneurysms*

GEORGES F. HADDAD, MD
Clinical Associate Professor of Neurosurgery, American
University of Beirut, Beirut, Lebanon
*Diagnosis and Management of Traumatic Intracranial
Aneurysms*

REGIS W. HAID, JR., MD
Atlanta Brain and Spine Care, Atlanta, Georgia
Treatment of Odontoid Fractures

STEPHEN J. HAINES, MD
Professor, Department of Neurosurgery, University of
Minnesota, Twin Cities, Minneapolis, Minnesota
Assessing Surgical Innovation

STEN HÅKANSON, MD, PhD
Former Head, Pediatric Neurosurgery, Karolinska
University Hospital, Stockholm, Sweden
Retrogasserian Glycerol Rhizolysis in Trigeminal Neuralgia

AKIRA HAKUBA, MD†
*Orbitozygomatic Infratemporal Approach to Parasellar
Meningiomas*

MARK G. HAMILTON, MD, FRCS(C)
Associate Professor of Neurosurgery, Departments of
Neurosciences, Pediatrics, and Surgery, University of
Calgary; Director, Division of Pediatric Neurosurgery and
Pediatric Neurosciences, Alberta Children's Hospital;
Co-Director, Surgical Neuro-oncology Program, Foothills
Hospital, Calgary, Alberta, Canada
*Surgical Management of Midbasilar and Lower Basilar
Aneurysms*

WINIFRED J. HAMILTON, PhD, SM
Assistant Professor, Departments of Medicine and
Neurosurgery, Baylor College of Medicine, Houston, Texas
Temporal Lobe Operations for Drug-Resistant Epilepsy

JOSEPH K. HAN, MD
Director of Rhinology and Sinus Surgery, Associate
Professor, Division of Rhinology and Endoscopic Sinonasal
Surgery, Department of Otorhinolaryngology–Head and
Neck Surgery, University of Virginia, Charlottesville, Virginia
Transnasal Endoscopic Repair of Cranionasal Fistulas

J. FREDERICK HARRINGTON, JR., MD
Assistant Professor of Neurosurgery, Department of
Clinical Neurosciences Program in Neurosurgery,
Brown Medical School; Surgeon-in-Charge, Spinal
Neurosurgery, Rhode Island Hospital, Providence,
Rhode Island
Surgical Management of Segmental Spinal Instability

---

†Deceased.

BRENT T. HARRIS, MD, PhD
Neuropathologist, Dartmouth-Hitchcock Medical Center,
Lebanon, New Hampshire
Frame-Based Stereotactic Brain Biopsy

GRIFFITH R. HARSH IV, MD
Professor of Neurological Surgery, Stanford Medical
School, Stanford, California
Surgical Management of Recurrent Gliomas

ROGER HARTL, MD
Assistant Professor, Department of Neurological Surgery,
Weill Cornell Medical College, New York, New York
*Surgical Techniques for Stabilization of the Subaxial
Cervical Spine (C3–C7)*

ADAM O. HEBB, MD
Resident, Department of Neurosurgery, University of
Minnesota, Twin Cities, Minneapolis, Minnesota
Assessing Surgical Innovation

CARL B. HEILMAN, MD
Associate Professor, Department of Neurosurgery, Tufts-
New England Medical Center, Boston, Massachusetts
Surgical Management of Glomus Jugulare Tumors

STEFAN HEINZE, MD
Neurosurgeon, Department of Neurosurgery, Philipps
University Marburg, Marburg, Germany
*Surgical Management of Aneurysms of the Vertebral and
Posterior Inferior Cerebellar Artery Complex*

DIETER HELLWIG, MD, PhD
Neurosurgeon, Department of Neurosurgery, Philipps
University Marburg, Marburg, Germany
*Surgical Management of Arachnoid, Suprasellar, and
Rathke's Cleft Cysts; Neuronavigation in Neuroendoscopic
Surgery*

STEPHEN J. HENTSCHEL, MD
Fellow, Department of Neurosurgery, The University of
Texas MD Anderson Cancer Center, Houston,
Texas
Surgical Management of Cerebral Metastases

JUHA HERNESNIEMI, MD, PhD
Professor and Chairman, Department of Neurosurgery,
University Hospital of Helsinki, Helsinki, Finland
*Surgical Management of Aneurysms of the Middle Cerebral
Artery; Surgical Techniques of Terminal Basilar and
Posterior Cerebral Artery Aneurysms*

SHIGERU HIRABAYASHI, MD, DMSc
Associate Professor, Saitama Medical School, Saitama, Japan
*Surgical Management of Ossification of the Posterior
Longitudinal Ligament*

PATRICK W. HITCHON, MD
Professor of Neurosurgery and Biomedical Engineering,
University of Iowa College of Medicine; Chief,
Neurosurgery Service, Veterans Administration Medical
Center, Iowa City, Iowa

*Diagnosis and Management of Traumatic Intracranial
Aneurysms; Ankylosing Spondylitis and Management of
Spinal Complications; Management Options in
Thoracolumbar Fractures*

BERND M. HOFMANN, MD
Neurosurgeon, Department of Neurosurgery, University of
Erlangen-Nuremberg, Erlangen, Germany
*Surgical Management of Convexity, Parasagittal, and
Falx Meningiomas*

BRIAN L. HOH, MD
Clinical Instructor of Surgery, Harvard Medical School;
Attending Neurosurgeon, Massachusetts General Hospital,
Boston, Massachusetts
*Management of Dissections of the Carotid and Vertebral
Arteries*

LANGSTON T. HOLLY, MD
Ruth and Raymond Stotter Chair in Neurosurgery,
Assistant Professor of Neurosurgery, UCLA School of
Medicine, Los Angeles, California
Image-Guided Spine Surgery

ROBERT N. N. HOLTZMAN, MD, PC
Associate Clinical Professor, Department of Neurological
Surgery, Columbia University School of Medicine,
New York, New York
*Surgical Management of Intracranial Aneurysms Caused by
Infection*

JOHN H. HONEYCUTT, JR., MD
Assistant Professor, Department of Neurosurgery,
University of Oklahoma, Oklahoma City, Oklahoma
*Surgical Management of Extracranial Carotid
Artery Disease*

EDGAR M. HOUSEPIAN, MD
Professor Emeritus, Clinical Neurological Surgery,
Columbia University College of Physicians and Surgeons;
Special Lecturer, Columbia Presbyterian Medical Center,
New York, New York
Surgical Management of Intraorbital Tumors

JASON H. HUANG, MD
University of Pennsylvania School of Medicine,
The Hospital of the University of Pennsylvania,
Philadelphia, Pennsylvania
Surgical Management of Sciatic Nerve Lesions

ALAN R. HUDSON, MD
President and CEO, Cancer Care Ontario, Toronto,
Ontario, Canada
Surgical Management of Peripheral Nerve Tumors

JAMES E. O. HUGHES, MD
Assistant Clinical Professor, Department of Neurological
Surgery, Columbia University School of Medicine,
Harlem Hospital Center, New York, New York
*Surgical Management of Intracranial Aneurysms
Caused by Infection*

MARK R. IANTOSCA, MD
Assistant Clinical Professor, University of Connecticut, Farmington; Director, Connecticut Children's Medical Center, Hartford, Connecticut
Cerebrospinal Fluid Shunting and Management of Pediatric Hydrocephalus

KEISUKE ISHII, MD, PhD
Associate Professor, Faculty of Medicine, University of Oita; Chief, Emergency Department, University Hospital of Oita, Oita, Japan
Surgical Management of Aneurysms of the Middle Cerebral Artery; Surgical Techniques of Terminal Basilar and Posterior Cerebral Artery Aneurysms

IVO P. JANECKA, MD, MBA
Senior Lecturer, Harvard Medical School, Brigham and Women's Hospital, Boston, Massachusetts
Anterior Midline Approaches to the Skull Base

MOHSEN JAVADPOUR, MB, BCh, FRCS(SN)
Consultant Neurosurgeon, Walton Centre for Neurology and Neurosurgery, Liverpool, England
Surgical Management of Cranial Dural Arteriovenous Fistulas

LOUIS G. JENIS, MD
Assistant Clinical Professor, Department of Orthopaedic Surgery, Tufts University School of Medicine; The Boston Spine Group, New England Baptist Hospital, Boston, Massachusetts
Surgical Management of Segmental Spinal Instability

DAVID H. JHO, BA
University of Illinois at Chicago College of Medicine, Chicago, Illinois
Endoscopic Transsphenoidal Surgery

HAE-DONG JHO, MD, PhD
Professor of Neurosurgery, Drexel University College of Medicine, Philadelphia; Director, Jho Institute for Minimally Invasive Neurosurgery, Allegheny General Hospital, Pittsburgh, Pennsylvania
Endoscopic Transsphenoidal Surgery

PATRICK JOHNSON, MD
Director, Institute for Spinal Disorders, Cedars-Sinai Medical Center, Los Angeles, California
Thoracoscopic Sympathectomy for Hyperhidrosis

FRANCIS G. JOHNSTON, MB, ChB
Consultant, St. George's Healthcare NHS Trust, London, England
Craniofacial Resection for Anterior Skull Base Tumors

ROBIN A. JOHNSTON, MD, FRCS
Honorary Senior Lecturer, University of Glasgow; Consultant Neurosurgeon, Institute of Neurological Sciences, Southern General Hospital, Glasgow, Scotland
Surgical Management of the Rheumatoid Cervical Spine

PETER JUN, MD
Department of Neurological Surgery, University of California, San Francisco, School of Medicine, San Francisco, California
Microsurgical Management of Anterior Communicating Artery Aneurysms

SILLOO B. KAPADIA, MD
Professor of Pathology and Surgery, Penn State College of Medicine, State College; Director of Surgical Pathology, Department of Anatomic Pathology, Milton S. Hershey Medical Center, Hershey, Pennsylvania
Anterior Midline Approaches to the Skull Base

AYSE KARATAS, MD
Department of Neurosurgery, University Hospital of Helsinki, Helsinki, Finland
Surgical Techniques of Terminal Basilar and Posterior Cerebral Artery Aneurysms

ANTHONY M. KAUFMANN, MD, BSc (Med), MSc, FRCS(C)
Associate Professor, Division of Neurological Surgery, University of Manitoba, Winnipeg, Manitoba, Canada
Microvascular Decompression Surgery for Hemifacial Spasm

MICHAEL KAZIM, MD
Associate Clinical Professor of Ophthalmology and Surgery, Columbia University College of Physicians and Surgeons; Associate Attending Physician in Opthalmology and Surgery, New York Presbyterian Hospital, New York, New York
Surgical Management of Intraorbital Tumors

DANIEL F. KELLY, MD
Professor of Neurosurgery, David Geffen School of Medicine, University of California; Director, UCLA Pituitary Tumor and Neuroendocrine Program; Co-Director of Clinical Brain Injury Program, UCLA Medical Center, Los Angeles, Harbor-UCLA Medical Center, Torrance, California
Surgical Management of Severe Closed Head Injury in Adults

PATRICK J. KELLY, MD
Joseph Ransohoff Professor of Neurosurgery; Chairman, Department of Neurosurgery, New York University, New York, New York
CT/MRI-Based Computer-Assisted Volumetric Stereotactic Resection of Intracranial Lesions

SANFORD KEMPIN, MD
Director of Clinical Research, Department of Medical Oncology, St. Vincent's Comprehensive Cancer Center, New York, New York
Disorders of the Spine Related to Plasma Cell Dyscrasias

SAAD KHAIRI, MD
Fellow, Institute for Spinal Disorders, Cedars-Sinai Medical Center, Los Angeles, California
Thoracoscopic Sympathectomy for Hyperhidrosis

ELENA A. KHUHLAEVA, MD, PhD
Chief Neurologist, Department of Pediatric Neurosurgery,
Burdenko Neurosurgical Institute, Moscow, Russia
*Surgical Management of Brain Stem, Thalamic, and
Hypothalamic Tumors*

DANIEL H. KIM, MD
Associate Professor, Director, Spinal Neurosurgery and
Reconstructive Peripheral Nerve Surgery, Stanford
University Medical Center, Stanford, California
*Surgical Approaches to the Cervicothoracic Junction;
Surgical Management of Peripheral Nerve Tumors*

DONG H. KIM, MD
Associate Professor, Department of Neurosurgery,
Dana-Farber Cancer Institute, Harvard Medical School;
Cerebrovascular and Skull Base Surgery, Brigham and
Women's Hospital, Boston, Massachusetts
*Perioperative Management of Severe Traumatic Brain
Injury in Adults; Surgical and Endovascular Management
of Aneurysms and Fistulas Involving the Cavernous Sinus;
Management of Unruptured Cerebral Aneurysms*

HIROYUKI KINOUCHI, MD, PhD
Associate Professor, Department of Neurosurgery, Akita
University School of Medicine, Akita, Japan
*Intraoperative Endovascular Techniques in the Management
of Intracranial Aneurysms*

RIKU KIVISAARI, MD
Radiologist, Resident in Neurosurgery, Department of
Neurosurgery, University Hospital of Helsinki, Helsinki,
Finland
*Surgical Management of Aneurysms of the Middle
Cerebral Artery*

DAVID G. KLINE, MD
Boyd Professor and Chair, Department of Neurosurgery,
Louisiana State University Health Science Center,
New Orleans, Louisiana
Surgical Management of Peripheral Nerve Tumors

SHIGEAKI KOBAYASHI, MD, PhD
Professor Emeritus, Department of Neurosurgery,
Shinshu University School of Medicine, Matsumoto,
Japan; Director, Komoro Kosei General Hospital,
Komoro, Japan
Surgical Management of Paraclinoid Aneurysms

DOUGLAS KONDZIOLKA, MD, FACS, FRCS(C)
Professor, Departments of Neurological Surgery and
Radiation Oncology, University of Pittsburgh School of
Medicine; Director, Specialized Neurosurgical Center,
UPMC-Presbyterian Hospital, Pittsburgh, Pennsylvania
Radiosurgery of Vestibular Schwannomas

ALEXANDER N. KONOVALOV, MD
Professor and Director, Burdenko Neurosurgical Institute,
Moscow, Russia
*Surgical Management of Brain Stem, Thalamic,
and Hypothalamic Tumors*

MARK D. KRIEGER, MD
Assistant Professor, Keck School of Medicine at the
University of Southern California, Childrens Hospital of
Los Angeles, Los Angeles, California
*Surgical Management of Growth Hormone–Secreting and
Prolactin-Secreting Pituitary Adenomas*

AJIT A. KRISHNANEY, MD
Resident, Departments of Neurosurgery and Orthopedic
Surgery, The Cleveland Clinic Foundation,
Cleveland, Ohio
Surgical Management of Cervical Spondylotic Myelopathy

JAMES T. KRYZANSKI, MD
Assistant Professor, Tufts University School of Medicine,
Neurosurgeon, Tufts-New England Medical Center,
Boston, Massachusetts
Distal Anterior Cerebral Artery Aneurysms

KAZUHIKO KYOSHIMA, MD, PhD
Department of Neurosurgery, Shinshu University School
of Medicine, Matsumoto; Medical Advisor, Neurosurgery,
Nadogaya Hospital, Kashiwa, Japan
Surgical Management of Paraclinoid Aneurysms

MAUREEN LACY, PhD
Assistant Professor of Psychiatry, The University of
Chicago, Chicago, Illinois
Surgical Management of Adult Hydrocephalus

SANTOSH D. LAD, MBBS, MS
Clinical Tutor, Department of Neurosurgery, Sultan
Qaboos University; Senior Consultant Neurosurgeon,
Head of Department of Neurosurgery, National
Neurosurgical Centre, Muscat, Sultanate of Oman
*Surgical Management of Fungal Infections of the Central
Nervous System*

JESUS LAFUENTE, MD, PhD
Senior Registrar, National Hospital for Neurology and
Neurosurgery, London, England
Innovations in Anterior Cervical Spine Surgery

FREDERICK F. LANG, MD, FACS
Associate Professor and Director of Clinical Research,
Department of Neurosurgery, The University of Texas MD
Anderson Cancer Center, Houston, Texas
Surgical Management of Cerebral Metastases

FRANÇOISE LAPIERRE, MD
Professor, Department of Neurosurgery, Poitiers University
Medical School; Chief Neurosurgeon, University Hospital,
Poitiers, France
Management of Cauda Equina Tumors

MICHAEL T. LAWTON, MD
Associate Professor, Department of Neurological Surgery,
University of California, San Francisco, San Francisco,
California
*Microsurgical Management of Anterior Communicating
Artery Aneurysms*

HOANG N. LE, MD
Fellow, Department of Neurosurgery, Stanford University
Medical Center, Stanford, California
Surgical Approaches to the Cervicothoracic Junction

KENDALL H. LEE, MD, PhD
Neurosurgery Resident, Dartmouth-Hitchcock Medical
Center, Lebanon, New Hampshire
Frame-Based Stereotactic Brain Biopsy

MAX C. LEE, MD
Fellow in Spine Surgery, Department of Neurosurgery,
Stanford University Medical Center, Stanford, California
Primary Reconstruction for Spinal Infections

ADAM I. LEWIS, MD
Jackson Neurosurgery Clinic, Jackson, Mississippi
*Surgical Management of Brain Stem Vascular
Malformations*

ROGER LICHTENBAUM, MD
Resident, Department of Neurosurgery, New York
University, New York, New York
*CT/MRI-Based Computer-Assisted Volumetric Stereotactic
Resection of Intracranial Lesions*

BENGT LINDEROTH, MD, PhD
Professor, Section of Functional Neurosurgery, Karolinska
Institute; Head, Section of Functional Neurosurgery,
Karolinska University Hospital, Stockholm, Sweden
*Retrogasserian Glycerol Rhizolysis in Trigeminal Neuralgia;
Spinal Cord Stimulation for Chronic Pain*

CHRISTER LINDQUIST, MD, PhD
Consultant Neurosurgeon, Director, Gamma Knife Center,
Cromwell Hospital, London, England
*Gamma Knife Surgery for Cerebral Vascular
Malformations, Tumors, and Functional Disorders*

MICHAEL J. LINK, MD
Department of Neurosurgery, Mayo Clinic, Rochester,
Minnesota
Surgical Management of Brain Stem Vascular Malformations

KENNETH LITTLE, MD
Chief Resident, Division of Neurosurgery, Duke University
Medical Center, Durham, North Carolina
*Spinal Infections: Vertebral Osteomyelitis and Spinal
Epidural Abscess*

ALI LIU, MD
Professor, Capital University of Medical Sciences; Chief
Doctor, The Gamma Knife Center, Beijing Neurosurgical
Institute, Beijing, China
*Surgical Management of Nonglomus Tumors of the Jugular
Foramen*

JAMES K. LIU, MD
Department of Neurosurgery, University of Utah School of
Medicine, Salt Lake City, Utah
*Surgical Management of Growth Hormone–Secreting and
Prolactin-Secreting Pituitary Adenomas*

GIORGIO LO RUSSO, MD
Chief, "Claudio Munari" Epilepsy Surgery Center,
Niguarda Hospital, Milan, Italy
Multilobar Resections in Epilepsy Surgery

CHRISTOPHER M. LOFTUS, MD
Professor and Chair, Department of Neurosurgery,
Temple University Hospital, Philadelphia,
Pennsylvania
*Surgical Management of Extracranial
Carotid Artery Disease*

S. SCOTT LOLLIS, MD
Division of Neurosurgery, Dartmouth Medical School,
Dartmouth-Hitchcock Medical Center, Lebanon,
New Hampshire
Entrapment Neuropathies of the Lower Extremities

DONLIN M. LONG, MD, PhD
Distinguished Service Professor, Department of
Neurosurgery, Johns Hopkins University, Johns Hopkins
Hospital, Baltimore, Maryland
*Management of Persistent Symptoms after Lumbar
Disc Surgery*

RUSSELL R. LONSER, MD
Staff Neurosurgeon, Surgical Neurology Branch,
National Institute of Neurological Disorders
and Stroke, National Institutes of Health, Bethesda,
Maryland
*Neurovascular Decompression in Surgical Disorders of
Cranial Nerves V, VII, IX, and X*

WOLF LÜDEMANN, MD
Consultant, International Neuroscience Institute (INI),
Hannover, Germany
Surgical Management of Craniopharyngiomas

L. DADE LUNSFORD, MD, FACS
Professor and Chair, Department of Neurological Surgery,
University of Pittsburgh School of Medicine; Chair,
Department of Neurological Surgery, UPMC-Presbyterian
Hospital, Pittsburgh, Pennsylvania
Radiosurgery of Vestibular Schwannomas

JOSEPH R. MADSEN, MD
Associate Professor of Surgery, Harvard School of
Medicine, Children's Hospital, Bringham and Women's
Hospital, Boston, Massachusetts
*Treatment of Intractable Epilepsy by Electrical Stimulation
of the Vagus Nerve*

SUBU N. MAGGE, MD
Assistant Professor, Tufts University School of
Medicine, Boston; Lahey Clinic, Burlington, Massachusetts
Microsurgery of Ruptured Lumbar Intervertebral Disc

ASHOK K. MAHAPATRA, MBBS, MS, MCh
Professor, Department of Neurosurgery, All India Institute
of Medical Sciences, New Delhi, India
*Surgical Management of Fungal Infections of the Central
Nervous System*

KHALID MAHLA, MD
Assistant, Faculty of Medicine R. T. H. Laennec, Université Claude Bernard Lyon 1; Assistant, Neurochirurgie "B", Hôpital Neurologique et Neurochirurgical Pierre Wertheimer, Lyon, France
Surgical Management of Intramedullary Spinal Cord Tumors in Adults

ROBERTO MAI, MD
"Claudio Munari" Epilepsy Surgery Center, Niguarda Hospital, Milan, Italy
Multilobar Resections in Epilepsy Surgery

GIULIO MAIRA, MD
Professor and Department Head, Department of Neurosurgery, Catholic University School of Medicine, Rome, Italy
Surgical Management of Lesions of the Clivus

DAVID G. MALONE, MD
Neurosurgeon, Oklahoma Spine and Brain Institute, Tulsa, Oklahoma
Cervical Laminoplasty

MITCHELL D. MARTINEAU, MS
Oklahoma Spine and Brain Institute, Tulsa, Oklahoma
Cervical Laminoplasty

ROBERT L. MARTUZA, MD
Professor of Surgery, Harvard Medical School; Chief, Neurosurgical Service, Massachusetts General Hospital, Boston, Massachusetts
Surgical Management of Olfactory Groove Meningiomas; Suboccipital Transmeatal Approach to Vestibular Schwannoma

JOHN E. McGILLICUDDY, MD
Professor of Neurosurgery and Orthopedics, University of Michigan, University of Michigan Hospitals, Ann Arbor, Michigan
Thoracic Outlet Syndrome

ARNOLD H. MENEZES, MD, FACS, FAAP
Professor and Vice Chairman, Department of Neurosurgery, Roy J. and Lucille A. Carter College of Medicine; Professor of Neurosurgery, University of Iowa Hospitals and Clinics, Iowa City, Iowa
Craniovertebral Abnormalities and Their Neurosurgical Management; Ankylosing Spondylitis and Management of Spinal Complications

ALI H. MESIWALA, MD
Maxine Dunitz Neurosugical Institute, Cedars-Sinai Medical Center, Los Angeles, California
Surgical Management of Moyamoya Disease in Adults

FREDRIC B. MEYER, MD
Professor and Chair, Department of Neurologic Surgery, Mayo Clinic College of Medicine, Rochester, Minnesota
Surgical Management of Lesions in Eloquent Areas of Brain

JONATHAN P. MILLER, MD
Resident, University Hospitals of Cleveland, Cleveland, Ohio
Surgical Management of Tumors of the Fourth Ventricle

JOHN MISLOW, MD
Resident, Department of Neurological Surgery, Harvard Medical School, Brigham and Women's Hospital, Boston, Massachusetts
Primary Reconstruction for Spinal Infections

KAZUO MIZOI, MD
Professor and Chairman, Department of Neurosurgery, Akita University School of Medicine, Akita, Japan
Intraoperative Endovascular Techniques in the Management of Intracranial Aneurysms

A. ALEX MOHIT, MD, PhD
Resident, Department of Neurological Surgery, University of Washington School of Medicine, Seattle, Washington
Craniofacial Resection for Anterior Skull Base Tumors

CHAD J. MORGAN, MD
Chief Resident, Department of Neurosurgery, University of Cincinnati College of Medicine, Cincinnati, Ohio
Percutaneous Stereotactic Rhizotomy in the Treatment of Intractable Facial Pain

PRAVEEN V. MUMMANENI, MD
Assistant Professor, Neurosurgery, Emory University, Atlanta, Georgia
Treatment of Odontoid Fractures

CLAUDIO MUNARI, MD[†]
Multilobar Resections in Epilepsy Surgery

AURANGZEB NAGY, MD
Department of Neurosurgery, University Medical Center, Las Vegas, Nevada
Surgical Management of Peripheral Nerve Tumors

DAVID W. NEWELL, MD
Executive Director, Swedish Neurological Institute, Seattle, Washington
Surgical Management of Moyamoya Disease in Adults

MIKA NIEMELÄ, MD
Professor and Chairman, Department of Neurosurgery, University Hospital of Helsinki, Helsinki, Finland
Surgical Techniques of Terminal Basilar and Posterior Cerebral Artery Aneurysms

DIMITRIOS C. NIKAS, MD
Division of Neurosurgery, Dartmouth Medical School, Dartmouth-Hitchcock Medical Center, Lebanon, New Hampshire
Entrapment Neuropathies of the Lower Extremities

LINO NOBILI, MD
"Claudio Munari" Epilepsy Surgery Center, Niguarda Hospital, Milan, Italy
Multilobar Resections in Epilepsy Surgery

[†]Deceased.

RICHARD B. NORTH, MD
Professor, Departments of Neurosurgery, Anesthesiology, and Critical Care Medicine; Director, Functional Spinal Neurosurgery, Department of Neurosurgery, Johns Hopkins University School of Medicine, Baltimore, Maryland
Spinal Cord Stimulation for Chronic Pain

W. JERRY OAKES, MD
Professor of Neurosurgery and Pediatrics, University of Alabama at Birmingham, Children's Hospital, Birmingham, Alabama
Tethered Cord Syndrome in the Adult

JOACHIM M. K. OERTEL, MD, PhD
Associate Professor of Neurosurgery, Hannover Medical School; Attending Neurosurgeon, Department of Neurosurgery, Hannover Norstadt Hospital, Hannover, Germany
Neuroendoscopic Approach to Intraventricular Tumors

CHRISTOPHER S. OGILVY, MD
Professor of Neurosurgery, Harvard Medical School; Attending Neurosurgeon, Director of Cerebrovascular Surgery, Massachusetts General Hospital, Boston, Massachusetts
Decompressive Craniectomy: Physiologic Rationale, Clinical Indications, and Surgical Considerations; Management of Dissections of the Carotid and Vertebral Arteries; Surgical Management of Intracerebral Hemorrhage; Surgical Management of Cavernous Malformations of the Nervous System

KENJI OHATA, MD
Associate Professor, Department of Neurosurgery, Osaka City University Graduate School of Medicine, Osaka, Japan
Orbitozygomatic Infratemporal Approach to Parasellar Meningiomas

ROBERT G. OJEMANN, MD
Professor, Department of Neurosurgery, Harvard Medical School; Visiting Neurosurgeon, Massachusetts General Hospital, Boston, Massachusetts
Surgical Management of Olfactory Groove Meningiomas; Suboccipital Transmeatal Approach to Vestibular Schwannoma; Surgical Management of Cavernous Malformations of the Nervous System

EDWARD H. OLDFIELD, MD
Chief, Surgical Neurology Branch, National Institute of Neurological Disorders and Stroke, National Institutes of Health, Bethesda, Maryland
Management of Cushing's Disease

S. BULENT OMAY, MD
Resident, Department of Neurosurgery, Yale University School of Medicine, New Haven, Connecticut
Approaches to Lateral and Third Ventricular Tumors

RICHARD K. OSENBACH, MD
Assistant Professor, Division of Neurological Surgery, Duke University Medical Center, Durham, North Carolina
Spinal Infections: Vertebral Osteomyelitis and Spinal Epidural Abscess

ROBERTO PALLINI, MD
Assistant Professor, Department of Neurosurgery, Catholic University School of Medicine, Rome, Italy
Surgical Management of Lesions of the Clivus

JON PARK, MD
Assistant Professor, Stanford University, Stanford, California
Surgical Approaches to the Cervicothoracic Junction

MICHAEL C. PARK, MD, PhD
Neurosurgery Resident, Department of Clinical Neurosciences Program in Neurosurgery, Brown Medical School, Rhode Island Hospital, Providence, Rhode Island
Surgical Management of Segmental Spinal Instability

FRANCESCO S. PASTORE, MD
Assistant Professor, Institute of Neurosurgery, Department of Neuroscience, University of Rome "Tor Vergata," Rome, Italy
Surgical Management of Low-Grade Gliomas

RANA PATIR, MS, MCh (Neurosurg)
Senior Consultant, Sir Ganga Ram Hospital, New Delhi, India
Surgical Management of Tuberculous Infections of the Nervous System

SANJAY J. PAWAR, MBBS, MS, MCh
Visiting Consultant Neurosurgeon, Wanless Hospital, Meeraj Medical College; Consultant Neurosurgeon, Poona Hospital, Ruby-Hall Hospital, Jahangir Hospital, Maharastra, India
Surgical Management of Fungal Infections of the Central Nervous System

SYDNEY J. PEERLESS, MD
Retired, Punta Gorda, Florida
Surgical Techniques of Terminal Basilar and Posterior Cerebral Artery Aneurysms

ISABELLE PELISSOU-GUYOTAT, MD, PhD
Head, Department of Emergency Neurosurgery, Neurological Hospital, Lyon, France
Surgical Management of Cerebral Arteriovenous Malformations

PAUL M. PELOSO, MD
Associate Professor, Department of Internal Medicine, University of Iowa Hospitals and Clinics, Iowa City, Iowa
Ankylosing Spondylitis and Management of Spinal Complications

PHILIPPE PENCALET, MD
Department of Neurosurgery, Hôpital Foch, Suresnes,
France
*Transbasal Approach to Tumors Invading the Skull Base;
Surgical Management of Endocrinologically Silent Pituitary
Tumors*

RICHARD PENN, MD
Professor of Neurosurgery, The University of Chicago,
Chicago, Illinois
Surgical Management of Adult Hydrocephalus

NOEL PERIN, MD
Director, Spine and Minimally Invasive Surgery,
Department of Neurosurgery, St. Luke's-Roosevelt
Hospital Center, New York, New York
*Surgical Management of Spinal Cord Tumors and
Arteriovenous Malformations*

MARK A. PICHELMANN, MD
Chief Resident Associate, Department of Neurologic
Surgery, Mayo School of Graduate Medical Education;
Chief Resident of Neurologic Surgery, Mayo Clinic
College of Medicine, Rochester, Minnesota
*Surgical Management of Lesions in Eloquent
Areas of Brain*

JOSEPH PIEPMEIER, MD
Professor, Yale University School of Medicine,
New Haven, Connecticut
Approaches to Lateral and Third Ventricular Tumors

JOHN M. D. PILE-SPELLMAN, MD
Professor, Departments of Radiology, Neurological Surgery,
and Neurology; Director, Academic Interventional
Neuroradiology; Vice-Chair of Research, Department of
Radiology, Colombia University School of Medicine,
New York, New York
*Surgical Management of Intracranial Aneurysms
Caused by Infection*

RICK J. PLACIDE, MD, PT
Spinal and Orthopaedic Surgeon, West End Orthopaedic
Clinic, Richmond, Virginia
*Surgical Management of Cervical Spondylotic
Myelopathy*

CHARLES E. POLETTI, MD
Hartford Hospital, Hartford, Connecticut
Open Cordotomy and Medullary Tractotomy

KALMON D. POST, MD
Department of Neurosurgery, Mount Sinai School of
Medicine, New York, New York
*Surgical Management of Spinal Cord Tumors and
Arteriovenous Malformations*

LARS POULSGAARD, MD
Associate Professor, University Clinic of Neurosurgery,
The Neuroscience Center, University of Copenhagen,
Copenhagen, Denmark
Translabyrinthine Approach to Vestibular Schwannomas

PATRICIA B. QUEBADA, MD
Resident, Section of Neurosurgery, Dartmouth-Hitchcock
Medical Center, Lebanon, New Hampshire
*Surgical Management of Chronic Subdural Hematoma in
Adults*

ALFREDO QUIÑONES-HINOJOSA, MD
Resident, Department of Neurological Surgery, University
of California School of Medicine, San Francisco, California
*Microsurgical Management of Anterior Communicating
Artery Aneurysms*

ANTONINO RACO, MD
Associate Professor of Neurosurgery, Department of
Neurolocal Sciences, "La Sapienza" Univeristy of Rome;
Policlinico Umberto I, Rome, Italy
*Surgical Management of Cerebellar Hemorrhage and
Cerebellar Infarction*

JOHN RATLIFF, MD
Assistant Professor, Department of Neurosurgery,
Rush University, Chicago, Illinois
Endoscopic and Minimally Invasive Surgery of the Spine

AFSHIN E. RAZI, MD
Assistant Professor, Department of Orthopaedic Surgery,
New York University School of Medicine; Attending
Physician, NYU Medical Center, Hospital for Joint
Diseases, New York, New York
*Surgical Management of Degenerative Lumbar Stenosis and
Spondylolisthesis*

JAAKKO RINNE, MD, PhD
Associate Professor of Neurosurgery, Faculty of Medicine,
University of Kuopio; Head of Division, Director,
Neurovascular Surgery Group, Department of
Neurosurgery, Kuopio University Hospital, Kuopio,
Finland
*Surgical Management of Aneurysms of the Middle Cerebral
Artery*

DAVID W. ROBERTS, MD
Professor of Surgery (Neurosurgery), Alma Hass Milham
Distinguished Chair in Clinical Medicine, Dartmouth
Medical School, Hanover; Chief, Section of Neurosurgery,
Dartmouth-Hitchcock Medical Center, Lebanon,
New Hampshire
*Frame-Based Stereotactic Brain Biopsy; Section of the
Corpus Callosum for Epilepsy*

JON H. ROBERTSON, MD
Professor and Chairman, Department of Neurosurgery,
University of Tennessee College of Medicine; Member,
Semmes-Murphey Neurologic and Spine Institute,
Memphis, Tennessee
*Transtemporal Approaches to the Posterior Cranial Fossa;
Surgical Management of Glomus Jugulare Tumors*

JACK P. ROCK, MD
Senior Neurosurgical Staff, Henry Ford Hospital,
Detroit, Michigan
Posterior Fossa Meningiomas

GERALD E. RODTS, JR., MD
Professor, Neurosurgery, Emory University, Atlanta, Georgia
Treatment of Odontoid Fractures

AXEL ROMINGER, MD
Treatment of Intractable Epilepsy by Electrical Stimulation of the Vagus Nerve

SETH I. ROSENBERG, MD
Clinical Assistant Professor, University of Pennsylvania, Philadelphia, Pennsylvania; Clinical Assistant Professor, University of South Florida; Sarasota Memorial Hospital, Lakewood Ranch Hospital, Venice Hospital, Sarasota, Florida
Vestibular Nerve Section in the Management of Intractable Vertigo

GUY ROSENTHAL, MD
Clinical Instructor, Department of Neurosurgery, Hebrew University Medical School, Hadassah University Hospital, Jerusalem, Israel
Penetrating Brain Injuries

SALVADOR RUIZ-GONZALEZ
Mexico City, Mexico
Neurosurgical Aspects of Neurocysticercosis

STEPHEN M. RUSSELL, MD
Assistant Professor, Department of Neurosurgery, New York University School of Medicine, New York, New York
Surgical Management of Tuberculum Sellae and Medial Sphenoid Ridge Meningiomas

SAMUEL RYU, MD
Senior Staff, Director, Center for Radiosurgery, Departments of Radiation Oncology and Neurosurgery, Henry Ford Hospital, Detroit, Michigan
Posterior Fossa Meningiomas

STEPHEN I. RYU, MD
Resident, Department of Neurosurgery, Stanford University School of Medicine, Stanford, California
CyberKnife Radiosurgery for Spinal Lesions

FRANCESCO SALA, MD
Attending Physician, Neurosurgeon, Department of Neurological Sciences and Vision, Verona University Hospital, Verona, Italy
Intraoperative Neurophysiology: A Tool to Prevent and/or Document Intraoperative Injury to the Nervous System

AMIR SAMII, MD, PhD
Associate Professor, Department of Neurosurgery, Medical School of Hannover; Vice Director, Department of Neurosurgery, International Neuroscience Institute (INI), Hannover, Germany
Surgical Management of Craniopharyngiomas

MADJID SAMII, MD, PhD
President, International Neuroscience Institute (INI), Hannover, Germany
Surgical Management of Craniopharyngiomas

PRAKASH SAMPATH, MD
Assistant Professor, Brown University, Rhode Island Hospital, Providence, Rhode Island
Surgical Management of Injuries of the Cervical Spine and Spinal Cord

RENE O. SANCHEZ-MEJIA, MD
Resident, University of California at San Francisco, San Francisco, California
Microsurgical Management of Anterior Communicating Artery Aneurysms

KEIJI SANO, MD
Emeritus Professor, Department of Neurosurgery, University of Tokyo; Director, Fuji Brain Institute Hospital, Fujinomiya City, Japan
Alternate Surgical Approaches to Pineal Region Neoplasms

IVANA SARTORI, MD
"Claudio Munari" Epilepsy Surgery Center, Niguarda Hospital, Milan, Italy
Multilobar Resections in Epilepsy Surgery

PAUL D. SAWIN, MD
Florida Neurosurgical Consultants, PA, Orlando, Florida
Surgical Techniques for Stabilization of the Subaxial Cervical Spine (C3–C7)

ALEXANDRA K. SCHMIDEK, MD
Division of Plastic Surgery, Department of Surgery, Harvard Medical School, Massachusetts General Hospital, Boston, Massachusetts
Surgical Management of Median Nerve Compression at the Wrist by Open Technique

HENRY H. SCHMIDEK, MD, FACS
Senior Neurosurgeon, Dartmouth-Hitchcock Medical Center, Dartmouth Medical School, Lebanon, New Hampshire
Surgical Management of Chronic Subdural Hematoma in Adults; Suppurative Intracranial Infections

HENRY W. S. SCHROEDER, MD, PhD
Professor of Neurosurgery; Director, Department of Neurosurgery, Ernst-Moritz-Arndt-Universität, Greifswald, Germany
Neuroendoscopic Approach to Intraventricular Tumors

DIRK MICHAEL SCHULTE, MD
Resident and Instructor, Department of Neurosurgery, Philipps University Marburg, Marburg, Germany
Surgical Management of Arachnoid, Suprasellar, and Rathke's Cleft Cysts; Neuronavigation in Neuroendoscopic Surgery

VOLKER SEIFERT, MD, PhD
Director, Klinik und Poliklinik für Neurochirurgie, Johann Wolfgang Goethe-Universität, Frankfurt, Germany
Anterior Approaches in Multisegmental Cervical Spondylosis

RICARDO SEGAL, MD
Senior Neurosurgeon, Department of Neurosurgery, Hadassah University Hospital, Jerusalem, Israel
Penetrating Brain Injuries

DILIP K. SENGUPTA, MD, PhD
Department of Orthopaedics, Spine Center, Dartmouth-Hitchcock Medical Center, Lebanon, New Hampshire
Ankylosing Spondylitis and Management of Spinal Complications

REWATI RAMAN SHARMA, MBBS, MS, DNB
Clinical Tutor, Department of Neurosurgery, Sultan Qaboos University; Chairman, Staff Development; Senior Consultant Neurosurgeon, National Neurosurgical Centre, Khoula Hospital, Muscat, Sultanate of Oman
Surgical Management of Fungal Infections of the Central Nervous System

JASON SHEEHAN, MD, PhD
Assistant Professor of Neurological Surgery and Neuroscience, University of Virginia, Charlottesville, Virginia
Gamma Knife Surgery for Cerebral Vascular Malformations, Tumors, and Functional Disorders

BASSEM SHEIKH, MD, FRCS, FKFU(NS)
Associate Professor, Department of Neurosurgery, King Faisal University, Dammam, Saudi Arabia; Consultant Neurosurgeon and Acting Chairman, Department of Neurosurgery, King Fahd Teaching Hospital, Al-Khobar, Saudi Arabia
Orbitozygomatic Infratemporal Approach to Parasellar Meningiomas

HU SHEN, MD
Senior Neurosurgeon, Department of Neurosurgery, Nanshan Hospital, Shenzhen, Guangdong, China
Surgical Management of Aneurysms of the Middle Cerebral Artery

MASATO SHIBUYA, MD, PhD
Clinical Professor, Nagoya University School of Medicine, Director, Chukyo Hospital, Nagoya, Japan
Surgical Management of Paraclinoid Aneurysms

PRISCILLA SHORT, MD
Clinical Associate in Neurosurgery, The University of Chicago Pritzker School of Medicine, Chicago, Illinois
Surgical Treatment of Neurofibromatosis

WILLIAM A. SHUCART, MD
Professor and Chair, Department of Neurosurgery, Tufts University School of Medicine, Chief of Neurosurgery, Tufts-New England Medical Center, Boston, Massachusetts
Distal Anterior Cerebral Artery Aneurysms

ADRIAN M. SIEGEL, MD
Department of Neurology, University Hospital of Zurich, Zurich, Switzerland
Section of the Corpus Callosum for Epilepsy

HERBERT SILVERSTEIN, MD
Clinical Professor of Otorhinolaryngology, University of Pennsylvania School of Medicine, Philadelphia, Pennsylvania; University of South Florida, Sarasota Memorial Hospital, Sarasota, Florida
Vestibular Nerve Section in the Management of Intractable Vertigo

NATHAN E. SIMMONS, MD
Assistant Professor, Section of Neurosurgery, Dartmouth-Hitchcock Medical Center, Lebanon, New Hampshire
Surgical Techniques in the Management of Thoracic Disc Herniations

MARC P. SINDOU, MD, DSc
Professor, Department of Neurosurgery, University of Lyon Medical School: Chairman, Department of Neurosurgery, Hospital Neurologique Pierre Wertheimer, Lyon, France
Microsurgical DREZotomy

ROBERT J. SINGER, MD
Neurosurgeon, Neurological Surgeons, PC, Nashville, Tennessee
Management of Dissections of the Carotid and Vertebral Arteries

EDWARD R. SMITH, MD
Instructor, Department of Neurosurgery, Harvard Medical School; Assistant Professor, Neurosurgery, Children's Hospital, Boston, Massachusetts
Decompressive Craniectomy: Physiologic Rationale, Clinical Indications, and Surgical Considerations

BRIAN E. SNELL, MD
Clinical Instructor, Department of Neurosurgery, Medical College of Wisconsin; Spinal Surgery Fellow, Froedtert Memorial Lutheran Hospital, Milwaukee, Wisconsin
Surgical Management of Extracranial Carotid Artery Disease

VOLKER K. H. SONNTAG, MD
Clinical Professor, Department of Neurosurgery, University of Arizona, Tucson; Vice Chairman, Division of Neurological Surgery, Barrow Neurological Institute; Director, Residency Program, Chairman, BNI Spine Section, Barrow Neurological Institute, Phoenix, Arizona
Surgical Techniques for Stabilization of the Subaxial Cervical Spine (C3–C7)

RENATO SPAZIANTE, MD
Professor of Neurosurgery and Chairman, University of Genoa Medical School; Chairman, Department of Neurosurgery, San Martino University Hospital, Genoa, Italy
Repair of the Sella Turcica after Transsphenoidal Surgery

ROBERT F. SPETZLER, MD, FACS
Division of Neurosurgery, University of Arizona College of Medicine, Tucson; Director, Barrow Neurological Institute, St. Joseph's Hospital, Phoenix, Arizona
Surgical Management of Midbasilar and Lower Basilar Aneurysms

BENNETT M. STEIN, MD
Bernardsville, New Jersey
Surgical Management of Spinal Cord Tumors and Arteriovenous Malformations

LADISLAU STEINER, MD, PhD
Professor of Neurological Surgery, University of Virginia, Charlottesville, Virginia
Gamma Knife Surgery for Cerebral Vascular Malformations, Tumors, and Functional Disorders

MELITA STEINER, MD
Research Professor of Neurosurgery, University of Virginia, Charlottesville, Virginia
Gamma Knife Surgery for Cerebral Vascular Malformations, Tumors, and Functional Disorders

MICHAEL P. STEINMETZ, MD
Resident, Departments of Neurosurgery and Orthopedic Surgery, The Cleveland Clinic Foundation, Cleveland, Ohio
Surgical Management of Cervical Spondylotic Myelopathy

BERTIL STENER, MD, PhD[†]
Technique of Complete Spondylectomy in the Thoracic and Lumbar Spine

MATEI STROILA, PhD
Assistant Professor, Department of Neursurgery, Lars Leksell Center for Gamma Surgery, University of Virginia Health System, Charlottesville, Virginia
Gamma Knife Surgery for Cerebral Vascular Malformations, Tumors, and Functional Disorders

NARAYAN SUNDARESAN, MD
Central Park Neurosurgery, New York, New York
Disorders of the Spine Related to Plasma Cell Dyscrasias

ULRICH SURE, MD
Neurosurgeon and Associate Professor, Department of Neurosurgery, Philipps University Marburg, Marburg, Germany
Surgical Management of Aneurysms of the Vertebral and Posterior Inferior Cerebellar Artery Complex

BROOKE SWEARINGEN, MD
Assistant Professor of Surgery, Harvard Medical School, Associate Visiting Neurosurgeon, Massachusetts General Hospital, Boston, Massachusetts
Transsphenoidal Approach to Pituitary Tumors

WILLIAM H. SWEET, MD, DSc, FACS[†]
Craniopharyngiomas: A Summary of Data; Cervicothoracic Ankylosing Spondylitis

TOSHIHIRO TAKAMI, MD
Lecturer, Department of Neurosurgery, Osaka City University Graduate School of Medicine, Osaka, Japan
Orbitozygomatic Infratemporal Approach to Parasellar Meningiomas

---
†Deceased.

PRAKASH NARAIN TANDON, MD, MS, FRCS
Emeritus Professor, All India Institute of Medical Sciences, New Delhi, India
Surgical Management of Tuberculous Infections of the Nervous System

EDWARD C. TARLOV, MD
Associate Professor, Department of Neurosurgery, Tufts University School of Medicine, Boston; Neurosurgeon, Lahey Clinic, Burlington, Massachusetts
Intraspinal Cerebrospinal Fluid Cysts; Microsurgery of Ruptured Lumbar Intervertebral Disc

RONALD R. TASKER, MD, FRCS(C)
Professor Emeritus, Department of Surgery, University of Toronto; Honorary Neurosurgeon, University Health Network, Toronto Western Hospital, Toronto, Ontario, Canada
Surgical Treatment of the Dyskinesias

LAURA TASSI, MD
"Claudio Munari" Epilepsy Surgery Center, Niguarda Hospital, Milan, Italy
Multilobar Resections in Epilepsy Surgery

JULIA K. TERZIS, MD, PhD
Professor of Surgery, Department of Surgery, Division of Plastic and Reconstructive Surgery, Eastern Virginia Medical School; Senior Surgeon, Sentara Norfolk General Hospital, Norfolk, Virginia
Surgical Management of Brachial Plexus Injuries in Adults

JOHN M. TEW, JR., MD
Professor, Department of Neurosurgery, University of Cincinnati College of Medicine; Medical Director, The Neuroscience Institute, Mayfield Clinic, Cincinnati, Ohio
Surgical Management of Brain Stem Vascular Malformations; Percutaneous Stereotactic Rhizotomy in the Treatment of Intractable Facial Pain

ISSADA THONGTRANGAN, MD
Fellow, Stanford University, Stanford, California
Surgical Approaches to the Cervicothoracic Junction

WUTTIPONG TIRAKOTAI, MD, MSc
Neurosurgeon, Siriraj Hospital, Mahidol University, Bangkok, Thailand, Clincal Fellow, Department of Neurosurgery, Philipps University Marburg, Marburg, Germany
Surgical Management of Arachnoid, Suprasellar, and Rathke's Cleft Cysts; Neuronavigation in Neuroendoscopic Surgery; Surgical Management of Aneurysms of the Vertebral and Posterior Inferior Cerebellar Artery Complex

GIUSTINO TOMEI, MD
Professor of Neurosurgery, Department of Surgical Sciences, University of Insubria-Varese, Varese, Italy
Transcallosal Approach to Tumors of the Third Ventricle

JAMES H. TONSGARD, MD
Associate Professor of Pediatrics and Neurology,
The University of Chicago Pritzker School of Medicine,
Chicago, Illinois
Surgical Treatment of Neurofibromatosis

JAMES C. TORNER, PhD
Professor, University of Iowa College of Public Health,
Iowa City, Iowa
Management Options in Thoracolumbar Fractures

NGUYEN VAN TUAN, MD
Associate Professor, University Formation Center;
Neurosurgeon, Bênh Viên Nhân Dân 115, Ho Chi Minh
City, Vietnam
Management of Cauda Equina Tumors

R. SHANE TUBBS, PA-C, PhD
Assistant Professor of Cell Biology and Neurosurgery,
University of Alabama at Birmingham, Children's
Hospital, Birmingham, Alabama
Tethered Cord Syndrome in the Adult

SERGIO TURAZZI, MD
Chief, Division of Neurosurgery, University Hospital of
Verona, Verona, Italy
Petroclival Meningiomas

FRANCIS TURJMAN, MD, PhD
Professor, Department of Neuroradiology, Laennec
University, Head, Interventional Radiology, Department
of Radiology, Neurological Hospital, Lyon, France
*Surgical Management of Cerebral Arteriovenous
Malformations*

PETER F. ULLRICH, JR., MD
Medical Director, NeuroSpine Center of Wisconsin,
Appleton, Wisconisn
*Anterior Lumbar Interbody Fusion: Mini-Open
Laparotomy Approach*

FELIX UMANSKY, MD
Professor of Neurosurgery, Hebrew University Medical
School; Professor and Chairman, Department of
Neurosurgery, Hadassah University Hospital, Jerusalem,
Israel
Penetrating Brain Injuries

JOHN C. VAN GILDER, MD
Professor, Department of Neurosurgery, Roy J. and
Lucille A. Carver College of Medicine, University of
Iowa Hospitals and Clinics, Iowa City, Iowa
*Craniovertebral Abnormalities and Their Neurosurgical
Management*

MARIOS D. VEKRIS
Lecturer in Orthopaedics, Ioannina University Medical
School, Attending in Orthopaedic Department,
University Hospital of Ioannina, Ioannina, Greece; Senior
Fellow in Microsurgery, Microsurgical Research Center,
Eastern Virginia Medical School, Norfolk, Virginia
Surgical Management of Brachial Plexus Injuries in Adults

PAUL VESPA, MD
Associate Professor , Director, Neurocritical Care Program,
Department of Neurology, Division of Neurosurgery,
David Geffen School of Medicine at UCLA, University of
California at Los Angeles, Los Angeles, California
Surgical Management of Severe Closed Head Injury in Adults

ROBERTO M. VILLANI, MD
Professor of Neurosurgery, Department of Neurological
Sciences, University of Milan, Milan, Italy
Transcallosal Approach to Tumors of the Third Ventricle

ANDRÉ VISOT, MD, AIHP, ACCA
Chief of Department of Neurosurgery, Hôpital Foch,
Suresnes, France
*Transbasal Approach to Tumors Invading the Skull Base;
Surgical Management of Endocrinologically Silent Pituitary
Tumors*

FRANK D. VRIONIS, MD, PhD
Associate Professor of Neurosurgery, ENT, and Oncology,
University of South Florida College of Medicine; Director,
Skull Base Oncology, H. Lee Moffitt Cancer Center and
Research Institute, Tampa, Florida
*Transtemporal Approaches to the Posterior
Cranial Fossa*

MICHEL P. WAGER, MD
Neurosurgeon, Poitiers University Medical School,
University Hospital, Poitiers, France
Management of Cauda Equina Tumors

M. CHRISTOPHER WALLACE, MD, MSc, FRCSC, FACS
Professor and Program Director, Division of Neurosurgery,
Faculty of Medicine, University of Toronto; Toronto
Western Hospital, Toronto, Ontario, Canada
*Surgical Management of Cranial Dural Arteriovenous
Fistulas*

CHUNG-CHENG WANG, MD, PhD
Professor, Capital University of Medical Sciences,
Director, Beijing Neurosurgical Institute, Beijing, China
*Surgical Management of Nonglomus Tumors of the Jugular
Foramen*

THOMAS N. WARD, MD
Associate Professor, Department of Neurology, Dartmouth
Medical School; Staff Neurologist, Dartmouth-Hitchcock
Medical Center, Lebanon, New Hampshire
Current Management of Cervical Dystonia

JOSEPH C. WATSON, MD
Assistant Professor, Albert Einstein College of Medicine;
Chief of Neurosurgery, Jacobi Medical Center and North
Central Bronx Hospital, Bronx, New York
Management of Cushing's Disease

HOWARD L. WEINER, MD
Associate Professor of Neurosurgery, New York University,
New York, New York
*CT/MRI-Based Computer-Assisted Volumetric Stereotactic
Resection of Intracranial Lesions*

MARTIN H. WEISS, MD
Professor of Neurology and Neurosurgery,
Department of Neurological Surgery, Keck School of
Medicine of University of Southern California, Los
Angeles, California
*Surgical Management of Growth Hormone–Secreting and
Prolactin-Secreting Pituitary Adenomas*

WILLIAM C. WELCH, MD, FACS, FICS
Professor, Departments of Neurological Surgery,
Orthopaedic Surgery, and Rehabilitation Science and
Technology, University of Pittsburgh; Chief, Neurological
Surgery, UPMC Health System, Pittsburgh, Pennsylvania
Thoracoscopic Sympathectomy for Hyperhidrosis

WALTER W. WHISLER, MD, PhD
Professor and Chairman Emeritus, Rush University
Medical School, Senior Attending Physician Emeritus,
Rush University Medical Center, Chicago, Illinois
Multiple Subpial Transection for Epilepsy

LOUIS A. WHITWORTH, MD
Assistant Professor, Department of Neurosurgical Surgery,
The University of Texas Southwestern, The University of
Texas Southwestern Medical Center at Dallas, Dallas, Texas
*Deep Brain Stimulation in the Management of Parkinson's
Disease and Disabling Tremor*

MARSHALL F. WILKINSON, MSc, PhD
Neurophysiologist, Inoperative Monitoring Program,
Health Sciences Centre, Winnipeg, Manitoba, Canada
Microvascular Decompression Surgery for Hemifacial Spasm

JONATHAN M. WINOGRAD, MD
Instructor in Surgery, Department of Surgery, Harvard
Medical School, Division of Plastic and Reconstructive
Surgery, Massachusetts General Hospital, Boston,
Massachusetts
*Surgical Management of Median Nerve Compression at the
Wrist by Open Technique*

MICHAEL L. WOLAK, MD, PhD
Department of Neurosurgery, Dartmouth-Hitchcock
Medical Center, Lebanon, New Hampshire
Cervicothoracic Ankylosing Spondylitis—Commentary

MICHAEL WOYDT, MD
Associate Professor, Neurosurgical Department,
University of Basel, Basel, Switzerland
Ultrasound in Neurosurgery

BAKHTIAR YAMINI, MD
Assistant Professor of Neurosurgery, The University
of Chicago Pritzker School of Medicine, Chicago,
Illinois
Surgical Treatment of Neurofibromatosis

MICHAEL J. YAREMCHUK, MD
Professor of Surgery, Harvard Medical School,
Chief of Craniofacial Surgery, Massachusetts General
Hospital, Boston, Massachusetts
Surgical Repair of Major Defects of the Scalp and Skull

DANIEL YOSHOR, MD
Assistant Professor, Department of Neurosurgery, Baylor
College of Medicine, Houston, Texas
Temporal Lobe Operations for Drug-Resistant Epilepsy

CHUN-JIANG YU, MD, PhD
Professor, Capital University of Medical Sciences;
Doctor, Department of Neurosurgery, Beijing Tiantan
Hospital, Beijing, China
*Surgical Management of Nonglomus Tumors of the Jugular
Foramen*

SETH M. ZEIDMAN, MD
Assistant Professor of Neurological Surgery and Neurology,
University of Rochester Medical Center, Rochester,
New York; Uniformed Services University of the Health
Sciences, Bethesda, Maryland
Circumferential Spinal Fusion (Cervical)

VASILIOS A. ZERRIS, MD, MPH, MMSc
Clinical Instructor, Brown University, Rhode Island
Hospital, Providence, Rhode Island
*Surgical Management of Injuries of the Cervical Spine and
Spinal Cord*

MICHAEL ZIMMERMANN, MD, PhD
Associate Professor, Department of Neurosurgery,
Johann Wolfgang Goethe University, Frankfurt,
Germany
*Anterior Approaches in Multisegmental Cervical
Spondylosis*

GIANLUIGI ZONA, MD, PhD
Attending Neurosurgeon, Department of Neurosurgery,
San Martino University Hospital, Genoa, Italy
Repair of the Sella Turcica after Transsphenoidal Surgery

PREFACE

In 1977 Dr. Sweet and I coedited a single volume entitled *Current Techniques in Operative Neurosurgery*, which reflected our own interests in a spectrum of neurosurgical procedures, with emphasis on those at the forefront of contemporary neurosurgical practice. Conceptually, we attempted in this and the subsequent three editions to provide the working neurosurgeon with information which would be useful when taking an adult patient with a particular brain, spine, or peripheral nerve problem to the operating room. The chapters provided an overview of the topic, a discussion of available options and results. In many cases, alternative surgical and nonsurgical options were included for dealing with a particular clinical situation. It was our goal to provide a single source that would allow a neurosurgeon to develop a surgical plan for the patient. The chapter references would be up-to-date and allow further immersion in the topic as needed. The success of these volumes, along with the recent translation of the fourth edition into Chinese, places *Operative Neurosurgical Techniques: Indications, Methods, and Results* among the most widely used neurosurgical texts worldwide. David W. Roberts has been added to the roster as a coeditor, and the current edition is dedicated to the memory of Dr. Sweet.

The fifth edition continues to reflect the same underlying vision for the book and attempts to keep up to date with the rapidly evolving changes in neurosurgery. The fifth edition consists of 168 chapters authored by 380 contributors representing neurosurgical services from 22 different countries. As scientific advances are being made worldwide, the book has attempted to reflect these contributions and their origins and to perpetuate the idea of an international text in neurosurgery. Approximately 40% of the chapters deal with material not previously addressed in this text, and, where appropriate, chapters published in earlier editions have been extensively rewritten. All the chapters have been reviewed to ensure that they reflect the current state of the art.

This edition could not have been accomplished without the enthusiastic participation of the contributors who, to the delight of the editors, completed their chapters in record time. To each of these individuals I extend my sincerest thanks. Every effort has been made to produce a product worthy of the contributions. This could only have been accomplished with the professionalism of Rebecca Schmidt Gaertner, Agnes Hunt Byrne, and Joan Sinclair at Elsevier, and of the staff at P. M. Gordon Associates. All deserve the sincerest thanks for a job well done, which I extend to them on behalf of the contributors and the editors.

Henry H. Schmidek, MD, FACS
Lebanon, New Hampshire

Color Plate

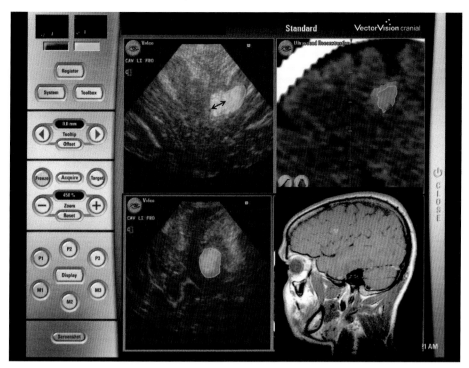

FIGURE 43-6 Left frontal subcortical cavernoma. Screen shot from a frameless neuronavigation system (FLNN). *Upper left:* Intraoperative ultrasound (IOUS) with high echogenic subcortical cavernoma (green: localization of cavernoma with FLNN) in coronal plane. *Upper right:* Reconstructed computed tomography image from ultrasound plane. *Lower left:* IOUS in sagittal plane. *Lower right:* Corresponding magnetic resonance image. Due to difference of 5 mm between FLNN and IOUS, localization of the cavernoma (*upper left, black arrow*) object was shifted in FLNN and navigation was successful.

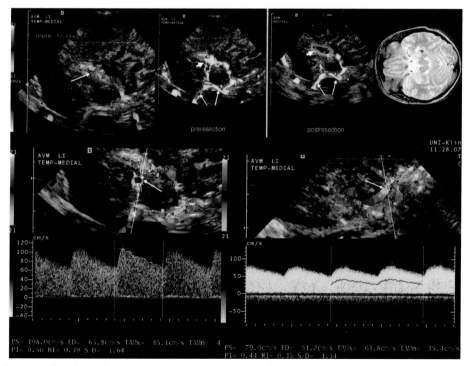

FIGURE 43-7 Left temporobasal arteriovenous angioma. *Upper left:* Localization of the AVM nidus in C mode (*arrow*); measurement of depth from the cortical surface (22.3 mm). *Upper middle and right:* Display of the angioarchitecture pre- and postresection in power mode and corresponding magnetic resonance image. Nidus and resection cavity, respectively (*arrowheads*) and posterior cerebral artery (P2 and P3 segment) with feeder vessels (*small arrows*). *Lower left:* Measurement of flow velocity in feeder vessel with triplex mode (angle corrected Doppler sample volume marked with *arrow*); at the bottom, spectral curve with elevated peak systolic flow of 108.0 cm/second and low resistance index of 0.39 are shown. *Lower right:* Triplex mode of draining vessel (sample volume, *arrow*) with flow away from nidus.

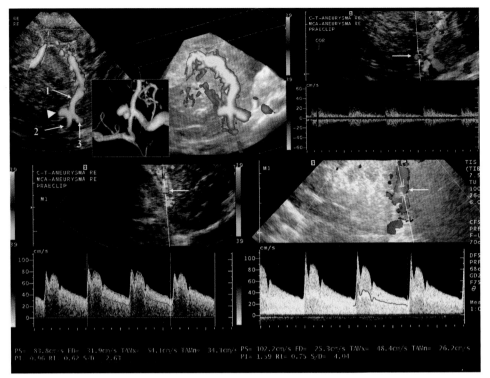

FIGURE 43-8 Aneurysm of the left carotid bifurcation. *Upper left:* Aneurysm (*arrowhead*) and bifurcation (1 = middle cerebral artery, 2 = anterior cerebral artery, 3 = carotid artery) in power mode (coronal plane, with corresponding 3-dimensional angiography). *Upper middle:* Intraoperative 3-dimensional ultrasound image of the aneurysm. *Upper right:* Triplex mode of the aneurysm with bichromatic display (*arrow*) and bidirectional Doppler signal (*bottom line*). *Lower left* (preclipping) and *lower right* (postclipping): Hemodynamic monitoring of middle cerebral artery with quantitative assessment of velocities due to angle-corrected Doppler sample volume (*arrows*). Postclipping there is only slight elevation of peak systolic flow (83.3 to 102.2 cm/second) and resistance index (0.67 to 0.73).

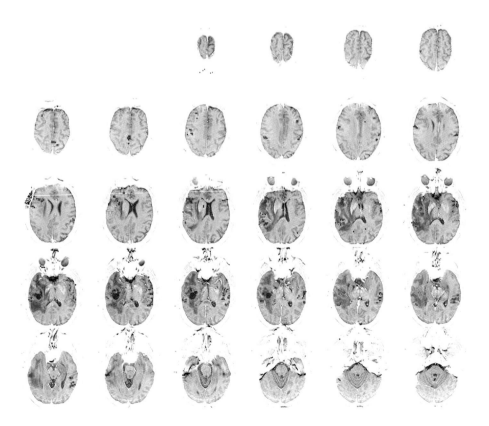

FIGURE 47-1 Functional MRI during a silent speech task in a patient with a glioblastoma of the left temporal glioblastoma (left and right are reversed).

CONTENTS

Section XIX
Surgery of the Peripheral Nervous System **2233**

Section XX
Safety Measures in Surgery **2325**

Section I

Introduction

1 Assessing Surgical Innovation

ADAM O. HEBB and STEPHEN J. HAINES

The assessment of the success of surgical intervention is an essential part of surgical practice; it has been practiced by the best surgeons since the emergence of the specialty. There is an important distinction to be made, however, between *continuous process improvement*, which all surgeons practice to one extent or another, and the *evaluation of surgical innovation*, which is the subject of this chapter.

Every good surgeon reviews every operation, searching for technical issues that can be changed to improve the conduct or outcome of the procedure. The complications and outcomes of a series of operations are routinely reviewed, and decisions are made about changes intended to reduce the risk of complications and improve outcome. This monitoring of surgical outcome may be performed by the surgeon or by the institution. The formality of this process varies, and specific suggestions for best practices in this regard are available.[1,2]

Much of the published clinical surgical literature is the report of such process improvement efforts. A series of patients is reviewed to identify factors that predict good outcome and that identify and reduce risk. Such reports can provide insight into process improvement efforts that may have helped the authors improve their outcomes and that generate ideas that the reader may choose to try in his or her own practice. They suffer, however, from many forms of bias; this means that the results are not necessarily generalizable to other practices.

Surgical innovation, on the other hand, is a process intended to produce a *generalizable* result. The surgeon who develops a new procedure, or a major technical refinement, and believes that this innovation can be broadly applied by surgeons with similar practices is obligated to provide evidence of safety and effectiveness that can be generalized to other surgical practices with confidence. The requirement for a more rigorous evaluation process derives from two factors: the *novelty* of the innovation (i.e., the effect on outcome is untested and uncertain) and the desire to *generalize* the result.

We strongly encourage all surgeons to engage regularly in well-planned, continuous process improvement, utilizing modern techniques and well-validated measures of outcome. Our focus in this chapter, however, is the evaluation of surgical innovation.

BACKGROUND

Surgical innovation is an active process of developing new techniques or strategies in order to improve outcome, increase patient satisfaction, reduce pain and suffering, or reduce the economic burden of a disease process. Surgical practice has developed from innovation largely through an unregulated process. Dynamic adaptation of techniques to a variety of clinical scenarios is inherent in surgery, and therefore surgical innovation is a natural extension of its practice. It is understandably difficult to distinguish natural evolution of surgical technique from surgical research. As pressure increases for institutional oversight of research and experimentation involving human subjects, and as peer-reviewed journals are requiring institutional review board (IRB) approval for publication of results, surgeons will need to participate in a paradigm to ethically and responsibly evaluate new techniques.

Although there is currently no agency corresponding to the Food and Drug Administration (FDA) for the technique and practice of surgery in the United States, Britain and Australia have developed such agencies. The Academy of Royal Medical Colleges (Britain) established a voluntary safety and efficacy register of new interventional procedures. The National Institute for Clinical Excellence is a component of the National Health Service for England and Wales, and its role is to "provide patients, health professionals, and the public with authoritative, robust, and reliable guidance on current 'best practice'."[3] Australia developed the Australian Safety and Efficacy Register for New Interventional Procedures—Surgical (ASERNIP-S), regulated by the Royal Australian College of Surgeons. Its mission is to "provide quality and timely assessments of new and emerging surgical technologies and techniques."[4] The American College of Surgeons has issued statements related to applying new surgical technology to the care of patients.[5,6] These statements give basic guidelines for the introduction of new equipment into surgical practice that would require a significant adaptation of surgical technique. They describe the need for controlled clinical trials and observation, with publication of the results of these initial trials in peer-reviewed journals.[6] Although these principles are generally applicable to surgical technique, these guidelines do not address surgical technique independent of new technology. Agencies that monitor the introduction of new techniques may also provide a means of accruing data on outcome and surgical complications.[7] The goals of these agencies are to monitor the introduction of new surgical techniques as well as to encourage innovation. As voluntary organizations, their recommendations do not have the force of law as is the case with drugs and devices in the United States.

Review agencies must determine a method of identifying procedures to review and a method of reviewing those procedures. Identification of procedures is the responsibility of the surgeon or of an overseeing party. These procedures are new if "a doctor no longer in a training post is using it for the first time in his or her NHS (National Health Service) clinical practice," as defined by the UK department of health.[8] Once a procedure has been deemed to require review, an advisory panel determines the requirements for approval. This review process generally involves a review of literature and available surgical options and results, with consultation with advisory surgeons. A consensus determines if the procedure is safe or requires further investigation.[9] Agencies that review these new procedures have not clearly defined the requirements of approval.

Defining exactly what constitutes a new procedure is difficult. A new procedure can be defined as "an intervention that is not yet viewed by the institution, community, or profession as meeting the accepted standards of safety, reliability, and familiarity with effects, side effects, and complications."[10] Given this description, Dandy's introduction of the third ventriculocisternostomy for treatment of hydrocephalus in 1922 was new. He described performing a craniotomy, sectioning of the optic nerve, and entering the lamina terminalis and subsequent opening of the floor of the third ventricle into the interpeduncular cistern.[11] Scarff later described a modification using a dental instrument passed through the lamina terminalis to blindly puncture the third ventricular floor.[12] Guiot then described an approach via the lateral ventricle through the foramen of Monroe, perforating the floor of the third ventricle under television control.[13] Jones and colleagues described their experience with a cannulated endoscope for the third ventriculocisternostomy.[14] Recently, a prospectively collected cohort was reported, with a follow-up of at least 3 years.[15] This progression of surgical technique is an excellent example of a novel procedure and its subsequent clinically relevant adaptations. Therefore, these clinically relevant adaptations of established procedures should also be considered "new" because they would have the potential of affecting the patient's surgical result. There is subjectivity to this definition that has allowed the development and evaluation of procedures without proper oversight and understanding of what constitutes a new procedure.

Over time, Dandy's innovation was refined to a well-accepted procedure. There are procedures that had similar beginnings that were abandoned after rigorous evaluation. An example in the general surgical literature is internal mammary artery ligation for the treatment of angina pectoris. This procedure was first introduced in 1939, and in 1958 a case series of 82 patients was reported. Fifty patients were followed for 2 to 6 months, and 34 of 45 patients who were still living were symptomatically improved.[16] Later, two randomized, double-blinded, sham-surgery controlled clinical trials did not demonstrate any difference between the ligation group and the sham-surgery group.[17,18] Thus the benefit was deemed a placebo effect.

PRINCIPLES OF THERAPEUTIC EVALUATION

There are a number of fundamental principles that guide the evaluation of new therapies, surgical or not. They can be classified into four large categories: (1) objective observation, (2) concurrent comparison, (3) equal prognostic allocation, and (4) rigorous conduct (Table 1-1).

Objective Observation

Everyone's baby is beautiful, in the parent's own eyes. The inability to evaluate objectively that which one creates is a

---

TABLE 1-1 ▪ Fundamental Characteristics of Evaluation of Innovation

Objective observation
Concurrent control
Equal prognostic allocation
Rigorous conduct

---

well-known human characteristic, and it applies to operations as well as children.[19] Special care must be taken to be objective in the evaluation of the outcome of a new intervention. Two crucial decisions confront the clinical investigator when determining how best to measure outcome: what to measure and how to measure it objectively.

The World Health Organization classified the "consequences of diseases" as impairments, disability, and handicaps.[20] Measurement of technical success in changing the impairment or disease process is an important outcome relevant to the surgeon. The physician equates the patient's disability with the impairment of the disease process; however, a surgical therapy may not address all components of the disease. Surgical therapies for Parkinson's disease, for example, may alleviate motor symptoms but not the cognitive decline. Therefore, motor scores would not well represent the patient's overall disability.[21] Patients are most concerned with relief of the disability and handicap the disease creates, and outcome criteria should be both health-centered and patient-centered.[22,23] Functional outcome measures that have had extensive validation (e.g., SF-36, FIM, the NIH Stroke Scale, and the Glasgow Outcome Scale) meet these criteria, can be more objectively applied than simple assessments (e.g., "excellent," "good," "fair," and "poor"), and should be incorporated into the evaluation of new surgical procedures.[24–30]

Although clinical investigators may have several unanswered questions concerning a new surgical technique, a study must be designed with one primary question. This will identify the primary outcome measure, and it will be used to determine the required number of participants and the feasibility of the study. This primary measure should have significant clinical importance for the patient and should be sensitive to the intervention. Patient survival would be an appropriate measure for a new treatment for glioblastoma, whereas a motor function score would be an appropriate measure for a therapy for spinal cord injury. Secondary outcome measures are important because they aid in explaining the primary result and may generate hypotheses for future studies.[31]

The outcome measures must be applied in a consistent and unbiased fashion. Blinding of patient, physician, and analyst is the classic technique. If blinding of patients and investigators is not possible, other techniques may be used to reduce observer bias. This includes independent evaluations (e.g., imaging studies or video recordings of clinical outcome), outcome assessment by physicians other than the treating surgeon, and data analysts who are not involved in the care of the patient.

Concurrent Comparison

Time changes things. The gradual accretion of multiple changes in medical care will lead to improvement of outcome over time even when the fundamental therapeutic intervention is not changed. This creates a high risk of false comparison when new procedures are compared to patients treated in an earlier period.[32] Sacks and colleagues demonstrated that trials using historical controls were more likely to conclude that the experimental treatment was better.[33] The outcome of a new procedure should therefore be evaluated concurrently with the outcome of a standard procedure. Historical controls have their own set of selection or referral biases, and their evaluation was conducted by other groups of investigators using different evaluation procedures. The intensity of follow-up may have a significant effect on outcome. The Hawthorne effect refers to the phenomenon that outcome may be biased even by simple observation rather than by a placebo effect. This concept comes from experiments of lighting conditions on worker productivity in the Hawthorne Works Plant of the Western Electric Company in Chicago. There was increased productivity regardless of how the lighting was varied, suggesting that worker productivity increased solely from observation of the workers.[34] Mismatching of surgical skill is also present with the use of historical controls. Concurrent controls minimize bias related to those factors that influence outcome and make it far easier to ensure that factors such as method of diagnosis, choice of outcome measurement tools, surgical expertise, supportive patient care, and method and intensity of follow-up are similar. Thus concurrent controls are most likely to provide the most reliable comparison between new treatments and the current state of the standard therapy.

Equal Prognostic Allocation

For any comparison to be valid, the patients receiving the treatments being compared must be equivalent in the factors that affect outcome (i.e., their prognosis must be equivalent). Using clinical judgment to allocate patients to treatment groups introduces multiple biases. These may include allocation based on disease severity, surgeon and patient preference, and urgency of treatment.[35] Study design techniques (e.g., matching in a case-control study) or stratification in a prospective cohort or randomized trial may allow allocation of patients so that *known* factors influencing outcome are equally distributed in the treatment and control groups. However, *unknown* factors might differentially affect the prognosis of one of the groups. The unique role of randomization is to equalize the likelihood that any factor, including unknown factors, will be present and acting on the groups of patients. Randomization provides protection against bias from things we don't even know about and from which we have no other method of protection.

Definitive surgical trials should be designed with true random allocation. Pseudo-randomization techniques (e.g., alternate allocation, or odd and even allocation by hospital or Social Security number) do not completely protect against bias. These techniques may be circumvented by biased clinical investigators. When randomization is simply not possible, a study design must ensure prognostic equivalence of treatment groups, including equalizing factors only suspected of having an influence.

One of the most obvious factors that can affect outcome is the skill and experience of the surgeon. Surgical evaluation must include measures of the technical success and of the complications rates of the surgeons, and they must incorporate safeguards to see that all patients are exposed to similar chances of technical success and complication. For example, to be eligible to participate in the North American Symptomatic Carotid Endarterectomy Trial (NASCET), surgeons had to demonstrate a perioperative rate of stroke and death of less than 6% in a minimum of 50 consecutive cases in 2 years.[36] This provides a means for surgeons not involved in the study to determine if they could offer patients the same benefit as measured in the study. Such a requirement was not required of surgeons participating in the International Subarachnoid Aneurysm Trial (ISAT), and therefore it is more difficult to determine the generalizability of the results.[37]

Rigorous Conduct

Many of the factors that can lead to biased (and therefore incorrect) results in assessing an operation relate to the conduct of the assessment rather than its design or analysis. These are inherently nonstatistical issues, and biases introduced through poor study conduct cannot be removed in analysis. Careful adherence to the study protocol in both experimental and control patients is essential. The diagnostic process must be identical. If patients are screened by CT, but only those allocated to the experimental arm get an MRI, the experimental group may have a much higher chance of detection of certain disease factors that could exclude them from the study or affect the outcome assessment. The follow-up procedures must be identical. If the experimental patients have more frequent visits, more lab tests, and more imaging, it is more likely that complications will be detected.

Critical to the introduction of a new technique to clinical practice is the protection of the patients who are the subject of initial attempts. Agich coined the term *regulatory ethics paradigm*, which refers to a set of principles to guide innovation.[38] Within this paradigm there should be early pursuit of formal research in order to determine the safety and efficacy of the new procedure.[39] However, the protocols of surgical innovation may deviate significantly from formal scientific methodology. Innovation demands a flexible system of oversight because it incorporates additional experience and undergoes dynamic change.

McKneally and Daar identified five elements of a regulatory ethics paradigm for surgical innovation: (1) the participant must be informed of the experimental nature of the treatment, (2) a much more complete discussion of potential risks is required than is customary for clinical informed consent to ordinary care, (3) participants must be told they are free to choose standard care rather than the experimental treatment, (4) a multidisciplinary institutional review board that includes representatives of the public must review and approve the protocol, and (5) the outcomes of the experiment, including all adverse events, must be reported to the review board.[10]

THE IDEAL EVALUATION PARADIGM

Ideal evaluation of a new surgical procedure would follow the same four phases now well defined for pharmaceutical innovation (Table 1-2).

TABLE 1-2 ▪ Ideal Evaluation Paradigm

Phase	Goal	When to Begin
Phase I	Assess feasibility of new technique, incorporate modifications	When first ready to apply to a patient
Phase II	Estimate efficacy and safety	When ready to teach a few other surgeons
Phase III	Definitive comparative trial	When ready to teach to many other surgeons
Phase IV	Monitoring of effectiveness in practice	After release into widespread practice

Phase I: Feasibility

A novel idea may be developed from an interaction with a single patient, in response to a systematic problem with treatment of a group of patients, or as a result of basic scientific research. An idea should prompt a standardized development pathway.[22] A systematic review of the disease process and its current management should be performed. Ideas may be further refined by discussion with peers, with cadaveric studies, or in collaboration with basic science research and possibly creation of an animal model for preclinical testing. A proposal with significant merit and background evidence of potential benefit to patients should be presented to a diverse group of peers and patient advocates. In North America, the IRB or research ethics board (REB) fulfills this role. In presentation of a proposed procedure to the review board, the procedure may be subdivided into component parts. Each component may be designated as standard or novel, with novel components requiring support from research. This support may be from literature review or from cadaveric or animal models, and should demonstrate likely procedure feasibility and effectiveness.[40]

The purpose of this phase of evaluation is to determine if the procedure can be done in the clinical environment, achieving the expected technical outcome without unexpectedly poor results. This phase I trial should be conducted on a strictly limited number of patients with fully informed consent and intense oversight. The trial must be prospective from the first patient and have well-defined outcome criteria. By definition of this phase, the primary outcome measure will be disease-centered rather than patient-centered. Outcome measures such as procedure success would be appropriate with careful monitoring for complications, patient morbidity, and mortality.

In this phase, unexpected issues may arise that require modification of the procedure, and possibly even more basic investigation before additional procedures are done. Although the oversight must be intense, it should also be flexible enough to allow modification and improvement of the procedure in order to avoid unnecessarily discontinuing a promising innovation.[41]

Phase II: Estimates of Surgical Risks and Benefits

When the surgeon has standardized a proposed intervention, and when the procedure is deemed by the institutional review process to have a potential benefit to patients and to be safe to implement, the next stage is to formally estimate the success rate and risk of the procedure. The innovator may recruit interested colleagues to replicate the technique. At this stage, a phase II trial should be conducted to evaluate the benefits and risks associated with the now standardized and reproducible innovation. This would take the form of a prospective case series in which the therapy is applied to a cohort of patients who may be followed to evaluate outcome and complications. The number of patients included in the phase II evaluation should be limited to the number required to get the required accuracy for estimates of success and risk, knowing that a definitive trial will follow if the phase II evaluation is successful. Specifics regarding the number of patients required are determined by the expected improvement in the primary outcome measure and the desired precision of the estimates of success and risk. In order to speed the pace of evaluation, it is common to choose a surrogate outcome for phase II trials. For example, instead of survival, studies of brain tumors often use image-determined measures of response because they can be assessed rapidly.[32] Surrogate measures do not always, however, precisely predict the actual response to the most desired outcome. For example, Olanow and colleagues demonstrated survival of fetal tissue grafts in a series of patients with Parkinson's disease but were unable to demonstrate a clinical benefit.[42]

Great care must be taken in choosing a comparison group for the treated patients in this phase of evaluation. It is quite easy to bias the selection of patients for entry into a phase II trial, and if the controls are not chosen in the same biased way, a false comparison can result. Biases introduced by using historical controls apply here, as do biases introduced by choosing a control population that differs prognostically from the treatment population. The use of large databases of patients with similar disease, from which prognostically stratified controls can be chosen, may be helpful in this phase of evaluation.[43-45] Some even go so far as to recommend randomization at this phase, although it is more common to reserve randomization for phase III. Clinician bias for selection of a subgroup of patients to apply the new procedure hinders application of randomized trial designs. In a survey after a failed randomized trial for minimally invasive surgery, surgeons reported a strong bias toward a particular procedure that was independent of surgical ability.[46]

Phase III: Definitive Comparative Trial

Phase I and II evaluations play the important roles of confirming feasibility, allowing for modification and improvement of the procedure, and providing *estimates* of safety and efficacy. Occasionally they may serve to identify a procedure so effective that no further evaluation is required before the procedure enters the standard neurosurgical armamentarium. This would undoubtedly have been the case had the surgical evacuation of acute epidural hematoma in a deteriorating patient been evaluated in this paradigm. The relentless natural history and the rapid and dramatic results of surgery would have provided data showing a therapeutic benefit so large that it would overcome any subtle or moderate bias in the cohorts. A phase III trial would not have been justifiable.

Most new procedures in the modern era, however, propose a degree of benefit that is relatively modest when compared with that of epidural hematoma evacuation. For example, carotid endarterectomy in symptomatic patients, considered a very effective procedure, reduced the ipsilateral stroke rate by 6.5% (22.2% to 15.7%) in patients with moderate (50% to 69%) stenosis.[47] Such differences can easily be overwhelmed by unanticipated bias, and they require a more sophisticated evaluation if there is to be enough confidence in their usefulness to make them part of standard care.

Therefore, in the ideal paradigm, the next phase of evaluation would be a randomized clinical trial (RCT) designed to study a generalizable population of patients operated on by surgeons with demonstrated technical expertise in the procedure. That group of surgeons should be chosen and trained in a manner that will permit the results to be generalized to the larger population of surgeons who may employ the procedure in the future.

Phase IV: Effectiveness after Implementation

Just as there is a period of postrelease surveillance for drugs, the *effectiveness* of a new surgical procedure (when put into common practice after its *efficacy* has been demonstrated in phase III) should be assessed in ongoing prospective cohort studies. A large literature of such studies in carotid endarterectomy has grown following the definitive studies of the last decade (e.g., Tan and colleagues, reference 48). The translation of new surgical techniques from clinical trials to community practice is not trivial. Clinicians involved in clinical trials are proficient in the technique before the initiation of the trial. The American College of Surgeons has published a statement on "guidelines for evaluation of credentials of individuals for the purpose of awarding surgical privileges in new technologies," which outlines the need for a "defined educational program in the technology, including didactic and practical elements," and that "maintenance of skills should be documented through periodic outcomes assessment and evaluation."[5] Although this practice may be enforced where specific devices are used, the individual surgeon decides when he or she is proficient enough to practice a new procedure. Follow-up studies on a regional level should be conducted to monitor outcome of a new procedure. This may take the form of an individual surgeon or group of surgeons monitoring the outcome of a procedure in their practice, or an institution monitoring surgical outcome measures for the purposes of credentialing surgeons. This monitoring of outcome also allows surgeons to share their individual or local results with a procedure in the informed consent process rather than only quoting the results of landmark trials.

OBSTACLES TO THE IDEAL EVALUATION

This ideal evaluation paradigm sets a standard that is difficult to meet. There are several barriers to the evaluation of new procedures with appropriate oversight. They fall into the large categories of technical difficulties with ideal study design in surgery, continuous procedural improvement, difficulty in distinguishing between minor modification of standard procedures and true innovation,[49] insufficient resources for ideal evaluation, lack of oversight, and poor understanding of the risks of inadequate evaluation.

Technical Difficulties with Ideal Study Design in Surgery

Ideal clinical trial designs attempt to eliminate all sources of bias. To this effect, patients and evaluators may be blinded to the treatment in order to eliminate placebo effect and observer bias, respectively. In a trial of a new pharmaceutical, a placebo or standard treatment arm with blinding is a very effective and ethical design. However, translating this to a surgical trial is fraught with difficulties. For instance, if proposed treatments have different approaches, such as craniotomy versus endovascular, researchers will not be able to blind patients. Where blinding of patients and surgeons is not possible, outcome assessment and data analysis by researchers not involved in the patients' treatment provides a good deal of bias protection.

In certain circumstances, placebo or sham surgeries can be performed. Sham surgery has been defended in order to prevent widespread acceptance of procedures that provide no clinical benefit.[50,51] Sham surgery may be appropriate for the definitive evaluation of certain operations in carefully selected and monitored circumstances; however, it should not be included in an initial trial design to test a new procedure because of the risks and costs associated with sham surgery.[52]

To eliminate patient selection bias, randomization of patients should be performed. This principle is also difficult to apply to surgical trials. Enrolled patients must be equally eligible for either therapy. This requirement often leads to exclusion of a large proportion of patients who are screened for the study. This was likely a significant cause for the exclusion of 7416 of 9559 patients screened in ISAT for surgical clipping vs. endovascular coiling.[37] Furthermore, because of the invasive nature of surgery, patients may be unwilling to subject themselves to randomization.[53]

Beyond the issues of blinding and randomization, however, technical issues for well-conducted prospective cohort studies are very similar to those of RCTs.

Continuous Procedural Improvement

Operations continuously improve. Surgeons repeatedly fiddle and tweak their procedures to make them better. Some use this as an argument against formal evaluation, on the grounds that the procedure at the time of the start of a trial is not the same as at its end. Although this is indeed a challenge, it does not invalidate the concept of formal procedural evaluation; in fact, it strengthens the argument. It would be inappropriate to recommend the widespread adoption of a procedure that had not reached a demonstrable level of efficacy. Further refinement and improvement of the procedure would make it easier, not harder, to demonstrate the level of efficacy present at the start of the evaluation. Innovators who claim that their procedure failed evaluation because the "current" or "modern" procedure had not been refined at the point of evaluation are essentially admitting that they recommended adoption, and therefore evaluation, of the procedure prematurely.

Distinguishing between Minor Modification of Standard Procedures and True Innovation

The current practice of surgery has largely developed through an informal and unregulated process. Fundamentally, it can be difficult to define when surgical innovation is research.[54] Surgical practice has evolved with small adaptations and numerous variations on procedures. There is a significant regional variation or "founder effect" of surgical technique that has developed from the influence of dominant surgeons teaching apprentice residents. Therefore, there is a lack of understanding among professionals of when a procedure is new or different enough to require institutional review. It would be impractical to obtain IRB approval before adapting a procedure to a patient who is clearly in need of an urgent treatment. Surgeons must respond urgently to surgical emergencies, and there may be no available surgical experience for a particular situation. In these circumstances, a colleague may be consulted to assist and perform the role of a peer review panel for a planned salvage technique. Carrying such an adaptation or new procedure to future patients for evaluation and subsequent publication of results does require oversight from an institutional review process because it constitutes surgical research.[49]

There are no clear guidelines here, but modifications that are expected to change outcomes or that require a new set of surgical skills represent changes that may pose a risk to the patient and should be treated as research rather than simple clinical variation. Referring back to the example of third ventriculocisternostomy, Dandy had developed a new procedure for hydrocephalus, a condition that had a devastating natural history. However, reintroduction of this procedure when ventriculoperitoneal shunting was standard therapy should have prompted a clinical trial to compare efficacy and risks.

Insufficient Resources for Ideal Evaluation

The introduction of a new drug follows a significant investment by the pharmaceutical industry, justified by the prediction that a successful drug will generate sales that will repay the investment and more. Operations that do not depend on unique devices have no such commercial investment value and therefore no reservoir of capital from which to pay for the optimal evaluation paradigm previously described. Although there is a theoretical large savings in future health care expense and increase in personal productivity when a successful operation is created, no mechanism exists to capture a portion of that economic benefit to support the evaluation of new procedures. This means that the evaluation of new procedures relies on funding from governmental or philanthropic sources, health care organizations that wish to promote quality care, and the volunteer efforts of surgeons. The costs of well-designed and well-conducted, large-scale clinical trials are measured in millions of dollars and are well beyond the limits that most sources can support.

Labeling new procedures as research may create a challenge for funding innovative techniques. Whereas insurers currently reimburse surgeons who dynamically alter their procedures (because it is hidden from regulatory bodies), protocols identified as research may require independent funding sources. In the absence of an affiliated company with a financial interest of having a device approved by the FDA, this funding may be unavailable for new surgical techniques.

Lack of Oversight

If an innovation paradigm is poorly designed, there will be a disincentive for surgeons to participate. Excessive regulatory paperwork or meetings may form an institutional barrier to the ideal evaluation, because these may exhaust the time resources of the surgeon. Therefore, surgeons willing and able to devote voluntary resources to such an evaluation may simply declare that the procedure is an innovation that does not require careful evaluation. This will lead to a lack of oversight, with haphazard and careless introduction of new procedures. However, a well-designed paradigm would encourage surgeons to participate in the intense oversight of the review process with an appropriate evaluation of new procedures.

Poor Understanding of the Risks of Inadequate Evaluation

Public and professional misunderstanding of medical science is also an obstacle in the proper evaluation of a new technology. Many physicians and most patients are unfamiliar with the many subtle ways in which bias creeps into the casual evaluation of therapeutic interventions. A patient's misunderstanding of study design may lead to fear that he or she will be denied proven therapy in a clinical trial. Media coverage of innovative surgical technique rarely emphasizes the unproven nature of its benefit; it more often miseducates patients, leading them to place pressure on the surgeon to provide the latest, yet untested, technique.

SURGICAL EVALUATION: A PRACTICAL APPROACH

A surgeon with a good, innovative idea for a procedure should ask a few simple questions to determine how the evaluation of that idea should proceed.

Is Formal Evaluation Necessary?

Certain procedures and scenarios do not require formal evaluation (e.g., interventions in situations where the natural history is uniformly poor or fatal and an intervention clearly benefits the patient). Such an intervention should be readily replicated by many surgeons. Examples may be drawn from all facets of clinical neurosurgery. The evacuation of a traumatic epidural hematoma in a deteriorating patient is an example where evaluation in a comparative study would be unethical. If one were to devise a treatment for glioblastoma that produced 50% 5-year survival, the effect would be so dramatic that further investigation would be unnecessary.

It is equally unnecessary to evaluate minor changes in technique for which there is no expectation of increased risk or better outcome. Changes are often made to shorten the time of operation, to make the procedure easier on the surgeon, or to decrease the cost of surgery. Formal evaluation of these aspects of patient care that are not expected to directly affect patient outcome is a waste of time and resources. These assessments should be shared with impartial colleagues and gain peer acceptance.

Bernstein and Bampoe outline five distinct clinical scenarios according to their need for regulation: (1) a new procedure that has never been performed, (2) a fairly new procedure that is part of an RCT, (3) an amendment to the technique of an established operation, (4) an amendment to other features of an established operation, and (5) a new procedure to an individual surgeon.[55] In the first category, it is clear that an urgent solution to an urgent clinical problem should not involve the IRB approval process. The Declaration of Helsinki recognizes this clinical scenario as one in which the surgeon must use his or her own clinical judgment to act in the best interest of the patient.[56] Alternatively, an elective procedure with preconceived application to a number of patients requires appropriate review before implementation. A procedure that is being evaluated within an RCT clearly requires IRB approval. Amendment to the technique or other features of an established operation represents a gray zone of the regulatory ethics paradigm. Surgeons may gradually adjust a procedure over time; however, if a significant preconceived change is planned, IRB approval should be sought. Finally, a surgeon who undertakes a procedure in which he or she is unfamiliar, but has been proven to be safe and effective, has the ethical obligation to seek adequate training and supervision. This is outside the realm of the regulatory ethics paradigm but falls directly into the purview of institutional quality assurance.

Can I Demonstrate That the Procedure Is Feasible?

If the procedure does not meet either of the above two extremes of effectiveness, its feasibility must be tested. This should be done by the innovator under the supervision of peers and impartial observers, such as members of a review board. A formal protocol with careful data collection should be followed on a predetermined small number of patients. The results should be reviewed by impartial observers. This constitutes the phase I feasibility analysis. As a result of this analysis, the procedure may be discarded, revised and re-evaluated, or it may be considered ready for the next phase of evaluation.

Am I Ready to Teach It to My Friends?

Once feasibility has been demonstrated, the innovator is usually ready to share the new procedure with close colleagues. This is also commonly the point at which the press is notified and public pressure for wide availability of the procedure must be resisted. The desire to teach the procedure to others should trigger a phase II evaluation. The surgical protocol, refined in phase I, is taught to several other surgeons who demonstrate technical competence. Appropriate controls are identified, and a carefully selected number of patients undergo the procedure. Dispassionate review of the resulting estimates of efficacy and safety may again lead to discarding

the procedure, refining the procedure, or moving to further evaluation.

Do I Believe That Many Surgeons Can Successfully Perform This Procedure?

By this time, most innovators are firmly convinced of the usefulness of their new operation. It is time for them to move aside and let less passionate surgeons carry out the definitive evaluation. This should not be a problem, because, by definition, many surgeons must be able to perform well a procedure appropriate for wide dissemination.

It is at this point that the difficult decision between randomized and nonrandomized prospective cohort studies usually must be made. For definitive comparison, no other experimental design is appropriate. Both study designs are valuable in surgical research, with each having specific strengths. The major differences between the two designs are randomization, ease of enrollment of patients, blinding, and use of concurrent controls. A randomized design attempts to equalize known and unknown prognostic factors, and therefore nonrandomized designs are prone to the bias introduced by selecting the therapy for the patient. It is not possible to identify all the factors that influence that clinical decision, and clinicians must be willing to apply either therapy to their patients for a randomized trial to be successful. Clinician bias will also affect study enrollment; patients will be more willing to undergo randomization if their clinician values the goals of the study. Blinding is used more commonly in randomized trials, and this will reduce the placebo effect. Concurrent controls should be used in both study designs; however, well-selected historical controls may be used in cohort trials with the risk of introducing bias.

In both designs, generalizability (and, hence, the impact of the research) will be limited if the study population differs significantly from a clinician's own practice. Table 1-3 summarizes the characteristics of each study design. Factors that will affect the decision between a randomized clinical trial and a prospective cohort trial may be grouped as factors related to the patient and population, disease, current standard therapy, or novel therapy (Table 1-4). A large target population facilitates randomization. Patients with surrogate decision makers demand special ethical considerations for participation in clinical trials, especially when randomization is involved.[56] These considerations are outside the scope of this chapter.

Factors relating to the disease itself influence the choice of study design. Randomized designs allow the equalization of unknown factors that are present in conditions with many poorly understood variables (e.g., aneurysmal subarachnoid hemorrhage, Parkinson's disease). The current standard therapy and the proposed novel therapy also have an impact; procedures that carry a very low risk or a very high benefit may be accepted more readily with cohort trial evidence than will procedures with high risk or moderate benefit.

The number needed to treat (NNT), the inverse of the absolute risk reduction, may be calculated for procedures as a measure of benefit. For example, the absolute risk reduction for ipsilateral stroke with carotid endarterectomy over medical management is 6.5% and 17% for moderate (50% to 69%) and severe (70% to 99%) stenosis, respectively.[47,57]

TABLE 1-3 ▪ Characteristics of Randomized Controlled Clinical Trials and Prospective Controlled Cohort Study

	Randomized Controlled Clinical Trial	Prospective Cohort Study
Concurrent controls	Built into design	If concurrent cohorts are studied
Allocation of bias: known factors	Can be controlled with good design	Can be controlled with good design
Allocation of bias: unknown factors	Risk equalized	Cannot control
Objective observation	Dependent on design and investigators	Dependent on design and investigators
Rigor of protocol conduct	Dependent on design and investigators	Dependent on design and investigators
Generalizability	Depends on design; generalizable only to population similar to that studied	Depends on design; generalizable only to population similar to that studied
Range of disease studied	Restricted to patients equally eligible for all procedures being compared	Can apply treatment to a wide range of patients, but comparisons possible only for patients equally eligible for all procedures being compared
Enrollment	Difficult	Easier
Cost	Dependent on design and investigators; not necessarily more expensive	Dependent on design and investigators; not necessarily less expensive

Therefore, the corresponding NNT to avoid 1 patient having an ipsilateral stroke are 15 and 6 patients, respectively. If the NNT is low (e.g., arbitrarily, less than 5), evidence of treatment benefit from cohort trial data would likely be convincing. In contrast, if the procedure has low clinical significance (e.g., titanium mesh cranioplasty vs. methylmethacrylate), a cohort trial may be better suited to provide data on outcomes such as patient satisfaction or infection rates.

A procedure that creates a high financial burden on the health care system should have strong evidence to support its use over a less expensive option; a randomized trial may be more appropriate here. Table 1-4 summarizes these considerations. Inspection will reveal that both study designs have significant issues with generalizability, duration of follow-up, study design, and protocol compliance. Indeed, the major problem with randomized trials at this stage is lack of acceptance by physicians and patients. Success of surgical clinical trials requires surgeons to be unbiased toward unproven therapies (i.e., have *equipoise*), and the explanation given to patients will have a great impact on their willingness to participate.[53] This is one of the few situations in which surgeons and patients often choose convenience over quality.

The timing of a definitive comparative trial is crucial. This stage must be conducted at a point when the procedure is standardized and a number of surgeons have become proficient but before it has gained public acclaim and is in widespread use. There is an inherent learning curve for new procedures, and if evaluated too early in development they may be needlessly discarded because of poor surgical results. However, rigorous evaluation must be performed before widespread acceptance. These concepts are summarized in Table 1-2.

GOOD SCIENCE IS THE BEST DEFENSE

New techniques will come under scrutiny of our patients, our peers, our institutions, and the public. As new techniques are developed, they are evaluated according to the paradigm of evidence-based medicine with increasing frequency. There are numerous examples of neurosurgical therapies that have been criticized and subsequently proven or disproven with well-designed trials. In the absence of

TABLE 1-4 ▪ Factors in Choosing a Study Design

	Randomized Controlled Clinical Trial	Prospective Controlled Cohort Study
Patient and Population Factors		
Size of target population	Large (atherosclerosis)	Small (pontine cavernomas)
Disease Factors		
Cofactors of disease	Multiple unknown factors (atherosclerosis)	Minimal unknown factors (epidural hematoma)
Current Standard Therapy Factors		
Available treatment	High risk (suprasellar craniopharyngioma)	Safe (cerebellar JPA)
Availability of surgeons willing to randomize	High (less bias toward one treatment)	Low (more bias toward one treatment)
Novel Therapy Factors		
Expected benefit	Small – moderate (NNT > 10)	Large (NNT < 5)
Clinical significance to patient	High (microvascular decompression)	Low (mesh cranioplasty)
Risk to patient	High (clival chordoma resection)	Low (transposition of ulnar nerve)
Cost of procedure	High (deep brain stimulation)	Low (aspiration of brain abscess)

NNT, number needed to treat (see text).

definitive data on patient outcome after carotid endarterectomy, there was concern that it was being performed too frequently[58]; however, clinical trials of carotid endarterectomy quantified the benefit in symptomatic and asymptomatic patients.[47,57,59,60] In contrast, fetal tissue transplantation for Parkinson's disease was shown to be of no benefit in one randomized, double-blinded, control trial,[42] and benefit was limited to younger patients in another trial.[61] When scrutinizing published data, the clinician must compare his or her patient population to the sample represented by the clinical trial. If the study population is too diverse or too narrow in scope, the results may not be applicable. Two studies that were criticized for overgeneralizing negative results are the ISAT trial and the EC/IC (extracranial/intracranial) Bypass Study Group trial.[37,62]

The neurosurgical community has an obligation to our patients, peers, and the payers of health care to provide data on the benefits and risks of surgical procedures before they become widely practiced. RCTs are the standard for evaluation of new pharmacologic agents and have also been used to evaluate surgical therapies. Well-designed observational studies with a concurrent control group may serve as a strong alternative study design for evaluation of new surgical therapies. This maximizes the generalizability of the study and avoids external or historical controls that may not be directly comparable to a contemporary study.

Surgical innovation has transformed from individuals developing techniques under the cloak of surgical creativity into a research endeavor requiring ethical oversight with protection of the interests of patients and objective evaluation of surgical outcome and complications. This regulation may be seen to hinder the development of new surgical techniques, because it will likely become unacceptable to publish a case series of a new technique that was not developed with an ethics review process. However, this regulation will reward the proper development of therapies that ultimately improve patient safety and outcome and that are more cost effective for the health system. As neurosurgeons, we must work in cooperation with our local review boards in the innovation of surgical techniques to ensure that proper protection is in place for our patients.

REFERENCES

1. Birkmeyer JD: Outcomes research and surgeons. Surgery 124:477–483, 1998.
2. Dziuban SW Jr, McIlduff JB, Miller SJ, et al: How a New York cardiac surgery program uses outcomes data. Ann Thorac Surg 58:1871–1876, 1994.
3. NICE: National Institute for Clinical Excellence. Available at: www.nice.org.uk, 2004.
4. Royal Australasian College of Surgeons: Australian Safety and Efficacy Register of New Interventional Procedures—Surgical. Available at: www.surgeons.org/asernip-s/, 2004.
5. American College of Surgeons: Statements on emerging surgical technologies and the evaluation of credentials. American College of Surgeons. Bull Am Coll Surg 79:40–41, 1994.
6. American College of Surgeons: Statement on issues to be considered before new surgical technology is applied to the care of patients. Committee on Emerging Surgical Technology and Education, American College of Surgeons. Bull Am Coll Surg 80:46–47, 1995.
7. Campbell B, Maddern G: Safety and efficacy of interventional procedures. BMJ 326:347–348, 2003.
8. Halligan A: The Interventional Procedures Program. Health Service Circular Department of Health United Kingdom HSC 2003/011:1–4, 2003.
9. Australian Safety and Efficacy Register of New Interventional Procedures—Surgical: ASERNIP-S Systematic Review Process. Available at: www.surgeons.org/asernip-s, 2001.
10. McKneally MF, Daar AS: Introducing new technologies: Protecting subjects of surgical innovation and research. World J Surg 27:930–934, 2003.
11. Dandy WE: An operative procedure for hydrocephalus. Johns Hopkins Hosp Bull 33:189–190, 1922.
12. Scarff JE: Treatment of obstructive hydrocephalus by puncture of the floor of the third ventricle. J Neurosurg 8:204–209, 1951.
13. Guiot G: Ventriculo-cisternostomy for stenosis of the aqueduct of Sylvius: Puncture of the floor of the third ventricle with a leucotome under television control. Acta Neurochir (Wien) 28:275–289, 1973.
14. Jones RF, Stening WA, Brydon M: Endoscopic third ventriculostomy. Neurosurgery 26:86–91, 1990.
15. Boschert J, Hellwig D, Krauss JK: Endoscopic third ventriculostomy for shunt dysfunction in occlusive hydrocephalus: Long-term follow up and review. J Neurosurg 98:1032–1039, 2003.
16. Kitchell JR, Glover RP, Kyle RH: Bilateral internal mammary artery ligation for angina pectoris: Preliminary clinical considerations. Am J Cardiol 1:46–50, 1958.
17. Dimond EG, Kittle CF, Crockett JE: Comparison of internal mammary artery ligation and sham operation for angina pectoris. Am J Cardiol 5:483–486, 1960.
18. Cobb LA, Thomas GI, Dillard DH, et al: An evaluation of internal-mammary-artery ligation by a double-blind technic. N Engl J Med 260:1115–1118, 1959.
19. Kerr AG: Emotional investments in surgical decision making. J Laryngol Otol 116:575–579, 2002.
20. Badley EM: An introduction to the concepts and classifications of the international classification of impairments, disabilities, and handicaps. Disabil Rehabil 15:161–178, 1993.
21. Stowe RL, Wheatley K, Clarke CE, et al: Surgery for Parkinson's disease: Lack of reliable clinical trial evidence. J Neurol Neurosurg Psychiatry 74:519–521, 2003.
22. Meakins JL: Innovation in surgery: The rules of evidence. Am J Surg 183:399–405, 2002.
23. Wright JG: Outcomes research: What to measure. World J Surg 23:1224–1226, 1999.
24. Jenkinson C, Lawrence K, McWhinnie D, et al: Sensitivity to change of health status measures in a randomized controlled trial: Comparison of the COOP charts and the SF-36. Qual Life Res 4:47–52, 1995.
25. Choi SC, Marmarou A, Bullock R, et al: Primary end points in phase III clinical trials of severe head trauma: DRS versus GOS. The American Brain Injury Consortium Study Group. J Neurotrauma 15:771–776, 1998.
26. Woischneck D, Firsching R: Efficiency of the Glasgow Outcome Scale (GOS) score for the long-term follow-up after severe brain injuries. Acta Neurochir Suppl (Wien) 71:138–141, 1998.
27. Panesar BS, Morrison P, Hunter J: A comparison of three measures of progress in early lower limb amputee rehabilitation. Clin Rehabil 15:157–171, 2001.
28. Wityk RJ, Pessin MS, Kaplan RF, et al: Serial assessment of acute stroke using the NIH Stroke Scale. Stroke 25:362–365, 1994.
29. Lyden P, Brott T, Tilley B, et al: Improved reliability of the NIH Stroke Scale using video training. NINDS TPA Stroke Study Group. Stroke 25:2220–2226, 1994.
30. Dodds TA, Martin DP, Stolov WC, et al: A validation of the functional independence measurement and its performance among rehabilitation inpatients. Arch Phys Med Rehabil 74:531–536, 1993.
31. Kestle JR: Clinical trials. World J Surg 23:1205–1209, 1999.
32. Haines SJ: Moving targets and ghosts of the past: Outcome measurement in brain tumour therapy. J Clin Neurosci 9:109–112, 2002.
33. Sacks H, Chalmers TC, Smith H Jr: Randomized versus historical controls for clinical trials. Am J Med 72:233–240, 1982.
34. Parsons HM: What happened at Hawthorne? Science 183:922–932, 1974.
35. Fletcher RH, Fletcher SW, Wagner EH: Clinical Epidemiology: The Essentials, 3rd ed. Baltimore: Williams & Wilkins, 1996.
36. Ferguson GG, Eliasziw M, Barr HW, et al: The North American Symptomatic Carotid Endarterectomy Trial: Surgical results in 1415 patients. Stroke 30:1751–1758, 1999.
37. Molyneux A, Kerr R, Stratton I, et al: International Subarachnoid Aneurysm Trial (ISAT) of neurosurgical clipping versus endovascular coiling in 2143 patients with ruptured intracranial aneurysms: A randomised trial. Lancet 360:1267–1274, 2002.

38. Agich GJ: Ethics and innovation in medicine. J Med Ethics 27:295–296, 2001.

39. National Commission: The Belmont Report: Ethical principles and guidelines of the protection of human subjects of research. Washington, DC: U.S. Government Printing Office, 1979.

40. Steiger HJ: How to control the risk of novel surgical procedures. Acta Neurochir Suppl 78:179–184, 2001.

41. Bull C, Yates R, Sarkar D, et al: Scientific, ethical, and logistical considerations in introducing a new operation: A retrospective cohort study from paediatric cardiac surgery. BMJ 320:1168–1173, 2000.

42. Olanow CW, Goetz CG, Kordower JH, et al: A double-blind controlled trial of bilateral fetal nigral transplantation in Parkinson's disease. Ann Neurol 54:403–414, 2003.

43. Florell RC, Macdonald DR, Irish WD, et al: Selection bias, survival, and brachytherapy for glioma. J Neurosurg 76:179–183, 1992.

44. Irish WD, Macdonald DR, Cairncross JG: Measuring bias in uncontrolled brain tumor trials: To randomize or not to randomize? Can J Neurol Sci 24:307–312, 1997.

45. Patchell RA, Tibbs PA, Walsh JW, et al: A randomized trial of surgery in the treatment of single metastases to the brain. N Engl J Med 322:494–500, 1990.

46. Ehrlich PF, Newman KD, Haase GM, et al: Lessons learned from a failed multi-institutional randomized controlled study. J Pediatr Surg 37:431–436, 2002.

47. Barnett HJ, Taylor DW, Eliasziw M, et al: Benefit of carotid endarterectomy in patients with symptomatic moderate or severe stenosis. North American Symptomatic Carotid Endarterectomy Trial Collaborators. N Engl J Med 339:1415–1425, 1998.

48. Tan LC, Sutton GL, Taffinder NJ, et al: Audit of 149 consecutive carotid endarterectomies performed by a single surgeon in a district general hospital over a 12-year period. Ann R Coll Surg Engl 78:340–344, 1996.

49. Reitsma AM, Moreno JD: Ethical regulations for innovative surgery: The last frontier? J Am Coll Surg 194:792–801, 2002.

50. Clark PI, Leaverton PE: Scientific and ethical issues in the use of placebo controls in clinical trials. Annu Rev Public Health 15:19–38, 1994.

51. Freeman TB, Vawter DE, Leaverton PE, et al: Use of placebo surgery in controlled trials of a cellular-based therapy for Parkinson's disease. N Engl J Med 341:988–992, 1999.

52. Albin RL: Sham surgery controls: Intracerebral grafting of fetal tissue for Parkinson's disease and proposed criteria for use of sham surgery controls. J Med Ethics 28:322–325, 2002.

53. Cook RC, Alscher KT, Hsiang YN: A debate on the value and necessity of clinical trials in surgery. Am J Surg 185:305–310, 2003.

54. Margo CE: When is surgery research? Towards an operational definition of human research. J Med Ethics 27:40–43, 2001.

55. Bernstein M, Bampoe J: Surgical innovation or surgical evolution: An ethical and practical guide to handling novel neurosurgical procedures. J Neurosurg 100:2–7, 2004.

56. World Medical Association: World Medical Association Declaration of Helsinki: Ethical principles for medical research involving human subjects. JAMA 284:3043–3045, 2000.

57. North American Symptomatic Carotid Endarterectomy Trial Collaborators: Beneficial effect of carotid endarterectomy in symptomatic patients with high-grade carotid stenosis. N Engl J Med 325:445–453, 1991.

58. Barnett HJ, Plum F, Walton JN: Carotid endarterectomy: An expression of concern. Stroke 15:941–943, 1984.

59. Benavente O, Moher D, Pham B: Carotid endarterectomy for asymptomatic carotid stenosis: A meta-analysis. BMJ 317:1477–1480, 1998.

60. Asymptomatic Carotid Atherosclerosis Study: Endarterectomy for asymptomatic carotid artery stenosis. JAMA 273:1421–1428, 1995.

61. Freed CR, Greene PE, Breeze RE, et al: Transplantation of embryonic dopamine neurons for severe Parkinson's disease. N Engl J Med 344:710–719, 2001.

62. The EC/IC Bypass Study Group: Failure of extracranial-intracranial arterial bypass to reduce the risk of ischemic stroke: Results of an international randomized trial. N Engl J Med 313:1191–1200, 1985.

Trauma to the Scalp, Skull, and Brain

2 Surgical Repair of Major Defects of the Scalp and Skull

MICHAEL J. YAREMCHUK

Major defects of the scalp and skull are most often the result of trauma or extirpation for tumor. Although a careful physical examination is paramount in the preoperative evaluation, in most cases computed tomography (CT) or magnetic resonance imaging (MRI) is performed to provide optimal definition of the real or anticipated defect and the status of the adjacent structures.

This chapter presents plastic surgical concepts and techniques used to reconstruct major defects of the scalp and skull. The first part addresses the reconstruction of the scalp; the second part covers the reconstruction of the skull.

SCALP

Anatomy of the Scalp

The scalp consists of five distinct anatomic layers. Listed from the most superficial to the deepest, these layers include: (1) the skin with its characteristic thick dermis; (2) the subcutaneous tissue; (3) the relatively rigid galea aponeurotica, which is continuous with the superficial musculoaponeurotic system, frontalis, occipitalis, and superficial temporal fascia; (4) underlying areolar tissue; and (5) skull periosteum. The rich vascular supply of the subcutaneous layer, in which there is an abundant communication of vessels, can result in significant blood loss when the scalp is lacerated. The relatively poor fixation of the galea to the underlying periosteum of the skull provides little resistance to shear injuries, resulting in large flaps or "scalping" injuries. This layer's resultant potential space also provides little resistance to hematoma or abscess formation. As a result, extensive fluid collections related to scalp injury tend to accumulate in the subgaleal plane.

Lacerations of the Scalp

The scalp wound should always be inspected for fractures. Because the scalp has a rich vascular supply, lacerations may result in significant blood loss, particularly in children. The large diameter of the scalp vessels often requires that they be individually clamped and ligated for control. Bleeding from a scalp wound can be controlled emergently until definitive care is provided with temporary pressure dressings, Raney clip placement of the wound edges, or an over-and-over continuous stitch with large sutures.

The rich intercommunicating blood supply of the scalp is such that one set of superficial temporal vessels alone may nourish the entire scalp. This rich vascularity allows the survival of large, narrow-pedicled avulsion flaps that would never survive anywhere else on the body. For that reason, almost all traumatic scalp flaps should be appropriately cleansed, minimally débrided, and anatomically replaced. Only the hair adjacent to the lacerated edges needs to be shaved to allow easier suture placement and removal. The subgaleal space is drained with a closed suction drainage system before the scalp is closed in layers. In general, the galea and the dermis are closed with 2-0 or 3-0 polyglycolic acid sutures before the skin is closed with running or interrupted 3-0 or 4-0 nylon sutures.

Wounds with Tissue Loss

The management of scalp wounds with soft-tissue loss is determined by the amount of soft-tissue lost and the type of tissue exposed.

Local Advancement (Galeal Scoring)

The surface area of the scalp adjacent to the defect can be enlarged considerably by galeal scoring to allow closure by advancement of the wound edge. Each cut, which is made at 1-cm intervals in a parallel or crosshatch fashion, allows the scalp to be stretched approximately 4 to 6 mm. This scoring maneuver requires a complete division of the substantial galeal layer (Fig. 2-1). Tissue loss of more than 1 to 2 cm may require extension of the laceration to allow greater undermining and scoring. Defects that are 3 cm in diameter can be routinely closed with this technique.

Skin Grafts

Wounds in which soft-tissue loss is so extensive that the skin edges cannot be approximated are closed with either skin grafts or flaps. Full-thickness skin grafts contain the epidermis and the complete thickness of dermis from the recipient area. Split-thickness grafts contain the epidermis and a variable thickness of the dermis. Grafts with a greater thickness of dermis contract less on the wound bed and provide more durable coverage. Thin grafts have the advantage of more rapid revascularization, so they are more likely to be successful. Thin grafts, however, tend to provide less durable coverage.

A skin graft may cover any scalp wound that has capillary circulation, which will ultimately provide a source of vascular ingrowth for that graft. For that reason, skull periosteum or any more superficial scalp layer will support a skin graft. Most scalp defects are closed with thin (0.010- to 0.014-inch thickness), "meshed" skin grafts.

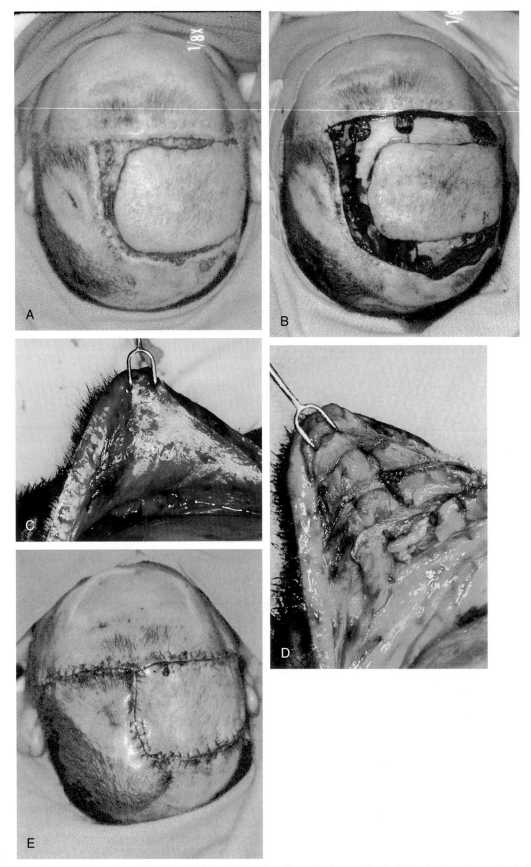

FIGURE 2-1 Scalp flaps can be enlarged considerably by galeal scoring. The galea is completely divided at 1-cm intervals. *A*, Defect before débridement. *B*, Defect after débridement. *C*, The appearance of galea before scoring. *D*, The appearance of galea after scoring. Note the increase in surface area. *E*, Resultant closure.

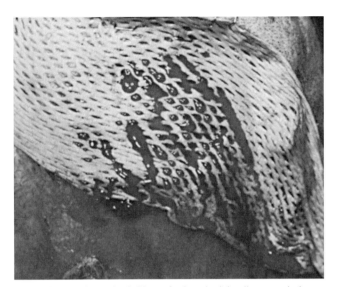

FIGURE 2-2 A meshed skin graft placed minimally expanded over a scalp wound. Note how perforations in the graft allow egress for drainage from the wound bed.

Meshed grafts are those that are mechanically perforated in a grid pattern, which allows them to be expanded and to conform to irregular surfaces. The perforations also provide egress for wound drainage. The resultant improved graft bed contact optimizes conditions for graft take (Fig. 2-2). For scalp defects, meshed grafts should not be perforated and expanded more than 1.5 times their normal size unless donor skin is in short supply. A widely expanded graft is less desirable because larger open areas take longer to epithelialize and provide poorer protective coverage.

Skin grafts are most easily harvested with an electric dermatome. The upper lateral thigh has skin of sufficient thickness to allow uncomplicated healing of the donor site. Donor site scarring in this area is usually covered with clothing.

To ensure optimal graft-bed interface for graft take, the graft should be immobilized to the scalp recipient site. A tie-over stent dressing or a quilt dressing in which the overlying dressing is sutured to the intact wound edges is most often used to achieve this immobilization.

Several flap designs allow closure of scalp wounds with significant soft-tissue loss. However, the wound should not be enlarged considerably to close a large traumatic wound emergently; rather, if the periosteum remains, a split-thickness skin graft should be applied. When scalp with periosteum is lost, a closed wound is obtained most expeditiously if, at the time of presentation, the outer table is drilled down to find bleeding points that can provide a bed for a split-thickness skin graft take. A meshed, nonexpanded, split-thickness skin graft is placed immediately at the time of the drilling. An older, well-proven technique involves removing the outer table of the skull to expose the diploë and treating the wound with wet dressings for 5 to 7 days, at which time luxuriant granulation tissue usually forms. This granulation tissue readily accepts a skin graft.

Another method involves making small drill holes 1 cm apart through the outer table down into the diploë space. Usually, granulation tissue arises from these holes and grows over the exposed calvarium to coalesce and form a suitable bed for skin grafting.

Recently, vacuum-assisted closure devices have been shown to hasten soft-tissue contraction as well as granulation tissue formation in various trunk and extremity wounds.[1] The role of such devices for treating wounds of the scalp and skull is promising but has not yet been defined.

Skin grafting directly onto bone is susceptible to breakdown after minimal trauma and leaves an area with alopecia and significant contour deformity. This problem can be corrected as a delayed reconstruction with advancement or rotational flaps after galeal scoring or with tissue expanders.

Flaps

Wounds with exposed vital structures or wounds that do not have exposed capillary circulation require flap coverage. Whereas skin grafts provide only thin coverage and depend on the wound bed for their revascularization and survival, flaps carry their own blood supply and provide soft-tissue bulk to the wound.

The two basic principles of flap coverage are: (1) to move available tissue with its intact circulation from an area of relative excess to the area of deficiency, and (2) to optimize vascularity of the flap. In the scalp, the lateral and posterior aspects are usually used as donor sites to avoid distortion of the forehead or frontal hairline. The flaps are designed to include axial vessels in their bases. Usually, the superficial temporal artery or the occipital artery provides the basic blood supply to these flaps. The flaps should be designed with respect to previous incisions, which may block vascular inflow to the flap. Although many types of rotation flaps are possible, their design requires considerable expertise and extensive mobilization of the scalp tissues. Usually most of the scalp must be degloved, and the galea should be scored to allow primary closure of the secondary defect.

Full-thickness skin coverage for the skull can usually be provided either by galeal scoring and direct advancement or by the creation of a bipedicle flap. As noted earlier, galeal scoring and advancement of wound edges usually close defects up to 3 or 4 cm in diameter. Defects larger than this can be closed by creating a bipedicle flap and by closing the secondary defect with a split-thickness skin graft on the skull periosteum. This can be considered equivalent to the situation of local advancement and placement of a relaxing incision (Fig. 2-3; see Case Report 1). Wounds too large to allow bipedicle flap coverage usually require coverage with a free tissue transfer (free flap).

Free Flaps

A free flap is one that is completely detached from the donor area and moved to another site on the body. After this movement, circulation to the flap is restored by the microsurgical anastomosis of flap and available recipient site vasculature. The superficial temporal artery or other branches of the external carotid system in the neck most often provide donor site vasculature for free tissue transfers used to reconstruct the scalp. The addition of free flaps to the reconstructive surgeon's armamentarium makes almost any size of wound reconstructable[2] (Fig. 2-4; see Case Report 2).

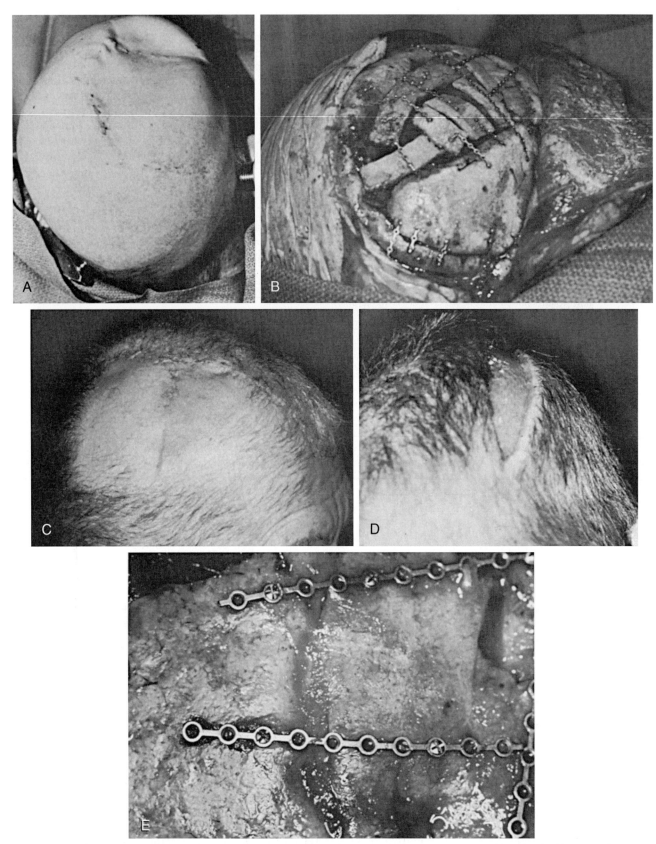

FIGURE 2-3 Scalp reconstruction and split cranial bone cranioplasty after removal of a recurrent meningioma that had been previously irradiated. A bipedicle flap was advanced to replace the unstable skin. The secondary defect was resurfaced with a skin graft. *A*, Intraoperative appearance from behind and above. Note that positioning allows access to and exposure of as much skull as possible. *B*, Reconstruction of a right temperoparietal defect from behind, with split cranial bone stabilized with microplates and screws. *C*, Postoperative appearance from the right side of the reconstruction site. *D*, Frontal postoperative appearance of a skin-grafted secondary defect after rotation of the bipedicle flap. *E*, Appearance of skull reconstruction at the time of reoperation, 2 years later.

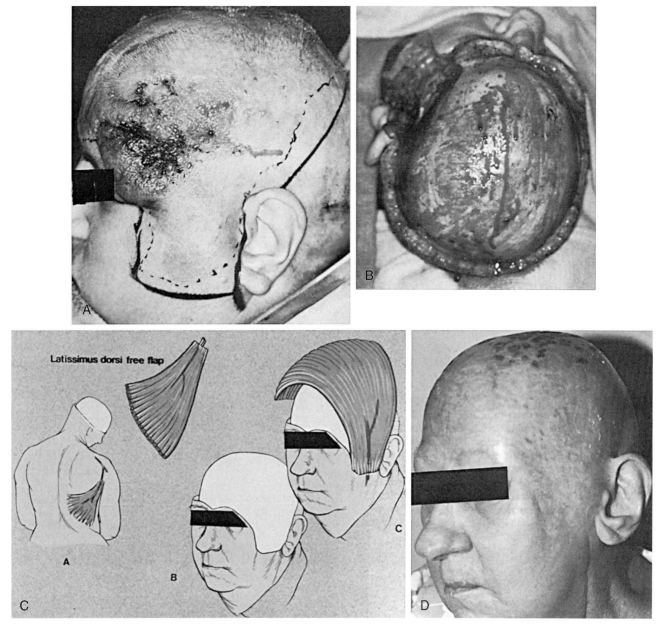

FIGURE 2-4 *A*, Preoperative lateral view of a scalp tumor. *B*, Intraoperative view of the defect from above and behind. *C*, A diagrammatic representation of the procedure. *D*, The postoperative result.

Tissue Expansion

Tissue expansion makes use of the long-observed principle that skin expands to accommodate itself to gradual stretching. In 1978, Radovan was the first to report successful clinical applications of this observation and to demonstrate prototypes of the expanders in clinical use today.[3–5] The expanders that are currently in use are silicone bags with self-sealing valves placed beneath the areas to be expanded.

Tissue expansion has become a preferred technique of scalp reconstruction because it provides hair-bearing skin for reconstruction. The distance between hair follicles does not increase to a clinically noticeable amount, and, unlike many rotation flaps, the resultant advancement flap created by the expansion process does not appreciably change the orientation of the hair follicles.

Tissue expanders are placed adjacent to the defect in a subgaleal pocket. Saline may be injected percutaneously through a one-way valve into the expander once or twice per week to increase the volume. The duration required to inflate the expander varies with each clinical situation, but it is usually between 4 and 8 weeks. At a second operation, the expander is removed, and the resultant scalp flap is used to close the defect.

Disadvantages of tissue expansion include the need for two or more operations, the interim deformity, and usually the fact that the expander cannot be placed in the acute setting. Tissue expanders are most often placed after the wound has been closed temporarily by simpler but less definitive techniques (Fig. 2-5; see Case Report 3).

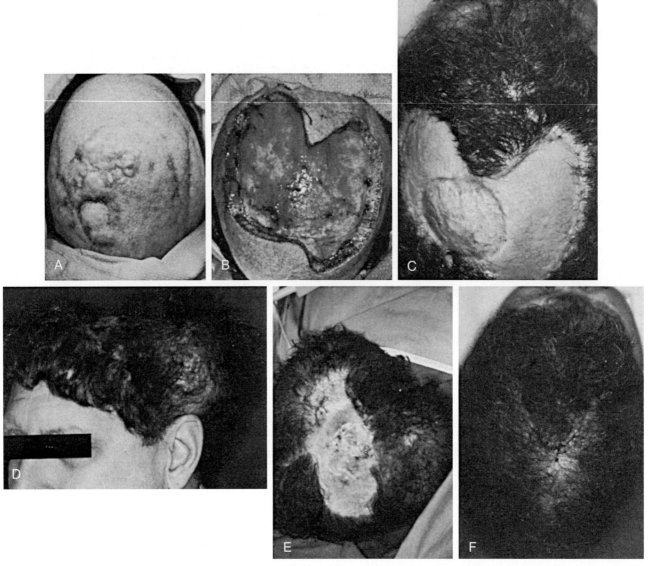

FIGURE 2-5 This patient underwent radical excision of a scalp cancer and staged reconstruction using tissue expansion. *A,* Preoperative appearance of a scalp tumor. *B,* An intraoperative view of the resultant scalp defect. *C,* Postoperative appearance after placement of a meshed split-thickness skin graft. The central area is where the outer table was removed and the split graft was placed on the diploë. *D,* Appearance with tissue expander in place. Scalp expansion and advancement were performed twice to close the defect. *E,* Intraoperative appearance during removal of a second set of expanders. *F,* Postoperative appearance after removal of the second set of expanders, flap advancement, and closure.

CASE REPORT 1

SCALP AND SKULL RECONSTRUCTION WITH A LOCAL FLAP AND CRANIAL BONE GRAFTS (See Fig. 2-3)

A 65-year-old woman was referred for treatment of a recurrent meningioma arising in the right parietal area. This patient had undergone high-dose radiation treatment for the lesion as well as extirpative surgery. Complications led to loss of the bone flap in this area. On preoperative examination, the patient was found to have extremely atrophic skin in the area of her previous surgery and radiation and a large parietal skull defect beneath it.

The patient's previous craniotomy scars were reopened, the recurrent tumor was removed, and a dural repair was performed. A separate bone flap in the occipital area was

harvested, and the inner table removed using the Midas Rex drill. The outer table of the occipital bone was returned to its anatomic position. The right parietal defect was repaired with the bone harvested from this flap, and fixation was provided with microplates and screws. At the time of closure, the unstable skin was excised and replaced with a sagittally oriented bipedicle flap, which was harvested in a supraperiosteal plane. The resultant defect located in the left parietal area was skin grafted with a meshed, split-thickness skin graft that was harvested from the left lateral thigh. This graft was meshed 1 to 1.5 times and placed nonexpanded on the secondary skull defect.

The patient's postoperative course was unremarkable. Two years later, another meningioma was found in an adjacent area. During this surgery the anterior aspect of the previous operative site was exposed to reveal complete healing of the previous reconstruction of the skull vault.

CASE REPORT 2
SCALP RECONSTRUCTION WITH A FREE TISSUE TRANSFER (See Fig. 2-4)

A 58-year-old previously healthy woman was referred with a 6-month history of a rapidly growing scalp tumor. The preoperative evaluation revealed no evidence of tumor spread beyond the scalp. A biopsy revealed that the tumor was an angiosarcoma.

The entire tumor, along with a 2-cm margin of grossly normal-appearing skin, was removed down to the outer table of the skull. In addition, a left-sided parotidectomy was performed. The defect was reconstructed with a latissimus dorsi muscle–free tissue transfer. The muscle was then covered with a split-thickness skin graft that was harvested from the left thigh.

The patient's postoperative course was unremarkable. Chemotherapy was administered postoperatively. The patient died of metastatic disease approximately 2.5 years after surgery.

CASE REPORT 3
SCALP RECONSTRUCTION WITH SKIN GRAFT AND TISSUE EXPANSION
(See Fig. 2-5)

A 47-year-old man was referred with a massive dermatofibrosarcoma protuberans carcinoma of the scalp, which had been treated 8 years previously with a topical solution. A preoperative evaluation revealed clinical and CT evidence that the tumor focally involved the outer table of the skull.

The lesion was excised together with a 2-cm margin of grossly normal-appearing tissue. Removal resulted in a defect down to the periosteum of 17×12 cm. Where the tumor was adjacent to the outer table, the outer table was excised to an area 8 cm^2. The wound was immediately closed by the placement of a meshed, split-thickness skin graft of approximately 0.014-inch thickness on the patient's periosteum and drilled-down outer table. This recipient site was dressed with Adaptic and saline-soaked gauze, which was immobilized by sewing the dressing to the intact scalp. The dressing was removed after 7 days, at which time the graft had almost completely taken. The area was observed for a recurrence for 1 year, but none occurred. During this time, small areas of skin graft breakdown occurred; these areas were managed with local dressing care. Approximately 1.5 years after radical removal of the tumor, two large tissue expanders were placed in the hair-bearing skin in the occipital and temporal areas. These expanders were gradually filled over the next 10 weeks, after which the expanders were removed and the resultant scalp flap was advanced. This action resulted in a remaining defect of approximately 8×10 cm. Two more tissue expanders were placed, and the expansion process was repeated. At the time of removal of the second set of expanders, the entire area of skin-grafted skull was resurfaced with hair-bearing skin.

SKULL
Anatomy of the Skull

The calvaria has three distinct layers in the adult: the hard internal and external laminae and the cancellous middle layer, or diploë. The bony vault has an average thickness of about 5 mm, but this varies considerably across areas and among individuals. Skull thickness lessens considerably in the elderly. The thickest area is usually the occipital, and the thinnest area is usually the temporal.

The calvaria is covered with periosteum on both the outer and inner surfaces. On the inner surface, it fuses with the dura to become the dura's outer layer. Unlike other areas of the skeleton, and perhaps because of the lack of functional stresses on the skull, the periosteum of the skull seems to have little osteogenic potential in the adult. Therefore, the loss or removal of the calvaria requires its replacement if its location is important from a protective or esthetic standpoint.

Esthetically, the frontal bone is the most important calvaria because only a small portion of it is concealed by hair-bearing scalp. In addition, it forms the roof and portions of the medial and lateral walls of the orbit. Displaced frontal fractures may therefore cause a visible deformity or globe malposition. The frontal bone also includes the frontal sinuses, which are paired structures that lie between the inner and outer lamellae of the frontal bone. The lesser thickness of the anterior wall of the frontal sinus makes this area more susceptible to fracture than the adjacent temperorbital areas.

Fractures of the Skull

Skull fractures should be considered after any craniofacial trauma. Bruises, lacerations, ocular injuries, brain impairment, or adjacent facial fractures should alert the physician to the possibility of skull fracture.

The radiographic examination is essential for the diagnosis. Plain films are limited by artifact secondary to suture lines, density overlap, and vessel grooves. For that reason, a CT scan has become the gold standard when evaluating injuries to the craniofacial skeleton and the intracranial structures.

Indications for Surgery

Surgery for skull fracture is indicated for three main reasons: (1) to address a dural tear or an associated brain injury, (2) to avoid early or late sinus dysfunction, or (3) to avoid deformity.

Surgical Technique for Frontobasilar Fractures
Exposure

The bicoronal incision provides ideal exposure to the frontobasilar region for both the neurosurgeon and the craniofacial surgeon. Neurosurgical exploration, if necessary, is usually conducted through this access under the control provided by a craniotomy and bone flap. The dural repair should provide a watertight seal. In addition to allowing a panoramic view to compare for symmetry, the coronal incision provides easy access to cranial bone grafts. The resultant scalp scar is usually hidden inconspicuously within the hair. Unless they are very extensive or preclude the use of a bicoronal approach, preexisting lacerations are rarely used for access to this area. The access provided by lacerations is often limited and usually requires their significant enlargement; the resultant long scar is often the most deforming sequela of the injury. We have been disappointed with the postoperative appearance of the eyebrow incision and therefore avoid its use.

Management of Frontal Sinus Injuries

Management of frontal sinus injuries has long been controversial for several reasons. Because such injuries are relatively rare, very few surgeons have extensive experience with this injury. The care of these injuries tends to be fragmented by different specialties, which also limits the experience by any one surgeon or surgical group. This fragmentation by specialization also results in varied criteria for evaluating the results of surgery. In addition, the infectious complications that may arise after treatment of these injuries do so many years later. Finally, the evaluation of esthetic results is quite arbitrary.

Our treatment algorithm is determined by the extent of the injury. Because the skeletal injury can be well documented by a preoperative CT scan, this imaging modality is important in the preoperative assessment. In any frontal sinus injury, the status of the brain, the anterior and posterior frontal walls of the sinus, the nasofrontal ducts, and the sinus mucosa must be considered. Injuries isolated to the anterior wall of the frontal sinus have a very low incidence of nasofrontal duct dysfunction.[6] Therefore, if the anterior wall displacement does not constitute an objectionable contour deformity, these injuries are observed but are not necessarily treated operatively. If a significant contour deformity exists, surgery can be undertaken to correct it. During the surgery, any devitalized sinus mucosa is

removed, the nasofrontal ducts are examined for patency, and fracture segments are replaced anatomically and stabilized in position.

Injuries extending into the adjacent supraorbital area have a much greater likelihood of nasofrontal duct injury and subsequent dysfunction.[6] These injuries are explored, and the frontal sinus is defunctionalized. To avoid frontal sinus mucocele formation, the walls of the sinus are drilled with a high-speed drill under constant irrigation to remove any sinus invaginations along venous channels that might later allow mucous formation.[7] The frontal sinus is further defunctionalized and isolated from the nasal cavity by obstruction of the nasofrontal ducts with contour-fit bone graft plugs. Finally, the sinus is obliterated with autogenous material. Craniofacial surgeons tend to obliterate the sinus with cancellous bone, whereas otolaryngologic surgeons usually employ autogenous fat.[8,9] The use of alloplastic materials[10] is controversial. The superiority of any one material has not been documented.

Injuries that include the posterior wall have the greatest potential for intracranial contamination with sinus contents. When the posterior wall is badly disrupted, it is removed, thus "cranializing" the frontal sinus. When cranialization is performed, care is taken to effectively seal the expanded intracranial cavity from the nasal cavity. This process may require reconstruction of the cranial base with bone grafts. Pericranial and galeal frontalis flaps may be particularly useful in providing a well-vascularized seal.[11]

Note that no attempts are made to restore nasofrontal duct or sinus function once concern exists for its compromise; rather, the sinus is defunctionalized by mucosal exenteration and sinus obliteration or cranialization.

Frontal Bone Reconstruction

The reconstructive goal in frontal bone reconstruction is to restore the fronto-orbital contour. In most cases, this can be

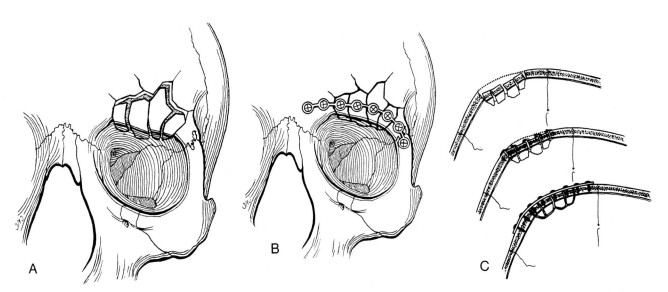

FIGURE 2-6 Miniaturized plates and screws are used to maintain 3-dimensional anatomic reduction of the fronto-orbital area. *A,* A comminuted supraorbital rim fracture. *B,* Fracture segments are anatomically reduced and stabilized with plates and screws. *C,* Axial view (*top*) of a supraorbital rim fracture showing resultant loss of projection (*dotted lines*). Fixation with interfragmentary wires (*middle*) does not restore the projection. Fixation with plates and screws (*bottom*) restores the projection. (From Yaremchuk MJ, Gruss JS, Manson PN [eds]: Rigid Fixation of the Craniofacial Skeleton. Boston: Butterworth Publishers, 1992.)

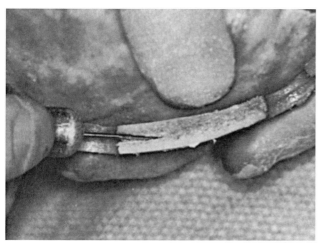

FIGURE 2-7 The bone flap is being split with a Midas Rex drill (Midas Rex Pneumatic Tools, Fort Worth, TX) using a C-1 bit.

performed in the acute setting. The creation of a surgically clean wound allows replacement of frontal bone fragments and acute bone grafting in most injuries. This process may require débridement of devitalized soft-tissue edges to allow primary wound healing and effective management of the sinuses, as noted previously.

The key to restoring fronto-orbital contour is the anatomic replacement of fracture segments in three dimensions. Interfragmentary wiring of fracture segments alone is usually inadequate because wiring allows bone fragments to sink posteriorly and inferiorly, thus losing projection. Bone loss at multiple sites (and particularly along craniotomy cuts) tends to aggravate this problem. In fact, surgical restoration of preinjury contour often requires fracture segment replacement without bone-to-bone contact. Such replacement can be accomplished only by stabilizing bone segments with plates and screws. The plates are bent to the appropriate shape and are fixed to a stable anatomic point. The fracture segments or bone grafts are then attached to the plates with screws (Fig. 2-6). Titanium has become a popular material for craniofacial plates because of its high strength and decreased artifact on CT and MRI studies compared with stainless steel or cobalt chromium (Vitallium).[12,13]

When autogenous bone grafts are required for replacement or augmentation, they are often harvested from the inner table of the bone flaps used to obtain neurosurgical access (Fig. 2-7; see Case Report 4 and Fig. 2-11).

CRANIOPLASTY

The most common indication for cranioplasty is the infectious loss of a bone flap after elective craniotomy. Cranioplasty may also become necessary in primary repair where bone replacement was not possible at the time of the acute post-traumatic reconstruction. Cranioplasty can only be performed after infection has been eradicated. Eradication of infection may require the removal of bone flaps used in elective procedures or of bone fragments replaced immediately after trauma. The resultant deformity is reconstructed after the clinical infection has been treated and the area remains clinically free of infection.

As is true of acute craniomaxillofacial reconstruction, the reconstructive goal in cranioplasty is to provide protection for the brain and to restore the preinjury appearance. The two major indications for cranioplasty are protection and esthetics. In addition, speech problems and hemiparesis may improve by cranial reconstruction, but the more vague symptoms related to the "syndrome of the trephined" are less reliably improved.[14,15] Skull defects larger than 2 or 3 cm should be considered for repair; however, this decision varies with location of the defect. Even small defects in the frontal area can be disturbing to the patient and can, therefore, be considered for repair. Defects of the temporal and occipital areas, which are covered by thick muscle, are usually not reconstructed.

Timing of Surgery

The incidence of infection is influenced by the timing of cranioplasty. A significant reduction in incidence of infection has been shown when 1 year is allowed to elapse between the initial injury or infection and the subsequent reconstruction.[16–18]

Bone cranioplasty has been advocated when the reconstruction is performed adjacent to sinus cavities or in areas in which previous infection occurred, despite a lack of objective evidence to support this contention.[15,19,20]

A recent review of the literature shows that a history of infection increases the incidence of infection after cranioplasty by an average of 14% and that cranioplasty in the frontal area causes twice the incidence of infection noted for all other areas (5%).[20,21] In reviewing their experience of 42 post-traumatic reconstructions of frontal defects in which both bone and acrylic were used, Manson and colleagues found that the material employed was not as important as the timing of reconstruction (i.e., more than 1 year after infection), eradication of communication between the cranial vault reconstruction and the nasal and frontal sinus cavities, and absence of any ethmoidal or frontal sinus inflammatory disease.[16] These data are consistent with our clinical observations. We prefer to delay cranioplasty for 1 year after control of infection, to treat all sinus disease before reconstruction, and to eradicate communication between the sinus cavities and the reconstruction. Bone is used when the potential for sinus communication or a history of recurrent infection exists; otherwise, most reconstructions are performed with alloplastic material.

Preparation for Cranioplasty

Before cranioplasty, poorly vascularized skin areas are revised, and residual frontal or ethmoidal sinus disease is eliminated. At surgery, the patient is positioned so that a panoramic view of the skull is possible and, if appropriate, the upper face can be draped into the field. This position allows the surgeon to compare the contralateral anatomy and to avoid unnatural transitions. Preinjury photographs may be helpful in certain situations. A skull model should be available to aid in the creation of complex curvatures and landmarks.

Old scars are usually incised for exposure, and the scalp flap is removed carefully from the underlying dura and brain. Any dural tears are repaired. Resection of the bone edge to identify normal dura, and establishment of a plane of dissection may be necessary. The freed bone edge is saucerized by removal of the outer table with rongeurs or a high-speed burr. This lip prevents the implant from slipping into the defect and provides a ledge for subsequent fixation.

Choice of Material for Cranioplasty

Cranioplasty is performed using autogenous bone or alloplastic implants.

Bone

Bone is preferred by many craniofacial surgeons because its revascularization and concomitant "creeping substitution" allows it to be incorporated into the host as a living graft. Conceptually, but not proven by objective data, this viability makes these reconstructions less susceptible to late infection. Bone cranioplasty has the disadvantages of requiring a donor site, being technically demanding to perform, and exhibiting variable resorption and therefore being prone to irregular contour. Furthermore, the strength of this cranioplasty has not been documented. Bone donor sites include the ribs; the calvaria; and, less commonly, the iliac crest.

Split ribs are useful when large defects are to be reconstructed and calvarial bone is in short supply. Split ribs are usually fitted into a shelf created in the adjacent intact skull. In the past, an interlocking "chain link"[19] technique was used for fixation, but most craniofacial surgeons now use a combination of plates and screws (Fig. 2-8).

Calvarial bone is the preferred donor site of most craniofacial surgeons. Clinical experience and several animal studies have shown that calvarial bone maintains its volume better than split rib or iliac crest. The calvarial bone is harvested in two ways. The outer table may be harvested from the intact skull. The parietal area usually serves as the donor site, because this area is usually accessible and the donor site contour deformity is hidden by the patient's hair (see Case Report 6 and Fig. 2-12).

Another technique for harvesting cranial bone is to perform a craniotomy and harvest a full-thickness piece of skull of appropriate size and curvature. The inner table is split from the outer table. A simple way to do this is with the aid of the Midas Rex drill and the C-1 bit (see Fig. 2-7). This thin bit is placed in the diploë between the two skull cortices. The outer cortex can be replaced, and the inner cortex is used for reconstruction of the defect. Most often, microplates and screws are used to stabilize this reconstruction.

Methyl Methacrylate

Today, the most commonly used material for cranioplasty is methyl methacrylate. Methyl methacrylate reconstruction

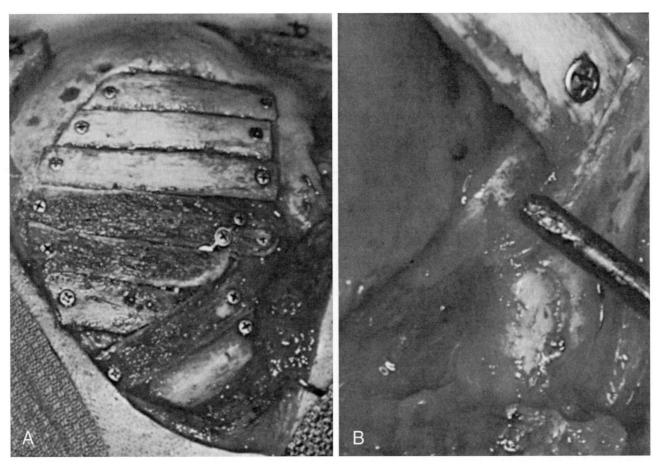

FIGURE 2-8 *A,* An example of a split-rib cranioplasty stabilized with plates and screws on the right frontotemporal area. *B,* A close-up view shows a ledge created by removing the outer table at the edge of the defect. This allows a ledge for the rib graft and ease of screw fixation.

has the advantages of ease of reconstruction and avoidance of donor site morbidity. The contour of this substance is stable. It is radiolucent and, therefore, does not affect postoperative radiologic imaging. It is not affected by temperature and is very strong. Methyl methacrylate is believed by some to be more susceptible to infection and late complications.[16,22] Cranioplasty kits are available that contain a single dose of 30 g of powdered polymer and 17 mL of liquid monomer. The elements are mixed with a spatula in a bowl. The mixing should be conducted under ventilation so that the person who is mixing the substance is not overcome by fumes. The mixing process takes about 30 seconds. The bowl is then covered to avoid evaporation of the monomer. Doughing time varies with the temperature and takes approximately 5 minutes at 72°F.

Shaping of the plastic implant is usually performed by placing the doughy mixture in a plastic sleeve provided in the cranioplasty kit. The sleeve containing the still pliable implant mixture is placed onto the skull defect and molded by digital compression. The molding process occurs under continuous irrigation to avoid thermal damage to the dura and brain. The molding time usually takes 6 to 8 minutes. The very exothermic polymerization process is allowed to take place away from the surgical field.

Some surgeons place a wire mesh into the skull defect. Methyl methacrylate is then cured directly on the mesh. This technique allows more risk for burn damage to the dura during the exothermic reaction; however, data from Manson and colleagues show that temperature rises less than 3°C when the implant is continuously irrigated.[16]

Complex curvatures, particularly in the supraorbital area, are created by adding material to an initial construct. Final adjustments can be made with a contouring burr on a high-speed drill. The implants may be secured with wires or, more simply and rapidly, with microscrews. The plate may be perforated to allow the dura to be tented up to it. This method reduces the potential for epidural collection. Perforations in the implant also allow for drainage and for soft-tissue ingrowth, which also aids in implant fixation (see Case Report 5).

Porous Materials

Newer implant materials have been developed to decrease the likelihood of postoperative infection after alloplastic cranioplasty. These materials exploit their porosity, allowing some degree of host incorporation as opposed to the fibrous encapsulation seen with smooth surfaced implants such as methyl methacrylate. Polyethylene (Medpor)[23] (Fig. 2-9) and polymethylmethacrylate/polyhydroxy methyl methacrylate (HTR)[24] have both been proven useful for cranioplasty. Both of these implant materials are strong and can be fixed to the intact skull with plates and screws.

Hydroxyapatite

Hydroxyapatite is a ceramic biomaterial that consists of calcium phosphate, a main constituent of bone. It can be manufactured synthetically or formed by chemically converting the naturally porous calcium carbonate skeleton of marine coral. Three forms of hydroxyapatite have been used for facial skeletal reconstruction. Block hydroxyapatite has been used as relatively small interposition grafts.[25] Ono and colleagues[26] found that computer-generated hydroxyapatite cranioplasty implants were extremely fragile because of the brittle nature of hydroxyapatite forms. Granular hydroxyapatite has been used as an onlay for orbitocranial defects. The problems with this material included slow cement consolidation and unpredictable volume restoration.[26] A powdered form of hydroxyapatite became available in 1996 (Bone Source, Leibinger Corp., Carrollton, TX). When mixed with water, the powder becomes a paste that is easily applied to regular surfaces. The paste sets in approximately 20 minutes. Hydroxyapatite cement has been shown to be osteoconductive, but because of its microporous nature (6 mm for Bone Source), minimal direct bony or vascular ingrowth occurs.[28] Because of its low flexural resistance, it has been primarily used for recontouring.

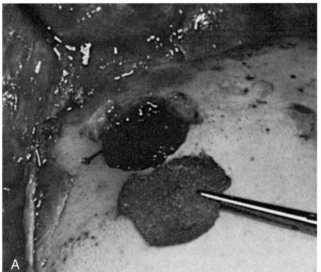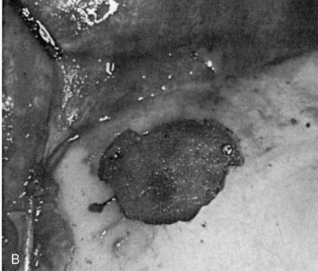

FIGURE 2-9 A 3-cm left frontal defect after removal of a benign bone tumor is reconstructed with a Medpor implant. *A,* An intraoperative view showing the defect and the implant. *B,* The implant is in place. A ledge was created in the frontal bone by removing the outer table in two places. A flange of Medpor was affixed to this ledge with microscrews.

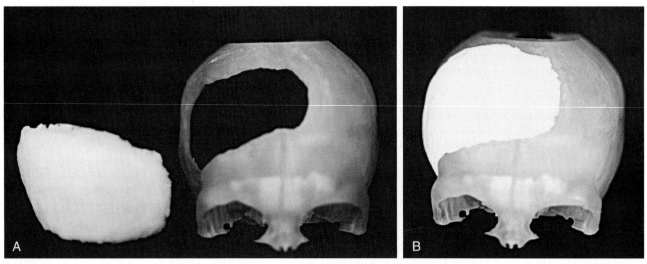

FIGURE 2-10 A 3-dimensional model of a skull defect with a CAD/CAM-generated polyethylene implant (*A*) adjacent to the skull and (*B*) fitted into the defect.

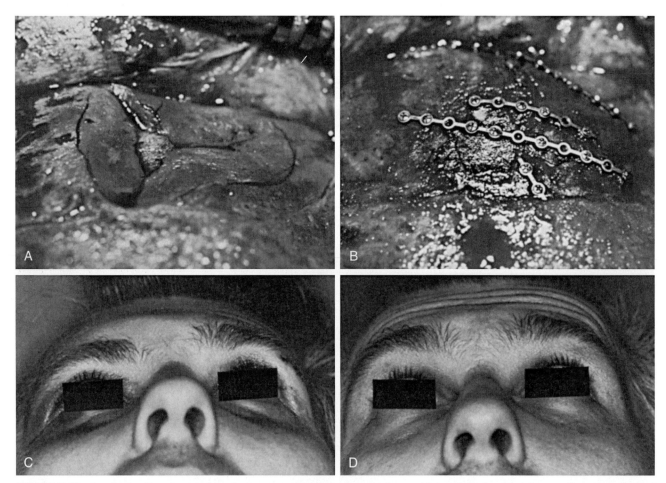

FIGURE 2-11 A patient with a frontal sinus fracture managed by open reduction and internal fixation. *A*, Intraoperative appearance of fracture as seen from above through the coronal approach. *B*, After reduction and fixation. Miniplates and screws were used for fixation. *C*, A preoperative worm's eye view. *D*, A postoperative worm's eye view.

When used to reconstruct defects, it is used with metallic mesh.[29,30] The appropriate role of hydroxyapatite for cranioplasty has not yet been defined.

Computer-Aided Design/Computer-Aided Manufacture (CAD/CAM)

CT imaging of skull defects provides digitized information that can be transferred to design software. Data describing the contour along the edge of the defect and the surface characteristics of the normal cranium surrounding the defect can be used to design a custom-fitted implant. The electronic data describing the newly designed prosthesis are then used by a computer-controlled manufacturing system to create a wax model, which is then cast; or it is used to directly mill raw material into the finished implant (Fig. 2-10).[31,32] Prefabricated implants of various materials, including HTR,[24] porous polyethylene,[33] and polymethylmethacrylate,[34] are available. The use of custom prefabricated implants can reduce operative time significantly.

CASE REPORT 4
FRONTAL BONE FRACTURE REPAIR

A 38-year-old man was referred with a frontal fracture 1 week after being involved in a motor vehicle accident (Fig. 2-11A to D). The patient had no neurologic symptoms, and a preoperative axial CT scan showed the fracture to be confined to the anterior wall of the frontal sinus. Surgery was performed through a bicoronal incision. The fracture segments were elevated, and the frontal sinus was explored. No injury to the nasofrontal ducts was found. The devitalized mucosa was removed, and the fracture segments were replaced anatomically and fixed in position with microplates and screws. The patient was discharged on the fourth postoperative day. His postoperative course has been unremarkable over the past 2 years.

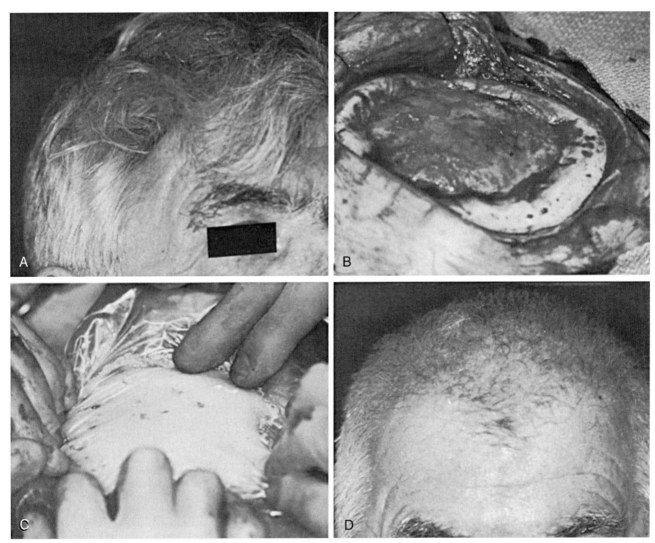

FIGURE 2-12 Acrylic cranioplasty. *A,* The preoperative appearance. *B,* An intraoperative view of the right frontoparietal defect. *C,* Molding of methyl methacrylate to the defect. *D,* The postoperative result.

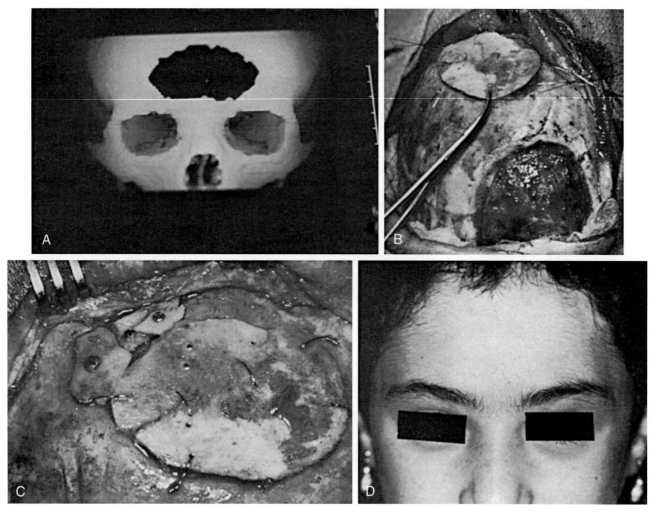

FIGURE 2-13   A frontal cranioplasty is performed with an outer table cranial bone. *A*, A preoperative 3-dimensional CT scan shows the frontal defect. *B*, An intraoperative view shows the donor site and the graft in position. *C*, A close-up view of the graft, which is stabilized with screws. The supraorbital rim was augmented with onlay grafts. *D*, The postoperative appearance.

CASE REPORT 5
ACRYLIC CRANIOPLASTY

A 65-year-old man was referred for cranioplasty (Fig. 2-12A to C). The patient had undergone tumor resection in the parietal area 1 year before, and postoperative infection required removal of the bone flap. The patient's previous surgical scar was incised. The scalp flap was dissected off to the dura, and an acrylic cranioplasty with methyl methacrylate was performed. The patient's postoperative course was unremarkable.

CASE REPORT 6
CRANIOPLASTY WITH CRANIAL BONE GRAFTS

A 10-year-old girl was referred from Armenia after having had an open skull fracture in an earthquake (Fig. 2-13). Emergency treatment consisted of débridement of bone fragments and soft-tissue closure. The patient had no neurologic abnormalities. The physical examination and CT scan revealed a large frontal defect. In addition, there were unrepaired fractures of the supraorbital rim, resulting in supraorbital depression on the left side. Surgery was performed through a bicoronal incision. The scalp flap was dissected away from the dura. A template of the defect was placed over the parietal area, and bone from the outer table of the skull was removed. This bone was transferred to the central frontal area to reconstruct the defect, and it was stabilized with microplates and screws. In addition, left supraorbital contour was restored by the placement of onlay grafts of outer table cranial bone. These grafts were fixed with microscrews and contoured in situ. The patient was discharged on the fifth postoperative day, and her postoperative course was unremarkable.

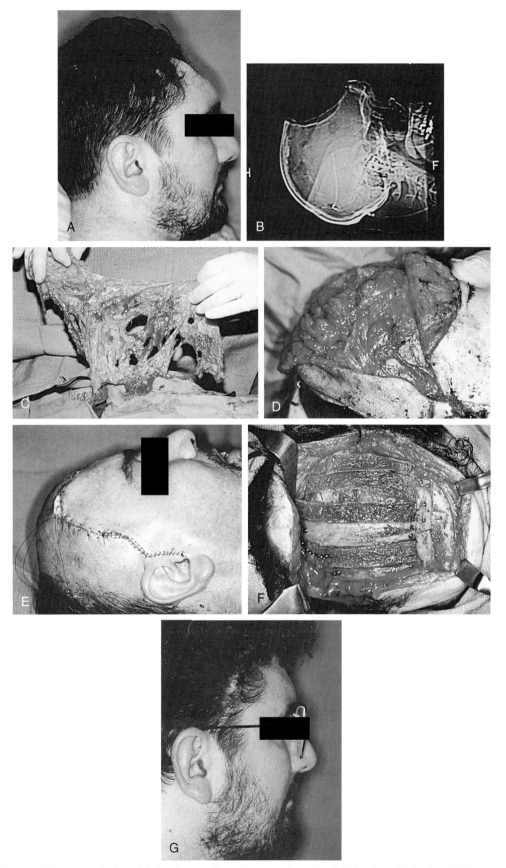

FIGURE 2-14 Repair of the traumatic frontal defect is complicated by a cerebrospinal fluid fistula and infection. *A,* The preoperative profile. *B,* Sagittal plane CT scan image of the defect. *C,* Harvest of an omental flap. *D,* Placement in defect. *E,* Postoperative view from the omental flap. *F,* Split rib grafts are in place. *G,* A late postoperative photograph showing restoration of the normal contour.

CASE REPORT 7
COMPOSITE SCALP AND SKULL RECONSTRUCTION WITH FREE TISSUE TRANSFER AND RIB GRAFTS

A 32-year-old man sustained an open frontal injury in a high-speed motor vehicle accident (Fig. 2-14A to G). He developed a cerebrospinal spinal fluid fistula and meningitis, necessitating lumbar drainage and intravenous antibiotics. The skull deformity persisted, and the overlying skin remained unstable. An omental free flap was used to cover the dura and fill dead space. Six months later, split rib grafts were used to restore the bone contour.

CONCLUSIONS

Reconstruction of the scalp and skull usually requires computerized image evaluation, in addition to careful clinical examination, to provide optimal definition of the real or anticipated defect and the status of the adjacent structures. The size and location of a soft-tissue defect will determine the complexity of procedures required for reconstruction. Alternatives include local tissues advancement, skin grafting, tissue expansion, and possibly the use of free tissue transfers. Skull reconstruction requires that the surgeon have facility with both carpentry, the use of alloplastic materials, and rigid fixation techniques.

REFERENCES

1. Argenta LC, Morykwas MJ: Vacuum-assisted closure: A new method for wound control and treatment: Clinical experience. Ann Plast Surg 38:563–577, 1997.
2. Urken ML, Catanlano PJ, Sen C, et al: Free tissue transfer for skull base reconstruction: An analysis of complications and a classification system for defining skull base defects. Arch Otolaryngol Head Neck Surg 119:1318–1325, 1993.
3. Nordstrom REA, Devine JW: Scalp stretching with a tissue expander for closure of scalp defects. Plast Reconstr Surg 75:578–581, 1985.
4. Radovan C: Breast reconstruction after mastectomy using the temporary expander. Plast Reconstr Surg 69:195–206, 1982.
5. Radovan C: Tissue expansion in soft tissue reconstruction. Plast Reconstr Surg 74:482–490, 1984.
6. Stanley RB Jr: Fractures of the frontal sinus. Clin Plast Surg 16:115–123, 1989.
7. Donald PJ: The tenacity of frontal sinus mucosa. Otolaryngol Head Neck Surg 87:557–566, 1979.
8. Donald PJ, Ettin M: The safety of frontal sinus fat obliteration when sinus walls are missing. Laryngoscope 96:190–198, 1986.
9. Wolfe SA, Johnson P: Frontal sinus injuries: Primary care and management of late complications. Plast Reconstr Surg 82:781–789, 1988.
10. Rosen G, Nachtigal D: The use of hydroxyapatite for obliteration of the human frontal sinus. Laryngoscope 105:553–555, 1995.
11. Gruss JS, Pollock RA, Phillips JH, Antonyshyn O: Combined injuries of the cranium and face. Br J Plast Surg 42:385–398, 1989.
12. Fiala TGS, Paige KT, Davis TL, et al: Comparison of artifact from craniomaxillofacial internal fixation devices: Magnetic resonance imaging. Plast Reconstr Surg 93:725–731, 1994.
13. Saxe AW, Doppman JL, Brennan MF: Use of titanium surgical clips to avoid artifacts seen on computed tomography. Arch Surg 117:978–979, 1982.
14. Grantham EG, Landis HP: Cranioplasty and posttraumatic syndrome. J Neurosurg 5:19–26, 1948.
15. Stula D: The problem of "sinking skin-flap syndrome" in cranioplasty. J Craniomaxillofac Surg 10:142–146, 1982.
16. Manson PN, Crawley WA, Hoopes JE: Frontal cranioplasty: Risk factors and choice of cranial vault reconstructive material. Plast Reconstr Surg 77:888–900, 1986.
17. Hammon WM, Kempe LG: Methyl methacrylate cranioplasty: 13 years experience with 417 patients. Acta Neurochir 25:69–76, 1971.
18. Rish BL, Dillon JD, Meirowsky AM, et al: Cranioplasty: A review of 1030 cases of penetrating head injury. Neurosurgery 4:381–386, 1979.
19. Munro IR, Guyuron B: Split-rib cranioplasty. Ann Plast Surg 7:341–346, 1981.
20. White JC: Late complications following cranioplasty with alloplastic plates. Ann Surg 128:743–751, 1948.
21. Woolf JI, Walker AE: Cranioplasty. Int J Surg 81:1–9, 1945.
22. Wofle SA: In discussion: Manson PN, Crawley WA, Hoopes JE. Frontal cranioplasty: Risk factors and choice of cranial vault reconstructive material. Plast Reconstr Surg 77:901–904, 1986.
23. Yaremchuk MJ: Facial skeletal reconstruction using porous polyethylene implants. Plast Reconstr Surg 111:1818–1827, 2003.
24. Eppley BL, Kilgo M, Coleman JJ: Cranial reconstruction with computer generated hard-tissue replacement patient-matched implants: Indications surgical techniques and long-term follow-up. Plast Reconstr Surg 109:864–871, 2002.
25. Holmes R, Hagler H: Porous hydroxyapatite as a bone graft substitute in cranial reconstruction: A histometric study. Plast Reconstr Surg 81:662, 1988.
26. Ono I, Tateshita T, Satou M, et al: Treatment of large complex cranial bone defects by using hydroxyapatite ceramic implants. Plast Reconstr Surg 104:339–347, 1999.
27. Byrd HS, Hobar PC, Shewmake K: Augmentation of the craniofacial skeleton with porous hydroxyapatite granules. Plast Reconstr Surg 91:15–26, 1993.
28. Matic D, Phillips JH: A contraindication for the use of hydroxyapatite cement in the pediatric population. Plast Reconstr Surg 110:1–5, 2002.
29. Burstein FD, Cohen SR, Hudgins R, et al: The use of hydroxyapatite cement in secondary craniofacial reconstruction. Plast Reconstr Surg 104:1270, 1999.
30. Constantino PD, Friedman CD, Jones K, et al: Experimental hydroxyapatite cement cranioplasty. Plast Reconstr Surg 90:174, 1992.
31. Wehmoller MW, Eufinge H, Kruse D, Massberg W: CAD by processing of computed tomography data and CAM of individually designed prostheses. Int J Oral Maxillofac Surg 24:90–97, 1995.
32. Eufinger H, Wehmoller MW, Machtens E, et al: Reconstruction of craniofacial bone defects with individual alloplastic implants based on CAD/CAM manipulated CT data. J Craniomaxillofac Surg 23:175–181, 1995.
33. Yaremchuk MJ: Acquired cranial deformities. In Mathes SJ: Plastic Surgery. Philadelphia: WB Saunders (in press).
34. Taub PJ, Rudkin GH, Clearihue WJ, Miller TA: Prefabricated alloplastic implants for cranial defects. Plast Reconstr Surg 111:1232–1240, 2003.

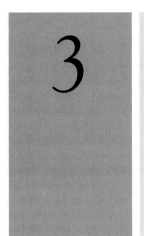

3

Perioperative Management of Severe Traumatic Brain Injury in Adults

IAN F. DUNN, KAI FRERICHS, ARTHUR L. DAY, and DONG H. KIM

INTRODUCTION

Traumatic brain injury (TBI) is responsible for nearly 2 million emergency department admissions in the United States, affecting 2% of the population per year. Approximately 250,000 of these patients require hospitalization; nearly 50% of those admitted will undergo surgical evacuation of a hematoma.[1] Mortality is 20%; another 35% have significant long-term neurologic deficits.[2] Given these demographics, there have been organized efforts to standardize assessment and care of the patient with head injury, with the International Data Bank and the Traumatic Coma Data Bank (TCDB) representing significant efforts to define the assessment of coma as well as identify the critical variables that can affect outcome.[3,4] Attempts to systematize care of patients with severe TBI have culminated in evidence-based guidelines issued by the joint task force between the Brain Trauma Foundation and the American Association of Neurological Surgeons.[5,6] The results of collaborative efforts such as these have focused management emphasis on both the primary injury, that which occurs from the initial traumatic insult, and secondary injuries, the pathophysiologic events occurring in subsequent minutes, hours, and days after the primary insult. In this chapter, we review the important considerations in the nonsurgical management of patients with severe TBI. We first note the classifications and assessment of severe TBI. Second, we focus on appropriate management strategies to avoid intracranial hypertension and cerebral ischemia. Last, we discuss overall medical optimization and possibilities for novel neuroprotective strategies.

INITIAL NEUROLOGIC ASSESSMENT

Glasgow Coma Scale

The examination begins with a careful assessment for external head trauma; the neurologic examination starts with the Glasgow Coma Scale (GCS) (Table 3-1). Developed in 1974 by Teasdale and Jennett, the GCS is the most widely used method of determining the severity of TBI. Included in the assessment are eye opening, verbal response, and motor response, giving a general gauge of the level of consciousness.[7] A well-documented prehospital GCS score is helpful, but situations in the field often complicate the GCS score calculation. Examples include pharmacologic paralysis required for intubation and significant facial trauma precluding accurate eye opening assessment. Any physiologic derangements at the time of assessment must also be considered. Conditions such as hypotension and hypoxia significantly impair the neural response to stimulation, leading to a GCS score that may not accurately reflect the extent of injury. When a patient has an endotracheal or tracheostomy tube in place and cannot give a verbal response, a GCS score of 1 is given for that section, with a T following to indicate the intubated status.

GCS scores of 3 to 8 indicate severe TBI and correlate significantly with outcome; the motor score is the most reproducible and carries the most prognostic information.[8] Nearly 80% of patients with an initial hospital GCS score of 3 to 5 have an eventual outcome of death, severe disability, or vegetative state; patients with an initial GCS score of 3 have a 65% mortality rate.[8-10] Additionally, patients with a GCS score decrease of 2 points or more between the field and the emergency department are more likely to require surgical intervention.[11]

TABLE 3-1 ▪ Glasgow Coma Scale

Eye opening (E)

Spontaneous	4
To speech	3
To pain	2
Not open	1

Verbal response (V)

Conversant	5
Confused	4
Nonsense	3
Sounds	2
Silence	1
Intubated	1T

Motor response (M)

To command	6
To pain	
Localizing	5
Withdrawal	4
Arm flexion	3
Arm extension	2
No response	1

GCS = E + V + M (range, 3 or 3T–15)

GCS, Glasgow Coma Scale.
From Teasdale G, Jennett B: Assessment of coma and impaired consciousness: A practical scale. Lancet 2:81–84, 1974.

Pupillary Examination

The pupillary examination is critical; a dilated pupil that fails to respond to light is evidence of ipsilateral uncal herniation until proven otherwise. Bilaterally dilated pupils may result from hypoxia, hypotension, bilateral nerve dysfunction, or severe irreversible brain stem injury. A change in the pupillary examination is the most reliable indicator in determining the side of a mass lesion and carries an 80% positive predictive value.

Motor Examination

Hemiparesis is also useful but can be confusing due to the Kernohan's notch phenomenon, a mass lesion may manifest with *ipsilateral* hemiparesis from compromise of the contralateral cerebral peduncle that is pushed against the contralateral tentorial edge.

PRIMARY AND SECONDARY TRAUMATIC BRAIN INJURY

Primary Brain Injury

Significant morbidity and mortality results not only from the original injury sustained during TBI, but also from ensuing pathophysiologic processes evolving over a period of hours to days,[12,13] prompting the differentiation between what has been termed *primary* and *secondary* brain injury. Primary brain injury, referring to the clinical sequelae resulting directly from the initial injury, can be broadly divided into focal and diffuse injuries (Table 3-2). Focal injuries include traumatic intracranial hematomas and contusions. Diffuse injuries comprise the clinical spectrum from concussion to posttraumatic coma or diffuse axonal injury (DAI). The particular injury depends on the nature of the force during injury (contact or inertial loading), the type of injury (rotational, translational, or angular acceleration), and the magnitude and duration of impact. While diffuse injuries were more common and account for nearly 60% of severe TBI in the TCDB, mortality rates are higher in focal injuries when compared to diffuse injuries (39% vs. 24%).[14] Because emergent surgical intervention may be required, the first critical step in the management of primary brain injury is the determination of the presence of a mass lesion by computed tomography (CT) scan.

Secondary Brain Injury

Although primary brain injury refers to a particular traumatic insult, secondary brain injury refers to cellular processes that take place over hours to days after the initial brain injury that compound the effects of the initial injury. Secondary brain injury results not only from the delayed effects of primary brain injury but also from aggravating factors such as hypotension, hypoxia, inadequate cerebral perfusion pressure (CPP), and intracranial hypertension.[15] Untreated, the ultimate result is cerebral ischemia, which can significantly compound the effects of the initial injury. Knowledge of the pathophysiologic basis, indications for monitoring, and the treatments available for cerebral ischemia and intracranial hypertension are of paramount importance to the neurosurgeon caring for patients with severe TBI.

CEREBRAL ISCHEMIA

Pathophysiology

Nearly 80% of patients who die after severe TBI have ischemic damage on gross autopsy.[16] Cerebral ischemia is defined as cerebral blood flow (CBF) which is inadequate to meet metabolic demands of the brain. While the brain constitutes only 2% to 3% of the body's weight, it consumes 25% of its oxygen and receives about 20% of its cardiac output. The brain is almost totally reliant on adequate blood flow; nearly 95% of the brain's metabolism is oxidative, and there is no significant oxygen storage capacity and limited glucose and glycogen reserves. As such, a discrete metabolic autoregulatory mechanism exists which couples cerebral blood flow (in units of mL/100 g/min) with the cerebral metabolic rate of oxygen ($CMRO_2$, measured in mL/100 g/min), so that adequate perfusion exists to support local metabolic needs. This relationship is codified by the Fick equation: $CMRO_2 = CBF \times AVDO_2$, where $AVDO_2$ (mL/dL) is the arteriovenous difference in oxygen and is measured by subtracting the jugular venous oxygen content ($S_{jv}O_2$) from the systemic arterial oxygen content. $CMRO_2$ in comatose patients is typically reduced from a normal value of 3.3 mL/100 g/min to 2.1 mL/100 g/min.[17] In physiologic conditions, changes in $CMRO_2$ are paralleled by changes in CBF, maintaining a constant $AVDO_2$. In circumstances of decreased CBF, as with systemic hypotension or deranged cerebral pressure autoregulation, $AVDO_2$ increases as the brain increases extraction of oxygen to avoid ischemia, and this change can be measured by noting the $S_{jv}O_2$. Normal oxidative cerebral metabolism is altered in patients with $S_{jv}O_2$ less than 50%, and neurologic deterioration and irreversible ischemic injury are correlated with values less than 20% to 30%. In one study, a single episode of $S_{jv}O_2$ reduced below 50% was tied to a twofold increase in poor outcome; two or more episodes carried a 14-fold increase in poor outcome in the same study.[18]

Cerebral Blood Flow and Cerebral Perfusion Pressure

A central tenet of cerebrovascular physiology is that a constant supply of metabolic substrates is maintained by a constant CBF over a range of CPPs, a concept known as pressure autoregulation and distinct from metabolic autoregulation. CPP is defined as the mean arterial pressure (MAP) minus the intracranial pressure (ICP). Normally, CBF is relatively constant in a range of CPPs between

TABLE 3-2 ▪ Types of Structural Primary Brain Injury

Focal	Diffuse
Hematoma	Concussion
Epidural	Multifocal contusion
Subdural	Diffuse axonal injury
Intracerebral	
Contusion	
Concussion	
Lacerations	

40 and 150 mm Hg. A dynamic system of arterial vasoconstriction and dilation exists to preserve CBF and oxygen delivery. At low perfusion pressures within this range, the arteriolar bed dilates to reduce cerebral vascular resistance and increase blood flow to normal levels. At higher perfusion pressures, arteriolar constriction occurs to protect the vascular bed from overperfusion. At perfusion pressures below the autoregulatory threshold, arterioles passively collapse and CBF decreases. At pressures above the autoregulatory limits, vessels are maximally dilated and CBF increases.

An important distinction in cerebrovascular physiology exists between CBF and cerebral blood volume (CBV). CBF is the physiologic parameter that governs cerebral perfusion and adequate oxygenation. CBV is the total intracranial blood content and is a major determinant of ICP by the Monro-Kellie doctrine. Importantly, CBV can be reduced while maintaining an adequate degree of CBF to control ICP.

Pressure autoregulation is lost in many patients after TBI.[19] Bouma and Muizelaar[20] reported in a series of 117 patients in which autoregulation was lost in 49% of patients. Even when pressure autoregulation is intact, the parameters at which autoregulation occurs were often shifted, with significant therapeutic implications. The lower limit of autoregulation may increase from the 40- to 50-mm Hg range to the 70- to 90-mm Hg range,[20–22] meaning that normally adequate perfusion pressures may cause ischemia in these patients, even when autoregulation is intact.

Given these findings, the clinician must assume that in patients with severe TBI, CBF has a linear relationship to CPP. Many local processes can affect CBF, including physical compression of vessels by mass lesions or local edema, reduced cerebral metabolism of oxygen, and post-traumatic vasospasm.[23,24] Nearly 33% of patients with severe TBI have CBF values near the ischemic threshold (<18 mL/dL), occurring most often with diffuse cerebral edema and acute subdural hematoma[25–27] within the first 24 hours after primary injury.[28,29] Many investigators have demonstrated a significantly higher mortality rate and worse outcomes among survivors when CBF was inadequate at any point during the first 7 days after injury.[19,30–33]

To prevent cerebral ischemia and maximize outcome, CPP must be closely monitored and maintained. Some authors report that CPP higher than 60 mm Hg maintains adequate levels of brain tissue PO_2 in patents with head injury, whereas others believe that a CPP of 70 mm Hg is required to prevent reduction in $S_{jv}O_2$.[34,35] Prospective studies have demonstrated a mean mortality rate of 21% in patients with severe TBI when CPP is maintained above 70 mm Hg, as compared with a 40% mortality rate in the Traumatic Coma Data Bank series.[36] Others have shown in retrospective analyses that mortality increased by 20% for each 10 mm Hg decrement in CPP below 80 mm Hg.[37] Although targets may differ among various authors, there is consensus that CPP less than 60 mm Hg is harmful.[5,6]

Systemic Contributors to Ischemia: Hypotension and Hypoxia

Adequate cerebral oxygenation is threatened by systemic hypotension and hypoxia. Miller and colleagues[38] and Marmarou and colleagues[39] showed a 150% increased risk of mortality in patients with severe TBI who had at least one episode of hypotension as defined by systolic blood pressure

less than 90 mm Hg when compared with patients without hypotension. Others have noted that mortality doubled in patients with TBI who had a single hypotensive episode (systolic blood pressure <90 mm Hg).[40]

Similarly, Stochetti and colleagues[41] showed that patients with severe TBI with hypoxic episodes before intubation had a 77% mortality rate, and 100% of survivors were severely disabled. In contrast, a 14.3% mortality rate and 4.8% severe disability rate were noted among survivors of severe head injury with no documented hypoxic episodes. More alarmingly, poor outcomes have been correlated even with a single episode of hypoxia.[8,41] Early intubation in patients with a GCS score of less than 9 was shown to improve outcome among 1092 patients with severe head injury.[42]

Monitoring

CPP calculation is the most routinely used parameter in treatments aimed at avoiding cerebral ischemia. Systemic arterial oxygen saturation and blood hematocrit are monitored as standard practice in all trauma patients. Other techniques available include direct brain tissue PO_2 (monitoring by fiberoptic catheter) and venous oxygenation sampling (by an internal jugular vein catheter directed toward the jugular bulb). Imaging modalities aimed at directly assessing CBF include such noninvasive techniques as transcranial Doppler sonography, xenon CT, and N_2O uptake as well as several techniques performed during surgery with brain exposed, such as laser Doppler flowmetry and laser flow flowmetry (reviewed in references 43 and 44).

Management Principles

The avoidance of cerebral ischemia is one of the pillars in the modern management of severe head injury. Management principles center on maintaining an adequate CPP and avoiding systemic hypotension, hypoxia, and anemia to ensure adequate CBF. The Brain Trauma Foundation currently supports maintaining a CPP higher than 60 mm Hg, whereas other centers advocate a CPP higher than 70 mm Hg.[6] In patients with inadequate CPP, systemic causes of hypotension such as cardiac or spinal cord injury, tension pneumothorax, and bleeding must be ruled out. Intravascular volume must also be assessed. Vasopressors are often necessary to maintain adequate CPP. The profiles of commonly used pressors are listed in Table 3-3. All listed agents are sympathomimetics; phenylephrine is probably the most commonly used.[45–48] Treatment with these agents, although clearly necessary, may be associated with complications such as pulmonary edema and/or expansion of preexisting hematomas or contusions[49] and as such they must they must be used with caution (see later discussion).

Anemia may also decrease tissue oxygenation, and the hematocrit deserves particular attention in the patient with head injury. Although an optimal value has not been established, reports suggest that brain tissue oxygen delivery begins to decrease at a hematocrit of less than 33%.[50] Most centers transfuse packed red blood cells for a hematocrit less than 30%. As with all trauma patients, a hematocrit refractory to blood transfusion should prompt a search for extracranial bleeding sources.

TABLE 3-3 ▪ Pressors and Cerebral Hemodynamics

Agent	MAP	CBF	ICP
Dopamine <2 µg/kg/min	↔	↔	↔/↓
Dopamine 2–6 µg/kg/min	↑	↔/↑	↑
Dopamine 7–20 µg/kg/min	↑	↔/↑	↓/↑
Phenylephrine	↑	↔	↔
Norepinephrine	↑	↔	↔
Epinephrine	↑	↔	↔
Dobutamine	↔/↑	↑	↔/↑

CBF, cerebral blood flow; ICP, intracranial pressure; MAP, mean arterial pressure.

INTRACRANIAL HYPERTENSION

Pathophysiology

The other pillar of modern management is attention to intracranial hypertension, a common complication of severe head injury. Nearly 50% of patients with head injury with intracranial mass lesions and 33% of patients with diffuse axonal injury have persistently elevated ICP.[51] ICP is determined by the contents of the intracranial vault, whose physiology is codified by the Monro-Kellie doctrine. The total volume available for intracranial contents (CBV, cerebrospinal fluid [CSF], and brain) is constant, and an increase in one compartment must be accompanied by a decrease in the other. An uncompensated increase in one or more compartments results in ICP higher than the normal range of 5 to 15 mm Hg.[52,53] In the absence of a mass lesion, increased ICP in severe TBI results from alterations in CSF flow, CBV, and the development of vasogenic and cytotoxic edema.[54,55] Resistance to absorption of CSF in traumatic subarachnoid hemorrhage may lead to an increase in overall CSF. An increase in CBV results from the loss of autoregulation in severe TBI, and vasogenic and cytotoxic edema result from a compromised blood-brain barrier and osmotic dysregulation in ischemic cells. Physiologic volume-buffering mechanisms exist and involve alterations of blood and CSF volume and include arteriolar vasoconstriction, increasing cerebral venous outflow, and downward CSF displacement through the foramen magnum or into expanded root sleeves. Once these mechanisms are exhausted, ICP increases in an exponential fashion (Fig. 3-1). In such states, small volumetric changes can lead to rapid and devastating neurologic deterioration. Another way of conceptualizing ICP and its relationship to volume is Marmarou's linear pressure-volume index in which the ICP and volume are plotted on a semilogarithmic curve whose slope is the pressure-volume index (PVI), or brain compliance, representing the amount of volume needed to change ICP 10-fold.[56,57] Sustained ICP readings of greater than 20 mm Hg are abnormal, ICP readings between 20 and 40 mm Hg represent moderate intracranial hypertension, and ICP readings greater than 40 mm Hg represent severe preterminal intracranial hypertension.[58]

The two principal consequences of elevated ICP are brain herniation and impaired cerebral perfusion (as noted by the formula CPP = MAP − ICP). The displacement or herniation of brain through openings in the dura and skull occurs in several patterns: subfalcine herniation, uncal herniation, central downward herniation, tonsillar herniation, and external herniation of brain through an open skull fracture. Of particular importance are uncal herniation and downward herniation. Uncal herniation is produced by medial displacement of the temporal lobe by lateral middle fossa or temporal lobe lesions in which the ipsilateral

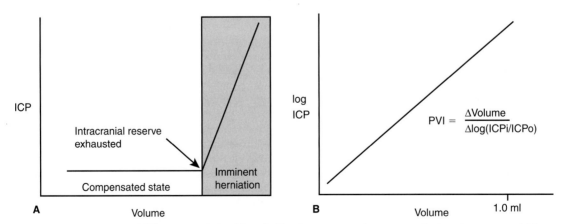

FIGURE 3-1 Intracranial pressure (ICP)-volume relationships. *A,* Classic pressure-volume curve depicts the exponential increase in ICP once compensatory mechanisms of handling additional intracranial volume are exhausted. In the patient with severe head injury, additional volume may take the form of increased cerebrospinal fluid from poor absorption, increased cerebral blood volume, vasogenic edema from a compromised blood-brain barrier, and cytotoxic edema. *B,* Pressure-volume index (PVI). Change in volume plotted against ICP before (ICPo) and after (ICPi) volume change in a logarithmic fashion. (From Marmarou A, Shulman K, Rosende RM: A nonlinear analysis of the cerebrospinal fluid system and intracranial pressure dynamics. J Neurosurg 48:332–344, 1978.)

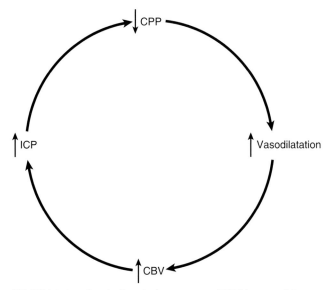

FIGURE 3-2 Cerebral perfusion pressure (CPP)-intracranial pressure (ICP) relationship in preserved autoregulation. CBV, cerebral blood volume. (From Rosner MJ: Introduction to cerebral perfusion pressure management. Neurosurg Clin N Am 6:761–763, 1995.)

oculomotor nerve, cerebral peduncle, reticular activating system, and possibly contralateral cerebral peduncle (Kernohan's phenomenon) are compromised. The resulting clinical syndrome involves coma, ipsilateral fixed and dilated pupil, and contralateral hemiparesis. Should the contralateral peduncle be compressed against the contralateral tentorial edge, ipsilateral motor function may also be compromised. Central or downward herniation may result from globally increased ICP and is defined by progressive caudal displacement of the brain stem through the foramen magnum. Basilar artery perforators are stretched and may hemorrhage (Duret's hemorrhages). The clinical syndrome may include Cushing's triad (arterial hypertension, bradycardia, and respiratory irregularity); coma is the result.

Increased ICP also compromises cerebral perfusion. Aside from the fact that increased ICP can decrease CPP, it is also true that a decrease in CPP can increase ICP. As CPP decreases, pial arterioles vasodilate and accommodate larger blood volumes (CBV), diagrammed in Rosner's[22] vasodilatory cascade (Fig. 3-2). This increased blood volume can increase ICP. When CPP is restored, pial arterioles can constrict and ICP will often decrease.

Monitoring

Consensus has emerged regarding indications for placing an ICP monitor in patients with TBI, based on the identification of groups at risk of developing intracranial hypertension. At highest risk are patients with a GCS score of less than 8 and an abnormal CT scan; as many as 60% of these patients develop elevated ICP readings.[59] Although patients with a GCS score of less than 8 with normal-appearing CT scans on admission have a 10% to 15% chance of developing elevated ICPs, there is a subgroup with a 60% chance of intracranial hypertension: those older than age 40, systolic blood pressure less than 90 mm Hg, and unilateral or bilateral motor posturing.[59–61] We place

ICP monitoring devices in all patients with GCS scores of less than 8, unless there is a coexisting coagulopathy. We also consider placement in some patients with GCS scores of more than 8 who are undergoing extensive anesthesia for extracranial surgery.

Ventriculostomy: Indications and Technique

Ventriculostomy permits drainage of CSF in addition to ICP monitoring and is especially indicated in patients with hydrocephalus and intraventricular hemorrhage or whenever intracranial hypertension is expected to be a significant problem. The risks of placement include a 5% hemorrhage rate[62] and a 5% to 10% infection rate, which can be minimized by appropriate placement and sterile technique. Infection may be further reduced by the use of antibiotic-impregnated catheters.[63] Current data do not support prophylactic catheter exchange to reduce infection rates (reviewed in reference 64).

We favor a right-sided ventriculostomy, avoiding the dominant hemisphere, unless this ventricle is collapsed. With the patient supine, the head is shaved widely and prepared in sterile fashion. Midline is always marked and careful attention paid to the position of the ipsilateral mid-pupillary line, tragus, and medial canthus. A small linear incision is carried down through skin to bone at the spot 10 cm back from the nasion and 3 cm lateral to the midline; this position may also be marked as the spot 1 to 2 cm in front of the coronal suture in the mid-pupillary line (Fig. 3-3). A twist drill is used to open the cranium. After the bony fragments are removed, the dura and pia are opened by abrading them gently with a to-and-fro twisting action of the drill. The hole must be drilled in the trajectory desired: if the skull is thick, it will influence the subsequent passage of the catheter. The catheter is directed toward the ipsilateral medial canthus in the mediolateral plane and the ipsilateral tragus in the anteroposterior plane. An alternative is to pass the catheter perfectly perpendicular to the skull surface. The catheter is then tunneled out through the skin through a separate stab incision to reduce the likelihood of infection. Even in the presence of a mass lesion or shift, the same landmarks and trajectory are used.

We never pass to a depth of more than 6 cm from the inner table. If the ventricle is not cannulated on the third attempt, the catheter is left in and a CT scan is obtained to check the position. An overly lateral placement risks internal capsule injury, and an overly deep catheter pass risks injury to critical brain stem structures.

Other Monitoring Devices: Indications and Technique

When we are not certain that intracranial hypertension will be a problem or when the ventricles are slitlike, an intraparenchymal monitor is placed. The scalp incision is made in the same location as for ventriculostomy, and a smaller drill bit is used. The dura is opened with a small stylet, and a fixation bolt screwed in to hold parenchymal fiberoptic catheter in place; the catheter itself is passed approximately 1 to 2 cm into the parenchyma. The hemorrhage and infection risks are lower than for ventriculostomy, but the disadvantages include drift of ICP readings over time and the inability to drain CSF therapeutically.

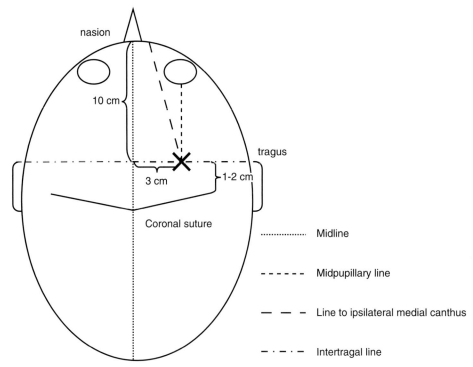

FIGURE 3-3 Ventriculostomy anatomy.

Management of Increased Intracranial Pressure

The goals of intracranial hypertension management are the maintenance of satisfactory CPP and the avoidance of intracranial herniation. The clinical justification for ICP reduction is that elevated ICP is an independent predictor of poor neurologic outcome in patients with severe head injury.[31,59,60,65] Although this management principle is well supported, the particular threshold at which treatment is initiated varies. Marmarou documented incrementally worse outcomes with increasing duration of ICP readings higher than 20 mm Hg.[39] Saul and Ducker and Contant and colleagues reported worse outcomes in patients with sustained ICP readings greater than 25 mm Hg.[65,66] More recently, Marshall and colleagues found that initial or sustained ICP readings higher than 20 mm Hg were effective predictors of poor neurologic outcome among patients with severe head injury.[34] The Brain Trauma Foundation[6] supports initiating treatment at ICP readings between 20 and 25 mm Hg, while preserving adequate CBF. A caveat in the rigid adherence to these oft-quoted values is that herniation may occur at ICP readings of less than 20 mm Hg, particularly with temporal lesions. Conversely, a therapeutic CPP target may be reached with ICP readings as high as 25 mm Hg. At our institution, we initiate treatment for ICP readings greater than 25 mm Hg, unless CPP is compromised at lower levels. We employ a stepwise approach, beginning with techniques to optimize venous outflow from the brain (head elevation), followed by pharmacotherapy and CSF drainage (Fig. 3-4).

Physical Positioning

We advocate elevating the head of the bed to 30 degrees and maintaining a neutral head position to maximize venous return from the brain and thereby reduce CBV. CBV is to be differentiated from CBF; CBV represents the

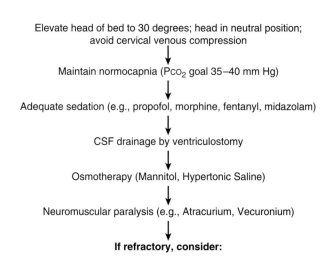

FIGURE 3-4 Stepwise protocol for intracranial pressure management. CSF, cerebrospinal fluid.

total amount of blood in the intracranial space and affects ICP, whereas CBF is the physiologic parameter that governs adequate brain tissue oxygenation. A reduction in CBV does not a priori suggest a reduction in CBF; it is possible to maintain adequate CBF and CPP while reducing CBV. Although some advocate keeping the head of the bed flat to maximize CPP,[67] other data have shown that CPP and CBF may be preserved and ICP reduced by elevating the head of the bed to 30 degrees.[68–70] In addition, raising the head of the bed more than 30 degrees significantly decreases the rate of pneumonia.

Avoidance of Hypoventilation: CO$_2$ Reactivity

CBF varies with CPP in pressure autoregulation and with CMRO$_2$ in metabolic autoregulation. Changes in arterial CO$_2$ also affect CBF and vascular caliber. For every mm Hg change in PaCO$_2$, the CBF changes 2% to 3%. These vascular effects are passively mediated through changes in pH in the perivascular space, not directly by PaCO$_2$.[71] Hypoventilation leads to an increase in PaCO$_2$, resulting in vasodilatation and an increase in CBF and ICP. Hyperventilation leads to a decrease in PaCO$_2$, arteriolar vasoconstriction, and a reduction in CBF and ICP.

Although pressure autoregulation may be deranged in severe head injury, CO$_2$ reactivity is preserved.[19,72] The routine measurement of PaCO$_2$ in patients with head injury is strongly recommended. Hypoventilation increases PaCO$_2$ and ICP, whereas PaCO$_2$ levels below 35 mm Hg may lower ICP but compromise CBF. The ideal PaCO$_2$ level in patients with head injury is normocapnia to avoid elevations in ICP from hypoventilation and decreased CBF and ischemia from hyperventilation.

Adequate Sedation and Analgesia: Neuromuscular Paralysis

Sedation and analgesia may blunt the sympathetic stimulation provided by pain from traumatic injury or agitation from brain injury, endotracheal irritation, or routine nursing care, all of which if untreated may increase ICP. An additional benefit of benzodiazepine sedation is the reduction of CMRO$_2$. The effects on MAP, CBF, and ICP of commonly used sedative and analgesic agents are shown in Table 3-4.[73–75] Narcotics (e.g., fentanyl, morphine) alone or in combination with short-acting benzodiazepines (e.g., midazolam) are commonly administered. The short-acting sedative-anesthetic propofol is being used with increasing frequency because its short half-life permits frequent neurologic examinations and because it appears to have superior effects on ICP reduction compared with narcotic-based regimens.[76] Propofol is a potent vasodilator, and careful attention must be paid to MAP and CPP during its administration.

When intracranial hypertension becomes severe, patients may require pharmacologic paralysis by neuromuscular blockade for maximal muscle relaxation. Agents with short durations of effect (atracurium lasts for 30–45 minutes and vecuronium lasts for 45–60 minutes) are preferred so that neurologic examinations may be conducted at frequent intervals.[77,78] Their effects on cerebrovascular hemodynamics and ICP in normal conditions are shown in Table 3-4. Neuromuscular paralysis is reserved when all standard treatments have been exhausted (see Fig. 3-4).

Occasionally observed in patients with severe head injury is the paradoxical sympathetic storm characterized by episodic hyperhidrosis, hypertension, hyperthermia, tachypnea, tachycardia, and posturing; this constellation is only suggested after mass lesions, seizure, toxic/metabolic derangements, and infection have been excluded. The prevailing view is that these symptoms represent disruption of autonomic function in the diencephalon and brain stem. A combination of small doses of morphine for sedation and appropriate α$_1$- and β-receptor blockade with labetalol is particularly effective in addressing the clinical manifestations of these occasional sympathetic outbursts.[79]

Cerebrospinal Fluid Drainage by Ventriculostomy

CSF drainage via an external ventricular drain or ventriculostomy is a highly effective and physiologic method of ICP reduction in patients with head injury. The utility of the ventriculostomy catheter, however, may be compromised in the presence of considerable brain edema and subsequent ventricular collapse. When a ventriculostomy is in place, we use it to drain CSF to its maximal capacity for increased ICP control before starting osmotherapy. When an intraparenchymal monitor is in place, however, osmotherapy may be instituted first. If large amounts of mannitol or hypertonic saline are required to control ICP, we replace the intraparenchymal device with a ventriculostomy if possible.

Osmotherapy

The osmotic diuretic mannitol is a mainstay in the control of elevated ICP. We prefer to administer this drug in 0.25- to 1-g/kg boluses and expect maximal reduction of ICP within 15 minutes of administration, with effects lasting as long as 4 hours. An osmotic diuretic, mannitol was commonly thought to reduce ICP by reducing intracranial water[80] but is now recognized to also expand plasma volume and decrease viscosity. CBF increases and ICP is decreased by autoregulatory vasoconstriction.[81–85] Furosemide (0.7 mg/kg), which can inhibit the production of CSF, may potentiate the effects of mannitol. When given together, a greater and more sustained decrease in ICP has been observed.[86]

TABLE 3-4 ▪ Cerebrovascular Profiles of Commonly Used Sedatives and Analgesics

Agent	MAP	CBF	ICP
Morphine (1–5 mg/hr)	↓	↔	↑
Fentanyl (25–100 µg/hr)	↓	↔	↑
Midazolam (0.05–5 µg/kg/min)	↓	↓	↔ / ↓
Propofol (0–100 µg/kg/min)	↓	↓	↓
Atracurium (20–50 mg/hr)	↔ / ↓	↔	↔
Vecuronium (4–10 mg/hr)	↔	↔	↔

CBF, cerebral blood flow; ICP, intracranial pressure; MAP, mean arterial pressure.
Data from references 73–76.

When using mannitol, intravascular volume status, serum osmolarity, sodium, and blood urea nitrogen and creatinine levels must be monitored for possible adverse effects. When the serum osmolarity is more than 320 mOsm, mannitol, particularly in large doses, may precipitate acute tubular necrosis.[87] With prolonged use, mannitol can also disrupt the blood-brain barrier, and it may pass into the brain parenchyma and cause a rebound effect, with subsequent increases in ICP.[87–89]

Two studies have demonstrated the effectiveness of mannitol in controlling ICP. A randomized, controlled trial comparing mannitol with barbiturates in the management of high ICP in patients with head injury showed superior ICP reduction, CPP preservation, and overall outcome in patients treated with mannitol.[90] A smaller study showed the superior effects of mannitol in ICP reduction, CPP preservation, and $S_{jv}O_2$ levels when compared with ventriculostomy drainage alone or hyperventilation.[91]

Hypertonic Saline Solutions

Hypertonic saline solutions may be used as an adjunct or alternative to mannitol. One advantage of these agents compared with mannitol is a lower risk of rebound intracranial hypertension and renal failure. In hyperosmolar concentrations, sodium chloride creates a gradient that drives water from its interstitial and intracellular compartments into the intravascular space,[92] reducing brain water and ICP. Hypertonic saline may also augment CBF and cardiac output, reducing secondary ischemia.

Data on the effectiveness of hypertonic saline solutions in the management of increased ICP in patients with head injury have been gathered only in small case series and controlled groups. Suarez and colleagues[93] reported that 23.4% saline in doses of 30 to 60 mL over 20 minutes can markedly reduce ICP when standard treatments fail. In smaller studies, 7.5% hypertonic saline was particularly effective in ICP reduction and CPP elevation in patients with severe TBI whose ICP was refractory to standard therapy.[94] Hypernatremia is commonly observed but usually resolves as renal free water clearance is reduced.[95] Potential adverse consequences include central pontine myelinolysis and seizures, as well as hypernatremia, congestive heart failure from fluid shifts, and coagulopathy.[96] At present, hypertonic saline use in the management of high ICP is primarily limited to patients in whom standard osmotherapy is ineffective.

Intracranial Hypertension Refractory to Standard Treatment: Other Measures to Consider

The measures that we described previously are routinely used to manage intracranial hypertension. When ICP begins to increase despite maximal treatment, other measures are considered such as hyperventilation, decompressive craniectomy, and barbiturate-induced burst suppression. Prolonged hyperventilation can actually be harmful, and barbiturate-induced burst suppression and decompressive hemicraniectomy have not been proven to be beneficial. Therefore, we use these measures in select situations only, after careful consideration and discussion with family members regarding the advantages and disadvantages of each. We also consider the practical consequences of these treatments, including increased costs that result from prolonged intensive care unit stays (when a patient is placed into a barbiturate coma, withdrawal of

ventilatory support cannot occur until the barbiturate level becomes low, which can take several days).

Barbiturates

Barbiturates potentiate the effects of γ-aminobutyric acid at γ-aminobutyric acid receptors and reduce $CMRO_2$ by globally inhibiting neuronal transmission. With an intact metabolic autoregulatory mechanism, a reduction in $CMRO_2$ may be accompanied by a corresponding decrease in CBF and CBV and a concomitant reduction in ICP. Barbiturates may also decrease ICP by limiting free radical–mediated lipid peroxidation and limiting resultant cerebral edema.[97,98]

The routine use of barbiturates as the prophylactic treatment of ICP is not indicated because two studies have shown no improvement in outcome.[90,99] In the study of Ward and colleagues,[99] more than half of the treated group developed clinically significant hypotension during pentobarbital administration. Nevertheless, barbiturates decreased ICP in two early studies.[90,100] In a prospective, randomized trial, Eisenberg and colleagues[101] showed that pentobarbital coma in patients with refractory intracranial hypertension had a 2:1 benefit in the control of ICP. In this trial, the recommended loading dose was 10 mg/kg over 30 minutes, followed by 5 mg/kg each hour for three doses. The maintenance dose was 1 mg/kg/hr. Plasma and CSF pentobarbital levels correlate poorly with physiologic effects, and pentobarbital dosing and effects are best followed by electroencephalographic monitoring, with dose titration to achieve burst suppression.[102]

The most frequently cited and clinically important side effects of barbiturate administration are hypotension and global oligemic hypoxia, followed by hypokalemia, respiratory depression, hepatic dysfunction, and renal dysfunction.[103,104] For these reasons, this treatment should only be used in conjunction with a Swan-Ganz catheter.

Hyperventilation

In addition to pressure and metabolic autoregulation, CO_2 reactivity is a potent vasoactive agent. Vascular caliber and CBF are highly responsive to changes in arterial CO_2; CBF changes 2% to 3% for each mm Hg of $PaCO_2$. Hypercarbia from hypoventilation leads to vasodilatation and increased CBF, and hypocarbia (hypoventilation) results in vasoconstriction and a lower CBF and a lower ICP. Although pressure and metabolic autoregulation is sometimes impaired in patients with severe head injury, observers have noted a trend toward preservation of CO_2 reactivity.[19,72] As such, hyperventilation was at one time routinely used as a prophylactic means of reducing intracranial hypertension. However, ICP reduction by hyperventilatory vasoconstriction carries with it the significant risk of inducing cerebral ischemia through inadequate CBF, particularly in the first 24 hours after injury when CBF is already severely compromised. These physiologic effects have been tied to outcome, with Muizelaar and colleagues[105] reporting an improved outcome at 3 and 6 months when prophylactic hyperventilation was *avoided* for 5 days after injury. The routine use of hyperventilation should therefore generally be avoided, but it remains a rapid method of reducing ICP in emergency situations with acute neurologic deterioration and impending herniation. In such situations, hyperventilation should be maintained only as long as necessary to initiate other treatments.

Decompressive Hemicraniectomy

Delayed decompressive hemicraniectomy, in which the bone is removed and the dura is opened to increase the size of the intracranial compartment, can lower ICP. The first large series of such an intervention was the bifrontal decompressive craniotomy reported by Kjellberg and Prieto[106] in 1971; outcomes, however, were generally poor. Gaab and colleagues[107] reported their prospective results of the use of bifrontal or hemicraniectomy with more stringent inclusion criteria, in which they excluded patients older than 40 years of age and those with a GCS score of less than 5. They reported a 14% mortality rate and a 38% rate of "full restitution." Polin and colleagues[108] reported favorable outcomes in 60% of patients undergoing a modified Kjellberg procedure within 48 hours of injury with a GCS score between 3 and 8 and intractable hypertension but with an ICP less than 40 mm Hg. Other studies without direct comparisons with patients who did not have the procedure have also noted favorable outcomes.[109–113] The particular timing and indications for intervention have yet to be codified.

Steroid Use

Class I data do not support the use of the steroids dexamethasone, methylprednisolone, and tirilazad to reduce ICP in patients with head injury. Side effects include gastrointestinal bleeding and hyperglycemia with no benefit in ICP reduction or outcome observed.[114–117]

MANAGEMENT PARADIGMS

The principal goal of severe TBI management is the limitation of secondary brain injury from cerebral ischemia. The avoidance of intracranial hypertension is essential to this goal and has as its physiologic basis the prevention of brain herniation and reduced CPP. This concept has led to what has been termed an *ICP-based approach* to patients with severe TBI, in which therapy centers on the maintenance of a normal ICP, with stepwise measures taken as shown in Figure 3-4.

Others have stressed the importance of *CPP-based management,* in which maintenance of a particular CPP is central to management rather than the avoidance of a particular ICP. The guiding physiologic underpinnings of this approach are that a decrease in CPP, whether by an increase in ICP or a decrease in MAP, leads to compensatory vasodilatation and an increase in CBV, which further increases ICP and, in turn, even further compromises CPP (see Fig. 3-2). Initial favorable outcomes[36] have led to the widespread adoption of CPP preservation in the management algorithms of severe TBI (BTF).[5,6] Although Rosner's original paper suggests maintaining a CPP of greater than 70 mm Hg,[36] other reports have failed to document added benefit of maintaining CPP at higher than 60 mm Hg. One report noted an increase in acute respiratory distress syndrome in their trial arm in which a CPP higher than 70 mm Hg was maintained in the patients.[118]

Given these considerations, the three cornerstones of an integrated management paradigm that monitors and controls both ICP and CPP include (1) rapid identification and potential management of intra- or extra-axial mass lesions,

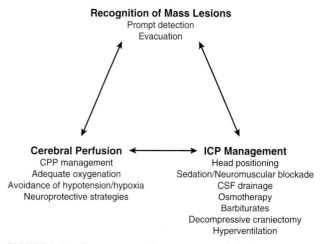

FIGURE 3-5 Cornerstones of severe traumatic brain injury management. CPP, cerebral perfusion pressure; CSF, cerebrospinal fluid; ICP, intracranial pressure.

(2) ICP monitoring and treatment of intracranial hypertension, and (3) CPP preservation and avoidance of cerebral ischemia (Fig. 3-5).

SYSTEMIC MEDICAL MANAGEMENT

Nutritional Support and Gastrointestinal Prophylaxis

The systemic response to multitrauma and severe TBI includes hypermetabolism, catabolism, and altered gastric voiding. Patients with severe head injury may need 140% of their normal caloric expenditures, whereas those in barbiturate coma may require between 100% and 120% of normal resting levels.[119] Enteral alimentation should be established as soon as possible, with a goal of full caloric replacement by the end of the first week after injury. Full caloric replacement through the seventh day after injury, with at least 15% of calories by protein, is correlated with improved outcome.[120,121] Orogastric tubes are preferred to the nasogastric route in the presence of skull base fractures or sinus disease. Long-term feeding may require placement of a percutaneous endoscopic gastrostomy tube or jejunal tube if gastric emptying is compromised. Although the enteral route decreases the risk of bacterial translocation and sepsis, parenteral nutrition may serve as a temporary route for nutritional support until gastroparesis resolves.

An appropriate nutritional regimen also includes gastric ulcer prophylaxis. Ulcers are common complications in patients in the intensive care unit, and the potential morbidity from hemorrhagic diathesis demands appropriate prophylaxis. Reduction of acid production by histamine type 2 antagonists or proton pump inhibitors are commonly used, but neutralizing gastric acid pH carries the theoretical risk of increasing nosocomial pneumonias. Sucralfate, which strengthens gastric mucosa, may avoid this risk.

Sodium Derangements

Hypernatremia and hyponatremia are common disorders, and nearly 60% of patients experience electrolyte abnormalities after head injury.[122] Careful distinction between the syndrome of inappropriate antidiuretic hormone secretion and cerebral salt wasting should be made in the patient with head injury; the former are euvolemic or volume expanded, whereas the latter is likely to be hypovolemic. Fluid restriction in syndrome of inappropriate antidiuretic hormone secretion may be complemented by demeclocycline use. Cerebral salt wasting may require the judicious use of hypertonic saline, should normal saline prove ineffective.

Diabetes insipidus from stalk dysfunction should also be considered in the patient with hypernatremia. Great care should be taken when administering large free water boluses, which may increase the risk of worsened cerebral edema. Desmopressin may be used to complement hypotonic therapy in such cases.

Intravenous Fluid Use

Isotonic saline (0.9% NaCl) remains the standard maintenance fluid in patients with head injury after initial resuscitation, with dextrose excluded from the solution if hyperglycemia becomes difficult to manage. Hypotonic fluids should be strictly avoided because they may exacerbate cerebral edema. The presence of syndrome of inappropriate antidiuretic hormone secretion, salt wasting, or diabetes insipidus may prompt more specific alterations in fluid administration.

Hyperglycemia

Elevated glucose levels are common in all intensive care unit patients, irrespective of the presence of diabetes. Patients with head trauma are no different, and this abnormality is thought to be related to a systemic surge in the sympathoadrenal axis. In fact, hyperglycemia has been correlated with the severity of injury and with poor outcome in patients with severe TBI.[123,124] We aggressively correct serum glucose higher than 150 mg/dL with either sliding scale insulin or insulin infusions, based on recent data demonstrating improved mortality and reduced infection rates in intensive care unit patients with tight glucose control.[125]

Seizure Prophylaxis

Between 4% and 53% of patients with TBI have at least one seizure,[126] with the onset described as either early or late, occurring either before or after the first 7 days of injury. Risk factors for long-term seizures include the presence of cortical contusions; depressed skull fracture; subdural, epidural, or intracranial hematoma; penetrating injury; or seizure within 24 hours of injury.[127,128] Because seizures may dramatically increase $CMRO_2$ and ICP, a large number of prevention studies in patients with head trauma have been conducted. To date, the current literature supports the use of phenytoin or carbamazepine to prevent seizures only within the first 7 days after injury.[129,130] Otherwise, seizures are managed as a first-time seizure in any other patient population.

Hyperpyrexia

Fever increases cerebral metabolism. In cases in which metabolic autoregulation is uncoupled and CBF does not match $CMRO_2$, significant secondary ischemia may result. Fever is a negative predictor of outcome in patients with head injury[131] and must be aggressively controlled with antipyretics and cooling blankets. Infectious sources should be aggressively investigated as in any other type of patient.

Deep Vein Thrombosis Prophylaxis

Patients with severe head injury are at high risk of deep venous thrombosis and pulmonary embolism. Prophylactic treatment by low-dose heparin or venous compression devices was shown to decrease the incidence of deep vein thrombosis in trauma patients.[132] More recent data demonstrate the safety of using subcutaneous heparin for deep vein thrombosis prophylaxis in patients with severe head injury.[133] Because of the high frequency of this complication in severe TBI, we have recently begun to routinely place temporary inferior vena cava filters in these patients. These devices have demonstrated efficacy and safety[134] and, when combined with compression devices and low-dose heparin, may prevent the significant morbidity and mortality associated with pulmonary emboli in this high-risk patient population. No definitive class I data support any particular preventative measure.

HYPOTHERMIA, NEUROPROTECTION, AND RESTORATIVE THERAPIES

Current clinical management of severe TBI has been appropriately guided by evidence-based algorithms to preserve normal physiology in the face of nervous system derangement. Future directions in brain injury management include the formulation of strategies to "protect" the head-injured brain from further secondary injury and to repair injured neural tissue. An early attempt at neuroprotection was cooling, or hypothermia, which produces proportionate reductions in energy production, use, $CMRO_2$, and CBF. Although early pilot studies demonstrated favorable outcomes in patients with head injury,[135,136] a multicenter, prospective, randomized, controlled trial failed to show improvement in outcome.[137] However, a follow-up study in a subgroup of patients who may have benefited is currently in progress.

Therapeutic strategies have also been developed to antagonize the glutamate excitotoxic pathway at the level of the N-methyl-D-aspartate receptor to reduce calcium entry into injured neurons, but no convincing effect on outcome has been demonstrated to date.[138,139] Tirilazad, a 21-aminosteroid that inhibits lipid peroxidation, and the free radical scavenger PEGSOD were both studied in large clinical trials, with no benefit to outcome reported.[117,140] Large clinical trials of compounds inhibiting calpains, calcium-activated proteolytic enzymes, and proapoptotic enzymes of the caspase family may be conducted in the future (reviewed in references 141 and 142).

Another exciting possibility is the stimulation of endogenous neurogenesis or engraftment of exogenous neural stem cells to repair damaged brain by cell replacement or growth factor release.[143–145] In the coming years, current TBI management paradigms will surely be complemented by highly selective neuroprotective and neurorestorative strategies to enhance the likelihood of meaningful functional recovery.

REFERENCES

1. Sosin DM, Sniezek JE, Waxweiler RJ: Trends in death associated with traumatic brain injury, 1979 through 1992: Success and failure. JAMA 273:1778–1780, 1995.
2. Consensus Conference. Rehabilitation of persons with traumatic brain injury. NIH Consensus Development Panel on Rehabilitation of Persons with Traumatic Brain Injury. JAMA 282:974–983, 1999.

3. Jennett B, Teasdale G, Galbraith S, et al: Severe head injuries in three countries. J Neurol Neurosurg Psychiatry 40:291–298, 1977.
4. Marshall LF, Becker DP, Bowers SA, et al: The National Traumatic Coma Data Bank. Part 1: Design, purpose, goals, and results. J Neurosurg 59:276–284, 1983.
5. The Brain Trauma Foundation. The American Association of Neurological Surgeons. The Joint Section on Neurotrauma and Critical Care: Guidelines for the management of severe head injury. J Neurotrauma 3:641–734, 1996.
6. The Brain Trauma Foundation. The American Association of Neurological Surgeons. The Joint Section on Neurotrauma and Critical Care: Trauma systems. J Neurotrauma 17:457–627, 2000.
7. Teasdale G, Jennett B: Assessment of coma and impaired consciousness: A practical scale. Lancet 2:81–84, 1974.
8. Choi SC, Narayan RK, Anderson RL, et al: Enhanced specificity of prognosis in severe head injury. J Neurosurg 69:381–385, 1988.
9. Narayan RK, Greenberg RP, Miller JD, et al: Improved confidence of outcome prediction in severe head injury: A comparative analysis of the clinical examination, multimodality evoked potentials, CT scanning, and intracranial pressure. J Neurosurg 54:751–762, 1981.
10. Fearnside MR, Cook RJ, McDougall P, McNeil RJ: The Westmead Head Injury Project outcome in severe head injury: A comparative analysis of pre-hospital, clinical and CT variables. Br J Neurosurg 7:267–279, 1993.
11. Servadei F, Nasi MT, Cremonini AM, et al: Importance of a reliable admission Glasgow Coma Scale score for determining the need for evacuation of posttraumatic subdural hematomas: A prospective study of 65 patients. J Trauma 44:868–873, 1998.
12. Hovda DA, Becker DP, Kayayama Y: Secondary injury and acidosis. J Neurotrauma 9(Suppl):S47–S60, 1992.
13. Chesnut RM, Marshall LF, Klauber MR, et al: The role of secondary brain injury in determining outcome from severe head injury. J Trauma 34:216–222, 1993.
14. Foulkes M, Eisenberg HM, Jane JA, et al: The Traumatic Coma Data Bank: Design, methods, and baseline characteristics. J Neurosurg 75(Suppl):S8–S13, 1991.
15. Andrews PJ, Piper IR, Dearden NM, Miller JD: Secondary insults during intrahospital transport of head-injured patients. Lancet 335:327–330, 1990.
16. Adams J, Graham D: The pathology of blunt head injury. In Critchley M, O'Leary J, Jennet B (eds): Scientific Foundation of Neurology. London: W Heineman, 1972.
17. Robertson C: Nitrous oxide saturation technique for CBF measurement. In Narayan RK, Wilbert JE, Povlishock JT (eds): Neurotrauma. New York: McGraw-Hill, 1996.
18. Gopinath SP, Robertson CS, Contant CF, et al: Jugular venous desaturation and outcome after head injury. J Neurol Neurosurg Psychiatry 57:717–723, 1994.
19. Fieschi C, Battistini N, Beduschi A, et al: Regional cerebral blood flow and intraventricular pressure in acute head injuries. J Neurol Neurosurg Psychiatry 37:1378–1388, 1974.
20. Bouma GJ, Muizelaar JP: Cerebral blood flow, cerebral blood volume, and cerebrovascular reactivity after severe head injury. J Neurotrauma 9(Suppl 1):S333–S348, 1992.
21. Gray WJ, Rosner MJ: Pressure-volume index. Part II: The effects of low cerebral perfusion pressure and autoregulation. J Neurosurg 67:377, 1987.
22. Rosner MJ: Introduction to cerebral perfusion pressure management. Neurosurg Clin N Am 6:761–773, 1995.
23. Obrist WD, Langfitt TW, Jaggi JL, et al: Cerebral blood flow and metabolism in comatose patients with acute head injury: Relationship to intracranial hypertension. J Neurosurg 61:241–253, 1984.
24. Weber M, Grolimund P, Seiler RW: Evaluation of posttraumatic cerebral blood flow velocities by transcranial Doppler ultrasonography. Neurosurgery 27:106–112, 1990.
25. Bouma GJ, Muizelaar JP, Choi SC, et al: Cerebral circulation and metabolism after severe traumatic brain injury: The elusive role of ischemia. J Neurosurg 5:685–693, 1991.
26. Jones T: Thresholds of focal cerebral ischemia in awake monkeys. J Neurosurg 54:773–782, 1981.
27. Schroder JL, Muizelaar JP, Kuta AJ, Choi SC: Thresholds for cerebral ischemia after severe head injury: Relationship with late CT findings and outcome. J Neurotrauma 13:17–23, 1996.
28. Bouma GJ, Muizelaar JP, Handoh K, Marmarou A: Blood pressure and intracranial pressure-volume dynamics in severe head injury: Relationship with cerebral blood flow. J Neurosurg 77:15–19, 1992.
29. Salvant JB Jr, Muizelaar JP: Changes in cerebral blood flow and metabolism related to the presence of subdural hematoma. Neurosurgery 33:387–393, 1993.
30. Robertson CS, Contant CF, Gokaslan ZL, et al: Cerebral blood flow, arteriovenous oxygen difference, and outcome in head injured patients. J Neurol Neurosurg Psychiatry 55:594–603, 1992.
31. Jaggi JL, Obrist WD, Gennarelli TA, Langfitt TW: Relationship of early cerebral blood flow and metabolism to outcome in acute head injury. J Neurosurg 72:176–182, 1990.
32. Bouma GJ, Muizelaar JP, Stringer WA, et al: Ultra-early evaluation of regional cerebral blood flow in severely head-patients using xenon-enhanced computerized tomography. J Neurosurg 77:360–368, 1992.
33. Kelly DF, Martin NA, Kordestani R, et al: Cerebral blood flow as a predictor of outcome following traumatic brain injury. J Neurosurg 86:633–641, 1997.
34. Juul N, Morris GF, Marshall SB, Marshall LF: Intracranial hypertension and cerebral perfusion pressure: Influence on neurological deterioration and outcome in severe head injury. The Executive Committee of the International Selfotel Trial. J Neurosurg 92:1–6, 2000.
35. Chan KH, Miller JD, Dearden NM, et al: The effects of changes in cerebral perfusion pressure upon middle cerebral artery blood flow velocity and jugular bulb venous oxygen saturation after severe brain trauma. J Neurosurg 77:55–61, 1992.
36. Rosner MJ, Rosner SD, Johnson AH: Cerebral perfusion pressure: Management protocol and clinical results. J Neurosurg 83:949–962, 1995.
37. McGraw CP: A cerebral perfusion pressure greater than 80 mmHg is more beneficial. In Hoff JT, Betz AL (eds): Intracranial Pressure VII. Berlin: Springer-Verlag, 1989.
38. Miller JD, Sweet RC, Narayan R, et al: Early insults to the injured brain. JAMA 240:439–442, 1978.
39. Marmarou A, Anderson RL, Ward JD, et al: Impact of ICP instability and hypotension on outcome in patients with severe head trauma. J Neurosurg 75:S59–S66, 1991.
40. Chesnut RM, Marshal LF, Klauber MR, et al: The role of secondary brain injury in determining outcome from severe head injury. J Trauma 34:216–222, 1993.
41. Stochetti N, Furlan A, Volta F: Hypoxemia and arterial hypotension at the accident scene in head injury. J Trauma 40:764–767, 1996.
42. Winchel RJ, Hoyt DB: Endotracheal intubation in the field improves survival in patients with severe head injury. Arch Surg 132:592–597, 1997.
43. Matz PG, Pitts L: Monitoring in traumatic brain injury. Clin Neurosurg 44:267–294, 1997.
44. Alvarez del Castillo M: Monitoring neurologic patients in intensive care. Curr Opin Crit Care 7:49–60, 2001.
45. von Essen C, Zervas NT, Brown DR, et al: Local cerebral blood flow in the dog during intravenous infusion of dopamine. Surg Neurol 13:181–188, 1980.
46. Myburgh JA, Upton RN, Grant C, Martinez A: A comparison of the effects of norepinephrine, epinephrine, and dopamine on cerebral blood flow and oxygen utilisation. Acta Neurochir Suppl (Wien) 71:19–21, 1998.
47. Berre J, De Backer D, Moraine JJ, et al: Effects of dobutamine and prostacyclin on cerebral blood flow velocity in septic patients. J Crit Care 9:1–6, 1994.
48. Robertson C: Critical care management of traumatic brain injury. In Winn HR (ed): Youmans Neurological Surgery, 5th ed. Philadelphia: WB Saunders, 2004.
49. Kroppenstedt SN, Kern M, Thomale UW, et al: Effect of cerebral perfusion pressure on contusion volume following impact injury. J Neurosurg 90:520–526, 1999.
50. Kee DB, Wood JH: Rheology of the cerebral circulation. Neurosurgery 15:125–131, 1984.
51. Becker DP, Miller JD, Ward JD, et al: The outcome from severe head injury with early diagnosis and intensive management. J Neurosurg 47:491–502, 1977.
52. Kellie G: On death from cold, and on congestions of the brain: An account of the appearances observed in the dissection of two of three individuals presumed to have perished in the storm of 3(rd) November 1821; with some reflections on the pathology of the brain. Trans Med Chir Soc Edinb 1:84–169, 1824.
53. Monro A: Observations Ion the Structure and Function of the Nervous System. Edinburgh: Creech & Johnson, 1823.

54. Marmarou A, Shulman K, Rosende RM: A nonlinear analysis of the cerebrospinal fluid system and intracranial pressure dynamics. J Neurosurg 48:332–344, 1978.

55. Marmarou A: Increased intracranial pressure in head injury and influence of blood volume. J Neurotrauma 9(Suppl 1):S327–S332, 1992.

56. Marmarou A: Pathophysiology of intracranial pressure. In Narayan RK, Wilberger JE, Povlishock JT (eds): Neurotrauma. New York: McGraw-Hill, 1996.

57. Marmarou A, Maset AL, Ward JD, et al: Contribution of CSF and vascular factors to elevation of ICP in severely head-injured patients. J Neurosurg 66:883–890, 1987.

58. Lundberg N, Troupp H, Lorin H: Continuous recording of the ventricular-fluid pressure in patients with severe acute traumatic brain injury: A preliminary report. J Neurosurg 22:581–590, 1965.

59. Narayan RK, Kishore PRS, Becker DP, et al: Intracranial pressure: To monitor or not to monitor? A review of our experience with severe head injury. J Neurosurg 56:650–659, 1982.

60. Marmarou A, Anderson RL, Ward JD: Impact of ICP instability and hypotension in outcome in patients with severe head trauma. J Neurosurg 75:s59–s66, 1991.

61. Eisenberg HM, Gary HE Jr, Aldrich EF, et al: Initial CT findings in 753 patients with severe head injury: A report from the NIH Traumatic Coma Data Bank. J Neurosurg 73:688–698, 1990.

62. Wiesmann M, Mayer TE: Intracranial bleeding rates associated with two methods of external ventricular drainage. J Clin Neurosci 8:126–128, 2001.

63. Zabramski JM, Whiting D, Darouiche RO, et al: Efficacy of antimicrobial-impregnated external ventricular drain catheters: A prospective, randomized, controlled trial. J Neurosurg 98:725–730, 2003.

64. Lozier AP, Sciacca RR, Romagnoli MF, Connolly ES Jr: Ventriculostomy-related infections: A critical review of the literature. Neurosurgery 51:170–181, 2002.

65. Saul TG, Ducker TB: Effect of intracranial pressure monitoring and aggressive treatment on mortality in severe head injury. J Neurosurg 56:498–503, 1982.

66. Contant CF, Robertson CS, Gopinath SP, et al: Determination of clinically important thresholds in continuously monitored patients with head injury [abstract]. J Neurotrauma 10(Suppl 1):S57, 1993.

67. Rosner MJ, Coley IB: Cerebral perfusion pressure, intracranial pressure, and head elevation. J Neurosurg 65:636–641, 1986.

68. Durward QJ, Amacher AL, Del Maestro RF, Sibbald WJ: Cerebral and cardiovascular responses to changes in head elevation in patients with intracranial hypertension. J Neurosurg 59:938–944, 1983.

69. Feldman Z, Kanter MJ, Robertson CS, et al: Effect of head elevation on intracranial pressure, cerebral perfusion pressure, and cerebral blood flow in head-injured patients. J Neurosurg 76:207–211, 1992.

70. Meixensberger J, Baunach S, Amschler J, et al: Influence of body position on tissue-pO2, cerebral perfusion pressure and intracranial pressure in patients with acute brain injury. Neurol Res 19:249–253, 1997.

71. Muizelaar JP, van der Poel HG, Li ZC, et al: Pial arteriolar vessel diameter and CO2 reactivity during prolonged hyperventilation in the rabbit. J Neurosurg 69:923–927, 1988.

72. Enevoldsen EM, Jensen FT: Autoregulation and CO2 responses of cerebral blood flow in patients with acute severe head injury. J Neurosurg 48:689–703, 1978.

73. Giffin JP, Cottrell JE, Shwiry B, et al: Intracranial pressure, mean arterial pressure, and heart rate following midazolam or thiopental in humans with brain tumors. Anesthesiology 60:491–494, 1984.

74. Moyer JH, Pontius R, Morris G, Hershber R: Effect of morphine and n-allylnormorphine on cerebral hemodynamics and oxygen metabolism. Circulation 15:379–384, 1957.

75. Sperry RJ, Bailey PL, Reichman MV, et al: Fentanyl and sufentanil increase intracranial pressure in head trauma patients. Anesthesiology 77:416–420, 1992.

76. Kelly DF, Goodale DB, Williams J, et al: Propofol in the treatment of moderate and severe head injury: A randomized, prospective double-blinded pilot trial. J Neurosurg 90:1042–1052, 1999.

77. Rosa G, Sanfilippo M, Vilardi V, et al: Effects of vecuronium bromide on intracranial pressure and cerebral perfusion pressure: A preliminary report. Br J Anaesth 58:437–440, 1986.

78. Rosa G, Orfei P, Sanfilippo M, et al: The effects of atracurium besylate (Tracrium) on intracranial pressure and cerebral perfusion pressure. Anesth Analg 65:381–384, 1986.

79. Do D, Sheen VL, Bromfield E: Treatment of paroxysmal sympathetic storm with labetalol. J Neurol Neurosurg Psychiatry 69:832–833, 2000.

80. Hartwell RC, Sutton LN: Mannitol, intracranial pressure, and vasogenic edema. Neurosurgery 32:444–450, 1993.

81. Barry KG, Berman AR: Mannitol infusion. III: The acute effect of the intravenous infusion of mannitol on blood and plasma volumes. N Engl J Med 264:1085–1088, 1961.

82. Brown FD, Johns L, Jafar JJ, et al: Detailed monitoring of the effects of mannitol following experimental head injury. J Neurosurg 50:423–432, 1979.

83. Israel RS, Marx JA, Moore EE, Lowenstein SR: Hemodynamic effect of mannitol in a canine model of concomitant increased intracranial pressure and hemorrhagic shock. Ann Emerg Med 17:560–566, 1988.

84. Kassell NF, Baumann KW, Hitchon PW, et al: The effects of high dose mannitol on cerebral blood flow in dogs with normal intracranial pressure. Stroke 13:59–61, 1982.

85. Muizelaar JP, Lutz HA 3rd, Becker DP: Effect of mannitol on ICP and CBF and correlation with pressure autoregulation in severely head-injured patients. J Neurosurg 61:700–706, 1984.

86. Pollay M, Fullenwider C, Roberts PA, Stevens FA: Effect of mannitol and furosemide on blood-brain osmotic gradient and intracranial pressure. J Neurosurg 59:945–950, 1983.

87. Feig PU, McCurdy DK: The hypertonic state. N Engl J Med 297:1444–1454, 1977.

88. Kaufmann AM, Cardoso ER: Aggravation of vasogenic cerebral edema by multiple-dose mannitol. J Neurosurg 77:584–589, 1992.

89. Shackford SR, Norton CH, Todd MM: Renal, cerebral, and pulmonary effects of hypertonic resuscitation in a porcine model of hemorrhagic shock. Surgery 104:553–560, 1988.

90. Schwartz ML, Tator CH, Rowed DW, et al: The University of Toronto head injury treatment study: A prospective, randomized comparison of pentobarbital and mannitol. Can J Neurol Sci 11:434–440, 1984.

91. Smith HP, Kelly DL Jr, McWhorter JM, et al: Comparison of mannitol regimens in patients with severe head injury undergoing intracranial monitoring. J Neurosurg 65:820–824, 1986.

92. Zornow MH: Hypertonic saline as a safe and efficacious treatment of intracranial hypertension. J Neurosurg Anesthesiol 8:175–177, 1996.

93. Suarez JI, Qureshi AI, Bhardwaj A, et al: Treatment of refractory intracranial hypertension with 23.4% saline. Crit Care Med 26:1118–1122, 1998.

94. Hartl R, Ghajar J, Hochleuthner H, Mauritz W: Hypertonic/hyperoncotic saline reliably reduces ICP in severely head-injured patients with intracranial hypertension. Acta Neurochir Suppl (Wien) 70:126–129, 1997.

95. Shackford SR, Fortlage DA, Peters RM, et al: Serum osmolar and electrolyte changes associated with large infusions of hypertonic sodium lactate for intravascular volume expansion of patients undergoing aortic reconstruction. Surg Gynecol Obstet 164:127–136, 1987.

96. Qureshi AI, Suarez JI: Use of hypertonic saline solutions in treatment of cerebral edema and intracranial hypertension. Crit Care Med 28:3301–3313, 2000.

97. Demopoulos HB, Flamm ES, Pietronigro DD, Seligman ML: The free radical pathology and the microcirculation in the major central nervous system disorders. Acta Physiol Scand Suppl 492:91–119, 1980.

98. Kassell NF, Hitchon PW, Gerk MK, et al: Alterations in cerebral blood flow, oxygen metabolism, and electrical activity produced by high dose sodium thiopental. Neurosurgery 7:598–603, 1980.

99. Ward JD, Becker DP, Miller JD, et al: Failure of prophylactic barbiturate coma in the treatment of severe head injury. J Neurosurg 62:383–388, 1985.

100. Marshall LF, Smith RW, Shapiro HM: The outcome with aggressive treatment in severe head injuries. Part II: Acute and chronic barbiturate administration in the management of head injury. J Neurosurg 50:26–30, 1979.

101. Eisenberg HM, Frankowski RF, Contant CF, et al: High-dose barbiturate control of elevated intracranial pressure in patients with severe head injury. J Neurosurg 69:15–23, 1988.

102. Winer JW, Rosenwasser RH, Jimenez F: Electroencephalographic activity and serum and cerebrospinal fluid pentobarbital levels in determining the therapeutic end point during barbiturate coma. Neurosurgery 29:739–741, 1991.

103. Schalen W, Messeter K, Nordstrom CH: Complications and side effects during thiopentone therapy in patients with severe head injuries. Acta Anaesthesiol Scand 36:369–377, 1992.

104. Cruz J: Adverse effects of pentobarbital on cerebral venous oxygenation of comatose patients with acute traumatic brain swelling: Relationship to outcome. J Neurosurg 85:758–761, 1996.

105. Muizelaar JP, Marmarou A, Ward JD, et al: Adverse effects of prolonged hyperventilation in patients with severe head injury: A randomized clinical trial. J Neurosurg 75:731–739, 1991.

106. Kjellberg RN, Prieto A Jr: Bifrontal decompressive craniotomy for massive cerebral edema. J Neurosurg 34:488–493, 1971.

107. Gaab MR, Rittierodt M, Lorenz M, Heissler HE: Traumatic brain swelling and operative decompression: A prospective investigation. Acta Neurochir Suppl (Wien) 51:326–328, 1990.

108. Polin RS, Shaffrey ME, Bogaev CA, et al: Decompressive bifrontal craniectomy in the treatment of severe refractory posttraumatic cerebral edema. Neurosurgery 41:84–92, 1997.

109. Guerra WK, Gaab MR, Dietz H, et al: Surgical decompression for traumatic brain swelling: Indications and results. J Neurosurg 90:187–196, 1999.

110. De Luca GP, Volpin L, Fornezza U, et al: The role of decompressive craniectomy in the treatment of uncontrollable post-traumatic intracranial hypertension. Acta Neurochir Suppl 76:401–404, 2000.

111. Meier U, Zeilinger FS, Henzka O: The use of decompressive craniectomy for the management of severe head injuries. Acta Neurochir Suppl 76:475–478, 2000.

112. Coplin WM, Cullen NK, Policherla PN, et al: Safety and feasibility of craniectomy with duraplasty as the initial surgical intervention for severe traumatic brain injury. J Trauma 50:1050–1059, 2001.

113. Albanese J, Leone M, Alliez JR, et al: Decompressive craniectomy for severe traumatic brain injury: Evaluation of the effects at one year. Crit Care Med 31:2535–2538, 2003.

114. Cooper PR, Moody S, Clark WK, et al: Dexamethasone and severe head injury: A prospective double-blind study. J Neurosurg 51:307–316, 1979.

115. Dearden NM, Gibson JS, McDowall DG, et al: Effect of high-dose dexamethasone on outcome from severe head injury. J Neurosurg 64:81–88, 1986.

116. Gudeman SK, Miller JD, Becker DP: Failure of high-dose steroid therapy to influence intracranial pressure in patients with severe head injury. J Neurosurg 51:301–306, 1979.

117. Marshall LF, Maas AI, Marshall SB, et al: A multicenter trial on the efficacy of using tirilazad mesylate in cases of head injury. J Neurosurg 89:519–525, 1998.

118. Robertson CS, Valadka AB, Hannay HJ, et al: Prevention of secondary ischemic insults after severe head injury. Crit Care Med 27:2086–2095, 1999.

119. Clifton GL, Robertson CS, Choi SC: Assessment of nutritional requirements of head-injured patients. J Neurosurg 64:895–901, 1986.

120. Rapp RP, Young B, Twyman D, et al: The favorable effect of early parenteral feeding on survival in head-injured patients. J Neurosurg 58:906–912, 1983.

121. Deutschman CS, Konstantinides FN, Raup S, et al: Physiological and metabolic response to isolated closed-head injury. Part 1: Basal metabolic state: correlations of metabolic and physiological parameters with fasting and stressed controls. J Neurosurg 64:89–98, 1986.

122. Piek J, Chesnut RM, Marshall LF, et al: Extracranial complications of severe head injury. J Neurosurg 77:901–907, 1992.

123. Young B, Ott L, Dempsey R, et al: Relationship between admission hyperglycemia and neurologic outcome of severely brain-injured patients. Ann Surg 210:466–473, 1989.

124. Lam AM, Winn HR, Cullen BF, Sundling N: Hyperglycemia and neurological outcome in patients with head injury. J Neurosurg 75:545–551, 1991.

125. van den Berghe G, Wouters P, Weekers F, et al: Intensive insulin therapy in the critically ill patients. N Engl J Med 345:1359–1367, 2001.

126. Frey LC: Epidemiology of posttraumatic epilepsy: A critical review. Epilepsia 44(Suppl 10):11–17, 2003.

127. Temkin NR, Dikmen SS, Winn HR: Management of head injury: Posttraumatic seizures. Neurosurg Clin N Am 2:425–435, 1991.

128. Yablon SA: Posttraumatic seizures. Arch Phys Med Rehabil 74:983–1001, 1993.

129. Glotzner FL, Haubitz I, Miltner F, et al: Seizure prevention using carbamazepine following severe brain injuries. Neurochirurgia (Stuttg) 26:66–79, 1983.

130. Temkin NR, Dikmen SS, Wilensky AJ, et al: A randomized, double-blind study of phenytoin for the prevention of post-traumatic seizures. N Engl J Med 323:497–502, 1990.

131. Jones PA, Andrews PJ, Midgley S, et al: Measuring the burden of secondary insults in head-injured patients during intensive care. J Neurosurg Anesthesiol 6:4–14, 1994.

132. Dennis JW, Menawat S, Von Thron J, et al: Efficacy of deep venous thrombosis prophylaxis in trauma patients and identification of high-risk groups. J Trauma 35:132–138, 1993.

133. Kim J, Gearhart MM, Zurick A, et al: Preliminary report on the safety of heparin for deep venous thrombosis prophylaxis after severe head injury. J Trauma 53:38–42, 2002.

134. Langan EM 3rd, Miller RS, Casey WJ 3rd, et al: Prophylactic inferior vena cava filters in trauma patients at high risk: Follow-up examination and risk/benefit assessment. J Vasc Surg 30:484–488, 1999.

135. Marion DW, Obrist WD, Carlier PM, et al: The use of moderate therapeutic hypothermia for patients with severe head injuries: A preliminary report. J Neurosurg 79:354–362, 1993.

136. Clifton GL, Allen S, Barrodale P, et al: A phase II study of moderate hypothermia in severe brain injury. J Neurotrauma 10:263–271, 1993.

137. Clifton GL, Miller ER, Choi SC, et al: Lack of effect of induction of hypothermia after acute brain injury. N Engl J Med 344:556–563, 2001.

138. Maas AI, Steyerberg EW, Murray GD, et al: Why have recent trials of neuroprotective agents in head injury failed to show convincing efficacy? A pragmatic analysis and theoretical considerations. Neurosurgery 44:1286–1298, 1999.

139. Morris GF, Bullock R, Marshall SB, et al: Failure of the competitive N-methyl-D-aspartate antagonist Selfotel (CGS 19755) in the treatment of severe head injury: Results of two phase III clinical trials. The Selfotel Investigators. J Neurosurg 91:737–743, 1999.

140. Young B, Runge JW, Waxman KS, et al: Effects of Pegorgotein on neurologic outcome of patients with severe head injury: A multicenter, randomized controlled trial. JAMA 276:538–543, 1996.

141. Ray SK, Banik NL: Calpain and its involvement in the pathophysiology of CNS injuries and diseases: Therapeutic potential of calpain inhibitors for prevention of neurodegeneration. Curr Drug Target CNS Neurol Disord 2:173–189, 2003.

142. Raghupathi R, Graham DI, McIntosh TK: Apoptosis after traumatic brain injury. J Neurotrauma 17:927–938, 2000.

143. Dash PK, Mach SA, Moore AN: Enhanced neurogenesis in the rodent hippocampus following traumatic brain injury. J Neurosci Res 63:313–319, 2001.

144. Riess P, Zhang C, Saatman KE, et al: Transplanted neural stem cells survive, differentiate, and improve neurological motor function after experimental traumatic brain injury. Neurosurgery 51:1043–1052, 2002.

145. Hagan M, Wennersten A, Meijer X, et al: Neuroprotection by human neural progenitor cells after experimental contusion in rats. Neurosci Lett 351:149–152, 2003.

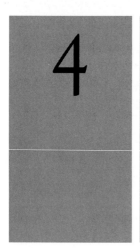

4 Surgical Management of Severe Closed Head Injury in Adults

JOSHUA R. DUSICK, DANIEL F. KELLY, PAUL VESPA, and DONALD P. BECKER

INTRODUCTION

Broadly defined, closed head injury encompasses all non-missile head injuries, including those associated with simple or compound skull fractures. Severe head injury usually refers to an initial postresuscitation Glasgow Coma Scale (GCS) score of 8 or less or a subsequent deterioration to a GCS score of 8 or less. Patients with a GCS score of 7 or less are in coma, defined by the International Coma Data Bank as an inability to obey commands, utter words, or open eyes; only a portion of patients with a GCS score of 8 fulfill these criteria for coma. Although this chapter is focuses on patients with severe traumatic brain injury (TBI), many of the concepts and treatment recommendations discussed here are highly relevant to patients sustaining moderate (GCS score, 9–13) or mild (GCS score, 14–15) head injuries. So-called talk and deteriorate patients comprise as many as one third of patients with severe head injury, the majority of whom have focal mass lesions, which typically accounts for their clinical deterioration.[1–3]

Overall, 25% to 45% of patients who sustain a severe nonpenetrating head injury require a craniotomy for evacuation of a hemorrhagic mass lesion, including epidural (EDH), subdural (SDH), and intracerebral hematomas (ICH).[4–6] In patients with moderate head injuries (GCS score, 9–13), on average, 3% to 12% will require hematoma evacuation, and in patients with mild injuries (GCS score, 14–15), less than 1% will require hematoma evacuation.[7] Diffuse brain injury often accompanies focal mass lesions in the patient with severe brain injury and has a significant impact on outcome.[8–10] Secondary insults such as hypotension, hypoxia, increased intracranial pressure (ICP), seizures, and hyperthermia can further hinder neurologic recovery.[11–16] Aggressive medical intervention aimed at preventing secondary injury and optimizing conditions for brain recovery plays a major role in managing patients with severe head injury.

Consequently, this chapter focuses on both surgical and perioperative critical care aspects of managing patients with severe closed head injury. The recommendations put forth here closely follow four sets of recently published guidelines sponsored by the Brain Trauma Foundation and the Joint Section on Neurotrauma and Critical Care including "Guidelines for the Management of Severe Head Injury,"[17] published in 1996, "Guidelines on Management and Prognosis of Severe Traumatic Brain Injury" and the updates on cerebral perfusion pressure (CPP) published in 2000[11,18–21] and 2003,[22] *Guidelines for Prehospital Management of Traumatic Brain Injury* published in 2000,[23] and the most recent guidelines on the surgical management of TBI published in 2004.[24]

Epidemiology

In the United States, trauma is the leading cause of death in individuals younger than 45 years of age and resulted in approximately 148,000 deaths in 1990.[25] The estimated incidence of TBI is 100 per 100,000 and results in 52,000 deaths per year, making it of major public health significance.[7,26] TBI is more than twice as common in men than women (77% of patients were male in the Traumatic Coma Data Bank (TCDB) cohort[27]) with the highest incidence between the ages of 15 and 24 years and in those 75 years and older.[28,29] The most common cause of head injury remains motor vehicle accidents, accounting for more than 50% of such injuries, followed by falls, which account for 20% to 30%.[29,30] The remainder is accounted for by acts of violence and sports-related injuries. Concomitant extracranial trauma, including facial, thoracic, abdominal, and orthopedic injuries, compounds as many as 70% of severe closed head injuries; 5% to 10% of patients also sustain a cervical spinal injury.[6,31–33]

Approximately 500,000 head injuries requiring admission to a hospital occur annually in the United States[34]; 50,000 of these patients die before reaching a medical facility. Of the 450,000 initial survivors, approximately 80% sustain minor injuries (GCS score, 13–15), 10% have moderate injuries (GCS score, 9–12), and 10% have severe brain injuries (GCS score, 3–8).[28] Given current survival and outcome data, another 15,000 to 20,000 of these patients will die after reaching the hospital, and approximately 50,000 will have some form of permanent disability.[27,35] Gennarelli and colleagues,[36] in assessing more than 49,000 trauma victims from 95 trauma centers in the United States, found that the overall mortality rate was three times higher in patients with head injury compared with those who did not sustain cranial trauma. Additionally, those patients surviving head injury frequently go on to experience long-term disability.[7,26] It has been estimated that the financial burden of TBI annually in the United States alone, in terms of loss of productivity and medical care costs, is approximately $100 billion.[7,37,38]

Alcohol intoxication is another factor affecting TBI. It was a contributing factor in 44% of all fatal motor vehicle accidents in the United States in 1993,[39] and 36% of victims of severe head injury in the TCDB cohort had blood alcohol levels of 100 mg% or higher.[40] In most reports, 25% to 50% of patients are intoxicated at the time of injury, with as many as 73% reported with detectable blood alcohol present.[35,41,42]

It appears that the incidence of fatal head injuries and nonfatal head injuries requiring hospitalization has decreased over the past 10 to 15 years. Although Kraus and colleagues[41] estimated the incidence to be 200 per 100,000 per year during the 1980s, resulting in as many as 75,000 deaths, more recent estimates in the late 1990s, as mentioned previously, indicate a 100 per 100,000 incidence and a death rate of 52,000.[29,43] Although these decreases in incidence and mortality may in part reflect differences in admission criteria[7] and reporting practices and methods of data collection, it appears likely that the implementation of new prevention and safety measures and the increased availability of emergency medical services and specialized trauma centers have resulted in real reductions over time. Nevertheless, head injury continues to be a major public health concern, with an estimated annual cost of care and rehabilitation of $9 to $10 billion and affecting 2.5 to 6.5 million individuals.[29] The prevention of these injuries and the care of these patients must continue to improve. In addition, these studies may underestimate the total impact that TBI has on our society because they do not include all patients with mild to moderate head injuries who do not require hospitalization but who nonetheless can suffer permanent disability such as subtle memory and cognitive deficits.[44]

Prognostic Indicators

In June 2000, the Brain Trauma Foundation and the American Association of Neurological Surgeons Joint Section on Neurotrauma and Critical Care published a comprehensive evidence-based review of both management of and prognostic indicators for TBI, based on the literature available up to 1999.[11,18–21] The factors shown in multiple studies to have consistent and significant effects on outcome after TBI included initial (postresuscitation) GCS score, age, pupillary diameter and light reflex, hypotension, and computed tomography (CT) scan features. The findings of studies published more recently have been in agreement with these prognostic indicators (Table 4-1).[15,45]

Glasgow Coma Scale

The initial GCS score, when obtained after resuscitation and not tainted by prehospital medications or intubation, is a powerful predictor of outcome as measured by mortality rates and Glasgow Outcome Scale scores. Although 85% to 90% of patients with a GCS score of 7 to 15 will survive and at least 75% will go on to have a functional survival (Glasgow Outcome Scale score, 4–5), of those with an initial GCS score of 3, only 20% will survive and 8% to 10% will have a functional recovery.[21]

Age

Patient age is also a strong independent factor for prognosis, not explained only by the increased frequency of systemic complications or intracerebral hematomas with age.[45] Children routinely fare better than adults because they

TABLE 4-1 ▪ Prognostic Indicators for Severe Traumatic Brain Injury

Indicator	Feature Supported by Class I and/or Strong Class II Evidence to Have ≥70% PPV
Early Indicators of Prognosis, per the Brain Trauma Foundation, 2000	
GCS score	Increasing probability of poor outcome with decreasing GCS score in a continuous, stepwise manner
Age	Increasing probability of poor outcome with increasing age in a stepwise manner
Pupillary diameter and light reflex	Bilaterally absent pupillary light reflex
Hypotension	SBP <90 mm Hg has 67% PPV for poor outcome and when combined with hypoxia a 79% PPV
	Poor outcome in 17% without hypotensive episode, 47% with early hypotension, 66% with late hypotension, and 77% for those with both
CT scan features	Presence of abnormalities on initial CT CT classification Compressed or absent basal cisterns Presence and extent of traumatic subarachnoid hemorrhage
Other Indicators Commonly Associated with Poor Outcomes	
Hypoxia	Presence of hypoxia significantly associated with worse prognosis Concurrent hypotension associated with further worsening in prognosis
Intracranial hypertension	Poor ICP control and increasing maximal ICP recorded significantly associated with worse prognosis Guideline is to treat at upper threshold of 20–25 mm Hg

CT, computed tomography; GCS, Glasgow Coma Scale; ICP, intracranial pressure; PPV, positive predictive value; SBP, systolic blood pressure.

appear to have greater reserve for neurologic recovery. Of patients older than age 50, at least 75% will have a poor outcome.[20]

Pupillary Diameter and Light Reflex

Unlike GCS and age, which are linear variables, the pupillary diameter and light reflex are difficult to study because of the various methods of measurement. Nevertheless, pupillary abnormalities clearly predict a worse prognosis. For example, bilaterally unreactive pupils were significantly associated with poor outcome in at least 70% of these patients.[19] When assessing the pupil, a few things should be considered. Direct orbital trauma should not be included in pupillary assessment. A pupil more than 4 mm is defined as dilated. A fixed pupil is defined as exhibiting no constrictor response to bright light.

Hypotension

Defined as a systolic blood pressure less than 90 mm Hg, hypotension occurring at any time after TBI through acute intensive care is a primary predictor of outcome and is the only one that is generally amenable to therapeutic modification. When combined with hypoxia, the positive predictive value for poor outcome is further increased. A single hypotensive episode leads to a doubling of mortality and a significant increase in morbidity. Additional episodes lead to even poorer outcomes. Close monitoring and aggressive treatment to prevent such episodes can lead to a significant improvement in outcomes.[11]

Computed Tomography Findings

The acute CT findings have proven consistently to predict outcome after TBI. All the following have been shown to have at least a 70% positive predictive value for predicting a poor outcome: the presence of any abnormalities on initial CT, poor CT classification (based on TCDB classification system or the classification system proposed by Lobato and colleagues[46]), the presence of compressed or absent basal cisterns, and the presence and extent of traumatic subarachnoid hemorrhage. Less significant than the others but also important are the presence and extent of midline shift.[18]

Hypoxia

In addition to the aforementioned prognostic indicators, there is good evidence from the TCDB and previous studies that hypoxia, at any time after TBI through acute intensive care, significantly predicts a poor outcome, especially in the setting of hypotension.[15] However, it has been more difficult to confirm a defining level in its measurement. It appears clear that apnea/cyanosis in the field or a PaO_2 less than 90 mm Hg by arterial blood gas significantly affects the outcome of these patients and should be avoided and aggressively treated.[23] Consistent with this, patients intubated in the field after severe TBI appear to have better outcomes.[47] Additionally, maximal ICP has been shown to be predictive of poor outcomes.

INITIAL PATIENT ASSESSMENT AND STABILIZATION

Stabilization of the victim of head injury ideally begins at the site of the accident by emergency medical personnel. Their tasks are numerous and vital and include securing the patient's airway, providing adequate oxygenation, initiating fluid resuscitation, stabilizing the cervical and thoracolumbar spine, assessing the patient's level of consciousness, obtaining an account of the accident, and providing safe and rapid transport to a qualified medical facility.

Once in the hospital, the initial evaluation and care of the patient should proceed in an expedient and systematic manner, with diagnostic and therapeutic maneuvers proceeding simultaneously. This approach is best facilitated by a designated trauma team, which has become the ideal model for acute management of the trauma victim. Given that many patients with severe brain injury have sustained multiple injuries, a thorough but brief general examination is mandatory. Life-threatening insults, such as tension pneumothorax, cardiac tamponade, or major vascular injuries with hypovolemic shock, take precedence over neurologic injury and are addressed immediately.

The National Research Council in 1966 pointed to serious inadequacies in the care of trauma patients that have subsequently led to major improvements in the way that we treat the injured patient.[206] Over the subsequent decades, several changes have been implemented with the goal of reducing preventable morbidity and mortality. Of significant impact was the widespread implementation of paramedical services since the late 1970s, which led to decreases in the deaths associated with head injury and traumatic injury in general. It is believed that this decrease was primarily the effect of improved prehospital care, specifically skilled paramedics who could provide rapid resuscitation and evacuation of patients, and this benefit has continued to demonstrate improved outcomes in the most recent reviews.[30,48]

More recently, the formation of regionalized trauma systems and implementation of the Advance Trauma Life Support course have further improved care of the injured. These systems have already been shown to decrease the time to the operating room for patients undergoing laparotomy or craniotomy or who are hypotensive and to decrease complications, length of hospital stay, and deaths.[49,50] These improvements have largely been attributed to increased efficiency and cumulative experience.

The Brain Trauma Foundation published a set of guidelines for prehospital management of TBI in 2000.[23] These guidelines supported the routine assessment and treatment by emergency medical personnel of hypoxemia, defined as apnea, cyanosis, or oxygen saturation less than 90%, and hypotension, defined as systolic blood pressure less than 90 mm Hg. The interventions advocated were aggressive fluid resuscitation, administration of supplemental oxygen and intubation. Intubation was recommended for all patients with an initial GCS score of less than 9, inability to maintain an adequate airway, and hypoxemia despite oxygen supplementation. However, the guidelines did not support the routine use of prophylactic hyperventilation, defined as 20 breaths per minute for adults, except when signs of cerebral herniation (extensor posturing; asymmetric, dilated, or unreactive pupils; or progressive neurologic deterioration) exist after correcting hypoxia and hypotension. Furthermore, the guidelines supported the implementation of organized trauma care systems for all regions that have protocols to direct paramedics to transport those patients with recognized severe TBI to a hospital capable of assessing and treating such patients.

ABCs of Trauma Resuscitation

Airway and Breathing

Because of the high rate of airway and oxygenation problems in patients with TBI and the poor outcome associated with hypoxia,[47] establishing a secure airway is a primary goal. Prompt intubation and mechanical ventilation is mandatory in all patients with a GCS score of 8 or less. In those with a GCS score of 9 to 13, intubation should be seriously considered, especially in the patient with multiple injuries who may have sustained other injuries that impair oxygenation, such as flail chest, hemothorax or pneumothorax, upper airway trauma, and cervical spinal cord injury. In addition, alcohol intoxication, common in the trauma patient, can impair protective airway reflexes. The establishment of a secure airway ensures adequate oxygenation during transport for diagnostic procedures and to the operating room.

Most victims of head injury can be intubated safely by the orotracheal route with inline stabilization of the cervical spine with strict maintenance of a neutral head position and slight or no axial traction. This method of intubation causes minimal movement of the potentially unstable cervical spine and has not been associated with new neurologic deficit.[51,52]

Oral endotracheal intubation in the patient with a head injury is best facilitated by rapid-sequence induction, using sedation, such as thiopental (3–5 mg/kg), and a short-acting paralytic agent, such as succinylcholine (1–2 mg/kg).[52,53] Despite the risk of transiently aggravating intracranial hypertension with the use of succinylcholine, this method of intubation appears to be the safest for most patients with acute brain injury.[53,54] In patients with major facial or upper airway trauma, cricothyroidotomy may be required, although the complication rate in the emergency setting may be as high as 32%.[53] The nasotracheal route of intubation is contraindicated in patients with possible anterior cranial base fractures, requires considerably more experience and time, and has a lower success rate and a higher complication rate than orotracheal intubation.[53] Once the patient is intubated, providing adequate sedation and paralysis is essential; "bucking" by the patient on the endotracheal tube and excessive motor activity should be prevented by sedation with either narcotics or short-acting benzodiazepines.

Circulation

Given the profound impact of hypotension on outcome after TBI, every attempt should be made to keep the patient's systolic blood pressure at more than 90 mm Hg at all times.[11] Aggressive fluid resuscitation with crystalloid, colloid, and, in some instances, packed red blood cells should be initiated. Simultaneous identification and control of hemorrhage are mandatory. If hypotension persists without obvious cause, a more in-depth search for causes of hypotension (cardiac tamponade, tension pneumothorax, intra-abdominal hemorrhage) should proceed. If necessary, an infusion of a vasopressor such as norepinephrine or dopamine may be started to help correct hypotension.

Coagulopathy

Coagulation abnormalities may occur in as many as 30% of victims of moderate and severe head injury, and coagulopathy has been associated with progressive hemorrhage in several studies.[55,56] When coagulopathy is present with a significantly elevated prothrombin time, partial thromboplastin time, international normalized ratio, or low platelet count (<75,000), fresh frozen plasma and/or platelets should be available in the operating room and transfused if hemostasis is problematic.[57] Disseminated intravascular coagulopathy is often associated with severe TBI.[58] If coagulopathy is suggested by excessive bleeding or by abnormalities of prothrombin time, partial thromboplastin time, or platelet count, a complete screen for disseminated intravascular coagulopathy should be undertaken.[58] If disseminated intravascular coagulopathy is confirmed by low fibrinogen level, elevated levels of fibrin degradation products, and prolonged thrombin time, then transfusion of platelets, cryoprecipitate, and fresh frozen plasma is indicated.[59] Surgery should not be delayed, however, while waiting for blood products, especially in the neurologically deteriorating patient.

Neurologic Assessment and Initial Resuscitation

The initial neurologic examination of the patient with severe brain injury is necessarily abbreviated and should focus on the level of consciousness, using the GCS, the patient's pupillary light reflexes, extraocular eye movements, lower brain stem reflexes when appropriate, and asymmetries of the motor examination. This initial neurologic survey, along with examination of the head, neck, and thoracolumbar spine, should take no longer than 5 minutes. Additional signs of severe cranial trauma should be sought, including manifestations of a basilar skull fracture such as hemotympanum, cerebrospinal fluid (CSF) otorrhea or rhinorrhea, mastoid ecchymosis (Battle's sign), or periorbital ecchymosis (raccoon eyes).

A depressed or deteriorating level of consciousness, pupillary abnormalities, and hemiparesis with or without abnormal posturing are the findings most frequently associated with a traumatic hematoma and, when noted, should heighten the urgency of evaluation. Although such signs are highly suggestive of a traumatic mass lesion, they can be falsely localizing and are seen in patients with diffuse brain injuries, as well.[60] Alcohol intoxication is another factor that frequently confounds early diagnostic efforts in the victim of head injury. In most people, however, a blood alcohol level of less than 200 mg/dL is insufficient to explain a decreased level of consciousness.[61] Because these factors make the neurologic examination unreliable in determining whether an intracranial lesion is present, a noncontrast axial CT is always indicated in patients sustaining a serious head injury.

Given the aggressive prehospital and emergency care that is common today, many critically ill trauma patients are intubated, sedated, and pharmacologically paralyzed before being seen by a neurosurgeon. Close cooperation and communication with the trauma surgeons and emergency physicians are essential to obtain information on the patient's initial neurologic status and to plan a coherent sequence of diagnostic and therapeutic procedures, especially in the patient who has sustained multiple injuries.

In a patient with a depressed or deteriorating level of consciousness or obvious localizing signs, it is reasonable to begin treating the presumptive brain injury even before a head CT is obtained with specific measures aimed at reducing or preventing intracranial hypertension. Such preemptive measures include use of additional sedation and neuromuscular blocking agents, mild hyperventilation to maintain the $PaCO_2$ at 30 to 35 mm Hg, intravenous (IV) bolus mannitol (1 g/kg), and anticonvulsant therapy. Because generalized seizures in the setting of increased ICP can have devastating consequences, appropriate patients should be given an IV loading dose of phenytoin (18 mg/kg) as early as possible. Rapid infusion of phenytoin of more than 50 mg/min is to be avoided because significant hypotension or arrhythmias may result.

Radiographic Spinal Evaluation

Cervical Injury Risk and Characteristics

Cervical spine injury is a relatively common occurrence after serious head injury with an incidence ranging from 4% to 8%.[31,62,63] Rigid cervical spine immobilization with a collar is thus essential for all trauma patients until appropriate radiographic studies are completed. According to a recent study by Holly and colleagues[31] of 447 patients with moderate or severe TBI who presented to two level I trauma centers, 5.4% had a concomitant cervical spine injury. Of these patients with cervical injuries, 62% had mechanical instability, 58% had a spinal cord injury, and 58% had high cervical spine injuries located between the occiput and C3. The two major risk factors associated with cervical injury were vehicle-related accidents (as passengers or pedestrians), and a GCS score of 8 or less. More than 90% of patients sustaining a cervical spine injury meet at least one of these criteria.

Spinal Imaging

Spinal radiographic evaluation of patients with moderate or severe TBI should include plain cervical radiographs from the occiput to the cervicothoracic junction (cross-table lateral, anteroposterior, and open-mouth [odontoid] views). Thin-cut CT scans should be obtained in cases in which the plain films poorly visualize the occiput-C3 region and/or the cervicothoracic junction. Radiographic studies of the thoracic and lumbar spine (including lateral and anteroposterior views) should also be obtained when indicated by mechanism of injury or physical examination. These views of the lower spine are preferably performed early in the evaluation process to minimize the time that a patient spends on a spine board, where pressure sores can develop rapidly, especially in patients in coma.

Flexion/Extension Radiographs

Controversy persists over the utility of obtaining cervical flexion/extension radiographs to evaluate for a ligamentous injury in comatose patients with TBI in whom the initial cervical plain films and CT are normal. The potential risk of an in-hospital cervical spinal cord injury in a patient with an undiagnosed unstable ligamentous injury is certainly of great concern. However, based on several recent studies totaling almost 600 patients with TBI in whom cervical flexion/extension radiographs were obtained, the risk of missing an occult unstable cervical injury with adequate prior static radiographs appears to be less than 1%.[64–67] Therefore, some advocate clearing the cervical spine and removing the collar after static plain radiographs and CT are confirmed to be normal.[67] An alternative, somewhat more prudent approach is to reserve the use of dynamic (flexion/extension) imaging for patients at relatively high risk, including those with vehicle-related injuries (including pedestrians struck by a vehicle) and those with a GCS score of 8 or less.[31]

Magnetic Resonance Imaging

Magnetic resonance imaging studies have been increasingly used as an alternative to flexion/extension films because of their ability to demonstrate soft-tissue injury and to better visualize the cervicothoracic junction.[68–70] However, interpretation of the images and what they indicate about cervical stability have not been adequately studied and remain a subject for future investigation.

DIAGNOSTIC PROCEDURES

Computed Tomography

The noncontrast axial CT scan is the imaging modality of choice for evaluation of a patient with head injury. It is performed in less than 10 minutes and clearly defines the location, extent, and type of intracranial lesion. With the lateral scout view and CT bone windows, skull fractures are usually well visualized, thus obviating skull radiographic studies.

The presence of a skull fracture on skull radiography, although highly suggestive of a traumatic hematoma, does not identify the type of intracranial injury. Skull fractures are seen in 66% to 100% of patients with EDH, with a lower incidence of fracture occurring in younger patients. In patients with SDH, skull fractures are seen 18% to 60% of the time, and most frequently are contralateral to the side of the hematoma. With ICH and cerebral contusions, skull fractures have been noted in 40% to 80% of cases.[71] The lack of specificity and time required to obtain skull films make them a wasteful endeavor when CT is readily available.

In situations in which CT is unavailable, emergency cerebral angiography can often demonstrate traumatic hematomas and a midline shift. If both CT and angiography are unobtainable, a rapidly deteriorating patient can undergo twist drill ventriculostomy followed by air ventriculography in the emergency department. A ventricular shift indicative of a mass lesion can usually be demonstrated.

Magnetic Resonance Imaging

Magnetic resonance imaging can clearly demonstrate traumatic hematomas, especially those that are subacute and appear isodense on CT. However, magnetic resonance imaging does not demonstrate acute blood as clearly as CT does, takes significantly longer than CT, is more expensive, and requires a ventilator with nonferromagnetic components for intubated patients. These factors make magnetic resonance imaging impractical for initial evaluation of the patients with severe head injury.

Exploratory Burr Holes

Fortunately, there are increasingly rare situations in which a patient is deteriorating so rapidly that diagnostic studies are unobtainable and placement of exploratory burr holes is indicated. Nonetheless, it is a procedure with which all neurosurgeons should be familiar. It is of value only if the surgeon is prepared to proceed with a formal craniotomy because acute traumatic hematomas cannot be dealt with adequately through burr holes.

The patient is placed supine with the brow up to provide access to both sides of the head (Fig. 4-1). The first burr hole should be made in the temporal region, immediately above the zygomatic arch, according to the following scheme based on the relative localizing value of neurologic findings: (1) ipsilateral to a dilated pupil, (2) contralateral to the most abnormal motor response, and (3) ipsilateral to the side of a skull fracture. Subsequent trephinations are then made in the parietal and frontal regions. The scalp incisions and burr holes should be placed to permit their incorporation into a formal craniotomy if a hematoma is encountered. When the procedure is completed on one side of the head, it should be repeated on the other side.

FIGURE 4-1 Positioning of exploratory burr holes, lateral view (*A*) and superior view (*B*). Placement begins in the temporal fossa, (1) ipsilateral to the suspected lesion, followed by trephinations in the frontal (2) and parietal (3) regions.

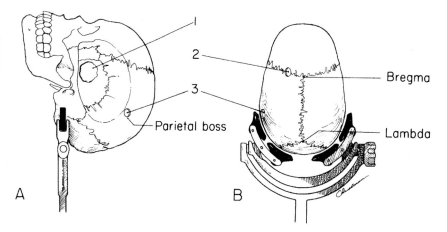

SURGICAL MANAGEMENT OF TRAUMATIC INTRACRANIAL HEMATOMAS

Indications for Surgery

In the recently published guidelines for surgical management of TBI,[24] it is notable that for all types of traumatic intracranial hematomas, including epidural, subdural, parenchymal, and posterior fossa mass lesions, there are insufficient data in the literature (up to year 2001) to support any treatment standards or guidelines. Given the lack of class I and II data, the recommendations put forth here constitute only treatment options, defined in the methodology of the guidelines as *unclear clinical certainty*. Although the abundant class III data derived from case series, case reports, and expert opinion may be considered relatively weak, the treatment recommendations for patients with intracranial hematomas are logical and clinically useful (Table 4-2).

The key factors in deciding whether to proceed with surgery for hematoma evacuation are the patient's overall clinical condition, neurologic status, and the CT findings. There is little debate in the surgical management of a rapidly deteriorating patient with a focal neurologic deficit harboring an expanding intracranial hematoma associated with significant mass effect and midline shift. For less obvious situations, controversy persists, but several reasonable statements can be made. In general, an SDH or EDH of more than 5 mm in thickness with a commensurate midline shift in a comatose patient (GCS score, ≤8) should be evacuated urgently. On the other hand, surgical decompression of a thin-rim SDH of 3 mm or less, associated with marked hemispheric swelling and a large midline shift, is unlikely to improve the patient's condition or reduce ICP.[57,71,72] Such patients are best managed medically, although a decompressive craniectomy (as discussed later) should be considered if control of ICP remains problematic. A CT scan should also be repeated, especially if the first scan was obtained within a few hours of injury or if there are other associated lesions, such as contusions, on the original CT that may have progressed in the interim.[56]

TABLE 4-2 ▪ Treatment Options for EDH, SDH, and ICH

If	Then
EDH	
>30 mL, regardless of GCS	Surgical evacuation
<30 mL *and* <15 mm thickness *and* <5 mm midline shift *and* GCS score >8 *without* focal deficit	Neurologic observation and serial CT scans
SDH	
>10 mm thickness *or* midline shift >5 mm, regardless of GCS score	Surgical evacuation
GCS score <9	ICP monitoring
<10 mm thickness and midline shift <5 mm if GCS score <9 and has decreased by ≥2 points between injury and hospital admission *and/or* asymmetric or fixed and dilated pupils *and/or* ICP >20 mm Hg	Surgical evacuation
ICH	
Progressive neurologic deterioration referable to lesion, refractory ICP, or mass effect on CT	Surgical evacuation
GCS score 6–8 *and* frontal or temporal contusions >20 mL *and* midline shift ≥5 mm *and/or* cisternal compression	Surgical evacuation
>50 mL volume	Surgical evacuation
No neurologic compromise, controlled ICP, no significant signs of mass effect on CT	Neurologic observation and serial CT scans

CT, computed tomography; EDH, epidural hematoma; GCS, Glasgow Coma Scale; ICH, intracerebral hematoma; ICP, intracranial pressure; SDH, subdural hematoma.

*When a surgical intervention is indicated, it should be undertaken as rapidly as possible. Decompressive procedures (subtemporal decompression, temporal lobectomy, and/or decompressive craniectomy) should be considered when there is refractory post-traumatic cerebral edema and resultant intracranial hypertension, diffuse parenchymal injury, and/or radiographic evidence for impending transtentorial herniation.

Adapted from Bullock MR, Chesnut R, Ghajar J, et al: Surgical management of traumatic brain injury, Neurosurgery (in press).

Although controversy remains regarding the indications for surgery for parenchymal injuries, the latest guidelines published in 2004 offer useful recommendations (see Table 4-2).[24] Part of the confusion and difficulty in defining guidelines lies in the diversity of lesions in question. Parenchymal lesions encompass several traumatic injuries including ICH, delayed traumatic ICH, contusions, lacerations, diffuse axonal injury, and infarctions. In addition, these can occur in any part of the brain, and thus their effect depends on the structures involved. In general, the decision to operate should be based on a spectrum of clinical and radiographic findings including GCS score, elevated ICP, neurologic deterioration, cisternal compression, midline shift, and lesion volume and location rather than any one of these factors alone. Those patients who deteriorate before surgery secondary to evolving parenchymal lesions tend to do worse, and thus operating on patients early is preferable to waiting for deterioration to prompt surgery. Several studies have shown that patients with a worsened clinical condition, delayed surgery, and larger hematoma volumes consistently had a poorer outcome and higher mortality.[73-77] Therefore, patients with parenchymal mass lesions and signs of progressive deterioration referable to the lesion, medically refractory intracranial hypertension, or signs of mass effect on CT should be surgically evacuated. In those patients with a GCS score of 6 to 8 with frontotemporal contusions with volumes greater than 20 mL (see Fig. 4-2 for estimation of hematoma volume by CT measurements) and midline shift 5 mm or more and/or cisternal compression on CT should undergo surgical decompression. Any patient with a lesion of more than 50 mL in volume should be operated on. In those patients with no evidence of neurologic compromise, increased ICP or mass effect can be treated nonoperatively with serial CT scans and close neurologic monitoring. Finally, in those patients with diffuse lesions with diffuse swelling and increased ICP, a decompressive craniectomy should be considered.

Finally, there are situations in which the dismal clinical status of the patient warrants a nonoperative course despite the presence of a radiographic surgical lesion. Although advanced age, low GCS score, and signs of herniation have some relationship with poor outcome, threshold values for these factors have not been defined. The recent guidelines clearly state that older patients who present with very low GCS scores are very unlikely to make a functional recovery; however, they do not go as far as to set a guideline regarding the withholding of surgical treatment for such patients. The decision not to offer surgical treatment to such patients thus lies in the surgeon's hands and should be based on these multiple factors of age, injury severity, evidence of irreversible brain stem injury, premorbid health and functional status, and effects of drugs and alcohol.[24]

Potential Operative Mass Lesions and Early Repeat Computed Tomography Scan

In patients with potential surgical lesions on the initial CT scan, it is best to repeat the study sooner rather than later, when the scan may then be prompted by irreversible neurologic deterioration. In a study by Oertel and colleagues[56] of 142 patients with moderate or severe head injury, progressive hemorrhage was found on the second CT scan in 42% of patients and 24% of those who underwent a craniotomy for hematoma evacuation did so after the second CT because of hematoma enlargement. By hematoma type, hemorrhagic progression was observed in 51% of intraparenchymal contusions, 22% of EDHs, and 11% of SDHs. Risk factors for hemorrhage progression included male gender, older age, time interval from injury to first CT scan, and partial thromboplastin time. Almost 50% of patients who had their first CT scan performed within 2 hours of injury had significant hemorrhagic progression seen on the second CT.

In another study by Stein and colleagues,[55] 44.5% of 337 consecutive patients sustaining a closed head injury had delayed or progressive lesions seen on a follow-up CT scan. Significant indicators of progressive injury included lower initial GCS score, cardiopulmonary resuscitation at the accident site, presence of an SDH on the first CT scan, and presence of coagulopathy. In another report, these same investigators found coagulopathy (elevated prothrombin time or partial thromboplastin time, or low platelet count) to be both common after head injury and significantly associated with delayed progression of hemorrhagic lesions on CT scan.[78] For patients with abnormal coagulation studies, the risk of development of a delayed insult on CT was 85% compared with 31% for those without such abnormalities. An additional clue to an evolving lesion is the presence of CT hypodense whorls within an acute hematoma, which can indicate hyperacute bleeding.[79,80]

These studies support early repeat CT scanning for patients not treated surgically if the initial CT reveals nonoperative intracranial hemorrhage, especially in those with coagulopathy or other identified risk factors. This concept of timely follow-up CT scans is particularly relevant today given that most injury victims are rapidly transported to a trauma center where they are typically imaged within 1 to 2 hours of injury when hemorrhagic lesions are still evolving. As a general rule, we recommend obtaining a second CT within 4 to 6 hours of the first CT if the first CT was obtained within 4 hours of injury and shows an initial nonoperative intracranial hemorrhage.

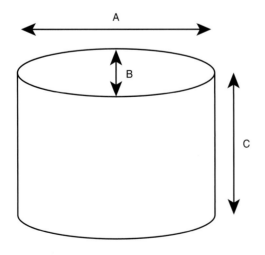

Estimated volume = (A × B × C)/2

FIGURE 4-2 Calculation of estimated intracerebral hematoma volume from dimensions measured on computed tomography.

Surgical Evacuation of Traumatic Hematomas

Basic Trauma Craniotomy

Relatively small, localized EDHs or contusions of the temporal pole occasionally can be evacuated through a vertical scalp incision and limited temporal craniotomy (Fig. 4-3). However, most traumatic injuries are best addressed through a generous frontotemporal parietal craniotomy that provides access to the frontal and temporal poles and the area along the vertex. Hemorrhage from bridging veins and from draining veins to the sagittal sinus can be seen and controlled, and fractures, dural lacerations, and vascular injuries at the skull base can be visualized and treated.

The patient should be positioned with the head turned almost 90 degrees to the side, supported on a donut or a similar headrest, with the head slightly elevated above the level of the heart. A bolster placed under the ipsilateral shoulder helps prevent positional obstruction of cranial venous outflow. If the cervical spine has not been radiographically cleared and a collar is still in place, the patient should be put in the lateral position to maintain the head and neck in neutral alignment.

After appropriate prophylactic antibiotics, such as cefazolin, have been given, the scalp incision is begun directly in front of the tragus, curved posteriorly above the helix of the ear, and continued in a question mark fashion from the parietal area toward the frontal midline, ending, if possible, behind the hairline (Fig. 4-4). In a patient who is deteriorating and has a known temporal fossa lesion, the temporal end of the incision should be opened and a limited temporal craniectomy performed immediately. The dura is opened and hematoma and contused brain are removed, thereby achieving prompt decompression and relief of increased ICP as well as compression of the midbrain at the tentorial incisura. The scalp incision can then be completed, and a large free bone flap, which extends to within 2 or 3 cm of the midline and curves low over the frontal region, can be elevated. Taking the medial craniotomy cut any closer to the midline gains little in exposure and increases the risk of

transgressing large venous tributaries near the sagittal sinus. In cases in which fractures cross the sagittal sinus, the surgeon and anesthesiologist should be prepared for major blood loss at the time that the bone flap is elevated. Resection of a portion of the lateral sphenoid wing may be necessary to provide adequate exposure of the middle fossa.

With a relatively thin SDH and underlying swollen brain, care must be taken when opening the dura to avoid a cortical laceration. In such cases, performing multiple individual slit openings in the dura can be used instead and thereby avoid marked brain herniation through the craniotomy defect. Otherwise, the dural opening should begin over the area of maximal clot thickness or in the anterior temporal region because if the brain begins to herniate through the exposure here, relatively silent cortex is affected (Fig. 4-5). Hematoma and cerebral contusions are evacuated, and the subdural space is explored (Fig. 4-6). A severely contused or pulped frontal or temporal pole should be resected while taking care to leave normal-appearing brain intact. An anterior temporal lobectomy in the case of severe midline shift, tentorial herniation, and unilateral swelling may improve the outcome in some patients.[81] Obtaining meticulous hemostasis with the use of bipolar electrocautery and hemostatic agents, such as Avitene, Surgicel, Fibrillar, thrombin-soaked Gelfoam, or Surgifoam, is essential in avoiding recurrent hematoma formation. Before dural closure, intraoperative ultrasound is helpful to look for the completeness of resection of intraparenchymal contusions.

After the intradural portion of the procedure is completed, the dura is closed primarily if brain swelling has resolved. If brain swelling persists, attempts at primary dural closure will only exacerbate intracranial hypertension. Instead the swollen brain should be simply covered with collagen sponge or an expanded duraplasty can be performed with pericranium or fascia lata. Additionally, generous subtemporal decompression can be performed in anticipation of further swelling. Multiple dural tacking sutures are placed around the craniotomy margin, and one or two are placed in the bone flap to prevent a postoperative EDH.

FIGURE 4-3 A limited craniectomy for a small epidural hematoma. The same exposure provides access to localized contusion of the temporal pole.

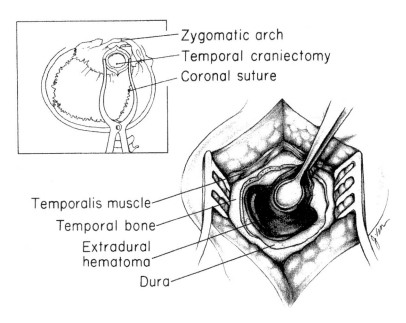

Zygomatic arch
Temporal craniectomy
Coronal suture
Temporalis muscle
Temporal bone
Extradural hematoma
Dura

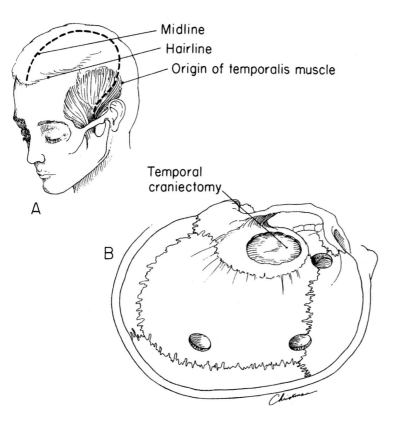

FIGURE 4-4 Placement of scalp incision (*A*) and burr holes (*B*) for a standard trauma craniotomy. Note the temporal craniectomy for initial decompression, followed by keyhole, frontal, and parietal burr holes.

The bone flap is secured preferably with titanium cranial miniplates and screws. The scalp is closed in two layers. Prophylactic antibiotics may be continued if a ventriculostomy is in place. Duration of prophylaxis is an area of some debate and is discussed later.

In the less common situations in which parietal, occipital, or interhemispheric posterior fossa lesions are present, the approach is modified accordingly.

Epidural Hematoma

The mortality rate for patients with acute EDH is directly related to the level of consciousness before surgery. In patients who present comatose with an acute EDH, the mortality rate is approximately 40%, whereas in those who are awake and alert without focal deficit before surgery, the mortality rate approaches zero.[24] For additional outcome data, see Table 4-3. Rapid diagnosis and urgent evacuation are the keys to optimizing outcome in patients with an acute EDH.

Because most epidural clots are located in the middle or frontal fossa or both, a standard frontotemporal craniotomy, as described earlier, is typically most appropriate. The initial burr hole should be placed over or near the area of maximal clot thickness, which is usually in the low temporal area. After rapidly widening this opening to a small craniectomy, accessible hematoma is removed to provide prompt ICP reduction (Fig. 4-7). A formal craniotomy is then completed, and the hematoma is removed with irrigation, suction, and cup forceps. An adequately sized craniotomy is essential so that all clot can be easily removed without brain retraction and so the epidural bleeding source, which in most cases is a branch of the middle meningeal artery, can be visualized. With EDHs resulting from petrous bone fractures, exposure

of the main trunk of the middle meningeal artery at or near the foramen spinosum is often necessary. This bleeding is usually easily controlled with bipolar coagulation, but packing the foramen spinosum with bone wax may be necessary. Dural bleeding from beyond the bony exposure can typically be controlled placing dural tacking sutures but in some instances requires additional bone removal. If the epidural hematoma is the only intracranial injury, the underlying dura is typically relaxed after clot evacuation. However, if the dura remains tense or has a bluish color suggestive of subdural blood or if there is an underlying contusion seen on CT, the subdural space should be inspected. This exposure can be initiated through a small linear incision and expanded as necessary. Alternatively, intraoperative ultrasound can be used to look for underlying parenchymal contusions. After achieving meticulous hemostasis in the epidural space with bipolar coagulation and hemostatic agents, circumferential and bone flap dural tacking stitches are placed followed by routine scalp closure (Fig. 4-8).

Subdural Hematoma

Rates of mortality and morbidity after an acute SDH are the highest of all traumatic mass lesions. This poor outcome results largely from associated parenchymal injuries and subsequent intracranial hypertension. Approximately 50% of patients have associated lesions.[82,83] For more outcome data, see Table 4-3.

A large frontotemporal parietal craniotomy, as described earlier, is usually required to remove an acute SDH and to treat associated parenchymal injuries. Exposure of the frontal and temporal poles and along the sagittal sinus is especially important. Again, an immediate temporal

FIGURE 4-5 *A,* The dural opening for evacuation of a subdural hematoma. The incision begins over the temporal lobe. *B,* Removal of clot.

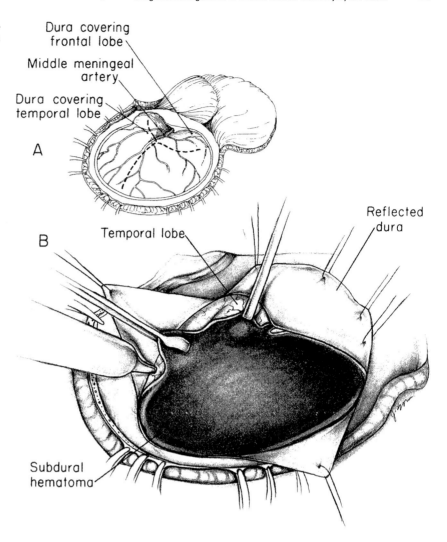

Dura covering
frontal lobe

Middle meningeal
artery

Dura covering
temporal lobe

A

B

Temporal lobe

Reflected
dura

Subdural
hematoma

craniectomy and partial clot removal should initiate the procedure before a craniotomy is performed.

After a generous dural opening, the clot is carefully removed with irrigation, suction, and cup forceps (see Fig. 4-5). The subdural space and cortical surface should be widely inspected for additional hematoma, bleeding, and surface contusions. Bleeding points on the cortical surface are coagulated with the bipolar coagulator, whereas more troublesome, diffuse oozing can often be controlled with hemostatic agents, such as thrombin-soaked Gelfoam or Surgifoam. Areas of cerebral contusion more than 1 to 2 cm in size with irreparably damaged brain, appearing purplish and mottled, should be removed with gentle aspiration and bipolar coagulation (see Fig. 4-6). In eloquent areas, such as along the dominant superior temporal gyrus and the central sulcus, a more limited removal of such contusions is prudent. If cautious bipolar coagulation is ineffective in controlling hemorrhage from draining veins along the sagittal sinus, tamponade with Gelfoam or Surgifoam is used. Small amounts of clot that cannot be visualized adequately, that require undue brain retraction for exposure, or that are adjacent to bleeding points along the sagittal sinus should be left undisturbed. A watertight dural closure should be attempted, followed by routine closure of the craniotomy.

Intracerebral Hematomas and Contusions

ICHs and contusions occur most frequently in the frontal and temporal lobes. Because they frequently are associated with other traumatic lesions, the standard trauma craniotomy usually is indicated. Ideally, the transcortical approach is via a limited cortical incision through already traumatized or otherwise noneloquent brain. If the hematoma is a considerable depth from the cortical surface according to the CT scan, ultrasound can be helpful for precise localization. After thorough clot removal, adjacent contused brain should be resected. In eloquent areas, less aggressive removal of injured parenchyma should be performed. After bipolar coagulation, placement of cotton balls soaked in half-strength hydrogen peroxide in the hematoma cavity is effective in achieving hemostasis, provided the ventricle has not been entered. After removal of the cotton balls, the hematoma bed is lined with Surgicel or Surgifoam, followed by routine closure.

In the previous decade, there was a move toward minimally invasive approaches for treatment of ICHs, although most of these refer to spontaneous rather than traumatic hemorrhages with the exception of a report by Fernandes and colleagues.[84] Evacuation by stereotactic catheter placement, endoscopic surgery, and through a small burr hole have all been described. Until further studies have been

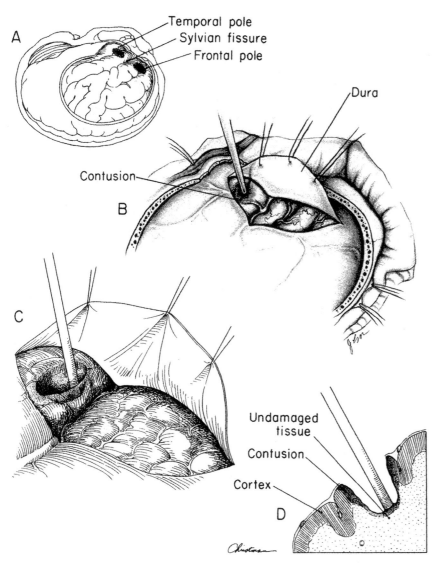

A

Temporal pole
Sylvian fissure
Frontal pole

Dura

Contusion

B

C

Undamaged
tissue
Contusion
Cortex

D

FIGURE 4-6 *A,* The usual location of contusions. *B,* The dural opening for access to contusions. *C,* Resection of contusion limited to damaged brain. *D,* Cross section of contusion resection.

TABLE 4-3 ▪ Overall Outcome for Traumatic Lesions and Factors (in Addition to Hypotension, Hypoxia, GCS, Pupillary Abnormalities, CT Grading, and Age) Associated with Poor Outcomes (GOS Score 1–3)

Lesion	Overall Outcome	Factors Associated with Poor Outcomes
EDH	10% mortality (36% for GCS score, 3–5); >90% functional recovery (GOS score, 4–5) if GCS score is 8–15	Associated lesions (especially, SDH) Hematoma volume: poor outcome in 6.2% with <50 mL and 24% with >50 mL Midline shift, cisternal compression, hyperacute bleeding Duration of brain herniation (anisocoria) before surgery: mortality increases from <17% to >56% with longer duration (>2°)
SDH	40%–60% mortality; 40% functional recovery	Hematoma volume/thickness: mortality 10% for <10 mm and 90% for >30 mm thickness Midline shift Increasing time from clinical deterioration to surgery: mortality increases from 47% to >80% with increasing duration
ICH or contusion	11%–30% mortality; 72.2% functional recovery	Presence of associated lesions (e.g., skull fracture, SDH) Associated edema, intracranial hypertension, and compression of cisterns/third ventricle Location of lesion Large volume and increasing number of lesions Increasing from clinical deterioration to surgery

CT, computed tomography; EDH, epidural hematoma; GCS, Glasgow Coma Scale; GOS, Glasgow Outcome Scale; ICH, intracerebral hematoma; SDH, subdural hematoma.
Adapted from Bullock MR, Chesnut R, Ghajar J, et al: Surgical management of traumatic brain injury, Neurosurgery (in press).

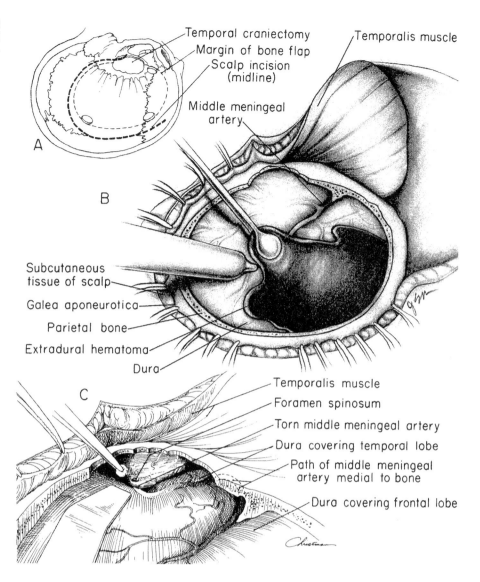

FIGURE 4-7 *A,* The scalp incision and bone flap for removal of a large extradural hematoma. *B,* Removal of the clot. *C,* Packing of the foramen spinosum.

Temporal craniectomy
Margin of bone flap
Scalp incision (midline)
Middle meningeal artery
Temporalis muscle

Subcutaneous tissue of scalp
Galea aponeurotica
Parietal bone
Extradural hematoma
Dura

Temporalis muscle
Foramen spinosum
Torn middle meningeal artery
Dura covering temporal lobe
Path of middle meningeal artery medial to bone
Dura covering frontal lobe

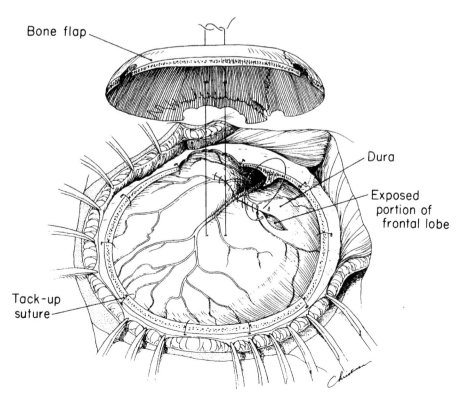

FIGURE 4-8 Closure of an exploratory dural incision and tacking up of the dura to the bone flap.

Bone flap

Dura

Exposed portion of frontal lobe

Tack-up suture

done to assess the effectiveness of these methods, these approaches should only be considered in patients in whom there appears to be an isolated ICH without associated lesions that would otherwise require a formal craniotomy to address.

Dural Tacking Sutures

Dural tacking sutures (also known as tenting sutures, hitch stitches, and sleeper sutures), designed to cinch the dura to the overlying bone or muscle to tamponade bleeding and prevent hematoma accumulation in the epidural space, were initially introduced by Walter Dandy to prevent postoperative hematoma accumulation, which was very common at the time he was operating.[85–87] They were successful in dramatically decreasing the number of postoperative hematomas and have been used routinely since that time. Today, however, with advances in hemostatic agents and anesthesia techniques, the utility of dural tacking stitches has been brought into question.[85–87] Both Swayne and colleagues[85] and Winston[86,87] have suggested that this practice is unnecessary. The former excluded trauma cases, whereas the later included them. Neither saw an increase in postoperative hematomas without the use of dural sutures. They did, however, include the use of tacking sutures in select cases in which hemostasis could not be adequately controlled by other means. This was decided on a suture-by-suture basis in the series of Swayne and colleagues and on all craniotomies for trauma and in those patients with coagulopathy in Winston's series. Based on these reports, it is likely that dural tacking sutures can be omitted from the routine craniotomy closure after removal of SDHs or parenchymal contusions if some degree of brain swelling persists resulting in obliteration of the epidural space. However, dural tacking sutures are still recommended if the brain is sunken away from the dural surface after clot evacuation, the epidural space is gapping around the bone edges after evacuation of all EDHs, and in any patient with epidural oozing and confirmed coagulopathy.

Intraoperative Brain Swelling: Medical and Surgical Options

Despite thorough hematoma removal, a significant minority of patients will have persistent intraoperative brain swelling. A systematic approach to finding the cause of swelling and controlling it is essential. The possibility of occult bleeding should be investigated with intraoperative ultrasound, although an evolving contralateral hematoma will likely not be identified by ultrasound. If one is confident that no other mass lesions exist based on the first CT and on intraoperative ultrasound, several medical and surgical options should be considered.

Medical Options

The endotracheal tube position should be assessed and an arterial blood gas should be obtained to ensure adequate oxygenation and that the P_{CO_2} is approximately 30 to 35 mm Hg or lower. Hyperventilation down to a $PaCO_2$ of 25 to 30 mm Hg can be instituted but prolonged hyperventilation should be avoided if possible. The head of the operating table should be elevated and rotation of the head and neck minimized. Marked arterial hypertension should be controlled, but even modest hypotension should be avoided. As these maneuvers are carried out, further sedation,

neuromuscular blocking agents, and mannitol should be given. In extremely recalcitrant cases, provided the patient is normovolemic and normotensive, metabolic suppression with high-dose pentobarbital or the ultrashort-acting agent propofol can be initiated. For pentobarbital, the loading dose is a 10-mg/kg IV bolus, given over 20 to 30 minutes. For propofol, a loading dose of 2 to 4 mg/kg should be given followed by an infusion of 4 to 8 mg/kg/hr. The advantage of propofol over pentobarbital is its very short half-life, which allows easy and rapid dose titration.[88] However, use of high-dose propofol (>5 mg/kg/hr) should not be extended beyond 48 to 72 hours, given the risk of propofol infusion syndrome, which can be associated with cardiac failure.[89,90]

Surgical Options

DECOMPRESSIVE CRANIECTOMY

At this juncture, if generalized brain swelling persists, simply closing the dura and replacing the bone flap will only serve to exacerbate intracranial hypertension. If not already in place, a ventriculostomy can be attempted to allow drainage of CSF. This may only result in minimal and brief brain relaxation but does provide a reliable ICP monitor.

Whether to perform a decompressive craniectomy (either hemicraniectomy or bifrontal craniectomy) for refractory intracranial hypertension has been a topic of much debate over recent decades. Early studies suggested this aggressive maneuver did not improve outcome.[71,91] Recently, however, numerous reports have supported its use in select cases. Although many studies have demonstrated reduction in ICP, improvement in CPP, improved midline shift, and improved appearance of basal cisterns after decompression,[92–98] others have failed to do so.[99] Additionally, the studies performed to date have been nonrandomized, retrospective series with considerable inherent bias. Mortality rates in these studies have ranged from 11% to 52%, poor outcomes (severe disability or persistent vegetative state) from 8% to 48%, and good outcomes (defined as good social rehabilitation or Glasgow Outcome Scale score of 4–5) from 19% to 68% of patients.[92–98,100–104] One of the more convincing reports supporting the use of craniectomy comes from Polin and colleagues[96] who compared their patients who underwent craniectomy with matched controls from the TCDB. They were able to demonstrate a significant improvement in good outcomes in the patients who underwent bifrontal decompressive craniectomy within 48 hours of injury over those patients who underwent decompressive craniectomy more than 48 hours after injury (46% vs. 0%) and over matched controls in the TCDB (37% vs. 15%). Others, such as Munch and colleagues,[99] Soukiasian and colleagues,[101] and Coplin and colleagues,[105] demonstrated no difference in survival as compared with patients treated with traditional craniotomy, yet the preoperative CT scans in the patients undergoing craniectomy showed worse injuries (e.g., a higher rate of absent basilar cisterns). With clinical evidence of more severe injury on CT, one would expect patients to do worse, yet with craniectomy, they did no worse than other patients, implying some survival benefit from the procedure.

The studies performed to date suggest that three factors largely dictate the success or failure of decompressive craniectomy: patient age, preoperative neurologic status, and timing of surgery. Regarding age, younger patients, particularly those younger than 50 years of age, appear to gain greater benefit than older patients from craniectomy. In fact, several pediatric studies have shown promising results with craniectomy in children with TBI, one of which is a randomized trial.[106–108] Preoperative neurologic status also appears to significantly affect the likelihood of clinical benefit; patients with evidence of brain stem dysfunction (e.g., nonreactive pupils), very low GCS score, and/or markedly elevated ICP are unlikely to benefit from craniectomy. Finally, there is evidence, as suggested by Coplin and colleagues[105] and Munch and colleagues,[99] that early craniectomy (within 48 hours of injury or at the time of initial hematoma evacuation) is more likely to benefit patients than delayed craniectomy when it is used as a salvage procedure after refractory intracranial hypertension and irreversible brain stem injury are already established.

At present, there is no agreed-upon best method of decompressive craniectomy. In general, sufficient bone removal is mandatory to avoid "strangulation" of herniating brain parenchyma and to ensure adequate brain stem decompression. If the initial craniectomy does not appear sufficient, additional bone removal should be performed, particularly down to the floor of the middle fossa. A generous duraplasty should also be performed with pericranium, fascia lata, bovine pericardium, or collagen sponge to allow room for the swollen brain to expand. The bone flap can be temporarily placed in an abdominal subcutaneous pocket or stored in a −70°C freezer for later insertion, avoiding a large and often problematic cranioplasty. A CT should be obtained promptly after the patient leaves the operating room to look for possible causes of brain swelling.

Clearly, the debate over the use of decompressive craniectomy, either as an initial surgical approach or later for refractory intracranial hypertension, will continue. Well-designed randomized studies are needed to determine the ideal timing, patient population, and the best surgical method for this procedure. Until then, the available evidence suggests decompressive craniectomy should be considered, especially within the first 48 hours of injury in younger patients with compressed or absent cisterns in whom their clinical examination does not show clear brain stem injury.

LOBECTOMY

An additional surgical alternative for refractory brain swelling is a lobectomy, typically an anterior temporal lobectomy. In one series of 10 patients treated in this manner for severe unilateral hemispheric swelling, seven of the patients recovered satisfactorily.[81] The major concern with this procedure is that it typically requires removal of radiographically normal-appearing (and perhaps functionally normal) brain. Given the promising results of decompressive craniectomy, which involves no normal brain removal, lobectomy should generally be reserved for instances in which the portion of brain to be removed is grossly abnormal with evidence of contusional injury.

Intracranial Pressure Monitoring

Before leaving the operating room, all patients with severe head injury should have an ICP monitor placed

because intracranial hypertension develops in 50% to 75% of patients.[109] ICP monitoring should also be considered in patients with moderate injuries (preoperative GCS score, 9–13), particularly in those who undergo evacuation of an acute subdural or intraparenchymal hematoma, those with multiple contusions, and patients with significant intraoperative brain swelling. A ventriculostomy is preferable over other monitoring devices because it permits drainage of CSF as an additional and effective means of treating increased ICP and is more accurate.[110] Typically, the catheter is placed through the nondominant frontal lobe into the frontal horn of the lateral ventricle from an entry point 1 to 2 cm anterior to the coronal suture and 2 to 3 cm lateral to the midline. However, if the trauma occurs over the dominant side, it is reasonable to place the catheter through the injured hemisphere, provided there is no effacement of the ventricle from swelling or residual mass effect. If the operative site was contaminated by an open depressed fracture or an ipsilateral slit ventricle is present, the contralateral ventricle is used. After placement, the catheter is tunneled at least 4 or 5 cm in the subgaleal space and externalized through a separate stab incision. When a ventricle cannot be cannulated, a fiberoptic subarachnoid or parenchymal monitor should be placed.

POSTOPERATIVE CRITICAL CARE

After removal of an intracranial hematoma in the patient with severe head injury, intensive postoperative care is essential to optimize recovery. The major focus of therapy is aimed at normalizing ICP and maintaining adequate CPP. Prompt recognition and treatment of secondary insults, including hypotension, hypoxia, seizures, hyperthermia, electrolyte disturbances, and infection, are also crucial in achieving the best possible outcome. Described in the following sections is a management regimen that incorporates the most recent findings concerning CPP, the modified use of hyperventilation, and other data that appear to have a significant impact on recovery after TBI.

Treatment Rationale

Cerebral Ischemia

Cerebral ischemia as documented by direct measurements of blood flow, inferred by the presence of hypotension or hypoxia, or confirmed by postmortem brain examination, is a common and ominous event after severe head injury.[111,112] Bouma and colleagues[111,113] have documented global ischemia, defined as a cerebral blood flow (CBF) of 18 mL/100 g/min or less, by the ^{133}Xe method or by stable xenon CT in approximately one third of patients with severe head injury who underwent CBF measurements within 6 to 8 hours of injury. Hypotension or hypoxia was documented in 57% of the patients with severe head injury in the TCDB cohort. A single episode of hypotension was associated with an 85% increase in mortality.[114] In a postmortem study of 112 head injury fatalities, Graham and colleagues[112] documented histopathologic evidence of ischemic brain damage in 88% of subjects. As the devastating effects of cerebral ischemia have become increasingly recognized as a major contributor to poor outcome, greater emphasis has been placed on identifying and correcting factors that diminish CBF.[72,111] Two of the most significant and easily manipulated factors that appear to have a direct impact on CBF are the CPP and the use of hyperventilation to lower ICP.

Cerebral Perfusion Pressure

CPP is defined as the difference between the mean arterial pressure and the ICP, which in normal subjects is in the range of 70 to 90 mm Hg. At significantly lower levels, compensatory autoregulatory mechanisms are overcome and cerebral ischemia results. At supraphysiologic CPP levels, cerebral vasoconstriction is overcome and hyperemia or even hemorrhage ensues.[115,116]

Because of the influence of CPP on CBF and the consistently poor outcomes associated with cerebral ischemia, CPP management has become an area of significant investigation. Intuitively, keeping the CPP above some threshold level, by ICP reduction and/or blood pressure support, should prevent ischemic episodes and improve outcomes. Unfortunately, defining that ideal threshold and proving its effectiveness has been difficult and the topic of much debate. The variable loss of pressure autoregulation after TBI is likely the cause of this difficulty. The 2000 guidelines for management of brain injury cited insufficient evidence to support a treatment standard or guideline on the topic and only put forth the option of maintaining CPP at a minimum of 70 mm Hg.[117]

In analyzing the pertinent literature, there does appear to be an improvement in outcome since the start of the so-called CPP era during which CPP was closely monitored and controlled. In the pre-CPP era, favorable outcome was seen in 43% to 60% of patients and mortality ranged from 30% to 38%. However, these series included children and two excluded victims of gunshot wounds. In the CPP era, in which only patients 15 years and older were included, the favorable outcome rate was 56% to 59% and the mortality rate was below 30%.[30] Although these numbers suggest an improvement in outcomes, other factors may also be contributing to this, namely general improvements in critical care, improved prehospital paramedical care, trauma resuscitation, and better understanding and prevention of poor prognostic indicators such as hypotension and hypoxia.

In the prospective, randomized study by Robertson and colleagues of 189 patients with severe TBI, no outcome benefit was derived from maintaining a CPP of more than 70 mm Hg and $PaCO_2$ at 35 mm Hg compared with a lower CPP goal of 50 mm Hg and routine use of hyperventilation to a $PaCO_2$ of 25 to 30 mm Hg. Notably in both treatment cohorts, episodes of jugular venous desaturation were promptly treated. This study emphasizes several important points: (1) strict maintenance of CPP at more than 70 mm Hg (as opposed to a lower threshold of 50 to 60 mm Hg) is not necessarily beneficial, (2) normalizing ICP is likely equally as important as CPP, and (3) use of moderate hyperventilation is not necessarily harmful if done in conjunction with jugular bulb saturation monitoring to avoid creating global hypoperfusion and ischemia.[118]

The precise threshold level above which to maintain CPP is also controversial. Estimates generally range from 55 to 70 mm Hg and have been compared by many indicators including outcome, brain tissue, and jugular bulb oxygen monitoring and CBF measurements.[117,119–121] Meixensberger and colleagues[121] showed that using brain tissue oxygen monitors to guide CPP management resulted in fewer ischemic episodes than simply keeping the CPP greater than 70 mm Hg. True ischemia after the initial 6 hours after injury is rare but consistently predictive of a poor prognosis.[111,122,123] CPP less than 70 mm Hg has been shown to be significantly associated with jugular venous desaturation to less than 50%, increased pulsatility on transcranial Doppler sonography, decreased brain tissue oxygen, and increased extracellular glutamate to excitotoxic levels, as measured by microdialysis.[115,124,125] In other words, decreased CPP is associated with both global and regional measures of ischemia. Rosner and colleagues[126] have even reported reduced mortality rates in patients treated with CPP of more than 80 mm Hg compared with historical controls. Conversely, some studies have failed to demonstrate an advantage of CPP targeted management over ICP targeted management, and others have shown hyperemia even at CPP of 70 to 100 mm Hg.[118,127] There is also debate as to whether induced hypertension with vasopressors is beneficial in CPP management. Although early studies suggested that it was safe and did not increase ICP,[117] Oertel and colleagues[128,129] showed that induced hypertension with phenylephrine was both generally ineffective in lowering ICP, as compared with hyperventilation and metabolic suppression, and that 62% of patients had an increase in ICP. In those patients with higher GCS scores, lower jugular bulb oxygen saturation, and higher ICP, however, increasing CPP was most safe and effective.

For the present, it appears prudent to recommend monitoring CPP and maintaining a minimum of 60 to 70 mm Hg, although some patients may tolerate CPP as low as 55 mm Hg. Additionally, monitoring for evidence of cerebral ischemia may help to better direct CPP management and more accurately predict the appropriate critical threshold for each individual patient.

Hyperventilation

Although aggressive hyperventilation in patients with head injury has traditionally been used to prevent and treat intracranial hypertension, the safety of this intervention has come under considerable scrutiny over the previous decade. Based on several studies suggesting that prolonged prophylactic hyperventilation causes an increase in cerebral ischemia and leads to worse outcomes, the 2000 guidelines for management and prognosis of severe TBI put forth the following recommendations: (1) in the absence of increased ICP, prolonged hyperventilation should be avoided after severe TBI, (2) the use of prophylactic hyperventilation during the first 24 hours after injury, when cerebral perfusion is lowest, should be avoided, and (3) in the setting of acute neurologic deterioration or intracranial hypertension refractory to alternative treatments, mild or moderate hyperventilation may be used, preferably with monitoring for cerebral ischemia such as jugular venous oxygen saturation, brain tissue oxygen monitoring, and CBF monitoring.[130]

However, many of the studies on which these guidelines were based instituted prolonged prophylactic hyperventilation in all patients with head injury, even in the first 24 hours after injury and in patients without increased ICP. Therefore, the poor outcomes and incidence of ischemia may have been increased compared with a protocol with more judicious use of hyperventilation based on specific patient parameters. As noted earlier, the study by Robertson and colleagues[118] demonstrates that moderate hyperventilation ($PaCO_2$ 25–30 mm Hg) can be done relatively safely and effectively provided a surrogate measure of CBF such as jugular bulb saturation monitoring is used to monitor for hyperventilation-induced ischemia. Two more recent studies using positron emission tomography and microdialysis have showed a tendency toward hypoperfusion with hyperventilation, but blood flows were not in the ischemic range.[131,132] Oertel et al,[128,133] in two studies, evaluated the effect of hyperventilation on ICP control and pulsatility index, as measured by transcranial Doppler ultrasound. Hyperventilation to an average $PaCO_2$ of 27 mm Hg was significantly associated with a reduction in ICP, with 77.2% of patients decreasing by at least 20% of baseline value. In no patient did the jugular venous oxygen saturation decrease to less than 55%. The greatest predictor of ICP reduction was a high prestudy $PaCO_2$ and hyperventilation was more effective than both metabolic suppression with propofol and induced hypertension. Additionally, they observed a significant decrease in pulsatility by transcranial Doppler in those patients with ICP greater than 30 mm Hg. Decreased pulsatility was also associated with a low GCS score and impaired CO_2 vasoreactivity, which is relatively common after TBI, especially with high ICP, low CPP, and early hypotension and hypoxia. Decreased pulsatility suggests decreased cerebral vascular resistance. Therefore, although previously thought to decrease blood flow, hyperventilation may actually improve cerebral microcirculation in some patients.

Although the debate about the safety and long-term outcomes of hyperventilation is not over, there is enough evidence to support the following general recommendation. Although its use in the first 24 hours after injury and its prolonged prophylactic use in all intubated patients with TBI should be avoided, hyperventilation therapy is effective in lowering ICP and may be used safely after the first day of injury in patients with refractory intracranial hypertension. The initial goal $PaCO_2$ for treatment should be 30 to 35 mm Hg, although more aggressive therapy as low as 25 mm Hg may be useful for some patients. In these patients, it is recommended that hyperventilation be used in conjunction with monitoring for cerebral ischemia (jugular bulb venous oxygen saturation, brain tissue oxygen, or CBF monitoring) to help guide therapy and avoid ischemia.

Management of Neurologic Injury

Physiologic Monitoring

Essential monitoring equipment for the patient with severe head injury includes an ICP monitor, central venous pressure (CVP) line, an arterial line, pulse oximetry, and end-tidal CO_2 monitoring. A Foley catheter and nasogastric or orogastric tube are also placed.

Additional modalities that provide further information on regional and global CBF and metabolism are being used increasingly in the neurosurgical intensive care unit. Methods such as transcranial Doppler sonography,

Kety-Schmidt-based CBF measurement with NO_2 or radioactive ^{133}Xe, Xe-CT, positron-emission tomography, and laser Doppler flowmetry provide estimated blood flow measurements, whereas surrogate markers such as brain tissue oxygen monitors, jugular bulb oximeters, and electroencephalography supply information from which the brain's oxygen supply can be indirectly assessed. Each method has its own merits and can be useful in various settings to aid in the management of the patient. The Lund group has shown improved survival with the implementation of a standardized protocol to optimize CBF using blood pressure adjustments, hyperventilation, and sedation.[134] Vespa[135] recently reviewed the literature pertinent to CBF monitoring and made the following recommendations regarding monitoring CBF both to guide management and as a prognostic indicator. Because the incidence of ischemia is the highest in the first 12 hours after TBI, CBF, or a surrogate thereof such as jugular bulb saturation monitoring, should be measured during this time in those patients with an initial GCS score of less than 9.[118] During the first 10 days in patients with persistent GCS scores of less than 9, regular monitoring can help detect hyperemia, which can help guide hemodynamic management, as well as vasospasm, which is common after TBI. CBF should be followed in all patients with intractable ICP and in those who experience neurologic deterioration during the initial 2 weeks. Extremes of CBF, either very low or very high, have been associated with poor outcomes and thus maintaining CBF in the normal range may improve outcomes, although there are only class III data to support this.[135]

One of the most common surrogate markers of cerebral ischemia currently in use, jugular bulb catheterization allows continuous recording of jugular venous oxygen saturation ($S_{jv}O_2$), which is reflective of global CBF.[72,136] This relatively simple global modality allows safer titration of hyperventilation and blood pressure manipulation to optimize ICP and CPP management.[128] However, focal brain regions, such as areas of pathology, may experience changes in oxygen tension that would be missed by global measurements.[137] Therefore, brain tissue oxygen monitors have been increasingly used to direct CPP management. By titrating CPP to keep oxygen tension above a threshold level, cerebral hypoxic events in at-risk areas may be prevented.[121,138] CBF measurements by the ^{133}Xe technique (or by stable xenon CT) are also commonly used and can also aid in the detection of ischemia and can be used with $S_{jv}O_2$ values to optimize CPP and $PaCO_2$, particularly when ischemia is suspected.[111,113,139] Transcranial Doppler measurements of middle cerebral artery flow velocity, when combined with cervical internal carotid flow velocity or CBF measurements, appear to allow differentiation between traumatic arterial spasm with ischemia versus hyperemia. Given that as many as 40% of patients with severe head injury have post-traumatic spasm, the use of serial transcranial Doppler measurements, if available, appears warranted in such patients,[140,141] especially in the setting of significant traumatic subarachnoid hemorrhage.

Additionally, continuous electroencephalographic monitoring, when available, may better facilitate detection and treatment of occult trauma-induced seizure activity, which has been shown to be very common.[142,143] The degree of electroencephalographic abnormality, as indicated by qualitative and as quantitative measures such as the percentage of alpha variability, has been useful in predicting poor outcome.[144–147] Conversely, the presence of normal electroencephalographic signs such as well-formed sleep potentials is predictive of a good outcome.[148,149] The ultimate utility of these technologies in the management of severe TBI remains to be proven, but initial experiences indicate such information helps further optimize therapy.

Cerebral Perfusion Pressure Management

To maintain CPP at or higher than 60 to 70 mm Hg, normovolemia is essential. Full-maintenance IV fluids are given at a rate of 1.5 mL/kg/hr of 5% dextrose in half-normal or normal saline. A CVP line or a Swan-Ganz catheter is placed to optimize fluid management. A Swan-Ganz catheter is recommended in patients older than 55 years of age, in those with known cardiac disease or chest or visceral injury, or when pressor agents or high-dose barbiturates are used. The CVP is maintained from 5 to 10 mm Hg or the pulmonary artery wedge pressure (PAWP) is kept at 10 to 14 mm Hg.

A maximal wedge pressure of 14 mm Hg is chosen because this level has been associated with maximal cardiac performance in previously healthy patients with subarachnoid hemorrhage without cardiac disease; increasing wedge pressure above 14 mm Hg did not improve cardiac or stroke volume indices.[150] In some patients, especially the elderly and those with cardiac disease or hypertension, higher filling pressures may be needed to achieve optimal cardiac output.

Additional fluids, in the form of colloid (250 mL of 5% albumin) or 0.9% normal saline boluses, are given as needed when the CVP drops below 5 mm Hg or the PAWP is less than 10 mm Hg. If the goal of maintaining CPP at 70 mm Hg is not being met with the CVP or PAWP in the desired range, then additional albumin is given. Once CVP is more than 10 mm Hg or PAWP is more than 14 and CPP is still less than 70 mm Hg, a pressor agent such as norepinephrine (Levophed) is recommended to achieve the CPP goal. Levophed infusion should not exceed 0.2 μg/kg/min. If urine output decreases to less than 0.5 mL/kg/hr, dopamine should be started and Levophed discontinued or decreased. When the cardiac index is less than 3.0 L/min/m², the cardiac inotropic agent dobutamine is highly effective in improving CPP. Some patients occasionally require more than one pressor to achieve adequate cerebral perfusion. In patients with acute intraparenchymal blood on CT scan, an upper limit for systolic blood pressure of 180 to 200 mm Hg is probably prudent, given the risk of worsening such hemorrhage with excessive hypertension. Patients with chronic hypertension, however, are likely to tolerate and, in fact, require higher systemic pressures to maintain adequate cerebral perfusion. Further measures to reduce ICP, which are outlined in the next section, also improve CPP.

Strict and frequent monitoring of total intake (crystalloid, colloid, blood products, parenteral nutrition, and tube feedings) and output (urine, nasogastric, CSF) are essential in maintaining a euvolemic state. Negative fluid balance is corrected by replacement of the fluid deficit every 2 hours. With intensive fluid management as described, the risk of pulmonary edema is significant. Careful clinical assessment and daily chest radiographs are mandatory, especially in elderly patients and in those with multiple injuries.

Intracranial Hypertension Management

An ICP of more than 20 mm Hg sustained for more than 5 minutes should be treated. In patients with temporal lobe or deep frontal lobe lesions in whom the risk of uncal herniation is greater, an ICP treatment threshold of 15 mm Hg may be warranted.

The treatment of intracranial hypertension should proceed in a stepwise manner. Routine preemptive measures exercised in all patients with severe head injury include maintenance of normothermia, head elevation to 30 degrees, and mild hyperventilation to a PaCO₂ of 30 to 35 mm Hg.[151] Seizure prophylaxis should be used for at least the first week after injury. Additional therapies to control ICP are used as needed, including sedation with narcotics, benzodiazepines, or propofol, neuromuscular blockade (e.g., vecuronium), and ventricular drainage, followed by bolus mannitol administration, and finally, in some select patients, induction of propofol or pentobarbital coma. As discussed previously, a decompressive craniectomy should also be considered when medical measures fail. When acute and sustained increases in ICP occur, rapid manual hyperventilation of the patient should be avoided because the PaCO₂ may drop dramatically, resulting in critical cerebral vasoconstriction and ischemia. If an S$_{jv}$O₂ monitor is in place, more liberal PaCO₂ reduction can be accomplished while monitoring for ischemia.

SEDATION

Sedative agents including narcotics, benzodiazepines, and propofol reduce pain (narcotics only) and agitation that might otherwise exacerbate intracranial hypertension. Short-acting narcotics such fentanyl and the short-acting benzodiazepine midazolam are good first-line agents. If effective in reducing ICP, a continuous infusion of fentanyl or midazolam can be started and titrated accordingly. If this is ineffective, a propofol infusion may be started typically in a range of 1 to 2 mg/kg/hr. If intracranial hypertension persists despite sedation and the patient is agitated, has increased motor tone, is shivering, or is resisting the ventilator, a neuromuscular blocking agent such as vecuronium is added to help control ICP. Alcohol withdrawal may also contribute to agitation and intracranial hypertension and is typically poorly controlled with narcotics. If withdrawal is suspected, lorazepam (Ativan), 5 mg IV every 6 hours, is administered empirically for 48 to 72 hours. Chlordiazepoxide (Librium) is an effective alternative.

VENTRICULAR CEREBROSPINAL FLUID DRAINAGE

When these initial measures are inadequate to control ICP or achieve an adequate CPP, ventricular drainage is used. In patients without significant agitation or motor activity, ventricular drainage can be used as the initial intervention to reduce ICP before narcotic administration. Ventricular drainage is titrated to control the ICP while avoiding overdrainage. If the transduced waveform is lost, the catheter should be checked for patency and flushed with preservative-free normal saline if necessary.

MANNITOL

If ventricular drainage is inadequate or a functioning ventriculostomy is not in place, bolus mannitol therapy is the next line of treatment for intracranial hypertension.

Mannitol removes extravascular water from the brain, acts as a fluid bolus to improve CPP, and is thought to reduce blood viscosity and thus improve cerebral oxygen delivery.[152] Because boluses of 0.25 g/kg have been shown to be equally effective in lowering ICP, as have larger doses, it is recommended that smaller doses be used first. For most adults, a 25-g bolus is effective in lowering ICP and for improving CPP and can be repeated as necessary. Serum osmolality should not be allowed to increase to above 310 mOsm/kg. Given that excessive mannitol use may result in acute oliguric renal failure, total daily doses of mannitol should not exceed 200 g; in patients with renal insufficiency, substantially lower doses are recommended.[153]

BLOOD PRESSURE MANIPULATION

When ICP remains elevated and CPP is 60 to 70 mm Hg or less, despite use of the aforementioned maneuvers, an attempt to increase CPP further to the range of 80 to 100 mm Hg can be made before resorting to metabolic suppressive therapy. Rosner[152] notes numerous patients who require a CPP considerably higher than 70 mm Hg before adequate ICP control is achieved. A corollary to the concept of a minimally acceptable perfusion pressure is that at an adequate CPP, modest intracranial hypertension appears to be well tolerated if clinical status and CT findings do not suggest impending herniation. The studies of Miller[72] and Rosner[152] support this idea. The precise level and duration of increased ICP that do not adversely affect outcome remain to be defined. Given the strong correlation between elevated ICP and poor outcome in the TCDB and numerous other reports, an aggressive attempt to maintain ICP at less than 20 mm Hg should still be made.[4,154,155] More aggressive hyperventilation to less than 30 mm Hg can also be considered in this situation but preferably with a jugular bulb catheter or a parenchymal oxygen probe in place to monitor for cerebral ischemia.

METABOLIC SUPPRESSIVE THERAPY

When all previously outlined measures fail to control ICP, barbiturate therapy can be considered in select patients, provided that it is not begun too late in the course of treatment.[72] Only one randomized study, performed by Eisenberg and colleagues,[156] demonstrated some benefit from the use of barbiturate coma in the patient with severe head injury. Indications for initiating barbiturate treatment have not been rigidly defined, and current reviews and guidelines on the subject state that there is insufficient evidence to support its use except as an extreme salvage approach.[157–160] However, it appears that a favorable outcome is most likely to occur in young patients who do not have evidence of brain stem injury and who have a Glasgow Motor Scale score of 4 or more before sedation and paralysis. Additionally, it appears that there may be selection bias in previous retrospective studies because barbiturate coma was only started in the patients with the most severe head trauma in the first place and would therefore be expected to have poor outcomes. Reasonable indications to begin high-dose barbiturates include 30 minutes of ICP more than 30 mm Hg with CPP less than 70 mm Hg or ICP more than 40 mm Hg despite CPP of 70 mm Hg, after all previously outlined measures to control ICP have been exhausted. Patients should be monitored closely because barbiturate coma can lead to complications such as pneumonia, sepsis,

and hemodynamic instability, especially in older patients and those with previous cardiac instability. Thus volume and hemodynamic status should be monitored with a Swan-Ganz catheter. In such patients, initiating therapy with lower doses is prudent. Pentobarbital administration begins with a 10-mg/kg loading dose over 30 minutes followed by 5 mg/kg/hr over the next 3 hours. Ideally, CPP should be maintained at higher than 70 mm Hg and vasopressors instituted rapidly if blood pressure decreases. A maintenance infusion of 1 to 3 mg/kg/hr is usually sufficient to maintain burst suppression on electroencephalography and reasonable control of ICP. Serum pentobarbital levels should be monitored; ICP control usually is achieved with serum levels of 30 to 50 mg/100 mL. Withdrawal of barbiturate therapy over several days can begin after ICP control has been achieved for 24 to 48 hours. It should be noted that pentobarbital levels could take several days to return to normal after withdrawing treatment.

PROPOFOL

An alternative metabolic suppressive agent to pentobarbital is high-dose propofol. The advantage of propofol over barbiturates is that it is ultrashort acting and can thus be rapidly titrated. The treatment threshold is the same as for barbiturates, i.e., burst suppression as demonstrated on electroencephalography. Oertel and colleagues[128] showed that a short (20–30 minutes) high-dose trial of metabolic suppression with propofol was more effective than induced hypertension but less effective than hyperventilation in reducing ICP. This study also indicates that propofol appears to be most effective for ICP reduction when CO_2 reactivity is intact and ICP is only moderately high. Kelly and colleagues,[88] in a randomized, prospective study, demonstrated improved mortality and 6-month outcomes in patients in whom propofol with morphine was used for sedation and ICP control as compared with morphine alone. Whether propofol is more effective than barbiturates is unclear at this point. Two potential problems with propofol are hyperlipidemia secondary to its lipid vehicle and propofol-infusion syndrome, which is characterized by myocardial failure, metabolic acidosis, rhabdomyolysis, and, in some cases, renal failure.[89,90] Given that the risk of this potentially fatal syndrome appears to be dose and duration dependent, it is recommended that propofol infusions of more than 5 mg/kg/hr not be continued for longer than 48 to 72 hours. With these cautions in mind, propofol can be a very useful and effective agent for short-term metabolic suppression and ICP control.

Delayed Neurologic Deficit, Refractory Intracranial Hypertension, and Recurrent Hematoma Formation

If control of intracranial hypertension becomes increasingly problematic in a given patient or if the patient otherwise worsens neurologically, the possibility of a new or reaccumulating intracranial hematoma must be investigated by a repeat CT scan. This procedure is especially important in patients who undergo a CT scan within a few hours of injury and in those patients with coagulopathy on admission. One must consider all of the following as potential sources of neurologic worsening: recurrent hematoma at the operative site, delayed ICH, traumatic cervical carotid dissection, and arterial vasospasm.

In a report by Bullock and colleagues,[161] recurrent hematoma requiring reoperation developed at the operative site in almost 7% of 850 patients who underwent craniotomy for evacuation of a traumatic hemorrhage. EDHs comprised 69% of these lesions, followed by SDHs and ICHs. Patients with postoperative hematoma had a higher incidence of alcohol intoxication and coagulopathy, were more likely to have received preoperative mannitol, and had significantly worse outcomes.

Delayed ICHs are also relatively common after severe closed head injury, occurring in 1.5% to 7% of patients.[71] As reported by Gentleman and colleagues,[162] development of a delayed ICH was almost always associated with persistent intracranial hypertension, clinical worsening, or failure to improve neurologically, and 80% became evident within 48 hours of injury.[163]

Carotid dissection typically occurs after severe blunt head and neck trauma and is usually manifested in a subacute manner within hours to days of injury. It is often heralded by a new hemiparesis in the absence of associated CT findings.

Significantly more common than carotid dissection, traumatic arterial spasm has a time course similar to that seen in patients with aneurysmal subarachnoid hemorrhage, usually occurring at least 3 days after injury. It is most likely to occur in patients with CT evidence of subdural, subarachnoid, intraventricular, or intraparenchymal hemorrhage.[140] When a repeat CT scan does not provide an explanation for the patient's neurologic deterioration, transcranial and cervical Doppler studies are indicated, followed by angiography in some cases. Ideally, transcranial Doppler studies are performed on a daily basis in patients with severe head injury to allow detection of increased flow velocities before the development of a delayed ischemic deficit.

Neurologic Assessment during the Postoperative Period

When narcotics, sedatives, and neuromuscular blocking agents are routinely used for ICP control, neurologic assessment is limited until such medications are withheld. After surgery, in patients whose ICP is easily controlled, these agents can be suspended early to permit clinical evaluation. However, in patients with problematic ICP, diffuse swelling, or poorly visualized cisterns on CT, little is gained by reversing such therapy shortly after surgery and marked exacerbations of ICP may develop. In such cases, a gradual weaning of these agents over a 24- to 48-hour period is recommended and only if the ICP treatment intensity significantly lessens.

Duration of Intracranial Pressure Monitoring

The criteria for how long to monitor ICP are not firmly established. Post-traumatic swelling, edema, and progression of hemorrhagic lesions typically are maximal within 48 to 96 hours of injury. However, delayed increases in ICP are not uncommon. In a series of 53 patients with severe head injury, 15 (31%) had a secondary increase in ICP occurring 3 to 10 days after injury.[164] In 6 of the 15 patients, the delayed increase in ICP was uncontrollable, resulting in death; only 2 patients had a good outcome. The most frequent initial diagnoses in these 15 patients were multiple contusions (7 patients) and acute SDH (5 patients). Possible explanations for the secondary increase in ICP

were available in only seven patients and included delayed ICH in three patients, vasospasm detected by transcranial Doppler in two patients, and hypoxia or hyponatremia in two others.

Discontinuation of ICP monitoring is reasonable in patients who maintain normal ICP without specific therapy or with only minimal sedation for at least 24 hours. Such patients should also show significant and steady clinical improvement to a GCS score of 9 or greater (unless a primary brain stem injury is evident) and demonstrate resolving lesions on follow-up CT scans, including visible cisterns. Even if these criteria are met, a longer period of observation may be warranted when the initial diagnosis is acute SDH or multiple contusions, in patients with significant vasospasm by transcranial Doppler studies, and in those patients with major systemic derangements. In addition, intraoperative ICP monitoring is strongly recommended in patients with severe head injury who require general anesthesia within 7 to 10 days of injury for an extracranial operation that cannot otherwise be delayed.

Ventriculostomy-Related Complications

Ventriculostomy placement is certainly not without risk, the most damaging complications being parenchymal injury, hemorrhage, and infection. The incidence of ventriculostomy-related hemorrhage was 1.4% in the series by Narayan and colleagues[165] and was related to presence of coagulopathy and the number of passes made during catheter placement. More recent reviews have shown similar rates of hemorrhage.[166–168] In patients with clotting abnormalities, placement of an ICP monitor should be deferred until such deficiencies are at least temporarily corrected.

Ventriculitis in association with ventricular catheter placement is a more frequent problem, being seen in 11% of general neurosurgical patients in the series by Mayhall and colleagues.[169] The risk of infection was thought to be related largely to the length of time that the catheter was in place. Ventriculitis developed in only 6% of patients if the catheter was removed within 5 days, whereas this complication developed in 18% of patients when the catheter was in place longer. However, a new series of 205 neurosurgical patients, including 76 with head injuries, reported by Winfield and colleagues[170] demonstrated no relationship between the duration of ICP monitoring and incidence of infection with as long as 2 weeks of monitoring. The overall infection rate was 7%, with an average monitoring time of 7 days. From their data and a review of the literature, they conclude that the duration of monitoring should be dictated by the clinical need to follow ICP, not the concern of infection. They also stress the need for prophylactic antibiotics and minimal manipulation and irrigation of the catheter system. This report is a welcome addition to the ventriculostomy literature given the significant time, cost, and risk to the patient that accompany catheter replacement, especially in those with small ventricles. Thus it appears reasonable to leave a ventriculostomy in place for as long as 2 weeks, provided prophylactic antibiotics are used, the catheter is tunneled several centimeters away from the insertion site, and CSF samples taken every 2 or 3 days show no evidence of incipient infection. No study has yet demonstrated an advantage of one antibiotic over another in appropriateness for prophylaxis. Various drugs have been used such as vancomycin, cefazolin, ampicillin, and nafcillin with gentamicin. There is some controversy on the appropriate duration of antibiotic prophylaxis in the literature. Although some studies have suggested continuing prophylaxis until the ventriculostomy is removed, some have shown no difference in infections between the use of peri-insertional antibiotics alone and prolonged prophylaxis.[171] The same study showed the risk factors for infection to be greater than 5 days of monitoring, ventriculostomy (as opposed to fiberoptic ICP monitor), CSF leak, systemic infection, and serial placements of ventriculostomy. Poon and colleagues,[172] in a prospective study, has showed that prolonged prophylaxis does reduce the rates of infection (from 11% to 3%) and that it also selected for more virulent and resistant organisms such as methicillin-resistant *Staphylococcus aureus* and *Candida*. If ventriculitis does develop, removal or changing of the catheter to another site is recommended, if it can be done safely, and the patient is placed on appropriate antibiotics. Prophylactic antibiotics are not routinely used for fiberoptic ICP monitors, which are not placed in the ventricle.

Postoperative Intracranial Infections

Osteomyelitis, subdural empyema, meningitis, and brain abscess are seen in 2% to 10% of patients after craniotomy for traumatic intracranial hematoma, with the highest incidence reported in patients with an associated open depressed fracture.[173] Perioperative prophylactic antibiotics and meticulous operative débridement and wound closure are essential to minimize this risk. Poor débridement and neglect of open injuries lead to a high risk of infection.[174] Once infection is diagnosed, broad-spectrum antibiotics are begun without delay, followed by more targeted therapy when cultures are available. In all cases of osteomyelitis and subdural empyema and in most cases of brain abscess, surgery is also indicated.

Post-traumatic Seizures

Early post-traumatic seizures, defined as occurring in the first week after injury, are seen in approximately 25% of patients with traumatic intracranial hematomas. Vespa and colleagues,[175] in a prospective study of 94 patients with moderate or severe TBI, confirmed this incidence but additionally noted that about half of the seizures were nonconvulsive and only diagnosed by evaluation of continuous electroencephalography. Therefore, in patients who are critically ill or comatose, the use of continuous electroencephalographic monitoring, if available, may be beneficial in diagnosing and treating nonconvulsive epileptic activity as well as supplying prognostic information.[142,145] Temkin and colleagues,[176] in a well-designed randomized study of patients with head injury with intracranial injury on CT scan or a GCS score of 10 or lower, demonstrated a significant beneficial effect with the use of prophylactic phenytoin during the first week after injury. A serum level in the high therapeutic range (15–20 μg/L) appears most effective. Haltiner and colleagues[177] confirmed the safety and efficacy of phenytoin in this setting. If early seizures do occur despite high therapeutic levels of phenytoin and an underlying cause, including electrolyte derangements (particularly hyponatremia), hypoglycemia, hypoxemia, and a new lesion on CT scan, has been excluded, administration of phenobarbital

should be started. Valproate, on the other hand, has no additional benefit over phenytoin and possibly increases mortality and thus should be avoided.[178]

Late post-traumatic epilepsy with onset after the first week of injury occurs in as many as 15% of patients with severe head injury and in approximately 35% of patients with intracranial hematomas. Early seizures also significantly increase the risk of late seizures. No randomized studies have shown a beneficial effect of prophylactic anticonvulsant therapy in controlling late seizures. In fact, numerous recent reports have recommended against routine prophylaxis after the first 7 days after injury.[179–181] If a patient should develop late post-traumatic epilepsy, he or she should be managed in accordance with standard approaches used in patients with new-onset seizures.[179]

Management of Systemic and Extracranial Complications

Hyperthermia

Hyperthermia, a general metabolic stimulant, has been associated with worse outcome after severe head injury. Conversely, the use of mild systemic hypothermia in patients with severe head injury yielded some promising early results in preliminary studies,[182–184] and a review of the literature by McIntyre and colleagues[185] indicated a possible beneficial effect of hypothermia that was most pronounced for hypothermia to 32°C to 33°C, duration of 24 hours, and a rewarming rate of 24 hours or less. These and other studies prompted a randomized multicenter trial of mild hypothermia (34°C) by Shiozaki et al,[186] which failed to show a benefit and actually increased infectious, hematologic, and metabolic complications as well as the use of neuromuscular blocking agents. A follow-up study by the same group also caused increased complications and failed to show a benefit of moderate hypothermia (31°C) in patients with ICP uncontrolled by mild hypothermia.[187] For the present, an aggressive attempt to maintain normothermia (core temperature <37.5°C) appears warranted; however, hypothermia should be avoided. A regimen using a combination of acetaminophen, cooling blankets, craniocervical ice packs, and ice water lavage is usually effective.

Hematologic, Electrolyte, and Nutritional Concerns

In the acute postoperative period, a complete blood count should be obtained at least once daily and packed red blood cells transfused if the hematocrit decreases to less than 30% to optimize cerebral oxygen delivery. Serum electrolytes, including calcium and magnesium, should be checked at least twice daily.

Hyponatremia lowers the seizure threshold and can exacerbate cerebral edema.[188] Low serum sodium is relatively common after head injury, occurring in 8% of patients with moderate or severe injuries in one study.[189] If serum sodium level decreases to less than 135 mmol/L, the maintenance IV infusion should be changed to normal saline. For hyponatremia less than 130 mmol/L, which typically begins several days after injury, IV urea and hypertonic saline have proved safe and rapidly effective in correcting this problem, whether it is attributed to the syndrome of inappropriate antidiuretic hormone or to cerebral salt wasting.[188,190,191]

Urea is effective because it is a potent osmotic diuretic and has the unique property of significantly increasing sodium resorption at the kidney. Forty grams of urea in 150 mL of normal saline is given over 2 hours and repeated every 8 hours. A significant increase in serum sodium is typically seen after two or three doses. Infusion of hypertonic saline (3%) is also an effective method of correcting significant hyponatremia but usually takes longer than urea and requires close monitoring of urine electrolytes. In cases in which urea or hypertonic saline alone does not correct the hyponatremia, Florinef (fludrocortisone), which reduces sodium loss in the urine, at a starting dose of 0.1 mg orally twice daily is often effective in maintaining sodium in the normal range. Most important, marked fluid restriction is not an option in these patients, in whom maintaining normovolemia is essential.

Magnesium levels should be carefully followed in patients with severe brain injury because low serum and low brain magnesium levels are frequently seen in these patients. Hypomagnesemia lowers the seizure threshold, frequently complicates alcohol withdrawal, and, in experimental TBI, hinders neurologic recovery.[192] Conversely, administration of IV magnesium after injury in a rat head injury model was shown to improve motor function significantly compared with saline-treated animals.[192] A randomized trial of magnesium in the treatment of severe head injury is under way, and early outcome data suggest that there is a therapeutic benefit from its use.[193] It appears reasonable and safe to maintain serum levels in the upper range of normal (1.8–2.2 mEq/L) with IV supplementation. Magnesium sulfate, 2 g every 4 hours, can be given as needed, provided renal function is normal.

Hyperglycemia is another common metabolic derangement seen early after both experimental and human TBI and is a significant predictor of poor outcome.[194] It is thought that high glucose levels enhance ischemia-mediated cell damage, probably through lactate accumulation.[194] Based on these data, hyperglycemia of more than 200 mg/dL should be treated with an insulin drip or sliding scale coverage, and enteral or parental nutrition withheld until 48 hours after injury to minimize early elevations in serum glucose. Dextrose should also be limited to 5% or less in IV fluids during this early postinjury phase.

Pneumonia

Pneumonia is a frequent and often serious complication after severe head injury, occurring in 41% of patients in the TCDB.[195] Aspiration at the scene of injury, impaired airway reflexes, prolonged intubation, and treatment with barbiturates make the patient with severe head injury highly predisposed to the development of pneumonia. A high index of suspicion must be maintained. In febrile patients who show new infiltrates on chest radiographs, an evolving leukocytosis, and sputum analysis showing copious white blood cells, empiric antibiotic treatment is indicated. Aggressive chest physiotherapy is an important adjunct to antimicrobial therapy. In patients with problematic ICP, chest percussion and nasotracheal suctioning should be preceded by IV lidocaine, as much as 100 mg/hr, to blunt the stimulation that may result in ICP spikes.[196]

An important contributing factor in the development of pneumonia in intubated neurosurgical patients appears to be the use of antacids or histamine type 2 (H_2) antagonists (cimetidine, famotidine, nizatidine, and ranitidine) for stress ulcer prophylaxis. In three randomized trials composed of more than 250 ventilator-dependent intensive care unit patients, including neurosurgical patients, the incidence of pneumonia averaged 31% in the patients treated with antacids, H_2 blockers, or both, whereas in patients treated with sucralfate, the incidence of pneumonia averaged 10%.[197] The frequency of clinically significant gastrointestinal hemorrhage using either method of ulcer prophylaxis was low in both groups, approximately 1% for the patients treated with an antacid and an H_2 antagonist and 2% for those patients treated with sucralfate. The higher rate of pneumonia in the patients treated with an H_2 antagonist or antacids is thought to be related to a higher gastric pH, which allows gastric colonization of aerobic gram-negative bacilli and subsequent oropharyngeal and tracheal colonization. Thus sucralfate is recommended as the initial ulcer prophylactic agent in the intubated patient with brain injury. When sucralfate is used, however, absorption of enterally administered medications may be impaired. In particular, this problem has been noted with anticonvulsants; consequently, the IV route of administration for such medication is preferable.

Thromboembolic Events

Deep vein thrombosis and pulmonary embolism are both relatively frequent and often devastating complications in patients with head injury and a high degree of suspicion for deep vein thrombosis and pulmonary embolism must be maintained. If a pulmonary embolism is suspected, a spiral CT angiogram or ventilation-perfusion ($\dot{V}/\dot{Q}$) scan should be obtained. In patients with intermediate probability or indeterminate scans in whom the clinical suspicion of pulmonary embolism is high, a pulmonary angiogram is indicated. If a pulmonary embolism or deep vein thrombosis occurring above the level of the knee is detected, an inferior vena cava filter is placed without delay.[196] The unacceptable risk of intracranial hemorrhage with full anticoagulation precludes such treatment in the patient with acute head injury for at least 10 days to 2 weeks after injury. However, the ideal timing for safe anticoagulation after head injury remains unclear.[196]

The incidence of these complications is reduced by the use of pneumatic compression stockings. In a study of both neurologic and neurosurgical patients treated with compression stockings, the incidence of clinically evident deep vein thrombosis was 2.3%, and for pulmonary embolism, the incidence was 1.8%.[198] More recently, Frim and colleagues[199] administered low-dose subcutaneous heparin to 138 consecutive neurosurgical patients requiring operation, including 58 patients with head injuries. The patients were treated with a regimen using perioperative compression stockings and subcutaneous heparin, 5000 units twice daily, starting on the first day after surgery. In these patients, there were no thromboembolic events and no postoperative hemorrhages. In the control group of 473 patients treated with only compression stockings during and after surgery, thromboembolic complications developed in 3.2% of patients, including 8 patients with deep vein thrombosis and 7 with PE. From this study, low-dose subcutaneous heparin in conjunction with compression stockings appears to be a safe and effective measure against thromboembolic events in the postoperative population with head injuries. However, in patients with abnormal coagulation studies or in those whose hemorrhagic lesions have not stabilized on CT scan, a delay in use of low-dose heparin is warranted.

Gastrointestinal Hemorrhage

Erosive gastrointestinal lesions are remarkably common after severe head injury. In one endoscopic study, 91% of such patients had gastritis within 24 hours of injury.[200] Significant gastrointestinal bleeding requiring transfusion or other intervention has been reported in 2% to 11% of patients with severe head injury.[201] Routine ulcer prophylaxis in all patients with severe head injury is warranted. Use of sucralfate is recommended because of the significantly lower incidence of associated pneumonia and equivalent ulcer prophylaxis compared with H_2 antagonists or antacids.[197]

SUMMARY AND FUTURE EFFORTS

Recent North American studies indicate that the overall rate of TBI is decreasing, likely in large part due to safety and prevention measures that have been implemented over the past two decades. Studies from North America, Europe, and elsewhere also demonstrate that long-term outcomes after severe TBI have also gradually improved over this period. Higher rates of functional survival are likely the result of multiple factors including (1) advances in prehospital care and emergency resuscitation, (2) better and more widespread use of trauma centers, (3) advances in critical care management of ICP and CPP and avoidance of other secondary insults, and (4) implementation of evidence-based treatment guidelines.[202,203] Additional studies over the past two decades have also shown that the key prognostic indicators for patients with head injury are age, postresuscitation GCS score, pupillary status, and CT findings as well as the potentially preventable secondary insults of hypotension, hypoxia, and ICP course.[4-6,11,18-21,27]

Although the surgical management of traumatic intracranial hematomas has not changed substantially over the past two decades, this most basic neurosurgical procedure remains one of the key tools in the armamentarium to preserve neurologic function and reduce ICP after head injury. Prompt and appropriate evacuation of intracranial hematomas in conjunction with timely medical therapies aimed at minimizing or preventing secondary insults is often highly effective and life saving. Functional neurologic recovery rates after evacuation of an acute EDH, SDH, or cerebral contusion/hematoma currently average 90%, 40%, and 70%, respectively (see Table 4-3). Further improvements in the surgical treatment of head injury will perhaps come from more widespread and earlier use of decompressive craniectomy for otherwise uncontrollable brain swelling.

Additional advances in neurocritical care and novel pharmacologic strategies are also needed to increase the rate of functional recovery after head injury.[186,187] Although no proven pharmacologic therapy has arisen from the multitude of clinical trials in head injury over the past two decades, much has been learned about how to better design and conduct such trials.[204,205] It is hoped that ongoing and future studies will further improve outcome after head injury.

REFERENCES

1. Ratanalert S, Chompikul J, Hirunpat S: Talked and deteriorated head injury patients: How many poor outcomes can be avoided? J Clin Neurosci 9:640–643, 2002.
2. Marshall LF, Toole BM, Bowers SA: The National Traumatic Coma Data Bank. Part 2: Patients who talk and deteriorate: Implications for treatment. J Neurosurg 59:285–288, 1983.
3. Lobato RD, Rivas JJ, Gomez PA, et al: Head-injured patients who talk and deteriorate into coma: Analysis of 211 cases studied with computerized tomography. J Neurosurg 75:256–261, 1991.
4. Alberico AM, Ward JD, Choi SC, et al: Outcome after severe head injury: Relationship to mass lesions, diffuse injury, and ICP course in pediatric and adult patients. J Neurosurg 67:648–656, 1987.
5. Becker DP, Miller JD, Ward JD, et al: The outcome from severe head injury with early diagnosis and intensive management. J Neurosurg 47:491–502, 1977.
6. Miller JD, Butterworth JF, Gudeman SK, et al: Further experience in the management of severe head injury. J Neurosurg 54:289–299, 1981.
7. Thurman D, Guerrero J: Trends in hospitalization associated with traumatic brain injury. JAMA 282:954–957, 1999.
8. Mataro M, Poca MA, Sahuquillo J, et al: Neuropsychological outcome in relation to the Traumatic Coma Data Bank classification of computed tomography imaging. J Neurotrauma 18:869–879, 2001.
9. Ono J, Yamaura A, Kubota M, et al: Outcome prediction in severe head injury: Analyses of clinical prognostic factors. J Clin Neurosci 8:120–123, 2001.
10. Lubillo S, Bolanos J, Cardenosa JA, et al: Diffuse axonal injury with or without an evacuated intracranial hematoma in head injured patients: Are they different lesions? Acta Neurochir Suppl 76:415–418, 2000.
11. The Brain Trauma Foundation. The American Association of Neurological Surgeons. The Joint Section on Neurotrauma and Critical Care: Hypotension. J Neurotrauma 17:591–595, 2000.
12. Sarrafzadeh AS, Peltonen EE, Kaisers U, et al: Secondary insults in severe head injury—Do multiply injured patients do worse? Crit Care Med 29:1116–1123, 2001.
13. Pilitsis JG, Rengachary SS: Complications of head injury. Neurol Res 23:227–236, 2001.
14. Wiedemayer H, Triesch K, Schafer H, et al: Early seizures following non-penetrating traumatic brain injury in adults: Risk factors and clinical significance. Brain Inj 16:323–330, 2002.
15. Jiang JY, Gao GY, Li WP, et al: Early indicators of prognosis in 846 cases of severe traumatic brain injury. J Neurotrauma 19:869–874, 2002.
16. Jeremitsky E, Omert L, Dunham CM, et al: Harbingers of poor outcome the day after severe brain injury: Hypothermia, hypoxia, and hypoperfusion. J Trauma 54:312–319, 2003.
17. The Brain Trauma Foundation. The American Association of Neurological Surgeons. The Joint Section on Neurotrauma and Critical Care: Guidelines for the management of severe head injury. J Neurotrauma 13:641–734, 1996.
18. The Brain Trauma Foundation. The American Association of Neurological Surgeons. The Joint Section on Neurotrauma and Critical Care: Computed tomography scan features. J Neurotrauma 17:597–627, 2000.
19. The Brain Trauma Foundation. The American Association of Neurological Surgeons. The Joint Section on Neurotrauma and Critical Care: Pupillary diameter and light reflex. J Neurotrauma 17:583–590, 2000.
20. The Brain Trauma Foundation. The American Association of Neurological Surgeons. The Joint Section on Neurotrauma and Critical Care: Age. J Neurotrauma 17:573–581, 2000.
21. The Brain Trauma Foundation. The American Association of Neurological Surgeons. The Joint Section on Neurotrauma and Critical Care: Glasgow Coma Scale score. J Neurotrauma 17:563–571, 2000.
22. The Brain Trauma Foundation. The American Association of Neurological Surgeons. The Congress of Neurological Surgeons. The Joint Section on Neurotrauma and Critical Care: Guidelines for the Management of Severe Traumatic Brain Injury: Cerebral Perfusion Pressure. New York: The Brain Trauma Foundation, 2003.
23. The Brain Trauma Foundation. Guidelines for Prehospital Management of Traumatic Brain Injury. New York: The Brain Trauma Foundation, 2000.
24. Bullock MR, Chesnut R, Ghajar J, et al: Surgical management of traumatic brain injury. Neurosurgery (in press).

25. Baker SP, O'Neill B, Ginsburg MJ, Li G: The Injury Fact Book 2nd ed. New York: Oxford University Press, 1992, pp 8–16.

26. Thurman DJ, Alverson C, Dunn KA, et al: Traumatic brain injury in the United States: A public health perspective. J Head Trauma Rehabil 14:602–615, 1999.

27. Marshall LF, Gautille T, Klauber MR, et al: The outcome of severe closed head injury. J Neurosurg 75(Suppl):S28–S36, 1991.

28. Kraus JF: Epidemiology of head injury. In Cooper PR (ed): Head Injury. Baltimore: Williams & Wilkins, 1993, pp 1–25.

29. Consensus Conference. Rehabilitation of persons with traumatic brain injury. NIH Consensus Development Panel on Rehabilitation of Persons with Traumatic Brain Injury. JAMA 282:974–983, 1999.

30. Kelly DF, Becker DP: Advances in management of neurosurgical trauma: USA and Canada. World J Surg 25:1179–1185, 2001.

31. Holly LT, Kelly DF, Counelis GJ, et al: Cervical spine trauma associated with moderate and severe head injury: Incidence, risk factors, and injury characteristics. J Neurosurg 96(3 Suppl):285–291, 2002.

32. Gentleman D, Teasdale G, Murray L: Cause of severe head injury and risk of complications. BMJ 292:449, 1986.

33. Vollmer DG, Torner JC, Jane JA: Age and outcome following traumatic coma: Why do older patients fare worse? J Neurosurg 75(Suppl):S37–S49, 1991.

34. Narayan RK, Michel ME, Ansell B, et al: Clinical trials in head injury. J Neurotrauma 19:503–557, 2002.

35. Rimel RW, Giordani B, Barth JT, et al: Moderate head injury: Completing the clinical spectrum of brain trauma. Neurosurgery 11:344–351, 1982.

36. Gennarelli TA, Champion HR, Sacco WJ, et al: Mortality of patients with head injury and extracranial injury treated in trauma centers. J Trauma 29:1193–1202, 1989.

37. Sosin DM, Sniezek JE, Waxweiler RJ: Trends in death associated with traumatic brain injury, 1979 through 1992: Success and failure. JAMA 273:1778–1780, 1995.

38. Karus JF: Epidemiology of Head Injury. In Cooper PR (ed): Head Injury. Baltimore: Williams & Wilkins, 1993, pp 1–25.

39. U.S. Department of Transportation, National Highway Traffic Safety Administration: 1994 Occupant Protection Idea Sampler. Washington, DC: U.S. Dept of Transportation, 1994.

40. Ruff RM, Marshall LF, Klauber MR, et al: Alcohol abuse and neurological outcome of the severely head injured. J Head Trauma Rehabil 5:21–31, 1990.

41. Kraus JF, McArthur D, Silverman TA, et al: Epidemiology of brain injury. In Narayan RK, Wilberger J, Povlishock JT (eds): Neurotrauma. New York: McGraw-Hill, 1996, pp 13–30.

42. Rimel RW, Giordani B, Barth JT, et al: Disability caused by minor head injury. Neurosurgery 9:221–228, 1981.

43. Collins JG: Types of injuries by selected characteristics. Vital Health Stat 10:1–68, 1990.

44. Guerrero JL, Thurman DJ, Sniezek JE: Emergency department visits associated with traumatic brain injury: United States, 1995–1996. Brain Inj 14:181–186, 2000.

45. Hukkelhoven CW, Steyerberg EW, Rampen AJ, et al: Patient age and outcome following severe traumatic brain injury: An analysis of 5600 patients. J Neurosurg 99:666–673, 2003.

46. Lobato RD, Cordobes F, Rivas JJ, et al: Outcome from severe head injury related to the type of intracranial lesion: A computerized tomography study. J Neurosurg 59:762–774, 1983.

47. The Brain Trauma Foundation. The American Association of Neurological Surgeons. The Joint Section on Neurotrauma and Critical Care: Resuscitation of blood pressure and oxygenation. J Neurotrauma 17:471–478, 2000.

48. Rudehill A, Bellander BM, Weitzberg E, et al: Outcome of traumatic brain injuries in 1,508 patients: Impact of prehospital care. J Neurotrauma 19:855–868, 2002.

49. O'Keefe GE, Jurkovich GJ, Copass M, et al: Ten-year trend in survival and resource utilization at a level I trauma center. Ann Surg 229: 409–415, 1999.

50. Peitzman AB, Courcoulas AP, Stinson C, et al: Trauma center maturation: Quantification of process and outcome. Ann Surg 230:87–94, 1999.

51. Rhee KJ, Green W, Holcroft JW, et al: Oral intubation in the multiply injured patient: The risk of exacerbating spinal cord damage. Ann Emerg Med 19:511–514, 1990.

52. Talucci RC, Shaikh KA, Schwab CW: Rapid sequence induction with oral endotracheal intubation in the multiply injured patient. Am Surg 54:185–187, 1988.

53. Delaney KA, Goldfrank LR: Initial management of the multiply injured or intoxicated patient. In Cooper PR (ed): Head Injury. Baltimore: Williams & Wilkins, 1993, pp 43–63.

54. Marsh ML, Dunlop BJ, Shapiro HM, et al: Succinylcholine: Intracranial pressure effects in neurosurgical patients. Anesth Analg 59:550–551, 1980.

55. Stein SC, Spettell C, Young G, et al: Delayed and progressive brain injury in closed-head trauma: Radiological demonstration. Neurosurgery 32:25–31, 1993.

56. Oertel M, Kelly DF, McArthur D, et al: Progressive hemorrhage after head trauma: Predictors and consequences of the evolving injury. J Neurosurg 96:109–116, 2002.

57. Aldrich EF, Eisenberg HM: Acute subdural hematoma. In Apuzzo MLJ (ed): Brain Surgery Complication Avoidance and Management. New York: Churchill Livingstone, 1993, pp 1283–1298.

58. Olson JD, Kaufman HH, Moake J, et al: The incidence and significance of hemostatic abnormalities in patients with head injuries. Neurosurgery 24:825–832, 1989.

59. Goodnight SH, Kenoyer G, Rapaport SI, et al: Defibrination after brain-tissue destruction: A serious complication of head injury. N Engl J Med 290:1043–1047, 1974.

60. Wilberger JE Jr, Rothfus WE, Tabas J, et al: Acute tissue tear hemorrhages of the brain: Computed tomography and clinicopathological correlations. Neurosurgery 27:208–213, 1990.

61. Jagger J, Fife D, Vernberg K, et al: Effect of alcohol intoxication on the diagnosis and apparent severity of brain injury. Neurosurgery 15:303–306, 1984.

62. Hills MW, Deane SA: Head injury and facial injury: Is there an increased risk of cervical spine injury? J Trauma 34:549–554, 1993.

63. Michael DB, Guyot DR, Darmody WR: Coincidence of head and cervical spine injury. J Neurotrauma 6:177–189, 1989.

64. Sees DW, Rodriguez Cruz LR, Flaherty SF, et al: The use of bedside fluoroscopy to evaluate the cervical spine in obtunded trauma patients. J Trauma 45:768–771, 1998.

65. Marciano FF, Apostolides PJ, Vishteh AG, et al: Cervical spine management in severe, nonpenetrating closed head injury: A prospective study [abstract]. Neurosurgery 41:740–741, 1997.

66. Harris OA, Moure FC, Chappell ET: Use of modified EAST practice parameters in clearing the cervical spine in the obtunded trauma patient: A prospective study [abstract]. J Neurosurg 94:413A–414A, 2001.

67. Davis JW, Kaups KL, Dunningham MA, et al: Routine evaluation of the cervical spine in head-injured patients with dynamic fluoroscopy: A reappraisal. J Trauma 50:1044–1047, 2001.

68. Albrecht RM, Kingsley D, Schermer CR, et al: Evaluation of cervical spine in intensive care patients following blunt trauma. World J Surg 25:1089–1096, 2001.

69. Crim JR, Moore K, Brodke D: Clearance of the cervical spine in multitrauma patients: The role of advanced imaging. Semin Ultrasound CT MR 22:283–305, 2001.

70. D'Alise MD, Benzel EC, Hart BL: Magnetic resonance imaging evaluation of the cervical spine in the comatose or obtunded trauma patient. J Neurosurg 91(1 Suppl):54–59, 1999.

71. Cooper PR: Post-traumatic intracranial mass lesions. In Cooper PR (ed): Head Injury. Baltimore: Williams & Wilkins, 1993, pp 275–329.

72. Miller JD: Evaluation and treatment of head injury in adults. Neurosurg Q 2:28–43, 1992.

73. Gallbraith S, Teasdale G: Predicting the need for operation in the patient with an occult traumatic intracranial hematoma. J Neurosurg 55:75–81, 1981.

74. Katayama Y, Tsubokawa T, Miyazaki S, et al: Oedema fluid formation within contused brain tissue as a cause of medically uncontrollable elevation of intracranial pressure: The role of surgical therapy. Acta Neurochir Suppl (Wien) 51:308–310, 1990.

75. Mathiesen T, Kakarieka A, Edner G: Traumatic intracerebral lesions without extracerebral haematoma in 218 patients. Acta Neurochir (Wien) 137:155–163, 1995.

76. Patel NY, Hoyt DB, Nakaji P, et al: Traumatic brain injury: Patterns of failure of nonoperative management. J Trauma 48:367–375, 2000.

77. Choksey M, Crockard HA, Sandilands M: Acute traumatic intracerebral haematomas: Determinants of outcome in a retrospective series of 202 cases. Br J Neurosurg 7:611–622, 1993.

78. Stein SC, Young GS, Talucci RC, et al: Delayed brain injury after head trauma: Significance of coagulopathy. Neurosurgery 30:160–165, 1992.

79. Greenberg J, Cohen WA, Cooper PR: The "hyperacute" extraaxial intracranial hematoma: Computed tomographic findings and clinical significance. Neurosurgery 17:48–56, 1985.

80. Rivas JJ, Lobato RD, Sarabia R, et al: Extradural hematoma: Analysis of factors influencing the courses of 161 patients. Neurosurgery 23:44–51, 1988.

81. Nussbaum ES, Wolf AL, Sebring L, et al: Complete temporal lobectomy for surgical resuscitation of patients with transtentorial herniation secondary to unilateral hemispheric swelling. Neurosurgery 29:62–66, 1991.

82. Jamieson KG, Yelland JD: Surgically treated traumatic subdural hematomas. J Neurosurg 37:137–149, 1972.

83. Howard MA 3rd, Gross AS, Dacey RG Jr, et al: Acute subdural hematomas: An age-dependent clinical entity. J Neurosurg 71:858–863, 1989.

84. Fernandes YB, Borges G, Ramina R, et al: Minimally invasive approach to traumatic intracerebral hematomas. Minim Invasive Neurosurg 44:221–225, 2001.

85. Swayne OB, Horner BM, Dorward NL: The hitch stitch: An obsolete neurosurgical technique? Br J Neurosurg 16:541–544, 2002.

86. Winston KR: Efficacy of dural tenting sutures. J Neurosurg 91:180–284, 1999.

87. Winston KR: Dural tenting sutures in pediatric neurosurgery. Pediatr Neurosurg 28:230–235, 1998.

88. Kelly DF, Goodale DB, Williams J, et al: Propofol in the treatment of moderate and severe head injury: A randomized, prospective double-blinded pilot trial. J Neurosurg 90:1042–1052, 1999.

89. Kang TM: Propofol infusion syndrome in critically ill patients. Ann Pharmacother 36:1453–1456, 2002.

90. Kelly DF: Propofol-infusion syndrome. J Neurosurg 95:925–926, 2001.

91. Cooper PR, Rovit RL, Ransohoff J: Hemicraniectomy in the treatment of acute subdural hematoma: A re-appraisal. Surg Neurol 5:25–28, 1976.

92. Gaab MR, Rittierodt M, Lorenz M, et al: Traumatic brain swelling and operative decompression: A prospective investigation. Acta Neurochir Suppl (Wien) 51:326–328, 1990.

93. Schneider GH, Bardt T, Lanksch WR, et al: Decompressive craniectomy following traumatic brain injury: ICP, CPP and neurological outcome. Acta Neurochir Suppl 81:77–79, 2002.

94. Whitfield PC, Patel H, Hutchinson PJ, et al: Bifrontal decompressive craniectomy in the management of posttraumatic intracranial hypertension. Br J Neurosurg 15:500–507, 2001.

95. Whitfield PC, Kirkpatrick PJ, Czosnyka M, et al: Management of severe traumatic brain injury by decompressive craniectomy. Neurosurgery 49:225–226, 2001.

96. Polin RS, Shaffrey ME, Bogaev CA, et al: Decompressive bifrontal craniectomy in the treatment of severe refractory posttraumatic cerebral edema. Neurosurgery 41:84–94, 1997.

97. Kunze E, Meixensberger J, Janka M, et al: Decompressive craniectomy in patients with uncontrollable intracranial hypertension. Acta Neurochir Suppl (Wien) 71:16–18, 1998.

98. Kontopoulos V, Foroglou N, Patsalas J, et al: Decompressive craniectomy for the management of patients with refractory hypertension: Should it be reconsidered? Acta Neurochir (Wien) 144:791–796, 2002.

99. Munch E, Horn P, Schurer L, et al: Management of severe traumatic brain injury by decompressive craniectomy. Neurosurgery 47:315–323, 2000.

100. Albanese J, Leone M, Alliez JR, et al: Decompressive craniectomy for severe traumatic brain injury: Evaluation of the effects at one year. Crit Care Med 31:2535–2538, 2003.

101. Soukiasian HJ, Hui T, Avital I, et al: Decompressive craniectomy in trauma patients with severe brain injury. Am Surg 68:1066–1071, 2002.

102. Guerra WK, Gaab MR, Dietz H, et al: Surgical decompression for traumatic brain swelling: Indications and results. J Neurosurg 90:187–196, 1999.

103. Guerra WK, Piek J, Gaab MR: Decompressive craniectomy to treat intracranial hypertension in head injury patients. Intensive Care Med 25:1327–1329, 1999.

104. De Luca GP, Volpin L, Fornezza U, et al: The role of decompressive craniectomy in the treatment of uncontrollable post-traumatic intracranial hypertension. Acta Neurochir Suppl 76:401–404, 2000.

105. Coplin WM, Cullen NK, Policherla PN, et al: Safety and feasibility of craniectomy with duraplasty as the initial surgical intervention for severe traumatic brain injury. J Trauma 50:1050–1059, 2001.

106. Taylor A, Butt W, Rosenfeld J, et al: A randomized trial of very early decompressive craniectomy in children with traumatic brain injury and sustained intracranial hypertension. Childs Nerv Syst 17:154–162, 2001.

107. Simma B, Tscharre A, Hejazi N, et al: Neurologic outcome after decompressive craniectomy in children. Intensive Care Med 28:1000, 2002.

108. Berger S, Schwarz M, Huth R: Hypertonic saline solution and decompressive craniectomy for treatment of intracranial hypertension in pediatric severe traumatic brain injury. J Trauma 53:558–563, 2002.

109. Miller JD, Dearden NM, Piper IR, et al: Control of intracranial pressure in patients with severe head injury. J Neurotrauma 9(Suppl 1): S317–S326, 1992.

110. The Brain Trauma Foundation. The American Association of Neurological Surgeons. The Joint Section on Neurotrauma and Critical Care: Recommendations for intracranial pressure monitoring technology. J Neurotrauma 17:497–506, 2000.

111. Bouma GJ, Muizelaar JP, Choi SC, et al: Cerebral circulation and metabolism after severe traumatic brain injury: The elusive role of ischemia. J Neurosurg 75:685–693, 1991.

112. Graham DI, Ford I, Adams JH, et al: Ischaemic brain damage is still common in fatal non-missile head injury. J Neurol Neurosurg Psychiatry 52:346–350, 1989.

113. Bouma GJ, Muizelaar JP, Stringer WA, et al: Ultra-early evaluation of regional cerebral blood flow in severely head-injured patients using xenon-enhanced computerized tomography. J Neurosurg 77:360–368, 1992.

114. Chesnut RM, Marshall LF, Marshall SB: Medical management of intracranial pressure. In Cooper PR (ed): Head Injury. Baltimore: Williams & Wilkins, 1993, pp 225–246.

115. Chan KH, Miller JD, Dearden NM, et al: The effect of changes in cerebral perfusion pressure upon middle cerebral artery blood flow velocity and jugular bulb venous oxygen saturation after severe brain injury. J Neurosurg 77:55–61, 1992.

116. Paulson OB, Strandgaard S, Edvinsson L: Cerebral autoregulation. Cerebrovasc Brain Metab Rev 2:161–192, 1990.

117. The Brain Trauma Foundation. The American Association of Neurological Surgeons. The Joint Section on Neurotrauma and Critical Care: Guidelines for cerebral perfusion pressure. J Neurotrauma 17:507–511, 2000.

118. Robertson CS, Valadka AB, Hannay HJ, et al: Prevention of secondary ischemic insults after severe head injury. Crit Care Med 27:2086–2095, 1999.

119. al-Rawi PG, Hutchinson PJ, Gupta AK, et al: Multiparameter brain tissue monitoring—Correlation between parameters and identification of CPP thresholds. Zentralbl Neurochir 61:74–79, 2000.

120. Chambers IR, Treadwell L, Mendelow AD: Determination of threshold levels of cerebral perfusion pressure and intracranial pressure in severe head injury by using receiver-operating characteristic curves: An observational study in 291 patients. J Neurosurg 94:412–416, 2001.

121. Meixensberger J, Jaeger M, Vath A, et al: Brain tissue oxygen guided treatment supplementing ICP/CPP therapy after traumatic brain injury. J Neurol Neurosurg Psychiatry 74:760–764, 2003.

122. Fandino J, Stocker R, Prokop S, et al: Cerebral oxygenation and systemic trauma related factors determining neurological outcome after brain injury. J Clin Neurosci 7:226–233, 2000.

123. Vespa PM, McArthur D, O'Phelan K, et al: Persistently low extracellular glucose correlates with poor outcome 6 months after human traumatic brain injury despite a lack of increased lactate: A microdialysis study. J Cereb Blood Flow Metab 23:865–877, 2003.

124. Menzel M, Soukup J, Henze D, et al: Brain tissue oxygen monitoring for assessment of autoregulation: Preliminary results suggest a new hypothesis. J Neurosurg Anesthesiol 15:33–41, 2003.

125. Vespa P, Prins M, Ronne-Engstrom E, et al: Increase in extracellular glutamate caused by reduced cerebral perfusion pressure and seizures after human traumatic brain injury: A microdialysis study. J Neurosurg 89:971–982, 1998.

126. Rosner MJ, Rosner SD, Johnson AH: Cerebral perfusion pressure: Management protocol and clinical results. J Neurosurg 83:949–962, 1995.

127. Asgeirsson B, Grande PO, Nordstrom CH: A new therapy of post-trauma brain oedema based on haemodynamic principles for brain volume regulation. Intensive Care Med 20:260–267, 1994.

128. Oertel M, Kelly DF, Lee JH, et al: Efficacy of hyperventilation, blood pressure elevation, and metabolic suppression therapy in controlling intracranial pressure after head injury. J Neurosurg 97:1045–1053, 2002.

129. Oertel M, Kelly DF, Lee JH, et al: Is CPP therapy beneficial for all patients with high ICP? Acta Neurochir Suppl 81:6768, 2002.

130. The Brain Trauma Foundation. The American Association of Neurological Surgeons. The Joint Section on Neurotrauma and Critical Care: Hyperventilation. J Neurotrauma 17:513–520, 2000.

131. Coles JP, Minhas PS, Fryer TD, et al: Effect of hyperventilation on cerebral blood flow in traumatic head injury: Clinical relevance and monitoring correlates. Crit Care Med 30:1950–1959, 2002.

132. Hutchinson PJ, Gupta AK, Fryer TF, et al: Correlation between cerebral blood flow, substrate delivery, and metabolism in head injury: A combined microdialysis and triple oxygen positron emission tomography study. J Cereb Blood Flow Metab 22:735–745, 2002.

133. Oertel M, Kelly DF, Lee JH, et al: Can hyperventilation improve cerebral microcirculation in patients with high ICP? Acta Neurochir Suppl 81:71–72, 2002.

134. Eker C, Asgeirsson B, Grande PO, et al: Improved outcome after severe head injury with a new therapy based on principles for brain volume regulation and preserved microcirculation. Crit Care Med 26:1881–1886, 1998.

135. Vespa P: Should I monitor cerebral blood flow in the neurointensive care unit. In Valadka AB and Andrews BT (eds): Neurotrauma: Evidence-Based Answers to Common Questions. New York: Thieme, 2005, pp 68–74.

136. Sheinberg M, Kanter MJ, Robertson CS, et al: Continuous monitoring of jugular venous oxygen saturation in head-injured patients. J Neurosurg 76:212–217, 1992.

137. Gupta AK, Hutchinson PJ, Al-Rawi P, et al: Measuring brain tissue oxygenation compared with jugular venous oxygen saturation for monitoring cerebral oxygenation after traumatic brain injury. Anesth Analg 88:549–553, 1999.

138. Kett-White R, Hutchinson PJ, Czosnyka M, et al: Multi-modal monitoring of acute brain injury. Adv Tech Stand Neurosurg 27:87–134, 2002.

139. Marion D, Obrist WD, Penrod LE, et al: Treatment of cerebral ischemia improves outcome following severe traumatic brain injury. Paper presented at the 61st Annual Meeting of the American Association of Neurological Surgeons, 1993, Boston.

140. Martin NA, Doberstein C, Zane C, et al: Posttraumatic cerebral arterial spasm: Transcranial Doppler ultrasound, cerebral blood flow, and angiographic findings. J Neurosurg 77:575–583, 1992.

141. Chan KH, Dearden NM, Miller JD, et al: Transcranial Doppler waveform differences in hyperemic and nonhyperemic patients after severe head injury. Surg Neurol 38:433–436, 1992.

142. Claassen J, Mayer SA: Continuous electroencephalographic monitoring in neurocritical care. Curr Neurol Neurosci Rep 2:534–540, 2002.

143. Scheuer ML: Continuous EEG monitoring in the intensive care unit. Epilepsia 43(Suppl 3):114–127, 2002.

144. Steudel WI, Kruger J: Using the spectral analysis of the EEG for prognosis of severe brain injuries in the first post-traumatic week. Acta Neurochir Suppl (Wien) 28:40–42, 1979.

145. Vespa PM, Boscardin WJ, Hovda DA, et al: Early and persistent impaired percent alpha variability on continuous electroencephalography monitoring as predictive of poor outcome after traumatic brain injury. J Neurosurg 97:84–92, 2002.

146. Synek VM: EEG abnormality grades and subdivisions of prognostic importance in traumatic and anoxic coma in adults. Clin Electroencephalogr 19:160–166, 1988.

147. Synek VM: Prognostically important EEG coma patterns in diffuse anoxic and traumatic encephalopathies in adults. J Clin Neurophysiol 5:161–174, 1988.

148. Hulihan JF Jr, Syna DR: Electroencephalographic sleep patterns in post-anoxic stupor and coma. Neurology 44:758–760, 1994.

149. Evans BM, Bartlett JR: Prediction of outcome in severe head injury based on recognition of sleep related activity in the polygraphic electroencephalogram. J Neurol Neurosurg Psychiatry 59:17–25, 1995.

150. Levy ML, Giannotta SL: Cardiac performance indices during hypervolemic therapy for cerebral vasospasm. J Neurosurg 75:27–31, 1991.

151. Feldman Z, Kanter MJ, Robertson CS, et al: Effect of head elevation on intracranial pressure, cerebral perfusion pressure, and cerebral blood flow in head-injured patients. J Neurosurg 76:207–211, 1992.

152. Rosner MJ: Pathophysiology and management of increased intracranial pressure. In Andrews BT (ed): Neurosurgical Intensive Care. New York: McGraw-Hill, 1993, pp 57–112.

153. Dorman HR, Sondheimer JH, Cadnapaphornchai P: Mannitol-induced acute renal failure. Medicine (Baltimore) 69:153–159, 1990.

154. Marmarou A, Anderson RL, Ward JD, et al: NINDS traumatic coma data bank: Intracranial pressure monitoring methodology. J Neurosurg 75(Suppl):S21–S27, 1991.

155. Marmarou A, Anderson RL, Ward JD, et al: Impact of ICP instability and hypotension on outcome in patients with severe head trauma. J Neurosurg 75(Suppl):S59–S66, 1991.

156. Eisenberg HM, Frankowski RF, Contant CF, et al: High-dose barbiturate control of elevated intracranial pressure in patients with severe head injury. J Neurosurg 69:15–23, 1988.

157. The Brain Trauma Foundation. The American Association of Neurological Surgeons. The Joint Section on Neurotrauma and Critical Care: Use of barbiturates in the control of intracranial hypertension. J Neurotrauma 17:527–530, 2000.

158. Cordato DJ, Herkes GK, Mather LE, et al: Barbiturates for acute neurological and neurosurgical emergencies—Do they still have a role? J Clin Neurosci 10:283–288, 2003.

159. Procaccio F, Stocchetti N, Citerio G, et al: Guidelines for the treatment of adults with severe head trauma (part II): Criteria for medical treatment. J Neurosurg Sci 44:11–18, 2000.

160. Roberts I: Barbiturates for acute traumatic brain injury. Cochrane Database Syst Rev 2:CD000033, 2000.

161. Bullock R, Hanemann CO, Murray L, et al: Recurrent hematomas following craniotomy for traumatic intracranial mass. J Neurosurg 72:9–14, 1990.

162. Gentleman D, Nath F, Macpherson P: Diagnosis and management of delayed traumatic intracerebral haematomas. Br J Neurosurg 3:367–372, 1989.

163. Sprick C, Bettag M, Bock WJ: Delayed traumatic intracranial hematomas—Clinical study of seven years. Neurosurg Rev 12 (Suppl 1):228–230, 1989.

164. Unterberg A, Kiening K, Schmiedek P, et al: Long-term observations of intracranial pressure after severe head injury: The phenomenon of secondary rise of intracranial pressure. Neurosurgery 32:17–24, 1993.

165. Narayan RK, Kishore PR, Becker DP, et al: Intracranial pressure: To monitor or not to monitor? A review of our experience with severe head injury. J Neurosurg 56:650–659, 1982.

166. Roitberg BZ, Khan N, Alp MS, et al: Bedside external ventricular drain placement for the treatment of acute hydrocephalus. Br J Neurosurg 15:324–327, 2001.

167. Guyot LL, Dowling C, Diaz FG, et al: Cerebral monitoring devices: Analysis of complications. Acta Neurochir Suppl (Wien) 71:47–49, 1998.

168. Rossi S, Buzzi F, Paparella A, et al: Complications and safety associated with ICP monitoring: A study of 542 patients. Acta Neurochir Suppl (Wien) 71:91–93, 1998.

169. Mayhall CG, Archer NH, Lamb VA, et al: Ventriculostomy-related infections: A prospective epidemiologic study. N Engl J Med 310:553–559, 1984.

170. Winfield JA, Rosenthal P, Kanter RK, et al: Duration of intracranial pressure monitoring does not predict daily risk of infectious complications. Neurosurgery 33:424–431, 1993.

171. Rebuck JA, Murry KR, Rhoney DH, et al: Infection related to intracranial pressure monitors in adults: Analysis of risk factors and antibiotic prophylaxis. J Neurol Neurosurg Psychiatry 69:381–384, 2000.

172. Poon WS, Ng S, Wai S: CSF antibiotic prophylaxis for neurosurgical patients with ventriculostomy: A randomised study. Acta Neurochir Suppl (Wien) 71:146–148, 1998.

173. Sande GM, Galbraith SL, McLatchie G: Infection after depressed fracture in the west of Scotland. Scott Med J 25:227–229, 1980.

174. Stephanov S: Brain abscesses from neglected open head injuries: Experience with 17 cases over 20 years. Swiss Surg 5:288–292, 1999.

175. Vespa PM, Nuwer MR, Nenov V, et al: Increased incidence and impact of nonconvulsive and convulsive seizures after traumatic brain injury as detected by continuous electroencephalographic monitoring. J Neurosurg 91:750–760, 1999.

176. Temkin NR, Dikmen SS, Wilensky AJ, et al: A randomized, double-blind study of phenytoin for the prevention of post-traumatic seizures. N Engl J Med 323:497–502, 1990.

177. Haltiner AM, Newell DW, Temkin NR, et al: Side effects and mortality associated with use of phenytoin for early posttraumatic seizure prophylaxis. J Neurosurg 91:588–592, 1999.

178. Temkin NR, Dikmen SS, Anderson GD, et al: Valproate therapy for prevention of posttraumatic seizures: A randomized trial. J Neurosurg 91:593–600, 1999.

179. The Brain Trauma Foundation. The American Association of Neurological Surgeons. The Joint Section on Neurotrauma and Critical Care: Role of antiseizure prophylaxis following head injury. J Neurotrauma 17:549–553, 2000.
180. Chang BS, Lowenstein DH: Practice parameter: Antiepileptic drug prophylaxis in severe traumatic brain injury. Report of the Quality Standards Subcommittee of the American Academy of Neurology. Neurology 60:10–16, 2003.
181. Schierhout G, Roberts I: Anti-epileptic drugs for preventing seizures following acute traumatic brain injury. Cochrane Database Syst Rev 4:CD000173, 2001.
182. Shiozaki T, Sugimoto H, Taneda M, et al: Effect of mild hypothermia on uncontrollable intracranial hypertension after severe head injury. J Neurosurg 79:363–368, 1993.
183. Marion DW, Obrist WD, Carlier PM, et al: The use of moderate therapeutic hypothermia for patients with severe head injuries: A preliminary report. J Neurosurg 79:354–362, 1993.
184. Clifton GL, Allen S, Barrodale P, et al: A phase II study of moderate hypothermia in severe brain injury. J Neurotrauma 10:263–273, 1993.
185. McIntyre LA, Fergusson DA, Hebert PC, et al: Prolonged therapeutic hypothermia after traumatic brain injury in adults: A systematic review. JAMA 289:2992–2999, 2003.
186. Shiozaki T, Hayakata T, Taneda M, et al: A multicenter prospective randomized controlled trial of the efficacy of mild hypothermia for severely head injured patients with low intracranial pressure. Mild Hypothermia Study Group in Japan. J Neurosurg 94:50–54, 2001.
187. Shiozaki T, Nakajima Y, Taneda M, et al: Efficacy of moderate hypothermia in patients with severe head injury and intracranial hypertension refractory to mild hypothermia. J Neurosurg 99:47–51, 2003.
188. Reeder RF, Harbaugh RE: Administration of intravenous urea and normal saline for the treatment of hyponatremia in neurosurgical patients. J Neurosurg 70:201–206, 1989.
189. Doczi T, Tarjanyi J, Huszka E, et al: Syndrome of inappropriate secretion of antidiuretic hormone (SIADH) after head injury. Neurosurgery 10:685–688, 1982.
190. Kelly DF, Laws ER, Fossett DT: Fluid and sodium abnormalities after transsphenoidal surgery for pituitary adenomas with emphasis on delayed hyponatremia: A review of 99 patients [abstract]. Paper presented at the Congress of Neurological Surgeons Annual Meeting, 1993, Vancouver.
191. Decaux G, Soupart A: Treatment of symptomatic hyponatremia. Am J Med Sci 326:25–30, 2003.
192. McIntosh TK: Pharmacologic strategies in the treatment of experimental brain injury. J Neurotrauma 9(Suppl 1):S201–S209, 1992.
193. Canavero S, Bonicalzi V, Narcisi P: Safety of magnesium-lidocaine combination for severe head injury: The Turin lidomag pilot study. Surg Neurol 60:165–169, 2003.
194. Young B, Ott L, Dempsey R, et al: Relationship between admission hyperglycemia and neurologic outcome of severely brain-injured patients. Ann Surg 210:466–473, 1989.
195. Piek J, Chesnut RM, Marshall LF, et al: Extracranial complications of severe head injury. J Neurosurg 77:901–907, 1992.
196. Chesnut RM: Medical complications of the head-injured patient. In Cooper PR (ed): Head Injury. Baltimore: Williams & Wilkins, 1993, pp 459–501.
197. Eddleston JM, Vohra A, Scott P, et al: A comparison of the frequency of stress ulceration and secondary pneumonia in sucralfate- or ranitidine-treated intensive care unit patients. Crit Care Med 19:1491–1496, 1991.
198. Black PM, Baker MF, Snook CP: Experience with external pneumatic calf compression in neurology and neurosurgery. Neurosurgery 18:440–444, 1986.
199. Frim DM, Barker FG 2nd, Poletti CE, et al: Postoperative low-dose heparin decreases thromboembolic complications in neurosurgical patients. Neurosurgery 30:830–833, 1992.
200. Brown TH, Davidson PF, Larson GM: Acute gastritis occurring within 24 hours of severe head injury. Gastrointest Endosc 35:37–40, 1989.
201. Epstein FM, Ward JD, Becker DP: Medical complications of head injury. In Cooper PR (ed): Head Injury. Baltimore: Williams & Wilkins, 1987, pp 390–421.
202. Elf K, Nilsson P, Enblad P: Outcome after traumatic brain injury improved by an organized secondary insult program and standardized neurointensive care. Crit Care Med 30:2129–2134, 2002.
203. Citerio G, Stocchetti N, Cormio M, et al: Application of guidelines for severe head trauma: Data from an Italian database. Eur J Emerg Med 10:68–72, 2003.
204. Imberti R: Why have recent trials of neuroprotective agents in head injury failed to show. Neurosurgery 53:241–242, 2003.
205. Maas A, Steyerberg EW, Murray GD, et al: Why have recent trials of neuroprotective agents in head injury failed to show convincing efficacy? A pragmatic analysis and theoretical considerations. Neurosurgery 44:1286–1298, 1999.
206. National Academy of Sciences and National Research Council. Accidental Death and Disability: The Neglected Disease of Modern Society [white paper]. Washington, DC: Division of Medical Sciences, National Academy of Sciences, National Research Council, September 1966.

5 Decompressive Craniectomy: Physiologic Rationale, Clinical Indications, and Surgical Considerations

CLARK CHEN, EDWARD R. SMITH, CHRISTOPHER S. OGILVY, and BOB S. CARTER

The management of increased intracranial pressure is a common clinical scenario in neurosurgery. Among the many available treatments for increased intracranial pressure, none remains more controversial than decompressive craniectomy. In this chapter we discuss the physiologic effects of decompressive craniectomy as it relates to the management of intracranial hypertension. We further review the indications of decompressive craniectomy in the context of malignant cerebral edema, especially in the setting of cerebral infarction, traumatic brain injury, aneurysmal subarachnoid hemorrhage, central venous thrombosis, encephalitis, intracerebral hematoma, and metabolic encephalopathies. Surgical considerations in the planning of decompressive craniectomy will also be discussed.

DECOMPRESSIVE CRANIECTOMY IN THE MANAGEMENT OF INTRACRANIAL HYPERTENSION

Intracranial Pressure Determines the Extent of Cerebral Oxygenation

Intracranial pressure, defined as the pressure within the cranial vault, represents the resistance that the heart must overcome in order to deliver blood to the cerebral parenchyma. One expression of this relationship is that CPP (cerebral perfusion pressure) = MAP (mean arterial pressure) – ICP (intracranial pressure). This relationship predicts that increased intracranial pressure results in cerebral ischemia in the absence of physiologic compensation. The initial response to this ischemia involves dilatation of cerebral vasculature in order to afford increased blood flow and, therefore, oxygen delivery. When intracranial pressure elevates past the point of inducing maximal vasodilatation, systemic hypertension is required to maintain cerebral perfusion. Elevation of intracranial pressure beyond the point where CPP is adequately maintained results in hypoxic brain injury.

The Monro-Kellie Doctrine

Despite being the product of several complex physiologic processes, intracranial pressure is fundamentally governed by a simple observation commonly referred to as the Monro-Kellie doctrine. The observation is that the matured cranial vault represents a rigid structure, the contents of which consist of the brain parenchyma, cerebrospinal fluid (CSF), and blood. Because the cranial vault offers little or no compliance, expansion in any of these compartments is expected to elevate intracranial pressure. The expansion can occur focally, as in the case of parenchymal hematoma, or globally, as in the case of diffuse cerebral edema. Compensatory mechanisms allow for initial volume expansion of one or more of the intracranial compartments without effects on intracranial pressure. However, after a certain volume threshold is surpassed, further volume expansion of the intracranial contents causes an exponential rise in intracranial pressure (Fig. 5-1).

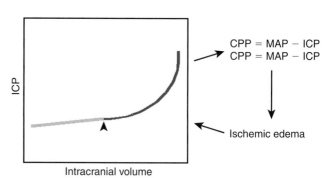

FIGURE 5-1 Feed-forward cycle for intracranial hypertension. Compensatory mechanisms allow for initial expansion of one or more of the intracranial compartments with minimal effects on intracranial pressure (*arrowhead*). However, after a certain volume threshold is surpassed, further volume expansion of the intracranial contents causes an exponential rise in intracranial pressure. As intracranial pressure increases beyond the limits of physiologic compensation, cerebral perfusion is compromised. Decreased oxygen availability disrupts cellular capacity for maintaining an osmotic differential across the cellular membrane, causing influx of water into the cell, which further elevates the intracranial pressure. The increased intracranial pressure, in turn, decreases cerebral perfusion, resulting in a feed-forward cycle for intracranial hypertension.

Pathophysiology of Intracranial Hypertension

As intracranial pressure increases beyond the limits of physiologic compensation, cerebral perfusion is compromised. Decreased oxygen availability diminishes the efficiency of cellular energy production by loss of oxidative phosphorylation. The resulting energy depletion disrupts cellular capacity for maintaining an osmotic differential across the cellular membrane, causing influx of water into the cells. This intracellular edema represents an expansion of the parenchymal compartment, which further elevates the intracranial pressure. The increased intracranial pressure, in turn, decreases cerebral perfusion, resulting in a feed-forward cycle for intracranial hypertension.

Regions of cerebral edema cause localized pressure against their surrounding tissues. Herniation occurs when this localized pressure becomes greater than the resistance of the surrounding tissues. Because of the high resistance of the cranial vault, parenchymal herniation inevitably occurs in a centrifugal manner, causing transgression against semirigid dural septa as well as herniation through compartments defined by these septa. Cellular injuries are incurred by direct pressure imposed by the herniating tissue. Injuries are also incurred as a result of venous hypertension and arterial insufficiency induced by distortion of the vascular anatomy. In addition, the pathways of normal cerebral spinal fluid flow are often obstructed, further exacerbating the escalation of intracranial hypertension. Ultimately, compression of the brain stem structures produces rapid neurologic deterioration if appropriate therapies are not instituted.

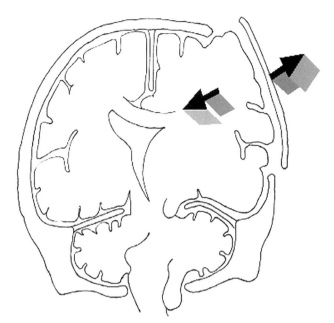

FIGURE 5-2 Mechanism by which decompressive craniectomy minimizes herniation syndromes. Because of the high resistance of the cranial vault, cerebral herniation inevitably occurs in a centrifugal manner, causing transgression against semirigid dural septa as well as herniation through compartments defined by these septa *(inward arrow)*. Decompressive craniectomies allow for outward herniation beyond boundaries previously defined by the cranial vault, allowing for centripetal herniation *(outward arrow)* and minimizing centrifugal compression of brain stem structures.

Management of Intracranial Hypertension

Strategies for management of intracranial hypertension fall into two general categories: to reduce the volume of the intracranial compartments and to remove the mechanical constraints imposed by the cranial vault. In the first approach, the parenchymal compartment is reduced either by the administration of osmotic agents (e.g., mannitol) or by partial lobectomies. The blood compartment is minimized by head positioning, hemodynamic optimization, or hyperventilation. The cerebrospinal fluid compartment is decreased by ventriculostomy drainage. The second approach utilizes large craniectomies in association with duratomies to decrease the resistive force of the cranial vault, allowing for outward herniation beyond boundaries previously defined by the cranial vault. The overall effects of decompressive craniotomies are to increase volume-buffering capacity of the cranial vault by allowing for centripetal herniation. The centripetal herniation in turn minimizes centrifugal compression of brain stem structures (Fig. 5-2). The effectiveness of craniectomy in the management of intracranial hypertension has been well documented in various experimental and clinical settings.[1–11] The magnitude of intracranial cerebral pressure reduction correlates with the size of the craniectomy and ranges from 15% to 85%.[4,8,11] Duratomy further enhances intracranial pressure reduction achieved by craniectomy, and some studies suggest that dural release allows for the maximal ICP reduction.[11–13] Although there

are concerns that decompressive craniectomy can exacerbate cerebral edema by decreasing interstitial tissue pressure in the decompressed region or by inducing venous congestion/arterial insufficiency by facilitating vascular distortion through centripetal herniation,[9,14,15] such concerns have not been substantiated by clinical observations.[11,16] Early clinical experiences with decompressive craniectomies were limited to severe traumatic head injuries that presented in extremis. These studies consisted of small case series and reported high morbidity and mortality.[17–19] For this reason, interest in decompressive craniectomy for trauma waned. Modern surgical techniques, refined postoperative care, and careful patient selection have yielded improved clinical outcome for decompressive craniectomies and have led to renewed interest in the procedure.

CLINICAL INDICATIONS OF DECOMPRESSIVE CRANIECTOMY

Criteria for decompressive craniectomy in the posterior fossa is reviewed elsewhere and will not be further discussed here. The following section will review the existing literature on the potential role of decompressive craniectomy in the treatment of intracranial hypertension secondary to malignant cerebral edema, traumatic brain injury, aneurysmal subarachnoid hemorrhage, central venous thrombosis, encephalitis, intracerebral hematoma, and metabolic encephalopathies.

Malignant Cerebral Infarction

Definition of Malignant Cerebral Infarction

The term *malignant cerebral infarction* refers to large territorial parenchymal infarctions with postischemic edema and associated uncal or axial brain stem herniation. The initial insult generally involves proximal occlusion of the middle cerebral artery (MCA), causing a greater than 50% infarct in the supplied territory.[20] Although accounting for only 7% to 15% of all strokes,[21,22] associated mortality in this subcategory ranges from 70% to 80% with maximal hyperventilation, osmotherapy, barbiturate suppression, and induced hypothermia.[23,24] These patients present clinically with rapid neurologic deterioration 2 to 4 days after initial onset of stroke, with gaze toward the side of infarction, contralateral hemiplegia, and progressive deterioration in consciousness.

Hemicraniectomy in the Treatment of Malignant Infarction

Hemicraniectomy refers to the removal of a large frontotemporal-parietal bone fragment. Several retrospective case series, as well as prospective nonrandomized clinical trials, have yielded compelling evidence that hemicraniectomy with duraplasty effectively controls the intracranial hypertension associated with malignant cerebral infarction and reduces associated mortality from 80% to 30%.[25–27] Some studies suggest that mortality can further be reduced to 10% by undertaking decompression within 24 hours of ictus.[28] One criticism of these reports, however, is that hemicraniectomies tend to be performed in younger patients, whose prognosis is generally more favorable irrespective of surgical intervention. The improvement in survival reported thus represents age bias in patient selection rather than effectiveness of surgical intervention. For instance, Wijdicks and Diringer showed that mortality associated with malignant infarction managed medically is approximately 40% in patients under age 60 and 90% in patients over age 60.[29] To address this issue, Holtkamp and colleagues retrospectively compared the survival rate of 24 patients older than 55 affected with malignant infarction. Twelve of the 24 patients underwent hemicraniectomy, and 12 were medically managed. The mean age, the age distribution, and the extent of infarct between the two groups were not statistically significant. According to this report, 8 of 12 patients (67%) who underwent hemicraniectomy survived, whereas only 3 of 12 patients (25%) who underwent maximal medical therapy survived.[27]

The most compelling argument for hemicraniectomy in malignant infarctions is that timing of surgery affects survival as well as length of intensive care unit stay. A retrospective analysis of 52 decompressions as stratified by time to surgery into groups intervened in under 6 hours from ictus, 6 hours after ictus, and no intervention showed mortalities of 8%, 36%, and 80%, respectively. The corresponding average length of intensive care stay was 12 days (range, 6 to 21 days), 18 days (4 to 56 days), and 7 days (2 to 18 days, shortened by fatality).[28] Similar data were reported by Schwab and colleagues, who retrospectively stratified 63 interventions into decompression within 24 hours (early, 31 patients) and after 24 hours (late, 32 patients) of initial injury. Mortality was 16% for early decompression and 34% for late decompression. The average length of intensive care stay was 7 days for early decompression and 13 days for late decompression.[26] In both reports, the baseline demographic distribution within the subcategories was comparable.

Radiologic Predictors of Malignant Cerebral Infarction

Benefits of early hemicraniectomy can only be attained with reliable detection of malignant cerebral infarction prior to clinical deterioration. Imaging modalities used for this purpose include magnetic resonance imaging (MRI) with diffusion weighted imaging (DWI), computed tomography (CT), ultrasound, and positron emission test (PET). Of these modalities, MRI with DWI offers the best correlation to stroke severity and long-term clinical outcome. Hyperacute MRI findings with DWI signals filling greater than 89 cm^3 volume is roughly 90% sensitive and 96% specific in predicting malignant cerebral infarction.[30] These values are superior to those reported for early (i.e., within 12 hours of ictus) CT findings of hypodensity in more than 50% of the MCA territory, hyperdense MCA, and diffusely attenuated corticomedullary contrast. The sensitivity and specificity of these CT findings in predicting malignant infarction are 60% and 70% to 90%, respectively.[31] The predictive power of MRI with DWI also compares favorably with those obtained using PET (99% sensitivity, 68% to 86% specificity).[32] Although 100% sensitivity and specificity in the prediction of malignant infarction have been reported using sonographic monitoring of midline shifts, these shifts tend to accompany rather than precede neurologic deterioration.[33]

Functional Recovery after Hemicraniectomy

As would be expected given the severity of initial insult, hemicraniectomy, though often life-saving in the context of malignant infarction, often leaves surviving patients with moderate to severe disability. A commonly used scale for physical disability in stroke patients is the Barthel index, which assesses the performance of specific tasks related to self-care and mobility. Although the index is limited in scope (e.g., it fails to consider the psychiatric, linguistic, and social aspects of the disability), its simplicity and widely accepted use allow for cross-comparison analysis of data from different studies. In this index, the maximal score is 100 (no disability) scaled in 5-point increments (Table 5-1). A score of 60 implies functional independence despite moderate disability, and scores of 60 to 99 imply mild to moderate disability.[34] A survey of existing literature revealed Barthel index scores ranging from 10 to 100 in patients who survived malignant cerebral infarct after hemicraniectomy. The mean Barthel index scores in the various series ranged from 55 to 70. A notable trend across all studies is that the Barthel index score is higher for younger patients. Fifty percent to 80% of all patients under age 60 who underwent craniectomy attained scores of 60 or more at follow-up (length of follow-up ranged from 3 to 27 months).[25,26,28,35–37] In contrast, 0% to 30% of patients over age 60 attained scores of 60 or more.[25,27,35,36] All of the patients who recovered sufficient function to attain a score of 90 or more were patients under the age of 45.

Another trend seen in some reports is that the subcategory of patients who underwent early decompression exhibited improved functional outcome. Cho and colleagues

TABLE 5-1 ▪ Functional Recovery as Measured by the Barthel Index and the Glasgow Outcome Scale

Barthel Index

Feeding	10
Bathing	5
Grooming	5
Dressing	10
Bowel	10
Bladder	10
Toilet use	10
Transfer	15
Mobility	15
Stairs	10

Glasgow Outcome Scale

Good recovery	5
Moderate disability	4
Severe disability	3
Vegetative	2
Dead	1

retrospectively examined the effect of early (i.e., within 6 hours of ictus) and late (i.e., more than 6 hours after ictus) decompression in a group of 42 patients, of whom 30 underwent early hemicraniectomy and 12 underwent late hemicraniectomy. The demographic distributions of the two groups were comparable; however, the mean Barthel score was 70 in the group that underwent early decompression (range of 60 to 80) and 53 in the group that underwent late decompression (range of 10 to 70). This difference was statistically significant.[28] Such improvement in outcome, however, was not observed in a study that compared Barthel scores of patients who underwent hemicraniectomy within 24 hours of injury and others who underwent hemicraniectomy more than 24 hours after injury (63 and 69, respectively).[26]

Despite achieving Barthel index scores that suggest functional independence, most patients who survived malignant infarction fail to reintegrate socially and also suffer from depression.[35] Although many indices have been developed to measure disability incurred in physical, social, emotional, and economic dimensions for the family and the patient, poor correlation is found among these indices. For instance, patients with objectively excellent functional recovery with poor social support may experience severe depression and may fail to integrate socially. As an abstract for these indices, two studies surveyed whether patients who survived the procedure (and their family members) would approve of the procedure in retrospect. In the 11 patients surveyed by Carter and colleagues, 6 (55%) replied yes, 3 (27%) were uncertain, and 2 (18%) answered no.[35] In 12 patients surveyed by Waltz and colleagues, 11 of 12 (96%) patients, as well as their relatives, approved of the procedure in retrospect.[25]

Functional Outcome for Right- versus Left-Sided Infarctions

Although hemispheric infarction of the dominant hemisphere and presentation of global aphasia is often cited as a poor functional prognostic indicator and reason against decompression, existing data are not strongly supportive of such a supposition. Waltz and colleagues compared the

functional outcome of 10 right-sided and 8 left-sided hemispheric infarcts treated with hemicraniectomy after a minimum of 7 months recovery. The two patient populations faced two distinct sets of challenges. Patients with right-sided hemispheric infarcts suffered from multimodal neglect and disturbance of incentives and concentration. Patients with left-sided (dominant) hemispheric infarcts tended to suffer deficits in verbal memory and reduced verbal expression.[25] Similar results have been reported by others.[26,36,38] Although there were no significant differences between the two populations in quality-of-life indices, there is historical resistance in performing dominant hemispheric hemicraniectomy.

Summary

Overall existing data suggest that decompressive hemicraniectomy represents an effective life-preserving measure in malignant cerebral infarction for all patients independent of age, initial presentation, and the side of hemispheric infarction. Patients under the age of 60 are more likely to gain meaningful functional recovery from this procedure. Maximal benefit from the decompression may be achieved with early intervention. Detailed discussions with the patient and the family must be undertaken to elucidate realistic expectations from the surgical intervention.

Traumatic Brain Injury

Management of Focal and Diffuse Traumatic Injuries

Traumatic brain injury represents a heterogeneous set of lesions suffered as a result of mechanical stress on the cerebral parenchyma. Essentially, these injuries are grouped into focal or diffuse subtypes. Focal injuries are macroscopically visible lesions limited to well-defined areas (e.g., contusions and hematomas). Diffuse injuries are associated with widespread cerebral dysfunction, manifesting in the form of regional or global cerebral edema. Intracranial pressure management is central in the treatment of both disease processes because it remains the most powerful prognostic measure of clinical outcome in traumatic brain injuries.[39-42] The defined boundaries of focal injuries facilitate surgical resection in the management of intracranial hypertension, although focal injuries are often accompanied by diffuse injuries. Management of diffuse injuries, on the other hand, relies on optimizing hemodynamic, metabolic, and osmotic parameters, as well as ventriculostomy drainage of CSF. According to current American Academy of Neurosurgical Society (AANS) and European Brain Injury Consortium recommendations, barbiturate-induced coma, hypothermia, and decompressive craniectomy represent second-tier treatments.

Decompressive Craniectomy in Traumatic Brain Injury

In contrast to malignant cerebral edema, the evidence supporting emergent decompressive craniectomy in trauma remains controversial. In animal studies using artificially induced intracranial lesions, craniectomy has been associated with increased cerebral edema, hemorrhagic infarcts, and cortical necrosis at the craniectomy sites.[9,14,15,43] On the other hand, decreased intracranial pressure, improved oxygen tension, and improved cerebral perfusion are also reported.[1,2,4,7,9] In one series, mortality was reduced by craniectomy, although all surviving animals remained comatose.[9] A review of the more than 30 studies published on the subject of decompressive craniectomy in the context of severe head trauma failed to demonstrate clear benefit.[44] The study designs are predominantly retrospective analysis with few prospective efforts. Most reports consist of a small number of patients or populations of heterogeneous pathology. Interpretations of these studies are confounded by the lack of randomized, contemporary comparison groups to control for the severity and type of head injury, criteria for patient selection, and intensity and timing of therapeutic intervention. Furthermore, because the studies were published over a span of 40 years, the results need to be interpreted in the context of evolving surgical techniques as well as the changes in critical care interventions. The difficulties facing retrospective analysis of studies with small sample size and without adequate control are illustrated by Cooper and colleagues.[18] The authors initially reported encouraging outcomes for hemicraniectomy as treatment for traumatic cerebral edema, with 40% overall survival.[45] Since the original report, however, prospective treatment of an additional 50 patients yielded only a 10% total survival rate.[18]

Despite these caveats, proponents of decompressive craniectomy often site three studies in support of the procedure. Polin and colleagues retrospectively analyzed 35 bifrontal decompressive craniectomies in patients suffering from intracranial hypertension and compared their outcome against 92 control patients selected from the Traumatic Coma Data Bank (TCDB). Patients with focal traumatic injuries were excluded from the study. Controls were matched in terms of sex, age, preoperative Glasgow Coma Scale (GCS) scores, and maximum preoperative intracranial pressure. Defining favorable recovery as Glasgow Outcome Score (GOS) scores of 4 or 5 (i.e., moderate disability and good recovery, respectively; see Table 5-1), 37% of the decompressed patients and 16% of the control patients showed favorable recovery ($p = 0.014$). Arguing that prolonged intracranial pressure elevation causes irreversible cerebral damage, the authors performed a subset analysis excluding patients with intracranial pressure of greater than 40 mm Hg and whose decompression was undertaken after 48 hours. In this analysis, favorable outcome for decompressed patients was 60% and 18% for control patients ($p < 0.0001$). The improved outcome was associated with reduction in intracranial pressure.[46]

Whitefield and colleagues retrospectively examined a series of 26 patients with refractory, post-traumatic intracranial hypertension who were treated with bifrontal decompressive craniectomy.[47] The results of maximal medical therapy were derived from the control group of a contemporary, randomized trial investigating the therapeutic effects of an N-methyl-D-aspartate (NMDA) antagonist on traumatic brain injury.[40] The authors argued that the demographic distribution and therapeutic intensities of the two groups were comparable. In both studies, favorable outcome was defined as a GOS score of 4 or 5 at 6 months follow-up. Sixty-one percent of the patients who underwent decompressive craniectomy attained favorable outcome, compared with 30% in the control group.[47] Improved outcome was associated with reduction in intracranial pressure.

Guerra and colleagues reported one of the few prospective series for surgical decompression. The patients were accrued starting in 1977 with a standard protocol. Initially, patients older than age 30 were excluded from the study. Patients younger than 40 were accepted starting in 1989, and patients under 50 were accepted starting in 1991. Patients with initial and persistent GCS score of 3, or bilaterally fixed and dilated pupils, were excluded from the study. In total, 57 patients underwent unilateral or bilateral hemicraniectomy for diffuse cerebral edema associated with intracranial hypertension. Fifty-eight percent ($n = 33$) of patients survived with a GOS score of 4 or 5. Nineteen percent of the patients ($n = 11$) died, 9% ($n = 5$) remained in persistent vegetative state, and 11% survived with severe neurologic deficit ($n = 6$).[6] These statistics represent favorable results when compared with the control group derived from the NMDA trial.

Decompressive Craniectomy in the Pediatric Population

The only randomized trial of decompressive craniectomy in the setting of traumatic brain injury was carried out in the pediatric population. Taylor and colleagues randomized children over the age of 12 months with post-traumatic intracranial hypertension and neurologic deterioration to conventional management and bitemporal craniectomy. Surgery was performed within 6 hours of deterioration. Twenty-seven patients were randomized to 13 craniectomies and 14 medical treatments. The intracranial pressure in the craniectomy group was significantly lower than that seen in the medical therapy group. Fifty-four percent of the patients who underwent craniectomy (7 out of 13) recovered with mild disability after 6 months, compared with 14% (2 of 14) of the medically managed group.[48] The difference in favorable outcome, although very suggestive, did not achieve statistical significance.

Summary

The indications for decompressive craniectomy in traumatic brain injury remain controversial. Most published reports suggest that intracranial pressure is reduced by craniotomies. Whether clinical course is altered by this intervention is a question that awaits definitive randomized trials. The picture emerging from recent reports, however, suggests that young patients with GCS scores greater than 4 may benefit from decompression when the intervention is performed early. Most studies to date have included a diverse study population suffering from a variety of cerebral injuries. Future studies that focus on distinct subpopulations may offer the best information regarding those subgroups of patients most likely to benefit from this procedure.

Aneurysmal Subarachnoid Hemorrhage

Aneurysm rupture leading to focal hematoma formation correlates with worsening clinical outcome in comparison to isolated subarachnoid hemorrhage.[49–51] Presumably, the local mass effect induced by hematoma formation initiates the feed-forward cycle of intracranial hypertension escalation. Accordingly, prompt reduction of intracranial hypertension is associated with reduced morbidity and mortality.[51,52] In this context, Smith and colleagues examined the effect of prophylactic hemicraniectomy at the time of aneurysm clipping in patients presenting with middle cerebral artery aneurysm rupture with associated Sylvian fissure or intra-parenchymal hematoma. In this series of 8 patients (5 patients presented with Hunt-Hess grade IV, 3 patients with Hunt-Hess grade V), prophylactic hemicraniectomy added 20 to 25 minutes to surgical time and was not associated with any complications. Postoperatively, all 8 patients experienced immediate reduction in intracranial pressure (mean preoperative ICP of 31.6 mm Hg, mean postoperative ICP of 13.1 mm Hg). All 5 Hunt-Hess grade IV patients (100%) recovered to good or excellent function (GOS score equivalent of 4 or 5). Of the 3 Hunt-Hess grade V patients, only 1 (33%) attained good outcome. Because the Hunt-Hess grading represent prognostic measure of clinical outcome, the results by Smith and colleagues can be compared with the expected outcome. For Hunt-Hess grades IV and V, the predicted percentage of patients who will attain good or excellent outcome are 53% and 15%, respectively. Although the sample size of the series is prohibitive to statistical analysis, the results suggest therapeutic efficacy of hemicraniectomy in aneurysm rupture with associated parenchymal hematoma.[53]

Cerebral Venous Sinus Thrombosis

The outflow of the blood from the cranial vault is determined primarily by the patency of the venous sinuses. Thrombosis of the sinuses is initially accommodated by recruitment of collateral venous drainage pathways. However, as these pathways are exhausted, the venous pressure approaches that of the arterial pressure. Cerebrospinal fluid resorption from arachnoid granulation is impaired by this venous congestion. Cerebral edema results when venous pressure overcomes the structural integrity of endothelial lining, resulting in transgression of fluid into the interstitial space. Further elevation of venous pressure can impair influx of blood, causing infarct with possible rupture of the low-resistance vasculature and hematoma formation. These events, in turn, initiate the cycle of escalating intracranial hypertension.

The standard treatment of venous thrombosis involves either anticoagulation or endovascular thrombolysis followed by anticoagulation.[54–57] Venous congestion further increases fragility of cerebral vasculature and can hamper hemostasis. For these reasons, surgical manipulation of the cerebral parenchyma (e.g., lobectomy or hematoma evacuation) is generally discouraged in this setting. To the extent that decompressive craniectomy allows for control of intracranial pressure without parenchymal manipulation, it represents a surgical option when medical therapies fail. To assess the efficacy of this option, Stefini and colleagues reported 3 patients who developed large hemorrhagic infarcts from dural sinus thrombosis and who developed signs of brain stem compromise (i.e., bilaterally fixed and dilated pupils) while on maximal medical therapy. All 3 patients were women between the ages of 40 and 50 years who underwent hemicraniectomy. Two patients underwent hemicraniectomy at the onset of clinical deterioration and recovered with mild disability. The third patient incurred fixed and dilated pupils for several hours before undergoing the procedure and remained severely disabled at 6 months

follow-up. The authors suggested that emergent decompression should be considered in the treatment of venous sinus thrombosis in patients who developed brain stem herniation while on maximal medical therapy.[58]

Encephalitis

Cerebral edema is the most common manifestation of encephalitis. Pathogenesis involves direct cellular damage by bacterial/viral toxin and breakdown of the blood-brain barrier. The onset usually takes the form of seizure; depressed consciousness; hemiplegia; and altered papillary response in the context of fever, systemic leukocytosis, and central nervous system leukocytosis. With severe cerebral edema, the feed-forward cycle of intracranial hypertension is initiated. Death and severe neurologic deficit have been described.[59]

Although cerebral edema secondary to encephalitis can be medically managed in most instances, the use of osmotic agents such as mannitol in the context of blood-brain barrier breakdown may hasten fluid shifts and aggravate brain edema.[60] Additionally, hypothermia and barbiturate-induced coma both are associated with systemic immune suppression.[61–63] These considerations have led to an interest in decompressive craniectomy as a treatment option. Schwab and colleagues reported a case series of 6 patients who developed signs of brain stem compression as a result of acute encephalitis and despite maximal medical treatment. The age distribution of this cohort was 24 to 39 years. All 6 patients had survived and recovered without neurologic deficit in subsequent follow-up.[64]

Intracerebral Hematomas

Intracerebral hematomas arise either from the spontaneous rupture of vessels whose structural integrity is impaired by hypertension, malformations, or tumor; or they may occur as a result of coagulopathy.[65] Although the indications for surgical evacuation remain controversial, recent evidence suggests that the subset of patients with large hematoma (>30 mL) who showed neurologic deterioration may benefit from evacuation.[66]

The role of craniectomy in conjunction with hematoma evacuation was retrospectively examined by Dierssen and colleagues. They reported the outcome of 31 patients with spontaneous intraparenchymal hematomas and acute neurologic deterioration treated by surgical evacuation and decompressive craniectomy; the mortality of this series was compared with another series of 20 patients treated only with evacuation. They found statistically significant improvement in mortality in the group with craniectomy (32% vs. 70%, $p = 0.005$).[67] Interpretation of this result, however, is difficult given the noncontemporary and non-matched nature of the two groups.

A major concern in combining craniectomy with hematoma evacuation lies in the risk of rehemorrhage. Fatal hemorrhage into surgically inaccessible glioma has been reported subsequent to hemicraniectomy.[68] Although gliomas and intracerebral hemorrhages represent two distinct disease entities, they have in common impaired integrity of cerebral vasculature. Allowance of centripetal herniation subsequent to craniectomy could impose mechanical stress on and contribute to the rupture of these friable vessels.

As such, meticulous hemostasis must be attained when considering craniectomy.

Metabolic Encephalopathies

Several metabolic diseases are associated with cerebral edema and elevated intracranial pressure. Although it is conceivable that medically resistant intracranial hypertension secondary to metabolic derangement could benefit from decompressive craniectomies (e.g., by allowing time for the underlying disease to be treated), the existing literature is limited in this regard. Survey of the literature reveals only one case where medically resistant cerebral edema secondary to Reye's syndrome was successfully treated with decompressive craniectomy.[69]

SURGICAL CONSIDERATIONS IN DECOMPRESSIVE CRANIECTOMY

A wide spectrum of surgical techniques has been reported for decompressive craniectomy. In general, these decompression techniques can be divided into three approaches: frontal approach, frontotemporal-parietal approach, and temporal approach.[70] All three approaches can be performed unilaterally or bilaterally. The removed bone fragment can be stored in the patient's abdominal subcutaneous fat. In thin patients, or in patients expected to undergo further abdominal surgery, cryopreservation in bone banks can be considered.

Frontotemporal-parietal Approach

Indications

Large frontotemporal-parietal craniectomy (hemicraniectomy) provides the most extensive decompression for unilateral lesions (e.g., middle cerebral artery infarcts) with contralateral or axial herniation. For diffuse cerebral edema, bilateral hemicraniectomy may be considered, with advance planning for reconstructive cranioplasty.

Surgical Technique

The patient is placed supine with head elevated and rotated 30 to 45 degrees. Vertex of the head is directed downward to bring the zygomatic arch to the uppermost plane. The skin incision can be in the form of a trauma flap, with the goal of exposing the following margins for craniectomy: anteriorly to the superior border of the orbital roof (avoiding entry into the frontal sinus); posteriorly to at least 2 cm posterior to the external meatus; medially to 2 cm lateral to the midline (avoiding the sagittal sinus); and inferiorly to the floor of the middle cranial fossa (Fig. 5-3). The temporalis muscle is reflected anteriorly. Burr holes are placed at the keyhole, the root of the zygoma, and along the planned craniectomy margin, and these are connected with a high-speed drill. The sphenoid wing is fractured and removed to the superior orbital fissure. The dural edges are tacked up to bony margins to prevent epidural hematoma formation. Duraplasty is performed using dural substitute after the dura is opened in a stellate manner. It is critical that dural closure be nonconstraining and loose to allow for further expansion of intracranial contents.

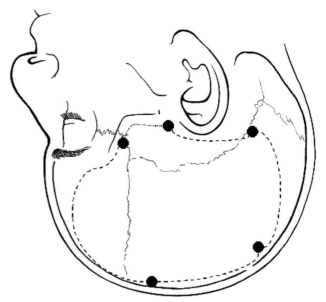

FIGURE 5-3   Hemicraniectomy. The skin incision can be in the form of a trauma flap with the goal of exposing the following margins for craniectomy: anteriorly to the superior border of the orbital roof (avoiding entry into the frontal sinus), posteriorly to at least 2 cm posterior to the external meatus, medially to 2 cm lateral to the midline (avoiding the sagittal sinus), and inferiorly to the floor of the middle cranial fossa. The temporalis muscle is reflected anteriorly. Burr holes are placed at the keyhole, the root of the zygoma, and along the planned craniectomy margin and connected with a high-speed drill. The sphenoid wing is fractured and removed to the superior orbital fissure. The dural edges are tacked up to bony margins to prevent epidural hematoma formation. Duraplasty is performed using dural substitute after dural is opened in a stellate manner.

Craniectomy Size and Margins

As would be expected, the size of the craniectomy directly correlates with the degree of cerebral expansion.[11–13] Moreover, smaller craniectomies are associated with infarcts and hemorrhages in the proximity of the craniectomy margin. Wagner and colleagues reported that these events were more commonly observed when the craniectomy diameter fell below 8 cm. Moreover, the mortality rate was significantly higher in decompression associated with pericraniectomy hemorrhage or infarcts.[43]

Munch and colleagues suggested that the lower margin of the craniectomy, relative to the middle fossa floor, directly correlates to the state of mesencephalic cisternal decompression.[44] Because compression of these cisterns is shown to impair clinical outcome, a larger craniectomy to the base of the cranium could minimize brain stem compression.[71] This hypothesis was tested by examining the relationship between the distance of the inferior craniectomy margin from the middle fossa floor with the rate of survival in patients who underwent hemicraniectomy for malignant cerebral infarction. Although the mean distance between craniectomy margin and the middle fossa was less in the survivors when compared with the nonsurvivors (1.7 cm vs. 2.3 cm), the difference did not reach statistical significance ($p = 0.27$).[72]

In summary, taking into consideration the dimensions of the cranial vault and the existing literature, recommendation of a 10- × 15-cm craniectomy, with the lower margin extending to less than 1 cm from the middle cranial fossa, appears reasonable in surgical planning of a hemicraniectomy.

Frontal Approach

Indications

Unilateral frontal craniectomy provides a moderate amount of decompression, and its use is limited to unilateral frontal contusions. Bifrontal craniectomy is the most widely used approach in the decompression of diffuse traumatic brain injury. The technique for bifrontal craniectomy as described by Polin and colleagues will be reviewed below.[46]

Surgical Technique

The patient is placed in the supine position with the head flexed 15 to 30 degrees. Bicoronal skin incision is planned to extend 3 to 5 cm posterior to the coronal suture. After the incision, the temporalis muscle is reflected inferiorly. Burr holes are made at the keyhole and at the root of the zygoma. A 3- to 4-cm temporal bone fragment is removed bilaterally. Burr holes are subsequently placed on either side of the sagittal sinus and along the posterior edge of the planned craniectomy. Bilateral craniectomies are performed, leaving a strip of bone covering the superior sagittal sinus. This bone is removed after the sinus is freed from its bony attachments. Bilateral dura openings are made into U-shaped flaps extending to the anterior one third of the sagittal sinus, followed by ligation of the sinus to maximize allowance for forward swelling. Duraplasty is performed using dural substitute and allowing for a generous dural expansion (Fig. 5-4).

Manipulation of the Sagittal Sinus

Some authors advocate preserving the strip of bone overlying the sagittal sinus, others argue that sagittal sinus ligation could contribute to increased venous pressure and aggravate cerebral edema.[6] There are currently no available data to substantiate or refute the merits of these suggestions. At our institution, we routinely ligate the superior sagittal sinus as well as sever the falx.

Temporal Approach

Indications

Bitemporal craniectomies have been described in the treatment of traumatic brain injury. The key advantage in this technique lies in avoiding manipulation of the sagittal sinus and injury to the cortical draining veins. The extent of decompression, however, is inferior to the bifrontal or frontoparieto-occipital craniectomy

Surgical Technique

In the temporal approach, the two sides are done sequentially, with decompression first of the side with more severe edema. The patient is placed in a semilateral to lateral position with the head placed such that the temporal base is perpendicular to the floor. A linear skin incision is made in the midtemporal region extending down to the floor of the middle fossa. The temporalis muscle is split and retracted. Burr holes are made at the root of the zygoma and 3 to 5 cm rostral to the zygomatic burr hole. A 3- to 5-cm fragment of the temporal bone is then removed. Dura is opened in a stellate manner and expanded with dura substitutes (Fig. 5-5).

Duraplasty

Generous duraplasty is a crucial portion of decompressive craniectomy. Most studies show that dural opening and expansion significantly contributes to intracranial pressure reduction. In the case of hemicraniectomy, craniectomy alone reduces intracranial pressure by approximately 15%. Further duraplasty reduces intracranial pressure by an additional 55%. How much dural opening and expansion is required for adequate decompression remains an unanswered question.

Lobectomy

In addition to craniectomy, resecting the noneloquent portions of the frontal or temporal lobe further enhance the volume buffering capacity of the cranial vault. The technique is appropriate in three situations: (1) where local regions of swelling and injury are identified and correspond to noneloquent functions, (2) where global swelling with volume expansion exceeds the capacity of the duraplasty or skin closure, and (3) when postoperative findings demonstrate persistent intracranial hypertension after adequate bone decompression.[28]

The efficacy of this approach was examined by Cho and colleagues. In their case series, 13 patients who exhibited persistent intracranial pressure of more than 30 mm Hg after hemicraniectomy for malignant cerebral swelling were studied. Eight of the 13 underwent temporal lobectomy and survived; the remaining 5 patients, whose families refused temporal lobectomy, died ($p < 0.001$). One concern with this

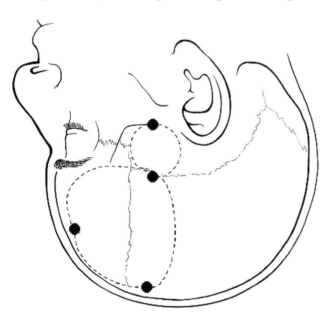

FIGURE 5-4 Frontal craniectomy. Bicoronal skin incision is planned to extend 3 to 5 cm posterior to the coronal suture. After the incision, the temporalis muscle is reflected inferiorly. Burr holes are made at the keyhole and the root of the zygoma. A 3- to 4-cm temporal bone fragment is removed bilaterally. Burr holes are subsequently placed on either side of the sagittal sinus and along the posterior edge of the planned craniectomy. Bilateral craniectomies are performed, leaving a strip of bone covering the superior sagittal sinus. This bone is removed after the sinus is freed from its bony attachments. Bilateral dura openings are made into U-shaped flaps extending to the anterior one third of the sagittal sinus, followed by ligation of the sinus to maximize allowance for forward swelling.

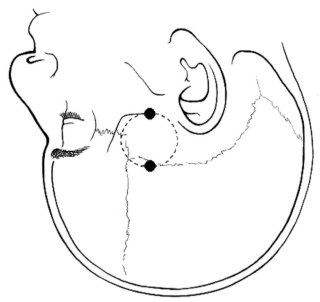

FIGURE 5-5 Temporal craniotomy. The two sides are done sequentially, with decompression of the side of worse edema first. The patient is placed in a semilateral to lateral position with the head placed such that the temporal base is perpendicular to the floor. A linear skin incision is made in the midtemporal region extending down to the floor of the middle fossa. The temporalis muscle is split and retracted. Burr holes are made at the root of the zygoma and 3 to 5 cm rostral to the zygomatic burr hole. A 3- to 5-cm fragment of the temporal bone is then removed. Dura is opened in a stellate manner and expanded with dura substitutes.

technique entails whether additional neurologic deficit is incurred as a result.[28] To address this concern, Litofsky and colleagues followed 20 patients with traumatic brain injury who underwent lobectomies without craniectomies. Of the 20, 11 (55%) recovered sufficient function to achieve a GOS of 4 or 5. Nine (45%) remained severely disabled or died. These statistics are no worse than those reported historically for craniectomy without lobectomy, suggesting that lobectomy is not associated with gross worsening of neurologic recovery.[73]

The guidelines for frontal and temporal lobectomies, as published by Litofsky and colleagues, are reviewed here.[73] Considerations of intraoperative findings should be undertaken so as to modify the application of these landmarks. For frontal lobectomy, posterior margin is marked by the coronal suture in the nondominant hemisphere and 2 cm anterior to the coronal suture in the dominant hemisphere. No more than 5 cm in depth of frontal lobe is resected. For temporal lobectomies, the anterior 5 cm of the temporal lobe is removed to visualize the incisura. A layer of cortex bordering the sylvian fissure is preserved to prevent disruption of the vasculature. In the dominant hemisphere, the superior temporal lobe is preserved to minimize disruption of speech functions.

To maximize cranial volume buffering capacity, suggestions have been made to evacuate infarcted tissues in the treatment of malignant cerebral swelling. Several authors have reported that the removal of necrotic tissue with hemicraniectomy can be performed without incurring additional neurologic deficit.[74–76] However, because the margins of ischemic penumbra are poorly defined, such an

approach is likely to damage viable tissue. The consensus in the current literature is to avoid cerebral necrotectomy unless necessary for dural closure.[36] However, this technique is widely employed for posterior fossa decompressions and warrants further study.

Cranioplasty

Replacement of the cranial bone flap generally takes place 6 weeks to 6 months after the initial injury to ensure the resolution of the primary process. In patients who suffer from postcraniectomy syndrome, however, earlier replacement should be considered. Symptoms of postcraniectomy syndrome include dizziness; fatigue; headache; apprehension; local tenderness; and focal neurologic deficits such as progressive hemiparesis/hemiplegia, hypoalgesia, hypoesthesia, astereognosis, and hemianopsia.[77,78] Complete reversal of these symptoms occurs after bone flap replacement. The pathogenesis of these symptoms likely involves cerebrospinal fluid pressure disequilibrium. In support of this hypothesis, Langfitt showed that the lumbar cerebrospinal fluid pressure in a patient with a large cranial defect is greater than in a patient with closed calvaria. This pressure differential is reversed after cranioplasty.[79]

Complications

Operative complications from decompressive craniectomy can be divided into four subcategories: (1) intracerebral hematoma, (2) extra-axial collections, (3) cerebrospinal fluid leakage, and (4) cranioplasty failure.

Intracerebral Hematoma

Intracerebral hematoma formation has been discussed previously; it results either from inadequate craniectomy, inadequate surgical hemastasis, or rupture of friable vessels during the process of centripetal herniation. Incidence of intracerebral hematoma postdecompression ranges from 3% to 40%, greater than 90% of these hematomas are clinically silent.[6,43,46]

Extra-axial Collections

The most common extra-axial collection seen postcraniectomy is that of epidural hygroma, which likely represents egress of cerebrospinal fluid from inadequate dural closure. This complication is reported in roughly 20% of all craniectomies and is easily treated with bedside drainage.[6] Subdural and epidural hematomas are seen in roughly 5% of all cases,[6,43,46] and most of these lesions are benign. Their etiologies include inadequate craniectomy, sharp craniectomy border, and vessel rupture from centripetal herniation.

Generally, the temporalis muscle does not impose sufficient resistance to centripetal herniation to warrant resection during decompressive craniectomy. Andre and colleagues, however, reported the case of a 55-year-old woman who underwent hemicraniectomy for malignant cerebral edema. Decompression was initially unsuccessful because of a massive temporal muscle hemorrhage. The hematoma imposed sufficient resistance to prevent centripetal herniation of the underlying parenchyma. Subsequent surgical exploration with muscle resection allowed for excellent recovery.[80]

Cerebrospinal Fluid Leak

Cerebrospinal fluid leak occurs in the context of inadequate dural closure in conjunction with inadequate galeal and skin closure, local infection, or hydrocephalus. Such leakage predisposes to meningitis and encephalitis. The incidence of these lesions ranges from 3% to 5%.[6,43,46]

Cranioplasty Failure

Cranioplasty failure occurs as a result of bone flap resorption or infection. This occurs in 2% to 6% of all reported cases. Cranioplasty is adversely affected by poor graft fixation and approximation, synthetic dural replacement that impairs angiogenesis, excessive bone waxing, poorly vascularized scalp flap, and infection.[46] Efforts should be made to avoid these situations (e.g., by careful efforts to free the bone edges of scar tissue). Autograft cranioplasty failure necessitates acrylic cranioplasty. In anticipation of such potential failure, a high-resolution head CT may be attained prior to craniectomy for the purpose of acrylic bone flap construction.

Seizure and Hydrocephalus

Postoperative seizure and shunt dependency are also reported with an incidence of 5% to 30%.[6,46,81] It is unclear whether they are the result of the decompression, the initial injury, or some combination of the two processes.

CONCLUSIONS

Intracranial hypertension is a common mechanism of neurologic injury for many disease processes. Because decompressive craniectomy provides an effective means of reducing intracranial pressure, it can be a life-preserving procedure. As such, neurosurgeons will be increasingly urged to perform these procedures. Although the selection criteria for this procedure remain in evolution, it appears that the best outcomes are achieved in young, otherwise healthy patients treated early in the disease process. The decision to pursue surgical intervention should take into consideration the severity of the initial insult, the likelihood of meaningful functional recovery, the premorbid lifestyle, the extent of social support, and family dynamics.

REFERENCES

1. Burkert W, Paver H: Decompressive trepanation in therapy refractory brain edema. Zentralbl Neurochir 50:318–323, 1988.
2. Burkert W, Plaumann H: The value of large pressure-relieving trepanation in treatment of refractory brain edema: Animal experiment studies, initial clinical results. Zentralbl Neurochir 50:106–108, 1989.
3. Dam Hieu P, Sizun J, Person H, et al: The place of decompressive surgery in the treatment of uncontrollable post-traumatic intracranial hypertension in children. Childs Nerv Syst 12:270–275, 1996.
4. Gaab M, Knoblich O, Fuhrmeister U, et al: Comparison of the effects of surgical decompression and resection of local edema in the therapy of experimental brain trauma: Investigation of ICP, EEG and cerebral metabolism in cats. Childs Brain 5:484–498, 1979.
5. Gower D, Lee K, McWhorter J: Role of subtemporal decompression in severe closed head injury. Neurosurgery 23:417–422, 1988.
6. Guerra W, Gaab M, Dietz H, et al: Surgical decompression for traumatic brain swelling: Indications and results. J Neurosurg 90:187–196, 1999.
7. Hatashita S, Hoff J: The effect of craniectomy on the biomechanics of normal brain. J Neurosurg 67:573–578, 1987.
8. Jourdan C, Convert J, Mottolese C, et al: Evaluation of the clinical benefit of decompression hemicraniectomy in intracranial hypertension not controlled by medical treatment. Neurochirugie 39:304–310, 1993.
9. Moody R, Ruamsuke S, Mullan S: An evaluation of decompression in experimental head injury. J Neurosurg 29:586–590, 1968.
10. Rinaldi A, Mangiola A, Anile C, et al: Hemodynamic effects of decompressive craniectomy in cold induced brain oedema. Acta Neurochir Suppl 51:394–396, 1990.
11. Yoo D, Kim D, Cho K, et al: Ventricular pressure monitoring during bilateral decompression with dural expansion. J Neurosurg 91:953–959, 1999.
12. Shapiro K, Fried A, Takei F, et al: Effect of the skull and dura on neural axis pressure-volume relationships and CSF hydrodynamics. J Neurosurg 63:76–81, 1985.
13. Gaab M, Rittierodt M, Lorenz M, et al: Traumatic brain swelling and operative decompression: A prospective investigation. Acta Neurochir Suppl 51:326–328, 1990.
14. Forsting M, Reith W, Schabitz W, et al: Decompressive craniectomy for cerebral infarction: An experimental study in rats. Stroke 26: 259–264, 1995.
15. Cooper P, Hagler H, Clark W, et al: Enhancement of experimental cerebral edema after decompressive craniectomy: Implications for the management of severe head injuries. Neurosurgery 4:296–300, 1979.
16. Coplin W, Cullen N, Policherla P, et al: Safety and feasibility of craniectomy with duraplasty as the initial surgical intervention for severe traumatic brain injury. J Trauma 50:1050–1059, 2001.
17. Venes J, Collins W: Bifrontal decompressive craniectomy in the management of head trauma. J Neurosurg 42:429–433, 1975.
18. Cooper P, Rovit R, Ransohoff J: Hemicraniectomy in the treatment of acute subdural hematoma: A re-appraisal. Surg Neurol 5:25–28, 1976.
19. Clark K, Nash T, Hutchison G: The failure of circumferential craniotomy in acute traumatic cerebral swelling. J Neurosurg 29:361–371, 1968.
20. von Kummer R, Meyding-Lamade U, Forsting M, et al: Sensitivity and prognostic value of early CT in occlusion of the middle cerebral artery trunk. Am J Neuroradiol 15:9–15, 1994.
21. Silver F, Norris J, Lewis A, et al: Early mortality following stroke: A prospective review. Stroke 15:492–426, 1984.
22. Ng L, Nimmannitya J: Massive cerebral infarction with severe brain swelling: A clinicopathological study. Stroke 1:158–163, 1970.
23. Schwab S, Horn M, Spranger M, et al: Therapeutic hypothermia after cerebral ischemia: Theoretical principles and possible clinical applications. Nervenarzt 65:828–835, 1994.
24. Berrouschot J, Sterker M, Bettin S, et al: Mortality of space-occupying ("malignant") middle cerebral artery infarction under conservative intensive care. Intensive Care Med 24:620–623, 1998.
25. Walz B, Zimmermann C, Bottger S, et al: Prognosis of patients after hemicraniectomy in malignant middle cerebral artery infarction. J Neurol 249:1183–1190, 2002.
26. Schwab S, Steiner T, Aschoff A, et al: Early hemicraniectomy in patients with complete middle cerebral artery infarction. Stroke 29:1888–1893, 1998.
27. Holtkamp M, Buchheim K, Unterberg A, et al: Hemicraniectomy in elderly patients with space occupying media infarction: Improved survival but poor functional outcome. J Neurol Neurosurg Psychiatry 70:226–228, 2001.
28. Cho D, Chen T, Lee H: Ultra-early decompressive craniectomy for malignant middle cerebral artery infarction. Surg Neurol 60:227–232, 2003.
29. Wijdicks E, Diringer M: Middle cerebral artery territory infarction and early brain swelling: Progression and effect of age on outcome. Mayo Clin Proc 73:829–836, 1998.
30. Arenillas J, Rovira A, Molina C, et al: Prediction of early neurological deterioration using diffusion- and perfusion-weighted imaging in hyperacute middle cerebral artery ischemic stroke. Stroke 33:2197–2120, 2002.
31. Manno E, Nichols D, Fulgham J, et al: Computed tomographic determinants of neurologic deterioration in patients with large middle cerebral artery infarctions. Mayo Clin Proc 78:156–160, 2003.
32. Dohmen C, Bosche B, Graf R, et al: Prediction of malignant course in MCA infarction by PET and microdialysis. Stroke 34:2152–2158, 2003.
33. Gerriets T, Stolz E, Konig S, et al: Sonographic monitoring of midline shift in space-occupying stroke: An early outcome predictor. Stroke 32:442–447, 2001.
34. Mahoney F, Barthel D: Functional evaluation: The Barthel Index. Md State Med J 14:61–65, 1965.
35. Carter B, Ogilvy C, Candia G, et al: One-year outcome after decompressive surgery for massive nondominant hemispheric infarction. Neurosurgery 40:1168–1175, 1997.

36. Rieke K, Schwab S, Krieger D, et al: Decompressive surgery in space-occupying hemispheric infarction: Results of an open, prospective trial. Crit Care Med 23:1576–1587, 1995.

37. Delashaw J, Broaddus W, Kassell N, et al: Treatment of right hemispheric cerebral infarction by hemicraniectomy. Stroke 21:874–881, 1990.

38. de Haan R, Aaronson N, Limburg M, et al: Measuring quality of life in stroke. Stroke 24:320–327, 1993.

39. Berger M, Pitts L, Lovely M, et al: Outcome from severe head injury in children and adolescents. J Neurosurg 62:194–199, 1985.

40. Juul N, Morris G, Marshall S, et al: Intracranial hypertension and cerebral perfusion pressure: Influence on neurological deterioration and outcome in severe head injury. The Executive Committee of the International Selfotel Trial. J Neurosurg 92:1–6, 2000.

41. Marshall L, Smith R, Shapiro H: The outcome with aggressive treatment in severe head injuries. Part I: The significance of intracranial pressure monitoring. J Neurosurg 50:20–25, 1979.

42. Pople I, Muhlbauer M, Sanford R, et al: Results and complications of intracranial pressure monitoring in 303 children. Pediatr Neurosurg 23:64–67, 1995.

43. Wagner S, Schnippering H, Aschoff A, et al: Suboptimum hemicraniectomy as a cause of additional cerebral lesions in patients with malignant infarction of the middle cerebral artery. J Neurosurg 94:693–696, 2001.

44. Munch E, Horn P, Schurer L, et al: Management of severe traumatic brain injury by decompressive craniectomy. Neurosurgery 47:315–322, 2000.

45. Ransohoff J, Benjamin M, Gage EJ, et al: Hemicraniectomy in the management of acute subdural hematoma. J Neurosurg 34:70–76, 1971.

46. Polin R, Shaffrey M, Bogaev C, et al: Decompressive bifrontal craniectomy in the treatment of severe refractory posttraumatic cerebral edema. Neurosurgery 41:84–92, 1997.

47. Whitfield P, Patel H, Hutchinson P, et al: Bifrontal decompressive craniectomy in the management of posttraumatic intracranial hypertension. Br J Neurosurg 15:500–507, 2001.

48. Taylor A, Butt W, Rosenfeld J, et al: A randomized trial of very early decompressive craniectomy in children with traumatic brain injury and sustained intracranial hypertension. Childs Nerv Syst 17:154–162, 2001.

49. Hayashi M, Marukawa S, Fujii H, et al: Intracranial hypertension in patients with ruptured intracranial aneurysm. J Neurosurg 46:584–590, 1977.

50. Hauerberg J, Eskesen V, Rosenorn J: The prognostic significance of intracerebral haematoma as shown on CT scanning after aneurysmal subarachnoid haemorrhage. Br J Neurosurg 8:333–339, 1994.

51. Bailes J, Spetzler R, Hadley M, et al: Management morbidity and mortality of poor-grade aneurysm patients. J Neurosurg 72:559–566, 1990.

52. Gambardella G, De Blasi F, Caruso G, et al: Intracranial pressure, cerebral perfusion pressure, and SPECT in the management of patients with SAH Hunt and Hess grades I-II. Acta Neurochir Suppl (Wien) 71:215–218, 1998.

53. Smith E, Carter B, Ogilvy C: Proposed use of prophylactic decompressive craniectomy in poor-grade aneurysmal subarachnoid hemorrhage patients presenting with associated large sylvian hematomas. Neurosurgery 51:117–124, 2002.

54. Smith·T, Higashida R, Barnwell S, et al: Treatment of dural sinus thrombosis by urokinase infusion. Am J Neuroradiol 15:801–807, 1994.

55. Kim S, Suh J: Direct endovascular thrombolytic therapy for dural sinus thrombosis: Infusion of alteplase. Am J Neuroradiol 18:639–645, 1997.

56. Horowitz M, Purdy P, Unwin H, et al: Treatment of dural sinus thrombosis using selective catheterization and urokinase. Ann Neurol 38:58–67, 1995.

57. Einhaupl K, Villringer A, Meister W, et al: Heparin treatment in sinus venous thrombosis. Lancet 338:597–600, 1991.

58. Stefini R, Latronico N, Cornali C, et al: Emergent decompressive craniectomy in patients with fixed dilated pupils due to cerebral venous and dural sinus thrombosis: Report of three cases. Neurosurgery 45:626–629, 1999.

59. Barnett G, Ropper A, Romeo J: Intracranial pressure and outcome in adult encephalitis. J Neurosurg 68:585–588, 1988.

60. Kaufmann A, Cardoso E: Aggravation of vasogenic cerebral edema by multiple-dose mannitol. J Neurosurg 77:584–589, 1992.

61. Bernard S, Buist M: Induced hypothermia in critical care medicine: A review. Crit Care Med 31:2041–2051, 2003.

62. Ward J, Becker D, Miller J, et al: Failure of prophylactic barbiturate coma in the treatment of severe head injury. J Neurosurg 62:383–388, 1985.

63. Sato M, Tanaka S, Suzuki K, et al: Complications associated with barbiturate therapy. Resuscitation 17:233–241, 1989.

64. Schwab S, Junger E, Spranger M, et al: Craniectomy: An aggressive treatment approach in severe encephalitis. Neurology 48:412–417, 1997.

65. Broderick J, Adams H, Barsan W, et al: Guidelines for the management of spontaneous intracerebral hemorrhage: A statement for healthcare professionals from a special writing group of the Stroke Council, American Heart Association. Stroke 30:905–915, 1999.

66. Kaya R, Turkmenoglu O, Ziyal I, et al: The effects on prognosis of surgical treatment of hypertensive putaminal hematomas through transsylvian transinsular approach. Surg Neurol 59:176–183, 2003.

67. Dierssen G, Carda R, Coca J: The influence of large decompressive craniectomy on the outcome of surgical treatment in spontaneous intracerebral haematomas. Acta Neurochir Suppl 69:53–60, 1983.

68. Goel A: Fatal tumoural haemorrhage following decompressive craniectomy: A report of three cases. Br J Neurosurg 11:554–557, 1997.

69. Ausman J, Rogers C, Sharp H: Decompressive craniectomy for the encephalopathy of Reye's syndrome. Surg Neurol 6:97–99, 1976.

70. Figaji A, Fieggen A, Peter J: Early decompressive craniotomy in children with severe traumatic brain injury. Childs Nerv Syst 19:666–673, 2003.

71. Toutant S, Klauber M, Marshall L, et al: Absent or compressed basal cisterns on first CT scan: Ominous predictors of outcome in severe head injury. J Neurosurg 61:691–694, 1984.

72. Wirtz C, Steiner T, Aschoff A, et al: Hemicraniectomy with dural augmentation in medically uncontrollable hemispheric infarction. Neurosurgical Focus 2:1–9, 1997.

73. Litofsky N, Chin L, Tang G, et al: The use of lobectomy in the management of severe closed-head trauma. Neurosurgery 34:628–632, 1994.

74. Nussbaum E, Wolf A, Sebring L, et al: Complete temporal lobectomy for surgical resuscitation of patients with transtentorial herniation secondary to unilateral hemispheric swelling. Neurosurgery 29:62–66, 1991.

75. Ivamoto H, Numoto M, Donaghy R: Surgical decompression for cerebral and cerebellar infarcts. Stroke 5:365–370, 1974.

76. Greenwood J: Acute brain infarctions with high intracranial pressure: Surgical indications. Johns Hopkins Med J 122:254–260, 1968.

77. Dujovny M, Aviles A, Agner C, et al: Cranioplasty: Cosmetic or therapeutic? Surg Neurol 47:238–241, 1997.

78. Schiffer J, Gur R, Nisim U, et al: Symptomatic patients after craniectomy. Surg Neurol 47:231–237, 1997.

79. Langfitt T: Increased intracranial pressure. Clin Neurosurg 16:436–471, 1969.

80. Andre C, Py M, Niemeyer-Filho P: Temporal muscle haematoma as a cause of suboptimal haemicraniectomy: Case report. Arq Neuropsiquiatr 61:682–686, 2003.

81. Yang X, Hong G, Su S, et al: Complications induced by decompressive craniectomies after traumatic brain injury. Chin J Traumatol 6:99–103, 2003.

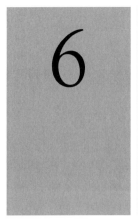

6

Surgical Management of Chronic Subdural Hematoma in Adults

PATRICIA B. QUEBADA and HENRY H. SCHMIDEK

INTRODUCTION

A *chronic subdural hematoma* (CSDH) is a common type of intracranial hemorrhage and is predominantly seen in the elderly. It typically consists of darkish red liquefied blood and blood breakdown products with an associated neomembrane and is located in the otherwise potential space between the arachnoid and dura. The space that the CSDH occupies is technically the intradural space. It is a disruption of the dural border cell layer from the deep pachymeninges.[1] Blood in this space provokes an inflammatory reaction, which results in an enveloping membrane surrounding the blood (Fig. 6-1). If this follows clearly dated trauma, a CSDH may become symptomatic days to weeks after the event. Most of the time, there is no clear traumatic history that precedes the discovery of a CSDH. In the cases in which there is no associated trauma, other etiologies have to be considered such as coagulopathy, arachnoid cysts, vascular malformations, metastatic cancer, meningiomas, or other neoplastic/inflammatory lesions.[2–8] People generally do well after surgical drainage of the CSDH, but the optimal surgical management is still debated.

PATHOPHYSIOLOGY

Although some CSDHs evolve from an acute subdural hematoma, most experimental models fail to produce an enlarging CSDH from an acute solid clot.[9,10] Acute subdural hematomas and CSDHs result from an acceleration/deceleration mechanism that results in tearing of the bridging veins. Yamashima and Friede[11] have shown an attenuation of the vascular walls as the vessel exits the subarachnoid space and enters the potential subdural space, explaining the propensity for the hemorrhage to collect in that space. The hematoma can expand rapidly, and, left untreated, it rapidly leads to a patient's demise. In 3% to 6% of cases of the hemorrhage, the patient's condition becomes compensated, and these represent the cases that evolve into CSDHs.[12]

An inflammatory process concomitant with a coagulation defect is now implicated in the development of a CSDH. A bleed triggers an inflammatory process that results in a deposition of fibrin, which is then followed by formation of neomembranes and neocapillaries.[13–16] Tissue plasminogen activator, which is found to be abundant on the neomembrane of the hematoma, converts plasminogen into plasmin,

subsequently producing large amounts of fibrinogen and fibrin degradation products. This liquefies the blood clot and increases the permeability of the capillaries. Neovascularization and hyperpermeability of the vessels have been related to the enlargement of CSDHs.

Recently, the role of interleukin-6 and -8 and vascular endothelial growth factor has been implicated in the pathogenesis of CSDHs, supporting the notion that this disorder is a self-perpetuating inflammatory and angiogenic process involving the dura. Within this inflammatory capsule forming around the hematoma in the subdural, the mast cells, eosinophils, neutrophils, monocytes, macrophages, and fibroblasts are activated, which produces these cytokines.[17,18]

The disruption of the coagulation cascade contributes to the expansion and slow growth of a CSDH. The CSDH is less associated with injury to the underlying brain but arises from repetitive low-pressure venous bleeding into the subdural space. This bleeding probably originates from vessels of the outer membrane of the hematoma fed by the middle meningeal artery. Analysis of the CSDH contents shows significant increased levels of markers of thrombin and thrombomodulin generation (TAT, F1 and 2), activation of the extrinsic coagulation pathway, and of fibrinolysis (D dimer) in the CSDH. Coagulation factors V and VII were also found to be lower in the hematoma than in the peripheral blood. The activation of these processes of coagulation and fibrinolysis within the hematoma precludes coagulation, organization, and resolution of the hematoma. Transmitted pulsation variation the hematoma cavity is reported to generate sinusoidal vessel injury.[19] Vessels then continue to bleed, encouraging hematoma growth.

These hematomas are most commonly located in the frontoparietal region over the cerebral convexities, where they may be unilateral or bilateral, but they may also occur at the cranial base, between the cerebral hemispheres, in the posterior fossa, or rarely in the spinal canal.

An alternate route to the formation of a CSDH is evolution from a subdural hygroma. After trauma or ventricular shunting, a rent occurs in the arachnoid and a one-way valve mechanism allows cerebrospinal fluid (CSF) to enter into the subdural space, producing a subdural hygroma. Subdural hygromas most commonly follow trauma or intracranial surgery with reduced intracranial pressure. The fluid of the subdural hygroma may originate from CSF,

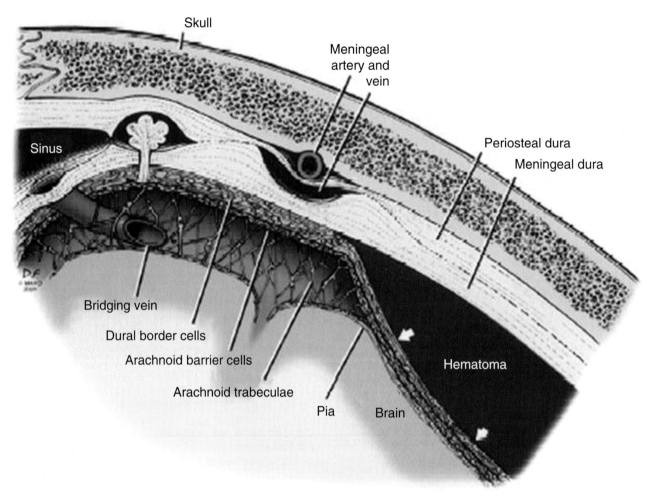

FIGURE 6-1 An artist's rendition of the pachymeningeal layers as described by Haines and colleagues.[1] The potential subdural space becomes a real subdural space when the dural border cell layer cleaves away from the inner meningeal layer (in this case, caused by hemorrhage), and subsequently a chronic intradural hematoma evolves. The prevalence of this lesion as a component of all spontaneously or trauma acquired subdural hematomas is unknown. (From Atkinson JL, Lane JI, Aksamit AJ: MRI depiction of chronic intradural (subdural) hematoma in evolution. J Magn Reson Imaging 17:485, 2003.)

but then this fluid may undergo modifications after membrane formation. The outer membrane consists of a plethora of capillaries susceptible to bleeding, eosinophils that secrete plasminogen inhibiting formation of platelet thrombus within the capillary lumen and contributing to lysis of existing clot.

Subdural hygromas are often bilateral and most often in the frontal and temporal regions. These lesions are usually clinically silent and often disappear within 3 months. In approximately one third of cases, the hygroma, which appears on computed tomography (CT) as an extra-axial collection of fluid with the density of CSF, enlarges on serial scans. The lesion then no longer has the characteristics of CSF but forms transitional lesions between hygroma and subdural hematoma. This occurs due to hemorrhage from the capillaries of the outer membrane and the transformation of the hygroma into a CSDH.[20,21]

Sometimes it is difficult to distinguish a CSDH arising from subdural hygromas from one associated with bleeding into an arachnoid cyst. Arachnoid cysts are intra-arachnoid cystic lesions filled with CSF, which are probably developmental in origin, and become symptomatic either with progressive enlargement or after minor trauma and hemorrhage into the cyst and the subsequent formation of a CSDH. These patients are significantly younger than other patients with CSDH and are characterized as presenting with signs of increased intracranial pressure.[22]

CLINICAL PRESENTATION

Several studies place the incidence of CSDHs at 1.72 to 13.1 per 100,000.[23,24] The variables that predispose to the development of a CSDH are being male, older than 70 years of age, cerebral atrophy, alcoholism with its attendant risk of repetitive trauma and coagulopathy, anticoagulation, and intracranial hypotension associated with CSF shunts or CSF leaks.[24-31] Trauma and antithrombotic therapy are the most frequent risk factors.[32]

The presentation of a patient on warfarin (Coumadin), often in combination with other anticoagulants, and a CSDH is a commonplace occurrence on a neurosurgical service. Warfarin depletes vitamin K–dependent factors and thus inhibits the intrinsic coagulation cascade. In a multivariate analysis of the risk factors involved in oral anticoagulant–related intracranial hemorrhages, Berwaerts and Webster[33] found the significant risk factors to be hypertension, an international normalized ratio (INR) on admission of more than 4.5, and the duration of anticoagulation. The incidence of CSDHs in patients on warfarin is reported as between 21% and 36%, and in 75% of spontaneous CSDHs, patients are found to be on anticoagulants.[34,35]

The clinical manifestations of a CSDH are protean, and an initial misdiagnosis is commonplace. One must maintain a high index of suspicion about this entity. There may not be a history of trauma and the complaints are often non-specific. The onset may be spontaneous, and in almost one half of patients, the precipitating event is unclear. The initial impression is sometimes that of a stroke or dementia, or the presentation is in the context of unexplained headache, seizures, focal weakness, and extrapyramidal or ophthalmologic findings. In the younger patient, the presentation is more commonly that of mass effect with symptoms and signs of increased intracranial pressure with a variable degree of motor deficit. In this group, one should consider the possibility of bleeding into an arachnoid cyst, whereas in the patient in the fourth decade and onward, these lesions are often present in association with anticoagulants or coagulopathy with an insidious decline of mentation and alertness.

CHRONIC SPINAL SUBDURAL HEMATOMAS

Chronic spinal subdural hematomas are very rare, with fewer than 30 cases reported in the literature.[36] This entity is more common in women, seen most frequently in the thoracolumbar spine, and more commonly found in those age 50 to 70.[37,38] It represents hemorrhage into the subdural space, which may be spontaneous, after lumbar puncture or spinal anesthesia, or is associated with anticoagulants or bleeding diathesis. These lesions are to be differentiated from hematomyelia and spinal epidural hemorrhage, which occur in similar circumstances.

Magnetic resonance imaging is the diagnostic study of choice for these lesions. The evolution of the blood clot in the spinal hematoma is similar to the evolution of intracranial hematomas.

The pathophysiology of this lesion is uncertain. Bridging veins, analogous to those that cause the subdural bleeding intracranially, do not exist in the spine. Some report that the source of the blood is primarily from a subarachnoid hemorrhage that has dissected into the subdural space.[39] This entity may also occur in conjunction with an intracranial CSDH with downward movement of blood from the cranial subdural space.

Chronic spinal subdural hematoma was first reported by Rader.[40] The patient in his case, as did some patients in subsequent cases, presented with severe, sudden-onset back pain and paraparesis. Most present with symptoms of spinal cord compression that can last from weeks to years. In addition, a rare case has also been reported of a chronic spinal subdural hematoma associated with bleeding into the CSF causing a hemosiderosis of the brain with resultant seizures, ataxia, hypoacusis, dementia, CSF xanthochromia, pleocytosis, and elevated protein levels.

Surgical drainage is the treatment of choice for these lesions.

RADIOGRAPHIC PRESENTATION

CT and magnetic resonance imaging are diagnostic of CSDH. On CT, the lesion(s) typically appears as a pericerebral fluid collection along the convexity with a convex outer border and irregular concave inner border. Difficulties arise in making the radiographic diagnosis of CSDH when the lesion is isodense with the adjacent brain tissue. This happens in approximately 25% of cases. Difficulty may also arise in the setting of marked cerebral atrophy in which a prominent subarachnoid space may mimic CSDH. It is in these cases that the magnetic resonance imaging unequivocally establishes the diagnosis.

The evolution of an extracerebral hematoma on CT imaging has been well described.[31,41–43] Density readings on the CT scans are measured in Hounsfield units. Initially, the acute blood is at 60 to 90 Hounsfield units, changing within 3 weeks to 30 Hounsfield units unless there are repetitive hemorrhages into the mass. Low-density CSDHs range from 0 to 25 Hounsfield units. The hematoma remains hyperdense for approximately 1 week. Afterward, it becomes isodense. After 3 weeks, approximately 75% of the hematomas are isodense. Hematomas are considered chronic after 2 to 3 weeks.

Nomura and colleagues[44] group CSDH into five types based on the CT appearance: high-density type, mixed-density type, layering type, isodense type, and low-density type. They suggest that the low-density hematoma is clinically stable with a low tendency to rebleeding in contrast to the layering- or mixed-type lesions, which are active and have a high concentration of fibrinogen and fibrinolytic activity predisposing to a tendency to rebleed (Fig. 6-2). All hypodense lesions were correlated with the "crankcase oil" appearance of the surgically evacuated fluid.[45]

Magnetic resonance imaging is the study of choice to demonstrate a CSDH, its extent, its intradural location, whether it is multicompartmentalized, and its probable age. The magnetic resonance imaging characteristics of an intracranial hematoma undergo a predictable series of changes on T1- and T2-weighted images. Acute hematomas have isointense to hyperintense signal relative to brain on T1 imaging and low signal relative to brain on T2 imaging. Hyperacute hemorrhages are isointense on T1 and T2 imaging. Early subacute hematomas are primarily hyperintense on T1 and hypointense on T2. Late subacute hematomas are hyperintense on T1 and iso- to hypointense on T2. In the chronic stage, the hematoma is hypointense on both imaging modalities. Blood products during the evolution of the hematoma are responsible for these imaging characteristics (Table 6-1). Due to the capillary-rich capsules around the hematoma, there is slight ring enhancement with intravenous gadolinium.

After examining 230 CSDHs, Tsutsumi and colleagues[25] classified these lesions into five groups according to the intensity of their appearance on T1-weighted magnetic

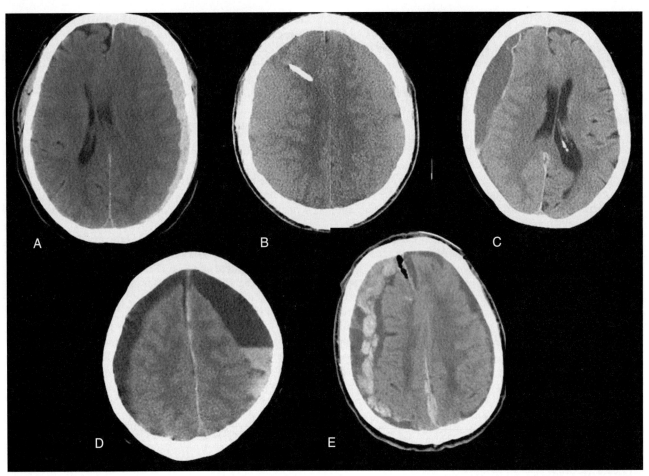

FIGURE 6-2   Appearance on computed tomography of subdural hematomas. *A*, High density; *B*, isodense; *C*, low density; *D*, layering type; and *E*, mixed density.

resonance images and correlated these categories with recurrence rates after surgery. The lesions are classified as high, mixed high/isointense, isointense, mixed isointense/low, and low (Fig. 6-3). The high-intensity group recurrence rate was reported as being 3.4% compared with an 11.6% recurrence rate in the non-high-intensity group.

PERIOPERATIVE MANAGEMENT

A CSDH is often seen in association with abnormalities of coagulation, and therefore the perioperative management of these issues are important. Specifically, in a recent report on coagulation defects in patients with a CSDH, Konig and colleagues found that of 114 patients studied, coagulation disorders were found in 42%: 13% of patients were alcoholics, 8% of patients were on acetylsalicylic acid and all of them had abnormalities in platelet aggregation, 15% of patients were on warfarin for atrial fibrillation after cardiac surgery, and 6% of patients had a history of hematologic or oncologic disease.

Assessment of the patient's coagulation status involves screening with a complete blood count, liver function tests, prothrombin time, INR, activated partial thromboplastin time, platelet count, and fibrinogen level. INR was found to be the best indicator for the presence of a coagulopathy. Recently, factor XIII has also been assayed because of

an association of a deficiency of this postoperative hemorrhage in neurosurgical cases. Factor XIII facilitates the final stage of the coagulation cascade, which involves the enzymatic cross-linking of the amino acid groups of lysine and glutamine residues of fibrin. If deficiencies are detected, prothrombin complex, fibrinogen, or antithrombin concentrate are administered to maintain a prothrombin time greater than 60%, the number of platelets greater than 100,000, fibrinogen greater than 1.5 g/L, and antithrombin III greater than 80%. A specific photometric is used to assay factor XIII, and activity between 60% and 140% is normal.

TABLE 6-1 ▪ Imaging Characteristics Affected by Blood Products during the Evolution of a Hematoma

Age of Hemorrhage	Blood Product	T1	T2
Hyperacute	Oxyhemoglobin	Isointense	Isointense-hyperintense
Acute	Deoxyhemoglobin	Isointense	Hypointense
Late subacute	Methemoglobin	Hyperintense	Isointense-hypointense
Chronic	Hemosiderin	Hypointense	Hypointense

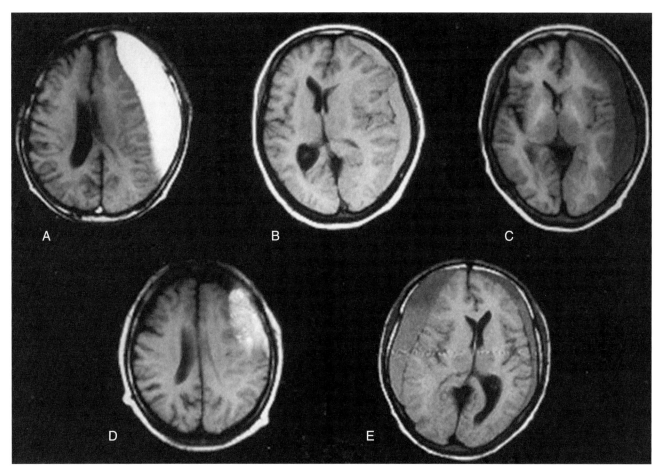

FIGURE 6-3   Magnetic resonance T1-weighted images demonstrate five types of chronic subdural hematoma: *A*, High intensity; *B*, isointense; *C*, low intensity; *D*, mixed high intensity and isointensity; and *E*, mixed isointense and low intensity. (From Tsutsumi K, Maeda K, Iijima A, et al: The relationship of preoperative magnetic resonance imaging findings and closed system drainage in the recurrence of chronic subdural hematoma. J Neurosurg 87:870–875, 1997.)

If rapid correction of a coagulopathy is required, the report of Boulis and colleagues[46] comparing the use of fresh frozen plasma (10–20 mL/kg) and factor IX complex concentrate in patients with warfarin-related CSDH is instructive. These authors find that there is an accelerated correction of coagulation in the factor IX group and a higher complication rate with those treated with fresh frozen plasma. In addition, factor IX is delivered in less volume load compared with fresh frozen plasma, a significant consideration in the elderly and those with heart disease. Correction of the anticoagulation is defined as achieving an INR of 1.5 or less.

The clinical effect of the vitamin K does not begin for approximately 8 hours after it is administered subcutaneously. It requires this interval for the liver synthesis of clotting factors to be initiated, the plasma factors II, VII, IX, and X to be replenished, and the INR to normalize. Under emergent or urgent situations, administering vitamin K intravenously has no advantage and has been associated with cardiovascular collapse.

Restarting anticoagulation after surgical evacuation of a CSDH remains an inaccurate process. The minimal

effective dose of warfarin has been studied in a variety of conditions, and the optimal risk/benefit appears to be at an INR of 2 to 3 for almost all conditions with the exception of mechanical heart valves, which require an INR of 3 to 4. In the absence of atrial fibrillation, bioprosthetic valves need no anticoagulation.[47] The general experience is that no adverse effects are encountered when warfarin is stopped for the surgical intervention. The decision to restart anticoagulation after an intracranial hemorrhage should take into consideration the risk of a thromboembolic complication while not receiving anticoagulation (0.016% per day) versus the risk of any further intracranial bleeding. Restarting warfarin after CSDH surgery has been reported as beginning anywhere from 3 days postoperatively in patients with mechanical heart valves to within weeks for the other conditions necessitating anticoagulation. When warfarin is restarted on day 3, therapeutic effectiveness is not achieved until day 5. It takes 36 to 48 hours for the warfarin to block the synthesis of the coagulation factors. In situations in which anticoagulation is critical, low-dose heparin is started early and discontinued when the therapeutic INR range is achieved.[34,48]

SURGICAL OPTIONS IN THE MANAGEMENT OF CHRONIC SUBDURAL HEMATOMA IN ADULTS

Although spontaneous resolution of chronic spinal subdural hematoma occurs and some have been evacuated by guided puncture, patients with an obvious neurologic deficit should undergo direct surgical evacuation. A CSDH in an asymptomatic or mildly symptomatic patient complaining of headache but otherwise neurologically intact is a commonplace referral to a neurosurgical service. The studies may show a unilateral or bilateral lesion, cerebral atrophy without brain shift, or evidence of increased intracranial pressure. Patients with this profile can be observed and monitored with serial CT scans, and the collection will often become smaller or disappear. Should there be an increase in the size of the CSDH and/or of the symptomatology, the patient should undergo surgical intervention.

An ongoing debate concerns optimal surgical management of a CSDH. Part of this is influenced by the preoperative perceptions of the collection in a given case and an attempt by neurosurgeons to tailor the procedure to the clinical and radiographic characteristics of these lesions. Those lesions that appear to contain recent clotted blood or loculated collections or are recurrences tend to have larger openings made in the skull, dura, and outer membrane combined with irrigation and drainage of the subdural space. When one attempts to assess the results of these operations, the meta-analysis by Weigel and colleagues[49] is of interest. This publication addresses the morbidity, mortality, recurrence, and cure rates of CSDHs based on a review of 48 publications culled from the literature on these subjects between 1981 and October 2001. Of these publications, no article provides class I evidence, six articles provide class II evidence, and the remainder provides class III evidence. Being evaluated are the relative merits of twist drill (skull opening as large as 5 mm), burr hole (5–30-mm opening), and craniotomy, with or without intraoperative irrigation and with or without postoperative closed system drainage. The authors conclude that twist drill and burr hole are the safest procedures, that craniotomy is associated with the lowest recurrence rate but a higher morbidity rate, and that drainage reduces the recurrence rate in both twist drill and burr hole cases. In addition, drainage and irrigation do not increase the risk of infection after surgery.

In the absence of compelling evidence supporting a particular approach, our general guidelines for the management of CSDH in adults reflect the following preferences:

- General or local anesthesia
- Use of preoperative prophylactic antibiotics
- Use of perioperative prophylactic anticonvulsants
- Linear incision centered on the lesion
- Initial burr hole in the most dependent (posteroinferior) part of the exposure
- Vigorous cauterization of the dura and the subdural hematoma's parietal membrane and opening into the collection; CSDH removed by evacuation or irrigation with warm normal saline until effluent is clear; the inner membrane is not usually disturbed
- Assessment of the characteristics of the subdural collection, whether hygromatous, classic "crankcase oil" CSDH fluid, component of fresh blood with clot

- Amount of drainage and how it corresponds to the anticipated size of the collection noted on the preoperative radiographic studies
- If needed, using the burr hole as a start, remove a 5-cm disc of bone (minicraniotomy) and widen the opening of the dura and subdural membrane if needed to allow emptying of loculated collections and clotted blood, irrigating the subdural space, and placing a drain under direct vision in the subdural space (directed frontally to remove air and residual subdural fluid) to remain in position for 24 to 72 hours
- Same approach for the second side in the case of bilateral collections
- Replacement of bone disc with miniplates from disc to skull
- Multilayer closure
- Serial postoperative CT scans beginning on day 1 and then as judged clinically appropriate

RECURRENCE OF CHRONIC SUBDURAL HEMATOMA AFTER SURGERY

The efficacy of the standard procedures for evacuation of a CSDH (i.e., twist drill, burr hole, or craniotomy, with or without irrigation and drainage of the subdural space) can be gauged by the symptomatic recurrence rate of the CSDH after these procedures. Among published series, these rates usually vary between 3.7% and 21.5%.[31,50–52] Sambasivan[31] reports a recurrence rate of 0.35% when the technique of craniotomy and subtemporalis marsupialization was used. The recurrences are higher in the presence of coagulopathy, intracranial hypotension, intracranial air seen on postoperative scans, alcoholism, seizures, CSF shunts, and cerebral atrophy; when magnetic resonance imaging does not demonstrate a high-intensity extracerebral collection on the T1-weighted images; and among those undergoing bilateral surgery.[44,51,53–59] Placing patients in the supine or upright position postoperatively seems to have no influence on the recurrence rate.[60] There have also been studies that show different recurrence rates depending on the hematoma density, internal architecture (homogeneous, laminar, separated, trabecular), or the intracranial extension. The recurrence rate was high for the separated type and low for the trabecular type. Moreover, an association between postoperative drainage and recurrence rate has been made. In those who had postoperative drains, those who had total drainage of greater than 200 mL had no recurrence, suggesting that those who do not drain greater than 200 mL over 5 days should be watched more closely for recurrence.[61] Those drains whose catheters were found to have a frontal location were also associated with a lower recurrence rate.[62] Interestingly, those with diabetes have been correlated with a lower recurrence rate. The blood of patients with diabetes reportedly has a higher osmotic pressure and has increased platelet aggregation. The hyperviscosity diminishes the rebleed rate.[57]

Symptomatic recurrence implies a reappearance of neurologic signs and/or symptoms and an increase in the volume of the CSDH on the operated side with compression of the brain on CT within weeks to months after surgery.

This needs to be distinguished from residual collections that are asymptomatic, do not demonstrate pressure effects on CT, and can be followed with serial studies until their complete or nearly complete resolution without surgical intervention.

Concerning the cases requiring reoperation, 20 articles were reviewed by Weigel and colleagues[49] that contain detailed data on the treatment of recurrences after twist drill, burr hole, and craniotomy. Data were found on 151 patients undergoing twist drill evacuation of CSDH in seven publications. Among these patients, 70% (106 patients) were successfully treated by the same technique, 24% (35 patients) underwent burr hole, and 6% underwent craniotomy. Among 229 patients in this series who underwent primary burr hole, 85% were subsequently successfully treated by the same procedure previously performed, 14% underwent craniotomy, and 1% died.

A variety of alternative approaches have been devised for the repeated accumulations of a CSDH. Among these particularly recalcitrant cases, which constitute approximately 1% of CSDH cases, the following tactics have been used: placement of an Omaya reservoir in the burr hole to allow the subdural space to be tapped repeatedly[63]; placement of a hollow screw in the hematoma[64]; replacement of hematoma with oxygen[65] insertion of a subdural peritoneal shunt (which may be removed after approximately 6 weeks); endoscopic exploration of the subdural space with a flexible, steerable endoscope through the burr hole to resect membrane and open compartmentalized collections[66,67]; and superselective embolization of branches of the ipsilateral middle meningeal artery to interrupt the vascularity of the subdural outer membrane and hence its propensity to bleed.[68,69] Each of these tactics has been found to have restricted use.

POSTOPERATIVE COMPLICATIONS

Although approximately 90% of patients make a good recovery after surgery for CSDH, mortality rates in different series have been reported of between 1% and 10%, which depend largely on the patient's preoperative clinical status. Approximately 10% of patients will have a permanent residual neurologic deficit. Among the other postoperative complications associated specifically with CSDH surgery are tension pneumocephalus, infection of the subdural space (1%–2% of cases) that has not been shown to be associated with a postoperative drain left in situ for as long as 72 hours, and intracranial hemorrhage on the contralateral side or intracerebrally.

Delayed clinical deterioration after evacuation of a CSDH raises a number of clinical diagnostic possibilities. However, in some of these cases, the postoperative imaging studies do not provide an adequate explanation of the findings, which may include aphasia and hemiparesis. In these patients, a dramatic improvement can follow short-term treatment with mannitol. The mechanism of this improvement remains problematic.

Perioperative seizure prevalence, morbidity, and anticonvulsant use in a surgically treated series of 98 patients with CSDH treated between 1987 and 1992 have been reported. The seizure prevalence for all these patients during hospitalization and follow-up was 20.4%, with a preexisting seizure disorder in 6.1%. In the latter group of patients, three fourths of the patients experienced an increase in the seizure frequency with the development of the CSDH. In 18.5% of this population, new seizure activity occurred in the absence of a previous seizure disorder. This study also documented the increased morbidity and mortality with these seizures due to respiratory complications, especially among the older patients in the study. New-onset seizures occurred in 2.4% of patients and 32% of those without perioperative anticonvulsant medicine. Even taking into account the undesirable side effects of the anticonvulsants, the complications are lower when they are used perioperatively in patients treated for a CSDH.

REFERENCES

1. Haines DE, Harkey HL, al-Mefty O: The "subdural" space: A new look at an outdated concept. Neurosurgery 32:11–20, 1993.
2. Guiffre R: Physiopathogenesis of chronic subdural hematomas: A new look at an old problem. Rev Neurol 5:298, 1987.
3. McKenzie CR, Rengachary SS, McGregor DH, et al: Subdural hematoma associated with metastatic neoplasms. Neurosurgery 27:619–625, 1990.
4. Munk PL, Robertson WD, Durity FA: Middle fossa arachnoid cyst and subdural hematoma: CT studies. J Comput Assist Tomogr 12:1073–1075, 1988.
5. Page AC, Mohan D, Paxton RM: Arachnoid cysts of the middle fossa predispose to subdural haematoma formation fact or fiction? Acta Neurochir Suppl 42:210–215, 1988.
6. Pozzati E, Tognetti F, Gaist G: Chronic subdural haematoma from cerebral arteriovenous malformation. Neurochirurgia 29:61–62, 1986.
7. Alimehmeti R, Locatelli M: Epidural B cell non-Hodgkin's lymphoma associated with chronic subdural hematoma. Surg Neurol 57:179–182, 2002.
8. Bergmann M, Puskas Z, Kuchelmeister K: Subdural hematoma due to dural metastasis: Case report and review of the literature. Clin Neurol Neurosurg 94:235–240, 1992.
9. Watanabe S, Shimada H, Ishii S: Production of clinical form of chronic subdural hematoma in experimental animals. J Neurosurg 37:552–561, 1972.
10. Apfelbaum R, Guthkelch A, Schulman K: Experimental production of subdural hematomas. J Neurosurg 40:336–346, 1974.
11. Yamashima T, Friede RL: Why do bridging veins rupture into the virtual subdural space? J Neurol Neurosurg Psychiatry 47:121–127, 1984.
12. Lee KS, Bae WK, Doh JW, et al: Origin of chronic subdural haematoma and relation to traumatic subdural lesions. Brain Inj 12:901–910, 1998.
13. Tanikawa M, Mase M, Yamada K, et al: Surgical treatment of chronic subdural hematoma based on intrahematomal membrane structure on MRI. Acta Neurochir 143:613–619, 2001.
14. Yamashima T, Yamamoto S: How do vessels proliferate in the capsule of a chronic subdural hematoma? Neurosurgery 15:672–678, 1984.
15. Vaquero J, Zurita M, Cincu R: Vascular endothelial growth-permeability factor in the granulation tissue of chronic subdural hematomas. Acta Neurochir 144:343–346, 2002.
16. Weigel R, Schilling L, Schmiedek P: Specific pattern of growth factor distribution in chronic subdural hematoma (CSH): Evidence for an angiogenic disease. Acta Neurochir 143:811–819, 2001.
17. Frati A, Dalvati M, Maimeu F: Inflammatory markers and risk factors for recurrence. J Neurosurg 100:24–32, 2004.
18. Shono T, Inamura T, Morioka T, et al: Vascular endothelial growth factors in chronic subdural hematomas. J Clin Neurosci 5:411–415, 2001.
19. Murakami H, Hirose Y, Sagoh M, et al: Why do chronic subdural hematomas grow slowly and not coagulate? Role of thrombomodulin in the mechanism. J Neurosurg 96:877–884, 2002.
20. Liu Y, Zhu S, Jiang Y, et al: [Clinical characteristics of chronic subdural hematoma evolving from traumatic subdural effusion]. Chung Hua Wai Ko Tsa Chih 40:360–362, 2002.
21. Lee KS: The pathogenesis and clinical significance of traumatic subdural hygroma. Brain Inj 12:595–603, 199.
22. Mori K, Yamamoto T, Horinaka N, Maeda M: Arachnoid cyst is a risk factor for chronic subdural hematoma in juveniles: Twelve cases of chronic subdural hematoma associated with arachnoid cyst. J Neurotrauma 19:1017–1027, 2002.

23. Fogelholm R, Waltimo O: Epidemiology of chronic subdural hematoma. Acta Neurochir 32:247–250, 1975.

24. Kudo H, Kuwamura K, Izawa I, et al: Chronic subdural hematoma in elderly people: Present status on Awaji Island and epidemiological prospect. Neurol Med Chir (Tokyo) 32:207–209, 1992.

25. Tsutsumi K, Maeda K, Iijima A, et al: The relationship of preoperative magnetic resonance imaging findings and closed system drainage in the recurrence of chronic subdural hematoma [see comment]. J Neurosurg 87:870–875, 1997.

26. Camel M, Grubb RL Jr: Treatment of chronic subdural hematoma by twist-drill craniotomy with continuous catheter drainage. J Neurosurg 65:183–187, 1986.

27. Fogelholm R, Heiskanen O, Waltimo O: Chronic subdural hematoma in adults: Influence of patient's age on symptoms, signs, and thickness of hematoma. J Neurosurg 42:43–46, 1975.

28. Hamilton MG, Frizzell JB, Tranmer BI: Chronic subdural hematoma: The role for craniotomy reevaluated. Neurosurgery 33:67–72, 1993.

29. McKissock L, Lond M, Richardson A: Subdural hematoma: A review of 389 cases. Lancet 2:1365–1369, 1960.

30. Svien H, Gelety J: On the surgical management of an encapsulated subdural hematoma. J Neurosurg 21:172–177, 1964.

31. Sambasivan M: An overview of chronic subdural hematoma: Experience with 2300 cases. Surg Neurol 47:418–422, 1997.

32. Asghar M, Adhiyaman V, Greenway MW, et al: Chronic subdural haematoma in the elderly—A North Wales experience. J R Soc Med 95:290–292, 2002.

33. Berwaerts J, Webster J: Analysis of risk factors involved in oral-anticoagulant-related intracranial haemorrhages. Q J Med 93:513–521, 2000.

34. Gonogunta V, Buxton N: Warfarin and chronic subdural haematomas. Br J Neurosurg 15:514–517, 2001.

35. Hylek E, Singer D: Risk factors for intracranial hemorrhage in outpatients taking warfarin. Ann Intern Med 120:897–902, 1994.

36. Abla AA, Oh MY: Spinal chronic subdural hematoma. Neurosurg Clin N Am 11:465–471, 2000.

37. Khosla V, Kak V, Mathuriya S: Chronic spinal subdural hematomas: Report of two cases. J Neurosurg 66:636–639, 1985.

38. Russell NA, Benoit BG: Spinal subdural hematoma: A review. Surg Neurol 20:133–137, 1983.

39. Vinters H, Barnett H, Kaufmann J: Subdural hematoma of the spinal cord and widespread subarachnoid hemorrhage complicating anti-coagulant therapy. Stroke 11:459–464, 1980.

40. Rader J: Chronic subdural hematoma of the spinal cord. N Engl J Med 252:374–376, 1955.

41. Bergstrom M, Ericson K, Lavender B: Variation with time of the attenuation values of intracranial hematomas. J Comput Assist Tomogr 1:57–63, 1977.

42. Naim-ur-Rahman: Chronic subdural hematoma: Correlation of computerized tomography with colour. Neuroradiology 29:40–42, 1987.

43. Zee CS, Go JL: CT of head trauma. Neuroimaging Clin N Am 8:525–539, 1998.

44. Nomura S, Kashiwagi S, Fujisawa H, et al: Characterization of local hyperfibrinolysis in chronic subdural hematomas by SDS-PAGE and immunoblot. J Neurosurg 81:910–913, 1994.

45. Kostanian V, Choi JC, Liker MA, et al: Computed tomographic characteristics of chronic subdural hematomas. Neurosurg Clin N Am 11:479–489, 2000.

46. Boulis N, Bobek M, Schmair A, Hoff J: Use of factor IX complex in warfarin-related hemorrhage. Neurosurgery 45:1113–1118, 1999.

47. Hemostasis and Thrombosis Task Force: Guidelines on Oral Anticoagulation, 3rd ed. Br J Haematol 101:374–387, 1998.

48. Kawamata T, Takeshita M, Kubo O, et al: Management of intracranial hemorrhage associated with anticoagulant therapy. Surg Neurol 44:438–443, 1995.

49. Weigel R, Schmiedek P, Krauss J: Outcome of contemporary surgery for chronic subdural haematoma: Evidence based review. J Neurol Neurosurg Psychiatry 74:937–943, 2003.

50. Miki T, Ikeda Y, Saito K, et al: Clinical Study of Recurrent Chronic Subdural Hematoma. New York: Springer-Verlag, 1993.

51. Oishi M, Toyama M, Tamatani S, et al: Clinical factors of recurrent chronic subdural hematoma. Neurol Med Chir (Tokyo) 41:382–386, 2001.

52. Mori K, Maeda M: Surgical treatment of chronic subdural hematoma in 500 consecutive cases: Clinical characteristics, surgical outcome, complications, and recurrence rate. Neurol Med Chir 41:371–381, 2001.

53. Asano Y, Hasuo M, Takahashi I, Shimosawa S: [Recurrent cases of chronic subdural hematoma—Its clinical review and serial CT findings]. No To Shinkei 44:827–831, 1992.

54. Cameron MM: Chronic subdural haematoma: A review of 114 cases. J Neurol Neurosurg Psychiatry 41:834–839, 1978.

55. Fukuhara T, Gotoh M, Asari S, Ohmoto T, Akioka T: The relationship between brain surface elastance and brain reexpansion after evacuation of chronic subdural hematoma. Surg Neurol 45:570–574, 1996.

56. Naganuma H, Fukamachi A, Kawakami M, et al: Spontaneous resolution of chronic subdural hematomas. Neurosurgery 19:794–798, 1986.

57. Yamamoto H, Hirashima Y, Hamada H, et al: Independent predictors of recurrence of chronic subdural hematoma: Results of multivariate analysis performed using a logistic regression model. J Neurosurg 98:1217–1221, 2003.

58. Cucchiara B, Kasner S: Atherosclerotic risk factors in patients with ischemic vascular disease. Curr Treat Options Neurol 4:445–453, 2002.

59. Park C, Choi K, Kim M: Spontaneous evolution of posttraumatic subdural hygroma into chronic subdural hematoma. Acta Neurochir 127:41–47, 1994.

60. Nakajima H, Yasui T, Nishikawa M, et al: The role of postoperative patient posture in the recurrence of chronic subdural hematoma: A prospective randomized trial. Surg Neurol 58:385–387, 2002.

61. Kwon TH, Park YK, Lim DJ, et al: Chronic subdural hematoma: Evaluation of the clinical significance of postoperative drainage volume. J Neurosurg 93:796–799, 2000.

62. Nakaguchi H, Tanishima T, Yoshimasu N: Relationship between drainage catheter location and postoperative recurrence of chronic subdural hematoma after burr-hole irrigation and closed-system drainage [see comment]. J Neurosurg 93:791–795, 2000.

63. Sato M, Iwatsuki K, Akiyama C, et al: [Use of Ommaya CSF reservoir for refractory chronic subdural hematoma]. No Shinkei Geka 27:423–428, 1999.

64. Emonds N, Hassler WE: New device to treat chronic subdural hematoma—Hollow screw. Neurol Res 21:7–8, 1999.

65. Aoki N: A new therapeutic method for chronic subdural hematoma in adults: Replacement of the hematoma with oxygen via percutaneous subdural tapping [see comment]. Surg Neurol 38:53–56, 1992.

66. Hellwig D, Kuhn TJ, Bauer BL, List-Hellwig E: Endoscopic treatment of septated chronic subdural hematoma. Surg Neurol 45:272–277, 1996.

67. Hellwig D, Heinze S, Riegel T, Benes L: Neuroendoscopic treatment of loculated chronic subdural hematoma. Neurosurg Clin N Am 11:525–534, 2000.

68. Mandai S, Sakurai M, Matsumoto Y: Middle meningeal artery embolization for refractory chronic subdural hematoma: Case report. J Neurosurg 93:686–688, 2000.

69. Takahashi K, Muraoka K, Sugiura T, et al: [Middle meningeal artery embolization for refractory chronic subdural hematoma: 3 case reports]. No Shinkei Geka 30:35–39, 2002.

7 Penetrating Brain Injuries

GUY ROSENTHAL, RICARDO SEGAL, and FELIX UMANSKY

HISTORICAL ASPECTS

The basic principles of the treatment of penetrating brain injuries (PBIs) have, to a large degree, developed from experience treating casualties of the wars of the twentieth century. The application of modern antiseptic techniques was first applied to head injuries sustained in combat during the Anglo-Boer war.[1] During World War I, Harvey Cushing, serving with the first expeditionary force in France, laid down the principles that serve as the basis for the treatment of penetrating head injuries and demonstrated that their implementation resulted in a decrease of mortality from 54% to 28%.[2,3] During World War II, introduction of antibiotics dramatically changed wound care in general and impacted care of PBI patients, dramatically reducing rates of infection.[4-7] Korean War experience emphasized the role of early evacuation of the patient with head injury.[8]

In the Vietnam conflict, a wealth of experience and data were obtained, often in a prospective fashion.[9] However, the only routine imaging techniques available during the Vietnam conflict were plain roentgenographs of the skull and angiography, and this undoubtedly affected the prevailing attitudes concerning treatment. Military medical doctrine at the time advocated the pursuit of all retained bone fragments even when this entailed repeat operation,[9] because fragments were thought to be associated with increased rates of infection and seizures. This dogma was later questioned when follow-up studies of Vietnam veterans with retained fragments failed to find increased rates of either infectious complications[10] or epilepsy.[11] The routine use of computed tomography (CT) scanning coincided with the Arab-Israeli conflict in Lebanon, and the utility of CT in guiding initial therapy was demonstrated. One of the results was a less aggressive initial surgical approach in the absence of mass effect; another was the questioning of the need to remove all fragments.[12,13] The Iran-Iraq war also led to a wealth of published data,[14,15] including reports on the vascular complications of penetrating head injury.[16] Data from bomb blasts in the Lebanon conflict[17] and, more recently, from terrorist bombings, have demonstrated that these injuries represent a particular challenge, combining elements of penetrating and blast injury.

BALLISTICS

The kinetic energy (KE) released by a missile fragment is related to its mass (M) and velocity (V) and may be estimated by the formula[18]:

$$KE = \frac{1}{2} M(V_{entry} - V_{exit})^2$$

This equation highlights the importance of missile velocity relative to mass, and is the theoretical basis for traditional classification schemes categorizing injuries as "low-velocity" or "high-velocity" wounds. The tendency of the surgeon to rely too heavily on such a classification and ascribe undue clinical significance to it has been pointed out.[19] In fact, no clear delineation exists in the literature between high- and low-velocity projectiles. The British draw the line at the speed of sound in air (1100 feet/second, 335 m/second), whereas American researchers define high velocity as between 2000 and 3000 feet/second (610 to 914 m/second).[19] Most modern high-velocity rifles surpass 2500 feet/second (762 m/second), whereas most handguns fire to a velocity of 800 to 1400 feet/second (244 to 427 m/second). Shrapnel typically has a velocity of 600 feet/second (183 m/second).[20] A missile's energy is greatest at the moment it is launched, and decays with time and distance. Therefore, it is the impact velocity of the projectile that more accurately reflects the true wounding potential of the missile. The actual energy delivered to tissue is determined not just by the kinetic energy available to the projectile (as expressed by the above equation) but also by the deformation and fragmentation of the missile itself.[21] Weapons and ammunition are designed to create friction-free flight in air but to enhance resistance to passage in tissue. Expansion, tumbling, yaw, and fragmentation all enhance energy delivery to the tissue.[18,20] Bone fragments driven into the brain may act as secondary missiles. Thus even a tangential missile strike can achieve a release of energy leading to significant injury to the brain.

From a clinical perspective, the neurosurgeon should not harbor preconceptions regarding any specific injuries. Military or hunting injuries from "high-velocity" weapons may mimic "low-velocity" injuries because of the large distance traveled by the projectile or because of protective military headgear.[22] A "low-velocity" injury from a handgun at short distance may result in a devastating injury.

PATHOPHYSIOLOGY

The biomechanical effects of a missile strike on tissue has been simulated and described by Harvey and colleagues[23] and, more recently, by Fackler and colleagues.[24] Carey utilized a cat model to study the wounding effects of a projectile through an intact skull.[25,26] First, a direct crush injury results in a permanent cylindrical cavity. Pressure waves resulting from kinetic energy transfer, termed *ordinary pressure waves*, are propelled radially from the missile path[25]; they create a temporary cavity lasting approximately 20 msec as the walls of the permanent cavity first expand, then contract. These ordinary pressure waves may result in stretch injury to adjacent tissues even at distances far removed from the projectile tract. A sonic pressure wave also occurs, but its significance in bullet injuries is minimized by its brevity (approximately 2 μsec).[27] Collapse of the temporary cavity is followed by extravasation of blood around the missile track, which may expand to occupy a much larger space than the initial cavity. The permanent cavity is often beet-shaped in a high-velocity injury, and carrot-shaped in a low-velocity injury. In perforating injuries, the exit wound is inevitably larger than the entrance wound; however, this rule does not hold true in short-range injuries.[20]

Animal models have been utilized to study the effects of a missile strike to the brain on the physiological parameters of intracranial pressure, mean arterial blood pressure (MABP), and cerebral perfusion pressure (CPP). In a monkey model, Crockard and colleagues[28] showed that a rapid rise in ICP immediately follows penetrating injury, peaking 2 to 5 minutes after injury and declining gradually thereafter. Carey and colleagues,[26] utilizing his feline model, demonstrated that a marked rise in MABP in the first minute after injury actually results in a short-lived rise in CPP; however, the rise in ICP is more sustained over time and larger in magnitude relative to baseline values than the rise in MABP, and it leads to a reduction in CPP. Levett and colleagues, using Crockard's model, showed that CPP values fell within 1 minute of injury to 41 mm Hg from a baseline of 90 mm Hg.[29] In this model, cerebral blood flow, as measured by the intracarotid xenon 133 injection method was also reduced to a level more than 50% below control values following penetrating injury. These pathophysiologic changes following PBI likely contribute to further neuronal damage and lend the theoretical justification for monitoring of ICP and CPP after PBI.

Carey and colleagues,[26] as well as others,[30] noted that severe respiratory changes occur after projectile injury, even when the missile is of low energy and the tract is distant from the brain stem. Carey hypothesized that the location of the medullary respiratory center (i.e., directly below the fluid-filled fourth ventricle) may make those neurons more susceptible to the ordinary pressure waves generated by a missile.[25] Above a certain level of energy, a missile often produces an apnea, which is fatal unless the animal is supported by mechanical ventilation.[26] The probable correlate in human injuries may be a significant factor responsible for mortality in PBI. In fact, Carey's experiments suggest that only a narrow window exists between the level of energy required for a missile to penetrate the skull and the level causing fatal apnea.[25]

INITIAL ASSESSMENT AND RESUSCITATION

The initial evaluation and stabilization of the patient with penetrating head injury must achieve multiple goals within a limited time. These include:

1. Initial stabilization, including airway, breathing, and circulation
2. Prevention of hypoxia
3. Prevention of hypotension
4. A brief initial neurologic evaluation, including the Glasgow Coma Scale (GCS), assessment of the pupils, and an evaluation for any focal deficit
5. Assessment of the cranium and face for external injuries

6. Concomitant evaluation by the trauma team for other life- or limb-threatening injuries

In many areas, initial care in the field is performed by well-trained prehospital personnel. Primary resuscitation is begun in the field and should include intubation in the comatose patient. Upon arrival in the trauma unit, a team including a general surgeon, anesthesiologist, and neurosurgeon should be involved in the initial evaluation and management. Any history available regarding mechanism of injury is valuable, and this can often be obtained from prehospital personnel. Importantly, these individuals often have details regarding the patient's neurologic status at the scene. This information needs to be clearly communicated to the trauma team on receipt of the patient to the trauma unit.

The rules delineated in advanced trauma life support apply to the patient with a PBI. Vital signs are obtained while the airway is secured as indicated. Any respiratory and circulatory instability are dealt with on arrival. Crystalloid or colloid fluids are given to restore intravascular volume as needed, and blood products are ordered as necessary. In addition to blood pressure and pulse, monitoring of oxygenation by pulse oximetry is useful in early detection of hypoxia. Blood is taken for laboratory tests, which should include arterial blood gas, complete blood count, electrolytes, and coagulation profile. A brief systemic survey is carried out, which usually includes a chest x-ray in the trauma unit. A cervical spine x-ray is usually performed, although it should be noted that some authors have questioned the utility of this exam in cases of civilian gunshot injuries.[31]

While these are being performed, a concomitant initial neurologic assessment is performed. This includes obtaining a GCS,[32] assessing pupillary size and reactivity, and noting any lateralizing signs. When recording the GCS, note needs to be taken of any sedating or paralyzing agents that may have been administered to the patient prior to arrival, as well as hemodynamic instability and prehospital intubation that affect the GCS for obvious reasons. The initial evaluation by the neurosurgeon should include an examination of the skull for external injuries, including entry and exit wounds as well as extruded brain tissue. Shaving may be necessary to adequately expose and inspect the cranium. In close-range injuries such as a suicide attempt or execution-style shooting, burn marks on the skin are often noted. Depressed fractures may be palpated, but care should be taken not to trigger uncontrollable bleeding when examining the region of the dural sinuses. The face and oral cavity should always be inspected, because the cranium can be accessed by projectiles through these routes. Any orbital penetration carries a high suspicion for intracranial involvement. If the injury involves the skull base, CSF rhinorrhea or otorrhea may be noted. An injury to the carotid may result in profuse bleeding and is often lethal.

INITIAL MEDICAL MANAGEMENT

Any evidence of brain herniation (e.g., unequal pupils) should be treated with prompt administration of mannitol (1.4 g/kg) if the patient is hemodynamically stable. This is accompanied by moderate hyperventilation to a P_{CO_2} of around 30 mm Hg. Tetanus toxin is administered to all PBI patients in the emergency department.

Anticonvulsants

Seizure may lead to acute deterioration; it is treated with an intravenous bolus of diazepam or lorazepam. It is appropriate to administer a loading dose of anticonvulsant medication intravenously to all patients with PBI, which is known to be associated with a higher rate of seizures than is nonpenetrating traumatic brain injury (TBI).[11,33–36] The rate of seizures after PBI has been reported as high as 30% to 50%, with 4% to 10% of seizures occurring within the first week after injury.[11,33] Temkin and colleagues[36] have demonstrated in a randomized trial the efficacy of phenytoin in reducing the incidence of seizures in the first week after head injury. Their study included patients with penetrating head injury. The use of anticonvulsant prophylaxis beyond 1 week is controversial. Salazar and associates[11] reported a seizure rate of 53% in their study of Vietnam veterans followed over a 15-year period, with 18% of patients having their first seizure more than 5 years after injury. Although no studies have demonstrated the efficacy of prophylactic anticonvulsants in preventing late seizures, the high rate of late epilepsy in this population leads many authors to recommend continuing prophylaxis for at least 1 year or more after injury.[37–40] There is no consensus regarding treatment beyond this point unless the patient has developed seizures.

Antibiotics

Initiation of prophylactic broad-spectrum antibiotic therapy is recommended in PBI. The rate of infection is high because of contamination from foreign objects, skin, hair, and bone fragments, which all may lodge in the wound tract. In the preantibiotic era, rates of infection were nearly 60%, as reported by Whitaker during World War I.[41] When penicillin was introduced in a successive fashion to the various theaters of war during World War II, reported rates of infection dropped to 6% to 13%.[4] More recent reports from the military and civilian literature, based on routine use of modern broad-spectrum antibiotics, document rates of infection between 1% and 11%, with a trend toward higher rates in the military setting.[10,14,42–51] Reports on causative organisms identify *Staphylococcus* species, *Streptococcus*, *Acinetobacter*, *Escherichia coli*, *Klebsiella*, and *Enterobacter* as the common organisms identified in cultures.[5,42,44,52] These reports are limited by methodologic difficulties, including a failure to perform anaerobic cultures routinely. Moreover, they do not uniformly distinguish between colonization and infection. Despite these limitations, the likelihood of infection by either gram-positive or gram-negative bacteria is clear and justifies the use of broad-spectrum antibiotics for prophylaxis.

Important risk factors for the development of infection include CSF leak,[42,53] air sinus wounds,[54] and wound dehiscence.[10,44]

The issue of which antibiotic regimen is best suited for prophylaxis is not settled. In a survey of American neurosurgeons, Kaufman and colleagues[55] reported the use of a cephalosporin by 87% of respondents, chloramphenicol by 24%, penicillin by 16%, an aminoglycoside by 12%, and vancomycin by 6%. We tend to favor the use of a broad-spectrum cephalosporin with blood-brain barrier penetration

to cover community-acquired gram-negative organisms as well as *Staphylococcus* and *Streptococcus* species. The issue of optimal duration of prophylaxis is also unsettled, with very little evidence in the literature to support a recommendation.[56] We generally treat patients for 5 days after injury, but vary our practice depending on the nature of the wound. Both the issues of choice of antibiotic and duration of treatment clearly merit a prospective randomized controlled study.

INITIAL IMAGING

Once the patient is stabilized and the initial neurologic evaluation completed, the patient is taken to CT. CT is the examination of choice because the extent of brain injury (including intracranial hematomas and air), the extent of bone injury (including in-driven bone chips), and the presence of foreign bodies are all easily identified. The wound tract is readily visualized, and the presence of cerebral edema is noted. The size of the ventricles and cisterns is also noted. The utility of CT in both the military and civilian settings has been well-documented.[12,13,57–59] Findings on the CT scan associated with poor prognosis include bihemispheric injury,[50,58,60–64] transventricular path of the projectile,[12] intraventricular hemorrhage,[61,64] diffuse cerebral edema, and effacement of cisterns.[65]

In rare cases, the patient is hemodynamically unstable because of abdominal or thoracic injuries, and must be taken urgently to the operating theater by the trauma team without CT scan. X-rays of the skull may help to define the projectile tract, the extent of bony injury, and the presence of intracranial air. In such circumstances the neurosurgeon's clinical judgment and experience are important and dictate further therapy. In some cases a conservative approach is warranted, which may include placement of an intracranial pressure (ICP) monitor until the patient is hemodynamically stable enough to proceed to CT. In the rare case when anisocoria is present, burr holes or an exploratory craniotomy may be undertaken with the aim of evacuating a life-threatening hematoma. Intraoperative ultrasound is useful to localize an intracerebral clot in such cases.

The role of cerebral angiography in PBI to identify traumatic intracranial vascular lesions is discussed in a separate section that follows. In cranial stab wounds, angiography should be performed immediately because a significant number of patients sustain vascular injury.[66] In other types of penetrating trauma, the exam can usually be postponed until after the patient has been stabilized and initial neurosurgical intervention is completed.

DECISION MAKING IN THE PATIENT WITH POOR PROGNOSIS

All patients with PBI should receive aggressive initial resuscitation and undergo CT scan. After stabilization and imaging, a decision concerning further therapy will need to be made. The most difficult clinical scenario exists when the postresuscitation GCS score is between 3 and 5. This occurs commonly, at least in the civilian setting, where between 38% and 81% of patients may present in this condition.[50,60,61,65,67] Published reports document poor rates of survival in patients with a GCS score of 3 to 5[50,60,61,63,65] and even lower rates of neurologically good outcomes.

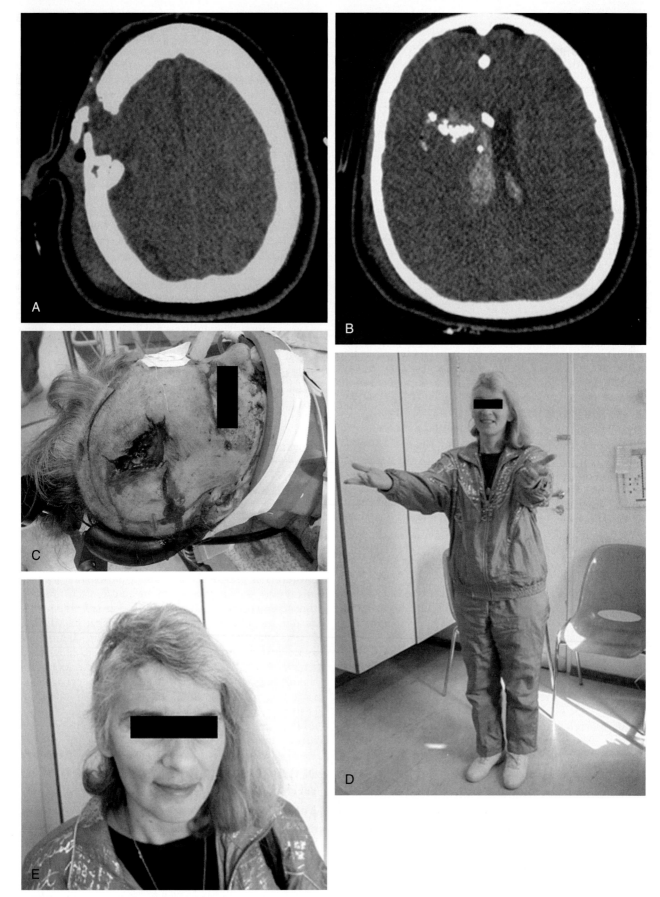

FIGURE 7-1 This 41-year-old female victim of a suicide bomber who detonated inside a bus had a GCS score of 6 on admission. CT revealing penetrating head injury with metal fragments and in-driven bone fragments in the ipsilateral frontal lobe and frontal horn of the lateral ventricle, as well as intraventricular blood (A, B). Extruding brain with outline of a possible question mark flap indicated (C). Instead, elongation of the existing wound was used for the craniotomy. No attempt was made to remove deeply located fragments. An intraventricular drain was placed. The patient regained consciousness and a left hemiparesis resolved (D). Excellent healing of scalp wound pending cranioplasty (E).

In the case of a patient who has a postresuscitation GCS score of 3 with dilated and nonreactive pupils without a mass lesion on CT, most neurosurgeons would agree that no surgical intervention is warranted.[58,68,69] Grahm and colleagues[60] prospectively studied 100 patients with gunshot wounds to the head in a civilian setting. They aggressively treated all patients with evidence of neurologic function after resuscitation, and found no satisfactory outcome in the group with a postresuscitation GCS score of 3 to 5. They concluded that no further therapy should be offered to a patient with a postresuscitation GCS score of 3 to 5 who did not have evidence of a large, surgically treatable hematoma on CT scan. In a study by Kaufman and colleagues involving two centers, the outcome of 412 patients presenting with a GCS score of 3 to 5 was evaluated. Of these, 4 had a neurologically good outcome.[63] In the study by Nagib and colleagues, 1 of 28 patients presenting with a GCS score of 3 to 5 had a favorable outcome.[50] Miner and colleagues, in their study of gunshot wounds in a pediatric population, found that decerebrate or decorticate posturing in children did not predict a poor outcome.[70] In military series, the results in patients with a GCS score of 3 to 5 is better, with rates of good outcome reaching 15% to 34%.[12,14] Thus it is important to keep in mind that, although few, some patients with a GCS score of 4 to 5, or even a GCS score of 3 with evidence of brain stem function, may have neurologically meaningful outcomes. Whether the tremendous societal costs incurred in the aggressive treatment of all patients in this group are justified, given the poor outcomes and low rates of survival, is an ethical dilemma well beyond the scope of this chapter. It is, however, a dilemma which the neurosurgeon treating the patient with PBI will inevitably encounter. Certainly no across-the-board recommendation can be made based on the current literature. Though each case will need to be considered individually, we concur with the view expressed by others[71] that an aggressive approach to treatment is warranted as long as some evidence of motor or brain stem function is demonstrated.

SURGICAL MANAGEMENT

The general guidelines of surgical treatment of penetrating injures of the head include:

1. Attaining adequate débridement of devitalized tissue
2. Removal of any mass lesions
3. Removal of accessible in-driven bone fragments and foreign bodies (but not at the expense of viable brain tissue)
4. Achievement of adequate hemostasis
5. Dural repair with watertight closure
6. Adequate closure of the scalp

All operative procedures for penetrating head injuries should begin with wide prepping and draping of the injured area to allow for adequate exposure. Thorough but gentle irrigation is used to flush out all tissues extruding from the wound site, including brain tissue. Two strategies are acceptable in planning the initial scalp incision. A large question-mark skin flap may be utilized, especially in cases where CT demonstrates a large hematoma. In cases where the entry site is punctuate, the skin flap may encompass it; this allows the necrotic edges to be excised and closed primarily.

When there is a large laceration at the entry site, this may be extended in lieu of a question-mark flap (Fig. 7-1). This may be preferable in cases where flap vascularity would otherwise be jeopardized. More extensive scalp injuries may require the use of rotation skin flaps for closure. Consultation with plastic surgery may be helpful in cases of extensive scalp injuries and should be undertaken prior to the initial incision in order to avoid difficulty with wound closure at the end of operation.

Adequate exposure of the bony defect is essential. The underlying dural injury often extends beyond the margins of the bone injury. A bone opening is recommended to extend beyond the limits of the visible bone injury until intact dura can be visualized. The same principle is utilized in cases when an underlying hematoma is present, but this may require the elevation of a larger bone flap if the clot is extensive. At the site of penetration, adequate débridement of the bony edges should be performed. Once the dura is exposed, herniating necrotic brain tissue is often noted extruding from the dural defect. This can be dealt with by irrigating with warm saline. The tract of penetration through the brain is flushed gently through the dural defect, removing necrotic tissue as well as any loose foreign objects within the necrotic cavity. At this point the dural defect may need to be extended to allow for adequate débridement of the injured brain. Blood clots are aspirated. A thorough exploration of the resulting cavity is undertaken. Accessible bone fragments and foreign bodies are removed. We recommend not continuing the exploration beyond this point even though preoperative CT may demonstrate deeper retained fragments. This is consistent with the approach advocating preservation of viable brain tissue over the removal of all retained fragments.[12,13] Meticulous hemostasis is accomplished, primarily using bipolar coagulation. Leaving hemostatic agents in the cavity should be avoided to the extent possible. Once hemostasis has been achieved, dural repair is undertaken. Any necrotic edges should be removed. Commonly, primary closure of the dura is not possible. Autologous grafts should be utilized in order to obtain a watertight closure. Temporalis fascia is probably the best option if accessible, followed by pericranium. If these are not available, a graft will need to be harvested, either fascia lata from the thigh or transversalis fascia from the abdomen. Allographic dura or cadaveric pericardium may be used only when the above-mentioned options are not practical. Artificial dural substitutes are not recommended.

Once dural closure is obtained, a decision regarding bone replacement needs to be taken. In cases where severe brain swelling cannot be controlled despite all operative and medical measures, the bone flap should not be replaced. In cases where replacement is feasible, sizeable retrieved bone fragments may be thoroughly cleaned and replaced at the site of defect. They can be assembled using miniplates or titanium wires and held in place with craniofix device (Fig. 7-2). Under no circumstances should a cranioplasty utilizing foreign materials be undertaken. A subgaleal drain should be inserted. The galea is closed with absorbable suture. The skin may be closed with nylon suture or skin stapler. As mentioned, some cases will require the use of a rotation flap to cover the wound. A skin graft may be needed to cover the resulting defect but should never cover the wound site (Fig. 7-3). The importance of this cannot be

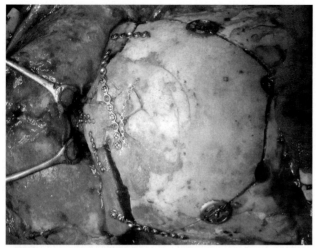

FIGURE 7-2 Bone fragments assembled with miniplates and held in place with craniofix device.

understated because the skin serves as a crucial barrier in preventing infection.

INTRACRANIAL PRESSURE MONITORING

Studies that include data on ICP after PBI indicate that intracranial hypertension is common after these injuries. Crockard studied ICP very early after PBI and found that high mortality was associated with elevated ICP.[72] Conversely, patients without elevated ICP did well. Nagib and colleagues[50] studied patients with civilian head injuries and found that patients with elevated ICP refractory to treatment measures invariably died. In contrast, the majority of patients in whom ICP responded to treatment survived, and those who did not have significant elevations of ICP had better outcomes. Miner and colleagues[70] studied a pediatric population and found that 75% of children with ICP above 40 mm Hg that was refractory to treatment died, whereas the rest were left with severe or moderate deficits. Patients with ICP controllable below 20 mm Hg had good outcomes or only moderate disability 6 months after injury. In our experience with PBI from bomb blasts, we also found an elevated mortality in patients with elevated ICP that is refractory to treatment[73] (Fig. 7-4). Patients in whom ICP responded to treatment had better outcomes (Fig. 7-5). Higher ICP values were seen in patients with intraventricular blood, brain edema, and large hematomas. Whether ICP monitoring improves outcome in PBI remains unresolved. We feel that PBI patients presenting with GCS scores below 8, intraventricular hemorrhage, significant brain edema, or significant intracerebral hematomas require ICP monitoring. Ventriculostomy remains the method of choice, because this allows therapeutic drainage of CSF. This is especially important when intraventricular blood is present. When prolonged drainage of CSF is required, catheter exchange at least every 5 to 7 days has been recommended,[74,75] although no prospective studies have documented the effectiveness of this measure. The ventriculostomy should always be tunneled, and we have found that long tunnels extending to the chest wall are useful in reducing rates of infection.[76] A recent report indicated that the use of a ventricular catheter

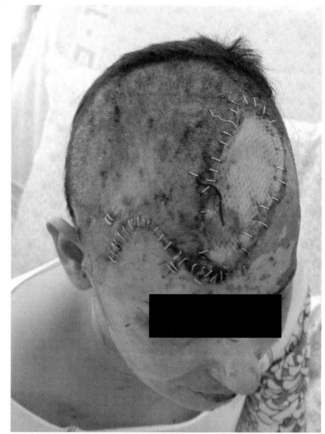

FIGURE 7-3 This 26-year-old female victim of a suicide bomber who detonated inside a bus had a GCS score of 15 on admission. The patient sustained a tangential injury with left frontal scalp avulsion and right epidural hematoma. A right frontal craniotomy and evacuation of the epidural hematoma was performed. A free skin graft was used to cover the scalp defect. Note that the incision for the craniotomy is not contiguous with the skin graft.

impregnated with rifampin and minocycline reduces the rate of infection in patients undergoing ventriculostomy, though no data pertaining specifically to the PBI setting were presented.[77] In cases where the ventricles cannot be cannulated, placement of an intraparenchymal ICP monitor is an acceptable alternative.

BONE FRAGMENTS

The need to remove all bone fragments has been a controversial issue in the surgical management of penetrating injuries of the brain. In the era when imaging was limited to plain roentgenographs of the skull, retained bone fragments were considered evidence of inadequate débridement and were thought to predispose to post-traumatic epilepsy and infection. United States military doctrine dictated removal of all retained fragments. Patients often underwent repeat operation to remove retained fragments.[9] During the Lebanon conflict, CT entered routine clinical use. The Israeli experience at the Rambam Medical Center in Haifa, to which most patients were evacuated (usually with transit times under 2 hours), led to a more conservative approach in the initial surgical management, with initial surgery limited to débridement, removal of large hematomas, dural repair, and ICP monitoring.[12] CT often demonstrated retained bone

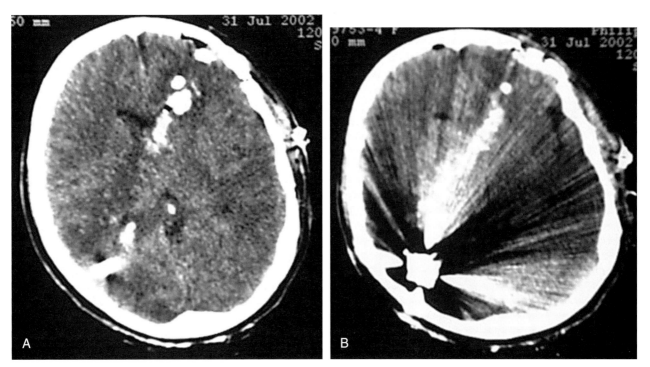

FIGURE 7-4   This 27-year-old female student, injured in a bomb blast inside a university cafeteria, had a GCS score of 7 on admission. The patient suffered a bihemispheric penetrating brain injury with transventricular trajectory (*A*). The projectile is lodged in the right parietal region (*B*). Blood is seen along the tract. The patient underwent surgical débridement and aggressive management of intracranial pressure (ICP), with measures including ventricular drainage and thiopental coma. Despite these efforts, the ICP rose on the third postinjury day above 70 mm Hg, and the patient expired on postinjury day 13.

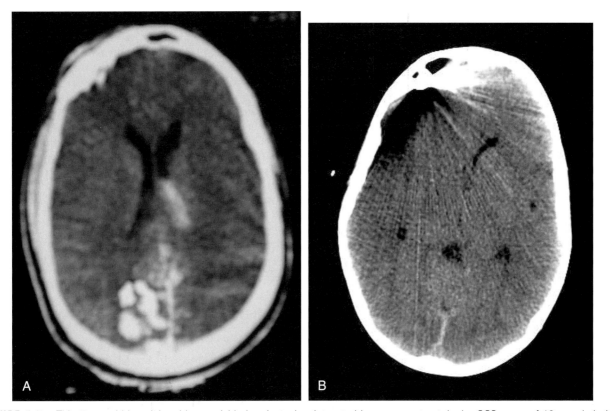

FIGURE 7-5   This 7-year-old boy, injured by a suicide bomber who detonated in an open street, had a GCS score of 12 on admission. Noncontrast CT reveals a penetrating injury with entrance in the right occipital region and hemorrhagic contusion of the calcarine cortex and white matter (*A*). A metal hexagonal nut is lodged in the ipsilateral frontal lobe (*B*). With ventricular drainage to help manage elevated ICP, the patient regained consciousness after 3 days. He had a transient left hemiparesis and sustained a permanent right homonymous hemianopsia. He underwent elective removal of the metal nut a year later and returned to normal function.

fragments, which were not pursued. This approach did not lead to an increase in the rate of infectious complications (8%) above accepted norms, nor was there any correlation between retained bone fragments and epilepsy.[12] Long-term follow-up from the Vietnam Head Injury Study (VHIS) helped clarify the issue. In an analysis of 1221 patients, only 37 cases of brain abscess were documented.[10] Although 11 of these patients had retained bone fragments, in all these cases additional risk factors for infection (e.g., CSF fistula, wound complications, air sinus injuries, or multiple surgical procedures) were present. Data from the VHIS also failed to find a relationship between retained bone fragments and epilepsy.[11] Based on these findings, we recommend that only easily accessible bone fragments should be removed at surgery, and that no potentially viable brain tissue be sacrificed to pursue distant fragments.

DURAL SINUS INJURIES

Injury to the dural sinus remains one of the most concerning injuries to the neurosurgeon treating penetrating head trauma. When an injury occurs in proximity to the midline of the cranial vault or the torcular Herophili, a high level of suspicion of dural sinus injury must be maintained. Digital exploration of the wound should be avoided, because this may exacerbate bleeding from the sinus by dislodging any tamponading fragments. When a venous sinus is injured, profuse bleeding may emanate from the wound; this should be treated immediately by a compressive bandage and elevation of the head to 30 degrees. CT is obtained as in all cases of PBI, and will often reveal either a foreign body or in-driven bone fragments adjacent to or perforating the sinus. Alternatively, the tract of a missile may transverse the sinus. Subdural blood often accompanies this injury. Before proceeding to the operating theater, preparations need to be made for the possibility of a massive hemorrhage. Blood products, including packed red blood cells and fresh frozen plasma, should be on hand in the operating room. The basic surgical approach is not different from that previously described for all penetrating injuries. Until good exposure has been achieved, the point of laceration of the dura should not be disturbed,[78] nor should any fragment already tamponading the injured sinus be removed. When the injury is bleeding actively, hemostasis can often be achieved by placing gelfoam and a brain cottonoid over the injured site. When the injury is more extensive, repair of the sinus may be necessary. The sinus should be clipped with a temporary vascular clip proximally and distally. This allows for a tear to be identified and repaired. When primary repair is possible, this is the preferred option. When the injury to the sinus is more extensive, a periosteal or muscle graft may be sutured into place to repair the defect.[79] If the injury involves only the anterior third of the superior sagittal sinus, ligation may be considered as an option, because the risks of reconstruction may outweigh the benefits. Reconstruction of the sinus with a vein graft or a silastic tube has been described[80] and may be necessary in cases of transection along the posterior two thirds of the superior sagittal sinus. However, the difficulty of performing such an operation under the challenging conditions of a penetrating injury should not be underestimated. The short-term patency of these grafts may be affected by the difficulty of

anticoagulating the PBI patient immediately after injury, and little information exists regarding the long-term patency of these grafts.

POSTOPERATIVE MANAGEMENT

The patient with PBI will require intensive care postoperatively in a neurosurgical or general ICU setting. Attention must be maintained to adequate oxygenation and stability of the blood pressure. This is especially important in the patient with multisystem injury. During the initial post-injury period, the intubated patient should be kept on adequate sedation with morphine, midazolam, or propofol. Sedation should only be stopped briefly on a once-daily basis to assess the neurologic status, and not at all when contraindicated as in the patient with severe respiratory failure or unstable ICP.

Treatment of elevated ICP in PBI patients includes moderate hyperventilation; CSF drainage; mannitol; hypertonic saline; and, in cases of refractory hypertension, barbiturate coma. These measures are the same as in nonpenetrating TBI. Questions remain whether the underlying physiologic measures responsible for ICP elevation are the same in PBI as opposed to nonpenetrating TBI. It has been suggested that failure of cerebral autoregulation plays an important role in the etiology of elevated ICP early after PBI.[72] Studies of effective treatment regimes for elevated ICP in PBI and their effect on outcome are yet to be done.

Coagulopathy is a concern following penetrating head injury. Risk factors for development of coagulopathy include the extent of brain injury,[61] massive blood loss in the multi-system-injured patient, acidosis, and hypothermia. Patients at risk should have fibrinogen levels, fibrin split products, and D dimers checked, in addition to routine studies of prothrombin time, activated partial thromboplastin time, and platelet count. The presence of disseminated intravascular coagulation (DIC) has been shown to be associated with risk of delayed intracranial hemorrhage, and it may impair hemostasis intraoperatively.[81] In the patient with DIC, plasma factors should be replaced until correction of the coagulation parameters is achieved. Recent reports have suggested that recombinant Factor VIIa (rFactor VIIa) may be efficacious in stabilizing patients with exsanguinating hemorrhage.[82–84] However, the published literature regarding the use of rFactor VIIa to correct coagulopathy in the neurosurgical population is limited.[85] Concerns exist, including thrombosis (most ominously, of the venous sinuses),[86] and caution is indicated until further studies are carried out.

POST-TRAUMATIC COMPLICATIONS
CSF Leakage

The variable most highly correlated with infection is acute or delayed CSF leakage. This has been corroborated by several authors, including Arendall and Meirowsky's evaluation of casualties from the Korean War.[54] Brandvold and colleagues reported the same finding in analyzing data from the Israeli experience in Lebanon,[12] as did Aarabi and colleagues in their experience with casualties from the Iran-Iraq War.[42] Meirowsky and colleagues,[53] analyzing data from the

Vietnam conflict, documented a 49.5% incidence of infection in patients who leaked CSF, as opposed to a rate of 4.6% in those who did not. Only half of patients experienced leaks from the wound site; the remainder had rhinorrhea or otorrhea from base-of-skull fractures or air sinus injury. Mortality in patients who leaked CSF was 22.8%, compared with 4.6% in those who did not leak. A majority (72%) of leaks appeared within 2 weeks after injury. The prompt treatment of CSF fistula is imperative. CSF drainage by ventricular or lumbar catheter is the first option. If there is a persistent leak from the skull base, craniotomy may be required. Preoperative imaging with thin-slice CT with intrathecal contrast media and coronal reconstructions is often helpful in defining the site of bony defect.[87,88] When not contraindicated by retained ferromagnetic fragments, MRI may also help to identify the site of CSF leakage.[89] An extradural search for the site of dural injury and bony defect is then undertaken. Primary dural repair is often not feasible; when it is not, options include placing a vascularized periosteal flap, plugging of the bony defect with fat or muscle together with fibrin glue, and oversewing the dura with a fascial graft. Unless contraindicated, patients should have a lumbar drain maintained for several days postoperatively.

Migration of Intracranial Fragments

Intracerebral migration of a metallic fragment is a rare complication of penetrating head injury.[90,91] When migration through the brain parenchyma occurs, neurologic deterioration may result.[92,93] Crossing of the midline has also been reported.[93] If migration has been documented, removal of the offending fragment is indicated to prevent further injury. Our preliminary experience suggests that neuronavigation systems are useful in planning the surgical approach to remove retained metallic fragments that have migrated.[73]

In the rare case when a fragment is lodged within the ventricular system, the risk of migration is high[94] and may lead to obstructive hydrocephalus.[95] Removal of such a fragment is warranted and may be assisted by judicious positioning of the patient preoperatively so that the fragment lodges in the occipital horn of the lateral ventricle.[94]

Post-traumatic Cerebrovascular Lesions

In PBI the vasculature may be damaged either directly by the projectile, or by shearing forces generated by the pressure wave of the expanding and contracting temporary cavity. In most cases a traumatic pseudoaneurysm results from complete disruption of the arterial wall with periarterial hematoma formation. In these false aneurysms, the defect is bound only by hematoma, fibrin, and surrounding brain tissue. In rare cases, a true traumatic intracranial aneurysm results from partial damage to the arterial wall. The incidence of post-traumatic intracranial aneurysms (TICA) in PBI is uncertain. Rates of incidence in penetrating missile wounds are reported between 3% and 8%.[16,96–98] The rate of vascular injury in stab wounds is much higher, and approached 35% in large series from South Africa.[66,99] These will be discussed in a following section. In PBI, traumatic aneurysms typically occur along the vessel's length and not at the bifurcation (as in berry aneurysms).

Most typically they occur along branches of the middle or anterior cerebral arteries, or the supraclinoid carotid artery[16,100] (Fig. 7-6). Angiogram is the diagnostic study of choice, and the varying reported rates of TICA may depend in part on the timing of the angiogram. There is no consensus regarding the optimal timing of angiography. Although some authors advocate angiography in the immediate postinjury period,[97] others note that these lesions may only become angiographically and clinically evident much longer after the initial insult.[100] Certainly, a negative angiogram performed soon after injury does not rule out the development of a TICA. If vessel spasm is noted on the angiogram, the study should be repeated because vasospasm may hide a vascular lesion. The clinician must maintain a high index of suspicion for post-traumatic vascular injury in PBI. Any patient who develops a delayed intracerebral or subarachnoid hemorrhage or has otherwise unexplained neurologic deterioration must be suspected of harboring a TICA. In cases where the projectile crosses two dural compartments, or involves the facial, orbital, or pterional regions, a higher rate of TICA has been reported.[96] We perform angiography in all such cases. Post-traumatic aneurysms have a high rate of repeat hemorrhage.[16,100] The rate of mortality in untreated post-traumatic aneurysms has been reported to be as high as 41%.[101] When a TICA is diagnosed, prompt therapy is indicated. The goal is exclusion of the lesion from the circulation. Today, we consider endovascular therapy an excellent first-line therapeutic option. In the rare case of a true aneurysm, coiling of the lesion will be possible (Fig. 7-7). In most cases, the TICA will need to be trapped either by endovascular coils or surgically. Most patients will tolerate the sacrifice of a distal branch of the middle or anterior cerebral artery, but in some cases a bypass procedure will be required.[102,103] When surgery is performed, proximal control is crucial because these lesions have a tendency to rupture and dissection may be difficult in the injured brain. As in standard aneurysmal surgery, the use of a cerebral protectant is useful.

CRANIOPLASTY

The patient with penetrating head injury will often have a bony deficit, ranging from a small entry site wound to a large skull defect. When the defect is large or presents a cosmetic deformity, a cranioplasty will need to be performed after the patient has recovered from the initial injury. In young children and infants, a growing skull fracture may result from a penetrating or tangential wound (Fig. 7-8). In general, we recommend waiting at least 3 months from the time of injury to the repair of a bony deficit to reduce the risk of infectious complications. By this time, the patient will usually have recovered from the initial injury and will be in better medical condition to undergo repeat surgery. In cases where a large bone flap is removed during initial surgery, it may be sterilized and preserved. When the patient is ready for cranioplasty, the original bone flap, after repeat sterilization, will usually achieve the best biologic and cosmetic result. Even in cases where bone has been fragmented, a good result can usually be attained with fixation of the fragments. When the autologous bone is unavailable, an adequate prosthesis can be made of methyl methacrylate and molded to fit the defect.

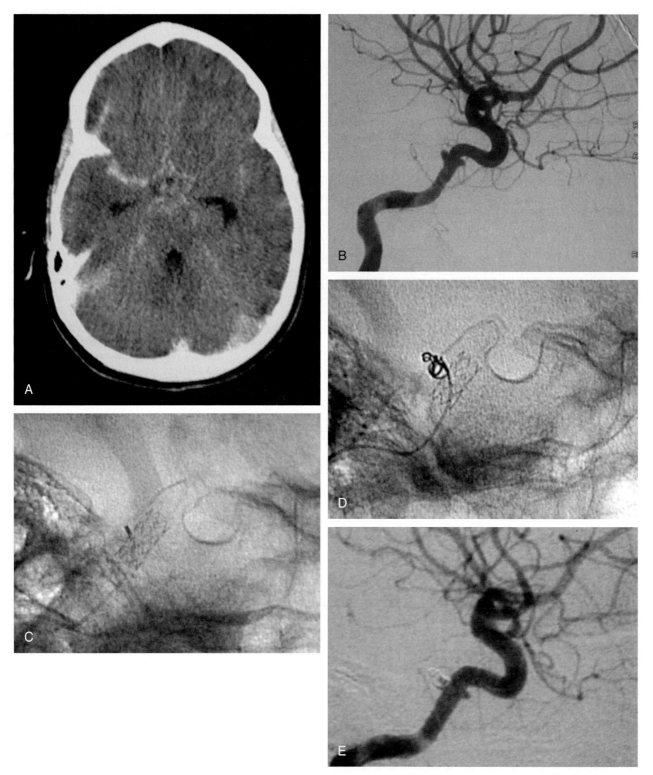

FIGURE 7-6   Penetrating injury of the intracavernous carotid artery in a 5-year-old child caused by an umbrella. Admission noncontrast CT demonstrates subarachnoid blood and mildly enlarged temporal horns (*A*). The angiogram reveals a carotid blowout syndrome (*B*). A fenestrated stent introduced by femoral catheterization allows passage of the microcatheter to the pseudoaneurysm (*C*) and embolization with detachable platinum coils (*D*), resulting in successful occlusion (*E*).

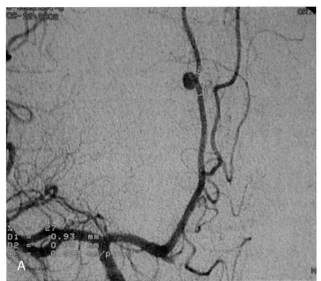

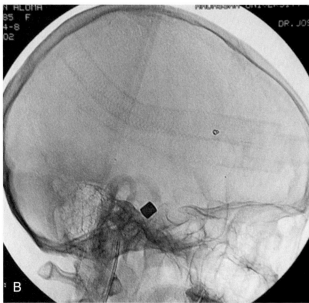

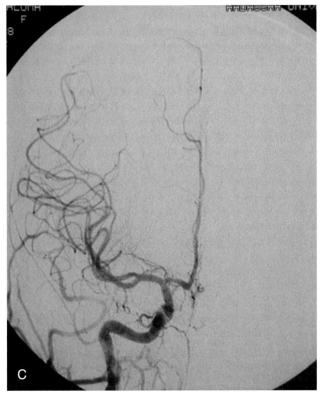

FIGURE 7-7   This 17-year-old female was injured by a suicide bomber who detonated inside a bus. The path of projectile crossed the midline. An angiogram was obtained and demonstrated a traumatic intracranial aneurysm of the pericallosal artery (*A*). The aneurysm was obliterated by embolization with detachable platinum coils through superselective catheterization (*B*). The projectile is seen lodged in the middle fossa floor. Post-treatment angiogram reveals successful obliteration of the aneurysm (*C*).

BOMB BLAST INJURIES

Penetrating head injuries from bomb blasts combine the effects of blast injury with penetrating shrapnel wounds. When a bomb is detonated, the transformation of a solid explosive into gas generates a highly pressurized wave of air that propagates radially from the site of the explosion at high speed, and this is followed by a wave of negative pressure.[104] A "blast front" is generated by the leading front of this massive air movement. The forces generated may be tremendous. As an example, a charge of 25 kg of TNT will result in a blast front with a 150 psi peak overpressure for 2 msec traveling at 3000 to 8000 m/second.[104]

Little experimental work has been done on the effects of blast on the brain. In a dog model of overpressure injury, perivascular hemorrhages were noted throughout the brain.[105] Our experience with terrorist bomb blasts, as well as the experiences of others[17,106] indicate that these injuries combine aspects of closed head injury, caused by blast effect, with penetrating injuries from shrapnel. The extent of injury will depend on a number of factors including the explosive power of the bomb, the distance of the injured patient from the site of detonation, the nature of the space in which the explosion occurred (closed or open), and the nature of the shrapnel within the bomb. The penetrating objects are likely comparable to low-velocity projectiles, at least in the

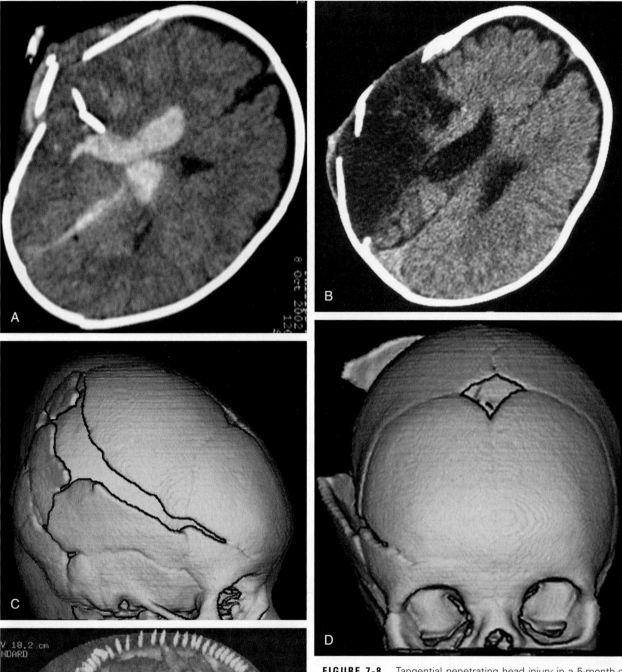

FIGURE 7-8 Tangential penetrating head injury in a 5-month-old child caused by a rubber bullet that produced a deep, in-driven bone fragment; brain laceration; and an intraventricular hematoma, as demonstrated on preoperative noncontrast CT (*A*). Emergency craniotomy with surgical débridement and removal of the in-driven bone fragment was performed. The unsuccessful dural repair and porencephaly communicating with the ventricle are demonstrated in a follow-up CT (*B*). Two months later, a growing skull fracture is noted in the CT with 3-dimensional reconstruction (*C, D*). A cranioplasty was performed using the bone fragments fixed with reabsorbable craniofix discs and placement of a cystoperitoneal shunt (*E*).

survivors who reach medical attention. Often, however, the relatively large mass of objects placed within terrorist bombs (bolts weighing up to 25 g have been recorded by our group) are a factor in enhancing tissue damage. Certainly, when a bomb is detonated in a closed space, injuries tend to be more severe and mortality is higher.[104]

Our experience with 23 patients with PBI sustained from terrorist bomb blasts treated over a 3-year period is summarized in the following. A variety of objects (e.g., ball bearings, metal bolts, hexagonal nuts, segments of metal rods, and nails [Fig. 7-9]) were placed in these bombs to maximize damage and penetrate the skull. The objects with larger mass often inflict greater damage within the brain and to the vasculature, and these may migrate within the brain parenchyma. The initial presentation of these patients is varied. In our series, 3 patients presented with a GCS score of 3 to 5, 6 patients presented with a GCS score of 6 to 9, 5 patients presented with a GCS score of 10 to 12, and 9 patients had a GCS score of 13 to 15. The initial surgical management of these injuries is the same as for other penetrating brain injuries, as described previously. Monitoring of the intracranial pressure is an important part of the management of these patients. In our series, mean ICP at insertion was 22.5 mm Hg, whereas peak ICP ranged from 12 to 70 and averaged 33.5 mm Hg. When elevations in ICP do not respond to treatment measures, prognosis is grim. Conversely, patients who respond well to therapy to decrease ICP can have good outcomes. Drainage of bloody CSF via ventriculostomy plays an important role in managing patients with intraventricular hemorrhage (Fig. 7-10). In our series, 3 patients died whereas 20 survived. Among the survivors, functional outcome as defined by the Glasgow Outcome Scale (GOS)[107] was generally good. Twelve patients achieved a GOS score of 5, 7 a GOS score of 4, and 1 patient had a GOS score of 3. In our series, 2 patients had documented migration of a metallic fragment as exemplified in Figure 7-11. Two patients developed a traumatic intracranial aneurysm. In the patients with documented migration,

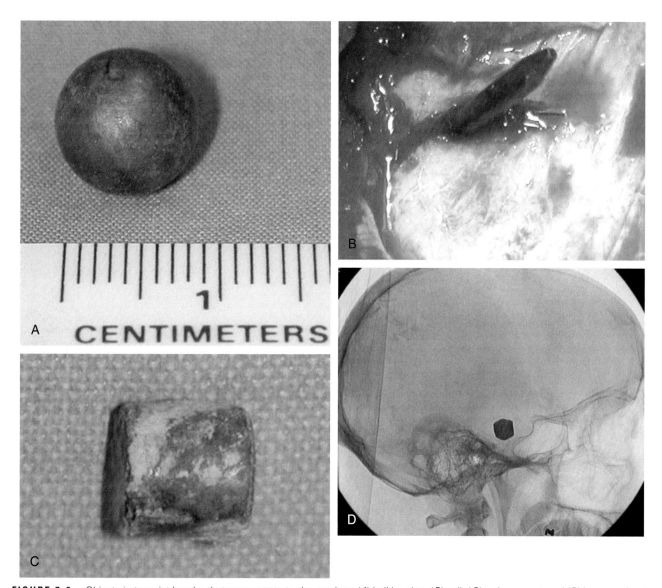

FIGURE 7-9   Objects in terrorist bombs that may penetrate the cranium: (A) ball bearing, (B) nail, (C) rod segment, and (D) hexagonal nut.

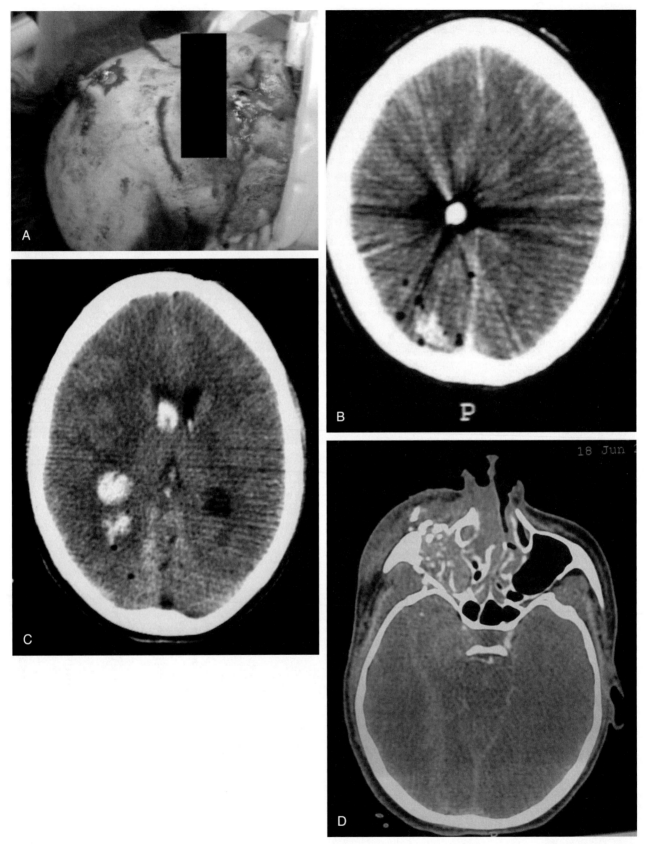

FIGURE 7-10   A 30-year-old female, injured by a suicide bomber who detonated inside a bus, GCS score of 7 on admission. Brain is seen extruding from a right frontal entry wound (*A*). Noncontrast CT demonstrates a metal ball bearing in the centrum semiovale (*B*), intracerebral and intraventricular hemorrhage (*C*), and injury to the maxillary sinus (*D*).

(Continued)

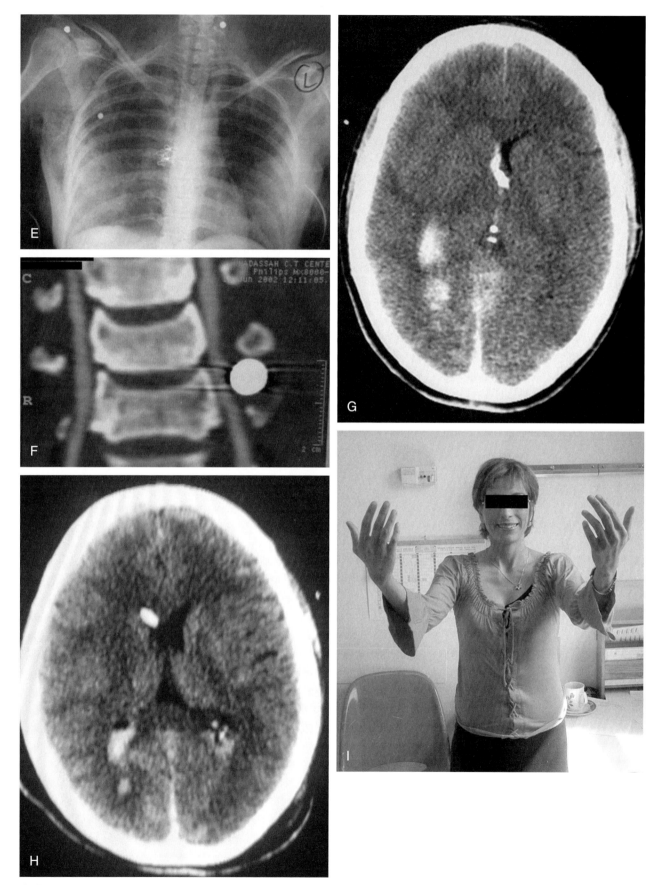

FIGURE 7-10 Cont'd   Chest x-ray reveals three ball bearings, one at the level of the left C5–6 foramen intertransversarium (*E*). CT-angiography with coronal reconstruction demonstrates close proximity of the ball bearing to the vertebral artery, but no impingement on the vessel (*F*). The patient was treated with surgical débridement and intraventricular drainage (*G*). One day postinjury CT demonstrates initial clearing of intraventricular blood (*H*). The patient did well (*I*) without removal of the ball bearings, which did not migrate in follow-up studies.

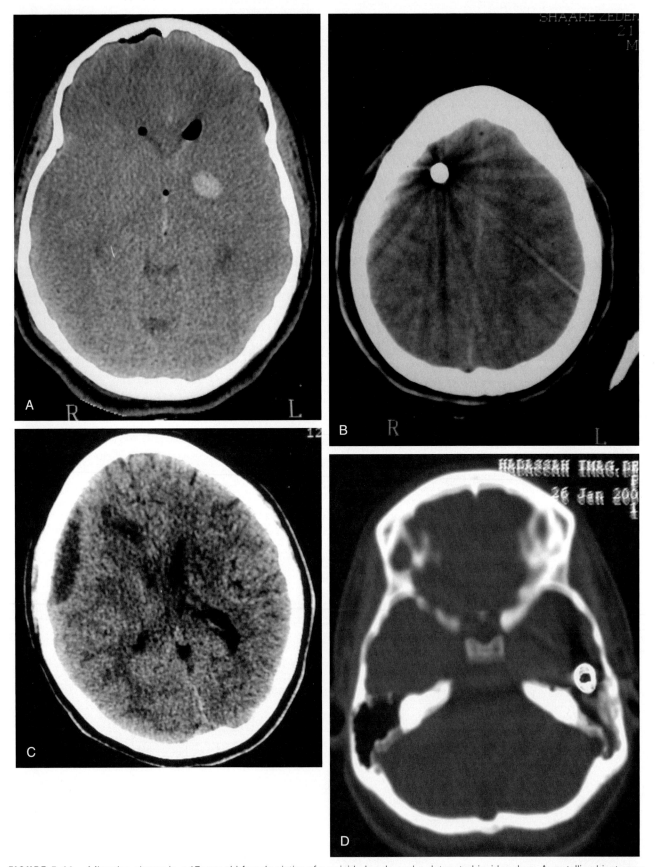

FIGURE 7-11   Migration shown in a 17-year-old female victim of a suicide bomber who detonated inside a bus. A metallic object penetrated through the left temporal squama, crossing to the contralateral hemisphere and lodging in the right frontal lobe as demonstrated on CT (*A*). Blood is seen in the left basal ganglia and air in the frontal horns (*B*). The patient was treated with surgical débridement and ventricular drainage and did well. One week later, a follow-up CT demonstrated a right subdural collection and a porencephalic cavity where the metal fragment had been located previously (*C*). Further images from the CT study reveal the metallic object in the floor of the left temporal fossa, close to the entry wound, just anterior to the tragus (*D*).

as well as in 2 others in which a large metallic fragment was accessible and was deemed to pose a potential risk, we removed these with the aid of an image-guided surgical navigation system (Fig. 7-12). In the 4 patients who underwent this operation, outcome was excellent without new neurologic deficits or other complications.

CRANIAL STAB WOUNDS

Stab wounds to the cranium are injuries caused with a weapon with a smaller impact area and wielded at low velocity in comparison with missile injuries.[66] Although knives are by far the most common weapon in assaults, even objects as innocuous as a pencil[108,109] or a sewing needle may penetrate the cranium.[110] The orbit is a common site for penetration into the cranial vault, especially in children[109,111,112] (Fig. 7-13). Because less kinetic energy is transmitted by a stab weapon, the injury is usually limited to the site of penetration. The site of penetration, its depth, and its trajectory are important factors in determining the extent of damage. Intracerebral hematoma and vascular injury are a common result. In two large series from South Africa, rates of vascular injury were between 31% and 35%.[66,99] Most often the patient will present with the weapon removed prior to arrival to a medical facility[66] (Fig. 7-14). In all cases, the radiologic evaluation should begin with a plain x-ray of the skull and CT. Both will demonstrate the characteristic "slot" fracture associated with a stab wound. CT will provide information regarding the extent and location of intracerebral hematoma, subarachnoid hemorrhage, and in-driven bone fragments. When the weapon is still embedded in the skull, angiography is essential[113,114] and should be obtained prior to any attempted removal. Approximately one third of patients will have a vascular injury.[99] In all cases, care must be taken in the removal of the penetrating object, because vigorous manipulation will often increase the damage to brain structures. Removal should only be performed in the operating theater[66,99,114] after the scalp incision and bone flap are completed. Cross-matched blood should be available in the operating room. The trajectory of removal must follow precisely that of the weapon's entry. In other respects, surgical management is similar to that for missile injuries, with débridement of the tract, removal of any hematomas or accessible bone chips, and watertight closure of the dura. In a large series of 330 patients, du Trevou and van Dellen[66] demonstrated the utility of early angiography in cranial stab wounds, and concluded that there is no advantage to delaying angiography as others had advocated.[99] The information gained from the angiogram can be utilized to achieve primary repair of the vascular lesion during the initial surgery or to expedite endovascular therapy. This is of paramount importance, given the high rates of mortality associated with a secondary bleed from a traumatic vascular lesion.[66]

Outcomes

Reported outcomes differ between civilian and military series, and will be considered separately. The most epidemiologically accurate data on civilian gunshot injuries has been reported by Siccardi and colleagues,[115] because they included all gunshot victims in their series, including those who expired at the scene. Patients who died underwent autopsy so that data were obtained concerning the extent of brain injury. Revealingly, 73% of patients died before reaching the hospital, and another 12% died within 3 hours of injury. All other civilian series reporting outcomes refer only to patients who survived to reach the emergency room, and their results must be viewed in the light of Siccardi's important findings. In recent series of civilian penetrating brain injuries, mortality rates varied from 51% to 75%.[50,58,60–62] Rates of mortality appear higher in self-inflicted injuries than in assaults, in most series.[50,60,61,115,116] Though rates of mortality are high in PBI, favorable outcome in survivors, defined as good recovery or moderate disability, is common (74%).[117]

In wartime reports, rates of mortality vary and may partly be related to transport times from the site of injury to a neurosurgically equipped facility. Presumably, long transport times bias data in the direction of decreased mortality, because many severely injured patients die in transit. In data from the Iran-Iraq war, as reported by Aarabi,[14] transport times averaged 49 hours. Mortality was 16% at 6 months. Good outcome was attained in 79% of patients in this series. In data from the Lebanon conflict, where median transport time from injury to tertiary-care facility averaged 2 hours, overall mortality was 26%.[12] Good outcome was reported in 62% of patients. In this report, as well as in data from the Vietnam conflict,[118] gunshot wounds to the head resulted in higher rates of mortality when compared with shrapnel injuries.

Important factors influencing outcome in both military and civilian head injuries include postresuscitation GCS score, age, and initial CT findings. The postresuscitation GCS score is perhaps the single most consistent factor among studies that is shown to influence outcome. Patients with a postresuscitation GCS score of 3 to 5 have extremely high rates of mortality in reported civilian series.[50,60,61,67,115,119] Reported rates of recovery, including moderate disability, have ranged from 0% to 9% in this group.[50,60,61,115,119] In fact, some authors have questioned the rationale for aggressive intervention in these patients, given the dismal prognosis.[60] The mortality rate of patients with a GCS score of 3 to 5 is high in military series as well.[12,14] In contradistinction, patients with postresuscitation GCS scores of 6 to 8 have outcomes from good recovery to moderate disability in 13% to 52% of cases, whereas those presenting with GCS score of 9 to 15 attain this result in 56% to 100% of cases, according to the published civilian literature.[50,60,61,115,119] The influence of age on outcome in PBI is less clear. Two studies demonstrate worse outcomes in patients over 49 years of age,[61,115] but in other reports no statistically significant relationship was found between age and outcome.[51,62]

The findings on initial CT scan are also correlated with outcome. Factors which have been reported to be associated with poor outcome include bihemispheric injury,[50,58,60–64] multilobar injury,[12,50,51,57,115] transventricular trajectory,[12] and intraventricular hemorrhage.[61,64] These are often devastating injuries. Siccardi and colleagues' data,[115] which included postmortem analysis of patients who died before CT could be performed, reported a mortality of 92% and 98% in patients with bihemispheric injuries and

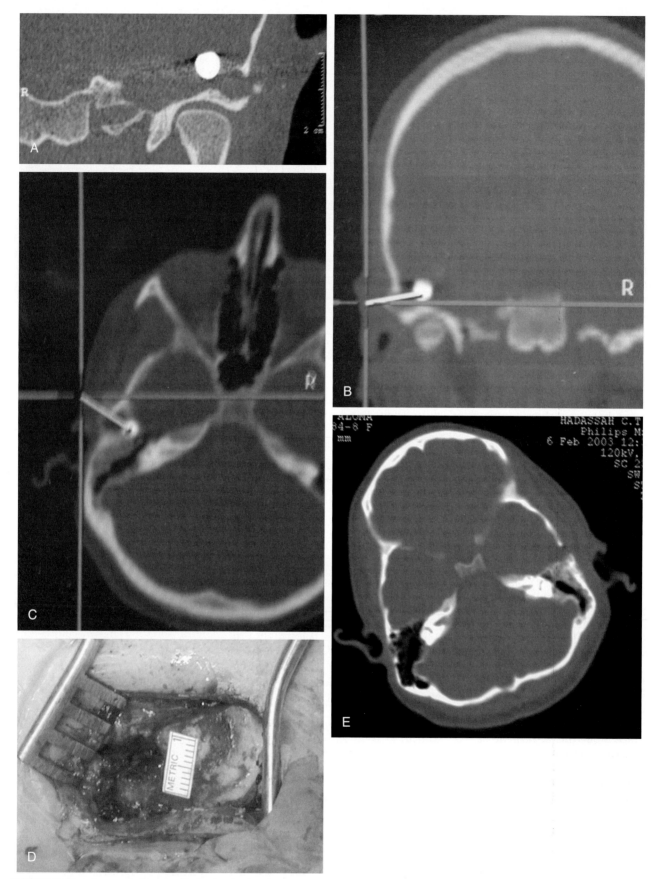

FIGURE 7-12   Removal of a metallic foreign body with the assistance of an intraoperative surgical navigation system in a 17-year-old female victim of a suicide bomber who detonated inside a bus (see Fig. 7-11). A coronal CT image demonstrates that the metallic object has migrated to the entry site in the middle temporal fossa just above the temporomandibular joint (*A*). Surgical planning with a navigation system (*B, C*), and exposure at surgery (*D*). Postoperative CT demonstrates the minimally invasive nature of the surgery (*E*). The removed object, a metal rod segment, is shown in Figure 7-9*C*. The patient has returned to normal function without neurologic deficit.

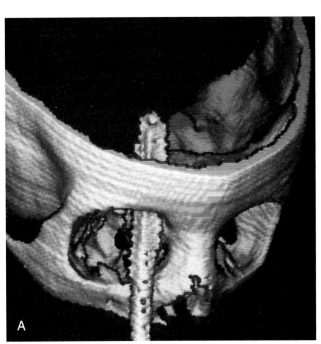
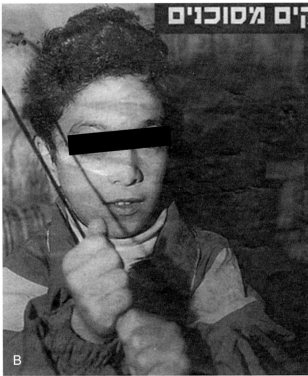

FIGURE 7-13   Three-dimensional reconstruction of the CT scan of a 6-year-old child with a skewer penetrating the frontal lobe through the orbit medial to the eye (*A*). Postoperative picture with the child holding the skewer (*B*).

intraventricular blood, respectively. Subarachnoid hemorrhage is another factor reported as a correlate of unfavorable outcome.[120] The presence of intracerebral hemorrhage has not been shown to be associated with worsened outcome.[12,120]

PLANNING FOR MASS CASUALTY SCENARIOS

It is our opinion that all secondary and tertiary care facilities with neurosurgical service should plan for the eventuality of a mass casualty event that may occur because of natural disaster, large-scale accidents, or terrorist incidents. When these occur, the strains on the medical system, including prehospital personnel, the medical staff, and the community in general, are enormous. Preparedness will often make a crucial difference in ensuring optimal care. The neurosurgeon needs to be involved in the advanced planning for these scenarios because, even under optimal circumstances in a tertiary care facility, the resources available to the neurosurgical department are inherently limited. The full scope of disaster preparedness is certainly beyond the scope of this chapter, but some useful caveats may be summarized.

When a mass casualty event occurs, the first step is to alert all available neurosurgical personnel to ensure their availability. Often the hospital has a disaster plan that may be activated at such a time. However, system failure under intense strain may occur, and it is prudent for the neurosurgical team to have a plan by which the neurosurgeon on call can easily contact the other team members in such

an eventuality. In a disaster with large numbers of casualties, triage plays a crucial role. The initial evaluation and triage as patients arrive at the emergency room is often made by the senior general surgeon or emergency room physician. A neurosurgeon needs to be on hand at this point, both to help guide appropriate triage of patients and to direct the resources of the neurosurgical team to the patients with head injury. The difficulty in ascertaining which patients have a significant head injury, let alone its severity, in a situation in which patients arrive in rapid succession to an emergency room strained to capacity, needs to be anticipated. As patients are being stabilized, the neurosurgical team will need to decide which casualties need to be taken to CT and in what priority. All information should be reported back to the initial triaging neurosurgeon so that he or she can continue to direct resources appropriately.

The next triage step, from the neurosurgical point of view, will usually occur at the CT scanner. In our experience, it is useful to have the most senior neurosurgeon available at this site because decisions regarding which patients proceed to the operating theater and in what order must be taken there. An appropriate neurosurgical team is then selected for each operation. A "second wave" of casualties from other medical facilities without neurosurgical capabilities needs to be anticipated, because patients are often triaged in the field or are taken to the nearest medical facility for stabilization (Fig. 7-15). Only by close cooperation with other specialties and thorough planning within the neurosurgical department can optimal care be achieved.

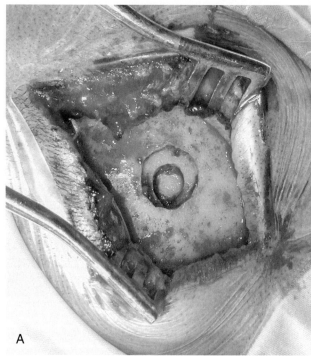

A

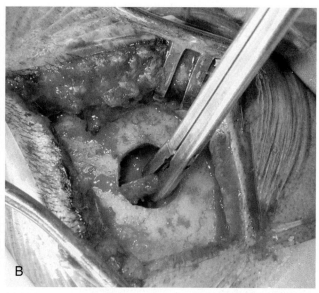

B

FIGURE 7-14   Circular depressed fracture resulting from an assault with a metal rod (*A*). Elevation (*B*) and repositioning (*C*) of the bone fragment.

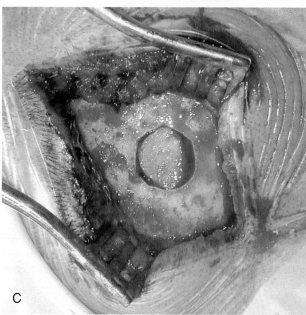

C

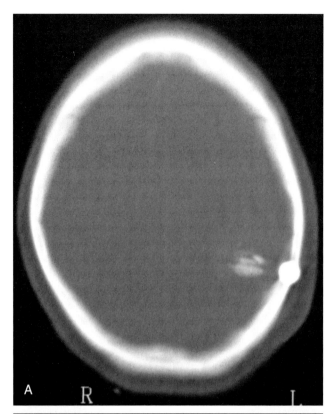

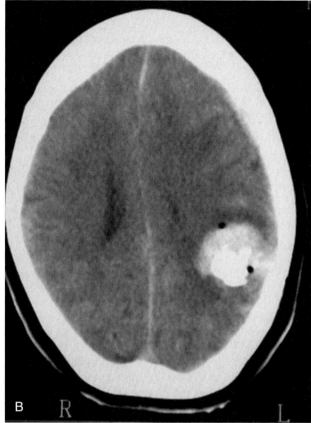

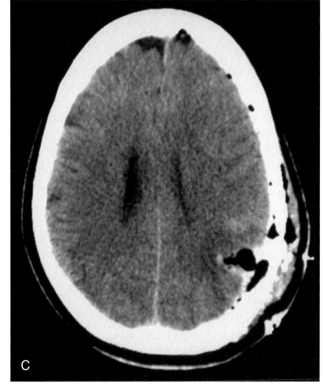

FIGURE 7-15 This 40-year-old woman was injured by a suicide bomber who detonated inside a bus. She was found at the scene with a GCS score of 15 and no overt signs of cranial injury and was transported to a hospital without neurosurgical facilities. CT scan with bone window reveals a round metal object lodged in the cranium, barely penetrating the inner table of the skull; secondary missiles in the form of fine bony fragments penetrate the brain (*A*). The CT demonstrates an intracerebral hematoma with mass effect (*B*). Following craniotomy and dural repair (*C*), the patient did well. The metal object was a ball bearing and is shown in Figure 7-9*A*.

REFERENCES

1. de Villiers J: The management of missile injuries of the head during the Anglo-Boer War. Br J Neurosurg 1:53–61, 1987.
2. Cushing H: A study of a series of wounds involving the brain and its enveloping structures. Br J Surg 5:558–684, 1918.
3. Cushing H: Notes on penetrating wounds of the brain. BMJ 1:221–226, 1918.
4. Slemon H: Forward neurosurgery in Italy. J Neurosurg 2:332–339, 1945.
5. Haynes W: Penetrating brain wounds: Analysis of 342 cases. J Neurosurg 2:365–378, 1945.
6. Martin J, Campbell E: Early complications following penetrating wounds of the skull. J Neurosurg 2:58–73, 1946.
7. Munslow R: Penetrating head wounds: Experiences from the Italian campaign. Ann Surg 123:180–189, 1946.

8. Lewin W: Missile head wounds in the Korean campaign: A survey of British casualties. Br J Surg 43:628–632, 1956.

9. Hammon W: Analysis of 2187 consecutive penetrating wounds of the brain in Vietnam. J Neurosurg 34:127–131, 1971.

10. Rish BL, Caveness WF, Dillon JD, et al: Analysis of brain abscess after penetrating craniocerebral injuries in Vietnam. Neurosurgery 9(5):535–541, 1981.

11. Salazar AM, Jabbari B, Vance SC, et al: Epilepsy after penetrating head injury. I: Clinical correlates: A report of the Vietnam Head Injury Study. Neurology 35(10):1406–1414, 1985.

12. Brandvold B, Levi L, Feinsod M, et al: Penetrating craniocerebral injuries in the Israeli involvement in the Lebanese conflict, 1982–1985: Analysis of a less aggressive surgical approach. J Neurosurg 72(1):15–21, 1990.

13. Levi L, Borovich B, Guilburd JN, et al: Wartime neurosurgical experience in Lebanon, 1982–1985. I: Penetrating craniocerebral injuries. Isr J Med Sci 26(10):548–554, 1990.

14. Aarabi B: Surgical outcome in 435 patients who sustained missile head wounds during the Iran-Iraq War. Neurosurgery 27:692–695, 1990.

15. Aarabi B: Causes of infections in penetrating head wounds in the Iran-Iraq War. Neurosurgery 25(6):923–926, 1989.

16. Aarabi B: Traumatic aneurysms of brain due to high velocity missile head wounds. Neurosurgery 22(6 Pt 1):1056–1063, 1988.

17. Levi L, Borovich B, Guilburd JN, et al: Wartime neurosurgical experience in Lebanon, 1982–1985. II: Closed craniocerebral injuries. Isr J Med Sci 26(10):555–558, 1990.

18. Hopkinson DA, Marshall TK: Firearm injuries. Br J Surg 54(5): 344–353, 1967.

19. Fackler ML: Gunshot wound review. Ann Emerg Med 28(2):194–203, 1996.

20. Dagi T, George E: Surgical management of penetrating missile injuries of the head. In Schmidek H, Sweet W (eds): Operative Neurosurgical Techniques, Indications, Methods, and Results, 3rd ed. Philadelphia: WB Saunders, 1995.

21. Cooper GJ, Ryan JM: Interaction of penetrating missiles with tissues: Some common misapprehensions and implications for wound management. Br J Surg 77(6):606–610, 1990.

22. Allen IV, Scott R, Tanner JA: Experimental high-velocity missile head injury. Injury 14(2):183–193, 1982.

23. Harvey E, Butler E, McMillen J, et al: Mechanisms of wounding. War Med 8:91–104, 1945.

24. Fackler ML, Bellamy RF, Malinowski JA: The wound profile: Illustration of the missile-tissue interaction. J Trauma 28(1 Suppl): S21–S29, 1988.

25. Carey M: Experimental missile wounding of the brain. In Levy M, Apuzzo M (eds): Neurosurgery Clinics of North America, vol 6. Penetrating Craniocerebral Injuries: Spectrum of Injury and Methods of Salvageability. Philadelphia: WB Saunders, 1995.

26. Carey ME, Sarna GS, Farrell JB, et al: Experimental missile wound to the brain. J Neurosurg 71(5 Pt 1):754–764, 1989.

27. Rosenberg W, Harsh G IV: Penetrating wounds of the head. In Wilkins R, Rengachary S (eds): Neurosurgery, 2nd ed. New York: McGraw-Hill, 1996.

28. Crockard H, Brown F, Calica A, et al: Physiological consequences of experimental cerebral missile injury and use of data analysis to predict survival. J Neurosurg 46:784–794, 1977.

29. Levett JM, Johns LM, Replogle RL, et al: Cardiovascular effects of experimental cerebral missile injury in primates. Surg Neurol 13(1):59–64, 1980.

30. Webster J, Gurdjian E: Acute physiological effects of gunshot and other penetrating wounds of the brain. J Neurophysiol 6:255–263, 1943.

31. Kennedy FR, Gonzalez P, Beitler A, et al: Incidence of cervical spine injury in patients with gunshot wounds to the head. South Med J 87(6):621–623, 1994.

32. Teasdale G, Jennett B: Assessment of coma and impaired consciousness: A practical scale. Lancet 2(7872):81–84, 1974.

33. Caveness WF, Meirowsky AM, Rish BL, et al: The nature of posttraumatic epilepsy. J Neurosurg 50(5):545–553, 1979.

34. Annegers JF, Hauser WA, Coan SP, et al: A population-based study of seizures after traumatic brain injuries. N Engl J Med 338(1):20–24, 1998.

35. Glotzner FL, Haubitz I, Miltner F, et al: Seizure prevention using carbamazepine following severe brain injuries. Neurochirurgia (Stuttg) 26(3):66–79, 1983.

36. Temkin NR, Dikmen SS, Wilensky AJ, et al: A randomized, double-blind study of phenytoin for the prevention of post-traumatic seizures. N Engl J Med 323(8):497–502, 1990.

37. Cooper P: Gunshot wounds of the brain. In Cooper P (ed): Head Injury, 3rd ed. Baltimore: Williams & Wilkins, 1993.

38. George E, Dagi T: Penetrating missile injuries of the head. In Schmidek H, Sweet W (eds): Operative Neurosurgical Techniques: Indications, Methods, and Results, 2nd ed. Orlando: Grune & Stratton, 1988.

39. Kaufman HH: Treatment of civilian gunshot wounds to the head. Neurosurg Clin N Am 2(2):387–397, 1991.

40. Saba M: Surgical management of gunshot wounds of the head. In Schmidek H, Sweet W (eds): Operative Neurosurgical Techniques: Indications, Methods, and Results, 2nd ed. Orlando: Grune & Stratton, 1988.

41. Whitaker R: Gunshot wounds of the cranium: With special reference to those of the brain. Br J Surg 3:708–735, 1916.

42. Aarabi B, Taghipour M, Alibaii E, et al: Central nervous system infections after military missile head wounds. Neurosurgery 42(3):500–507; discussion 507–509, 1998.

43. Taha JM, Haddad FS, Brown JA: Intracranial infection after missile injuries to the brain: Report of 30 cases from the Lebanese conflict. Neurosurgery 29(6):864–868, 1991.

44. Aarabi B: Comparative study of bacteriological contamination between primary and secondary exploration of missile head wounds. Neurosurgery 20(4):610–616, 1987.

45. Benzel EC, Day WT, Kesterson L, et al: Civilian craniocerebral gunshot wounds. Neurosurgery 29(1):67–71; discussion 71–72, 1991.

46. Byrnes DP, Crockard HA, Gordon DS, et al: Penetrating craniocerebral missile injuries in the civil disturbances in Northern Ireland. Br J Surg 61(3):169–176, 1974.

47. Helling TS, McNabney WK, Whittaker CK, et al: The role of early surgical intervention in civilian gunshot wounds to the head. J Trauma 32(3):398–400, 1992.

48. Hubschmann O, Shapiro K, Baden M, et al: Craniocerebral gunshot injuries in civilian practice: Prognostic criteria and surgical management: Experience with 82 cases. J Trauma 19(1):6–12, 1979.

49. Lillard PL: Five years experience with penetrating craniocerebral gunshot wounds. Surg Neurol 9(2):79–83, 1978.

50. Nagib MG, Rockswold GL, Sherman RS, et al: Civilian gunshot wounds to the brain: Prognosis and management. Neurosurgery 18(5):533–537, 1986.

51. Suddaby L, Weir B, Forsyth C: The management of .22 caliber gunshot wounds of the brain: A review of 49 cases. Can J Neurol Sci 14(3):268–272, 1987.

52. Carey M, Young H, Mathis J, et al: A bacteriological study of craniocerebral missile wounds from Vietnam. J Neurosurg 34:145–154, 1971.

53. Meirowsky AM, Caveness WF, Dillon JD, et al: Cerebrospinal fluid fistulas complicating missile wounds of the brain. J Neurosurg 54(1):44–48, 1981.

54. Arendall RE, Meirowsky AM: Air sinus wounds: An analysis of 163 consecutive cases incurred in the Korean War, 1950–1952. Neurosurgery 13(4):377–380, 1983.

55. Kaufman HH, Schwab K, Salazar AM: A national survey of neurosurgical care for penetrating head injury. Surg Neurol 36(5):370–377, 1991.

56. Antibiotic prophylaxis for penetrating brain injury. J Trauma 51(2 Suppl):S34–S40, 2001.

57. Shoung HM, Sichez JP, Pertuiset B: The early prognosis of craniocerebral gunshot wounds in civilian practice as an aid to the choice of treatment: A series of 56 cases studied by computerized tomography. Acta Neurochir (Wien) 74(1–2):27–30, 1985.

58. Clark WC, Muhlbauer MS, Watridge CB, et al: Analysis of 76 civilian craniocerebral gunshot wounds. J Neurosurg 65(1):9–14, 1986.

59. Cooper PR, Maravilla K, Cone J: Computerized tomographic scan and gunshot wounds of the head: Indications and radiographic findings. Neurosurgery 4(5):373–380, 1979.

60. Grahm TW, Williams FC Jr, Harrington T, et al: Civilian gunshot wounds to the head: A prospective study. Neurosurgery 27(5):696–700; discussion 700, 1990.

61. Kaufman HH, Makela ME, Lee KF, et al: Gunshot wounds to the head: A perspective. Neurosurgery 18(6):689–695, 1986.

62. Jacobs DG, Brandt CP, Piotrowski JJ, et al: Transcranial gunshot wounds: Cost and consequences. Am Surg 61(8):647–653; discussion 653–654, 1995.

63. Kaufman H, Levy M, Stone J, et al: Patients with Glasgow Coma Scale scores 3, 4, 5 after gunshot wounds to the brain. In Levy M, Apuzzo M (eds): Neurosurgery Clinics of N Amer, vol 6. Philadelphia: WB Saunders, 1995.

64. Shaffrey ME, Polin RS, Phillips CD, et al: Classification of civilian craniocerebral gunshot wounds: A multivariate analysis predictive of mortality. J Neurotrauma 9(Suppl 1):S279–S285, 1992.

65. Aldrich EF, Eisenberg HM, Saydjari C, et al: Predictors of mortality in severely head-injured patients with civilian gunshot wounds: A report from the NIH Traumatic Coma Data Bank. Surg Neurol 38(6):418–423, 1992.

66. du Trevou MD, van Dellen JR: Penetrating stab wounds to the brain: The timing of angiography in patients presenting with the weapon already removed. Neurosurgery 31(5):905–911; discussion 911–912, 1992.

67. Mancuso P, Chiaramonte I, Passanisi M, et al: Craniocerebral gunshot wounds in civilians: Report on 40 cases. J Neurosurg Sci 32(4):189–194, 1988.

68. Brierbrauer K, Tindall S: Gunshot wounds to the head and spine, Part I. Contemp Neurosurg 9(20):1–5, 1987.

69. Brierbrauer K, Tindall S: Gunshot wounds to the head and spine, Part II. Contemp Neurosurg 9(21):1–6, 1987.

70. Miner ME, Ewing-Cobbs L, Kopaniky DR, et al: The results of treatment of gunshot wounds to the brain in children. Neurosurgery 26(1):20–24; discussion 24–25, 1990.

71. Kelly D, Nikas D, Becker D: Diagnosis and treatment of moderate and severe head injuries in adults. In Youmans J (ed): Neurological Surgery. Philadelphia: WB Saunders, 1996.

72. Crockard HA: Early intracranial pressure studies in gunshot wounds of the brain. J Trauma 15(4):339–347, 1975.

73. Rosenthal G, Segal R, Umansky F: Unpublished data. 2004.

74. Mayhall CG, Archer NH, Lamb VA, et al: Ventriculostomy-related infections: A prospective epidemiologic study. N Engl J Med 310(9):553–559, 1984.

75. Paramore CG, Turner DA: Relative risks of ventriculostomy infection and morbidity. Acta Neurochir (Wien) 127(1–2):79–84, 1994.

76. Rosenthal G, Umansky F: Unpublished data. 2004.

77. Zabramski JM, Whiting D, Darouiche RO, et al: Efficacy of antimicrobial-impregnated external ventricular drain catheters: A prospective, randomized, controlled trial. J Neurosurg 98(4):725–730, 2003.

78. Meirowsky AM: Wounds of dural sinuses. J Neurosurg 10(5):496–514, 1953.

79. Cooper P: Depressed skull fracture. In Apuzzo M (ed): Brain Surgery: Complication Avoidance and Management, 1st ed. New York: Churchill Livingstone, 1993.

80. Donaghy RM, Wallman LJ, Flanagan MJ, et al: Saggital sinus repair: Technical note. J Neurosurg 38(2):244–248, 1973.

81. Kaufman HH, Moake JL, Olson JD, et al: Delayed and recurrent intracranial hematomas related to disseminated intravascular clotting and fibrinolysis in head injury. Neurosurgery 7(5):445–449, 1980.

82. Dutton RP, Hess JR, Scalea TM: Recombinant factor VIIa for control of hemorrhage: Early experience in critically ill trauma patients. J Clin Anesth 15(3):184–188, 2003.

83. Eikelboom JW, Bird R, Blythe D, et al: Recombinant activated factor VII for the treatment of life-threatening haemorrhage. Blood Coagul Fibrinolysis 14(8):713–717, 2003.

84. Bouwmeester FW, Jonkhoff AR, Verheijen RH, et al: Successful treatment of life-threatening postpartum hemorrhage with recombinant activated factor VII. Obstet Gynecol 101(6):1174–1176, 2003.

85. Park P, Fewel ME, Garton HJ, et al: Recombinant activated factor VII for the rapid correction of coagulopathy in nonhemophilic neurosurgical patients. Neurosurgery 53(1):34–38; discussion 38–39, 2003.

86. Siegel LJ, Gerigk L, Tuettenberg J, et al: Cerebral sinus thrombosis in a trauma patient after recombinant activated factor VII infusion. Anesthesiology 100(2):441–443, 2004.

87. Manelfe C, Cellerier P, Sobel D, et al: Cerebrospinal fluid rhinorrhea: Evaluation with metrizamide cisternography. AJR Am J Roentgenol 138(3):471–476, 1982.

88. Ozgen T, Tekkok IH, Cila A, et al: CT cisternography in evaluation of cerebrospinal fluid rhinorrhea. Neuroradiology 32(6):481–484, 1990.

89. el Gammal T, Brooks BS: MR cisternography: Initial experience in 41 cases. AJNR Am J Neuroradiol 15(9):1647–1656, 1994.

90. Bearcroft PW, Freer CE: CT of a peripatetic intracranial foreign body. Neuroradiology 37(7):542–544, 1995.

91. Alessi G, Aiyer S, Nathoo N: Home-made gun injury: Spontaneous version and anterior migration of bullet. Br J Neurosurg 16(4):381–384, 2002.

92. Zafonte RD, Watanabe T, Mann NR: Moving bullet syndrome: A complication of penetrating head injury. Arch Phys Med Rehabil 79(11):1469–1472, 1998.

93. Duman H, Ziyal IM, Canpolat A: Spontaneous subfalcial transcallosal migration of a missile to the contralateral hemisphere causing deterioration in neurological status: Case report. Neurol Med Chir (Tokyo) 42(8):332–333, 2002.

94. Milhorat TH, Elowitz EH, Johnson RW, et al: Spontaneous movement of bullets in the brain. Neurosurgery 32(1):140–143, 1993.

95. Furlow L, Bender M, Teuber H: Movable foreign body within the cerebral ventricle. J Neurosurg 4:380–386, 1947.

96. Aarabi B: Management of traumatic aneurysms caused by high-velocity missile head wounds. Neurosurg Clin N Am 6(4):775–797, 1995.

97. Amirjamshidi A, Rahmat H, Abbassioun K: Traumatic aneurysms and arteriovenous fistulas of intracranial vessels associated with penetrating head injuries occurring during war: Principles and pitfalls in diagnosis and management: A survey of 31 cases and review of the literature. J Neurosurg 84(5):769–780, 1996.

98. Rahimizadeh A, Abtahi H, Daylami MS, et al: Traumatic cerebral aneurysms caused by shell fragments: Report of four cases and review of the literature. Acta Neurochir (Wien) 84(3–4):93–98, 1987.

99. Kieck CF, de Villiers JC: Vascular lesions due to transcranial stab wounds. J Neurosurg 60(1):42–46, 1984.

100. Haddad FS, Haddad GF, Taha J: Traumatic intracranial aneurysms caused by missiles: Their presentation and management. Neurosurgery 28(1):1–7, 1991.

101. Fleischer AS, Patton JM, Tindall GT: Cerebral aneurysms of traumatic origin. Surg Neurol 4(2):233–239, 1975.

102. Batjer H, Giller C, Kopitnik T, et al: Intracranial and cervical vascular injuries. In Cooper PR (ed): Head Injury, 3rd ed. Baltimore: Williams & Wilkins, 1993.

103. Spetzler RF, Owen MP: Extracranial-intracranial arterial bypass to a single branch of the middle cerebral artery in the management of a traumatic aneurysm. Neurosurgery 4(4):334–337, 1979.

104. Kluger Y: Bomb explosions in acts of terrorism: Detonation, wound ballistics, triage and medical concerns. Isr Med Assoc J 5(4):235–240, 2003.

105. Young M: Mechanics of Blast Injuries in War Medicine: Washington, DC: U.S. Government Printing Office, 1945.

106. Sviri GE, Guilburd JN, Soustiel JF, et al: Penetrating head injuries caused by a new weapon, the side dome. Mil Med 164(10):746–750, 1999.

107. Jennett B, Bond M: Assessment of outcome after severe brain damage. Lancet 1(7905):480–484, 1975.

108. Bursick DM, Selker RG: Intracranial pencil injuries. Surg Neurol 16(6):427–431, 1981.

109. Ildan F, Bagdatoglu H, Boyar B, et al: The nonsurgical management of a penetrating orbitocranial injury reaching the brain stem: Case report. J Trauma 36(1):116–118, 1994.

110. Ashkenazi E, Mualem N, Umansky F: Successful removal of an intracranial needle by an ophthalmologic magnet: Case report. J Trauma 30(1):114–115, 1990.

111. Di Roio C, Jourdan C, Mottolese C, et al: Craniocerebral injury resulting from transorbital stick penetration in children. Childs Nerv Syst 16(8):503–506; discussion 507, 2000.

112. Matsumoto S, Hasuo K, Mizushima A, et al: Intracranial penetrating injuries via the optic canal. AJNR Am J Neuroradiol 19(6):1163–1165, 1998.

113. Bullock R, van Dellen JR: Acute carotid-cavernous fistula with retained knife blade after transorbital stab wound. Surg Neurol 24(5):555–558, 1985.

114. van Dellen JR, Lipschitz R: Stab wounds of the skull. Surg Neurol 10(2):110–114, 1978.

115. Siccardi D, Cavaliere R, Pau A, et al: Penetrating craniocerebral missile injuries in civilians: A retrospective analysis of 314 cases. Surg Neurol 35(6):455–460, 1991.

116. Levi L, Linn S, Feinsod M: Penetrating craniocerebral injuries in civilians. Br J Neurosurg 5(3):241–247, 1991.

117. Prognosis in penetrating head injury. J Trauma 52:544–586, 2001.

118. Rish BL, Dillon JD, Weiss GH: Mortality following penetrating craniocerebral injuries: An analysis of the deaths in the Vietnam Head Injury Registry population. J Neurosurg 59(5):775–780, 1983.

119. Levy ML, Masri LS, Levy KM, et al: Penetrating craniocerebral injury resultant from gunshot wounds: Gang-related injury in children and adolescents. Neurosurgery 33(6):1018–1024; discussion 1024–1025, 1993.

120. Levy ML, Rezai A, Masri LS, et al: The significance of subarachnoid hemorrhage after penetrating craniocerebral injury: Correlations with angiography and outcome in a civilian population. Neurosurgery 32(4):532–540, 1993.

Surgical Management of Trauma Involving the Skull Base and Paranasal Sinuses

FRANZ XAVER BRUNNER

Traffic accidents commonly cause trauma to the midface and frontal skull base. In many cases there are post-traumatic functional deficits, deformities, and stressful psychosocial problems accompanying facial distortions. The availability of microsurgical reconstruction techniques using tissue adhesive, preserved dura, resorbable materials, and thin rigid titanium plates for osteosynthesis puts more demand on the quality of surgery in maxillofacial and skull base trauma. By means of miniplate and microplate osteosynthesis, secure stabilization of the midface can be achieved after even extensive fractures of the midface or the floor of the anterior cranial fossa. This procedure is considered a satisfactory operative treatment in terms of cosmetic and functional results. As a rule, sealing of the frontal skull base should be performed before repairing the fractures of the midface. The postoperative results depend on the extent of the primary bone or soft-tissue lesions. To achieve satisfactory results in operative treatment, a team approach is necessary.

MECHANISMS OF INJURY

Most midfacial fractures occur in men and are related to high-impact forces usually sustained in motor vehicle accidents, industrial accidents, fistfights, aggravated assaults, sports injuries, and falls. Direct injuries lead to skull base and Le Fort maxillary fractures. In many cases, isolated depressed pieces of bone occur in addition to multiple fractures of the glabellar area and the anterior walls of frontal sinuses combined with skull base fractures.

In cars without airbags, head-on collisions account for approximately half of all motorist injuries. The driver who fails to use lap and shoulder seat belts is likely to be thrown face-first into the windshield in such a collision. In a broadside collision without airbag protection on the driver's side, bony injuries to the temporal skull area and zygomatic and nasal bones may occur, whereas midfacial fractures are less likely.

Because of expanded airbag protection, the absolute number of cases suffering severe facial and skull base injuries in Europe are falling; this is reflected in the statistics of the ENT Department of Augsburg. However, the number of cases needing surgical treatment in centers of excellence is still significant. Traumatologic statistics of the ENT Department of Würzburg from 1986 to 1988 show 58 cases of anterior skull base fractures. In comparison, the traumatologic statistics of the ENT Department of Augsburg

from 2000 to 2002 show 76 patients had to be treated with rhinosurgical duraplasty or combined rhinosurgical-neurosurgical duraplasty in a similar 3-year period.

ANATOMIC AND PATHOPHYSIOLOGIC ASPECTS AND FRACTURE CLASSIFICATIONS

The maxillary bones consist of a body and four processes: (1) frontal, (2) zygomatic, (3) palatine, and (4) alveolar. The body contains the maxillary sinus. All paranasal sinuses are air-filled extensions of the nasal cavity, which is developed in the bones of the skull.

The anterior group comprises the frontal sinus, the maxillary sinus, and the anterior ethmoidal cells. The posterior group comprises the posterior ethmoidal cells and the sphenoidal sinus. The sinuses are classified according to drainage rather than to the actual anatomic distribution. The sinuses vary widely in their positions during development so that the distinction between anterior and posterior may be misleading. The anterior group of sinuses drains into the middle *nasal* meatus, whereas the posterior group drains posteriorly into the sphenoethmoidal recess.

The fully developed maxillary sinus usually extends from the first premolar to the second molar tooth. The sinus reaches up to the floor of the orbit, occupying practically the whole body of the maxillary bone. The ostium lies in the medial wall. Additionally, a small accessory ostium may be anterior and inferior to it.

The frontal sinus occupies the space in the frontal bones between the inner and the outer tables. The sinus is not present at birth; it develops until the age of 5 years, when the air cells extend above the level of the supraorbital ridge. The fully developed frontal sinus may extend to the outer orbital angle, cranially into the frontal bone for a distance of several centimeters, and posteriorly above the roof of the orbit. The frontal sinuses are rarely symmetric and usually are separated from each other by a thin, bony plate. The roof of the orbit forms the floor of the frontal sinus; it contains the supraorbital nerve, which runs toward the inner orbital angle, and has attached to it, more medially, the trochlea nerve of the superior oblique muscle.

The ethmoidal cells, although divided into two groups, must be regarded as one cell system from the point of view of development and treatment. In contrast to the other sinuses, the ethmoidal cells consist of many small air-filled cells that do not have a regular symmetry or fixed number. They lie in the upper part of the lateral wall of the nose. Located laterally is the orbital periosteum; located inferiorly is a part of the maxillary air sinus; and superiorly, the cells meet at the apex. Although it lies in the anterior part, the frontal sinus may be considered to be a superior anatomic structure.

The two sphenoidal sinuses occupy the body of the sphenoid bone. The sphenoidal sinuses may vary widely in shape and position. The ostium is high on the anterior wall of the sinus. In most skulls, pneumatization extends inferiorly below the pituitary fossa, which bulges into the sinus. At the outer anterior angle where the roof and the lateral wall meet, the optic foramen, which contains the optic nerve, is in close relation to the sphenoidal sinus. The lateral wall is in contact with the cavernous sinus and the carotid artery.

All sinuses are lined by ciliated mucous membranes; these are richly provided with glands, which are found mainly around the ostium. The cilia are constantly beating to reach toward these openings.

The bony structures of the midface are connected to the skull base by four vertical bony buttresses. The nasomaxillary or anterior buttress comprises the anterior part of the alveolus, the pyriform aperture, and the nasal process of the maxilla through the anterior lacrimal crest to the superior orbital rim and frontocranial attachment. The lateral buttress extends from a bony crest of the maxilla above the anterior molar teeth to the zygomatic process of the frontal bone superiorly and the zygomatic arch laterally. Posteriorly, the pterygomaxillary buttress joins the maxillary tuberosity to the cranial base through the pyramidal process of the palatine bone and the medial pterygoid plate of the sphenoid. Finally, there is an important median buttress or frontoethmoidal vomerine pillar connecting the frontal bone to the median palatine suture and containing thinner and thicker parts of the bony nasal septum.

Fractures of the frontal sinuses are mainly fissures of the anterior walls, but in severe cases they may involve the inner table and the dura. Serious effects may be expected if the fracture extends into the cribriform area with tearing of the dura. Maxillary fractures involve the middle third of the face, in which both maxillae are pushed backward. Initially, swelling obscures the displacement. If this swelling is not recognized quickly and reduced, an ugly "dishface" deformity occurs.

Zygomatic fractures result from a blow or kick to the cheekbone. This type of fracture generally leads to an inward and downward displacement, which is commonly combined with a fracture of the orbital floor. Usually, there is an immediate diplopia, periorbital swelling, and enophthalmos. The affected eye lies at a lower level when compared with the contralateral one.

The Le Fort classifications (Figs. 8-1 through 8-3) of midfacial fractures are still evolving and may continue to do so. Although midfacial fractures occur only rarely in a pure Le Fort form, and often present as comminuted fractures, the classification system provides useful means for analysis and communication (see Fig. 8-1B). In approximately 50% of all cases, the so-called Le Fort maxillary fractures are combined with fractures of the frontal skull base. The Le Fort I fracture (see Fig. 8-1A) is a transverse, low maxillary fracture involving a traumatic separation of the palate from the body of the maxilla. Le Fort II or pyramidal fractures (see Fig. 8-2A) are the most common of the three types; the fracture line passes through the nasal bones and across the frontal process of the maxilla and the lacrimal bones, descending through the infraorbital rim and through the lateral inferior wall of the maxillary sinus. Le Fort III fractures (see Fig. 8-3A) represent the most severe form of maxillary and craniofacial injury and result in a separation of the facial skeleton from the skull base. These fractures occur in approximately 20% of cases. In Le Fort III injuries, the fracture line originates high on the nasal bones, crosses the upper part of the frontal processes of the maxilla and lacrimal bones, and passes through the lamina papyracea and ethmoid sinuses. In the orbit, the fracture line passes posterior to the inferior orbital fissure. Combination fractures refer to Le Fort fractures on the same side of the face (e.g., Le Fort I and Le Fort III fractures). These fractures are uncommon and are often confused with nasal, nasomaxillary, and zygomatic fractures.

Isolated crush fractures within the nasal area or anterior wall of the frontal sinus, or so-called central midfacial fractures (see Fig. 8-1C) without malocclusion, are often caused by impact forces (e.g., horse kick or a blow from a foreign body) and are associated with fractures of the anterior skull base. The varieties of the different fractures of the anterior skull base or the *rhinobase* have been classified by Escher[1] as follows (see Fig. 8-2):

- Type 1, the extended rhinobase fracture, is a frontal crush fracture. These fractures are normally treated by both neurosurgeons and rhinosurgeons.
- Type 2, the localized fracture, is normally a small fracture, often a microgap or a dura tear. The areas of predilection are the lamina cribrosa, crista galli, posterior area of the ethmoidal walls, and roof of sphenoid sinus.
- Type 3 typically consists of rhinobasal fractures with posterior displacement of the viscerocranium. As a consequence of the depression and compression of the viscerocranium that accompanies this posterior shift, a crush fracture of the rhinobase is often caused as well, particularly within the roof of the ethmoidal cell system.
- Type 4 are fronto-orbital fractures within the rhinobase. The fracture gap runs from the lateral frontal area to the roof of the orbit. Dural tears and brain prolapse are often difficult to diagnose because of the natural packing caused by the orbital contents.

DIAGNOSIS AND INDICATIONS FOR SURGERY

The diagnosis and treatment of frontobasal injuries *in many cases* requires an interdisciplinary approach and should take into account potential lesions of the midfacial region, orbit, paranasal sinuses, and intracranial cavity. The upper paranasal sinuses, the posterior wall of the frontal sinus, the roof of the ethmoidal cells, and the sphenoid sinus are directly adjacent to the frontal skull base. Even without soft-tissue lesions of the face, fractures of the frontal skull base have to be considered indirect open wounds. Lacerations of

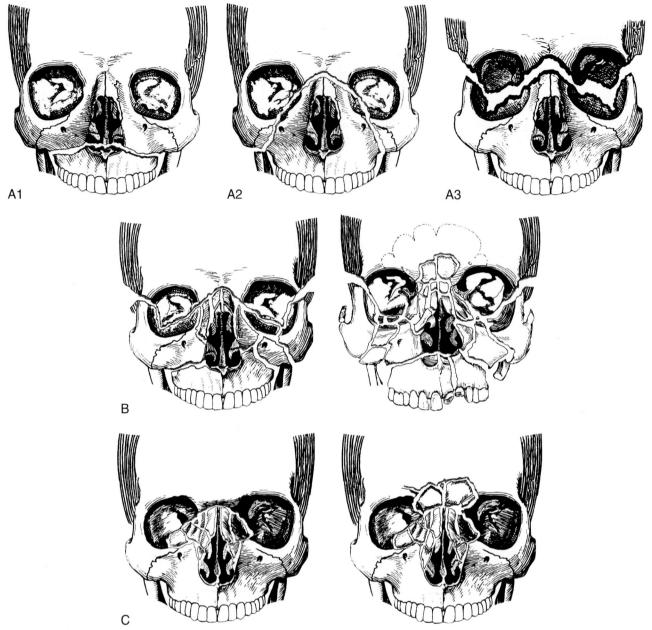

FIGURE 8-1   *A,* Le Fort fractures. *B,* Comminuted Le Fort fractures. *C,* Central midfacial fractures without malocclusion.

nasal mucosa and the mucous membranes of the paranasal sinuses are always present in these cases, and a high risk exists for ascending infection to lead to involvement of the endocranium. Cerebrospinal fluid (CSF) leakage from the nose or nasopharynx demands localization of the site of the leak and subsequent surgical repair, even if the leak stops spontaneously. The cicatricial healing of dural lesions in areas of the skull base that are in contact with the nose or paranasal sinuses (i.e., the rhinobase) normally does not adequately seal the cranial cavity. Because bacterial flora normally exist in the nose and paranasal sinuses at all times, intracranial complications such as meningitis, encephalitis, and brain abscess can develop years after the trauma. Therefore, the leak has to be definitively sealed by an appropriate duraplasty, a conclusion enunciated during World War II.

As a consequence, nearly every case of frontal skull base fracture requires some form of operative intervention. Current concepts for treatment of midface and frontal skull base injuries have evolved since 1927, based on the work of various surgeons.[2–9] These principles remain valid:

1. Closure of open or indirectly open fractures is necessary; fractures of the frontal skull base must be sealed to avoid endocranial complications.
2. The management of soft-tissue lesions and facial bone fractures should take into account all esthetic and functional aspects during primary treatment.

Spinal fluid leakage may remain clinically undetected for some time before complications occur. Diagnostic procedures include head-down positioning and jugular vein compression, the use of glucose test strips, and the measurement

Type 1   Type 2

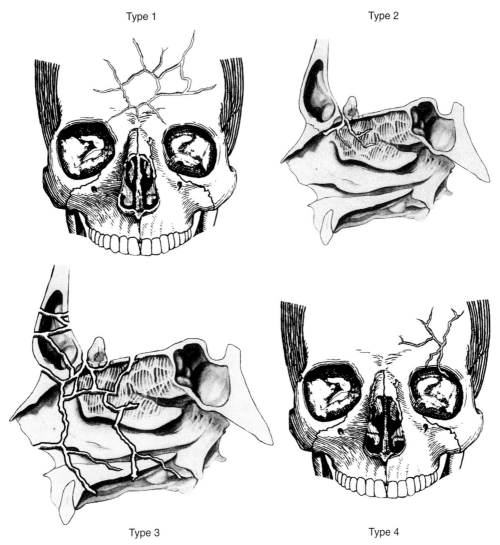

Type 3   Type 4

FIGURE 8-2   Escher classification of frontal skull base fractures.

of β_2-transferrin and the albumin-to-prealbumin ratio. For the diagnosis of CSF leak, β_2-transferrin is a highly sensitive parameter, but the procedure used to measure this element is time consuming and needs at least 1.5 mL of fluid and a lot of experience on the part of the examiner. In particularly difficult cases, the leak can be localized by injecting fluorescin into the lumbar canal. After decongestion in the nasal cavity, the yellow-stained CSF may be detected endoscopically with a special blue filter.[10] Methods using intralumbar injections of ^{131}I albumin, [169]Y, or ^{111}In do not produce reliable results.

Preoperative radiologic examinations with coronal computed tomography (CT) scans are of major importance. Although ordinary x-ray studies of the skull in the anteroposterior, lateral, semiaxial, and basal projections sufficiently demonstrate the extent of the fractures and possibly existing pneumatoceles, modern CT scans provide improved resolution of even tiny fractures without increased exposure to radiation. The use of a shoulder device and a gantry deviation of 20 degrees enables coronal scans even in cases in which overstretching of the head would cause a dangerous increase of intracranial pressure.

Most CSF leaks (see Fig. 8-3) result from dural injury at the ethmoidal roof. The second most common cause of CSF leakage is a fracture of the posterior wall of the frontal sinus. Only rarely is the dural defect located at the sphenoid area in the region of the tuberculum sellae, the anterior wall of the sella, or the planum sphenoidale. With extensive comminuted injuries of the anterior skull base, the frontal sinus, the roof of the ethmoidal cells, and the sphenoid sinus may all be involved concurrently. The absence of intracranial air does not prove that the dura is intact. In the author's experience, in 75% of all cases, air is resorbed after 48 hours, even after a large bony fracture gap.

Among the 58 patients suffering from an anterior skull base fracture that were treated in the ear, nose, and throat clinic of Würzburg from 1986 to 1988 (Table 8-1), the most common defect was located in the area of the ethmoidal roof and at the junction between the posterior wall of the frontal sinus and the ethmoidal roof (Fig. 8-4). Thirty-one patients showed defects only in the form of bony gaps, and 27 patients had a bony defect greater than 0.5 cm². The size of the defect of the skull base, as revealed in coronal CT scans, was compared with the lesion found during surgery. A dural

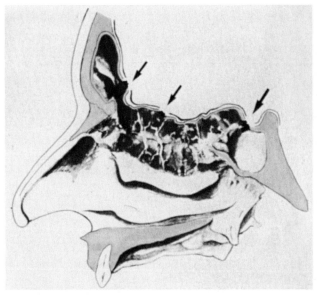

FIGURE 8-3 Common sites of frontal skull base fractures.

lesion existed in 92.4% of the cases in which the CT scan had shown a gap greater than 2 mm and in all cases with a gap greater than 4 mm.

OPERATIVE TREATMENT

The timing of surgical treatment depends on the patient's general condition, the type of injury involved, and the requirements of the specialties involved. Serious bleeding demands emergency surgery, even without complete pre-operative diagnostic evaluation. If the patient is in poor general condition, the definitive treatment of the fractures may be delayed for hours, days, or weeks. In these cases, emergency procedures can be of only short duration. Bleeding is stopped by nasal and pharyngeal packing, and soft-tissue lesions are closed adequately by suturing mucosa, subcutaneous tissue, and skin wounds. In most of these cases, tracheostomy cannot be avoided. Soft-tissue lesions of the face should be closed within 12 hours, however. Nasal fractures should be treated within the first 5 days. Midfacial fractures should be reduced and stabilized within the first 2 to 3 weeks. Duraplasty should be performed as soon as possible in cases that combine comminuted fractures of the posterior wall of the frontal sinus with extensive CSF rhinorrhea. Duraplasty of localized fractures in the area of

TABLE 8-1 ■ Statistics on Traumatology 1986 to 1988 (Ear, Nose, and Throat Clinic of Würzburg)		
Localization of Anterior Skull Base Fractures	Size of Defect (No. = 58) (%)	(%)
Posterior wall of frontal sinus	6 (10, 3) gap	31 (53)
Posterior wall of frontal sinus +		27 (47)
roof of ethmoid cells	21 (36, 2) > 0, 5 cm²	
Roof of ethmoid cells	24 (41, 4)	
Roof of ethmoid cells +		
sphenoid sinus	7 (12, 1)	

the ethmoidal roof and sphenoid sinus roof can be performed as a delayed second procedure. In these cases, high-dose antibiotic coverage should be given for at least 1 week, and a constant follow-up of the trauma patient has to be maintained. After having completed clinical and radiologic examinations, surgical approaches and techniques should be discussed in a joint meeting with all relevant disciplines to plan surgery in which neurosurgeons, rhinosurgeons, and maxillofacial surgeons cooperate.

Rhinosurgical Approach to the Frontal Skull Base

The classic epidurotransethmoidal rhinosurgical approach for the closure of CSF leaks localized in the median and paramedian frontal skull base and sphenoidal region has been favored by various specialists. Using this approach, via a Killian (eyebrow) or bilateral Killian incision (Fig. 8-5A), defects of the ethmoidal roof and the sella-sphenoidal planes can be closed. Fractures of the posterior wall of the frontal sinus can be sealed using an osteoplastic approach involving temporary removal of the anterior wall of the frontal sinus (Fig. 8-5B). The area is cut out earlier as a cone-shaped lid, then later repositioned exactly by osteosynthesis. One disadvantage of this method of approaching the skull base, in cases of laterally situated fractures of the posterior wall of the frontal sinus, is that painful irritation of the supra-trochlear and supraorbital nerves can appear in the months and years after surgery. This approach cannot be recom-mended for extensive and comminuted fractures of the posterior wall of the frontal sinus and the whole frontal skull base with brain herniation, intracranial bleeding, and hematoma.

If the only problems are preexisting facial and frontal wounds, and the patient is in good general condition, an approach to the anterior skull base by widening the pre-existing wounds (if necessary) is preferable. The wounds have to be cleaned and closed exactly from inside out after beginning with repair of the dural defect.

In cases of localized fractures of the ethmoidal cell system or sphenoid sinus roof, with bone defects below 0.5 × 0.5 cm, the endonasal approach using the microscope (a procedure similar to the transsphenoidal approach to the sella) or the endoscopic rhinosurgical technique as primary or delayed second procedure may be indicated. To be success-fully performed, however, these procedures require an expe-rienced surgeon.

Rhinosurgical Closure of Dural Lesions

As just noted, the first step consists of closing the defect within the anterior skull base. In a rhinosurgical approach, the patient's fascia lata, fascia of the temporalis muscle, or preserved fascia lata is used. A generously sized graft under-mines the defect, allowing the surgeon to close it without tension. A double layer of fascia transplants attached with fibrin glue is even more efficient (Fig. 8-6). Sealing CSF leaks tightly within the area of the roof or posterior wall of the sphenoid sinus often presents a major problem. Draf and Samii[6,9] describe the sealing technique of Kley, which uses a "tobacco-pouch" consisting of fascia lata filled with gelatin sponges. It can be recommended to cover the tobacco-pouch

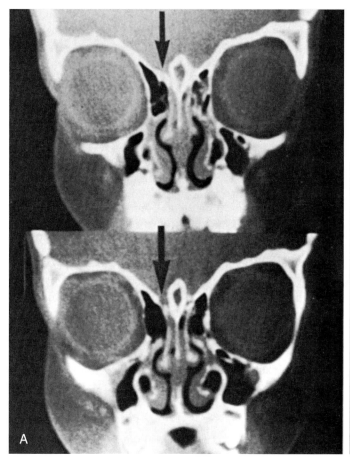

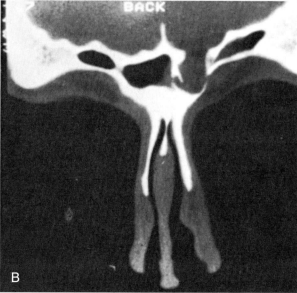

FIGURE 8-4 *A*, Coronary computed tomography (CT) scan showing localized fracture of the ethmoid roof. *B*, Coronary CT scan showing large fracture of the posterior wall of the frontal sinus.

packing with fibrin glue and glue it in (Fig. 8-7). Provided that a small leak within the roof or posterior wall of the sphenoid sinus can be totally visualized under the microscope, merely a cover of fascia lata coated with fibrin glue is sufficient. In cases without malocclusion and with an intact lateral bone frame, the easiest way to induce osteosynthesis is by putting back the conic bone lid, which was removed earlier, using resorbable sutures or resorbable plates and screws.

Combined Neurosurgical and Rhinosurgical Procedures

The management of major intracranial fragment dislocations and multiple dural tears should incorporate a combined intracranial and extracranial transfrontal approach. According to Samii and Draf,[9] this procedure was described first by Unterberger and involved division of the olfactory fibers in cases requiring bilateral exposure of the cribriform plate because of the necessity of elevating the dura. This technique, however, can be modified by stopping the intracranial approach before reaching the olfactory fibers. Exposure and sealing of posteriorly situated dural lesions can be performed without dissection by subcranial preparations similar to the techniques developed by Tessier[11,12] for craniofacial surgery. After coronal incision, periosteal

flaps based frontally or laterally are created, if necessary (Fig. 8-8A). The supraorbital nerves are then exposed if a bony supraorbital canal exists. The next step provides laterally an exposure of the frontozygomatic junction by moving exactly frontally and inferiorly along the fascia of the temporal muscle. The bony supraorbital rims are then identified. The bony orbital roofs (Fig. 8-8B) are stripped subperiosteally, and this process is continued to the complete medial and lateral wall of the orbit. Then the nasal bones and the fracture lines of the lamina papyracea are identified. After removal of the fragments of the anterior areas of the lamina papyracea and coagulation of the anterior ethmoidal artery, the anterior and medial parts of the ethmoidal roof can be identified. By removing bony fragments in this area by an extradural rhinosurgical approach, the areas of the posterior ethmoid roof and sphenoidal sinus usually can be surveyed carefully and dural tears can be sealed.

In severe craniofacial injuries and midfacial fractures, the incidence of involvement of the skull base with concomitant major dural tears is significantly high. Regarding functional and esthetic results, treatment consisting of primary urgent neurosurgical exploration, combined with rhinosurgical and maxillofacial reconstruction, produces the best results. The major advantage of this method is the possibility of an early one-stage craniofacial reconstruction, avoiding extreme frontal lobe retraction and damage to the

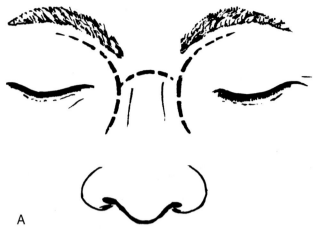

A

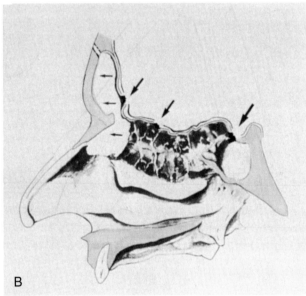

B

FIGURE 8-5   *A*, Rhinosurgical exposure of the frontal skull base via the bilateral eyebrow (Killian) incision. *B*, Osteoplastic rhinosurgical approach.

olfactory fibers. Reduction of telecanthus, decompression of the optic nerve, and meticulous reconstruction of the bony structures of the midface and frontal skull base can be performed in a one-session procedure.

Extensive fractures and depressions within the area of the frontal bone are often associated with vast crush fractures of the posterior wall of the frontal sinus. In these cases, dura lesions and subdural hematomas are common; these problems require primary or secondary interdisciplinary involvement of a neurosurgeon.

The surgical approach chosen in these cases is a frontal or frontotemporal bone lid type of craniotomy. An intradural or an extradural approach may also be used. In cases of excessively large crush defects of the posterior wall of the frontal sinus, the reconstruction is no longer possible. Partial or total cranialization of the frontal sinus may then be necessary (Fig. 8-9A). Tears of the dura are mended using sutures or fibrin glue. Bony edges at the transition of the former frontal sinus with the tabula interna of the os frontale have to be smoothed down to avoid a bony overhang and to give the brain and the dura the chance to use up the newly

gained space completely. The mucosa of the frontal sinus must be entirely removed. For sealing the area toward the nose and the ethmoid roof, a pedicle flap consisting of periosteum and muscle and periosteum, fibrin glue, bone meal, and bone chips of the wall of the former frontal sinus, minus all mucosa, is used (Fig. 8-9B).

If fracture lines involve only the superior parts of a large frontal sinus, partial cranialization is performed by removing the upper fragments only and pushing the mucosa downward (Fig. 8-10). If the parietotemporofrontal bone of one side is markedly involved, and the posterior wall of the frontal sinus of only one side is crushed, it suffices merely to conceal the injured frontal sinus, approaching it laterally. This technique, combining rhinosurgical and neurosurgical treatment, has been used successfully in many cases.

Optic Nerve Decompression

In severe craniofacial-frontobasal injuries, the optic nerve is quite often damaged. Recommendations in the literature for management of traumatic injuries to the nerve include expectant management, medical therapy, surgical treatment, and medical therapy combined with surgical decompression. Traditional surgical approaches to optical nerve decompression are a neurosurgical or craniotomy approach; extranasal transethmoidal approach; intranasal, transorbital, or transantral microscopic approach; and endonasal endoscopic approach. Levin and colleagues[18] report the results of visual outcome of a total of 133 patients with traumatic optic neuropathy. Visual acuity increased in 32% of the surgery group, 57% in the untreated group, and 52% of the steroid group. Although the surgery group had more patients whose initial vision was so poor as to produce no light perception, no clear benefit could be found for either corticosteroid therapy or optic canal decompression surgery. Therefore, it seems clinically reasonable to decide to treat or not to treat on an individual patient basis.

Wang and co-workers[19] reported on 61 consecutive cases presenting visual loss after facial trauma between 1984 and 1996 that were assessed for outcome. There was no significant difference in improvement of visual acuity in patients treated with surgical versus nonsurgical methods; however, 83% of patients without orbital fractures had improvement, compared with 38% of patients with orbital fractures ($p < 0.05$). Consequently, patients who sustain penetrating trauma may have a worse prognosis than do those with blunt trauma.

The establishment of flash-evoked visual-evoked potentials (VEPs) and the electroretinogram (ERG) are reliable electrophysiologic methods, which may help gather specific information as to whether the visual pathway is intact. In cases of blunt trauma, the conservative treatment of choice is the methylprednisolone-megadose regimen (30 mg Urbason/kg bodyweight IV and 5.4 mg/kg bodyweight/hour IV for the following hours). Recovery of VEP from no response to abnormal wave, or abnormal wave to normal VEP, are both indicators of relatively good visual prognosis but cannot predict return to normal.

Surgical decompression of the orbital compartment, in combination with conservative steroid treatment, is absolutely indicated in cases of retrobulbar hematoma. This treatment is also indicated in cases where CT and MRI

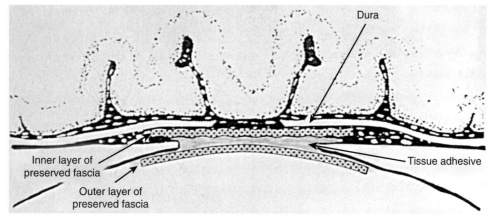

FIGURE 8-6   Rhinosurgical closure of dural leaks. This technique uses two layers of fascia and tissue adhesive.

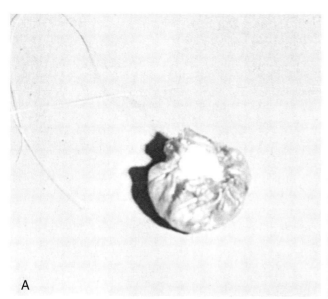

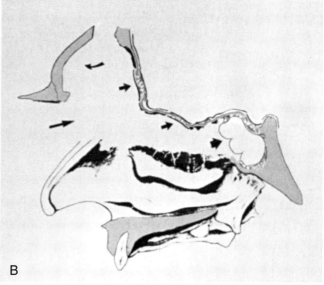

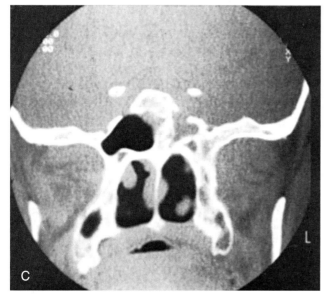

FIGURE 8-7   *A*, Tobacco-pouch technique, according to Kley. *B*, Osteoplastic approach. The tobacco pouch is fixed with fibrin glue. *C*, X-ray control study 1 year after surgery showing tight seal of the sphenoidal roof.

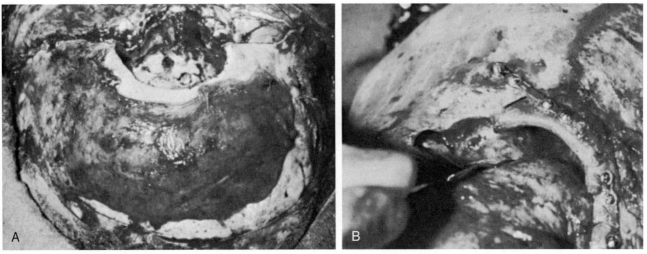

FIGURE 8-8   *A,* Rhinosurgical approach to the frontal skull base using a coronary incision. The anterior wall of the frontal sinus is sawn out, and a laterally based periosteal flap is created. *B,* Exposure of the orbital roof.

scans show bone fragment dislocation into the orbit with contact to the retrobulbar part of the optical nerve, or in cases of fragmentations of the bony optic canal combined with blindness caused by local swelling and blood flow disturbance.

If surgical decompression, even in unconscious patients, seems to be helpful, regarding all clinical and electrophysiological data, as well as CT and MRI findings, surgery should be performed as soon as possible. Figure 8-11 shows the preoperative CT scan of a patient with a severe skull base fracture involving the optic canal; a dislocation of a bony fragment via sphenoidal sinus is visible. Because there was complete blindness in the left eye, surgical decompression was performed via transseptal microscopic approach as an emergency procedure. Postoperatively, conservative treatment with soludecortin-pentoxiphyllin infusions was performed according to the regime for the treatment of Bell's palsy described by Stennert,[20] and visual acuity improved to 0.5 clear by 6 months postoperatively.

Drainage of the Frontal Sinus and the Ethmoidal Cell System

In most cases of midfacial and anterior skull base fractures, the frontal sinus and ethmoidal cell system remains pneumatized. To avoid the development of mucoceles or inflammation, a wide, fully epithelialized access to the frontal sinus, the ethmoidal cells, and the nose has to be created.

In cases of a primary crush fracture of the upper bony septum associated with corresponding lesions of the mucosa, the construction of a median drainage route by resection of the upper parts of the bony nasal septum can be suggested. In cases without major fractures in the upper parts of the septum, this method should not be applied to avoid further instability in the area of the forehead-nose pillar, which has to be reconstructed. Because there is already a bony crush within the area of the nose and glabella, any further bony destabilization should be avoided.

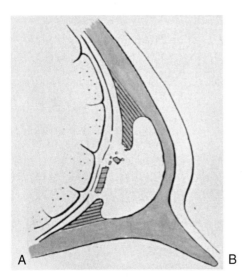

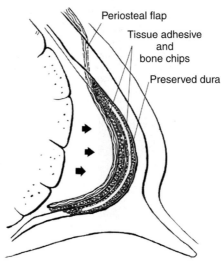

Periosteal flap

Tissue adhesive and bone chips

Preserved dura

FIGURE 8-9   *A,* Extensive fracture of the posterior wall of the frontal sinus. *B,* Situation after complete cranialization.

FIGURE 8-10 *A*, Fractures within the superior or lateral parts of the posterior wall of the frontal sinus. *B*, Situation after partial cranialization.

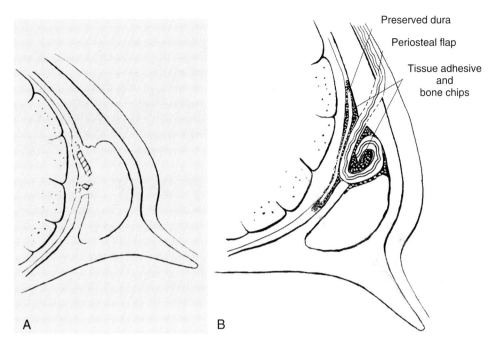

Preserved dura

Periosteal flap

Tissue adhesive and bone chips

A   B

In these cases, the author prefers a local mucosal flap. This rotating flap (Fig. 8-12) is created using the mucosa of the middle parts of the middle concha, which is tipped sideways and cranially, thereby epithelializing the access to the frontal sinus and ethmoidal cells before osteosynthesis of the forehead-nose pillar. Because of the anatomically narrow passages, bone must be reduced in the area of the nasofrontal junction. Nevertheless, it is important to avoid extensive thinning to achieve a stable bony union. Fibrin glue is used for the attachment of the mucosa-periosteal flap of the frontal parts of the middle turbinate.

Endoscopic Surgical Techniques

Endoscopic management of facial and skull base fractures has lagged behind endoscopic surgery in other areas of the body, but more and more is gaining credibility. With the

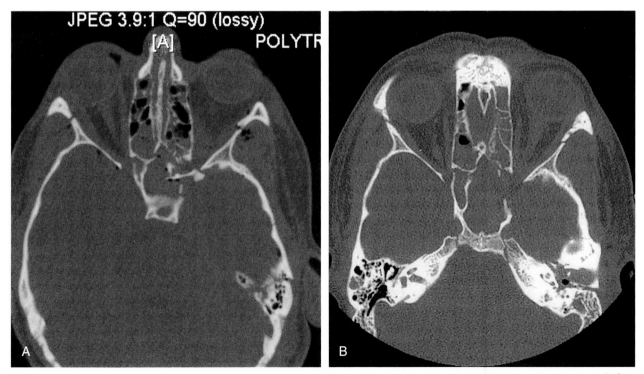

FIGURE 8-11 *A*, Preoperative CT of a skull base fracture involving the roof of ethmoid cells, sphenoidal sinus, and optic canal. *B*, Same patient after removal of bone fragments and optical nerve decompression.

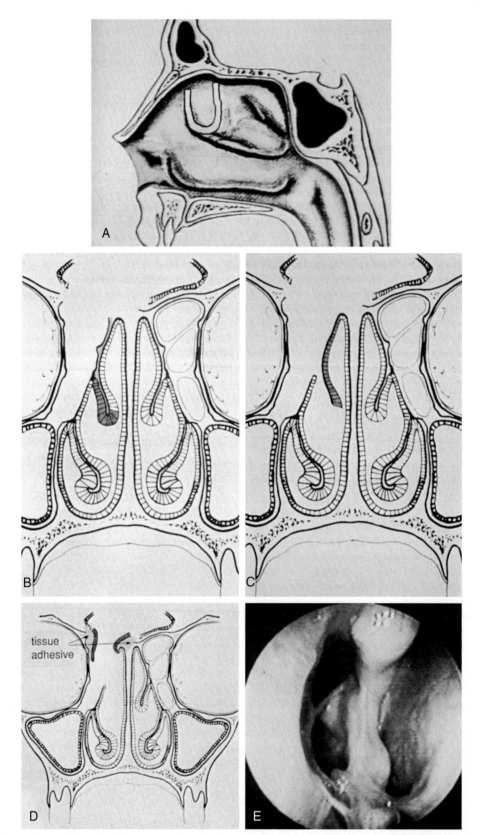

FIGURE 8-12   Operative technique involving the creation of a rotating flap using the middle turbinate. *A,* Superiorly based mucosal flap. *B* and *C,* Bony lamella and inferior and lateral parts of the mucosa are removed. *D,* The mucosal flap is turned upward. The flap and free mucosal transplant are fixed with fibrin glue. *E,* Endoscopic control 8 weeks after surgery. Wide and fully epithelialized frontal sinus and ethmoid cavity openings are visualized.

development of improved instrumentation for fracture reduction and stabilization, and increasing surgical skills, open approaches may come to be reserved for only the most complicated cases.

DEVELOPMENT OF OSTEOSYNTHESIS

In the past, the treatment of fractures of the frontomaxillary area (i.e., the so-called interorbital space[4]) and the sealing of fractures of the frontal skull base were commonly osteoclastic procedures. Loss of bony structures created visible and disturbing facial defects, however.

Secondary correction required considerable effort (e.g., using the implantation of bone or cartilage or individually prepared plates of tantalum). These types of correction were possible only in a few cases. Wiring has been the standard procedure for stabilizing fractured facial bones, but it has not always given satisfactory results. Wiring promotes readaptation of bony fragments but cannot achieve a stable 3-dimensional reconstruction of the frontomaxillary area in cases of multiple fractures.

Clinical observations made it obvious that wiring of the frontomaxillary area could not prevent secondary dislocations of the affected bones by the forces present at the time of the repair and during the period of any intermaxillary fixation. Repositioning the maxilla and its wire suspension to the zygomatic process of the frontal bone also creates pressure on the rebuilt osseous nasal or frontomaxillary complex. In the case of the frontomaxillary complex, deforming pressure is exerted toward the back and the side. Despite intermaxillary fixation, pressure transferred by the masticatory muscles acts in the same manner. In general, in these cases, wiring of the osseous fragments of the interorbital space cannot prevent traumatic bony telecanthus and a traumatic saddle-nose deformity.

Based on the investigations of Michelet and associates[13] and Champy and colleagues,[14] various bone plates were developed in many clinics, such as those created by Luhr.[15] Developing bone plate osteosynthesis for facial bone was continued in the basic investigations of Perren and co-workers[16] in the surgical treatment of fractures of the extremities. Thin bone plates were used primarily for osteosynthesis of the zygomatic bone.

To create a bone plate fixation able to withstand any normal functional loads, an anatomic and clinical study[7] was initiated in 1979 in the ear, nose, and throat clinic of the University of Würzburg. These investigations first tried to define which sizes and forms of the plates and screws might be ideal for use in the frontomaxillary area. The thickness of the bone in the areas to be considered for plate osteosynthesis were measured on adult skulls and skull pieces, using the skull collections of the departments of anatomy of the universities of Würzburg and Innsbruck. Measuring instruments used were dental calipers, which are normally used in maxillofacial orthopedics and orthodontic techniques. With these instruments, the deep-seated and usually inaccessible bone in the area of the nasal roof could be measured within a precision of 0.1 mm.

As in most of the skulls, the calvaria had already been separated, permitting the thickness of the anterior walls of the frontal sinuses and of the skull caps also to be measured. Forty-five skulls and 21 right or left halves or skull pieces

were studied. Significant differences between the right and the left sides were not found.

In the medial part of the nasal bone and up to the roof of the nose, the bone has a mean thickness of 1.5 to 4.2 mm. The thickness of the bony wall of the frontal process of the maxilla increases similarly to its upper areas. Mean values of 2.1 mm were found inferiorly, whereas mean values of 3.2 mm were found superiorly. Consequently, the superior parts of the osseous base of the bony nose seem to be thick enough to allow fixation of bone plates with screws 5 to 7 mm long (e.g., the miniplate system).

The mean thickness of the anterior wall of the frontal sinus varies from 1.75 to 2.42 mm. The differences are caused by bone crests at the back of the bone, which usually arise from the interfrontal septum.

The mean thickness of the calvarial bones in the specimens studied was 5.5 mm, making it suitable for bone plate fixation in every case. The bone of the anterior wall of the frontal sinus also seems to be generally suitable for bone plate osteosynthesis, although sites less than 2 mm thick are too thin to allow satisfactory miniplate osteosynthesis; therefore, in these areas, microplate osteosynthesis is preferable. Elsewhere, all bones of the supraorbital and infraorbital rims with a mean thickness of more than 5 mm were found to allow miniplate fixation.

Figure 8-13 shows all sites of the upper cranial and facial skeleton at which miniplate or microplate bone fixation might be considered. In essence, bony walls that are at least 2 mm thick should provide sufficient retention only for microscrews. Miniplate osteosynthesis, however, requires bone at least 3 mm thick.

Resorbable materials, plates, and screws composed of a copolymer of 82% polylactic acid and 18% polyglycolic acid have been successfully used in the reconstruction of pediatric craniofacial deformities for several years. Eppley and colleagues,[21] as well as Weingart and co-workers,[22] did not see serious complications such as infection, overlying soft-tissue reactions, reconstructive instability, or underlying osteolysis around the screws during postoperative periods of several years. Bhanot and co-workers[23] tested the resorbable system in three patients with frontal sinus fractures, two patients with midfacial fractures, two patients with mandibular defects, and two patients with laryngeal fractures; they found no disadvantage as far as rigidity of fixation, functional results, and complications in comparison with traditional plating systems. In our own experience, resorbable plates appear to be safe; easy to contour and apply; and allow stable fixation of bone fragments in areas without dislocation risk, probably because of the activity of the masticatory muscles. If long-term results remain favorable, the use of resorbable material may be a promising method also for stabilization of bone fragments of the forehead and frontal skull base.

CLINICAL EXPERIENCES

Most midfacial fractures are associated with frontal skull base fractures. Cases of maxillary fractures with malocclusion (i.e., Le Fort II or III fractures) are treated in cooperation with colleagues from a department of maxillofacial surgery. The first step of the operation is the rhinosurgical removal of any debris in the sinuses and the sealing of the frontal

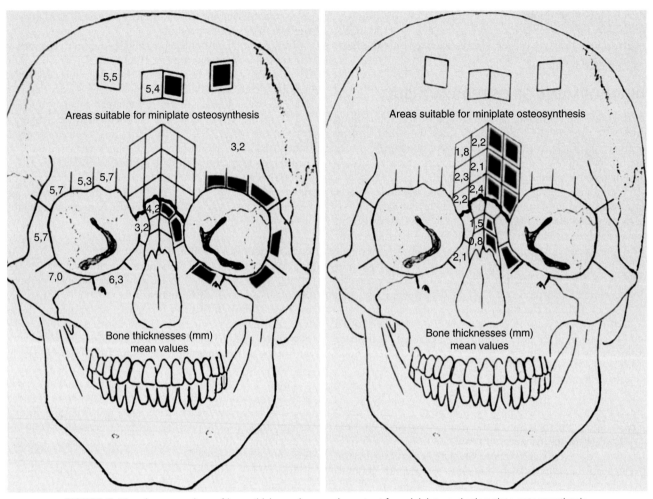

FIGURE 8-13   Average values of bone thickness in areas important for miniplate and microplate osteosynthesis.

skull base, as needed. After this step is completed, reconstruction of the osseous base of the nose follows, with stable osteosynthesis performed by the ear, nose, and throat surgeon.

In contrast to Champy's vitallium miniplates, titanium minisystems and microsystems are easier to handle. The versatility of these systems is a product of their better design and construction. Their design is also more variable and allows anatomic reconstruction to be carried out even in those cases having spatially irregular points of fixation. Further, because the quality of the titanium material is excellent, it allows the surgeon to bend the material over edges much more easily than with Champy's vitallium plates. The titanium plate can be formed quickly and without difficulty, so that it is even possible to reconstruct a previously prominent and angular nose. The osseous infraorbital rim can be readily joined to a bone plate framing the osseous nose. Repositioning the maxilla to the frontal bone, with its wire fixation to the zygomatic process, cannot damage an initially performed stable reconstruction of the nose using plates (Fig. 8-14). The stability provided by such plates is a real improvement in comparison to the former wiring technique.

In cases of single-piece fractures in the glabellar area, if the bone of the anterior wall of the frontal sinus is thick enough, two or three 5-mm screws give sufficient stability to hold the reconstructed osseous frame of the nose in place. The fragments of superior parts of the osseous nose can usually be fixed with 7- or 5-mm screws.

It is more difficult to reconstruct multiple fractures of the glabellar area because they are often associated with multiple fractures of the anterior wall of the frontal sinus. Solid osseous structures are needed for a stable reconstruction of the osseous base of the nasofrontal area, but they are generally located beyond the frontal sinus in the lateral or superior frontal bone. Such repairs require superior fixation in the calvaria (Fig. 8-15). In these cases, reconstruction of the anterior wall of the frontal sinus is best performed as a combination osteosynthesis. First, the fragments of the anterior wall of the frontal sinus are readapted with wires or microplates and microscrews before they are elevated so that they act as a lid. Following this step, definite fixation and stabilization can be performed by miniplate osteosynthesis.

Therefore, osteoplastic treatment of fractures of the osseous nasofrontomaxillary area with miniplate and microplate osteosynthesis allows three advantages: (1) a stable medial fixation of the maxilla to the frontal bone, (2) an effective treatment for traumatic telecanthus, and (3) prevention of a bony saddle-nose deformity.

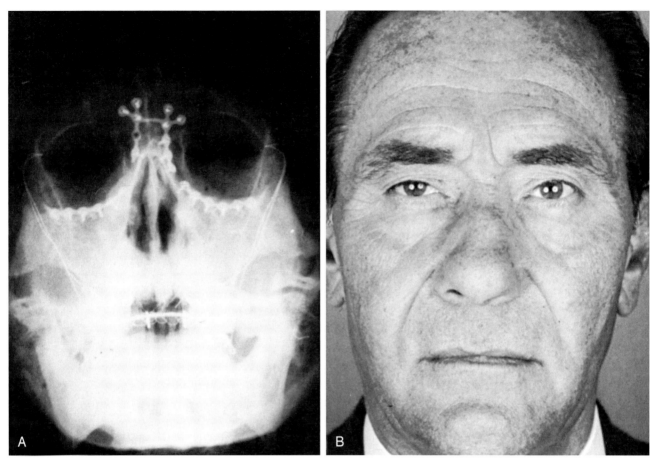

FIGURE 8-14 Radiologic and clinical example of miniplate osteosynthesis after Le Fort III fracture combined with a localized fracture of the ethmoidal roof; strong fixation of the medial bony midfacial fractures to the anterior wall of the frontal sinus.

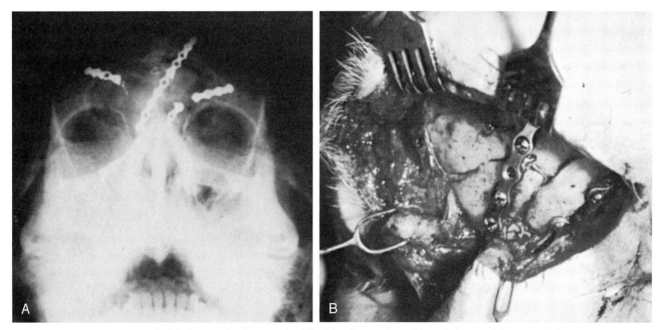

FIGURE 8-15 Radiologic and clinical example of a central midfacial and comminuted frontal sinus wall fracture. *A*, Osteosynthesis using wires and miniplates with fixation to the calvarium. *B*, Situation 9 months later. Bony healing is complete, and the material used for osteosynthesis can be removed.

With a stable bone plate osteosynthesis of the osseous nasofrontomaxillary complex, the osseous base of the nose is restructured as a well-fixed medial osseous block. This block acts as a solid foundation against any lateral traction arising from the more laterally situated suspension of the maxilla to the zygomatic process of the frontal bone. Similarly, this solid medial osseous block prevents redislocation produced by the masticatory muscles. Another advantage of this step is that it prevents the occurrence of a dish-face deformity, as was commonly seen in the past. Thus a good esthetic result is achieved, and satisfactory function is also possible. In patients with these conditions, tracheotomy often can be avoided. The osseous base of the nose that has been reconstructed by bone plates is usually so stable that nasal intubation is generally possible after rhinosurgical treatment. If nasal intubation is performed, it is preferable that the procedure be completed by the ear, nose, and throat surgeon.

The advantage of bone plate maxillofacial osteosynthesis is the stable fixation of bony fragments. This method allows better healing of the overlying soft tissues and especially prevents excessive tissue shrinkage and scar formation. The author's experience has also been that tiny fragments of the anterior wall of the frontal sinus with a bone thickness less than 1 mm do not heal, and these are completely resorbed when the bone plates is removed. To avoid inflammatory complications, it is preferable in these cases to use the biggest bone pieces only (having a wall thickness of at least 2.5 mm) to reconstruct the anterior wall of the frontal sinus. For fixation of the fragments, micro-osteosynthetic material is preferable.

As long as good frontal sinus drainage is gained, it is not necessary to remove the mucosa of the back part of the big bone pieces used for osteosynthesis. Remaining gaps can be closed by using titanium micromesh in combination with bone chips or adapted bone transplants from the skull (Fig. 8-16). The free bone transplants are adjusted using wires or micro-osteosynthetic material. The edges of the transplants are formed in such a way as to create broad bony contact areas. Gaps are filled with bone meal and fibrin glue. These reconstruction techniques are better performed after a primary coronal incision has been selected.

POSTOPERATIVE PROGRESS, PROBLEMS, AND COMPLICATIONS, AND SECONDARY RECONSTRUCTIVE TECHNIQUES

Even with extensive experience with osteosynthesis, it is not possible to prevent screws from having contact with the mucosa of the upper paranasal sinuses and thus allow infection to spread from the mucosa to the bone. Therefore, it seems to be important to carry out careful postoperative management of the nasal region, including decongestion and frequent suctioning of the nose, combined with cortisol and other inhalation aerosols, to reduce inflammation of the soft tissues.

All nonresorbable osteosynthetic material should be removed after bony consolidation has taken place. Before discharge from the hospital, the patient and family have to be instructed to attend follow-up examinations on a regular basis and to be certain that osteosynthetic material is removed

at a later date. All patients with paranasal sinus surgery after trauma, especially those with osteosynthetic material above the frontal or ethmoidal sinus, should be registered in an osteosynthesis chart and asked to attend follow-up examinations.

Important diagnostic procedures in these follow-up examinations at 1 week; then 3 weeks; and, later, yearly periods are endoscopy of the nose and paranasal sinuses using various items of optical equipment (e.g., a flexible endoscope; ultrasound; and the conventional x-ray study, CT scan, or MRI study).

From 1980 to 1983, 73 patients with fractures of the central and lateral viscerocranium and of the rhinobase were treated in the ear, nose, and throat clinic of Würzburg using miniplate osteosynthesis. The results using this method are satisfying in both esthetic and functional aspects. Postoperative follow-up studies showed that an astonishingly high percentage of patients remained without any complaints, even those who suffered from extensive crush fractures and the loss of precious mucosa. Fifteen patients were found to have rhinitis sicca, and 13 showed recurrent mucopurulent sinusitis. Accompanying edema of the upper and lower eyelids, which is a sign of a threatening orbital complication, was found in 6.8% of all cases. To date, only two patients had a true complication of menacing pyesis.

Early complications usually are caused by penetration of ascending infection from the nasal and sinus mucosa along the screws, reaching the frontal bone and thus creating frontal sinus empyema, a subperiosteal abscess, or osteitis within the frontal area. Late complications are caused by scar formation in the area of the newly created frontal sinus opening. Following blocking of the drainage, mucoceles and secondary inflammatory reactions may develop months or even years later; if one fails to diagnose and treat them at an early stage, meningitis, frontal bone osteitis, or subdural or brain abscess can occur (Fig. 8-17).

Different opinions exist as to whether nonresorbable osteosynthetic material may remain permanently or must always must be removed. In Germany, because there are still serious disadvantages, nearly all metal implants are removed after bony consolidation takes place. This approach creates additional costs, however. Reasons for removal of the material are at first cosmetic. Usually after a few months, because of a thin cover of soft tissue, plates and screws within the face and the skull can be palpated by the patient and become disturbing foreign bodies. Chromium, nickel, cobalt, and a few other alloys have proved to be potential causes of cancer in animal studies. It cannot be denied that leaving metallic (or other) foreign material within the human body may cause cancer.

Because even the so-called Titan alloys may be corroded in vivo, and because high concentrations of titanium oxide (up to 2000 parts per million) were commonly found in the localized areas of Titan implants, especially those within soft tissue, all kinds of Titan material should be removed, as far as possible, even if a few manufacturers have claimed that the removal of the so-called "pure Titan" is not absolutely necessary. Exceptions have to be considered concerning the elderly or patients with tumors. Metallic implants covering nasal sinuses should always be removed 6 to 9 months after bony consolidation, because at least one of the screws has contact with the mucosa of the nasal sinus. Thus an infection

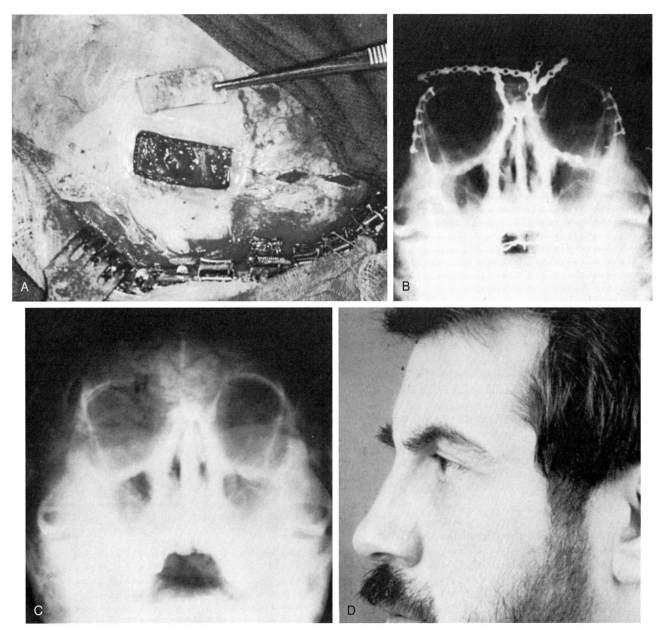

FIGURE 8-16　Radiologic and clinical example of adapted bone transplants from the skull. *A*, Removal of a piece of split skull from the parietotemporal area. *B*, Reconstruction using miniplates and wires. *C*, Radiologic control 10 months after surgery, with the free bone transplant completely healed. *D*, Clinical situation 1 year after surgery.

within the nasal sinus may easily reach a screw and cause an acute large osteolytic infection of the frontal bone and adjacent skull bone or even initiate an endocranial complication as well.

In the case of allergic reactions, the metallic implants have to be removed immediately. In the author's practice, two such cases were observed, one occurring 4 months after a midfacial osteosynthesis with titanium plates (Fig. 8-18) and another occurring 6 months after refixation of a frontonasal osteotomy lid with a chromium-cobalt plate. In both cases, punctiform, itching, pimple-like skin irritations occurred, starting in the face within the area covering the osteosynthesis material and causing severe itching, foreign body sensation, and malaise. In both cases, shortly after that time, pruritic skin eruptions could also be found on the entire body and extremities. After removal of the osteosynthetic material, the skin irritations disappeared completely. In both cases, an epicutaneous skin test showed the specific sensitization.

Ionomer bone cement was used for several years in Europe and proved to be a good material for secondary reconstructive surgery (e.g., the reconstruction of the frontonasal or supraorbital bone defects as well as for the roof of the skull). Although pure acrylates have the disadvantage of producing heat during polymerization, ionomer cement remains at an almost constant temperature. Because of cases of lethal neurotoxic reactions in skull base surgery in 1996 in Belgium, France, and Austria, probably caused by lysis of cemental frame work in contact with liquor, this material was taken out of practice.[17]

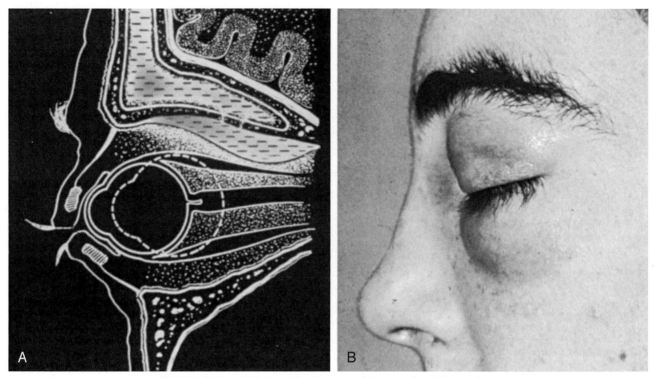

FIGURE 8-17   Orbital complication caused by ascending inflammation.

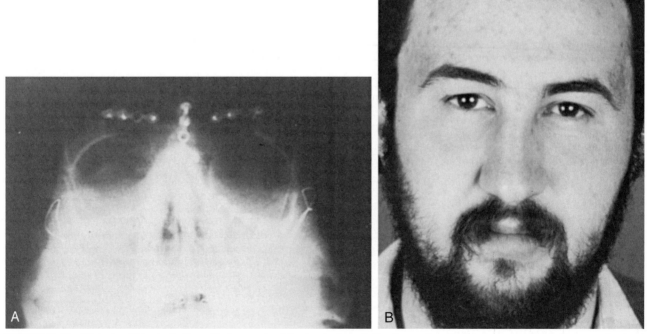

FIGURE 8-18   Clinical and histologically verified example of foreign body and allergic reactions to titanium material. *A,* Osteosynthesis of the left infraorbital rim and anterior wall of the frontal sinus using titanium miniplates and screws. *B,* Allergic reaction 4 months after surgery.

CONCLUSIONS

Surgical experience in Europe, and the author's personal work in the area of anterior skull base and midfacial trauma in Würzburg and Augsburg ENT Departments, proved that closing traumatic dural tears offers protection against primary and secondary meningitis resulting from ascending infection.[24] The use of the operative microscope, well-tolerated implants, fibrin glue, miniosteosynthesis and microosteosynthesis, and cooperation among all participant specialists guarantee a high quality of functional and esthetic results in most cases. The result of the surgery, however, depends on the extent of *primary* bone and soft tissue destruction. Therefore, in cases in which only emergency treatment is possible, insufficient functional and esthetic results may occur and require secondary treatment.

Acknowledgments

Thanks are due to all colleagues and staff members of the Head Clinic of the University of Würzburg between 1983 and 1996; and colleagues of the ENT Department Zentralklinikum of Augsburg, Germany since 1996, especially to Professor Roosen, Department of Neurosurgery, Wuerzburg; Professor Reuther, Department of Maxillofacial Surgery, Wuerzburg; Professor Grumme, Department of Neurosurgery, Augsburg; Professor Solymosi and colleagues from Department of Neuroradiology, University of Wuerzburg; Professor Kretzschmar and Dr. Roesler, with colleagues from the Department of Neuroradiology, Zentralklinikum Augsburg, for cooperation and preparing excellent x-rays, MRIs, and CT scans; as well as Dr. Guenzel, senior resident, and Dr. Julia Tegeler, resident of the ENT Department of Augsburg.

REFERENCES

1. Escher F: Clinical classification and treatment of frontobasal fractures. In Hamberger CA, Wersäll J (eds): Disorders of the Skull Base Region. Proceedings of the Tenth Nobel Symposium Stockholm, August 1968. Stockholm: Almquist & Wiksell; New York: Wiley, 1969, pp 343–352.
2. Teachenor FR: Intracranial complications of fracture of skull involving frontal sinus. JAMA 88:987–989, 1927.
3. Cairns H: Injuries of the frontal and ethmoidal sinuses with special reference to cerebrospinal rhinorrhoea and aeroceles. J Laryngol 52:589, 1937.
4. Converse JM, Smith B, Wood-Smith D: Orbital and naso-orbital fractures. In Converse JM (ed): Reconstructive Plastic Surgery. Philadelphia: WB Saunders, 1977, pp 748–793.
5. Dingman RO, Converse JM: The clinical management of facial injuries and fractures of the facial bones. In Converse JM (ed): Reconstructive Plastic Surgery. Philadelphia: WB Saunders, 1977, pp 599–747.
6. Draf W, Samii M: Fronto-basal injuries-principles in diagnosis and treatment. In Samii M, Brihaye J (eds): Traumatology of the Skull Base. Berlin: Springer, 1983, pp 61–69.
7. Brunner FX, Kley W, Plinkert K: Anatomical studies and a correlative management of facial skeleton and skull base injuries with bone plate fixation. Arch Otorhinolaryngol 245:61–68, 1988.
8. Raveh J, Vuillemin T: The surgical one-stage management of combined cranio-maxillo-facial and frontobasal fractures. J Craniomaxillofac Surg 16:160–172, 1988.
9. Samii M, Draf W: Surgery of the Skull Base. Berlin: Springer, 1989, pp 114–158.
10. Oberascher G: Cerebrospinal fluid otorrhoea-rhinorrhea: The Salzburg concept of cerebrospinal fluid diagnosis. Laryngol Rhinol Otol (Stuttg) 67:375–381, 1988.
11. Tessier P: Relationship of craniostenoses to craniofacial dysostoses, and to faciostenoses: A study with therapeutic implications. Plast Reconstr Surg 48:224–237, 1971.
12. Tessier P: Definitive plastic surgical treatment of the severe facial deformities of craniofacial dysostosis: Crouzon's and Apert's diseases. Plast Reconstr Surg 48:419–442, 1971.
13. Michelet FX, Deymes J, Dessus B: Osteosynthesis with miniaturized screwed plates in maxillo-facial surgery. J Maxillofac Surg 1:79–84, 1973.
14. Champy M, Loddé JP, Schmitt R, et al: Mandibular osteosynthesis by miniature screwed plates via a buccal approach. J Craniomaxillofac Surg 6:14–21, 1978.
15. Luhr HG: Indications for use of a microsystem for internal fixation in craniofacial surgery. J Craniomaxillofac Surg 1:35–52, 1990.
16. Perren SM, Russenberger M, Steinemann S, et al: A dynamic compression plate. Acta Orthop Scand 125(Suppl):29–41, 1969.
17. Helms J, Geyer G: Alloplastic materials in skull base reconstruction. In Sekhar LN, Janecka IP (eds): Surgery of Cranial Base Tumors: A Color Atlas. New York: Raven Press, 1993, pp 461–469.
18. Levin LA, Beck RW, Joseph MP, et al: The treatment of traumatic optic neuropathy: The international optic nerve trauma study. Ophthalmology 107(5):814, 2000.
19. Wang BH, Robertson, BC, Girotto JA, et al: Traumatic optic neuropathy: A review of 61 patients. Plast Reconstr Surg 107(7):1655–1664, 2001.
20. Stennert E: Bell's palsy: A new concept of treatment. Arch Otorhinolaryngol 225(4):265–268, 1979.
21. Eppley BL, Sadove AM, Havlik RJ: Resorbable plate fixation in pediatric craniofacial surgery. Plast Reconstr Surg 100(1):1–7, 1997.
22. Weingart D, Bublitz R, Michilli R, Class D: Resorbable osteosynthesis material in craniosynostosis surgery. Mund Kiefer Gesichtschir 5(3):198–201, 2001.
23. Bhanot S, Alex JC, Lowlicht RA, et al: The efficacy of resorbable plates in head and neck reconstruction. Laryngoscope 112(5):890–898, 2002.
24. Winkler J, Bogdan U, Becker G, et al: Surgical intervention and heparin-anticoagulation improve prognosis of rhinogenic/otogenic and posttraumatic meningitis Acta Neurol Scand 89:293–298, 1994.

9

Management of Cerebrospinal Fluid Leaks

T. FORCHT DAGI

Cerebrospinal fluid (CSF) fistula is a serious, frustrating, and potentially fatal condition whose successful management requires a fundamental understanding of the anatomy and pathophysiology of the problem. Until recently, the management of this condition was almost exclusively neurosurgical. Over the past decade, however, otolaryngologists skilled in functional endoscopic sinus surgery have contributed considerably to the surgical armamentarium, and the endoscopic approach is considered by some of those surgeons to have become the standard of care.[1] Although the endoscopic approach may be well-suited to the majority of cases encountered in otolaryngologic practice, it does not exhaust the techniques with which the neurosurgeon must be conversant in view of the full range of anatomic and pathophysiologic conditions confronted in neurosurgical practice. This chapter, therefore, addresses both the traditional neurosurgical approaches and the newer endoscopic techniques. In addition, it reviews the use of glues, engineered tissues, and tissue substitutes in the management of CSF fistulas.

The evolution of current thinking is best reviewed from a historical perspective.

HISTORICAL OVERVIEW

The correlation of post-traumatic rhinorrhea with leakage of CSF was made in the 17th century by a Dutch surgeon, Bidloo the Elder.[2,3] Cases in which apparently nontraumatic CSF rhinorrhea resulted from increased intracranial pressure were then reported by Miller in 1826[4] and by King in 1834.[5] The full significance of CSF fistulas was not elucidated until 1884, however, when Chiari[6] demonstrated a fistulous connection between a pneumatocele in the frontal lobes and the ethmoid sinuses of a patient who died of meningitis following rhinorrhea. The introduction of roentgenography enabled the diagnosis of a fistula to be made in vivo through the detection of intracranial air,[7] ultimately leading to the development of pneumoencephalography as a diagnostic procedure[8] and, less directly, to the refinement of surgical techniques for the repair of CSF fistulas.[9,10]

Despite a number of early attempts, successful repair was not consistently achieved until the mid-1930s. In 1937, Cairns[11] published a series of cases demonstrating that CSF leaks could be repaired by the extradural application of fascia lata. The actual need for surgical intervention was regarded as unproven, however, and the indications remained controversial until the latter part of World War II.

By 1944, Dandy[12] advocated surgical repair of any CSF leak within 2 weeks of onset to prevent meningitis. In British neurosurgery, Lewin's review of the British combat experience and of a large series of basilar skull

fractures[13,14] became the basis for the adoption of aggressive operative management as the standard of care. Lewin demonstrated that the cessation of an active leak did not itself eliminate the risk of meningitis, because the possibility of intermittent communication with the contaminated extracranial space persisted unless repaired. By the mid-1950s, it became virtually axiomatic to operate on all CSF fistulas, except for some that had a well-understood cause and that closed spontaneously within several days of onset.

The recent enthusiasm for extradural endoscopic approaches to the skull base reflects both the elegance of endoscopic technology and the relative safety of extradural techniques. In fact, Cairns and Dandy both advocated the extradural approach because of its safety. As intradural surgery became safer in the years following World War II, the extradural approach was supplanted, at least among neurosurgeons.[15] Evidence upon which to base a consensus regarding the more successful operative route has yet to be collected.

The introduction of minimally invasive approaches to CSF fistulas, whether microscopic or endoscopic, has simultaneously facilitated the extradural approach and blurred the distinction between truly extradural and intradural repair.[1,16–18] For purposes of this discussion, endoscopic repair is considered extradural when it is intended to patch or plug a fistula from outside in, and is considered intradural when it is intended to facilitate the localization or repair of a fistula by placing a plug or graft intradurally.[19,20]

The primary danger of CSF leakage has been framed in terms of the potential for meningitis, and the primary indication for treatment has been driven by the rarity of spontaneous and permanent cessation of the leak. Recent years have witnessed an increasing appreciation for the inherent complexity of this problem. Why should some leaks stop and others not? Why should some recur? Why should 20% or more of repairs that are done come to failure? With these questions in mind, the principle promoted by Lewin[13] (i.e., the idea that *all* cranial CSF fistulas, without exception, be repaired surgically unless they resolve spontaneously within 5 days or a week) has come under increasing scrutiny. The observations that have led to a reconsideration of the Lewin principle are as follows:

1. Some fistulas seem to heal spontaneously with time and stay closed, especially if external CSF drainage is used as an adjunctive maneuver.
2. A recurrence rate of 6% to 25% and a not inconsequential historical operative morbidity and mortality accompany the various forms of reparative surgery.

3. The incidence and severity of meningitis in otherwise uncomplicated CSF leaks may be diminished by treatment with antibiotics.[3,21-29]

CONVENTIONS AND DEFINITIONS

The term *rhinorrhea* is used to describe fluid dripping from the nose. *Otorrhea* is used to describe fluid dripping from the ear. These terms are intended to indicate the site of the *drip*, rather than the site of the *fistula* or the leak. CSF leaking through temporal bone fractures, for example, can easily reach the nasopharynx through the eustachian tube and mimic a leak through the cribriform plate. There is no specific term to describe leaks from the spinal subarachnoid space.

Transcranial CSF leaks fall into two major categories: *traumatic* leaks and the so-called *spontaneous* or nontraumatic leaks. The traumatic group, in turn, is divided into two groups: *acute or early* leaks that present within 1 week of injury and *delayed* leaks that occur months or years later. The nontraumatic group is also divided into subsets, including leaks associated with intracranial mass lesions; leaks associated with congenital defects of the skull base; leaks associated with osteomyelitis, osteonecrosis, and other causes of bony erosion; leaks associated with focal cerebral atrophy[5]; and leaks associated with an ill-defined group of acquired hernias, meningoceles, and meningeal diverticula perforating pneumatized bone in the anteromedial middle fossa.[30] Nontraumatic fistulas are divided again into high-pressure and low-pressure categories.[5,31] There is good reason to apply an analogous nosology to the traumatic group as well.[25] Iatrogenic or postoperative leaks are usually included in the category of traumatic fistulas.

Spinal CSF leaks can be classified similarly. Most spinal CSF leaks are postoperative and therefore traumatic. A number of rare congenital anomalies can give rise to meningopleural or meningoperitoneal fistulas.[32] The distinction between high-pressure and low-pressure fistulas is particularly important in the management of spinal leaks. In children with spinal dysraphism or other anomalies, the leak may be the first expression of hydrocephalus or shunt failure.[33,34]

CAUSE AND EPIDEMIOLOGY

Traumatic Leaks

The most common cause of CSF leaks is head trauma, particularly basilar skull fracture.[35] In Lewin's series of 100 patients with head injury,[13] 7% had basal skull fractures and 2% had CSF leaks. A CSF leak was detected in 2.8% of 1250 head injuries and in 11.5% of the basilar fractures studied by Brawley.[22] In another study of 1077 skull fractures, including a particularly large proportion of high-speed road traffic accidents, 20.8% of 168 basilar skull fractures had an acute CSF leak.[36] The association of incidence with high speed, although not rising to the level of a correlation, is certainly suggestive. The incidence in cases of penetrating missile injuries is comparable: in 1133 cases, 101 (8.9%) developed a CSF fistula. The proportion is somewhat higher with transventricular penetration.[37]

Thus CSF leaks occur in approximately 3% of all head injuries; 5% of cases with craniofacial trauma; 9% of high-energy penetrating injuries; and 12% to 30% of basilar skull fractures, depending on the accelerative forces involved. Traumatic CSF leaks typically begin within 48 hours, and it is estimated that 95% of them will be evident within 3 months of injury.[38,39]

In childhood, the incidence of traumatic CSF leaks is far lower at 1% or less of closed head injuries.[40] This disparity may be caused by differences in fragility between the adult and the pediatric skull, as well as by the lack of development of the air sinuses in children. As a rule, the frontal sinuses become visible between the 4th and 12th year, and they are always detected by the 15th year. These sinuses are often asymmetric until age 20 years. The ethmoids are present at birth, enlarge by age 3 years, and are fully formed by age 16 or 17 years. The cavity of the sphenoid sinus is usually recognizable by age 4 years and is fully developed by puberty. In the pediatric age range, the interpretation of sinus x-ray studies is often difficult because of small size, variations in development, and normal calcification and clouding.[35]

Spontaneous Leaks

The term *spontaneous leak* is a 19th century misnomer that has persisted and entered into common use. If it is to have any useful meaning, the term should be restricted to leaks explained neither by trauma nor by any other cause. The literature allows far broader license.

Because there have been few, if any, collected series of nontraumatic leaks rigorously studied, there are insufficient data to extrapolate quantitative estimates of incidence or cause.[31] Tumors and increased intracranial pressure (ICP) are highly correlated with nontraumatic leaks. Anecdotal series suggest that pituitary tumors are the most common neoplastic cause of spontaneous CSF leaks. Increased ICP may be present or absent. Because of the structures eroded by sellar masses, such leaks generally present as rhinorrhea.[33,41,42] Other presentations, including a serous otitis media, have also been reported.[43-45] On the other hand, there is an intriguing report of pituitary hyperemia in the context of nontraumatic CSF leak masquerading as pituitary adenoma in three patients. After surgical repair of the leak, the magnetic resonance imaging (MRI) abnormalities, including an enlarged pituitary resembling pituitary tumor, reverted to normal.[45]

Postoperative Leaks

Large, annoying, and potentially dangerous subgaleal collections of CSF were common before the modern era of neurosurgery. In retrospect, they probably represented the most visible manifestations of altered postoperative CSF flow characteristics, increases in intracranial pressure, or unrecognized or untreated hydrocephalus, in some *combination*. These collections often leaked through the incision. In consequence, postoperative incisional CSF leaks were understood to be common neurosurgical complications. Attempts to prevent this complication were focused on careful dural closure, buttressing the suture line, multiple-layer incisional repair, and other techniques for reconstruction and reinforcement of violated tissue planes and compartments, and especially the air sinuses after frontal and posterior fossa surgery. All of these technical details were important, but none was as important as control of intracranial pressure and CSF dynamics postoperatively and the improvement in postoperative management contributed by serial sectional imaging.

Although more radical approaches to cerebellopontine angle lesions, to tumors straddling the nasopharynx and the anterior and middle fossae, and to the skull base as a whole appear to have increased the prevalence of CSF leaks of all types, an accurate estimate of the incidence of incisional CSF leaks is difficult to provide. A recent study reports a 12% incidence (10 patients) in 85 posterior fossa procedures, but this figure may not pertain to other types of craniotomy.[46]

In large series CSF fistula occurs in 1.4% to 22% of operations for cerebellopontine angle tumor. The wide range may reflect the fact that it often proves necessary to report results encompassing many years and spanning important variations in technique in order to achieve significance.[46–50] The incidence of leakage has been reduced by careful technique, including waxing and plugging mastoid air cells as they are opened and placing a graft of adipose tissue in the opened porus acusticus.[51–54] The use of endoscopy to inspect the craniectomy site for unsealed air sinuses has also been advocated.[55] Several recent series demonstrate that the incidence can be reduced below 11%, and that much lower rates are achievable, but that the incidence of leak seems relatively consistent irrespective of surgical approach (e.g., posterior fossa, transmastoid, or middle fossa).[46,48–51,54] It is noteworthy that rhinorrhea, a classic false localizing sign in this setting, may be the presenting sign in up to 50% of leaks.[46]

In transsphenoidal approaches to the pituitary, leaks occur in 1.4% to 6.4%.[56–58] In a small series reporting outcomes after the endoscopic transnasal transsphenoidal approach, the incidence was 14% (1/7).[59]

Frontal, ethmoid, and sphenoid surgeries have always entailed the risk of inadvertent skull dural penetration. Endoscopic techniques were developed to improve visualization in the hope of reducing complications associated with blind instrumentation. It is not immediately obvious that the prevalence of CSF fistula has changed substantially, however. Estimates of incidence range from 0.002% to 2.9%.[60,61] The latter figure was derived from a study explicitly designed to maximize the likelihood of diagnosing occult leaks using β-trace protein (prostaglandin D synthase) analysis and a 6-month follow-up.[61]

PNEUMOCEPHALUS

Intracranial air, a pathognomonic sign of CSF fistula after trauma or spontaneous rhinorrhea (but not pathognomonic after surgery), is demonstrable in approximately 20% of patients with CSF leaks.[62] Pneumocephalus is post-traumatic in 75% of these patients and is spontaneous, or otherwise unexplained, in 10%.[63]

MENINGITIS

Meningitis occurs in approximately 20% of acute post-traumatic leaks and in 57% of delayed leaks.[35] Although these figures vary, meningitis occurs more commonly in the delayed post-traumatic group. The incidence of meningitis in nontraumatic CSF leaks has not been well documented. Anecdotally, copious, continuous leakage of the high-pressure

type is less likely to be associated with meningitis than is intermittent leakage.[31] The overall risk of meningitis associated with traumatic CSF leaks of all types is on the order of 25%.[1,14,64–67] In neurosurgical postoperative leaks, the incidence of meningitis can be calculated to be on the order of 20%, but this figure is admittedly complicated by the problem of distinguishing aseptic from bacterial meningitis, and by the complexity introduced by factors such as steroid administration, chronic illness, and immunosuppression that might impair wound healing and predispose to both leaks and meningitis. The high incidence of delayed infection in military penetrating head injuries is demonstrably correlated to CSF fistulas, actively leaking or not.[68,69]

DEFINING AND LOCALIZING A FISTULA

The management of CSF leaks involves three steps[1]: (1) confirming that the leaking fluid is really CSF,[2] (2) delineating the site of the fistula, and (3) defining its mechanism.[3]

Clinical Evidence to Confirm the Presence of Cerebrospinal Fluid

Glucose

The presence of glucose in clear leaking fluid has been used historically to differentiate CSF from nasal secretions and other sources of serous or serosanguinous drainage. The concentration of glucose in CSF equals or exceeds 50% of the serum concentration except as follows[1]: during meningitis,[2] after subarachnoid hemorrhage, or under other unusual circumstances.[3] The glucose concentration in nasal secretions, in contrast, is 10 mg/dL or less.[70]

Quantitative measurements of glucose concentration are diagnostic. *Qualitative* spot tests, such as those provided by chemical testing strips (e.g., Clinistix, Dextrostix, Uristix, or Tes-Tape), are *not* definitive for two reasons.[1] First, the glucose oxidase test on which they are based is too sensitive, turning positive at values less than 20 mg/100 mL of glucose.[2] Second, normal nasopharyngeal secretions often elicit false-positive reactions even in the absence of glucose.[71,72] Thus, although a *negative* glucose oxidase reaction effectively eliminates the possibility of CSF rhinorrhea, a *positive* result does not diagnose it unequivocally.

Reservoir Sign

It is widely held that true CSF leaks produce quantities of fluid sufficient for collection and quantitative analysis at some time in their course. The reservoir sign, the ability of a patient to produce CSF at will by positioning the head in a certain way, is generally taken to be quite specific for a fistula with pooling in the sphenoid sinus.[30] Although Dandy[12] believed that this sign would differentiate leakage through the frontal sinus from ethmoidal and sphenoidal leaks, it is not reliably localizing.

Target Sign

The target sign refers to the pseudochromatographic pattern produced by the differential diffusion of CSF admixed with blood or other serosanguinous fluid on filter paper or bedclothes. CSF migrates further, creating a bull's-eye stain with blood in the center. This is a convenient but unreliable sign, because whenever watery nasal secretions and blood are mixed, the same phenomenon occurs.

Headache

CSF leaks can be accompanied by high-pressure or low-pressure headaches. Intermittent high-pressure leaks are characterized by *high* CSF pressure headaches that are relieved by the sudden discharge of fluid and that build up again over time. Normal-pressure leaks, in contrast, are characterized by postural *low* CSF pressure headaches, relieved by reclining or otherwise allowing pressure in the subarachnoid space to rise to normal levels.

Other Confirmatory Evidence

The finding of unusually low opening pressure in the lumbar subarachnoid space is corroborative evidence for CSF leak. Unilateral or bilateral *anosmia* is associated with defects or leaks in the region of the cribriform plate and the fovea ethmoidalis. Olfaction may be preserved, however, in cases of spontaneous CSF rhinorrhea with congenital defects of the cribriform fossa.[31,64] *Optic nerve* lesions point to the tuberculum sella, the sphenoid sinus, and the posterior ethmoids as the likely site of injury. Impaired *vestibular function, facial nerve palsy,* and *cochlear damage* accompany fractures in the temporal bone.

Imaging Techniques

Imaging techniques are used to detect intracranial air, fractures and defects in the skull base, mass lesions, and hydrocephalus, and to demonstrate flow through fistulas or skull defects.[73] Plain films, multiplanar tomography, computed tomography (CT), and MRI have been used to delineate the anatomy and pathology of the skull base, sinuses, and calvaria. Stains, contrast agents, and radioactive tracers are injected into the ventricular or lumbar subarachnoid space to prove that leaking fluid is CSF and to show, directly or by inference, the location of the leak.

Radiographic data must be interpreted in the context of clinical findings. As always, *positive* data obtained from radiography are helpful, but *negative* data are often meaningless.

Plain Radiography and Computed Tomography

Plain films and CT are examined for evidence of fracture; air/fluid levels in the frontal, ethmoidal, and sphenoid sinuses; intracranial air; chronic increased intracranial pressure; erosion of bone by tumor or infection; congenital anomalies; and penetrating objects. Although multiplanar tomography provided exquisite detail of bony anatomy, it is of historical interest only, having been supplanted by high-resolution thin-slice CT with overlapping cuts.[74] Contrast cisternography in conjunction with CT provides dynamic information about flow patterns of CSF.[75] Similar information is also obtainable from MRI with appropriate software.[76] MRI also provides superb detail of soft tissue pathology at the skull base and in the nasopharynx.

Tracers

The categorical proof of CSF fistula is the ability to retrieve extracranially a tracer substance injected into the CSF. The nonradioactive substances injected into the CSF historically have included methylene blue, phenolsulfonphthalein, indigo carmine, and fluorescein.[77,78] Only indigo carmine and fluorescein remain in common use for intraoperative visualization: the others proved unacceptably toxic.[5]

In the presence of an active leak, cotton pledgets placed along the anterior roof of the nose, the posterior roof and the sphenoethmoid recess, and the middle meatus and below the posterior end of the inferior turbinate can be used to confirm that a leak exists. When differentially stained or contaminated by radioactive isotopes, they indicate the location of the leak.[29] The following procedure has been recommended to localize a leak with fluorescein:*

1. A spinal tap is performed.
2. Ten milliliters of spinal fluid are withdrawn after measuring the opening pressure.
3. The fluid is mixed with 0.5 mL of 5% fluorescein.
4. The mixture is slowly reinjected intrathecally.
5. The patient assumes a recumbent position for about 30 minutes, the time depending on the size of the leak.
6. The pledgets are removed and examined under ultraviolet illumination.

The findings are interpreted in Table 9-1. In addition, the middle ear is examined for evidence of staining, an indication of leakage.

In the presence of an active leak, tracer methods are sensitive and reasonably specific. With slow, low-volume, or intermittent leaks, tracer methods may give false-negative results.

The use of intrathecal fluorescein injection is quite controversial. Although otolaryngologists continue to recommend and utilize it routinely, neurosurgeons have become wary of its use because of reports of transverse myelitis and other serious adverse events.[79] Indigo carmine is preferred by most neurosurgeons, not only because of its safety record but also because it is more visible than fluorescein to the unaided eye. This characteristic makes it useful to check for the presence of CSF fistulas intraoperatively, when ultraviolet illumination may not be readily available.[30]

Radioactive tracers require less skill to detect. It is easier to detect minute amounts of radioactivity than to distinguish faint color on pledgets stained by bloody fluid or mucus. [131]I (RISA) was widely used for cisternography in the past. It has been replaced by ^{111}In DTPA, an isobaric tracer that combines improved physical properties, fewer adverse reactions, better imaging quality, and shorter half-life (2.8 days). [169]Yb DTPA and ^{99m}Tc albumin have also

TABLE 9-1 ▪ Interpretation of Nasal Pledget Staining

Location of Stain	Probable Site of Fistula
Anterior nasal	Cribriform plate or anterior ethmoidal roof
Posterior nasal or sphenoethmoidal	Posterior ethmoid or sphenoid sinus
Middle meatus	Frontal sinus
Below posterior end of inferior turbinate	Eustachian tube (middle fossa)
Behind tympanic membrane	Not accurately predicted

*Caveat: Fluorescein has been associated with severe adverse reactions in this application, see below.

been approved for CSF imaging, but these tracers suffer from suboptimal imaging characteristics and half-lives (32 days and 6 hours).

Isotope cisternography is an effective method by which to demonstrate the existence of a CSF leak, but it becomes inaccurate for purposes of localization when "flooded" by a high-volume leak. The tracer saturates the pledgets and contaminates surrounding tissues with radioactivity so that differential localization becomes impossible.[35,80,81]

The importance of the timing of radioactive contamination is insufficiently appreciated. Active leaks can be documented by contamination of accurately placed pledgets within 0.5 to 2 hours. Slow or intermittent leaks can sometimes be detected by leaving the pledgets in longer or by replacing them over 6 to 48 hours. The danger lies in overinterpretation or misinterpretation of the data. There are two confounding mechanisms. First, the isotope can be absorbed into the bloodstream from the CSF and undergo secondary secretion into the nasopharynx.[82] Second, there exists an alternate pathway for isotope secretion, first recognized in normal dogs and subsequently documented in normal human volunteers, involving active transport from the CSF and passage via the olfactory nerves, or passive lymphatic drainage leading to contamination of nasopharyngeal secretions.[83]

The accuracy of faintly positive tests can be improved slightly by calculating a radioactivity index (RI) ratio. This ratio compares the radioactivity in counts per minute of an exposed pledget with that of 1 mL of blood, as follows:

$$\text{RI ratio} = \text{RI}_{\text{pledget}} / \text{RI}_{1\text{ mL blood}}$$

An RI ratio less than 0.3 is normal. Canine studies suggest that the ratio is at least five times greater in the presence of a leak. In the canine model, the RI ratio of nasal activity to CSF is 1:14 when measured 2 to 5 hours after cisternal injection of radiosotope. The RI ratio of nasal activity to blood is 1:2 to 3 when measured 2 to 5 hours after intravenous injection of radioisotope. Thus the RI ratio of CSF to blood is 4.6:7. The significance of tracer substances that appear in low concentrations only 5 hours or more after injection should be carefully weighed.

Two additional points deserve mention. First, it has been suggested that tracer injected into the cervical subarachnoid cistern can be forced through a slow, intermittent, or low-pressure leak by raising the CSF pressure with saline or artificial CSF delivered via a constant infusion pump.[84] Second, scans carried out 24 and 48 hours after injection of isotopes can help define the mechanism of a leak by detecting defects in CSF absorption and circulation.

Cisternography

Early attempts at demonstrating CSF leaks by injecting air or iophendylate (Pantopaque) into the subarachnoid space failed to produce consistently satisfactory images. The combination of high-resolution CT and metrizamide, or of other form of cisternography with water-soluble contrast agents, yields excellent visualization of *active* leaks. Smaller fistulas have been demonstrated through stressing the barriers to CSF flow by having the patient cough or carry out a Valsalva maneuver.[35] For maximal contrast enhancement, cisternal injections can be performed via C1–C2 punctures. Overlapping views in both the coronal

and the axial planes are required.[74] Direct coronal studies are preferable to reconstructed images. The risk of provoking seizures and aseptic or chemical meningitis following cisternography should be kept in mind.

A newer and safer technique utilizes MRI technologies to visualize CSF flow.[76,85–88] A full discussion of the technique is outside the scope of this chapter, but heavily T2-weighted fast spin–echo studies with fat suppression and video reversal of the images are reported to yield sensitivity, specificity, and accuracy of 0.87, 0.57, and 0.78, respectively, in a study in which 65% of patients eventually underwent surgical exploration.[86]

MR remains less effective than CT in demonstrating bony anatomic detail. It is absolutely reasonable to require both for diagnostic purposes and in conjunction with the preoperative planning.[89–94]

Immunologic Methods

Immunologic methods differentiate between proteins in CSF and those in nasopharyngeal secretions.[95,96] Irjala and colleagues[97] have described the use of an immunofixation technique for the identification of microaliquots (100 μL) of CSF by demonstrating two electrophoretically characteristic bands of transferrin. The B1 fraction consists of normal transferrin and sometimes two variant fractions. The B2 fraction characteristic of CSF contains smaller amounts of neuraminic acid. This method is not subject to contamination from other body fluids (e.g., tears or nasal secretions). The immunofixation method could theoretically be used for localization of the leak by differential suction techniques in the nasopharynx, but large-scale clinical trials of this method have yet to be reported. Another surrogate marker for CSF is β-trace protein (prostaglandin β synthase), as reported by Arrer and colleagues.[98] The β-trace protein test is reported to offer an overall accuracy of 95.7%, a specificity of near 100%, and a sensitivity of 91.2%.[99]

ANATOMIC CONSIDERATIONS: SITES OF LEAKAGE

Trauma

CSF leak can occur wherever the dura is lacerated during an injury. It is more likely to persist or recur, rather than close spontaneously, where a meningeal hiatus is maintained by bony spicules, by dura entrapped in the edges of a fracture, or by herniating brain and leptomeninges. Avulsion of the olfactory fibrils can result in a dural fistula through the cribriform plate even without a fracture, particularly in the elderly or where the tissue around the ethmoidal roof has been thinned. Post-traumatic fistulas are often complex and multiple.

Spontaneous

Nontraumatic leaks are usually confined to a single region where an anatomic defect is demonstrable, but exceptions have been noted.[100] It is usually easier to demonstrate the defect than the leak. High-pressure leaks that act as safety valves for hydrocephalus occur where the skull is thinnest, usually the cribriform fossa and the sellar region. This is the case, for example, in Crouzon's disease and osteopetrosis (Albers-Schönberg disease).

The middle fossa can be the site of CSF leaks that are direct in that they do not cross the inner ear. Such fistulas have been described mainly in conjunction with a pneumatized temporal fossa. Pulsatile CSF forces induce additional thinning of the bone and enlargement of the pits and small bony defects that are normally present. The leptomeninges and brain herniate, thinning the dura and leading to rupture of the arachnoid. The leak may be constant or intermittent depending on several factors, such as the underlying intracranial pressure, whether an arachnoid diverticulum is created, and whether brain tissue temporarily obliterates the leak. A similar sequence of events has been postulated to explain CSF leaks in the empty sella syndrome[30] and in focal atrophy.[31]

Indirect fistulas through the temporal bone are the most elusive. In *extralabyrinthine fistulas* the defect is in the *middle fossa* in the region of the tegmen tympani. In *intra-labyrinthine fistulas*, CSF escapes into the labyrinth through the subarachnoid space of the *posterior fossa*. In either case, the leak can present as otorrhea or, when the tympanic membrane is intact, as rhinorrhea.[62] The possibility of temporal bone dysplasia should be investigated whenever a patient with severe hearing loss develops unexplained or recurrent meningitis.[30,35,101] For example, in the Mondini malformation (i.e., unreactive ear with a shortened cochlear coil, dilated semicircular canal system, and widened inner ear vestibule), it is hypothesized that a widened, patent cochlear aqueduct allows CSF to pass from the subarachnoid space to the inner ear via a leak in the oval window. Other proposed routes include defects of the scala tympani; of the footplate of the stapes; or of the thin, bony plate separating the internal auditory canal and the inner ear vestibule and perforated by nerve fibers innervating the utricular and saccular maculas.[102–104]

HIGH-PRESSURE VERSUS LOW-PRESSURE LEAKS

When a CSF leak is the manifestation of increased intracranial pressure from mass effect or from hydrocephalus, the underlying cause must be treated before the leak can be effectively repaired. The existence of increased intracranial pressure can be inferred from several sources. Skull films and CT scans disclose signs of pressure, mass effect, and tumors. Radiographic signs suggestive of defective circulation and absorption of CSF include periventricular lucencies, enlarged temporal horns, a disproportionately plump third ventricle narrowed at the massa intermedia, and an empty sella. Extracerebral collections of CSF can represent the so-called fifth ventricle phenomenon, a hydrocephalus variant. Other concomitants of high-pressure leakage include papilledema and optic atrophy; pallor of the optic disc; enlarged central scotoma or subtle binasal visual field cuts; a history of headaches worse in the morning or while recumbent, relieved by a gush of fluid; variable or intermittent diplopia; intermittent clonus or pyramidal tract signs reversing spontaneously after leakage; and a history of granulomatous meningitis, subarachnoid hemorrhage, head trauma, or some other event that might adversely affect the circulation of CSF.

Infants with incisional leaks after fresh meningomyelocele repair can be assumed to have hydrocephalus, especially if there is an accompanying Dandy-Walker malformation.

In contrast to other cases of postoperative leak, in which the temporizing maneuvers discussed subsequently are often effective, CSF shunting is generally required.

INITIAL MANAGEMENT

The initial management of CSF leaks is intended to confirm the existence of a leak, to slow or stop the leak, and to prevent meningitis. Usually, these ends can be satisfied simultaneously.

Antibiotics

Antibiotics have not been proven effective in changing the incidence of meningitis in post-traumatic or postoperative CSF leaks. In traumatic leaks, they are no longer recommended routinely.[15–17,21,36,105–109] For postoperative leaks, however, prophylactic antibiotics are commonly, if not universally, employed. There is some theoretical justification for distinguishing between the two situations. Several principles are useful to keep in mind when prescribing prophylactic antibiotics[108,110]:

1. Patients should not be kept on antibiotics indefinitely in the hope that a leak will seal; a trial of conservative therapy is reasonable, but the end point should be decided a priori.
2. Wide-spectrum antibiotics are not desirable for prophylaxis; the most specific antibiotic capable of eliminating the potential pathogens should be used.
3. Patients of different ages and in different locations harbor different vulnerabilities because of changes in nasopharyngeal and environmental flora; thus, *Haemophilus influenzae* is a common cause of meningitis in children and in the elderly, whereas diplococcus is more common in healthy adults.
4. Patients can develop meningitis even while on prophylactic antibiotics; after the usual investigations are carried out, the antibiotics are changed to cover the appropriate organisms and sensitivities.
5. Bactericidal antibiotics should be chosen when possible.

Intensive Care

The admission to intensive care units of patients with CSF leak was universally advocated in the older literature. This admission may certainly be warranted in some cases of trauma or spontaneous high-pressure leaks, but it is not always needed for recurrent or postoperative leaks. A great deal depends on the adequacy of staffing in a given institution; on intensivist, nursing, and house staff coverage; and on specific aspects of nursing policy affecting the type of care and interventions that can be offered in various locations. One consideration to keep in mind is that opportunistic infections arising in intensive care units are usually caused by resistant organisms and are often highly recalcitrant to treatment with the usual antibiotics.

Position

The preferred elevation for patients with cranial leaks is between 45 and 70 degrees. Patients with a spinal leak should be kept flat if at all possible.

EXTERNAL DRAINAGE OF CEREBROSPINAL FLUID

External drainage of CSF has been used in various forms for many years. External ventricular drainage[111,112] has been replaced in most centers by continuous lumbar drainage, first described in 1963.[113] Since then, lumbar drainage has been found useful in controlling and sometimes curing CSF leak of every cause.[23–25] McCoy[114] provided theoretical justification for the initial management of CSF fistulas with CSF diversion by demonstrating that granulation can seal the fistulas, provided that the leakage has stopped. Lumbar drainage should be considered, therefore, whenever positioning alone does not eliminate, or at least significantly diminish, a leak within 24 hours.

Technique

A 19-gauge catheter is threaded percutaneously through a 17-gauge Touhy needle inserted into the lumbar subarachnoid space between L4–L5 and L2–L3. Aside from increased attention to sterile technique, there is no difference from standard lumbar puncture procedure. After 10 to 20 cm have been threaded rostrally, the needle is removed over the catheter. If there is any significant resistance to passage, the needle and the catheter should be removed as a unit. *Under no circumstances should the catheter be withdrawn through the needle once the tip has protruded,* because the needle tip may shear the catheter, leaving the tip irretrievably lost in the subarachnoid space or in the subcutaneous tissue. The proximal end of the catheter is connected via the appropriate adapters to a closed, sterile drainage system. Prepackaged kits for epidural anesthesia generally provide all the necessary catheters, needles, and fittings. Specialized drainage kits for lumbar CSF drainage are also marketed commercially. In their absence, a blood transfusion pack connected to the catheter with intravenous tubing can be used for collection. Antibiotic ointment may be placed at the skin entry site. A waterproof, occlusive dressing should be applied, with the catheter coiled and taped to relieve strain and to prevent disconnection.

Prevention of Infection with Indwelling Subarachnoid Catheters

The infection rate with indwelling catheters can be prohibitive, ranging in some series as high as 10% or more.[115] The risk is lower with lumbar catheters.[26] Infection can be reduced by prophylactic antibiotics (potentially, by two thirds[115]) and by externalization of the catheter through an extended subcutaneous tunnel.[116] *Staphylococcus* species and other skin flora are the major threat: antibiotics should be chosen to reflect the sensitivities of local pathogens.

Prophylaxis is continued for 8 to 24 hours after the catheter is withdrawn. Daily samples of CSF are obtained; cultured; examined by Gram stain; and analyzed for cell count and differential, glucose, and protein. The presence of a catheter does not, of its own accord, lower the CSF glucose or evoke a major leukocytotic reaction; the cell count and glucose concentration remain quite stable in uninfected CSF over 4 to 9 days. Any persisting variation of 2 standard deviations or more from the cumulative average cell count

and glucose concentration over several days is cause for concern and careful reexamination of the CSF for signs of opportunistic infection.[117] So too would be the emergence of any clinical signs or symptoms of meningeal irritation.

External drainage has been maintained in large series for 10 days without infection. Longer durations have been reported in exceptional cases.[25] By analogy with central venous access lines, it may be wise to change catheters if drainage is continued beyond 7 days.

How Long to Drain

The data on which these recommendations are made are empirically derived. Drainage should be continued for 3 to 5 days after stoppage of the leak to allow healing. If leakage recurs, operative repair is indicated. If the underlying problem is increased intracranial pressure or hydrocephalus, implantation of a drain acts purely as a temporizing maneuver: no "cure" is effected. Similarly, the patient whose leak is not controlled by external drainage should be considered for early operation. In Findler's series of 50 patients,[29] drainage of 350 to 420 mL daily was continued for an average of 10 days, with a leak recurrence rate of 14%. There was an additional 8% incidence of delayed leak at the site of lumbar puncture.

As a rule, acute post-traumatic and postoperative normal-pressure leaks respond to external drainage. Transitory high-pressure leaks also respond, so long as the pressure elevation recedes over the duration of the drainage. Delayed and recurring leaks cannot be definitively managed by drainage.

Pharmacologic Adjuvants to Drainage

Pharmacologic agents such as acetazolamide (Diamox) that retard the production of CSF may be helpful in reducing CSF pressure after the drain has been removed.[118] They are temporizing agents only. They do not serve as definitive treatments for the fistulas, nor as definitive treatments for altered states of intracranial pressure.

Complications

High CSF protein concentrations predispose against a successful drainage. If, for technical reasons, patency of the drainage catheter cannot be maintained, repetitive lumbar punctures through a large needle (18 gauge) often afford almost the same benefit.

Calcaterra[18] records one case of fatal postoperative suboccipital hemorrhage attributed to overdrainage of CSF in an elderly patient. Similar complications have followed spinal anesthesia.[119–121] Overdrainage of CSF can also cause life-threatening pneumocephalus.[64,122–124] The CSF pressure should be lowered, and may even be lowered substantially, but should not be reduced to less than 0 through negative pressure.

The acute reduction of CSF pressure can also precipitate headache, nausea, and vomiting. This reaction can be prevented, according to Findler and colleagues,[29] by gradually lowering the pressure and increasing the drainage over several days. An accidental siphon effect can be avoided by relating the height of the drainage valve or the drainage bag to the level of the ventricular system rather than the bed. In this way, the pressure column remains constant as the bed is raised and lowered or as the patient is moved. Most commercial systems incorporate a micropore filtered air port to prevent siphonage. Improvised systems are generally unable to include such a port, and positioning becomes critical.

There has been long-standing concern regarding the possibility of inducing meningitis by retrograde migration of bacteria into an open fistula under the influence of negative CSF pressure induced by an external drain.[5] This seems to be an extremely rare complication, avoidable by maintaining a low but steady positive pressure in the CSF.

Catheters should not be removed forcibly. If a catheter resists withdrawal, the advantages of removal under direct vision in the operating room should be seriously weighed. After removal of the catheter, the tip is examined to ensure that no part of it has been left behind. An unused catheter should be available for comparison because the indwelling catheter may be distorted or elongated during withdrawal. It is prudent to note the condition of the catheter in the medical record, and to follow up any unusual findings with sectional imaging studies.

If the catheter is not intact, an effort should be made to locate and identify the retained segment. Although most catheters are intended to be radiopaque, they are easily missed on plain x-ray studies and are better visualized on CT.

There are two strong indications for retrieval of a broken catheter tip: (1) infection in the region of the tip, and (2) radicular pain or paresis associated with juxtaposition of the retained catheter to an appropriate root. In most cases, the retained fragment can be ignored safely. If symptoms in the region point to possible catheter involvement at some future time, sectional imaging studies should be obtained and the matter weighed anew.

Dural-cutaneous fistulas can occur at the site of catheter insertion, particularly in the setting of a high-pressure leak. Most such fistulas stop spontaneously or seal with a single stitch. Low-pressure or normal-pressure leaks can also be sealed by an injection of 10 to 20 mL of autologous blood as an epidural blood patch. This technique is favored by anesthetists and obstetricians for the treatment of low-pressure, "spinal" headaches. The technique has been shown by a number of studies to improve over natural history[125–129] with a success rate of 93%.[130,131]

Epidural blood patching has resulted in symptomatic mass effect, hemorrhagic complications,[132] and infection. Surgical repair of the dura may still be needed. External lumbar drainage is contraindicated in the context of increased intracranial pressure from a mass in the posterior fossa because of the danger of precipitating herniation through the foramen magnum.

OPERATIVE MANAGEMENT

Timing of Surgery

The debate regarding the timing of surgery revolves around three issues:

1. Most CSF leaks stop spontaneously and do not recur.
2. Surgery is neither universally successful nor without hazard.
3. Modern antibiotics have significantly reduced the morbidity from any infection that may develop while waiting for the leaks to stop, or that may ensue should a leak recur.

Acute Post-traumatic Leaks

Some types of leak have relatively high probability of sealing spontaneously. Most acute post-traumatic leaks stop within 10 days of injury: in Mincy's classic series[3] of 54 cases of rhinorrhea in frontal fossa injury, 35% had stopped within 24 hours, 68% within 48 hours, and 85% within 1 week. Similar numbers emerge even from series of complex craniofacial injuries.[39] The use of lumbar drainage may further increase the rate of sealing.

There are three classic indications for surgical intervention: (1) a bout of meningitis, (2) pneumocephalus, or (3) an active leak (persistent or recurring). Lewin's insistence on surgery for virtually all leaks was based on the threat of meningitis. There is no evidence that early surgical repair offers any significant improvement over natural history in patients with acute post-traumatic leaks that cease spontaneously within the first week after injury.

Most leaks or dural tears associated with midface fractures stop permanently when the facial fractures are reduced.[39,133] Meningitis is relatively uncommon in dural tears associated with facial fractures despite the fact that the incidence of dural laceration in facial fractures (43%) is higher than in closed head injuries (7%) and that CSF leak occurs far more commonly (36%).[133]

Postoperative Leaks

Most postoperative incisional leaks also stop spontaneously or with lumbar drainage, particularly if the incision is reinforced or oversewn and underlying abnormalities of intracranial pressure are addressed.

Postoperative rhinorrhea and otorrhea are less likely to seal. If position and lumbar drainage do not stop the leak within 48 hours, or if the leak stops and recurs, most authors favor re-exploration of the wound and direct repair of the fistula. The air sinuses are usually implicated in these cases.

In the series by Spaziante and colleagues[57] of 140 transsphenoidal operations, 4 of 6 leaks stopped with lumbar drainage alone. Ciric[58] estimates that 2% of transsphenoidal cases require reoperation for CSF leak. The statistics in series of posterior fossa lesions is more variable,[46,48–50] with reoperation required in 75% of one well-documented series.[49]

Indications for Surgical Intervention

Prompt surgical intervention may be indicated under the following circumstances:

1. Acute traumatic or postoperative leaks that recur or persist after 10 to 13 days of conservative management, including external drainage
2. Proven intermittent or delayed leaks
3. High-pressure leaks acting as a "safety valve" for hydrocephalus
4. Leaks associated with erosion, destruction, disruption, or severe comminution of the skull base or of the paranasal sinuses
5. Leaks associated with congenital dysplasias of the brain, skull base, orbit, or ear, particularly after a bout of meningitis
6. Leaks caused by high-energy missile wounds

7. Postoperative rhinorrhea and otorrhea that cannot be controlled by position and drainage, especially when the air sinuses have been violated as part of the operative route
8. High-volume leaks through the petrous bone and the sella are particularly recalcitrant to conservative management

Operative Techniques

There are three major operative approaches currently in use. Often combined, they are as follows: (1) craniotomy, including intradural and extradural techniques; (2) extracranial extradural, endoscopic or not, with degrees of complexity ranging from simple packing to complicated mucoperiosteal grafts; and (3) CSF shunting procedures.

Table 9-2 summarizes current techniques and their applications. Endoscopic technologies are becoming increasingly sophisticated. When 3-dimensional endoscopic visualization becomes available, the application of endoscopic techniques may broaden.

Craniotomy

Anterior Fossa

In the anterior fossa, the two approaches that are most used are the *intracranial extradural* and the *intracranial intradural*. The intracranial extradural approach has several limitations:

1. Dural tears are virtually inevitable in the course of dissection.
2. Areas of cerebral tissue herniation into bony defects cannot be easily visualized.
3. Permanent dural repair is not reliably achieved.

For these reasons, the intracranial intradural route is generally preferred when craniotomy is indicated.

Steroids, anticonvulsants, and prophylactic antibiotics are given preoperatively. The patient is positioned supine in a three-point or four-point frame or on a cerebellar head rest with body flexed, knees bent, nose at the midline, and head hyperextended with the malar eminences uppermost. A Doppler probe monitors for air emboli during the procedure; arterial and central venous access is obtained. A bicoronal scalp flap is turned. A bone flap is elevated ipsilateral to the leak for a unilateral exposure, and bilaterally otherwise. Although in some situations satisfactory access can be obtained from a unilateral exposure, a full exploration of the anterior fossa generally requires a bifrontal flap. Surgeons experienced in neuroendoscopy may find that a more limited approach suffices. Should the frontal air sinus be entered, the mucosa is stripped from both the flap and the sinus, the sinus is packed with bacitracin-soaked Gelfoam sponge, and a pericranial flap reflected from the scalp is sutured over open sinus to the dura. Instruments used to close the sinus are considered contaminated and replaced.

The intracranial intradural approach allows a full exposure of the anterior fossa. A satisfactory exposure results in the demonstration of both sphenoid wings, both cribriform fossae, and both orbital roofs. The middle fossa is usually out of reach. The exposure should extend as far posteriorly as possible. The anterior clinoids should be visualized. If the leak is to be repaired in conjunction with the definitive

TABLE 9-2 ▪ Operative Approaches to CSF Leaks

Procedure	Indications
Intracranial, intradural exploration	1. Acute or delayed traumatic leak from anterior or middle fossae 2. Anterior fossa leak with extrasellar intracranial mass 3. Congenital anomaly of brain 4. Definable dysplasia of the anterior or middle fossae 5. Postoperative leak after anterior or middle fossa surgery 6. Complex penetrating or through-and-through injuries involving cerebral tissue as well as extracranial structures 7. When craniotomy is indicated for other reasons 8. Whenever a significant dural hiatus is demonstrable
Extracranial, extradural approach Transseptal, transsphenoidal, or transethmoidal *Open* or *endoscopic* With tissue transfer, placement of fat plug or muscle pledget, injection of fibrin or other glues, applications of engineered tissue or tissue substitutes	1. Clearly defined "spontaneous" leaks from the anterior fossa, including the cribiform fossa and fovea ethmoidalis 2. Postoperative leaks after treatment of sellar and parasellar lesions
Primary repair of facial fractures *Sinus repair and ablation as necessary*	1. Le Fort II or III fracture with dural tear or CSF leak but without evidence of gross bony disruption of the skull base or significant cerebral contusion 2. Complex facial fractures involving orbit or air sinuses in which the initial leak has spontaneously sealed, without evidence of gross bony disruption of the skull base or significant cerebral contusion
Osteoplastic sinusotomy *Repair of posterior sinus wall or cranialization of sinus and packing*	1. Leaks associated with simple fractures through the posterior wall of the frontal sinus without evidence of comminution of the skull base or significant cerebral contusion
Ventricular or lumboperitoneal shunting	1. Carried out in conjunction with anatomic repair of a fistula or resection of a space-occupying mass in the face of hydrocephalus 2. Small leaks that cannot be identified

resection of an intracranial mass, other considerations may govern the exposure conjointly. Dehydrating agents and the drainage of CSF facilitate retraction.

The fistula is often betrayed by a palpable or visible dural defect or by a contusion, adhesion, or herniation of cerebral tissue. An obvious fistula is sealed by inserting a plug of abdominal fat and then covering the defect with a free or reflected flap of dura. The dura can be obtained from the adjacent bone or from the falx cerebri, depending on the location of the fistula. Alternatively, a free patch of pericranium, temporalis fascia, fascia lata, or lyophilized dura can be sutured to the surrounding dura and, if needed, used to reinforce a plug of fat. Fat forms a more durable plug than does muscle: muscle fibroses and shrinks, whereas fat remains viable by recruiting a blood supply from adjacent tissues. Simple dural laceration can often be sutured primarily. A dural patch graft may be inserted when necessary. Dural grafts should be harvested from autologous tissue (e.g., temporalis fascia, pericranium, fascia lata, or transversalis fascia) or from commercially prepared cadaver tissue (e.g., dura, pericardium, or amniotic sac).

Synthetic dural substitutes have been found wanting in the past. These substitutes have been implicated in secondary leaks at the suture site and as foci for secondary or persistent infection. Newer biomaterials may address these issues but should be subjected to rigorous outcome-based analysis when adoption is considered (see following section on Biomaterials and Tissue Substitutes).

If no discrete fistula is visualized, the entire floor of the frontal fossa (including both cribriform plates) and the limbus sphenoidale are invested with a large free pericranial graft. Sutures are placed to maintain approximation rather than to obtain a watertight seal. The vector of CSF pressure tends to approximate the graft to the dura and stop the leak. Although dural substitutes have been used to repair dural defects (with the limitations noted), there is usually enough pericranium available for this purpose to obviate the need for synthetic grafts.

Middle Fossa

For leaks from the middle fossa, the temporal floor must be thoroughly inspected. This is most efficiently done with an intradural approach. An extradural dissection runs the additional risk of damaging the facial nerve by inadvertent traction on the geniculate ganglion during exposure and dissection.

Craniotomy is the preferred route to the floor of middle fossa. Leaks involving the petrous bone and the posterior margins of the temporal fossa are often better approached from an extradural approach or a combined exposure. The principles of repair are identical to those in the anterior fossa. Free pericranial grafts are easier to manipulate than are dural flaps in the middle fossa. Additionally, because the middle fossa is bounded by venous sinuses, reflecting a flap of any substantial size is impossible. Because only a unilateral exposure can be obtained in the middle fossa, it is particularly important to identify the site of the leak preoperatively.

Air can be insufflated through specially designed tubes that seal the nares and occlude the posterior pharynx during surgery. By flooding the field with saline, it is sometimes possible to identify, by the bubbles, a fistula that would not otherwise be evident.[66] As a rule, it is simpler and more prudent to cover the entire anterior or middle fossa with a graft than to count on this technique.

Posterior Fossa

CSF does not leak from the posterior fossa except when fractures extend through the petrous bone, after surgery, and

in conjunction with some rare congenital anomalies. Otorrhea from petrous fractures rarely presents a problem because it typically stops spontaneously or after a course of external CSF drainage. The same holds true for rhinorrhea emanating in the posterior fossa and presenting as a false localizing sign.

Postoperative CSF leaks can present as rhinorrhea or otorrhea, or as trickles through the suture line, with or without an incisional collection. Leakage through the suture line may be self-limiting and may not lead to other serious complications, but it should not be regarded as normal.

Postoperative leaks through the mastoid or through the temporal bone can be quite challenging. It is standard technique to wax or to otherwise seal any opened mastoid air cells intraoperatively. This task can be facilitated endoscopically.[48–50,66] Some surgeons also recommend plugging the porus acusticus with fat when it has been enlarged for tumor removal. Watertight closure of the dura is achieved using a dural graft, and other precautions are routinely deployed as well.[47–53]

In the event of a persistent leak, re-exploration of the incision is indicated.[47–53] Some surgeons prefer an extradural approach via mastoidectomy, particularly for recalcitrant cases. When the ear is nonfunctional, this approach, combined with an obliteration of the inner and middle ear, ensures the maximal likelihood of detection and obliteration of the site of leakage. The approach does not address the problem of altered CSF dynamics, however.

For the so-called "spontaneous" leaks, such as those associated with the Mondini malformation, the extradural approach is generally adopted. These are complex cases, and multiple layer closures may be required.[134]

Although most incisional leaks after posterior fossa surgery can be repaired by oversewing the wound and draining CSF, an incisional leak should be understood to reflect a condition of altered CSF dynamics and increased intracranial pressure. Should leakage recur, or should the wound bulge with subgaleal CSF after drainage is discontinued, permanent CSF diversion should be considered. In children particularly, but also in adults, increasing the dose of corticosteroids and adopting a slower taper than usual may reduce the pressure and allow tissue barriers to reestablish.

Closure

A routine craniotomy closure is carried out. The patient is nursed in the head-up position for 3 to 5 days postoperatively, and is treated with laxatives and stool softeners to prevent straining. All heavy labor and lifting are prohibited for 3 months.

Lumbar Drainage

Lumbar drainage is not generally carried out after craniotomy because it is hoped that the CSF pressure will compress the graft onto the dura surrounding the fistula and create a seal. In extracranial extradural approaches, drainage of CSF helps create a seal and promotes healing.

Combined Craniotomy and Reduction of Facial Fractures

Most CSF leaks associated with fractures of the midface can be managed definitively by reducing the facial fracture.

Complex fractures impacted into the skull base often require reduction via craniotomy before realignment of the facial fracture. No definitive rules can be given for these injuries; treatment must be carefully individualized and often requires a team approach using professionals skilled in ear, nose, and throat surgery; dental surgery; ophthalmology; plastic surgery; and neurosurgery.[39]

Extracranial and Endoscopic Approaches

Aside from the classic transsphenoidal operations, the extracranial approaches to the skull base are often performed by a team involving otolaryngology (and, sometimes, other specialties). All the surgical disciplines interested in the skull base have begun exploring the benefits of endoscopy, either as a stand-alone technique or as an adjunct to open surgery. Lesser invasive approaches confer obvious advantages but depend for their success on the ability to localize and seal the leak or leaks with certainty. The easier the identification, the more focal the leak, and the more room to maneuver from below, the better are the odds of successful endoscopic intervention. Even so, remarkably complex procedures have been carried out with endoscopic visualization[1,21,22,135]

The endoscopic approach is a subset of the extracranial, extradural approach to CSF fistula. Although not identical, the guiding principles for the endoscopic and the nonendoscopic techniques are close enough to be considered together. This section focuses on the techniques of sealing a CSF fistula via the extracranial route rather than on the techniques of endoscopic surgery per se.

Indications

There are four situations for which the extracranial approach is particularly well adapted:

1. Discrete and definable normal pressure leaks through the cribriform plate or adjacent ethmoid labyrinth
2. Fractures that abut on an air sinus, particularly when the bony defect is limited to the cranial wall of that sinus
3. Postoperative leaks after transsphenoidal surgery
4. Leaks through the oval window, petrous bone, or other parts of the ear

Special Techniques

Intrathecal dye injected at the beginning of the procedure helps to visualize the leak intraoperatively. Indwelling catheters are often used: saline or artificial CSF can be injected intrathecally to distend the subarachnoid space and provoke an intermittent leak, and CSF can be drained postoperatively to encourage approximation of the flap and dural packing. Neuronavigational techniques and intraoperative sectional imaging may also be of value in particularly complex cases.

The key to the extradural approach is to identify and seal the leak or leaks with some combination of dural graft or substitute, bone or bone substitute, and packing. Lasting reconstruction of a dural barrier is the primary goal. Although the insertion of bone or bone substitute to reconstitute the skull base and hold the dural graft in place is not universally practiced, it is strongly advocated by some.[136] There is a view that reinforcement with bone is unnecessary because the air sinus below the leak should in any event be packed, a maneuver that serves both to reinforce the dural repair and to maintain the graft in position. The packing acts as a seal in its own right and serves to hold mucoperiosteal, periosteal, free fascia lata, or other grafts against the dura. A bone graft serves the same purpose, in theory, but it can be difficult to place and does not in and of itself act as a substantial barrier to CSF flow, unlike the ablated sinus packed with fat or muscle. Adipose tissue is generally preferred over muscle; anecdotally, it seems less likely to fibrose and is easier to harvest. Some centers have substituted cancellous iliac crest for fat. Others advocate attaching a graft with fibrin glue, packing the sinuses temporarily, and forgoing sinus ablation.[136,137] Irrespective of the choice of packing material, the mucosa of the sinus must be stripped to avoid mucocele formation if it is to be ablated.

Transfrontal extradural procedures can be carried out either through a forehead incision or via a bicoronal incision. There is one important advantage to the bicoronal incision: should it be necessary to obtain a more generous view of the frontal fossa, a craniotomy can be carried out without difficulty. This eventuality should be considered and discussed with the patient before surgery. The anterior wall of the frontal sinus is removed with a Stryker saw or the Midas Rex with the C1 attachment, following a template obtained from a 72-inch sinus film. The posterior wall is fully exposed: the mucosa is resected, and enough bone is removed to display the dural defect. The dura can be patched or sutured primarily. Depending on the extent of damage, the fragments of the posterior wall can be replaced or totally removed, thereby cranializing the frontal sinus. In either case, the sinus is ablated with fat or bone, and the frontal wall is restored.

Endoscopic techniques have been adapted to each of these approaches. The learning curve is high for endoscopic manipulation. In the event that a leak can be pinpointed, and the necessary tissue manipulation achieved, endoscopic procedures have the advantage of reduced hospitalization and, quite often, better visualization. In most cases 3-dimensional visualization is lost and the field of view is limited. Still, once the technique has been mastered, endoscopy offers remarkable versatility.[136–140] Three-dimensional endoscopy is just beginning to enter the market and may prove very useful in this application.

Depending on the angle required, the width of the desired window, the site of the leak, and the surgeon's preference, the sphenoid sinus and the sella can be approached trans-septally via a sublabial or a transnasal route, or transethmoidally via an external rhinotomy incision. The first approach is more familiar to neurosurgeons; but the transethmoidal approach is shorter, gives a wider exposure, permits more complete resection of the sphenoid septae, and overcomes some of the difficulties of endoscopic visualization of the lateral extensions of the sphenoid sinus, where spontaneous leaks are known to arise.[137] This is an important consideration in reoperation for CSF leak after transsphenoidal surgery, for example. The leak can often be sealed by reconstructing the sellar floor and packing the ethmoid or sphenoid sinus. A flap of mucoperiosteum can be elevated with or without the underlying cartilage and folded over the dural defect, sometimes after the interposition of free fascia lata graft. The wider the view, the easier the procedure.[136–143]

The endoscopic endonasal approach is still very useful. When used to seal CSF leaks in the parasellar area,[138–141] mucoperiosteum from the inferior turbinate serves as a convenient source of tissue.[138] Dural defects up to 10×10 mm have been successfully repaired, and Van Den Abbeele and colleages have successfully addressed even complex congenital malformations of the skull base by this route.[143]

If an open extracranial approach to the cribriform fossa and fovea ethmoidalis is preferred, these structures are best approached through a curved naso-orbital incision and a complete ethmoidectomy. A flap rotated from the middle turbinate or the septum is used to cover the cribriform plate and the ethmoid roof from below. The posterior ethmoidal artery is a landmark situated directly anterior to the optic nerve.

Extracranial techniques, whether open or endoscopic, carry a lower morbidity than does craniotomy, and these techniques also avoid anosmia. Endoscopic transfacial approaches are aesthetically preferable to open transfacial approaches. Extracranial techniques are sometimes successful in situations in which multiple craniotomies have failed; however, they do not permit a wide visual inspection of the orbitofrontal cortex or of the floor of the anterior fossa.

Glues, Tissue Substitutes, Engineered Biomaterials, and Other Technical Considerations

Parasellar leaks have been treated by injecting fibrin glue transmucosally under CT guidance.[142] The use of tissue glue to reduce the need for sinus ablation has been mentioned. From an historical perspective, the management of CSF leaks has drawn heavily upon the innovative use of glues, tissue substitutes, polymers, and engineered biomaterials to overcome the challenges of obtaining a permanent seal with reduced morbidity in relatively inaccessible areas.

After initially disappointing results with various forms of oxidized cellulose, sheet rubber, synthetic membranes, and gutta percha in the years following World War II, neurosurgeons returned to the use of autologous fascia and pericranium, or cadaver dura or pericardium, or similar human tissue for use as dural substitutes. Early tissue glues were also disappointing.

There was a round of enthusiasm for methyl methacrylate; for a time, it was hailed as the panacea for CSF leaks.[62,144] Long-term outcomes, however, were disappointing. Methacrylate was found to shrink; the leaks recurred. If infection set in, the plug became a septic nidus. The so-called "super-glues," or cynanoacrylates, which are chemically related to methacrylate, also proved problematic, although they were more successful when used to adhere packing or supporting tissue in place rather than to create an adhesive layer between dura and patch.[145–149]

More importantly, it has become evident that the concept behind the use of methacrylate was faulty: it is the dura, not the bone, that requires repair. Leaks seal when the dural fistula is closed. Except in rare instances, the bony structures do not require reinforcement. When they do, however, autologous bone or cartilage is preferable to foreign material. Should the underlying problem be hydrocephalus or increased intracranial pressure, the leak will not permanently stop until the intracranial pressures are adequately controlled.

Tissue Adhesives and Sealants

It was hoped that tissue adhesives might overcome some of the problems associated with obtaining a durable seal, especially in relatively inaccessible areas, and act as tissue sealants: they did not. The first generation of acrylic-based compounds proved particularly disappointing. In addition to carrying a risk of meningitis and of neural toxicity, particularly to the optic apparatus, they formed a barrier between layers of tissue, inhibiting granulation and preventing fibroblastic proliferation from fusing one layer to the next. With time, tissue adhesives became porous and resulted in recurring leaks.[146–149] More recently, the use of autogenous or prepackaged fibrin clot adhesives has prompted a reconsideration of the role of tissue adhesives. Initial tests of Bioglue have been promising.[150] Fibrin-based adhesives may be worth investigating in conjunction with relatively porous engineered tissue substitutes such as acellular cadaveric dermal matrix (ACDM), which is processed from human cadaver skin (AlloDerm, Life Cell Corp., Branchburg, NJ).[151] An excellent review of tissue adhesives is offered by Preul and colleagues.[152]

Use of Cerebrospinal Fluid Shunts

High-pressure leaks cannot be sealed without reducing the intracranial pressure. The primary pathology must be treated first, either by resection of the space-occupying lesion or by reduction of CSF volume and flow in hydrocephalus. Nonetheless, several types of recalcitrant fistulas have been successfully treated with lumboperitoneal shunts.[153–154]

CSF shunting can be attempted in normal-pressure leaks when other means of repair have failed, or when, after exhaustive investigation, the site of the leak cannot be delineated. Lumboperitoneal shunting has been advocated as the only treatment needed for small leaks that cannot be visualized.[84,155] This empirical approach assumes that the resistance to flow through the shunt will be less than the resistance to passage through the fistula. With shunt malfunction, the leak may recur. Moreover, tension pneumocephalus can occur when air is aspirated intracranially through an open fistula under negative pressure.[62,122,123] The treatment for this complication is ligation of the shunt, initially, and replacement of the valve with a higher pressure unit once the mass effect has been treated and the air resorbed.

Treatment of Spinal Cerebrospinal Fluid Leaks

Although the treatment of spinal CSF leaks does not fit neatly into a discussion of cranial fistula, the great majority of the issues and principles are very similar, if not identical. Spontaneous spinal CSF leaks rarely occur outside the setting of spinal dysraphism or unusual spinal anomalies. Some rare leaks have been attributed to bone spurs at the skull base or cervical spine.[156] There is a rare and relatively young population subject to recurrent leaks at multiple sites without explanation,[157] or with unusual abnormalities such as "nude nerve roots" in which the nerve root sleeve is absent at multiple levels.[158] Another category, documented in three patients, is characterized by new onset of daily headaches and C1–C2 retrospinal fluid collections. The collections did not correlate with the sites of leakage in the lower cervical spine.[159] Spontaneous leaks of this nature have responded to the percutaneous injection of fibrin sealants after epidural blood patches failed.[160] Leaking meningeal diverticula and ill-defined connective tissue syndromes have also been implicated in spontaneous leaks.[32,34,161,162] These leaks tend to occur at the cervicothoracic junction or the thoracic spine. Many leaks are self-limiting; some have required surgical intervention. The diagnosis of these cases requires considerable persistence. CT-myelography has been reported as the study of choice.[32]

Traumatic leaks occur after penetrating injury, after surgery, after lumbar puncture, and after spinal anesthesia. Leaks that are less explicable as truly *traumatic*, at least in the sense that an episode of dural penetration cannot always be demonstrated with certainty, occur after multiple epidural injections with steroid preparations.

Intraoperative observations suggest that the dura may both thicken and thin after multiple steroid injections. The dura is sometimes gossamer-thin and almost porous. The CSF that leaks from this location more accurately *seeps* than *leaks*. Multiple sites of leakage and recurrences are recognized when the dura is thin, even without a history of epidural steroid injections.[157] Epidural fat grafts seem to contain this seepage in many, but not all, cases. The dura is easily torn during operative manipulation in this setting.

The prevalence of postoperative leaks is becoming well documented.[163,164] Age, complexity of surgery, and especially reoperation are risk factors. In reoperation for herniated thoracic discs, for example, the incidence is approximately 7% (1/15).[164]

Prevention of postoperative leaks is far preferable to cure. Dural defects should be closed in a watertight fashion whenever possible. The dura should not be closed under tension; a graft, taken from the lumbodorsal fascia, can be inserted if necessary. Dural flaps should be studiously avoided; they embody the potential to act as ball valves. Closure of the fascial and superficial layers should not be left to inexperienced surgeons.

Much has been said regarding the importance of intraoperative Valsalva maneuvers in detecting small meningeal tears and proving the adequacy of dural repair. Although the emergence of CSF obviously implies that satisfactory repair has not been achieved, the absence of CSF with increase in intrathoracic pressure does not eliminate the possibility of a delayed leak.

For patients undergoing elective repair of spinal anomalies (e.g., spinal lipomas associated with dysraphism), or in other situations in which the skin or subcutaneous tissue is defective, consideration should be given to rotating a generous myocutaneous flap. This technique is also useful when there is a recurrence of CSF leak with breakdown of the wound edges, or when difficulty with wound healing can be anticipated, or in the face of infection. Despite the dictum that infection should be cleared before a graft is applied, the myocutaneous flaps seem to survive rotation onto a clean but infected base, and even seem to facilitate healing in chronically infected wounds.

Other principles of management are analogous to those already described for transcranial leaks. In meningomyeloceles and other dysraphic states, the repair of the leak becomes part of the repair of the anomaly. Increased intracranial pressure must be controlled before the leak stops. Except in open injuries, transcutaneous leaks, and obvious anomalies, the site of the leak may be quite difficult to determine.[130] Isotope cisternography and CT-myelography are usually accurate in active leaks.[165] Most uncomplicated traumatic leaks seal within several days, so long as there is no ball-valve dural defect to resist healing. Certain maneuvers may be helpful: incisional leaks should be initially repaired by resuturing the wound and applying an abdominal binder over a pressure pad to increase resistance to CSF flow. External CSF drainage from the cervical subarachnoid space via C1–C2 is another alternative. The Touhy needle and drainage catheter must be inserted under fluoroscopy. Although the cervical subarachnoid catheters are more likely to kink, no other major difficulties have been encountered. If the leak persists over 10 days and if the intracranial pressure is normal, re-exploration of the wound should be weighed.

A number of other techniques have been reported in the management of spinal leaks. Three are mentioned as additions to the surgeon's armamentarium, although they cannot be recommended as a routine: (1) an infusion of 100 mL of 20% mannitol every 4 hours for 7 days and positioning in a head-down attitude for 1 week,[166] (2) insertion of a fat plug through a limited midline durotomy for small rents of the anterior and lateral thecal walls,[167] and (3) the use of tissue adhesives to seal the dura.[168] It is particularly important not to confuse an infected serous exudate with a delayed spinal CSF leak. It is necessary to re-explore a recalcitrant postoperative leak to determine what tissue layers need to be repaired for the leak to be contained.

CONCLUSIONS

The large number of solutions to the problem of CSF leak attests to the difficulty of the problem. CSF leaks can be managed only after the mechanisms of causation, the anatomic origin, and the pathophysiology have been understood. Both extradural and intradural approaches are effective in the appropriate setting. A team approach may be advisable for complex lesions at the skull base.

Leaks that decompress increased intracranial pressure do not stop until the pressure is reduced. The usefulness of CSF diversion should be kept in mind. A long duration of follow-up is necessary before the possibility of recurrence can be dismissed absolutely.

REFERENCES

1. Schlosser RJ, Bolger WE: Nasal cerebrospinal fluid leaks: Critical review and surgical considerations. Laryngoscope 113(2):255–265, 2004.
2. Bidloo the Elder, quoted in Morgagni: De Sedibus et Causis Morborum, 1, 15, art 21.Cited in Lewin W: Cerebrospinal fluid rhinorrhea in non-missile head injuries. Clin Neurosurg 12:237–252, 1966.
3. Mincy JE: Post-traumatic cerebrospinal fluid fistula of the frontal fossa. J Trauma 6:618–622, 1966.
4. Miller C: Case of hydrocephalus chronicus with some unusual symptoms and appearances on dissection. Trans Med Chir Soc Edinb 2:243–248, 1826.
5. Ommaya AK: Spinal fluid fistulae. Clin Neurosurg 23:363–392, 1975.
6. Chiari H: Ueber einem Fall von Luftansammlung in den Ventrikeln des menchichen Gehirns. Z Heilkd 5:383–390, 1884.

7. Luckett WH: Air in the ventricles of the brain, following a fracture of the skull: Report of a case. Surg Gynecol Obstet 17:237–240, 1913.
8. Wilkins RH: Neurosurgical Classics. New York and London: Johnson Reprint Corporation, 1965, pp 242–256.
9. Grant FC: Intracranial aerocele following fracture of the skull: Report of a case with review of the literature. Surg Gynecol Obstet 36: 251–255, 1923.
10. Dandy WE: Pneumocephalus (intracranial pneumatocele or aerocele). Arch Surg 12:949–982, 1926.
11. Cairns H: Injuries of the frontal and ethmoidal sinuses with special reference to cerebrospinal fluid rhinorrhea and aeroceles. J Laryngol Otol 52:589–623, 1937.
12. Dandy WE: Treatment of rhinorrhea and otorrhea. Arch Surg 49: 75–85, 1944.
13. Lewin W: Cerebrospinal fluid rhinorrhea in closed head injuries. Br J Surg 42:1–18, 1954.
14. Lewin W: Cerebrospinal fluid rhinorrhea in nonmissile head injuries. Clin Neurosurg 12:237–252, 1966.
15. Eden K: Traumatic cerebrospinal rhinorrhoea: Repair of a fistula by a transfrontal intradural operation. Br J Surg 29:299–303, 1941.
16. Dohlman G: Spontaneous cerebrospinal rhinorrhoea: Case operated by rhinologic methods. Acta Otolaryngol (Stockh) 67(Suppl):20–23, 1948.
17. McCabe NF: The osteo-mucoperiosteal flap in repair of cerebrospinal fluid rhinorrhea. Laryngoscope 86:537–539, 1976.
18. Calcaterra TC: Extracranial surgical repair of cerebrospinal rhinorrhea. Ann Otol 89:108–116, 1980.
19. Wormald PJ, McDonogh M: "Bath-plug" technique for the endoscopic management of cerebrospinal fluid leaks. J Laryngol Otol 111: 1042–1046, 1997.
20. Sethi DS, Chan C, Pillay PK: Endoscopic management of cerebrospinal fluid fistulae and traumatic cephalocoele. Ann Acad Med Singapore 25:724–727, 1996.
21. Appelbaum E: Meningitis following trauma to the head and face. JAMA 173:116–120, 1968.
22. Brawley B, Kelly W: Treatment of skull fractures with and without cerebrospinal fluid fistula. J Neurosurg 26:57–61, 1967.
23. Einhorn A, Mizrahia EM: Basilar skull fractures in children: Incidence of CNS infection and the use of antibiotics. Am J Dis Child 132:1121–1124, 1978.
24. Krayenbuhl HA: Questions and answers. Clin Neurosurg 14:23–24, 1967.
25. Leech PJ, Patterson R: Conservative and operative management for cerebrospinal leakage after closed head injury. Lancet 1:1013–1016, 1973.
26. Vourc'h G: Continuous cerebrospinal fluid drainage by indwelling spinal catheter. Br J Anaesth 35:118–120, 1963.
27. Aitken RR, Drake CG: Continuous spinal drainage in the treatment of postoperative cerebrospinal-fluid fistulae. J Neurosurg 21:275–277, 1964.
28. McCallum J, Maroon JC, Janetta PJ: Treatment of postoperative cerebrospinal fluid fistulas by subarachnoid drainage. J Neurosurg 42:434–437, 1975.
29. Findler G, Sahar A, Beller AJ: Continuous lumbar drainage of cerebrospinal fluid in neurosurgical patients. Surg Neurol 8:455–457, 1977.
30. Kaufman B, Nulsen FE, Weiss MH, et al: Acquired spontaneous nontraumatic normal-pressure cerebrospinal fluid fistulas originating from the middle fossa. Radiology 122:379–387, 1977.
31. Ommaya AK, Di Chiro G, Baldwain M, Pennybacker JB: Nontraumatic cerebrospinal fluid rhinorrhoea. J Neurol Neurosurg Psychiatry 31:214–225, 1968.
32. Scievink WI, Meyer FB, Atkinson JJ, Mokri B: Spontaneous spinal cerebrospinal fluid leaks and intracranial hypotension. J Neurosurg 84:598–605, 1996.
33. Droste DW, Krauss JK: Oscillations of cerebrospinal fluid in nonhydrocephalic persons. Neurol Res 19:135–138, 1997.
34. Schievink WI, Morreale VM, Atkinson JL, et al: Surgical treatment of spontaneous spinal cerebrospinal fluid leaks. J Neurosurg 88:2430–2436, 1998.
35. Park JI, Strelzow VV, Friedman WH: Current management of cerebrospinal fluid rhinorrhea. Laryngoscope 93:1294–1300, 1983.
36. Dagi TF, Meyer FB, Poletti CA: The incidence and prevention of meningitis after basilar skull fracture. Am J Emerg Med 3:295–298, 1983.
37. Meirowsky AM, Caveness WF, Dillon JD, et al: Cerebrospinal fluid fistulas complicating missile wounds of the brain. J Neurosurg 54:44–48, 1981.

38. Zlab MK, Moore GF, Daly DT, et al. Cerebrospinal fluid rhinorrhea: A review of the literature. Ear Nose Throat J 71:314–317, 1992.
39. Bell RB, Dierks EJ, Homer L, Potter BE: Management of cerebrospinal fluid leak associated with craniomaxillofacial trauma. J Oral Maxillofacial Surg 62(6):676–684, 2004.
40. Shulman K: Later complications of head injuries in children. Clin Neurosurg 19:371–380, 1971.
41. Nutkiewicz A, DeFeo DR, Kohut RI, Fierstien S: Cerebrospinal fluid rhinorrhea as a presentation of pituitary adenoma. Neurosurgery 6:195–197, 1980.
42. Haran RP, Chandy MJ: Symptomatic pneumocephalus after transsphenoidal surgery. Surg Neurol 48:575–578, 1997.
43. Landy LB, Graham MD, Kartush JM, LaRouere MJ: Temporal bone encephalocele and cerebrospinal fluid leaks. Am J Otol 17:461–469, 1996.
44. Piziak VK, Gilliland PF, Boyd G, et al: Pituitary tumor initially seen as serous otitis media. JAMA 251:3131–3132, 1984.
45. Mokri B, Atkinson JL: False pituitary tumor in CSF leaks. Neurology 55(4):573–575, 2000.
46. Magliulo G, Sepe C, Varacalli S, Fusconi M: Cerebrospinal fluid leak management following cerebellopontine angle surgery. J Otolaryngol 27(5):258–262, 1998.
47. Horowitz NH, Rizzoli HV: Postoperative Complications of Intracranial Surgery. Baltimore: Williams & Wilkins, 1982, p 76.
48. Becker SS, Jackler RK, Pitts LH: Cerebrospinal fluid leak after acoustic neuroma surgery: A comparison of the translabyrinthine, middle fossa, and retrosigmoid approaches. Otol Neurotol 24(1): 107–112, 2003.
49. Sanna M, Taibah A, Russo A, et al: Perioperative complications in acoustic neuroma (vestibular schwannoma) surgery. Otol Neurotol 25(3):379–386, 2004.
50. Selesnick SH, Liu JC, Jen A, Newman J: The incidence of cerebrospinal fluid leak after vestibular schwannoma surgery. Otol Neurotol 25(3): 387–393, 2004.
51. Shen T, Friedman RA, Brackmann DE, et al: The evolution of surgical approaches for posterior fossa meningiomas. Otol Neurotol 25(3): 394–397, 2004.
52. Montgomery WW: Surgery for acoustic neurinoma. Ann Otolaryngol 82:428–444, 1973.
53. Ojemann RG: Microsurgical suboccipital approach to cerebellopontine angle tumors. Clin Neurosurg 25:461–479, 1978.
54. Khrais TH, Falcioni M, Taibah A, et al: Cerebrospinal fluid leak prevention after translabyrinthine removal of vestibular schwannoma. Laryngoscope 114(6):1015–1020, 2004.
55. Valtonen HJ, Poe DS, Heilman CB, Tarlov EC: Endoscopically assisted prevention of cerebrospinal fluid leak in suboccipital acoustic neuroma surgery. Am J Otol 18:381–385, 1997.
56. Horowitz NH, Rizzoli HV: Postoperative Complications of Intracranial Surgery. Baltimore: Williams & Wilkins, 1982, pp 123–124.
57. Spaziante R, de Divitiis E, Cappabianca P: Reconstruction of the pituitary fossa in transsphenoidal surgery: An experience of 140 cases. Neurosurgery 17:453–458, 1985.
58. Ciric I: Comment on Spaziante et al. Neurosurgery 17:458, 1985.
59. Aust MR, McCaffrey TV, Atkinson J: Transnasal endoscopic approach to the sella turcica. Am J Rhinol 12(4):283–287, 1998.
60. Castillo L, Verschuur HP, Poissonnet G, et al: Complications of endoscopically guided sinus surgery. Rhinology 34(4):215–218, 1996.
61. Bachmann G, Djenabi U, Jungehulsing M, et al: Incidence of occult cerebrospinal fluid fistula during paranasal sinus surgery. Arch Otolaryngol Head Neck Surg 128(1):11299–11302, 2002.
62. Bakay L, Glasauer FE: Head Injury. Boston: Little, Brown, 1980, p 280.
63. Markham JW: The clinical features of pneumocephalus based upon a survey of 284 cases with report of 11 additional cases. Acta Neurochir 16:1–78, 1967.
64. Hubbard JL, Thomas JM, Pearson BW, Laws ER: Spontaneous cerebrospinal fluid rhinorrhea: Evolving concepts in diagnosis and surgical management based on the Mayo Clinic experience from 1970 through 1981. Neurosurgery 16:314–321, 1985.
65. Flanagan JC, McLachlan DL, Shannon GM: Orbital roof fractures: Neurologic and neurosurgical considerations. Ophthalmology 87:325–329, 1980.
66. Ray BS, Bergland RM: Cerebrospinal fluid fistula: Clinical aspects, techniques of localization, and methods of closure. J Neurosurg 30:399–405, 1969.
67. Jamieson KG, Yelland JDN: Surgical repair of the anterior fossa because of rhinorrhea, aerocele, or meningitis. J Neurosurg 39:328–331, 1973.

68. Anonymous: Management of cerebrospinal fluid leaks. J Trauma 51(Suppl 2):S29–S33, 2001.

69. Bernal-Sprekelsen M, Bleda-Vazquez C, Carrau RL: Ascending meningitis secondary to traumatic cerebrospinal fluid leaks. Am J Rhinol 14:257–259, 2000.

70. Kosoy J, Trieff N, Winkelmann P, et al: Glucose in nasal secretions. Arch Otolaryngol 95:225–229, 1975.

71. Healy CE: Significance of a positive reaction for glucose in rhinorrhea. Clin Pediatr 8:239, 1969.

72. Kirsch AP: Diagnosis of cerebrospinal fluid rhinorrhea: Lack of specificity of the glucose oxidase Tes-Tape. J Pediatr 71:718, 1967.

73. Ghoshhajra K: Radiologic techniques for identification and localization of cerebrospinal fluid fistulae. Semin Neurol 2:115–125, 1982.

74. Levy JM, Christensen FK, Nykamp PW: Detection of a cerebrospinal fluid fistula by computed tomography. AJR Am J Roentgenol 131:344–345, 1978.

75. Ahmadi J, Weiss MH, Segali HD, et al: Evaluation of cerebrospinal fluid rhinorrhea by metrizamide computed tomographic cisternography. Neurosurgery 16:54–60, 1985.

76. Matsumura A, Anno I, Kimura H, et al: Diagnosis of spontaneous intracranial hypotension by using magnetic resonance myelography: Case report. J Neurosurg 92(5):873–876, 2000.

77. Strauss H: Fluorescein als indikator fuer die nierenfunktion. Berliner Klin Wchschr 50:2226–2227, 1913.

78. Fox N: Cure in a case of cerebrospinal rhinorrhea. Arch Otolaryngol 17:85–86, 1933.

79. Mahaley MS, Odom GL: Complications following intrathecal injections of fluorescein. J Neurosurg 25:298, 1966.

80. Staab EV, Shirkhoda A: Cerebrospinal fluid scanning. Clin Nucl Med 6:103–109, 1981.

81. Coletti PM, Siegel ME: Posttraumatic lumbar cerebrospinal fluid leak: Detection by retrograde In-111-DTPA myeloscintigraphy. Clin Nucl Med 6:403–404, 1981.

82. Hasegawa M, Watanabe I, Hiratsuka H, et al: Transfer of radioisotope from CSF to nasal secretion. Acta Otolaryngol (Stockh) 95:359–364, 1983.

83. Di Chiro G, Stein SC, Harrington T: Spontaneous cerebrospinal fluid rhinorrhea in normal dogs: Radioisotope studies of an alternate pathway of CSF drainage. J Neuropathol Exp Neurol 31:447–453, 1972.

84. Spetzler RF, Wilson CB: Management of recurrent CSF rhinorrhea of the middle and posterior fossa. J Neurosurg 49:393–397, 1978.

85. El Jamel MS, Pidgeon CN, Toland J, et al: MRI cisternography and the localization of CSF fistulae. Br J Neurosurg 8:433–437, 1994.

86. El Gammal T, Sobol W, Wadlington VR, et al: Cerebrospinal fluid fistula: Detection with MR cisternography. Am J Neuroradiol 19(4):627–631, 1998.

87. Moayeri NN, Henson JW, Schaefer PW, Zervas NT: Spinal dural enhancement on magnetic resonance imaging associated with spontaneous intracranial hypotension: Report of three cases and review of the literature. J Neurosurg 88(5):912–918, 1998.

88. Shetty PG, Schroff MM, Sahani DV, Kirtane MV: Evaluation of high-resolution CT and MR cisternography in the diagnosis of cerebrospinal fluid fistula. Am J Neuroradiol 19:633–639, 1998.

89. Lloyd MNH, Kimber PM, Burrows EH: Post-traumatic cerebrospinal fluid rhinorrhea: Modern high-definition computed tomography is all that is required for the effective demonstration of the site of leakage. Clin Radiol 49:100–103, 1994.

90. Zapalac JS, Marple BF, Schwade ND: Skull base cerebrospinal fluid fistulas: A comprehensive diagnostic algorithm. Otolaryngol Head Neck Surg 126:669–676, 2002.

91. Bernal-Sprekelsen M, Bleda-Vazquez C, Carrau RL: Ascending meningitis secondary to traumatic cerebrospinal fluid leaks. Am J Rhinol 14:257–259, 2000.

92. Marshall AH, Jones NS, Robertson IJA: An algorithm for the management of CSF rhinorrhea illustrated by 36 cases. Rhinology 37:182–185, 1993.

93. Bateman N, Jones NS: Rhinorrhoea feigning cerebrospinal fluid leak: Nine illustrative cases. J Laryngol Otol 114:462–464, 2000.

94. Meco C, Oberascher G: Comprehensive algorithm for skull base dural lesion and cerebrospinal fluid fistula diagnosis. Laryngoscope 114(6):991–999, 2004.

95. Ricchetti A, Burkhard PR, Rodrigo N, et al: Skull base cerebrospinal fluid fistula: A novel detection method based on 2-dimensional electrophoresis. Head & Neck 26(5):464–469, 2004.

96. Oberascher G, Arrer E: First clinical experience with (beta)2-transferrin in cerebrospinal fluid oto- and rhinoliquorrhea. HNO 34:151–155, 1986.

97. Irjala K, Suonpaa J, Laurent B: Identification of CSF leakage by immunofixation. Arch Otolaryngol 105:447–448, 1979.

98. Arrer E, Meco C, Oberascher G, et al: (Beta)-trace protein as a marker for cerebrospinal fluid rhinorrhea. Clin Chemistry 48:939–941, 2002.

99. Bachmann G, Nekic M, Michel O: Clinical experience with beta-trace protein as a marker for cerebrospinal fluid. Ann Otol, Rhinol Laryngol 109(12 Pt 1):1099–1102, 2000.

100. Schlosser RJ, Bolger WE: Management of multiple spontaneous nasal meningoencephaloceles. Laryngoscope 112:980–985, 2002.

101. Parisier SC, Briken EA: Recurrent meningitis secondary to idiopathic oval window CSF leak. Laryngoscope 86:1503–1515, 1976.

102. Nenzelius C: On spontaneous cerebrospinal otorrhea due to congenital malformations. Acta Otolaryngol (Stockh) 39:314–328, 1951.

103. Bottema T: Spontaneous cerebrospinal fluid otorrhea. Arch Otolaryngol 101:693–694, 1975.

104. Rice WJ, Waggoner LG: Congenital cerebrospinal fluid otorrhea via defect in the stapes footplate. Laryngoscope 77:341–349, 1967.

105. Ignelzi RJ, VanderArk GD: Analysis of the treatment of basilar skull fractures with and without antibiotics. J Neurosurg 43:75–78, 1975.

106. Eljamel MS, Foy PM: Acute traumatic CSF fistulae: The risk of intracranial infection. Br J Neurosurg 4:381–385, 1990.

107. Choi D, Spann B: Traumatic cerebrospinal fluid leakage: Risk factors and the use of prophylactic antibiotics. Br J Neurosurg 10:571–575, 1996.

108. Hilary AB: Prophylactic antibiotics for post-traumatic cerebrospinal fluid fistula: A meta-analysis. Arch Otolaryngol Head Neck Surg 123:749–752, 1997.

109. Bernal-Sprekelsen M, Bleda-Vazquez C, Carrau RL: Ascending meningitis secondary to traumatic cerebrospinal fluid leaks. Am J Rhinol 14:257–259, 2000.

110. Dagi TF, Ojemann RG, Zervas NT: Incidence and prevention of infection after neurosurgical operations. In Thompson RA, Green JR (eds): Infectious Diseases of the Central Nervous System. Jamaica, NY: Spectrum Publications, 1984, pp 155–173.

111. Ingraham FD, Campbell JB: An apparatus for closed drainage of the ventricular system. Ann Surg 114:1096–1098, 1941.

112. White RJ, Dakters JG, Yashon D, et al: Temporary control of cerebrospinal fluid volume and pressure by means of an externalized valve-drainage system. J Neurosurg 30:264–269, 1969.

113. Vourc'h G: Continuous cerebrospinal fluid drainage by indwelling spinal catheter. Br J Anaesth 35:118–120, 1963.

114. McCoy G: Cerebrospinal rhinorrhea: A comprehensive review and a definition of the responsibility of the rhinologist in the diagnosis and treatment. Laryngoscope 73:1125–1157, 1963.

115. Wyler AR, Kelly WA: Use of antibiotics with external ventriculostomies. J Neurosurg 37:185–187, 1972.

116. Friedman WA, Vries JK: Percutanous tunnel ventriculostomy: Summary of 100 procedures. J Neurosurg 53:662–665, 1980.

117. Dagi TF, Ondra SL: The role of artificial intelligence systems in neurosurgical intensive care. International Congress on Trends in Neurosurgery, Diagnostic and Surgical Perspectives, Vienna, Austria, May 14–17, 1986.

118. Carrion E, Hertzog JH, Medlock MD, et al: Use of acetazolamide to decrease cerebrospinal fluid production in chronically ventilated patients with ventriculopleural shunts. Arch Dis Child 84:68–71, 2001.

119. Brownridge P: Spinal anesthesia revisited: An evaluation of subarachnoid block in obstetrics. Anaesth Intensive Care 12:334–342, 1984.

120. Rudehill A, Gordon E, Rahn T: Subdural haematoma: A rare but life-threatening complication after spinal anaesthesia. Acta Anaesthesiol Scand 27:376–377, 1983.

121. Benzon HT: Intracerebral hemorrhage after dural puncture and epidural blood patch: Nonpostural and noncontinuous headache. Anesthesiology 60:258–259, 1984.

122. Ikeda K, Nakano M, Tani E: Tension pneumocephalus complicating ventriculoperitoneal shunt for cerebrospinal fluid rhinorrhea: Case report. J Neurol Neurosurg Psychiatry 41:319–322, 1978.

123. Little JR, McCarty CS: Tension pneumocephalus after insertion of ventriculoperitoneal shunt for aqueductal stenosis. J Neurosurg 44:383–385, 1976.

124. Jooma R, Grant DN: Cerebrospinal fluid rhinorrhea and intraventricular pneumocephalus due to intermittent shunt obstruction. Surg Neurol 20:231–124, 1983.

125. Katz J: Treatment of a subarachnoid-cutaneous fistula with an epidural blood patch. Anesthesiology 60:603–604, 1984.

126. Digiovanni AJ, Galbert MW, Wahle WM: Epidural injection of autologous blood for post-lumbar puncture headache. I: Additional clinical experiences and laboratory investigation. Anesth Analg 51:226–228, 1972.

127. Crawford JS: Experiences with epidural blood patch. Anaesthesia 35:513–515, 1980.

128. Casement BA, Danielson DR: The epidural blood patch: Are more than two ever necessary? Anesth Analg 63:1033–1035, 1984.

129. Rosenberg PH, Heavner JE: In vitro study of the effect of epidural blood patch on leakage through a dural puncture. Anesth Analg 64:501–504, 1985.

130. Harrington H, Tyler HR, Welch K: Surgical treatment of post-lumbar puncture dural CSF leak causing chronic headache. J Neurosurg 57:703–707, 1982.

131. Sencakova D, Mokri B, McClelland RL: The efficacy of epidural blood patch in spontaneous CSF leaks. Neurology 57(10): 1921–1923, 2001.

132. Reynolds AF, Hameroff SR, Blitt CD, et al: Spinal subdural epiarachnoid hematoma: A complication of a novel epidural blood patch technique. Anesth Analg 59:702–703, 1980.

133. O'Brien MD, Reade PC: The management of dural tear resulting from mid-facial fracture. Head Neck Surg 6:810–818, 1984.

134. da Cruz MJ, Ahmed SM, Moffat DA: An alternative method for dealing with cerebrospinal fluid fistulae in inner ear deformities. Am J Otol 19:288–291, 1998.

135. Kelley TF, Stankiewicz JA, Chow JM, et al: Endoscopic closure of postsurgical anterior cranial fossa cerebrospinal fluid leaks. Neurosurgery 39:743–746, 1996.

136. Bolger WE, McLaughlin K: Cranial bone grafts in cerebrospinal fluid leak and encephalocele repair: A preliminary report. Am J Rhinol 17(3):153–158, 2003.

137. Mortuaire G, Louis E, Pellerin P: Sphenoidal cerebrospinal fluid rhinorrhea: An original surgical approach. J Craniofac Surg 15(3): 458–463, 2004.

138. Yessenow RS, McCabe BF: The osteo-mucoperiosteal flap in repair of cerebrospinal fluid rhinorrhea: 20-year experience. Otolaryngol Head Neck Surg 101:555–558, 1989.

139. Hughes RGM, Jones NS, Robertson IJA: The endoscopic treatment of cerebrospinal fluid rhinorrhea: The Nottingham experience. J Laryngol Otol 111:125–128, 1997.

140. Jho HD, Carrau RL, Ko Y, Daly MA: Endoscopic pituitary surgery: An early experience. Surg Neurol 47:213–223, 1997.

141. Gjuric M, Goede U, Keimer H, Wigand ME: Endonasal endoscopic closure of cerebrospinal fluid fistulas at the anterior cranial base. Ann Otol Rhinol Laryngol 105:620–623, 1996.

142. Fraioli B, Pastore FS, Floris R, et al: Computed tomography-guided transsphenoidal closure of postsurgical cerebrospinal fluid fistula: A transmucosal needle technique. Surg Neurol 48:409–413, 1997.

143. Van Den Abbeele T, Elmaleh M, Herman P, et al: Transnasal endoscopic repair of congenital defects of the skull base in children. Arch Otolaryngol Head Neck Surg 125(5):580–584, 1999.

144. Jakoby RK: The use of a methylmethacrylate seal in spinal fluid otorrhea and rhinorrhea. J Neurosurg 18:614–615, 1961.

145. Papini RPG, Niranjan NS: Superglue sealant for persistent leakage of cerebrospinal fluid. Plast Reconstr Surg 91:371–372, 1993.

146. Lehman RAW, Hayes GJ, Martins AN: The use of adhesive and lyophilized dura in the treatment of cerebrospinal rhinorrhea. J Neurosurg 26:92–95, 1967.

147. VanderArk GD, Pitkethly DT, Ducker TB, et al: Repair of cerebrospinal fluid fistulas using a tissue adhesive. J Neurosurg 33:151–155, 1970.

148. Maxwell JA, Goldware SI: Use of tissue adhesive in the surgical treatment of cerebrospinal fluid leaks: Experience with isobutyl-2 cyanoacrylate in 12 cases. J Neurosurg 39:332–336, 1973.

149. Mickey BE, Samson D: Neurosurgical applications of the cyanoacrylate adhesives. Clin Neurosurg 29:429–444, 1982.

150. Kumar A, Maartens NF, Kaye AH: Reconstruction of the sellar floor using Bioglue following transsphenoidal procedures. J Clin Neurosci 10(1):92–95, 2003.

151. Agag RL, Granick MS, Omidi M, et al: Neurosurgical reconstruction with acellular cadaveric dermal matrix. Ann Plastic Surg 52(6):571–577, 2004.

152. Preul MC, Bichard WD, Spetzler RF: Toward optimal tissue sealants for neurosurgery: Use of a novel hydrogel sealant in a canine durotomy repair model. Neurosurgery 53(5):1189–1198; discussion 1198–1199, 2003.

153. Greenblatt SH, Wilson DH: Persistent cerebrospinal fluid rhinorrhea treated by lumboperitoneal shunt: Technical note. J Neurosurg 38:524–526, 1973.

154. Bret P, Hor F, Huppert J, et al: Treatment of cerebrospinal fluid rhinorrhea by percutaneous lumboperitoneal shunting: Review of 15 cases. Neurosurgery 16:44–47, 1985.

155. Spetzler RF: Commentary on Bret P, et al. Neurosurgery 16:47, 1985.

156. Vishteh AG, Scievink WI, Baskin JJ, Sonntag VK: Cervical bone spur presenting with spontaneous intracranial hypotension: Case report. J Neurosurg 89:483–484, 1998.

157. Schievink WI, Maya MM, Riedinger M: Recurrent spontaneous spinal cerebrospinal fluid leaks and intracranial hypotension: A prospective study. J Neurosurg 99(5):840–842, 2003.

158. Schievink WI, Jacques L: Recurrent spontaneous spinal cerebrospinal fluid leak associated with "nude nerve root" syndrome: Case report. Neurosurgery 53(5):1216–1218; discussion 1218–1219, 2003.

159. Schievink WI, Maya MM, Tourje J: False localizing sign of C1-C2 cerebrospinal fluid leak in spontaneous intracranial hypotension. J Neurosurg 100(4):639–644, 2004. Erratum appears in J Neurosurg 100(6):1135, 2004.

160. Schievink WI, Maya MM, Moser FM: Treatment of spontaneous intracranial hypotension with percutaneous placement of a fibrin sealant: Report of four cases. J Neurosurg 100(6):1098–1100, 2004.

161. Schrijver I, Schievink WI, Godfrey M, et al: Spontaneous spinal cerebrospinal fluid leaks and minor skeletal features of Marfan syndrome: A microfibrillopathy. J Neurosurg 96(3):483–489, 2002.

162. Schievink WI, Gordon OK, Tourje J: Connective tissue disorders with spontaneous spinal cerebrospinal fluid leaks and intracranial hypotension: A prospective study. Neurosurgery 54(1):65–70; discussion 70–71, 2004.

163. Dickman CA, Rosenthal D, Regan JJ: Reoperation for herniated thoracic discs. J Neurosurg 91(2 Suppl):157–162, 1999.

164. Regan JJ, Aronoff RJ, Ohnmeiss DD, Sengupta DK: Laparoscopic approach to L4-L5 for interbody fusion using BAK cages: Experience in the first 58 cases. Spine 24(20):2171–2174, 1999.

165. Gass H, Goldstein AS, Ruskin R, et al: Chronic postmyelogram headache: Isotopic demonstration of dural leak and surgical cure. Arch Neurol 25:108–170, 1971.

166. Rosenthal JD, Hahn JF, Martinez GJ: A technique for closure of leak of spinal fluid. Surg Gynecol Obstet 140:948–950, 1975.

167. Mayfield FH, Kurokawa K: Watertight closure of the spinal dura mater: Technical note. J Neurosurg 43:639–640, 1975.

168. Papadakis N, Mark VH: Repair of spinal cerebrospinal fluid fistula with the use of a tissue adhesive: Technical note. Neurosurgery 6:63–65, 1980.

10 Transnasal Endoscopic Repair of Cranionasal Fistulas

JOSEPH K. HAN, JAMES A. BURNS, and CHARLES W. GROSS

Cerebrospinal fluid (CSF) rhinorrhea presents a major challenge in management. Difficulties in diagnosis and localization add to the complexity of the problem, and management varies with etiology and site. Immediate measures must be taken to repair the defect because the risk of meningitis can reach 20% to 40%.[1,2] Since its first report by Dohlman in 1948,[3] extracranial repair of CSF rhinorrhea has evolved considerably. Several recent reports describe endoscopic cranionasal fistula repair with success rates reaching 88% to 100% with the first procedure.[4–10] We have recently presented our 10 years of experience with 92 patients at the University of Virginia, which had an overall success rate of 94%.[11]

With an increasing number of neurosurgical and otolaryngologic procedures being performed, as well as increased amount of head trauma in modern society, the number of cranionasal fistulas has increased, allowing refinement of techniques for transnasal endoscopic repair. Because these techniques (diagnostic and surgical) have evolved to produce a higher success rate and lower morbidity than the external approach, the endoscopic approach is now considered by many to represent the standard of care.

This chapter describes the pertinent anatomy, pathophysiology, and manifestations of cranionasal fistulas, as well as current methods of diagnosis and localization. The endoscopic repair of cranionasal fistula is detailed.

PATHOPHYSIOLOGY

Leakage of CSF occurs when arachnoid, dura, bone, and mucosal epithelium are violated, and there is a connection between the subarachnoid space and the nasal cavity. There are traumatic and nontraumatic etiologies of craniofacial fistula (Table 10-1).[12]

TABLE 10-1 ▪ Causes of Cerebrospinal Fluid Rhinorrhea

Traumatic	Atraumatic
Nonsurgical	**High-Pressure Flow**
Blunt trauma	Intracranial tumors
Projectile trauma	Hydrocephalus
Surgical	**Low-Pressure Flow**
Craniotomy	Bony erosion
Paranasal sinus surgery	Sellar atrophy
Tumor ablation	Olfactory atrophy
	Congenital anomalies
	Idiopathic

Traumatic Cerebrospinal Fluid Rhinorrhea

The roofs of the ethmoid and the cribriform plate are the most common sites of CSF rhinorrhea because dura is tightly adherent to bone in these areas.[13] Also, the lateral cribriform plate is easily fractured because it is the thinnest area of the ethmoid roof, particularly where the anterior ethmoid artery creates a natural dehiscence. Fractures through the frontal sinus and anterior ethmoid roof drain into the anteriosuperior aspect of the nasal vault, whereas fractures through the posterior ethmoid roof and sphenoid roof drain to the posteriosuperior aspect of the nasal vault. Cerebrospinal fluid may also enter the nasal vault by way of the eustachian tube by traveling through the middle ear space from the dural defect surrounding the petrous portion of the temporal bone (Fig. 10-1).

Cerebrospinal fluid may appear immediately after the nonsurgical trauma or at some later time. Delayed leaks

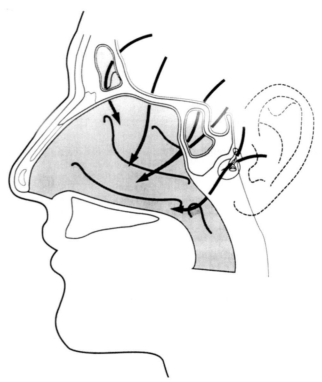

FIGURE 10-1 Common pathways of cerebrospinal fluid (CSF) drainage presenting as CSF rhinorrhea. (From Papay FA, Maggiano H, Dominquez S, et al: Rigid endoscopic repair of paranasal sinus cerebrospinal fluid fistulas. Laryngoscope 99:1195–1201, 1989.)

may be caused by delayed increase in intracranial pressure after the trauma, by lysis of clot in an area of fracture, by resolution of soft-tissue edema, or by loss of vascularity with necrosis of soft tissue around the wound. In addition, the dura may herniate, and with continued pulsations and physiologic changes in CSF pressure the herniation may progress with eventual dehiscence and CSF leak.[14,15]

Also nonsurgical trauma, which was previously the most common cause for CSF rhinorrhea, has now been surpassed by iatrogenic causes. Iatrogenic causes for CSF rhinorrhea account for 51% to 58% of cases, whereas nonsurgical traumatic CSF rhinorrhea accounts for 10% to 20% of all cases of CSF rhinorrhea.[1,18,19] Iatrogenically caused CSF rhinorrhea may follow intracranial and extracranial surgery. Postoperative rhinorrhea occurs in 3% to 6% of cases after trans-sphenoidal hypophysectomy, ethmoidectomy, and anterior skull base tumor ablation.[16] The most common site for iatrogenic injury following an ethmoidectomy is the lateral wall of the cribriform plate, because it has the thinnest bone in the ethmoid roof and because the dura is closely adherent to the cribriform plate. Although the percentage of postoperative CSF rhinorrhea has not increased, the total number of such cases has increased because of the increasing number of advanced skull base surgical procedures and functional endoscopic sinus surgery procedures being performed at present. In contrast to most cases of nonsurgical traumatic CSF rhinorrhea, which usually have a small defect in the dura, iatrogenic causes can have portions of the bone and dura absent secondary to the procedure; therefore, iatrogenic CSF rhinorrhea is less likely to resolve spontaneously than is traumatic CSF leak. In the latter case, the CSF leak resolves spontaneously in 53% of patients within 5 days of trauma.[17]

Nontraumatic Cerebrospinal Fluid Rhinorrhea

The majority of cases of nontraumatic cerebrospinal fluid rhinorrhea are of idiopathic origin, and only a small percentage of cases are from tumors or congenital causes.[18] Both idiopathic CSF rhinorrhea and tumor can be associated with elevated intracranial pressure leading to continued erosion and weakening of bone with the eventual development of a cranionasal fistula.[20] Tumors may also cause CSF rhinorrhea through direct erosion of bone. Idiopathic CSF rhinorrhea has been associated with pseudotumor cerebri (benign intracranial hypertension), which are often seen in obese females.[21] Patients with pseudotumor cerebri may commonly have an empty sella syndrome. An empty sella syndrome that occurs because of an absent portion of the diaphragma sellae is a congenital lesion, whereas a spontaneous empty sella is associated with pituitary gland atrophy.[14]

Low-pressure rhinorrhea likely results from normal intermittent physiologic elevations of CSF pressure. Normal intracranial pressure, which is 5 to 15 mm of H_2O, can undergo normal physiologic elevations to 80 mm H_2O spontaneously every few seconds.[21,22] This increase in CSF pressure in general is not by itself able to erode or fracture bone. However, the presence of sudden, short-lived, marked increases in intracranial pressure because of coughing or straining may be an important precipitating factor in the development of spontaneous CSF rhinorrhea in those instances where there is a preexisting weakness in the skull base.[14] In these patients there is often a history of remote head trauma.

DIAGNOSIS

Symptoms of cranionasal fistula include unilateral watery rhinorrhea, salty taste, and headaches. Twenty percent of patients with cranionasal fistula present with meningitis as their initial manifestation, with the risk of meningitis in the first 3 weeks after trauma being 3% to 11%.[16]

Paramount in the diagnosis of cranionasal fistula is the clear demonstration that extracranial CSF exists. In cases where the rhinorrhea is profuse, the diagnosis is obvious. However, diagnosis is more difficult when the drainage is minimal, intermittent, or nonexistent. When CSF rhinorrhea is a direct result of endoscopic sinus surgery, the intraoperative presence of a clear fluid draining from the roof of the nasal cavity and washing away blood is pathognomonic of a CSF leak. The presence of β_2-transferrin in the fluid is a highly accurate way of determining the presence of CSF because it is only present in the CSF, aqueous humor, and perilymph.[9,10] This is not only a highly specific test but is also quite sensitive because only 1.0 mL of fluid is required to perform the test.

Radiographic studies can assist in determining the precise location of the cranionasal fistula, in possibly identifying the underlying cause, and in measuring the size of the anterior skull base defect. There are several radiographic imaging studies that have been used for the diagnosis of cranionasal fistula, including 3-dimensional multidetector high-resolution computed tomography (HRCT), magnetic resonance imaging (MRI), CT cisternography, and radionuclide cisternography.[1] Of these radiographic studies, HRCT is the most sensitive (87%) and accurate (87%) in detecting skull-based defects; however, this study does not establish if there is leakage at the site of the fistula. MRI has a sensitivity of 78%. Although MRI is less sensitive, it is helpful in delineating the defect and in identifying a herniated soft tissue mass such as a cephalocele (Fig. 10-2). Traditional CT cisternography employed a CT scan with coronal thickness of 3 to 5 mm following administration of intrathecal iohexal or other low-osmolar, nonionic, iodine contrast media.[10] The low sensitivity for this type of CT cisternography (33%) is brought about because extravasations of the dye through the cranionasal fistula have to be present at the time of the study to demonstrate the leak and localize the site (Fig. 10-3). However, if a 1-mm sliced CT is used for the CT cisternography, the sensitivity for the CT cisternography is likely to be similar to the HRCT and will further demonstrate a leakage of CSF, when present. CT image guidance can also be used to identify the site of a craniofacial fistula, and can be used to localize the site of the craniofacial fistula at operation to repair the fistula.

The clinical localization of cranionasal fistulas has improved dramatically with the use of endoscopes. One of the main advantages of the endoscopic repair of cranionasal fistulas is the excellent field of magnified visualization, which allows exact localization of the leak.[4,9,10] Although fluorescein is routinely used to aid in the localization of CSF leaks, it must be used with caution. Intrathecal fluorescein

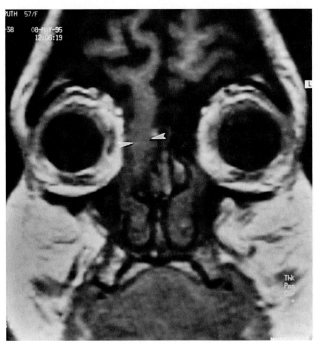

FIGURE 10-2   Coronal T2-weighted magnetic resonance imaging scan showing a cephalocele presenting through the ethmoid roof defect. The cranionasal fistula measured 2.2 × 1 cm. (From Burns JA, Dodson EE, Gross GW: Transnasal endoscopic repair of cranionasal fistulae: A refined technique with long-term follow-up. Laryngoscope 106:1080–1083, 1996.)

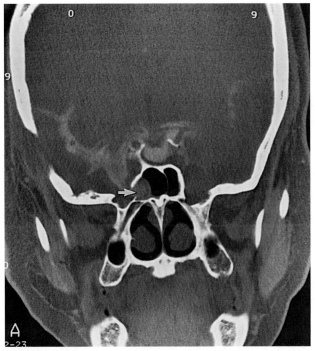

FIGURE 10-3   A coronal computed tomography scan showing cranionasal fistula in the sphenoid sinus with Iohexol dye collecting in the sphenoid sinus *(arrow)*. (From Burns JA, Dodson EE, Gross GW: Transnasal endoscopic repair of cranionasal fistulae: A refined technique with long-term follow-up. Laryngoscope 106:1080–1083, 1996.)

is administered through a lumbar puncture. Ten mL of CSF is withdrawn, mixed with 0.05 mL of 10% fluorescein (injectable, not ophthalmic preparation), and slowly reinjected into the lumbar subarachnoid space. After a 20- to 30-minute diffusion throughout the CSF, the bright yellow-green fluorescein dye can be seen readily with the rigid nasal endoscope if a CSF leak is present. A Valsalva maneuver can enhance the flow of CSF through a defect for better visualization. Because iohexal and fluorescein can be given simultaneously, CT cisternography and rigid nasal endoscopy can work in a complementary fashion to precisely localize the cranionasal defect.[23–25] The complications of intrathecal fluorescein include lower extremity weakness, seizures, and cranial nerve deficits,[26] although several large series of endoscopic repairs using fluorescein for localization did not experience these problems.[4,5,7,10] Most adverse reactions are associated with much higher doses of fluorescein, and even those complications rarely produce permanent neurologic sequelae.

MANAGEMENT

The intracranial repair of CSF rhinorrhea was initially described by Dandy in 1926.[27] Although the intracranial approach is often preferred by neurosurgeons, its disadvantages include anosmia, intracerebral hemorrhage, retraction-related brain edema, and a success rate of about 60% after the first attempt.[20] By contrast, several studies have reported success rates of 86% to 100% for closure of cranionasal fistula using the endoscopic approach on the first attempt.[4,9,10,28] Without the craniotomy-related problems, and with the additional advantage that using the endoscopic approach provides, intraoperative leaks can be treated as soon as the problem is recognized.[29]

REPAIR OF SPECIFIC SITES

Sphenoid Sinus

With the patient under general anesthesia, and after administration of a prophylactic dose of a third-generation cephalosporin, the nasal cavities and sphenoid sinus are injected with a solution of 1% lidocaine with 1:100,000 epinephrine. Diagnostic nasal endoscopy is performed with or without intrathecal injection of fluorescein. An endoscopic sphenoidotomy is then accomplished through the transethmoid approach. Some surgeons prefer a midline transseptal approach. This opening is enlarged only to the point of adequate exposure, to provide maximal support for a graft. It is important to preserve as much of the face of the sphenoid sinus as possible to prevent extrusion of the graft. The bony defect is exposed, and mucosa is removed from the sinus (Fig. 10-4). Some surgeons remove as much mucosa from the sinus as possible, whereas others remove only mucosa adjacent to the defect.

A fat graft is harvested from the abdomen with either dermis or rectus fascia. The graft is then trimmed and placed into the sphenoid, with fascia or dermis placed over the site of the defect. Tissue glue is applied at the opening, and then great care is taken to place dermal or fascial tissue over the opening. Additional tissue glue is then used to seal the graft. The face of the sphenoid and ethmoid cavity

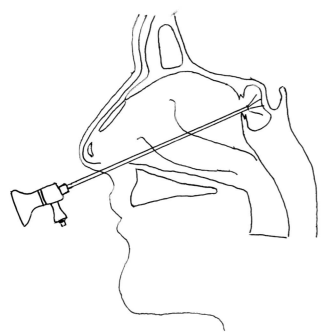

FIGURE 10-4 Sagittal view showing the sphenoidotomy opening viewed with an endoscope for a sphenoid sinus fistula.

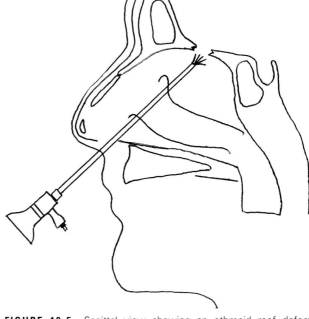

FIGURE 10-5 Sagittal view showing an ethmoid roof defect as viewed by an endoscope after performing a standard total ethmoidectomy.

is packed firmly with Gelfoam, and Surgicel is placed around the Gelfoam to keep the graft and packing in place.

Failure in the endoscopic repair of the sphenoid sinus cranionasal fistula is likely to occur in the lateral recess of the sphenoid sinus[30] and is likely caused by poor visualization of the fistula. Either a sublabial transeptal approach or a widened transethmoid approach can be used to provide better visualization. The repair of the lateral sphenoid sinus fistula is similar to the one described; however, the anterior wall of the sphenoid sinus has to be widened, and repair of the widened bony defect will likely need a cartilage or bone graft, which can be taken from the septum.

Ethmoid Roof and Cribriform Plate

The repair of cranionasal fistula in the ethmoid roof or the cribriform area is identical to repair of the sphenoid sinus fistula in the use of general anesthesia, local anesthetic/vasoconstrictor, perioperative antibiotics, and diagnostic nasal endoscopy. If not previously accomplished, a partial or complete ethmoidectomy is performed to expose defects in the anterior skull base. If the CT image guidance system is available, this can be used to aid in locating the fistula intraoperatively. This is especially useful in those cases when fluorescein is not used. Failure to exactly identify the site of the defect will likely result in failure of the operation.[1,18,28] After the site of the fistula is identified, any remaining adjacent mucosa is removed to expose the bone as a graft recipient site (Fig. 10-5). It is important to remove the mucosa surrounding the defect, because residual mucosa prevents adhesion of the graft. Mucosal grafts are used as simple or complex grafts in most instances. The mucosal graft may be harvested from the turbinate, septum, or nasal floor of the opposite nasal cavity and prepared on a back table. The mucosa is removed from the underlying bone, trimmed to

the appropriate size, and placed over the defect, followed by the application of fibrin glue.

For defects larger than 0.5 cm in diameter, bone or cartilage graft should be used. The bone can be part of a composite graft consisting of turbinate bone, submucosal tissue, and mucosa that was removed from one side of the resected turbinate. The denuded side of the composite graft is placed against the defect and held in place with fibrin glue. A free bone graft can also be placed on the intracranial side (underlay graft) of the bony defect and positioned between the dura and the skull base. In this case, a neuro-otologic elevator is used to elevate the dura off the anterior skull base, thereby creating an epidural space. The bone or cartilage graft is then carefully inserted through the skull defect to lie in the epidural space (Fig. 10-6). A free mucosal graft is then placed over the bone graft and covered with fibrin glue. Additional support to hold the graft in place is established with Gelfoam first and then followed by Surgicel.

Repair of ethmoid roof and cribriform fistulas varies based on the size of the defect. In general, we favor free tissue grafts as opposed to pedicled grafts. This approach is favored by Mattox and Kennedy,[4] but Yessenow and McCabe[29] have achieved good results using pedicled grafts. For defects less than 0.5 cm in diameter, a free mucosa graft is used. For defects larger than 0.5 cm in diameter, a composite graft with rigid support from turbinate bone or septal bone is used. Although there is no limitation for endoscopic repair of sphenoid sinus fistula in regards to the size of the bony defect, a ethmoid roof defect greater than 1.5 cm has been considered a relative contraindication to endoscopic repair.[31] However, several recent cases of cranionasal fistulas with an ethmoid roof defect greater than 2 cm in diameter were repaired endoscopically with no recurrence of CSF rhinorrhea.

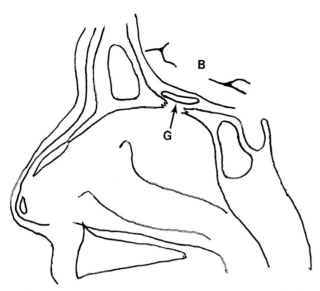

FIGURE 10-6 Schematic representation of placement of a free composite graft through an ethmoid roof defect. The graft lies in the epidural space. B, brain; G, graft.

Factors that might affect the recurrence of CSF rhinorrhea after endoscopic repair include types of graft, use of a lumbar drain, and placement of grafts. There is no statistical difference in results based on the type of grafts used (e.g., free vs. pedicled flap, mucosa vs. temporalis fascia, or muscle vs. fat), the use of lumbar drain, or the position of the graft (overlay vs. underlay graft).[18] Factors that do contribute to the success or failure of the endoscopic repair of cranionasal fistula are the surgeon's lack of experience, failure to locate the fistula intraoperatively, and increased CSF pressure.[1,18]

Cephaloceles

Sphenoid and ethmoid roof cephaloceles are managed by removing the mucosa from the mass and reducing the mass through the bony defect by direct manipulation or by using bipolar cautery. The mass is resected if its size precludes easy manipulation or if there is incomplete mucosal removal. After closure of the dura, if possible, composite grafts are used as previously described. Figure 10-7 shows the endoscopic view of a large ethmoid roof encephalocele. Excision of this lesion created a cranionasal fistula measuring 2.2 × 1 cm. The fistula was successfully repaired endoscopically with use of a free composite turbinate graft, showing that even very large skull base defects can be managed endoscopically.

POSTOPERATIVE CARE

After the procedure, patients are kept at bed rest with the head of the bed elevated. While on bed rest, deep venous thrombosis precaution is taken, intravenous antibiotics are continued while the patient is in the hospital, and stool softeners are prescribed to reduce straining. If a lumbar drain is used, it is removed on the second postoperative day. Packing is removed after 48 hours, and the patient is usually discharged from the hospital after an additional 24 hours of observation. The average hospital stay ranges from 2 to 4 days. Patients are instructed to avoid heavy lifting or strenuous activity for 4 to 6 weeks.

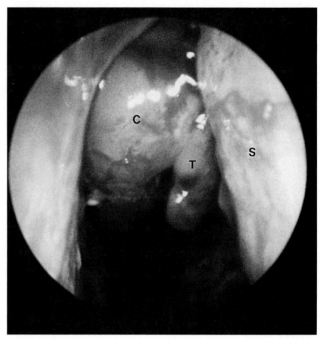

FIGURE 10-7 Endoscopic view of large cephalocele originating through an ethmoid roof cranionasal fistula. The resultant defect measured 2.2 × 1 cm. S, septum; T, middle turbinate; C, cephalocele. (From Burns JA, Dodson EE, Gross GW: Transnasal endoscopic repair of cranionasal fistulae: A refined technique with long-term follow-up. Laryngoscope 106:1080–1083, 1996.)

CONCLUSIONS

The growing number of patients with cranionasal defects has provided ample experience with this endoscopic algorithm. By using a consistent technique for each location and defect size, the success rate for closure is optimized. Precise localization afforded by the rigid nasal endoscope avoids the use of huge grafts or flaps and preserves normal nasal structure and function. The transnasal endoscopic approach effectively repairs cranionasal fistulas with excellent long-term results.

REFERENCES

1. Zapalac JS, Marple BF, Schwade ND: Skull base cerebrospinal fluid fistulas: A comprehensive diagnostic algorithm. Otolaryngol Head Neck Surg 126:669–676, 2002.
2. Church CA, Chiu AG, Vaughan WC: Endoscopic repair of large skull base defects after powered sinus surgery. Otolaryngol Head Neck Surg 129:204–209, 2003.
3. Dohlman G: Spontaneous cerebrospinal rhinorrhea. Acta Otolaryngol 67(Suppl):20–23, 1948.
4. Mattox DE, Kennedy DW: Endoscopic management of cerebrospinal fluid leaks and cephaloceles. Laryngoscope 100:857–862, 1990.
5. Papay FA, Benninger MS, Levine HL, et al: Transnasal transseptal endoscopic repair of sphenoidal cerebral spinal fluid fistula. Otolaryngol Head Neck Surg 101:595–597, 1989.
6. Levine HL: Endoscopic diagnosis and management of cerebrospinal fluid rhinorrhea. Oper Tech Otolaryngol Head Neck Surg 2:282–284, 1991.
7. Papay FA, Maggiano H, Dominquez S, et al: Rigid endoscopic repair of paranasal sinus cerebrospinal fluid fistulas. Laryngoscope 99:1195–1201, 1989.
8. Stankiewicz JA: Cerebrospinal fluid fistula and endoscopic sinus surgery. Laryngoscope 101:250–256, 1991.
9. Dodson EE, Gross CW, Swerdloff JL, Gustafson LM: Transnasal endoscopic repair of cerebrospinal fluid rhinorrhea and skull base defects: A review of 29 cases. Otolaryngol Head Neck Surg 111:600–605, 1994.

10. Burns JA, Dodson EE, Gross GW: Transnasal endoscopic repair of cranio-nasal fistulae: A refined technique with long-term follow-up. Laryngoscope 106:1080–1083, 1996.
11. McMains KC, Gross CW, Kountakis S: Presented at the Southern Section meeting of the Triological Society, Orlando, FL, 2004.
12. Ommaya AK, Dichuro G, Baldwin M, et al: Nontraumatic cerebrospinal fluid rhinorrhea. J Neurol Neurosurg Psychiatry 31:214–225, 1968.
13. Calcaterra TC: Diagnosis and management of ethmoid cerebrospinal rhinorrhea. Otolaryngol Clin North Am 18:99–117, 1985.
14. Applebaum EL, Chow JE: CSF leaks. In Cummings CW (ed): Otolaryngology: Head and Neck Surgery, 2nd ed. St. Louis: CV Mosby, 1993, pp 965–974.
15. McCormack B, Hunt CE, Sofer S: Extracranial repair of cerebrospinal fluid fistulae: Techniques and results in 37 patients. Neurosurgery 27:412–417, 1998.
16. Loew F, Loh KK: Traumatic, spontaneous and postoperative CSF rhinorrhea. Adv Tech Stand Neurosurg 11:169–171, 1984.
17. Friedman JA, Ebersold MJ, Quast LM: Post-traumatic cerebrospinal fluid leakage. World J Surg 25:1062–1066, 2001.
18. Zweig JL, Carrau RL, Celine SE, et al: Endoscopic repair of cerebrospinal fluid leaks to the sinonasal tract: Predictors of success. Otolaryngol Head Neck Surg 123:195–201, 2003.
19. Dodson EE, Gross CW, Swerdloff JL, et al: Transnasal endoscopic repair of cerebrospinal fluid rhinorrhea and skull base defects: A review of 29 cases. Otolaryngol Head Neck Surg 111:600–605, 1994.
20. Park JI, Strelzow VV, Friedman WH: Current management of cerebrospinal fluid rhinorrhea. Laryngoscope 93:1294–1300, 1983.
21. Schlosser RJ, Bolger WE: Nasal cerebrospinal fluid leaks. J Otolaryngol 31:S28–S37, 2002.
22. VonHaeke NP, Craft CB: Cerebrospinal fluid rhinorrhea and otorrhea: Extracranial repair. Clin Otolaryngol 8:317–345, 1983.
23. Chow JM, Goodman D, Mafee MF: Evaluation of CSF rhinorrhea by computerized tomography with metrizamide. Otolaryngol Head Neck Surg 100:99–105, 1989.
24. Luotonen J, Jokinen K, Laitinen J: Localization of a CSF fistula by metrizamide CT cisternography. J Laryngol Otol 100:955–958, 1986.
25. Schaefer SD, Briggs WH: The diagnosis of CSF rhinorrhea by metrizamide CT scanning. Laryngoscope 90:871–875, 1980.
26. Moseley JI, Carton CA, Stern WE: Spectrum of complications in the use of intrathecal fluorescein. J Neurosurg 48:765–767, 1978.
27. Dandy WE: Pneumocephalus (intracranial pneumatocele or aerocele). Arch Surg 12:949–982, 1926.
28. Lanza DC, O'Brien DA, Kennedy DW: Endoscopic repair of cerebrospinal fluid fistulae and encephaloceles. Laryngoscope 106:1119–1125, 1996.
29. Yessenow RS, McCabe BF: The osteo-cutaneous flap in repair of cerebrospinal fluid rhinorrhea: A 20-year experience. Otolaryngol Head Neck Surg 101:555–558, 1989.
30. Mehendale NH, Marple BF, Nussenbaum B: Management of sphenoid sinus cerebrospinal fluid rhinorrhea: Making use of an extended approach to the sphenoid sinus. Otolaryngol Head Neck Surg 126:147–153, 2002.
31. Hughes RG, Jones NS, Robertson IJ: The endoscopic treatment of cerebrospinal fluid rhinorrhea: The Notthingham experience. J Laryngol Otol 111:125–128, 1997.

Section III

Orbit

11 Transcranial Approach to Lesions of the Orbit

ANTONIO G. CARRIZO and ARMANDO BASSO

The orbit is an anatomic region located between the facial structures, paranasal sinuses, and skull base that is occupied by the organs of sight and their adnexa. From the surgical viewpoint, it represents a field shared by ophthalmology, neurosurgery, maxillofacial surgery, and ear-nose-throat surgery, each with its own techniques for orbital approach.[1]

The orbit can be considered as a quadrangular pyramid that may be approached by its open base or by one of its four walls resected in a transient or permanent way. In the anteroposterior direction, three sections may be discerned: one anterior, ample, and superficial with regard to the base; another intermediate; and the last posterior, deep, and narrow with many vascular, nervous, and muscular structures, making access to this section the most complex of the three.[1,2]

The anatomic structure of the orbital contents encompasses three areas: the periosteal, located between the periorbita and the bone; the muscular cone, which encloses the intricate components of the apex; and the area limited by the preceding two, mainly occupied by orbital fat. Primary space-occupying lesions that develop in these divisions tend to remain confined within them, requiring a different access for each compartment.[1,3]

Selecting the most suitable surgical treatment for orbital tumors requires a thorough knowledge of the diverse surgical approaches as well as their advantages, indications, limitations, and contraindications. The main considerations are the location and size of the lesion, its apparent site of origin, its routes of propagation, and its probable histological status. Such features are gleaned from clinical evaluation and complementary examinations. Current technologies allow accurate anatomic localization and earlier, more reliable diagnosis than former methods, resulting in improved treatment planning.[1,3]

SURGICAL APPROACHES TO THE ORBIT

Historically, the earliest approaches were anterior orbitotomies. One of the pioneers of this technique was the German ophthalmologist Bartisch, who described a kind of subtotal exenteration with preservation of eyelids in 1583. In 1744, Thomas Hope reported one of the first orbital interventions that spared the eyeball. Herman Knapp described the transconjunctival approach through the upper eyelid in 1874.[4]

The so-called transpalpebral access was reported by Rollet (1907, 1924), Elschnig (1927), Golovine (1930),[3,4] and Benedict (1949).[2] In fact, the skin incision is performed on the superior orbital rim. This technique remains virtually unchanged.[3,4]

In 1940, Davis[5] described the removal of optic nerve gliomas through an incision along the inferior orbital rim. Callahan adapted this approach in 1948 to other tumor types.[6]

Philip Gustav Passavant in Frankfurt was the first to use a lateral approach to the orbit for a vascular malformation in 1866, the same year that Wagner described its application to the removal of foreign bodies. However, this technique is associated with Krönlein's name based on his complete description in 1888 for the excision of a dermoid cyst. Later, multiple modifications were advanced, mainly concerning the cutaneous incision. The most widely adopted is Berke's (1954),[7] which uses Swift's horizontal incision.

The earliest craniotomy to remove an intracranial tumor causing exophthalmos was carried out by Durante in Rome in 1887.[3] In 1941, Walter Dandy[8] published his landmark paper advancing the transcranial approach to the orbit as the procedure of choice, which he regarded as superior to "that performed by ophthalmologists." This route was used during the same decade by Naffziger for decompressive purposes, as well as by Poppen (1943)[9] and Love and Benedict (1945)[10] for tumor removal.

In 1913, Frazier[11] described an approach to the hypophyseal region by means of frontal craniotomy and resection of the superior orbital rim at the anterior portion of the roof, with later replacement. This technique, which allows minimal cerebral retraction, fell into disuse with improvement in anesthetic techniques but later proved extremely valuable for gaining access to the orbital apex after the work of Johnson and Tym (1961) and Bachs (1962)[3] and, more recently, that of Jane and colleagues,[12] Maroon and Kennerdell,[13] Leone and Wissinger,[14] and Santoro, Salvati, and Vangelista.[38]

REGIONAL SURGICAL ANATOMY OF THE ORBIT

The orbital cavity is generally visualized as a quadrangular pyramid in its anterior part and a cone in its posterior. The inner wall is formed by the lacrimal and ethmoid bones, along with the body of the sphenoid bone, and the zygomatic bone and the greater wing of the sphenoid form the lateral wall. The floor consists of the zygomatic, the maxillary, and the palatine bones. The roof, finally, is formed by the horizontal portion of the frontal bone and by the lesser wing of the sphenoid bone.[15] The depth of the orbital cavity ranges from 42 to 50 mm, with a maximal base width of approximately 40 mm and a height of 35 mm.[16]

The optic canal, actually a tubular cavity lying in the deepest portion of the orbit, is sculpted in the base of the minor sphenoid wing at an angle of approximately 37 degrees with regard to the sagittal axis. It measures, on average, 5 to 10 mm long, 4.5 mm wide, and 5 mm high. The thickness of the roof varies from 1 to 3 mm, and it merges backward into the falciform process, a sheet of dura mater covering the optic nerve.[13,17]

The superior orbital fissure, through which the intracranial dura mater joins the periorbita, is delimited by the minor sphenoid wing along its superointernal margin and by the major wing along its inferolateral border. It allows passage of the oculomotor and ophthalmic nerves, as well as exit of the ophthalmic vein, which drains into the medial sector of the cavernous sinus.[16,17]

The intracranial portion of the optic nerve, whose cross section is 4 × 6 mm and whose length is 10 to 15 mm, is flattened in the horizontal direction. The intracanalicular portion of the nerve is 10 to 12 mm long, and its section is circular, almost 5 mm in diameter (Figs. 11-1 and 11-2). The intraorbital segment extends from 25 to 30 mm and presents an oval section, measuring 6 to 4 mm, whose major vertical axis lies at the exit from the optic foramen.[13,17]

The meninges and subarachnoid space accompany the optic nerve up to the sclera. At the orbital apex, the pia mater and the arachnoid fuse in the dorsal, medial, and ventral portions with the dura mater and the anulus of Zinn, partially occluding the subarachnoid space. The anulus of Zinn, a fibrous band that attaches the optic nerve at the orbital apex, receives the insertion of the levator palpebralis and extraocular muscles, with the exception of the minor oblique. The anulus is in close contact with the optic nerve dorsally but separates from it in its lateral and inferior portions, creating a space between the two heads of the lateral rectus muscle, forward to the basal sector of the superior orbital fissure. This opening is termed the *oculomotor foramen* and is traversed by the superior division of the oculomotor nerve innervating the superior rectus and levator palpebralis, the nasociliary branch of the ophthalmic nerve, the abducens, and the inferior division of the oculomotor nerve.[13,18]

Through the superior orbital fissure but outward from the oculomotor foramen, the frontal and lacrimal branches of the ophthalmic nerve, as well the sympathetic nerves, are directed inward, just below the periorbita, to gain entry into the orbit. The ciliary ganglion is located external to the optic nerve, emerging from the nasociliary branch of the ophthalmic nerve, which crosses the optic nerve superiorly to proceed toward the medial orbital wall.[19]

The ophthalmic artery arises from the anteromedial or superomedial surface of the internal carotid artery at its exit from the cavernous sinus (occasionally emerging from the intracavernous portion) and crosses the optic canal laterally and inferiorly with respect to the optic nerve. In turn, the central retinal artery arises from the ophthalmic artery and crosses the dura mater of the nerve 5 to 20 mm behind the eyeball. The ophthalmic artery then crosses above (in 82.5% of cases) or below (in 17.5%) the optic nerve, according to Rengachary and Kishore,[20] proceeding forward parallel to the internal orbital wall to reach the trochlea, where it divides into its two terminal branches, frontal (or supratrochlear) and nasal. Its collateral branches comprise the ocular (central retinal, short, and long posterior ciliary and collaterals to the optic nerve), orbital (lacrimal, superior, and inferior muscular and branches to the orbital periosteum and areolar tissue), and extraorbital (anterior and posterior ethmoidal, supraorbital, and medial palpebral) branches.[17,21]

The superior and inferior ophthalmic veins drain the orbit. These veins lack valves and anastomose several times with one another and with external tributaries. The much more developed superior ophthalmic vein passes over the lateral rectus muscle and drains into the cavernous sinus. The inferior ophthalmic vein receives the veins from the medial wall and from the floor of the orbit and divides into two branches, one draining toward the pterygoid plexus through the inferior orbital fissure and the other reaching the superior ophthalmic vein just before traversing the superior orbital fissure.[17,22]

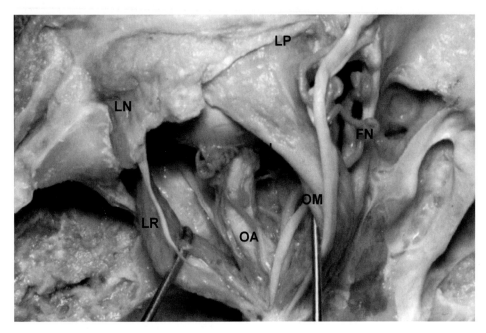

FIGURE 11-1 Microsurgical dissection of the orbital apex as observed during a superolateral approach between the levator palpebrae muscle (LP) and the lateral rectus muscle (LR), showing the optic nerve (ON), the ophthalmic artery (OA), the division of the oculomotor nerve (OM), and the frontal and lacrimal branches of the ophthalmic nerve (FN, LN).

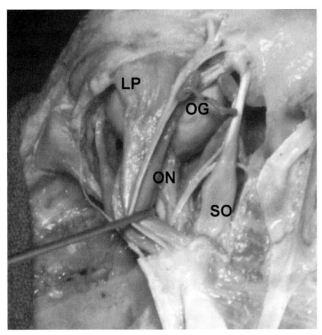

FIGURE 11-2 Anatomic view of a superomedial approach to the orbital apex between the levator palpebrae (LP) and the superior oblique muscle (SO) that allows direct access to the optic nerve (ON) and posterior pole of the ocular globe (OG).

DIAGNOSIS OF ORBITAL LESIONS

Before the widespread availability of computed tomography, orbital lesions were studied by means of plain radiography, orbitography with positive contrast, orbital phlebography, and echography. Data provided by these methods were indirect and poorly characteristic, so that a thorough knowledge of the patient's clinical history and physical examination was crucial for a presumptive diagnosis and for determination of the surgical indication, usually exploration, decompression, or biopsy.

Computed tomography scanning had a great impact on the diagnosis of orbital disease, greater perhaps than that on the field of neurologic diagnosis, and led to earlier diagnosis, more accurate lesion localization, closer delineation of lesion extension, and determination of the status of the orbital walls and neighboring areas.[1,23] In tomographic imaging, the bone structure of orbital walls, the eyeball, the optic nerve, and the extraocular muscles are clearly outlined in contrast to the low-density backdrop of the orbital fat. As a rule, space-occupying lesions also are depicted sharply against adjacent structures and may enhance with endovenous contrast.[23]

An optic nerve glioma is commonly observed on axial computed tomography scan as a spindle-shaped thickening of the optic nerve (Fig. 11-3), with a rounded, enlarged section on coronal views.[24] Meningiomas involving the optic nerve sheath present diverse tomographic features, such as diffuse thickening of the optic nerve image that expands toward the apex, occasionally accompanied by a negative shadow of the optic nerve in its interior or, at other times, by tubular calcification of the enlarged sheath (tram-track sign). Another image typical of meningioma is that of an extensive lesion surrounding the optic nerve and presenting irregular borders[24–26] (Fig. 11-4).

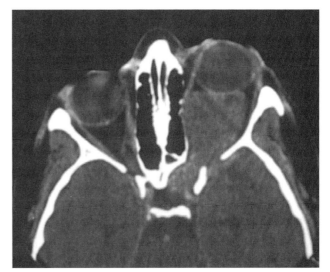

FIGURE 11-3 An axial computed tomography scan of an optic nerve glioma with intracranial extension through an enlarged optic foramen.

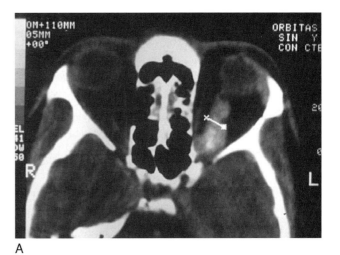

A

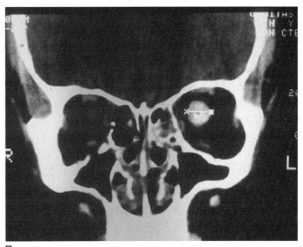

B

FIGURE 11-4 *A,* Axial computed tomography scan of a calcified optic nerve sheath meningioma. *B,* Coronal view in the same patient.

Cavernous hemangiomas are characterized by well-defined, rounded images that enhance with contrast. These must be distinguished from neurinomas, which are similar in aspect and location but more elongated and heterogeneous in structure.[1,23,27] Orbital roof lesions include osteomas, dysplasias, aneurysmal bone cysts, and osteolytic lesions such as cholesteatomas, mucoceles, histiocytosis X, and metastases, all of which are clearly visualized in bone algorithm images.[1,24]

The incorporation of magnetic resonance imaging has enriched orbital diagnosis by allowing lateral incidence, parasagittal oblique views in the direction of the optic nerve, weighting at different times, and fat saturation techniques, in addition to axial and coronal sections. Magnetic resonance imaging provides greater anatomic detail of normal structures and better comparative delineation of the pathologic process (Fig. 11-5).[23,28]

Magnetic resonance imaging is of special interest in the study of optic nerve disease, often distinguishing whether the lesion is attached to the nerve or arises from the nerve itself or from its meningeal sheath. Gadolinium enhancement commonly and accurately delineates tumoral extension, mainly toward the endocranium. In the case of meningiomas, this spreading is observed more frequently than expected (Fig. 11-6). Another finding in perioptic meningiomas is that of perioptic arachnoid cyst anterior to the tumoral obstruction; this finding must be differentiated from true arachnoid cysts of the optic nerve.[23,26,29,30]

In orbital schwannomas, a correlation of magnetic resonance imaging and pathology findings can be made: Cavity changes of heterogeneous signal intensity on T2-weighted images correspond to soft and friable structures in the pathologic findings.[31]

T2-weighted magnetic resonance imaging of an optic nerve glioma shows a fusiform area of high signal intensity with a central linear core of lower signal intensity

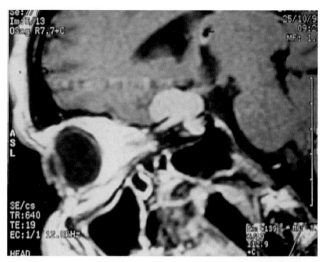

FIGURE 11-6 A T1-weighted magnetic resonance imaging scan with an oblique view along the optic nerve course shows a foraminal meningioma.

corresponding with circumferential, perineural glial proliferation, which seems to be a feature of orbital optic gliomas in neurofibromatosis.[32]

Digital subtraction angiography is mainly indicated in vascular lesions or highly vascularized tumors. It has been increasingly replaced by computed tomography and magnetic resonance angiography.

SURGICAL TECHNIQUE

Transcranial Approach to the Orbit

The orbital approach by means of craniotomy is the most complex and demanding route. It is reliably indicated in cranio-orbital disease, including sphenoid wing or anterior fossa meningiomas with orbital extension, fronto-orbital fibrous dysplasia, chondromas, chondrosarcomas, and large epidermoid cysts, as well as in bone lesions arising from the orbital roof, most commonly osteomas and aneurysmal bone cysts. In such cases, frontal or frontotemporal craniotomy is performed according to lesion extension, with tumor resection including the roof and, occasionally, the lateral wall of the orbit, followed by plastic reconstruction of invaded orbital walls, and, if necessary, of compromised dura mater.[1]

The primary types of intraorbital tumors that should be approached via the transcranial route are those arising in the orbital apex or the superointernal quadrant of the orbit. In our experience, optic nerve sheath meningiomas, optic nerve gliomas, neurinomas, intraconal cavernous hemangiomas, inflammatory pseudotumors, perioptic metastases, vascular malformations, and lymphangiomas represent most of such lesions.[1]

Since 1985, we have performed supraorbital craniotomy for primary tumors of the orbital apex. In sheath meningiomas, optic gliomas, and other tumors types extending toward the intracranial cavity, this procedure is followed by extradural decompression of the optic canal and exploration of the optic nerve by the intradural route. In meningiomas, an anular or cufflike tumoral growth may be observed

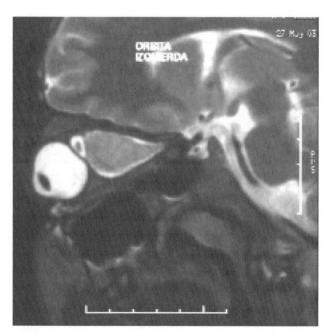

FIGURE 11-5 A T2-weighted magnetic resonance imaging oblique view of an optic nerve glioma in a child.

extending from the orbit and surrounding the intracranial segment of the optic nerve. In optic nerve gliomas, it is advisable to carry out prechiasmatic section of the nerve to avoid tumor extension toward the optic chiasm. Such combined extradural and intracranial procedures can be performed only by the transcranial route because the other approaches to the orbit prove insufficient.[33,34]

Supraorbital Craniotomy

Under general anesthesia and with endotracheal intubation, the patient is placed supine, with the head slightly extended to allow separation of the frontal lobe from the orbital roof by the effect of gravity. The sagittal axis of the skull is rotated 10 degrees toward the contralateral side. A strip of scalp is shaved along the line of incision.

Bearing cosmesis in mind, we use a hemicoronal incision behind the hairline, starting in front of the tragus and extending upward and forward, crossing the midline. The cutaneous flap is raised and dissected from the pericranium and from the temporal muscle aponeurosis, including the superior branch of the facial nerve in the folded planes. We use an incision through the eyebrow for the superior orbitotomy without bone resection, but we do not use it for supraorbital craniotomy, as it was proposed.[35]

A sickle-shaped incision with a lower concavity is made in the periosteum. The incision continues toward the lateral orbital rim, dissects the flap up to the superior orbital rim, and then proceeds toward the periorbita. The supraorbital nerve is released from the notch and, if a bony bridge exists, it is sectioned with a fine chisel (Fig. 11-7).

The most anterior portion of the temporal muscle is dissected, and a burr hole is made in the temporal fossa, behind the zygomatic process of the frontal bone, exposing the dura mater of the anterior fossa in its upper portion and the periorbita in its lower portion, both separated by the orbital roof. A second opening is made immediately above the orbital rim in the superointernal angle, outside the glabella. Because this opening usually crosses the frontal sinus, standard precautions are required. Both openings may be connected with a craniotome. Otherwise, a third frontal burr hole is made,

equidistant from the first two and approximately 4 to 5 cm from the orbital rim. This opening is connected to the former two with a Gigli saw.[1,12]

From the lateral burr hole first described, a Gigli saw or an oscillating saw is passed toward the lateral rim, which is then sectioned. From this same opening, while the dura mater and the periorbita are protected with small spatulas, the orbital roof is sectioned with a fine chisel directed toward the midline. From the medial frontal opening, the superior orbital rim and the orbital roof are sectioned with the chisel directed laterally and posteriorly toward the osteotomy previously performed. The frontal bone flap is then easily raised, together with the superior orbital rim and the anterior and wider sector of the orbital roof, exposing the frontal dura mater and the periorbita (Fig. 11-8).[1,12,13]

In apical tumors, it is necessary to complete bone resection of the orbital roof and the upper margin of the optic canal using a high-speed drill with a diamond bit.[1,13]

The surgical microscope and self-retaining retractors are placed with only minimal frontal displacement. The use of spatulas on the meninges is avoided. The periorbita frequently opens during osteotomy and flap elevation maneuvers; should the periorbita remain intact, an anteroposterior incision is made medially to the levator palpebralis muscle.[13,21]

Next, the inner and superior rectus muscles are explored by microsurgical technique until the optic nerve is located. This method carries the least risk of causing irreversible ophthalmoplegia.[21,22]

In optic nerve gliomas, the nerve is often extremely thickened in its distended meningeal coverings, showing regular contours. In these cases, the lesion is dissected laterally, the anterior portion from behind the eyeball and the posterior one at the level of the anulus of Zinn, followed by opening of the frontobasal dura mater to explore the optic nerve along its intracranial course. The nerve is then resected from the prechiasmatic level toward the optic canal, including the foraminal portion.[1,13,21]

In sheath meningiomas presenting as diffuse thickening, the dural sheath may be opened anteroposteriorly, and the tumor may be dissected jointly with the invaded sheath by following the subarachnoid space. In few cases, particularly

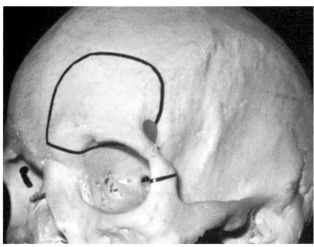

FIGURE 11-7 Diagram of a supraorbital craniotomy is outlined on a skull.

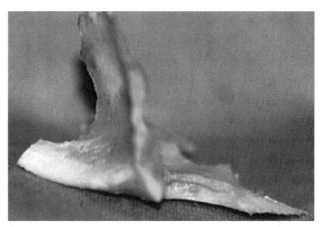

FIGURE 11-8 Surgical photograph of a supraorbital bone flap, including the superior orbital rim and the anterior part of the orbital roof.

in lesions located anteriorly, sight preservation may be achieved, provided that careful dissection is carried out and vascularization is spared in the nerve and retina. When the tumoral mass is larger, is not clearly restricted to the nerve course, and exhibits micronodular infiltration of the muscles at the apex, the eye is most likely amaurotic. Thus it is advisable to resect this type of mass with the nerve because the latter cannot be spared from the former. In such cases, it is essential to perform intracranial exploration of the optic nerve, which may be surrounded by tumor extending through the optic canal.[1]

In neurinomas and cavernous hemangiomas, the procedure is often simpler. Once the lesion has been located, it is dissected by microsurgical technique and may be removed because attachment to critical structures is unusual. In rare cases, we have found hourglass neurinomas extending toward the middle cerebral fossa through a markedly enlarged superior orbital fissure that required resection by a combined intracranial and intraorbital procedure.[1,22]

Transcranial Approach with Resection of the Orbital Roof

Tumors invading or arising from the orbital roof demand a technique differing from the one used for purely intraorbital lesions. We resort to a frontal or frontotemporal craniotomy, according to lesion extension. When marked hyperostosis is present, as in pterional meningioma, fibrous dysplasia, or osteoma, the procedure begins with a gradual resection of the pathologic bone with burrs, drills, and gouges before the bone flap is raised, so that the dura mater is protected by that bony sector during such maneuvers. It often is necessary to continue bone resection toward the roof and lateral orbital wall, leaving the orbital contents amply exposed. In meningiomas that extend toward the anterior clinoid process, a clinoidectomy and decompression of the optic canal are performed. In purely osseous lesions, this stage ends with total removal of the lesion.[27,36]

In sphenoid wing meningiomas, it is essential to proceed with dural opening and resection of invaded dura mater, as well as the attached meningioma en plaque. Occasionally, in a large intradural tumor with temporal or frontotemporal extension that projects toward the sylvian fissure, tumoral dissection proceeds from the cerebral cortex and along the internal carotid and middle cerebral arteries using microsurgical technique.[27]

The final step is to perform plastic reconstruction of the resected dura mater with pericranium. Lyophilized dura mater produced good results in some of our earlier patients but was abandoned after some cases of Creutzfeldt-Jakob disease associated with its use were reported in the literature.[27] The roof and, at times, the lateral wall of the orbit are reconstructed with methyl methacrylate. Initially, we carried out plastic reconstruction with costal autografts, but the procedure proved protracted and tedious because graft modeling was highly complex and the cosmetic results were suboptimal.[27]

In the case of malar involvement by the hyperostosis, mostly seen early in our series, we proposed a transmalar approach by means of a separated incision. At present, we use an orbitozygomatic approach as described by different authors.[37,38]

COMPLICATIONS

In primary intraorbital tumors lacking intracranial extension operated on by the diverse methods described, no mortality or neurologic complications, such as seizures, hemipareses, or sensory disorders, occurred. Infrequently, signs of intracranial hypotension or pneumocephalus may be detected during the first 48 postoperative hours in patients operated on transcranially.

In tumors extending toward the apex, mainly optic nerve gliomas and sheath meningiomas, most patients presented with subtotal ophthalmoplegia and ptosis immediately after surgery, followed by nearly entire remission within 2 to 3 months. Although amaurosis of the corresponding eye is the rule in gliomas and most meningiomas, in a few cases of spared sight, preservation of useful sight was achieved with the technique described. In other histologic forms, the cosmetic and functional results were most satisfactory, barring transient inflammatory pseudoptosis in the upper eyelid. Neither cerebrospinal fluid collection nor leaks were observed; no infectious processes occurred.[27]

With sphenoid wing meningiomas, the most crucial complications occurred in the earlier cases of the series, mainly in the internal third of the wing. They consisted mostly of contralateral hemiparesis or hemiplegia in 4%, seizures in 3%, and transient disorders of consciousness in 4% of the cases. The mortality rate in these cases was 2%. Almost invariably, such complications resulted from damage to the internal carotid or middle cerebral arteries in the course of dissection. However, these undesirable effects have been avoided during the past two decades owing to improvements in microsurgical technique and instruments, such as the ultrasonic aspirator.[27]

Our experience is based on a series of 628 operative cases of orbital disease from 1974 to the present (Table 11-1). The surgical techniques used are presented in Table 11-2. Although this a neurosurgical series, most cases were resolved by superior orbitotomy, although the transcranial approach was necessary in 25.11% of patients with primary intraorbital disease. Including tumors extending secondarily to the orbit increased the incidence of craniotomies to 41.71% of all interventions.

In primary intraorbital tumors, Berke lateral orbitotomy was performed in 11.53% and inferior orbitotomy in 4.76% of patients. In 10 patients, a superolateral approach by means of a Kocher-Stallard incision was used, and in 27 patients, inferolateral transmalar access was used, nine with large primary tumors and 18 with tumors extending to the orbit, mostly pterional meningiomas from the start of our series. Early in the series, exenteration was required in 13 patients with advanced malignant tumors. At present, more conservative management is preferred.[39,40] In eight patients with paranasal sinus tumor with orbital invasion, a transantral approach was used.[1] Revision surgery, using the initial or an alternative route, was necessary in 21 patients.

The diversity of procedures used in our series is the result of a systematic and thorough evaluation of the patient's clinical history and of complementary examinations to select the most suitable treatment for each particular case.[1,13,21]

TABLE 11-1 ▪ Surgical Experience with Orbital Tumors (1974–2004)

Tumor Type	Number
Primary Orbital Tumors	
Mucocele	118
Cholesteatoma	63
Meningioma	42
Neurinoma	33
Cavernous hemangioma	32
Lacrimal gland tumor	31
Lymphoma	22
Inflammatory pseudotumor	17
Sarcoma	15
Optic nerve glioma	14
Localized bone lesion	13
Hydatid cyst	13
Miscellaneous	29
Subtotal	442
Propagated Orbital Tumors	
Sphenoid ridge meningioma	145
Metastasis	18
Paranasal sinus carcinoma	7
Fibrous dysplasia	6
Chondroma, chondrosarcoma	4
Miscellaneous (e.g., reticulosarcoma, Ewing's sarcoma, metastasis)	6
Subtotal	186
Total	628

PRIMARY INTRAORBITAL MENINGIOMAS

Primary intraorbital meningioma was a condition rarely diagnosed before the development of modern neurodiagnostic tools. At present, the widespread use of magnetic resonance imaging allows better diagnosis and thus primary intraorbital meningioma is the tumor more frequently operated by the transcranial approach in our series. Most of the meningiomas that affect the orbit are secondary to intracranial sources, such as olfactory groove, basofrontal, and sphenoidal wing meningiomas.[41,42] We found 42 primary intraorbital meningiomas and 145 sphenoid wing meningiomas during the same period. The management of a primary

TABLE 11-2 ▪ Surgical Approaches to Orbital Tumors

	Primary Tumors		Propagated Tumors		Total	
	No.	%	No.	%	No.	%
Superior orbitotomy	219	49.54			219	34.87
Transcranial approach	111	25.11	151	81.18	262	41.71
Lateral orbitotomy	51	11.53	9	4.83	60	9.55
Inferior orbitotomy	21	4.75			21	3.34
Exenteration	13	2.94			13	2.07
Superolateral	10	2.26			10	1.59
Inferolateral	9	2.03	18	9.67	27	4.29
Transantral approach	8	1.80	8	4.30	16	2.54
Total	442	100	186	100	628	100

intraorbital meningioma is controversial. The following treatment modalities have been proposed:

1. Conservative, nonsurgical.
2. Fine needle aspiration biopsy.
3. Biopsy and decompression of the optic nerve by lateral orbitotomy.
4. Complete or partial excision with sparing of the optic nerve by the transcranial approach.
5. Excision of the nerve and tumor.
6. Enucleation or exenteration of the globe and orbital contents.
7. Radiotherapy.

Based on our frequent findings of an intracranial extension of primary intraorbital meningioma, our policy has been to perform a total or subtotal removal of the tumor, sparing the optic nerve, if the patient presented with useful vision preoperatively (Fig. 11-9).

Our series comprises 42 consecutive patients (37 women and five men) operated on between 1976 and 2004. According to Craig and Gogela classification, we found 26 optic nerve sheath meningiomas, 14 of the foraminal type, one extradural, and one bilateral.[25,43] Forty-five operations were carried out. Since 1980 we have used fronto-orbital craniotomy

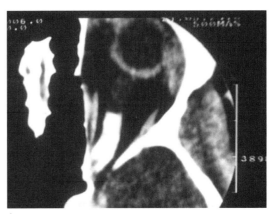

A

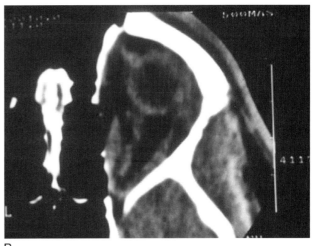

B

FIGURE 11-9 *A,* Axial computed tomography scan shows a calcified optic nerve sheath meningioma. *B,* Postoperative computed tomography scan of the same patient shows the resection of the lesion. Useful vision was preserved in the patient.

followed by microsurgical resection of the intraorbital and intracranial components of the tumor. Lateral orbitotomy was performed in three cases. Early in the series, two patients with exorbitism were exenterated.

Our results were as follows: There was no mortality in our series. Six recurrences were documented. In nine patients with useful vision preoperatively, the same vision was maintained in six patients, improved in two patients with foraminal meningiomas, and worsened in one patient.

Radiotherapy is indicated as a primary treatment by some authors.[44] We indicated radiotherapy as complementary treatment after recurrence in three patients. Recently, radiosurgery became available in our center and was used in one patient after one transcranial and two lateral approaches. This patient presented an exophytic meningioma and even now has useful vision.

SCHWANNOMAS

It is classically accepted that orbital schwannomas derive from sensitive branches of the ophthalmic nerve and exceptionally from branches of the oculomotor nerves. Frequently they are located in the orbital apex, obscuring the optic nerve, and can be confused with optic nerve gliomas or sheath meningiomas. The surgical approach is selected according to the location and extension of the lesion.[45,46] Of our 33 cases, 21 lesions were located in the orbital apex, two of them extended toward the medial cranial fossa and other one to the cavernous sinus through an enlarged superior orbital fissure adopting an hourglass configuration (Fig. 11-10). These patients were treated by means of a supraorbital craniotomy, which, in the three latter patients, extended to the temporal region.

In seven cases, schwannomas were located laterally, and a lateral orbitotomy through a Smith-Berke or a Stallard incision was performed. Five tumors were located below the optic nerve and were operated on by a inferolateral approach that included removal of the malar bone and its reposition after resection of the tumor.[47]

CAVERNOUS HEMANGIOMA

The approach to this well-circumscribed rounded lesion is determined by its location. We treated 32 of these lesions; 19 of them were intraconal, in the orbital apex and were operated on transcranially (Fig. 11-11), eight were located in the lateral part of the intraconal space and could be resected by a lateral approach, and five inferiorly located were operated on using a transmalar approach that allows excellent exposure of the inferolateral aspect of the orbit.[48–50]

Typically, there is a clear plane of cleavage that allows an easy dissection of the lesion from the surrounding structures and a clean en bloc resection.[1,21] We did not find any indication for a contralateral pterional approach for this lesion.[51]

OPTIC NERVE GLIOMA

This lesion occurs principally in children in the first decade of life, many of them with neurofibromatosis 1, but can also be found sporadically in young adults. Considered as a hamartoma by some authors, it appears to be a true neoplasm

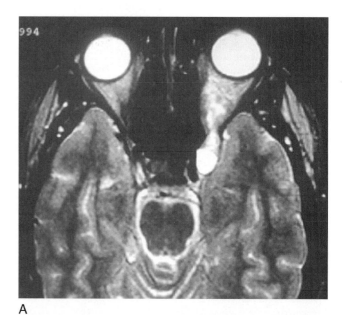

A

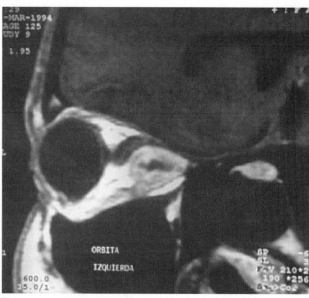

B

FIGURE 11-10 *A,* Axial magnetic resonance imaging demonstrating a dumbbell neurinoma occupying the orbital apex and the cavernous sinus, trespassing an enlarged superior orbital fissure. *B,* Oblique view in the same patient.

that characteristically shows early growth followed by stability in many patients.[52] Even regression was observed in those with neurofibromatosis 1.[53] Because of its indolent course, many authors propose conservative management, although the visual prognosis is fair, with visual loss usually occurring between 1 and 6 years after the diagnosis of optic glioma.[54,55]

We treated surgically 14 patients harboring pilocytic astrocytomas of the intraorbital optic nerve, differentiating them from the chiasmatic gliomas. All the patients were blind or almost blind at the time of surgery. None of them had neurofibromatosis 1. We employed the technique described previously, the main step being the resection of the prechiasmatic portion of the nerve and preservation of the anterior knee (also known as Wilbrand's knee) of the contralateral nerve.

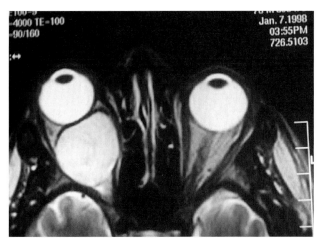

FIGURE 11-11 T2-weighted magnetic resonance imaging axial view of an intraconal cavernous hemangioma.

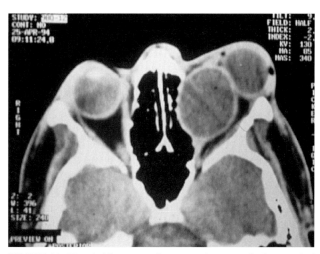

FIGURE 11-12 Axial computed tomography scan of a huge apical hydatid cyst that had to be removed with a supraorbital craniotomy.

Even with this technique, we observed two intracranial extensions, 3 and 20 years after surgery in two young women. In the case of early recurrence, which was reoperated on, the patient eventually died due to hypothalamic involvement 5 years after diagnosis, in spite of its well-differentiated histology.

Based on our experience, we disagree with conservative management of a distant sporadic optic nerve glioma, which we do not consider as being an inoffensive lesion.

MISCELLANEOUS

The other orbital lesion that we treated via the transcranial route was idiopathic orbital inflammation in its local form, formerly known as orbital pseudotumor, located in the orbital apex.[56]

Mixed tumors of the lacrimal gland are usually operated on using a superior orbitotomy without bone resection, except in cases with involvement of the lacrimal fossa, especially found in some patients with malignant transformation. In this case, we resected the tumor and the eroded bone and performed a plastic reconstruction with methylmethacrylate.[57]

Different vascular malformations are found in the orbit. They can be classified according to hemodynamic concepts as type I (no flow) lesions that have essentially little connection with the vascular system, as venous lymphatic malformations, previously known as lymphangiomas; type II (venous flow) lesions distensible with direct and rich communication with the venous system, as orbital varices, and not distensible with minimal connection with the venous system; and type III (arterial flow) that corresponds to arteriovenous malformations. We have found these lesions frequently associated with intracranial arteriovenous malformations. With this pathology, the transcranial approach allows exposure of the ophthalmic artery and the superior ophthalmic vein and is clearly indicated.[58]

Metastases are mainly found in older patients; sometimes they present with enophthalmos instead of the classic exophthalmos.[59] We do not use the transcranial route in these patients to avoid intracranial dissemination. The same is true for infectious or parasitic pathology, except in two cases of extensive intraconal apical hydatid cysts (Fig. 11-12).

SUMMARY

The choice of the most suitable surgical treatment for space-occupying orbital lesions is made based on tumor location, size, apparent site of origin, propagation routes, and probable histologic type.

Superior orbitotomy, the technique most frequently used, is mainly indicated in frontoethmoidal mucoceles, dermoid cysts, and lacrimal gland tumors. Lateral orbitotomy allows access to the lateral quadrants of the orbital cavity, where cavernous hemangiomas, neurinomas, inflammatory pseudotumors, and metastases may develop.

We found fewer indications for inferior orbitotomy, which is used in rare lesions such as some lymphomas and metastases. For tumors originating in ethmoid cells or the maxillary sinus, a transantral approach is indicated.

Less frequently, larger lesions require extended approaches (e.g., superolateral or inferolateral) according to tumor topography. Such techniques are used mainly for removal of hydatid cysts or huge cavernous hemangiomas or neurinomas.

The transcranial approach to the orbit is indicated for cranio-orbital meningioma of the sphenoid wing and for anterior cranial fossa disease with orbital extension (fronto-orbital fibrous dysplasia, chondroma, chondrosarcoma, aneurysmal bone cyst, osteoma, and large epidermoid cysts). Primary intraorbital tumors requiring a transcranial approach are those located in the apex or the superointernal quadrant that are large or extend posteriorly. The most common lesions are optic nerve sheath meningiomas, optic nerve gliomas, cavernous hemangiomas, neurinomas, inflammatory pseudotumors, vascular malformations, lymphangiomas, hemangiopericytomas, and perioptic metastases. The transcranial route is the only one that allows decompression of the optic canal and intracranial exploration of the optic nerve along its prechiasmatic course.

REFERENCES

1. Basso A, Carrizo A, Kreutel A: Transcranial approach to lesions of the orbit. In Schmidek H, Sweet W (eds): Operative Neurosurgical Techniques. Philadelphia: WB Saunders, 1995, pp 205–212.
2. Benedict W: Surgical treatment of tumors and cysts of the orbit. Am J Ophthalmol 32:765–773, 1949.

3. Brihaye J: Neurosurgical approaches to orbital tumors. In Krayenbuhl H (ed): Advances and Technical Standards in Neurosurgery, vol 3. Wien/New York: Springer-Verlag, 1976, pp 103–121.

4. Duke-Elder S: Systems of Ophthalmology, vol 13, part II. London: Henry Kimpton, 1974, pp 774–1230.

5. Davis F: Primary tumors of the optic nerve. Arch Ophthalmol 23:735–821, 1940.

6. Vergez A: Les voies temporales d'abord de l'orbite. Arch Ophtal (Paris) 18:294–343, 1958.

7. Berke R: A modified Kronlein operation. Arch Ophthalmol 51:609–632, 1954.

8. Dandy W: Orbital tumors. New York: Oskar Piest, 1941, pp 154–160.

9. Poppen J: Exophthalmos. Am J Surg 64:64–79, 1943.

10. Love J, Benedict W: Transcranial removal of intraorbital tumors. JAMA 129:777–784, 1945.

11. Frazier C: An approach to the hypophysis through the anterior cranial fossa. Ann Surg 57:145–152, 1913.

12. Jane J, Park T, Pobereskin L, et al: The supraorbital approach: Technical note. Neurosurgery 11:537–542, 1982.

13. Maroon J, Kennerdell J: Surgical approaches to the orbit. J Neurosurg 60:1226–1235, 1984.

14. Leone C, Wissinger J: Surgical approaches to diseases of the orbital apex. Ophthalmology 95:391–397, 1988.

15. Reese A: Tumors of the Eye. New York: Hoeber Medical Division, 1963, pp 562–570.

16. Casper D, Linda Chi T, Trokel S: Orbital Disease: Imaging and Analysis. New York: Thieme, 1993, pp 64–79.

17. Doxanas M, Anderson R: Clinical Orbital Anatomy. Baltimore: Williams & Wilkins, 1984, pp 153–169.

18. Shields J: Diagnosis and Management of Orbital Tumors. Philadelphia: WB Saunders, 1989, pp 8–10.

19. Towsend D: Orbital surgical techniques. In Albert D, Jakobiec F (eds): Principles and Practice of Ophthalmology, vol 3. Philadelphia: WB Saunders, 1994, pp 1890–1895.

20. Rengachary S, Kishore P: Intraorbital ophthalmic aneurysms and arteriovenous fistulae. Surg Neurol 9:35–40, 1978.

21. Housepian E: Microsurgical anatomy of the orbital apex and principles of transcranial orbital exploration. Clin Neurosurg 25:556–573, 1977.

22. Housepian E, Trokel S: Tumors of the orbit. In Youmans J (ed): Neurological Surgery, vol 3. Philadelphia: WB Saunders, 1973, pp 1275–1296.

23. Lindblom B, Truwit C, Hoyt W: Optic nerve sheath meningioma: Definition of intraorbital, intracanalicular and intracranial components with magnetic resonance imaging. Ophthalmology 99:560–566, 1992.

24. Jakobiec F, Depot M, Kennerdell J: Combined clinical and computed tomographic diagnosis of orbital glioma and meningioma. Ophthalmology 91:137–155, 1984.

25. Wright J, Call N, Liaricos S: Primary optic nerve meningioma. Br J Ophthalmol 64:553–558, 1980.

26. Muller-Forell W, Pitz S: Orbital pathology. Eur J Radiol 49:105–142, 2004.

27. Abe T, Kawamura N, Homma H, et al: MRI of orbital schwannoma. Neuroradiology 42:466–468, 2000.

28. Warner M, Weber A, Jakobiec F: Benign and malignant tumors of the orbital cavity including the lacrimal gland. Neuroimag Clin North Am 6:123–142, 1996.

29. Mafee M, Goodwin J, Dorodi S: Optic nerve sheath meningioma: Role of MR imaging. Radiol Clin North Am 37:37–58, 1999.

30. Akor C, Wojno T, Newman N, et al: Arachnoid cyst of the optic nerve: Report of two cases and review of the literature. Ophthal Plast Reconstr Surg 19:466–469, 2003.

31. Gunduz K, Shields C, Gunalp I, et al: Orbital schwannomas: Correlation of magnetic resonance imaging and pathological findings. Graefes Arch Clin Exp Opthalmol 241:593–597, 2003.

32. Seiff S, Brodsky M, MacDonald G, et al: Orbital optic glioma in neurofibromatosis. Arch Ophthalmol 105:1689–1692, 1987.

33. Basso A, Carrizo A, Kreutel A, Tomecek F: Primary intraorbital meningiomas. In Schmidek H (ed): Meningiomas and Their Surgical Management. Philadelphia: WB Saunders, 1991, pp 311–323.

34. Basso A, Carrizo A: Sphenoid ridge meningiomas. In Schmidek H (ed): Meningiomas and Their Surgical Management. Philadelphia: WB Saunders, 1991, pp 233–241.

35. Cutney C, Bernardino C, Buono L, et al: Transorbital craniotomy through a suprabrow approach: A case series. Orbit 20:107–117, 2001.

36. Margalit N, Lesser J, Moche J, et al: Meningiomas involving the optic nerve: Technical aspects and outcomes for a series of 50 patients. Neurosurgery 53:523–532, 2003.

37. Ducic Y: Orbitozygomatic resection of meningioma of the orbit. Laryngoscope 114:164–170, 2004.

38. Santoro A, Salvati M, Vangelista T, et al: Fronto-temporo-orbito zygomatic approach and variants. Surgical technique and indications. J Neurosurg Sci 47:141–147, 2003.

39. Goldberg R, Kim J, Shorr N: Orbital exenteration: Results of an individualized approach. Ophthal Plast Reconstr Surg 19:229–236, 2003.

40. Ugurlu S, Bartley G: Evolution of en orbital apex tumor over a decade. Ophthal Plast Reconstr Surg 20:75–77, 2004.

41. Cantore W: Neural orbital tumors. Curr Opin Ophthalmol 11:367–371, 2000.

42. Volpe N, Gausas R: Optic nerve and orbital tumors. Neurosurg Clin N Am 10:699–715, 1999.

43. Farah S, Konrad H, Huang D, et al: Ectopic orbital meningioma: A case report and review. Ophthal Plast Reconstr Surg 15:463–466, 1999.

44. Mashayekhi A, Shields J, Shields C: Involution of retinochoroidal shunt vessel after radiotherapy for optic nerve sheath meningioma. Eur J Ophthalmol 14:61–64, 2004.

45. Schick U, Bleyen J, Hassler W: Treatment of orbital schwannomas and neurofibromas. Br J Neurosurg 17:541–545, 2003.

46. Weisman R, Kikkawe D, Moe K, Osguthorpe J: Orbital tumors. Otolaryngol Clin North Am 34:1157–1174, 2001.

47. Gonul E, Timurkaynak E: Inferolateral microsurgical approach to the orbit: An anatomical study. Minim Invasive Neurosurg 42:137–141, 1999.

48. Schick U, Dott U, Hassler W: Surgical treatment of orbital cavernomas. Surg Neurol 60:234–244, 2003.

49. Otto C, Coppit G, Mazzoli R, et al: Gaze-evoked amaurosis: a report of five cases. Ophthalmology 110:322–326, 2003.

50. Rios Dias G, Velasco Cruz A: Intraosseus hemangioma of the lateral orbital wall. Ophthal Plast Reconstr Surg 20:27–30, 2004.

51. Hassler W, Meyer B, Rohde V, et al: Pterional approach to the contralateral orbit. Neurosurgery 34:552–554, 1994.

52. Dutton J: Gliomas of the anterior visual pathway. Surv Ophthalmol 38:427–452, 1994.

53. Astrup J: Natural history and clinical management of optic pathway gliomas. Br J Neurosurg 17:327–335, 2003.

54. Balcer L, Liu G, Heller G, et al: Visual loss in children with neurofibromatosis type 1 and optic pathway gliomas: Relation to tumor location by magnetic resonance imaging. Am J Ophthalmol 131:442–445, 2001.

55. Hollander M, FitzPatrick M, O'Connor S, et al: Optic nerve gliomas. Radiol Clin North Am 37:59–71, 1999.

56. Demirci H, Shields C, Shields J, et al: Orbital tumor of the older adult population. Ophthalmology 109:243–248, 2002.

57. Sadick H, Riedel F, Naim R, et al: Benign mixed tumors of the lacrimal gland. Clinical diagnosis and surgical management. ORL J Otorhinolaryngol Relat Spec 65:295–299, 2003.

58. Rootman J: Vascular malformations of the orbit: Hemodynamic concepts. Orbit 22:103–120, 2003.

59. Shields C, Stopyra G, Marr B, et al: Enophthalmos as initial manifestation of occult, mammogram-negative carciphoma of the breast. Opthalmic Surg Lasers Imaging 35:56–57, 2004.

12 Surgical Management of Intraorbital Tumors

JEFFREY N. BRUCE, MICHAEL KAZIM, and EDGAR M. HOUSEPIAN

SURGICAL MANAGEMENT OF INTRAORBITAL TUMORS

To optimize results from surgical management of intraorbital tumors, the objectives of the operation must be clearly understood. These objectives are derived from a clear understanding of the nature of the pathologic process and the details of the regional anatomy to allow a rational decision regarding approach and technique. The transcranial neurosurgical approach to the orbit is of greater advantage when dealing with disease processes that span the orbital and intracranial spaces. It also affords superior access to the apical portion of the optic nerve and to the medial and lateral superior quadrants of the orbital apex.

The great variety of tumors and other mass lesions that occur behind the eye and cause proptosis are of interest to several surgical disciplines, and access to a multidisciplinary team can be valuable when contemplating surgical management. Ophthalmic surgeons can deal with many of these problems by one of a number of direct orbital approaches. The otolaryngologist can gain access to pathologic conditions arising within sinuses bordering the superior, medial, and inferior margins of the orbit. The neurologic surgeon has access to those tumors that involve both the intracranial and the intraorbital space. With the advent of modern neurosurgery, which allows safe access to the orbit by the cranial route, the neurosurgical literature began to reflect an increasing application of the transcranial orbital exploration to a large number of orbital problems.[1-5]

As one might expect, this encroachment on a traditionally ophthalmologic field led to a period of justifiable controversy regarding the proper approach to orbital problems.[6-10] Fortunately, the rapid development of diagnostic radiologic procedures has provided a means of more precisely defining the nature and extent of a lesion and has brought a rational basis to the surgical approach to orbital surgery.

SURGICAL ANATOMY

The purpose of surgical anatomy is to describe and define significant anatomic interrelationships and to correlate the anatomy with clinical and surgical considerations.[11-14]

The Orbit

The surgeon must be oriented to the medial obliquity of the apex of the orbit (Fig. 12-1).

The 5- to 10-mm long optic canal enters the intracranial cavity medial to the anterior clinoid process, beneath which lies one of the two roots of the lesser wing of the sphenoid bone. This root forms the lateral wall of the optic canal and the medial margin of the superior orbital fissure. The lateral margin of the superior orbital fissure is bordered by the greater wing of the sphenoid bone, and, together with the frontosphenoid process of the zygomatic bone, it forms the lateral wall of the orbit. The roof of the orbit and the floor of the anterior cranial fossa are, of course, one and the same, and the orbital plate of the maxillary bone forms both the floor of the orbit and the roof of the maxillary sinus. The medial wall of the orbit is formed by the lacrimal bone and the fragile lamina papyracea, which covers the ethmoid sinuses, and closer to the apex, the sphenoid sinus. The frontal sinus, to a variable extent, fills that portion of the frontal bone forming the supraorbital rim.

Optic Nerve

Starting at the chiasmal end, the optic nerve has a flattened horizontal oval shape and measures approximately 4 × 6 mm (Fig. 12-2).

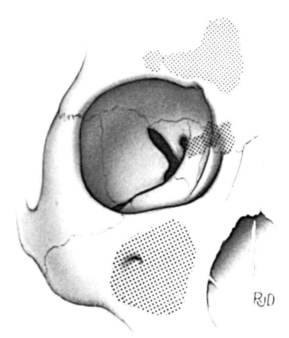

FIGURE 12-1 The integrity of the bony orbit and the size and shape of its fissures and foramina can be defined by plain skull radiographs and computed tomography bone windows. The frontal, ethmoidal, and maxillary sinuses are shown in diagrammatic fashion. Attention is directed to one of the two roots of the lesser wing of the sphenoid, which lies beneath the anterior clinoid and forms the lateral margin of the optic canal in the medial margin of the superior orbital fissure.

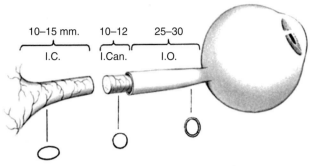

FIGURE 12-2 The dimensions and contours of the intracranial (I.C.), intracanalicular (I.Can.), and intraorbital (I.O.) portions of the optic nerve.

After it enters the cranial end of the optic canal, it is circular and 5 mm in diameter, and continues to the globe as a 6 × 4-mm vertically oval structure. A pial membrane, carrying the blood supply, accompanies the nerve from the chiasm throughout its entire course to the sclera. The intracranial arachnoid, in like fashion, continues as a discrete structure through the optic canal and fuses with the pia at the globe. There are loose trabeculations in the subarachnoid space. At the apical orbital portion of the nerve, however, the pia and arachnoid are fused dorsomedially and ventrally with the dura and the fibrous anulus of Zinn, tethering the optic nerve and partially occluding the subarachnoid space but not obliterating its continuity. Normally, the intraocular pressure is slightly higher than the intracranial pressure; therefore, it is most likely that the papilledema found in conditions producing increased intracranial pressure is directly related to this continuity of the subarachnoid space from the cranial cavity to its termination at the lamina cribrosa.

Periorbita

The intracranial dura extends into and lines the optic canal, and at the orbital exit of the canal, it splits into an outer periosteal (or periorbital) layer and an inner layer that accompanies the optic nerve to the globe, where it fuses with the arachnoid, pia, and sclera (Fig. 12-3).

To remove the optic nerve from the globe to the chiasm, as in cases of optic nerve glioma and meningioma, it is therefore necessary to section the anulus of Zinn and its fibrous attachment to the nerve. The periorbital dura also is continuous with the intracranial dura at the superior orbital fissure and, of course, lines the inferior orbital fissure as well as the other foramina, becoming continuous with the periosteum of the skull at these sites. Anteriorly, the periorbita is continuous with the periosteum at the orbital margin; structural modifications in the periorbita enclose the lacrimal gland and fix the pulley of the superior oblique tendon.

This confluence of the periorbita with the intracranial dura at the superior orbital fissure may serve as a route of entry of en plaque meningioma. Arachnoidal rests at this border zone may be the source of intraorbital meningiomas that appear to arise from the periorbita. Resection of a meningioma invading the superior fissure cannot be achieved without a risk of injury to the oculomotor nerves passing therein. Primary optic nerve sheath meningiomas can be defined preoperatively and safely removed by the transcranial approach.

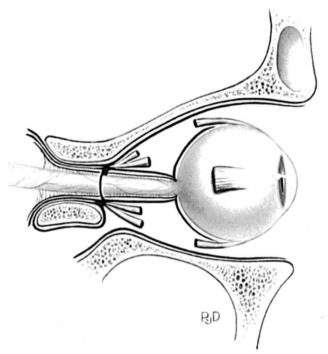

FIGURE 12-3 The membranes investing the optic nerve and lining the intracranial cavity, optic canal, and orbit. A double-layered intracranial dura is seen extending through the optic canal and superior orbital fissure. The inner layer continues in the orbit as Schwann's dural sheath. The outer layer forms the periorbita beyond the anulus of Zinn. There is a continuous subarachnoid space that extends from the intracranial space to the junction of the pia, arachnoid, and dura at the scleral margin. This space is partially obliterated at the anulus of Zinn.

When these tumors occur at the extreme apex, where the dural sheath of the optic nerve is fused with the origins of the extraocular muscles at the anulus of Zinn, total excision can be achieved without injury to these structures if they have not been invaded by the tumor.

Meningiomas may have a propensity for more rapid growth in children; therefore, more aggressive management may be advisable in children if there is microscopic residual tissue at the anulus of Zinn or the superior orbital fissure. In older patients, microscopic residual tissue within the muscle cone may be acceptable because the tumors grow more slowly. The anulus of Zinn provides no barrier against extension of a tumor through the optic nerve (Fig. 12-4), and routine monitoring of the canal for hyperostosis, together with computed tomography (CT) or magnetic resonance imaging (MRI), must be performed to detect the presence of intracanalicular tumors.

Muscle Cone and Anulus of Zinn

The fibrous anulus tendineus (anulus of Zinn), previously described, serves as the origin of six of the seven extraocular muscles (see Fig. 12-4).

Superiorly, the superior rectus muscle arises from the anulus, which, at this point, is fused with the leptomeninges and dura of the optic nerve. The origin of the levator palpebrae is medial and superior to that of the superior rectus muscle. More medial and inferior to this are the origins of the medial rectus and superior oblique muscles. Although it is firmly fused to the optic nerve dorsally, the anulus of Zinn

The orbital cavity is drained principally by the superior and inferior ophthalmic veins. Both of these valveless channels have extensive anastomoses with each other as well as with external tributaries. The superior ophthalmic vein passes through the superior orbital fissure to drain into the cavernous sinus. The inferior ophthalmic vein, which primarily drains a network of channels on the medial wall and floor of the orbit, divides; one branch drains the pterygoid plexus through the inferior orbital fissure, and the other joins the superior ophthalmic vein before it enters the superior orbital fissure. These extensive communications between the pterygoid plexus and the angular and deep facial veins accommodate minor alterations in venous drainage; however, occlusion of the superior ophthalmic vein may result in severe orbital venous congestion, chemosis, and proptosis.

Orbital Nerves

When the orbit is unroofed from above, the frontalis nerve usually is visible through the thin periorbita. Once the periorbita is opened, the surgeon finds the frontalis nerve overlying the levator and superior rectus muscles. In the same plane but closer to the apex lies the fine trochlear nerve. The trochlear nerve, the frontalis branch of the fifth nerve, and its lacrimal branch pass through the superior orbital fissure in that order and lie within the periorbita but over the extraocular muscles (Fig. 12-5).

The remaining nerves traversing the superior orbital fissure enter the orbit and the muscle cone through the so-called oculomotor foramen between the two heads of the lateral rectus muscle in the following order: the superior

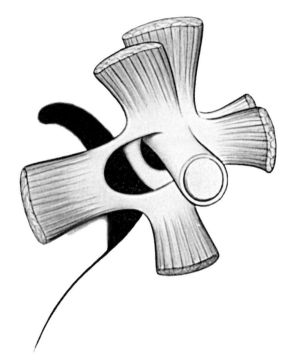

FIGURE 12-4 The anulus of Zinn is a fibrous band giving rise to the origins of six of the seven extraocular muscles. This fibrous tissue is in continuity with the dural sheath of the optic nerve. The two heads of the lateral rectus loop around that portion of the superior orbital fissure known as the oculomotor foramen.

loops widely around the nerve, laterally and inferiorly, giving rise to the lateral rectus muscle, which has its origin from two heads; the inferior rectus derives its origin from the inferior head, and the space between the two heads of the lateral rectus muscle is known as the oculomotor foramen. Thus it is evident that this arrangement separates the portal of entry of the nerves, arteries, and veins into essentially three spaces: the optic foramen, the superior orbital fissure, and the oculomotor foramen.

Arterial Supply and Venous Drainage

The ophthalmic artery arises from the internal carotid artery at its emergence from the cavernous sinus, passes on the medial side of the anterior clinoid, and runs in a split layer of dura beneath the optic nerve as it enters the orbital cavity through the optic foramen.[12] On entering the orbit, it curves over the lateral margin of the optic nerve, gives off the central retinal branch, which perforates the dural sheath approximately 10 mm from the optic foramen, and then, within several millimeters, enters the nerve obliquely approximately 1.0 cm behind the globe. After giving off the central retinal branch, the ophthalmic artery crosses medially forward, giving off two long posterior ciliary arteries and six or eight short posterior ciliary arteries, and then anastomoses freely with the external carotid circulation. Two small branches of the ophthalmic artery supply the ocular muscles at their origin near the anulus.

Although obstruction of the central retinal artery results in loss of vision, obstruction of the ophthalmic artery may not if the arterial anastomoses are sufficient to preserve blood flow to the retina and choroidal circulation.

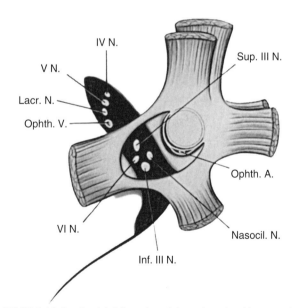

FIGURE 12-5 Partial obliteration of the subarachnoid space of the optic nerve at the anulus of Zinn is shown and the medial origin of the levator muscle is evident. The ophthalmic artery (Ophth. A.) enters the orbit through the optic canal. The trochlear (IV N.), frontalis (V N.), and lacrimal nerves (Lacr. N.) and the ophthalmic vein (Ophth. V.) enter through the superior orbital fissure and thus lie within the periorbita but outside the muscle cone, whereas the superior division of the oculomotor nerve (Sup. III N.), the abducens nerve (VI N.), nasociliary nerve (Nasocil. N.), and the inferior division of the oculomotor nerve (Inf. III N.) enter the muscle cone through the oculomotor foramen and lie within the muscle cone.

division of the oculomotor nerve, which supplies the superior rectus and levator muscles; the nasociliary branch of the ophthalmic nerve; the sixth nerve; and the inferior division of the third nerve. The nasociliary nerve crosses over the optic nerve to reach the medial wall of the orbit. The ciliary ganglion lies lateral to the optic nerve. The inferior division of the oculomotor nerve crosses beneath the optic nerve to reach the medial and inferior rectus muscles.

Because of this arrangement, it is clear that the optic nerve can be approached directly through the medial compartment, between the medial rectus and the levator muscles, without fear of injury to the nerve supply of any extraocular muscle (Fig. 12-6).

The trochlear nerve rarely can be spared. When optic nerve resection is the objective, however, there is little functional or cosmetic consequence of fourth nerve section.

Careful dissection through the lateral compartment, between the lateral and superior rectus and levator muscles, allows access to solitary neurofibromas, which most frequently arise from branches of the long ciliary nerves lying lateral to the optic nerve.

Tumors or mass lesions that arise external to the muscle cone are most likely to cause proptosis without limitation of extraocular movements or loss of vision. Some tumors within the muscle cone cause proptosis without causing neurologic or ophthalmologic deficits; however, tumors that crowd the apex are most likely to lead to dysfunction of one or more of the extraocular muscles or their nerve supply, causing specific deficits.

A clear understanding of orbital apical anatomy should help the surgeon approach the apical region safely and provides a basis for understanding the surgical limitations imposed by specific pathologic conditions.

DIAGNOSIS

When an orbital pathologic entity is suspected and, in particular, when unilateral exophthalmos exists, a logical sequential workup should follow the clinical examination.

Magnetic resonance imaging with fat suppression is now widely available and provides excellent definition of orbital pathology.[15–17] Fat suppression eliminates T1-associated bright signals, which can obscure intraorbital pathology. Gadolinium-enhanced magnetic resonance imaging is superior to CT for resolution of soft-tissue structures and is the best modality for demonstrating orbital apex lesions as well as the intracranial extension of gliomas and meningiomas.

CT has effectively supplanted the use of skull and orbital radiographs. Because of the contrast with orbital fat, CT is useful in defining orbital pathologic processes and is best used to image bony anatomy.[18] A well-performed study shows normal orbital anatomy, including the size and position of the globe, optic nerve, and extraocular muscles. The size and extent of a meningioma, optic glioma, or neurofibroma can be defined preoperatively. Most of these tumors enhance with contrast. CT scanning with bone windows offers the best definition of destructive or invasive pathology of the bony margins of the orbit and is also available with 3-dimensional reconstructions.

Orbital angiography has a limited place in defining vascular lesions in the orbit and is required with less frequency now that a combination of noninvasive studies is available. Angiography can be useful when highly vascular tumors are suspected or to identify tumors that might benefit from embolization.

CASE SELECTION

When a thoughtful sequential diagnostic workup has been completed, the location and extent of the pathologic process can be defined. Is a tumor present at all? If so, is it confined within the muscle cone? Does it arise from the optic nerve, or is it medial to or lateral to the optic nerve? Is the optic canal enlarged or hyperostotic? Is the bony integrity of the orbit violated? Are the fissures normal? Is the process erosive or destructive? Does the pathologic process extend to or from a sinus or arise from or enter the cranial cavity?

The clinical diagnosis of optic nerve glioma can be made with a high degree of accuracy. For optic nerve glioma confined to a single optic nerve, primary treatment is excision via the transcranial approach.[19] The ideal surgical candidate is a patient with a glioma of a single optic nerve who has disfiguring proptosis and poor vision in the involved eye. The rationale for the transcranial orbital approach is based on the conclusion that a wide excision, from the globe to the chiasm, is necessary to ensure total removal. A simple orbital resection too often leaves residual tumor in the apical stump of the transected, tumor-bearing nerve, thereby risking chiasmal extension.

Surgical indications are more complicated for tumors extending beyond a single nerve.[20,21] Surgical resection would not be considered for multicentric optic glioma, but exophytic chiasmal glioma should be excised. The decision

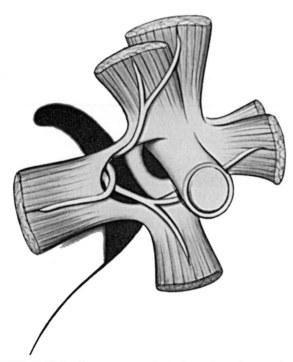

FIGURE 12-6 The nerve supply to the extraocular muscles is shown entering through the oculomotor foramen. A medial superior approach to the optic nerve between the lateral and medial rectus muscles provides direct access, with minimal chance of injury to this nerve supply to the extraocular muscles.

making for patients with chiasmal gliomas but intact vision is even less clear but probably should consider conservative management, at least as long as mass effect is not symptomatic. The role of radiotherapy is controversial; however, there is convincing evidence from our own large case series that astrocytoma of the optic nerve is a benign but often progressive process, similar to pilocytic astrocytoma of childhood in other locations. Our experience suggests that, in many cases, radiotherapy effectively arrests the course and improves proptosis and vision.[22]

The risks of radiation therapy to growth and maturation in infants and young children younger than the age of 5 years are more problematic. Initial treatment with chemotherapy, allowing for the deferral of radiotherapy in these cases, is recommended, although long-term results await further analysis.[20,23]

Primary meningiomas of the optic nerve most often produce visual impairment with minimal proptosis. When a meningioma of the optic nerve or orbit is responsible for nonfunctional vision, transcranial exploration is the preferred approach, although some studies advocate radiation as an initial treatment for these patients in an effort to preserve useful visual function for the longest length of time.[24,25] Meningiomas also frequently arise between the optic nerve and carotid artery and involve both the cranial and orbital cavities. The transcranial approach allows direct and safe access to the apical and intracanalicular part of the optic nerve.[17,26] Tumors occurring distal to the orbital apex and close to the globe may be explored by a direct approach.

Tumors involving the lateral periorbita from arachnoidal rests near the superior orbital fissure are frequently associated with multicentric or en plaque lesions on the cranial side of the superior orbital fissure. Pterional and skull base approaches are desirable in these circumstances, both for exposure and to facilitate radical resection of tumor and involved bone.

A microsurgical technique is essential for the successful removal of solitary neurofibromas, which usually are found lateral to the optic nerve. Although the transcranial approach provides better access to the most apical lesions, more anteriorly located lesions can also be accessed via lateral canthotomy (Krönlein's operation). In view of the relative difficulty in making this diagnosis clinically, the latter approach may be advantageous.

Osteomas and other bony lesions arising from the posterior ethmoid region can be defined and the transcranial approach selected for primary removal because of their medial epiperiorbital location. Reconstruction is important for these patients to prevent cerebrospinal fluid (CSF) leak and encephaloceles.

Obviously, encephaloceles must be treated by a neurosurgical approach, and some dermoid cysts and hemangiomas of the orbit also can be treated neurosurgically. Lesions such as ossifying fibromas and aneurysmal bone cysts that border both the orbit and the cranial cavity can be best approached transcranially.

The vast majority of problems arising within the orbit can be dealt with more simply by a direct approach, including the most common mucoceles and most hemangiomas and lymphangiomas. Similarly, malignant processes of the orbit may require extensive skull base approaches for en bloc resection and orbital exenteration. Finally, the surgeon dealing with proptosis must be aware of the very common nonsurgical causes, such as pseudotumor and thyrotoxicosis, which are generally diagnosed by preoperative noninvasive imaging.

Under some conditions in which clinical parameters have not firmly established the surgical indications and particularly when a lymphoid lesion is suspected, a fine needle aspiration biopsy can be useful for directing management decisions.[27] This technique is limited by sampling error and cytologic misinterpretation and can be complicated by orbital hemorrhage or globe perforation.

PREOPERATIVE MANAGEMENT AND ANESTHESIA

General anesthesia is used in all cases of transcranial orbital exploration. The principles of neuroanesthesia are adhered to, and there are no special anesthetic requirements for exploring the orbit. Dexamethasone is used as an intraoperative and postoperative adjunct to reduce postoperative edema. Mannitol is used intraoperatively to reduce intraocular tension as well as intracranial tension so that a suitable surgical field is obtained without unnecessary retraction. Placement of a lumbar spinal drain for CSF removal can be useful for brain relaxation.

AIDS TO SURGERY

Besides deserving credit for systematizing the preoperative workup in patients with orbital tumors, neurosurgery also can claim contributions to improved instrumentation and techniques for operating within the orbit. Maroon and Kennerdell[28] have described the advantages of neurosurgical techniques in an ophthalmologic lateral approach to the orbit. Magnification with a microscope is mandatory when operating on the fine and attenuated structures within the orbit. Similarly, cottonoids and controlled suction are indispensable, as is the use of malleable retractors. Bipolar coagulation has materially added to the safety of operating within the orbit by either the cranial or the direct orbital approach. The CO_2 and Nd-YAG lasers can be valuable adjuncts for tumor removal.[17] The CO_2 laser can be mounted on surgical microscope and targeted with a micromanipulator. The shallow depth of energy penetration facilitates vaporization of tumor tissue while sparing deeper normal anatomic structures.

Additionally, the routine use of stereotactic navigational systems in neurosurgery has extended to patients with orbital tumors. Preoperative volumetric magnetic resonance scans can be registered with a number of commercial stereotactic systems to facilitate navigation, operative approaches, localization of tumor, and verification of extent of resection.

OPERATIVE PROCEDURE[13,17,28,29]

It may not be necessary to include an orbital osteotomy along with a craniotomy to gain access to the apex of the orbit. It is most important, however, to plan a flap that is medial to allow a medial orbital approach to the optic nerve when dealing with primary tumors of the optic nerve. The frontotemporal approach, which is so useful for most invasive tumors of the lateral orbit, such as sphenoid wing meningiomas, does not provide sufficient medial exposure for surgery on optic nerve tumors.

Exposure

The patient is placed supine on the operating table and a Mayfield three-point headholder or a similar device is used to secure the head. The head is extended to allow the frontal lobe to fall away from the orbital roof. A bicoronal incision is made 1 to 2 cm behind the hairline extending from the tragus on the ipsilateral side to the superior temporal line on the contralateral side. A smaller incision extending to the midline can be used if the orbital rim is not going to be removed and if medial exposure is not needed. The incision is carried down to the pericranium, but the temporalis muscle and fascia are allowed to remain intact. It is preferable to leave the pericranium attached to the scalp to preserve its blood supply during the course of the operation. It can be easily dissected free and left attached to its vascularized pedicle at the end of the operation when it is needed for reconstruction. If the lateral orbital rim and zygoma are to be removed or exposed, the temporalis fascia should be brought forward with the scalp flap to ensure that the frontal branches of the seventh nerve are preserved. The scalp flap is brought forward far enough to expose the frontal bone so that the inferior portion of the craniotomy provides exposure of the floor of the anterior fossa. The extent of the craniotomy should be anticipated to decide whether the galeal dissection must extend to the orbital rim because it will be associated with considerable postoperative ecchymosis and swelling. In addition, there may be injury to the supraorbital vessels and nerve. However, if the supraorbital rim is to be removed, the scalp flap should be brought lower to expose the supraorbital rim so that the periorbital fascia, which is continuous with the pericranium, can be freed up from the orbital roof. This dissection must avoid damage to the supraorbital nerve as it exits through the supraorbital foramen. A fine osteotome or rongeur may be needed to unroof the foramen if the nerve is completely enclosed by bone.

After placement of a small burr hole in the posterolateral portion of the frontal bone, a craniotome is used to turn a craniotomy flap extending to the floor of the anterior fossa and just ipsilateral to the sagittal sinus (Fig. 12-7). A simple median frontal craniotomy is sufficient for the majority of the exposures that are required in the orbit.

For lesions extending beyond the orbit itself, modifications of the simple frontal craniotomy can be made depending on the required degree of exposure. If the orbital lesion extends anteriorly, the supraorbital rim may be removed. When removing the orbital rim, it is desirable to include as much of the orbital roof with it as possible to minimize the orbital defect to be repaired at the conclusion of the operation. This can be done by drilling an opening in the orbital roof and using an oscillating saw or Gigli saw threaded through the opening to make a cut through the orbital rim both medially and laterally. For cosmetic purposes, the width of the cut should be small so that a noticeable gap is not left when the rim is replaced at the end of the operation. Additionally, holes for titanium miniplates should be drilled before making the cut through the orbital rim to facilitate realignment of the rim at the time of closure. If the lesion extends laterally in the orbit or into the cavernous sinus or parasellar area through the optic foramen or superior orbital fissure, then a frontotemporal exposure

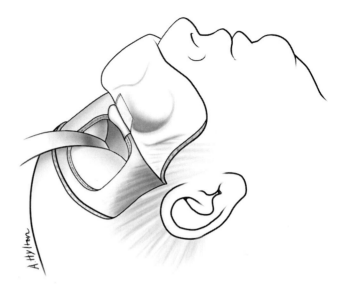

FIGURE 12-7   The coronal incision and low mediofrontal craniotomy flap is used in exposing the floor of the anterior fossa. Drainage of cerebrospinal fluid from a spinal drain before beginning the epidural approach to the orbital roof minimizes the need for frontal retraction.

is necessary. This is done by incising the temporalis muscle and reflecting it forward with the scalp flap to expose the inferior temporal area. The craniotomy should include the temporal bone and pterion. When the cavernous sinus is involved, the lateral wing of the sphenoid bone is drilled off, unroofing the optic foramen and superior orbital fissure and removing the anterior clinoid process.

If the lesion extends medially into the ethmoid sinus and a wide exposure is needed, an orbitoethmoidal osteotomy can be used by making cuts through the supraorbital rim, frontonasal suture, and the contralateral, medial orbital rim. The frontal craniotomy in this situation must extend across the midline, exposing the sagittal sinus. Although this opening invariably sacrifices the ipsilateral olfactory nerve, the contralateral olfactory nerve should be preserved if possible. When the olfactory nerve is cut at its sheath, the ensuing dural opening must be repaired primarily. To complete the orbitoethmoidal osteotomy, additional cuts are made through the cribriform plate and orbital roof. An osteotome is used to release the final attachment through the ethmoidal bone.

If the frontal sinus is opened with the craniotomy, as is often the case, the mucosa is exenterated and the sinus obliterated with either a fat graft from the patient's abdomen or with portions of pericranium, temporalis muscle, or temporalis fascia. At the end of the procedure, a flap of vascularized pericranium is brought over the frontal sinus defect and sutured to the dura, cordoning off the sinus.

After the craniotomy, the orbital roof is exposed extradurally with careful preservation of the dura to minimize the possibility of CSF leaks and infection. The frontal lobe is gently retracted extradurally, and the orbit is unroofed with a high-speed cutting drill. Depending on the location of the lesion, it may be necessary to drill out the optic foramen. In this situation, a diamond drill bit is used under copious irrigation to avoid heat injury to the nerve. Once the orbit is exposed, the lesion may be removed using microsurgical techniques.

If the orbit is being explored for optic glioma, it is advisable to open the dura and inspect the intracranial optic nerve before proceeding with the orbital unroofing. In so doing, the removal of CSF from the chiasmatic cistern aids in the development of an excellent operative field without the need for spinal drainage or excessive retraction. If the tumor is found to extend into the chiasm, indicating that gross total resection cannot be achieved, the procedure can be discontinued after a biopsy specimen is obtained. Once the tumor is identified within the nerve but not extending to the chiasm, the optic nerve is cut perpendicular to its direction at the chiasm. Hemostasis of the fine pial circulation is achieved with Surgicel or other hemostatic material. If the tumor is not seen in the intracranial space, the optic nerve should not be sectioned until pathology is identified within the orbit.

An extradural approach is desirable for orbital exploration because the underlying brain remains protected by the dura during gentle retraction. In addition, it protects the olfactory nerve and bulb from avulsion. Because the dura inserts at the cribriform fossa lateral to the olfactory nerve, epidural retraction avoids injury in this location. Malleable self-retaining retractors are shaped and curved to expose the entire anterior fossa up to the clinoid. Moist cottonoids are placed at the lateral margins of the exposure to advance the epidural dissection, allow irrigation, and facilitate suctioning.

The orbital unroofing is begun with a chisel or a high-speed burr. Once a small opening is made in the midportion of the floor of the anterior fossa, the remainder of the resection is facilitated by the use of fine, double-action mastoid or infant Leksell rongeurs (Fig. 12-8). The canal can be unroofed, if required, with a drill. The orbital unroofing does not need to come closer than 1 cm to the orbital rim anteriorly; it should extend approximately 1.5 cm from the medial margin and should be extended laterally to within 0.5 cm of the lateral orbital margin. This unroofing must be carried through the optic canal.

The periorbita is usually thin and transparent. When there is a significant orbital mass, the intraorbital structures are attenuated and blanched and may be difficult to see. The periorbita is incised in a cruciate fashion with a no. 11 blade. The vertical limb is placed lateral or medial to the levator and superior rectus muscles, depending on whether a lateral or medial approach to the orbit is planned. The frontalis nerve usually is visible through the periorbita because it lies over these muscles. It serves to approximate their location. The trochlear nerve lies beneath the periorbita but outside the muscle cone. It lies close to the apex, is extremely fine, and cannot be easily spared if the optic nerve is to be resected. There is, of course, no functional or cosmetic consequence to fourth nerve section in a blind eye.

Approach to the Medial Orbit

A medial approach to the optic nerve is preferred when dealing with meningioma or optic glioma (Fig. 12-9). The primary advantage of this approach relates to preservation of the nerve supply to extraocular muscles. The third (oculomotor) nerve, after it enters the orbit through the superior orbital fissure and oculomotor foramen lateral to the optic nerve, sends branches over the nerve to supply

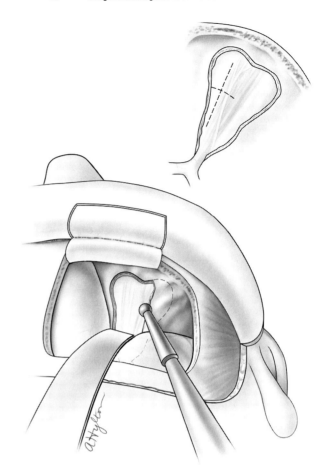

FIGURE 12-8 The thin orbital roof is entered with a chisel or burr. The extent of orbital unroofing is outlined. The unroofing is completed with fine double-action and Leksell rongeurs. The optic canal is opened as illustrated. The frontalis nerve can be seen through the thin periosteum and is a landmark indicating the course of the levator and superior rectus muscles, otherwise seen with difficulty. The dura is incised medial or lateral to these structures as indicated.

the underbelly of the levator and superior rectus muscles and beneath the nerve to the inferior and medial rectus muscles. A medial approach to the optic nerve thus can be made without traversing the course of these nerves to the extraocular muscles. Small malleable retractors are individually bent to retract the levator and superior rectus complex laterally and anteriorly. The tumor is approached by blunt dissection through residual orbital fat. Magnification and gentle handling of tissues are essential to this portion of the procedure. Both optic gliomas and primary optic nerve sheath meningiomas are fairly firm encapsulated tumors, and a plane of dissection is started directly on the tumor capsule. Gentle retraction and the placement of moist cottonoids allow the development of a plane entirely around the tumor capsule, which is not adherent to the surrounding residual areolar tissue. This tissue separates and protects the normal neurovascular structures, which thus can be spared during tumor removal.

The junction of the tumor and the posterior margin of the globe is readily found. At this point, the nerve is transected between two fine mosquito forceps, which are used to clamp the tumor-bearing optic nerve. Use of this technique avoids injury to the posterior margin of the globe

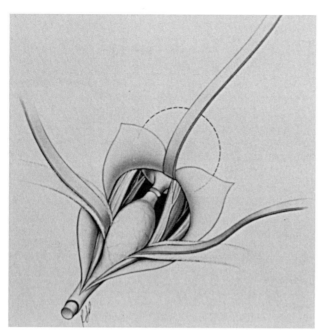

FIGURE 12-9   Narrow malleable retractors and cottonoid pledgets are used to retract gently the orbital structures. The preferred approach to the optic nerve is shown.

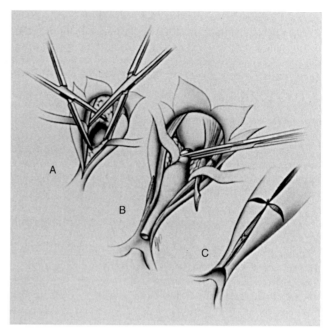

FIGURE 12-10   The technique of sectioning the levator. The anulus of Zinn cannot be opened without performing this maneuver. After resecting a tumor-bearing optic nerve from the globe to the chiasm, the origin of the levator muscle is resutured. This maneuver is useful in some cases of optic glioma and meningioma. (From Housepian EM, Marquardt MD, Behrens M: Orbital tumors. In Wilkins RH, Renganchary SS [eds]: Neurosurgery, vol 1. New York, McGraw-Hill, 1985.)

and the sclera. After the nerve is sectioned, the distal clamp is removed and any bleeding from the cut margin is carefully electrocoagulated with bipolar cautery. The proximal clamp can be used as a handle for further tumor dissection toward the apex.

In the case of optic nerve glioma, to remove the tumor in one piece from the globe to the chiasm (Fig. 12-10), the origin of the levator muscle, which inserts at the anulus of Zinn medial to the superior rectus, must be sectioned. Only in this way can the anulus of Zinn be opened from above to remove the canalicular portion of the optic nerve tethered at the orbital end of the canal. The origin of the levator muscle then can be resutured after the tumor is removed. This maneuver is difficult, and in young infants, the structures are small and the exposure limited, making the procedure more difficult. The optic nerve can be sectioned with curved scissors at the extreme apex and the orbital specimen removed. At this juncture, the ophthalmic artery is sometimes severed, but the bleeding can be controlled with bipolar electrocautery. The intracranial portion of the nerve then can be removed as a second specimen. To accomplish this, the epidural retractors must be removed and placed intradurally again, reexposing the intracranial optic nerve so that it can be pulled through the canal. If the surgeon believes that there may be a small amount of residual glioma at the canalicular face of the anulus, brief electrocoagulation on an angled nerve hook can be used safely and may limit recurrence. A small pledget of temporalis muscle placed within the canal will prevent the flow of CSF into the orbital space in the immediate postoperative period.

When dealing with a primary optic nerve sheath meningioma however, it is mandatory to unroof the optic canal, open the intracanalicular dura, section the origin of the levator at the anulus of Zinn, and open the anulus. This approach permits inspection at high magnification and gross total removal of the entire intracanalicular tumor with the optic nerve from the orbit close to the globe, back to the cranial end of the optic nerve near the chiasm. The anulus and levator origin should then be resutured with fine atraumatic silk or synthetic suture. Unlike the situation with optic nerve gliomas, electrocoagulation of residual meningioma at the orbital apex or in the canal is not an acceptable technique and will lead to recurrence.

There is ample histopathologic evidence of the primary intraorbital origin of optic nerve meningiomas. Cushing and Eisenhardt[1] described a psammomatous meningioma arising at Schwann's sheath and growing into the optic nerve. Although it is not clearly defined, it may represent the origin of some nerve sheath meningiomas. These tumors have been shown to traverse the optic canal by microscopic spread along the subarachnoid space or within the nerve, without producing enlargement or hyperostosis of the optic canal.

Lateral Orbital Approach

The transcranial orbital approach to the lateral superior quadrant of the orbit can be used for some cases of suspected solitary neurofibroma believed to arise from the long ciliary nerves. They are thus found in a position lateral to the optic nerve. In these cases, the periorbital opening is made lateral to the superior rectus insertion (Fig. 12-11), and, using the techniques described for orbital exploration with malleable retractors and cottonoids, a plane is developed directly on the tumor capsule. Efforts are made to separate the loose areolar tissue from the tumor itself and minimize dissection within this tissue. To achieve exposure of the lateral quadrant,

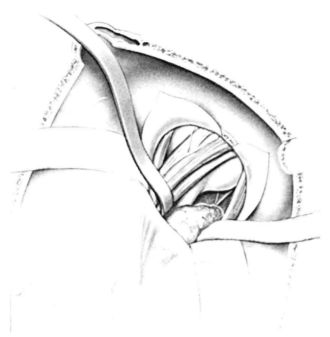

FIGURE 12-11 The lateral transcranial orbital approach to an apical neurofibroma. Dissection in the areolar tissue is avoided, and cottonoid pledgets and narrow, shaped, malleable retractors are used to define a plane directly on the tumor capsule. Injury to the extraocular nerve supply is avoided in this way.

the superior rectus muscle is retracted medially. If the tumor is large, it can be broken into several pieces for removal. Efforts should be made to avoid the extreme apex in the lateral approach to minimize the chance of injury to the third and sixth cranial nerves.

The Berke modification of Krönlein's operation may provide good access to pathologic processes in the lateral quadrant of the orbit.[6] The application of neurosurgical techniques, as described by Maroon and Kennerdell,[28] and adherence to strict microsurgical technique should allow safe access to the lateral apex and minimize the possibility of injury to the sixth nerve. This approach is not recommended for primary optic nerve tumors, however, because of the anatomic configuration of the nerve supply to the extraocular muscles, as described previously.

Closure and Reconstruction

Once removal of the tumor is complete and before retraction is released, cottonoids are carefully removed and the apical bed is inspected for hemostasis. Bipolar electrocoagulation should be used sparingly to achieve this. Extensive electrocauterization behind the globe should be avoided because it can injure the retinal blood supply as well as the autonomic nerves and result in pupillary dilatation and corneal anesthesia. When the field is dry, all retractors and cottonoids are removed, the origin of the levator resutured, if it has been sectioned, and the periorbita closed loosely by approximating the four corners.

With small orbital roof defects, the vascularized pericranium flap is usually sufficient to provide support and no further reconstruction is needed. If the orbital defect is large, reconstruction is needed to avoid enophthalmos or

pulsating exophthalmos. We generally prefer to reconstruct the orbital defect with a piece of bone from the inner table of the craniotomy flap plated to the orbital rim (Fig. 12-12). Although defects may be repaired with titanium mesh, autologous bone is generally preferred because there is decreased risk of infection and less interference with postoperative radiographic imagining.

If the ethmoid sinus is entered during the exposure, it must be covered with vascularized tissue. A pericranium flap is most convenient for this purpose and should be developed and separated from the scalp while preserving its blood supply anteriorly. If the olfactory nerve has been sacrificed, the pericranium should be sutured back behind the area of the closure of dural sleeve, completely covering it. If the dura has been torn or has been purposely opened to remove an intradural lesion, a watertight dural repair is needed to prevent CSF leakage. If the dural opening is small, this can be accomplished primarily, but a larger opening must be covered with a patch taken from either the pericranium or temporalis fascia.

The craniotomy flap is secured with titanium miniplates. The orbital rim is replaced first and is secured with plates or wire. The galea and skin are closed as separate layers. A subgaleal Hemovac is placed and brought out through a separate stab incision to remain in place for 24 hours. A snug head wrap will discourage the accumulation of any subcutaneous or subgaleal fluid collection. If the spinal drain has been used, it is removed immediately unless there has been a significant

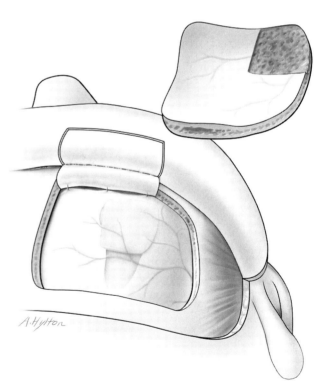

FIGURE 12-12 On completion of tumor removal, the periorbita is closed with one or several fine atraumatic sutures. A bridge formed from a split thickness of bone taken from the craniotomy flap is placed at the orbital roof defect to avoid postoperative pulsation of the globe. Dural tenting sutures are then placed, and any defect in the frontal sinus repaired and a flap of pericranium sutured to the dura to cover the bony defect.

dural repair with potential for CSF leakage postoperatively. Depending on the completeness of the dural closure, the drain may be left on continuous drainage (5–10 mL/hr) for as long as 5 days to allow the leaks to seal.

Tarsorrhaphy

Before extubation and after the head dressing has been applied, temporary tarsorrhaphy should be performed in all cases of orbital exploration when optic nerve function has been sacrificed. In other cases, the lids are not closed to allow monitoring of vision. The procedure is simple and atraumatic (Fig. 12-13). The lids are washed with a cotton ball, and the cornea and conjunctiva are irrigated with saline. Sterile towels are placed to keep the sutures sterile. A double-ended 6-0 suture is used to place a horizontal mattress with two rubber band bumper guards. The thin skin of the lid is protected with the bumpers and makes removal of the tarsorrhaphy simple. In principle, the suture should pass through the tarsal plate posterior to the anterior extension of the orbicularis muscle (gray line) of both lids. Care should be taken to see that there are no inverted lashes before the suture is tied. When the tarsorrhaphy is completed, an ophthalmic ointment is used to lubricate the cornea and conjunctiva. A pledget of nonstick gauze is placed over the eye; fluffy cotton balls then are used to gently diffuse the pressure when taped to the head dressing. It is important

for the surgeon to remove the tarsorrhaphy dressing daily to inspect the eye for signs of irritation and to reapply ophthalmic ointment. The tarsorrhaphy is left in place until the peak edema period has passed. It is advisable to remove the pressure dressing 1 day before the tarsorrhaphy suture is removed. In this way, if pressure has been removed prematurely and the eye begins to bulge, the cornea will be protected.

POSTOPERATIVE CARE

Intraoperative antibiotics are used routinely and dexamethasone is administered in high doses through the fourth postoperative day and then tapered over the ensuing week. With care in hemostasis, blood transfusion should not be required. Anticonvulsant therapy can be used, although there is usually little retraction injury to the orbital brain surface.

Complications

Transcranial exploration should be a relatively benign procedure. There is, however, transient palsy of the levator and superior rectus muscles in all cases. This may be complete or partial. Improvement is usually seen from within several days to 3 to 6 weeks, and recovery is complete by 3 months. Ptosis and limitation of extraocular movement can, however, be a permanent accompaniment to the removal of orbital tumors by any approach. Blindness may occur in any orbital exploration, even when the optic nerve is preserved. Postoperative keratitis is an infrequent but recognized complication. Seizures are rarely seen in the postoperative period. Recurrence of glioma within the orbit occurred in only one case. In this instance, tumor was seeded by earlier Krönlein's operation.

SUMMARY

The diagnostic techniques that are currently available have vastly improved the ability to predict the nature, precise location, and extent of tumors of the orbit. Familiarity with the variety of diseases that occur in the orbit and that can produce proptosis is essential for the neurosurgeon involved in the management of patients with orbital disease. A clear understanding of the regional anatomy will allow the surgeon to plan his or her surgical approach based on rational surgical objectives. The availability of a multidisciplinary team composed of surgeons experienced in ophthalmology and neurosurgery provides the best opportunity for successful management of these tumors.

REFERENCES

1. Cushing H, Eisenhardt L: Meningiomas. Springfield, IL: Charles C Thomas, 1938.
2. Matson D: Unilateral exophthalmos in childhood. Clin Neurosurg 5:116, 1958.
3. Van Buren J, Poppen J, Horrax G: Unilateral exophthalmos: A consideration of symptom pathogenesis. Brain 80:139, 1957.
4. Love J, Benedict W: Transcranial removal of intraorbital tumors. JAMA 121:777, 1945.
5. Dandy W: Results following transcranial attack on orbital tumors. Arch Ophthalmol 25:191, 1941.
6. Berke RN: A modified Krönlein operation. Trans Am Acad Ophthalmol Otolaryngol 51:193–231, 1953.

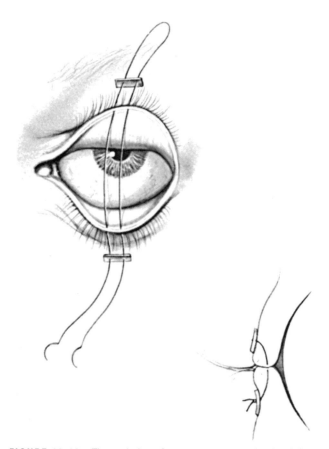

FIGURE 12-13 The technique for temporary tarsorrhaphy. A fine double-ended atraumatic suture is placed through the tarsal plate of each lid. Small rubber bumpers prevent maceration of the thin skin of the lid.

7. Davis F: Primary tumors of the optic nerves. Arch Ophthalmol 23:735, 1940.
8. Jackson H: Orbital tumors. Proc Soc Med 38:587, 1945.
9. Reese AB: Expanding lesions of the orbit. Trans Ophthalmol Soc U K 91:85–104, 1971.
10. Spencer W: Primary neoplasms of the optic nerve and its sheaths: Clinical features and current concepted pathogenetic mechanisms. J Am Ophthalmol Soc 70:490, 1972.
11. Zide B, Jelks G: Surgical Anatomy of the Orbit. New York: Raven Press, 1985.
12. Rhoton AL Jr: The orbit. Neurosurgery 51(4 Suppl):S303–S334, 2002.
13. Natori Y, Rhoton AL Jr: Transcranial approach to the orbit: Microsurgical anatomy. J Neurosurg 81:18–86, 1994.
14. Housepian EM: Microsurgical anatomy of the orbital apex and principles of transcranial orbital exploration. Clin Neurosurg 25:556–573, 1978.
15. Bilaniuk LT, Schenck JF, Zimmerman RA, et al: Ocular and orbital lesions: Surface coil MR imaging. Radiology 156:669–674, 1985.
16. Haik BG, Saint Louis L, Bierly J, et al: Magnetic resonance imaging in the evaluation of optic nerve gliomas. Ophthalmology 94:709–717, 1987.
17. Kazim M, Bruce J: Neurogenic tumors. In Bosniak S (ed): Ophthalmic Plastic and Reconstructive Surgery. Philadelphia: WB Saunders, 1996, pp 983–993.
18. Jakobiec FA, Depot MJ, Kennerdell JS, et al: Combined clinical and computed tomographic diagnosis of orbital glioma and meningioma. Ophthalmology 91:137–155, 1984.
19. Housepian EM: Surgical treatment of unilateral optic nerve gliomas. J Neurosurg 31:604–607, 1969.
20. Alshail E, Rutka JT, Becker LE, Hoffman HJ: Optic chiasmatic-hypothalamic glioma. Brain Pathol 7:799–806, 1997.
21. Astrup J: Natural history and clinical management of optic pathway glioma. Br J Neurosurg 17:327–333, 2003.
22. Housepian EM, Bruce JN, Habif D: Current concepts in the diagnosis and treatment of optic gliomas. Contemp Neurosurg 14:1–6, 1992.
23. Kato T, Sawamura Y, Tada M, et al: Cisplatin/vincristine chemotherapy for hypothalamic/visual pathway astrocytomas in young children. J Neurooncol 37:263–270, 1998.
24. Saeed P, Rootman J, Nugent RA, et al: Optic nerve sheath meningiomas. Ophthalmology 110:2019–2030, 2003.
25. Turbin RE, Thompson CR, Kennerdell JS, et al: A long-term visual outcome comparison in patients with optic nerve sheath meningioma managed with observation, surgery, radiotherapy, or surgery and radiotherapy. Ophthalmology 109:890–900, 2002.
26. Margalit NS, Lesser JB, Moche J, Sen C: Meningiomas involving the optic nerve: technical aspects and outcomes for a series of 50 patients. Neurosurgery 53:523–533, 2003.
27. Kennerdell JS, Dekker A, Johnson BL, Dubois PJ: Fine-needle aspiration biopsy. Its use in orbital tumors. Arch Ophthalmol 97:1315–1317, 1979.
28. Maroon JC, Kennerdell JS: Surgical approaches to the orbit. Indications and techniques. J Neurosurg 60:1226–1235, 1984.
29. Jane JA, Park TS, Pobereskin LH, et al: The supraorbital approach: Technical note. Neurosurgery 11:537–542, 1982.

Section IV

Anterior Skull Base

13

Transbasal Approach to Tumors Invading the Skull Base

ANDRÉ VISOT, ANNE BOULIN, PHILIPPE PENCALET, and
STEPHAN GAILLARD

For many years, the total removal of tumors invading the middle area of the skull base was considered impossible, because they were considered inaccessible by most surgical teams. Exploratory surgery successively approached these cases through narrow exposures, and tumor removal was often incomplete. The transbasal approach to the anterior skull base was first applied for the correction of craniofacial malformations such as hypertelorism or craniofacial dysostosis.[1] It was then adapted for the surgical removal of basal tumors. Several modifications have subsequently been proposed with effective results.[2–4] However depending on the extension and invasion of these basal tumors, their surgical removal can still present a true challenge.

GOALS WITH THE TRANSBASAL APPROACH

The primary goal with the transbasal approach is complete removal of the tumor. Some basal tumors are located at the middle, but most extend laterally toward the orbital walls, the lesser and greater sphenoid wings, and the middle fossa. The second goal is to free the cranial nerves and to open the optic foramens, the sphenoidal fissures, and even the foramen rotundum and foramen ovale areas that cannot be reached through narrow anterior approaches. If it is necessary to expose the anterior and possibly the middle fossae, an anterior subdural and extradural approach is required. Anosmia, which often is present before the procedure, is the only side effect. Procedures that conserve structures of the cribriform area and the olfactory placode have been described, but their use depends on the tumor's origin.[5]

HAZARDS OF THE TRANSBASAL APPROACH

The most important complication of the transbasal approach is the creation of a communication between the subarachnoid spaces and the upper air-filled cavities of the face (Fig. 13-1). The resection of an ethmoidosphenoidal tumor widely opens the frontal and the sphenoid sinuses and the ethmoid air cells. The floor of the nasal fossa and the pharyngeal or cavum mucosa can be reached through the cranial approach. Meningeal tears and dural defects occur frequently, resulting in pneumatocele, cerebrospinal fluid (CSF) leak, ascending infection, and meningitis.

The three structures between the intradural spaces and the air-filled cavities of the face are the dura, the bone involved by the tumor, and the rhinopharyngeal mucosal plane. After tumor removal, these structures must be repaired

carefully to prevent complications. The dura must be closed tightly (which may require a pericranial graft), and the base of the skull must be reconstructed to eliminate a dead space that can lead to meningocele or encephalocele, postoperative extradural hematomas, or postoperative infections (Fig. 13-2).[6] The mucosal plane must be preserved or

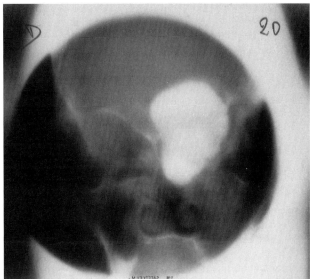

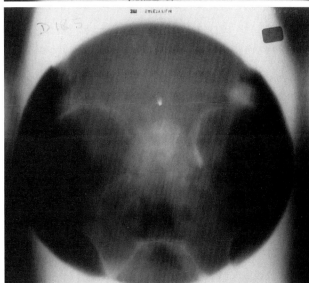

FIGURE 13-1 Resection of the ethmoidal osteoma will lead to the wide opening of the upper air cavities of the face. Preoperative (*top*) and postoperative (*bottom*) aspects.

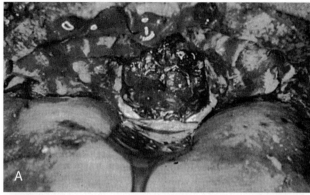

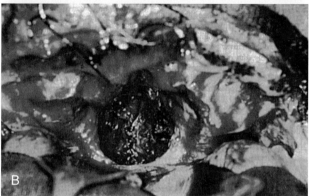

FIGURE 13-2 *A,* Intraoperative view of an ethmoidosphenoidal chordoma responsible for extradural compression of both optic nerves. The orbital roofs are partially removed. *B,* After the tumor has been removed, a large dead space extends to the nasal fossae and the deeper aspects of pharyngeal mucosae. Note the free optic nerves.

reconstructed for the closure of the nasal fossa. Living tissue is necessary to feed the bone grafts used for the repair of the skull base. When these rules are strictly applied, the transbasal approach remains a benign and effective procedure.

The preoperative imaging includes computed tomography (CT) scan and magnetic resonance imaging (MRI) without and with injection. These two neuroradiologic examinations give additional information: CT scan, especially in axial and coronal slices and with osseous windows, can provide the best study of the skull base. Three-dimensional bone reconstruction may be useful. MRI is much more helpful for analysis of the brain, optic nerve, and nonosseous adjacent structures. Angio MRI gives information on the vascular structures and the vascular supply.

In some cases, these studies can be preparatory for conventional angiogram and embolization of feeding arteries with microparticles or glue (Fig. 13-3). This preoperative imaging is equally important for comparison with subsequent postoperative imaging studies to detect residual or recurrent pathology.[7]

SURGICAL TECHNIQUES

Preparation

Preoperative autotransfusion is used routinely in the month before surgery. Prophylactic antibiotic therapy is strongly recommended and is started with anesthesia induction and continued for 24 hours.

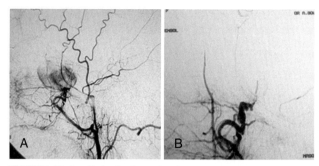

FIGURE 13-3 Embolization of a basal meningioma (*A*) preoperative and (*B*) postoperative aspects.

The patient is placed in the dorsal decubitus position with the head in a three-point headrest. In some cases the patient's head is not kept in a fixed position, so that the head can be repositioned during surgery. The operating microscope should be used near the neurovascular structures or around the cranial nerves, particularly the optic nerves.

Because the frontal lobe must be retracted to expose the base of the skull, mannitol and continuous intraoperative lumbar drainage are used routinely. Because the procedure may be a very long one, the anesthesiologist must keep the patient is normothermic status. Blood losses are carefully replaced, and strict hemostasis is applied at each step.

Mucosal Plane

Preserving the mucosal plane is always difficult. With a surgical approach from above, the sinus mucosa is dissected at the end of the procedure after tumor removal. Depending on the kind of tumor, the mucosa may be involved by the disease. In noninvasive tumors, the sinus mucosa is usually preserved, but this plane disappears in the ethmoidal area where the nasal fossae are widely opened and the turbinates visible. The best solution for closure of this area is a large anterior pericranial flap prepared at the beginning of the surgical procedure. This flap is cut along the temporal crests, as far as necessary, and turned anteriorly (Fig. 13-4); its supraorbital vascularization is preserved. At the end of the procedure, it is turned down to close the nasal fossae and the basal defect, and its posterior edge is affixed to the

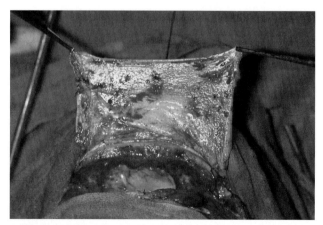

FIGURE 13-4 A large anterior pericranial flap is raised at the beginning of the operation; it will close the basal defect and may be considered a "new mucosal plane."

farthest limits of the subfrontal dura. A bone graft is inserted in the basal defect, and its posterior edge is sutured to the farthest limits of the subfrontal dura. Insertion of a bone graft in the basal defect is often sufficient to ensure a perfect closure without a posterior fixation of this "new mucosal plane".[8,9]

Exposing the Skull Base

A bicoronal incision is made just behind the hairline. The scalp is turned forward, taking care not to injure the frontotemporal branch of the facial nerve. The pericranial incision follows both temporal crests laterally to reach or overlap the coronal sutures, preserving a large anterior pericranial flap, which is curved upward. If more lateral exposure is necessary, the temporalis muscle is dissected from the temporal fossa and retromalar area to the zygomatic arch. A bifrontal free bone flap is lifted up with a supraorbital inferior margin, without attention to the size of frontal sinuses. If these sinuses are wide, their posterior walls and mucosae are removed, and their ostia are closed with bone grafts. After the subfrontal dura is dissected, the anterior fossa is exposed. This dissection is fairly easy, except for the area of both olfactory grooves. Sometimes it is possible to avoid meningeal tears by doing a primary resection of the crista galli and cutting the olfactory nerves one by one. The dissection must reach the posterior limits of the anterior fossa, the posterior edge of the lesser sphenoid wings, the tuberculum sellae, and the base of the anterior clinoid processes. A partially invaded dura or a tumor growing through the meninges into the intradural spaces may cause some problems. The subfrontal and intracerebral parts of the tumor are removed through a classic intradural approach before the subfrontal dura around the basal insertion of the tumor is dissected.

Meningeal Repair

After exposure of the base, the dura is closed before the base is resected and the upper air-filled cavities are opened. There are three possible repair situations:

1. The dura is preserved, but there are a few meningeal tears in the area of the olfactory grooves. The tears can be sutured with tiny sutures, but strengthening the dura at the middle with another material is advisable (Fig. 13-5).
2. There is a true dural defect, which must be closed with a dural substitute more than twice the size of the defect. This substitute is sutured to the dura at the farthest margins of the anterior fossa.
3. The defect is exceptionally large, and the posterior dura has totally disappeared in front of the optochiasmatic cistern; in this case, it is impossible to suture the dural substitute posteriorly. This often occurs in tumors invading the posterior aspect of the anterior base up to the tuberculum sellae. In such cases, the graft is sutured only laterally and folded like a leaf of a book on the posterior third of the skull base. A few weeks or months later, the subfrontal dura will be totally reconstituted, and a new extradural transbasal approach will allow the removal of the invaded base and the tumor invading the nasal fossae without any intraoperative CSF leak.

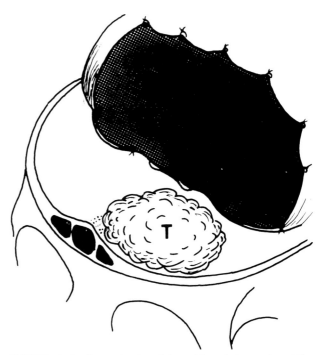

FIGURE 13-5 Strengthening of the subfrontal dura at the midline with a pericranial graft. T, tumor.

The choice of the material for the dura substitute depends on many variables. The material must be thick enough to prevent leaks and ascending infection, it must be supple enough to permit brain reexpansion, and it must revascularize rapidly for quick adherence and to feed the bone grafts used to reconstruct the skull base. A pericranial autograft is preferred to prosthetic materials or fascia lata. This kind of pericranial graft is routinely used in almost all cases.

A pericranial autograft has the same properties as periosteum. For a thicker graft and to preserve the anterior pericranium (covering the bifrontal free flap at the end of the procedure), the graft should be taken from the biparietal area through the same scalp incision. If necessary, the sample can be as large as the entire subfrontal dura. Its periostic aspect is placed toward the basal reconstruction.

The following steps in the removal of a tumor invading the anterior skull base and developed intracranially and extracranially depend on the quality of the dural repair. Two-step operations are strongly recommended when a watertight repair of the subfrontal dura is not obtained after intracranial tumor removal. A 2- or 3-month waiting period is necessary to ensure the watertight closure of the dura. During this waiting period, a piece of inert material (Silastic) is inserted between the base and the pericranial graft (Fig. 13-6); it protects the grafts against hypothetical tumor invasion and makes the second extradural approach easier, at which time the tumor is removed.

Such a pericranial graft may also be used to close a clival dural defect (Fig. 13-7).

Removal of the Basal Tumor

The difficulties in removing a basal tumor depend on the location, extension, and consistency of the tumor.

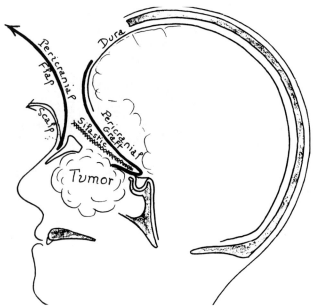

FIGURE 13-6 Two-step operation. During the waiting time, a piece of inert material is inserted between the pericranial graft and skull base, repairing the subfrontal dura and the remaining basal tumor (multiple crosses).

All kinds of rongeurs and drills can be used to remove the involved bone.

Tumors in the ethmoid area can be easily removed, because there are no structures that can be injured. The nasal fossae are quickly reached, where the turbinates and septal mucosae are identified and preserved if they are not invaded by tumor.

In the sphenoidal area, the first step is to identify both optic nerves. Partial resection of the orbital roofs is the first step after the periorbit has been separated through an orbital approach. When the supraorbital foramens are closed, resection of their lower rims helps to preserve the supraorbital

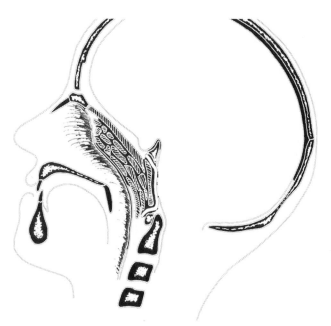

FIGURE 13-7 Repair of a clival dural defect. The graft is applied to the bone reconstruction.

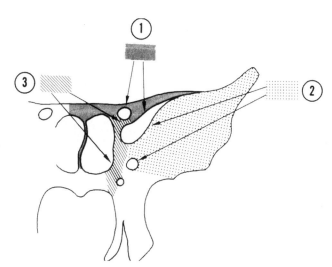

FIGURE 13-8 (1) Vertical attack, (2) medial attack, and (3) lateral attack of the optical canal.

vessels and nerves. The optic canals are then opened, and the extradural part of the optic nerves is identified. A first gross extradural debulking is realized between the optic nerves. After intratumoral resection, the margins of both orbits and the entire body of the sphenoid are then resected, if necessary, down the pharyngeal and sinus mucosae. The medial rim of the sphenoidal fissure can be opened from the midline (Fig. 13-8), and the foramen rotundum and the vidian canal in the root of the pterygoid can be reached.

Laterally, if the tumor involves the lesser and greater wings of the sphenoid, resection of the orbital roof is extended to the temporal dura so that the lesser wing and the upper margin of the sphenoidal fissure disappear. Working between the sphenoidal fissure and the optic foramen, the anterior clinoid process in progressively removed.

This resection must be done very carefully because of the proximity of the internal carotid artery and the insertion of the small circumference of the tentorium just below the dura. Resection of the greater wing, between the periorbit and the temporal dura, is now easy and opens the inferior margin of the sphenoidal fissure, leading toward the floor of the middle fossa, the foramen rotundum, and the foramen ovale (see Fig. 13-8). At the end of this procedure, all upper cranial nerves are free. Posteriorly on the midline, it is possible to reach the clivus after the tuberculum sellar area and the vertical part of the sella floor have been removed. Some bleeding may occur in this area, because the dura of the sella is usually vascularized. Proceeding downward, the clivus is removed and the clival dura dissected to the anterior margin of the foramen magnum, which is opened. If dissection of the pharyngeal mucosa follows, the precervical space, the anterior arch of the atlas, and even the bodies of C2 and C3 can be reached (Fig. 13-9). After the wide dissection, the base of the skull looks very different: the bony tissue has disappeared and the soft tissues of the orbits are attached only to the frontal and temporal dura by the optic nerves and sphenoidal fissures, and between them there is a large dead space bounded by the rhinopharyngeal mucosae. The extent of the basal resection depends on the kind of tumor.

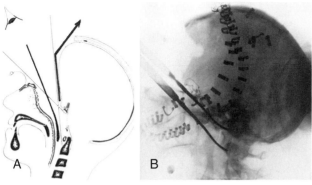

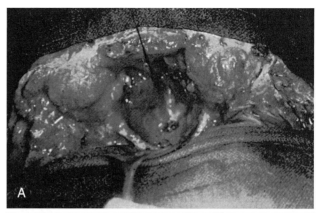

FIGURE 13-9 *A,* Through the transbasal approach, it is possible to reach the clivus, the anterior arch of the atlas, and the bodies of C1 and C2. Notice the preservation of the pharyngeal mucosae. *B,* An intraoperative radiogram. The tips of the instruments are located at the anterior margin of the foramen magnum and the body of C2.

Repair of the Skull Base

Repair of the skull base is not necessary if the basal defect is relatively small. However, reconstruction of the bony plane prevents the risk of CSF leak; it protects the intracranial structures during transfacial or ear-nose-throat operations if necessary. The repair of the skull base must definitely be performed in three situations: a large medial dead space, a large lateral orbital removal (thereby avoiding enophthalmos and pulsation of the eyeball), and an extension of the resection toward the orbitofrontal rim, the supraorbital margins, and the frontal area (for cosmetic reasons).

Autogenous bone is the best material for closure when the air-filled cavities of the face have been widely opened. Grafts can be taken from the iliac bone, where it is possible to obtain a large specimen in one procedure. The iliac graft has the additional advantage that it provides cancellous rather than cortical bone. Grafts taken from the vault, using the inner table of the bone flap (or extracted posteriorly if the bifrontal flap is involved by disease) are increasingly being used. Bone dust is also an excellent material that may be harvested with partial-thickness burr holes behind the posterior margin of the bifrontal free flap.

When the whole anterior fossa has been resected medially and laterally, after the medial walls and the roofs of the orbits have been repaired with two single grafts or one modeled graft, the dead space should be packed with cancellous bone. A cortical graft can be used to close the ethmoidosphenoidal area. It should be implanted between the nasion and the clivus, beneath the horizontal portion of the sellar floor. If the clivus has also been removed, the graft should be applied as a near-vertical graft, fitted between the floor of the sella and the anterior margin of the foramen magnum or the anterior arch of the atlas. The optic nerve must remain completely free. At the end, bone dust should be packed intracranially to provide a tight a closure (Fig. 13-10). Such reconstruction is required after resection of bone lesions, particularly in extensive fibrous dysplasia. Commonly, however, the basal repair is much easier; a bone graft is fitted in the basal defect, above the pericranial flap and closing the nasal fossae (Fig. 13-11), after which bone dust is packed to suppress the dead space below the pericranial graft reconstructing the subfrontal dura.

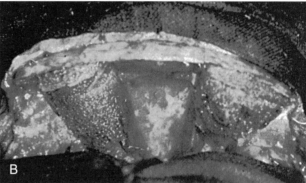

FIGURE 13-10 *A,* Extensive removal and basal reconstruction in a case of fibrous dysplasia. Intraoperative view of the removal of the entire anterior fossa. The upper orbital margins, roofs, and medial walls; the ethmoid; the body and lesser wings of the sphenoid; and the anterior clinoid processes have all been resected. Medially, this resection leads to the nasal fossae and pharyngeal mucosae. Both optic nerves are totally free, and the sphenoidal fissures are opened. *B,* Intraoperative view of the reconstruction. Both upper orbital margins have been repaired with a single wired split rib graft. Note the large medial graft between the reconstruction of both orbits.

Closure

The bifrontal free flap is replaced using dural suspensions and cranioplasty of the burr holes. If the tumor has also invaded a part of the flap, the pathologically involved bone must be resected and a cranioplasty performed at the same stage. A bone autograft is preferred to prosthetic material (the possible need for such reconstruction must be anticipated when grafts are being obtained).

If not used for closure of the nasal fossae and repair of the mucosal plane (two-step operations), the anterior pericranial flap is turned down to cover the bifrontal free flap. Two drains are placed before the scalp is sutured: one extradurally in the subfrontal area and the other in the parietal area where the pericranial graft was extracted.

LIMITATIONS OF THE TRANSBASAL APPROACH AND COMBINED APPROACHES

First described for basal osteotomies in craniofacial malformations, the subfrontal approach was successfully applied for the removal of bony lesions or extracranial/intracranial tumors destroying or invading the anterior skull base. Two aspects of this pathologic process must be considered: the

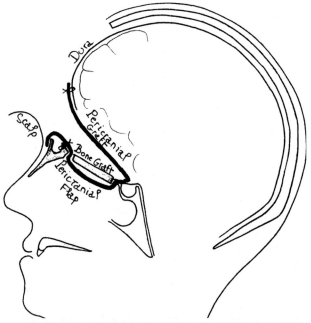

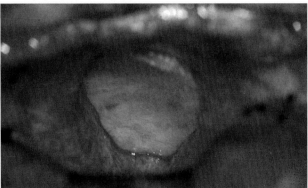

FIGURE 13-11 Basal repair. A bone graft is fitted into the defect above the pericranial flap, which is also used for the closure of the frontal sinuses.

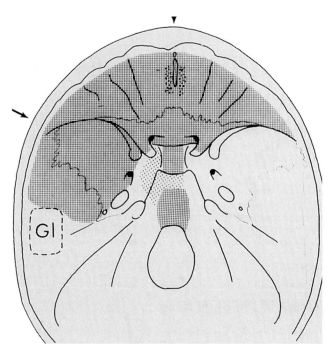

FIGURE 13-12 Limits of basal resection through the transbasal approach.

possibilities for resection of bone and the tumoral limits that can be reached. Bone resection does not present problems. The entire anterior fossa and the largest part of the middle fossa can be resected. It is possible to free vessels and nerves that enter through the optic canals, the sphenoidal fissures, the foramen rotundum, and the foramen ovale (Fig. 13-12). The posterior limit is the petrous bone, which can be reached through a posterolateral approach. Resection of a pathologic anterior and middle basal tumor involving the greater sphenoidal wing preserves all upper cranial nerves except for the olfactory tracts.

Problems arise when the adjacent soft tissues are involved. In the orbital area, the transbasal approach provides an excellent exposure. The anterior and inferomedial aspects of the cavernous sinus may be reached extradurally, but, except for a few encapsulated lesions, its involvement is one of the limitations of the single transbasal approach. Inferiorly, the removal of a medial tumor extends laterally to the maxillary sinuses. Posteriorly, the possibilities for removing the clivus through different anterior approaches are summarized in Figure 13-13: the transcervical[10] and transoral approaches provide access only to its lower half; the

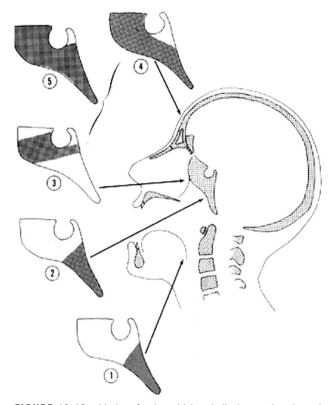

FIGURE 13-13 Limits of sphenoidal and clival resection through anterior approaches: (1) Transcervical approach, (2) transoral approach, (3) rhinoseptal approach, (4) transbasal approach, (5) combination of transbasal and rhinoseptal approaches.

rhinoseptal route is convenient for gaining access to the sella and the upper half of the clivus on the midline, but this approach remains narrow and lateral structures are not visible. The transbasal approach allows an extended resection of the clivus except below the sella. Therefore, depending on the location and main extension of the tumor, the transbasal approach can be modified or combined with another surgical approach.

Many modifications have been proposed to enlarge the posterior visual field and decrease the frontal brain retraction; all these approaches enlarge the bony resection or osteotomies toward the middle face and orbits.[2,3,11] Depending on their extent, they are called subfrontal, subfrontoextradural, frontonasal, fronto-orbitonasal, and extended basal approach. Another possibility that remains is the combination, in a one-step procedure, of the transbasal and a transfacial approaches, particularly for inferior and lateral facial extensions of the tumor (Fig. 13-14). Combined rhinoseptal route and transbasal approach is very helpful with sphenoidal tumors that involve both the anterior cranial base and the posterior clival area (Fig. 13-15). This combination is particularly useful and successful with chordomas and chondromas.

INDICATIONS FOR THE TRANSBASAL APPROACH

A transbasal approach is not necessary to gain access to all tumors at the skull base. Its use depends on the exact anatomic location of the lesion. The transbasal approach should be used to increase the chances for total removal of a tumor. Table 13-1 summarizes cases in which this approach seemed absolutely necessary.

Diagnosis of a tumor invading the skull base does not routinely lead to a uniform treatment strategy. The choice of complete removal, decompression, or radiotherapy without surgery must be based on the histologic characteristics and extent of the lesion. These features must be assessed during the preoperative examination.

If the nature of the lesion is unknown, rhinoseptal biopsy or fibroscopy is suggested for diagnosis. Biopsy prevents errors. Some invasive adenomas and sphenoidal mucoceles are often confused, clinically and radiologically, with destructive chordomas.

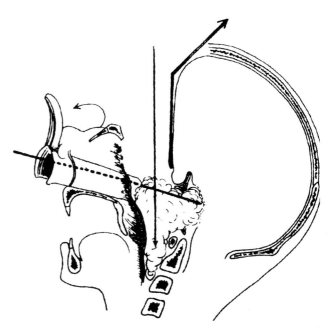

FIGURE 13-15 Combination of a rhinoseptal and transbasal approach in a one-step procedure.

Lesions involving the skull base can be classified into three groups: tumors of intracranial origin, such as meningiomas, primary bone tumors, and tumors of rhinopharyngeal origin, the latter of which are usually malignant.

Meningiomas

Meningiomas invade the skull base in three different ways (Figs. 13-17 and 13-18). First, the anterior fossa can be ruptured at its weakest point, the ethmoidal area and cribriform plates, as with intranasal extension of olfactory meningiomas, in which no true bone invasion occurs.[12,13] Second, with an en plaque meningioma[12,14,15] the dural tumor is less important than hyperostosis, which is not single reaction

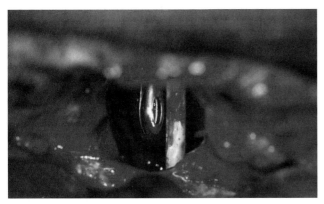

FIGURE 13-14 Instruments introduced by the facial route are visible through the skull base by the transbasal approach.

TABLE 13-1 ▪ Cases in Which a Transbasal Approach Was Used (to December 2003)

Case Type	No. of Patients
Meningiomas	73
Fibrous dysplasia	63
Malignant ear-nose throat tumor	33
Chordoma	80
Olfactory placode tumor	10
Chondroma	7
Ossifying fibroma	6
Nasopharyngeal fibroma	6
Cylindroma	5
Osteoma	5
Osteoblastoma	
Sarcoma	4
Hemangiopericytoma	1
Craniopharyngioma	1
Osteopetrosis	1
Sphenoethmoidal encephalocele (see Fig. 13–16)	1
Total	239

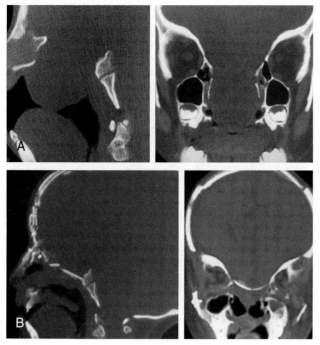

FIGURE 13-16 Ethmoidosphenoidal encephalocele. *A,* Preoperative aspect. *B,* Postoperative aspect: the skull base has been closed with a pericranium graft and with bone extracted from the cranial vault.

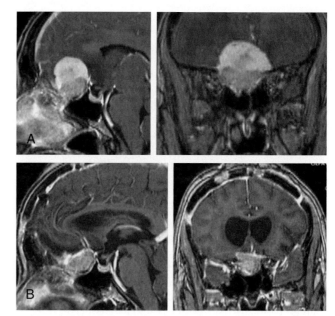

FIGURE 13-18 MRI in a case of basal meningioma. *A,* Preoperative aspect. *B,* After a first intracranial approach and before a transbasal surgery waiting for the dura to be made watertight.

but a true tumoral invasion of bone. Hyperostosis is responsible for the entire clinical syndrome and compression of the optic nerve into the optic canal. The dural plaque as well as the bone must be removed to avoid recurrence. A pterional location is not an indication for the transbasal approach. This approach is necessary and useful, however, when the lesion overlaps the optic canal and involves the sphenoidal area medially. Third, a bone reaction may be found close to the basal insertion of some en masse meningiomas. The pathologic features of such a reaction are difficult to confirm, but it may be a true invasion that will result in the basal malignancy recurring several years after the intracranial part has been removed. Basal invasion by a meningioma must be removed along with the intradural mass in one or two stages, depending on the size of the dural defect and the duration of the intracranial procedure.[13]

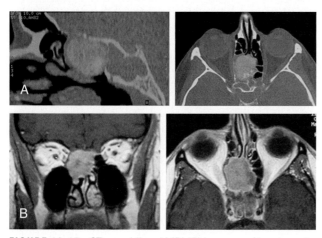

FIGURE 13-17 CT scan (*A*) and MRI (*B*) in a case of basal meningioma.

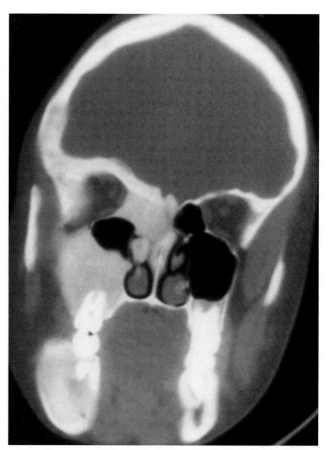

FIGURE 13-19 Basal and orbital fibrous dysplasia.

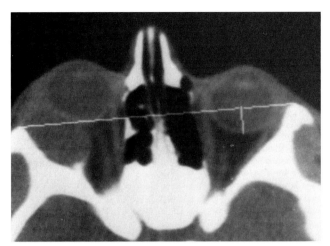

FIGURE 13-20 Medial compact sphenoidal fibrous dysplasia with stenosis of the optic canals.

Primary Bone Tumors Involving the Skull Base

Bone tumors include many kinds of lesions: some are malignant, such as sarcomas or metastases, whereas many are benign, such as osteomas, osteoblastomas, hemangiomas, ossifying fibromas, or fibrous dysplasia.

The natural history of fibrous dysplasia is uncommon and usually progressive; it can be acute, especially in young patients with fibrocystic-type fibrous dysplasia (Figs. 13-19 to 13-21).[8] Our experience suggests that surgery is required if the fibrous dysplasia is progressive or if the area of the optic foramen is involved.

Some bone tumors are difficult to classify, because their pathologic potential is doubtful. Some of these tumors are malignant, but their malignancy is local and it is often impossible to make a total removal. Examples of these tumors include giant cell tumors, chondromas, and chordomas.[15,16] Surgery is advised for chondromas, because radiation therapy is ineffective. These tumors are more or less encapsulated, and they probably can be removed almost completely, even

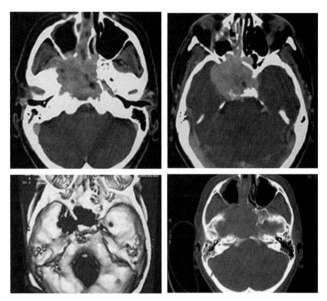

FIGURE 13-22 Basal osteosarcoma.

when they reach into the cavernous sinus. With chordomas, an aggressive surgical strategy[16] is indicated; the transbasal approach (alone or combined with a transphenoidal route) was useful in 15% of our cases for achieving the most complete removal of the tumor. Chordomas remain a real challenge for the neurosurgeon, and combined approaches are often necessary.

Complementary irradiation with proton beam or gamma knife, rather than conventional radiation therapy, is recommended and gives the patient the best chance for long-term survival.

Tumors of Rhinopharyngeal Origin

Among the rhinopharyngeal tumors that involve the skull base, very few are benign (i.e., benign olfactory placode or

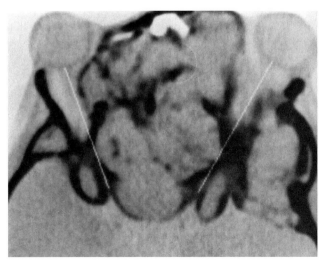

FIGURE 13-21 Huge fibrocystic fibrous dysplasia with hypertelorism.

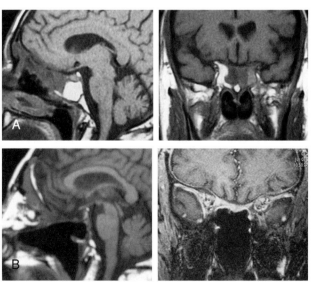

FIGURE 13-23 *A,* Preoperative aspect of an ethmoidosphenoidal adenocarcinoma. *B,* Postoperative aspect 6 years after transbasal transfacial surgery and radiotherapy for ethmoidosphenoidal adenocarcinoma.

nasopharyngeal fibroma).[17,18] These tumors usually are malignant carcinomas or epitheliomas, and the surgical strategy must be adapted. If the tumor extends toward the anterior fossa, the intracranial approach is suggested, combined with a transfacial route. Extensive removal in these cases is more important than reconstruction. Unfortunately, when a patient with this kind of tumor is seen by the neurosurgeon, it is often too late to accomplish a complete removal of all tumorous tissue. These patients must be seen very early in the course of tumor development, and to do so requires close cooperation between neurosurgical ear-nose-throat and maxillofacial teams (Figs. 13-22 and 13-23A and B).

REFERENCES

1. Tessier P, Guiot G, Derome P: Orbital hypertelorism. II: Definite treatment of orbital hypertelorism by craniofacial or by extracranial osteotomies. Scand J Plast Reconstr Surg 7:39, 1973.
2. Cophignon J, George B, Marchac D, et al: Voie transbasale élargie par mobilisation du bandeau fronto-orbitaire médian. Neurochirurgie 29:407, 1989.
3. Seckhar LN, Nanda A, Synderma CN, et al: The extended frontal approach to tumors of the anterior middle and posterior skull base. J Neurosurg 76:198–206, 1992.
4. Kawamaki K, Yamanouchi Y, Kubota C: An extensive transbasal approach to frontal skull-base tumors. J Neurosurg 74:1011–1013, 1991.
5. Spetzler RF, Herman JN, Beals S, et al: Preservation of olfaction in anterior craniofacial approaches. J Neurosurg 79:48, 1993.
6. Solero CL, DiMecco F, Sampath P: Combined anterior craniofacial resection for tumors involving the cribriform plate: Early postoperative complications and technical considerations. Neurosurgery 47:1084–1092, 2000.
7. Wallace RC, Dean BL, Beals SP: Posttreatment imaging of the skull base. Semin Ultrasound CT MR 24:164–181, 2003.
8. Derome PJ, Visot A, Akerman M, et al: Fibrous dysplasia of the skull. Neurochirurgie 29(Suppl 1):1–114, 1983.
9. Derome PJ, Visot A: Osseous lesions of anterior and middle base. In Seckhar LN, Janecka IP (eds): Surgery of Cranial Base Tumors. New York: Raven Press, 1993, pp 809–817.
10. Stevenson GC, Stoney RJ, Perkins RK et al: Transcervical, transclival approach to the ventral surface of the brainstem for removal of a clivus chordoma. J Neurosurg 24:544, 1966.
11. Chang DW, Robb GL: Microvascular reconstruction of the skull base. Semin Surg Oncol 19(3):211–217, 2000.
12. Derome P, Akerman M, Anquez L, et al: Les tumeurs sphenoethmoidales: Possibilités d'exérèse et réparations chirurgicales. Rapport de la Société Française de Neurochirurgie de Langue Française. Neurochirurgie 15(Suppl 1):1, 1972.
13. Derome PJ, Visot A: Bony reaction and invasion in meningiomas. In Al-Mefty O (ed): Meningiomas. New York: Raven Press, 1991, pp 169–177.
14. Castellano F, Guidetti B, Olivecrona H: Pterional meningiomas en plaques. Neurosurgery 9:188–196, 1952.
15. Visot A, Tessier P: Around the optic nerves in benign osseous tumors and malformations of the sphenoidal area. In Whitaker LA (ed): Craniofacial Surgery. Bologna. Monduzzi ed., pp 197–200, 1997.
16. Crockard HA, Cheeseman A, Steel T et al: A multidisciplinary team approach to skull base chondrosarcomas. J Neurosurg 95:184–189, 2001.
17. DeMonte F, Ginsberg LE, Clayman GL: Primary malignant tumors of the sphenoidal sinus. Neurosurgery 46:1084–1092, 2000.
18. Bentz BG, Bilsky MH, Shah JP, et al: Anterior skull base surgery for malignant tumors: A multivariate analysis of 27 years of experience. Head Neck 25(7):515–520, 2003.

14 Anterior Midline Approaches to the Skull Base

IVO P. JANECKA and SILLOO B. KAPADIA

INTRODUCTION

Comprehensive oncologic management of neoplasms involving the cranial base is an expanding field. Surgery has emerged as the primary modality of treatment for most tumors in this region, either as a single modality (for benign tumors) or in combination with irradiation and chemotherapy (for most malignant tumors). As with most tumors, the control of the primary site is one of the most important determinants of the ultimate outcome of treated patients, and thus a 3-dimensional tumor resection with histologically clear margins is the primary goal of cranial base oncologic surgery. Extensive resections must be balanced with an acceptable functional and esthetic morbidity. Gross central nervous system involvement or internal carotid encasement in a patient with poor collateral cerebral circulation is considered a relative contraindication to oncologic surgery.

Neoplastic growth affecting the anterolateral skull base often originates from central and paracentral craniofacial anatomic structures (dura, orbit, ethmoid, sphenoid and maxillary sinus, pterygoids, infratemporal fossa, clivus, etc.). Histologically this group of tumors includes a great diversity of cell origin.

The surgical approach to such tumors should accommodate the following features: (1) tumor-specific predilectional neoplastic growth; (2) when feasible, protection of key anatomic structures such as the internal carotid artery (ICA), the optic nerves, and the content of the cavernous sinus and the superior orbital fissure; (3) the best cosmetic result; (4) the stability of the craniovertebral junction.

The principal goal of an anterolateral approach to the skull base is to achieve an unobstructed view of the midline and paramedian skull base region. Strictly midline lesions of the anterior cranial fossa are treated with craniofacial resection using a low (basal) subfrontal combined with a midfacial translocation approach. For small clival (central) skull base lesions, a transoral approach may be satisfactory. For larger lesions, we have combined that with midfacial translocation. Midline lesions extending laterally can be resected through various units of the facial translocation system of approaches.

Anatomic Considerations

The intimate relationship of the skull base to the cranial as well as facial structures requires tissue displacement of one or both of these compartments to reach the desired section of the skull base. It is important to consider the effects of surgery on the normal but surgically manipulated tissues so as to select the most optimal approach. Any operative tissue displacement produces alterations in the anatomy and physiology of

affected structures. Such changes have variable consequences when they occur in the neurocranium or the facial viscerocranium. For example, facial swelling is usually self-limiting, with minimal long-term consequences for the patient. Similar edema, however, may be very deleterious when it involves the neurocranium.

The anterolateral skull base constitutes the floor of the anterior and middle cranial fossa. The proximate paranasal sinuses (ethmoid, sphenoid) with the nasal cavity and the orbits are intimate components of this skull base section.

The proximity of the face to the anterior cranial base gives this region a unique significance. The craniofacial skeleton gives protection to the organs of olfaction and vision and provides support for the configuration of the soft-tissue facial anatomy. This arrangement, however, hinders a direct surgical approach to the cranial base for tumors and requires planning of incisions and osteotomies that respect not only function but esthetics as well.

Anterolateral skull base approaches permit visualization of the surgical anatomy of the skull base that may extend from the ipsilateral temporomandibular joint and geniculate ganglion through trigeminal nerve branches of V3 and V2 as well as the ICA to the cavernous sinus, inferior and superior orbital fissures, and both anterior clinoids with corresponding optic nerves.

DIAGNOSTIC EVALUATION

Several essential issues guide our evaluation of cranial base neoplasms: (1) tumor biology and its extent, (2) tumor composition, (3) relationship of the tumor to the ICA and its importance to cerebral circulation (Fig. 14-1).

Tumor biology is best determined by preoperative histologic evaluation obtained after biopsy. New endoscopic instrumentation permits access to many skull base sites for direct visualization and tissue biopsy, or an open biopsy can be performed. The tumor extent determines the potential for surgical resection of the neoplasm. This is currently best determined by multiplanar CT as well as MRI. Both tests are also very useful in assessing the character of the lesion in terms of its vascular, bony, or soft-tissue content. The location of the ICA, its contribution to the tumor vascularity, as well as the relationship of this vessel to the tumor perimeter are assessed by MRI, MR angiography, or invasive angiography. The tolerance of the patient to temporary occlusion of the ICA can be evaluated with a series of tests known as temporary balloon occlusion test and xenon blood flow studies.[1] These tests permit us to estimate the risk of neurologic deficit with a permanent occlusion in the ICA.

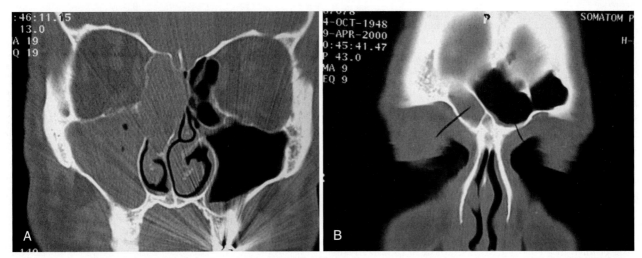

FIGURE 14-1   Imaging diagnostic evaluation. *A*, Coronal CT, bone algorithm, demonstrating a mass (a squamous cell carcinoma) in the right ethmoid sinus with involvement of the cribriform plate, medial orbital wall, and extending into the right maxillary sinus. *B*, Tumor extension into the right frontal sinus.

For orbital or periorbital tumors, a detailed neuro-ophthalmologic evaluation is valuable. Not only must the precise level of visual acuity, extent of visual fields, and ocular mobility be ascertained, but the completeness of function or the degree of dysfunction of the superior orbital fissure structures, optic nerve, and lacrimal apparatus should be known as well.

Endocrinologic evaluation is necessary preoperatively and in the follow-up period for tumors of the sellar or parasellar region.

SELECTED TUMORS

Carcinoma

Carcinoma that involves the anterior cranial base originates primarily in the paranasal sinuses, the nose and nasopharynx, or occasionally as a metastatic disease. Carcinoma of the nose and sinuses makes up less than 1% of all malignancies. It carries an overall 30% 5-year survival rate. In general, the prognosis of a patient with a carcinoma is very much related to the histologic type. Anaplastic carcinoma must be differentiated from lymphoma and melanoma with leukocyte common antigen and S-100 protein. Anaplastic carcinoma appears to be a separate entity from poorly differentiated squamous cell carcinoma, which still exhibits some squamous differentiation. It is found more often in women, with occurrence on the left side predominant. Among these patients, 33% develop cervical metastases, but only 70% of these have obvious evidence of bone destruction on radiographs. The survival of patients with anaplastic carcinoma varies with the site of origin. If it occurs in the nose, the 5-year survival rate is 40%. If it originates in the sinuses, the 5-year survival rate decreases to 15% (see reference 2).

The signs and symptoms common to most malignancies in the sinus-nose region include nasal obstruction, discharge, epistaxis, facial pain, as well as swelling, proptosis, or cervical node metastases.

The nasal passages and the sinuses are intimately related, permitting tumor to spread easily from one cavity to the other. Therefore, ethmoid sinuses are often involved secondarily by tumor spread from the nasal cavity or the maxillary sinus. This is reflected in the fact that isolated ethmoid carcinomas compose no more than 5% to 20% of all carcinomas involving the ethmoid sinus. The initial symptoms are usually insidious and trivial, accounting for a significant delay of diagnosis from the onset of symptoms. Sixty to seventy-five percent of patients with malignant tumors of the ethmoid sinuses do not survive for 5 years. The ethmoid sinus is closely related to the orbit. Both the orbit and the ethmoid sinus are simultaneously involved in 60% of malignant sinus neoplasms, and 45% of the patients are likely to require orbital exenteration. Most sinus tumors arise from the mucous membrane lining that is in continuity with the mucosa of the remaining sinuses, nasopharynx, and lacrimal draining system. The respiratory mucosa of the ethmoid sinus gives rise to two types of neoplasm. The first is squamous cell carcinoma, arising from the metaplastic epithelium. Of all malignant neoplasms of the sinuses, 75% to 95% will be squamous cell carcinomas, and the ethmoid sinus is the second most common site for this neoplasm. The second is a glandular tumor, arising from mucous glands. The submucosal glands give rise to adenocarcinomas or adenoid cystic carcinomas. Adenocarcinoma occurs most frequently in the ethmoid sinus, and its behavior is similar to that of squamous cell carcinoma. There is some suggestion that this tumor is found more frequently among workers in woodworking industries than in the population in general.[3] The lymphatic drainage from the ethmoid sinus is into the superior cervical chain and the retropharyngeal nodes. The incidence of metastases at the time of diagnosis is low, but 25% to 35% of patients will eventually develop metastatic disease. Distant metastases may occur in up to 18% of the cases.[4]

Esthesioneuroblastoma

This is a rare tumor originating from the olfactory epithelium and represents 3% of all intranasal neoplasms. It was originally described by Berger and Luc.[5] This tumor has been identified under different terms, for example, olfactory neuroblastoma, esthesioneurocytoma, and olfactory esthesioneuroblastoma.

It arises from cells of neural crest origin and resembles childhood neuroblastoma. The tumor does contain neurosecretory granules and is linked to other neural crest tumors, such as carcinoid, chemodectoma, and pheochromocytoma. It occurs most frequently in the third decade of life and is more common in males. Unilateral nasal obstruction and epistaxis are the most common symptoms. The tumor may fill the nose and paranasal sinuses and involve the cribriform plate.

A staging system has been proposed by Kadish and colleagues that recognizes three stages[6]:

Stage A: Tumor involves only nasal cavity.
Stage B: Tumor extends also to sinuses.
Stage C: Tumor extends beyond stage B.

However, correlation of tumor extent with prognosis has not been as accurate as the relationship of clear surgical margins.

Esthesioneuroblastoma is known to have a slow but insidious malignant course, and death comes from local recurrence, intracranial invasion, and/or metastatic disease. Differential diagnosis must exclude lymphoma, melanoma, and metastatic neuroblastoma. The characteristic histologic picture includes a fibrillary intercytoplasmic background that on electron microscopy is identified as representing neuronal cell processes. The 5-year survival rate is approximately 50%, with a median survival of 58 months. When the cranial base is invaded, the survival rate drops to about 40%. Long-term recurrence has also been observed 10 to 20 years after the original diagnosis. This tumor is characterized by local persistence and recurrence. There is a 20% to 40% potential that this tumor will metastasize into cervical lymph nodes, lungs, and bones. The current modality of treatment includes a radical resection of the area involved that includes the cribriform plate with or without the attached dura followed by a full course of irradiation and possibly chemotherapy as well.

Nasopharyngeal Carcinoma

Nasopharyngeal carcinoma is a rare tumor among non-Chinese patients, with an incidence of 1 in 100,000 among the North American population as compared with 2 in 100,000 among Chinese, especially those living in the Canton province of the People's Republic of China. Several etiologic factors have been implicated in the development of nasopharyngeal carcinoma, for example, the Epstein-Barr virus and numerous external inhalation as well as dietary carcinogens. The male-to-female ratio heavily favors male patients (3:1), with an average age of onset of 45 years.

Clinically, the tumor appears to arise primarily at the superior or lateral aspect of the nasopharynx. The symptomatology often includes epistaxis, nasal and eustachian tube obstruction, and eventual cranial nerve neuropathies (the fifth cranial nerve is most commonly involved). Histologically, these tumors are predominantly poorly differentiated carcinomas with a high propensity for metastatic regional spread, so that at the time of diagnosis, 50% of patients are expected to have regional disease. In the diagnostic evaluation, direct nasopharyngoscopy and biopsy, as well as a CT scan and MRI, provide for full assessment of the primary site. Irradiation is still considered a primary therapeutic modality for the nonkeratinizing squamous cell carcinoma of the primary site and the regional lymph node

draining area.[7] The cure rate, however, varies tremendously depending on the histologic type of the tumor, stage of the disease, and subsequent therapy. The most frequent recurrence of nasopharyngeal carcinoma is in the neck (42%), as reported in a series of 219 cases by Yan and colleagues in 1983 (see reference 8). Reirradiation of recurrent nasopharyngeal carcinoma gives a 5-year cure rate of only 14%, with a high chance of radiation-induced complications. It is important prognostically to separate patients with metastatic nasopharyngeal carcinoma in the neck on the basis of their response to the primary irradiation. If metastatic neck nodes disappeared completely following irradiation, the recurrence rate was only 13%. If nodes persisted throughout the course of irradiation, the recurrence rate was 91%.

With the advent of new approaches to the nasopharynx, surgery is becoming a therapeutic option for the treatment of resectable recurrent nasopharyngeal cancer with expected survival of over 50% (5 years). For tumors with very poor response to the primary radiotherapy (e.g., keratinizing squamous cell carcinoma, adenoid cystic carcinoma), surgery should be considered as the initial treatment.

Fibrous Dysplasia

Fibrous dysplasia is a progressive benign fibro-osseous lesion. Its natural growth is one of gradual expansion beyond its bony margins with concomitant displacement of surrounding soft tissue. It was first described by Lichtenstein in 1938 (see reference 9). It may be placed into three categories on the basis of its clinical presentation. The monostotic form represents a localized disease to one osseous structure and is the most frequent form (up to 70%). A polyostotic form involves several bones but usually on the same side of the body. Here the frequency ranges from 30% to 50%. The third form is disseminated, in which numerous bones are involved, along with the possibility of extraskeletal developments such as skin pigmentation and precocious puberty. The incidence ranges from 3% to 30%. These individual clinical forms retain their categorization during the course of the disease and do not seem to change from, for example, the monostotic to the polyostotic form. Fibrous dysplasia is more common in females. In the head and neck region (0.5% of all head and neck tumors), it is the maxilla, frontal bone, mandible, and parietal and temporal bones that are most frequently involved. It is of interest that the progression of the disease is often limited after completion of skeletal maturation.[10]

The clinical symptomatology usually includes swelling at the tumor site with displacement of surrounding soft tissues. For example, diplopia, when present, is usually caused by mechanical displacement of the globe. If the cribriform plate is directly involved, alteration in olfaction can be perceived. Histologic verification can be considered in addition to the clinical and radiographic examination. In the differential histologic diagnosis, fibrous dysplasia may mimic meningioma, and sarcoma is also a possibility. Radiographically, a sclerotic form manifests itself with dense bone. The cystic and pagetoid forms are distinguished radiographically from each other by the greater amount of fibrous component in the former.

Fibrous dysplasia can be treated by surgical resection when functional or esthetic deformity warrants it.[11] Full preoperative evaluation should include CT scan, with and without contrast, in the axial and coronal planes with bone algorithms.

Osseous reconstruction of the surgical defect is necessary only when the tumor involves key aspects of the craniofacial skeleton. Autogenous bone graft or alloplastic materials can be used. In the orbital region, most of the fibro-osseous lesions involve the orbital roof. Prolonged ocular displacement by the tumor often produces a secondary concavity in the orbital floor. This must be taken into account, since after orbital tumor removal superiorly, the globe may not return to the expected normal level. Secondary bone grafting of the deformed orbital floor may have to be considered.

Juvenile Angiofibroma

Juvenile angiofibroma is a relatively rare tumor occurring primarily in adolescent boys. The site of origin of the tumor is thought to be the medial pterygoid region. Clinically, the tumor has the potential to involve the nasopharynx, nose, infratemporal fossa, sphenoid, orbit, middle cranial fossa, and cavernous sinus. There is a preferential growth through preformed anatomic fissures and foramina. The symptomatology is one of nasal obstruction with episodes of nasal hemorrhage that can be profound. The diagnostic evaluation usually consists of CT scan and MRI as well as angiography. The CT scan demonstrates classical widening of the pterygopalatine fossa. MRI is assuming a greater importance in the diagnosis of this tumor, its extent, as well as the degree of its vascularity. Angiography determines the blood supply to this lesion, which originates primarily in the external carotid system, usually the internal maxillary or the ascending pharyngeal artery. There may be additional blood supply from the internal carotid system. In the differential diagnosis, angiomatous polyp, pyogenic granuloma, and hemangioma are included in the benign group. Carcinoma, rhabdomyosarcoma, and chordoma should be considered among the malignant tumors.[12]

The primary treatment has been surgical through a transfacial or transpalatal approach, or, for extensive cases, craniofacial resection. Because of its vascularity and potential for a recurrence, a complete removal of this tumor should be attempted. The need for preoperative embolization can be determined at the time of the diagnostic angiography as well as from the appearance of tumor vascularity on the MRI scan. However, the potential complications from embolization must be considered and its advantage weighed against the potential risks. Recurrent tumors are usually treated again with surgery (if accessible) or irradiation. Hormonal therapy, originally thought to be beneficial, has not proved to be of significant value. Histologically, this tumor is composed of fibrous stroma and multiple vascular channels without a definite layer of muscularis in the vessel walls.[13]

Careful postoperative and long-term evaluation of patients with juvenile angiofibromas is important. MRI provides the best modality of clinical assessment. Harrison published a personal series of 44 patients treated by surgical removal in whom there was a 23% incidence of recurrence.[14] These 10 patients with recurrent tumor received another operation. Of these 10 patients, 3 developed a second recurrence that was subsequently treated successfully with irradiation.

Chordomas

Chordomas are tumors that are thought to arise from remnants of the notochord, which is the embryonic precursor of the axial skeleton. Chordomas constitute only 1% of all intracranial tumors, and 30% to 40% of all chordomas arise in the skull base area. Chordomas may involve the sphenoethmoidal area, the petrosphenoid synchondrosis, and the cavernous sinus region, the upper, middle, or lower clivus. The symptoms produced depend on the location of the tumor. Patients may develop cranial nerve palsies, brain stem compression, or merely a nasal or nasopharyngeal mass with nasal airway obstruction.

There are two histologic types of chordoma. The chondroid variety demonstrates a cartilaginous matrix histologically and is associated with a much better long-term survival. Patients with chondroid chordoma may live as long as 20 to 30 years. The regular variety of chordoma is associated with a poorer prognosis (5-year survival rate of 30% to 50%). Death is usually caused by local recurrence of tumor. Metastasis to distant sites occurs in about 10% of patients and is more common with longer survival periods. Chordomas are relatively radioresistant to standard radiotherapy and do not respond to chemotherapy.

During the last 10 years, two new developments in the treatment of chordomas have occurred that may change the prognosis for cranial base chordomas. First, the advances in cranial base surgery have allowed a more complete resection of chordomas from difficult regions such as the clivus, the petrous apex, and the cavernous sinus. Second, irradiation with high-energy particles, such as proton beams (Bragg peak) or helium ions, has permitted the delivery of large amounts of radiation to a restricted area. The effects of both of these advances will require many years to evaluate, since chordomas are slow-growing tumors. The current management principle consists of surgical removal and postoperative irradiation.[15–17]

Chondrosarcoma

Since the bones of the cranial base are derived from a cartilaginous matrix through endochondral ossification, 60% to 70% of chondrosarcomas involve the cranial base skeleton. Such tumors may involve any area of the cranial base but have a predilection for the petrosphenoid synchondrosis.

The prognosis of chondrosarcomas in general depends on the histologic grade, which is worse in patients with a poorly differentiated tumor. The majority of cranial base chondrosarcomas are low grade, locally confined for many years. They recur repeatedly after local resection and metastasize rarely.

Similar to the management of skull base chordomas, our present management consists of tumor resection. Irradiation is administered to patients with residual tumor or high-grade chondrosarcoma.

Osseous Meningiomas

Meningiomas of the cranial base area are often associated with hyperostosis of the cranium. In 30% to 50% of cases, such hyperostosis is due to actual tumor invasion into the bone. In the others, it occurs as a reaction to the tumor resulting from increased vascularity. A patient with a hyperostotic bony reaction or tumor may have either a carpetlike "meningioma en plaque" or a globular "meningioma en masse" involving the dura, the periorbita, and the paranasal sinuses. Osseous meningiomas may be discovered when a patient presents with signs and symptoms caused by a globular tumor. With the en plaque variety, such osseous involvement is often the reason for neurologic symptoms, commonly proptosis, extraocular muscle palsies, and visual loss.

Failure to remove the osseous portion of the tumor will result in eventual progression of symptoms. Regrowth of osseous tumor is often slow, permitting conservative surgery in many patients.

SURGERY

Several basic principles, well utilized in other surgical areas, are applicable to cranial base tumor surgery. One is simplicity. Even in complex cranial base surgery, the simplicity and thus the proper sequential logic of the procedural steps should be high on the priority list. The second principle is exposure. It is essential that adequate surgical access to the tumor be achieved with good visualization to allow its complete removal and preservation of uninvolved anatomic structures. In particular, the blood supply to the overlying skin and surrounding muscles must be respected during exposure and tumor resection, so as to have adequate and viable soft tissue available for reconstruction. The cranial nerves, if free of neoplastic growth, are preserved or reconstructed following tumor removal.

Craniofacial Resection

This procedure is performed for neoplasms involving the midline anterior cranial base. For example, tumors involving the ethmoid sinuses and cribriform plate would be encompassed by this procedure.

A bicoronal incision is used with removal of the craniofacial skeleton (Fig. 14-2). This incision outlines the distal end of the frontoparietal scalp flap used for the exposure of the cranium. It is based inferiorly on supraorbital and supratrochlear vessels and laterally on branches of the superficial temporal arteries. It is a broad-based flap. It can include all the layers of the scalp, including the underlying pericranium,

or it can be raised at the galeopericranial plane. Anterolateral extensions of this bicoronal incision, in front of each ear, permit reflection of the flap over the face (a greater rotational arch was achieved) and thus unhindered exposure to the cranium, the roof of the orbit, and both zygomatic arches. The frontalis branch of the facial nerve is preserved and reflected inferiorly in a fascial layer with the overlying scalp flap. The supraorbital neurovascular pedicle can be dissected out of its foramen or groove on each side and preserved. The nasion is well exposed, permitting access to both medial orbital walls. Loss of the sense of smell is always a consequence of this approach.

In addition to the bicoronal scalp flap for superior exposure, inferior facial incisions are made (see Fig. 14-2). Several options are available, from a purely midline "face-splitting" incision (from the nasion through the upper lip) to a paramedian incision, a modification of a lateral rhinotomy incision. It is also possible to avoid direct facial skin incisions by performing what is referred to as a "degloving" procedure (a horizontal mucosal incision from one maxillary tuberosity to the other in the gingivolabial sulcus with elevation of all the soft tissues of the face including the nose). This approach, however, provides wide surgical access only at the level of the incision and significantly narrows at the skull base. Optimal visualization at the skull base is not achieved in the majority of cases. Also, reconstruction of the skull base, if needed, is difficult with this approach.

The "exposure osteotomies," done in a zigzagging fashion, are performed with the intent to remove, as a free graft, the supraorbital bar, usually from one supraorbital nerve to the other. The facial bony segments are displaced following osteotomies, with the attached soft tissues. They may extend from one medial orbit across the nasion to the opposite orbit (usually to the level of the superior orbital nerve on the opposite side). If the orbital content is involved with the tumor, then it becomes part of the specimen. Before tumor extirpation, when needed, the ICA is isolated in the neck. The craniotomy used in this approach is a bifrontal craniotomy. After dural elevation from the anterior cranial fossa, tumor extent is appropriately assessed with preservation of as many uninvolved anatomic structures as possible including cranial nerves and the carotid artery.

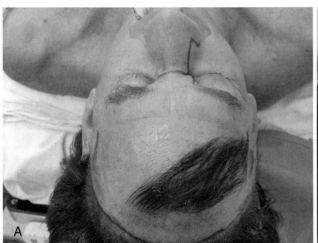 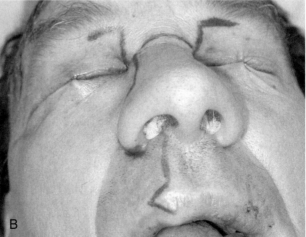

FIGURE 14-2 Incisions. *A,* Midfacial incisions. *B,* Bicoronal and midfacial incisions.

The planning for 3-dimensional tumor resection should include the natural anatomic boundaries to tumor progression. These include dura, one or both medial walls of the orbit, the cribriform plate, and the nasal septum. A portion of the frontal bone, corresponding to the upper boundary of the interorbital space, is usually removed with the specimen. If the frontal sinus is not involved by the tumor, it is possible to replace the most anterior portion of this bone.

Midfacial Split and Midfacial Translocation

Midfacial split provides a direct access and a unified surgical field at the central cranial base. It is performed utilizing bilateral facial osteotomies and soft-tissue mobilization. It extends in the sagittal plane from the anterior cranial fossa floor and sphenoid sinus to the level of C1. In the axial plane, the surgical reach extends between medial orbits superiorly, through the plane between V2 to the level of the palate. If the tumor demands wider exposure, an extended facial translocation with palatal split can be utilized.[18]

Incision consists of either a midline or a paramedian nasal incision with supraorbital extensions. If needed, it may continue inferiorly through the upper lip. The uninvolved nasal septum is reflected with one of the lateral composite tissue components. Facial soft tissues are elevated from the nasomaxillary bones to both infraorbital foramina.

The upper end of the nasal incision is extended laterally below the medial eyebrows, exposing the superior and medial orbital rims. Elevation of the periorbita reveals the anterior and posterior ethmoid foramina; cauterization of the ethmoid vascular pedicles is performed. Inferiorly, the nasolacrimal duct is identified and preserved (or repositioned for subsequent dacryocystorhinostomy).

Bone cuts are made from the medial orbit on one side to the other, through the nasion followed by LeFort I osteotomy. Vertical maxillary cuts are made just medial to the infraorbital nerves. The osteotomies in the medial and inferior orbit are then connected. A midline nasal osteotomy completes bony disassembly if a central nasal incision is used; if a paramedian nasal incision is selected, the entire nasal-midfacial complex is rotated laterally as a composite flap on a single soft-tissue pedicle. Nasal cavities and maxillary sinuses are now widely exposed, allowing resection of the medial maxillary walls. Nonessential nasal septum and vomer can be removed or dislocated to one side, providing direct access to the nasopharynx, sphenoid sinus, and clivus.

For more inferior exposure, the procedure is modified (by omitting the LeFort I osteotomy and separating the maxillary segment from the pterygoid plates posteriorly) and splitting the hard palate in the midline. Each hemipalate (still attached to its vascular pedicle and the rest of the maxilla) is then rotated laterally and retracted. The soft palate can also be divided in the midline, giving access to the entire oronasopharynx and C1–C4 area.

If further inferior exposure is needed, a tranoral-transmandibular approach can be selected.[19] For more lateral access, an extended facial translocation[18,20] can be added.

Facial Translocation

This approach to the skull base has undergone a significant evolution since its original description in 1989 and now comprises a system of approaches based on a principle of facial disassembly along embryonic planes of fusion.[18,20,21] Due to its modular design, it permits great versatility of design and accommodates the surgical needs for limited as well as complex procedures at the skull base. The operative manipulation of cranial base anatomy and pathology, crucial for oncologic surgery, can be tailored with this system of approaches very precisely to a specific skull base tumor. Maximum preservation and functional and esthetic reconstruction of craniofacial anatomy is an integral part of this procedure.

The current underlying principle of skull base approaches is to minimize brain retraction while maximizing skull base visualization reflected in disassembly and displacement of craniofacial bony and soft-tissue anatomy while preserving the intactness of the brain. This concept facilitates 3-dimensional tumor resection, tumor margin verification, and functional reconstruction with appropriate esthetic concerns. Facial translocation approach to the skull base through its great versatility contributes to this goal.

In general, surgical treatment of lesions located anterior to the neuroaxis should be done through an anterior approach. This requires selection of a transfacial approach because of the anteroinferior anatomic relationship of the facial viscerocranium to the cranial base.

The advantages of the facial translocation system of approaches include the following:

1. Facial anatomy has developed through the embryonic fusion of nasofrontal, maxillary, and mandibular processes. Normally, the fusion takes place in the midline or in the paramedian region, thus logically presenting optimal lines of "separation" of facial units for a surgical approach, permitting the least consequential displacement.
2. The primary blood supply to the "facial units" is through the external carotid system, which also has a lateral-to-medial direction of flow, thus ensuring viability of displaced surgical units.
3. The midface contains multiple "hollow" anatomic spaces (oronasal cavity, nasopharynx, paranasal sinuses) that facilitate the relative ease of surgical access to the central skull base.
4. Displacement of facial units for an approach to the cranial base offers much greater tolerance to postoperative surgical swelling, as opposed to similar displacement of the content of the neurocranium.
5. Reestablishment of the normal anatomy, following repositioning of the facial units during the reconstructive phase of surgery, has a high degree of functional as well as aesthetic achievement.

However, there are some disadvantages:

1. Contamination of the surgical wound with oropharyngeal bacterial flora.
2. The need for facial incisions with subsequent scar development.
3. Emotional considerations for the patient related to "surgical facial disassembly."
4. The potential need for supplementary airway management (postoperative endotracheal intubation, temporary tracheostomy).

The listed disadvantages are of much lesser consequence to the patient when viewed from the perspective of the procedure's overall safety, tumor control potential, and the facilitation of excellent reconstructive options.

In the past, several surgeons worked on achieving additional oncologic exposure of the facial viscerocranium. Barbosa[22] expanded exposure for the treatment of maxillary sinus cancer and Altemir[23] did the same for the nasomaxillary area access.

Operative Technique

Modular craniofacial disassembly is the principle of the facial translocation approach to the skull base. It is based on the creation of composite facial units that are designed along key neurovascular anatomy and esthetic lines. The individual units merge into larger composites without compromising their function. It is possible to attach eponyms to the technical variations of facial translocation for ease of communication and comparison. Thus we can recognize "mini," "standard," "expanded" (vertically, medially, posteriorly), and "bilateral" facial translocation procedures.[24] Complementary craniotomies or craniectomies are added to these approaches as necessary to assist with 3-dimensional tumor resection.

Minifacial translocation–central is designed to reach the medial orbit, sphenoid and ethmoid sinuses, and the inferior clivus. The port of entry is through the displaced ipsilateral nasal bone, the nasal process of the maxilla, and the medial orbital rim (with an attached medial canthal ligament, the lacrimal duct, and the skin). The skin incision is made along the lateral aspect of the nose and the inferior aspect of the medial eyebrow with a triangular design at the level of the medial canthal ligament to limit potential scar contracture. Osteotomies create a rectangular window with a lateral extent being just medial to the inferior orbital nerve. The entire unit is displaced laterally for surgical exposure. Closure is accomplished with replacement of this composite unit (skin, bone, mucosa). Rigid fixation of the bone is accomplished with microplating. The perimeter of this approach can be further augmented with endoscopic instrumentation.

Minifacial translocation–lateral opens the infratemporal fossa. The incisions run from the inner canthus horizontally in the inferior fornix of the lower eyelid through the lateral canthus to the preauricular area. Here, it joins vertical temporal and preauricular incisions. The frontal branches of the facial nerve are temporarily disconnected through entubulation (see later). The temporalis muscle is reflected inferiorly after displacement of the zygomatic arch–malar eminence. The head of the mandible, when needed, may be either displaced or resected.

Standard facial translocation achieves surgical access to the anterolateral skull base. The ipsilateral facial skin (including the lower eyelid) is displaced laterally and inferiorly with the attached underlying maxilla (with or without the hard palate). The nasal incision may extend inferiorly to include an upper lip split. Superior incision continues from the nose to the inferior fornix of the lower eyelid, and again through the lateral canthus horizontally to the preauricular area. In some cases (more anterior tumors), it is possible to conclude the horizontal canthal incision about 1.5 cm beyond the lateral orbital rim after identifying and preserving the most anterior frontal branch of the facial nerve. This point then serves as the point of rotation of the displaced composite unit, providing sufficient surgical space for some paracentral tumors. When the entire extent of the horizontal temple incision is needed, the frontal branches of the facial nerve are identified with a nerve stimulator, placed in silicone tubings, and transected (entubulation). During the reconstruction, only these transected tubings are reconnected, approximating the facial nerve branches, and providing a stable, enclosed milieu for nerve regeneration. Osteotomies correlate to LeFort I or II or the midpalatal lines when the entire maxilla is being displaced. The inferior orbital nerve is electively sectioned along the floor of the orbit, tagged, and repaired at the end of the procedure. Rigid fixation is achieved with mini- and microplates. With this technique of facial translocation, good exposure of the anterolateral skull base is achieved, especially when the infratemporal fossa is involved as well.

Extended facial translocation–medial incorporates the standard translocation unit plus the nose and the medial one half of the opposite face (up to the infraorbital nerve). It can be rotated at the LeFort I level or include the ipsilateral palate and upper lip split. The skin incisions are similar to the standard technique, except that the paranasal incision is made on the contralateral side. The surgical exposure includes the ipsilateral infratemporal fossa and the central and paracentral skull base bilaterally. The entire clivus is accessible, as are the optic nerves, both precavernous ICAs, and the nasopharynx. The wide communication with the infratemporal fossa allows the placement of the temporalis muscle flap for vascularized reconstruction of any skull base defect. Bony fixation of craniofacial osteotomies is done with miniplates and a lag screw for the palate. The occlusal plane is reestablished with the help of an orthognathic splint prefabricated preoperatively. In addition, a full palatal splint is attached to the contralateral stable palate for additional stability and protection of the palatal incision. Temporary silicone intranasal stents are inserted, as are bilateral lacrimal stents.

Extended facial translocation–medial and inferior includes the aforementioned procedure with an inferior extension via mandibular split. The lower lip split incision is performed in a zigzagging fashion to conform to the tension lines of the skin with a horizontal extension into the upper neck. Mandibular osteotomy is performed just medial to the mental foramen. Usually an interdental space is found wide enough to permit placement of a reciprocating saw for the osteotomy. This is performed in a step fashion, which then permits more stable reconstructive reapproximation of the bone. Before performing the osteotomy, it is wise to select an appropriate miniplate for eventual fixation, contour it to the mandible, and create drill holes. This maneuver assists in the reestablishment of a normal occlusion during reconstruction. This extended translocation procedure adds a significant inferior as well as upper cervical surgical access.

Bilateral facial translocation combines complete right and left basic translocation units with or without palatal split. The exposure incorporates both infratemporal fossae, central and the entire paracentral skull base. Both distal cervical ICAs are in view, as is the full clivus. The palatal split permits a reach to the level of C2–C3. If further inferior extension is

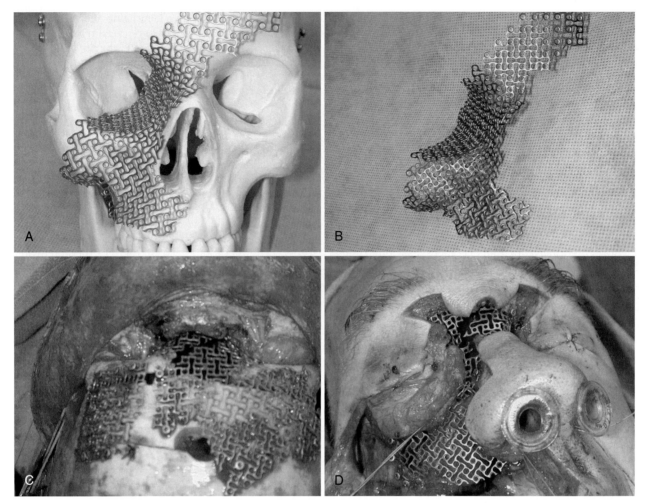

FIGURE 14-3   Reconstruction. *A,* Titanium meshed used for osseous substitution is molded on a skull model. *B,* Molded titanium implant retains its shape. *C,* Inserted titanium mesh-cranial view. *D,* Inserted titanium mesh-facial view.

needed, a mandibular split can be added so a vertical reach to C3–C4 is accomplished. A single temporalis muscle flap is sufficient for the coverage of the surgical defect at the skull base.

Reconstruction

The repair of any dural defect is performed with a pericranial graft harvested posterior to the bicoronal incision. In addition, a pericranial flap, based on supraorbital vessels, is utilized to enclose the cranial cavity and complete the separation of the cranial cavity from the extracranium. The reestablishment of external craniofacial bony continuity is done by replacing any skeleton displaced for exposure. Any surgical defect can be augmented with a split cranial bone graft or a titanium mesh (see Fig. 14-3; Fig. 14-4 and 14-5). The most inferior portion of cranial base defects (floor of cranial fossae) is usually not bone grafted. Further soft-tissue repair may include regional muscle transposition (temporalis) or free muscle–skin flap transfer (rectus abdominis or latissimus dorsi myocutaneous flaps).

COMPLICATIONS

Complications of a craniofacial resection can be categorized into fatal and nonfatal groups. Terz and colleagues reported an 11% fatal complication rate in their group of 28 patients. The three deaths in this series resulted from pulmonary embolus, brain injury, and tracheal abscess. In the nonfatal complication group, reported by the same investigators, there were several CSF leaks, meningitis, and osteomyelitis of the bone flap, for a 35% nonfatal complication rate.[25]

Careful attention to even minor details during the preoperative evaluation, the operation, and the postoperative period can often prevent major complications. For instance, when severe lower cranial nerve dysfunction is expected, a temporary tracheostomy and gastrostomy can prevent aspiration pneumonia and malnutrition. Since many of the initial postoperative problems are neurologic, cardiac, or respiratory, the patient should be observed in a unit with facilities for neurologic and cardiorespiratory intensive care. Because of the close collaboration among neurosurgery, otolaryngology, and plastic surgery, the incidence of postoperative problems following extensive cranial base surgery has been greatly reduced.[26]

ADJUVANT THERAPY

External beam irradiation is usually administered as an adjuvant treatment to patients with malignant cranial base neoplasms. The value of such combined therapy (surgery and irradiation) for extensive skull base tumors is unproven

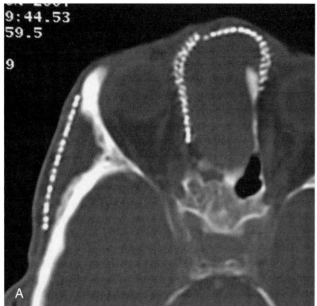

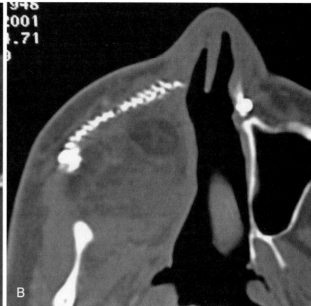

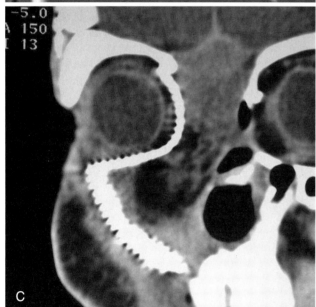

FIGURE 14-4 Postoperative imaging at 1 year. *A,* CT, bone algorithm, demonstrating implanted titanium mesh-midline face. *B,* CT, bone algorithm, demonstrating implanted titanium mesh-right maxilla, with underlying transferred temporalis muscle used for vascularized reconstruction. *C,* CT, bone algorithm, demonstrating implanted titanium mesh-coronal view.

at this time in the absence of prospective controlled trials. However, such combined modalities have become a standard in head and neck surgery for extensive neoplasms (T3–T4).

High-energy focused radiation, with proton beams or helium ions, has been used to treat cranial base chordomas and chondrosarcomas with encouraging results.[17]

Although benign tumors such as meningiomas and neurilemmomas have been considered radioresistant, recent reports suggest that recurrent or residual tumors can be treated with external beam irradiation, reducing their growth rates.[27] However, the deleterious effects of irradiation (carcinogenesis, normal tissue growth retardation) must be kept in mind.

For small benign lesions (<2.5 cm), such as meningiomas or acoustic neurilemmomas, stereotactically focused cobalt radiation has been used. Such "gamma knife" treatments

appear to be effective in arresting the growth of tumors in many cases and offer an alternative to surgical treatment.[28]

In general, chemotherapy for cranial base tumors has not been successful. It is hoped that biologic modifiers will offer greater benefit in the future.

CONCLUSIONS

The management of complex cranial base neoplasms by a team approach, combined with other therapeutic advances, has greatly improved the outlook for these patients in the past 10 years. The next decade will witness the consolidation of such advances and the conduction of cooperative and prospective clinical trials to assess further the efficacy of such aggressive approaches in controlling neoplastic disease at the skull base. Patients with extensive cranial base neoplasms often need considerable help with psychologic,

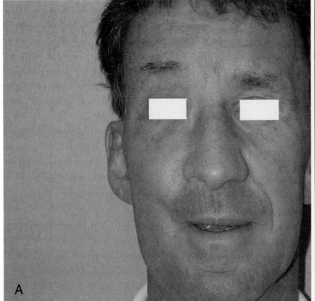

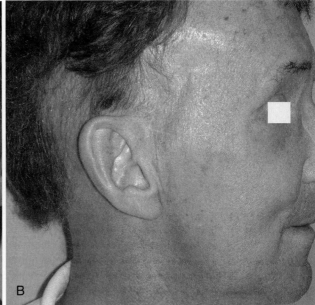

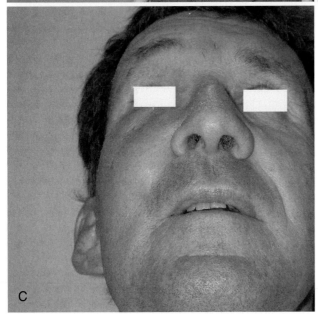

FIGURE 14-5 Postoperative patient's appearance at 1 year. *A,* Frontal view. *B,* Lateral view. *C,* Base view.

social, and financial problems. Such problems are best handled with the assistance of psychology, nursing, and social service departments.

The oncologic benefit of cranial base surgery is continuously being assessed. The percentage of patients living disease free after cranial base surgery for malignant disease has increased to 60% to 65% at 5 years. This "overall" percentage (all histologies, all sites) reflects not only the slow biologic aggressiveness of some tumors (e.g., chondrosarcomas, adenoid cystic carcinomas) but also the high aggressiveness of others (e.g., squamous cell and anaplastic carcinomas). Most encouraging is that primary cranial base surgery (done as the initial treatment) has a significantly greater chance of oncologic success than "salvage" procedures following failure of other therapeutic modalities (e.g., non–skull base surgery, radiotherapy).

For most benign tumors, cranial base surgery is the only therapeutic modality and has a high degree of effectiveness.

Acknowledgment

This chapter has been adapted with permission from Nuss DW, Janecka IP: Cranial base tumors. In Myers EN, Suen JY (eds): Cancer of the Head and Neck. Philadelphia: WB Saunders, 1996; and from Janecka IP, Tiedemann K (eds): Skull Base Surgery. Philadelphia: Lippincott-Raven Publishers, 1997.

Supported in part by the Foundation for Surgical Research and Education and the Health Research International.

REFERENCES

1. deVries EJ, Sekhar LN, Janecka IP, et al: Elective resection of the internal carotid artery without reconstruction. Laryngoscope 98:960–966, 1988.
2. Helliwell TR, Yeoh LH, Stell PM: Anaplastic carcinoma of the nose and paranasal sinuses: Light microscopy, immunochemistry, and clinical correlation. Cancer 58:2038–2045, 1986.
3. Roush GC: Epidemiology of cancer of the nose and paranasal sinuses: Current concept. Head Neck Surg 2:3–11, 1979.
4. Rice DH: Benign and malignant tumors of the ethmoid sinus. In Mattox DE (ed): The Otolaryngologic Clinics of North America. Philadelphia: WB Saunders, 1985, p 113.

5. Berger L, Luc R: L'esthesioneuroepitheliome olfactif. Bull Assoc Fr Etude Cancer 13:410–420, 1924.
6. Kadish S, Goodman M, Wang CC: Olfactory neuroblastoma: A clinical analysis of 17 cases. Cancer 37:1571–1576, 1976.
7. Hu YH, Yin WB, Li CL et al: Assessment of the method and result of radiotherapy for nasopharyngeal carcinoma. Chin J Radiol 10:467, 1965.
8. Yan JH, Hu YH, Gu XZ: Radiation therapy of recurrent nasopharyngeal cancer. Acta Radiol Oncol 22:23, 1983.
9. Lichtenstein L: Polyostotic fibrous dysplasia. Arch Surg 36:874–898, 1938.
10. Feldman MD, Rao VM, Lowry LD, Kelly M: Fibrous dysplasia of the paranasal sinuses. Otolaryngol Head Neck Surg 95:222–225, 1986.
11. Janecka IP, Housepian E: Craniofacial approach to ossifying fibromas. Laryngoscope 95:305–306, 1985.
12. Duvall AJ, Moreano AE: Juvenile nasopharyngeal angiofibroma: Diagnosis and treatment. Otolaryngol Head Neck Surg 97:534–540, 1987.
13. Antonelli AR, Cappiello J, DiLorenzo D, et al: Diagnosis, staging and treatment of juvenile nasopharyngeal angiofibroma. Laryngoscope 97:1319–1325, 1987.
14. Harrison DF: The natural history, pathogenesis, and treatment of juvenile angiofibroma. Arch Otolaryngol Head Neck Surg 113:936–942, 1987.
15. Derome PJ, Viscot A, Monteil JP, Maestro JL: Management of cranial chordomas. In Sekhar LN, Schramm VL (eds): Tumors of the Cranial Base: Diagnosis and Treatment. New York, Futura Publishing, 1987, pp 607–622.
16. Raffel C, Wright DC, Gutin PA, Wilson CB: Cranial chordomas: Clinical presentation and results of operative and radiation therapy in twenty six patients. Neurosurgery 17:703–710, 1985.
17. Suit HD, Goitein M, Munzenrider J: Definitive radiation therapy for chordoma and chondrosarcoma of the base of the skull and cervical spine. J Neurosurg 56:377–385, 1982.
18. Janecka IP, Tiedemann K (eds): Skull Base Surgery. Philadelphia: Lippincott-Raven, 1998.
19. Krespi YP, Sisson GA: Transmandibular exposure of the skull base. Am J Surg 148:534–538, 1984.
20. Janecka IP, Sen Ch, Sekhar LN, Arriaga M: Facial translocation: A new approach to the cranial base. Otolaryngol Head and Neck Surg 103:413–419, 1990.
21. Janecka IP: A new approach to the cranial base. Proceedings of the XIV World Congress of Otolaryngology, Head and Neck Surgery, Madrid, Spain, September 10–15, 1989. Amsterdam: Kugler & Ghedini Publisher, 1990.
22. Barbosa J: Surgery of extensive cancer of paranasal sinuses. Arch Otolaryngol 73:129–138, 1961.
23. Altemir FH: Transfacial access to the retromaxillary area. J Maxillofac Surg 14:119–182, 1986.
24. Janecka IP: Classification of facial translocation approach to the skull base. Otolaryngol Head Neck Surg 112:579–585, 1995.
25. Terz JJ, Young HF, Lawrence W Jr: Combined craniofacial resection for locally advanced carcinoma of the head and neck: Carcinoma of the paranasal sinuses. Am J Surg 140:618–624, 1980.
26. Janecka IP, Sen C, Sekhar LN, et al: Cranial base surgery: Results in 183 patients. Otolaryngol Head Neck Surg 110:539–546, 1994.
27. Wallner KE, Sheline GE, Pitts LH, et al: Efficacy of radiation for incompletely excised acoustic neurilemmomas. J Neurosurg 67:858–863, 1987.
28. Noren G, Arndt J, Hindmarsh J: Stereotactic radiosurgery in cases of acoustic neurinomas: Further experiences. Neurosurgery 13:12–22, 1983.

15 Orbitozygomatic Infratemporal Approach to Parasellar Meningiomas

KENJI OHATA, BASSEM SHEIKH, ALAA EL-NAGGAR, TAKEO GOTO, TOSHIHIRO TAKAMI, and AKIRA HAKUBA[†]

Lesions located high in the parasellar region and the interpeduncular fossa are challenging and often difficult to approach, as a result of both the deep position and the surrounding vital structures that obscure the view. In 1977, we developed a new surgical approach, the orbitozygomatic infratemporal approach,[1] consisting of an orbitozygomatic osteotomy, a fronto-temporo-orbital craniotomy, and removal of the posterolateral wall of the orbital bone and major sphenoid wing lateral to the foramen spinosum. This approach provides a good exposure of the infratemporal fossa, permits access obliquely upward to the parasellar region and the interpeduncular fossa, and permits safe manipulation of parasellar and interpeduncular lesions via the shortest distance.[2–4]

OPERATIVE TECHNIQUE

The patient is placed in the supine position with the thorax elevated 30 degrees to facilitate venous drainage. By using a three-pin headholder, the head is rotated to the side opposite the lesion without creating excessive torsion of the neck, so that the right pterion is the highest in the surgical field.

A bicoronal scalp incision is made to gain sufficient exposure of the zygomatic arch and superior and lateral orbital margins, starting at the inferior end of the base of the earlobe, running along the anterior margin of the ear cartilage, extending upward and forward, and running within the hairline to a level 3 cm above the upper margin of the contralateral zygomatic arch. The superficial layer of deep temporal fascia is incised and reflected with the skin flap to avoid the injury of the frontal branch of the facial nerve. The skin flap is reflected farther anteriorly with the frontal pericranium to expose the orbitozygomatic complex, cutting the supraorbital notch for the preservation of the right supraorbital nerve.[5,6] To preserve the temporal and zygomatic branches of the facial nerve, the fascia covering the temporomandibular joint capsule is carefully pulled away, and the periosteum covering the outer surface of the zygomatic arch is incised vertically just in front of the tuberculum articulare. The entire outer surface of the zygomatic arch from its frontal process to its pedicle is then fully exposed subperiosteally. The superior and lateral orbital margins are then exposed, maintaining continuity of the pericranium and the periorbita. The superior and lateral periorbita are separated from the superior and lateral posterior walls of the orbit.

Multiple burr holes are made, the first of which, in the lateral frontal bone just behind the frontal process of the zygomatic bone, is the key burr hole. The second burr hole is at the pterion, the third in the temporal bone just above the pedicle of the zygomatic process, the fourth in the squamous suture about 3 cm above the zygomatic arch, the fifth in the coronal suture about 6 cm above the zygomatic arch, and the sixth in the frontal bone 3 cm above the orbital ridge (Fig. 15-1). The anterior and posterior ends of the zygomatic arch are then cut using a sagittal saw, and it is retracted downward hinged on the masseter muscle.

The second, third, fourth, fifth, and sixth burr holes are then connected with a craniotome (see Fig. 15-1). Using a reciprocating saw, osteotomy of the lateral and superior walls of the orbit is performed from the inferior orbital fissure. The orbital content is protected by a spatula during this osteotomy. The frontotemporal bone flap and the orbitozygomatic flap are kept in saline solution containing an antibiotic. While protecting the periorbita and the dura mater with self-retaining retractors with spatulas, the remaining major sphenoid wing lateral to the foramen spinosum, forming the posterolateral orbital wall and the anterolateral part of the middle fossa, and the posterior portion of the orbital roof lateral to the superior orbital fissure, are divided, using either a sagittal saw or small chisel (see Fig. 15-1). The remaining medial part of the minor sphenoid wing is then partially removed with an air drill and a bone rongeur. The bone fragments are kept in the saline solution to be replaced at the end of the procedure.

The exposed frontotemporal dura mater is opened in semicircular fashion, from the medial superior orbital margin to the midportion of the inferior temporal region. Alternatively, in a combined orbitozygomatic epidural and subdural approach,[7–9] an inverted T-shaped dural incision is made along the sylvian fissure to the superior surface of the optic nerve sheath forward with a short vertical incision at the distal sylvian fissure. The orbital contents are retracted medially downward by retracting the anterior dural fringe forward.

The operative microscope is now introduced, and either a trans-sylvian approach or a subtemporal approach can be taken with minimal retraction of the brain. In the trans-sylvian approach, the sylvian fissure is widely opened, with

†Deceased.

FIGURE 15-1 *A,* Location of the burr holes and the extent of craniotomy. The first burr hole, made at the frontal bone just behind its zygomatic process, is the "key burr hole." The second burr hole is made at the pterion, the third on the temporal bone just above the pedicle of the zygomatic arch, the fourth in the squamous suture, the fifth in the coronal suture, and the sixth in the frontal bone 3 cm above the orbital ridge. *B,* An orbitozygomatic osteotomy. The zygoma has been well exposed down to the zygomaticofacial canal. The supraorbital canal has been opened by a chisel to prevent its nerve from stretching. The osteotomy of the lateral and superior wall of the orbit is done from the inferior orbital fissure using a reciprocal saw. The orbital content is protected with a spatula during this procedure (the temporal muscle is not drawn). *C,* Osteotomy of the greater sphenoid wing. The dura mater of the frontal base and temporal pole are retracted to expose the greater and lesser sphenoid wings. The line of osteotomy passes 5 to 10 mm lateral to the lateral margin of the superior orbital fissure. (From Oheta K, Baba M: Orbitozygomatic infratemporal approach. In Hakuba A [ed]: Surgical Anatomy of the Skull Base. Tokyo: Miawa Shoten, 1996, pp 1–35.)

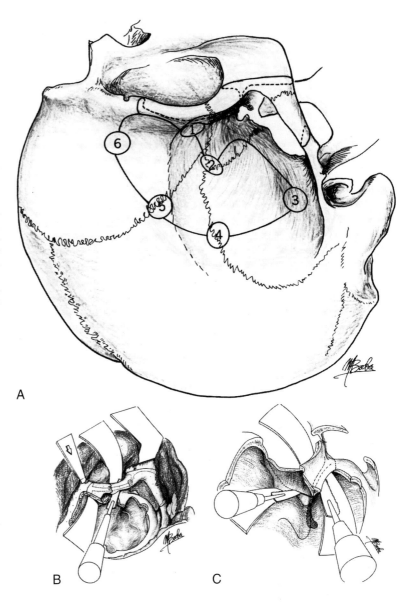

A

B   C

preservation of the bridging veins coming from the tip of the temporal lobe. The parasellar region as well as the interpeduncular fossa can be reached at a short distance through the space formed via this approach.

When the tumor is invading the cavernous sinus (CS),[5] the CS is explored by a combined orbitozygomatic infratemporal epidural and subdural approach, which has been described elsewhere.[7–9] The periosteal reflection, which is continuous with the periorbita, is divided at the superior and inferior margins of the superior orbital fissure by sharp dissection using either microscissors or a knife; then the temporal dura propria, forming the superficial layer of the CS, can be separated from the content of the superior orbital fissure (Fig. 15-2A). The lateral part of the anterior clinoid process is shelled out, leaving a thin layer of its cortical bone. The optic canal is then opened along its length. The cortical bone of the anterior clinoid process and the optic strut are removed by a bone-cutting forceps and a small diamond drill (Fig. 15-2B). The dural incision passes along the sylvian fissure to the superior surface of

the optic nerve sheath forward, then turns laterally at a right angle (Fig. 15-2C). It passes backward at a right angle and runs along the medial part of the distal carotid ring, then along the carotid artery 2 mm away from the artery (Fig. 15-2D). Opening of the medial triangle (Hakuba's triangle, which is a triangle in the subdural space) starts from the distal ring along the medial side of the triangle to the posterior clinoid process and turns laterally at a right angle along the posterior side of this triangle to the dural entrance of the third cranial nerve. The lateral dural fringe of the medial triangle is elevated. Then the remaining outer layer of the CS is separated farther backward from the inner layer of the lateral wall of the CS consisting of the nerve sheaths of the third through fifth cranial nerves (Fig. 15-2E), and the entire CS is unveiled (Fig. 15-2F). Bleeding from the CS is easily controlled by elevating the head side of the table, and the opened venous pathway in the CS is immediately sealed off by insertion of either a fibrinogen-soaked oxidized cellulose sponge or a collagen sponge into the CS, and a bipolar coagulation. Because the intracavernous

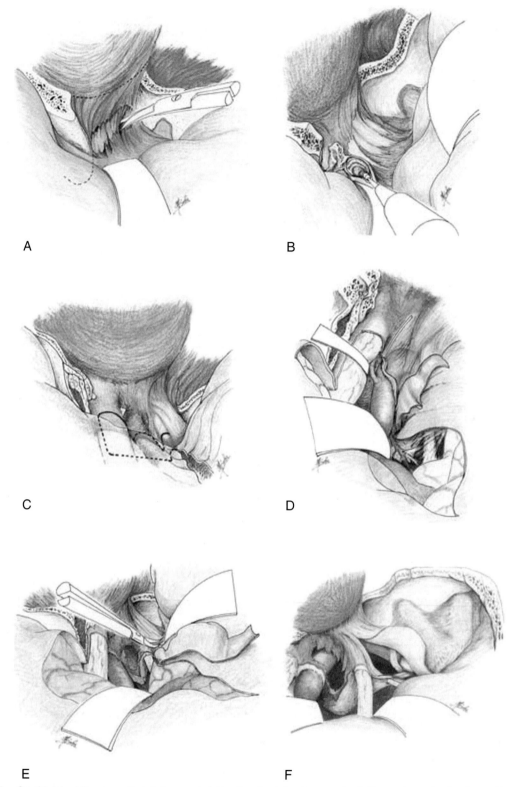

A

B

C

D

E

F

FIGURE 15-2 Combined orbitozygomatic infratemporal epidural and subdural approach. *A,* The periosteal reflection, which is continuous with the periorbita, is divided at the superior and inferior margins of the superior orbital fissure. Then the temporal dura propria, forming the superficial layer of the cavernous sinus (CS), can be separated from the content of the superior orbital fissure. *B,* The cortical bone of the anterior clinoid process and the optic strut are being removed by a bone curette and a small diamond drill, respectively. *C,* Dural opening around the paracavernous region. The dotted line shows the dural incision that passes along the sylvian fissure to the superior surface of the optic nerve sheath forward and is then turned laterally at a right angle. *D,* Dural incision passes backward at a right angle and runs along the medial part of the distal carotid ring and then along the carotid artery. *E,* Peeling off the temporal dura propria, the dural incision runs along the medial side to the posterior clinoid process and finally along the posterior side of the medial triangle (Hakuba's triangle) to the dural entrance of the oculomotor nerve. *F,* Finally, the CS is opened so as to expose the internal carotid artery. (From Oheta K, Baba M: Orbitozygomatic infratemporal approach. In Hakuba A [ed]: Surgical Anatomy of the Skull Base. Tokyo: Miawa Shoten; 1996, pp 1–35.)

internal carotid artery (ICA) has its own dural sheath,[10] the plane between the ICA and the tumor is usually found relatively easily, and the tumor is freed from the ICA if it is not invasive. When the artery is torn during dissection, 8-0 monofilament nylon interrupted sutures are applied while trapping this segment of the artery between two temporary clips at both C3 and either C5 or the intrapetrous portions of the ICA, with intravenous administration of barbiturates for brain protection[8] (pentobarbital 4 mg/kg as the initial dose, followed by 2 mg/kg/hour).

CLOSURE OF THE OPENED PARANASAL SINUS AND DURAL DEFECT

If laceration of the paranasal sinus mucosa is large, it is better to open this sinus wall maximally, and the mucosa of the opened sinus should be removed entirely to prevent postoperative sinusitis and empyema. The opened sinus is closed with a piece of the abdominal fat fixed with fibrin glue. If the laceration of the sinus mucosa is small, the defect is closed by application of a small piece of the temporal muscle. If the mucosa is intact, the bony defect is closed simply with insertion of either a sheet of the temporal fascia or the fascia lata in the epidural space. The dural defect developed by tumor removal is closed by a free pericranial graft. For watertight closure of the dura mater, fibrin glue is applied after approximation of the margins of the graft to the edges of the dura mater using interrupted 6-0 monofilament nylon sutures. Miniplates are used for adequate bone closure to fix the bone flaps to bone edges.

Summary of Cases

Between 1977 and 2000, 124 cases were treated using the orbitozygomatic approach either alone or combined with other approaches, such as the oticocondylar approach[11] or transpetrosal approach.[7] These cases included 28 parasellar meningiomas, 20 pituitary adenomas, 19 basilar tip aneurysms, 12 trigeminal neurinomas, 11 chordomas, 5 internal carotid aneurysms, 13 craniopharyngiomas, 3 CS cavernomas, and 13 other lesions (Table 15-1). Of 28 parasellar meningiomas, 12 patients were men and 16 women. Ages ranged from 35 to 76 years (mean of 53.2 years). Total removal of the tumor was accomplished in 21 cases, subtotal

TABLE 15-1 ▪ Summary of Cases Accessed with Orbitozygomatic Approach

Pathology	No. of Cases
Parasellar meningioma	28
Pituitary adenoma	20
Basilar tip aneurysm	19
Trigeminal neurinoma	12
Chordoma	11
Craniopharyngioma	13
IC aneurysm	5
CS cavernoma	3
Others	13
Total	124

CS, cavernous sinus; IC, internal carotid.

TABLE 15-2 ▪ Surgical Outcome of 28 Parasellar Meningiomas Removed by Orbitozygomatic Approach

Grade	No. of Cases
Excellent	9
Good	15
Fair	3
Poor	1

removal in 6, and partial removal in 1. Postoperative bacterial meningitis and either an epidural or a subdural hematoma was seen in three cases, wound infection in two, and pneumonia in one. In the cases of the tumors involving the CS, impairment of extraocular movement was seen postoperatively in five cases, trigeminal nerve injury in four, and ipsilateral blindness in two. There was no mortality, but four patients developed disturbance of their conscious level (severely disabled in one case and moderately disabled in three). The operative results were classified as follows: excellent, when the patients have no neurologic deficit; good, when the patients have normal activity in daily life with minor neurologic dysfunction; fair, when the patients are moderately disabled but independent with major neurologic deficit; and poor, when the patients are severely disabled and totally dependent. The operative results were excellent in 9 and good in 15 patients (Table 15-2). Three of the remaining four patients were fair postoperatively as a result of bacterial meningitis in one; hypothalamic damage, which had been seen preoperatively, in one; and a combined epidural and subdural hematoma in one. The last one was poor because of a postoperative epidural hematoma. Two representative cases are described briefly.

CASE REPORT 1

The right orbitozygomatic infratemporal approach with a combined epidural and subdural (medial triangle) approach was used on a 57-year-old, right-handed man with a large right parasellar meningioma who had total ophthalmoplegia after partial removal of the tumor in the past (Fig. 15-3). A large tumor occupied the entire CS with encasement of the intracavernous segment of the right ICA. The tumor extended backward subdurally behind the upper clivus with marked compression of the pons and extended inferiorly into the right sphenoid sinus. All the cranial nerves were encased and invaded by the tumor in the CS and had to be sacrificed and removed with the tumor. The intracavernous ICA was carefully dissected out and preserved. The upper basilar artery and its tributaries, which were displaced backward and partially encased, were also well preserved, with total removal of the tumor (Fig. 15-4). The patient had moderate left hemiparesis, which lasted 2 weeks postoperatively; he was neurologically intact except for permanent total ophthalmoplegia at 4 months.

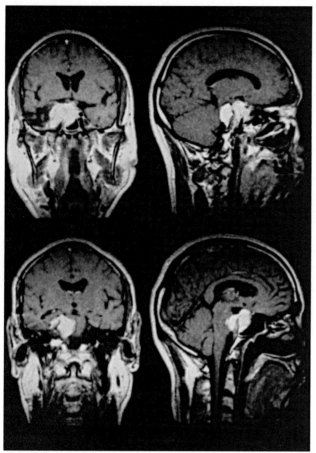

FIGURE 15-3 Case 1: Preoperative T1-weighted magnetic resonance imaging scan with contrast of a right parasellar meningioma that was partially removed previously. The tumor is encasing the right internal carotid artery and extending to the sphenoid sinus anteriorly. It also extends posteriorly, compressing the pons.

CASE REPORT 2

A 57-year-old woman presented with progressive visual deterioration of the left eye. Radiologic study showed a large left parasellar meningioma (Fig. 15-5). A left orbitozygomatic approach was used for total removal of the tumor. The tumor was engulfing the ICA, but it could be easily separated from it because of the presence of arachnoid space between the artery and the tumor. The tumor extended into the left optic canal and compressed the optic nerve. The canal was opened for excision of that part of the tumor. The anterior part of the lateral wall of the CS was invaded by the tumor, but intracavernous structures were not involved by the tumor. The pituitary stalk was shifted and flattened by the tumor. All these structures were preserved, and total removal of the tumor was achieved (Fig. 15-6; see also Fig. 15-5). Postoperatively the patient showed mild left oculomotor palsy, which improved gradually.

DISCUSSION

Radical removal of parasellar meningiomas usually involves difficult surgical procedures.[12] With the orbitozygomatic infratemporal approach, the working distance to the lesions in the parasellar region and the interpeduncular fossa is about 3 cm shorter and the angle to the lesions about 1 to 3 cm lower than with either the pterional or the subtemporal approach. With the combined orbitozygomatic infratemporal epidural and medial triangle approach, the intracanalicular portion of the optic nerve is well exposed, so that much more space can be obtained between the optic nerve and the carotid artery. With this combined approach, the parasellar region, including the CS, and the interpeduncular fossa can be accessed in the shortest possible distance with minimal retraction of the temporal lobe.[2–4] Manipulation of the vital structures is much easier and safer, even with large parasellar meningiomas, than with the conventional operative approaches.

In the orbitozygomatic infratemporal approach, wide exposure of the parasellar lesions can be obtained exclusively by aggressive posterior temporal lobe retraction, which may be at risk of temporal lobe contusion. Surgical strategy should consider the preoperative imaging study of the venous system. The contusion is avoidable by preservation of temporal venous drainage. In the cases of parasellar meningiomas invading the medial sphenoid ridge,

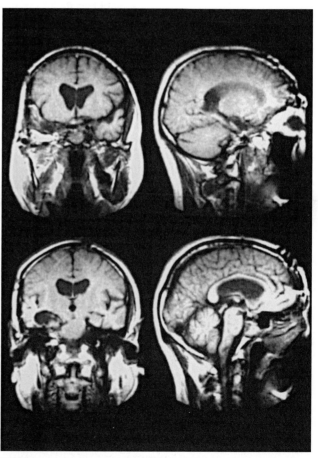

FIGURE 15-4 Case 1: Postoperative study showing the complete removal of the tumor. The sphenoid sinus is repaired with a vascularized temporal musculofascial flap.

FIGURE 15-5 Case 2: (*Top*) Preoperative study of; coronal and axial T1-weighted magnetic resonance imaging scan with contrast injection showing the parasellar meningioma encasing the internal carotid artery and extending to the interpeduncular cistern. (*Bottom*) Postoperative study after total excision of the meningioma.

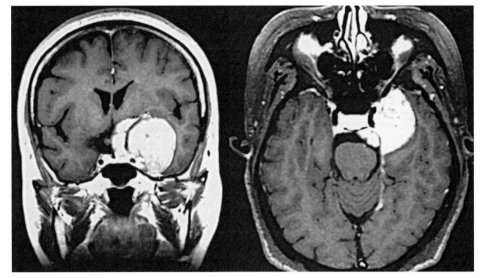
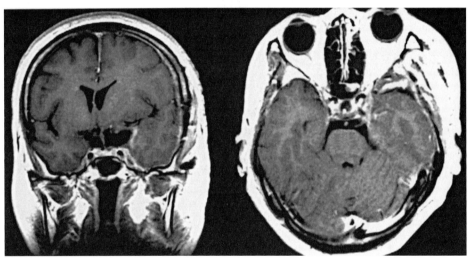

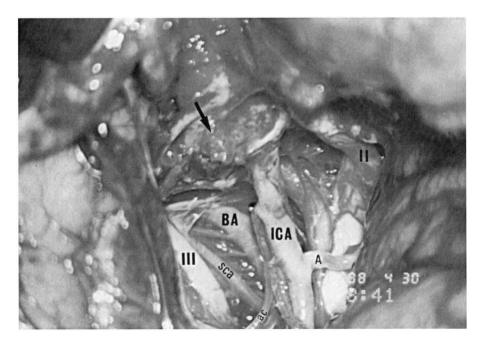

FIGURE 15-6 Case 2: Operative photograph after total excision of the tumor via the orbitozygomatic infratemporal approach with resection of the anterior clinoid process and opening the medial triangle to remove the tumor, involving the lateral wall of the cavernous sinus (CS). Notice the presence of the accessory middle cerebral artery (ac) in this case. The lateral wall of the CS is sealed with fibrin glue-soaked collagen sponge (*arrow*). A, anterior cerebral artery; BA, basilar artery; ICA, internal carotid artery; II and III, second and third cranial nerves; sca, superior cerebellar artery.

the sphenoparietal sinus is usually occluded by tumor and collateral flow via cortical veins is well developed, so that safe posterior temporal lobe retraction is possible after transecting the sylvian vein at its orifice to the sphenoparietal sinus. If the sphenoparietal sinus is patent, an extradural orbitozygomatic approach should be taken for preservation of the venous drainage of the sylvian vein to the pterygoid venous plexus. Peeling off of the temporal dura propria from the inner layer of medial wall of the cavernous sinus is feasible down to the dural entrance of the trochlear nerve.[13] In cases of retrochiasmatic parasellar meningioma in which either the superficial or deep sylvian vein is draining directly into the CS without efficient transcortical collateral circulation, the orbitozygomatic approach risks its damage. In such cases, we select the combined anterior and posterior transpetrosal approach.

The petrosal portion of the ICA, 1 cm long, is epidurally exposed with removal of the petrosal apex at the posterior portion of the trigeminal impression medial to the great petrosal nerve groove by using an air drill. Therefore, when parasellar tumors extend into the CS, the intracavernous portion of the procedure is performed relatively safely while trapping the intracavernous portion of the ICA between its petrosal and C3 portions if necessary.[14] Because the petrosal bone is removed, both medial to the petrosal ICA and anterior to the internal auditory meatus and cochlea, a transzygomatic preauricular transpetrosal approach[9] can be readily carried out. Therefore, parasellar tumors extending into the posterior fossa can be totally removed at one stage with this combined epidural and subdural approach.

If the sphenoparietal sinus is not involved by the parasellar meningiomas, the venous drainage from the sylvian vein should be preserved. Sphenoparietal sinus runs within the dura propria of the temporal lobe and drains usually into the pterygoid venous plexus through the foramen ovale. Preservation of the venous drainage can be done by using the described combined orbitozygomatic epidural and subdural approach, in which the dura propria of the temporal lobe forming the outer layer of the lateral wall of the CS medial to the foramen rotundum and ovale is separated from the inner layer consisting of the dural sheaths of the third and fourth cranial nerves and the first and second branches of the fifth cranial nerve. This dura propria is elevated and retracted backward together with the lateral leaf of the medial triangle opened along its medial and posterior sides. By this means, the infratemporal approach to the interpeduncular fossa can be taken via the temporopolar epidural space without cutting the temporopolar bridging veins.

To preserve the peripheral facial nerve in such low craniotomies, it is necessary to know its topographic anatomy.[15] After exiting from the stylomastoid foramen, the facial nerve crosses the posterior margin of the mandible about 2 cm below the inferior base of the earlobe and enters the parotid gland from behind, where it is situated between the superficial and deep portions of the gland. The branches leave the gland at its superior, anterior, and inferior borders, forming a pattern of rami located superficial to Bichat's fat pad and underneath the facial muscles, entering them from their deep surface. The temporal and zygomatic rami cross the zygomatic arch about 2 cm anterior to the anterior margin of the external auditory canal. Therefore, it is safe to make the skin incision along the anterior margin of the ear cartilage.

The temporal and zygomatic rami of the ipsilateral facial nerve are usually well preserved by elevating the superficial temporal fascia together with the skin flap and subperiosteally dissecting the zygomatic arch and zygomatic bone.

CONCLUSIONS

An orbitozygomatic infratemporal approach to the parasellar region, including the CS, and interpeduncular fossa has been presented and evaluated. We believe that an orbitozygomatic infratemporal approach may provide a better anatomic assessment of the lesions in the parasellar region and interpeduncular fossa and their surrounding structures than the conventional approach. This operation, however, is technically more demanding because familiarity with the use of chisels and sagittal saw, in addition to microsurgical techniques, is essential to its execution.

REFERENCES

1. Hakuba A, Liu SS, Nishimura S: The orbitozygomatic infratemporal approach: A new surgical technique. Surg Neurol 26:271–276, 1986.
2. Chanda A, Nanda A: Anatomical study of the orbitozygomatic transsellar-transcavernous-transclinoidal approach to the basilar artery bifurcation. J Neurosurg 97:151–160, 2002.
3. Lemole GM Jr, Henn JS, Zabramski JM, et al: Modifications to the orbitozygomatic approach [Technical note]. J Neurosurg 99:924–930, 2003.
4. Sindou MP: Working area and angle of attack in three cranial base approaches: Pterional, orbitozygomatic, and maxillary extension of the orbitozygomatic approach. Neurosurgery 51:1526–1527, 2002.
5. Ammirati M, Spallone A, Ma J, et al: An anatomical study of the temporal branch of the facial nerve. Neurosurgery 33:1038–1043, 1993.
6. Ohata K, Baba M: Orbitozygomatic infratemporal approach. In Hakuba A (ed): Surgical Anatomy of the Skull Base. Tokyo, Miwa Shoten, 1996, pp 1–35.
7. Hakuba A: Surgical approaches to the cavernous sinus via the medial triangle: Report of an aneurysm at the C4–C5 junction of the internal carotid artery [Japanese]. Geka Shinryo 26:1385–1390, 1965.
8. Hakuba A, Matsuoka Y, Suzuki T, et al: Direct approaches to vascular lesions in the cavernous sinus via the medial triangle. In Dolenc VV (ed): The Cavernous Sinus. New York: Springer-Verlag, 1987, pp 272–284.
9. Hakuba A, Tanaka K, Suzuki T, et al: A combined orbitozygomatic infratemporal epidural and subdural approach for lesions involving the entire cavernous sinus. J Neurosurg 71:699–704, 1989.
10. Ohata K, Hakuba A, Branco SJ: Development of the meninges: Application to microneurosurgery [Japanese]. In Ishii R (ed): Surgical Anatomy for Microneurosurgery. Tokyo, SIMED Publications, 1997, pp 58–64.
11. Ohata K, Baba M: Otico-condylar approach. In Hakuba A (ed): Surgical Anatomy of the Skull Base. Tokyo, Miwa Shoten, 1996, pp 37–75.
12. Day JD: Cranial base surgical techniques for large sphenocavernous meningiomas [Technical note]. Neurosurgery 46:754–759, 2000.
13. Takami T, Ohata K, Nishikawa M, et al: Transposition of the oculomotor nerve for resection of a midbrain cavernoma [Technical note]. J Neurosurg 98:913–916, 2003.
14. Bruder N, Ravussin P, Young WL, et al: Anesthesia for surgery of intracranial aneurysms. Ann Fr Anesth Reanim 13:209–220, 1994.
15. Millesi H: Extratemporal surgery of the facial nerve—palliative surgery. In Krayenbuhl H, et al (eds): Advances and Technical Standards in Neurosurgery, vol 8. Vienna: Springer-Verlag, 1980, pp 180–308.

SUGGESTED READINGS

Hakuba A, Nishimura S, Jang BJ: A combined retroauricular and preauricular transpetrosal-transtentorial approach to clivus meningiomas. Surg Neurol 30:106–116, 1988.
Hakuba A, Nishimura S, Shirakata S, et al: Surgical approaches to the cavernous sinus: Report of 19 cases [Japanese]. Neurol Med Chir 22:295–306, 1982.

16 Surgical Management of Olfactory Groove Meningiomas

ROBERT G. OJEMANN and ROBERT L. MARTUZA

In their classic monograph published in 1938, Cushing and Eisenhardt[1] described the origin, symptomatology, pathology, and surgical treatment of olfactory groove meningiomas based on careful observations in 29 patients. They clearly described the principles of surgical management, including internal decompression of the tumor before attempting to dissect the capsule, possible involvement of the anterior cerebral arteries, and repair of the defect in the floor of the frontal fossa with a fascial graft.

The clinical presentation, radiographic features, and surgical management of olfactory groove meningiomas have been previously discussed as part of several publications on meningiomas.[2–11] This chapter is based on those publications, a review of the literature, and our personal experience with this tumor.

SURGICAL ANATOMY

Olfactory groove meningiomas arise in the midline of the anterior fossa over the cribriform plate of the ethmoid bone and the area of the suture joining this structure and the sphenoid bone. The tumor may involve any of the area from the crista galli to the planum of the sphenoid bone and may be symmetric around the midline or extend predominantly to one side. The tumor may cause hyperostosis in the bone where the tumor is attached and may grow through the bone into the ethmoid sinus.

The primary blood supply comes from branches of the ethmoidal, meningeal, and ophthalmic arteries through the midline of the base of the skull. The A2 segments of the anterior cerebral arteries are usually separated from the tumor by a rim of cerebral tissue or arachnoid. In large tumors, these arteries may be involved with the tumor capsule. Frontopolar and small branches of the anterior cerebral arteries may be adherent into the posterior and superior tumor capsule and can be taken with the tumor.[5]

With small tumors or with tumors predominantly growing toward one side, the olfactory nerves are displaced laterally on the surface of the tumor, and preserving at least one of these nerves may be possible. When the tumor is large, the olfactory nerve is so adherent and spread out on the capsule of the tumor that it cannot be saved. The optic nerves and chiasm may be displaced downward and posteriorly and can be separated from the tumor.

CLINICAL PRESENTATION

These tumors usually grow slowly, gradually compress the frontal lobe, and cause edema in the adjacent cerebral tissue. In Bakay's[12] series of 36 patients seen between 1950 and 1983, the complaints that led to evaluation in 19 patients were failing vision in 12, dementia in 3, headache in 3, and urinary incontinence in 1.

In 19 patients seen from 1975 through 1992 by one of us (R.G.O.), 14 were women and 5 were men, ranging in age from 24 to 73 years, with 3 older than 70 years of age.[7] The complaints that led to evaluation in 17 patients were mental or personality change in 8, visual loss in 4, visual and mental symptoms in 1, headache and visual loss in 2, headache in 1, and seizure in 1. In two patients, the tumor was asymptomatic and was found on computed tomography (CT) scanning conducted for evaluation of a sinus problem. Many patients had a history of headache, but it was usually not this symptom that led to evaluation. Because of the ability of the cerebral tissue to adapt to slow compression and the relative lack of focal functional cortical regions in the adjacent frontal lobe tissue, these meningiomas can often grow large before causing symptoms. Even when symptoms begin, the patient, family, and colleagues tend to ignore mild and subtle symptoms.

Anosmia had not been an important symptom. Cushing and Eisenhardt[1] reported that loss of the sense of smell was possibly the primary symptom in only 3 of 29 patients, and they questioned the reliability of the records in this regard. In the series of R.G.O., one patient reported on questioning that loss of sense of smell was the first symptom and, in retrospect, had been present for approximately a year before subtle changes in personality were noted. In Bakay's[12] series, all symptomatic patients had anosmia on examination, but in none was it a symptom that led to the diagnosis. He noted that patients are not usually concerned when they gradually lose their sense of smell over a long period of time.

EVALUATION OF RADIOLOGIC STUDIES IN PLANNING THE OPERATION

For many years, the diagnosis of olfactory groove meningiomas was established by CT, and angiography was used to define the general relationship of the anterior cerebral arteries and the blood supply to the tumor. Magnetic resonance imaging (MRI) with gadolinium enhancement is now the preferred radiologic study, because it shows the extent of the tumor in all directions, the relationship of the tumor to the underlying ethmoid and sphenoid sinuses, the amount of edema in the surrounding brain, and, in many patients, the relationship of the optic nerves and anterior cerebral arteries to the tumor capsule (Figs. 16-1 and 16-2). Magnetic resonance (MR) angiography has been used but usually has added little essential information. Preoperative embolization has not been indicated in these patients.

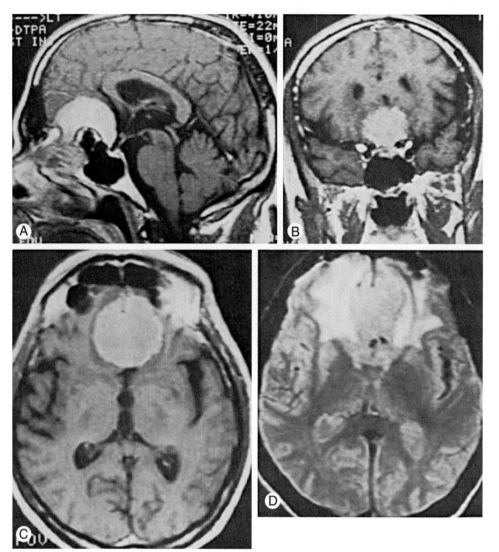

FIGURE 16-1   An olfactory groove meningioma in a 59-year-old man who presented with a 3-year history of subtle changes in personality and mental function. Magnetic resonance images: *A,* Sagittal image (T1) after gadolinium enhancement. This midline view shows the antero-posterior and superior extent of the tumor. There is an unusual projection of bone containing an extension of the air sinus that leads into the base of the tumor. The posteroinferior edge of the tumor is lying on the tuberculum and projects down between the optic nerves. There appears to be a cerebrospinal fluid cistern on the posterior surface of the tumor. The anteroinferior tumor edge projects into the cribriform plate region. *B,* Coronal image (T1) after gadolinium enhancement. This image through the posterior edge of the tumor shows the tongue of tissue projecting down between the internal carotid arteries and over the optic nerves. Other coronal images show that the lateral extent of the tumor has not extended into the air sinuses. *C,* Axial image (T1) after gadolinium enhancement. The lateral extent of the tumor is defined. Edema or gliotic reaction in the adjacent brain surrounds the tumor. *D,* Axial image (T2) without enhancement. The extent of the edema in tissue adjacent to the tumor is defined. The relationship of the A2 segments of the anterior cerebral arteries to the tumor capsule is visible. At operation, the A2 segment of the anterior cerebral artery was separated from the superoposterior capsule by a thin layer of gliotic tissue, and in the midportion of the posterior capsule, the artery was in an arachnoid cistern and loosely adherent to the capsule with small arterial branches. Total removal of the tumor was accomplished, and the patient made a full recovery. Figures 16-3 to 16-9 refer to the surgical treatment of this tumor.

GENERAL ASPECTS OF SURGICAL MANAGEMENT

The objective of the operation is total removal of the olfactory groove meningioma, including the dural attachment, the involved bone, and tumor extension into the ethmoid sinus with preservation and improvement of neurologic function. In most patients with olfactory groove meningiomas, complete removal can be done with low morbidity and good recovery of function. However, in the rare patients in whom total removal carries a significant risk because of

involvement of the major anterior cerebral artery branches, some tumor should be left, and the patient should be followed with periodic MRI scans. Radiation therapy or radiosurgery may be used if the tumor starts to grow.

Age alone does not contribute to the decision for surgery. Of 19 patients in the series of R.G.O., 9 were in their seventh decade and 3 in their eighth.[7] In patients older than 70 years of age with meningiomas, surgery was done if general health was reasonable and neurologic disability was worsening.[13] The incidence of operative morbidity has been low in this group of patients.

FIGURE 16-2 An olfactory groove meningioma in a 47-year-old woman who had a computed tomography (CT) scan to evaluate a sinus problem. There were no neurologic symptoms. *A* and *B*, CT images with contrast show the enhancing lesion in the posterior midline of the floor of the frontal fossa with extension to the right side. There is significant edema in the right frontal lobe. *C* and *D*, Magnetic resonance images (T_1) with gadolinium enhancement. The midline image (*C*) shows the posterior placement of the tumor, the separation from the region of the anterior cerebral arteries, and the chiasm. The image to the right of the midline (*D*) shows the proximity of the right optic nerve to the tumor. Figures 16-10 to 16-12 refer to the surgical treatment of this tumor.

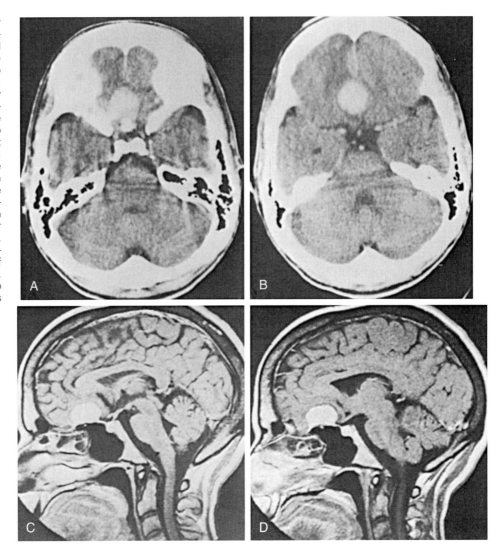

On examination, the sense of smell is usually absent, but if it is still present, as it may be in a small tumor, the patient should be warned about the loss of this function. This symptom is more troublesome after acute loss than it is after gradual loss associated with compression from the tumor. Because olfaction is an important part of the appreciation of flavors, the patient should also be warned that the overall sense of taste may be altered.

In most patients, steroids have been started before operation because of edema. Usually this is only for a 48-hour period preoperatively; however, if edema is abundant and the clinical situation is amenable, steroids may be started 5 to 7 days before surgery. When the patient arrives in the operating room, intravenous antibiotics are given and continued during the operation and for 24 hours afterward.

After induction of anesthesia and insertion of a catheter into the bladder, 10 to 20 mg of furosemide (Lasix) are given, and during the operative exposure, 100 g of mannitol are administered intravenously. Cooperation of a skilled neuroanesthesiologist helps reduce operative morbidity and mortality. A lumbar and subarachnoid drain may also

benefit in exposure and minimize retraction but should not be used in the presence of significant cerebral edema.

BIFRONTAL APPROACH

General Considerations

For patients with large tumors (see Fig. 16-1), we prefer a bifrontal craniotomy. This approach is associated with the least amount of retraction on the frontal lobes, it gives direct access to all sides of the tumor, and it allows decompression of the tumor while the surgeon is working along the base of the skull to interrupt the blood supply. There is no problem from ligation of the anterior aspect of the superior sagittal sinus or coagulation of a few very anterior draining veins in this region. If the frontal sinus is appropriately handled, there should be no complication from entering the sinus.

Hassler and Zentner[14] reported that in 1938 Tonnis described a midline fronto-orbital approach with division of the anterior sagittal sinus and falx and preservation of frontal brain tissue. A bifrontal approach for large tumors is also used by El Gindi,[15] Logue,[16] Long,[17] MacCarty and associates,[18] McDermott and Wilson,[19] Ransohoff and Nockels,[20] and Symon.[21] Various alternative approaches have been suggested, ranging from minimally invasive endoscopic approaches for some tumors as described by Jho and Alfieri,[22] to more extended procedures often involving orbital osteotomies as described by Moore[23] and Fliss[24,25] and their colleagues.

Operative Technique

The patient is carefully placed in the supine position with the knees slightly flexed and the head elevated, slightly extended, and held with the Mayfield-Kees three-point skeletal fixation headrest. Both the anterior cranium and an area of the abdomen are sterilely prepared. A bicoronal incision is made behind the hairline through the galea, and care is taken to preserve the pericranial tissue (Fig. 16-3). The skin along the posterior aspect of the incision is elevated approximately 2 cm, and the pericranial tissue is then incised. This step provides extra pericranial tissue to cover the open frontal sinus floor of the anterior fossa and to use to patch the convexity dura as needed. The skin flap and the pericranial tissue are then turned down together. The temporalis muscle is opened to expose the bone just below the anterior end of the superior temporal line. Burr holes are placed at this point and on each side of the sagittal sinus anterior to the skin incision. The dura is separated from the bone using a Penfield No. 3 dissector. The bone flap may be cut in one piece. For the bone cut just above the supraorbital ridge, the craniotome is used to make a cut on each side as far medially as possible. Usually, this maneuver leaves 1 cm or less of bone in the midline. Because of the irregular bone projecting from the inner table of the skull in this area, cutting completely across the area is usually not possible. The outer table is cut with a small burr on a high-speed air drill, and then the inner table is broken as the bone is elevated and

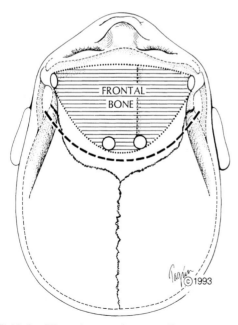

FIGURE 16-3 Bifrontal approach to an olfactory groove meningioma. The position of the skin incision (*dashed line*), burr holes, and free bone flap (*dotted line*) are outlined. (Copyright © 1993, Edith Tagrin.)

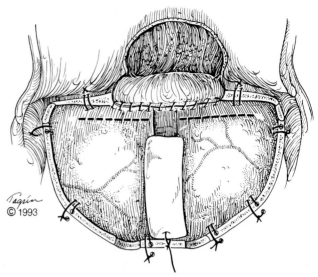

FIGURE 16-4 The opening over the frontal sinus has been covered with a flap of pericranial tissue sutured to the adjacent dura. Before this step, the mucosa of the frontal sinus was removed, and the sinus was packed with Gelfoam soaked with an antibiotic solution. (Copyright © 1993, Edith Tagrin.)

the free bone flap is removed. An alternate method is to cut a right frontal bone flap first and then free the sagittal sinus and cut a second bone flap across the midline to the left side. This is particularly useful when the dura is tightly adherent to the bone.

The frontal sinuses are almost always entered. The mucosa is removed, and the sinuses are rinsed with antibiotic irrigation and packed with adipose tissue removed from a small abdominal incision. A vascularized flap of pericranial tissue from the back of the skin flap is turned down over the sinus and sewn to the adjacent dura (Fig. 16-4). Sutures are placed along the edge of the craniotomy to control epidural bleeding.

The dural incision is made over each medial inferior frontal lobe just above the anterior edge of the craniotomy opening. This incision need not extend more than 3 to 4 cm to each side and is carried medially near the edge of the sagittal sinus (see Fig. 16-4), thereby allowing good exposure yet protecting most of both frontal lobes during the operation. Bridging veins from the anterior frontal lobe to the midline area are coagulated and divided. The frontal lobes are carefully retracted, the sagittal sinus is divided between two 0-silk sutures, and the falx is cut (Fig. 16-5). The frontal lobes are then carefully retracted laterally and slightly posteriorly with the Greenberg self-retaining retractor system. The tumor will come into view in the midline and at times grow into the region of the crista galli and falx. The cerebral cortex is carefully separated from the tumor capsule by division of arachnoid and small vascular attachments. The self-retaining retractors are repositioned.

The anterior capsule of the tumor is then opened, and a biopsy is performed. The anterior and midline portions of the tumor are then removed. The attachments of the tumor in the midline along the base of the frontal fossa are gradually divided, interrupting the blood supply that enters the tumor through numerous openings in the bone in this area (Fig. 16-6). These feeding arteries are occluded with coagulation and, occasionally, bone wax. Monopolar coagulation

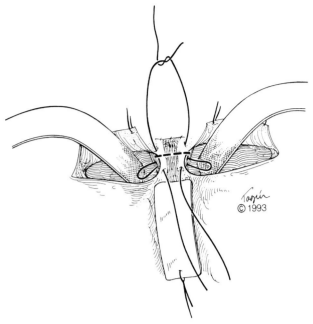

FIGURE 16-5 Ligation of the anterior sagittal sinus. (Copyright © 1993, Edith Tagrin.)

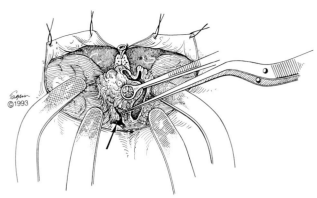

FIGURE 16-7 The capsule of the meningioma is being displaced into the area of internal decompression, and attachments to the frontal lobe are being divided. Minimal retraction is required on the frontal lobe. The frontopolar artery is often adherent to the tumor and may have to be divided. (Copyright © 1993, Edith Tagrin.)

on a coated Penfield No. 4 can be a very effective method of occluding the arteries as they come out of the bone.

The dissection along the base is alternated with internal decompression of the tumor. The ultrasonic aspirator and/or cautery loops are very effective in performing decompression. The capsule now can be reflected into the area of the decompression with minimal pressure on the adjacent frontal lobes (Fig. 16-7). Self-retaining retractors keep the frontal lobes from falling into the decompression area. Great care is taken during the dissection of the posterior portion of the capsule, which is reflected anteriorly while the surgeon looks for the pericallosal branch of the anterior cerebral artery complex. Usually, a rim of cerebral cortex or arachnoid separates the main trunk of the arteries from the tumor, although occasionally the artery may be embedded in the tumor. The frontopolar branch and other small branches are often adherent to the tumor or enter the capsule and may need to be divided (see Fig. 16-7). Symon[21] states,

and we agree, that occluding these arteries does not cause a problem. Following the tumor capsule back to the sphenoid wing and then working medially usually enables the surgeon to identify the anterior clinoid processes and then the optic nerves. At times, seeing the optic nerves may be difficult because of the posterior and inferior compression and the thickened arachnoid. However, under magnification, the tumor can be reflected off the optic nerves (Fig. 16-8). A tongue of tumor may grow down over the dura on the tuberculum (see Fig. 16-1). Once the bulk of the tumor has been removed, the dural attachment is totally excised (Fig. 16-9). If the bone is not involved, removal of the dura is all that is necessary, and the area is covered with a sheet of gelatin sponge.

If hyperostosis is present, should it be removed? This area contains many of the feeding arteries, and Symon[21] stated that the recurrence rate of these tumors was so low that extensive removal of the hyperostosis and entering the ethmoid sinus are not usually indicated. We agree that an extensive resection of bone is not usually needed, but an area of hyperostosis should be drilled off to a point where

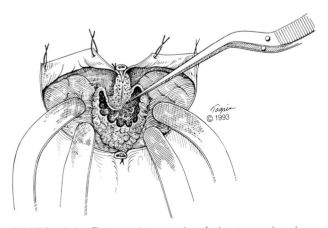

FIGURE 16-6 The anterior capsule of the tumor has been removed, and internal decompression has been started. The blood supply coming through the midline of the frontal fossa is being occluded. (Copyright © 1993, Edith Tagrin.)

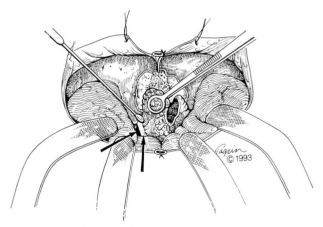

FIGURE 16-8 The capsule of the meningioma has been followed along the floor of the anterior fossa to the region of the anterior clinoid after detachment of most of the base. The left optic nerve and internal carotid artery (*arrows*) have been exposed. The tumor is being separated from the arachnoid over the nerve. (Copyright © 1993, Edith Tagrin.)

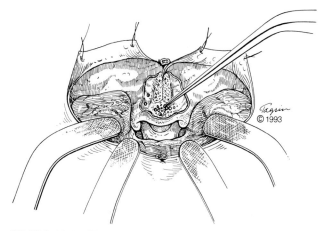

FIGURE 16-9 The tumor has been removed. Multiple holes are visible in the bone where the arterial blood supply entered the tumor. (Copyright © 1993, Edith Tagrin.)

a thin layer of bone is left. We recommend covering the area with an additional piece of adipose tissue held in place with Surgicel and Tisseal if the ethmoid sinus is thought to have been entered.

A special problem occurs if the tumor has grown through the bone into the ethmoid sinus. This occurs in approximately 15% of patients.[26,27] After removal of the involved bone and tumor, the defect is repaired. Long[17] uses several compressed thicknesses of gelatin sponge and fascia lata. Turazzi and colleagues[28] use a pediculated galeopericranial flap. Obeid and Al-Mefty[29] use a vascularized pericranial flap, which we also use, and stress that when recurrence does occur it is the result of incomplete resection of involved bone.

The convexity dura is closed with a free graft of pericranial tissue. The dura and graft are covered with gelatin sponge, and the bone flap is secured with titanium burr hole covers, miniplates, and miniscrews. The operative area is then thoroughly irrigated with antibiotic solution before closure.

UNILATERAL SUBFRONTAL APPROACH
General Considerations

For small tumors (see Fig. 16-2), a right subfrontal approach is usually used unless the tumor is located predominantly on the left side. The approach is from laterally over the orbital roof, with elevation of the frontal lobe. Kempe[30] described this approach, in which the patient's head was turned approximately 60 degrees to the side opposite the craniotomy. Symon[21] uses a unilateral approach for tumors of moderate size, with the head vertically positioned, and he may resect part of the frontal lobe, as does Logue.[16] McDermott and Wilson[19] also use a unilateral subfrontal approach for smaller tumors. We have found that with appropriate positioning and use of osmotic diuretics and a spinal drain, frontal lobe resection is generally not necessary.

Some neurosurgeons use this approach for all olfactory groove meningiomas. Solero and colleagues[31] reported using a unilateral frontal craniotomy and resection of part of the frontal lobe. Seeger[32] combines a bifrontal craniotomy with a unilateral basal approach and partial division of the falx. Hassler and Zentner[14] described a pterional approach as a modification of Seeger's technique. Obeid and Al-Mefty[29] use a unilateral or bifrontal exposure. Babu and colleagues[33]

prefer a unilateral frontal craniotomy with orbital osteotomy. Mayfrank and Gilsbach[34] use a unilateral frontal craniotomy with an interhemispheric approach. Paterniti and colleagues[35] Turazzi and colleagues[28] describe their pterional approach. Yasargil and Abdulraaf[36] usually use a pterional approach; however, when there is extensive bone and mucosal sinus involvement requiring cranial bone repair, a bifrontal approach is used. Sekhar and Tzortzidis[37] describe a combined frontotemporal craniotomy and half-frontal craniotomy with an orbital osteotomy, with most of the tumor dissection done subfrontally.

Operative Technique

The patient is carefully placed in the supine position with the right shoulder slightly elevated. The head is elevated and rotated approximately 60 degrees to the opposite side and held with the Mayfield-Kees skeletal fixation headrest.

The skin incision is made just above the zygomatic process behind the anterior hairline and extends medially to end near the midline at the hairline (Fig. 16-10). If the incision is too far forward or extends below the zygomatic process, the frontal branch of the facial nerve may be injured. The skin, underlying temporalis muscle, and pericranial tissue are turned down together, exposing the anterior and lateral inferior frontal and anterior temporal bone. The temporalis muscle may be cut to expose the zygomatic process. A burr hole is placed just below the anterior end of the superior temporal line (see Fig. 16-10), which allows exposure of the floor of the anterior fossa. Depending on the surgeon's preference, other burr holes are placed as needed. We commonly use two others, as illustrated in Figure 16-10. A free bone flap is then cut. The lateral portion of the sphenoid wing is removed, as is the bone over the antero-superior temporal region. After drill holes are made around the craniotomy opening, dural sutures are placed to control epidural bleeding. The dura is then opened over the inferior

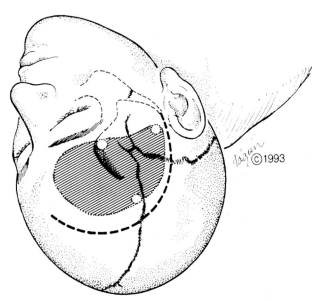

FIGURE 16-10 Right subfrontal approach to an olfactory groove meningioma. The position of the head, skin incision (*dashed line*), burr holes, and bone flap are visible. (Copyright © 1993, Edith Tagrin.)

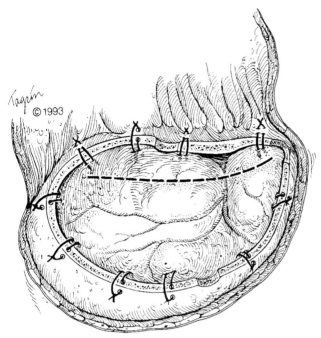

FIGURE 16-11   The skin and pericranial tissue have been turned down together. The bone flap has been elevated, and bone has been removed from the lateral sphenoid wing and over the temporal region. The dural incision is shown (*dashed line*). (Copyright © 1993, Edith Tagrin.)

frontal and anterior temporal region (Fig. 16-11). Draining veins from the anterior temporal lobe along the sphenoid wing are divided, if necessary.

The frontal lobe is carefully elevated over the orbital roof, bringing the tumor into view (Fig. 16-12). The brain is protected, and self-retaining retractors are placed. The olfactory

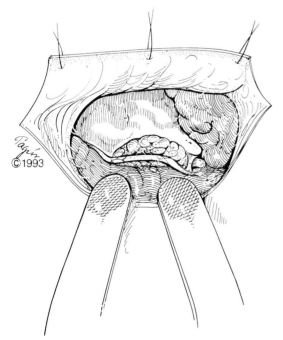

FIGURE 16-12   Exposure of the olfactory groove meningioma from the lateral subfrontal approach. The olfactory nerve is adherent to the tumor. The optic nerve is exposed posterior to the tumor. (Copyright © 1993, Edith Tagrin.)

nerve may be displaced laterally and be densely involved with the surface of the tumor. The posterior capsule is explored and the relationship of the optic nerve defined.

The principles of tumor removal are the same as described for the bifrontal approach. The tumor is internally decompressed, the blood supply is occluded along the base, and the tumor capsule is carefully withdrawn into the area of decompression, dividing attachments as they are encountered. Because these tumors are smaller, preserving the olfactory nerve on one side may be possible. Care is then taken to define the position of the optic nerves. The handling of the area of attachment of the tumor and the closure are the same as described for the bifrontal operation.

IMMEDIATE POSTOPERATIVE MANAGEMENT

Steroid dosages are usually tapered over 4 to 7 days, depending on the patient's neurologic status and the extent of cerebral edema. Antibiotics are continued for 24 hours after surgery. How long anticonvulsant medication should be continued has not been established. If no history of seizures exists, we usually taper anticonvulsant medication after 3 months. If a seizure disorder has been present, anticonvulsants are continued for 6 months to 1 year, and an electroencephalogram is performed to exclude an active focus before tapering off medication. There is considerable difference of opinion about this point.

COMPLICATIONS

The incidence of reported complications has been low since the advent of microneurosurgical techniques.[2–11,14,18,20] The major potential complications include worsening of mental function due to frontal lobe retraction or anterior cerebral artery injury, visual loss, cerebrospinal fluid leak, infection, and postoperative seizures. A cerebrospinal fluid leak through the ethmoid sinus can be closed through a transethmoidal repair.

In several series of patients treated since 1970, the operative mortality rate has also been low. Bakay[12] reported 1 death due to surgery in 11 patients, Symon[21] had no deaths in 18 patients, MacCarty and colleagues[18] reported 1 death in 27 patients, and Ransohoff and Nockels[20] had 2 deaths in 33 patients. In a personal series, R.G.O. noted 1 death occurred in 19 patients because of a pulmonary embolus.[7] Hassler and Zentner[14] had 1 death in 11 patients, also because of a pulmonary embolus. Turazzi and colleagues[28] reported 1 death in 37 patients.

RESULTS

In most patients with olfactory groove meningioma, the tumor can be completely removed and the patient can resume a nearly normal life. In the personal series of R.G.O., disturbance in mental function and personality changes that were present before surgery recovered or improved.[7] This was also the finding of Tarazzi and colleagues.[28]

Patients with preoperative visual symptoms usually recover after surgery. In none of our patients was the vision worse, and headache was usually relieved.

MacCarty and colleagues[18] reported that the survival rate was higher for olfactory groove meningiomas than for any other meningioma sites. Data regarding recurrence were not given. Symon[21], though not giving a specific figure, reported a very low recurrence rate. Chan and Thompson[38] reported no recurrence during a 9-year average follow-up. Ransohoff and Nockels[20] had no recurrence in patients with benign meningiomas. For benign meningiomas, we have not had a recurrence in our patients to date, and this result has been documented in most patients by follow-up MRI or CT.

MANAGEMENT OF PATIENTS WITH ASYMPTOMATIC OLFACTORY GROOVE MENINGIOMAS

With the increasing use of CT and MRI for evaluation of sinus problems and other diseases, an asymptomatic lesion occasionally is found. When evaluating such a patient, the neurosurgeon must consider the size of the lesion, the presence or absence of edema in the adjacent brain, the lesion's proximity to the optic nerves, the age and general health of the patient, and the patient's psychologic response to the presence of the tumor.

We have treated two patients with olfactory groove meningiomas in whom the lesion was found during evaluation for a sinus problem. One is illustrated in Figure 16-2. Surgery was recommended and performed because of edema in the adjacent brain structure and the proximity of the lesion to the optic nerves. Both patients made a full recovery.

REFERENCES

1. Cushing H, Eisenhardt L: Meningiomas: Their Classification, Regional Behaviour, Life History, and Surgical End Results. Springfield, IL: Charles C Thomas, 1938.
2. Ojemann RG: Meningiomas of the basal parapituitary region: Technical considerations. Clin Neurosurg 27:233–262, 1980.
3. Ojemann RG: Surgical management of meningiomas of the tuberculum sellae, olfactory groove, medial sphenoid wing and floor of the anterior fossa. In Schmidek HH, Sweet WH (eds): Operative Neurosurgical Techniques. New York: Grune & Stratton, 1982, pp 869–889.
4. Ojemann RG: Meningiomas: Clinical features and surgical management. In Wilkins RH, Rengachary SS (eds): Neurosurgery. New York: McGraw-Hill, 1985, pp 635–654.
5. Ojemann RG: Olfactory groove meningiomas. In Al-Mefty O (ed): Meningiomas. New York: Raven Press, 1991, pp 383–394.
6. Ojemann RG: Surgical management of olfactory groove and medial sphenoid wing meningiomas. In Schmidek HH (ed): Meningiomas and Their Surgical Management. Philadelphia: WB Saunders, 1991, pp 242–259.
7. Ojemann RG: Management of cranial and spinal meningiomas. Clin Neurosurg 40:321–383, 1993.
8. Ojemann RG: Surgical management of anterior basal meningiomas. In Schmidek HH, Sweet WH (eds): Operative Neurosurgical Techniques, 3rd ed. Philadelphia: WB Saunders, 1995, pp 393–402.
9. Ojemann RG: Supratentorial meningiomas: Clinical features and surgical management. In Wilkins RH, Rengachary SS (eds): Neurosurgery. New York: McGraw-Hill, 1996, pp 873–890.
10. Ojemann RG, Swann KW: Meningiomas of the anterior cranial base. In Sekhar LN, Schramm VSS (eds): Tumors of the Cranial Base: Diagnosis and Treatment. Mount Kisco, NY: Futura, 1987, pp 279–294.
11. Ojemann RG, Swann KW: Surgical management of olfactory groove, suprasellar and medial sphenoid wing meningiomas. In Schmidek HH, Sweet WH (eds): Operative Neurosurgical Techniques, 2nd ed. Orlando, FL: Grune & Stratton, 1988, pp 531–545.
12. Bakay L: Olfactory meningiomas: The missed diagnosis. JAMA 251:53–55, 1984.
13. McGrail KM, Ojemann RG: The surgical management of benign intracranial meningiomas and acoustic neuromas in patients 70 years of age and older. Surg Neurol 42:2–7, 1994.
14. Hassler W, Zentner J: Pterional approach for the surgical treatment of olfactory groove meningiomas. Neurosurgery 25:942–947, 1989.
15. El Gindi S: Olfactory groove meningioma: Surgical techniques and pitfalls. Surg Neurol 54:415–417, 2000.
16. Logue V: Surgery of meningioma. In Symon L (ed): Operative Surgery: Neurosurgery. London: Butterworth, 1979, pp 138–173.
17. Long DM: Meningiomas of the olfactory groove and anterior fossa. In Long DM (ed): Atlas of Operative Neurosurgical Technique, vol 1: Cranial Operations. Baltimore: Williams & Wilkins, 1989, pp 238–241.
18. MacCarty CS, Piepgras DG, Ebersold MJ: Meningeal tumors of the brain. In Youmans JR (ed): Neurological Surgery, 2nd ed. Philadelphia: WB Saunders, 1982, pp 2936–2966.
19. McDermott MW, Wilson CB: Meningiomas. In Youmans JR (ed): Neurological Surgery, 4th ed. Philadelphia: WB Saunders, 1996, pp 2782–2825.
20. Ransohoff J, Nockels RP: Olfactory groove and planum meningiomas. In Apuzzo MLJ (ed): Brain Surgery Complication Avoidance and Management. New York: Churchill Livingstone, 1993, pp 203–219.
21. Symon L: Olfactory groove and suprasellar meningiomas. In Krayenbuhl H (ed): Advances and Technical Standards in Neurosurgery, vol 4. Vienna: Springer-Verlag, 1977, pp 67–91.
22. Jho HD, Alfieri A: Endoscopic glabellar approach to the anterior skull base: A technical note. Minim Invasive Neurosurg 45:185–188, 2002.
23. Moore CE, Ross DA, Marentette LJ: Subcranial approach to tumors of the anterior cranial base: Analysis of current and traditional surgical techniques. Otolaryngol Head Neck Surg 120:387–390, 1999.
24. Fliss DM, Zucker G, Cohen A, et al: Early outcome and complications of extended subcranial approach to the anterior skull base. Laryngoscope 109:153–160, 1999.
25. Fliss DM, Gil Z, Spektor S, et al: Skull base reconstruction after anterior subcranial tumor resection. Neurosurgical Focus 12:1–7, 2002.
26. Derome PJ, Guiot G: Bone problems in meningiomas invading the base of the skull. Clin Neurosurg 25:435–451, 1978.
27. DeMonte F: Surgical treatment of anterior basal meningiomas. J Neurooncol 29:239–248, 1996.
28. Turazzi S, Cristofori L, Gambin R, Bricolo A: The pterional approach for microsurgical removal of olfactory groove meningiomas. Neurosurgery 45:821–825, 1999.
29. Obeid F, Al-Mefty O: Recurrence of olfactory groove meningiomas. Neurosurgery 53:534–542, 2003.
30. Kempe LG: Operative Neurosurgery, vol 1. New York: Springer-Verlag, 1968, pp 104–108.
31. Solero CL, Giombini S, Morello G: Suprasellar and olfactory meningioma: Report of a series of 153 personal cases. Acta Neurochir (Wien) 67:181–194, 1983.
32. Seeger W: Microsurgery of the Cranial Base. New York: Springer-Verlag, 1983.
33. Babu R, Barton A, Kasoff SS: Resection of olfactory groove meningiomas: Technical note revisited. Surg Neurol 44:567–572, 1955.
34. Mayfrank L, Gilsbach JM: Interhemispheric approach for microsurgical removal of olfactory groove meningiomas. Br J Neurosurg 10:541–545, 1996.
35. Paterniti S, Fiore P, Levita A, et al: Venous saving in olfactory groove meningioma surgery. Clin Neurol Neurosurg 101:235–237, 1999.
36. Yasargil MG, Abdulraaf SI: Comment on reference 28. Neurosurgery 45:825–826, 1999.
37. Sekhar LN, Tzortzidis F: Resection of tumors by the fronto-orbital approach. In Sekhar LN, deOliveira EP (eds): Cranial Microsurgical Approaches and Techniques. New York: Thieme, 1999, pp 61–75.
38. Chan RC, Thompson GB: Morbidity, mortality and quality of life following surgery for intracranial meningiomas: A retrospective study in 257 cases. J Neurosurg 60:52–60, 1984.

17

Surgical Management of Tuberculum Sellae and Medial Sphenoid Ridge Meningiomas

VALLO BENJAMIN and STEPHEN M. RUSSELL

Tuberculum sellae and medial sphenoid ridge meningiomas present difficult technical challenges to the neurosurgeon because of their close proximity to the anterior visual pathways, arteries of the anterior circulation, and the hypothalamus. Much has been written about these tumors, but little new information has been added to Cushing and Eisenhardt's classic work with regard to their study of anatomy, behavior, and classification.[1] Great strides, however, have been made in microneurosurgical techniques that enable resection of these tumors with a modest rate of morbidity and mortality when compared with the pioneering efforts of Cushing and earlier surgeons. In this chapter, we discuss the surgical management of tuberculum sellae and medial sphenoid ridge meningiomas. These tumors are discussed separately because of differences in their anatomic relationship to the surrounding vital structures as well as technical considerations.

TUBERCULUM SELLAE MENINGIOMA

Pathologic Anatomy and Classification

Cushing performed the first complete removal of a tuberculum sellae meningioma in 1916, but he did not report it until 1929. In 1938, Cushing and Eisenhardt reported 28 cases of tuberculum sellae meningioma and proposed a classification of four stages according to size.[1] In their often-quoted text, Cushing and Eisenhardt used the term *suprasellar* in their description of tumors arising from the tuberculum sellae dura. This term has led to much confusion in the literature, because subsequent publications have included tumors arising from different locations, such as the medial sphenoid ridge (or clinoidal), optic foramen, olfactory groove, and planum sphenoidale, under the rubric of suprasellar. We believe that tuberculum sellae tumors should and can be distinguished in most cases from these other suprasellar tumors.

The tuberculum sellae is a slight bony elevation in front of the pituitary fossa that measures several millimeters in height and width. Tumors arising from this region are usually 2 to 4 cm in diameter at the time of clinical presentation. Because of the relatively small dimensions of the tuberculum sellae, the dural attachment of these tumors often extends anteriorly to the sphenoid limbus (anterior border of prechiasmatic sulcus) and posteriorly to involve the diaphragm sellae.

It is not useful to subclassify further tumors arising within these boundaries, because with continued growth, all cause elevation of the optic nerves and chiasm and produce the same clinical picture. Although we recognize that the microscopic point of tumor origin may be at either the tuberculum or diaphragma sellae, we refer to these tumors as *tuberculum sellae meningiomas*.

Cushing and Eisenhardt subclassified tuberculum sellae tumors into four groups: (1) initial stage, (2) presymptomatic, (3) favorable for surgery, and (4) late or essentially inoperable.[1] They not only recognized tuberculum sellae meningiomas as a distinct clinical entity but also clarified the importance of tumor growth in relation to the anterior visual pathways and the potential for surgical resection. The introduction of the operating microscope allowed neurosurgeons to better understand the relationship of tumor with its surrounding structures.

Although meningiomas may invade bone and cause hyperostosis, they predominantly arise and grow in the "subdural space," remaining outside the arachnoid (epi-arachnoid). As tumors grow, the arachnoid of the floor of the chiasmatic cistern is pushed up and stretched over the tumor. With continued growth, the tumor encroaches on adjacent cisterns and becomes involved with various layers of arachnoid. The walls of the arachnoid cisterns provide a natural barrier between the meningioma and the arteries and nerves that course within the subarachnoid space.

The optic nerves are displaced and stretched superiorly and laterally by the tumor. Because the nerves are fixed at the optic foramen, they become angulated and compressed at this site. These tumors may grow eccentrically and involve one optic nerve to a greater degree than the other, and one or both of the nerves may be completely enveloped by tumor. The internal carotid arteries (ICAs) are displaced laterally but usually less than the optic nerves, and tongues of tumor may insinuate themselves between these two structures. Large tumors may completely encase the carotid vessels. Generally the anterior cerebral arteries (ACAs), which are located dorsal to the optic chiasm, are stretched, but on rare occasions they may be encased by tumors larger than 4 cm. With further growth, tumor extends behind the sella turcica into the interpeduncular cistern. The pituitary stalk is usually displaced posteriorly. Extremely large tumors may compress the third ventricle and cause hydrocephalus. Rarely, tumors can extend into the cavernous sinus (CS).

Tuberculum sellae tumors may spill over the planum sphenoidale. These tumors are distinguished from growths arising primarily from the planum, because they elevate the anterior visual pathways, whereas the planum sphenoidal tumors depress the anterior visual pathways. Likewise, olfactory groove meningiomas also depress the anterior visual pathways. Medial sphenoid ridge meningiomas displace the optic apparatus medially and are discussed later.

Clinical Presentation

Tuberculum sellae meningiomas constitute 4% to 10% of intracranial meningiomas.[1-3] The actual incidence is difficult to ascertain because in most series, the tumor has not been distinguished from other so-called suprasellar tumors. As with meningiomas in other locations, tuberculum sellae meningiomas occur much more frequently in women than men, usually presenting in the 30s and 40s.

With tuberculum sellae meningiomas and other so-called suprasellar meningiomas, visual failure was the most common complaint in 93% to 100% of patients.[4-6] The incidence of headache, the second most common symptom, varied from 12% to 45%.[3,5,7] In 1984, Symon and Rosenstein reviewed their series of 101 patients with so-called suprasellar meningiomas and reported that the most common signs on admission were visual field defects (100%), loss of visual acuity (99%), and optic atrophy (85%).[5] Papilledema, Foster-Kennedy syndrome, and oculomotor nerve palsy were rare findings. Signs of hypothalamic-hypophyseal dysfunction are also reported to be rare.[3,5] Mental changes, anosmia, neurologic deficits, and seizures are uncommon, and their incidence may, in part, reflect series with more heterogeneous tumor locations. In the senior author's own experience with 23 patients who were operated on from 1983 to 2003, all patients presented with visual deterioration, whereas none demonstrated motor deficits, endocrinopathy, or cognitive dysfunction.[8]

Cushing and Eisenhardt called attention to the chiasmal syndrome produced by tuberculum sellae meningioma. They noted a tendency toward bitemporal field defects, but more commonly the fields were asymmetric, and one eye often was blind. This situation occurred in adult patients with optic atrophy and a normal sellae on plain skull x-ray study. However, a prechiasmal syndrome, in which incongruity and asymmetry of the field defects are a common finding when the chiasm is displaced upward and posteriorly, may be technically more applicable to these tumors. The most common pattern of vision loss is gradual or rapid progressive visual loss in one eye, followed by gradual decrease in the acuity of the contralateral eye. Diagnosis is delayed for an average of 2 years from the onset of symptoms to diagnosis.[9,10] The visual disturbance is often misdiagnosed as retrobulbar neuritis. Pregnancy may aggravate the symptoms. The prompt diagnosis of these lesions requires a high index of suspicion by an ophthalmologist, particularly in elderly patients with failing vision and optic atrophy.

Preoperative Evaluation

Magnetic resonance imaging (MRI) with gadolinium enhancement is the diagnostic study of choice because it provides the 3-dimensional information of the tumor's anatomy and relationship with surrounding structures, including the brain, anterior visual pathways, arteries of the anterior circulation, and extent of dural origin (Fig. 17-1).

Gadolinium-enhanced MRI allows tumors arising from the tuberculum sellae to be distinguished from other so-called suprasellar tumors with a greater degree of accuracy than does computed tomography (CT). It may be difficult, however, to distinguish between a pituitary macroadenoma with suprasellar extension and a tuberculum sellae meningioma with intrasellar extension in certain cases. The imaging characteristics that are consistently seen in MRI studies of tuberculum sellae meningiomas but that are absent in those of pituitary macroadenomas are homogeneous enhancement with gadolinium, a suprasellar epicenter, a tapered dural base,[11] and normal sella dimensions.

The typical CT scan shows a densely enhancing round mass in the midline above the sella extending laterally and anteriorly. CT scanning is reserved for patients with suspected hyperostosis of the skull base, which is best appreciated with a CT scan with bone windows.

Cerebral angiography is not helpful and has been largely replaced by MRI and MR angiography. Elevation of both anterior cerebral arteries is the most common finding. The intracranial portion of the ICA may be displaced laterally, and rarely a tumor blush may be seen. These angiographic findings are often indistinguishable from the findings of a pituitary adenoma with suprasellar extension.

All patients should be examined by a neuro-ophthalmologist preoperatively to document visual acuity and to perform visual field examination. If hypothalamic-hypophyseal dysfunction is present, a complete series of endocrinologic studies should be obtained, and the patient should have a consultation with an endocrinologist.

Patient Selection and Decisions in Management

Optimal treatment of tuberculum sellae meningiomas is total surgical removal, including the dura and invaded bone, if possible. Conventional or stereotactic radiation therapy is not advocated for initial treatment because of the tumor's location next to the optic apparatus. However, radiation therapy may be an adjuvant treatment for recurrent or residual tumor that is deemed surgically inaccessible or in an elderly or medically compromised patient. Preoperative embolization is not feasible, because the tumor's arterial supply originates from the internal carotid circulation.

These tumors may be approached through three cranial bone openings: the bifrontal, unilateral frontal, and pterional. Advocates of the subfrontal approach believe it provides maximal exposure of the sellar region. Disadvantages include the risk of damage to the olfactory nerve and the potential for infection and cerebrospinal fluid (CSF) rhinorrhea as a result of opening of the frontal sinus. Others recommend removing the supraorbital arch with the subfrontal approach for optimal exposure of the sella. We resect tuberculum tumors via a pterional craniotomy. This approach does not jeopardize the olfactory nerves, and it does not subject the patient to the risks of CSF rhinorrhea or infection from transgression of the frontal sinus. Generous removal

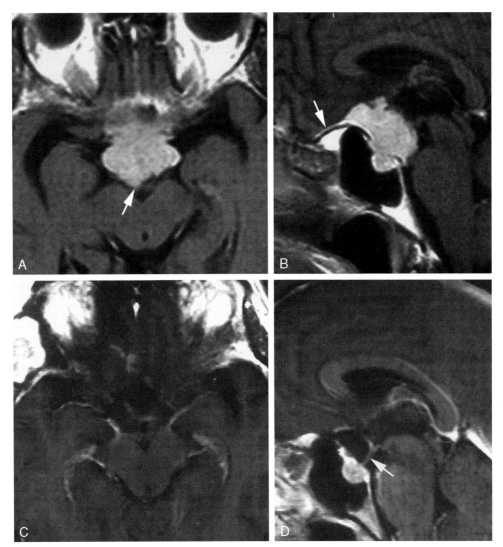

FIGURE 17-1   MRI with gadolinium enhancement in a patient with a 4 × 4 × 3 cm tuberculum sella meningioma. Representative axial (A) and sagittal (B) images obtained preoperatively demonstrate the tumor compressing the optic apparatus, extending into the sella, and compressing the interpeduncular cistern (arrow in A). A dural tail can be identified on the sagittal image extending anteriorly over the planum sphenoidale (arrow in B). This patient underwent a right pterional craniotomy and microsurgical resection of her tumor (see Fig. 17-2). Postoperative axial (C) and sagittal (D) images with gadolinium confirmed a gross total resection. Preservation of the pituitary stalk (arrow in D) and gland can be seen on the sagittal image. This patient has remained free of recurrence for 4 years, as documented with serial MRIs.

of the sphenoid ridge extradurally and a wide dissection of the sylvian fissure allows closest access to the suprasellar region with less brain retraction compared with the subfrontal approach. The only disadvantage is that the undersurface of the ipsilateral optic nerve and chiasm are not as well visualized as with the subfrontal approach. In our opinion, this minor disadvantage does not warrant exposing the patient to the risks and potential complications of a bifrontal craniotomy with anosmia. Generally the craniotomy flap is on the side of the nondominant hemisphere. If the tumor extends eccentrically between the optic nerve and carotid artery on one side, however, we approach the lesion from the ipsilateral side. This approach permits optimal surgical exposure for resection with no significant risk of injury to either the carotid artery or the optic nerve. If one eye is blind, the approach is from the amblyopic side, which permits optimal exposure for decompression of the less involved optic nerve.

Surgical Technique

At surgery, steroids, anticonvulsants, and a broad-spectrum antibiotic are administered. Although a spinal drain may be used, with opening the sylvian and suprasellar cisterns an adequate volume of CSF can be released. For this reason we do not routinely use a spinal drain for these tumors. The patient is placed in the supine position, and the operating table is flexed to place the head above the level of the heart to facilitate venous drainage. The head is rotated 35 degrees, bringing the medial half of the sphenoid ridge to a vertical position. To minimize brain retraction and achieve maximal exposure of the skull base, the head is extended approximately 25 degrees. It is secured in position with a three-pin fixation device.

We use a standard pterional craniotomy, as described by Yasargil.[12] The incision is started at the zygomatic arch, less than 5 mm anterior to the tragus to avoid injury to the frontal branch of the facial nerve, which courses over the zygomatic arch more anteriorly. The incision curves upward and forward within the hairline and loops backward for 1 or 2 cm on the opposite side of the midline. This approach provides adequate cranial exposure and keeps the incision off the forehead. The plane of dissection during reflection of the scalp flap is between the two layers of the true temporalis muscle fascia at the fat pad to avoid injury to the frontal nerve branch, which courses in the superficial fascia. The temporalis muscle and its true fascia are incised by electrocautery and reflected inferiorly and posteriorly over the ear.

A burr hole is made at the frontozygomatic suture. The second hole is made in the squama of the temporal bone just behind the greater wing of the sphenoid. The greater sphenoid wing is then thinned with a high-speed drill and removed with a rongeur, and a free frontotemporal bone flap is cut with the craniotome. The remaining portion of the sphenoid wing is drilled out extradurally to allow an unobstructed exposure of the skull base. The dura is then opened parallel to the skull base and reflected posteriorly to expose the sylvian fissure.

From this point on, the operating microscope is used. The arachnoid of the sylvian fissure must be opened widely to expose the tumor through the fissure, rather than from underneath the frontal and temporal lobes. The distal fissure is opened first and then dissected proximally. A single retractor is used to elevate the frontal lobe and expose the tumor. Temporal lobe retraction is not needed in the majority of cases. Exposed brain is covered with rubber Penrose drains, which we have found to be helpful in preventing cortical injury.

Surgical resection of a tuberculum sellae tumor is depicted in sequential intraoperative photographs in Figure 17-2. After the tumor has been exposed, high-power magnification is used to identify the optic nerves, which are located on the anterolateral surface of the tumor. With large tumors, the optic nerves may be difficult to identify because these nerves have either been thinned by extreme compression, or have been covered by a sheath of tumor.

The dural feeders to the tumor attachment are coagulated before debulking the tumor. These vessels travel along the planum sphenoidale and the lesser wing of the sphenoid. Generally the safest point to start internal decompression is in the midline, at the anterior limit of the tumor. The optic nerves are least likely to be injured at this point. If, however, the patient has long-standing blindness in one eye with optic atrophy, the nerve may be sectioned at its entrance into the optic canal to facilitate tumor removal and preservation of the intact contralateral optic nerve.

The overlying arachnoid is cut with microscissors, and conventional suction and bipolar coagulation are adequate for debulking the interior of the tumor. The ultrasonic aspirator may be difficult to use, because it requires an awkward angle. A laser is not used because of the close proximity and varied location of vessels that may be inadvertently injured. During the initial decompression, a 2- to 3-mm carpet of tumor should be cauterized and left at the dural attachment. This avoids troublesome bleeding from the bone that may result when tumor and involved dura are stripped off the skull. This residual tumor will be removed at the end of the operation.

The interior of the tumor is gutted, leaving an outer rim of tumor tissue. The contralateral optic nerve and carotid artery are easy to decompress with the pterional approach. The operation should begin with dissection of these structures. The surgeon then proceeds in a circumferential fashion to remove tumor from underneath the optic chiasm. The tumor on the ipsilateral carotid artery and optic nerve is removed last, because visualization of these structures is less optimal with the pterional approach.

At this point, most of the tumor will have been removed; this relaxes the arachnoid–tumor interface and facilitates dissection. Dissection of the tumor from the carotid arteries and optic nerves is performed by grasping the tumor with microbipolar forceps and gently pulling it away from these structures while cauterizing (using low power and continuous Ringers lactate irrigation) and shrinking the tumor. The bits of cauterized tumor are removed piecemeal with microdissectors. The interface between tumor and arachnoid should be identified using high-power magnification. The surgeon should avoid violating the arachnoid membrane as much as possible and perform the dissection in the plane between the tumor and the arachnoid to preserve vessels and nerves that lie in the subarachnoid space. Angled microdissectors, angled bipolar forceps, and dental mirrors are helpful in removing tumor from the undersurface of the ipsilateral carotid artery and optic nerve. After decompression of the optic apparatus and carotid arteries, the pituitary stalk, which has a reddish orange color, is identified and preserved. Removal of the most posterior aspect of the tumor exposes the arachnoid of the interpeduncular cistern (Liliequist's membrane). Extension into the optic foramen may require drilling of the anterior clinoid and the optic canal for additional exposure.

After the tumor has been removed, the dural attachment and remnants of tumor at the base of the skull should be coagulated and, if possible, resected. Involved bone should be removed using a small carbide cutting burr. If the sphenoid sinus is entered, the defect is repaired with an appropriate piece of temporalis muscle, which is secured in position with autologous fibrin glue.

At the conclusion of the procedure, the dura is closed, and the remaining closure is handled in a routine manner. A subgaleal drain is left in place for 24 hours. After surgery, the patients should be monitored for diabetes insipidus. We closely follow urine volume and specific gravity as well as serum electrolytes and osmolarity. Steroids are slowly tapered, and the patients should be followed closely for pituitary dysfunction. A postoperative MRI scan is crucial for determining the completeness of surgical resection (see Fig. 17-1).

Results

A summary of contemporary operative series of tuberculum meningiomas appears in Table 17-1.[8,10,13–16] A review of various recent reports on tuberculum sellae meningiomas demonstrates operative mortality rate ranging from 0% to 9%. Higher mortality rates were recorded before 1970, particularly in older series, when catastrophic vascular injury was frequent. A considerable increase in the rates of mortality, morbidity, and failure of visual improvement occurs in cases in which the tumor size exceeds 3 cm. Postoperative morbidity is common in all series and includes visual loss, diabetes insipidus, panhypopituitarism,

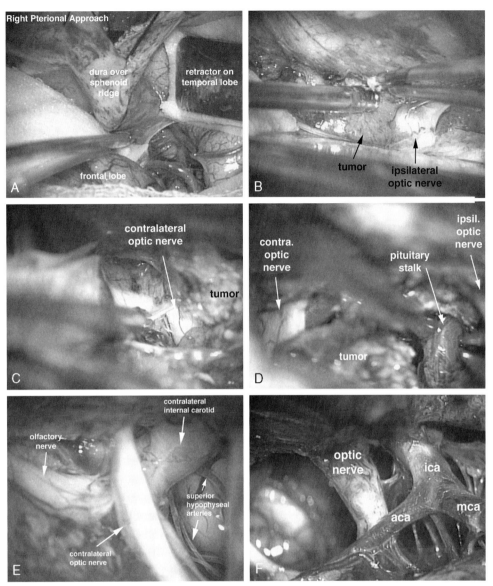

FIGURE 17-2 Serial intraoperative photomicrographs of a tuberculum sella meningioma being resected via a right pterional approach. *A,* Following craniotomy, the dura is opened in a curvilinear fashion and draped over the sphenoid ridge. The sylvian fissure is split widely, and before the tumor resection, a retractor is placed on both the frontal and temporal lobes. A piece of Penrose drain covered with a cottonoid is placed under the retractor to protect the cortical surface. *B,* Early in the tumor resection, the ipsilateral optic nerve is uncovered (*arrow*). Tumor underneath this nerve is left untouched, to be removed later in the procedure. *C,* After resecting the anterior portion of the tumor, the contralateral optic nerve is also identified. Following its identification, tumor is then removed from both above and below this nerve, exposing the contralateral ICA and its medial branches. *D,* Once the contralateral optic nerve has been fully decompressed, the tumor is removed from along the chiasm and then deep in the midline, exposing the pituitary stalk that is displaced posteriorly by the tumor. *E,* View of the region surrounding the contralateral optic nerve following resection. The contralateral ICA, olfactory nerve, and superior hypophyseal arteries are preserved. *F,* View of the region surrounding the ipsilateral optic nerve following resection. The ipsilateral ICA, ACA, and MCA, along with their lenticulostriate branches, are preserved. Though not seen in this postoperative image, the ipsilateral olfactory nerve and pituitary stalk were not damaged during the exposure and tumor resection.

anosmia, rhinorrhea, meningitis, cerebral infarction, and diencephalic dysfunction.

The percentage of patients with suprasellar meningioma having complete excision has varied from 44% to 98%. Recurrence rates, when reported, are generally less than 10%. Tumor recurrence is related to incomplete surgical resection. The most commonly cited reason for incomplete resection was to avoid major vascular injury.

With regard to visual function, except for patients with total blindness, improvement of visual acuity was the rule,

even in cases of long-term duration. The reported rate of visual improvement was 42% to 80%. Best results were obtained in patients who had been operated on within 1 year of the onset of visual symptoms. Postoperative visual deterioration can occur and may be due to a variety of problems, including inadequate tumor decompression, direct surgical trauma or compromise of vascular supply to the optic apparatus, and postoperative suprasellar hematoma.

In the senior author's series of 23 consecutive patients over a 19-year period, the average tumor diameter was 3.2 cm,

TABLE 17-1 ▪ Contemporary Studies of Tuberculum Sellae Meningiomas in the Peer-Reviewed Literature*

Series	Year	No. of Patients	Average Size (cm)	Average Follow-up	Mortality (%)	Gross Total Resection (%)	Improved Vision (%)	Recurrence (%)
Ojemann et al[13]	1995	23	NA	NA	0	44	67	NA
Raco et al[14]	1999	69	3–9	>3 yr	7	91	NA	NA
Ohta et al[15]	2001	33	NA	10.7 yr	NA	63	42	20
Fahlbusch and Schott[16]	2002	47	1–4	4.3 yr	0	98	80	4
Goel et al[10]	2002	70	NA	46 mo	3	84	70	1
Jallo and Benjamin[8]	2002	23	3.2	9.3 yr	9	87	55	4

NA, not available.
  *Patients without tuberculum sellae meningiomas were excluded.

and all patients underwent resection via a pterional approach.[8] Twenty patients had total tumor removal, and 3 had subtotal tumor resections. There was one regrowth in the subtotal tumor removal group, and there were no recurrences in the total tumor removal group. Patients were observed for a mean follow-up time of 9.3 years (range, 3 to 19 years). Visual acuity improved in 55%, was unchanged in 26%, and worsened in 19% of patients. Two of the oldest patients died from pulmonary complications, resulting in a mortality rate of 9%.

MEDIAL SPHENOID RIDGE MENINGIOMA

Pathologic Anatomy and Classification

Cushing and Eisenhardt were the first to describe medial sphenoid ridge meningiomas accurately.[1] They distinguished between global tumors, which are somewhat spherical in shape, and hyperostosing (en plaque) tumors, which are flat and cause bony invasion and reaction along the entire ridge. Medial sphenoid ridge tumors may grow from any point along the ridge and were divided into four groups: (1) deep or clinoidal third, (2) middle third or alar, (3) outer third or pterional, global, and (4) outer third or pterional, hyperostosing. Only global meningiomas arising from the deep or clinoidal third of the sphenoid ridge (i.e., medial sphenoid ridge tumors) will be discussed here. These tumors present a much more complex and difficult surgical problem than do lateral sphenoid ridge meningiomas, because they invariably involve the arteries of the anterior circulation, anterior visual pathways, and other cranial nerves. Although some medial sphenoid ridge meningiomas invade the CS, a separate category of meningiomas originate within the CS. Pure CS meningiomas, which present with extraocular motor nerve palsies, involve the visual pathways to a much smaller degree and require different management; thus they are excluded from this discussion. Small tumors of the optic foramen, which are often discovered early in their course and do not involve the carotid artery, are not considered within the medial sphenoid ridge group. Such lesions are classified as meningiomas of the optic canal, foramen, or sheath.

Cushing and Eisenhardt's original description of medial sphenoid ridge meningiomas was based on the relationship of the tumor to the bony ridge. We place more emphasis on the tumor's relationship to the various arachnoid cisterns,

vascular structures, and optic apparatus to understand the gross pathologic anatomy and develop a strategy for their surgical resection. In large tumors that occupy the entire length of the ridge, it may be difficult to distinguish between lateral and medial origins of growth preoperatively. Tumors that involve the carotid artery and other vessels are considered to be true medial ridge meningiomas.

Medial sphenoid ridge meningiomas arise from the dura over the frontal and temporal aspects of the lesser sphenoid wing as well as the anterior clinoid. With large growths, the dural attachment extends to the petroclinoid fold and tentorium. Involvement of the dura of the tuberculum sellae and cavernous sinus is less frequent. As described previously with tuberculum sellae tumors, meningiomas arising from the medial sphenoid ridge grow in the "subdural space" but remain outside the arachnoid. Despite the complete encirclement of the cranial nerves and arteries by the growing neoplasm, the arachnoid membranes and constant flow of CSF in the basal cisterns form a separable interface around these structures. Less commonly, tumor is directly adherent to these structures. This may occur with large and neglected tumors. The intracavernous cranial nerves and carotid artery lack an arachnoid investment, as does the initial 2- to 3-mm segment of the intracranial ICA as it arises from the CS. Tumor may adhere at these sites. This arachnoid–CSF interface is also absent in patients who have had previous surgeries, because it is disrupted at the time of the first procedure.

The carotid artery and optic nerve are displaced medially by the tumor. With further growth, the tumor ultimately engulfs the ICA and middle cerebral artery (MCA), the ACA, and their central perforating branches. The tumor can be divided into an anteromedial and a posterolateral section in relation to the arterial tree. The small perforators are always in a cleft of arachnoid between the anterior and posterior portion of the tumor. With large growths, the ipsilateral optic nerve and chiasm may be paper thin, displaced medially, and often engulfed by the tumor.

Tumor may extend into the orbit through the optic foramen and superior orbital fissure. With extremely large growths, the tumor grows anteriorly into the frontal fossa, elevating the frontal lobe, and posteriorly over the tentorium and posterior clinoid region, and it may extend into the posterior fossa. The dura of the petroclinoid fold and lateral wall of the CS is frequently involved and, less commonly, the CS itself.

Clinical Presentation

Sphenoid ridge meningiomas account for approximately 20% of supratentorial meningiomas, of which fewer than half arise from the medial ridge.[17] There is a preponderance of middle-aged women in all series. The onset of symptoms is insidious, usually developing over a 2-year period. In our series of 35 patients and in other series, visual loss is the most common presenting complaint.[18,19] Vision loss is usually unilateral and may often progress to blindness, but it is infrequent in the contralateral eye. Visual field abnormalities are variable, depending on the involvement of the chiasm and the optic tract. Funduscopic examination commonly reveals optic atrophy and, less frequently, contralateral papilledema (Foster-Kennedy syndrome). Oculomotor dysfunction and facial hypoesthesia occur when tumor involves the CS and superior orbital fissure. Exophthalmos is due to tumor extension into the orbit and CS. Headache and orbital pain may precede visual symptoms by many years. Intellectual deterioration and changes in cognition are frequently observed, particularly in elderly patients in whom the tumor is on the same side as the dominant cerebral hemisphere. Hemiparesis, aphasia, and seizures are seen less frequently.

Diagnostic Studies

MRI with gadolinium contrast is the best preoperative examination to delineate accurately the tumor and its dural attachment as well as its extension into the orbit, CS, and tentorial incisura (Fig. 17-3). MRI also defines the relationship between tumor and major intracranial arteries[20] and is the procedure of choice in postoperative follow-up. The position of the optic nerve and chiasm can be seen on T_1-weighted images, particularly in tumors less than 3 cm in size. T_2-weighted images best delineate the amount of cerebral edema. A CT scan with bone windows is performed on patients in whom MRI demonstrates invasion of bone and hyperostosis of the skull base.

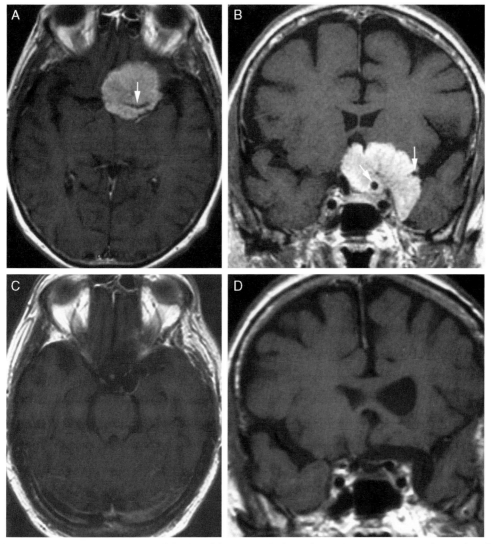

FIGURE 17-3 A representative patient with a medial sphenoid ridge meningioma that underwent a gross total resection. Preoperative axial (*A*) and coronal (*B*) MR images with enhancement demonstrating a meningioma arising from the medial third of the sphenoid ridge with extensive arterial encasement (*arrows*). This patient underwent a left-sided pterional craniotomy and microsurgical resection of her tumor. Postoperative axial (*C*) and coronal (*D*) MR images with enhancement documented a gross total tumor resection.

Cerebral angiography should be performed in tumors larger than 3 cm to determine the status of the intracranial arteries and define the blood supply to the tumor. With tumors smaller than 3 cm, preoperative angiography is not necessary. When indicated, cerebral angiography should include selective internal and external carotid catheterization to evaluate the anterior cerebral circulation and the dural blood supply of the tumor. Angiography shows elevation and stretching of the ICA, MCA, and ACA on the anteroposterior and lateral views. In large tumors, segmental narrowing or irregularity of the vessels may be seen, but complete vessel occlusion is rare. The ICA often supplies blood to the neoplasm through the recurrent meningeal artery (a branch of the ophthalmic artery) and through the cavernous branches from the inferior lateral trunk (the ramus sinus cavernosi). The extracranial dural blood supply includes the middle meningeal artery, the artery of the foramen rotundum, and the accessory meningeal and deep temporal arteries, which can be demonstrated by superselective catheterization of the external carotid artery. Embolization of the external carotid blood supply helps minimize blood loss in large and hypervascular tumors.

When dissection of the CS is contemplated, a preoperative temporary balloon occlusion test with neurologic monitoring and xenon/CT measurements of cerebral blood flow helps define the risk of ICA occlusion.[21] Neurologic deficits produced by test occlusion are an indication that the patient is at high risk for cerebral infarction if the carotid artery were to be occluded. Those who clinically tolerate temporary occlusion but who have reductions in cerebral blood flow in the range of 15 to 35 mL/100 g/minute are at moderate risk for cerebral infarction should permanent occlusion of the carotid be necessary.

As with tuberculum sellae meningiomas, documented visual field and acuity examinations are mandatory in the preoperative evaluation of these patients. A thorough general medical evaluation is important, especially in elderly patients, because these operations are lengthy and may require induced hypotension when hypervascular tumors are resected.

Patient Selection and Decisions in Management

Many surgeons who have become cautious as a result of the high morbidity and mortality rates of radical resections of medial sphenoid ridge meningiomas have been content with partial removal. However, partially resected tumors frequently recur and have been treated with repeated surgery and radiation therapy. Repeat surgery is associated with significantly higher rates of morbidity and mortality because the tumor adheres to vital structures. Tumors may regrow despite radiation therapy, and in our experience, radiation is less effective if a large amount of tumor is left behind.[22] Al-Mefty and Sekhar have advocated aggressive surgical resection of these tumors with dissection of the CS.[19,21] It is not clear whether in the long term the patient benefits most from more extensive surgery, with its increased risk of morbidity, or whether a radical removal of tumor, leaving the intracavernous portion behind, followed by radiation therapy, is the best treatment.

We attempt a gross total resection of the intracranial portion of the tumor. The initial procedure is the best

opportunity for cure. We believe that dissection of tumor from the CS is not warranted in patients with intact third nerve function for fear of permanent damage to this nerve. In this instance, patients should be observed or receive adjuvant stereotactic radiation therapy (e.g., gamma knife) to the small portion of tumor left behind. Patients with small benign irradiated tumors can survive for many years with no evidence of regrowth.[22,23] In elderly patients and in those with poor medical health, a less radical excision is acceptable.

Surgical Technique

The cranial exposure is similar to that outlined in the section on tuberculum sellae meningiomas. More temporal fossa exposure is needed for resection of medial sphenoid ridge meningiomas, and more of the greater sphenoid wing is removed. Extensive cranial base exposures (orbitozygomatic infratemporal approach) have been described for these tumors, but in our experience, it has not been necessary to use these approaches.

The frontal and temporal lobes are often compressed by large tumors. The sylvian fissure must be opened widely to avoid brain retraction. After a wide microdissection of the sylvian fissure and exposure of the tumor, the vascularized dura surrounding the lateral tumor attachment on both sides of the sphenoid ridge is thoroughly coagulated with bipolar forceps. This maneuver significantly reduces the blood supply to the neoplasm and helps reduce blood loss. Excision of the meningioma, however, should not be started at the base of the tumor, because the ICA and its branches are difficult to visualize and are at risk of injury there. The surgical strategy is first to identify branches of the MCA in the sylvian fissure and follow the branches into the tumor to the carotid bifurcation. While keeping constant surveillance of the arterial tree, the tumor is gutted and removed piecemeal. Surgical removal of a medial sphenoid ridge tumor is depicted with sequential intraoperative photographs in Figure 17-4. The tumor located anterior and lateral to the arterial tree, which is usually larger, should be removed first, to expose and protect the MCA, ICA, and ACA. The arachnoid covering this portion of the tumor is incised with microscissors, and the tumor surface is coagulated at a safe distance from these major vessels and their small branches. The tumor interior is then removed in a piecemeal fashion using suction and bipolar cautery. Microdissection is used to free the tumor from the arachnoid enveloping the sylvian vessels. With large tumors, the involved intracranial arteries may supply the tumor directly. In this case, these small vessels are dissected within the tumor and coagulated and cut on the tumor side of the arachnoid, leaving a coagulated stump on the parent artery. This approach avoids thrombosis of the parent vessel and tearing the feeder from the parent vessel. If tumor directly involves the adventitia of the ICA, small coagulated bits of tumor may be left on the vessel without significant risk of recurrence. The MCA, ICA, and ACA are exposed. The origins of the posterior communicating artery and the anterior choroidal artery are then identified and followed distally.

After resection of tumor located anterior and lateral to the arterial tree, the remaining tumor, which is posterior and medial to the M1 segment of the MCA and A1 segment

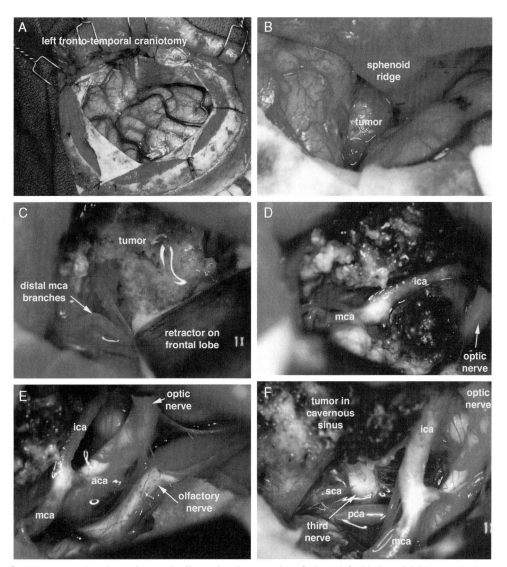

FIGURE 17-4 Serial intraoperative photomicrographs illustrating the resection of a large left-sided medial ridge meningioma using a pterional approach (*A*). The sylvian fissure is split widely, exposing tumor between the frontal and temporal lobes (*B*). Retractors are used to protect the brain during tumor removal. After the distal MCA branches are identified, they are exposed proximally by progressive tumor removal (*C* and *D*). A thin layer of tumor adherent to these arteries and their lenticulostriate perforators can be left in place and removed later in the procedure when the tumor has been mostly decompressed. Tumor is removed underneath the ipsilateral optic nerve and ICA through the optic-carotid space, from between the optic nerves, and from between the ICA and third nerve (*E*). Following tumor resection, the preserved intracranial arteries and cranial nerves can be identified (*F*). In this patient, residual tumor is left within the CS. PCA, posterior communicating artery; SCA, superior cerebellar artery.

of the ACA and the ICA, is removed. The neoplasm can be freed from these vessels using minimal bipolar coagulation, because the tumor is now devascularized as a result of its detachment from the sphenoid ridge. After exposure of the carotid artery and its major branches, the optic pathways are cleared of neoplasm. The optic nerve is best identified at its fixed point at the optic foramen. The optic system is invariably elevated, rotated, and displaced medially by tumor. The tumor is carefully separated from the optic nerve, and traction is applied to pull it gently away from the arachnoid of the optic and chiasmatic cisterns, rather than retracting the visual structures. The superior hypophyseal arteries coursing medially from the carotid artery supply blood to the optic nerves and should be preserved. When the tumor extends into the optic canal, the dura over

the canal and the anterior clinoid process is excised widely and the roof and lateral wall of the orbit are shaved away with a small cutting burr. Diamond burrs are not used because of heat production and the excessive manual pressure required for their use. The dural sleeve of the optic nerve is opened with a number 11 scalpel and microscissors under high magnification, and the intraorbital tumor is removed.

Tumor extending along the tentorium is reached by gentle lateral retraction of the medial temporal lobe. If the neoplasm extends beyond the tentorial edge into the posterior fossa, the tentorium is coagulated and sectioned behind the tumor. The fourth cranial nerve is exposed and preserved, if possible. The tumor is then removed from the upper clival region. If the tumor extends into the CS, this portion of the tumor is left behind, and a decision about further treatment is made at a later date.

Finally, the remaining fragments of neoplasm attached to the sphenoid ridge are removed. The involved dura is thoroughly coagulated or excised. If the sphenoid sinus is entered, it is repaired with a graft of temporalis fascia, which is secured over the defect with fibrin glue. At the conclusion of the procedure, the dura is closed and the craniotomy is closed in routine fashion. A subgaleal drain is left in place for 24 hours. Postoperatively, patients should be closely monitored in an intensive care unit.

Results

Cushing and Eisenhardt noted that "the crux of the removal lies in freeing the growth from its entanglement with the vessels at the carotid bifurcation," and they cautioned surgeons about the hazards of entering the carotid field.[1] Injury to the major vessels of the anterior circulation has been the major cause of operative mortality and morbidity in all subsequent surgical series, even after the advent and routine use of the operating microscope. The surgical morbidity for medial sphenoid ridge meningioma includes hemiplegia, hypothalamic infarction, aphasia, neurovegetative disorders, visual loss, and diplopia. In one study, 23% of surviving patients were severely impaired.[17] More recent reports have shown improvement in the rates of operative mortality and morbidity and chances for cure (Table 17–2).[19,24–27] The rate of recurrence for medial sphenoid ridge meningioma is one of the highest for intracranial meningiomas.[28] Recurrence is related to residual tumor that is left behind at the time of initial surgery. In the study conducted by Mirimanoff and colleagues,[29] the rate of recurrence or progression was 34% at 5 years and 54% at 10 years for medial ridge tumors compared with 3% and 25% at 5 and 10 years for convexity meningiomas.

Although most patients present with visual abnormalities, there are minimal data concerning visual function after resection of these tumors. In one series, among 20 of the 24 patients who presented with visual disturbances, only 2 had visual improvement after tumor removal.[19] The author concludes that "recovery of vision in clinoidal meningiomas is poor." In contemporary series, 8% to 75% of patients with medial sphenoid ridge meningioma had an improvement in visual function after resection.

In the senior author's personal series of 35 patients with medial sphenoid ridge global tumors with a mean diameter of 4.5 cm, 24 tumors (69%) were completely removed and 9 tumors (25%) had radical resections.[30] A radical resection was defined as no intradural tumor, but residual left in the CS, orbit, sella, or sphenoid sinus. All growths involved the anterior circulation, and 11 (31%) had invaded the CS. There were neither surgical mortalities nor cerebral infarctions, although one patient had a transient hemiparesis. There was one permanent third nerve injury. With a mean follow-up of 12.8 years, asymptomatic tumor regrowth was noted in three (9%) patients on serial MRI. Five (14%) patients were given postoperative radiation therapy, three to control regrowth and two for subtotal tumor removals. No additional tumor growth was noted after radiation therapy, with these patients remaining neurologically stable. With respect to visual outcome, 22 (63%) patients were improved, 10 (28%) were unchanged, and 3 (9%) worsened after surgery.

Intraoperative Complications and Their Management

The major intraoperative complications of surgery for tuberculum sellae and medial sphenoid ridge meningioma are optic nerve and vascular injury. Blindness and worsening of vision can occur from excessive surgical manipulation or devascularization of the optic nerve and chiasm. High-power magnification should be used to identify and preserve enveloping arachnoid and blood vessels supplying the optic apparatus. Manipulation is minimized during tumor removal by applying countertraction to the surrounding chiasmatic arachnoid rather than to the nerves.

Injury to major vessels can occur from sharp dissection, a cautery loop, excessive coagulation, and possibly from use of the ultrasonic aspirator. Partially injured vessels may cause postoperative hemorrhage. Major bleeding is controlled with temporary vascular clips. A Sundt clip or 10-0 suture may be applied to the site of the injury, if necessary.

SUMMARY

Tuberculum and diaphragma sellae meningiomas are clinically and anatomically indistinguishable and should be collectively termed as tuberculum sellae meningiomas.

TABLE 17-2 ▪ Contemporary Studies of Medial Sphenoid Ridge Meningiomas in the Peer-Reviewed Literature*

Series	Year	No. of Patients	Average Size (cm)	Average Follow-up	Mortality (%)	Gross Total Resection (%)	Improved Vision (%)	Recurrence (%)
Al-Mefty[19]	1990	24	NA	57 mo	8	89	8	4
Risi et al[26]	1994	34	NA	23 mo	6	59	32	21
Puzzilli et al[25]	1999	28	NA	54 mo	15	NA	51	26
Day[27]	2000	6	>5	3 mo	0	66	NA	NA
Lee et al[24]	2001	14	3.7	37 mo	0	87	75	0
Russell and Benjamin[30]	2003	35	4.5	12.8 yr	0	69	63	9

NA, not available.
*Patients without medial ridge meningiomas were excluded.

A pterional craniotomy with microsurgical dissection of the sylvian fissure allows access to these tumors with minimal neurologic and ophthalmologic morbidity. Gross total tumor removal can be achieved in the majority of patients, providing an acceptable progression-free survival. Preoperative visual dysfunction is the rule, and the majority of patients experience improvement in visual acuity following resection.

Resection of medial sphenoid ridge meningiomas has been associated with significant operative morbidity and mortality secondary to vascular injury. However, preoperative recognition of consistent unilateral involvement of the anterior cerebral circulation, with meticulous intraoperative preservation of these major arteries and their branches, can provide a successful and judicious microsurgical excision of these tumors. Because of their slow growth and the availability of advanced methods of radiotherapy, the surgeon must weigh the wisdom of attempted complete tumor removal in cases with invasion into the CS, orbit, and bone, with its associated risks of major neurologic morbidity and mortality.

Acknowledgment

The authors would like to thank Paul McCormick for his contribution to previous editions of this chapter.

REFERENCES

1. Cushing H, Eisenhardt L: Meningiomas: Their Classification, Regional Behavior, Life History, and Surgical End Results. Springfield: Charles C Thomas, 1938.
2. Kadis GN, Mount LA, Ganti SR: The importance of early diagnosis and treatment of the meningiomas of the planum sphenoidale and tuberculum sellae: A retrospective study of 105 cases. Surg Neurol 12:367–371, 1979.
3. Solero CL, Giombini S, Morello G: Suprasellar and olfactory meningiomas. Report on a series of 153 personal cases. Acta Neurochir (Wien) 67:181–194, 1983.
4. Andrews BT, Wilson CB: Suprasellar meningiomas: The effect of tumor location on postoperative visual outcome. J Neurosurg 69:523–528, 1988.
5. Symon L, Rosenstein J: Surgical management of suprasellar meningioma. Part 1: The influence of tumor size, duration of symptoms, and microsurgery on surgical outcome in 101 consecutive cases. J Neurosurg 61:633–641, 1984.
6. Finn JE, Mount LA: Meningiomas of the tuberculum sellae and planum sphenoidale. A review of 83 cases. Arch Ophthalmol 92:23–27, 1974.
7. Al-Mefty O, Holoubi A, Rifai A, et al: Microsurgical removal of suprasellar meningiomas. Neurosurgery 16:364–372, 1985.
8. Jallo GI, Benjamin V: Tuberculum sellae meningiomas: Microsurgical anatomy and surgical technique. Neurosurgery 51:1432–1439; discussion 1439–1440, 2002.
9. Grisoli F, Diaz-Vasquez P, Riss M, et al: Microsurgical management of tuberculum sellae meningiomas. Results in 28 consecutive cases. Surg Neurol 26:37–44, 1986.
10. Goel A, Muzumdar D, Desai KI: Tuberculum sellae meningioma: A report on management on the basis of a surgical experience with 70 patients. Neurosurgery 51:1358–1363; discussion 1363–1354, 2002.
11. Taylor SL, Barakos JA, Harsh GR, et al: Magnetic resonance imaging of tuberculum sellae meningiomas: Preventing preoperative misdiagnosis as pituitary macroadenoma. Neurosurgery 31:621–627; discussion 627, 1992.
12. Yasargil MG: Microneurosurgery, vol I. New York: Georg Thieme, 1984, pp 215–227.
13. Ojemann RG, Thornton AF, Harsh GR: Management of anterior cranial base and cavernous sinus neoplasms with conservative surgery alone or in combination with fractionated photon or stereotactic proton radiotherapy. Clin Neurosurg 42:71–98, 1995.
14. Raco A, Bristot R, Domenicucci M, et al: Meningiomas of the tuberculum sellae. Our experience in 69 cases surgically treated between 1973 and 1993. J Neurosurg Sci 43:253–260; discussion 260–262, 1999.
15. Ohta K, Yasuo K, Morikawa M, et al: Treatment of tuberculum sellae meningiomas: A long-term follow-up study. J Clin Neurosci 8(Suppl 1):26–31, 2001.
16. Fahlbusch R, Schott W: Pterional surgery of meningiomas of the tuberculum sellae and planum sphenoidale: Surgical results with special consideration of ophthalmological and endocrinological outcomes. J Neurosurg 96:235–243, 2002.
17. Fohanno D, Bitar A: Sphenoidal ridge meningioma. Adv Tech Stand Neurosurg 14:137–174, 1986.
18. Bonnal J, Thibaut A, Brotchi J, et al: Invading meningiomas of the sphenoid ridge. J Neurosurg 53:587–599, 1980.
19. Al-Mefty O: Clinoidal meningiomas. J Neurosurg 73:840–849, 1990.
20. Young SC, Grossman RI, Goldberg HI, et al: MR of vascular encasement in parasellar masses: Comparison with angiography and CT. AJNR Am J Neuroradiol 9:35–38, 1988.
21. Sekhar LN, Sen CN, Jho HD, et al: Surgical treatment of intracavernous neoplasms: A four-year experience. Neurosurgery 24:18–30, 1989.
22. Barbaro NM, Gutin PH, Wilson CB, et al: Radiation therapy in the treatment of partially resected meningiomas. Neurosurgery 20:525–528, 1987.
23. Peele KA, Kennerdell JS, Maroon JC, et al: The role of postoperative irradiation in the management of sphenoid wing meningiomas. A preliminary report. Ophthalmology 103:1761–1766; discussion 1766–1767, 1996.
24. Lee JH, Jeun SS, Evans J, et al: Surgical management of clinoidal meningiomas. Neurosurgery 48:1012–1019; discussion 1019–1021, 2001.
25. Puzzilli F, Ruggeri A, Mastronardi L, et al: Anterior clinoidal meningiomas: Report of a series of 33 patients operated on through the pterional approach. Neuro-oncol 1:188–195, 1999.
26. Risi P, Uske A, de Tribolet N: Meningiomas involving the anterior clinoid process. Br J Neurosurg 8:295–305, 1994.
27. Day JD: Cranial base surgical techniques for large sphenocavernous meningiomas [Technical note]. Neurosurgery 46:754–759; discussion 759–760, 2000.
28. Mathiesen T, Lindquist C, Kihlstrom L, et al: Recurrence of cranial base meningiomas. Neurosurgery 39:2–7; discussion 8–9, 1996.
29. Mirimanoff RO, Dosoretz DE, Linggood RM, et al: Meningioma: Analysis of recurrence and progression following neurosurgical resection. J Neurosurg 62:18–24, 1985.
30. Russell S, Benjamin V: Sphenoid ridge meningiomas: Classification, microsurgical anatomy, operative nuances, and long term surgical outcomes in 60 consecutive patients. Part I: Medial ridge tumors [Abstract]. Congress of Neurological Surgeons, Denver, Co, 2003.

18

Sphenoid Ridge Meningiomas

ARMANDO BASSO, ANTONIO G. CARRIZO,
and JULIO ANTICO

Meningiomas that grow from any point along the sphenoid ridge constitute approximately 14% to 20% of intracranial meningiomas.[1,2] These tumors represent a complex and difficult surgical problem, because they can involve arteries of the anterior circulation, anterior visual pathways, and oculomotor nerves.[1] For sphenoid ridge meningiomas, higher morbidity, mortality, and recurrence rates have been observed than for meningiomas in other locations.[1–4] Two main types can be recognized according to their presentation: nodular and en plaque.[3] The nodular meningioma is an encapsulated tumor of variable size that displaces or encircles intracranial arteries or cranial nerves. Generally, this tumor has a dural site of implantation through which it receives its blood supply. Meningioma en plaque has distinct characteristics that make it a different pathologic entity from the nodular type of sphenoidal meningioma. In the en plaque tumors, the pathologic cells fill the haversian canals and may spread into not only the pterion, orbital walls, and malar bone, but also the zygomatic, temporal, and middle cranial fossae.[3–5] In this way, these tumors produce typically a hyperostotic reaction of these structures, which causes exophthalmos and temporal bowing. Less frequently, conversely, an osteolytic lesion can be found. In addition, an intracranial meningomatous plaque is always present.[3,5]

According to Cushing and Eisenhardt,[3] the nodular or globoid meningiomas are classified depending on their site of implantation along the sphenoid wing as inner third, middle third, or outer third tumors. Tumors from the inner third are subdivided into sphenocavernous tumors (implanted in the external wall of the cavernous sinus [CS]) and clinoidal tumors (implanted on the corresponding clinoid process and projecting toward the anterior cranial fossa).[1,6] Tumors from the middle third of the sphenoid ridge (alar meningiomas) occur less frequently and are difficult to diagnose early. Nodular meningiomas from the outer third of the sphenoid ridge, or sphenotemporal meningiomas, cause neurologic symptoms primarily because of compression of adjacent structures. In large tumors that occupy the entire length of the bony ridge, it is difficult to establish the exact site of origin of the tumor; this difficulty could explain the different classifications that have been proposed for sphenoid wing meningiomas.[3] Petit-Dutaillis divided them into lesser wing and greater wing meningiomas.[3] Bonnal and colleagues[4,7] classified these tumors into five groups. Al-Mefty[6] distinguished three subgroups of clinoidal meningiomas on the basis of the presence or absence of an interfacing arachnoidal membrane between the cerebral vessels and the neoplasm. Sekhar and Altschuler[8] described five grades of intracavernous meningioma according to the extent of CS and internal carotid artery (ICA) involvement. The diversity of presentation of sphenoid ridge meningiomas and their complexity make surgical treatment a challenge that varies from case to case. If all the possibilities of presentation described were taken into consideration, almost a dozen types of sphenoid ridge meningiomas would have to be accepted, but such exhaustive classification is not practical for the analysis of a clinical series. For our presentation, we follow the classic Cushing division of these tumors, subdividing those of the deep or inner third into clinoidal and sphenocavernous varieties.[1]

ANATOMIC CONSIDERATIONS

The sphenoidal wings belong to various regions and are anatomically complex: The posterior edge of the lesser wing represents the limit between the middle and the anterior skull base fossae and is related to the orbit, the sylvian fissure, and the tip of the temporal lobe. The external face of the greater wing is in the temporal and zygomatic fossae, next to the temporal muscle. The lesser wing is part of the roof of the orbit, and the greater wing belongs to the external wall. These compartments communicate through the optic canal, where the optic nerve and the ophthalmic artery pass, and through the superior orbital fissure. The oculomotor nerve, the first division of the trigeminal nerve, and the ophthalmic vein pass through this fissure connecting the orbit with the CS.[1] An understanding of the microsurgical anatomy of this structure is essential for the management of sphenocavernous meningiomas. In certain cases, the CS can be considered the limit of resection.

The lateral, superior, and posterior walls are constituted by two dural layers, whereas the medial wall is formed by a single layer. The ICA lies within the CS surrounded by a venous plexus; the main intracavernous branches of the ICA are the meningohypophyseal trunk and the inferolateral trunk. At the exit of the ICA from the CS, two fibrous rings that represent the dura enclosing the anterior clinoid process can be observed. These fibrous rings are important landmarks for the access of the intracavernous ICA, after resection of the clinoid process. The lateral wall of the CS has a thick outer layer, which continues the dura of the middle cranial fossa, and a thinner layer, which encloses cranial nerves III, IV, V-1, and V-2. The sixth cranial nerve and the sympathetic trunk cross the CS lateral to the ICA.[8]

The orbit and skull also communicate by the leptomeningeal sheath, which accompanies the optic nerve along its orbital course to the posterior pole of the ocular globe. This sheath is a direct prolongation of the inner layer of the dura and leptomeningeal layers of the skull. The outer layer of the dura is in continuity with the periorbita, which is similar in its histologic structure, throughout the optic canal and the superior orbital fissure. Meningiomas are the tumors most frequently located in this region. They have a tendency either to involve the meninges, bone, periorbit, and muscles or to displace and compress brain and orbital contents.[1]

CLINICAL PRESENTATIONS

In early stages, sphenoid ridge meningiomas produce characteristic findings for each location from which they arise; however, detection of the site of origin of these lesions is difficult when the tumor has enlarged beyond a certain stage of development.[3,9]

Inner Third Sphenoid Wing Meningiomas

Clinoidal and sphenocavernous meningiomas are distinct varieties of tumor. Clinoidal meningiomas produce a progressive decrease in visual acuity and changes in the visual fields beginning with ipsilateral nasal hemianopsia. As the tumor grows, a superior temporal field defect occurs, and eventually the eye may become blind. Primary optic atrophy may be evident on the side of the tumor, and in tumors producing increased intracranial pressure, the contralateral optic disc may be swollen and edematous (Foster Kennedy syndrome).[1,3,6]

In patients with sphenocavernous meningiomas, oculomotor palsies occur frequently and usually start as abducens palsy. The symptoms slowly evolve and result in total ophthalmoplegia with hypesthesia in the distribution of the ophthalmic branch of the trigeminal nerve, which is secondary to the nerve's compression along the lateral wall of the CS. Exophthalmos may occur, owing to venous compression within the CS; this condition may be more evident with tumor progression toward the orbital apex.[1]

Middle Third or Alar Meningiomas

Meningiomas of the middle third of the sphenoid ridge are characteristically larger than those in the inner third before detection. Middle third tumors initially produce increased intracranial pressure, headache, and papilledema, which is more evident on the side of the lesion. Dysfunction of the olfactory nerve, contralateral homonymous hemianopsia, personality changes, visual and olfactory hallucinations, contralateral facial palsy, hemiparesis, and seizures are other symptoms that occur as the tumor increases in size.[2,3]

External Third or Pterional Meningiomas

Meningiomas en plaque are predominantly bony growths that must be differentiated from the globoid tumor, which has a far greater degree of intracranial involvement. The pterional meningioma produces a slowly evolving proptosis. This proptosis is caused by: (1) hyperostosis of the orbital walls, (2) the presence of an intraorbital tumor, (3) periorbital tumor infiltration, or (4) venous stasis secondary to ophthalmic vein compression when the tumor enters the CS. Another characteristic of these tumors, probably related to venous stasis and to obstruction of lymphatic drainage, is chronic palpebral edema. Skull deformities may be caused by

temporal bone hyperostosis, and, in some cases, the temporal muscle is infiltrated by the tumor. As with inner third meningiomas, loss of visual acuity occurs gradually, and blindness may develop in advanced cases of pterional meningioma. Diplopia is not a constant symptom, but when present it is probably related to mechanical changes within the orbit and, less frequently, to involvement of the oculomotor nerves and muscles. Epiphora, photophobia, and focal or generalized seizures may also occur. Early and frequent symptoms of globoid pterional meningioma include hemicranial headaches, seizures, contralateral hemiparesis, and increased intracranial pressure. This tumor behaves as either a temporal or a frontal mass. Signs of orbital involvement are not constant but are similar to those found in the en plaque variety.[1,3,5,9]

RADIOGRAPHIC STUDIES

Approximately 90% of sphenoid ridge meningiomas are diagnosed by the use of conventional radiographic studies. Lateral, inclined posteroanterior, and axial views for the skull base and temporo-orbital projections of the optic canals are used. Radiologic features of sphenoid ridge meningiomas include focal hyperostosis, sclerosis, and erosion at the area of tumor attachment. These lesions are seen mainly in the internal table of the skull. Other features may include widening of the vascular grooves, the sphenoparietal sinus, and the superior orbital fissure, as well as narrowing of the optic canal, and, rarely, enlargement of the foramen spinosum with hypertrophy of the middle meningeal artery. Although hyperostosis may not be present radiographically in a small percentage of inner and middle third meningiomas, it is an almost constant finding in the pterional en plaque meningioma (Fig. 18-1). This finding must be differentiated from fibrous dysplasia. In fibrous dysplasia, the hyperostotic alterations can be larger and tend to cross the midline more frequently than in the case of sphenoid ridge meningiomas. Bone becomes several times thicker, and alterations are more evident in the external table and diploë. Widening of the vascular grooves may also be seen.[1,5,10,11]

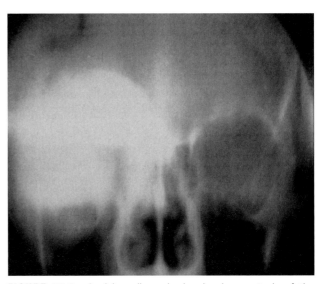

FIGURE 18-1 A plain radiograph showing hyperostosis of the right sphenoid wing.

Although hypocycloidal tomography has been almost completely replaced by computed tomography (CT) to delineate these lesions, it was used to determine precisely the tumor's bony extension and the appearance of the superior orbital fissure and to examine the optic canal for evidence of encroachment. This information is used to determine the possible limits of the surgical procedure.

Cerebral gammagraphic studies with ^{99m}Tc, ^{113}In, or ^{197}Hg yield positive results in 90% of meningiomas. In meningiomas of the sphenoid ridge, frontotemporal, retro-orbital, and supraorbital uptake is observed, overlapping skull base activity. Gammagraphic studies provide information about the intracranial tumors, peritumoral edema, and bony invasion by the tumors.[9] These data are scarcely useful today, compared with those furnished by current neuroimaging methods.

Cerebral Arteriography

Selective catheterization of the ICA and external carotid artery was used in most meningiomas of the sphenoid ridge before surgery. These meningiomas act radiologically as temporal or frontotemporal masses. The anterior cerebral artery shows anteroposterior displacement toward the opposite side, which is usually mild in character and is related to the tumor's volume. The slow-growing mass may allow the brain to adapt to the volume changes. On the anteroposterior view of the carotid arteriogram, the middle cerebral artery (MCA) is not parallel to the sphenoid wing, but rather the M1 and M2 segments of the MCA curve to surround the meningioma, indicating its site of attachment. Clinoidal meningiomas show an elevation of the horizontal segment of the MCA, and alar meningiomas show inversion of the sylvian elbow. In pterional meningiomas, the second segment of the MCA is inwardly displaced. In subfrontal locations, the sylvian triangle is displaced backward on the lateral projections. In pretemporal tumor locations, the sylvian triangle is elevated. On frontotemporal locations, the sylvian triangle is displaced upward and backward. When tumors are well vascularized, the tumor stain of the mass is seen (see Fig. 20-6), and by selective catheterization, contributions to the tumor's blood supply by the ICA and external carotid artery can be determined.[10,11]

Selective study of the ophthalmic artery demonstrates the presence of an intraorbital mass by staining, blush, or vessel displacement. Partial feeding of intracranial tumor in inner varieties can be seen from an ophthalmic branch, which passes through the superior orbital fissure. In other cases, additional vascularization is found through the anterior meningeal artery, anterior ethmoidal branch, and ophthalmic branches. A preponderant supply from the intracavernous carotid artery is also found through the meningohypophyseal trunk and inferolateral trunk in sphenocavernous meningiomas. A well-developed superficial temporal artery in the external carotid system is observed in most cases, especially when the temporal muscle is invaded. Some cases show an enlarged middle meningeal artery feeding the lesion. Highly vascular tumors can be embolized preoperatively (a portion irrigated by the external carotid artery system), allowing tumor resection without excessive blood loss.[1,9–11]

At present, magnetic resonance angiography (MRA) and CT angiography are replacing digital subtraction angiography in the preoperative evaluation of this pathology except in cases in which embolization is desired.

Computed Tomography

CT shows the different planes and compartments occupied by the tumor. CT scans must be performed in axial and coronal projections. The significant thickening of the roof and the lateral wall of the orbit that is common in hyperostotic pterional meningiomas is best appreciated with bone algorithms. This thickening can extend to the malar bone and anterior part of the middle cranial fossa. Osteolytic lesions are rare. Meningiomatous plaque will probably appear as a thin hyperdense image overlapping the adjacent bone that typically shows a marked enhancement with the contrast media; in other cases, the intradural component develops a nodular configuration. The orbit can be examined to determine the conditions producing exophthalmos: hyperostosis, periorbital infiltration by tumor, or intraorbital nodular tumor. Evidence of bone involvement by middle third sphenoid ridge meningiomas is usually less clear. The tumor can be seen as a well-defined mass demonstrating homogeneous enhancement with contrast agents. Edema of the temporal lobe and centrum semiovale can often be seen on the CT scan. This edema is attributed to middle cerebral vein and sphenoparietal sinus compression or occlusion, findings that can be verified by cerebral arteriography. With the use of CT scans, inner third sphenoid ridge meningiomas may be clearly categorized into clinoidal tumors and sphenocavernous tumors. Clinoidal tumors are almost always associated with hyperostosis of the anterior clinoid process or of the whole lesser wing of the sphenoid, with narrowing of the optic canal and, less frequently, of the superior orbital fissure. Characteristically the tumor mass grows predominantly upward, is subfrontal, has well-defined boundaries, and is rounded in shape. Sphenocavernous tumors are attached mainly to the external wall of the CS, are anteroposteriorly oriented, and extend toward the posterior fossa through the free margin of the tentorium or anteriorly through the superior orbital fissure into the orbital apex, usually as a diffuse infiltration instead of as a well-defined mass. Hyperostosis is usually a less prominent feature of this tumor than in clinoidal tumors.[1,2]

Magnetic Resonance Imaging

Magnetic resonance imaging (MRI) cannot demonstrate bony architecture as well as CT. Intracranial calcifications noted on skull films or CT can be missed by MRI. MRI surpasses CT, however, in demonstrating normal and pathologic intracranial anatomy.

Meningiomas may have signal intensity similar to that of brain tissue on T1-weighted and T2-weighted sequences. The signal intensities of meningiomas vary widely, and some are hyperintense on T2-weighted images because there are several histologic varieties of meningiomas. Usually, syncytial and angioblastic meningiomas present higher signal intensity on T2-weighted images than transitional cell or fibroblastic meningiomas. Meningiomas tend to enhance uniformly after gadolinium injection. There may be some lack of homogeneity in the appearance of meningiomas related to calcifications and cyst formations, which can appear in some cases. Sphenoidal wing meningiomas are prone to causing hyperostosis of adjacent bone. The hyperostosis, most commonly involving the greater and lesser sphenoid wings and clinoid processes, is not as well seen as with CT, as mentioned before.

MRI can identify the position of the ICA, MCA, and other vessels by flow void, and it can define the relationship of the ICA to the tumor better than digital subtraction angiography. A few meningiomas have visible vessels within them, seen as small curvilinear flow voids.

Gadolinium enhancement allows good anatomic definition of the CS. It is also useful in defining the extent of the meningiomatous plaque, which on CT scan can be difficult to distinguish from the adjacent hyperostosis and the thickening of adjacent dura (dura tail sign). In cases of parasellar or CS meningioma, the ICA may be encased and may become narrowed or occluded.

At present, MRA may be considered an important complement of MRI, which can be performed simultaneously. It can replace digital subtraction angiography in the preoperative assessment of sphenoidal meningiomas. It is generally not a satisfactory method of showing tumor vascularity; however, the circle of Willis and large intracranial vessels are well depicted.

TREATMENT

Surgery is the primary treatment for meningiomas. Although it is difficult in most sphenoid ridge meningiomas, radical excision of the tumor is the aim of surgical intervention.[6,8,12] Meningiomas of the sphenocavernous or clinoidal type that involve the inner third of the sphenoid ridge present problems different from those of tumors of the outer third of the sphenoid ridge.[1,6,8] Sphenocavernous meningiomas arise from the external wall of the CS, involve the oculomotor or trigeminal nerve, penetrate the CS, and constrict the ICA in a ringlike fashion. In these cases, total resection of the tumor is impossible. A resection of the nodular portion and coagulation of the wall of the CS (Simpson II grade) is advised in patients whose ocular motility is not definitely altered. Conversely, excision of the nodular part, microsurgical carotid dissection, and resection of the tumor's osteodural attachment (Simpson I grade) are possible in patients with a pure clinoidal tumor.[1,13] Patients with pterional meningiomas en plaque have proptosis, frontotemporal bowing, and palpebral edema. The tumor, which originates in the pterion, spreads to proliferate in the dura, periorbital tissues, and zygomatic fossa. In these cases, complete resection can be performed except if the CS or the orbital apex is infiltrated by the lesion. Some classic papers propose that no surgical intervention be undertaken in patients with slow-growing tumors that are not life-threatening.[14] Guiot and co-workers[15,16] recommended surgery to preserve vision, to effect orbital decompression, and to reduce proptosis except in cases of periorbital meningiomas, in which a complete resection is possible. More recently, some authors proposed a radical resection of these tumors, including the intracavernous component together with the encased ICA, with or without saphenous vein graft reconstruction.[17–19] There is no unanimous agreement with this attitude, and the matter is still open to debate.

SURGICAL TECHNIQUE

Pterional Meningiomas

In pterional meningiomas, surgery is performed with the head slightly elevated, to improve the venous return, and positioned 30 to 45 degrees away from the side of the lesion. A frontotemporal approach is used through a hemicoronal incision concealed behind the hairline. This approach permits a wide superior orbital edge exposure and allows one to obtain a pericranial graft, which may be used to close the dura later during the operation. The thickened pterion is resected starting with burr holes and rongeurs, then high-speed drills are used to remove the hyperostosis progressively, excising the roof and lateral wall of the orbit and carrying the surgery into the floor of the middle cranial fossa. The superior orbital fissure is decompressed, as is the optic canal, if necessary. All of the bone in this area can be resected (Figs. 18-2 and 18-3). Once the involved bone has been removed, a frontal craniotomy is performed enlarging the dural exposure as necessary, according to the extension of the tumor.[1,5]

At the end of the bone resection, a wide exposure of the superior and lateral compartments of the orbit is obtained. Next the orbital contents are explored. Three principal appearances are possible: (1) diffuse thickening of periorbital tissue, (2) nodular tumor formation, or (3) micronodular infiltration of the elements of the apex. Total excision is probable with the first two possibilities but not when the tumor has infiltrated the structures at the orbital apex.[1]

After opening of the dura of the anterior cranial fossa, the intracranial tumor mass is identified. If a small plaque of tumor is attached to thickened dura and covers the sphenoid ridge, dura and tumor are resected en bloc. Alternatively the tumor mass may be nodular and extend deeply into the sylvian fissure, displacing the temporal lobe and, to a lesser degree, the frontal lobe. Microsurgical techniques allow the careful dissection of tumor from the MCA and its branches. The ICA and optic nerve may be hidden by the lesion if the tumor has grown medially. Intradural tumor excision should be performed in a piecemeal fashion with the use of bipolar coagulation, microdissection, and

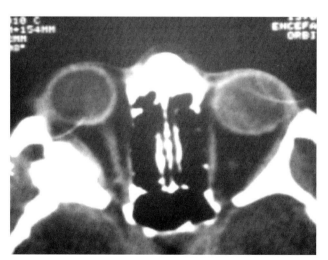

FIGURE 18-2 A CT scan with an axial view of a hyperostosing en plaque meningioma.

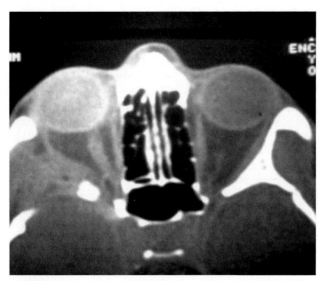

FIGURE 18-3   A postoperative CT scan of the patient in Figure 18-2 showing the extent of bone resection.

ultrasonic aspiration. The infiltrated dura is resected to its medial limits. In the past, we have used dermal grafts from the buttocks to replace resected dura; however, this technique is bothersome and time-consuming. We have also used lyophilized dura for the same purpose. This material is relatively rigid, and its use presents more potential problems, such as the delayed development of Creutzfeldt-Jakob disease, so we also abandoned its use.[20,21] We have used a periosteal flap fashioned from the tissues in the proximity of the craniotomy to close the dura. The periosteal graft is sutured to the dural defect and can then be further sealed, to obtain a watertight closure, with either fibrin glue or cyanoacrylate. No cerebrospinal fluid (CSF) leaks, collections of other fluids, or infections have occurred when we have used this technique to close the dura. At the beginning of our series, bony reconstruction was achieved with ribs that have been harvested, then split longitudinally through their cancellous portion. Each cortical fragment was fashioned to the bony defect and lateral wall of the orbit and was attached to the neighboring bone with stainless-steel sutures. The use of methyl methacrylate has shortened the surgical procedure significantly by eliminating the need to harvest the rib grafts and to fashion several pieces of rib to the defect. If the pterional defect is small, it can be covered with the temporal muscle alone; however, if it is larger, it can also be repaired with either rib grafts, as initially in our series, or methyl methacrylate.[1,5,9] We have not used iliac bone graft as has been proposed.[22,23]

A different strategy is necessary for tumors that have spread to the zygomatic fossa and lower segments of the orbit or for tumors directly invading the malar bone. We have used an inferolateral access to the orbit instead of enlarged transcranial approaches at the beginning of our series.[22,23] The transmalar approach is performed through a subciliary incision made in the lower lid that is extended horizontally for approximately 3 cm. The subcutaneous plane is dissected from the orbicular muscle, exposing the lateral and inferior orbital rim, where the periosteum is divided. After the periosteal incision, the malar bone is widely exposed. A medial and anterior osteotomy is performed following the maxillozygomatic suture, using an

oscillating saw; another osteotomy is made posteriorly and laterally in the zygomatic arcade, and another is made superiorly on the malar articulation with the fronto-orbital process. The malar bone is removed in one piece, exposing the orbital inferolateral sectors and the zygomatic fossa. Tumoral tissue is extirpated up to the apex, reaching the site of the transcranial access. When the malar bone is normal, it is replaced using titanium low-profile bone plates and screws at the osteotomy sites to restore the form of the orbital cavity. When the malar bone is macroscopically infiltrated by tumor, the area can be reconstructed with rib grafts or with methyl methacrylate. After routine closure, temporary tarsorrhaphy is performed to protect the eye.[1,5,9] At present, thanks to earlier diagnosis, malar invasion is rarely found, and this technique is used only rarely.

Inner and Middle Third Meningiomas

Inner third sphenoid ridge meningiomas are subclassified into clinoidal and sphenocavernous tumors.[1,6,8] The clinoidal tumors have a dural attachment on the upper part of the anterior clinoid process, whereas the sphenocavernous tumors are attached in the sphenocavernous angle. For operations on tumors of this location, the patient is placed in a supine position, and the head is slightly raised and turned 45 degrees to the side opposite the lesion. A pterional or frontopterional craniotomy is recommended. Depending on the tumor size, the lesser wing of the sphenoid is resected to the superior orbital fissure, allowing exposure of the lesion with a minimum of brain retraction. After the dura has been opened, the tumor capsule is identified and coagulated with a bipolar unit. The capsule is opened, and the bulk of the tumor is removed with the use of curets, scissors, bipolar coagulation, ultrasonic aspirator, or the carbon dioxide laser. The site of dural implantation is identified, and the tumor's feeding vessels are coagulated. These vessels are almost always meningeal branches from the internal maxillary artery and intracavernous branches of the ICA that supply the tumor. The supraclinoidal ICA and the MCA trunk and its branches must be handled carefully to avoid injury. The grade I Simpson technique of radical extirpation of a clinoidal meningioma is nearly always possible (Figs. 18-4 and 18-5). This technique involves complete macroscopic excision of the tumor and its osteodural implant. For sphenocavernous tumors with which a neurologic deficit has occurred because of abnormalities of ocular movements, extracavernous extirpation with coagulation of the dural attachment is advised (Simpson II technique).[11,24] In sphenocavernous meningiomas with CS invasion, complete ophthalmoplegia, and involvement of the trigeminal nerve, radical surgery is necessary to extirpate the lesion. In these cases, after the lesser wing of the sphenoid has been resected, one must unroof the orbit, remove the anterior clinoid process, open the optic canal, and approach the CS through its superior wall to reach the intracavernous nodular portion of the meningioma.[25] The tumor is then removed with an ultrasonic aspirator or vaporized with the carbon dioxide laser. This technique does not guarantee that the tumor will not recur as a result of meningiomatous cells lying in the dural base.[26] CSF leakage and infection can be avoided by the use of a watertight closure of the dura, which may involve the use of pericranium and fibrin glue.[1,9]

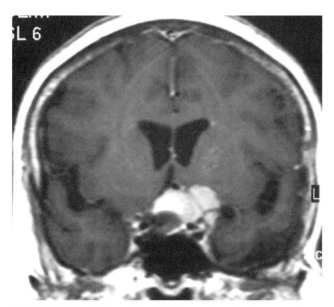

FIGURE 18-4 A T1-weighted MRI scan of a clinoidal meningioma with encasement of the internal carotid artery.

RESULTS

In the past 30 years, 145 patients with sphenoid ridge meningiomas have been treated at the Hospital Santa Lucia, Buenos Aires, Argentina. This hospital is the regional ophthalmologic and neurosurgical institute that deals with tumors of the skull base and of the visual system. Of the 145 patients, 51 had meningiomas of the inner third of the sphenoid ridge, 35 had meningiomas of the middle third of the sphenoid ridge, and 59 had meningiomas at the pterion. Patients included 116 women and 29 men, with ages ranging between 23 and 79 and a mean age of 48.7 years.

Immediately after surgery, the patients were classified into one of four categories according to their results: good (no sequelae), fair (minor sequelae), poor (severe sequelae), or death. Of the patients with inner third meningiomas, 41 patients (80.39%) had good results, 4 had fair results, 2 had poor results, and 4 died. In the middle third type,

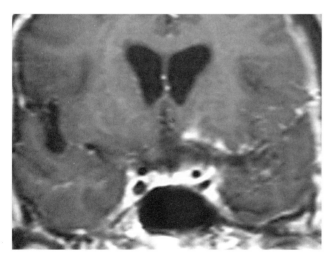

FIGURE 18-5 A postoperative MRI scan of the case in Figure 18-4 demonstrating complete resection sparing the internal carotid artery.

24 patients (68.57%) had good results, 6 had fair results, 3 had poor results, and 2 died. In the pterional type, 53 patients (89.83%) had good results, 5 (8.47%) had fair results, 1 had poor results, and no one died. Of the entire patient group, 81.37% had good results, and an overall operative mortality rate of 4.13% was noted. These results are consistent with other reports that consider the surgical technique and stress the difficulties involved in the radical resection of spheno-cavernous angle meningiomas, especially in relation to the supraclinoid ICA and its branches. Of the six deaths in our series, four resulted from a cerebral infarction as a consequence of a carotid or sylvian lesion, and the other two were from irreversible postoperative cerebral edema. This series spanned a long period of time, and most complications and deaths occurred at the beginning of the series. The use of microsurgical techniques has improved mortality and morbidity rates in our experience as well as in other series from the literature.[8,15,27,28] The main causes of fair and poor results were extraocular muscle dysfunction (generally partial or transient), persistent exophthalmos, hemiparesis, and, less frequently, visual impairment.

Tumor recurrence is an important issue, mainly for the inner third location. From our experience and according to most authors, meningiomas from the skull base are associated with the highest rate of tumor recurrence.[29] This high recurrence rate is due to the particular anatomic characteristics of skull base meningiomas, especially those located at the sphenoid ridge, with their wide base of dural attachment, invasion of the CS, invasion of the underlying bone, and propagation of the tumor through the foramina and fissures of the skull base into the orbit and zygomatic fossa. Seventy-three of our patients (62 women and 11 men) were followed for 9 to 30 years postoperatively. Among these patients, 29 had inner third meningiomas, 11 had middle third meningiomas, and 33 had external third meningiomas. Seven recurrences were found in the first group (24.13%), two were found in the second group (18.18%), and six were found in the third group (18.18%). These findings represent a 20.54% recurrence rate at 10 years for the 73 patients who underwent surgery for meningiomas of the sphenoid ridge. Fourteen of the patients with recurrences had repeat surgery, and all of them received radiotherapy, which seems to halt the growth of the tumor.[30] The mean time of tumor recurrence was 6.7 years after surgery.

For recurrent meningiomas, repeat surgery is the most effective treatment. Alternative treatments, such as radiosurgery, high-energy radiotherapy, hormone therapy, and ultraselective catheterization for local injection of cytostatic drugs, can also be used as adjuvants.

RADIOSURGERY

Meningiomas represent roughly 20% of all intracranial tumors[31] and in particular they are the most frequent benign tumor.[32] Although they may develop at any meningeal site, their proclivity is recognized for the meninges of the skull base where 50% of cases occur.[31] Because these tumors are histologically benign, radical surgery is considered as the treatment of choice, thus achieving a definitive cure. As a result of their implantation features in the meninges, not always visible during surgery, and the surgical difficulties presented by their vicinity and at times involvement with critical neurovascular structures, skull base meningiomas represent a challenge for modern neurosurgery, even when carried out by the most expert and able hands. For these reasons, long-term follow-up studies have demonstrated a high potential for recurrence and/or of incomplete resection, leading to conflicting reports.[33,34] Although there is no widespread agreement on the indication of radiotherapy for meningiomas,[35] this modality has been used especially in recurrent or partially resected tumors, to gain additional tumoral control. In this sense, radiosurgery has been called upon in the last few years to reach this goal, thus achieving excellent results in terms of disease control.

Gamma Knife Surgery

Radiosurgery is a technique introduced by Lars Leksell in 1951. Leksell demonstrated that by applying a single dose of radiation one could selectively destroy an intracerebral tissue while preserving the remainder of the adjacent tissue. Leksell's idea conceived the use of radiation in a manner very different from radiotherapy, both in its application and in its radiobiologic effect. In radiotherapy, the tissue is exposed to a diffuse field of radiation and the desired effect is obtained as a result of the differences in radiobiologic properties between the pathologic tissue and the normal tissue, only limited by the tolerance of the latter to an accumulated dose of radiation. In radiosurgery, the radiation is delivered in a single session, at a biologically effective dose that affects a target volume, carefully defined, inducing minimal damage to the surrounding normal tissue. On analyzing the two situations, it may be readily inferred that with radiotherapy a lesion in normal tissue could not be created, as is done in thalamotomy or pallidotomy used for the treatment of Parkinson's disease. The superior effectiveness of single-dose treatment may be especially demonstrated by the radiosurgical effect on benign tumors, an effect impossible to achieve with fractionated treatments.

Radiobiology of Radiosurgery

In his work, *The Radiobiology of Radiosurgery*, Larson[36] attempted to demonstrate the beneficial effect of radiosurgery on benign tumors starting from two unquestionable principles of radiobiology: (1) Malignant tumors habitually present in their population hypoxic, radioresistant cells that benefit with fractional treatments, and (2) there are differences in the dose/response ratio of early- and late-responder tissues to radiant effects. In that work, he explains the effect of radiosurgery in which several radiation beams converge onto a point, stereotactically defined, delivering a biologically effective dose that leads to thrombosis of small vessels and death of reproductive cells. Within the target volume the dose in radiosurgery is high and nonhomogeneous, so that there is greater variation as a result of radiobiologic effects expected after fractionated treatment. This is because both normal glial cells and benign tumors respond belatedly to the effects of x-ray and gamma radiation. Meningiomas are tumors that rarely invade cerebral tissue, so that both the tumor and the adjacent normal tissue are late responders to radiant effects. Because of its considerable gradient, radiosurgery exposes them to different doses; thus tumors may be destroyed efficiently without undue risk to adjacent normal structures.

Rationale for Radiosurgery

As employed for the control of meningiomas, radiosurgery has the following goals:

1. To arrest tumoral growth
2. To avoid new damage induced by tumoral growth
3. To achieve tumoral control without inducing additional damage by the treatment itself

Radiosurgery is a therapeutic option when:

1. There is tumoral recurrence after incomplete surgical resection
2. Partial resection is performed to avoid neurologic morbidity.
3. There is high potential risk because of patient age or status
4. It is desired to reduce the adverse effects of cerebral irradiation

For a comparison of microsurgery and radiosurgery, see Table 18-1.

Gamma Knife Surgery for Meningiomas of the Anterior Skull Base

Meningiomas of the Sphenoidal Wing (Spheno-orbital Meningiomas)

These tumors make up roughly 18% of all intracranial meningiomas.[37] Because the sphenoid bone forms the lateral and posterior walls of the orbit, meningiomas in this region involve periorbital structures. The orbital component of spheno-orbital meningiomas usually displaces rather than invades the orbital contents, and the nerves that course through the CS and the superior orbital fissure are quite resistant to tumoral compression. Once these tumors have gained entry to the orbit by the posterior vertex, they compress the optic nerve, with subsequent functional damage. The vicinity of these tumors to the optic pathway requires special care at the time of planning to give them an optimal dose for their control, avoiding exposure of these delicate structures to a toxic dose. There are sufficient data to limit the dose received by the optic apparatus to 8 Gy[38], in a single fraction. In some cases, when the nerve was previously subjected to prolonged tumoral compression, this dose should be even smaller (6 Gy). It has been demonstrated that with a dose at the margin of the tumor as low as 9 Gy, tumor growth may be effectively controlled. Habitually, an optimal dose at the tumor margin is considered to range from 12 to 14 Gy (Figs. 18-6 to 18-8).

TABLE 18-1 ▪ Microsurgery/Radiosurgery Comparison

Microsurgery	Radiosurgery
Prevents tumor growth only in case of total resection	Tumor remains in place but reduced, or at least does not increase in volume
Limits for microsurgery are carotid artery and cranial nerve involvement, and tumor extension	Limits for radiosurgery are vicinity of optic apparatus and large tumor volume

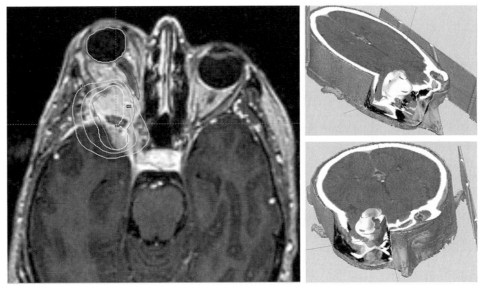

FIGURE 18-6 Spheno-orbital meningioma. (*Left*) MRI scan of gamma knife treatment planning. (*Right*) 3-Dimensional image.

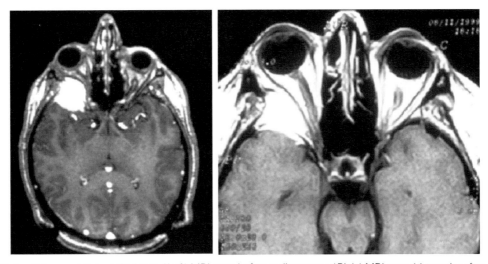

FIGURE 18-7 Spheno-orbital meningioma. (*Left*) MRI scan before radiosurgery. (*Right*) MRI scan 14 months after treatment.

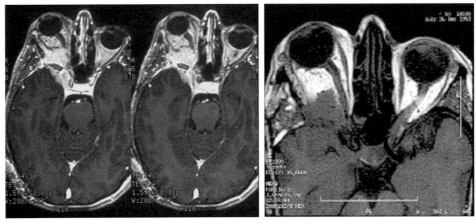

FIGURE 18-8 Spheno-orbital meningioma. (*Left*) MRI scan before radiosurgery. (*Right*) MRI scan 4 years after treatment.

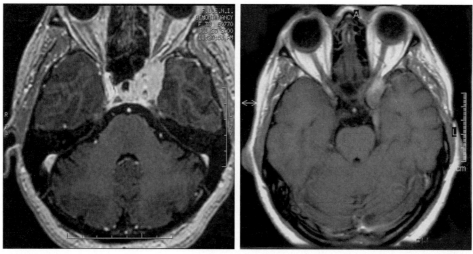

FIGURE 18-9 Sphenoidal ridge meningioma. (*Left*) MRI scan before radiosurgery. (*Right*) MRI scan 2 years after treatment. Note the tumor shrinkage and the optic tract liberation.

Meningiomas of the Internal Third of the Sphenoidal Wing

Meningiomas at this location may be located next to the optic nerve in its exit from the optic foramen or at the anterior portion of the chiasm, as mentioned earlier. Besides, at this location the tumor may approach the cranial nerves that course along the wall of the CS (third, fourth, fifth, and sixth). These nerves can tolerate a higher dose that the optic nerve, on the order of 15 Gy for the third, fourth, and sixth nerve and 13 Gy for the fifth cranial nerve. With respect to vascular lesions, although there are data about an occlusion of the carotid artery 14 months after radiosurgical

treatment,[11] the dose delivered to the artery was 36 Gy, much greater than the one necessary for efficient tumoral control (Fig. 18-9).

Meningiomas of the Cavernous Sinus

The same precautions as for the previous locations are relevant because of their proximity to the same structures (Figs. 18-10 to 18-14).

Tumoral Response to Treatment

Although there are response times within a range of 4 to 20 months, in most cases tumoral control is observed at a

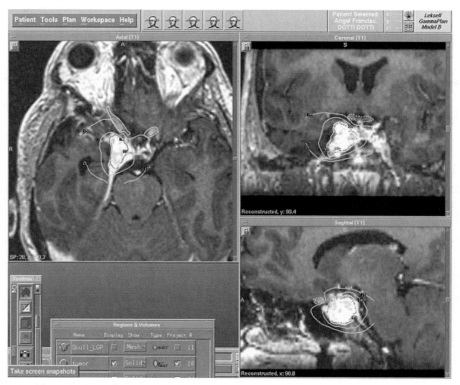

FIGURE 18-10 CS meningioma. Gamma knife treatment planning, avoiding delivering a toxic dose to the optic chiasm.

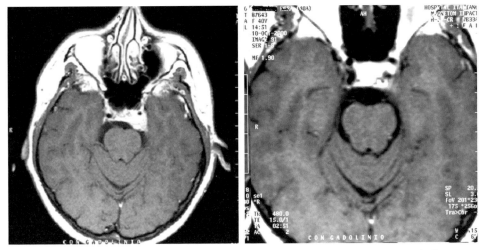

FIGURE 18-11 (*Left*) CS meningioma. (*Right*) MRI control scan 30 months after gamma knife surgery.

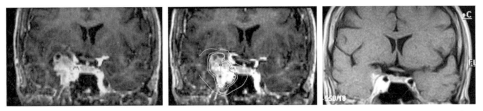

FIGURE 18-12 (*Left*) CS meningioma. (*Center*) Gamma knife surgery planning. (*Right*) MRI control scan after 2 years.

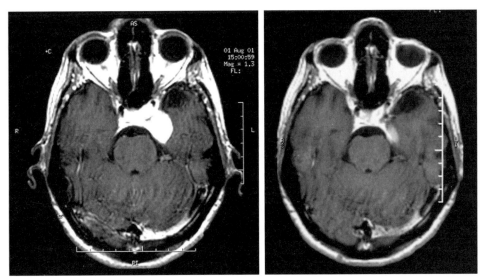

FIGURE 18-13 (*Left*) CS meningioma. (*Right*) MRI control scan 2 years after gamma knife surgery.

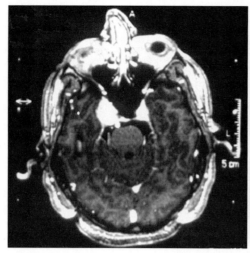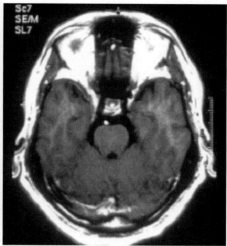

FIGURE 18-14 (*Left*) CS meningioma on date of gamma knife surgery. (*Right*) MRI control scan 2 years after treatment.

half-time of 12 months. In most series[39] and also in our population (132 cases), control is achieved in approximately 90% of cases, including growth arrest and reduction of tumoral volume.

CONCLUSIONS

The ideal objective within the best strategies for the management of skull base meningiomas is to obtain tumoral control minimizing the risk of additional morbidity induced by the therapeutic procedure. This may not always be achieved by microsurgical resection alone. In the search for therapeutic alternatives, gamma knife radiosurgery has proven to be a safe and effective option to reach these goals.

REFERENCES

1. Basso A, Carrizo A: Sphenoid ridge meningiomas. In Schmidek H (ed): Meningiomas and Their Surgical Management. Philadelphia: WB Saunders, 1991, pp 233–241.
2. Benjamin V, McCormack B: Surgical management of tuberculum sellae and sphenoid ridge meningiomas. In Schmidek H, Sweet W (eds): Operative Neurosurgical Techniques, 3rd ed, vol 1. Philadelphia: WB Saunders, 1995, pp 403–413.
3. Cushing H, Eisenhardt L: Meningiomas: Their Classification, Regional Behavior, Life History, and Surgical End Results. Springfield, IL: Charles C Thomas, 1938, pp 298–319.
4. Bonnal J, Sedan R, Paillas J: Problemes cliniques, évolutifs et thérapeutiques souleves par les meningiomes envahissant la base du crane. Neurochirurgie 7:l08–117, 1961.
5. Carrizo A, Basso A, Dickman G, et al: Combined approach to spheno-orbital tumors [Abstract]. 7th International Congress of Neurological Surgery, Munich, 1981, p 36.
6. Al-Mefty O: Clinoidal meningiomas. In Al-Mefty O (ed): Meningiomas. New York: Raven Press, 1991, pp 427–443.
7. Bonnal J, Thibaut A, Brotchi J, Born J: Invading meningiomas of the sphenoid ridge. J Neurosurg 53:587–599, 1980.
8. Sekhar L, Altschuler E: Meningiomas of the cavernous sinus. In Al-Mefty O (ed): Meningiomas. New York: Raven Press, 1991, pp 445–459.
9. Basso A, Carrizo A, Kreutel A, et al: La chirurgie des tumeurs spheno-orbitaires. Neurochirurgie 24:71–82, 1978.
10. Brihaye J, Hofman G, Francois J: Les exophtalmies neurochirurgicales. Neurochirurgie 14:188–487, 1968.
11. Guyot J, Vouyouklakis D, Pertuiset B: Meningiomes de l'arete sphenoidale. Neurochirurgie (Paris) 13:571–584, 1967.
12. Cook A: Total removal of large global meningiomas at the medial aspect of the sphenoid ridge. J Neurosurg 34:107–113, 1971.
13. Simpson D: The recurrence of intracranial meningiomas after surgical treatment. J Neurol Neurosurg Psychiatry 20:22–39, 1957.
14. Castellano F, Guidetti B, Olivecrona H: Pterional meningiomas en plaque. J Neurosurg 9:188–196, 1952.
15. Guiot G, Tessier P, Godon A: Faut-il operer les meningiomes en plaque de l'arete sphenoidale? Neurochirurgie 14:293–304, 1970.
16. Derome P, Guiot G: Bone problems in meningiomas invading the base of the skull. Clin Neurosurg 25:435–451, 1978.
17. Sekhar L, Moller A: Operative management of tumors involving the cavernous sinus. J Neurosurg 64:879–889, 1986.
18. Sekhar L, Sen C, Jho H: Saphenous vein graft bypass of the cavernous internal carotid artery. J Neurosurg 72:35–41, 1990.
19. Fukushima T, Diaz Day J: Surgical management of tumors involving the cavernous sinus. In Schmidek H, Sweet W (eds): Operative Neurosurgical Techniques, 3rd ed. Philadelphia: WB Saunders, 1995, pp 493–510.
20. Lane K, Brown P, Howell D, et al: Creutzfeldt-Jakob disease in a pregnant woman with an implanted dura mater graft. Neurosurgery 34:737–740, 1994.
21. Yamada S, Aiba T, Endo Y, et al: Creutzfeldt-Jakob disease transmitted by cadaveric dura mater graft. Neurosurgery 34:740–744, 1994.
22. Pellerin P, Lesoin F, Dhellemes R, et al: Usefulness of the orbitofronto-malar approach associated with bone reconstruction for frontemporosphenoid meningiomas. Neurosurgery 15:715–718, 1984.
23. Mickey B, Close L, Schaefter S, et al: A combined frontotemporal and lateral infratemporal fossa approach to the skull base. J Neurosurg 68:678, 1988.
24. Cophignon J, Lucena J, Clay C, et al: Limits to radical treatment of spheno-orbital meningiomas. Acta Neurochir Suppl 28:375–380, 1979.
25. Dolenc V: Microsurgical removal of large sphenoidal bone meningiomas. Acta Neurochir Suppl 28:391–396, 1979.
26. Adegbite A, Khan M, Paine K, Tan L: The recurrence of intracranial meningiomas after surgical treatment. J Neurosurg 58:51–56, 1983.
27. Konovalov A, Fedorov S, Faller T, et al: Experience in the treatment of the parasellar meningiomas. Acta Neurochir Suppl 28:371–372, 1979.
28. Pompili A, Derome P, Visot A, Guiot G: Hyperostosing meningiomas of the sphenoid ridge. Surg Neurol 17:411–416, 1982.
29. Philippon J, Bataini J, Cornu P, et al: Les meningiomes recidivants. Neurochirurgie 32(Suppl 1):l–84, 1986.
30. Barbaro N, Gutin P, Wilson C, et al: Radiation therapy in the treatment of partially resected meningiomas. Neurosurgery 20:525–527, 1987.
31. Salazar OM: Ensuring local control in meningiomas. Int J Radiat Oncol Biol Phys 15:501–504, 1988.
32. Newman SA, Meningiomas: A quest for the optimum therapy. J Neurosurg 80:191–194, 1994.
33. Mirabell R, Linggood RM, de la Monte S, et al: The role of radiotherapy in the treatment of subtotally resected benign meningiomas. J Neurooncol 13:157–164, 1992.

34. Guidetti B, Ciappetta P, Domenicucci M: Tentorial meningiomas: Surgical experience with 61 cases and long-term results. J Neurosurg 69:183–187, 1988.
35. Goldsmith BJ, Wara WM, Wilson CB, Larson D: Postoperative irradiation for subtotally resected meningiomas. J Neurosurg 80:195–201, 1994.
36. Larson DA, Flickinger J, Loeffler J: The radiobiology of radiosurgery. Int J Radiat Oncol Biol Phys 25:557–561, 1993.
37. MacCarty CS: Meningiomas of the sphenoidal ridge. J Neurosurg 36:114–120, 1972.
38. Tishler RB, Loeffler JS, Lunsford LD, et al: Tolerance of cranial nerves of the cavernous sinus to radiosurgery. Int J Radiat Oncol Biol Phys 27:215–221, 1993.
39. Roche PH, Regis J, Dufour H, et al: Gamma knife radiosurgery in the management of cavernous sinus meningiomas. J Neurosurg 93 (Suppl 3):68–73, 2000.

19 Surgical Management of Tumors Involving the Cavernous Sinus

TAKANORI FUKUSHIMA and J. DIAZ DAY

Until 1965, when Parkinson's landmark article describing the direct surgical approach to carotid-cavernous fistulas was published, little reference was made in the neurosurgical literature to direct operative attack on lesions of the cavernous sinus.[1] This lack of information was largely a result of the inability in the premicrosurgical era to address effectively the extreme risks of significant hemorrhage and damage to the cranial nerves in the region. This anatomic locale has long been considered a true "no man's land" for direct surgical approaches. The modern era of microneurosurgery has realized expanded capabilities in microsurgical technique and has fostered the work of several neurosurgeons who have made great strides in effectively approaching this region with reduced morbidity.[2–14] In particular, the work of Dolenc should be recognized for the development of his combined epidural and subdural approach, which has become the standard method used to treat lesions in this region.[6]

INDICATIONS

The indications for direct operative attack on neoplastic lesions arising in or involving the cavernous sinus have been a matter of recent debate. New forms of therapy, such as stereotactic radiosurgery, are providing alternatives in our armamentarium for treating these difficult tumors.[15–17] A firmer set of indications for operative intervention has been evolving. We briefly consider the presently acceptable indications for a direct operation on these lesions.

The presence of a mass in the cavernous sinus, of course, does not itself constitute an indication for a direct operation. Many variables must be taken into account, including the age and medical condition of the patient, imaging characteristics, adjacent structures involved, time course of the process, and functional severity of symptoms. Many patients, because of poor medical condition or refusal to undergo surgery, may not be candidates for intracavernous microsurgery. Recent reports have demonstrated that stereotactic radiosurgery presents a viable alternative in patients with small intracavernous meningiomas.[17] Most patients who are able to undergo general anesthesia and who harbor lesions that appear to be amenable to a total resection are offered an operation. Most of these patients have lesions that are consistent with benign tumors of the region (e.g., neurinomas, cavernous hemangiomas, pituitary adenomas, dermoids, chordomas, and chondrosarcomas). These tumors are well-encapsulated masses that are dissectible from the surrounding structures.

Patients with apparent meningiomas of the cavernous sinus, although their tumors are benign, are placed in a separate category for indications for operation. Patients who are able to undergo surgery who have debilitating symptoms, such as rapid visual loss or painful ophthalmoplegia, are offered an immediate operation. The goal of such an operation is decompression of the involved structures, with a total resection attempted only when circumstances are favorable. Patients with asymptomatic, small meningiomas are followed up with serial scans until they show enlargement of the mass or neurologic symptoms. A few patients with minimal symptoms who have tumors that typically are treated conservatively are offered an operation. The reason for this decision is that the size of the tumor and lack of invasion into critical structures makes the resection easier. These decisions rely on the judgment of the surgeon experienced with tumors in this area.

Difficult decisions are made in cases in which cavernous sinus involvement occurs by extensions of malignant processes from the paranasal sinuses and pharynx. Procedures treating such disorders are palliative because of the characteristically aggressive nature of these tumors, such as squamous cell carcinoma. En bloc resection of the cavernous sinus and adjacent areas may represent merely a heroic effort on the patient's behalf, with little realistic chance of long-term survival. Localized malignancies are an entirely different prospect in most cases. Local invasion by chordomas or chondrosarcomas can be effectively resected almost totally in many cases, with long-term recurrence-free survival, even though these tumors are incurable.[13]

Regardless of the process, surgery for these lesions is a formidable undertaking. As experience with these lesions advances, the indications will change according to technologic developments and growing surgical capabilities. This discussion outlines the methods for operative intervention when such an approach is deemed appropriate.

SURGICAL ANATOMY

Recent work focusing on the microsurgical anatomy of the cavernous sinus and its adjacent structures has made a critical contribution to our understanding and capabilities in dealing with neoplasms involving the cavernous sinus.[7,18–22] The individual surgeon's facility with the anatomic details of this complex region cannot be overemphasized as a basis for successful surgical therapy. The anatomy as presented in conventional texts, though an important initial basis, provides insufficient knowledge for the neurosurgeon operating in this region. An intimate comprehension of the multiple entry corridors and their specific anatomic substrates and boundaries is critical to the safe implementation of these procedures. Adequate preparation, including judicious use of the cadaver dissection laboratory, enhances the chances for a successful approach to these lesions.

The cavernous sinus is a tetrahedron-shaped space that is bounded on all sides by dura mater. It is located on either side of the sella turcica at the convergence of the anterior fossa, middle fossa, sphenoid ridge, and petroclival ridge. The contents of the sinus are contained within a membranous structure. Inferiorly and medially, this membrane consists of a periosteal layer of dura that covers the middle fossa and sella turcica. The superior and lateral portion of this outer cavernous membrane is contiguous with the connective tissue sheaths of cranial nerves III, IV, and V. This "true," or outer, cavernous membrane contains the structures within the cavernous sinus. A heavy venous plexus with connections to the ophthalmic veins, the pterygoid plexus, the superior and inferior petrosal sinuses, the basilar venous plexus, and the superficial middle cerebral veins via the sphenoparietal sinus is contained in the space. The internal carotid artery (ICA) and its branches, accompanied by a sympathetic plexus of nerves, pass through the sinus. Also, cranial nerve VI travels through the cavernous sinus to enter the superior orbital fissure under the ophthalmic division of cranial nerve V.

The anatomy of the intracavernous carotid artery deserves special attention. The artery enters the cavernous sinus, piercing the true cavernous membrane, at the foramen lacerum. It is surrounded here by a thickening of this connective tissue, which forms a fibrous ring around the artery. The artery then bends anterosuperiorly toward the superior orbital fissure. Just distal to this bend, the meningohypophyseal trunk typically arises on the superomedial side. This trunk has three branches: (1) the tentorial (Bernasconi-Cassinari), (2) the dorsal meningeal, and (3) the inferior hypophyseal arteries, all of which display some variability. The carotid artery usually gives rise to the artery of the inferior cavernous sinus on its lateral side as it courses anteriorly. This vessel traverses the sinus, usually crossing over cranial nerve VI, and anastomoses with several branches of the internal maxillary artery. These anastomoses include: (1) the recurrent meningeal artery at the superior orbital fissure, (2) the artery of the foramen rotundum, (3) the accessory meningeal artery at the foramen ovale, and (4) the middle meningeal artery at the foramen spinosum. The tentorial artery is absent from the meningohypophyseal trunk in some cases, and in these situations, a marginal tentorial artery is typically found arising from the artery of the inferior cavernous sinus.[19] In a few patients (~10%), branches off the medial side of this segment (known as McConnell's capsular arteries) supply the capsule of the pituitary gland.[19]

The artery makes another bend in the anterior portion of the cavernous sinus superomedially. This segment of the artery exits the cavernous sinus and pierces the enveloping membrane. The membrane in this region is called the carotico-oculomotor membrane, because it spans the gap between the oculomotor nerve in the medial wall of the cavernous sinus and the carotid artery.[19,23] This loop is then completed in the extracavernous, extradural space under

the anterior clinoid process. This loop has been designated the siphon segment, or clinoidal segment, and continues posteriorly a short distance before piercing the dura. Here, it is surrounded by a fibrous ring of dura, and the ophthalmic artery typically originates just inside this fibrous dural ring.[23–25]

The ICA has been assigned nomenclature that divides it into several segments by different authors. We have been using the system described by Fischer in 1938, which numbers the segments beginning from the carotid bifurcation.[26] We make a small modification to the original system with regard to numbering the petrous carotid segment (Fig. 19-1). The C1 segment begins at the carotid bifurcation and extends to the origin of the posterior communicating artery. C2 is the ophthalmic segment described by Day, stretching from the posterior communicating artery to the fibrous dural ring.[23] The extradural, extracavernous clinoid segment is given the designation of C3. C4 is the true intracavernous segment of the artery and is delimited by the caroticooculomotor membrane anteriorly and the origin of the meningohypophyseal trunk posteriorly. From the meningohypophyseal trunk, the artery is designated as C5 until it has passed under the trigeminal nerve. The intrapetrous portion begins at the point at which V3 crosses over the artery and extends to its entrance into the carotid canal in the infratemporal fossa. This segment is designated as C6.

Crucial to the surgeon's understanding of the relevant surgical anatomy of the cavernous sinus is a thorough working knowledge of the multiple triangular entry corridors into the region. The various entry points have been described by various authors and were brought together into a unified geometric construct of the region in 1986 by Fukushima.[7] This scheme is illustrated in Figure 19-2.

ANTERIOR TRIANGLE

The anterior triangle describes an epidural space that contains the C3 portion of the ICA. It is exposed by removal of the anterior clinoid process, either intradurally or extradurally. The boundaries of the triangle are the extradural optic nerve, the fibrous dural ring, and the medial wall of the superior orbital fissure.[4–6,27] The C3 carotid segment enters this space by piercing the carotico-oculomotor membrane. It is important to bear in mind the proximity of the oculomotor nerve, which runs in the medial wall of the superior orbital fissure, thus in apposition to the lateral boundary of this space.

MEDIAL TRIANGLE

The medial triangle is delimited by the intradural carotid artery, the posterior clinoid process, the porus oculomotorius, and the siphon angle of the carotid artery.[9] This space is the primary corridor of access to the C4 portion of the carotid and thus is used for the direct approach to most intracavernous aneurysms. This space is also critical in terms of exposure for most intracavernous tumors.

SUPERIOR TRIANGLE

The medial and lateral boundaries of the superior triangle are cranial nerves III and IV, respectively.[7] The posterior margin is the edge of the dura along the petrous ridge. This triangle is the entry corridor used to locate the meningohypophyseal trunk.

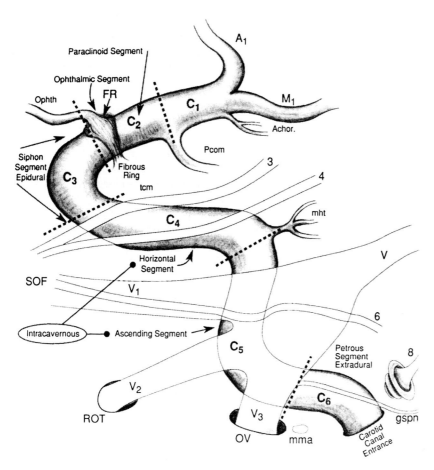

FIGURE 19-1 Illustration of the segmental nomenclature of the intracranial internal carotid artery. The divisions are indicated by the *dashed lines.* C1 begins at the bifurcation and extends to the origin of the posterior communicating artery (Pcom). C2 extends to the fibrous dural ring, making C1 and C2 the two intradural segments of the vessel. C3 corresponds to the extradural, extracavernous carotid siphon segment, which is delimited by the fibrous dural ring and the carotico-oculo-motor membrane. C4 is truly intracavernous and extends to the origin of the meningohypophyseal trunk (mht). The C5 segment is mainly inferior to the trigeminal complex and extends from the meningohypophyseal trunk to the posterolateral fibrous ring, at which point the carotid artery becomes extracavernous. The C6 segment is the horizontal intrapetrous carotid artery. gspn, greater superficial petrosal nerve; mma, middle meningeal artery; SOF, superior orbital fissure; V2, mandibular division of trigeminal complex; V3, maxillary division of trigeminal complex. (Modified from Fischer E: Die Lagabweichrugan der vorderen Hirnarterie in Gefassbild. Zentralb Neurochir 3:300–312, 1938.)

LATERAL TRIANGLE

Described by Parkinson in 1965, the lateral triangle is a very narrow space that is delimited by the trochlear nerve medially and by the ophthalmic division of the trigeminal nerve laterally.[1] Again, the dura of the petrous ridge forms the posterior margin. This triangle can be opened to expose cranial nerve VI as it crosses the C5 segment of the carotid artery.

POSTEROLATERAL TRIANGLE

The posterolateral triangle, first described by Glasscock in 1968, describes the location of the horizontal intrapetrous carotid artery.[28] Exposure of the artery in this space is a critical maneuver in gaining proximal control of the carotid artery. The foramen ovale, foramen spinosum, posterior border of the mandibular division of the trigeminal nerve,

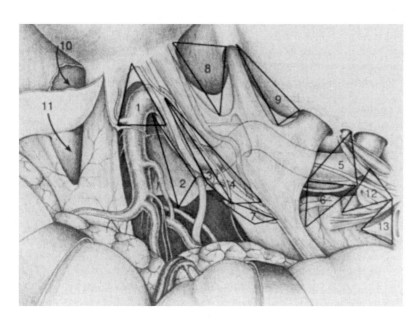

FIGURE 19-2 A geometric construct of the entry corridors to the cavernous sinus region. 1, anterior triangle; 2, medial triangle; 3, superior triangle; 4, lateral triangle; 5, posterolateral triangle; 6, posteromedial triangle; 7, posteroinferior triangle; 8, anterolateral triangle; 9, far lateral triangle; 10, anterior tip of the cavernous sinus route; 11, extended transsphenoidal route; 12, premeatal triangle; 13, postmeatal triangle.

and cochlear apex define this space. Removal of the bone of this triangle exposes approximately 10 mm of the C6 segment of the carotid artery.[29]

POSTEROMEDIAL TRIANGLE

The posteromedial triangle describes the anterior petrous projection of a volume of bone that can be removed to make a window in the petrous apex to the posterior fossa. First described by Kawase and colleagues, this space is delimited by the cochlea, the porus trigeminus, and the posterior border of V3 at the posterior apex of the posterolateral triangle.[30,31] If this triangle is used to make a window in the petrous bone, the anterior brain stem and root of the trigeminal nerve can be reached without encountering neural or vascular structures in the bone.

POSTEROINFERIOR TRIANGLE

The porus trigeminus, posterior clinoid, and entrance to Dorello's canal define this triangle. An incision in this area exposes the petrosphenoidal ligament (Gruber's ligament), which forms the roof of Dorello's canal. Cranial nerve VI can be observed in this space making the first of its two bends, the second occurring as it crosses the intracavernous carotid artery.

ANTEROLATERAL TRIANGLE

The anterolateral triangle is defined by the area between the first and second divisions of the trigeminal nerve as they exit the middle cranial fossa. The anterior border of the triangle is an imaginary line drawn from the lateral edge of the superior orbital fissure to the medial lip of the foramen rotundum. This space is the entry point for exposure of the superior orbital vein and cranial nerve VI and is used to gain access to carotid-cavernous fistulas.[32]

LATERALMOST TRIANGLE (LATERAL LOOP)

Analogous to the anterolateral triangle, this space is bounded by V2, V3, and an imaginary line from the foramen rotundum to the foramen ovale. Lateral extensions of cavernous sinus tumors are also reached through this route. In some patients, the sphenoidal emissary foramen and vein are found here, communicating the cavernous sinus with the pterygoid venous plexus.[19]

ANTERIOR TIP OF THE CAVERNOUS SINUS

This entry corridor is affected through an anterior transbasal approach to the cavernous sinus, which exposes the apical portion of the region. Bilateral exposure of the carotid siphon and the C4 segment is obtained through this strategy.

BACK OF THE CAVERNOUS SINUS

Through an extended transsphenoidal approach, the posteroinferior aspect of the cavernous sinus is appreciated from the underside. The bilateral C4 segments are seen after wide removal of the sellar floor toward the carotid eminence. This exposure is useful in cases of large pituitary adenomas that extend into the cavernous sinus.

PREMEATAL TRIANGLE

The premeatal triangle is used to help define the location of the cochlea from the middle fossa angle of view. The boundaries are the medial lip of the internal acoustic meatus,

the intrapetrous carotid genu, and the geniculate ganglion. The cochlea is located in the basal portion of this triangle. This triangle is important in cases in which the petrous apex is removed through the extradural middle fossa approach.[29]

POSTMEATAL TRIANGLE

The postmeatal triangle delimits the volume of bone located between the internal auditory canal (IAC) and the superior semicircular canal and is used to maximize bone removal of the petrous apex through an extradural middle fossa approach.[29] The boundaries are the geniculate ganglion, the lateral lip of the internal acoustic meatus, and the posterior end of the arcuate eminence.

A thorough working knowledge of these triangular entry corridors is a reasonable prerequisite to operating in the region. Because of the complicated anatomy and the potential for difficult hemostasis, this construct organizes the region in such a way that provides an anatomic foundation for the operative principles outlined herein.

Table 19-1 presents a morphometric analysis from our laboratory of the critical relationships between the major landmarks of the cavernous sinus (unpublished data). These measurements provide a gauge of the areas to be encountered through each of the triangular entry corridors to the region.

ANESTHETIC AND MONITORING TECHNIQUES

The ability of modern neuroanesthesia to facilitate operative procedures by providing increased relaxation of neural tissue and pharmacologic protection against ischemia has realized great improvements. Several maneuvers are used in our cases to help maximize exposure while minimizing retraction of the brain. Administration of osmotic diuretic agents is routine at the beginning of each surgery. We infuse 20% mannitol solution (0.5 mg/kg) along with furosemide (20–40 mg) at the time of skin incision. Further relaxation is attained by maintenance of end-tidal carbon dioxide in the range of 25 to 30 mm Hg. In some cases, these maneuvers alone may not be adequate to provide adequate relaxation, necessitating the use of cerebrospinal fluid (CSF) drainage. This procedure is performed either through a ventricular catheter or a lumbar drain. We rarely use lumbar drainage of CSF in our cases, mainly because of personal preference. Patients with significant elevation of intracranial pressure are not well served by insertion of a lumbar drain at the beginning of the operation. The safest and least complicated method is insertion of a catheter into the frontal horn of the lateral ventricle; this provides ample and accurate drainage of CSF throughout the operation.

Neurophysiologic monitoring is routinely used in all cases. The specific configuration is tailored to each case, taking into consideration the operative approach and the neural and vascular structures likely to be compromised. Somatosensory evoked potentials and electroencephalographic data are always recorded when there is a potential for temporary occlusion of the carotid artery. When the operative approach involves exposure of any part of the facial nerve, facial nerve monitoring is employed.[33] We are also interested in using the technique of extraocular muscle electrodes implanted to monitor the oculomotor, trochlear,

TABLE 19-1 ▪ Morphometric Analysis of the Anatomical Triangles of the Cavernous Sinus (No. = 30 Sides)

Triangle	Border Length (mm)	± SD	Range (mm)
Anterior			
Posterior (fibrous ring length)	6.30	1.01	5.0–8.0
Medial	6.88	1.52	4.5–9.0
Lateral	8.72	1.00	6.5–9.8
Medial			
Posterior	5.41	1.24	3.6–7.2
Medial	10.63	1.28	8.2–12.5
Lateral	8.04	0.93	6.0–10.0
Superior			
Posterior	7.61	1.94	5.8–9.5
Medial	8.73	1.65	5.9–10.2
Lateral	10.48	2.34	6.9–12.8
Lateral			
Posterior	6.94	2.78	3.5–8.0
Medial	10.48	2.34	6.9–12.8
Lateral	11.79	2.52	7.0–13.3
Anterolateral			
Anterior	5.83	1.22	4.2–7.4
Medial	10.63	2.29	7.2–15.1
Lateral	10.36	2.51	5.9–15.0
Lateralmost			
Anterior	10.53	2.58	7.0–15.9
Medial	10.03	2.43	6.7–13.8
Lateral	7.54	3.13	4.0–11.0
Posterolateral			
Medial	20.06	3.15	15.0–25.8
Lateral	14.42	2.52	9.5–19.0
Posterior	13.90	2.14	10.8–17.5
Posteromedial			
Anterior	13.90	2.14	10.8–17.5
Posterior	8.66	2.02	7.5–12.5
Lateral	9.48	2.22	7.8–13.2
Premeatal			
Anterior	8.09	1.57	5.0–9.2
Medial	10.72	1.89	8.0–14.0
Lateral	13.11	2.02	9.5–16.5
Postmeatal			
Medial	13.11	2.02	9.5–16.5
Lateral	14.39	1.84	10.0–16.0
Posterior	12.99	3.73	9.2–18.5

SD, standard deviation.

and abducens nerves.[34] It shows promise in the preservation of those structures. Visual and brain stem auditory evoked potentials have not found much application in our cases of tumors involving primarily the cavernous sinus.

Before planned occlusion of the carotid artery, a suppressive agent (e.g., propofol) is administered to the point of electroencephalographic burst suppression. Burst suppression is then maintained for the entire period of occlusion. Even with burst suppression, the best results are obtained when occlusion time is minimal. Any attenuation of response is an indicator that tolerance to occlusion may be limited, and preservation of the evoked potentials predicts tolerance to ischemia induced by occlusion. However, this is not always the case.

One addition to our armamentarium is a cerebral blood flow monitor, which is used intraoperatively.[35] The flow probe is applied directly to the pial surface and is capable of measuring flow through those vessels. We place the flow probe in an area known to be supplied by the occluded vessel and follow cerebral blood flow before and during the occlusion. Blood flow that drops below 30 mL/100 g/minute is unlikely to be tolerated and also gives information regarding the availability of collateral flow to the area being monitored.

SURGICAL APPROACHES

The cavernous sinus region may be approached through several different corridors. The appropriate choice of surgical approach is dictated mainly by the extent and character of involvement of adjacent structures. Some lesions are fairly well confined within the bounds of the cavernous sinus and require only a straightforward dissection of the region. Other lesions require the combination of two or more standard approaches to gain adequate access the lesion. Others are best handled by some variation of one of the standard approaches, and this is a point that we wish to emphasize. Because of the high potential for morbidity associated with these operations, we approach each lesion individually, tailoring our approach according to the exposure expected to be necessary. Maneuvers that put particular structures at unnecessary risk and lengthen operating time are not used.

Surgical strategy is dictated mainly by the specific entry corridors to the cavernous sinus expected to be used to resect the lesion. The cavernous sinus can be divided into four separate quadrants. Lesions involving the anteromedial region are approached via the anteromedial and anterolateral triangles. Because these two triangles are exposed extradurally, in selected cases (e.g., neurinoma of V2), opening the dura might not be necessary in resecting such a lesion. This concept similarly applies to lesions located in the anterolateral quadrant, approached via the lateral loop and posterolateral triangles (Fig. 19-3A). More posterior lesions, involving the posteromedial and posterolateral regions of the cavernous sinus, usually require exposure through the medial, superior, and lateral triangles (see Fig. 19-3B). These triangles, though possible to open through an extradural route, are typically entered intradurally. Masses confined mainly to the posterolateral quadrant of the region are best approached laterally through the middle fossa (see Fig. 19-3C). Lesions involving more than one of these four areas, for example, a mass with extensive posterior cavernous involvement with extension into the posterior fossa, may require a combined approach for adequate exposure (see Fig. 19-3D). This type of lesion requires a combined strategy via an anterolateral and middle fossa transpetrosal approach. Many lesions require more than one of the standard approaches for satisfactory exposure, and the experience and judgment of the surgeon are necessary to adequately plan the procedure. We outline the standard approaches to intracavernous neoplasms used in our practice and discuss the general indications for their use.

Frontotemporal Epidural and Subdural Approach to the Cavernous Sinus

Dolenc is credited with the initial development and use of the combined epidural and subdural frontotemporal approach (anteromedial transcavernous approach), originally used to directly approach intracavernous aneurysms.[4,6] This technique has become the standard by which lesions within the

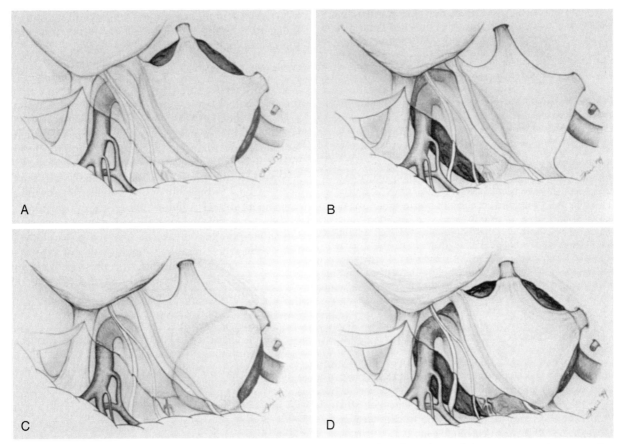

FIGURE 19-3 *A*, Tumors with their primary component located in the anterolateral quadrant of the cavernous sinus can often be approached exclusively through an extradural route to open the anterolateral and far lateral triangles. The mass illustrated may also require exposure via the posterolateral or posteromedial triangles but still remain extradural. *B*, This tumor is located in the posteromedial and antero-medial quadrants, which would require intradural exposure and dissection via the medial, superior, and lateral cavernous triangles. The antero-medial component could be resected via an extradural exposure of the anterior triangle. *C*, Masses with their greatest bulk in the posterolateral quadrant of the cavernous sinus are best handled via a lateral approach, again entirely extradural. *D*, Extensive lesions that involve all quadrants of the cavernous sinus and extend to the posterior fossa or the para/suprasellar regions require a combined approach for adequate exposure.

cavernous sinus are approached. This strategy effectively exposes lesions confined to the cavernous sinus and those with extension to the supratentorial compartment. Lesions with extension into the petroclival area and the posterior fossa are not well exposed by this approach. The method is, however, easily combined with a more lateral approach (e.g., middle fossa transpetrosal) to gain access to such posterior extensions of tumor. Dolenc's combined epidural and subdural strategy has been modified in several ways.[27,36–38] These modifications largely center around the bone flap used and the extent of extradural bone removal at the skull base. The following discussion presents these modifications as alternatives to the basic approach; the modifications are selected on the basis of the exposure expected to be necessary.

Positioning

After induction of general endotracheal anesthesia, the patient is placed in the supine position on the operating table. The table is flexed approximately 30 degrees, and the patient's legs are propped up on one or two pillows. The Mayfield pin headrest is applied with the two-pin arm on the dependent side. We place the posteriormost pin at the inion and rotate the arm such that the anterior pin comes

to rest on the body of the mastoid. The single pin is placed inside the hairline, near the contralateral pupillary line. The head position is fixed and is rotated approximately 30 degrees, with the vertex oriented slightly downward (Fig. 19-4). When in the proper orientation with respect to rotation, the malar eminence is the highest point of the head. We call this position the "head-hanging" position. The back of the table is then tilted such that the head is at, or slightly above, the level of the heart. The patient is now ready for the final skin preparation and draping.

Incision and Flap Elevation

We use three different methods of initial scalp incision and elevation, the choice of which depends mainly on the amount of inferior-to-superior exposure desired. Also, three different methods of craniotomy are used, again depending on the degree of inferior-to-superior exposure necessary.

SINGLE-LAYER TECHNIQUE

The standard one-layer technique is used when the requirement for extradural bone removal is minimal, and a limited inferior-to-superior viewing angle will be necessary. Also, this technique does not include the creation of a vascularized

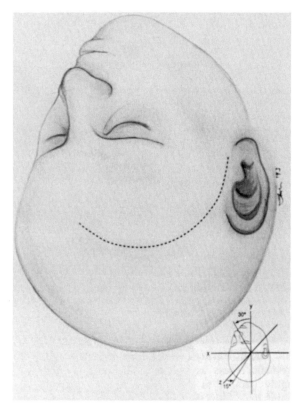

FIGURE 19-4 Head position for the standard frontotemporal approach to the cavernous sinus. The head-hanging position is demonstrated with the head turned 30 degrees and tilted downward approximately 15 degrees. This position is also used for the temporopolar approach.

pericranial flap for use at closure. We begin the incision just anterior to the tragus at the level of the zygoma root and proceed superiorly, inside the hairline. The incision curves gently forward, ending in the midline. The temporalis muscle and fascia are incised. Particular attention is paid to the area around the zygoma root. The temporalis muscle is freed from its attachment to the zygoma root, which yields increased elevation of the muscle anteriorly. Use of monopolar cautery in this area should be restrained because of the proximity of the frontalis branch of the facial nerve. The pericranium medial to the superior temporal line is elevated with the temporalis muscle and fascia. This myocutaneous flap is elevated anteriorly to expose the frontozygomatic recess and is held in place with large hooks.

HALF-AND-HALF TECHNIQUE

The half-and-half method is used when vascularized pericranial flap is desired and obtaining a high degree of inferior-to-superior exposure is not necessary. After the skin incision has been made, the flap is elevated medial to the superior temporal line in two layers by sharp dissection of the areolar connective tissue layer between the pericranium and the galea. Care must be exercised to avoid damaging the supraorbital nerve, which lies adherent to the inner surface of the galea and can be mistakenly included in the pericranial layer. At the superior temporal line, the pericranium is incised. The temporalis muscle and fascia are then elevated with the scalp and reflected anteriorly, just as in the single-layer technique. The pericranium is then elevated

from the bone to the supraorbital rim and reflected anteriorly. We protect this flap by wrapping it in wet gauze, and we keep it moist during the operation.

TWO-LAYER TECHNIQUE

The two-layer technique is used when increased inferior-to-superior trajectory is necessary, because this technique results in reflection of the temporalis muscle inferiorly and laterally. This method rotates the muscle away from the orbital rim and frontozygomatic recess, thus preventing the muscle mass from creating an obstruction when the microscope is radically rotated to obtain a more rostral view. The skin incision is typically started slightly more inferiorly, exposing the entire zygomatic root. Beginning medially, the galeal layer is elevated from the pericranium, and the areolar bands, which span the two layers, are sharply divided. Again, the supraorbital and supratrochlear nerves must be preserved with the galeal layer. As the superior temporal line is reached, the areolar connective tissue that is continuous with the pericranial layer is elevated with the galea, which exposes bare temporalis fascia. The critical step in this maneuver is handling the temporal fat pad. This fat pad consists of superficial and deep components. The superficial fat pad is surrounded by the loose areolar connective tissue overlying the temporalis fascia and contains the frontalis branches of the facial nerve. The fat pad is elevated with the areolar tissue and the galeal layer. The galeal layer is elevated to expose the supraorbital rim, lateral orbital rim, and entire zygomatic process, which is covered by fascia. The deep fat pad is situated over the inferior portion of the temporalis muscle as it passes under the zygomatic arch and is covered by fascia. This pad of fat is left in place and retracted with the muscle (Fig. 19-5).

The temporalis muscle is now elevated, and monopolar cautery is used as necessary. This elevation is begun anteriorly at the lateral orbital rim, and the periosteum is incised so as to leave a cuff for reattachment of the fascia. The muscle is elevated without any incision being made in this structure

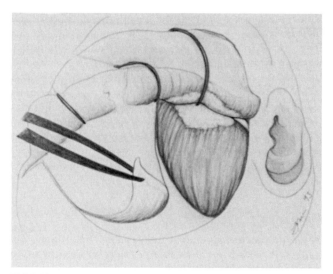

FIGURE 19-5 The two-layer scalp flap technique is illustrated, preserving the frontalis branches of the facial nerve by splitting the superficial and deep temporal fat pads. This technique preserves a vascularized periosteal flap, which is used in closure of the skull base. Note the preservation of the supraorbital nerve.

and is reflected inferiorly and posteriorly. The vascularized pericranial flap is next elevated and reflected anteriorly as described earlier for the half-and-half technique.

Craniotomy and Extradural Bone Removal

As with the elevation of the skin flap, the degree of inferior-to-superior exposure and the posterior limits of the expected dissection determine the type of bone flap to be used. A routine pterional bone flap is sufficient for masses limited to the anterior and anterolateral cavernous sinus. Tumors with much more extensive involvement posteriorly and those that escape the confines of the region require a more generous cranial opening for adequate exposure.

FRONTOTEMPORAL CRANIOTOMY

This is the most frequently used bone flap and provides satisfactory exposure in most cases. Two or three burr holes are made, preferably with the pediatric-sized burr hole drill bit. The first hole is placed in the keyhole area in an attempt to straddle the sphenoid ridge. The second hole is placed directly posterior, just below the superior temporal line, at the posterior limit of the exposed bone. The third hole is optional and is placed inferiorly, in the temporal squama, just above the floor of the middle fossa. Typically, the flap is made with a more generous frontal exposure than that typically used for an anterior circulation aneurysm. The dimensions are usually approximately 7 to 8 cm by 5 cm, centered one third above and two thirds below the superior temporal line. The temporal squama remaining inferiorly is removed, resulting in a flat angle of view along the middle fossa floor. The dura is then tacked to the posterosuperior bone margin with fine suture through obliquely drilled wire-pass holes.

With a generous frontal extension toward the midline, the frontal sinus is frequently encountered. An open frontal sinus must be handled properly to avoid an annoying complication from a CSF leak or postoperative infection. We recommend use of a high-speed drill and a diamond burr to exenterate the mucosa of the sinus. This procedure must be meticulously performed to avoid formation of a mucocele. Next, the ostia are carefully occluded, usually with a piece of temporalis muscle, and the sinus is then packed with fat. The packed sinus will be covered with pericranium, or other fascia, at the conclusion of the procedure.

TRANSZYGOMATIC CRANIOTOMY

After the galeal layer is reflected by use of the two-layer technique, the periosteum of the zygomatic process and the lateral orbital rim is incised and elevated. We make this incision in such a way that leaves a cuff of tissue for later reapproximation. The temporalis muscle is freed from the temporal squama and of its attachment to the inner surface of the zygoma. The zygoma is now cut with a sagittal or reciprocating saw (Fig. 19-6). The anterior cut is made parallel to the lateral orbital rim, beginning at the frontozygomatic suture, leaving as little bone overhanging the frontozygomatic recess as possible. The posterior cut is made roughly parallel to the surface of the temporal squama through the root of the temporal zygomatic process, and care is taken to avoid invasion of the temporomandibular joint. This technique results in what we call a "T-bone" cut and maximizes inferior temporalis muscle retraction, resulting

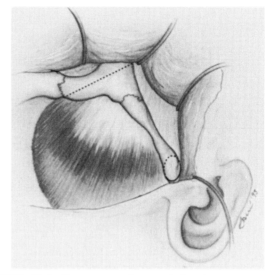

FIGURE 19-6 The osteotomies used for the transzygomatic craniotomy are demonstrated. This method results in what is called a T-bone cut, maximizing inferior temporalis retraction.

in an increased ability to gain an inferior-to-superior view. A frontotemporal craniotomy is now made as described earlier. The remaining temporal squama is removed to obtain a flat viewing angle along the middle cranial fossa floor.

ORBITOZYGOMATIC CRANIOTOMY

This craniotomy technique results in maximal inferior-to-superior trajectory and allows the widest access to the cavernous sinus up toward the brain base. The scalp flap must be made in two layers, and elevation of the pericranium is extended to include the periorbital fascia. The periorbital fascia is elevated from the midline superiorly to the inferolateral aspect of the orbit. This tissue must be freed to a depth of approximately 1.5 cm inside the orbit. If the supraorbital nerve travels through a supraorbital foramen, freeing the nerve is necessary. By use of a small osteotome, the bone of the foramen is removed in a wedge to free the nerve and allow forward reflection with the pericranium.

Two burr holes are then made, one in the keyhole area and the second about 5 cm posteriorly, inferior to the superior temporal line. Next, the thick bore that connects the anterior temporal base to the orbital wall is drilled away. Then, a cut is made with the craniotome beginning at the posterior burr hole, proceeding inferiorly toward the middle fossa floor, then curving upward over the temporal line to meet the pterional burr hole (Fig. 19-7). A sagittal or reciprocating saw is now used to cut the zygoma root parallel to the squamosal surface, as described earlier (Fig. 19-8). The next cut is made roughly parallel to, and several millimeters above, the zygomaticomaxillary suture, cutting into the lateral wall of the orbit. The medial supraorbital rim is cut and continued posteriorly several millimeters into the orbital roof. The orbital wall is next incised, either with the sagittal saw or a small osteotome, from medial to lateral, thus freeing the supraorbital and lateral orbital rims (Fig. 19-9). The final cut made is through the articulation of the zygomatic and sphenoid bones from posterior. These bone incisions free the flap as a single unit (Fig. 19-10). Sometimes the flap needs to be freed from some remaining attachment

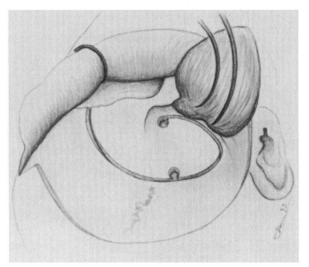

FIGURE 19-7 The initial craniotome osteotomy is illustrated, extending through the medial orbital rim.

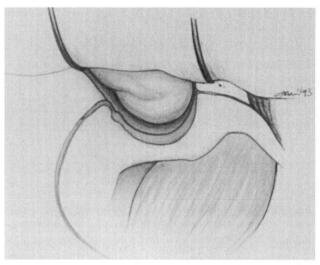

FIGURE 19-9 Intraorbitally, the osteotomy is made at a depth of approximately 10 to 15 mm. The zygoma is incised just superior to the zygomaticofrontal foramen (shown) and the zygomaticomaxillary suture.

of the sphenoid wing; this is easily accomplished via fracturing of that remaining attachment.

Extradural Bone Removal

Extradural removal of bone at the cranial base provides several advantages. Primarily, reduction of cranial base bone volume reduces the degree of necessary retraction of neural structures. Second, removal of bone surrounding neural structures as they pass through bone canals results in mobility of these structures without impingement against bone surfaces, which may result in pressure-induced ischemia. Third, transposition of neural and vascular structures from their bone canals results in wider corridors of access. In this chapter, we describe the technique for maximal removal of the anterolateral base; however, the extent of removal of the cranial base is individualized for each case. Risk is associated with every degree of bone removal at the skull base,

and for this reason, determination of the exposure for each particular case is an important step in surgical planning.

The initial step in this procedure is reduction of the sphenoid wing. The dura is elevated and retracted with 4-mm, tapered retractors. Under constant irrigation, the sphenoid wing is reduced with a high-speed drill. Initially, the wing is flattened down to the level of the meningo-orbital artery as it joins the dura at the superior orbital fissure apex. Bone irregularities of the frontal floor are reduced with a diamond burr, resulting in a smooth contour of the orbital roof. The superior orbital fissure is skeletonized to expose approximately 10 mm of periorbital fascia, and the foramen rotundum is unroofed to the infratemporal peripheral branches to expose 5 to 8 mm of V2. When lateral cavernous exposure is desired, the foramen ovale is similarly unroofed to mobilize V3. The orbit may now be skeletonized, leaving only a thin shell of bone adherent to the periorbital fascia. The meningo-orbital artery, typically at

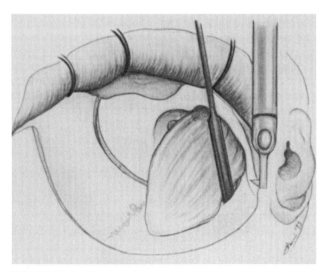

FIGURE 19-8 The root of the zygomatic process is cut parallel to the surface of the temporal squama to prevent any obstructing process to maximal inferior temporalis retraction.

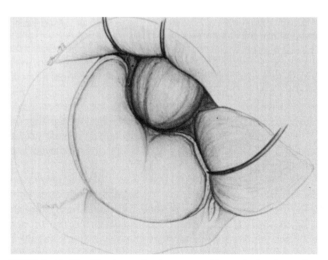

FIGURE 19-10 The bone flap is removed in a single piece after first fracturing any remaining attachment at the sphenoid ridge.

the superior orbital fissure apex, is coagulated and divided. The adhesion of the dura at the superior orbital fissure apex is divided approximately 4 to 5 mm. This goal can be achieved without risk to cranial nerves III and IV.

The next stage of extradural bone removal, optic canal unroofing, is the most technically demanding. It is helpful to first locate the exit point of the nerve from the optic canal. A very short segment (about 1 mm) can be identified as it spans the gap between bone and dura. On the medial side, care must be taken to avoid entering the sphenoid sinus, which lies just medial to the optic canal. If the sinus is opened, it must be carefully exenterated of its mucosa and packed with either muscle or fat. The sinus may likewise be entered on the lateral side when the surgeon drills between the optic canal and anterior clinoid, while reducing the optic strut.

The anterior clinoid process is next removed on the lateral side of the optic canal. Optimal technique is critical because the anterior clinoid process is surrounded by the optic nerve, ICA, and contents of the superior orbital fissure.

Under constant cooling from irrigation, the anterior clinoid process is hollowed out with the diamond drill. This structure must never be removed in a single piece. The sides are thinned to the point at which the sides can be lightly fractured and dissected free from the dura. The very tip of the anterior clinoid is usually removed with the aid of small alligator forceps, and the small (1 to 2 mm) tip is gently twisted free after careful dural dissection. When the anterior clinoid is hollowed out, the surgeon must be ever cognizant of the relative positions of the optic nerve, the carotid artery, and the superior orbital fissure contents. The optic nerve is medial; the carotid artery, anterior and inferior; and cranial nerve III, lateral in the medial superior orbital fissure wall. At times, this removal is complicated by the presence of a bridge between the anterior and posterior clinoid processes, forming a caroticoclinoidal foramen. Under such circumstances, completing the resection of this structure intradurally may be necessary. Occasionally, with final removal of the anterior clinoid, bleeding from the cavernous sinus occurs, typically from disruption from the carotico-oculomotor membrane. This bleeding is controlled by packing one or two small pieces of Surgicel in the defect.

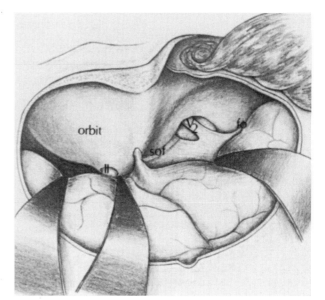

FIGURE 19-11 This figure illustrates the view of the anterior and middle cranial base at the completion of the extradural bone dissection to unroof the maxillary division of the trigeminal (V2), the superior orbital fissure (sof), and the optic nerve (II). fo, foramen ovale.

Bipolar cautery should not be used because it is ineffective, and current may spread to the oculomotor nerve.

Next, the full anterolateral cranial base is skeletonized, and the neural structures become capable of being mobilized, after being freed from the constraints of their respective bone foramina (Fig. 19-11). Hemostasis is attained with the use of bone wax and monopolar cautery. Monopolar cautery should be used only in areas that do not have underlying sensitive structures. A typical example is in the middle fossa in the region of the tegmen tympani. Heat transfer through bone here can damage cranial nerve VII or the hearing apparatus.

When extradural exposure of the intrapetrous carotid artery is desired, it is appropriately exposed in the postero-lateral triangle (Fig. 19-12). The dura must be elevated from the middle cranial fossa to expose the greater superficial petrosal nerve running in the major petrosal groove.

FIGURE 19-12 The dura propria is reflected from the outer cavernous membrane to expose the trigeminal complex (V1–V3), the trochlear, and the oculomotor nerves. With extradural resection of the anterior clinoid process, the carotid siphon is well exposed (C3). The extradural exposure of the intrapetrous carotid artery (C6) exposes approximately 10 mm of the vessel in the middle fossa. MMA, middle meningeal artery.

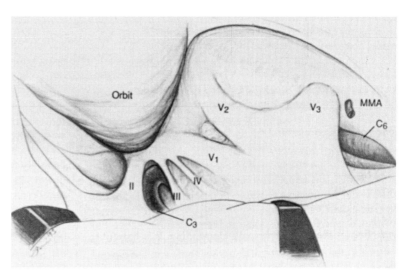

The middle meningeal artery must be coagulated and divided as it exits the foramen spinosum. This vessel is usually surrounded by a plexus of veins, which must be effectively coagulated. With the greater superficial petrosal nerve exposed, the landmarks delineating the position of the carotid artery are apparent because the artery lies under the nerve and is running parallel, toward V3. Drilling is begun posterior to V3, just medial to the foramen spinosum. The greater superficial petrosal nerve is typically divided near V3 and reflected posteriorly for greater exposure of the ICA. Bone over the artery is removed from the tensor tympani muscle lateral to bone that lies under V3. The greatest danger in this procedure is violation of the cochlea, which lies 1 to 2 mm from the carotid genu. Excessive bone removal posterior to the carotid genu carries significant risk for cochlear violation.

INTRADURAL TRANSCAVERNOUS DISSECTION

Neoplastic lesions that escape the bounds of the cavernous sinus typically require intradural exposure of adjacent regions. In these cases, the cavernous sinus may be opened through the medial, superior, and lateral triangles via an intradural dissection. This intradural approach to the cavernous sinus begins with opening of the dura using a T-shaped incision. The incision starts at the anterior frontal corner of the exposure and curves downward, close to the posterior bone margin, toward the anterior temporal corner. A cut is then made along the dura that covers the sylvian fissure and proceeds toward the optic nerve dura, completing the T. The dural flaps are retracted forward and tacked down with fine suture.

Arachnoid dissection usually begins with splitting of the sylvian fissure. Dividing the anterior 3 to 4 cm is sufficient in most cases and provides adequate retraction of the frontal and temporal lobes while minimizing retractor pressure. It is often necessary to coagulate and divide the bridging veins of the temporal tip to mobilize the temporal lobe satisfactorily. The arachnoid surrounding the optic nerve and intradural carotid artery is then sharply divided, and damage to small perforating arteries is carefully avoided. Arachnoid division continues posteriorly to the tentorial edge, dividing the membrane of Liliequist to expose the oculomotor nerve as it enters the porus oculomotorius. The lateral dural wall of the cavernous sinus is now visible at this point of the dissection from the anterior margin of the middle fossa to the tentorial edge posteriorly.

The medial triangle of the cavernous sinus is readily opened at its apex after the carotid artery has been sharply liberated of its attachment at the fibrous dural ring. The dura over the triangle can then be incised toward the posterior clinoid, a procedure that produces a tremendous amount of bleeding, except when the region is filled with tumor. Bleeding is controlled by judicious packing with Surgicel. Medial and posterior packing can be fairly generous to close off the connections to the basilar venous plexus and inferior petrosal sinus. Lateral packing must be more modest to avoid compression of cranial nerve III.

Dissection of the superior triangle is best performed after opening of the medial triangle and liberation of cranial nerve III by opening the porus oculomotorius, reflecting the dura from the outer cavernous membrane over cranial nerve III, and incising the outer cavernous membrane to free the nerve. The triangle can then be entered medial to

cranial nerve IV. This triangle contains the meningohypophyseal trunk, which is subject to compression by overzealous packing of the space to control hemorrhage. Vigorous packing posteriorly and laterally can also result in compression of cranial nerve VI. Analogous to the maneuver made to open this triangle, the lateral triangle is similarly opened by reflecting the middle fossa dura from the true cavernous membrane over cranial nerve IV and continuing to the trigeminal first branch and semilunar ganglion. The lateral triangle can then be entered and cranial nerve VI exposed as it crosses over the intracavernous carotid artery. Packing for hemostasis in this triangle must avoid compression of the carotid artery and cranial nerve VI.

At the completion of the dissection, the anteromedial, anterolateral, and posteromedial quadrants of the cavernous sinus are exposed. The posterolateral portion is usually incompletely exposed via this dissection because of obstruction by the trigeminal complex. Intradurally, cranial nerve III is visible from the interpeduncular fossa to its entrance into the superior orbital fissure. Cranial nerve IV is seen from near its entrance into the incisural edge, crossing the cavernous sinus to enter the superior orbital fissure on top of cranial nerve III. Lateral to the trochlear nerve, in the lateral triangle, deflection of the ophthalmic division of the trigeminal nerve exposes cranial nerve VI crossing the intracavernous carotid artery. Incision of the incisural edge between the porus trochlearis and the porus trigeminus widely opens the posteroinferior triangle and Dorello's canal. Tumor is resected by use of the techniques outlined in the subsequent section on Special Techniques of Intracavernous Surgery.

CLOSURE

Closure in these procedures is at times complicated. The goal of closure at the skull base is complete separation of the intradural compartment from extradural structures. A watertight dural closure is critical to the successful avoidance of postoperative complications secondary to CSF leakage and contamination, and fascial patch grafts are used as necessary to meet this goal. Even the most meticulous closure has the potential for small leaks. Therefore, all potential routes of communication should be closed off with autologous fat grafts and fascial barriers. As discussed earlier, opened paranasal sinuses must be exenterated of mucosa to avoid mucocele formation. Then, any ostia are obliterated and the sinus is occluded with muscle or fat. The fat or muscle graft is then best sealed from the dural closure by covering with an additional vascularized pericranial flap, and strategically placing tacking sutures prevents migration. We use titanium plates for securing the bone flap because of the superior cosmetic results obtained.

Anterolateral Temporopolar Transcavernous Approach

This approach provides access to the cavernous sinus from a more lateral trajectory than the standard frontotemporal method.[36] The technique makes use of extradural retraction of the frontal and temporal lobes, both to protect the cortical surface and to preserve the venous drainage of the temporal tip. The extensive extradural dissection provides a very wide corridor of access to the cavernous sinus region, as well as wide access to the infrachiasmatic and upper clival areas.

In contrast to the standard frontotemporal approach, the cavernous sinus triangles are opened from an extradural route, using minimal intradural dissection.

Integral to the basis of this technique is an understanding of the anatomy of the lateral wall and roof of the cavernous sinus. The dura covering the cavernous sinus, on the undersurface of the temporal lobe, is adherent to the outer cavernous membrane. The outer (or "true") cavernous membrane is formed by the connective tissue sheaths of cranial nerves III, IV, and V and is continuous with periosteum at the bone margins. This membrane envelops the structures in the cavernous sinus. Thus the dura can be elevated from the outer cavernous membrane with minimal hemorrhage if no large tears are created in this membrane. The ability to expose the cavernous sinus in this way is the key element of this approach.

Closure typically requires a vascularized pericranial flap; therefore, the two-layer scalp flap technique is necessary. The incision is a generous frontotemporal incision, beginning at, or just below, the root of the zygomatic process. Either of the three bone flaps described earlier may be used for this approach. Again, the degree of inferior-to-superior trajectory that will be required dictates the use of the transzygomatic or orbitozygomatic flaps. Extradural bone removal proceeds as outlined earlier. The novel aspects of the approach begin when extradural bone removal is complete and the dura is ready to be opened.

Beginning at the superior orbital fissure apex, the meningo-orbital fibrous band is coagulated and divided. The temporal dura is retracted posteriorly. Elevation of the dural margin begins at the superior orbital fissure and extends laterally to the foramen ovale. At the junction of the periorbital fascia and dura, the cleavage plane is sharply developed, and the connective tissue fibrils bridging the dura and the outer cavernous membrane are divided, as the dura is retracted posteriorly. In this way, the dura is reflected from the outer cavernous membrane toward the petrous ridge (see Fig. 19-12). If this maneuver is performed properly, little bleeding occurs from the cavernous sinus. Cavernous sinus bleeding from small tears in the outer cavernous membrane is stopped by packing small pieces of Surgicel into the openings. The anteromedial limit in dural elevation is the tentorial edge, which is handled after the dura is opened.

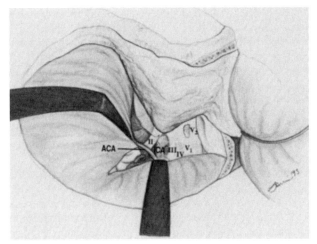

FIGURE 19-13 The dura is opened in an L-shaped incision to expose the sylvian fissure and intradural internal carotid artery. The sylvian fissure is split approximately 2 cm for additional retraction. ACA, anterior cerebral artery; CA, carotid artery.

The dura is now ready to be opened. An L-shaped incision is made beginning along the dura covering the sylvian fissure, approximately 5 cm from its attachment to the carotid artery. The incision is extended through optic nerve sheath dura and is then carried medially across the tuberculum sellae for 2 to 3 cm (Fig. 19-13). The retractors are replaced to provide posterior retraction on both the frontal and temporal lobes, and the fibrous dural ring surrounding the carotid artery is sharply freed from the vessel. The lateral portion of this fibrous ring is met by the tentorial edge, formed by a fold in the dura. The two layers composing this fold are then split. This maneuver elevates the temporal dura from the outer cavernous membrane over the medial triangle and effectively frees the medial margin of temporal dura, resulting in full lateral and posterior retraction. Some arachnoidal dissection around the porus oculomotorius is typically a prerequisite to this move. At this juncture, the structures of the lateral wall of the cavernous sinus should be plainly visible through the thin veil of the outer cavernous membrane, from the sella to the trigeminal third division. The medial, superior, and lateral triangles are well delineated (Fig. 19-14).

FIGURE 19-14 The opening of the fibrous dural ring and the porus oculomotorius with splitting of dural leaves composing the tentorial edge are shown. This maneuver allows lateral retraction of this dural edge and opening of the medial triangle. This also leads into the opening of the superior triangle in similar fashion. PCom A, posterior communicating artery; ICA, internal carotid artery.

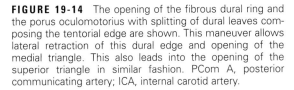

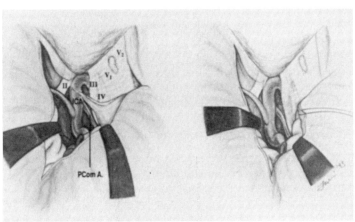

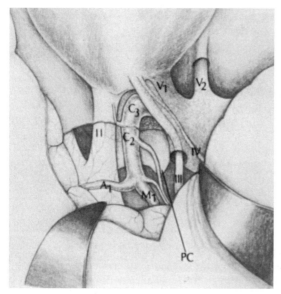

FIGURE 19-15 The final exposure of the anteromedial and posteromedial cavernous sinus via the temporopolar approach.

The sylvian fissure is usually split to decrease the required retractor pressure, even though the degree of frontal and temporal lobe retraction is somewhat lessened with this approach. No more than the anterior 1 to 2 cm of the fissure need be split in most cases. During the dissection, it will be clear that the temporal tip bridging veins need not be sacrificed with this approach because the temporal dura is retracted with the temporal lobe, obviating sacrifice of these vessels. The arachnoid is opened over the optic nerve and chiasm, as well as the carotid artery to expose the A1 and M1 segments (Fig. 19-15). The medial and anterolateral portions of the cavernous sinus are exposed at this point of the dissection, and tumor resection may proceed.

At the conclusion of the procedure, dural closure must be performed in as complete a manner as possible. Closure requires the use of a pericranial or fascial graft, and if any bone sinuses were opened during the extradural bone removal, these must be exenterated and packed with a fat or muscle graft. A problem area of closure is that around the optic nerve. The incision in the optic nerve sheath dura is not closed with suture because of the risk of damage to the nerve from compression or direct trauma. Fascial patch grafts are used to close the incision around the nerve, and then fat is placed around the nerve area. The fascial graft is tacked such that it will prevent migration of the fat graft, and the area is finally sealed with fibrin glue. For superior cosmetic results, the bone flaps are secured with one of the titanium plating systems.

Lateral Approach to the Posterior Cavernous Sinus Region (Rhomboid Approach)

Although the posterior cavernous sinus region may be reached strictly through an anterior trajectory, the exposure is narrow, and cranial nerve V is an obstacle to adequate vision. This narrow corridor provides limited access to the posteroinferior triangle and region surrounding the porus trigeminus.

For this reason, a more lateral and posterior approach is indicated, either subtemporal or transpetrosal, that provides a wider operative corridor and access inferolateral to the trigeminal complex. The extradural middle fossa transpetrosal approach provides such exposure through a subtemporal route and is easily combined with the frontotemporal approach.[29–31,39,40] At our institution, we call this method the rhomboid approach, named for the complex of middle fossa floor landmarks that delineate the anterior transpetrosal window of bone through which the posterior cavernous sinus and petroclival areas are exposed. When bone removal through this approach is maximized, near-total resection of the petrous apex results.[29]

Avoidance of complication from this technique depends mainly on an intimate knowledge of the internal anatomy of the petrous bone and the relationships between internal structures and surface landmarks. The major potential complications of the procedure are hearing loss resulting from cochlear or bone labyrinth violation and compromise of facial nerve integrity and function. In an attempt to simplify the technique, we have devised a geometric construct of key middle fossa landmarks that delineates the volume of bone to be resected. This construct helps to locate, and thus avoid, internal structures of the petrous pyramid.[29]

The approach is performed with the head in the 90-degree lateral position, through a 4-cm by 4-cm temporal craniotomy centered two thirds anterior and one third posterior over the external auditory meatus. When performed in combination with a frontotemporal approach, a more generous temporal extension of the craniotomy must be made that reaches posterior to the root of the zygomatic process. The head is rotated about 60 degrees toward the contralateral side, either initially or by later rotation of the table. Middle fossa dural elevation begins posteriorly and laterally, over the petrous ridge, and continues anteromedially to the foramen ovale. Dura is elevated in this manner to avoid traction on the greater superficial petrosal nerve (GSPN), which may result in facial nerve compromise. The GSPN lies in the major petrosal groove of the middle fossa floor and is covered by a thin layer of periosteum. The middle meningeal artery and surrounding venous plexus are coagulated and divided near the artery's exit from the foramen spinosum. The dura is then separated from the trigeminal complex at the foramen ovale, continuing posteriorly toward the porus trigeminus. Tapered retractors are used to retract the dura medially and posteriorly to expose the entire middle fossa floor (Fig. 19-16).

At this juncture, the landmarks necessary to begin the bone dissection are identifiable. The volume of bone that will be resected corresponds to a rhomboid-shaped complex of landmarks of the middle fossa floor. This geometric construct is defined by: (1) the intersection of the GSPN and V3, (2) the intersection of lines projected along the axes of the GSPN and the arcuate eminence, (3) the intersection with the petrous ridge, and (4) the porus trigeminus. Obliquely projecting this construct through the petrous bone to the inferior petrosal sinus delimits the volume of petrous bone that has no neural or vascular structures.

Bony resection begins with the exposure of the IAC. By use of a high-speed diamond drill, the IAC is found 3 to 4 mm deep to the middle fossa floor along the bisection axis between lines projected along the GSPN and the

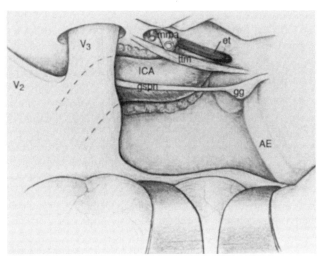

FIGURE 19-16 This middle fossa floor is exposed via the extended middle fossa approach. The landmarks to begin the extradural bone removal are visible at this point in the procedure. AE, arcuate eminence; et, eustachian tube; gg, geniculate ganglion; gspn, greater superficial petrosal nerve; ICA, internal carotid artery; mma, middle meningeal artery; ttm, tensor tympani muscle; V2 and V3, mandibular and maxillary divisions of trigeminal complex.

arcuate eminence. We call this bisection axis Brackmann's line, and drilling begins along its midpoint. The entire length of the IAC is exposed. Next, the GSPN is uncovered lateral to the facial hiatus, until the geniculate ganglion is exposed. A thin shell of bone is left over the ganglion for protection. The GSPN is sectioned near V3 and reflected laterally to increase intrapetrous carotid exposure. The carotid is exposed in the posterolateral triangle from V3 to the tensor tympani muscle. Then, the bone between the IAC and carotid can be safely removed to expose posterior fossa dura (Fig. 19-17). Great care must be taken to avoid the cochlea during this portion of bone dissection.

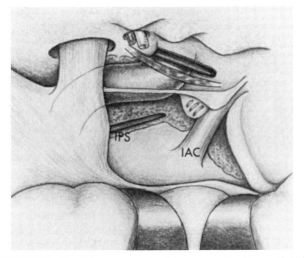

FIGURE 27-17 After the extradural bone resection is completed, the posterior fossa dura to the level of the inferior petrosal sinus (IPS) is exposed. The internal auditory canal (IAC) is skeletonized approximately 270 degrees. The posterior cavernous sinus is exposed via this route by elevating and medially translocating the trigeminal complex, opening the outer cavernous membrane inferior to the trigeminal ganglion.

The cochlea is located in the base of the premeatal triangle, which is defined by the carotid genu, the geniculate ganglion, and the medial lip of the internal auditory meatus.[29] Resection of apical petrous bone is continued inferiorly to the level of the inferior petrosal sinus. The apical bone inferior to the trigeminal ganglion can be removed by coring out of the petrous apex. The wedge of bone remaining that lies lateral to the IAC can be removed, to result in an almost 270-degree exposure of the IAC. This lateral wedge of bone is defined by the postmeatal triangle, which is bounded by the geniculate ganglion, the arcuate eminence, and the lateral lip of the internal auditory meatus. It is often helpful to blue-line the superior semicircular canal during removal of this bone to avoid entering the vestibule.

With the bone dissection complete, the posterior and inferolateral cavernous sinus can be widely reached. The limits of this exposure are the foramen of Dorello medially and the inferior petrosal sinus below. The trigeminal complex can be completely freed of dura and then elevated or retracted medially. This exposure provides visualization of the C5 and C6 portions of the carotid artery. A prerequisite to this maneuver for increasing the exposure of the posterior cavernous sinus is extradural liberation of the V2 and V3 divisions in their respective bone canals. Elevation of the trigeminal complex in this way allows full exposure of the posterior cavernous sinus and complete petrous apex resection extradurally under direct vision (unpublished data).

The dura is opened at the porus trigeminus above the superior petrosal sinus. This incision is carried laterally as far as the arcuate eminence and exposes the superior surface of the tentorium. A parallel incision is then made inferior to the superior petrosal sinus. The superior petrosal sinus is ligated with small vascular clips and divided at its medial aspect. The retractors can then be placed on the undersurface of the tentorium, and the temporal lobe is retracted more superiorly under its protection. The trigeminal root is also liberated from its dural attachment at the porus trigeminus. Mobilizing the trigeminal complex medially and superiorly provides a corridor to the posterior cavernous sinus and the entrance of cranial nerve VI into Dorello's canal. To expose the intracavernous carotid artery, it is necessary to open the outer cavernous membrane between the trigeminal ganglion and the posterolateral fibrous ring surrounding the carotid's entrance to the cavernous sinus at the foramen lacerum. In this way, the intracavernous carotid can be exposed to the crossing point of cranial nerve VI. This strategy provides full access to the posterolateral quadrant of the cavernous sinus, and tumor resection may proceed. The main venous connections of the posterolateral cavernous sinus are to the pterygoid venous plexus via the sphenoidal emissary, the inferior petrosal sinus, and the basilar venous plexus. Effective hemostasis is obtained via packing oxidized cellulose in the direction of these venous connections.

Closure requires the use of a vascularized musculofascial flap fashioned from the temporalis muscle and fascia. This flap is laid across the middle fossa floor and the petrous bone defect. Attaining a watertight dural closure in the posterior fossa dura is very difficult; therefore, it is often helpful to place a fascial graft in the defect in the petrous apex supported by a fat graft.

SPECIAL TECHNIQUES OF INTRACAVERNOUS SURGERY

Intracavernous Tumor Resection

Proper instrumentation is one of the major assets to successful resection of cavernous sinus neoplasms. A full array of dissectors, including microring curets, is useful. A wide selection of cottonoids is also necessary for protection of neural and vascular structures and dissection of tumor. An extremely useful tool is a pressure-attenuable suction tip that is invaluable for working around delicate structures to prevent damage induced by traction. The pressure-adjustable sucker is used for retraction and dissection as well as suction of blood and CSF. Proper instrumentation is key to application of the technical principles of tumor resection in this region.

The techniques used for resection of these tumors vary, depending on the degree of invasiveness and adherence to neural and vascular structures. Tumors such as trigeminal neurinomas that are well encapsulated and nonadherent can be relatively uncomplicated to remove. After exposure of tumor capsule through one of the triangular entry corridors, tumor debulking is performed with suction, ring curets, and alligator biopsy forceps. Developing a plane between tumor capsule and the neural and vascular structures is usually possible within the confines of the cavernous sinus. This dissection is typically performed by use of a combination of fine dissectors and long, thin cottonoids. The capsule is dissected free, continually collapsing solid tumor at the periphery into the center. Adjacent entry corridors may need to be utilized to completely free the tumor capsule. Usually, tumor is primarily resected from one or two triangular spaces, and adjacent portals are entered to dissect tumor and to push or sweep the mass toward the primary route of resection. When the capsule is freed, it is removed from the cavernous sinus, and hemostasis is attained with judicious use of Surgicel packing. This same general technique is used for any well-encapsulated, nonadherent tumor.

Invasive and adherent tumors present an entirely different surgical challenge. In these cases, the outcome with regard to morbidity depends mainly on the judgment and experience of the surgeon. Attempts at dissection of tumor from cranial nerves often result in damage either directly or from interruption of the nerves' blood supply. In some cases, when the cranial nerves have already been rendered nonfunctional by tumor invasion, the nerves can be resected with tumor to gain a more complete resection. This possibility is always considered and discussed with the patient before surgery.

Tumors such as meningiomas are approached initially with the primary intent of interrupting the blood supply to the tumor. These tumors can be quite tenacious and invasive, qualities that can prevent total resection without significant morbidity. Invasion of the intracavernous carotid artery may require a bypass procedure for total tumor resection. The dural origin and surrounding margin are resected in cases in which a complete resection is performed.

Invasive, malignant processes, such as squamous cell cancer, involve a very extensive procedure for removal. In these cases, the affected cavernous sinus and adjacent structures are removed en bloc. This procedure requires wide exposure of the cavernous sinus and adjacent regions as well as a bypass procedure to permit resection of the affected carotid artery.

Techniques of Hemostasis

Complete hemostasis throughout the surgical procedure is one of the primary determinants of the success or failure of any direct approach to the cavernous sinus. The potential for tremendous bleeding from the cavernous sinus requires familiarity and practice with certain techniques before such a surgical undertaking. A complete understanding of the anatomy and the elements of the triangular entry corridors is requisite to maintaining a dry operative field. Compulsive hemostasis begins with the skin incision and is maintained until final skin closure.

Preparation for the maintenance of hemostasis begins with the selection of instruments and the arrangement of materials by the scrub nurse. Bipolar cautery forceps should be available in a wide range of lengths and tip sizes. We prefer to use high settings during the initial phases of the operation to treat bleeding from scalp and muscle more effectively. As structures vulnerable to damage from the spread of heat or current are neared, the settings are reduced. Monopolar cautery is used frequently during the initial phases of these operations and is very useful to stop bleeding from bone at the skull base. When the bone of the middle fossa floor and sphenoid ridge is drilled, hemostasis is attained by several methods. Bone wax is judiciously used to seal off bleeding from porous bone. In addition to monopolar cautery, a high-speed drill, fitted with a diamond burr, cauterizes bone when used without irrigation. Bone bleeding at the skull base can often be persistent; therefore, patience and effective use of these techniques are necessary.

As the foramina of the cranial nerves are approached, the technical strategy changes. Heat and current from the monopolar cautery can spread for several millimeters through bone and can damage the nerves. Bone bleeding around neural foramina is controlled more with bone wax than with cautery or the diamond drill. Bleeding from the cavernous sinus also occurs via tiny rents in the cavernous membrane when the dura is separated from the margins of the foramina. This bleeding can be controlled by packing tiny pieces of Surgicel into the open cavernous membrane and covering for 1 or 2 minutes with a small cottonoid. Coagulating the Surgicel for 1 to 2 seconds with the bipolar after it is packed in the hole is sometimes helpful. Bleeding can occur from a tear in the cavernous membrane during the final stages of removal of the anterior clinoid process. Though possible to remove without bleeding, more frequently, the carotico-oculomotor membrane develops a small tear that can bleed profusely. A small piece of Surgicel suffices when packed into the opening and covered with a cottonoid for 1 to 2 minutes. An important principle in hemostatic technique in the cavernous sinus is patience. Much is gained by packing an area, moving to another area to work, then coming back later to the original bleeding site.

The geometric construct describing the entry corridors to the cavernous sinus region serves as a foundation for effective hemostasis. Knowledge of the nature and communications of the venous plexus residing within each triangle, as well as the proximity of anatomic structures, is critical.

In cases of tumor resection, the tumor mass often tamponades the cavernous venous plexus. Surgicel packing for hemostasis then begins after the tumor mass is removed from the area. In the anterior triangle, lateral and medial packing must be conservative because of the position of cranial nerve III and the optic nerve. Anteroinferior packing is less constrained; however, constriction of the carotid siphon must obviously be avoided. The anterolateral triangle typically contains the anastomosis of the superior orbital vein with the cavernous venous plexus and, therefore, can produce brisk bleeding when opened. The main concern in this triangle is avoidance of overpacking in the direction of cranial nerve VI, because the abducens nerve is entering the superior orbital fissure on its underside. The lateralmost triangle can also produce significant bleeding if a sphenoid emissary vein is present beside the mandibular branch that exits the foramen ovale. This sphenoid emissary is seen only in a few patients; however, when present, it can be quite large.

The medial cavernous triangle can bleed tremendously when opened. Packing must be conservative laterally, in the direction of cranial nerve III; however, inferomedial packing can be quite generous. Here, the cavernous sinus communicates with the basilar venous plexus along the clivus and the inferior petrosal sinus. Therefore, a large amount of Surgicel may be packed in their direction without compromise of any vital structures. The superior triangle does not have such an area that may be so generously packed. The meningohypophyseal trunk is found in this triangle and is vulnerable to overzealous packing. The lateral triangle is the space entered to expose cranial nerve VI as it crosses over the C4 segment of the carotid artery. Surgicel placement must be modest, except in the inferomedial direction toward the clivus.

Exposure of the intrapetrous carotid artery in the posterolateral triangle does not usually produce significant bleeding. This segment of the carotid is, however, often covered by a venous plexus that is an extension of the cavernous venous plexus. This plexus must be coagulated with bipolar cautery before work with this segment begins. The posteromedial triangle similarly is not a major concern for significant hemorrhage. When bone deep in this space is removed, the inferior petrosal sinus is encountered and must be occluded. Also, deep drilling to the clivus usually results in encountering the basilar venous plexus, which must be packed and coagulated. The posteroinferior triangle can also produce a fair amount of hemorrhage from connections with the basilar venous plexus and inferior petrosal sinus. In the floor of this space runs Dorello's canal and cranial nerve VI. Hemostasis in this space must be performed carefully to avoid compression of this structure.

Closure Techniques

Avoidance of complications in these procedures includes meticulous attention to dural closure to prevent CSF leakage and subsequent contamination. Judicious use of fascial grafts is important in meeting this goal. Typically, abdominal fat and rectus fascia are harvested in these cases for dural closure and sealing of opened paranasal sinuses. In areas of difficult dural closure, such as around the optic nerve, fat grafts are placed and secured with fine sutures tamponading

them against the open area. This arrangement is then covered with a layer of fibrin glue to hasten the fibrotic process. Muscle or fat is also tacked to areas where it is impossible to attain tight apposition of dural edges. Also, at the corner areas of complex dural incisions, fat or muscle is used to completely plug any small holes. Fibrin glue is applied to the entire dural surface at the completion of dural closure.

As discussed, open paranasal sinuses commonly result from extensive removal of bone at the skull base. Any open sinus must be meticulously exenterated of any mucosa. We prefer to use a high-speed drill fitted with a diamond burr for this purpose. The heat generated by the drill provides extra assurance of destroying any mucus-producing epithelial cells. Ostia are then occluded with muscle or bone wax to prevent communication with bacteria-laden adjacent sinus cavities. The sinus is then packed with autologous fat. We then cover the opening to the packed sinus with a vascularized pericranial flap and carefully tack the edges to adjacent surfaces to prevent migration.

The ultimate cosmetic result of these procedures is partially dependent on the proper reattachment of the bone flap, especially in cases in which a transzygomatic or orbitozygomatic flap has been used. One of the titanium plating systems now available provides superior cosmetic results over those obtained with wire or suture. We prefer to use one of the low-profile systems, especially at points where only skin is covering the bone surface to be approximated.

Another cosmetic consideration relates to the reattachment of the temporalis muscle. If the muscle is not supported in some manner along the superior temporal line, it tends to sink into the temporal fossa, resulting in a poor appearance. To combat this, oblique wire-pass holes are made along the superior temporal line before the bone flap is replaced. The superior edge of the muscle can then be sutured to the superior temporal line, maintaining its position during the healing process.

Skull Base Carotid Bypass Procedures

Invasive tumors often require sacrifice of the ICA if they are to be completely removed. Balloon test occlusion is performed before surgery to determine tolerance to occlusion of the involved ICA.[41] Patients who tolerate occlusion without incident may be treated without bypass, thus avoiding the potential major complications of thromboembolic sequelae and anticoagulation associated with these procedures. In cases in which occlusion is not tolerated, the carotid flow can be preserved by performing a bypass procedure.[8,18,20,42,43] This procedure was first performed in 1986 by Fukushima to treat a giant intracavernous aneurysm.[7,8,44] Over time, the procedure has evolved to include three variations. The most common form is a bypass between the C3 and C6 segments of the carotid. The second important variation is an anastomosis from the high cervical portion of the ICA to the C3 segment.[8,45]

The C3-to-C6 bypass procedure requires exposure of those two segments in sufficient length to perform the anastomosis procedure. The C3 portion is exposed in the anterior triangle through removal of the anterior clinoid process and detachment of the fibrous dural ring. The C6 segment is exposed in the posterolateral triangle.[46] It is usually helpful to free the dura from the posterior trigeminal complex, as discussed earlier, to gain several additional millimeters of exposure. Clips can then be placed to trap the intracavernous carotid segments. A saphenous vein graft is harvested from the upper thigh and prepared for anastomosis. Any loose adventitia is stripped from the vein, and tributaries are ligated with fine suture. The graft is flushed with heparinized saline solution, and proper orientation is maintained by marking either end of the graft. The distal anastomosis is then performed, either end to end or end to side, with 8-0, 9-0, or 10-0 suture. Suture selection depends on the wall thickness of both the graft and the carotid artery. Control of carotid flow is maintained either by a temporary clip near the genu or by exposure in the neck. The proximal anastomosis is performed between the origins of the ophthalmic artery and the posterior communicating artery. In some cases, the anastomosis may be performed in an end-to-end fashion if the tumor resection leaves a carotid stump including the ophthalmic origin or the ophthalmic artery is taken with tumor resection in the orbit. The anastomosis is performed under electroencephalographic burst suppression induced by barbiturates. Patients are given low-dose heparin therapy for several days postoperatively, and they are then given aspirin or warfarin (Coumadin) for approximately 3 months.

In cases of en bloc cavernous sinus resection, resecting carotid artery well into the infratemporal fossa and petrous bone may be necessary. In this case, the carotid is bypassed from the high cervical segment, near the origin at the carotid bifurcation. Saphenous vein is again harvested from the upper thigh in an appropriate length. The graft is anastomosed in end-to-end fashion and tunneled through the infratemporal fossa to enter the cranial vault subtemporally. The proximal end is then anastomosed to the C3 segment as outlined earlier.

SUMMARY

Direct operative treatment of intracavernous neoplasms has realized great strides in the past decade. Several experienced centers have had success with treating these patients more aggressively, while limiting morbidity. Advances in microsurgical technique, neuroanesthesia, imaging techniques, neurovascular reconstruction, and microanatomic knowledge have all provided significant contributions to the successful surgery of these lesions. However, the therapeutic approach to these difficult tumors is still debated. The appropriate role of surgery in the overall management of these patients is still evolving as we continue to refine our management strategies.

The techniques and strategies outlined in this chapter have evolved over an experience with these lesions, beginning in 1983. This series encompasses 146 cases of cavernous sinus neoplasms. Forty-eight cases in the series, patients who had benign encapsulated tumors, such as neurinomas, had the most satisfying results. Total resection in this group of patients is almost always a realistic expectation, with a minimum of morbidity. The most common lesion treated was meningioma, accounting for 72 cases. As experience has accumulated, a less aggressive approach has been taken with meningiomas of the cavernous sinus because of our inability to remove these tumors completely without the risk of cranial nerve morbidity. Treating patients with invasive tumors

has also contributed the most to our understanding of the important variables involved in revascularization of the ICA. Balloon test occlusion with measurement of cerebral blood flow is currently the best tool for determining the need for revascularization.

We anticipate that direct surgery will continue to figure prominently in the treatment of these tumors, although it is increasingly combined with adjuvant therapies that present less risk to the cranial nerves while increasing the effectiveness of treatment. The indications for these procedures are still evolving as different centers gain wider experience with direct surgery, stereotactic radiosurgery, and endovascular techniques. Clearly, much room for improvement remains in the overall results of treating these difficult lesions.

REFERENCES

1. Parkinson D: A surgical approach to the cavernous portion of the carotid artery: Anatomical studies and case report. J Neurosurg 23:474–483, 1965.
2. Al-Mefty O, Smith RR: Surgery of tumors invading the cavernous sinus. Surg Neurol 30:370–381, 1988.
3. Cioffi FA, Bernine FP, Punzo A, et al: Cavernous sinus meningiomas. Neurochirurgia (Stuttg) 30:40–47, 1987.
4. Dolenc V: A combined epi- and subdural direct approach to carotid-ophthalmic artery aneurysms. J Neurosurg 62:667–672, 1985.
5. Dolenc VV, Kregar R, Ferluga M, et al: Treatment of tumors invading the cavernous sinus. In Dolenc VV (ed): The Cavernous Sinus: Multidisciplinary Approach to Vascular and Tumorous Lesions. Wien: Springer-Verlag, 1987, pp 377–391.
6. Dolenc VV: Cavernous sinus masses. In Apuzzo MLJ (ed): Brain Surgery: Complication Avoidance and Management. New York: Churchill Livingstone, 1993, pp 601–614.
7. Fukushima T: Direct operative approach to the vascular lesions in the cavernous sinus: Summary of 27 cases. Mt Fuji Workshop Cerebrovasc Dis 6:169–189, 1988.
8. Fukushima T, Day JD, Tung H: Intracavernous carotid artery aneurysms. In Apuzzo MLJ (ed): Brain Surgery: Complication Avoidance and Management. New York: Churchill Livingstone, 1993, pp 925–944.
9. Hakuba A, Matsuoka Y, Suzuki T, et al: Direct approaches to vascular lesions in the cavernous sinus via the medial triangle. In Dolenc VV (ed): The Cavernous Sinus. Wien: Springer-Verlag, 1987, pp 272–284.
10. Hakuba A, Suzuki T, Jin TB, Komiyama M: Surgical approaches to the cavernous sinus: Report of 52 cases. In Dolenc VV (ed): The Cavernous Sinus. Wien: Springer-Verlag, 1987, pp 302–327.
11. Lesoin F, Jomin M, Boucez B, et al: Management of cavernous sinus meningiomas: Report of twelve cases and review of the literature. Neurochirurgia (Stuttg) 28:195–198, 1985.
12. Lesoin F, Jomin M: Direct microsurgical approach to intracavernous tumors. Surg Neurol 28:17–22, 1987.
13. Sekhar LN, Ross DA, Sen C: Cavernous sinus and sphenocavernous neoplasms. In Sekhar LN, Janecka IP (eds): Surgery of Cranial Base Tumors. New York: Raven Press, 1993, pp 521–604.
14. Sephernia A, Samii M, Tatgiba M: Management of intracavernous tumours: An 11-year experience. Acta Neurochir Suppl (Wien) 53:122–126, 1991.
15. Barbaro NM, Gutin PH, Wilson CB, et al: Radiation therapy in the treatment of partially resected meningiomas. Neurosurgery 20:525–528, 1987.
16. Carella RJ, Ransohoff J, Newall J: Role of radiation therapy in the management of meningioma. Neurosurgery 10:332–339, 1982.
17. Duma CM, Lunsford LD, Kondziolka D, et al: Stereotactic radiosurgery of cavernous sinus meningiomas as an addition or alternative to microsurgery. Neurosurgery 32:699–705, 1993.
18. Al-Mefty O, Khalil N, Elwany MN, Smith RR: Shunt for bypass graft of the cavernous carotid artery: An anatomical and technical study. Neurosurgery 27:721–728, 1990.
19. Harris FS, Rhoton AL: Anatomy of the cavernous sinus: A microsurgical study. J Neurosurg 44:169–180, 1976.
20. Sekhar LN, Burgess J, Akin O: Anatomical study of the cavernous sinus emphasizing operative approaches and related vascular and neural reconstruction. Neurosurgery 21:806–816, 1987.

21. Umansky F, Elidan J, Valarezo A: Dorello's canal: A microanatomical study. J Neurosurg 75:294–298, 1991.
22. Umansky F, Nathan H: The lateral wall of the cavernous sinus with special reference to the nerves related to it. J Neurosurg 56:228–234, 1982.
23. Day AL: Aneurysms of the ophthalmic segment. J Neurosurg 72:677–691, 1990.
24. Perneczky A, Knosp E, Borkapic P, Czech T: Direct surgical approach to infraclinoidal aneurysms. Acta Neurochir (Wien) 76:36–44, 1983.
25. Perneczky A, Knosp E, Czech T: Para- and infraclinoidal aneurysms. Anatomy, surgical technique and report on 22 cases. In Dolenc VV (ed): The Cavernous Sinus. Wien: Springer-Verlag, 1987, pp 252–271.
26. Fischer E: Die Lagabweichrugan der vorderen Hirnarterie in Gefassbild. Zentralb Neurochir 3:300–312, 1938.
27. Dolenc V, Skrap M, Sustersic J, et al: A transcavernous-transsellar approach to the basilar tip aneurysms. Br J Neurosurg 1:251–259, 1987.
28. Glasscock ME: Exposure of the intra-petrous portion of the carotid artery. In Hamberger CA, Wersall J (eds): Disorders of the Skull Base Region: Proceedings of the Tenth Nobel Symposium, Stockholm, 1968. Stockholm: Almqvist & Wicksell, 1969, pp 135–143.
29. Day JD, Fukushima T, Giannotta SL: Microanatomical study of the extradural middle fossa approach to the petroclival and posterior cavernous sinus region: Description of the rhomboid construct. Neurosurgery 34:1009–1016, 1994.
30. Kawase T, Shiobara R, Toya S: Anterior transpetrosal-transtentorial approach for sphenopetroclival meningiomas: Surgical method and results in 10 patients. Neurosurgery 28:869–876, 1991.
31. Kawase T, Toya S, Shiobara R, Mine T: Transpetrosal approach for aneurysms of the lower basilar artery. J Neurosurg 63:857–861, 1985.
32. Mullan S: Treatment of carotid-cavernous fistulas by cavernous sinus occlusion. J Neurosurg 50:131–144, 1979.
33. Traynelis VC, Gantz BJ: Intraoperative facial nerve monitoring. In Loftus CM, Traynelis VC (eds): Intraoperative Monitoring Techniques in Neurosurgery. New York: McGraw-Hill, 1994, pp 157–163.
34. Moller AR: Monitoring techniques in cavernous sinus surgery. In Loftus CM, Traynelis VC (eds): Intraoperative Monitoring Techniques in Neurosurgery. New York: McGraw-Hill, 1994, pp 141–157.
35. Carter LP: Continuous monitoring of cortical blood flow. In Loftus CM, Traynelis VC (eds): Intraoperative Monitoring Techniques in Neurosurgery. New York: McGraw-Hill, 1994, pp 53–61.
36. Day JD, Giannotta SL, Fukushima T: Extradural temporopolar approach to lesions of the upper basilar artery and infrachiasmatic region. J Neurosurg in press.
37. Fujitsu K, Kuwabara T: Zygomatic approach for lesions in the interpeduncular cistern. J Neurosurg 62:340–343, 1985.
38. Hakuba A, Tanaka K, Suzuki T, Nishimura S: A combined orbitozygomatic infratemporal epidural and subdural approach for lesions involving the entire cavernous sinus. J Neurosurg 71:699–704, 1989.
39. Hitselberger WE, Horn KL, Hankinson H, et al: The middle fossa transpetrous approach for petroclival meningiomas. Skull Base Surg 3:130–135, 1993.
40. House WF, Hitselberger WE, Horn KL: The middle fossa transpetrous approach to the anterior-superior cerebellopontine angle. Am J Otol 7:1–4, 1986.
41. Horton JA, Jungreis CA, Pistoia F: Balloon test occlusion. In Sekhar LN, Janecka IP (eds): Surgery of Cranial Base Tumors. New York: Raven Press, 1993, pp 33–36.
42. Linskey ME, Sekhar LN, Sen C: Cerebral revascularization in cranial base surgery. In Sekhar LN, Janecka IP (eds): Surgery of Cranial Base Tumors. New York: Raven Press, 1993, pp 45–68.
43. Sekhar LN, Sen CN, Jho HD: Saphenous vein bypass of the cavernous internal carotid artery. J Neurosurg 72:35–41, 1990.
44. Spetzler RF, Fukushima T, Martin N, Zabramski JM: Petrous carotid-to-intradural carotid saphenous vein graft for intracavernous giant aneurysm, tumor, and occlusive cerebrovascular disease. J Neurosurg 73:496–501, 1990.
45. Miyazaki S, Fukushima T, Fujimaki T: Resection of high-cervical paraganglioma with cervical-to-petrous internal carotid artery saphenous vein bypass: Report of two cases. J Neurosurg 73:141–146, 1990.
46. Glasscock ME III, Smith PG, Whitaker SR, et al: Management of aneurysms of the petrous portion of the internal carotid artery by resection and primary anastomosis. Laryngoscope 93:1445–1453, 1983.

20 Surgical and Endovascular Management of Aneurysms and Fistulas Involving the Cavernous Sinus

IAN F. DUNN, DILANTHA B. ELLEGALA, SEAN P. CULLEN, DONG H. KIM, and ARTHUR L. DAY

ANATOMY AND TERMINOLOGY

The cavernous segment (CavSeg) of the internal carotid artery (ICA) has classically been defined as the segment that begins as the vessel emerges from the carotid canal at the foramen lacerum and ends as the artery penetrates the dura near the anterior clinoid (AC) process to enter the subarachnoid space. The CavSeg has been divided into five parts: (1) the posterior vertical portion, (2) the posterior bend, (3) the horizontal portion, (4) the anterior bend, and (5) the anterior vertical portion.[1,2]

Extradural removal of the AC exposes a segment of the carotid artery that is neither within the cavernous sinus nor the subarachnoid space (Fig. 20-1).[1,3] This vessel segment, herein called the clinoidal segment (ClinSeg), corresponds with the distal part of the anterior vertical portion of the CavSeg. Although some anatomists believe that this segment is invested by a collar of the cavernous sinus dura, it nevertheless exists as a clinically distinct and relevant portion of the ICA.[4] The ClinSeg is delineated distally (or superiorly) by dural reflections from the roof of the AC that extend medially toward the optic nerve and canal. The point where the ICA penetrates this dural plane to enter the subarachnoid space is known as the dural ring, upper ring, or Perneczky's ring.

Proximally, the ClinSeg is delineated by a thin extension of the periosteum covering the undersurface of the AC. This membrane, extending from the ICA to the oculomotor nerve and called the carotid-oculomotor membrane or membranous ring (also called the proximal ring), separates this segment from the cavernous sinus. An anatomic study by Seone and colleagues[4] suggests that this membrane may actually form a collar through which the ICA penetrates the roof of the cavernous sinus. Venous tributaries in this collar may indicate that the ClinSeg is technically intracavernous. In practice, however, the ClinSeg represents a distinct portion of the supracavernous ICA with specific clinical and surgical implications.

Vascular lesions of the intracavernous carotid artery can be broadly divided into two groups: nonfistulous arterial aneurysms and carotid-cavernous fistulas (CCFs).

NONFISTULOUS ARTERIAL ANEURYSMS

Cavernous sinus region aneurysms classically account for approximately 3% to 5% of all angiographically identified intracranial aneurysms, and approximately 15% of all aneurysms originating from the ICA.[2,5] The incidence may actually be considerably higher, as most lesions are small, never produce symptoms, and therefore remain undetected. Intracavernous aneurysms may be divided into four types based on their genesis and clinical course: (1) saccular, (2) fusiform, (3) infectious, and (4) traumatic.

Saccular and Fusiform Aneurysms

The numerous similarities between fusiform and saccular intracavernous aneurysms allow them to be discussed as a single clinical entity. Most intracavernous aneurysms are saccular and are believed to arise from defects in the vessel wall at the site of actual or vestigial branches. The intracavernous branches, most commonly thought to act as origin for such aneurysms, are the meningohypophyseal trunk, the inferolateral trunk, and McConnell's capsular arteries. Intracavernous aneurysms are much more common in women, and symptoms, when present, generally begin in the fifth and sixth decades.[6,7] Several clinical investigations have demonstrated clearly different natural histories and treatment options between those aneurysms arising from the anterior vertical segment of the cavernous carotid artery (within the ClinSeg) and those arising from the more proximal ICA (within the CavSeg); each are considered separately.[6–9]

Cavernous Segment Aneurysms

The hemodynamic forces exerted on the ICA as it courses in the cavernous sinus usually produce an aneurysm that burrows anteriorly and laterally beneath the sphenoid ridge, toward the superior orbital fissure. Most remain asymptomatic until reaching giant proportions (approximately 2.5 cm), at which point symptoms are caused by local mass effect against adjacent structures and may include isolated or combined deficits of the oculomotor, trochlear, abducens,

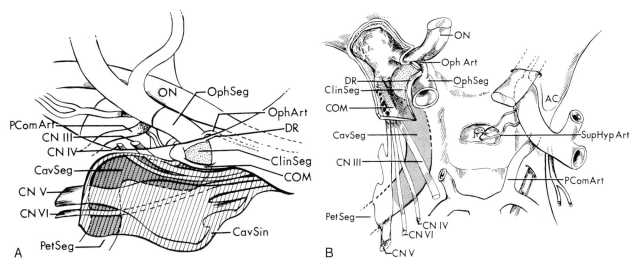

FIGURE 20-1   Cavernous sinus anatomy and terminology. Lateral (*A*) and dorsal (*B*) views. Note the two portions of the carotid artery considered to be within the cavernous sinus: (1) the cavernous segment (CavSeg) lies within the large venous channel of the cavernous sinus (CavSin) and (2) the clinoidal segment (ClinSeg), which corresponds to the anterior vertical segment of the cavernous carotid artery. Both segments lie below the dural ring and outside the subarachnoid space. AC, anterior clinoid process; CN III, oculomotor nerve; CN IV, trochlear nerve; CN V, trigeminal nerve; CN VI, abducens nerve; COM, carotid-oculomotor membrane; DR, dural ring; ON, optic nerve; OphArt, ophthalmic artery; OphSeg, ophthalmic segment; OS, optic strut; PComArt, posterior communicating artery; PetSeg, petrous segment; SupHypArt, superior hypophyseal artery.

trigeminal, and sympathetic nerves (Fig. 20-2A).[6,7] Subarachnoid hemorrhage (SAH) or epistaxis is rare because the aneurysm is covered by the venous structures within the sinus and by the overlying dura and surrounding bony structures in addition to its own arterial wall.

In the symptomatic patient, computed tomography (CT) or magnetic resonance imaging invariably demonstrates a round or oblong anterior extradural parasellar mass expanding anteriorly toward the superior orbital fissure and laterally into the middle cranial fossa, beneath the sphenoid ridge and AC (see Fig. 20-2B).[6,9] The definitive diagnosis can be established by CT-, magnetic resonance imaging-, or catheter-based arteriography. When treatment is being considered, studies should include careful assessment of the ipsilateral external carotid artery (ECA) and its distal branches for potential donor vessels, in the event that carotid ligation and extracranial-intracranial bypass are considered (see Fig. 20-2C).[10,11] Intraluminal thrombosis often occurs in large lesions and can cause an underestimation of the lesion's true size unless correlated with CT or magnetic resonance imaging.

When symptoms are mild and confined to oculomotor or trigeminal dysfunction in the typical 65-year-old woman, aggressive intervention is sometimes not advised because many patients will have a benign clinical course.[12] Visual loss (rare with this lesion type) or severe intractable facial pain are stronger indications for therapeutic intervention. SAH and epistaxis are neurologic emergencies and should be treated promptly and aggressively. Treatment options, when indicated, include proximal vessel ligation (common carotid artery or ICA), generally using detachable coils or balloons with/without a simultaneous bypass procedure,[4] direct clipping, and endovascular coiling with ICA preservation.[5] Treatment considerations are outlined in Figure 20-3.

PROXIMAL LIGATION

With the advent of endovascular techniques, common carotid artery ligation is rarely performed. ICA ligation is the preferred option for most patients with true symptomatic intracavernous aneurysms, provided that the risks of distal ischemia can be lowered to acceptable levels.[13] In most cases, proximal ICA ligation alone achieves aneurysmal thrombosis. Trapping should be performed in cases presenting with bleeding (SAH or epistaxis) to completely exclude the lesion from the circulation or when the aneurysm and its compressive symptoms persist after proximal ligation.

When ICA ligation is contemplated, the surgeon should have a high degree of certainty that flow to the ipsilateral hemisphere will be well maintained via collateral channels. Ischemic symptoms may be delayed for hours or days afterward and may occur despite a well-tolerated Matas test or trial ICA balloon occlusion test under local anesthesia.[10,14,15] To more accurately assess ischemic risks, most patients should be subjected to a trial balloon occlusion test. After intravenous hydration, a balloon is inflated high in the cervical ICA to arrest flow in the vessel for a brief (15 to 30 minutes) interval.[16] A clinically successfully trial (no new hemispheric symptoms) may be further confirmed by a brief period of induced systemic hypotension.[17] A cerebral blood flow study (single photon emission CT [SPECT] or Xe-CT) done thereafter provides quantitative and qualitative esti-mations of sufficient collateral channels (Fig. 20-4).[10,15,17] ICA ligation carries a 5% risk of ischemic complications even in patients who had tolerated test occlusion but results in a very high rate of aneurysm thrombosis.

If no significant clinical or hemispheric blood flow changes occur during the balloon occlusion test, the artery can usually be safely ligated without the need for surgical

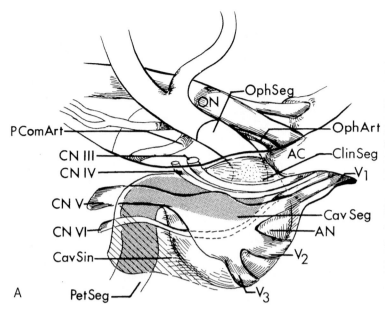

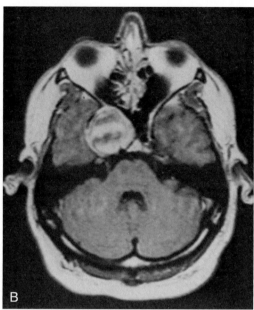

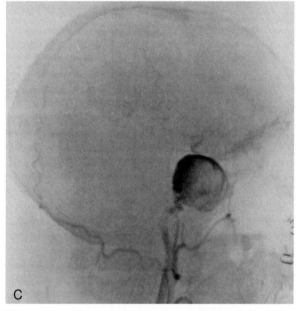

FIGURE 20-2 True cavernous aneurysm. *A,* Lateral view (schematic): The cavernous segment (CavSeg) (*shaded area*) has an intimate association with the cranial nerves within the cavernous sinus (CavSin). Aneurysms (AN) of this segment invariably present with clinical deficits related to compression of these structures. AC, anterior clinoid process; CN III, oculomotor nerve; CN IV, trochlear nerve; CN V, trigeminal nerve (three divisions: V1 to V3); CN VI, abducens nerve; ON, optic nerve; OphArt, ophthalmic artery; OphSeg, ophthalmic segment; PComArt, posterior communicating artery; PetSeg, petrous segment. *B,* A computed tomography scan in 30-year-old man with facial pain and complete cavernous sinus syndrome. Note the giant aneurysm in the right parasellar area, burrowing beneath the sphenoid ridge toward the superior orbital fissure. *C,* This preoperative arteriogram (lateral view) demonstrates a giant intracavernous aneurysm with delayed filling of the intracranial carotid artery.

(Continued)

flow augmentation.[17,18] A parent vessel occlusion that includes the entire aneurysm neck prevents both anterograde and retrograde flow into the lesion. Many patients with symptomatic CavSeg aneurysms are elderly, and the option of endovascular ligation eliminates the need for general anesthesia or an intracranial procedure, while providing excellent relief of compressive symptoms. Patients with

longer life expectancies or those with marginal blood flow values are treated with acute ICA ligation combined with an extracranial-intracranial arterial bypass, using the superficial temporal artery as the donor source.[19]

Patients with poor collateral circulation (clinical intolerance to trial balloon occlusion or obvious focal decreases in flow on SPECT or Xe-CT) cannot undergo acute ICA

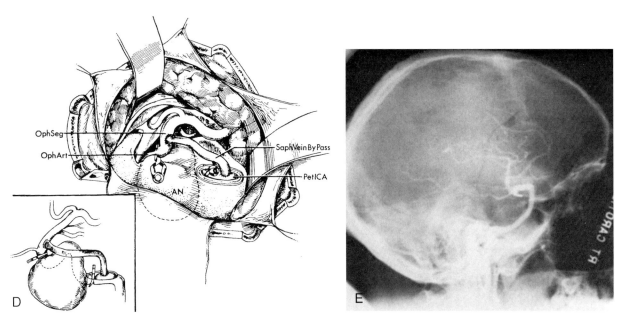

FIGURE 20-2 Cont'd   *D*, A petrosal to supraclinoidal carotid artery bypass (schematic): The petrous carotid artery has been exposed by drilling off the bone just posterior and slightly lateral to the foramen ovale. A saphenous vein graft spans over the bulging aneurysm, connecting the petrous and ophthalmic segments of the internal carotid artery. The aneurysm is thereafter trapped (insert) by clips on the distal petrous and clinoidal segments of the carotid artery. The contents of the cavernous sinus are not disturbed by the procedure. *E*, Postoperative arteriogram (lateral view). Note the excellent filling of the distal carotid artery from the short segment bypass. The patient subsequently had complete resolution of clinical symptoms other than mild abducens palsy apparent to extreme lateral gaze.

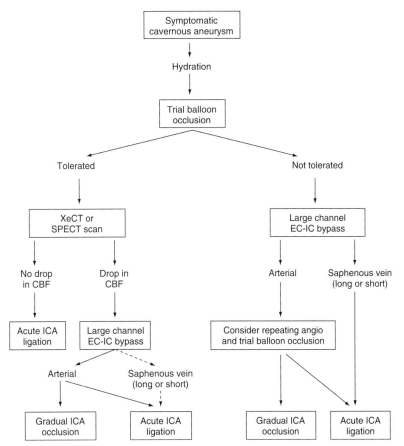

FIGURE 20-3   Treatment algorithm for internal carotid artery (ICA) ligation. Angio, angiography; CBF, cerebral blood flow; EC-IC, extracranial-intracranial; SPECT, single photon emission computed tomography; XeCT, xenon computed tomography.

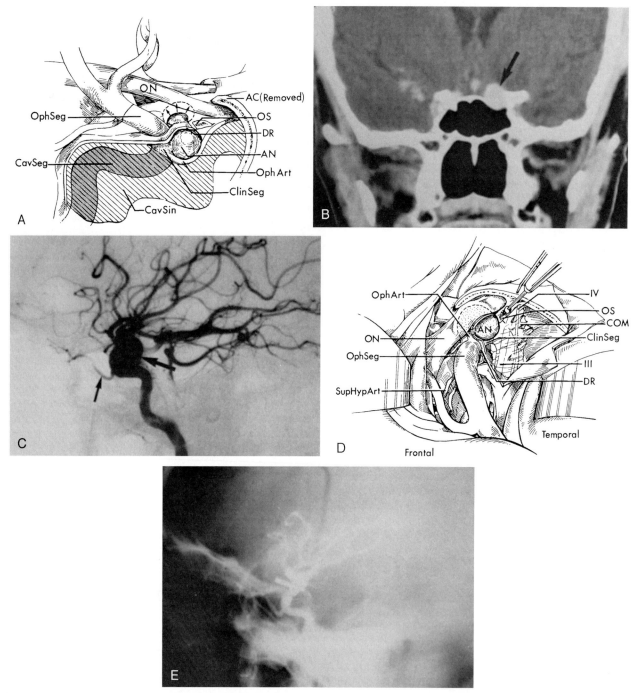

FIGURE 20-4   Clinoidal segment aneurysm. *A,* Operative view (schematic). Note the aneurysm (AN) arising in the clinoidal segment (ClinSeg) in conjunction with a similar origin of the ophthalmic artery (OphArt). Clinoidal segment aneurysms project above the plane of the cranial nerves within the cavernous sinus (CavSin) and present with either visual loss from optic nerve (ON) compression or subarachnoid hemorrhage after extension through the dura into the subarachnoid space (*arrows*). AC, anterior clinoid process; DR, dural ring; OS, optic strut; OphSeg, ophthalmic segment. *B,* A computed tomography scan of a clinoidal segment aneurysm (*arrow*). Note the aneurysm arising below and medial to the anterior clinoid process, indicating its origin within the clinoidal segment. *C,* A preoperative arteriogram (lateral view). Note the origin of the ophthalmic artery (*small arrow*) and the clinoidal segment aneurysm (*large arrow*) well below the plane of the anterior clinoid process, from the anterior vertical portion of the cavernous carotid artery (ClinSeg). Note the superior bulging of the aneurysm out of the clinoidal segment into the subarachnoid space. This lesion should prompt strong considerations for simultaneous cervical internal carotid artery exposure and intradural rather than extradural AC removal. *D,* Operative exposure (schematic) of the clinoidal segment aneurysm. Note that the entire lesser wing of the sphenoid bone, including the AC, has been removed. The roof, side, and floor of the optic canal have been drilled away, as has the optic strut, to completely define the dural ring and carotid-oculomotor membrane (COM). The dura adjacent to the ring is then sectioned circumferentially to allow mobilization of the internal carotid artery and to allow unimpeded clip placement on the aneurysm neck without compromise of the parent vessel lumen. III, oculomotor nerve; IV, trochlear nerve; SupHypArt, superior hypophyseal artery. *E,* Postoperative arteriogram demonstrates excellent patency of the internal carotid artery, with complete obliteration of the aneurysm. Note the proximal origin of the ophthalmic artery.

ligation without a high risk of stroke. A long saphenous vein or radial artery graft, connecting the ECA to a major middle cerebral artery trunk and combined with a trapping procedure, provides immediate flow replacement. In our experience, such procedures have higher risks and lesser long-term patency than do superficial temporal artery–middle cerebral artery anastomoses.[20] Obviously, the decision to use either of these options should be weighed carefully against the patient's symptoms and the natural history of the untreated lesion.

ICA ligation can also be combined with a short-segment saphenous vein bypass that spans the isolated CavSeg.[21–23] During this procedure, a frontotemporal scalp and temporalis flap is turned and combined with extensive removal of much of the greater sphenoid wing, the entire lesser sphenoid wing, and the AC. After the sylvian fissure is widely split, the temporal lobe is mobilized and retracted to expose the middle fossa floor. The dura is then opened laterally and stripped medially until the foramen spinosum and greater superficial petrosal nerve are identified. After the middle meningeal artery is coagulated and cut, bone posterior and lateral to the foramen ovale is drilled off to expose the petrous ICA. A short-segment saphenous vein bypass connecting the petrous ICA with the ophthalmic segment of the vessel is then performed, combined with trapping of the vessel segment harboring the aneurysm (see Fig. 20-2D, E).

The advantages of the short-segment petrosal bypass are theoretically compelling and include the benefits of a short length graft, the replacement of the sacrificed vessel with another that maintains normal flow directions intracranially, and avoidance of direct manipulation of the nerves within the cavernous sinus. This procedure is technically more difficult than convexity bypass procedures, however, and the exposure is often substantially limited by the bulging aneurysm. In addition, elderly patients often have arteriosclerotic intracranial vessels that do not respond well to temporary clipping or end-to-side anastomosis. In general, we reserve this procedure for younger patients in good medical health and without significant arteriosclerosis.

DIRECT CLIPPING

Direct clipping of CavSeg aneurysms can be performed, but the procedure is severely limited by the lesion's size, shape, associated arteriosclerosis and thrombosis, and morbidity to cranial nerves. The difficulty in reconstructing the ICA lumen while in the middle of a large venous channel makes this approach prohibitive in most instances.[24,25]

ANEURYSM COILING WITH AND WITHOUT STENTING

By the time they become symptomatic, CavSeg aneurysms often have very large necks that communicate widely with the parent vessel. This anatomic feature reduces the chances that the lesion can be endovascularly excluded from the circulation without parent vessel compromise. Detachable devices are most effective in eliminating cavernous sinus aneurysms when the parent vessel is simultaneously sacrificed.[26] Coil embolization alone is most effective when the aneurysm is small and/or its neck is narrow.[27–29] Larger lesions are more likely to have wider necks and be less amenable to this technology. The recent addition of intra-arterial stents, placed inside the parent vessel through which coils can be deployed into the

aneurysm lumen, has expanded the endovascular surgeon's ability to successfully treat these lesions.[30] Since smaller intracavernous aneurysms are invariably asymptomatic and have no demonstrable risk of bleeding, endovascular treatment is generally not warranted.

Clinoidal Segment Aneurysms

ClinSeg aneurysms have been identified as a distinct entity with very different clinical and anatomic features from those arising on more proximal intracavernous portions.[8,9] These lesions arise in the interval between the carotid-oculomotor membrane and the dural ring, from the anterior vertical segment of the intracavernous ICA, often in association with an ophthalmic or superior hypophyseal artery origin within this segment. With enlargement, hemodynamic forces project the aneurysm fundus superiorly against the overlying dura, AC, and optic strut.

Because ClinSeg aneurysms originate below the ICA's penetrance into the subarachnoid space, small ClinSeg aneurysms are usually asymptomatic. Because of their superior projection, the cranial nerves within the cavernous sinus are usually not affected by the lesion's growth, although small lesions may project into the optic canal and cause optic nerve compression and visual loss. With enlargement (≥1 cm), ClinSeg aneurysms may erode through the dura into the subarachnoid space, at which time they mimic ophthalmic segment lesions (see Fig. 20-4A). SAH from an "intracavernous" aneurysm is almost always attributable to this variant.

Unlike ophthalmic segment aneurysms, the neck of ClinSeg lesions is located below the dural ring, making preoperative recognition essential for safe treatment planning. Focal erosion of the optic strut or AC, as demonstrated best on CT, often marks the lesion's proximal origin (see Fig. 20-4B).[8] CT angiography may provide delineation of the aneurysm's location in relation to the optic strut. On arteriography, ClinSeg aneurysms invariably originate below the plane of the ophthalmic artery (see Fig. 20-4C). Two clinical variations, based on site of aneurysm origin and direction of projection from the ClinSeg, have been clarified. One originates from the anterior lateral surface of the ClinSeg and may extend upward into, through, or medial to the AC. This type may cause optic nerve compression either within the optic canal extradurally or within the subarachnoid space after penetrating the dura. The other originates from the medial ClinSeg surface and may erode through the lateral sphenoid sinus wall to produce epistaxis or into the lateral sella beneath the diaphragma sella to mimic a pituitary tumor. Once exceeding 1 cm, either type may produce SAH, as the likelihood that the aneurysm has eroded through the dural roof of this segment and is projecting into the subarachnoid space is much higher.

TREATMENT

Asymptomatic lesions smaller than 1 cm should probably be observed unless the ClinSeg is to be exposed for other reasons. Larger or symptomatic lesions can be clipped in most cases, with preservation of ICA patency. Because proximal control of the ClinSeg lies within the cavernous sinus, the operative field should include sterile preparation of the cervical carotid bifurcation region. When the aneurysm has bled, we routinely open the neck incision because the intracranial exposure necessary to clip the aneurysm carries significant risks of intraoperative rupture.

Adequate exposure of ClinSeg aneurysms begins with extensive extradural removal of the lateral sphenoid ridge and posterior orbital roof (see Fig. 20-4D). Because ClinSeg aneurysms are adherent to and may actually erode through the AC, the most medial extent of the lesser wing of the sphenoid bone is not removed extradurally. The dura is opened, and the sylvian fissure is widely split, allowing the subarachnoid extension of the aneurysm to be directly visualized. The AC is then removed using an intradural approach. The optic canal roof and lateral wall are also carefully drilled away with a diamond drill, and the dural sheath overlying the optic nerve is opened to allow its mobilization. Finally, the optic strut is drilled down flush to the wall of the sphenoid sinus. Any bleeding from the sinus can be controlled easily with Gelfoam or Surgicel.

After the optic nerve has been freed and the branches of the ophthalmic segment have been identified, the dural attachments of the ICA at the dural ring are sectioned circumferentially, providing unimpeded clip access to the ClinSeg. The anterolateral type is usually best obliterated with a gently curved clip, whereas the medial type invariably requires a right-angled fenestrated clip that encircles the ICA. We routinely use intraoperative arteriography to document that the clip is in the proper position and that the ICA is patent before the wound is closed (see Fig. 20-4E).

Care should be taken to avoid injury to the oculomotor nerve (which sits at the lateral edge of the carotid-oculomotor membrane), either during the exposure or as the clip blades are being advanced to secure the proximal aneurysm neck. The oculosympathetic fibers exit the ICA in the ClinSeg, and extensive dissection often results in a mild ptosis and miosis. Bone defects into the basal sinuses are often encountered while drilling the optic strut. To prevent postoperative cerebrospinal fluid rhinorrhea, these must be recognized and repaired, usually with a combination of muscle, Gelfoam, and tissue adhesive or methyl methacrylate. Surgical exposure to allow direct clipping of ClinSeg aneurysms can be safely performed in most patients, with only slightly higher operative risks than those associated with ophthalmic segment lesions.

Many of these lesions are amenable to endovascular treatment with coils, often without a stent, as their necks are usually quite narrow. Although no reports detail the long-term outcome of endovascular treatment of ClinSeg aneurysms, the lower mortality and morbidity with these methods should be carefully weighed against the risks and recovery period entailed in an open operative procedure.

INFECTIOUS ANEURYSMS

Infectious aneurysms may affect the cavernous ICA either by septic embolization or by extension of an adjacent septic focus within the venous sinus or skull base.[31] Ultimately, the arteritis produced by the infection may lead to arterial thrombosis, aneurysm formation, or arterial rupture. The primary treatment of such lesions is appropriate antimicrobial drugs, with aggressive intervention reserved for persistent symptomatic lesions. When necessary, therapy should generally include endovascular techniques, using the same precautions to prevent stroke as for the saccular variety.

TRAUMATIC NONFISTULOUS ANEURYSMS

Traumatic ICA aneurysm formation after closed head injury occurs predominantly in the intracavernous portion of that vessel. This type of aneurysm may also develop after penetrating injuries to the orbit or brain when the wall of the cavernous carotid artery is injured. The typical patient initially presents with a skull fracture of the anterior skull base, accompanied by unilateral blindness, anosmia, or other cranial neuropathies.[12] The aneurysm itself may not be symptomatic initially. Others may be heralded by unexplained arterial bleeding after parasphenoidal procedures that disrupt the ICA or one of its branches.[32–34] Massive epistaxis may develop immediately when nasal packing is removed or may occur later after the patient has been discharged seemingly free of problems. If epistaxis does occur, almost 50% of patients die before a diagnosis is established or adequate treatment is rendered.[34–36]

Aggressive therapy should be strongly considered after angiographic identification because the mortality rate with lesions presenting with epistaxis is so high. Surgical trapping with simultaneous intracranial and cervical carotid ligation or balloon occlusion at the site of the arterial injury accelerates thrombosis and lessens the chances of collateral circulation development. Extracranial-intracranial bypass surgery, using an arterial donor to obviate need for systemic anticoagulation, should be considered when time and the patient's clinical state and anatomy permit.

CAROTID-CAVERNOUS FISTULAS

Fistulous diversion of arterial flow in the region of the cavernous sinus can produce various clinical signs, including exophthalmos, orbital or cephalic bruit (or both), ocular pulsations, headache, chemosis, extraocular palsies, or visual failure.[35,37–39] Catastrophic complications such as SAH, epistaxis, or severe orbital bleeding are uncommon in untreated lesions and generally occur when venous drainage has been diverted away from the venous sinuses into adjacent parenchymal veins.[40,41] The pattern of venous drainage is a major determinant of the signs and symptoms produced by the fistula, regardless of the site or size of the arterial injury. The multiple venous outflow channels from the cavernous sinus allow the arterialized blood to be diverted anteriorly into the ipsilateral, contralateral, or bilateral orbital venous system or into parenchymal veins within the brain.[42]

CCFs can be categorized based on pathologic, hemodynamic, and arteriographic criteria, including (1) post-traumatic versus spontaneous (dependent on the presence or absence of head injury temporally related to onset), (2) high flow versus low flow (the size of the arteriovenous communication), (3) direct versus indirect (dural) arterial flow directly from the ICA or from dural branches of the ICA or ECA, and (4) typical versus atypical (venous drainage into the dural sinuses or through parenchymal veins).[37,38,43,44] The options and results of intervention are determined by a composite assessment of each of these criteria. Because some fistulas have unusual arterial feeding patterns or venous drainage, complete arteriography, including bilateral selective external and internal carotid injections and at least one vertebral injection, should be performed before treatment selection.

Barrow's classification scheme has become a common and practical grading system for CCFs (Table 20-1).[37]

High-flow fistulas are usually post-traumatic in origin, although a few develop after intracavernous aneurysm rupture.[37,38,44] The typical patient is a young man with a pronounced and rapidly progressive cavernous sinus syndrome appearing shortly after a significant head injury.[12] The arterial supply to the fistula originates directly from the cavernous ICA, and distal carotid flow is often impaired. Venous drainage proceeds forward through the ipsilateral superior ophthalmic vein into the orbit. Spontaneous thrombosis of the fistula or of adjacent veins is rare, and most cases require aggressive intervention.

Low-flow fistulas typically arise in middle-aged or elderly women, are invariably spontaneous in origin, and usually coexist with a previous venous sinus thrombosis. Symptoms are usually mild and rarely evolve to a full-blown exophthalmos and panophthalmoplegia syndrome so characteristic of the high-flow variety.[37,38,44] Arterial supply to the fistula originates from dural branches of the ICA or ECA, and blood flow into the hemisphere is normal. Because arterial inflow is low and there is already some impedance to venous outflow from previous sinus thrombosis, spontaneous regression is frequent, especially when compared with high-flow lesions.[37,40,43–45]

The goals of therapy for a CCF include preservation of vision, elimination of the bruit, and restoration of the orbit and its contents to normal while avoiding cerebral ischemic complications. The ideal treatment should obliterate the fistula while maintaining patency of the carotid artery. Endovascular techniques have greatly facilitated the treatment of many of these lesions with relatively low morbidity and mortality; such methods include both arterial and venous-side occlusion and are generally considered first before any open surgical intervention is contemplated.

High-Flow Fistulas

Endovascular Procedures

Detachable balloon or coil systems have been the procedure of choice for most high-flow CCFs because they offer the advantages of direct fistula occlusion without an open cervical or intracranial procedure, sparing the cavernous region from surgical manipulation.[37,38,46,47] Angiography characteristically demonstrates early and dense opacification of the enlarged cavernous sinus and poorer-than-expected opacification of the cerebral arterial system (Fig. 20-5A). Although the high-flow, high-pressure shunt often makes the exact point of arteriovenous communication difficult to demonstrate, these factors greatly facilitate the ease and safety of passing a flow-directed detachable balloon directly into the fistula (see Fig. 20-5B).

In this fistula type, blood flow from the ipsilateral ICA is already largely diverted directly into the venous system without contributing substantially to brain perfusion. If simultaneous ICA sacrifice is required, it is generally well tolerated as long as the fistula is simultaneously obliterated.[48,49] If the balloon is detached below the fistula or if ipsilateral proximal carotid thrombosis occurs from any other cause, several major problems are created, including (1) persistence of the fistula (now filled retrograde from intracranial communications), (2) cortical steal (flow from collaterals that were supplying the distal hemisphere is now diverted toward the

TABLE 20-1 ■ Barrow Classification for Carotid Cavernous Fistula

Type A	Direct high-flow shunts between ICA and CS
Type B	Dural shunts between meningeal branches of ICA and CS
Type C	Dural shunts between meningeal branches of ECA and CS
Type D	Dural shunts between both ICA ECA and CS

CS, cavernous sinus; ECA, external carotid artery; ICA, internal carotid artery

fistula), and (3) limited transarterial catheter access. In such circumstances, the fistula is still treatable by exposing the ClinSeg intracranially, temporarily clipping the ICA below the ophthalmic artery origin, and passing a catheter through the wall of the ClinSeg toward the fistula. When the temporary clip is released, retrograde flow will carry the catheter toward the fistula, where balloons or coils may be deployed. Trial inflation, monitored with transocular and transcranial Doppler and direct observation of the pulsating sinus, will confirm proper balloon placement and shunt obliteration. Once the fistula and its effects disappear, a permanent clip is left in place on the ClinSeg.

Direct Surgical Intervention

Using adjunctive hypothermia and circulatory arrest, Parkinson[49,50] exposed the intracavernous carotid artery through the lateral cavernous sinus wall. Dolenc and others[22–24] also described a direct operative approach to high-flow CCF, using the same exposure described for petrous-to-supraclinoid ICA bypass for intracavernous aneurysms. During such procedures, the ICA is very difficult to distinguish from the surrounding arterialized veins, and identification of the exact fistula site can be extremely tedious. Because of the technical difficulties of these approaches and their associated morbidity to the cranial nerves and brain, direct procedures should be restricted to those rare circumstances in which endovascular techniques are not applicable.[51,52]

Low-Flow Fistulas

Transarterial Procedures

Most spontaneous fistulas are low-flow, low-pressure dural shunts that receive blood from several sources. The ECA frequently supplies this type of fistula, primarily through terminal meningeal branches of the internal maxillary artery and also from other contributing branches including the ascending pharyngeal and pterygopalatine arteries.[36,37] The inferolateral and the meningohypophyseal trunks are the usual sources when the ICA supplies the fistula. Contralateral arterial dural contributions are also frequent.

The more benign symptoms, lesser likelihood of major visual complications, and greater tendency for spontaneous thrombosis justify conservative management of most spontaneous fistulas. Because the fistula originates from multiple, smaller dural branches of the ICA or ECA, detachable coil or balloon techniques have little or no value. When intervention is indicated, particulate embolization with polyvinyl alcohol or other agents introduced into the ECA have produced good results with low risks.[37,44–46] Occasionally, the hemodynamic changes caused by partial ECA embolization

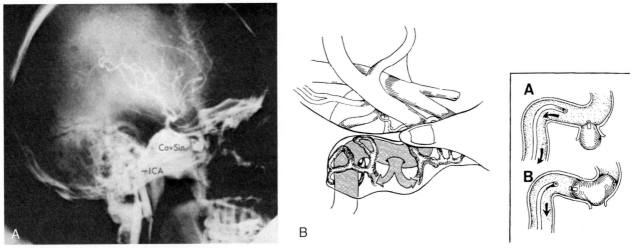

FIGURE 20-5   High-flow carotid cavernous fistula. *A,* A preoperative arteriogram (lateral view) in a young man who developed the subacute onset of a bruit and cavernous sinus syndrome after a closed head injury. Note the large arteriovenous fistula between the carotid artery (ICA) and the cavernous sinus (CavSin). *B,* Detachable balloon treatment of high-flow carotid-cavernous fistula (schematic). Note the tear in the carotid artery, with arterial flow proceeding directly into adjacent veins. A balloon-tipped, flow-directed catheter is passed into the fistula and the balloon is detached, preserving the carotid lumen (insert *A*) or occluding the carotid lumen (insert *B*).

are adequate to lead to spontaneous resolution of the entire fistula. ICA feeder embolization is more difficult and obviously more hazardous, and embolic procedures within this vessel should probably be delayed until all treatments through the ECA have been maximally exercised.

Transvenous Approaches

Thrombogenic materials, introduced into the cavernous sinus directly through Parkinson's triangle or indirectly through a draining vein (e.g., the superior ophthalmic vein) or sinus (e.g., the petrosal sinuses, clival plexus) can effectively thrombose these lesions with low morbidity, high likelihood of ICA preservation, and higher incidence of obliteration than transarterial techniques.[53–57]

Although venous drainage of a spontaneous CCF is usually through the ipsilateral lateral ophthalmic veins, variations are not uncommon. Arterialized outflow proceeding through parenchymal veins places these lesions at risk of hemorrhage, and more aggressive intervention is warranted (Fig. 20-6A). Using a frontotemporal craniotomy, the lateral wall of the cavernous sinus may be exposed, along with the arterialized draining veins bridging the subarachnoid space. The fistula, usually readily apparent within the dura, is coagulated with low-power bipolar cautery (see Fig. 20-6B).

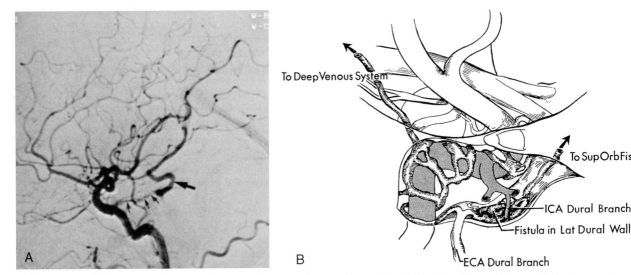

FIGURE 20-6   Low-flow carotid cavernous fistula. *A,* A preoperative arteriogram (lateral view) in a 55-year-old man who had a recent severe headache suggestive of subarachnoid hemorrhage. Note the small dural fistula in the region of the cavernous sinus (*multiple small arrows*), with venous drainage (*large arrow*) bridging the tentorium and subarachnoid space to enter the deep venous system (atypical variant). *B,* A schematic representation of a dural fistula on the lateral cavernous sinus dural wall. Note the potential arterial filling from both the external and internal carotid dural branches. Venous drainage usually proceeds anteriorly into the ophthalmic veins (typical variant). In the actual case (*A*), the dura containing the fistula and the vein draining into the parenchyma were coagulated. Subsequent arteriography confirmed the complete obliteration of the fistula. ECA, external carotid artery; ICA, internal carotid artery; Lat, lateral; SubOrbFiss, superior orbital fissure.

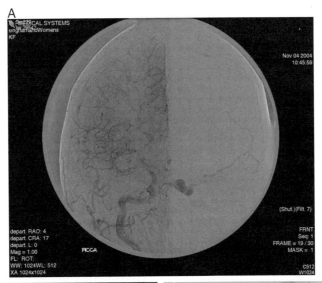

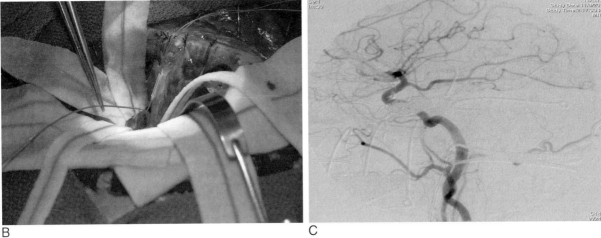

FIGURE 20-7 *A,* Cavernous-carotid fistula with venous outflow to the sphenoparietal sinus and superficial temporal vein. *B,* At surgery, the sylvian fissure is split exposing the superficial temporal vein as it enters the sphenoparietal sinus. *C,* An angiocatheter is introduced into the superficial temporal vein and advanced into the cavernous sinus for transvenous coiling of the carotid-cavernous fistula.

The veins exiting the sinus into parenchyma are also coagulated and sectioned, thus restricting any residual sinus arterialization from reaching weaker parenchymal veins. Figure 20-7 demonstrates the treatment of a CCF using combined open and endovascular surgical techniques.

Stereotactic Radiosurgery

Several reports have indicated that dural arteriovenous fistulas may resolve after stereotactic-focused radiation (radiosurgery), including several small series of lesions in the cavernous sinus area.[58–60] Such treatments generally require months or years to effect obliteration but may be considered in select cases in which the fistula is well circumscribed and other options are inadvisable.

REFERENCES

1. Inoue T, Rhoton AL, Jr, Theel D, Barry ME: Surgical approaches to the cavernous sinus: A microsurgical study. Neurosurgery 26:903–932, 1990.
2. Sahs AL, Perret GE, Locksley HB, Nishioka H: Intracranial Aneurysms and Subarachnoid Hemorrhage: A Cooperative Study. Philadelphia: JB Lippincott, 1969, pp 37–108.
3. Cawley CM, Zipfel GJ, Day AL: Surgical treatment of paraclinoid and ophthalmic aneurysms. Neurosurg Clin N Am 9:765–783, 1998.
4. Seone E, Rhoton AL, de Oliveira E: Microsurgical anatomy of the dural collar (carotid collar) and rings around the clinoidal segment of the internal carotid artery. Neurosurgery 42:869–886, 1998.
5. Locksley HB: Natural history of subarachnoid hemorrhage, intracranial aneurysms, and arteriovenous malformation. J Neurosurg 25:219–239, 1966.
6. Linskey ME, Sekhar LN, Hirsch W, et al: Aneurysms of the intracavernous carotid artery: Clinical presentation, radiographic features, and pathogenesis. Neurosurgery 26:71–79, 1990.
7. Kupersmith MJ, Hurst R, Berenstein A, et al: The benign course of cavernous carotid artery aneurysms. J Neurosurg 77:690–693, 1992.
8. Day AL, Knego RS, Masson RL: Aneurysms of the Clinoidal Segment: A Clinicoanatomic Study. Paper presented at the American Association of Neurological Surgeons Annual Meeting, April 1993, Boston.
9. al-Rodhan NR, Piepgras DG, Sundt TM, Jr: Transitional cavernous aneurysms of the internal carotid artery. Neurosurgery 33:993–996, 1993.
10. Linskey ME, Sekhar LN, Horton JA, et al: Aneurysms of the intracavernous carotid artery: A multidisciplinary approach to treatment. J Neurosurg 75:525–534, 1991.
11. Serbinenko FA, Filatov JM, Spallone A, et al: Management of giant intracranial ICA aneurysms with combined extracranial-intracranial anastomosis and endovascular occlusion. J Neurosurg 73:57–63, 1990.
12. Day AL, Rhoton AL, Jr: Aneurysms and arteriovenous fistulae of the intracavernous carotid artery and its branches.

In Youmans JR (ed): Neurological Surgery. Philadelphia: WB Saunders, 1990, pp 1807–1830.

13. Drake CG, Peerless SJ, Ferguson GG: Hunterian proximal arterial occlusion for giant aneurysm of the carotid circulation. J Neurosurg 81:656–665, 1994.

14. Pozzati E, Fagioli L, Servadei F, Gaist G: Effect of common carotid ligation of giant aneurysms of the internal carotid artery. J Neurosurg 55:527–531, 1981.

15. Linskey ME, Jungreis CA, Yonas H, et al: Stroke risk after abrupt internal carotid artery sacrifice: Accuracy of preoperative assessment with balloon test occlusion and stable xenon-enhanced CT. Am J Neuroradiol 15:829–843, 1994.

16. Polin RS, Shaffrey ME, Jensen ME, et al: Medical management in the endovascular treatment of carotid-cavernous aneurysms. J Neurosurg 84:755–761, 1996.

17. Lewis AI, Tomsick TA, Tew JM, Jr: Management of 100 consecutive direct carotid-cavernous fistulas: Results of treatment with detachable balloons. Neurosurgery 36:239–244, 1995.

18. Barnett DW, Barrow DL, Joseph GJ: Combined extracranial-intracranial bypass and intraoperative balloon occlusion for the treatment of intracavernous and proximal carotid artery aneurysms. Neurosurgery 35:92–97, 1994.

19. Fox AJ, Vinuela F, Pelz DM, et al: Use of detachable balloons for proximal artery occlusion in the treatment of unclippable cerebral aneurysms. J Neurosurg 66:40–46, 1987.

20. Diaz FG, Ausman A, Pearce JE: Ischemic complications after combined internal carotid artery occlusion and extracranial-intracranial anastomosis. Neurosurgery 10:563–570, 1982.

21. Sekhar LN, Linskey ME, Sen CN, Altschuler EM: Surgical management of lesions within the cavernous sinus. Clin Neurosurg 37:440–489, 1991.

22. Sekhar LN, Sen CN, Jho HD: Saphenous vein graft bypass of the cavernous internal carotid artery. J Neurosurg 72:35–41, 1990.

23. Spetzler RF, Fukushima T, Martin N, Zabramski JM: Petrous carotid-to-intradural carotid saphenous vein graft for intracavernous giant aneurysm, tumor, and occlusive cerebrovascular disease. J Neurosurg 73:496–501, 1990.

24. Dolenc VV: Direct microsurgical repair of intracavernous vascular lesions. J Neurosurg 58:824–831, 1983.

25. Diaz FG, Ohaegbulam S, Dujovny M, Ausman JI: Surgical alternatives in the treatment of cavernous sinus aneurysms. J Neurosurg 71:846–853, 1989.

26. van der Schaaf IC, Brilstra EH, Buskens E, Rinkel GJ: Endovascular treatment of aneurysms in the cavernous sinus: A systematic review on balloon occlusion of the parent vessel and embolization with coils. Stroke 33:313–318, 2002.

27. Higashida RT, Halbach VV, Dowd C, et al: Endovascular detachable balloon embolization therapy of cavernous carotid artery aneurysm: Results in 87 cases. J Neurosurg 72:857–863, 1990.

28. Guglielmi G, Vinuela F, Briganti F, Duckwiler G: Carotid-cavernous fistula caused by ruptured intracavernous aneurysm: Endovascular treatment by electrothrombosis with detachable coils. Neurosurgery 31:591–596, 1992.

29. Guglielmi G, Vinuela F, Dion J, Duckwiler G: Electrothrombosis of saccular aneurysms via endovascular approach. Part 2: Preliminary clinical experiences. J Neurosurg 75:8–14, 1991.

30. Felber S, Henkes H, Weber W, et al: Treatment of extracranial and intracranial aneurysms and arteriovenous fistulae using stent grafts. Neurosurgery 55:631–638, 2004.

31. Rout D, Sharma A, Mohan P, Rao VRK: Bacterial aneurysms of the intracavernous carotid artery. J Neurosurg 60:1236–1242, 1984.

32. Lister JR, Sypert GW: Traumatic false aneurysm and carotid-cavernous fistula: A complication of sphenoidotomy. Neurosurgery 5:473–475, 1979.

33. Robbins JB, Fitz-Hugh GS, Jane JA: Intracranial carotid catastrophes encountered by the otolaryngologist. Laryngoscope 86:893–902, 1976.

34. Baviszski G, Killer M, Knosp E, et al: False aneurysm of the intracavernous carotid artery: Report of 7 cases. Acta Neurochir (Wien) 139:37–43, 1997.

35. Handa J, Handa H: Severe epistaxis caused by traumatic aneurysm of cavernous carotid artery. Surg Neurol 5:241–243, 1976.

36. Liu MY, Shih CJ, Wang YC, Tsai SH: Traumatic intracavernous carotid aneurysm with massive epistaxis. Neurosurgery 17:569–573, 1985.

37. Barrow DL, Spector RH, Braun IF, et al: Classification and treatment of spontaneous carotid-cavernous sinus fistulas. J Neurosurg 62:248–256, 1985.

38. DeBrun GM, Vinuela F, Fox AJ, et al: Indications for treatment and classification of 132 carotid cavernous fistulas. Neurosurgery 22:285–289, 1988.

39. Martin JD, Jr, Mabon RF: Pulsating exophthalmos: Review of all reported cases. JAMA 121:330–334, 1943.

40. Dohrmann PJ, Batjer HH, Samson D, Suss RA: Recurrent subarachnoid hemorrhage complicating a traumatic carotid cavernous fistula. Neurosurgery 17:480–483, 1985.

41. Lee SH, Burton CV, Chan GH: Posttraumatic ophthalmic vein arterialization. Surg Neurol 4:483–484, 1974.

42. Bickerstaff ER: Mechanisms of presentation of carotico-cavernous fistulae. Br J Ophthalmol 54:186–190, 1970.

43. Peeters FLM, Kroger R: Dural and direct cavernous sinus fistulas. Am J Radiol 132:599–606, 1979.

44. Vinuela F, Fox AJ, DeBrun GM, et al: Spontaneous carotid-cavernous fistulas: Clinical, radiological, and therapeutic considerations. J Neurosurg 60:976–984, 1984.

45. Newton TH, Hoyt WF: Dural arteriovenous shunts in the region of cavernous sinus. Neuroradiology 1:71–81, 1970.

46. Berenstein A, Kricheff II, Ransohoff J: Carotid-cavernous fistula: Intraarterial treatment. AJNR Am J Neuroradiol 1:449–457, 1980.

47. DeBrun GN, LaCour P, Vinuela F, et al: Treatment of 54 traumatic carotid-cavernous fistulas. J Neurosurg 55:678–692, 1981.

48. Tomsick TA, Tew JM, Lukin RR, Johnson JK: Balloon catheters for aneurysms and fistulae. Clin Neurosurg 31:135–164, 1983.

49. Parkinson D: Carotid cavernous fistula: Direct approach and repair of fistula and preservation of the artery. In Morley TP (ed): Current Controversies in Neurosurgery. Philadelphia: WB Saunders, 1976, 237–249.

50. Parkinson D: Carotid cavernous fistula: Direct repair with preservation of carotid. J Neurosurg 38:99–106, 1973.

51. Tu YK, Liu HM, Hu SC: Direct surgery of carotid-cavernous fistulae and dural arteriovenous malformations of the cavernous sinus. Neurosurgery 41:798–805, 1997.

52. Day JD, Fukushima T: Direct microsurgery of dural arteriovenous malformation type carotid-cavernous sinus fistulas: Indications, technique, and results. Neurosurgery 41:1119–1124, 1997.

53. Mullan S: Experiences with surgical thrombosis of intracranial berry aneurysms and carotid cavernous fistulae. J Neurosurg 41:657–670, 1974.

54. Mullan S: Treatment of carotid-cavernous fistulae by cavernous sinus occlusion. J Neurosurg 50:131–144, 1979.

55. Miller NR, Monsein LH, Debrun GM, et al: Treatment of carotid-cavernous fistulas using a superior ophthalmic vein approach. J Neurosurg 83:838–842, 1995.

56. Klisch J, Huppertz HJ, Spetzger U, et al: Transvenous treatment of carotid cavernous and dural arteriovenous fistulae: Results for 31 patients and review of the literature. Neurosurgery 53:836–856, 2003.

57. Cheng KM, Chan CM, Cheung YL: Transvenous embolisation of dural carotid-cavernous fistulas by multiple venous routes: A series of 27 cases. Acta Neurochir (Wien) 145:17–29, 2003.

58. Chandler HC, Jr, Friedman WA: Successful radiosurgical treatment of a dural arteriovenous malformation: Case report. Neurosurgery 33:139–142, 1993.

59. Barcia-Salorio JL, Soler F, Barcia JA, Hernandez G: Radiosurgery of carotid-cavernous fistulae. Acta Neurochir Suppl (Wien) 62:10–12, 1994.

60. Guo WY, Pan DH, Wu HM, et al: Radiosurgery as a treatment alternative for dural arteriovenous fistulas of the cavernous sinus. Am J Neuroradiol 19:1081–1087, 1998.

21 Craniofacial Resection for Anterior Skull Base Tumors

GAVIN W. BRITZ, A. ALEX MOHIT, and
FRANCIS G. JOHNSTON

SUMMARY

Tumors of the anterior skull base represent a group of diverse lesions that share complexity of surgical access. Craniofacial approaches are often necessary for complete resection of these lesions. These approaches can be classified as transsphenoidal, transoral, and transfacial. The transsphenoidal route provides good access to the sellar region and the rostral clivus. Transoral approaches include palatal sparing, transpalatal, LeFort I osteotomy, and extended maxillotomy. These approaches provide the necessary access from the anterior rim of the foramen magnum that can be extended rostrally by division of the palate and with LeFort osteotomy. The transfacial approach provides good access to the paranasal sinuses and the rostral clivus. These surgical approaches, in combination with transcranial approaches, provide the means for complete resection of anterior skull base tumors.

Skull base tumors are by definition tumors that arise from or are located in the bony structures at the base of the brain. They may originate from a variety of extracranial or intracranial tissues, or directly from the skull base. The usual extracranial sources include areas such as the paranasal sinuses, nasopharynx, and surrounding connective tissues whose tumors secondarily invade the skull base. The intracranial sources include basal meningiomas, pituitary tumors, and metastatic tumors that erode into the base of the skull. Osteosarcomas, chordomas, and chondrosarcomas are tumors that originate directly from the skull base.

Despite this diversity in origin, these tumors behave rather uniformly: they are frequently benign or only locally malignant, they rarely metastasize, and they prove refractory to radiation therapy or chemotherapy; thus radical surgical resection is the treatment of choice in their management.[1] This procedure ideally involves an en bloc surgical resection of the tumor,[2–4] although this has often been limited to partial removals because of the many problems encountered in the treatment of skull base tumors.[5]

Several advances have occurred that have significantly altered the management of these tumors. Newer imaging techniques, such as computed tomography reconstructions of the skull base and magnetic resonance imaging, have led to improved delineation of the tumors, thus aiding in the preoperative evaluation and surgical planning (Figs. 21-1 and 21-2). Improvements in neuroanesthesia have allowed for greater control in the management of intraoperative cerebral swelling, thus improving the ultimate outcome.

In surgical treatment, the rate-limiting step in achieving the goal of radical surgical resection has been obtaining access to and exposure of these tumors. These tumors are difficult to approach, in that they lie ventral to the brain and posterior to the facial skeleton and aerodigestive system. Advances in surgical techniques, however, have resulted in the development of several different approaches that often involve a multidisciplinary team including neurosurgeons, plastic surgeons, maxillofacial surgeons, and otolaryngologists. The various approaches are used to obtain access to and exposure of skull base tumors in different locations, based on preoperative imaging studies and surgical planning. More recently, with the advent of surgical navigational systems, surgical planning has further evolved to include both preoperative and intraoperative computerized visualization of these tumors.[6]

The surgical management and choice of the surgical approach to skull base tumors depends largely on the location of the tumor. Each approach provides various angles and degrees of access along the skull base. This chapter concentrates on the management of anterior skull base tumors using the direct midline ventral approaches to these tumors in the region of the clivus. These approaches are particularly

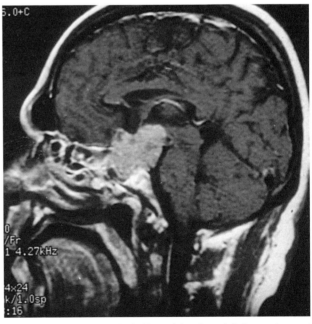

FIGURE 21-1 A sagittal T1-weighted gadolinium-enhanced magnetic resonance imaging scan demonstrating a chordoma that involves the superior clivus, the sphenoid sinus, and the sellar region with a suprasellar extension.

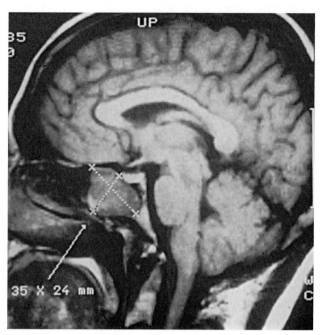

FIGURE 21-2 A sagittal T1-weighted gadolinium-enhanced magnetic resonance imaging scan demonstrating a chordoma that originates in the clivus and involves the sphenoid and ethmoid sinuses. Asterisks outline the lesion.

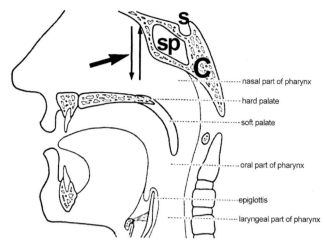

FIGURE 21-3 A schematic representation of the extent of access and exposure (*vertical arrows*) to the sphenoid sinus (sp), sellar region (s) and superior clivus (C), which is possible with a transsphenoidal route.

attractive, because they are unencumbered by cranial nerves or major blood vessels.[7] Direct midline ventral approaches can be transnasal, transoral, or transfacial, and are modified according to the location of the tumor.

The transnasal or transsphenoidal route provides good access to the sellar region and rostral third of the clivus but is limited in more extensive lesions in that region.[7,8] The purely transoral route provides a direct approach to the anterior rim of the foramen magnum.[7,9] This route can then be modified by extending the approach with various maneuvers to improve the access to and exposure of tumors in the anterior skull base. Dividing the soft or hard palate in the transpalatal approach allows for access to the lower and middle third of the clivus.[10,11] The Le Fort I osteotomy with mobilization of the hard palate and maxilla inferiorly allows for visualization of the whole clivus.[1,12,13] An extended maxillotomy combines a Le Fort I osteotomy with splitting of the hard and soft palate, and allows for exposure of the whole clivus and the craniocervical junction.[7,14] In the transfacial approach, removal of the midface gives access to the paranasal sinuses and upper two thirds of the clivus.[12,15] These various approaches can also be combined with intracranial approaches, if necessary, to obtain a complete tumor resection.

TRANSSPHENOIDAL APPROACH

Lesions involving the sellar region and the upper third of the clivus can be surgically treated using the sublabial-rhinoseptal-transsphenoidal approach[8] (Fig. 21-3). This approach is simply an extension of pituitary surgery, which is now widely performed. After oral intubation, the head is placed on a headrest slightly extended, with the surgeon next to the chest and positioned perpendicular to the plane

of the imaging intensifier to allow for the correct intraoperative orientation. An antiseptic is then applied to the nose and mouth, and the surrounding area is draped with sterile towels. The sphenoid sinus can be approached by either the sublabial or the rhinoseptal route; we prefer the latter approach and describe it here.

After infiltration with local anesthetic containing 1:200,000 epinephrine and 0.5% lidocaine at the junction between the skin and the mucosa of the right naris, which is retracted with a Senn retractor, an incision is made into the mucosa to the nasal septum. A mucoperichondrial plane is then developed between the nasal mucosa and the septum and followed posteriorly to the posterior boundary of the cartilaginous septum, where the bony septum derived from the superior portion of the vomer and the inferior portion of the perpendicular plate of the ethmoid is identified. A speculum is then introduced and opened, fracturing the inferior portion of the perpendicular plate of the ethmoid and allowing for visualization of the midline and both sides of the anterior wall of the sphenoid sinus, with its keel-like appearance. Confirmation of location should be obtained with the imaging intensifier, which should confirm access and exposure to the sellar region through the sphenoid sinus, and the upper third of the clivus. The operating microscope is then introduced and used for the rest of the procedure.

The anterior wall of the sphenoid sinus is then opened with a 1-mm Kerrison punch, either starting at the ostia of the sinus located laterally, or after fracturing the wall with a small osteotome. The sinus is opened to the lateral, superior, and inferior aspect of the sella. The mucosa of the sinus is then stripped and removed, and bleeding is controlled with coagulation. The direction of approach can then be adjusted with angulation of the speculum and correlation of the image on the image intensifier. After the angle of approach has been decided, the speculum is advanced into the sinus directed toward the area of interest and then opened. Care should be taken not to use force to open the speculum, because fractures of the sphenoid bone can occur. Occasionally, tumors may have eroded through the anterior wall of the sphenoid sinus, and then the sinus is opened around the tumor.

The remainder of the operation depends largely on the surgical goals and the location of the tumor. Using the microscope, lesions in the midline involving the sphenoid sinus, sellar region, and rostral clivus can be removed. Lesions within the sella or that have involved the sella may require opening of the anterior wall of the sella. This is performed with a small osteotome placed on the sella wall to initiate the opening, which is then extended with a 1-mm Kerrison punch. The opening is extended laterally to the cavernous sinus, inferiorly to the sellar floor, and superiorly to the intercavernous sinus. This exposure of the sellar region allows for a good decompression of the optic chiasm, and patients presenting with chiasmal compression can be expected to have some improvement in vision.[8] In situations in which the dura has been violated, such as when the tumors have involved the dura or when the dura has been inadvertently opened, human-derived fibrin glue (Tisseel; Immuno AG, Vienna, Austria) should be placed over the defect. Continuous lumbar cerebrospinal fluid (CSF) drainage should also be done for 5 days after surgery to facilitate repair and help prevent a CSF leak.

TRANSORAL APPROACHES

The various transoral approaches allow the surgeon access to the whole clivus and craniocervical junction, and are ideally situated to expose midline extradural lesions. Depending on the type of transoral procedure, different regions along this plane can be accessed, and these different approaches are individually described. However, common to all the approaches is the need to perform the procedure through the mouth; the palatal-sparing transoral approach, described first, serves as an example for the general approach to transoral procedures.

Transoral (Palatal-Sparing) Approach

The palatal-sparing transoral approach provides access to the anterior rim of the foramen magnum and thus is ideally suited to midline lesions in and around the basion (Fig. 21-4). Because the procedure is done through the mouth, the first step is to ensure that this is possible. To place the required instruments in the mouth, an interdental distance greater than 25 mm is required.[16] In patients with diseases of the mouth or jaw (e.g., temporomandibular disease) in whom this gap cannot be obtained, median mandibular splitting with a midline glossotomy is required, allowing the tongue halves to be retracted laterally and inferiorly and thus making the operation feasible.[17,18] It is also important preoperatively to assess the oral cavity and, if necessary, advise dental extractions before surgery; sepsis can arise from the teeth, leading to wound abscess and even death from sepsis.[16] Gum guards can also be used to prevent damage to the teeth from the retractor systems.[16]

It is not necessary to perform a preoperative tracheotomy in all patients, and it should be reserved for patients with preoperative bulbar palsies and those who will require prolonged airway care.[19] A fiberoptic nasotracheal airway should be placed, with the patient awake if the cervicomedullary junction is compromised by the mass. A nasogastric tube or feeding tube is placed at this time to allow for aspiration of gastric contents during the early postoperative phase, and

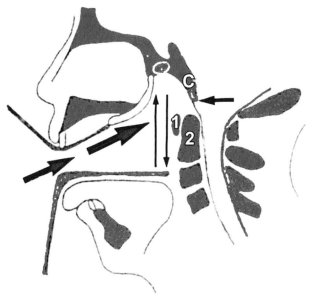

FIGURE 21-4 A schematic representation of the extent of access and exposure (*vertical arrows*) to the inferior clivus (C), the anterior foramen magnum (*small arrow*), the anterior arch of the atlas (1) and the body of the axis (2), which is possible with a palatal-sparing transoral approach (*large arrows*).

for nutritional support before the patient can initiate oral feedings. The patient is then placed on the Mayfield horseshoe in mild extension, and the mouth is prepared with povidone-iodine solution. In this approach, the soft palate need not be split but instead is retracted into the nasopharynx with passage of a Jacques catheter intranasally and sutured in the region of the uvula.[20] A retractor system is then placed; we prefer the Crockard self-retaining retractor system (Codman & Shurtleff; Johnson & Johnson, Randolph, MA; Figs. 21-5 and 21-6), which allows for retraction of the tissues without the need for stay sutures.

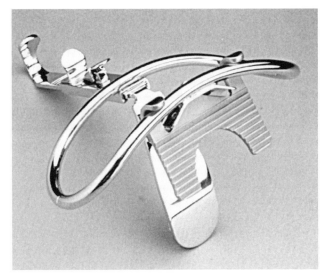

FIGURE 21-5 A photograph of the Crockard self-retaining retractor system, which allows for retraction of the tissues without the need for stay sutures. (Codman & Shurtleff; Johnson & Johnson, Randolph, MA).

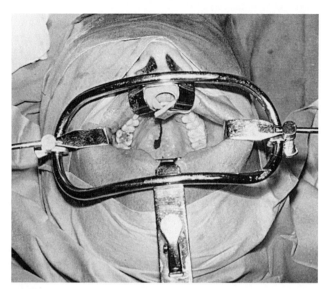

FIGURE 21-6 An intraoperative photograph demonstrating the Crockard self-retaining retractor system in use allowing for retraction of the soft tissues during transoral surgery.

The posterior pharyngeal wall is then palpated, and the anterior tubercle of the atlas is identified as a landmark. After infiltration of local anesthetic containing 1:200,000 epinephrine and 0.5% lidocaine into the median raphe, the posterior pharyngeal wall is incised. The longus colli and longus capitus muscles are then reflected laterally to expose the anterior longitudinal ligament, the caudalmost clivus, the anterior arch of C1, and the anterior surface of C2. To prevent injury to the hypoglossal nerves, the eustachian tubes, or the vertebral arteries, it is important to remain within 1.5 cm of the midline on each side. The caudalmost clivus, the anterior arch of C1, and the odontoid can then be removed with a high-speed drill, allowing for removal of the tumor and decompression of the neural system, depending on the tumor's location. A pulsatile tectorial membrane signifies completion of the extradural decompression. The longus colli and longus capitis muscles and the posterior pharyngeal wall are then closed with absorbable suture. At the end of all transoral procedures, the mandible should be moved to assess for temporomandibular joint dislocation, which can easily be corrected at the operation, but if missed necessitates another anesthetic.[16]

The subarachnoid space can be entered from this transoral approach to facilitate removal of intradural lesions in the region of the craniocervical junction.[21] Inadvertent entry may also occur in extradural lesions such as large clival chordomas, because the dura may be invaded by the tumor, or it may be damaged as the tumor is removed.[16] Because postoperative CSF leakage, often complicated by infection, is the most serious sequela of transoral surgery, this is to be avoided at all costs, and methods have been designed to minimize this complication. First, in all intradural tumors and all situations in which the potential exists for violation of the dura, a large-bore lumbar catheter should be inserted to allow for postoperative CSF drainage. One should allow for a CSF drainage rate of 10 to 20 mL/hour. This should be continued for at least 5 days to decrease hydrostatic pressure and allow wound healing.[20,21] It has also been

suggested that conversion to a lumbar-peritoneal shunt should be done after 5 days in patients with large dural defects,[21] although that is not our practice. The reason for this drainage is that dural closure in this region is difficult, often impossible, and drainage allows for healing to occur without continuous CSF pressure on the wound. In addition to lumbar drainage, repairing the defect with two layers of Lyodura, one layer inside and the other on the outside of the defect, held together with human-derived fibrin glue (Tisseel), aids in preventing postoperative CSF leak. The use of rotational flaps, either pharyngeal or sternocleidomastoid muscle, has also been described to prevent and treat CSF leaks after transoral surgery.[16,22] The postoperative complication of tongue swelling can also be avoided by carefully ensuring that the tongue is free from the retractors and is coated with 1% hydrocortisone before and after surgery.

After surgery, the patient should not be permitted oral intake for at least 3 to 5 days to allow for healing of the posterior pharyngeal wall; the oral intake can then be gradually increased from clear fluids to solids over a period of 2 to 3 days. Nutritional support should be provided with intravenous fluids and enteral feeds through the nasogastric tube or feeding tube that was placed after intubation. In those patients who underwent tracheotomy, the nasotracheal tube should be left in place for at least the first 24 hours to minimize the chance of upper airway obstruction from postoperative swelling.

Transpalatal Approach

The transpalatal approach is essentially an extension of the transoral procedure described already. However, with the additional splitting of the hard and soft palates, access to a longer rostral-to-caudal field is provided that includes the lower half of the clivus, the anterior arch of C1, and the anterior surface of C2. This approach, however, remains limited in its lateral extent. Several variations in the transpalatal approach have been described; here we discuss the one with which we are most familiar.

The mucosa over the hard palate is incised from approximately 4 cm from the junction of the hard and soft palate, and then extended into the soft palate down toward the base of the uvula. At the base of the uvula the incision is then pushed off the midline to one side to preserve the base of the uvula. The hard palate is then removed, providing visualization of the vomer, which may then be removed. The Crockard self-retaining retractor system is then inserted, and the operation continues as described in the palatal-sparing transoral approach, except that access is improved to include the lower half of the clivus, allowing for the removal of tumors that also involve this structure. A two-layer closure is then performed, with an absorbable suture to close the muscle and one to close the mucosa.

The potential complications of this procedure are similar to those of the palatal-sparing approach described earlier, although the additional splitting of the hard and soft palate produces some further potential problems. Oronasal fistulas may occur, particularly at the junction of the hard and soft palates.[16] These require secondary suturing and almost always heal over time.

Velopharyngeal dysfunction is more of a problem, and patients present with nasal regurgitation. That patients with purely extradural lesions and those without lower cranial nerve palsies have a much lower incidence of this problem may explain its pathogenesis. First, integrity of the posterior pharyngeal wall and the soft palate is necessary during phonation and swallowing to form a barrier between the nasopharynx and oropharynx.[21] With removal of a large amount of bone—and thus posterior pharyngeal wall support— such as in resection of the more extensive intradural tumors, patients have a higher incidence of this complication.[21] Posterior pharyngeal flaps, Teflon injections into this area,[21] and a "bone baffle"[23] have been described to provide more support in this area. Second, patients who have neurogenic swallowing problems as demonstrated on swallowing studies also have a higher incidence of this problem, reflecting the need for muscle coordination in the oropharynx and nasopharynx. Despite an improved understanding of its pathogenesis, patients with velopharyngeal dysfunction still present a serious problem that should be studied further.

Le Fort I Osteotomy

The Le Fort I osteotomy was first described for the removal of a nasopharyngeal tumor in 1867 and now is a common operation in the realm of maxillofacial surgery.[24] Anatomically, a direct line of vision to the entire clivus without obstruction by intervening soft tissues is obtained by displacing the maxilla inferiorly (Fig. 21-7). This prompted the use of this approach for access to the clivus, and it was described in the transclival surgical treatment of aneurysms of the vertebrobasilar system with good results.[13] At the same institution, this procedure was used to treat midline skull base tumors.[1] This approach is ideally suited for both intradural

and extradural midline lesions that can involve the whole clivus, because the whole clivus is exposed with this approach.

As with other transoral procedures, oral or nasotracheal intubation may be performed, with tracheotomies reserved for patients with compromised airways or severe bulbar palsies. All patients have a lumbar drain placed that is opened after surgery to allow for CSF drainage if dural violation occurs. The patient is then placed supine on a Mayfield headrest with the head elevated 15 degrees. After preparing the mouth with povidone-iodine solution, an incision is made above the mucogingival reflection extending from one upper molar to other, with the soft tissues reflected back subperiosteally to expose the maxilla. At this stage, the compression plates used to fixate the maxilla to the face at the end of the operation are marked off. This is important because precise relocation is necessary to prevent postoperative malocclusion. A standard Le Fort I osteotomy is then performed using a sagittal saw to cut through the malar buttresses to the maxillary tuberosities (Fig. 21-8). This exposes the nasal floor and pterygomaxillary fissure. The nasal septum is then divided from the maxilla in the midline, a curved chisel is used to separate the lateral pterygoid laminae from their maxillary attachments, and the maxilla is fractured downward[1] (Fig. 21-9). The blood supply to the maxilla is preserved with the greater palatine arteries and the mucosal supply of the faucial pillars.

The nasal mucosa is then stripped to expose the nasal septum and vomer. This is followed by removal of the inferior turbinates and the vomer. A modified Dingman gag is then inserted that retracts the cheeks laterally and the maxilla downward, exposing the posterior pharyngeal wall[1] (Figs. 21-10 and 21-11). This allows for exposure from the middle ethmoids to the anterior arch of the atlas, with the whole clivus between these structures. After infiltration of local anesthetic containing 1:200,000 epinephrine and 0.5% lidocaine into the median raphe, the posterior

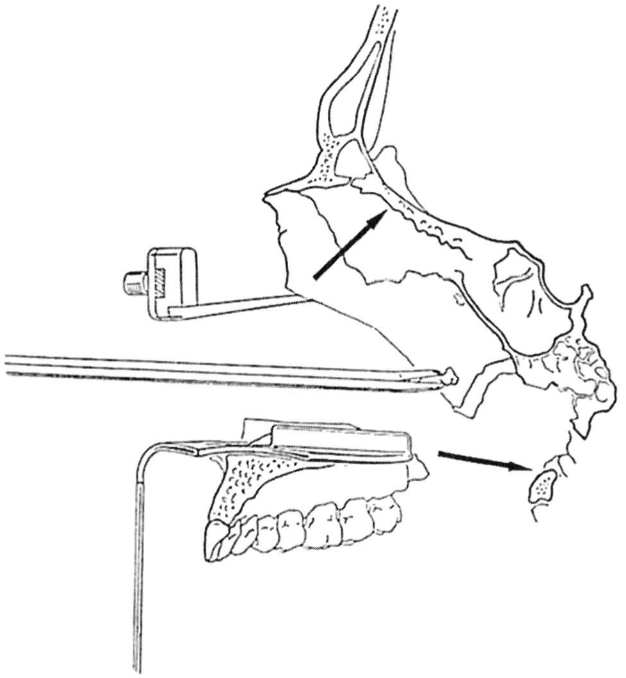

FIGURE 21-7 A schematic representation of the extent of access and exposure (*arrows*) to the sphenoid sinus, sellar region, whole clivus, anterior foramen magnum, and upper cervical spine, which is possible with a Le Fort I maxillotomy surgical approach.

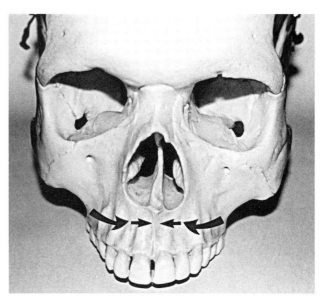

FIGURE 21-8 A photograph demonstrating a standard Le Fort I osteotomy (*arrows*), which is performed with a sagittal saw cutting through the malar buttresses to the maxillary tuberosities, exposing the nasal floor and a pterygomaxillary fissure.

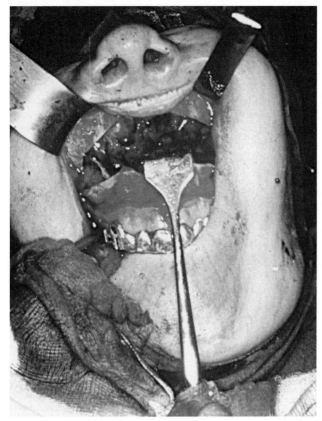

FIGURE 21-9 An intraoperative photograph taken after the nasal septum has been divided from the maxilla in the midline. A chisel is used to separate the lateral pterygoid laminae from their maxillary attachments, which then allows the maxilla to be fractured downward.

pharyngeal wall is incised and reflected laterally to expose the whole clivus and the anterior arch of the atlas. Depending on the location of tumor, the high-speed drill can be used to remove the clivus to obtain access to the tumor, which can then be removed. In tumors that require an intradural exposure, the dura is opened with a small-bladed knife.

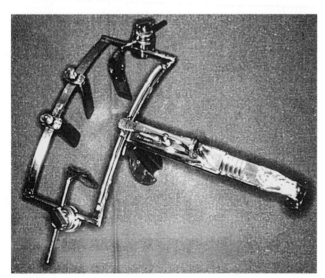

FIGURE 21-10 A photograph of a modified Dingman gag that is used during the Le Fort I osteotomy, thus allowing for retraction of the cheeks laterally and the maxilla downward, exposing the posterior pharyngeal wall.

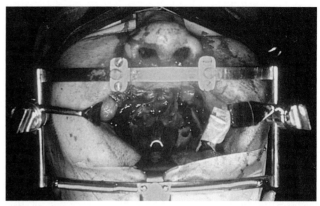

FIGURE 21-11 An intraoperative photograph with the modified Dingman gag in use demonstrating the exposure of the posterior pharyngeal wall.

At completion of tumor removal, the dura is often difficult to close primarily and thus can be repaired with Lyodura as described earlier, with lumbar drainage continued after surgery. The posterior pharyngeal wall is then repaired with absorbable suture. The maxilla is secured with minicompression plates and the mucosa repaired with absorbable suture. The postoperative course is as described earlier.

Extended "Open-Door" Maxillotomy

One disadvantage of the Le Fort I osteotomy is that the down-fractured maxilla may impede access to the craniocervical junction. This may be important if tumors involve the craniocervical junction in addition to the clivus, and thus require a larger area of access. Patients may also have an abnormal anatomic relationship between the clivus and craniocervical junction, impeding exposure. In these situations, the extended or "open-door" maxillotomy as described by Harkey and colleagues[25] and by James and Crockard[26] is indicated. In this procedure, the Le Fort I osteotomy is combined with midline sagittal splitting of the maxilla and soft palate and their lateral displacement, thus allowing for exposure from the sphenoid to the third cervical vertebra.[27]

The decision whether to institute orotracheal or nasotracheal intubation or to perform a tracheotomy is made as described earlier, as is the decision whether to provide lumbar drainage. The patient is then placed supine on a Mayfield headrest with the head mildly extended to allow for access to the palate. After the mouth has been prepared with povidone-iodine solution, an incision is made above the mucogingival reflection extending from one upper molar to other, with the soft tissues reflected back subperiosteally to expose the maxilla. As with the standard Le Fort I procedure, the compression plates used to fix the maxilla to the face at the end of the operation are marked off to ensure precise relocation. A midline sagittal incision is then made into the palatal mucoperiosteum and alveolar margin and is reflected off the underlying bone laterally. Care must be taken to ensure vascularity of the maxilla by not stripping the mucoperiosteum too far laterally. A standard Le Fort I osteotomy is then performed with a sagittal saw to cut through the malar buttresses to the maxillary tuberosities. This exposes the nasal floor and pterygomaxillary fissure. The nasal septum is then divided from the maxilla in the midline, and a curved chisel is used to separate the lateral pterygoid laminae from their maxillary attachments, after which the maxilla is fractured downward.[1] The nasal mucosa is then stripped to expose the nasal septum and vomer, and the inferior turbinates and vomer are removed. A Crockard retractor system is then inserted to permit exposure of the middle ethmoids, the entire clivus, and the craniocervical junction. After infiltration of local anesthetic containing 1:200,000 epinephrine and 0.5% lidocaine into the median raphe, the posterior pharyngeal wall is incised and reflected laterally. A high-speed drill is used to remove the clivus and associated bone necessary for access, and the tumor is resected. In intradural tumors, the dura is opened and then repaired with Lyodura as already described, with lumbar drainage continued after surgery. The posterior pharyngeal wall is then repaired with absorbable suture. The two halves of the maxilla are secured with miniplates, and the maxilla is secured with minicompression plates at the predetermined locations. The mucosa is repaired with absorbable suture. The postoperative course is as described earlier for the other transoral procedures.

TRANSFACIAL APPROACH

In tumors beneath the midface that include the anterior skull base, the transfacial route can be used to gain access with appropriate maxillectomy and ethmoidectomy. Exposure of the midface is the initial step in using the transfacial routes and can be done either by a lateral rhinotomy (Weber-Fergusson incision) or by using the midface degloving technique made popular by Conley, Price, and colleagues,[15,28,29] but originally described by Casson and associates in 1974.[30] The advantage of using the midface degloving technique in the transfacial route for treating tumors in and around the sphenoid sinus and clivus is that the exposure and access are superior to those with the traditional procedures that require facial incisions that can leave unsightly scars. Although the lateral exposure is less generous with the degloving technique than with the Weber-Fergusson incision, the bilateral exposure is an advantage in larger midline lesions such as in clival tumors.[15] Because of the advantages of the degloving approach in midline anterior skull base tumors, this approach is discussed as described by Price, Conley, and colleagues.[15,28,29]

Under general anesthesia, an oral endotracheal tube is placed and secured in the midline. A tarsorrhaphy is performed to prevent irritation of the eye, and topical cocaine is inserted on pledgets intranasally and 1:200,000 epinephrine injected into the junction between the skin and the mucosa of the nose, gingival sulcus, and canine fossae. The nasal tip is separated from the nasal dorsum by intercartilaginous incisions, and the incision is continued around the pyriform margin to complete a circumvestibular release. A sublabial incision is then made that extends from the molars on each side. The soft tissues of the face and the nasal tip are then elevated subperiosteally to expose the inferior orbital rims to their lateralmost extent. The upper lip and nasal columella, nasal tip, and alar cartilages are then retracted over the nose to the infraorbital rim. Osteotomy of the infraorbital foramen is then performed, allowing for preservation of the infraorbital complex.

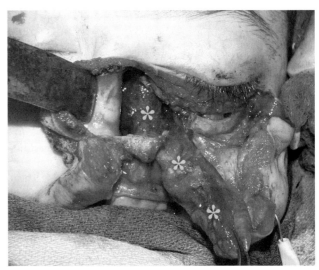

FIGURE 21-12 An intraoperative photograph demonstrating the exposure obtained through a midface degloving approach. In this patient a meningioma involving the ethmoid sinuses and the superior nasal cavity is resected. Asterisks demarcate the lesion.

The medial and inferior portions of the orbit are then freed and extended laterally to mobilize the face further.

The maxillary antrum is then entered and the anterior wall removed on both sides to provide access to the ethmoids (Fig. 21-12). Osteotomies are then performed over the superior and inferior pyriform margins, allowing for completion of a medial maxillectomy. The nasal septum is exposed and released to the cribriform plate after ethmoidectomy and sphenoidotomy have been performed. After removal of the posterior wall of the maxillary antrum and the ascending process of the palatine process, the nasopharynx, sphenoid sinus, and clivus are exposed. Tumor removal can then proceed, with the lateral limit of the dissection being the coronoid process of the mandible, and posteriorly the carotid arteries on the lateral aspect of the sphenoid sinus. The inferior resection is limited by the palate, although this can be extended by performing a palatectomy or maxillectomy if required.

On closure, the face is reapproximated anatomically, with the nasal tip repositioned with a transfixation suture and one placed at the base of the columella. The vestibular skin is then sutured to the pyriform margin, the frenulum carefully approximated, and the sublabial incision sutured. Packing is inserted into the cavity with antibiotic-saturated petroleum jelly, and rhinoplastic taping is applied.

CONCLUSIONS

Skull base tumors are rare tumors that originate from a variety of tissues, extracranially, intracranially, or directly from the skull base. Radical surgical resection is the treatment of choice in their management, because they are frequently benign or only locally malignant, and are refractory to radiation therapy or chemotherapy.

These tumors are difficult to treat surgically, lying ventral to the brain and posterior to the facial skeleton and aerodigestive system; however, advances in surgical techniques involving the creation of multidisciplinary surgical teams have improved outcomes. Surgical management and choice of surgical approach to skull base tumors depends largely on the location of the tumor, with each approach providing various angles and degrees of access along the skull base. For anterior skull base tumors the direct midline ventral approaches are particularly attractive, because they are unencumbered by cranial nerves or major blood vessels.

The transnasal or transsphenoidal route provides good access to the sellar region and rostral third of the clivus. The transoral route provides a direct approach to the anterior rim of the foramen magnum, and may then be modified to improve access and exposure. Dividing the soft or hard palate in the transpalatal approach allows for access to the lower and middle third of the clivus. A Le Fort 1 osteotomy with mobilization of the hard palate and maxilla inferiorly allows for visualization of the whole clivus, and this can be further modified by splitting the hard and soft palates, allowing for exposure of the entire clivus and the craniocervical junction. In the transfacial approach, removal of the midface permits access to the paranasal sinuses and upper two thirds of the clivus. Another important aspect of these direct midline ventral approaches is that they can also be combined with various intracranial approaches to facilitate a more complete removal of tumor.

REFERENCES

1. Uttley D, Moore A, Archer DJ: Surgical management of midline skull-base tumors: A new approach. J Neurosurg 71:705–710, 1989.
2. Cheesman AD, Lund VJ, Howard DJ: Craniofacial resection for tumors of the nasal cavity and paranasal sinuses. Head Neck Surg 8:429–435, 1986.
3. Westbury G, Wilson JSP, Richardson A: Combined craniofacial resection for malignant disease. Am J Surg 130:463–469, 1976.
4. Boyle JO, Shah KC, Shah JP: Craniofacial resection for malignant neoplasms of the skull case: An overview. J Surg Oncol 69:275–284, 1998.
5. Shah JP, Galicich JH: Craniofacial resection for malignant tumors of the ethmoid and anterior skull base. Arch Otolaryngol 103:514–517, 1977.
6. Golfinos JG, Fitzpatrick BC, Smith LR, Spetzler RF: Clinical use of a frameless stereotactic arm: Results of 325 cases. J Neurosurg 83:197–202, 1995.
7. Crockard HA: Transclival surgery. Br J Neurosurg 5:237–240, 1991.
8. Laws ER, Jr: Transsphenoidal surgery for tumors of the clivus. Otolaryngol Head Neck Surg 92:100–101, 1984.
9. Mullan LI, Naunton R, Hekmat-Panah J, et al: The use of an anterior approach to ventrally placed tumors in the foramen magnum and vertebral column. J Neurosurg 24:536–543, 1966.
10. Pasztor E, Vajda J, Piffko P: Transoral surgery for craniocervical space occupying process. J Neurosurg 60:276–281, 1984.
11. Crockard HA: Anterior approaches to lesions of the upper cervical spine. Clin Neurosurg 34:389–416, 1988.
12. Kyoshima K, Matsuo K, Kushima H, et al: Degloving transfacial approach with Le Fort I and nasomaxillary ostiotomies: Alternative transfacial approach. Neurosurgery 50:13–20, 2002.
13. Archer DJ, Young S, Uttley D: Basilar aneurysms: A new transclival approach via maxillotomy. J Neurosurg 67:54–58, 1987.
14. Harkey HL, Crockard HA, Stevens JM, et al: The operative management of basilar impression in osteogenesis imperfecta. Neurosurgery 27:782–786, 1990.
15. Price JC, Holliday MJ, Johns ME, et al: The versatile midface degloving approach. Laryngoscope 98:291–295, 1988.
16. Crockard HA, Johnston F: Development of transoral approaches to lesions of the skull base and craniocervical junction. Neurosurg Q 3:61–82, 1993.
17. Arbit E, Patterson RH, Jr: Combined transoral and median labiomandibular glossotomy approach to the upper cervical spine. Neurosurgery 8:672–674, 1981.
18. Delgado TE, Garrido E, Harwick RD: Labiomandibular transoral approach to chordomas in the clivus and upper cervical spine. Neurosurgery 8:675–679, 1981.
19. Crockard HA: The transoral approach to the base of the brain and upper cervical cord. Ann R Coll Surg Engl 67:321–325, 1985.
20. Spetzler RF, Selman WR, Nash CL, et al: Transoral microsurgical odontoid resection and spinal cord monitoring. Spine 4:506–510, 1979.
21. Crockard HA, Sen CN: The transoral approach for the management of intradural lesions at the craniovertebral junction: A review of 7 cases. Neurosurgery 28:88–98, 1991.
22. Kennedy DW, Papel I, Holliday N: Transpalatal approach to the skull base. Ear Nose Throat J 65:48–58, 1986.
23. Bonkowski JA, Gibson RD, Snape L: Foramen magnum meningioma: Transoral resection with a bone baffle to prevent CSF leakage. J Neurosurg 72:493–496, 1990.
24. Moloney F, Worthington P: The origin of the Le Fort 1 maxillary osteotomy: Cheever's operation. Oral Surg 39:731–734, 1981.
25. Harkey HL, Crockard HA, Stevens JM, et al: The operative management of basilar impression in osteogenesis imperfecta. Neurosurgery 27:782–786, 1990.
26. James D, Crockard HA: Surgical access to the base of the skull and upper cervical spine by extended maxillotomy. Neurosurgery 29:411–416, 1991.
27. Anand VK, House JR, 3rd, al-Mefty O: Management of benign neoplasms invading cavernous sinus. Laryngoscope 101:557–564, 1991.
28. Conley J, Price JC: Sublabial approach to the nasal and nasopharyngeal cavities. Am J Surg 138:615–618, 1979.
29. Price JC: The midfacial degloving approach to the central skull base. Ear Nose Throat J 65:46–53, 1986.
30. Casson PR, Bonnano PC, Converse JM: The midface degloving procedure. Plast Reconstr Surg 53:102–113, 1974.

22 Transtemporal Approaches to the Posterior Cranial Fossa

FRANK D. VRIONIS, GALE GARDNER, JON H. ROBERTSON, and JASON A. BRODKEY

Traditional approaches to the posterior cranial fossa do not permit direct access to complex lesions of the lateral skull base, cerebellopontine angle (CPA), or clivus. To circumvent brain retraction and allow for complete resection, approaches have been developed that position the dissection both lateral and anterior to the brain stem and cerebellum. All of these skull base approaches are combinations and variations of transtemporal bone routes (Table 22-1 and Fig. 22-1). Unlike craniotomies performed elsewhere, entry to the posterior fossa through the temporal bone poses special problems for the surgeon if the internal carotid artery (ICA), sigmoid sinus (SS), cranial nerves VII and VIII, and the specialized structures for hearing and balance are to be preserved. Despite the widely varied nomenclature, often only subtle differences exist between these approaches. It is imperative that the location, type, and extent of the lesion dictate the type of the approach. Tailored approaches to the lesion instead of standard ones are recommended for minimal disruption of normal structures. In this respect, transtemporal approaches represent an anatomic continuum of temporal bone dissection, with frequent overlaps and minor discrepancies or differences between the various approaches. The complicated nomenclature has arisen because skull base tumors tend to extend into different anatomic compartments, often necessitating combined approaches. Because of the overlap of neurosurgery and otology in this area, collaboration of neurosurgeons and otologists is mandatory.

This chapter is divided into three sections: Anterior Transpetrosal Approaches, describing anterior approaches within the temporal bone through the middle cranial fossa; Posterior Transpetrosal Approaches, for those that are situated more posteriorly through the mastoid process; and Combined Approaches. We define the external auditory canal (EAC) as the dividing structure between the anterior and posterior approaches. We divide each approach into sections, giving a brief historical perspective, indications, surgical technique, and complications and disadvantages.

ANTERIOR TRANSPETROSAL APPROACHES

Anterior transpetrosal approaches are based on a standard subtemporal extradural middle fossa approach. We divide the anterior approaches into three types: (1) middle fossa approach, (2) extended middle fossa approach (anterior petrosectomy), and (3) middle fossa transtentorial approach. The middle fossa approach provides a subtemporal extradural exposure of the middle fossa floor designed for removing acoustic neuromas situated laterally within the internal

TABLE 22-1 ▪ Temporal Bone Approaches

Anterior Approaches
Middle cranial fossa
Extended middle cranial fossa
Middle cranial fossa transtentorial

Posterior Approaches
Retrolabyrinthine—presigmoid
Retrolabyrinthine—retrosigmoid
Retrolabyrinthine—transsigmoid
Transotic
Translabyrinthine
Infralabyrinthine
Transcochlear
Transcanal-infracochlear

Combined Approaches
Petrosal
Infratemporal fossa

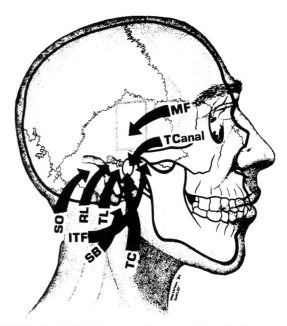

FIGURE 22-1 Multiple approach routes through the temporal bone to the posterior fossa. ITF, infratemporal fossa; MF, middle fossa; RL, retrolabyrinthine; SB, skull base; SO, suboccipital; TC, transcochlear; T Canal, transcanal; TL, translabyrinthine.

auditory canal (IAC). For more extensive tumors, the extended middle fossa approach provides additional exposure of the petrous apex and supraclival region. With the addition of division of the tentorium, the middle fossa transtentorial approach provides access to the middle clival region and posterior fossa as well as the posterior cavernous sinus.

Middle Fossa Approach

House developed the middle fossa access to the IAC and adjacent structures in 1961 in an effort to remove foci of labyrinthine otosclerosis.[1–3] Although he used this approach briefly for the removal of acoustic tumors, he soon directed his efforts to a translabyrinthine approach. Fisch has further refined the middle fossa approach.[4,5]

Several techniques for localization of the IAC have been described. House's technique identifies the greater superficial petrosal nerve (GSPN), follows it to the geniculate ganglion (GG), and then proceeds along the labyrinthine segment of the facial nerve to the IAC.[2] Another popular method described by Fisch uses the superior semicircular canal (SSC) as the primary landmark.[5] Using this method, once the SSC is identified, the meatal plane overlying the IAC is located in a 60-degree plane centered over the SSC ampulla. Garcia-Ibanez and Garcia-Ibanez[6] advocate a technique beginning at the bisection of the angle between the GSPN and the arcuate eminence. The medial "safe" part of the IAC is first identified and is followed laterally. Because of the wide variations in anatomy[4,6] and small working space, no single technique can ensure avoidance of injury to important structures. Careful dissection and a detailed understanding of the regional anatomy are important for success. Image-guided navigation through the temporal bone has been introduced as an accurate alternative method to localize the IAC without the need to expose the GG or the SSC.[7,8]

Indications

The middle fossa approach is best suited for lesions situated lateral within the IAC that have limited extension into the CPA (<1 cm) and where hearing preservation is the goal.[2,9] It is especially useful when preoperative computed tomography (CT) of the temporal bone demonstrates close proximity of the posterior semicircular canal (PSC), common crus, or vestibule to the posterior lip of the IAC. In those circumstances, retrosigmoid approaches are less preferable and the middle fossa approach becomes the hearing-preservation approach of choice. Tumors that are medial in position and do not extend to the fundus of the IAC are best approached by posterior approaches (e.g., retrosigmoid approach).

The middle fossa approach provides access to the labyrinthine segment of the facial nerve without sacrificing hearing. Thus decompression of the facial nerve in trauma or Bell's palsy, or resection of facial nerve tumors can be accomplished. This approach also permits selective sectioning of the vestibular nerve fibers for Ménière's disease. In theory, it could also be used to expose the horizontal portion of the ICA, eustachian tube, and temporomandibular joint (TMJ). Other indications include advanced otosclerosis, nerve section for tinnitus, facial nerve repair and facial nerve neuroma, repair of middle fossa encephaloceles, and cerebrospinal fluid (CSF) leaks through the tegmen.[2]

Surgical Approach

The patient is positioned supine on the operating table with the head turned opposite the side of the tumor.[2,4,6,9,10] Facial and auditory nerve monitoring is used. An incision is planned that begins at the level of the zygoma just anterior to the tragus and extends superiorly to approximately the superior temporal line. We prefer an S-shaped incision curving first anteriorly then posteriorly to allow for greater spreading of the soft tissues.

The temporalis muscle is divided and reflected anteriorly. A 4- by 5-cm bone flap is planned approximately two thirds anterior to the EAC and one third posterior. The inferior margin should be placed as close to the middle fossa floor as possible. A subtemporal craniectomy is performed. The dura is then elevated from the middle fossa floor from a posterior to anterior direction. This direction of dissection helps avoid inadvertent elevation of the GSPN and subsequent traction injury to the GG and facial nerve. Injury to the GSPN can produce a dry eye secondary to loss of lacrimal gland innervation. In approximately 16% of cases the GG is not covered by bone and inadvertent injury can occur.[4] To maintain a visible plane of dissection, a self-retaining brain retractor is used. Some retractors are limited to only 4 to 5 cm of spread, and thus too wide a craniotomy can impair the capability of the retractor to elevate the dura adequately.

Several landmarks must be identified before bone removal can begin over the IAC: (1) the middle meningeal artery, (2) the arcuate eminence, (3) the GSPN, and (4) the facial hiatus (Fig. 22-2). The first landmark is typically the middle meningeal artery at the foramen spinosum. This can be obliterated and divided if necessary. The foramen may be rarely duplicated or absent. It marks the anterior limit of the dural elevation. As dural elevation continues, the arcuate eminence, a rounded elevation of the petrous bone, can be identified. It is usually produced by the underlying SSC. Lateral to the arcuate eminence is the tegmen tympani, a thin lamina of bone that forms the roof of the tympanic cavity. The GSPN originates from the GG, exits through the petrous bone at the facial hiatus, and runs extradurally in an anteromedial direction toward the trigeminal ganglion. The GSPN serves as a landmark for the lateral margin of the horizontal segment of the petrous carotid artery. Care should be taken at this stage not to apply force to the floor of the middle fossa, because the bone over the carotid artery and the area of the tegmen can be quite thin and even dehiscent in up to 20% of cases.[4] The arcuate eminence is drilled until the dense bone of the SSC is encountered. The SSC is visualized with a bluish hue through the bone, the so-called blue line. In approximately 15% of cases, however, the arcuate eminence is absent, and in 50% of cases where it is present it is rotated in relationship to the SSC.[11]

Once the key landmarks have been identified, the IAC can be localized using two key angles. Traditionally, the GSPN-SSC angle (120 degrees)[6] and the SSC-IAC angle (60 degrees)[12] have been used. Unfortunately, these angles have been shown to be quite variable,[10] and in one study the GSPN-SSC angle ranged from 90 to 135 degrees and the SSC-IAC angle from 34 to 75 degrees.[4] Thus simply relying on angles can lead to inadvertent injury to the SSC and hence loss of hearing. House's technique places the facial nerve at risk, because it is this structure that is first identified

FIGURE 22-2 Middle fossa approach to the internal auditory canal. The illustration depicts the facial nerve, geniculate ganglion, and greater superficial petrosal nerve (GSPN). The petrous carotid artery is shown as a *dotted structure* under the GSPN. The tegmen is opened, and the head of the malleus, the incus, and the stapes are seen. Anteriorly, the branches of the trigeminal nerve (V1, V2, V3) are depicted. LSC, lateral semicircular canal; SSC, superior semicircular canal.

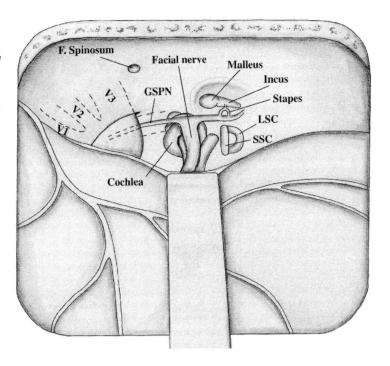

and followed to the IAC.[2] Fisch's technique places the SSC at risk. Orientation can be aided by removal of the tegmen and identification of the head of the malleus. This can help predict the location of the GG and IAC because these structures are usually collinear, at the expense of risking a CSF leak through the middle ear.[2] None of these techniques is fail-safe, and the best method of localizing the IAC is what the surgeon finds most comfortable in his or her own experience.

Once the IAC has been identified, exposure proceeds from lateral to medial until the entire IAC has been exposed along its superior surface. A safer technique is to begin medially, exposing first the porus acousticus and then working laterally, taking advantage of the larger margin for error in the region of the porus.[9,10] At the fundus of the IAC, the vertical crest (Bill's bar), a bone spicule that separates the superior vestibular nerve from the facial nerve, is identified. Finally, the dura over the IAC is opened, first posteriorly over the superior vestibular nerve to avoid facial nerve injury.

In the case of vestibular schwannomas, the tumor can be removed by separating the superior vestibular nerve and tumor away from the facial nerve. The tumor is usually delivered posteriorly away from the facial nerve. Small hooks are necessary to palpate the limits of the IAC and gently free the tumor, particularly its inferolateral portion where the view is especially obscured. The approach carries a higher risk to the facial and cochlear nerves when the tumor less commonly arises from the inferior vestibular nerve. Closure of the IAC defect is accomplished with a small free graft of temporalis muscle.

Complications and Disadvantages

The middle fossa approach requires retraction of the temporal lobe, and therefore potential injury can occur (e.g., aphasia, hemiparesis, seizure). There is potential for CSF leak

through unwaxed air cells or through the middle ear, if the tegmen is opened. Careful hemostasis and tenting sutures can lessen the risk of postoperative hematoma (e.g., epidural hematoma).

As with any temporal bone approach, high-speed drilling can potentially cause injury to the underlying neurovascular structures as a result of the vibration and heat from the drill. Using a diamond burr with continuous-suction irrigation lessens this risk.

Specifically with the middle fossa approach, during drilling of bone over the facial nerve there is a small margin for error, and inadvertent injury to the nerve, which is in the most superficial plane of the surgical field, can occur. The SSC, cochlea, and petrous portion of the carotid artery are obvious structures at risk with this approach. Also, the working zone is quite restricted, making this a somewhat technically demanding approach. If major bleeding occurs in the posterior fossa, control may necessitate conversion to a middle fossa transtentorial or to a translabyrinthine approach.

Extended Middle Fossa Approach— Anterior Petrosectomy

The traditional middle fossa approach works well for lesions in the IAC[2,3]; however, the exposure is limited. For that reason, extensions of the middle fossa approach have been developed to permit wider access to the petrous apex, clivus, and posterior fossa. The extended middle fossa approach involves a petrous apex resection in addition to the temporal craniotomy described for the middle fossa approach.[13] The horizontal segment of the carotid artery and the cochlea limit the inferior exposure to the level of the inferior petrosal sinus. The TMJ, ossicles, and petrous carotid artery laterally, the trigeminal ganglion anteriorly, and the SSC and vestibule posteriorly represent the limits of the extended middle fossa approach.

Indications

The anterior petrosectomy provides access to the petrous apex and superior clival region. It provides access to the posterior fossa past the carotid artery and trigeminal and facial nerves. Although the extended middle fossa approach is considered a hearing-preservation approach, it can provide additional exposure in the posterior fossa by sacrificing the SSC and labyrinth, and thus hearing.[13,14] Sacrifice of the cochlea improves visualization of the lateral extreme of the IAC, the medial wall of the tympanic cavity, and the jugular foramen if needed.

This approach permits resection of vestibular schwannomas that extend more medially in the CPA. Meningiomas and chordomas of the anterior CPA and clivus can be resected through this approach, as well as lesions of the petrous apex (i.e., cholesterol granulomas, cholesteatomas, petrositis). Lesions of the petrous carotid artery, posterior cavernous sinus, basilar artery, and anterior brain stem can also be approached.

Surgical Approach

A temporal craniotomy is performed, similar to the middle fossa approach. Occasionally, a zygomatic osteotomy is added for exposure of the middle fossa floor. The middle meningeal artery, foramen ovale, GSPN, and arcuate eminence are identified. The petrous carotid artery can be exposed at this point by drilling bone along the course of the GSPN (see Fig. 22-2). This area is also known as the posterolateral or Glasscock's triangle.[15] The boundaries of Glasscock's triangle are, laterally, a line extending from the foramen spinosum to the arcuate eminence; medially, the GSPN; and at the base, the third division of the trigeminal nerve (V3). Medial to this triangle is Kawase's or the posteromedial triangle, which consists of the bone in the area of the petrous apex. Drilling this bone provides access to the clivus and the infratentorial compartment.[16] Kawase's triangle is defined laterally by the GSPN, medially by the petrous ridge, and at the base, by the arcuate eminence. The cochlea represents the posterolateral limit of exposure within Kawase's triangle.

The IAC is identified by one of the means described in the previous section. Once the IAC is identified, bone is removed, exposing the canal widely and the dura of the posterior fossa. The otic capsule bone is particularly dense and lighter in color than the remaining bone of the petrous apex. To identify the cochlea, Miller and colleagues[17] advocate drilling bone along an imaginary line extending from the tip of the vertical crest to the junction of the petrous carotid artery and cranial nerve V3 until the cochlea is identified. With this exposure, the dura along the medial temporal lobe and infratentorially to the level of the inferior petrosal sinus can be exposed. The superior petrosal sinus (SPS) can be clipped and divided. A dural incision can be extended across the SPS and then inferiorly into the posterior fossa. Occasionally, the dura over Meckel's cave is divided to mobilize the trigeminal nerve anteriorly and increase exposure of the petroclival region.

Complications and Disadvantages

Complications are similar to those with the standard middle fossa approach. Because of the additional bone removal at the petrous apex, potential injury to the carotid artery and trigeminal nerve are possible. The disadvantage of this approach is the rather limited exposure of the posterior fossa. The main advantage of this approach compared with posteriorly based approaches (e.g., translabyrinthine, transcochlear), when used to remove petrous apex lesions, is hearing preservation.

Middle Fossa Transtentorial Approach

This approach was first reported by Kawase and colleagues[16] in 1985 for approaching aneurysms of the midbasilar artery through the petrous pyramid. In 1991, Kawase and colleagues[18] applied this approach for resection of petroclival meningiomas that extended into the parasellar region (sphenopetroclival meningiomas). This approach uses a combination of the extended middle fossa approach with the addition of intradural resection of the tentorium to allow wider posterior fossa exposure. It is in many ways similar to the subtemporal transtentorial approach, with the added advantage of drilling the anterior petrous ridge.

Indications

The middle fossa transtentorial exposure can be accomplished with an anterior or posterior petrosectomy or a combined petrosal approach.[13,18–20] It is suitable for meningiomas extending along the superior and middle clivus or along the posterior wall of the petrous ridge, which can have long dural attachments. Hearing is preserved with this approach, as with all middle fossa approaches. It also permits resection of tumors that extend to the parasellar region and posterior cavernous sinus. It is particularly attractive for small tumors in the petroclival region, laterally located pontine lesions (cavernous malformations, gliomas), or basilar trunk aneurysms. Compared with the extended middle fossa approach, it provides wider posterior fossa exposure because of sectioning of the tentorium.

Surgical Approach

The extent of petrous pyramid resection is similar to that obtained by the extended middle fossa approach. The dura is opened above and below the SPS. Cranial nerves IV and V are identified. The SPS is clipped between cranial nerves V and VII, with care taken to avoid sacrificing the petrosal vein. The tentorium is cut until the tentorial notch is seen. The tentorium can then be tented open with retention sutures, exposing the petroclival region from cranial nerves III through VII.[19] The inferomedial triangle of the cavernous sinus can be visualized, mobilization of the trigeminal nerve can be accomplished by opening Meckel's cave, and Dorello's canal is seen through this exposure.

Complications and Disadvantages

This approach carries the additional risk of injury to cranial nerve IV as a result of the tentorial incision. Furthermore, the degree of retraction and thus the risk of possible injury to the temporal lobe may be slightly higher than in the middle fossa or extended middle fossa approaches.

POSTERIOR TRANSPETROSAL APPROACHES

Most of these approaches involve a certain degree of mastoid resection, positioning the surgical corridor inferior to the middle fossa approaches. There are wide variations among these approaches, although often portions of approaches are used in combination to create more extensive exposure (e.g., presigmoid approach as part of the petrosal approach).

Retrolabyrinthine Approaches

Presigmoid Approach

The retrolabyrinthine presigmoid approach was first described by Hitselberger and Pulec[21] in 1972, and was popularized by Silverstein and Norrell[22] in 1977 and by House and associates[23] in 1984. It is performed through the mastoid air cells, with elevation of a dural flap between the labyrinth and the SS. The concept of this procedure is based on its allowing entry into the CPA anterior to the SS, thus lessening the need for cerebellar retraction. It was originally described as being useful for partial sectioning of the fibers of the sensory roots of cranial nerve V for trigeminal neuralgia. It has been used for selective sectioning of the vestibular division of cranial nerve VIII for treatment of vertigo and for endolymphatic duct surgery. It can be used, on occasion, to remove small acoustic tumors in cases in which preservation of hearing is desirable. The major advantage of this approach is that it provides direct access to the CPA without sacrificing hearing and without extensive cerebellar retraction. Its major disadvantage is the limited exposure, which can be compromised even further by a large dominant SS or when the mastoid air space is contracted ("crowded mastoid").

Transsigmoid Approach

This approach can be used as part of any posterior transpetrosal approach. Exposure is increased by ligating the SS, usually between the superior and inferior petrosal sinuses or between superior anastomotic vein (vein of Labbé) and the SPS. Thus the superior anastomotic vein drains retrograde into the transverse sinus and into the opposite jugular system. A preoperative angiogram or magnetic resonance venogram is essential to ensure patency of the torcular. In general, a nondominant sinus in the presence of a patent torcular can be sacrificed in selected cases. Temporary clipping across the SS is recommended to assess for the presence of temporal lobe or cerebellar swelling. The SS can be opened and packed with Surgicel and its lumen sutured, or it can be ligated and clipped. Cadaver and angiographic studies show that the incidence of unilateral transverse sinus is rather infrequent (2.5%), and absence of any communication at the torcular is even rarer.[24,25] Despite this, given the catastrophic results of ligating a unilateral SS, a preoperative arteriogram or magnetic resonance venogram is recommended.

Retrosigmoid (Suboccipital) Approach

The retrosigmoid approach, also known as the lateral suboccipital approach, is not a true transtemporal approach. This approach is most familiar to neurosurgeons and has been the traditional exposure used for resection of tumors of the CPA.[26,27] This approach provides wide entry into the posterior fossa with maximal exposure for tumors such as vestibular schwannomas. Using this approach, the neurovascular structures of the temporal bone are avoided at the expense of cerebellar retraction. The development of monitoring techniques using evoked-response methods has greatly increased the practicality of this approach.

INDICATIONS

Most tumors in the CPA can be approached through a suboccipital craniotomy (i.e., vestibular schwannomas, meningiomas, epidermoids). Cranial nerves V to XI can be visualized with this exposure. Tumors with extension into the petroclival region or with significant spread anterior to the brain stem are not optimally treated with this exposure because of the need for increased cerebellar retraction and a long surgical corridor. This exposure can be combined with other transpetrosal approaches to provide maximal supratentorial and infratentorial exposure for extensive lesions of the CPA.

SURGICAL APPROACH

This approach can be done with the patient sitting, lateral, or three fourths prone. An incision is made approximately 2 cm posterior to the mastoid tip, extending cephalad to slightly above the transverse sinus and caudally into the suboccipital musculature. The asterion is a useful landmark for the junction of the transverse and sigmoid sinuses. It represents the crossing of the lambdoid, parietomastoid, and occipitomastoid sutures, and it can be palpated as a depression in the bone. A burr hole is placed immediately medial to the asterion, and a craniectomy or "silver-dollar" craniotomy can be performed such that the edges of the transverse and sigmoid sinuses and their junction are clearly identified. In difficult reoperative cases, a line drawn from the root of the zygoma to the inion can reliably locate the course of the transverse sinus.[28] Bone removal can include the posterior lip of the foramen magnum as well as the upper cervical lamina. The arachnoid at the foramen magnum should be opened first to permit CSF egress and facilitate cerebellar retraction.

In the case of vestibular schwannoma resection, the tumor is immediately visualized. The facial nerve usually lies anterior to the tumor. For tumors that extend into the IAC, the porus is drilled until the dura over the IAC is seen. In a cadaver study, the amount of posterior IAC canal that can be safely unroofed averaged 5.9 mm (range, 4–8 mm). The best available way to avoid critical labyrinthine structures during the suboccipital approach is to use preoperative high-resolution CT. A line is drawn on axial CT images from the medial aspect of the SS to the fundus of the IAC. If this line crosses any labyrinthine structures, the risk of injury and hearing loss during drilling of the IAC significantly increases.[29]

COMPLICATIONS AND DISADVANTAGES

This exposure requires a certain amount of cerebellar retraction, and thus cerebellar edema or hematoma can occur. This is especially true for large tumors requiring lengthy surgery. If the surgeon maintains gentle retraction (1–2 cm), these types of complications can usually be avoided. Other complications include CSF leak and postoperative incisional pain attributed to adherence of the suboccipital muscles to the dura. The incisional pain can be lessened by either replacing the bone flap in the case of a craniotomy, or performing a cranioplasty to fill the bone defect.

The incidence of CSF leak may be lessened by identifying and waxing small air cells in the IAC with the use of an endoscope. In 9% of cases, a high jugular bulb may make drilling of the meatus through the retrosigmoid approach impossible and is associated with increased risk of bleeding and air embolism.[30] As previously mentioned, loss of hearing can occur during drilling of the posterior aspect of the IAC.

Translabyrinthine Approach

The first report of a translabyrinthine approach was in 1904 by Panse,[31] who advocated this approach for its shortest distance to the CPA. In 1961, William House[3] described the middle fossa approach for resection of vestibular schwannomas located laterally in the IAC with minimal CPA extension. Because of limited exposure, incidence of facial paresis, need for temporal lobe retraction, and limited control of vascular structures, House[32] introduced the translabyrinthine approach for resection of vestibular schwannomas. This was a more lateral approach and gave direct control of the facial nerve by drilling through the labyrinth. He emphasized the vertical crest (Bill's bar) at the lateral end of the IAC as a landmark. Differentiation between the superior and inferior vestibular nerves was more readily apparent with this approach.

Variations of the translabyrinthine approach have been described for more extensive exposure of the SS with mobilization of the jugular bulb as well as drilling out of the infralabyrinthine air cells to increase access for large tumors.[33] Furthermore, there is evidence that in rare cases hearing preservation may be possible with the translabyrinthine approach, such that in one case ablation of all three semicircular canals with preservation of the cochlea and saccule left the patient with useful, though decreased hearing.[34] Another variation of the translabyrinthine approach is the addition of a suboccipital approach with a partial labyrinthectomy, such that only those elements that are required for visualization of Bill's bar and the lateral IAC are removed.[35]

One advantage of the translabyrinthine compared with the middle fossa approach is that after drilling the labyrinth, the tumor is encountered together with the superior and inferior vestibular nerves. Thus the facial nerve, being anterior, is well protected. This is in contrast to the middle fossa approach, where the facial nerve is immediately beneath the dura. The advantage of the translabyrinthine approach over the suboccipital approach is the lack of cerebellar retraction. Thus for large tumors when surgery is expected to be long, this approach minimizes the chance of postoperative cerebellar edema, hematoma, or infarction. Its main disadvantage is the added surgical time for the labyrinthectomy and the need for sacrificing hearing.

Indications

The objective of the translabyrinthine approach is to expose the IAC and CPA through the labyrinth without entering the middle ear. Larger tumors occupying the IAC and CPA can be approached. Hearing and vestibular function are sacrificed by definition. Therefore, it is indicated only in those vestibular schwannomas with nonserviceable hearing (i.e., speech reception threshold >50 db and speech discrimination score <50%). It is an ideal approach for vestibular neurectomy for intractable vertigo when hearing is lost. For patients with normal hearing, this approach is contraindicated.

Surgical Approach

The patient is positioned supine with the head turned opposite to the side of the tumor. A retroauricular C-shaped skin incision is made, and an anteriorly based periosteal flap is elevated and preserved.[36]

A simple mastoidectomy is first accomplished by removing the mastoid cortex from the mastoid tip inferiorly, to the supramastoid crest superiorly, and to the posterior wall of the EAC anteriorly. The SS is visualized and skeletonized to the level of the jugular bulb. The angle between the middle fossa dura above, the posterior fossa dura below, and the SS is called the sinodural angle. After exposure of the sinodural angle, the SS and the transverse and superior petrosal sinuses are identified.

The mastoid antrum is then entered and the short process of the incus in the fossa incudis is identified. This provides a useful landmark for the lateral semicircular canal (LSC), which is found immediately below. The solid angle is located medial to the mastoid antrum and houses the three semicircular canals (Fig. 22-3). The air cells are then removed inferiorly to the level of the digastric groove. The air cells posterior to the LSC are removed and the posterior semicircular canal, located between the LSC and the posterior fossa plate, is exposed. The vertical segment of the facial nerve is then located within the fallopian canal by removing the remaining inferior mastoid and retrofacial air cells. The facial nerve passes from the external genu at the inferior surface of the LSC to the stylomastoid foramen, located just anterior to the digastric ridge. The facial nerve is skeletonized only to facilitate exposure of the jugular bulb and foramen, and it is otherwise left within the dense bone of the fallopian canal. The SSC is identified by following the sinodural angle through the supralabyrinthine air cells. The final area of posterior exposure is removal of the middle, posterior, and sigmoid plates, completing the subtotal petrosectomy. The roughly triangular area of bone bounded by the SS, SPS, and bony labyrinth (i.e., solid angle) is known as Trautmann's triangle. This bone is drilled to expose the presigmoid posterior fossa dura.

After the retrofacial air cells, the jugular bulb is exposed next. At this point in the exposure, the tympanic and mastoid segments of the facial nerve mark the anterior limit, the jugular bulb the inferior limit, the SS the inferior limit, and the middle cranial fossa the superior limit of the dissection.

The LSC, PSC, and SSC are removed, as well as the bone over the posterior fossa, revealing the endolymphatic sac. Next, the vestibule is opened and completely exposed beneath the facial nerve. Bone is removed over the medial and posterior vestibule until the nerves to the superior, lateral, and inferior ampullas are exposed. These nerves define the superior and inferior limits of the IAC. Bone removal continues over the IAC until a transparent shell remains. The transverse crest separating the superior and inferior division of the vestibular nerves can be seen through the thinned bone.

The facial nerve is then identified by palpation of the vertical crest (Bill's bar). Care should be taken when removing bone from the superior wall of the IAC, because the

FIGURE 22-3 Basic drawing depicting critical structures of the temporal bone as seen by posterior transmastoid approaches. The solid angle, housing the three semicircular canals, is shown. The facial recess anterior to the facial nerve (*hatched area*) is illustrated. Opening the facial recess provides access to the middle ear structures, ossicles, and round and oval windows. LSC, lateral semicircular canal; PSC, posterior semicircular canal; SPS, superior petrosal sinus; SSC, superior semicircular canal.

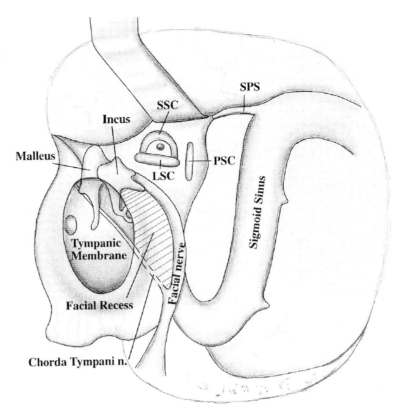

facial nerve is superficial under the dura and can be injured. Once the facial nerve has been skeletonized, the remaining bone over the IAC is removed. The dura over the IAC can then be opened for tumor removal or vestibular neurectomy.

The wound is closed by placing a free muscle graft over the malleus, incus, and attic. To gain access to the middle ear, the facial recess is sometimes opened. The facial recess is a triangular area defined superiorly by the fossa incudis, medially by the facial nerve, and inferiorly by the chorda tympani (see Fig. 22-3). In this situation, a muscle plug is placed to close the opening of the eustachian tube. The cavity is filled with fat graft and the periosteal flap is closed. The skin is closed tightly and a pressure dressing is applied.

Complications and Disadvantages

The main disadvantage of the translabyrinthine approach is the inadequate exposure of the tentorium, petroclival area, and foramen magnum. Thus, for large posterior fossa tumors, especially meningiomas with broad-based tentorial attachment, the translabyrinthine approach by itself is inadequate. Also, it may be difficult to control vascular structures (e.g., anterior inferior cerebellar artery) if inadvertent injury occurs.

The main complication with this approach seems to be a high incidence of CSF leak (up to 30% in some series, usually in the 10% to 20% range).[37] Access to the eustachian tube through the middle ear (facial recess) or the epitympanum can lessen the risk of CSF leak but involves additional exposure and drilling. Placing a free muscle graft over the attic, filling the operative cavity with fat graft, and closing with a periosteal graft, decreases the chance of CSF leak.

In a series from the House Ear Clinic of 166 large (>4 cm) vestibular schwannomas resected using the translabyrinthine approach, complete resection was achieved in 95% of cases, with acceptable facial nerve function at 2 years in 75% and good function in 42% (see reference 38). Vascular complications, which included infarct or hematoma, occurred in 4.8%, CSF leak in 9.6%, and meningitis in 8.3%. There were no deaths. Most incidents of meningitis were aseptic and due to blood products or emulsified fat in the posterior fossa from the fat graft.

Transotic Approach

The transotic approach was developed by Fisch[37] in response to the limitations of the translabyrinthine approach. Unlike the posteriorly directed translabyrinthine approach, the transotic approach permits more extensive temporal bone resection, and positions the dissection both anterior and posterior to the facial nerve, giving excellent visualization of the anterior CPA and petrous apex. The early description included transposition of the facial nerve and had similarities with the transcochlear approach of House and Hitselberger.[39] Unfortunately, the rate of facial nerve paralysis was unacceptable and modifications followed such that the facial nerve is not transposed but left in situ in the fallopian canal.[37,40]

Indications

The indication for this approach is essentially identical to that for the translabyrinthine approach. It was designed for vestibular schwannomas up to 2.5 cm in size,[37,38] although it can certainly be used for larger schwannomas and other lesions, such as meningiomas, hemangiomas, arachnoid cysts, and mucosal cysts, involving the IAC.[41] In contrast to the translabyrinthine approach, the transotic approach circumvents the problem of a high jugular bulb because of the anterior exposure obtained.

This approach may be useful for large vestibular schwannomas because it provides an additional corridor anterior to the facial nerve compared with the translabyrinthine approach. Less extensive petrosectomies (e.g., translabyrinthine) are probably adequate for most vestibular schwannomas. Its other main advantage is the obliteration of the eustachian tube, resulting in a decreased chance for CSF leak.

Surgical Approach

The surgical approach is similar to the transcochlear approach, with the important difference that the facial nerve is not mobilized (Fig. 22-4). It involves blind sac closure of the EAC, exenteration of the otic capsule including the cochlea, and exposure of the jugular bulb and petrous carotid artery. The additional exposure is obtained by drilling the bone anterior to the tympanic and mastoid segments of the facial nerve. The facial nerve from its entrance into the IAC to its exit at the stylomastoid foramen is exposed, yet remains within bone, thus reducing the potential risk for injury.[37,41]

Complications and Disadvantages

The original transotic approach was associated with a high incidence of facial nerve paralysis secondary to transposition of the facial nerve.[38] The modification of leaving the facial nerve within the fallopian canal reduced this risk.[40] In Fisch and Mattox's[37] series of 73 patients, for tumors less than 1.4 cm, all patients had normal facial nerve function at

2 years after surgery. For tumors measuring 1.5 to 2.5 cm, facial nerve function was normal in 61% at 2 years. CSF leak was contained subcutaneously in 4% and was transient in 3%, and no patient required revision. Removal of all of the middle ear mucosa and pneumatic air cells related to the middle ear space, and obliteration of the eustachian tube orifice combined with dural closure and filling of the defect with fat, lessen the chances for CSF leak.[41] In their series, meningitis occurred in 1%, and death in 1%. A disadvantage of this approach is that it adds operative time compared with other procedures (e.g., translabyrinthine approach).

Transcochlear Approach

In 1976, House and Hitselberger[39] described the transcochlear approach. This approach is a forward extension of the translabyrinthine approach in which the facial nerve is mobilized and the cochlea removed. This exposure essentially removes the entire petrous bone, giving maximal transpetrous exposure.

The operative field given by the transcochlear approach is limited by the EAC canal wall and middle ear, and though more anterior than the translabyrinthine approach, still remains posteriorly directed. The modified transcochlear approach was developed to give additional anterior exposure by removing the EAC and the tympanic membrane.[38] It also offered more extensive exposure and circumferential control of the petrous ICA.[42–46] Some authors also include resection of the glenoid fossa, joint capsule, and meniscus, and partial resection of the posterior aspect of the zygomatic arch.[45] Others combine it with a neck dissection,[47] and some describe extended exposures including tentorial section for supratentorial exposure.[48]

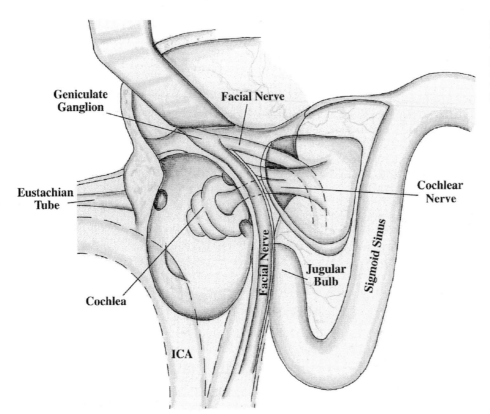

FIGURE 22-4 Exposure of the temporal bone as seen during a transcochlear approach. The cochlea is shown. The internal carotid artery (ICA) is shown anterior and inferior to the cochlea. The facial nerve lies in its canal (not transposed).

Indications

This approach was designed for large tumors in the CPA extending anterior to the IAC along the superior two thirds of the clivus, as well as for aneurysms of the middle and lower basilar artery. Its main advantage is the broadness of the exposure, giving the surgeon a parallel triangular view of the middle clivus. The addition of the modified transcochlear approach gives the surgeon a more direct and most laterally directed approach to the CPA, and circumferential exposure of the petrous ICA. This is important for selected cases in which a carotid bypass is required. It can be combined with resection of the mandibular condyle, closure of the EAC, zygomatic osteotomy, and drilling of the floor of the middle cranial fossa for tumors extending into the infratemporal fossa and nasopharynx.

Surgical Approach

The initial exposure for this approach is similar to that for the translabyrinthine approach. A curvilinear C-shaped retroauricular skin incision is made and the skin of the cartilaginous EAC is everted and sewn shut (see Fig. 22-4). A musculoperiosteal flap from the mastoid process is used medially as a second layer of closure.[45] The skin of the bony EAC and tympanic membrane were initially left in place, but removal of this bone improves access to the midline without increasing morbidity. The entire osseous EAC can be removed without affecting the function of the mandibular condyle in the glenoid fossa.

A mastoidectomy is performed exposing the canal wall inferiorly. The middle and posterior fossa plates along with the SS are then skeletonized. The facial nerve is skeletonized from its entrance into the IAC to its exit from the stylomastoid foramen. The facial recess is opened. The middle ear space and epitympanum are entered, and the ossicles can then be removed. In the original description, the middle ear was not removed.[39] The chorda tympani is then sectioned inferiorly at its origin from the descending portion of the facial nerve. Drilling is continued into the retrofacial air cells. The GSPN is then divided just anterior to its origin at the GG. The facial nerve can then be mobilized from its bony canal and transposed posteriorly. This invariably results in facial nerve paralysis because it disrupts the blood supply to the GG. Obviously, it is best to leave the facial nerve within the canal, if possible. If transposition is necessary, then anterior transposition by mobilizing the mastoid segment and the nerve exiting at the stylomastoid foramen is safer.

Next, the cochlea is removed, including the bony septum between the basal turn and the ICA (see Fig. 22-6). The jugular bulb is also exposed completely. Care should be taken not to injure the underlying neurovascular structures, namely, cranial nerves IX through XI near the jugular bulb and foramen, as well as the facial nerve in the dura of the IAC.

The complete petrosectomy gives exposure from the SPS superiorly to Meckel's cave, and to the inferior petrosal sinus and jugular bulb inferiorly. The osseous removal extends anteriorly to the petrous carotid artery and TMJ, and medially to the clivus. The dura is opened in a triangular manner parallel to the SPS, inferior petrosal sinus, and SS, to the IAC. It can also be opened on both sides of the IAC. This exposes the CPA widely.

Complications and Disadvantage

The main disadvantage of this approach is that hearing is sacrificed. The extensive mobilization of the facial nerve places it at risk, and most patients have a significant facial nerve paralysis. Although it usually improves after surgery, facial nerve function infrequently exceeds grade III on the House-Brackmann grading scale, and the nerve often is permanently impaired. Section of the GSPN can result in an ipsilateral dry eye. There is also a risk of CSF leak and meningitis. Resection of the mandibular condyle can result in TMJ dysfunction.

Infralabyrinthine Approach

Indications

In 1985, Gherini and co-workers[49] advocated the infralabyrinthine approach for the surgical management of cholesterol granulomas of the petrous apex and CPA. The purpose of this approach is to permit access to that portion of the petrous apex that is inferior to the labyrinth. As such, it is valuable in decompression of a cholesterol granuloma of the petrous apex. It can also be useful in conjunction with the suboccipital approach for resection of meningiomas of the petrous ridge with extension into the temporal bone, but without involvement of the labyrinth, hearing is therefore preserved.[47,50]

Surgical Approach

In this approach, a simple mastoidectomy is first performed. The middle and posterior fossa plates along with the SS are then skeletonized. At this point, the PSC and LSC can be identified and protected. The facial nerve is identified and skeletonized along its mastoid segment and left in its bony canal. A communication between the labyrinth superiorly and the jugular bulb inferiorly is then developed until the petrous apex is entered. The bulb can be skeletonized and its superior portion carefully dissected to free it of its adjacent bony covering. It is then packed inferiorly with bone wax so that additional exposure is obtained. In the case of a cholesterol granuloma, on opening the cavity, drainage of dark, thick fluid, sometimes under pressure, occurs. Cultures are obtained and the opening into the cavity is widened to approximately 0.5 to 1 cm to provide permanent drainage.

Complications and Disadvantages

If the jugular bulb is high in position, access below the labyrinth and above the bulb can be limited. A careful preoperative evaluation using high-resolution CT is useful.[29,30] Measuring the distance between the labyrinth and jugular bulb on coronal images can be particularly useful; a distance of less than 1 cm was found to be inadequate for satisfactory drainage of cholesterol granulomas.[50] In those instances, another approach is recommended (e.g., transcanal-infracochlear; see later).

Other complications include injury to the facial nerve, carotid artery, jugular bulb, and labyrinth. Obviously, the opening made for drainage of the cholesterol granuloma may scar and the granuloma may recur.

Transcanal-Infracochlear Approach

The transcanal part of the approach was first described by Farrior[51,52] in 1984.

Indications

This approach is used for access to the petrous apex in cases where hearing preservation is a goal and the jugular bulb is positioned high, limiting exposure through an infralabyrinthine approach. Because this approach is directed cephalad, it provides dependent drainage for cholesterol granulomas of the petrous apex. In addition, the drainage is to a well-aerated region near the eustachian tube.

Surgical Approach

The transcanal-infracochlear approach uses a C-shaped retroauricular skin incision similar to that used for the translabyrinthine and infralabyrinthine approaches. The soft tissues are reflected forward and the ear canal is transected just medial to the bony cartilaginous junction. The anterior, inferior, and posterior portions of the ear canal skin are lifted superiorly to the level of the umbo. Bone is removed from over the anterior, inferior, and posterior portions of the bony canal wall, effectively achieving near-total removal of the tympanic bone and enlargement of the canal. The thin bone over the TMJ is preserved. The carotid artery is then skeletonized anterior and inferior to the eustachian tube orifice. Bone is then removed from between the ICA and internal jugular vein without actually exposing the jugular bulb. The region of the facial nerve is identified using continuous electrical monitoring, but the nerve is not exposed. Inferiorly, the cholesterol granuloma sac is identified, opened for drainage, and irrigated.

Complications and Disadvantages

The complications are similar to those with the translabyrinthine approach except that injury to the cochlea, carotid artery, and jugular bulb is possible. This approach provides only limited exposure of the petrous apex, and therefore is useful only in the specific indications of drainage of a cholesterol granuloma or petrous apicitis.

COMBINED APPROACHES

Petrosal Approach

The petrosal approach is also referred to as the combined suprainfratentorial approach because it combines both supratentorial and infratentorial exposures to give wide anterior access to the CPA and ventral brain stem. The first reported transtentorial exposure was in 1896 by Stieglitz and colleagues,[53] in which a CPA tumor was approached through a supramastoid-suboccipital exposure. Several authors followed with modifications of the occipital flap with a suboccipital craniectomy, including ligation of the SS for wider exposure,[54] combined occipitotemporal craniotomy with or without ligation of the lateral sinus[55] and reapproximation of the lateral sinus,[56] and other approaches,[57,58] including the addition of a mastoidectomy.[59,60]

The petrosal approach was popularized by Malis,[60] who described ligation of the SS between its junction with the superior anastomotic vein and the SPS for increased exposure. Spetzler and colleagues[61] operated on 83 patients with the petrosal approach and sacrificed the SS in 50% of cases. Al-Mefty and colleagues[62] described the petrosal approach in detail, emphasizing an extensive petrous resection and directing the approach more laterally, thus lessening the operative distance to the clivus. They also stressed the importance of preserving the venous sinuses.

Indications

The petrosal approach includes a combined temporal craniotomy with a posterior fossa craniectomy-craniotomy for supratentorial and infratentorial exposure. Crucial to this approach is sectioning of the tentorium. With the addition of an extensive petrous resection, the anterior surface of the brain stem can be approached to the level of the inferior one third of the clivus. The lowest portion of the clivus is often obscured by the jugular tubercle. The petrosal approach provides access to lesions in the CPA and petroclival junction (upper two thirds of the clivus) such as meningiomas, trigeminal schwannomas, epidermoids, or chondrosarcomas. For lesions of the lower one third of the clivus and the foramen magnum, the far lateral transcondylar approach provides better access.

Surgical Approach

The patient is placed in a lateral position. The incision begins approximately 1 cm anterior to the ear and is directed posteriorly in a gentle curve to the postauricular area approximately 2 cm posterior to the mastoid process. The temporalis fascia and muscle are elevated and reflected anteriorly on a pedicle.

A mastoidectomy is first accomplished with preservation of the labyrinth and exposure of the mastoid segment of the facial nerve. A combined temporo-occipital bone flap is then raised (Fig. 22-5). The transverse and sigmoid sinuses have been previously identified during the mastoidectomy. This gives exposure along the middle fossa floor, transverse and sigmoid sinuses, and suboccipital dura. The dura can then be opened on the inferior aspect of the temporal lobe, and anterior or posterior to the SS. After opening the dura over the temporal lobe and the presigmoid dura, the SPS is clipped and divided. The tentorium can be divided in three different directions (Fig. 22-6). The first cut is done posteriorly along the transverse sinus to allow for retraction of

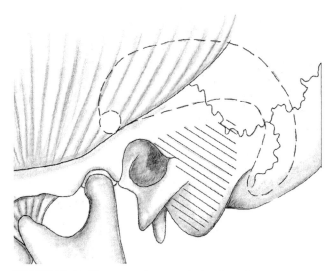

FIGURE 22-5 The petrosal approach. Outline of the craniotomy (*interrupted line*) and mastoidectomy (*hatched area*). The asterion and external auditory canal are shown.

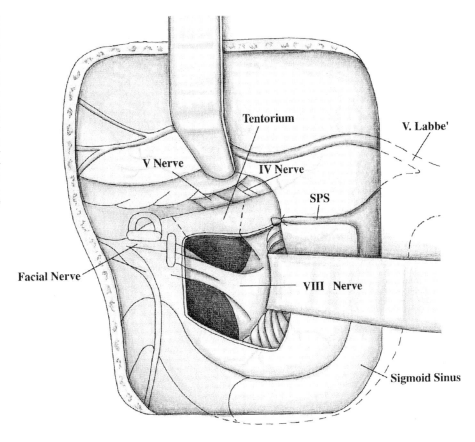

the transverse-sigmoid sinus junction posteriorly, thus enlarging the presigmoid corridor. The second cut is aimed medially toward the free edge to identify and protect the trochlear nerve. The third cut is parallel to the petrous pyramid and the SPS. This allows resection of the lateral tentorial leaflet and view of the supratentorial and infratentorial compartments. Ipsilateral cranial nerves IV through X are well visualized (Fig. 22-7). A retractor can be placed to retract the temporal lobe superiorly and another one to retract the transverse and sigmoid sinuses posteriorly. If the surgeon decides to work through the retrosigmoid corridor, a cerebellar retractor can be placed. Care must be taken to avoid injury to the superior anastomotic vein. In certain cases, the presigmoid avenue is limited and ligation and division of the SS can provide maximum anterior exposure of the CPA.

Wound closure begins with reapproximation of the dura. A dural defect usually remains after suturing. Any opened air cells are waxed. The mastoid antrum is sealed with fascia or muscle and an autologous fat graft is used to fill the petrosectomy defect. Alternatively or additionally, the posterior temporalis vascularized flap can be used to cover the petrosectomy defect to prevent CSF leak. The inner table from the craniotomy can be shaped and anchored with miniplates for a more cosmetic mastoid appearance. Spinal drainage can be used for several days after surgery depending on preference.

Complications and Disadvantages

Typical complications as described earlier for any intracranial approach may be encountered. In addition, there is potential for injury to the sinuses and for significant blood loss and air embolism, if that occurs. Specific to this approach is the potential for injury to the superior anastomotic vein, which provides significant venous drainage to the temporal lobe. Hence, edema and venous infarction are a possibility. During drilling of the petrous apex, injury to the semicircular canals (especially the posterior one) and facial nerve may occur.

Infratemporal Fossa Approach

The infratemporal fossa approach, developed by Fisch[63] in 1977, is a craniotemporocervical approach for exposure of the lateral inferior skull base. This approach is divided into three exposures, types A, B, or C, depending on the amount of anterior exposure required. The type A approach is similar to the combined lateral skull base approach reported by Gardner and colleagues[64] in 1977. With the type A exposure, a subtotal petrosectomy with transposition of the facial nerve is accomplished for exposure of the apical and infralabyrinthine temporal bone as well as the mandibular fossa and posterior infratemporal fossa. The type B exposure gives additional exposure of the clivus and horizontal segment of the ICA. The type C approach is an anterior extension of the type B approach, giving exposure of the infratemporal fossa, pterygopalatine fossa, parasellar region, and nasopharynx. With most indications for the type C approach, the surgeon can use a more anterior, preauricular pterional type of incision with a zygomatic osteotomy and subtemporal craniectomy.[65]

Indications

According to Fisch,[63] the type A approach is useful for lesions involving the jugular foramen (e.g., class C and D

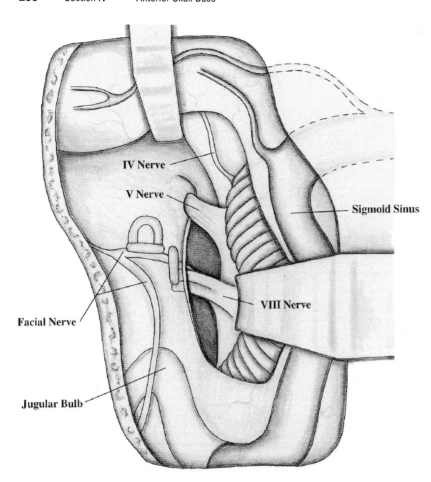

IV Nerve

V Nerve

Sigmoid Sinus

VIII Nerve

Facial Nerve

Jugular Bulb

FIGURE 22-7 The petrosal approach. The presigmoid retrolabyrinthine corridor is shown. Exposure is obtained after sectioning the tentorium. The trochlear, trigeminal, facial, and vestibulocochlear nerves are seen.

glomus jugulare tumors), lesions of the petrous apex, lower cranial nerve schwannomas, high cervical and petrous carotid artery lesions, and certain infratemporal fossa lesions. The type B approach is indicated for lesions of the petrous apex and clivus. The type C approach is best for lesions such as juvenile nasopharyngeal angiofibroma and nasopharyngeal carcinoma, or those involving the pterygopalatine fossa, cavernous sinus, and nasopharynx.

Surgical Approach

The details of these approaches have been well described by Fisch[5] and are summarized here. The skin incision is an extension of the standard C-shaped retroauricular incision. The skin and periosteal flap is reflected anteriorly with transection and closure of the EAC. Next, the great vessels (carotid artery, jugular vein) and nerves of the neck (glossopharyngeal, vagus, spinal accessory, and hypoglossal) are exposed (Fig. 22-8). The posterior belly of the digastric muscle is divided near its insertion at the mastoid process. The external carotid artery and its branches are ligated and transected above the lingual artery. The ICA is followed to the carotid foramen. Next, a subtotal petrosectomy is done by exposing the temporal bone and reflecting the sternocleidomastoid muscle away from the mastoid tip. The operation proceeds with removal of the EAC, mastoidectomy with complete mobilization of the facial nerve for anterior transposition, exposure, and possible ligation of the SS, removal of the styloid process for exposure of the ICA,

obliteration of the eustachian tube, and exposure of the infratemporal fossa. This includes anterior translocation of the mandible. The exposure obtained with this approach spans from the middle ear, mastoid, and upper neck, exposing the posterior portion of the infratemporal fossa.

The type B approach includes exposure of the ICA from the neck to the cavernous sinus. To expose the horizontal segment of the ICA, the middle meningeal artery is divided and the eustachian tube is sacrificed. By sacrificing the eustachian tube at this point and preserving the middle ear cleft, hearing can be preserved. The approach to the clivus requires division of cranial nerve V3 and complete removal of the bony eustachian tube.

The type C approach adds anterior exposure to the type B approach. The nasopharynx can be entered by removing the lateral pharyngeal wall behind the medial pterygoid process. Exposure here gives visualization of the vomer, opposite inferior turbinate, and pharyngeal end of the opposite eustachian tube. The pterygopalatine fossa is exposed by removing the pterygoid process. To expose the parasellar region, the zygoma and basal portion of the sphenoid are removed. The ipsilateral sphenoid and maxillary sinus are opened. For complete exposure of the cavernous sinus, the maxillary nerve is divided and the bone at the floor of the middle fossa is removed for extradural elevation of the temporal lobe.

We have used a combination of middle fossa and infratemporal fossa approaches for treating en plaque meningiomas of the temporal bone (Fig. 22-9). This particular combination

FIGURE 22-8 Exposure is obtained by an infratemporal fossa approach type A. The sternocleidomastoid muscle (SCM) and posterior belly of the digastric muscle are shown. Cranial nerves IX, X, XI, and XII are shown in the neck. The external auditory canal (EAC), malleus, and incus have been removed. The facial nerve has been transposed anteriorly. EAC, external auditory canal.

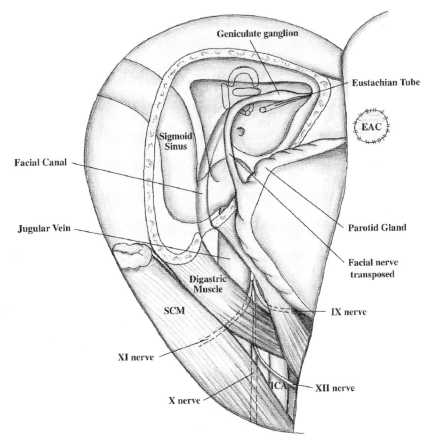

FIGURE 22-9 Combined middle fossa–infratemporal fossa approach. Adjacent structures are shown. The facial nerve is displaced, and the internal carotid artery is exposed. (From Gardner G, Robertson JH, Clark C: Transtemporal approaches to the cranial cavity. Am J Otol 6(Suppl):118, 1985.)

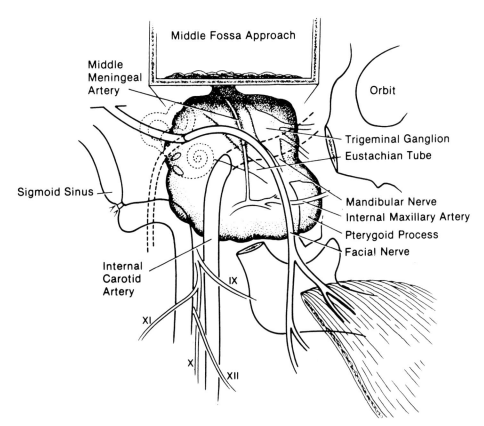

of approaches is a logical extension of either individual approach when both areas are involved pathologically. This approach could be of value in providing wider access to the petrous carotid artery.

Complications and Disadvantages

According to Fisch and Mattox,[5] transposition of the facial nerve always results in some paresis, but the average recovery of function (to House-Brackmann grade II) was 80%. A conductive hearing loss is common in all infratemporal fossa approaches because of removal of the tympanic membrane and ossicles. Tachycardia can occur after removal of glomus jugulare tumors. Preoperative laboratory evaluation of suspected glomus tumors should include blood vanillylmandelic acid levels and possible use of alpha-adrenergic blockers. With the additional exposure of the eustachian tube, ascending infection can occur even with subsequent primary closure of the eustachian tube. CSF leaks and meningitis can obviously occur. Fisch and Mattox[5] recommend obliteration of the wound with muscle rather than free fat graft to aid in closure of the eustachian tube. For the type C approach, the major risks include hearing loss, which occurs in most, and loss of mandibular function as a result of translocation of the mandibular condyle and resection of the articular disc and glenoid fossa during exposure. Initially there may be limitation in jaw opening, but this eventually resolves. Resection of cranial nerves V2 and V3 usually results in facial and tongue anesthesia; this generally improves over 9 months.[5]

SUMMARY

The ability to approach the posterior cranial fossa in a variety of ways is advantageous because it allows the neurosurgeon more options to reach and treat tumors in this area. The ability to drill away selected segments of the temporal bone, without major sacrifice of function, to achieve access for surgical procedures presents a continuing and exciting challenge to both neurosurgeons and their otologic colleagues.

Acknowledgment

Portions of this chapter are reproduced with permission from Brodkey J, Vrionis FD: Surgical approaches through the temporal bone. In Robertson JT, Coakham H, Robertson JH (eds): Cranial Base Surgery: Management, Complications and Outcome. Edinburgh: Churchill Livingstone, 2000.

REFERENCES

1. Parry RH: A case of tinnitus and vertigo treated by division of the auditory nerve. Laryngology 19:402–406, 1904.
2. House WF: Middle cranial fossa approach to the petrous pyramid: A report of 50 cases. Arch Otolaryngol 78:406–469, 1963.
3. House WF: Surgical exposure of the internal auditory canal and its contents through the middle cranial fossa. Laryngoscope 71:1363–1385, 1961.
4. Arsistegui M, Cokkeser Y, Saleh E, et al: Surgical anatomy of the extended middle fossa approach. Skull Base Surg 4:181–188, 1994.
5. Fisch U, Mattox D: Infratemporal fossa approach type B. In Fisch U, Mattox D (eds): Microsurgery of the Skull Base. New York: Thieme, 1988, pp 286–343.
6. Garcia-Ibanez E, Garcia-Ibanez JL: Middle fossa vestibular neurectomy: A report of 373 cases. Otolaryngol Head Neck Surg 88:486–490, 1980.
7. Vrionis FD, Robertson JH, Foley KT, et al: Image-interactive orientation in the middle cranial fossa approach to the internal auditory canal: An experimental study. Comput Aided Surg 2:34–41, 1997.
8. Vrionis FD, Foley KT, Robertson JH, et al: Use of cranial surface anatomic fiducials for interactive image-guided navigation in the temporal bone: A cadaveric study. Neurosurgery 40:755–764, 1997.
9. Brackmann DE: Middle fossa approach for acoustic tumor removal. Clin Neurosurg 38:603–618, 1990.
10. Parisier SC: The middle cranial fossa approach to the internal auditory canal: An anatomic study stressing critical distances between surgical landmarks. Laryngoscope 87(Suppl):1–19, 1977.
11. Kartush JM, Kemink JL, Graham MD: The arcuate eminence, topographic orientation in middle cranial fossa surgery. Ann Otol Rhinol Laryngol 94:25–28, 1985.
12. Fisch U, Mattox D: Transtemporal supralabyrinthine approach. In Fisch U, Mattox D (eds): Microsurgery of the Skull Base. New York: Thieme, 1988, pp 418–454.
13. Shiobara R, Ohira T, Kanzaki J, et al: A modified extended middle cranial fossa approach for acoustic tumors: Results of 125 operations. J Neurosurg 68:358–365, 1988.
14. King TI: Combined translabyrinthine-transtentorial approach to acoustic nerve tumors. Proc R Soc Med 63:780–782, 1970.
15. Glasscock ME: Middle fossa approach to the temporal bone. Arch Otolaryngol 90:41–53, 1969.
16. Kawase T, Toya S, Shiobara S, et al: Transpetrosal approach for aneurysms of the lower basilar artery. J Neurosurg 63:857–861, 1985.
17. Miller CG, van-Loveren HR, Keller JT, et al: Tranpetrosal approach: Surgical anatomy and technique. Neurosurgery 33:461–469, 1993.
18. Kawase T, Shiobara R, Toya S: Anterior tranpetrosal-transtentorial approach for sphenopetroclival meningiomas: Surgical method and results in 10 patients. Neurosurgery 28:869–876, 1991.
19. Kawase T, Shiobara R, Toya S: Middle fossa transpetrosal-transtentorial approaches for petroclival meningiomas: Selective pyramid resection and radicality. Acta Neurochir (Wien) 129:113–120, 1994.
20. Megerian CA, Chiocca EA, McKenna MJ, et al: The subtemporal-transpetrous approach for excision of petroclival tumors. Am J Otol 17:773–779, 1996.
21. Hitselberger WE, Pulec JL: Trigeminal nerve (posterior root) retrolabyrinthine selective section: Operative procedure for intractable pain. Arch Otolaryngol 96:412–415, 1972.
22. Silverstein H, Norrell H: Retrolabyrinthine surgery: A direct approach to the cerebellopontine angle. In Silverstein H, Norrell H (eds): Neurological Surgery of the Ear. Birmingham, AL: Aesculapius, 1977, pp 318–340.
23. House JW, Hitselberger WE, McElveen J, et al: Retrolabyrinthine section of the vestibular nerve. Otolaryngol Head Neck Surg 92:212–215, 1984.
24. Vrionis FD, Robertson JH, Heilman CB, et al: Asterion meningiomas. Skull Base Surg 8:153–161, 1998.
25. Durgun B, Ilglt ET, Cizmeli MO, et al: Evaluation by angiography of the lateral dominance of the drainage of the dural venous sinuses. Surg Radiol Anat 15:125–130, 1993.
26. Cushing H: Tumors of the Nervus Acousticus and the Syndrome of the Cerebellopontine Angle. New York: Hafner, 1917, pp 296–306.
27. Dandy WE: Operation for total extirpation of tumors in the cerebellopontine angle. Bull Johns Hopkins Hosp 33:344–355, 1922.
28. Day JD, Kellog JX, Tschabitscher M, et al: Surface and superficial surgical anatomy of the posterolateral cranial base: Significance for surgical planning and approach. Neurosurgery 38:1079–1084, 1996.
29. Yokoyama T, Uemura K, Ryu H, et al: Surgical approach to the internal auditory meatus in acoustic neuroma surgery: Significance of preoperative high-resolution computed tomography. Neurosurgery 39:965–970, 1996.
30. Shao KN, Tatagiba M, Samii M: Surgical management of high jugular bulb in acoustic neurinoma via retrosigmoid approach. Neurosurgery 32:32–37, 1993.
31. Panse R: Ein Gliom des Akustikus. Arch Ohrenheilkd 61:251–255, 1904.
32. House WF: Transtemporal bone microsurgical removal of acoustic neuromas. Arch Otolarygol 80:599–756, 1964.
33. Naguib MB, Saleh E, Cokkeser Y, et al: The enlarged translabyrinthine approach for removal of large vestibular schwannomas. J Laryngol Otol 108:545–550, 1994.
34. McElveen JT, Wilkins RH, Erwin AC, et al: Modifying the translabyrinthine approach to preserve hearing during acoustic tumour surgery. J Laryngol Otol 105:34–37, 1991.
35. Feghali JG, Kantrowitz AB: Transcranial translabyrinthine approach to vestibular schwannomas. J Laryngol Otol 107:111–114, 1993.

36. Fisch U, Mattox D: Tranlabyrinthine approach. In Fisch U, Mattox D (eds): Microsurgery of the Skull Base. New York: Thieme, 1988, pp 546–576.

37. Fisch U, Mattox D: Transotic approach to the cerebellopontine angle. In Fisch U, Mattox D (eds): Microsurgery of the Skull Base. New York: Thieme, 1988, pp 74–127.

38. Briggs RJS, Luxford WM, Atkins JS, Hitselberger WE: Translabyrinthine removal of large acoustic neuromas. Neurosurg 34:785–792, 1994.

39. House WF, Hitselberger WE: The transcochlear approach to the skull base. Arch Otolaryngol 102:334–342, 1976.

40. Gantz BJ, Fisch U: Modified transotic approach to the cerebellopontine angle. Arch Otolaryngol 109:252–256, 1983.

41. Browne JD, Fisch U: Transotic approach to the cerebellopontine angle. Otol Clin North Am 25:331–346, 1992.

42. Sanna M, Mazzoni A, Saleh EA, et al: Lateral approaches to the median skull base through the petrous bone: The system of the modified transcochlear approach. J Laryngol Otol 108:1036–1044, 1994.

43. De La Cruz A: The transcochlear approach to meningiomas and cholesteatomas of the cerebellopontine angle. In Brackmann DE (ed): Neurological Surgery of the Ear and Skull Base. New York: Raven Press, 1982, pp 353–360.

44. Sekhar LN, Estonillo R: Transtemporal approach to the skull base: An anatomical study. Neurosurgery 19:799–808, 1986.

45. Horn KL, Hankinson HL, Erasmus MD, et al: The modified transcochlear approach to the cerebellopontine angle. Otolaryngol Head Neck Surg 104:37–41, 1991.

46. Sanna M, Mazzoni A, Gamoletti R: The system of the modified transcochlear approaches to the petroclival area and the prepontine cistern. Skull Base Surg 6:237–248, 1996.

47. Gardner G, Robertson JH, Clark C: Transtemporal approaches to the cranial cavity. Am J Otol 6(Suppl):114–120, 1985.

48. Thedinger BA, Glasscock ME, Cueva RA: Transcochlear transtentorial approach for removal of large cerebellopontine angle meningiomas. Am J Otol 13:408–415, 1992.

49. Gherini SG, Brackmann DE, Lo WWM, et al: Cholesterol granuloma of the petrous apex. Laryngoscope 95:659–664, 1985.

50. Brodkey JA, Robertson JH, Shea JJ, et al: Cholesterol granulomas of the petrous apex: Combined neurosurgical and otological management. J Neurosurg 85:625–633, 1996.

51. Giddings NA, Brackmann DE, Kwartler JA: Transcanal infracochlear approach to the petrous apex. Otolaryngol Head Neck Surg 104:29–41, 1991.

52. Farrior JB: Anterior hypotympanic approach for glomus tumor of the infratemporal fossa. Laryngoscope 94:1016–1020, 1984.

53. Stieglitz L, Gerster AG, Lilienthal H: A study of three cases of tumor of the brain in which operation was performed: One recovery, two deaths. Am J Med Sci 111:509–531, 1896.

54. Naffziger HC. Brain surgery with special reference to exposure of the brainstem and posterior fossa: The principle of intracranial decompression, and the relief of impactions in the posterior fossa. Surg Gynecol Obstet 46:241–248, 1928.

55. Fay T: The management of tumors of the posterior fossa by a transtentorial approach. Surg Clin North Am 10:1427–1459, 1930.

56. Bailey P: Concerning the technique of operation for acoustic neurinoma. Zentralbl Neurochir 4:1–5, 1939.

57. Samii M, Ammirati M, Mahran A, et al: Surgery of petroclival meningiomas: Report of 24 cases. Neurosurgery 24:12–17, 1989.

58. Tarlov E. Surgical management of tumors of the tentorium and clivus. In Schmidek HH, Sweet WH (eds): Operative Neurosurgical Techniques: Indications, Methods, and Results, vol 1. New York: Grune & Stratton, 1977, pp 381–388.

59. Malis LI: Surgical resection of tumors of the skull base. Neurosurgery 1:1011–1021, 1985.

60. Malis LI: The petrosal approach. Clin Neurosurg 37:528–540, 1991.

61. Spetzler RF, Hamilton MG, Daspit CP: Petroclival lesions. Clin Neurosurg 41:62–82, 1994.

62. Al-Mefty O, Fox JL, Smith RR: Petrosal approach for petroclival meningiomas. Neurosurgery 22:510–517, 1988.

63. Fisch U: Infratemporal fossa approach to tumors of the temporal bone and base of the skull. J Laryngol Otol 92:949–967, 1978.

64. Gardner G, Cocke EW, Robertson JT, et al: Combined approach surgery for removal of glomus jugulare tumors. Laryngoscope 87:665–688, 1977.

65. Vrionis FD, Cano W, Heilman CB: Microsurgical anatomy of the infratemporal fossa as viewed laterally and superiorly. Neurosurgery 39:777–786, 1996.

Craniopharyngiomas and Pituitary Tumors

23

Stereotactic Radiosurgery for Pituitary Adenomas and Craniopharyngiomas

ERIK-OLOF BACKLUND

This chapter deals exclusively with radiosurgical treatment (stereotactic single-dose irradiation) of pituitary tumors, using the gamma knife (GK) (Elekta Instrument, Stockholm). The GK technique is described in Chapter 40 of this volume. Moreover, an excellent account on its use in the pituitary region is given in one of the articles quoted later in this chapter.[1]

In radiosurgery, other types of irradiation units are also used, for example, dedicated linear accelerators and generators for heavy particles. Examples of the latter used with pituitary tumors are the early clinical studies using proton beams, a technique already pioneered during the 1960s.[2]

ORIGINAL STUDIES

Lars Leksell, professor of neurosurgery at the Karolinska Institute in Stockholm from 1960 to 1974, invented the GK. Working with Dr. Leksell, the author initiated the first clinical trials with the GK in pituitary tumors. After Leksell's retirement, the author was appointed chief of the stereotactic service at the Karolinska, including the GK unit. In 1967, a young man with a craniopharyngioma was the first patient in history treated with GK,[3] whereas the second patient had a nonactive adenoma. Apart from these, most GK procedures during this period were thalamotomies performed for pain.

The GK was designed primarily for precision radiolesioning, to be a tool for functional operations.[4] It was obvious, however, that (parts of) the anterior pituitary also represented tissue volumes of appropriate size for radiolesioning. Thus receiving early attention as a project were not only intrasellar adrenocorticotropic hormone (ACTH)–producing adenomas,[5] but also growth hormone (GH)–producing adenomas of limited size.

A "cluster" irradiation technique, using a number of irradiation fields or isocenters, adjacent to or overlapping each other, was tried in macroadenomas and in craniopharyngiomas.[6,7] Moreover, the possibilities of using the GK for "gamma-hypophysectomy" in cancer patients as a pain-relieving procedure were early discussed, and a pilot study was performed.[8]

CURRENT PRACTICE

The treatment of pituitary adenomas often involves techniques beyond microsurgery. Thus GK irradiation is a valuable complement to surgical adenomectomy. The practice of using microsurgery and additional GK irradiation is generally improving the overall results with these tumors. In craniopharyngiomas, intracavitary irradiation with short-range β-irradiation represents the principally most notable change from the previous practice with surgery as the first-line method of treatment. Extensive evidence about this approach has been accumulated. In this chapter, the current state of the art with respect to the role of the GK in the treatment of pituitary adenomas and craniopharyngiomas is presented, along with the most current references.

ADENOMAS

Adrenocorticotropic Hormone–Producing Tumors

The first study during the 1970s on stereotactic radiosurgery in the treatment of Cushing's disease gave spectacular results, with an eventual high cure rate, in some cases only after additional adrenalectomy.[9] The irradiation design of this study was "prospective," with "staged lesioning" of the anterior pituitary lobe, that is, one to four intrasellar isocenters used stepwise, over a period (sometimes) of months, to obtain a cluster configuration of the radiation field. Nevertheless, these results did not set the stage for other trials on GK irradiation as a primary treatment method in Cushing's disease. Instead, the general treatment practice over the subsequent years was the use of adrenalectomy as the first-line treatment.

There were at least two obvious reasons for this decision. First, the very rewarding initial results of the pilot study were followed by a late pituitary insufficiency in 12/22 of these cases, 4 months to 7 years after completed GK procedure(s).[10] The other reason was that the responsible endocrinologists were often spellbound by the increasing sophistication of the transsphenoidal surgical adenomectomy, often implying immediate cure, a requisite in those patients with Cushing's disease, for whom the disease is an acute threat.

Three recent studies on GK treatment in Cushing's disease from centers of special excellence are summarized here. Sheehan and co-workers report on 43 patients unsuccessfully treated by surgery.[11] No patients with Nelson's syndrome are included in this selection. The tumor area is irradiated with two to six isocenters at doses to the margin of 3.6 to 30 Gy (mean 20 Gy), 30% to 50% of the maximum dose. Normal 24-hour urinary free-cortisol level was achieved in 63% of patients at an average of 1 year after GK irradiation (mean, 7 months; range, 3–48 months).

Surprisingly, there is no obvious dose-response correlation with respect to the biochemical outcome. In one case hypocortisolism was seen after 35 months, and in three other cases recurrent disease occurred after an initial satisfactory response. These relapses came 19, 37, and 38 months after treatment, surprisingly not correlated with radiation doses (25, 13.8, and 3.6 Gy to the tumor margin, respectively). Two of four patients in whom the whole sella was irradiated developed hypothyroidism, but in one patient, previous conventional radiotherapy may have contributed to this outcome. About 2 years after treatment (range, 8–5 months), five patients had new hormone deficiencies. The tumor volume decreased after treatment in 73% of cases, notably not significantly correlated with endocrine outcome, a finding previously confirmed.[12]

In a Japanese study, 25 patients with hypercortisolism (6 with Nelson's syndrome) were followed for more than 2 years (mean, 5.3 years) after GK irradiation, used either as primary or adjuvant treatment after surgery.[13] The overall results showed "a complete response near 30%, a total response rate of 85%, and a tumor control rate of 100%." The smaller the tumor, the better was the response. The best results were obtained after "a maximum dose of 55 Gy and a margin dose of more than 40 Gy." Serum ACTH was "decreased" in 85%, "normalized" in 35%, and "significantly decreased" in 60%. The hormone levels remained essentially unchanged in three patients. No side effects were reported. In the six patients with Nelson's syndrome, the endocrine response was less favorable (33%), although satisfying tumor control was achieved.

The third report is from the Mayo Clinic, where 11 patients with ACTH-producing adenomas after adrenalectomy underwent GK treatment.[14] Nine had documented tumor growth, hyperpigmentation, and elevated ACTH level before treatment, five of those with tumor growth despite prior radiotherapy. The median follow-up was 37 months (range, 22–74 months). At follow-up, the ACTH levels had decreased a median of 66%, in four patients to normal levels. Complications were found in three patients (diplopia, blindness, endocrine deficiency, and asymptomatic temporal lobe necrosis), but all three patients had had previous conventional radiotherapy (median dose 50 Gy).

Growth Hormone–Producing Tumors

Thirty acromegalic patients constitute the case material in a recent prospective study.[15] Twenty-seven had had previous unsuccessful surgery, but in three, GK irradiation was the primary treatment. Multiple (range, 3–11) isocenters were used, with a mean margin dose to the tumor of 20 Gy, and a maximum of 8 Gy to the optic apparatus. Follow-up studies were made after a mean of 46 months (range, 9–96 months). Mean GH levels gradually decreased, to less than 2.5 μg/L in 11 (37%). The rate of persistent elevated levels was 70% at 5 years (Kaplan-Meier method). Hormone deficiencies were seen in two patients present before the GK treatment in these cases. Tumor shrinkage was found in around 60%, and in none was further tumor growth observed. No patient developed visual deficits.

In a Chinese study from 1993 to 1997, 68 acromegaly patients were treated with GK as the primary procedure.[16] The tumor margin dose (50% to 90% isodose level) was

18 to 35 Gy (mean, 31.3 Gy). Normalization of the hormone levels was seen in 23 of 58 patients followed for 12 months, and in 25 of 26 followed for more than 36 months. The dose to the optic apparatus was planned not to exceed 10 Gy. However, one patient, with an excellent hormonal response and tumor shrinkage, had reduced visual acuity after 1 year. Notably, the visual pathways in this case had been given a dose of 12 Gy. There were no other obvious adverse effects. A radiation dose of 30 Gy to the tumor periphery was considered necessary for an optimal result. With regard to the vulnerable surroundings, this "marginal" dose is critical, particularly when a GH-producing tumor, most often larger than those producing ACTH, is planned for GK treatment. The result with the aforementioned patient who developed late-onset reduced vision is suggestive. Currently used maximum dose levels to the optic pathways approximate 8 Gy.

Tumor extension into the cavernous sinus is a special challenge. This is addressed in a recent Japanese study, where a smaller series of nine patients with GH-secreting tumors were critically assessed.[17] In eight patients, previous surgery had failed and octreotide been used to compensate for this. By an average dose of 20 Gy to the tumor periphery, all tumors were well controlled within 12 to 69 months (mean, 42 months). Half of the patients had normal GH and insulin-like growth factor-1 values at 36 months.

The importance of octreotide medication as an influence on the radiation response was confirmed recently.[18] When evaluating a series of 19 acromegaly patients with unsatisfactory results after surgery who were subsequently treated with GK with good overall outcome, the authors found in retrospect that ongoing octreotide medication during the radiosurgical procedure seemed to diminish the radiation effects. Thus in patients in whom octreotide is used, a regime involving a medication gap of 2 weeks before the GK procedure is recommended.

An excellent review on the current opportunities for controlling acromegaly was published in 2002.[19] Therapies including "somatostatin analogue, lanreotide, Gamma Knife radiosurgery, and pegvisomant" were compared, with the following conclusion: "Although it does not appear that Gamma Knife radiosurgery results in significant higher cure rates or fewer complications, it does provide a notable improvement in delivery compared with conventional radiation."

Prolactin-Producing Tumors

Two recent studies are reviewed here, one in which GK irradiation was used as primary treatment of prolactinomas, and another in which it was used for patients with previous unsuccessful surgery and/or failed medical treatment.

In the first study, 164 patients with prolactinomas received a tumor margin dose of 9 to 35 Gy (mean, 31.2 Gy).[20] The optic apparatus was exposed to less than 10 Gy. The tumors were of limited size, the mean diameter being 13.4 mm. Of 128 cases that were followed for 33.2 months (range, 6–72 months), tumor control was achieved in all but 2 cases, and clinical cure occurred in 67 patients. Of 108 patients who were followed for more than 2 years, 31 (29%) had elevated prolactin (PRL) values that were normalized with bromocriptine administration. Nine female patients considered infertile before treatment became pregnant and gave birth to normal children. No adverse vision effects were seen. Five women in whom "empty sella" was assumed to have been caused by the irradiation had a premature menopause.

The second study is retrospective. Twenty patients had GK irradiation of small tumors (or tumor remnants), up to a tissue volume of 6.5 cm³, located in the adjacent cavernous sinus.[21] The margin dose was 21.1 Gy (range, 20–35 Gy), and 5 to 19 isocenters were used. The dose to the optic apparatus was less than 9 Gy. After a mean follow-up of 27.8 months (range, 6.2–47.1 months), five patients had normal PRL levels and dopamine agonists could be discontinued. Another 11 patients had results almost as good, and in only 4 was treatment considered a failure. In comparison with similar studies, the overall results in this series are strikingly good. The authors' own interpretation is that no "salvage cases" were included. Moreover, the rewarding effect of the GK treatment were less pronounced in patients receiving dopamine agonist medication, so that the authors recommend GK irradiation only after discontinuation of these drugs.

Nonfunctional Adenomas and Gamma Knife Treatment—Some Crucial Questions

Apart from the studies cited earlier, with specific attention to hormone-producing tumors, a steadily increasing number of publications discuss GK treatment in nonsecreting pituitary adenomas. Although surgical removal of these tumors may be successful, the number of patients with incompletely resected tumors is still high; this presents a challenge for the GK technique, which is obviously superior to any conventional postoperative radiotherapy. The accumulated experience in such cases can be condensed to several main questions, among which the following merit particular attention:

1. What does the GK offer regarding "tumor bulk reduction," particularly in recurrent and/or residual nonfunctioning adenomas?[22,23]
2. Is magnetic resonance (MR) volumetry the method of choice for quantifying tumor bulk reduction?[24]
3. When and why might any postradiation pituitary insufficiency appear?[25]

Tumor Bulk Reduction in Nonfunctioning Adenomas

In one of the recent series referred here,[22] the results clearly prove the usefulness of the GK in recurrent nonfunctioning adenomas. All 42 patients, treated by GK between 1987 and 2001, had had previous treatments including transsphenoidal resections (58), craniotomies (16), and radiotherapy (9). The recurrent tumors showed suprasellar growth in 7 patients and cavernous sinus ingrowth in 24. Evidence-based practice was followed with respect to the irradiation parameters, and a mean dose of 32 Gy (range, 20–70 Gy) was given to the tumor center and 16 Gy (mean, range 10–34 Gy) to the tumor periphery. The maximum dose to the optic apparatus was 8.5 Gy in all cases. After a follow-up of 31.2 months (range, 6–102 months), the tumors were very well controlled. None had developed a new endocrine deficiency: 18 tumors were found to be smaller, 23 unchanged in size, and 1 enlarged. Notably, 23/24 tumors with intracavernous

growth were well controlled. Of 18 patients who had had visual disturbances before the GK treatment, 14 were unchanged, 2 were improved, and 2 worsened, in 1 accompanied by tumor enlargement. Notably these two cases had had radiotherapy before the GK treatment.

With a median follow-up period of 43 months (range, 16–106 months), another study[23] included 32 patients with nonfunctioning adenomas treated by GK after one or more previous tumor resections. Of these 32 patients, 67% had enlarging tumors before the GK procedure. The radiation parameters and the results were essentially the same as in the previous study. The tumor growth control rates at 2 and 5 years were 97%. However, in this series, in contrast to the previous one, no patient had impaired visual function after the GK treatment, although here also two patients had had prior radiotherapy. Another difference with this series was that new endocrine deficits were found in 5 of 18 patients with normal function or partial insufficiency before the GK treatment.

Volumetry

In a study on patients with nonfunctioning adenomas treated by GK after previous surgery,[24] sequential MR measurements of the residual tumor volume were made annually. After a follow-up of 28 to 86 months, using the Leksell stereotactic system and the Gamma Plan software (Elekta Instruments), 72 complete examinations had been performed in 30 patients. The patient's head was placed in the stereotactic localizer box without rigid fixation, and the MR imaging sequences were identical with those used for the dose planning. The technique has been found to be very reliable and offers a sophisticated follow-up protocol for any kind of tumor treated by GK; it is particularly valuable when treating intrasellar nonfunctioning pituitary adenomas, in which, for example, endocrinologic tests may give too little information about possible clinically suspected recurrences.

Chances of Postirradiation Pituitary Insufficiency

The enduring and important questions about the risk for anterior lobe insufficiency after GK treatment[10] are again thoroughly discussed in a recent publication.[25] Two subgroups were selected from a larger series of GK-treated adenoma patients (both functioning and nonfunctioning). The two groups were followed for a median of 5 years. Group 1 (N = 30) comprised those who had post-treatment hypopituitarism at follow-up, and those in group 2 (N = 33) were normal. All except 4 patients (in group 2) had functioning tumors, and the GK irradiation was the only treatment in 29 (10 in group 1, 19 in group 2).

Analysis of the results from the very ambitious follow-up protocol led to the conclusions that gonadotropic and thyrotropic failures should not be expected if the mean dose to the pituitary is lower than 15 Gy, but such insufficiencies appear in 50% of patients if a mean dose of 17 Gy is used. Accordingly, to save the adrenocorticotropic function the mean dose should not exceed 18 Gy. Moreover, in any case of pituitary insufficiency after GK treatment, one must establish whether the patient had received prior conventional radiotherapy. A noxious effect from this must always be considered contributory in cases of eventual anterior lobe failure.

The authors also direct attention to the role of (an unintentional) radiation load to the pituitary stalk as potentially causative in the appearance of the anterior lobe deficits. Confirmatory evidence regarding this role may be found in an ongoing study in which GK lesioning of the pituitary stalk is performed with the aim of achieving pituitary ablation, as a cancer pain-relieving measure.[26]

Summary: Adenomas

The early enthusiasm over the theoretical possibility of a radically new mode of pituitary adenoma treatment using the GK has been moderated by the contemporary progress of transsphenoidal microsurgery and, importantly, the limitation that any curative effect in the hormone-producing tumors would occur only after a certain latency (on the order of weeks to months), which is not acceptable in, for example, patients with "acute" Cushing's disease. Even sophisticated surgery has its limitations, and as soon as the GK became commercially available, various projects on pituitary irradiation were gradually resumed worldwide. It was realized that radiotherapy before GK treatment must be considered contributory to late-appearing adverse radiation effects. Attention to such knowledge and a strict adherence to established protocols makes GK irradiation safe and effective in selected pituitary adenoma cases, for example, as additional treatment following incomplete surgery.

CRANIOPHARYNGIOMAS

Therapeutic Problem Defined

In clinical reports on craniopharyngioma surgery, varying rates of removal are reported. The proposal that any craniopharyngioma may be removed by surgery now seems to be in a state of decline. Radical removal of a large tumor with a polymorphic structure is often a formidable surgical undertaking. In the short term, the results after such extensive surgery may seem acceptable, but published series in which the number of patients and the length of the observation time allow firm conclusions to be drawn include 20% (or more) of cases that are "fundamentally hopeless," that is, impossible to cure in the long term, regardless of surgical radicality. This must be seriously considered when management alternatives are discussed.

Most craniopharyngiomas are cystic, often with a solitary cyst, occasionally of more than 100 mL volume. Of the total tumor bulk, in multicystic tumors most of the mass may be cystic, with the solid part being a relatively small part of the tumor's total volume. The threat that a craniopharyngioma poses is most often related to the total volume of the tumor. Thus treatment of the cyst (or cysts) should be a first step of management.

Stereotactic intracystic injection of radioactive (β-emitting) colloids induces permanent cyst shrinkage or even cyst disappearance (Figs. 23-1 and 23-2). Moreover, the

AC 13 yrs: *Y-90 June 94*

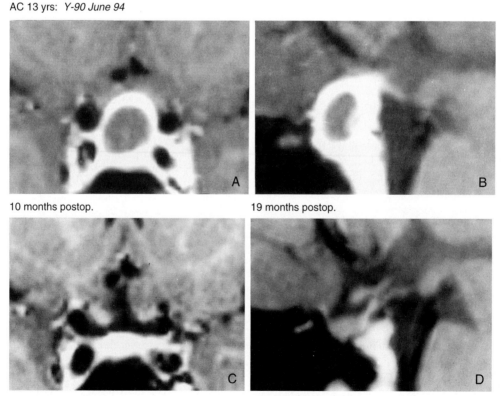

10 months postop.

19 months postop.

FIGURE 23-1   Case AC: This 13-year-old girl had suffered from headaches for 6 months and diplopia for 2 months. Weakness of the left sixth nerve was found, but visual acuity and fields were normal. Endocrine function was essentially normal, although serum prolactin was slightly elevated. Stereotactic puncture with injection of yttrium-90 (local anesthesia) was performed in June 1994. *A* and *B*, Preoperative anteroposterior and lateral magnetic resonance (MR) images (with gadolinium) before the operation. *C* and *D*, Postoperative MR images 10 and 19 months after the yttrium-90 injection, respectively. The anatomy appears completely normal. Ten years after the operation, the patient was symptom-free, had attended normal school with credit, and was leading a normal life as a senior's assistant.

MD 46 yrs, Jan 95: *Y-90*

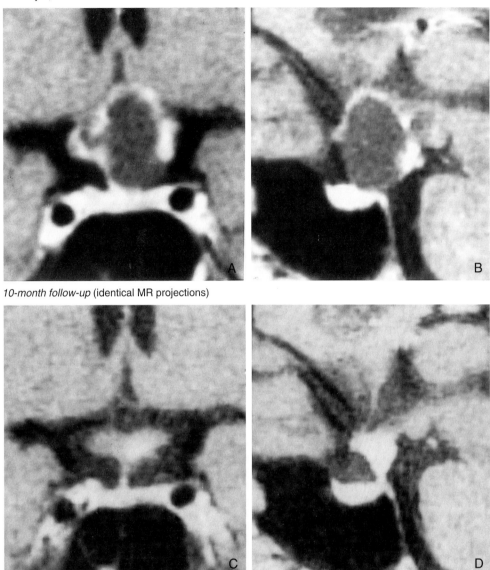

10-month follow-up (identical MR projections)

FIGURE 23-2 Case MD: In January 1995, this 46-year-old woman had had headaches for 2 months, rapidly deteriorating vision, and bitemporal field defects. Simultaneously, she had increased her fluid intake, but endocrine tests were essentially normal, except for a slight elevation in serum prolactin. *A* and *B*, MR showed a monocystic craniopharyngioma with a minor tumor nodule in the posterior wall. Stereotactic intracystic treatment with yttrium-90 caused a rapid improvement of vision. *C* and *D*, Postoperative MR 10 months later revealed an almost completely collapsed cyst. The nodule was considered for GK treatment, but because the clinical situation remained unchanged and the patient was leading a normal life, this had not yet been performed 9 years after the cyst treatment.

possibility of obliterating solid tumor parts with the GK was also shown early. The principles and practices of this technique have very little in common with conventional external irradiation, which still is recommended occasionally after subtotal microsurgical removal.

The value of a combination of conservative microsurgery and GK radiosurgery has been emphasized,[27] although, in the author's experience, tumor remnants or recurrences of appropriate size and shape for the GK (i.e., solid tumor parts) are fewer than expected. However, the currently used computerized dose planning may allow a widening of the indications.[1,28]

Multimodality Therapeutic Approach

The treatment in any craniopharyngioma case should be tailored to the requirements of the individual anatomy of the tumor. This means that a logical approach would be a multimodality treatment protocol in which four therapeutic options may be included, alone or in combination[29]:

1. Microsurgery
2. Stereotactic puncture of a cyst or cysts, with injection into the cysts of an obliterating substance, such as radioactive ^{90}Y (yttrium-90) as a colloidal solution

3. GK radiosurgery with stereotactically directed single-dose irradiation

4. In a few selected cases, often as a last resort, conventional radiation therapy, for example, using a linear accelerator

Crucial therapeutic decisions should be made by matching these therapeutic options with the individual tumor appearance.

The four therapeutic options have been used, alone or in combination, by the author since the early 1960s. The first 43 consecutive, unselected patients with no prior therapy have been reported in detail after a follow-up of 10 to 23 years.[30,31]

The results obtained with this multimodality protocol indicate that an optimal management in any case of craniopharyngioma should include two elements.

First, a detailed computed tomography–MR study of the tumor anatomy should be done, with the primary aim of disclosing cysts that are suitable for intracavitary irradiation. The proportions between solid and calcified tumor components, soft-tissue parts, and cystic compartments should be quantified, with the specific aim of assessing the relative bulk effect of each of these components as a basis for the individual treatment design.

Second, intracystic irradiation should be the first-line therapy if more than 50% of the total bulk of the tumor is cystic and there are not more than three cysts. Open craniotomy with microsurgical removal of monocystic tumors, especially if they are huge, may be difficult to justify today, even if this procedure can be performed with very little risk. The intracavitary isotope treatment must never be forgotten as a superior therapeutic alternative. Moreover, this treatment does not require shunting or drainage procedures, such as the insertion of reservoir devices for bleomycin installation, which is far from being innocent.

Recent Clinical Experience

Three recent series can serve as examples of the value of stereotactic alternatives in craniopharyngiomas. In one series, 31 consecutive adult craniopharyngioma patients were given GK irradiation, in 6 as primary treatment.[1] The other 25 had these prior therapies: excision (4), partial excision (19), biopsy (1), intracystic irradiation (2), Ommaya reservoir (3), ventriculoperitoneal shunt (9). Two had postoperative radiotherapy (50 and 59 Gy, respectively). Tumor volumes up to 28 cm^3 were irradiated, with a mean dose of 12.2 Gy (range, 9.5–16 Gy) to the tumor periphery, and a mean dose to the optic apparatus of 8 Gy (range, <7.2–12.5 Gy). In an average follow-up period of 36 months, tumor control was achieved in 87%, and 84% had "fair to excellent" clinical outcome.

Results comparable with the aforementioned, obtained when similar indications and the same techniques are used, are reported in another two excellent recent papers.[32,33]

Summary: Craniopharyngiomas

A low-risk, simple, cost-effective curative procedure should define the optimal treatment for a patient with a craniopharyngioma. The intrinsic safety of stereotactic methods must never be disregarded. Moreover, in human and economic terms, a stereotactic procedure, routinely performed under local anesthesia only, involves a much shorter hospital stay and time away from work for the patient than does an open operation.

The complete spectrum of surgical alternatives, microsurgery as well as stereotaxy, should be available in any modern department, making it possible for the surgeon to make the choice of treatment freely, and in relation to the specific problems of each patient. This is a prerequisite for progress in craniopharyngioma surgery.

REFERENCES

1. Chung WY, Pan DH, Shiau CY, et al: Gamma knife radiosurgery for craniopharyngiomas. J Neurosurg 93(Suppl 3):47–56, 2000.
2. Linfoot JA, Lawrence JH, Born JL, et al: The alpha particle of proton beam in radiosurgery of the pituitary gland for Cushing's disease. N Engl J Med 269:597–601, 1963.
3. Backlund EO: Stereotaxic treatment of craniopharyngiomas. In Hamberger CA, Wersäll J (eds): Nobel Symposium 10: Disorders of the Skull Base Region. Stockholm: Almqvist & Wiksell, 1969, pp 237–244.
4. Leksell L: Stereotaxis and Radiosurgery: An Operative System. Springfield, IL: Charles C Thomas, 1971.
5. Thorén M, Rähn T, Hall K, et al: Treatment of pituitary dependent Cushing's syndrome with closed stereotactic radiosurgery by means of Co-60 gamma radiation. Acta Endocrinol 88:7–17, 1978.
6. Backlund EO, Bergstrand G, Hierton-Laurell U, et al: Tumor changes after single dose irradiation by stereotactic radiosurgery in "nonactive" pituitary adenomas and prolactinomas. In Szikla G (ed): Sterotactic Cerebral Irradiation. New York: Elsevier/North-Holland, 1979, pp 199–206.
7. Backlund EO: Solid craniopharyngiomas treated by stereotactic radiosurgery. In Szikla G (ed): Stereotactic Cerebral Irradiation. New York: Elsevier/North-Holland, 1979, pp 271–281.
8. Backlund EO, Rähn T, Sarby B, et al: Closed stereotaxic hypophysectomy by means of Co-60 gamma radiation. Acta Radiol 11:545–555, 1972.
9. Rähn T, Thorén M, Hall K, et al: Stereotactic radiosurgery in Cushing's syndrome: Acute radiation effects. Surg Neurol 14:85–92, 1980.
10. Degerblad M, Rähn T, Bergstrand G, et al: Long-term results of stereotactic radiosurgery to the pituitary gland in Cushing's disease. Acta Endocrinol 112:310–314, 1986.
11. Sheehan JM, Vance ML, Sheehan JP, et al: Radiosurgery for Cushing's disease after failed transsphenoidal surgery. J Neurosurg 93:738–742, 2000.
12. Ganz JC, Backlund EO, Thorsen F: The effects of gamma knife surgery of pituitary adenomas on tumor growth and endocrinopathies. Stereotact Funct Neurosurg 61 (Suppl 1):30–37, 1993.
13. Kobayashi T, Kida Y, Mori Y: Gamma knife radiosurgery in the treatment of Cushing's disease, long-term results. J Neurosurg 97(Suppl 5):422–428, 2002.
14. Pollock BE, Young WF Jr: Stereotactic radiosurgery for patients with ACTH-producing pituitary adenomas after prior adrenalectomy. Int J Radiat Oncol Biol Phys 54:839–841, 2002.
15. Attanasio R, Epaminonda P, Motti E, et al: Gamma-knife radiosurgery in acromegaly: A 4-year follow-up study. Clin Endocrinol Metab 88:3105–3112, 2003.
16. Zhang N, Pan L, Wang EM, et al: Radiosurgery for hormone-producing pituitary adenomas. J Neurosurg 93(Suppl 3):6–9, 2000.
17. Fukuoka S, Ito T, Takanashi M, et al: Gamma knife radiosurgery for growth hormone-secreting pituitary adenomas invading the cavernous sinus. Stereotact Funct Neurosurg 76:213–217, 2001.
18. Landolt AM, Haller D, Lomax N, et al: Octreotide may act as a radioprotective agent in acromegaly. J Clin Endocrinol Metab 85:1287–1289, 2000.
19. Melmed S, Vance ML, Barkan AL, et al: Current status and future opportunities for controlling acromegaly. Pituitary 5:185–196, 2002.
20. Pan L, Zhang N, Wang EM, et al: Gamma knife radiosurgery as a primary treatment for prolactinomas. J Neurosurg 93(Suppl 3):10–13, 2000.
21. Landolt AM, Lomax N: Gamma knife radiosurgery for prolactinomas. J Neurosurg 93(Suppl 3):14–18, 2000.

22. Sheehan JP, Kondziolka D, Flickinger J, et al: Radiosurgery for residual or recurrent nonfunctioning pituitary adenoma. J Neurosurg 97(Suppl 5): 408–414, 2002.
23. Pollock BE, Carpenter PC: Stereotactic radiosurgery as an alternative to fractionated radiotherapy for patients with recurrent or residual nonfunctioning adenomas. Neurosurgery 53:1086–1094, 2003.
24. Wowra B, Stummer W: Efficacy of gamma knife radiosurgery for nonfunctioning pituitary adenomas: A quantitative follow-up with magnetic resonance imaging-based volumetric analysis. J Neurosurg 97(Suppl 5):429–432, 2002.
25. Vladyka V, Liscak R, Novotny J Jr, et al: Radiation tolerance of functioning pituitary tissue in gamma knife surgery for pituitary adenomas. Neurosurgery 52:309–316, 2003.
26. Hayashi M, Taira T, Chernov M, et al: Gamma knife surgery for cancer pain—pituitary gland-stalk ablation: A multicenter prospective protocol since 2002. J Neurosurg 97(Suppl 5):433–437, 2002.
27. Inoue HK, Fujimaki H, Kohga H, et al: Basal interhemispheric supra- and/or infrachiasmal approaches via superomedial orbitotomy for hypothalamic lesions: Preservation of hypothalamo-pituitary functions in combination treatment with radiosurgery. Childs Nerv Syst 13:250–256, 1997.

28. Leber KA, Berglöff J, Pendl G: Dose-response tolerance of the visual pathways and cranial nerves of the cavernous sinus to stereotactic radiosurgery. J Neurosurg 88:43–50, 1998.
29. Backlund EO: Treatment of craniopharyngiomas: The multimodality approach. Pediatr Neurosurg 21(Suppl 1):82–89, 1994.
30. Backlund EO, Axelsson B, Bergstrand CG, et al: Treatment of craniopharyngiomas: The stereotactic approach in a ten to twenty-three years' perspective. I: Surgical, radiological and ophthalmological aspects. Acta Neurochir 99:11–19, 1989.
31. Sääf M, Thorén M, Bergstrand CG, et al: Treatment of craniopharyngiomas: The stereotactic approach in a ten to twenty-three years' perspective. II: Psychosocial situation and pituitary function. Acta Neurochir 99:97–103, 1989.
32. Chiou SM, Lunsford LD, Niranjan A, et al: Stereotactic radiosurgery of residual or recurrent craniopharyngioma, after surgery, with or without radiation therapy. Neurooncol 3:159–166, 2001.
33. Pollock BE, Natt N, Schomberg PJ: Stereotactic management of craniopharyngiomas. Stereotact Funct Neurosurg 79:25–32, 2002.

24

Endocrinologic Approach to the Evaluation and Management of the Patient Undergoing Surgery for a Pituitary Tumor

JESSICA KOCH DEVIN and LEWIS S. BLEVINS, JR.

Pituitary tumors, unlike other intracranial neoplasms, pose a unique challenge to neurosurgeons because of their location adjacent to important structures and because they originate from a hormone-producing gland. Not only are pituitary tumors associated with mass effects, such as visual field abnormalities, cranial nerve palsies, and hormone deficiencies, but they also may cause increased morbidity due to excess hormone secretion. The neurosurgeon's task in the management of these tumors is not only to decompress the tumors and relieve mass effects, but also to preserve pituitary function and to attempt to resolve any syndromes that have occurred due to hormone hypersecretion.

In this chapter we will review the nonsurgical aspects of pituitary tumors so that neurosurgeons and other health care providers can better understand the nuances of the endocrine approach to the patient with a newly diagnosed tumor and the management of these patients in the perioperative and postoperative periods. A thorough understanding of this information will prepare the neurosurgeon to interact with the team of professionals usually involved in the management of these often complex patients.

PREOPERATIVE ENDOCRINE EVALUATION AND MANAGEMENT OF PATIENTS WITH PITUITARY TUMORS

Pituitary tumors account for 15% of all intracranial neoplasms. Whereas as many as 27% of autopsied pituitaries have been demonstrated to harbor a small pituitary tumor, clinically apparent tumors are evident in approximately 18 per 100,000 persons.[1] Nonfunctioning or clinically silent tumors make up approximately one third of all pituitary adenomas; a majority of these are gonadotroph adenomas. Prolactinomas account for roughly 30% of all pituitary tumors. Adrenocorticotrophic hormone (ACTH)–secreting and growth hormone (GH)–secreting neoplasms account for 15% and 20% of pituitary tumors, respectively, and thyrotropin (TSH)-secreting tumors account for 1%.[2-4]

Between 70% and 90% of patients with pituitary macroadenomas have deficiencies in one or more pituitary hormones at the time of presentation. The rates are much lower in cases of microadenomas.[3] The most common deficiencies involve GH and the gonadotropins, but clinically important ACTH and TSH deficiencies also occur.[5] Central diabetes insipidus (DI) is present in only about 2% of patients with pituitary tumors at the time of presentation.[3] The critical endocrinologic issues in the preoperative period that must be addressed to proceed with treatment planning include determining whether a tumor is functional and if there are any anterior or posterior pituitary hormone deficiencies that require immediate attention and treatment.

Hypopituitarism

The symptoms and signs of hypopituitarism are often vague and nonspecific. We usually recommend screening tests rather than dynamic tests to evaluate the adequacy of pituitary function before surgery. This approach saves both time and money and is designed to permit the identification of patients who require the initiation of hormone replacement in the preoperative period. We include assessment of the serum free thyroxine (T_4) level, serum TSH, and the low-dose ACTH (cosyntropin; Cortrosyn) stimulated cortisol secretion in all patients with pituitary tumors. Other studies, including serum insulin-like growth factor-1 (IGF-1), serum prolactin (PRL), serum luteinizing hormone (LH) and follicle-stimulating hormone (FSH) levels, and serum testosterone and estradiol levels, are done when clinically indicated. In most cases, however, a full investigation is conducted to ascertain the baseline pretreatment function of the pituitary gland. Table 24-1 addresses the signs and symptoms of hypopituitarism, along with the diagnosis and treatment pertinent to each hormone deficiency.

Central Adrenal Insufficiency

The low-dose ACTH stimulation test has become the dynamic test of choice when evaluating patients at risk for central adrenal insufficiency. The pool of endogenous ACTH stored within the pituitary gland is approximately 600 µg. It is no surprise, then, that the standard dose of ACTH, 250 µg, would overwhelm the adrenal glands.

TABLE 24-1 ▪ **Diagnosis and Treatment of Hypopituitarism**

Deficiency	Signs and Symptoms	Diagnosis	Treatment
Growth hormone (GH)	Fatigue, weight gain, decreased exercise endurance, poor sense of well-being, osteoporosis, hyperlipidemia	• Arginine-GHRH-stimulated GH < 9.5 μg/L • Screening serum IGF-1 below the normal range or in lower quartile of the lower range • Acipomox-GHRH stimulated GH < 11 μg/L	• Daily SC injections, starting at 0.4 mg/day • Titrate at 6- to 8-week intervals to IGF-1 within upper half-normal age and sex-specific range • Contraindicated in presence of tumor
ACTH	Nausea, anorexia, weight loss, fatigue and malaise; hyponatremia and hypoglycemia; hypotension unresponsive to fluids or pressors	• Serum cortisol in AM <5 μg/dL • Low-dose ACTH stimulated cortisol < 18 μg/dL at 30 minutes • Hypoglycemia-induced cortisol < 20 μg/dL	• Oral hydrocortisone 15–30 mg/day, in divided doses, with two thirds given in the AM *or* • Dexamethasone 0.125 to 0.375 mg qhs
TSH	Weight gain, fatigue, constipation, menorrhagia, cold intolerance, dry skin, bradycardia, delayed relaxation phase of deep tendon reflexes	Serum free T_4 in lower quartile of normal range or below the lower limit of normal	• 0.8 μg/pound ideal body weight of oral L-thyroxine • 25–50 μg qd in elderly or those with cardiovascular disease • Titrate dose to serum free T_4 in upper one half of normal range
LH, FSH	Mood swings, impotence, vaginal dryness, hot flashes, decreased libido, osteoporosis	• LH, FSH • Serum free testosterone in men • Serum estradiol in women	• Cyclic estrogen and progesterone in premenopausal women • Testosterone injections, gel, and patches; titrate to free testosterone in upper one half normal range • Not replaced preoperatively

ACTH, adrenocorticotropic hormone; FSH, follicle-stimulating hormone; GHRH, growth hormone–releasing hormone; IGF-1, insulin-like growth factor-1; LH, luteinizing hormone; TSH, thyrotropin.

Patients with partial ACTH deficiency will secrete enough ACTH to maintain their adrenal glands, such that they will provide an adequate cortisol response when exposed to this supraphysiologic stimulus. The standard Cortrosyn test may thus underdiagnose hypoadrenalism. The 1 μg used in the low-dose test provides a much more physiologic stimulus. In fact, normal individuals respond similarly to the 1- and 250-μg doses. Studies have shown that the results from the 1-μg dose test better correlate with the results from the insulin-induced hypoglycemia test.[6]

The low-dose ACTH stimulation test is performed by adding 250 μg of ACTH to 250 mL of 0.9% saline and then removing 1 mL of this solution for intravenous injection. A serum cortisol level is obtained 30 minutes after injection. A cortisol level less than 18 μg/dL indicates compromised adrenal function in patients with pituitary diseases and identifies patients who should be treated with glucocorticoids before surgery.[6]

Replacement for adrenal insufficiency should begin as soon as the diagnosis is made. An acceptable short-term outpatient regimen would involve the administration of hydrocortisone, 15 to 30 mg/day in divided doses until the day of surgery. Alternatively, patients could be treated with dexamethasone 0.25 mg orally at bedtime.[2,7]

Central Hypothyroidism

Measurement of the serum TSH is of limited value in patients with pituitary tumors, because the result in patients with central hypothyroidism may be low, normal, or even slightly elevated. We do, however, believe it is useful to measure TSH in patients with pituitary tumors to identify the occasional patient with severe primary hypothyroidism who presents with modest hyperprolactinemia, as well as lactotroph and thyrotroph hyperplasia, thus mimicking a pituitary tumor. Free T_4 levels that are either in the lower quartile of the normal range or else below the lower limit of the normal range should prompt the initiation of L-thyroxine replacement before surgery. Appropriate treatment will decrease the likelihood of perioperative morbidity due to hypothyroidism. Perioperative problems encountered in untreated hypothyroid patients include delayed clearance of anesthetic agents, electrolyte abnormalities, poor responses to factors that increase ventilatory drive, neuropsychiatric disturbances, ileus, and a bleeding diathesis.

Thyroid hormone replacement is best accomplished by providing oral L-thyroxine on a daily basis. If hormone replacement is required, it is most important to provide glucocorticoid replacement, if needed, before thyroid replacement so as to avoid precipitation of an adrenal crisis secondary to increased metabolism of cortisol.[2] Although there are numerous caveats to the proper dosing of thyroid hormone, in general, suitable replacement can be accomplished by administering 0.8 μg of L-thyroxine per pound of ideal body weight. Older patients and those with established or suspected cardiovascular disease should be started on 25 to 50 μg daily. If hypothyroidism is severe and the need for surgery is deemed urgent, and there are no contraindications to rapid replacement, then L-thyroxine,

200 to 400 μg, should be administered intravenously on one occasion. Thereafter, 85% of the calculated oral daily dose can be administered intravenously on a daily basis until the patient is taking oral medications.

Central Hypogonadism

Hypogonadism can often be detected by obtaining a careful history from the patient with pituitary disease. LH, FSH, free testosterone levels in men, and estradiol levels in women, are often useful to confirm clinically suspected sex steroid deficiency. Treatment is rarely necessary before surgery. Furthermore, oral estrogen replacement may contribute to the risk of perioperative deep vein thrombosis and, thus, treatment should be withheld until after surgery.[2]

Growth Hormone Deficiency

Finally, an IGF-1 (somatomedin-C) level is useful as a screening tool for GH deficiency. Treatment is not indicated before surgery, because GH is contraindicated in the presence of any tumor or malignancy.

Hormone Hypersecretion

Prolactinoma

The serum PRL level should be determined in all patients with pituitary tumors. Several clinically important disorders may account for hyperprolactinemia. Box 24-1 outlines the

---

BOX 24-1	*Differential Diagnosis of Hyperprolactinemia*

Pituitary Tumors

Prolactinoma
GH/PRL-secreting adenoma
Acidophil stem adenoma

Drugs

Antihypertensives (methyldopa, reserpine, verapamil)
Antipsychotics (phenothiazines, butyrophenones)
Antidepressants (tricyclics)
Narcotics (morphine and heroin)
Metoclopramide
Oral contraceptives (estrogen)

Pituitary Stalk Disorders

"Stalk effect" secondary to sellar mass
Infiltrative disease:
   Langerhans cell histiocytosis
   Sarcoidosis
   Tuberculosis
   Metastatic disease (breast, lung, lymphoma)
Stalk Section:
   Iatrogenic secondary surgery
   Basal skull fracture
   Facial trauma

Miscellaneous

Idiopathic
Hypothyroidism
Chronic disease (liver and renal)
Physiologic (stress, pregnancy, nursing, exercise, sleep)
Neurogenic (spinal cord tumors and chest wall injury)

---

differential diagnosis of hyperprolactinemia. Prolactinomas account for 30% to 50% of all endocrinologically active pituitary neoplasms. The majority of these tumors are microadenomas, and they are more common in women. Macroadenomas are more common in men. The risk of progression from a microadenoma to a macroadenoma has been estimated to be approximately 7% over a 6-year period. Estrogen administration and pregnancy may lead to rapid and dramatic growth of these tumors.[4] The signs and symptoms associated with hyperprolactinemia are displayed in Table 24-2.

Prolactin levels are weakly correlated with the size of the pituitary tumor. PRL levels in excess of 200 μg/L almost always indicate the presence of a prolactinoma, regardless of the size of the pituitary tumor. Microprolactinomas are often associated with PRL levels less than 150 μg/L. A macroadenoma associated with a PRL level in this range is usually either a tumor that secretes prolactin or a tumor producing the "stalk effect," by interfering with the delivery of the PRL-inhibitory factor, dopamine, to the normal lactotrophs. A diagnosis of severe primary hypothyroidism should be considered in all patients with hyperprolactinemia. All amenorrheic women with hyperprolactinemia should be evaluated for pregnancy unless they are castrated. The clinical laboratory should be asked to dilute the sample for measurement of the serum PRL to avoid the scenario known as the "hook effect." On account of the characteristics of the radioimmunoassay test for prolactin, patients with very high serum PRL levels may be misidentified as having normal or low PRL levels if the samples sent for PRL measurement are not diluted at the time of testing.[4]

Cushing's Disease

ACTH-secreting pituitary tumors (Cushing's disease) account for approximately 70% to 80% of all cases of Cushing's syndrome and for 15% of all pituitary adenomas in adults. Most patients harbor microadenomas; only 10%

TABLE 24-2 ■ Clinical Features of the Pituitary Tumor Endocrinopathies

Disorder	Signs and Symptoms
Cushing's disease	Moon facies, buffalo hump, supraclavicular fullness, purple striae, central obesity, proximal muscle weakness, ecchymosis, osteopenia, hypertension, insulin resistance
Acromegaly	Skeletal and soft-tissue overgrowth, carpal tunnel syndrome, hyperhidrosis, hypertension, congestive heart failure, obstructive sleep apnea, insulin resistance, increased prevalence of colorectal cancer
TSH adenoma	Goiter, moist skin, palmar erythema, weight loss, resting tachycardia, palpitations, menstrual irregularities, insomnia, fine tremor, brisk deep tendon reflexes
Prolactinoma	Menstrual irregularities in females, infertility, decreased libido, impotence, galactorrhea, weight gain

TSH, thyrotropin.
Adapted from reference 4.

to 20% of patients have macroadenomas.[2,4] Table 24-2 outlines the clinical signs and symptoms suggestive of Cushing's syndrome.

Screening tests that are useful when an evaluation for Cushing's disease is warranted include a 24-hour urine free cortisol (UFC), the overnight 1-mg dexamethasone suppression test, and a salivary cortisol profile to assess the diurnal secretion of cortisol. A 24-hour UFC result that is greater than three times the upper limit of normal for the assay performed is highly suggestive of a diagnosis of hypercortisolism. Results that are elevated to a lesser degree require confirmatory tests. The specificity of the overnight 1-mg dexamethasone suppression test is approximately 70%; therefore, an 8 AM serum cortisol greater than 5 μg/dL following the administration of 1 mg dexamethasone at 11 PM the preceding night should prompt the performance of confirmatory tests. Loss of the diurnal variation of cortisol secretion, as demonstrated by measurements of the salivary cortisol at different times throughout the 24-hour period, indicates a high likelihood of pathologic hypercortisolism. Confirmatory tests, such as the dexamethasone-suppressed corticotropin-releasing hormone (CRH) stimulation test and the formal 2-day low-dose dexamethasone suppression test, should be conducted by a qualified endocrinologist.[2,4]

A plasma ACTH level must always be measured to narrow the differential diagnosis of hypercortisolism. A high or inappropriately normal plasma ACTH level suggests either a pituitary or ectopic source of ACTH secretion. Tests used to distinguish between the two include inferior petrosal sinus sampling, the formal 2-day high-dose dexamethasone suppression test, the overnight metyrapone test, and the CRH stimulation test. These tests should be conducted and interpreted by an endocrinologist.[4] Box 24-2 details the differential diagnosis of Cushing's syndrome.

Approximately 10% of normal individuals with no obvious evidence of pituitary disease will be found to have inhomogeneous regions in their pituitary glands on magnetic resonance imaging (MRI) thought to represent a small pituitary tumor. Pituitary-dedicated MRI is able to detect a tumor in approximately two thirds of patients with

---

BOX 24-2 *Differential Diagnosis of Cushing's Syndrome*

ACTH Dependent

Pituitary
ACTH-secreting pituitary adenoma
Corticotroph hyperplasia, secondary to CRH-producing tumor

Ectopic
Bronchial carcinoid
Thymic carcinoid
Small cell bronchogenic carcinoma
Medullary thyroid carcinoma
Pheochromocytoma

ACTH Independent

Benign adrenal adenoma
Primary pigmented nodular dysplasia (Carney complex)
Adrenocortical carcinoma
Macronodular adrenal hyperplasia

Iatrogenic

Cushing's disease. Thus patients with clinical and biochemical features of hypercortisolism with suspected microadenomas and or "normal pituitary" findings on MRI should be further evaluated with the aforementioned tests so as to correctly diagnose their underlying disease process.[4]

Acromegaly

Growth hormone–secreting pituitary tumors account for 10% to 20% of all pituitary tumors. Macroadenomas are seen in 75% of patients. Successful therapy of this disease is important; the overall survival is decreased by an average of 10 years in patients with active disease when compared with age-matched controls. These patients are also at risk for morbidity due to cardiac hypertrophy, hypertension, sleep apnea, and development of other neoplasms such as colon carcinoma. Normal life expectancy can be restored by reducing GH levels to less than 2.5 μg/L and normalization of the IGF-1 level.[4,8] Table 24-2 discusses the clinical signs and symptoms characteristic of acromegaly.

In most cases, measurement of the serum IGF-1 level is sufficient to make a diagnosis in the proper clinical setting. Not only is the oral glucose suppression test valuable in confirming the diagnosis of inappropriate secretion of GH, but it may also provide a presurgical assessment of GH suppression by glucose for comparison with postoperative values.[2] The test is performed by oral administration of 75 g glucose solution and measurement of serum GH levels at 30-minute intervals for 2 hours. In normal individuals, GH levels fall below 2 μg/L when the standard radioimmunoassay is used and to less than 1 μg/L when the ultrasensitive immunoradiometric or immunochemiluminometric assays are used. Results exceeding these cutoffs in the clinical scenario of acromegalic features and a pituitary tumor confirm a diagnosis of acromegaly due to a GH-secreting pituitary tumor. The preoperative evaluation should also include serum PRL, TSH, ACTH, and alpha subunit level, in that 30% to 40% of these tumors are plurihormonal (i.e., they secrete more than one hormone).[4]

Gonadotroph Adenomas

Gonadotroph adenomas account for 70% of the nonfunctioning or clinically silent pituitary tumors. The differential diagnosis of nonfunctioning pituitary tumors is given in Box 24-3. The measurements of FSH, LH, and alpha subunit levels permit one to detect identify the rare functional gonadotroph adenomas. Pituitary hyperplasia, in the setting of elevated LH and FSH levels secondary to gonadal failure, may mimic a pituitary tumor. An elevated LH and FSH in a hypogonadal patient with a pituitary mass lesion accompanied by other pituitary hormone deficits is good clinical evidence in support of a diagnosis of a gonadotroph adenoma. Additionally, the alpha subunit level is often elevated in patients with gonadotroph adenomas.[1,4]

Hyperthyroidism

Thyrotropin adenomas account for 1% to 2% of all pituitary tumors.[3,4] A vast majority of these tumors are macroadenomas. Affected patients are usually hyperthyroid and have a diffuse goiter. Features of thyrotoxic Grave's disease including ophthalmopathy, pretibial myxedema, and acropachy are absent.[9,10] Clinical features suggestive of a TSH adenoma are illustrated in Table 24-2.

BOX 24-3 *Nonfunctional Pituitary Adenomas*

Gonadotropin-Secreting Pituitary Tumor

Null-Cell Adenoma

Clinically Silent Hormone-Producing Adenoma

Benign Neoplasms

Craniopharyngioma
Meningioma
Chordoma
Germ cell tumor
Rathke's cleft cyst

Malignant Neoplasms

Lymphoma
Metastatic disease (breast and lung)
Pituitary carcinoma

Infiltrative Diseases

Sarcoidosis
Lymphocytic hypophysitis
Granulomatous hypophysitis

These tumors are characterized biochemically by increased serum free T_4 concentrations and an inappropriately normal or elevated serum TSH level. Most of the tumors secrete TSH alone or in combination with the alpha subunit, and some may also secrete PRL and GH. Thus a baseline evaluation should consist of measurements of the serum concentrations of TSH, free T_4, free T_3, alpha subunit, PRL, and GH.[4]

It is important to distinguish patients with TSH-secreting adenomas from those with isolated pituitary resistance or generalized resistance to thyroid hormone. These disorders may also present with elevated thyroid hormone levels and inappropriately normal or elevated TSH levels. A useful method to confirm the presence of a TSH-secreting tumor is to calculate the molar ratio of alpha subunit to TSH: (alpha subunit [nmol/L])/(serum TSH [μIU/L]) $\times$ 10. This ratio is equimolar in patients with pituitary resistance or hyperthyroidism; however, the ratio exceeds 1.0 in approximately 80% of patients with TSH-secreting adenomas.[1,4]

PERIOPERATIVE ENDOCRINE EVALUATION AND MANAGEMENT OF PATIENTS WITH PITUITARY TUMORS

Transsphenoidal or transcranial surgery is a great time of change for patients with pituitary tumors. Successful resection of hormone-secreting tumors can result in prompt changes in physiology that often need medical attention. Injury to the anterior pituitary may result in hypopituitarism, whereas injury to the posterior pituitary or stalk may result in DI. Preexisting hypopituitarism may improve or even resolve. Furthermore, there are potential immediate complications of pituitary surgery. All treating physicians must be on the alert to identify and treat these as promptly as possible to decrease the risks of permanent morbidity and mortality. A team approach to the perioperative evaluation and management of the patient having pituitary surgery is ideal, so that patients are offered the best health possible during this phase of their illness.

Nonendocrine Morbidity and Mortality

Complications of pituitary surgery are, fortunately, somewhat rare. Because of their seriousness, treated patients must be evaluated for them on an ongoing basis both during and after their hospitalization for surgery. Complications of transsphenoidal surgery, quoted in a series of 185 operations involving 165 patients, included nasal perforation (7.6%), permanent DI (3.8%), donor site hematoma (2.2%), residual tumor hemorrhage (1.6%), ophthalmoplegia (1.1%), loss of vision (1.1%), meningitis (0.5%), and sinusitis (0.5%).[11] Other studies have showed that the rate of complications is higher when the surgical procedures are performed by inexperienced neurosurgeons.[12] Furthermore, vascular catastrophe may result from injury to the carotid arteries and even the vertebrobasilar system. We have seen at least one or more instances of thrombotic cerebrovascular accident, myocardial infarction, and deep vein thrombosis with pulmonary embolism. Visual loss is usually permanent, yet we have seen an occasional young patient who has regained sight. The presence of postoperative headache and fever should include an evaluation for meningitis and sinusitis in addition to the usual causes of fever in patients postoperatively. Meningitis and sinusitis often develop after hospital discharge; thus it is important for treating physicians to include them in the differential diagnosis when patients call from home complaining of headaches, systemic symptoms, lassitude, and fever.

Tension pneumocephalus is an interesting but unfortunate complication of transsphenoidal surgery. This disorder often presents with change in mental status, headache, seizure, cranial nerve palsy, hypertension, and bradycardia. Risk factors include obstructive sleep apnea, positive pressure ventilation, resection of large sellar masses, postoperative cerebrospinal fluid leak, and insertion of a lumbar subarachnoid drain. The long-term outcome is usually favorable pending prompt recognition and treatment of this rare complication.[13]

Central Diabetes Insipidus

Polyuria is not uncommon after pituitary surgery. The differential diagnosis of polyuria should include central DI, hyperglycemia, diuresis characteristic of patients with acromegaly, and the diuresis of intraoperative and postoperative fluids.

Central DI is a polyuric state that results from an absolute or relative deficiency of arginine vasopressin (AVP). Ninety percent of the magnocellular neurons in the supraoptic and paraventricular nuclei, or their projections to the posterior pituitary, must be lost or damaged before DI becomes clinically apparent. The incidence of DI following pituitary surgery is 10% to 20% in patients with surgery limited to the sella. Postoperative DI may be seen in as many as 60% to 80% of patients with larger tumors and particularly in those with marked suprasellar extension of their tumors.[3,14] Postoperative DI is usually temporary but may be permanent in 3% of all patients who develop this disorder. Although most patients who have DI for more than 6 months after surgery can be expected to suffer from a permanent form of the disorder, occasional patients do indeed enjoy late resolution of their polyuric state.[2]

The cardinal features of DI include polyuria, defined as the passage of more than 30 mL of urine per kilogram of body weight in a 24-hour period, dehydration or plasma hyperosmolarity, and subsequent thirst with resultant polydipsia. In most cases, the polyuria is abrupt and characterized clinically by the passage of more than 200 to 300 mL of urine per hour. The polyuria is often accompanied by a corresponding rise in the serum sodium toward 145 mEq/L and a decline in the urine specific gravity to less than 1.005. A rise in the urine specific gravity in the setting of a normal serum sodium and polyuria should prompt consideration of hyperglycemia and glucosuria with an osmotic diuresis as the cause of the polyuria. Treating physicians should be aware that hypernatremia may also result from adipsic hypernatremia, renal dysfunction and nephrogenic DI, osmotic diarrhea, uncontrollable hyperhidrosis, mannitol administration, and the overzealous use of hypertonic saline.[3,14]

Diabetes insipidus after pituitary surgery can exhibit one of three patterns: transient, permanent, or triphasic. In most affected patients, the onset of DI is within 24 to 48 hours of surgery. Transient DI accounts for 50% to 60% of all cases following pituitary surgery. It is characterized by an abrupt onset of polyuria and polydipsia within the first postoperative day and typically resolves within several days to weeks. Minor injury to the neurohypophysis during surgery that leads to inhibition of AVP release probably accounts for this disorder.[3,14]

Permanent DI has an abrupt onset but does not resolve within 6 months and requires lifelong treatment. This form of the disorder is thought to be due to direct damage to either the neurohypophyseal stalk or the hypothalamus. It is most often seen in patients who have had extensive resections of the sellar contents and trauma to suprasellar structures. Some patients may notice an improvement in their symptoms over several years.[3,14]

The triphasic pattern or response is characterized by an initial phase consisting of polyuria and polydipsia, followed by an interphase consisting of a period of antidiuresis and often hyponatremia, and a third phase characterized by permanent or prolonged DI. Figure 24-1 illustrates the triphasic pattern of postoperative DI. The first phase, during which the patient experiences an abrupt increase in urine volume coupled with a fall in urine osmolality, lasts approximately 4 to 5 days. This phase is believed to be due to injury-related neuronal shock and inhibition of AVP release. The interphase typically lasts 5 to 7 days and occurs approximately 1 week after surgery. In this time period urine output abruptly decreases and urine osmolality rises. Severe hypotonic hyponatremia may occur. The urine sodium excretion is usually greater then 40 mEq/L and the serum uric acid is usually low, reflective of renal losses. Symptoms may include nausea, headache, anorexia, and, rarely, obtundation and seizures. These nonspecific manifestations often first become apparent after hospital discharge, and treating physicians should be aware of this complication to direct an appropriate evaluation. The interphase is believed to result from the leakage of AVP from injured and dying magnocellular neurons. The final phase of DI occurs when the neurons have fully degenerated and AVP deficiency becomes clinically apparent because of a resultant deficiency of AVP-producing neurons. Occasional patients enjoy resolution of their interphase without experiencing DI, because a sufficient number of functioning neurons withstand the surgical insult and respond appropriately to changes in plasma osmolarity.[3,14]

The treatment of perioperative DI most commonly involves the administration of aqueous vasopressin (Pitressin) followed by DDAVP (desmopressin acetate, a synthetic analogue of AVP). We prefer to use aqueous vasopressin for the short-term in-hospital management of DI, particularly when it is expected that the DI may be transient. Most patients require a dose of 5 units SC every 6 to 8 hours. We do not write standing orders for aqueous vasopressin but instead choose to administer the drug on an as-needed basis after repeated confirmation that DI persists and ongoing therapy is required.

In patients who still have DI before anticipated discharge, and especially when the interphase of the triphasic response is not expected, we may choose to use subcutaneous DDAVP to control the polyuria. A single dose of DDAVP often exerts an immediate effect and often lasts as long as 8 to 16 hours. A 1-µg dose of DDAVP administered subcutaneously is almost always sufficient to control symptoms. The dose can be adjusted as indicated based on the clinical response.

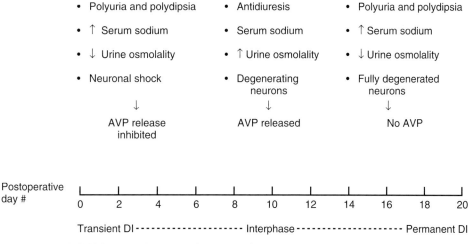

FIGURE 24-1 The triphasic pattern of postoperative diabetes insipidus.

TABLE 24-3 ▪ **Treatment of Central Diabetes Insipidus**

Formulation	Dosage	Use	Advantages	Disadvantages
Vasopressin (Pitressin)	5 units SC q6–8h prn	Postoperative transient DI	• Immediate bioavailability • Short duration of action	• Reaction at injection site • Anti-AVP antibodies
DDAVP, SQ	1 µg SC prn	Postoperative	Immediate bioavailability	Reaction at injection site
DDAVP, spray	10 µg/spray; 1 spray qhs to 1 spray bid	Maintenance medication	Ease of administration	Delivers fixed dose
DDAVP, Rhinal tube	5 µg qhs, up to 20 µg/day in divided doses	Maintenance medication	Allows for variable dosing	• Formulation requires refrigeration • Administration more complex
DDAVP, oral tablets	0.1 to 0.3 mg PO bid-tid	Maintenance medication	• Ease of administration • Alternative when nasal route not feasible	• Erratic bioavailability • May require large doses to achieve effect

AVP, arginine vasopressin; DDAVP, desmopressin acetate; DI, diabetes insipidus.

Lower doses are often needed in the elderly patient, whereas some younger patients require 2 µg to resolve polyuria. Once again, we do not permit administration of a subsequent dose until there is sufficient evidence that DI persists. This approach allows one to identify patients with transient DI. Patients with DI should be permitted free access to water so that they can ingest water in response to thirst and defend against dehydration. Symptoms and signs should always guide vasopressin replacement so as to avoid overtreatment and the danger of hyponatremia.

If DI persists at the time of discharge, and once nasal packs have been removed, patients may change to the DDAVP nasal spray or the calibrated rhinal tube formulation. An adequate initial dose via the rhinal tube formulation is 5 µg given intranasally at bedtime. The dose can then be titrated up by 5-µg increments to a total of 20 µg/day, usually in two divided doses. The nasal spray delivers a dose of 10 µg per spray; most patients require one spray at bedtime, although some may also require a dose in the morning for effective control of symptoms. DDAVP tablets are rarely used to treat central DI because of their erratic bioavailability and the need for large dose requirements. A typical dosage regimen would be 0.1 to 0.3 mg orally two to three times a day. Potential side effects of DDAVP therapy include nausea, diarrhea, and abdominal cramps. Table 24-3 outlines the different treatments available for DI.

One of the great dangers facing the patient who is discharged with a prescription for DDAVP is the triphasic response. We have seen patients who entered the interphase and continued their DDAVP and, as a result, developed severe life-threatening hyponatremia. For this reason, patients must be educated about the signs and symptoms of hyponatremia, asked to periodically hold their dose of DDAVP to permit return of polyuria, and to consider a postoperative visit 7 to 10 days after surgery to reassess their fluid and electrolyte status. Refer to Box 24-4 for an example of appropriate patient discharge instructions for patients who have undergone pituitary surgery.

Postoperative Hyponatremia

Postoperative hyponatremia can be due to several clinically important disorders. A reasonable differential diagnosis would include an isolated interphase of the so-called triphasic response, syndrome of inappropriate antidiuretic hormone as a result of infection, central nervous system trauma or meningitis, overzealous administration of hypotonic fluids or DDAVP, and cerebral salt wasting. Other important endocrine disorders that should be considered include pseudo-hyponatremia due to hyperglycemia, hypothyroidism, and most importantly in these patients, cortisol deficiency as a result of central adrenal insufficiency. Glucocorticoids inhibit the synthesis and secretion of AVP, and thus glucocorticoid deficiency can result in elevated levels of AVP. Hypothyroidism decreases cardiac output and free-water clearance. Cerebral salt wasting is characterized by a natriuresis and hypovolemia and is most commonly associated with subarachnoid disease.[3,7]

The treatment of postoperative hyponatremia is guided by a careful consideration of the differential diagnosis and consideration of the final diagnosis. Glucocorticoids or L-thyroxine might be all that is required to remedy the hyponatremia. Cerebral salt wasting is treated by aggressive volume replacement with saline and the transfusion of whole blood if anemia is present.

Most cases of inappropriate vasopressin release respond to fluid restriction. We typically restrict the oral and intravenous intake of fluids to 500 mL less than the estimated 24-hour urine output. Severe symptomatic hyponatremia associated with a rapid decline in serum sodium to less than 120 mmol/L requires immediate treatment. Hypertonic saline should be administered at a rate no greater than 0.01 mL/kg body weight per minute to allow for a serum sodium concentration correction at a rate no greater than 0.5 mmol/L/hour until serum sodium concentration is at least 120 mmol/L. It may be reasonable to raise the serum sodium at a rate of 1 to 2 mmol/L per hour in patients with acute symptomatic hyponatremia and marked central nervous system symptoms. Normal saline in combination with furosemide may be administered judiciously in some patients when there are little if any symptoms attributed to the hyponatremia. We prefer fluid restriction as the sole approach to management when the serum sodium concentration exceeds 125 mEq/L. The fluid restriction is lifted when the serum sodium exceeds 132 mEq/L or when there is clinical evidence of DI. The sudden occurrence of DI heralding the third phase of

<table>
<tr><td>

BOX 24-4 *Discharge Instructions for Patients Who Have Undergone Pituitary Surgery*

</td></tr>
</table>

Your physicians have determined that it is reasonably safe to discharge you from the hospital following transsphenoidal pituitary surgery. Several important situations may arise, however, following discharge, and you should be aware of these. The following general guidelines are provided to promote your health and safety.

Headache, facial, and sinus pain are not uncommon following pituitary surgery. As you may have noted, the pain and discomfort typically improve on a daily basis following surgery. If you should experience a worsening of your pain or discomfort, please contact your neurosurgeon immediately.

Worsening headache, fever, chills, yellowish green nasal discharge, and neck stiffness may all signify an infectious process complicating your surgery. You should notify your neurosurgeon, endocrinologist, or primary physician immediately should any of these symptoms and signs develop.

Persistent bloody, clear watery, or yellowish green nasal discharge should prompt an immediate call to one of your physicians.

Development of abnormalities in your vision should prompt an urgent call to your neurosurgeon, neuro-opthalmologist, or any other one of your physicians.

Chest pain or discomfort, shortness of breath, swelling of one or both of your legs, and passage of dark black tarry stools may represent medical complications in patients who undergo surgery of any type. Contact your physicians should any of these symptoms or signs occur.

Some patients develop disorders of salt and water metabolism following pituitary surgery. Headache, nausea, vomiting, confusion, impaired concentration, and muscle aches might be due to hyponatremia (low blood sodium levels). This disorder typically occurs 7 to 10 days after surgery and is more common in patients who have had surgery for Cushing's disease. If you develop these symptoms, contact your endocrinologist or one of your other physicians immediately. Excessive urination, thirst, and the need to ingest large quantities of fluids might be related to the onset of diabetes insipidus or diabetes mellitus. These disorders put you at risk for dehydration. The symptoms require urgent evaluation and determination of the underlying cause so that appropriate treatment may be given. Thus, if these symptoms develop, contact your endocrinologist or one of your other physicians immediately.

You may or may not have been prescribed hormones at the time of discharge. If so, you should take these medications, without interruption, as prescribed by your physician. Adjustments in your glucocorticoid hormone dosage may be required if you become ill. In general, you should double your dose of glucocorticoids if you have fever greater than 100.5°F. If you are unable to take your medications by mouth because of nausea, you should go to the nearest emergency room to receive intravenous stress-dose steroids. Additionally, you may be asked to withhold your dose of glucocorticoid replacement at the time of your first postoperative follow-up visit. Above all, contact your physicians if you have any questions whatsoever about any of these matters or if you should become ill.

In general, the first postoperative follow-up visit will be scheduled to occur 4 weeks after surgery. If problems develop before that time, you will be asked to return to the office for evaluation. Subsequent follow-up is tailored to the individual needs of each patient and in part depends on the diagnosis, presence of residual disease, likelihood of recurrent disease, extent and type of hormonal disorders, and other complications of pituitary disease. In most cases, lifelong follow-up is necessary. You should ensure that you receive appropriate follow-up by physicians knowledgeable regarding the diagnosis and management of pituitary disorders.

the triphasic response may result in rather dramatic and potentially dangerous rapid increases in the serum sodium concentration. Therapy with aqueous vasopressin is often required to control the rate of rise of the serum sodium concentration, even in patients who still have hyponatremia. We recommend avoidance of DDAVP in this setting until it can be determined whether the DI will persist.

Treatment of Presumed Central Adrenal Insufficiency

All patients undergoing pituitary surgery, including those with documented central adrenal insufficiency, should be treated as if their hypothalamic-pituitary-adrenal (HPA) function either has been or will remain compromised. We recommend intravenous injection of hydrocortisone, 50 mg, on the morning of surgery and at the time of anesthesia induction. We also recommend the administration of hydrocortisone, 50 to 100 mg, at the conclusion of the procedure. Thereafter, we administer hydrocortisone, 50 mg, at 8-hour intervals for 1 to 2 days. Provided the patient is recuperating satisfactorily, we aim to decrease the hydrocortisone dose to 25 mg IV every 8 hours on postoperative day 2 or 3. Once patients are able to take oral medications, and provided their postoperative course is uncomplicated, we prescribe hydrocortisone 20 mg PO each morning and 10 mg PO taken in the middle of the afternoon. All patients, with the notable exception of those with Cushing's syndrome for whom surgery has failed, are discharged on this dose of hydrocortisone. Our patients are asked to withhold their hydrocortisone for 24 hours just before their first postoperative visit to permit a laboratory assessment of the adequacy of their adrenal reserve.[2,7]

The Patient with Hormone Hypersecretion

Hyperthyroidism

Most patients with TSH-secreting adenomas require attention to their hyperthyroid state before surgery to decrease the likelihood of thyroid storm. Methimazole and propylthiouracil are both antithyroid drugs that inhibit the production of thyroid hormone. One to three months of therapy are usually required to normalize thyroid hormone levels. Beta blockers and steroids are often necessary in patients with severe or refractory hyperthyroidism to minimize the potential for cardiac arrhythmias, congestive heart failure, and other consequences of thyroid storm.[3]

Cushing's Disease

The overall reported complication rate for pituitary surgery ranges from 3.3% to 9.3%. Patients with Cushing's disease are prone to several complications, and the reported complication rate ranges from 10% to 20%. Postoperative deep vein thrombosis occurs in 3.8% of patients with Cushing's. We encourage our patients to become mobile as soon as possible following surgery to prevent venous stasis. The use of low-molecular-weight heparin is standard unless there are any particular contraindications to this form of prophylaxis. Some groups also institute prophylactic aspirin therapy in the postoperative period.[15]

Cushing's patients are at increased risk for infections as a result of their relative degree of immunosupression due to hypercortisolemia and coexisting glucose intolerance. Importantly, patients with hypercortisolism may fail to manifest a febrile response to an infection. Thus a high index of suspicion is warranted when these patients have nonspecific complaints in the postoperative period.[15]

Patients with marked hypercortisolism who enjoy a dramatic fall in their cortisol levels after surgery are at risk for respiratory failure due to *Pneumocystis carinii* pneumonitis. Respiratory difficulty within the first couple of weeks should prompt an appropriate evaluation for this rare yet treatable complication; other respiratory complications that should be considered include pneumonia, pulmonary embolus, and volume overload.

Most patients also have diabetes mellitus that is exacerbated by the stress of surgery and the concomitant administration of glucocorticoids. The administration of short-acting and long-acting insulin is often required to normalize the blood glucose concentration. Attainment of normoglycemia promotes better wound healing, decreases the risk of an osmotic diuresis and dehydration, and decreases the likelihood of a perioperative infection. Metformin should be discontinued 48 hours before surgery in those patients treated with this drug. Other complications unique to these patients include poor wound healing and an increased risk of bleeding from the surgical site. Postoperative hyponatremia occurs in 10% of patients with Cushing's disease.

Finally, it is a common but not universal practice to administer perioperative glucocorticoids, as described earlier, to patients with Cushing's to treat an anticipated state of relative hypocortisolemia or central adrenal insufficiency following successful resection of an ACTH-secreting pituitary adenoma.[16]

Acromegaly

Occasional patients with acromegaly have diabetes mellitus as a consequence of GH hypersecretion. Many of them have glucose intolerance that is unmasked by the stress of surgery and the administration of supraphysiologic doses of glucocorticoids. These patients often require relatively high doses of insulin to normalize their serum glucose levels. Most patients with acromegaly who enjoy a rapid lowering of their GH levels will experience a diuresis of several liters of fluid beginning on the first postoperative day. Often, these patients are mistakenly thought to have DI. They require careful attention to the status of their fluid and electrolyte status to prevent the inappropriate administration of DDAVP. Approximately 80% of patients with acromegaly have sleep apnea.[17] This disorder may complicate the recovery from anesthesia and also the later postoperative period if nocturnal hypoventilation is not recognized and treated.

POSTOPERATIVE ENDOCRINE EVALUATION AND MANAGEMENT OF PATIENTS WITH PITUITARY TUMORS

Several important issues must be addressed in the postoperative phase of the evaluation and management of patients with pituitary tumors. First and foremost on the minds of the patient, the neurosurgeon, and other members of the health care team is whether the pituitary tumor has been successfully resected. One must also determine whether there is any evidence of clinically important hypopituitarism or DI that requires hormone replacement therapy. Furthermore, it is imperative to determine if any particular syndromes of hormone hypersecretion have resolved and also whether additional treatment may be indicated. We typically initiate the process of the postoperative evaluation 4 to 6 weeks after surgery unless there is a compelling reason to evaluate the patient sooner.[2,3]

Residual Tumor

We prefer to conduct a postoperative MRI scan to determine the degree of residual tumor at least 6 to 12 weeks after surgery. This delay permits resolution of any edema and other postoperative changes and facilitates recognition of residual tumor. Biochemical assessments guide our decisions regarding the timing of postoperative MRI scans in patients with hormonally active neoplasms. For example, a patient with a history of a microadenoma and Cushing's disease who demonstrates continued evidence of remission does not necessarily require a postoperative MRI. Depending on the clinical scenario, degree of residual tumor, adjuvant therapies, and the proliferative marker MIB-1 Labeling Index, we arrange for MRI assessment of the sella at 6- to 12-month intervals for a few years and then every couple of years thereafter. Patients with a history of hormonally active neoplasms do not undergo repeat imaging unless they have biochemical evidence of recurrent disease. Patient with a history of a nonfunctional adenoma are studied periodically throughout their lives because of the ever-present risk of tumor recurrence.

Hypopituitarism

Pituitary function may improve in patients with pituitary tumors following surgery. On the other hand, it may also worsen depending on whether there has been vascular or mechanical injury to the pituitary stalk or the gland itself. Those with panhypopituitarism rarely enjoy resolution of their hormone deficits. Arafah and colleagues reported recovery of pituitary function in several patients with pituitary adenomas.[7] Specifically, they noted recovery of TSH secretion in 57% of affected patients, recovery of ACTH secretion in 38%, recovery of gonadotropin secretion in 32%, and recovery of GH secretion in 5% of patients with preoperative hormone deficiencies.[5]

The incidence of postoperative hypopituitarism is much higher in patients previously treated with radiotherapy and in those who have undergone second surgical procedures. Hypopituitarism may occur in as many as two thirds of patients with a history of cranial irradiation. The incidence of GH deficiency is nearly 100% within 5 years of irradiation. ACTH, TSH, and gonadotropin deficiencies have been observed in 84%, 49%, and 96% of patients, respectively, within 8 years of the administration of radiotherapy. Thus one of the key issues in the postoperative evaluation of the pituitary tumor patient is centered on the repeat evaluation of these patients at risk for delayed consequences of therapy. We recommend evaluation of patients who have received radiotherapy at 6-month intervals for the first several years and then annually for at least 10 years.[5] Please refer to Table 25-1 for a brief summary of the following information about the diagnosis and treatment of the anterior pituitary hormone deficiencies.

Central Adrenal Insufficiency

Determination of whether a postoperative patient has central adrenal insufficiency is one of the most important tasks for clinicians when there is a history of pituitary tumor. There is considerable controversy about the most appropriate test of the sufficiency of the HPA axis, because several good diagnostic tests are available.

Early-morning serum cortisol levels, obtained 24 hours after the last dose of hydrocortisone or other steroid replacement dose, are sometimes useful to identify patients who need a definitive test of the HPA axis. A serum cortisol level less than 5 µg/dL indicate a high likelihood of central adrenal insufficiency, whereas a cortisol level greater than 15 µg/dL suggests the presence of a normal HPA axis. All patients with values within these extremes require dynamic tests before empiric steroids can be safely discontinued. Some physicians routinely assess serum cortisol levels in patients immediately after surgery and before hospital discharge. We have, however, seen a few patients develop adrenal insufficiency following discharge after having cortisol levels that were interpreted to reflect adequate pituitary and adrenal function. Because there is no anticipated harm in providing replacement-dose hydrocortisone for a period of 4 to 6 weeks, we typically conduct our evaluation at the first postoperative visit. Some patients may require retesting 3 to 6 months later.[2,12,16,18–20]

Several dynamic tests are available to assess the integrity of the HPA axis. The most commonly used tests include the standard and low-dose ACTH stimulation tests, the insulin-induced hypoglycemia test, and the overnight metyrapone test. Dynamic tests should not be performed until at least 4 weeks after surgery, because the presence of pituitary edema in the early postoperative period may interfere with pituitary function. Additionally, testing earlier than this may underdiagnose ACTH deficiency of recent onset, given that adrenal atrophy may not yet have occurred secondary to the recent loss of endogenous ACTH. Patients should continue on typical replacement doses of glucocorticoids until dynamic testing can be accomplished.[16,18,19]

The low-dose ACTH stimulation test has become the dynamic test of choice in our practice. In most patients, we proceed straight to this test rather than simply assessing the random or early-morning serum cortisol level. A serum cortisol level in excess of 18 µg/dL 30 minutes after the intravenous injection of 1 µg of ACTH defines a normal response. In this setting, empiric replacement doses of glucocorticoids can be abruptly discontinued. When the cortisol response is borderline (14–18 µg/dL) and the clinical picture is not consistent with adrenal insufficiency, we will consider performance of an insulin-induced hypoglycemia test. In patients with other pituitary hormone deficits or a history of irradiation, we simply assume those with borderline results require continued treatment for partial adrenal insufficiency.[6]

The insulin-induced hypoglycemia test and the overnight metyrapone test both provide assessment of the entire hypothalamic pituitary unit. The insulin-induced hypoglycemia test provides a stress paradigm, and many believe it to be the most appropriate test for the diagnosis of central adrenal insufficiency. The overnight metyrapone test relies on the principle of negative feedback. Because metyrapone is difficult to obtain commercially, we rarely use it in our practice. Additionally, corticotropin-releasing hormone administration can distinguish whether central adrenal insufficiency is due to hypothalamic or pituitary injury. Those with pituitary insufficiency will fail to respond to CRH, whereas those with hypothalamic insufficiency will indeed manifest a response to this secretagogue. This test is expensive and is rarely used outside of the research setting.[2,21,22]

The insulin-induced hypoglycemia test is performed by administering insulin to cause symptomatic hypoglycemia. Regular human insulin, 0.1 to 0.15 U/kg body weight, is administered intravenously. Patients with acromegaly often require a second dose of insulin if they do not become hypoglycemic within the first 30 minutes of the test. Patients are monitored for signs and symptoms of hypoglycemia, which must occur for the test to be valid. Blood glucose, serum cortisol, and plasma ACTH levels are evaluated at 30, 45, 60, and 90 minutes after insulin injection. A rise in the serum cortisol to greater than 20 µg/dL indicates an intact HPA axis. This test is contraindicated in patients with low baseline cortisol levels, as well as those patients with a history of ischemic heart disease and seizure disorders. Because of the potential for injury to the patient, a physician or other qualified health care provider must remain in attendance throughout the test.[2,21,22]

Metyrapone inhibits adrenal 11β-hydroxylase, the enzyme that catalyzes the conversion of 11-deoxycortisol to cortisol. In this setting, cortisol levels fall and the normal hypothalamic pituitary unit will respond by secreting a burst of ACTH that leads to increased adrenal steroid production. The overnight single-dose metyrapone test makes use of 30 mg/kg PO taken at midnight. Serum cortisol and 11-deoxycortisol levels are measured at 8 AM the very next morning. A normal response is characterized by an appropriate assay-specific rise in the serum 11-deoxycortisol level.[21,22]

Lifelong glucocorticoid replacement is recommended for patients with documented central adrenal insufficiency. Because the production of adrenal mineralocorticoids is under regulation of the renin-angiotensin system, patients with central adrenal insufficiency do not require concomitant treatment with mineralocorticoids. We prefer to use hydrocortisone in divided doses of 15 to 30 mg daily, with two thirds of the daily dose administered upon arising in the morning and one third administered in the middle of the afternoon. Dexamethasone 0.125 to 0.375 mg administered orally at bedtime is a suitable alternative form of replacement therapy. We often find it necessary to administer dexamethasone to those patients with persistent symptoms of hypocortisolemia despite standard doses of hydrocortisone replacement. Although prednisone in doses of 3 to 5 mg/day taken on arising probably represents adequate replacement therapy, we rarely use this drug in our own practice. Patients with adrenal insufficiency are advised to obtain and wear a Medic-Alert bracelet or other form of jewelry stating that they have adrenal insufficiency and require steroids. We also educate patients regarding the appropriate adjustment of their steroid doses to compensate for various physical stressors such as injury, illness, and invasive medical procedures.[2]

Central Hypothyroidism

The assessment of the hypothalamic-pituitary-thyroid axis following pituitary surgery is straightforward. We simply measure the serum free T_4 levels to assess the adequacy of thyroid hormone production in patients with pituitary diseases. Dynamic tests are not required. The serum TSH is of little value, because the etiology of central hypothyroidism is the secretion of inappropriate amounts of biologically active TSH. Patients with central hypothyroidism have been shown to have biologically ineffective TSH, impairment in the diurnal variation of TSH secretion, failure of pulsatile secretion of TSH, and a decrease in the mass of TSH secreted over the course of the day. Each of these circumstances will lead to central hypothyroidism, even in the setting of "normal" TSH levels as determined by a random TSH radioimmunoassay.[23]

Low free T_4 levels and levels in the lower quartile of the normal range in patients with clinical symptoms of hypothyroidism should be prompt empiric L-thyroxine replacement. We also favor treatment of patients who had normal free T_4 levels before surgery and who show a significant decline postoperatively of their free T_4 levels to the lower part of the normal range. In patients with preoperative central hypothyroidism, we prefer to discontinue the thyroxine at the first postoperative visit and reassess in 6 weeks only if other tests indicate a high likelihood of normal pituitary function. Decisions about L-thyroxine replacement should always take into consideration the overall sense of well-being of the patient. We have seen patients with mid-range normal free T_4 levels who will complain of fatigue and an increased need for sleep. These patients often enjoy relief of their symptoms following the initiation of empiric L-thyroxine replacement.[2,3]

The volume of distribution of L-thyroxine is estimated by the lean body mass. Thus dosing is dependent on the ideal body weight, with slight upward adjustments for marked obesity. As previously outlined, satisfactory initial L-thyroxine replacement can be accomplished by administering 0.8 µg of L-thyroxine per pound of ideal body weight, though older patients and those with established or suspected cardiovascular disease should be started on 25 to 50 µg/day. Patients taking oral estrogens may ultimately require a higher dose. We assess the efficacy of therapy in our patients by reassessing their clinical responses to treatment and by measuring their serum free T_4 levels 6 to 8 weeks after the initiation of treatment and following any change in dosage. TSH levels are not reliable indicators of adequate replacement, because these patients have pituitary disease and in fact developed hypothyroidism as a consequence of impaired TSH secretion. Our main goal of treatment is to dose L-thyroxine so that patients are free of symptoms of both hypothyroidism and hyperthyroidism. We aim to treat such that the free T_4 level will remain in the upper one half of the normal range.[2,3]

Central Hypogonadism

The resumption of cyclic menses in women following pituitary surgery is generally indicative of a normal hypothalamic-pituitary-gonadal axis. Serum estradiol and FSH levels should be measured if cyclic menses does not resume within 3 months of surgery. If clinically indicated, replacement therapy with cyclic estrogen and progesterone should be prescribed for premenopausal women.[2,3] Treatment is often indicated to preserve bone mineral density, libido, sexual function, and to maintain an overall sense of well-being. Considerable controversy exists about the appropriateness and indications of hormone replacement therapy in older women.

In men, self-reports of libido and erectile function are not reliable indicators of the sufficiency of the hypothalamic-pituitary-gonadal axis. Measurements of the serum total or free testosterone and LH levels are often required to determine if central hypogonadism is present. Testosterone replacement can be accomplished by regular intramuscular injections and also by the application of patches and gels to the skin. Benefits of treatment include maintenance of and improvements in muscle mass, preservation of bone mineral density, improvements in libido and sexual function, and improvements in overall sense of well-being. It is prudent to measure a serum prostate-specific antigen and to perform a digital rectal examination of the prostate gland to screen for prostate disease in men over the age of 40 before initiating treatment and then annually thereafter in men receiving testosterone replacement. We aim to treat patients such that their free testosterone levels are maintained in the age-specific normal range.[2]

Growth Hormone Deficiency

Growth hormone deficiency can result in a number of non-specific complaints in patients with a history of pituitary surgery. These often include fatigue, weakness, decreased exercise tolerance, and moodiness. Patients may develop osteoporosis, decreases in muscle mass, increases in body fat, weight gain, an abnormal lipid profile, and other biochemical cardiovascular risk factors. Many patients may not present with classical features of GH deficiency until one or more years after pituitary surgery. We have seen several patients who presented for what they suspected was a late recurrence of their Cushing's disease, only to discover that the cause of their presenting symptoms was GH deficiency.

The likelihood of GH deficiency increases in the setting of multiple pituitary hormone deficiencies. Patients with three or more hormone deficits almost always have GH deficiency. Importantly, approximately 45% of patients with a history of pituitary disease and otherwise normal pituitary function have GH deficiency as defined by standard dynamic tests of pituitary function.[1]

Serum IGF-1 levels are a useful screening test in the evaluation of patients with suspected GH deficiency. IGF-1 results that are either low or in the lower quartile of the normal range should prompt the performance of dynamic tests to confirm a suspected diagnosis of GH deficiency. The combination arginine–growth hormone–releasing hormone (GHRH) stimulation test is the most commonly used dynamic test to assess GH reserve. GHRH directly stimulates GH release from the anterior pituitary, whereas arginine decreases hypothalamic somatostatin release, leading to a consequent rise in GH secretion. Arginine as a sole provocative agent should be used in patients with suspected hypothalamic or pituitary stalk injury. Although insulin-induced hypoglycemia is considered to be the gold standard test to assess GH reserve, this test has largely been supplanted by the arginine-GHRH stimulation test as a result of its safety and ease of administration. The combined acipomox-GHRH test, currently under clinical investigation, may be an excellent alternative to these other tests. Acipomox, a nicotinic acid derivative, reduces free fatty acid levels—an effect that, in turn, leads to an increase in the magnitude of the GH response to GHRH. GH levels greater than 9.5 µg/L in response to the arginine-GHRH test are considered normal. GH levels in excess of 11 µg/L in the acipomox-GHRH test indicate normal pituitary reserve. A GH level of 5 µg/L serves as a cutoff point when using a single provocative agent.[24]

Growth hormone replacement is accomplished by the daily subcutaneous injection of recombinant human growth hormone. In most patients, we initiate treatment with a dose of 0.4 mg/day. The dose is titrated upward to achieve a serum IGF-1 level in the middle to upper one half of the age- and sex-specific normal range. Women taking oral estrogens often require higher doses, as do younger patients. Older patients often require lower doses. Stepwise titration of the dose at 6- to 8-week intervals usually avoids the uncommon side effects of fluid retention, arthralgias, and nerve entrapment syndromes. GH replacement is contraindicated in the presence of an active malignancy. Treatment should not begin until completion of therapy directed at the pituitary tumor. There is no compelling evidence that restoration of GH levels to the normal range would result in progressive growth of residual pituitary tumor.

Central Diabetes Insipidus

A careful clinical history should be conducted to identify patients who may have developed DI in the postoperative period. Furthermore, those patients with established DI should be evaluated to determine if their treatment is effective and if continued treatment is even necessary. The aforementioned protocol of periodic assessment of the need for continued therapy as determined by patients and their responses to withholding a dose of medication often results in appropriate and timely self-discontinuance of DDAVP. Most patients who still have DI are well aware of their disease and will report a resurgence of polyuria if their dose of DDAVP is withheld for more than 12 hours.

For patients in whom it is not clear if DI is present, a water deprivation test may be useful in making a definitive diagnosis and in distinguishing central DI from primary polydipsia and nephrogenic DI. Because this test can be dangerous and is contraindicated in patients with hypertonic hypernatremia, it should be conducted and supervised by an endocrinologist. Patients are asked to refrain from the ingestion of water and other similar beverages for a specified amount of time before the onset of the test. Body weight, urine volume and osmolality, and plasma sodium and osmolality are evaluated on an hourly basis. The test is terminated when any of the following events occur: the body weight decreases by more than 5%, the plasma sodium concentration exceeds 145 mEq/L, or two or more successive urine osmolalities differ by less than 10%. At the termination of the test, 1 µg DDAVP is administered subcutaneously, and urine volume and osmolality are measured at 30, 60, and 120 minutes following the injection. An increase in urine

osmolality by 50% from the baseline value characterizes a response to DDAVP, and, in the clinical context of dehydration with polyuria, strongly suggests a diagnosis of central DI. An increase in the urine osmolality by less than 50% usually suggests the presence of nephrogenic DI, although some patients with severe central DI may demonstrate only a partial response to DDAVP. Primary polydipsia is suspected when a therapeutic trial of DDAVP is helpful in treating the polyuria but is associated with a decline in serum sodium concentration.[14] Figure 24-2 illustrates the aforementioned testing process.

The pharmacologic management of the patient with chronic DI has been summarized in Table 24-3. Patients may note an increased vasopressin dose requirement in the setting of an upper respiratory infection, during a period of allergic rhinitis, and during pregnancy. We advise patients to avoid activities and habits that may lead to the irresponsible ingestion of large amounts of water while being treated with DDAVP. Some of these situations include ingestion of numerous glasses of water to comply with diet recommendations, ingestion of large amounts of beer at parties, and ingestion of water to treat a dry mouth due to mouth breathing during vigorous prolonged exercise. Severe symptomatic hyponatremia has resulted in each of these situations.

Hormone Hypersecretion

Prolactinoma

Although most patients with prolactinomas are now treated with medications, surgery is often performed in the following situations: when the patient does not tolerate medical therapy or does not desire to take lifelong medications, when a patient has a tumor that is largely cystic, when a woman with a macroprolactinoma desires pregnancy, and in the setting of pituitary apoplexy. Restoration of a normal serum PRL and return of normal gonadal function are the goals in the surgical

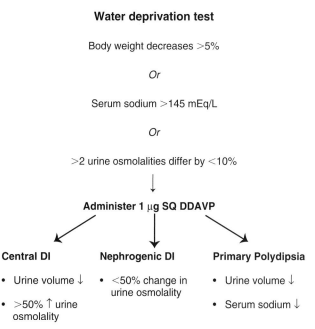

FIGURE 24-2 Diagnosis of diabetes insipidus.

treatment of a prolactinoma.[2–4] In general, surgery is successful in 76% of patients who have preoperative PRL levels less than 200 µg/L and in 46% of patients who have PRL levels greater than 200 µg/L.[25]

Although the PRL level can be measured the morning after surgery, with a level at this time near the lower limit of detectability ensuring a 90% chance of long-term remission, we favor reassessment at the first postoperative visit. Serum PRL levels that remain within the normal range for at least 6 months usually indicate that a patient has been rendered disease free. Stable modest hyperprolactinemia, with PRL levels in the range of 20 to 70 µg/L and in the absence of any residual tumor on pituitary MRI, usually reflects damage to the pituitary stalk that occurred during surgery. This is especially true if there is also evidence of hypopituitarism.[1,25]

Successful normalization of the serum PRL is often accompanied by cessation of galactorrhea as well as resumption of cyclic menses in women and resolution of hypogonadism in men. Some patients with persistent hypogonadism despite normalization of their PRL levels suffer from central gonadotropin deficiency as a result of their underlying pituitary disease. The overall recurrence rate of hyperprolactinemia of 5% to 10% dictates that patients be followed annually to reassess their serum PRL concentrations and gonadal functions.[25] Table 24-4 summarizes the surgical success rates and the criteria for a cure pertinent for each of the hormonally active pituitary tumors.

Cushing's Syndrome

Surgery results in remission in approximately 90% of patients with Cushing's disease and microadenomas and in 65% of those patients with macroadenomas. If a pituitary tumor is not identified at surgery, the failure rate is as high as 40%.[26–28] Other causes of failure to achieve remission include misdiagnosis of the syndrome of ectopic ACTH hypersecretion, incomplete resection of invasive tumor, failure to recognize multiple adenomas, and corticotroph hyperplasia.

Although there are no consensus criteria for predicting long-term outcome, a postoperative cortisol level less than 3.6 µg/dL strongly suggests and predicts a long-term remission.

In most patients treated successfully, serum and urine cortisol levels usually fall to low or undetectable levels within the first 1 to 2 days after surgery. These patients require glucocorticoid replacement, because the remaining normal corticotroph cells of the anterior pituitary have been profoundly suppressed, resulting in a period of transient central adrenal insufficiency. Steroid replacement is usually required for 6 to 18 months until the normal corticotrophs recover their function.[2,3,15,16,29] Generally speaking, a more rapid recovery of the HPA axis suggests recurrent disease. In some patients, the development of central adrenal insufficiency after surgery is delayed by several weeks. For this reason, we do not deem a surgery a true failure for a patient until after the first postoperative visit and sometimes not until we have followed him or her for 6 months. Unless failure is obvious or expected based on the presence of known or suspected residual or invasive tumor, we discharge patients on hydrocortisone 20 mg in the morning and 10 mg in the middle of the afternoon. Patients are asked to withhold their dose of hydrocortisone for 24 hours before the first postoperative visit to permit testing.

The initial postoperative laboratory assessment of the patient with a history of Cushing's disease involves determination of the plasma ACTH and serum cortisol. A plasma cortisol less than 3.6 µg/dL suggests remission.[2] These patients are continued on hydrocortisone for presumed central adrenal insufficiency. A value between 3.6 and 7.2 µg/dL suggests a probable cure. These patients are selected for a low-dose ACTH stimulation test to determine if they require continued steroid therapy. If they demonstrate an adequate cortisol response, a 24-hour urine is collected to assess their cortisol production rates. A serum cortisol value between 7.2 and 14.5 µg/dL is equivocal and requires discontinuation of steroids and collection of a 24-hour urine for cortisol. A level greater than 14.5 µg/dL suggests failure to render the patient disease free and also prompts discontinuation of steroids and collection of urine. Patients with both normal and elevated urine cortisol excretion rates probably have residual disease.[3,16] Imaging studies should be done to assess for residual tumor in those patients

---

TABLE 24-4 ▪ Criteria for a Cure and Surgical Success Rates Following Initial Surgery for Hormone Secreting Pituitary Tumors

Tumor	Surgical Success Rate	Criteria for a Cure
Prolactinoma	• 76% of patients with preoperative PRL levels <200 µg/L • 46% of patients with preoperative PRL levels >200 µg/L	Serum PRL levels within the normal range for 6 months following surgery
Cushing's disease	• 96% of patients with microadenomas • 65% of patients with macroadenomas	• Serum postoperative cortisol level <3.6 µg/dL • Low-dose ACTH stimulated cortisol <18 µg/dL
Acromegaly	• 85% to 90% of patients with microadenomas • 50% of patients with macroadenomas	• Nadir GH during OGTT <1.0 µg/L • Normal age- and sex-referenced IGF-1 level • Serum GH <2 µg/L during the early postoperative period
TSH-secreting adenoma	40% of patients	Suppressed TSH level measured 1–7 days following surgery

ACTH, adrenocorticotropic hormone; GH, growth hormone; IGF-1, insulin-like growth factor-1; OGTT, oral glucose tolerance test; PRL, prolactin; TSH, thyrotropin.

who had demonstrable tumors before surgery. Pathology specimens should be reviewed to determine if there is any confirmation of the suspected preoperative diagnosis. Inferior petrosal sinus sampling and various dynamic tests may be necessary to determine the precise reason that a patient may have failed surgery.

Decisions regarding the need for adjuvant therapy are based on the aforementioned results and the careful consideration of the patient's desire for additional treatment. Some patients who have achieved eucortisolemia choose long-term follow-up instead of additional therapy. Most will enjoy beneficial changes in their health as a result of a reduction in their cortisol levels. These patients should be offered treatment at the time of recurrence of hypercortisolism to limit morbidity and to preserve their health. Development of a strategy for treatment of residual or recurrent hypercortisolism should ideally involve endocrinologists, neurosurgeons, radiation oncologists, and neuroophthalmologists. Decisions about whether to perform repeat surgery, administer radiotherapy, administer steroid biosynthesis inhibitors, or proceed with bilateral adrenalectomy depend on many issues, whose full discussion is beyond the scope of this chapter.

Patients deemed to be in remission at the time of the first postoperative visit are followed at 3- to 6-month intervals. Periodic laboratory tests include serum cortisol and plasma ACTH levels, ACTH stimulation tests, and 24-hour urine cortisol determinations. Once the HPA axis recovers and cortisol production returns to normal, a 24-hour urine cortisol is collected every 3 to 4 months for several years to detect recurrence at the earliest possible time. Recurrence can be expected in as many as 15% of those who had microadenomas and 33% of those with a history of macroadenomas.[26,27] Patients will occasionally present in between scheduled visits for repeat evaluation when they suspect a recurrence. During this period of follow-up, patients will experience weight loss, improvements in body composition and strength, and improvement in their mood and overall sense of well-being. In most, hypertension, diabetes, and hyperlipidemia either resolve or greatly improve. Bone mineral density can improve dramatically over a period of several years.

Steroid "withdrawal" can be seen in patients in remission of Cushing's disease. This syndrome is characterized by symptoms of adrenal insufficiency despite eucortisolemia. Symptoms often include diffuse arthralgias and myalgias, weight loss, weakness, fatigue, and depression and may last for 2 to 4 months. These symptoms can be attributed to a relative "insufficiency" of cortisol levels following the excessive values characteristic of Cushing's disease. Typically, serum cortisol results are greater than 15 μg/dL, and the cortisol response to insulin-induced hypoglycemia is normal. If the syndrome should occur, patients should be reassured that their symptoms are temporary. Antidepressant medications may be of benefit. Physical activity should be strongly encouraged. Glucocorticoid therapy is ill-advised and should be provided only if symptoms are absolutely intolerable.[22]

Acromegaly

Remission following initial surgery can be expected in 85% to 90% of acromegalic patients with microadenomas and in one half of those with macroadenomas.[30–32] Recurrences are seen in approximately 6% of patients at 10 years, and

10% at 15 years after surgery.[33] In most patients who enter remission, and even in some who enjoy marked reductions in GH secretion, symptoms attributed to GH excess improve dramatically. Signs of an unsatisfactory outcome of initial surgery include an elevated (>10 μg/L) preoperative GH value, dural invasion by the tumor, mixed GH-PRL-secreting tumors and the presence of extrasellar extension.[8] Patients suffering from gigantism are known to be particularly refractory with respect to recurrence.[17]

The indicators of successful treatment of acromegaly have been revised over the past several decades. At present, they include restoration of normal pulsatile GH secretion, a normal GH response to the oral glucose tolerance test (nadir GH < 1.0 μg/L), and a normal age- and sex-referenced IGF-1 level.[8]

Growth hormone values obtained within the first week after surgery are highly predictive of both the long- and short-term outcome of surgery.[8] A random serum GH value of less than 2 μg/L within the early postoperative period suggests a high likelihood of remission. In a retrospective study of 68 patients, a mean serum GH less than 2 μg/L during the first postoperative week was found to have a 77% specificity and a predictive value of 97% for remission with regard to the surgical outcome as evaluated 3 months later. The specificity was 83%, and the predictive value for remission increased to 94% when surgical outcome was evaluated at 60 months.[34] Measuring the serum IGF-1 level immediately following surgery is generally not recommended, because this value may not return to normal for several months.[8] Thus we typically wait until the first postoperative visit to measure GH and IGF-1 levels. An oral glucose tolerance test is performed in patients with an IGF-1 level in the upper part of the normal range accompanied by an inappropriate normal or elevated GH level. Patients in remission are followed at 3- to 6-month intervals for several years and then annually thereafter. Patients with either residual or recurrent disease are considered for repeat surgery, radiotherapy, medical therapy, or a combination of these modalities.

Hyperthyroidism

In general, 40% of patients with TSH-secreting adenomas enjoy successful resection of their tumors with normalization of thyroid hormone levels. Prognostic variables indicating a higher likelihood of remission include the presence of a microadenoma, the absence of tumor invasion, a short duration of symptoms, and the presence of mild hyperthyroidism.[9]

The specific criteria for a cure following pituitary surgery for a TSH-secreting adenoma have not been rigorously defined. Some have proposed the measurement of serum TSH and free T_4 levels 1 to 7 days after surgery. Patients who have had successful resections of their pituitary tumors would be expected to have low TSH levels as a result of suppression of their normal thyrotroph cells due to the preexisting hyperthyroidism. Persistent or recurrent elevations in TSH, alpha subunit, and the free T_4 and T_3 levels suggest residual or recurrent disease.[9] Thyroid hormone levels take several weeks to fall in successfully treated patients, because the serum half-life of thyroxine is 7 to 8 days. Free T_4 and T_3 levels, therefore, are not reliable indicators of remission in the early postoperative period.[3]

MEDICAL MANAGEMENT OF HORMONE-SECRETING PITUITARY TUMORS

Medical management of hormonally active pituitary tumors is often necessary because of the inability to resect invasive tumors completely and the delay in response to subsequent radiotherapy. Furthermore, some patients are not candidates for surgical intervention and must be treated medically to decrease morbidity secondary to hormone hypersecretion.

Cushing's Disease

Several different drugs are available to lower the cortisol levels in patients with Cushing's disease. Medical treatment for Cushing's disease is most commonly chosen in cases of failure of all other treatment modalities, in preparation for surgery to relieve extreme symptoms, or in the interval between radiotherapy and the development of eucortisolemia. Table 24-5 summarizes the medical treatments available for the treatment of hypercortisolemia.

Ketoconazole

Ketoconazole, an imidazole derivative with antimycotic properties, inhibits several of the cytochrome P450 enzymes involved in cortisol synthesis. It may also act as an antagonist of the glucocorticoid receptor and impair ACTH release from pituitary adenoma cells. It is the most effective medication available and is usually the first drug we prescribe when the need for medical management has been established. Ketoconazole is successful in normalizing urinary free cortisol levels in 70% to 100% of patients. A beneficial response is usually noted within the first week of initiating treatment. Effective doses generally range from 400 to 1200 mg/day in two to three divided doses. Liver function test (LFT) abnormalities occur in 15% of patients, and marked hepatocellular injury occurs in 1 of 15,000 patients. Other side effects include skin rash, nausea, dyspepsia, gynecomastia, hypogonadism, and hypocalcemia. The drug is contraindicated in pregnancy, and one must be cognizant of drug interactions because it affects the cytochrome P450 enzymes.[26,35] Ketoconazole must be discontinued for 4 to 6 weeks when it is necessary to reestablish the need for ongoing medical therapy, for example, in patients who have received radiotherapy. We usually will not arrange for ketoconazole withdrawal and reassessment until we see 24-hour urine cortisol results in the lower half of the normal range while the patient is taking 400 mg/day.

Aminoglutethimide

Aminoglutethimide is an antiseizure medication that inhibits the conversion of cholesterol to pregnenolone, the initial step of steroid hormone synthesis. Nearly half of all patients treated with this drug enjoy normalization of their cortisol levels. Effective doses range from 250 to 2000 mg/day. Aminoglutethimide may be used in combination with ketoconazole to obtain a full response. The medication is generally not well tolerated at first; low-grade fever and rash occur in approximately 18% of patients, and dizziness, somnolence, and lethargy are reported in 30% of patients. Tolerance to these side effects develops with continued treatment.[26,35]

Metyrapone

Metyrapone, a pyridine derivative, blocks the conversion of 11-deoxycortisol to cortisol, the final step in cortisol synthesis. This drug elicits a good response in 85% of patients, although 25% may require significant dosage increases secondary to increased levels of plasma ACTH overriding the enzyme blockade. Effective doses range from 750 mg/day to 2000 mg/day. The main side effects, seen in 70% of women, include acne and hirsutism. Other side effects include edema, hypokalemia, nausea, rash, dizziness, lethargy, and ataxia. The hirsutism, edema, and hypokalemia are due to 11-hydroxylase inhibition and subsequent accumulation of adrenal androgens and mineralocorticoids.[26,35]

Mitotane

Mitotane, structurally related to the pesticide DDT, blocks 11β-hydroxylase as well as cholesterol side chain cleavage enzymes. Its metabolites disrupt mitochondrial function in the zona fasciculata and reticularis, ultimately leading to mitochrondrial destruction and adrenocortical cell death. The medication is effective in approximately 80% of patients, although long-term remission is maintained in only 30% of patients following discontinuation of therapy. Higher response rates are seen in patients with Cushing's disease

---

TABLE 24-5 ▪ Medical Management of Cushing's Disease

Drug	Mechanism	Dosage	Side Effects	Efficacy
Ketoconazole	• Cytochrome P450 adrenal enzyme inhibitor • Impairs release of ACTH	400–1200 mg PO daily	Transaminitis, skin rash, nausea, gynecomastia, hypogonadism, hypocalcemia	70% to 100% of patients
Aminoglutethimide	Inhibits cholesterol conversion to pregnenolone	250–2000 mg PO daily	Low-grade fever, rash, dizziness, lethargy	50% patients
Metyrapone	Inhibits 11β-hydroxylase, blocking conversion of 11-deoxycortisol to cortisol	750–2000 mg PO daily	Acne, hirsutism, edema, hypokalemia, dizziness, rash, lethargy, ataxia	85% of patients
Mitotane	• Metabolites are adrenolytic • Inhibits 11β-hydroxylase and cholesterol side chain cleavage	2000–4000 mg PO daily	Increased LDL, transaminitis, hypouricemia, adrenal insufficiency	80% of patients

ACTH, adrenocorticotropic hormone; LDL, low-density lipoprotein.

who receive concomitant pituitary irradiation. Doses range from 2 to 4 g/day, and treatment is commonly limited by gastrointestinal side effects, as well as dizziness and gynecomastia. Lab abnormalities, which may be a result of therapy, include dramatic increases in low-density lipoprotein cholesterol, abnormal liver function tests (LFTs), and hypouricemia. Adrenal insufficiency can also occur and requires treatment. Hydrocortisone is the recommended replacement therapy when adrenal insufficiency occurs, because mitotane accelerates the metabolism of halogenated steroids such as dexamethasone. Mineralocorticoid therapy is generally not needed, because mitotane does not affect the zona glomerulosa. The clinical efficacy of mitotane must be monitored by 24-hour urinary free cortisol, because mitotane reduces urinary 19-hydroxycorticosteroids.[26,35]

Other Medications

Other medications less commonly prescribed include etomidate, mifepristone, and octreotide. Etomidate is the most potent inhibitor of 11β-hydroxylase; the usual dose is 0.3 mg/kg/hour. Its use is typically restricted to hospitalized patients, who must be monitored for excessive sedation and adrenal insufficiency. Mifepristone is a progesterone and glucocorticoid antagonist that may be used to reverse psychosis, major vegetative depression, and suicidal ideation in patients with hypercortisolism. It is an FDA-approved drug that is used to terminate pregnancy. Effective doses range from 5 to 20 mg/kg/day. ACTH and cortisol levels increase in patients with tumors that have functional glucocorticoid receptors due to loss of negative feedback. Side effects include relative adrenal insufficiency, hypoglycemia, and eosinophilia. Octreotide, a somatostatin analogue, inhibits the secretion of ACTH. It normalizes cortisol levels in only a minority of patients, although it is more successful in patients with an ectopic ACTH source.[35]

General Approach

A reasonable drug with which to initiate medical therapy is ketoconazole, at a dose of 200 mg PO twice daily. A 24-hour urinary free cortisol collected 1 week after the initiation of therapy will determine if any dose adjustments are necessary. LFTs may be checked at monthly intervals for 3 months and then every month thereafter. Ketoconazole should be discontinued if LFTs reach a value three times the upper limit of normal. Aminoglutethimide is usually the next drug prescribed when ketoconazole is ineffective or must be discontinued; it may also be used in combination with ketoconazole. Therapy is generally initiated at 125 mg PO twice daily and increased at weekly intervals based on 24-hour urinary free cortisol levels. Slowly increasing the dose seems to limit the side effect of sedation. Metyrapone is our third drug of choice, at a starting dose of 250 mg PO three times daily. This drug can also be used in combination with either ketoconazole or aminoglutethimide. Once again, 24-hour urinary free cortisol levels are used to guide any dosage adjustments.[35]

Mitotane is typically reserved for patients with adrenocortical carcinoma and those with ACTH-dependent forms of Cushing's syndrome who prefer a medical adrenalectomy to surgical excision and for patients who are high surgical risk and who have failed all other forms of medical therapy. Treatment is initiated at 500 mg PO at bed time and escalated

at weekly intervals by 500 mg/week until a maximum daily dose of 4 g is reached. Side effects occur less frequently when 50% of the dose is administered at bedtime and the other 50% divided between breakfast and lunch. After 3 months, or when patients begin to experience side effects, the dose is lowered to 2 g daily. Therapy may be withdrawn 6 to 9 months following the initiation of therapy to assess the need for continued therapy, provided that normalization of urinary cortisol secretion has been achieved.[35]

Medical therapy may be used in patients who are pregnant or desire pregnancy. Ketoconazole is teratogenic, and mifepristone is an FDA-approved abortifacient. Mitotane will result in destruction of the fetal adrenal glands and thus must be avoided in pregnancy as well.[35]

Acromegaly

Uncontrolled acromegaly is associated with a two- to three-fold increased mortality. Thus, medical therapy must be instituted to normalize IGF-1 levels when surgery fails and while awaiting the beneficial effects of radiotherapy. Pharmacologic therapy is often used either following surgery or as the first-line therapy for unresectable tumors or in patients who are not surgical candidates.[36,37] The past 10 years have seen major advances in the medical management of acromegalic patients, and it is now possible to control IGF-1 levels in nearly all patients. Somatostatin analogues, dopamine agonists, and the new GH receptor antagonist pegvisomant are widely available, and there is now sufficient clinical experience with these drugs to permit their routine use in acromegalic patients. The major advantages of these drugs are the low frequency of administration and the sustained suppression of GH and IGF-1 in patients in whom adequate suppression occurs. The major disadvantages are cost, especially if long-term treatment is needed, and the inability of the drugs to induce an amount of tumor shrinkage sufficient to relieve any mass effects. An overview of the medical management of acromegaly is provided in Table 24-6.

Somatostatin Analogues

Somatostatin is a ubiquitous inhibitory hormone. Hypothalamic somatostatin inhibits GH secretion from somatotrophs of the anterior pituitary. Pharmacologic manipulation and truncation of the native molecule have led to the development of somatostatin analogues that can be used to lower GH secretion from tumoral somatotrophs in patients with acromegaly. Several different preparations of somatostatin analogues are available, including a short-acting preparation of octreotide that is administered subcutaneously, a long-acting depot form of octreotide LAR (long-acting repeatable) that is administered intramuscularly, and lanreotide SR (slow release) that is administered intramuscularly.

Octreotide is 45 times more potent and has a longer half-life than somatostatin. The short-acting preparation has a maximal suppressive effect on GH that occurs between 2 and 6 hours after injection. GH levels rise between injections given every 8 hours, but with continued treatment this rise is lessened. The frequency of injections has been a problem for some patients and may lead to noncompliance. The short-acting preparation has a role in assessing patient

TABLE 24-6 ▪ **Medical Management of Acromegaly**

Drug	Mechanism	Dosage	Side Effects	Efficacy
Octreotide LAR	Somatostatin analogue	10–40 mg IM q4wk	Asymptomatic cholesterol gallstones, abdominal pain, nausea, diarrhea, fat malabsorption	• Normalizes GH: 56% of patients • Normalizes IGF-1: 66% of patients
Lanreotide 30 mg (LAN30)	Somatostatin analogue	30 mg IM q7–14 days	Asymptomatic cholesterol gallstones, abdominal pain, nausea, diarrhea, fat malabsorption	• Normalizes GH: 49% of patients • Normalizes IGF-1: 48% of patients
Lanreotide 60 mg (LAN60)	Somatostatin analogue	60 mg IM q4wk	Asymptomatic cholesterol gallstones, abdominal pain, nausea, diarrhea, fat malabsorption	• Normalizes GH: 65% pts • Normalizes IGF-1: 63% pts
Pegvisomant (Somavert)	GH receptor antagonist	40 mg SC loading dose, followed by 10–30 mg/day SC	Elevated liver function tests	• Normalizes IGF-1: 97% of patients

GH, growth hormone; LAR, long-acting repeatable; IGF-1, insulin-like growth factor-1.

tolerance to somatostatin analogues; it may be given as a 2-week course before initiation of depot analogue therapy. It also may be useful when rapid lowering of GH levels is needed.[36]

Octreotide LAR causes a rise in drug levels approximately 7 to 14 days after injection, and levels then remain elevated for an average of 24 days. Steady-state conditions are usually achieved after two to three injections. GH levels rise and fall in response to changing octreotide levels. The usual starting dose of octreotide LAR is 20 mg, with titration down to 10 mg or up to 30 or 40 mg based on the response of GH and IGF-1 levels. Monthly drug administration allows for overlap between injections to maintain sufficiently high octreotide levels. The dose interval may be extended longer than 4 weeks in some patients.[32,36] Fifty-six percent of patients treated with octreotide LAR adequately suppress their GH levels, and 66% adequately suppress their IGF-1 levels. Success is more likely to occur in patients with pretreatment levels of GH less than 20 μg/L.[31] IGF-1 levels are further suppressed after the first 3 to 6 months of treatment, whereas GH levels remain constant. GH levels obtained after 3 months of octreotide LAR treatment and IGF-1 levels obtained after 6 months of treatment are the best predictors of ultimate achievement of safe GH levels and normal IGF-1 levels, respectively.[38]

Lanreotide SR has a shorter duration of action than octreotide LAR and must be administered as a 30-mg intramuscular dose every 7 to 14 days. Nearly one half of patients treated with lanreotide SR adequately suppress their GH levels, and 48% adequately suppress their IGF-1 levels.[32,36,39] Lanreotide 60 mg is a relatively new preparation that proposes to suppress GH and IGF-1 levels for up to 28 days. The main difference between the 30-mg and 60-mg formulations consists of the amount of microparticles contained in the vials; all components of the two formulations are essentially identical.[39]

In a prospective open multicenter study in which the 60-mg dose was administered to 92 patients with active acromegaly (adjuvant treatment in 60 patients and primary treatment in 30 patients) with a median follow-up of 34 months, IGF-1 levels were normalized in 65% of patients and GH levels fell to less than 2.5 μg/L in 63% of patients and to less than 1 μg/L in 25% of patients. Similarly to the experience with octreotide LAR, IGF-1 levels were further suppressed after the first 3 to 6 months of treatment, whereas the GH levels remained constant. There was a progressive increase in the rate of IGF-1 normalization, such that 49% of patients showed normalization at 12 months, 69% at 24 months, and 77% at 36 months. At 12 months, 46% of patients showed a GH level less than 2.5 μg/L, 68% did so at 24 months, and 81% did so at 36 months. Patients starting from a higher basal GH level achieved a greater percentage in GH suppression. In contrast, this phenomenon was not seen with the basal IGF-1 level. There was no tachyphylaxis observed throughout the study. Shortening the interval between injections to 21 days further improved GH and IGF-1 suppression. There was no substantial improvement in GH or IGF-1 suppression in poorly sensitive patients after increasing the dose or shortening the interval between injections. Conversely, the same level of IGF-1 and GH suppression could be maintained in highly sensitive patients by prolonging the interval between injections up to 75 days.[39]

Symptoms and signs of acromegaly improve in 64% to 74% of patients treated with depot somatostatin analogue therapy. Approximately 30% of patients treated with somatostatin analogues as adjuvant or primary therapy show tumor shrinkage, most commonly in the range of 20% to 50%, and usually within the first year of treatment. Studies have demonstrated that both microadenomas and macroadenomas may regress after a period of at least 24 weeks of therapy.[31] The effect of treatment on tumor size has been shown to correlate with the size of the adenoma; patients with macroadenomas enjoy a higher rate of tumor shrinkage than those patients with microadenomas or remnant tumors.[38] Nearly one half of those patients receiving somatostatin analogues as primary therapy have tumor regression. It is important to note, however, that in the presence of tumor mass effects, the degree of shrinkage is not felt to be clinically significant and surgery is mandatory for decompression.[32]

Somatostatin analogues have been well studied with respect to their efficacy as primary versus adjuvant therapy.

Studies have shown that, when used as primary therapy, these drugs normalize IGF-1 levels in 60% of patients and suppress GH in 50% of patients. These results are similar to those achieved when the drugs are used as adjuvant therapy. Some have postulated that many patients with GH-secreting microadenomas could be treated successfully with primary somatostatin therapy alone. However, cost-benefit analysis does make this strategy unattractive, especially given the cure rate following surgery for microadenomas. Nevertheless, given these comparable rates of success in adjuvant versus primary treatment groups, there may be a role for primary somatostatin analogue therapy in certain groups of patients who show a low cure rate following transsphenoidal surgery (TSS), such as the elderly or those with large invasive tumors, in those patients who are unfit for or refuse surgery, or in those who have no adenoma visible upon MRI.[32]

The question of the benefits of preoperative pharmacotherapy for acromegalic patients has been raised recently. Theoretically, the shrinkage of tumor with medical therapy before surgery may facilitate their complete resection. This hypothesis has been examined in a controlled, randomized, blinded manner. Summarizing 14 studies, 55% to 89% of patients with macroadenomas enjoyed control of their disease if short-term treatment with a somatostatin analogue was administered before surgery. This is significantly higher than the reported 48% cure rate for macroadenomas with surgery alone. Additionally, 23% to 100% of these patients enjoyed more than 20% tumor shrinkage.[30]

Preoperative medical therapy may have additional clinical benefits. It may lessen soft-tissue swelling, therefore making intubation easier. It also may improve hemodynamic function and aid in the control of diabetes. Optimizing cardiovascular status is an important consideration in these patients, given that it is the primary determinant of morbidity and mortality in acromegaly, responsible for 60% of deaths. Improvement in cardiovascular function has been reported with somatostatin analogue therapy. In patients who achieve disease control, a reduction in left ventricular mass as well as posterior and septal wall has been seen as early as 1 week following therapy. It has also been shown that 3 to 6 months of therapy decreases the incidence of cardiac arrhythmias in patients with acromegaly. The net long-term effect of somatostatin analogues on glucose intolerance is still unclear, although glucose control before surgery is certainly appealing, given that diabetic patients are at increased risk for poor wound healing and increased susceptibility to infection.[30]

The side effects associated with somatostatin analogue therapy include increased risk for asymptomatic cholesterol gallstone development in 25% of patients. The routine use of surveillance ultrasonography in asymptomatic patients, however, is not warranted. Short-term effects, which often resolve with continued treatment, include abdominal pain, diarrhea, fat malabsorption, nausea, and flatulence.[31,32]

Pegvisomant

Pegvisomant (Somavert) is an analogue of human GH that has been mutated to bind to the GH receptor, block the access of native GH to the receptor, and prevent functionally correct dimerization of the receptor and subsequent activation of signal transduction pathways. The drug has no direct effect on GH-secreting tumors, because it blocks GH action at the level of the target tissue. This drug is the preferred agent in patients resistant to or intolerant of somatostatin analogues. Many physicians now administer this drug as first-line therapy in the management of acromegalic patients in whom surgery has failed.[36,40]

Treatment is initiated with a loading dose of 40 mg of pegvisomant injected subcutaneously followed by daily therapy. The initial daily dose is 10 mg, and the dose can be titrated up to 40 mg/day depending on the clinical response to treatment. IGF-1 levels should be checked every 4 to 6 weeks after the initiation of therapy, and at least every 6 months after IGF-1 levels have normalized. Serum GH concentrations are not reliable indicators of disease activity, because the pegvisomant molecule cross-reacts with most GH assays.[41]

In one 12-week study, serum IGF-1 levels were normalized in 10%, 39%, 75%, and 82% of patients treated with placebo, 10, 15, or 20 mg/day of pegvisomant, respectively.[41] Another 12-week randomized double-blind study reported success rates of IGF-1 normalization in 54%, 81%, and 89% of patients receiving 10, 15, and 20 mg/day of pegvisomant. The mean serum concentration of IGF-1 decreased from baseline by 26% in the 10 mg/day group, by 50% in the 15 mg/day group, and by 62.5% in the 20 mg/day group. The onset of action is rapid, with 75% or more of the maximal reduction in serum IGF-1 concentrations occurring within 2 weeks after initiation of therapy and remaining sustained through the 12 week course of treatment.[40] In studies of longer duration, normalization of IGF-1 levels was observed in 97% of 90 patients treated for more than 12 months with doses up to 40 mg/day. Pegvisomant has thus been shown to be the most successful medical therapy for normalizing serum IGF-1 values; however, unlike the somatostatin analogues, it has no effect on tumor size. Although there are no data to suggest that GH-secreting tumors will increase in size during treatment with pegvisomant, the drug does not have any activity directly against these tumors, and patients should, therefore, undergo regular pituitary MRI scans to assess for disease progression. Although combination therapy with pegvisomant and somatostatin receptor analogues is feasible, it is very costly and there is little experience with this approach to date.[36]

The major adverse effect of pegvisomant is related to the development of abnormal LFTs in 1% to 2% of treated patients. Elevations in the transaminases are usually not associated with increases in the levels of serum total bilirubin and alkaline phosphatase. These elevations do not appear to be related to the dose of pegvisomant. If baseline LFTs are normal, then treatment with pegvisomant may commence with monthly monitoring of LFTs during the first 6 months of treatment and periodically thereafter. If baseline LFTs are greater than three times the upper limit of normal, a comprehensive workup to establish the cause of liver dysfunction should be initiated before consideration of treatment with pegvisomant.[41]

Dopamine Agonists

Dopamine agonists are worth consideration in the treatment of acromegaly. Dopamine agonists bind to the D_2 dopamine receptors in the pituitary and suppress GH secretion. Only 20% of patients are able to achieve a GH level less than 5 μg/L, and only 10% are able to achieve a normal IGF-1 level. Cabergoline is the most effective dopamine agonist used in the treatment of acromegaly. Therapy for 3 to 40 months has been shown to normalize IGF-1 levels in 35% of 48 patients with pure GH-secreting tumors and to suppress GH levels to less than 2 µg/L in 44% of patients. Patients with combined GH- and prolactin-secreting tumors typically have higher success rates, with approximately 50% showing IGF-1 normalization and 56% showing GH suppression.[36] Lower baseline GH and IGF-1 levels have been associated with greater efficacy. Side effects of dopamine agonists include nausea, vomiting, abdominal spasms, sleep disturbances, fatigue, and transient postural hypotension. Studies have shown that 10% to 20% of somatostatin-resistant patients have further suppression of GH and IGF-1 levels with the addition of a dopamine agonist to their somatostatin analogue therapy.[32]

Monitoring Medical Therapy

Patient monitoring during medical therapy should ideally include periodic assessment of signs and symptoms of acromegaly, IGF-1 levels, and GH levels, as well as an annual MRI for the first several years after the start of therapy, unless the tumor is known to be progressive, in which case more frequent monitoring is advised. When evaluating the efficacy of medical therapy, it should be understood that other conditions can affect IGF-1 levels. Conditions that increase IGF-1 include adolescence and pregnancy. Conditions that decrease IGF-1 levels include malnutrition, poorly controlled diabetes mellitus, liver disease, and end-stage renal disease. Attainment of a normal IGF-1 level does not necessarily indicate complete restoration of control of GH secretion.[36] Therefore, GH levels must be monitored as well except in patients receiving pegvisomant therapy. Patients whose IGF-1 levels have normalized yet who do not show evidence of GH suppression after glucose administration may be at higher risk for disease recurrence and should be followed more closely. Conversely, even though a substantial drop in GH allows for significant improvement in clinical symptoms, the patient should still be considered to have residual tumor activity if the IGF-1 level remains elevated.[42]

Prolactinomas

The goals of the treatment of prolactinomas are threefold: control tumor growth, abolish galactorrhea, and restore gonadal function. Observation may be the most appropriate course of action in women whose hyperprolactinemia is not accompanied by bothersome symptoms or hypogonadism, and who do not desire pregnancy. Approximately 10% to 20% of microprolactinomas may spontaneously resolve, both morphologically and hormonally, over a period of 10 years.[42] Medical therapy is often selected as first-line therapy in patents with prolactinomas, even in those with tumor-related mass effects. Additionally, dopamine agonists are often used postoperatively to treat patients with residual tumor.

Dopamine is the naturally occurring hypothalamic-derived PRL inhibitory factor. It acts at the D_2 receptors on the lactotroph cell membrane. Available dopamine agonists include bromocriptine (Parlodel) and cabergoline (Dostinex).[25] Bromocriptine is usually started at a dose of 1.25 mg/day and may be gradually increased to a dose of 20 mg/day for larger tumors. Most patients require dosing

two to three times a day to treat their disorder effectively. Side effects, seen in 20% to 40% of patients, include headache, postural hypotension, nausea, and drowsiness. Approximately 10% to 20% of patients may fail to demonstrate an acceptable response to treatment.[42]

Cabergoline has a longer half-life and greater D_2 receptor affinity than bromocriptine. It has been shown to be more effective than bromocriptine in normalizing PRL levels. It has the drawback of being more expensive, but it is better tolerated and has fewer, though similar, side effects. Both drugs are probably safe during pregnancy. A single dose of cabergoline has a duration of action of up to 14 days and may be administered at a dose of 0.25 mg to 1.5 mg once or twice a week. Patients who have not responded in the past to bromocriptine have been known to respond to cabergoline.[43]

Verhelst and colleagues summarize the efficacy of cabergoline in a prospective study with 455 patients on a mean dose of 0.5 mg/week of cabergoline who were followed for a median of 28 months.[43] Ninety-nine of these patients were initially treated with bromocriptine and switched to cabergoline without a wash-out period. This dosage was effective in normalizing PRL levels in 86% of patients. The probability of reaching a normal PRL level was higher in patients with microadenomas than in patients with macroadenomas (93% versus 77%). There was a weak but significant correlation between the basal PRL level and the nadir PRL level.

With respect to tumor volume, a greater than 50% decrease was seen in 31% of these patients and a 25% to 50% decrease was seen in 16% of patients. Altogether, 67% of patients demonstrated some degree of tumor shrinkage. Visual field abnormalities normalized in 70% of patients.[43]

Seventy percent of these patients in whom bromocriptine failed to normalize PRL levels experienced success with cabergoline. These patients, as a group, however, were less likely to achieve normal PRL levels with cabergoline than were the patients who had not previously been on bromocriptine (70% versus 88%). These patients also required a higher dosage of cabergoline at a median of 1.5 mg/week. Only 3.9% of patients discontinued the study because of intolerance of cabergoline; the majority of these patients had been intolerant of bromocriptine.[43]

Thyrotropin-Secreting Adenomas

Medical treatment is often necessary for patients with TSH-secreting adenomas. Dopamine agonists and somatostatin analogues are useful and are directed against the pituitary tumor. A host of drugs are available to control persistent hyperthyroidism in those who do not fully respond to surgery and medical therapy.

D_2 receptors are expressed in some TSH-secreting adenomas. However, only approximately 20% of patients respond to bromocriptine in a sustained fashion, and tumor shrinkage in seen in only approximately one third of patients. Treatment has also been associated with escape from the inhibitory effects of the drug.[9,10,44]

Somatostatin receptors are less numerous in TSH-secreting tumors than in those that secrete GH. However, TSH-secreting adenomas have proven to be quite responsive to treatment with octreotide. Octreotide, 50 to 750 µg two or three times daily, is effective in improving the status of approximately 92% of patients. Complete normalization of TSH occurs in 79% of patients, and tumor shrinkage occurs in 75%. Long-term studies demonstrate escape from therapy in approximately 10% of cases and the development of treatment resistance in 4%.[9] Hypothyroidism may occur when therapy produces too profound a fall in TSH. Reducing the dose of octreotide to restore euthyroidism is unwise, because it may allow tumor escape and recurrence of hyperthyroidism. Treatment with L-thyroxine is warranted in this situation.[10]

Acknowledgments and Caveats

We are grateful to John Schefter, Ph.D. for his kind and expert editorial assistance in the process of revision and review of this treatise.

Disclaimer

The recommendations herein are meant to be construed as a general guide to the endocrinologic evaluation and management of patients with pituitary tumors. The selection and appropriation of therapy and subsequent follow-up for each and every patient must be individualized. Drug doses, therapeutic approaches, and follow-up schemes recommended in this treatise should be carefully considered and verified by the treating physician because of individual patient variability and a multitude of caveats in the management of these complex patients.

REFERENCES

1. Blevins LS, Jr, Shore D, Weinstein J, et al: Clinical presentation of pituitary tumors. In Krisht AF, Tindall GT (eds): Pituitary Disorders: Comprehensive Management. Baltimore: Lippincott Williams & Wilkins, 1999, pp 145–161.
2. Vance ML: Perioperative management of patients undergoing pituitary surgery. Endocrinol Metab Clin North Am 32:355–365, 2003.
3. Singer PA, Sevilla LJ: Postoperative endocrine management of pituitary tumors. Neurosurg Clin N Am 14:123–138, 2003.
4. Simard MF: Pituitary tumor endocrinopathies and their endocrine evaluation. Neurosurg Clin N Am 14:41–54, 2003.
5. Lissett CA, Shalet SM: Management of pituitary tumours: Strategy for investigation and follow-up. Horm Res 53:65–70, 2000.
6. Thaler LM, Blevins LS, Jr: The low dose (1 µg) adrenocorticotropin stimulation test in the evaluation of patients with suspected central adrenal insufficiency. J Clin Endocrinol Metab 83:2726–2729, 1998.
7. Arafah BM, Hlavin ML, Selman WR: Pituitary adenomas: Perioperative endocrine management. In Krisht AF, Tindall GT (eds): Pituitary Disorders: Comprehensive Management. Baltimore: Lippincott Williams & Wilkins, 1999, pp 51–60.
8. Kreutzer J, Vance ML, Lopes MB S, et al: Surgical management of GH-secreting pituitary adenomas: An outcome study using modern remission criteria. J Clin Endocrinol Metab 86:4072–4077, 2001.
9. Sanno N, Teramoto A, Osamura RY: Thyrotropin-secreting pituitary adenomas: Clinical and biological heterogeneity and current treatment. J Neurooncol 54:179–186, 2001.
10. McCutcheon IE, Oldfield EH: Thyroid-stimulating hormone-secreting pituitary tumors. In Krisht AF, Tindall GT (eds): Pituitary Disorders: Comprehensive Management. Baltimore: Lippincott Williams & Wilkins, 1999, pp 267–280.
11. Woollons AC, Balakrishnan V, Hunn MK, et al: Complications of transsphenoidal surgery: The Wellington Experience. Aust N Z J Surg 70:405–408, 2000.
12. Jane JA, Jr, Thapar K, Kaptain GJ, et al: Pituitary surgery: Transsphenoidal approach. Neurosurgery 51:435–444, 2002.
13. Sawka AM, Aniszewski JP, Young WF, Jr, et al: Tension pneumocranium, a Rrare complication of transsphenoidal pituitary surgery: Mayo Clinic Experience 1976–1998. J Clin Endocrinol Metab 84:4731–4734, 1999.
14. Reeves WB, Andreoli TE: The antidiuretic hormone: Physiology and pathophysiology. In Krisht AF, Tindall GT (eds): Pituitary Disorders: Comprehensive Management. Baltimore: Lippincott Williams & Wilkins, 1999, pp 79–98.
15. Semple PL, Laws ER, Jr: Complications in a contemporary series of patients who underwent transsphenoidal surgery for Cushing's disease. J Neurosurg 91:175–179, 1999.
16. Inder WJ, Hunt PJ: Glucocorticoid replacement in pituitary surgery: Guidelines for perioperative assessment and management. J Clin Endocrinol Metab 87:2745–2750, 2002.
17. Thapar K, Laws ER, Jr: Growth hormone-secreting pituitary tumors: Operative management. In Krisht AF, Tindall GT (eds): Pituitary Disorders: Comprehensive Management. Baltimore: Lippincott Williams & Wilkins, 1999, pp 243–258.
18. Dökmetas HS, Çolak R, Kelestimur F, et al: A comparison between the 1-µg adrenocorticotropin (ACTH) test, the short ACTH (250 µg) test, and the insulin tolerance test in the assessment of hypothalamo-pituitary-adrenal axis immediately after pituitary surgery. J Clin Endocrinol Metab 85:2713–3719, 2000.
19. Courtney CH, McAllister AS, McCance DR, et al: Comparison of one week 0900 h serum cortisol, low and standard dose Synacthen tests with a 4 to 6 week insulin hypoglycaemia test after pituitary surgery in assessing HPA axis. Clin Endocrinol 53:431–436, 2000.
20. Gleeson HK, Walker BR, Seckl BR, et al: Ten years on: Safety of short Synacthen tests in assessing adrenocorticotropin deficiency in clinical practice. J Clin Endocrinol Metab 88:2106–2111, 2003.
21. Courtney CH, McAllister AS, McCance DR, et al: The insulin hypoglycemia and overnight metyrapone tests in the assessment of the hypothalamic-pituitary-adrenal axis following pituitary surgery. Clin Endocrinol 53:309–312, 2000.
22. McKenna TJ: Perioperative evaluation and management. In Blevins LS, Jr (ed): Cushing's Syndrome. Boston: Kluwer Academic Publishers, 2002, pp 279–299.
23. Mönig H, Stracke L, Arendt T, et al: Blunted nocturnal TSH surge does not indicate central hypothyroidism in patients after pituitary surgery. Exp Clin Endocrinol Diabetes 107:89–92, 1999.
24. van Dam PS, Dieguez C, Cordido F, et al: Diagnosis of growth hormone deficiency after pituitary surgery: The combined acipimox/GH-releasing hormone test. Clin Endocrinol 58:156–162, 2003.
25. Frankel RH, Tindall GT: Prolactinomas. In Krisht AF, Tindall GT (eds): Pituitary Disorders: Comprehensive Management. Baltimore: Lippincott Williams & Wilkins, 1999, pp 199–207.
26. Graham KE, Samuels MH: Cushing's disease. In Krisht AF, Tindall GT (eds): Pituitary Disorders: Comprehensive Management. Baltimore: Lippincott Williams & Wilkins, 1999, pp 209–224.
27. Arginteanu MS, Post KD: Cushing's disease: Operative management. In Krisht AF, Tindall GT (eds): Pituitary Disorders: Comprehensive Management. Baltimore: Lippincott Williams & Wilkins, 1999, pp 225–234.
28. Weil RJ, Allen GS: Transsphenoidal surgery for Cushing's disease. In Blevins LS, Jr (ed): Cushing's Syndrome. Boston: Kluwer Academic Publishers, 2002, pp 265–278.
29. Imaki T, Tsushima T, Hizuka N, et al: Postoperative plasma cortisol levels predict long-term outcome in patients with Cushing's disease and determine which patients should be treated with pituitary irradiation after surgery. Endocr J 48:53–62, 2001.
30. Ben-Shlomo A, Melmed S: Clinical review 154: The role of pharmacotherapy in perioperative management of patients with acromegaly. J Clin Endocrinol Metab 88:963–968, 2003.
31. Bevan JS, Atkin SL, Atkinson AB, et al: Primary medical therapy for acromegaly: An open, prospective, multicenter study of the effects of subcutaneous and intramuscular slow-release octreotide on growth hormone, insulin-like growth factor-1, and tumor size. J Clin Endocrinol Metab 87:4554–4563, 2002.
32. Freda PU: Clinical review 150: Somatostatin analogs in acromegaly. J Clin Endocrinol Metab 87:3013–3018, 2002.
33. Swearingen B, Barker FG II, Katznelson L, et al: Long-term mortality after transsphenoidal surgery and adjunctive therapy for acromegaly. J Clin Endocrinol Metab 83:3419–3426, 1998.
34. Valdemarsson S, Ljunggren S, Bramnert M, et al: Early postoperative growth hormone levels: High predictive value for long-term outcome after surgery for acromegaly. J Intern Med 247:640–650, 2000.
35. Kason TK, Blevins LS, Jr: The medical management of Cushing's syndrome. In Blevins LS, Jr (ed): Cushing's Syndrome. Boston: Kluwer Academic Publishers, 2002, pp 334–341.
36. Clemmons DR, Chihara K, Freda PU, et al: Optimizing control of acromegaly: Integrating a growth hormone receptor antagonist into the treatment algorithm. J Clin Endocrinol Metab 88:4759–4767, 2003.
37. Melmed S, Jackson I, Kleinberg D, et al: Current treatment guidelines for acromegaly. J Clin Endocrinol Metab 83:2646–2651, 1998.

38. Cozzi R, Attanasio R, Montini M, et al: Four-year treatment with octreotide-long-acting repeatable in 110 acromegalic patients: Predictive value of short-term results. J Clin Endocrinol Metab 88:3090–3098, 2003.

39. Attanasio R, Baldelli R, Pivonello R, et al: Lanreotide 60 mg, a new long-acting formulation: Effectiveness in the chronic treatment of acromegaly. J Clin Endocrinol Metab 88:5258–5265, 2003.

40. Trainer PJ, Drake WM, Katznelson L, et al: Treatment of acromegaly with the growth-hormone-receptor antagonist Pegvisoment. N Engl J Med 342:1171–1177, 2000.

41. Full prescribing information: Somavert, Pharmacia Corporation, 2003.

42. Chandler WF, Barkan AL, Schteingart DE: Management options for persistent functional tumors. Neurosurg Clin N Am 14:139–145, 2003.

43. Verhelst J, Abs R, Maiter D, et al: Cabergoline in the treatment of hyperprolactinemia: A study of 455 patients. J Clin Endocrinol Metab 84:2518–2522, 1999.

44. Iglesias P, Díez JJ: Long-term preoperative management of thyrotropin-secreting pituitary adenoma with octreotide. J Endocrinol Invest 21:775–778, 1998.

25 Transsphenoidal Approach to Pituitary Tumors

BROOKE SWEARINGEN

Though originally described almost 100 years ago, the transsphenoidal approach remains the optimal technique for removal of pituitary and other sellar tumors. A Viennese otolaryngologist, Victor Schloffer, initially described the lateral transfacial approach to the sphenoid in 1907.[1] This was modified by Halstead and then Cushing, who adopted the sublabial approach in 1910.[2] The endonasal approach was described by Otto Hirsch, based on the intranasal sphenoidotomy devised by Hajek.[3] Technical advances, including intraoperative lateral fluoroscopy, were introduced by Guiot and colleagues,[4] and with the microsurgical removal of the first microadenoma for Cushing's disease by Jules Hardy, reported in 1962 (see reference 5), pituitary surgery entered the modern era.

PREOPERATIVE EVALUATION

Endocrine Evaluation

A preoperative endocrine evaluation by an experienced pituitary endocrinologist will serve to define both conditions of hormone excess and possible hormone deficiency. Correction of hypoadrenalism or hypothyroidism preoperatively will improve surgical and anesthetic risk. Marked elevations in prolactin level (>200–250 ng/mL) are virtually diagnostic of a prolactinoma and may obviate the need for surgery, given the efficacy of dopamine agonist therapy. Postoperatively, the patient will again require complete hormone evaluation to monitor for any surgically induced hormone insufficiency.

Imaging

Preoperative imaging is best accomplished using high-field-strength magnetic resonance imaging (MRI). Coronal and sagittal T1-weighted images with and without gadolinium best define sellar anatomy and the relationship of sellar tumors to surrounding structures, especially the cavernous sinus and optic chiasm. Most pituitary tumors, even large macroadenomas, can be safely removed via the transsphenoidal approach, but unfavorable anatomy-extensive middle fossa growth through the cavernous sinus or a "dumbbell" shape will make the transsphenoidal approach more difficult and less likely to achieve a satisfactory result. T2-weighted images may indicate if the abnormality is cystic, suggesting a Rathke's cleft cyst, cystic adenoma, or craniopharyngioma. The location of the carotid arteries can be best determined on the coronal images. Though usually splayed laterally by a large macroadenoma, they are occasionally ectatic and displaced medially into the sella. Preoperative computed tomography (CT) scanning can demonstrate tumor calcification, and coronal reconstructions will help define the bony anatomy of the sphenoid septations. These preoperative MR and CT images can also be incorporated into neuronavigational devices for intraoperative localization, if these are to be used.

OPERATIVE TECHNIQUE

Recent reviews have summarized variations in the technique used by experienced pituitary surgeons.[6,7] Our own approach is as follows.

Patient Positioning and Preparation

The patient is placed in a semirecumbent position with the neck flexed toward the left shoulder so that the midline axis of approach is aligned with the surgeon's field of view. The head is elevated slightly higher than the right atrium to decrease venous bleeding. The surgeon stands at the right shoulder of the patient, looking up into the nasopharynx. Some surgeons prefer to stand directly at the head of the patient, facing caudally from above. This position tends to increase both venous and intracranial pressure, facilitating delivery of the suprasellar tumor, but increasing venous hemorrhage. The head is supported on a soft gel donut or horseshoe headrest and taped securely in place. Some surgeons prefer to immobilize the head using the Mayfield headrest, and skeletal fixation is necessary if navigational devices are to be used intraoperatively. The lateral fluoroscope is positioned to give a coplanar view of the sella, or the navigational workstation is positioned for ease of view. The retropharynx is packed with soft gauze to prevent blood from pooling. The perinasal skin is prepared with antiseptic solution and the nasal mucosa is sprayed with oxymetazoline (Afrin), and a prophylactic antibiotic is administered. The right lower quadrant of the abdomen is prepared for harvesting a fat graft. Stress dose steroid coverage is routinely provided with 4 mg of dexamethasone or 100 mg of hydrocortisone, unless the patient has Cushing's disease, when postoperative steroids are withheld until dexamethasone (0.5 mg daily) is begun on the first postoperative day.

Approach

There are three commonly used routes of access to the sphenoid: the direct endonasal, the submucosal tunnel via an anterior mucosal incision, or the sublabial approach (Fig. 25-1). We have found that in almost all cases a direct endonasal approach through the nostril provides adequate visualization with minimal tissue dissection, for either conventional microscopic or endoscopic approaches.

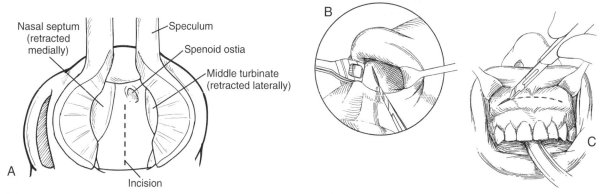

FIGURE 25-1   The three transsphenoidal approaches to pituitary tumors. *A,* Direct endonasal approach. *B,* Submucosal tunnel via an anterior mucosal incision. *C,* Sublabial approach. (*B* and *C* from Laws ER Jr: Transsphenoidal approach to pituitary tumors. In Schmidek HH, Sweet WH: Operative Neurosurgical Techniques. Indications, Methods, and Results, 3rd ed. Philadelphia: WB Saunders, 1995, p 285.)

Using a long hand-held nasal speculum and the operative microscope under low power, we infiltrate the mucosa overlying the intersection of the posterior septum and rostrum of the sphenoid with 0.25% lidocaine with epinephrine 1:400,000 (Fig. 25-2). A linear incision is made in the mucosa and the posterior septum fractured and deviated to the opposite side. As the septum is deviated, the contralateral mucosa over the rostrum is elevated and retracted as well. A self-retaining speculum is then placed with the leaves of the speculum on either side of the small remnant of the fractured bony septum. Orientation in the sagittal plane can be confirmed using the fluoroscope or navigational device, as well as with intranasal anatomic landmarks including the location of the sphenoid ostia, marking the superiormost extent of the sphenoidotomy, and the trajectory provided by the middle turbinate. Correct midline orientation is provided by the location of the keel of the rostrum. A midline approach is crucial to prevent inadvertent damage to perisellar structures, especially the cavernous sinus, carotid artery, and optic canal. If the anatomic landmarks are unclear and the septum is preserved, it is possible to identify the cartilaginous septum anteriorly, using an anterior hemitransfixion incision, and follow it back to the sphenoid rostrum through a submucosal tunnel. The septum itself can be fractured posteriorly and not removed, to help prevent a "saddle-nose" deformity.[8] The mucosa in the opposite nostril

is left intact since it will remain attached to the septum, and this will help prevent a postoperative septal perforation.

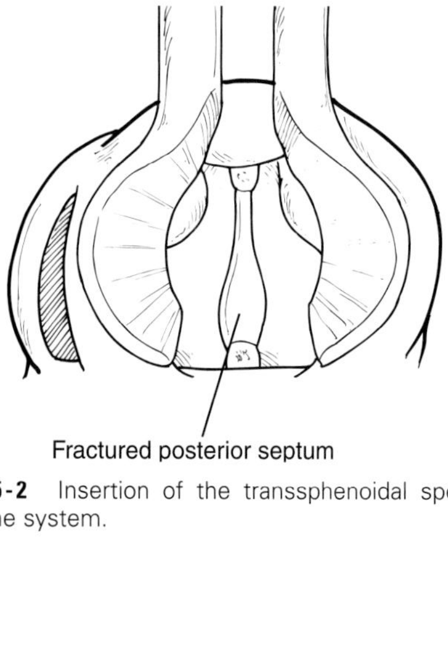

In those patients with small nostrils, where an endonasal approach does not provide adequate direct visualization, the sublabial approach can offer a wider field of view. In this approach, we prefer to begin with a unilateral anterior hemitransfixion incision, to identify the anterior septal cartilage and develop a submucosal tunnel. The upper lip is then retracted, and the gingiva is infiltrated with local anesthetic with epinephrine. The mucosa is incised from one incisor to the other and elevated from the maxilla until the nasal spine is reached. Use of the electrocautery against the maxilla should be avoided for fear of damaging the nervous supply to the front teeth and gums with resultant numbness. The inferior margin of the pyriform aperture is dissected free of mucosa bilaterally. The nasal mucosa can then be stripped at the aperture, connecting the gingival incision to the submucosal tunnel. We prefer to strip the mucosa from the septum on the left, transect the nasal spine using a small osteotome, and sweep the anterior septum to the right with the right-sided mucosa attached. It is then possible to fracture the posterior septum and place a self-retaining speculum, again using the keel of the rostrum to obtain correct midline orientation. Any septal bone or cartilage removed can be saved to aid in reconstruction of the sellar floor.

With the self-retaining speculum in place (Fig. 25-3), the rostrum of the sphenoid is now visualized. The sphenoid can be entered by fracturing the anterior wall with an osteotome and removed by grasping with forceps, but we prefer to drill into the sphenoid sinus with a high-speed diamond-tipped drill. Bony removal is carried back to the edges of the leaves of the speculum. The exposed sphenoid mucosa is then cauterized. We do not routinely exenterate the entire mucosa from the sphenoid, although some have argued that exenteration will minimize the risk of a postoperative mucocele. After incising the mucosa, the face of the sella can often be visualized, depending on the position of the sphenoid septations. Knowledge of the bony anatomy of the sphenoid is useful in maintaining the correct orientation.[9,10] This anatomy can be determined from preoperative CT or MR scanning. Septations within the sphenoid are inconstant and variable, but by correlating their intraoperative position with preoperative imaging studies, correct midline orientation can be maintained. The sphenoid may

FIGURE 25-2   Insertion of the transsphenoidal speculum after fracturing the system.

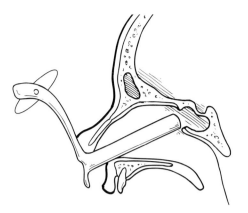

FIGURE 25-3 Positioning of the pituitary speculum after opening into the sphenoid.

be incompletely pneumatized, especially in children, which will require drilling a channel to achieve an open pathway to the sella. The sphenoid mucosa overlying the bony face of the sella is then cauterized. The face of the sella is often deficient, especially when the sella is expanded by a large tumor. Thinned bone can sometimes be outfractured using a small bone curet. Usually, the bone is drilled down to dura using a diamond-tipped drill.

Endoscopic Visualization

The successful development of the endoscopic approach for sinus surgery by the otolaryngologist has led to its application in pituitary surgery as well.[11] Use of the endoscope allows a wider field of view, and lateral visualization is possible with angled scopes.[12,13] This may aid in the removal of large tumors with significant lateral extent. The optics available on the video monitor are not equivalent to that obtainable with the best conventional operating microscopes, however, and depth of field is absent since visualization is monocular. The approach used for endoscopic resection is similar to the direct transnasal approach described earlier, although many surgeons skilled in endoscopy do not use the self-retaining speculum and work directly through the nasal channel, minimizing tissue trauma even further. The sphenoid ostium can be visualized endoscopically and enlarged. The endoscope can then be placed into the sphenoid, with visualization of the sella and surrounding anatomy. Some endoscopists prefer to introduce working instruments through the other nostril, while others work alongside the endoscope. The results for secretory adenomas with defined criteria for remission appear similar between endoscopic and open microsurgical techniques. For larger tumors, endoscopic approaches may improve visualization of the tumor's lateral extent, although a well-designed study comparing extent of resection will in practice be difficult to achieve. Combined techniques, using microsurgical techniques for tumor removal followed by endoscopic inspection for tumor remnants, offer the benefits of both approaches.

Tumor Removal

Correlating the preoperative sagittal MRI with the intraoperative fluoroscopy is useful to plan the dural opening. If the sella is partially empty, the dural opening should be planned

sufficiently inferiorly on the face of the sella to allow entrance into tissue, not into the suprasellar cistern. With larger tumors this is less important, although entry into the anterior recess of the suprasellar cistern along the superior margin of the sella may still cause cerebrospinal fluid (CSF) leakage. Cystic fluid or CSF can sometimes be identified through the dura as a bluish tint. The dural face of a small sella, explored for a microadenoma, may contain venous channels or the intercavernous (circular) sinus. It is worth planning the dural opening to allow cauterization of these channels if possible, since the search for a microadenoma requires absolute hemostasis. We prefer an X-shaped dural opening with bipolar cauterization of the dural leaflets, although others prefer a cruciate opening or a rectangular window (Fig. 25-4). Biopsy of the dura from this window has been suggested as a means of assessing dural invasion by the tumor.[14] Before making the dural incision, we pierce it with a spinal needle to help ensure that the proposed incision is not over the carotid canal or an ectatic carotid artery, although evaluation of the flow voids on the preoperative MRI may render this step superfluous.

With a large macroadenoma, tumor will be seen immediately upon opening the dura. The tumor is entered inferiorly using ring curets, and the tumor fragments are removed piecemeal using cup forceps. It is usually safer to divide the tumor bluntly by curettage rather than biting it away with cup forceps, as undue traction on a tenacious tumor may damage surrounding structures. The tumor is removed inferiorly back to the dorsum, and then out laterally to either cavernous sinus. Dissection is continued superiorly, up the lateral walls, until the attenuated diaphragm prolapses into the field. Removal of large tumors can be difficult if the tumor does not deliver itself or is of fibrous consistency. Delivery of the suprasellar tumor can sometimes be achieved by injecting 20 to 30 mL of intracranial air via a lumbar subarachnoid catheter. Using the lateral fluoroscope for visualization, a side-angled curet can also be introduced into the suprasellar space in an attempt to carefully sweep down residual suprasellar tumor. A staged resection can sometimes be beneficial for situations in which the suprasellar remnant does not descend during the initial procedure, since CSF pulsation over time may slowly force it into the sella where it can be resected at a second procedure.[15–17] The normal pituitary is usually flattened posteriorly against the diaphragm or dorsum. It can be recognized by its more yellow color and firmer consistency, and should be left

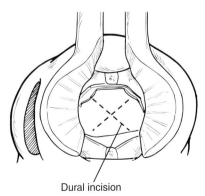

Dural incision

FIGURE 25-4 X-shaped dural incision with bipolar cauterization of the dural leaflets.

intact if possible. Adenomas are usually soft and reddish gray, although growth hormone–secreting tumors can be almost white. Tumors are sometimes very firm and vascular, and these can be difficult both to remove and to separate from the compressed normal gland.

When exploring for a microadenoma, normal gland is usually seen upon opening the dura. If the tumor has been visualized on the preoperative MRI, it can be approached by dissecting through the gland in the appropriate direction with a blunt probe, and then removed with a small ring curet. In Cushing's disease, unfortunately, the MRI often does not reveal the location of the tumor, and some have advocated intraoperative ultrasonography to aid in localization.[18] In these cases we begin by hemisecting the gland transversely. Multiple biopsy specimens are then sent for frozen-section analysis, beginning on the side suggested by the lateralization of the inferior petrosal sinus sampling. (Since lateralization data are not always correct, both sides of the gland may require inspection.) If the tumor is identified, that portion of pituitary is then removed. Since these microadenomas may be extraordinarily small, we have found it useful to prepare intraoperative cytologic smears for pathologic analysis when tiny fragments of suspect tissue are seen. The tissue is smeared between two sterile microscope slides and placed immediately into 95% alcohol fixative. This avoids repetitive handling and subsequent loss of these minute fragments.

Hemostasis must be meticulous, since the accumulation of even a small postoperative hematoma can be problematic in a confined space. Usually, transient packing with Surgical or Oxycel cotton will suffice. Injecting a slurry of Avitene or FloSeal into the tumor bed is sometimes helpful.[19] Bleeding from a large tumor will often cease as the tumor is completely removed. For difficult cases in which significant residual cavernous sinus or suprasellar tumor remains, a prolonged period of packing may be required. The use of intraoperative imaging before closure can sometimes detect the presence of an unsuspected hematoma.

Reconstruction of the Sella and Control of Cerebrospinal Fluid Leakage

Careful dissection and curettage will minimize the risk of a CSF leak, but intraoperative leakage is not uncommon. With a large macroadenoma, the diaphragm may be attenuated and leakage can occur. The anterior recess of the suprasellar cistern can be entered despite a careful dural opening, with leakage from the superior dural margin. Removal of extensive portions of the normal gland during an exploration for Cushing's disease will often lead to leakage, since damage to the diaphragm occurs when adherent normal gland is dissected from it. Packing the tumor bed with autologous fat harvested from a small right lower quadrant abdominal incision is usually sufficient to control the leak.[20] Others have successfully used muscle, fascia lata, lyophilized dura, and collagen sponge; moreover, some have argued that packing is often unnecessary for small sellas if no leak is seen.[21–24] The fat is then buttressed in place and the floor of the sella reconstructed. If bone or cartilage from the septum is available, this can be used as a strut to hold the fat in place and to reconstruct the bony floor. Thin, flexible titanium mesh can easily be cut to fit the sellar opening and the edges embedded in the margins of the bony defect. We use

this routinely, since we now rarely resect the nasal septum. Others have reconstructed the floor of the sella using a silicon strut, bioabsorbable plates, or tissue derived from the turbinate.[25–27] The construct can be coated with fibrin sealant if needed. We do not routinely pack the sphenoid sinus but will do so if the repair is tenuous. A lumbar drain can be placed if needed.

If the direct transnasal approach has been successful with minimal mucosal dissection, the septum can be returned to the midline, and nasal packing is not needed. If a submucosal tunnel was created or extensive mucosal dissection was required, the unoperated nostril is packed using a foreshortened nasal airway as a stent and the side of the approach with an expandable foam sponge (Merocel). The packing, if used, is removed on the first postoperative morning. If the sublabial approach was required, the gingival incision is closed with interrupted absorbable sutures and the nares are packed as described.

INTRAOPERATIVE IMAGING AND NAVIGATION

The navigational techniques that have gained widespread use in intracranial neurosurgery have also been used in the transsphenoidal approach. Reports in the literature find that the navigational devices are especially helpful in cases of reoperation or where normal anatomic landmarks have been destroyed, and may also be beneficial when used in combination with the endoscopic approach.[28–30] Direct comparison between fluoroscopic and navigational guidance suggests that the degree of accuracy is similar, although registration error leads to some navigational inaccuracy (within 3 mm).[31] Navigational devices offer a more 3-dimensional representation, instead of the unidimensional sagittal plane seen with conventional fluoroscopy.

Intraoperative MRI has also been used in pituitary surgery, with generally favorable results.[32] Some authors have reported finding residual tumor requiring further resection in a significant proportion (66%) of patients.[33] Others have reported that intraoperative imaging will demonstrate residual tumor in many patients, but that further resection is only possible in a smaller number (34%).[34] Our own experience with a low-field-strength magnet (0.12 T Odin PoleStar) suggests that intraoperative imaging is useful primarily in cases of large suprasellar tumors in which the diaphragm does not prolapse, since the images may suggest where to concentrate further attempts at resection. Often, however, failure to achieve complete resection in invasive macroadenomas is at least as much a function of the limitations of the exposure and unfavorable tumor anatomy as it is ignorance of the location of tumor remnants.

POSTOPERATIVE CARE

Patients are managed postoperatively in conjunction with the neuroendocrinologist. Daily serum sodium determinations are necessary to monitor for the development of diabetes insipidus or syndrome of inappropriate antidiuretic hormone secretion (SIADH), with determination of the urine specific gravity and careful recording of intake and output. Patients with acromegaly may excrete relatively large amounts of urine because they clear free water as their growth hormone levels fall; this has to be distinguished from true diabetes insipidus. Since the risk of developing SIADH is present for 7 to 10 days postoperatively, biweekly (outpatient) sodium determinations are continued during this period. Visual fields and acuity are monitored at the bedside. Perioperative prophylactic antibiotics are continued for 24 hours. Maintenance steroid coverage is continued until fasting cortisol levels are proven to be satisfactory. The patients are usually discharged within 24 to 48 hours. Follow-up endocrine testing and MRI scanning are then performed at 8 to 12 weeks.

Transsphenoidal surgery has been proven safe and effective in the management of sellar lesions, with acceptably low risks when the surgeon follows accepted surgical and anatomic principles.[35,36]

REFERENCES

1. Schloffer H: Erfolgreiche Operation eines Hypophysentumors auf nasalem Wege. Wien Klin Wochenschr 20:621–624, 1907.
2. Cushing H: Surgical experiences with pituitary disorders. JAMA 63:1515–1525, 1914.
3. Hirsch O: Endonasal method of removal of hypophyseal tumors. JAMA 55:772–774, 1910.
4. Guiot G, Arfel G, Brion S, et al: Adènomes Hypophysaires. Paris: Masson, 1958.
5. Hardy J: L'exérèse des adénomes hypophysiares par voie transsphénoidale. Union Médicale du Canada 91:933–945, 1962.
6. Jane JA, Jr, Thapar K, Kaptain GJ, Maartens N, Laws ER, Jr: Pituitary surgery: Transsphenoidal approach. Neurosurgery 51:435–442, 2002.
7. Ciric I, Rosenblatt S, Zhao JC: Transsphenoidal microsurgery. Neurosurgery 51:161–169, 2002.
8. Tindall GT, Collins WF, Jr, Kirchner JA: Unilateral septal technique for transsphenoidal microsurgical approach to the sella turcica: Technical note. J Neurosurg 49:138–142, 1978.
9. Bergland RM, Ray BS, Torack RM: Anatomical variations in the pituitary gland and adjacent structures in 225 human autopsy cases. J Neurosurg 28:93–99, 1968.
10. Rhoton AL, Jr: The sellar region. Neurosurgery 51:S335–S374, 2002.
11. Cappabianca P, de Divitiis E: Endoscopy and transsphenoidal surgery. Neurosurgery 54:1043–1050, 2004.
12. Jho HD, Alfieri A: Endoscopic endonasal pituitary surgery: Evolution of surgical technique and equipment in 150 operations. Minim Invasive Neurosurg 44:1–12, 2001.
13. Cappabianca P, Cavallo LM, Colao A, et al: Endoscopic endonasal transsphenoidal approach: Outcome analysis of 100 consecutive procedures. Minim Invasive Neurosurg 45:193–200, 2002.
14. Landolt AM, Schiller Z: Surgical technique: Transsphenoidal approach. In Landolt AM, Vance ML, Reilly PL (eds): Pituitary Adenomas. New York: Churchill Livingstone, 1996, pp 315–331.
15. Abe T, Iwata T, Kawamura N, et al: Staged transsphenoidal surgery for fibrous nonfunctioning pituitary adenomas with suprasellar extension. Neurol Med Chir (Tokyo) 37:830–835, 1997.
16. Nishizawa S, Yokoyama T, Ohta S, Uemura K: Surgical indications for and limitations of staged transsphenoidal surgery for large pituitary tumors. Neurol Med Chir (Tokyo) 38:213–219, 1998.
17. Saito K, Kuwayama A, Yamamoto N, Sugita K: The transsphenoidal removal of nonfunctioning pituitary adenomas with suprasellar extensions: The open sella method and intentionally staged operation. Neurosurgery 36:668–675, 1995.
18. Ram Z, Shawker TH, Bradford MH, Doppman JL, Oldfield EH: Intraoperative ultrasound-directed resection of pituitary tumors. J Neurosurg 83:225–230, 1995.
19. Ellegala DB, Maartens NF, Laws ER, Jr: Use of FloSeal hemostatic sealant in transsphenoidal pituitary surgery: Technical note. Neurosurgery 51:513–515, 2002.
20. Spaziante R, de Divitiis E, Cappabianca P: Reconstruction of the pituitary fossa in transsphenoidal surgery: An experience of 140 cases. Neurosurgery 17:453–458, 1985.
21. Sonnenburg RE, White D, Ewend MG, Senior B: Sellar reconstruction: Is it necessary? Am J Rhinol 17:343–346, 2003.
22. Kelly DF, Oskouian RJ, Fineman I: Collagen sponge repair of small cerebrospinal fluid leaks obviates tissue grafts and cerebrospinal fluid diversion after pituitary surgery. Neurosurgery 49:885–889, 2001.
23. Cappabianca P, Cavallo LM, Esposito F, Valente V, de Divitiis E: Sellar repair in endoscopic endonasal transsphenoidal surgery: Results of 170 cases. Neurosurgery 51:1365–1371, 2002.
24. Tindall GT, Woodard E, Barrow DL: Pituitary adenomas: General considerations. In Apuzzo MLJ (ed): Brain Surgery. New York: Churchill Livingstone, 1993, pp 269–276.
25. Kaptain GJ, Vincent DA, Laws ER, Jr: Cranial base reconstruction after transsphenoidal surgery with bioabsorbable implants. Neurosurgery 48:232–233, 2001.
26. El Banhawy OA, Halaka AN, El Dien AE, Ayad H: Sellar floor reconstruction with nasal turbinate tissue after endoscopic endonasal transsphenoidal surgery for pituitary adenomas. Minim Invasive Neurosurg 46:289–292, 2003.
27. Kabuto M, Kubota T, Kobayashi H, et al: Long-term evaluation of reconstruction of the sellar floor with a silicone plate in transsphenoidal surgery. J Neurosurg 88:949–953, 1998.
28. Elias WJ, Chadduck JB, Alden TD, Laws ER, Jr: Frameless stereotaxy for transsphenoidal surgery. Neurosurgery 45:271–275, 1999.
29. Sandeman D, Moufid A: Interactive image-guided pituitary surgery. An experience of 101 procedures. Neurochirurgie 44:331–338, 1998.
30. Cappabianca P, de Divitiis E: Image guided endoscopic transnasal removal of recurrent pituitary adenomas. Neurosurgery 52:483–484, 2003.
31. McCutcheon IE, Kitagawa RS, Demasi PF, Law BK, Friend KE: Frameless stereotactic navigation in transsphenoidal surgery: Comparison with fluoroscopy. Stereotact Funct Neurosurg 82:43–48, 2004.
32. Martin CH, Schwartz R, Jolesz F, Black PM: Transsphenoidal resection of pituitary adenomas in an intraoperative MRI unit. Pituitary 2:155–162, 1999.
33. Bohinski RJ, Warnick RE, Gaskill-Shipley MF, et al: Intraoperative magnetic resonance imaging to determine the extent of resection of pituitary macroadenomas during transsphenoidal microsurgery. Neurosurgery 49:1133–1143, 2001.
34. Fahlbusch R, Ganslandt O, Buchfelder M, Schott W, Nimsky C: Intraoperative magnetic resonance imaging during transsphenoidal surgery. J Neurosurg 95:381–390, 2001.
35. Ciric I, Ragin A, Baumgartner C, Pierce D: Complications of transsphenoidal surgery: Results of a national survey, review of the literature, and personal experience. Neurosurgery 40:225–236, 1997.
36. Barker FG, Klibanski A, Swearingen B: Transsphenoidal surgery for pituitary tumors in the United States, 1996–2000: Mortality, morbidity, and the effects of hospital and surgeon volume. J Clin Endocrinol Metab 88:4709–4719, 2003.

26 Complications of Transsphenoidal Microsurgery

IVAN S. CIRIC

INTRODUCTION

Transsphenoidal microsurgery is a well-established neurosurgical procedure that is routinely employed by neurosurgeons for a variety of pathologic processes involving the sphenoid bone region, sella, and the suprasellar space. Although this procedure dates back some 100 years,[1] it was not until Hardy reintroduced the procedure in the early 1960s that this technique took hold and eventually evolved into one of the safest neurosurgical procedures known to our specialty. The main moving force behind the ever-increasing popularity of transsphenoidal microsurgical technique in the second half of the twentieth century was the introduction of the operating microscope by Hardy.[2] The operating microscope affords not only magnification and coaxial illumination, but it also allows for a 3-dimensional viewing of a small and deep operative field. In fact, the 3-dimensional viewing of the operative field with the operating microscope is the single biggest advantage of microscope-based microsurgery, including transsphenoidal microsurgery over endoscopic-based microsurgery.[3,4,5,6] These two techniques, however, should not be exclusionary but complementary. The main advantage of the endoscope is its ability to look around beyond the visual field of the surgeon.

Despite the significant advances made in the understanding of the anatomic principles of transsphenoidal microsurgery, and the steady improvement in the technical aspects of the operation (e.g., the introduction of intracranial navigation), transsphenoidal microsurgery is still associated with significant complications.[7] Although complications associated with transsphenoidal microsurgery may not be very common, they can be devastating. The purpose of this chapter is to introduce the reader to possible complications associated with transsphenoidal microsurgery, to make some suggestions as to how to avoid these complications, and to discuss possible treatment options of these complications.

ANATOMIC PRINCIPLES

Transsphenoidal microsurgery is essentially a midline procedure. Veering off the midline can be associated with significant morbidity. Even though one may approach the sphenoid sinus from one side of the nasal septum, the sphenoid sinus should be opened in its entirety so as to expose the sella completely. Furthermore, it should also be recognized that the pituitary gland is an extra-arachnoid structure, because of which the overwhelming majority of pituitary adenomas, regardless of their size and extent, are also extra-arachnoid. Thus the ultimate goal of transsphenoidal microsurgery is to execute the operation without penetrating the arachnoid membrane of the diaphragma sellae. In the majority of cases this can be accomplished.

If one imagines the brain as surrounded by a double-membranous sac (i.e., the dura mater and the arachnoid), the transsphenoidal microsurgical operation should be executed outside the inner brain sac. Although pituitary adenomas do not penetrate the arachnoid membrane (which they push ahead as they grow), they do not respect the dura, which they invade and penetrate. This is especially true of giant prolactinomas and of approximately half of the growth hormone–secreting tumors. This has a significant implication in terms of possible complications associated with this procedure.

There may be a few exceptions to this anatomic principle. For example, it has been reported that some of the ACTH-secreting pituitary adenomas may be situated high on the intermediate lobe or the stalk, above the arachnoid of the diaphragma sella.[8] Such an anatomic configuration is relatively rare. Another anatomic principle is that pituitary adenomas commence within the anterior lobe, which they gradually distend as they continue to grow. Consequently, in very large pituitary adenomas (both secreting and nonsecreting), the residual normal anterior pituitary may be relegated to a very thin layer of anterior pituitary tissue surrounding the adenoma. This layer is usually represented by a fine line of enhancement around the pituitary macroadenoma that can be seen, at least partially, on the T1-infused MRI images.

COMPLICATIONS

Anesthetic Complications

The main anesthetic complications specific to transsphenoidal microsurgery are those that relate to airway obstruction. A patient undergoing transsphenoidal microsurgery should not be prematurely extubated postoperatively (i.e., before the patient regains full control of respiratory and swallowing functions). This is especially true in acromegalic patients who commonly suffer from sleep apnea.[9,10] In some patients, this will require that the patient remain intubated for an extended period postoperatively before being allowed to awaken and be extubated. It is also important to have the endotracheal tube secured in such a way that it will not dislodge intraoperatively, inasmuch as the anesthesiologist may have no control at all of the airway because of the surrounding drapes.

Complications of Positioning

The patient is positioned supine with the bridge of the nose parallel to the operating room floor. In patients with macroadenomas, we allow for some extension (e.g., 20 to 30 degrees) of the patient's head. The approach to the operative field is from the patient's right-hand side. Thus the head is tilted slightly toward the left shoulder while still maintaining an upright position of the face. Preoperatively, the patient is asked to place the head and neck in accordance with the position of the head and neck during surgery. Any forceful tilting of the neck, also a potential occlusion of the jugular outflow, must be avoided. A 3-point fixation clamp is used to secure the head to the operating table, inasmuch as even the slightest motion intraoperatively could prove disastrous. In addition, appropriate navigational attachments can be secured to the 3-point fixation clamp.

A preoperative navigational protocol MRI is carried out several days or even weeks preoperatively. The patient's head and tumor are then registered utilizing external anatomic landmarks such as the tragus on either side, the tip of the nose, the nasion, and a prominent area on the forehead that can be identified on the computer-generated images and that is at a certain distance from the nasion in the midline. It is usually not necessary to have more than 4 or 5 such external anatomic landmarks as fiducials to obtain a very accurate 3-dimensional representation of the patient's head and sellar tumor with a margin of error no greater than 1 mm in the vicinity of the sella.[11] The main advantage of utilizing external anatomic landmarks as fiducials is that the preoperative navigational protocol MRI can be obtained days prior to surgery, thereby saving considerable time in the preoperative preparations on the day of surgery.

In contrast to intraoperative fluoroscopy, which allows for vertical orientation only, intracranial navigation offers both vertical as well as horizontal orientation. This is important, especially when operating on recurrent tumors or in conjunction with extended transsphenoidal approaches. Intraoperative MRI may be useful in assessing the completeness of tumor removal; however, the surgeon should always be guided by his or her surgical instincts and experience as to when to stop the operation. No surgeon should go beyond his or her level of comfort when deciding whether to discontinue an operative procedure, regardless of what the intraoperative MRI may reveal.

Approach Complications

There are three main ways of reaching the sphenoid sinus. The first, and presently least practiced approach, is the sublabial ororhinoseptal approach; the second is the rhinoseptal-submucous approach; and the third is the direct transnasal approach.

The ororhinoseptal approach can be associated with postoperative numbness in the upper lip and upper midline teeth. The latter occurs especially if the maxillary spine is removed, and in the process the alveolar nerves are injured, be it in the process of bone removal or by using electrocautery. This is, however, the only approach during which nasal mucosa may not be penetrated at all. The nasal mucosal sacs are exposed on either side of the septum from below. The nasal mucosal sac on one side is then separated from the cartilaginous septum, while the opposite one is displaced together with the nasal cartilage to the contralateral side. A bilateral posterior submucous dissection is subsequently carried out on either side of the bony septum. This brings the surgeon directly onto the sphenoid rostrum without the need to open either of the two nasal mucosal sacs. This can be difficult to accomplish in a number of patients, especially in those with a significant septum deviation. Penetration of the nasal mucosal sac on one side will usually not result in a nasal septum defect. A nasal septum defect, on the other hand, will occur if there is a bilateral opposing tear present in the medial nasal mucosa. A nasal septum defect can be bothersome: if very small, it may result in a whistling noise; or if large, it may produce encrustations around the septal defect. The best way to prevent a nasal septum defect utilizing this approach is not to dissect the nasal mucosa on both sides of the cartilaginous septum and thereby avoid bilateral tears. When a tear is present, it should be repaired if possible utilizing 3-0 Vicryl sutures.

The rhinoseptal approach is similar to the ororhinoseptal approach in that it too can result in a septum defect; however, the incidence of septal defects utilizing this approach is considerably less. The incision into the nasal mucosa is usually carried out just behind the junction of the medial skin of the nares on one side and the adjacent medial mucosa. A submucous tunnel is then developed on the ipsilateral side, and the nasal cartilage is again dislocated to the contralateral side before a posterior tunnel is developed on that side. During both the ororhinoseptal approach and the rhinoseptal approach, the inferior part of the bony septum is removed. The advantages of these techniques are that they allow the less experienced surgeon to follow the midline toward the sphenoid rostrum, and it also provides for autogenous bony material to be used at the time of the closure of the sella.

The least traumatic route for the patient is the direct transnasal approach. The speculum is introduced into the nasal cavity on one side and opened just anterior to the sphenoid rostrum. Utilizing spot checks with the navigational probe, the surgeon can determine the best place to open the posteromedial nasal mucosa. This requires a little more experience in order to identify the midline. The surgeon should always strive to expose both sides of the sphenoid rostrum by dislocating the posterior portion of the bony septum across the midline and by identifying the characteristic appearance of the sphenoid rostrum, also confirming the midline with the navigational probe. By introducing a speculum, the surgeon further displaces the midline nasal mucosa and the underlying septum toward the opposite side. The speculum is locked just anterior to the sphenoid rostrum. This approach is not associated with a nasal septum defect. The main complications associated with this approach are those that relate to a failure to recognize the midline and that involve a veering off toward the cavernous sinus. A less experienced surgeon should probably use either the ororhinoseptal approach or the rhinoseptal approach, which readily identify the midline even without the help of intracranial navigation. The direct transnasal approach is also preferred in recurrent tumors because of the adherence of the medial nasal mucosac to the residual septum and to the opposite mucosal sac.

In all three approaches, intracranial navigation allows the surgeon to proceed in the appropriate direction (i.e., toward the sphenoid rostrum). There have been reports of surgeons getting lost in terms of the vertical orientation and reaching too high toward the cribriform plate; this can lead to serious complications such as CNS injury, cerebrospinal fluid leak, or meningitis. Intracranial navigation will also allow for horizontal orientation as to the midline. The surgeon may lose the appreciation for the midline if intracranial navigation either is not used or if it is incorrectly interpreted. Veering from the midline toward one side or the other can result in complications such as entering the orbits, injuring the cavernous sinuses and the anatomic structures contained within, or a possibly fatal hemorrhage caused by an injury to the carotid artery. Should the surgeon lose orientation during the approach, in spite of using intracranial navigation, it is probably better to stop and back out and come back some other day with no harm done, or to consult a senior colleague with more experience with the procedure.

None of the three approaches should be associated with any significant bleeding. If there is significant bleeding present, the surgeon has probably penetrated the nasal mucosa into the nasal cavity. In contrast, a bloodless field usually indicates that the surgeon is in the proper intermucosal plane, heading along the midline toward the sphenoid rostrum. We prefer not to inject xylocaine during the direct transnasal approach because it may distort the anatomy. Placing the speculum into the nasal cavity toward the sphenoid rostrum is usually not associated with any significant bleeding, especially after the speculum is opened. The posteromedial nasal mucosa can then be opened, utilizing either bipolar or monopolar coagulation and blunt or sharp dissection, until the opposite side of the slope of the sphenoid rostrum has been identified and the speculum advanced so it can lock on either side of the rostrum.

Sphenoidal Complications

After the speculum is locked in place anterior to the sphenoid rostrum, and the same is clearly identified under the operating microscope, the sphenoid rostrum is removed. It is advisable to revisit the preoperative imaging as to the configuration and location of the sphenoid sinus septi before the same are removed. Failure to do so can also result in the surgeon veering toward one side of the sphenoid sinus, with the potential of an inappropriate unilateral opening of the sella and injury to the cavernous sinus. The use of the navigational probe will prove helpful in identifying the entire extent of the sphenoid sinus before the septi are removed. A horizontal septum that divides the sphenoid sinus into an upper and lower compartment can be especially confusing because it may mimic the inferior surface of the planum, thus limiting the exposure. The use of the navigational probe will again reveal the true anatomic configuration of the sphenoid sinus and allow the surgeon to remove such a horizontally positioned sphenoid sinus septum.

Monopolar coagulation can be used outside the sphenoid sinus but never inside the sphenoid sinus because there may be a breach in the sphenoid bone with exposure of the dura that covers either the carotid arteries or the optic nerves. The speculum can be introduced into the widely opened anterior wall of the sphenoid sinus; however, great care must be exercised not to open the speculum forcefully and

create a fracture of the sphenoid bone that could result in injury to the optic nerves or to the carotid artery. When viewing the sphenoid sinus through the microscope, it should be remembered that the superolateral aspects of the sphenoid sinus posteriorly are represented by the inferomedial wall of the optic nerve canal; and that the anterolateral aspect of the anterior sella wall, especially inferiorly, is represented by the so-called carotid tubercle, behind which is situated the carotid canal. Consequently, the bone over these areas should be left intact. It is probably better to remove the sphenoid sinus mucosa in its entirety to avoid the formation of a postoperative sphenoid sinus mucocele.

Sellar Complications

The anterior wall of the sella should preferably be opened from the medial border of one cavernous sinus to the other. The cavernous sinuses usually reveal themselves as a change in the appearance of the exposed dura. Whereas the dura of the anterior sella wall has a grayish appearance, the medial border of the cavernous sinus will have a bluish hue. In less experienced hands, and especially in patients with invasion of the tumor into the cavernous sinus or in patients with recurrent adenomas, the position of the cavernous sinus may be more difficult to determine. Consequently, the use of intracranial navigation is of considerable help in locating the position of the cavernous sinuses. Preferably, the anterior sella dura should be opened first below the equator of the exposure so as not to injure a pronounced anterior arachnoid recess. This recess may be partially obliterated by the intrasellar pathology, only to open once the intrasellar pathology has been removed. This will then result in a CSF fistula. In order to avoid this, it is preferable to inspect the preoperative MRI for such an anterior arachnoid recess or a partially empty sella before proceeding with opening of the anterior dura superiorly.

With the anterior sella dura opened and the intrasellar contents exposed, it is not uncommon to see a thin layer of residual normal anterior pituitary draping over the actual pathology. This layer has to be incised, and perhaps a portion of it even excised, in order to reach the pathology. In accordance with standard microsurgical principles, it is always of benefit to first decompress the lesion internally before proceeding with the separation of the slacked tumor surface from the surrounding structures. Intermittent internal decompression and separation of the tumor surface from the surrounding structures is the most common way to proceed. In pituitary tumors, the separation of the tumor surface from the surrounding structures should preferably be started along the sellar floor, working alternatively toward either medial cavernous sinus walls, then proceeding along the medial walls of the cavernous sinus on either side until the reflection of the arachnoid membrane sloping toward the dura ring of the diaphragma sella is encountered, first on one and then on the other side. At no time should the medial wall of the cavernous sinus be penetrated. Adhering to this anatomic/surgical principle will certainly avoid intracavernous complications such as injury to the carotid artery and the surrounding cranial nerves.

Once the intrasellar portion of the tumor has been freed from the surrounding structures, including posteriorly between the pseudocapsule of the tumor and the posterior lobe (usually covered by a thin layer of areolar tissue), the removal of the suprasellar tumor portion can proceed. Again, the surgeon works from lateral to medial, alternating from both sides. The separation should always be between the tumor and the arachnoid membrane of the diaphragma sella, which is often covered by a very thin layer of residual normal anterior pituitary. This layer should be preserved. The separation can be accomplished by holding onto the tumor pseudocapsule while separating the overlying arachnoid with a variety of microdissectors, loop curettes, and perforated microsuction tips (preferably using 5 French microsuction tips). This technique will eventually result in an inversion of the arachnoid membrane and the ability of the surgeon to finally free the tumor pseudocapsule from the overlying layer of tissue represented by a thin layer of residual normal anterior pituitary and arachnoid. The main anatomic/surgical principle here is to avoid penetrating the arachnoid membrane: penetrating the arachnoid in search of more tumor significantly increases the possibility of serious morbidity. Penetration through the arachnoid membrane can result in an injury to the optic nerves and chiasm, to the carotid arteries and branches, or to the hypothalamus; it also will result in a CSF leak, which creates the possibility of meningitis. In short, avoidance of penetration through the arachnoid membrane overlying a pituitary adenoma will provide for a smooth and uncomplicated postoperative course. In contrast, significant penetration through the arachnoid membrane can be associated with grievous complications previously described.

Complications of Closure

Our closure technique includes placement of an autologous fat graft into the tumor bed cavity without overpacking it. Overpacking can cause pressure against the optic nerves and chiasm, which should be avoided. If there is evidence of a significant intraoperative CSF leak, an autologous fascia should also be harvested and placed directly underneath the diaphragma sella. We prefer to mix the fascia-fat graft with pulverized Surgicel, which allows for the construct to adhere to the diaphragma sella and also provides for additional hemostasis. The anterior sella wall is then reconstructed with a fragment of the bony septum, preferably placed precisely between the dura and the bony openings of the sella. If such bony fragment is not available, an appropriately thin-cut layer of bone can be obtained from a fibular allograft. If this is not possible, the intrasphenoidal fat graft should be held in place with fibrin glue. If, in the judgment of the surgeon, it is necessary to place a lumbar subarachnoid drain in order to further promote the healing of the graft, this is done as well.

Endocrine Complications

Postoperative anterior or posterior pituitary insufficiencies are rare following transsphenoidal microsurgery. They tend to occur more commonly following removal of microadenomas, when radical surgery is performed to achieve endocrine cure. It is very rare to see a patient with a postoperative anterior-posterior pituitary insufficiency following a gross total removal of a pituitary macroadenoma. This is despite the fact that the residual normal anterior pituitary may be

relegated to a very thin layer of tissue stretched along the diaphragma sella and along one side of the sella, and despite the fact that the posterior lobe and the stalk may never have been identified during surgery. Avoidance of removal of even the thinnest layer of residual normal anterior pituitary from the undersurface of the diaphragma sella will be sufficient in the majority of cases to prevent the postoperative occurrence of an anterior pituitary insufficiency.

DISCUSSION

A national survey conducted to evaluate complications of transsphenoidal surgery revealed that these complications are relatively rare.[7] The survey also revealed that a greater experience with the operation is associated with a statistically significant lower incidence of complications. That suggests that transsphenoidal surgery should be done as a programmatic and collaborative effort between several specialties including neurosurgery; endocrinology; anesthesiology; and, in some instances, otolaryngology (Tables 26-1 and 26-2).

The use of intracranial navigation has proven reliable and useful,[11] especially in patients with recurrent tumors. Absence of intracranial navigation can result in a faulty trajectory, be it during microsurgical or endoscopic approach. The end result of such a misdirected approach may be disastrous, with penetration through the cribriform plate resulting in brain injury, hemorrhage, or spinal fluid leak. For less experienced surgeons, the transnasal-submucous approach is probably preferable inasmuch as it allows the surgeon to follow a midline structure such as the nasal septum, although this may at times be deviated. In more experienced hands, the direct transnasal approach is the commonly

---

TABLE 26-1 ▪ Percentage of Operations, in Three Experience Groups, Resulting in Each Complication of Transsphenoidal Pituitary Surgery in the National Survey

Complication	% of Operations Resulting in Complication[a]		
	<200[b]	200–500	>500
Anesthetic complications	3.5	1.9	0.9
Carotid artery injury	1.4	0.6	0.4
Central nervous system injury	1.6	0.9	0.6
Hemorrhage into residual tumor bed	2.8	4.0	0.8
Loss of vision	2.4	0.8	0.5
Ophthalmoplegia	1.9	0.8	0.4
Cerebrospinal fluid leak	4.2	2.8	1.5
Meningitis	1.9	0.8	0.5
Nasal septum perforation	7.6	4.6	3.3
Postoperative epistaxis	4.3	1.7	0.4
Postoperative sinusitis	9.6	6.0	3.6
Anterior pituitary insufficiency	20.6	14.9	7.2
Diabetes insipidus	19.0	NA[c]	7.6
Death	1.2	0.6	0.2

[a]Estimation by participating neurosurgeons.
[b]Number of previous operations.
[c]NA, not applicable.
From Ciric I, Ragin A, Baumgartner C, Pierce D: Complications of transsphenoidal surgery: Results of a national survey, review of the literature, and personal experience. Neurosurgery 40:227, 1997.

TABLE 26-2 ▪ Association between Experience and Respondents' Estimation of Percentage of Operations Resulting in Specific Complications

Complication	Spearman Correlation	P
Anesthetic complications	−0.36	0.001
Carotid artery injury	−0.56	<0.001
Central nervous system injury	−0.33	<0.001
Hemorrhage into residual tumor bed	−0.30	<0.001
Loss of vision	−0.51	<0.001
Ophthalmoplegia	−0.57	<0.001
Cerebrospinal fluid leak	−0.17	<0.001
Meningitis	−0.49	0.003
Nasal septum perforation	−0.16	<0.001
Postoperative epistaxis	−0.56	<0.001
Postoperative sinusitis	−0.30	<0.001
Anterior pituitary insufficiency	−0.16	<0.001
Diabetes insipidus	−0.18	<0.001
Death	−0.61	<0.001

From Ciric I, Ragin A, Baumgartner C, Pierce D: Complications of transsphenoidal surgery: Results of a national survey, review of the literature, and personal experience. Neurosurgery 40:228, 1997.

chosen route, especially in recurrent tumors. A bloody operative field is usually an indication that the surgeon has veered off into the nasal cavities. In contrast, a bloodless field usually signifies a proper intermucosal trajectory.

Good care should be exercised to identify preoperatively the sphenoid sinus anatomy, especially as far as the position of the sphenoid sinus septa is concerned. Failure to do so can result in a misdirected trajectory toward one or the other side of the sella, with the potential of injury to the cavernous sinuses. It is always useful to expose anatomic landmarks such as the planum and the clivus because they signify the boundaries of the sella. The lateral extension of the sella can easily be obtained with the navigational probe. Monopolar coagulation should never be used inside the sphenoid sinus, because there may be a spontaneous breach present in the bony walls of the sphenoid sinus with the dura of the optic nerve canals exposed, and this may lead to a heat injury of the optic nerve.[12] Recognition of the position of the optic nerve canals in relationship to the sphenoid sinus, and also the position of the carotid arteries, is important prior to opening the sella.

It is preferable not to use an 11-blade knife or similar pointed instrument intrasellarly, because it could inadvertently penetrate the medial wall of the cavernous sinus and injure the carotid artery.[13] This was, indeed, the situation in a single case in our series of carotid artery injury: an 11-blade knife was used to attempt to resect a portion of the anterior sella dura adjacent to the cavernous sinus containing what appeared to be some invasion of a growth hormone–secreting pituitary microadenoma.

A pituitary surgeon with considerable experience may attempt to enter the medial wall of the cavernous sinus if there is evidence, either on the preoperative studies or intraoperatively, that the tumor had penetrated through the medial wall of the cavernous sinus and extended into the cavernous sinus in a dumbbell-shaped fashion. Such tumor invasion is usually associated with formation of a pseudo-fibrotic plane around the soft tumor within the

cavernous sinus. Thus such tumor extension can be removed, in some instances. Such a maneuver is associated with a much higher risk of injury to the carotid arteries or the surrounding cranial nerves. If an injury to the carotid artery occurs, the surgeon can pack the operative field with Surgicel/Gelfoam/moist Telfa cotton pads, apply gentle pressure to the construct, and ask the anesthesiologist to lower the mean arterial pressure in the hope of stemming the tide of hemorrhage. This is more often than not possible. A carotid-cerebral angiogram should then be obtained in order to identify the site of the fistula and decide where the fistula should be occluded, utilizing balloon occlusion technique and with or without trapping of the carotid artery.[14] A trial with balloon occlusion should be carried out with EEG recordings. Given good collateral circulation with no change in the EEG recordings, the balloon occlusion may then be completed in a permanent fashion. On the other hand, if there is evidence of a lack of collateral circulation, a superficial temporal-middle cerebral artery bypass may be necessary prior to occlusion of the fistula.

It is evident from this discussion that such an involved treatment of an injury to the carotid artery is best avoided by following the previously described principles. It is also obvious that such treatment requires an operative team experienced with these techniques and an operating room that is set up for such a complex surgical endeavor.

Intrasellar and suprasellar complications tend to occur when there is a failure on part of the surgeon to recognize the arachnoid or the diaphragma sella as it comes into view. Clearly, breach of the arachnoid increases the complication rate significantly. The surgery should never exceed his or her level of comfort in terms of how much tumor is removed. In this regard, availability of an intraoperative MRI, although useful in experienced hands, may be of detriment to the patient in less experienced hands. Recognition of significant residual tumor tissue on the intraoperative MRI does not mean that the surgeon must proceed with the removal of the residual tumor tissue if the surgical judgment is that this should not be done. On the other hand, deliberate inadequate removal of the tumor can also be associated with complications. For example, if the suprasellar tumor is disturbed by a timid surgeon who eventually decides not to proceed with its removal, the surgical manipulations in the suprasellar tumor can result in hemorrhage and edema and significant optic nerve and chiasm compression leading to loss of vision postoperatively.[15,16] Consequently, it is very important for the surgeon to decide as he or she proceeds whether the next layer of tumor should be addressed surgically. This may require the gentlest manipulation of this residual tumor in order to assess its consistency and vascularity before making the final decision in this regard.

It is probably better and safer for the patient if the surgeon decides to leave a portion of the suprasellar tumor unscathed, as opposed to manipulating the tumor vigorously only to back out and not remove it. On balance, however, a gross total tumor removal is always associated with better results than is an incomplete tumor removal. This brings us back to the issue of experience with this procedure. Perhaps it is better for a neurosurgeon who does not perform this operation on a regular basis to refer large and complex pituitary adenomas to a center where this procedure is done on a regular basis by an experienced team.

CONCLUSIONS

Transsphenoidal microsurgery is a well-established and, by and large, a safe operative procedure; however, significant complications can occur during the operation. To avoid these complications, the surgeon should adhere to certain anatomic/surgical principles. Less-experienced surgeons should exercise great caution when deciding to proceed with transsphenoidal surgery in a given patient. Transsphenoidal microsurgery should be done on a programmatic basis rather than on an ad hoc, sporadic basis.

REFERENCES

1. Schoffler H: Ergolgreiche Operations eines Hypophysentumors auf nasalem Wege. Wien Klin Wochenschr 21:621, 1907.
2. Hardy J: Transsphenoidal removal of pituitary adenomas. Union Med Can 91:933–945, 1962.
3. Apuzzo MLJ, Heifetz M, Weiss MH, Kurze T: Neurosurgical endoscopy using the side-viewing telescope: Technical note. J Neurosurg 16:398–400, 1977.
4. Cappabianca P, Cavallo LM, Colao A, et al: Endoscopic endonasal transsphenoidal approach: Outcome analysis of 100 consecutive procedures. Minim Invasive Neurosurg 45:1–8, 2002.
5. Cappabianca P, Cavallo LM, Colao A, de Divitiis E: Surgical complications of the endoscopic endonasal transsphenoidal approach for pituitary adenomas. J Neurosurg 97:293–298, 2002.
6. Jho HD, Carrau RL, Ko Y: Endoscopic pituitary surgery. In Wilkins RH, Rengachary SS (eds): Neurosurgical Operative Atlas. Park Ridge, IL: American Association of Neurological Surgeons, 1996, pp 1–12.
7. Ciric I, Ragin A, Baumgartner, Pierce D: Complications of transsphenoidal surgery: Results of a national survey, review of literature, and personal experience. Neurosurgery 40:225–237, 1997.
8. Mason RB, Nieman L, Doppman J, Oldfield E: Selective excision of adenomas originating in or extending into the pituitary stalk with preservation of pituitary function. J Neurosurg 87:343–351, 1997.
9. Goldhill DR, Dalgleish JG, Lake RHN: Respiratory problems and acromegaly. Anesthesiology 37:1200–1203, 1982.
10. Young ML, Hanson CW III: An alternative to tracheostomy following transsphenoidal hypophysectomy in a patient with acromegaly and sleep apnea. Anesth Analg 76:446–449, 1993.
11. Ciric I, Rosenblatt S, Zhao JC: Transsphenoidal microsurgery. Neurosurgery 51:161–169, 2002.
12. Renn WH, Rhoton AL Jr: Microsurgical anatomy of the sellar region. J Neurosurg 43:288–298, 1975.
13. Ahuja A, Guterman LR, Hopkins LN: Carotid cavernous fistula and false aneurysm of the cavenous carotid artery: Complications of transsphenoidal surgery. Neurosurgery 31:774–779, 1992.
14. Britt RH, Silverberg GD, Prolo DJ, Kendrick MM: Balloon catheter occlusion for cavernous carotid artery injury during transsphenoidal hypophysectomy. J Neurosurg 55:450–452, 1981.
15. Ciric I, Mikhael M, Stafford T, et al: Transsphenoidal microsurgery of pituitary macroadenomas with long-term follow-up results. J Neurosurg 59:395–401, 1983.
16. Decker RE, Chalif DJ: Progressive coma after the transsphenoidal decompression of a pituitary adenoma with marked suprasellar extension: Report of two cases. Neurosurgery 28:154–157, 1991.

27 Endoscopic Transsphenoidal Surgery

HAE-DONG JHO and DAVID H. JHO

Neuroendoscopy was first implemented almost a century ago for choroid plexus surgery in a patient with hydrocephalus; its advancement since has been sluggish, with only sporadic reports in the literature until recent years. With the advent of ventricular shunt systems, general enthusiasm for ventricular endoscopy declined, and was only just revived for third ventriculostomies in selected patients with obstructive hydrocephalus. Yet a few neurosurgeons continued to expand the use of neuroendoscopy to include ventricular tumor surgery, intra-axial brain surgery with stereotactic guidance, extra-axial intracranial surgery, endoscope-assisted microsurgery, endonasal transsphenoidal surgery, and spinal surgery. These advances were accompanied by concurrent technological developments in endoscopic optics, video imaging systems, endoscopic accessory attachments for neurosurgical applications, compatible frameless stereotaxis or computer image–guided systems, and suitable neuroendoscopic surgical instruments. As neuroendoscopic surgical technique and equipment have evolved together, the addition of neuroendoscopy to the repertoire of the modern neurosurgeon has become increasingly practical. Of note, general interest has grown in recent years for the use of neuroendoscopy in endonasal transsphenoidal pituitary surgery. Although Guiot and colleagues[1] first reported the use of an endoscope in sublabial transsphenoidal surgery in 1963, common use of neuroendoscopy in pituitary surgery only came about as of late with the present ongoing development of commercially available neuroendoscopic equipment.

The initial use of sinonasal endoscopy began in Europe three decades ago, and its introduction to the United States two decades ago, sparked an evolution in surgical techniques. Endoscopic sinus surgery rapidly replaced conventional sinus surgery, and sinonasal endoscopy brought radical changes in the concepts of pathophysiology and treatments of sinonasal ailments.[2] Rather than stripping the infected sinus mucosa (as done in conventional sinus surgery), endoscopic sinus surgery aimed to restore physiologic mucous drainage merely by eliminating obstructive pathoanatomy, and it came to be called *functional endoscopic sinonasal surgery*. Interest developed in the use of endoscopy for transsphenoidal surgery with advances in sinonasal endoscopy. Current use of sinonasal endoscopy in transsphenoidal surgery ranges from guidance during simple biopsy of a sellar lesion, to aid during insertion of transsphenoidal retractors for the microscopic removal of pituitary adenomas, to adjunct visualization during microscopic surgery, and for sole endoscopic pituitary tumor surgery.[3–10]

Traditional microscopic transsphenoidal surgery utilizes a sublabial or transfixional transseptal approach, but neuroendoscopy has facilitated the use of the endonasal route in pituitary surgery. Even though the removal of pituitary tumors completely through endoscopic visualization via an endonasal route has been a relatively recent development, the use of the endonasal approach itself was first reported in 1909 by Hirsch, who performed his first pituitary surgery in Vienna by approaching the sella though an endonasal route with multiple-staged sinonasal operations.[11] Although his first endonasal transsphenoidal surgery was successful, Hirsch subsequently converted to a transseptal submucosal approach, likely because of a fear of surgical infection through the wide communication made between the nasal and the cranial cavities. The use of the endonasal approach was revisited in 1987 by Griffith and Veerapen, when they inserted a transsphenoidal retractor through the natural nasal airway to the sphenoidal rostrum for microscopic pituitary surgery.[12] In 1994, Cooke and Jones reported the lack of sinonasal and dental complications when an endonasal route was adopted for microscopic pituitary surgery.[13]

This chapter describes endoscopic endonasal transsphenoidal surgery, which is not merely endoscope-assisted microscopic surgery, but is rather an operation done completely with an endoscope without any transsphenoidal retractor or nasal speculum, eliminating the need for postoperative nasal packing.[14–21] Endoscopic transsphenoidal surgery utilizes an endonasal route to the rostrum of the sphenoidal sinus, and an anterior sphenoidotomy about 1 to 1.5 cm in size. The physical nature of an endoscope, with its optics at the tip and slender shaft, allows easy access to the sella through the natural nasal air pathway via a nostril. The wide-angled panoramic view, angled-lens views, and a close-up zoom-in view provide optical advantages and distinct visualization at the surgical target site. The application of this endonasal endoscopic surgery has expanded to the surgical treatment of midline pathologies at the anterior cranial fossa, pterygoid fossa, clivus or posterior fossa, as well as for pathologies around the optic nerve and in the cavernous sinus. Endoscopic endonasal techniques can apply to any lesion within approximately 2 cm of the midline skull base, from the crista galli anteriorly to the foramen magnum posteriorly.[22–30]

PREOPERATIVE MANAGEMENT AND SURGICAL INDICATIONS

As with microscopic pituitary surgery, all patients with pituitary adenomas undergo formal endocrine evaluations preoperatively and postoperatively. Neurophthalmology evaluation is also required preoperatively, and follow-up visual examination is performed postoperatively for patients with positive preoperative visual findings. Magnetic resonance (MR) imaging of the brain with and without contrast enhancement is the main diagnostic test for pituitary adenomas. Occasionally a computed tomography (CT) scan of the brain is obtained when an MR scan cannot be done for patients with claustrophobia or extreme obesity. Bone windowed CT scans, axial and coronal views, can disclose the bony anatomy of the paranasal sinuses in detail; however, MR information for the paranasal sinuses is enough in most patients. Hypopituitarism is treated preoperatively, particularly for hypocortisolism and/or hypothyroidism.

Surgical indications for patients with pituitary adenomas who might undergo endoscopic transsphenoidal surgery are similar to those for conventional microscopic transsphenoidal surgery. Patients with hormonally inactive pituitary adenomas are operated on when the tumors cause symptomatic compression of the optic nerve system, hypopituitarism, pituitary apoplexy, or severe frontotemporal headaches. Patients with hormonally active pituitary adenomas causing acromegaly, hyperthyroidism, and Cushing's disease are operated on as the primary mode of treatment. Patients with prolactinomas are operated on only when they do not respond to dopaminergic medications, develop intolerable side effects to the medications, or choose against dopaminergic medications. Other mass lesions at the pituitary fossa are operated on for a simple biopsy or for resection. Contrary to conventional microscopic surgery, a large suprasellar tumor can be directly visualized, enhancing the chance for total resection. If further exploration at the planum sphenoidale is required for the suprasellar portion of the tumor, it can be done easily by extending bony exposure rostrally. This endoscopic transsphenoidal approach can therefore reduce the need of a transcranial approach for pituitary adenomas.

We have not yet encountered a patient whose nostril or nasal airway was too small or narrow to undergo endoscopic transsphenoidal surgery. Patients with Cushing's disease often have a narrow nasal airway because of swollen hypertrophic mucosa, which also tends to bleed easily. Among our patients who have undergone endoscopic transsphenoidal surgery, two patients with Cushing's disease required a two-nostril technique: an endoscope was inserted through one nostril and the surgical instruments were inserted through the other. Reoperation by endoscopic techniques for patients who have undergone previous transsphenoidal surgery is relatively easy because an anterior sphenoidotomy has already been done as part of the previous surgery, and submucosal dissection is not required. Reoperation can be performed as many times as indicated.

PERTINENT SINONASAL ANATOMY

To perform endoscopic pituitary surgery, the functional physiology and anatomy of the sinonasal cavity must be well understood. In the paranasal sinus, mucociliary movement is orchestrated by the delivery of mucus flow to the sinus ostia. From the sinus ostia, nasal mucosal ciliary movement is also directed to establish the physiologic flow of mucus toward the nasopharynx. When the tract of physiologic mucus flow is interrupted mechanically or functionally, the paranasal sinuses retain stagnant mucus, which can easily become infected, causing sinusitis. The confluence of the draining mucus from the frontal sinus, anterior ethmoidal sinus, and maxillary sinus is located anteriorly at the middle meatus. Mucosal drainage of the posterior ethmoidal sinus and sphenoidal sinus occurs at the sphenoethmoidal recess, which is located between the posterolateral aspect of the middle turbinate and the rostrum of the sphenoidal sinus. Any pathology interrupting this mucus flow is detrimental to the sinuses.

The endoscopic pituitary surgery described here does not involve complex anatomy because the approach occurs in the area between the middle turbinate and the nasal septum. However, the sinonasal anatomy located anteriorly and laterally to the middle turbinate is important for sinonasal function, and those structures should not be traumatized or disrupted. Anterolateral to the middle turbinate is the uncinate process, behind which is a groove called the hiatus semilunaris. Along the posterorostral bank of the hiatus semilunaris is the ethmoidal bullae. As mentioned earlier, the mucus from the frontal sinus and anterior ethmoidal air cells drains to the hiatus semilunaris. The maxillary sinus ostium is located at the caudal end of the hiatus semilunaris just lateral to the middle turbinate. During endoscopic endonasal pituitary surgery, the normal anatomy must be maintained or well restored.

To minimize disruption of the sphenoidal sinus mucosa, the mucosal removal is made only at the anterior sphenoidotomy hole and the anterior wall of the sella. When a pituitary tumor is removed, reconstruction is made at the anterior wall of the sella. The sphenoidal sinus is left as a naturally air-filled cavity, and no foreign surgical material is left in the sphenoidal sinus. The middle turbinate is placed back in its medial position so as not to block the mucus drainage through the maxillary sinus ostium. The same is true at the posterior mucus drainage channel at the sphenoethmoidal recess. When an anterior sphenoidotomy is made, attention must be paid not to disrupt the normal mucus drainage channel.

The posterior septal artery arises from the sphenopalatine branch of the internal maxillary artery and passes to the posterior nasal septum at the inferior medial aspect of the posterior middle turbinate. When surgical access is obtained between the middle turbinate and nasal septum for an anterior sphenoidotomy, the posterior septal artery must often be coagulated and divided to prevent unwanted intraoperative or postoperative nasal bleeding. Delayed copious nasal bleeding after transsphenoidal surgery usually arises from rebleeding of the posterior septal artery. When the sphenoidal sinus is entered with an endoscope, the complex anatomy is visualized in a panoramic fashion. The clival indentation is seen at the bottom midline, the bony protuberances covering the internal carotid arteries are lateral to the clival indentation, the sella is at the center, the cavernous sinuses are seen lateral to the sella, the tuberculum sella is at the top, and the bony protuberances of the optic nerves are seen laterally.

Surgical landmarks for endoscopic endonasal pituitary surgery consist of the nasopharynx and the inferior margin of the middle turbinate. The nasopharynx is always a good landmark to use to confirm the middle turbinate. The extended line along the inferior margin of the middle turbinate leads to the region 1 cm inferior to the sellar floor.

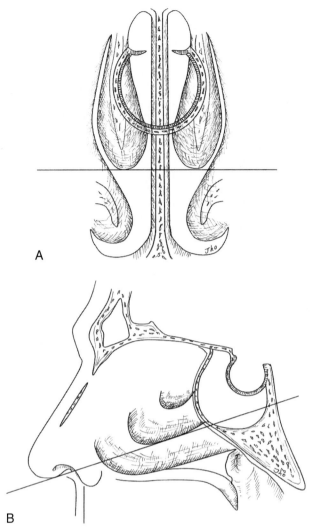

A

B

FIGURE 27-1 These schematic drawings (*A*, coronal, and *B*, sagittal views) of the sinonasal cavity demonstrate the anatomic landmarks leading to the sella. The line drawn along the inferior margin of the middle turbinate leads to the clivus about 1 cm inferior to the floor of the sella. The nasopharynx is the first surgical landmark. The middle turbinate is confirmed in reference to the nasopharynx. Because the superior turbinate can mimic the middle turbinate, the middle turbinate has to be confirmed in reference to the nasopharynx. These surgical landmarks are so consistent that intraoperative fluoroscopic C-arm imaging has not been necessary.

Although the sphenoidal sinus ostium is occasionally visible under the endoscope, it may not always be easily identifiable. Thus the sphenoidal sinus ostium cannot be used as a consistent surgical landmark. Anterior sphenoido-tomy approximately 1.5 cm in size is performed at the rostrum of the sphenoidal sinus at a location rostral to an extended line from the inferior margin of the middle turbinate (Fig. 27-1A and B).

OPTICAL ADVANTAGES OF AN ENDOSCOPE

Wide-Angled Panoramic View

As transsphenoidal pituitary surgery began to evolve in the twentieth century, one major advance was the adoption of

the operating microscope in the 1960s. The use of the endoscope for pituitary tumor resection represents another significant advancement. Whereas the operating microscope provides a magnified view of a limited portion of the sella through a narrow corridor revealed by the transsphenoidal retractor, an endoscope can physically enter into the sphenoidal sinus and provide a wide-angled panoramic view with zooming capability. An operating microscope renders a tubular parallel beam view, but an endoscope shows a diverging, flask-shaped, wide-angled view (Fig. 27-2A to D). This wide-angled panoramic view is particularly useful for pituitary tumor surgery because it allows excellent anatomic visualization at the posterior wall of the sphenoidal sinus. However, it must be recognized that the endoscopic view renders a fish-eye effect, with maximum magnification at the center, relative contraction at the periphery, and visualization of a wide anatomic area. In the well-pneumatized sphenoidal sinus, the sella is readily recognizable at the center of the surgical view, and a panoramic image of the surrounding anatomy at the posterior wall of the sphenoidal sinus is revealed under direct endoscopic view. Unless the sella is unpneumatized, or the patient is a complicated reoperation case, the use of fluoroscopic roentgenogram is not necessary because endoscopic visualization can adequately reveal the distinct surgical anatomy.

Angled-Lens View

The angled-lens endoscopic view provides direct visualization of the anatomic corners such as the suprasellar area or toward the cavernous sinus. These views can be of great assistance even if an endoscope is only used as an adjunctive tool during conventional microscopic surgery. Operating under an angled-lens endoscopic view requires specially designed surgical tools and advanced endoscopic surgical skills, particularly for the 70-degree-lens endoscope. As an angled-lens endoscope is rotated toward the surgical target, various anatomic corners can be visualized from the floor of the sella to the medial wall of the cavernous sinus and toward the suprasellar region. A fiberoptic endoscope can sometimes be used to inspect anatomic corners involving curved routes. This angled view is advantageous when large suprasellar macroadenomas are to be removed. This view also allows clear visualization at the medial wall of the cavernous sinus when the lateral margin of a sellar tumor abutting the cavernous sinus is dissected away or when tumor tissue invading the cavernous sinus is to be removed under direct visualization. Although pituitary adenomas invading the cavernous sinus are generally regarded as inoperable, the endoscopic techniques allow safe access to the cavernous sinus for tumor removal. Angled views allow for direct surgical access to the pterygoid fossa, anterior cranial fossa, clivus, and posterior cranial fossa, in addition to the cavernous sinus (Fig. 27-3A and B).

Close-up Internal View

When tumor resection is accomplished, an endoscope can be advanced into the sella or suprasellar area close to the surgical target. This close-up view, in liaison with zooming of the camera, enhances the magnification of the surgical site. For microadenoma removal, the close-up view is utilized

FIGURE 27-2 These schematic drawings demonstrate a comparison between the microscopic and the endoscopic exposure at the posterior wall of the sphenoidal sinus during transsphenoidal pituitary surgery. *A, B,* Microscopic view is confined at the very small limited area of the sella due to a straight narrow tubular vision. *C, D,* Endoscopic exposure discloses the wide area of the posterior wall of the sphenoidal sinus because of the wide-angled nature of the endoscopic optical characteristics. The center is maximally magnified, whereas the periphery is contracted with a panoramic view because of the fish-eye effect of an endoscope lens. Endoscopic view demonstrates the sella (S) at the center, cavernous sinuses (Cs) laterally, the cavernous carotid arteries (Ca) inferolaterally, clivus (Cl) inferiorly, tuberculum sella (Ts) superiorly, and optic nerves (O) superolaterally.

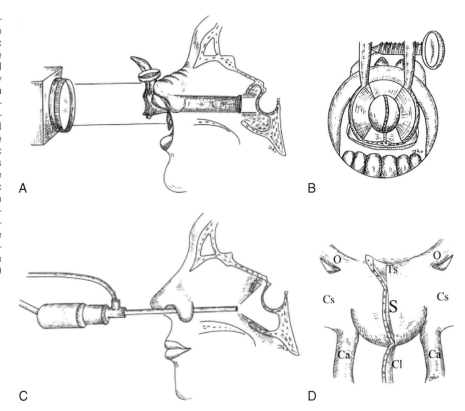

to confirm that the normal margin of the pituitary tissue is well exposed at the tumor resection site. For macroadenomas, an endoscope can be advanced into the tumor resection cavity to visualize the internal anatomy at the resection cavity. When a 30-degree angled endoscope is inserted into the cavity and rotated through a full revolution, it can visualize the entire circumference of the cavity. Often a minute amount of tumor residue is revealed at the hidden corners, assisting in completion of removal. These close-up magnified views thus enhance complete tumor removal in microadenomas as well as in macroadenomas.

PHYSICAL ADVANTAGES OF AN ENDOSCOPE

Endoscopes can be subdivided into two categories: fiberoptic flexible endoscopes and rod-lens rigid endoscopes. The number of fiberoptic fibers in most flexible endoscopes is approximately 10,000, although new flexible endoscopes carrying up to 50,000 fibers are being developed. Thus the image quality of the flexible endoscope is still inadequate for pituitary surgery, and its use is limited to occasional inspection at deep curved anatomic regions. Three-mm or 4-mm rod-lens endoscopes can be used for primary visualization during pituitary surgery because they provide clear video images. Four-mm rod-lens endoscopes provide full-screen, high-quality images in contrast to the smaller, inferior quality images provided by 3-mm rod-lens endoscopes. The basic endoscopes used by the authors are 4-mm rod-lens endoscopes with 0-, 30-, or 70-degree lenses. As previously mentioned, the slender physical shape of the endoscope shaft, with the visualizing lens at the tip, allows navigation

through a narrow anatomic space and eliminates the need to traumatically retract a straight tubular surgical corridor. Surgical incision, septal mucosal dissection, or removal of the nasal septum is unnecessary; therefore, postoperative nasal packing is also not necessary. The occurrence or amount of postoperative bloody nasal discharge is very minimal, and postoperative comfort of the patient is related to the minimal anatomic disruption during surgery.

SURGICAL PROCEDURE

Surgical Instruments

Appropriate surgical equipment is necessary to perform adequate endoscopic pituitary surgery. Attempting an endoscopic operation of this nature with a borrowed otolaryngologic endoscope will result in much frustration. Endoscopic surgical techniques are quite different from those of microscopic surgery. Being well-trained in microscopic surgery does not preclude the need for practice in endoscopy. The required surgical instruments are endoscopes with 0-, 30-, and 70-degree lenses (Fig. 27-4A); and their appendages, including a video-imaging system and light source connections, an endoscope lens-cleansing device, a rigid endoscope holder, and various other surgical instruments specifically designed for endoscopic pituitary surgery. The length of an endoscope must be 18 cm or longer. When an 18-cm-long endoscope was used for removal of a posterior fossa tumor through an endonasal transclival approach, it proved to be marginally short and restricted the surgeon's operating space between the endoscopic appendages and the patient's face.

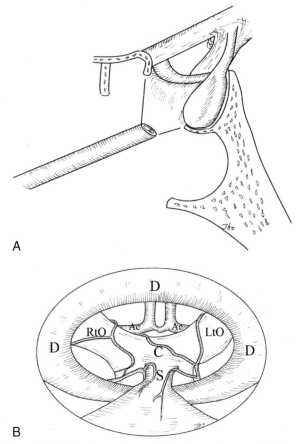

A

B

FIGURE 27-3 These schematic drawings show angled views toward the suprasellar region with 30-degree-lens endoscope. *A,* The 30-degree-lens endoscope is directed toward the suprasellar region. *B,* The 30-degree-lens endoscopic view discloses the anterior cerebral artery (Ac), optic chiasm (C), diaphragma sella (D), left optic nerve (LtO), right optic nerve (RtO), and pituitary stalk (S).

An endoscopic lens-cleansing device is required to cleanse the lens so that the surgeon can operate without interruption (Fig. 27-4B). The device consists of a disposable irrigation tube, which is passed through a battery-powered motor. The irrigation tube is connected into a saline bag, which is hung on a pole, and this motor-powered irrigation device is controlled by a foot pedal to flush saline forward. When the foot pedal is released, the motor reverses its rotary direction and draws the saline back for 1 to 2 seconds. The forward flow of irrigation saline cleans the lens, and the reverse flow clears water bubbles at the tip of the endoscope. Although this device is not ideal, it helps the surgeon significantly in the task of keeping the endoscope lens clean.

An appropriate endoscope holder is another piece of essential equipment required to perform this operation efficiently (Fig. 27-5A and B). The holder must provide rigid fixation of the endoscope, and its holding terminal must be compact and slender so as to render adequate operating space around the endoscope shaft needed for the surgeon to maneuver surgical instruments. Two different types of endoscope holders are currently in the process of development. One is a simple, manual holder with multiple joints that can be tightened by hand. The other is a holder with joints that are tightened or released by a single button powered by nitrogen gas. The latter, although more expensive, will be

a promising and convenient device once fully developed. An endoscope holder is mounted to the operating table or to various neurosurgical head-holding devices. Endoscope holders not only provide steady video imaging on a video monitor but also allow a surgeon to use both hands freely. Fluoroscopic guidance, which was used in earlier patients, is no longer used in routine pituitary surgery. Such guidance is rarely but occasionally used for anterior or posterior cranial fossa surgery; and for pituitary tumor patients, in whom complexity of the sinonasal anatomy is anticipated.

Among surgical instruments, a monopolar suction coagulator (No. 8 French or No. 9 French cannula), a bipolar suction coagulator (No. 8 French or No. 9 French cannula), and a single-bladed bipolar coagulator are useful tools for hemostasis. They are all disposable, and the monopolar suction coagulator is malleable and insulated. The malleable monopolar is useful in bloodless preparation of the nasal cavity for anterior sphenoidotomy. The bipolar suction coagulator and single-bladed bipolar coagulator have two cables for producing bipolar functioning: the single-bladed bipolar has one electrode at the core and the other at the shell. These bipolar instruments are used for dural or intradural hemostasis. Suction cannulas with variously curved tips (No. 5 French and No. 7 French cannulas) are used for sellar operations. Titanium microclips have been used as a dural suturing device, but further development is required for ideal endoscopic dural suturing. Other instruments used include a micropituitary rongeur, pituitary rongeur, ethmoid rongeurs, high-speed drill, micro-Kerrison rongeurs, pituitary ring curettes, Jannetta 45-degree microdissector, single-bladed Kurze scissors, and a specially designed septal breaker. A slender high-speed drill is useful when the sphenoidal sinus is small and not well pneumatized.

Myths in Sinonasal Surgery

In early patients, topical application of a vasoconstrictor and local infiltration of lidocaine with epinephrine were used with the belief that intraoperative and postoperative bleeding would be reduced. Sometimes a piece of polytetrafluoroethylene (Teflon) or Gelfoam sponge was also left at the middle meatus in the hope that it would minimize postoperative bleeding and mucosal adhesions. However, these ineffective practices were gradually eliminated from our technique as experience accumulated. When the topical use of a vasoconstrictor and local injection of lidocaine with epinephrine were completely eliminated, postoperative nasal bleeding markedly decreased. The use of vasoconstrictors may lessen bleeding intraoperatively, but postoperative nasal bleeding was increased, presumably because of inadequate intraoperative hemostasis during the active vasoconstriction phase and rebound vasodilatation when the vasoconstrictor effects wore off postoperatively. Meticulous hemostasis using monopolar coagulation at the rostrum of the sphenoidal sinus, without the masking effect of intraoperative vasoconstrictors, is the key to minimizing the incidence of postoperative nasal bleeding. When we performed careful hemostasis at the rostrum mucosa and anterior sphenoidotomy site, the placement of a Teflon or Gelfoam sponge was also unnecessary.

When an anterior sphenoidotomy was performed, care was taken not to strip off the mucosa at the sphenoidal sinus.

FIGURE 27-4 *A,* The sinonasal endoscopes used in our endonasal pituitary surgery are 4 mm in diameter and 18 cm in length with 0-degree, 30-degree, and 70-degree angled lenses. The object below the three endoscopes is the sheath of the endoscope lens-cleansing device (Endoscrub R, Xomed-Treace, Bristol-Myers Squibb, Jacksonville, FL). The endoscope-cleansing device is a tool for cleaning the lens without removing the endoscope from the surgical field. *B,* This battery-powered device cleanses the lens (by foot pedal control) with forward irrigation of the saline solution followed by brief reverse flow.

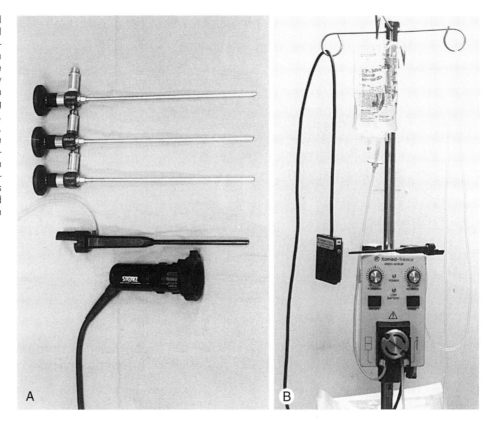

When the sphenoidal mucosa is stripped from the sinus cavity, not only can the resultant excessive bone bleeding interfere with the operation, the healing of the sinus is nonphysiologic. When the bony opening of an anterior sphenoidotomy is made, only the corresponding mucosa at the anterior sphenoidotomy hole is opened to enter the sphenoidal sinus. Minimal mucosa at the anterior wall of the sella is removed using electrocoagulation, with the remaining mucosa of the sphenoidal sinus kept intact as much as possible. When a pituitary tumor operation is finished,

FIGURE 27-5 *A,* Our manual endoscope holder consists of a combination of a Greenberg retractor mounting system and our own custom-made distal joint. *B,* It provides rigid fixation of the endoscope so that the surgeon can have continuous, stable video images while having both hands free to use surgical instruments.

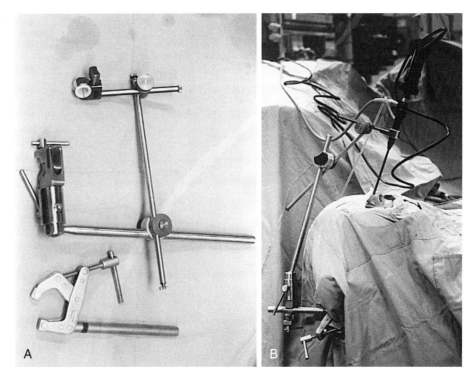

the anterior wall of the sella is reconstructed. The sphenoidal sinus is left intact without any packing, and these precautions allow physiologic healing of the open sphenoidal sinus with normal mucosal lining.

Because the nasal cavity cannot be conventionally prepared with an antiseptic solution, we prescribed postoperative oral antibiotic regimens empirically for 5 days in our early patients. Subsequently, postoperative antibiotic treatment has been completely abandoned without any evidence of increased infection. We still swab the nasal cavity with an antiseptic solution during surgical preparation, but even this practice may not be truly necessary.

Positioning

The patient is positioned supine with the torso elevated about 20 degrees, and the head is positioned with the forehead-chin line set horizontally. The level of the head is placed a little higher than that of the heart, with the intent that the cavernous sinus venous pressure stays low to minimize venous bleeding. The horizontally leveled head positioning allows the surgeon to access the middle turbinate easily and naturally when the endoscope is inserted at 25 degrees cephalad.[28] When the anterior cranial fossa is to be explored, the head is extended approximately 15 degrees.[27] Conversely, the head is flexed by 15 degrees when the clival or posterior fossa region is to be explored.[29] The head is rotated toward the surgeon at 10 to 20 degrees. A head pin fixation device can be used but is not necessary. The hip and knee joints are gently flexed for patient comfort, and a soft pillow is placed underneath the knee joints. A Foley catheter is inserted in selected patients who are expected to undergo longer operating hours or for the possible anticipated occurrence of diabetes insipidus. Fluoroscopic C-arm imaging is not used except in patients with anterior fossa or posterior fossa tumors or in patients with complex sinonasal anatomy. Ophthalmic eye ointment is placed on the cornea and conjunctiva. The eyelids are closed and sealed with soft vinyl adhesives. The oropharynx is packed with a 2-inch gauze roll to prevent the accumulation of blood at the perilaryngeal area during surgery, which may cause aspiration at the time of extubation.

The video monitor is placed a few feet away from the patient's head to face the surgeon directly. The lens-cleansing motor is placed next to the video monitor, and the scrub nurse is positioned adjacent to the surgeon. The entire face, nasal cavity, and abdominal wall are prepared and draped in an aseptic manner. When fat graft material is required to fill the tumor resection cavity, an appropriate amount of the abdominal fat tissue is obtained through a 1- to 2-cm infraumbilical transverse skin incision. Clindamycin is mixed with the endoscope's irrigation fluid. For the intraoperative antibiotic regimen, 2 g of cefazolin is given intravenously in the operating suite before the start of the operation.

Surgical Approaches

An endoscopic endonasal approach to the sella can be made by a paraseptal, middle meatal, or middle turbinectomy approach.[24,27] The paraseptal approach is the least traumatic of the three approaches; thus it has been most commonly used in our practice. The surgical technique described here involves the paraseptal approach. The paraseptal approach is made between the nasal septum and the middle turbinate. The middle turbinate is squeezed laterally, and the nasal septum is fractured away contralaterally at the sphenoidal rostrum. The fractured nasal septum is pushed away by submucosal dissection at the contralateral side of the sphenoidal rostrum. The paraseptal approach to the anterior cranial fossa accesses the anterior skull base directly under fluoroscopic C-arm guidance between the nasal septum and the middle turbinate. The middle meatal approach is made lateral to the middle turbinate; it provides direct access to the anterior aspect of the cavernous sinus and optic nerve by a posterior ethmoidectomy. This approach also allows access to the unilateral anterior cranial fossa by an anterior ethmoidectomy. When a larger operating space is required, the middle turbinectomy approach can be used by resection of the middle turbinate. Although it provides a wider corridor to the sella, lack of the middle turbinate structure can be problematic when a supportive structure is required for skull base reconstruction.

Surgical Technique of Endoscopic Transsphenoidal Pituitary Surgery

The entire face, nasal cavity, and abdominal wall are prepared and draped in an aseptic manner once the patient is positioned. As the nasal cavity is prepared with cotton swabs, the size of the nasal airway can be probed to determine which nostril is to be used. The nasal septum is usually somewhat deviated to one side, and thus the nostril with the wider nasal airway can be selected for the surgical approach. The size of the nasal airway can also be anticipated in advance by reviewing an axial MR scan of the nasal cavity. When both nasal cavities are comparable in size, the contralateral nostril is used in patients with microadenomas that are located laterally. Because the endonasal approach is a few degrees off from the midline, it is relatively easy to visualize the contralateral side of the sella and the cavernous sinus. For the intranasal portion of this operation, the endoscope is used with one hand and the surgical instrument is used with the other. When the anterior sphenoidotomy is complete, the endoscope can be mounted to the endoscope holder. When the endoscope is held in the hand, the palm and last three digits are generally used to stabilize the endoscope shaft, and the index finger and thumb are used to steer the video camera to maintain anatomic orientation of the video image. This endoscope grip will naturally keep the endoscope at a 25-degree incline and allows for continuous steering of the video camera for maintaining correct orientation of the video image. When the patient's head is positioned horizontally with the forehead-chin line parallel to the floor, the middle turbinate is easily visualized at the tip of the endoscope when it is inserted into the nasal cavity.

An endoscope is inserted with the inclined angle of the endoscope shaft at about 25 degrees, which has proven to be a comfortable and easy position for the surgeon who stands at the side of the patient. When the middle turbinate is identified, four to six $1/2 \times 3$-inch cotton patties are inserted between the middle turbinate and the nasal septum to widen the space in between (Figs. 27-6A and B and 27-7A and B). The cotton patties must be pushed down to the rostrum of

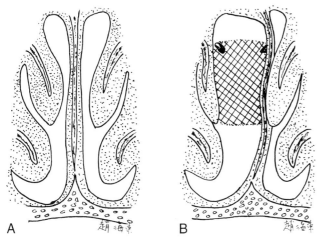

FIGURE 27-6 These schematic drawings demonstrate the area where an anterior sphenoidotomy is going to be made. *A,* The consistent landmark leading to the floor of the sella is the inferior margin of the middle turbinate. *B,* The inferior margin of the middle turbinate leads to the area that is approximately 1 cm below the floor of the sella in the sphenoidal sinus.

the sphenoidal sinus. The anterior sphenoidotomy should range from the inferior margin of the middle turbinate to the sphenoidal sinus ostia, which is about 1 to 1.5 cm rostral from the inferior margin of the middle turbinate. The consistent anatomic landmark for an anterior sphenoidotomy is the inferior margin of the middle turbinate. Although the sphenoidal sinus ostia may be visualized directly (Fig. 27-7C), its identification is not necessary for performing an anterior sphenoidotomy. When the sphenoidal sinus is entered near the level of the inferior margin of the middle turbinate, any further rostral exposure can be easily made relative to the exposed sellar floor. When an anterior sphenoidotomy is first attempted rostrally, the surgeon may erroneously enter the anterior cranial fossa because the superior turbinate can sometimes mimic the middle turbinate. Therefore, the middle turbinate must be confirmed in reference to the nasopharynx. The inferior margin of the middle turbinate is located just rostral to the nasopharynx in a sagittal plane. The inferior margin of the middle turbinate then leads to the clival indentation at approximately 1 cm below the level of the sellar floor.

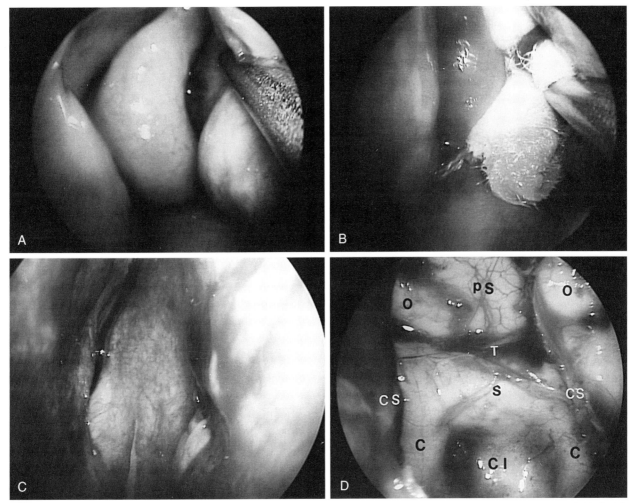

FIGURE 27-7 *A,* Under the 0-degree endoscope, the right-sided middle turbinate is exposed at the center of the surgical field. *B,* A few cotton patties, $\frac{1}{2} \times 3$ inches, are inserted between the middle turbinate and the nasal septum in front of the rostrum of the sphenoidal sinus. *C,* The rostrum of the sphenoidal sinus is exposed. Bilateral sphenoidal ostia are visible on either side. An anterior sphenoidotomy is made about 1.5 to 2 cm in size with ethmoidal rongeurs and Kerrison rongeurs or a high-speed drill. *D,* When the endoscope is advanced into the sphenoidal sinus, a panoramic view of the sphenoidal sinus demonstrates the clival indentation (CI), internal carotid arteries (C), sella (S), cavernous sinuses (CS), tuberculum sella (T), planum sphenoidale (PS), and optic protuberances (O).

Care must be taken not to traumatize the mucosa in the nasal cavity while surgical instruments are being inserted and removed. The degree of surgical trauma to the nasal mucosa is a crucial factor in determining the amount of postoperative nasal bleeding. When a sharp-edged surgical instrument is inserted, the instrument tip must be guided by direct endoscopic visualization. The insertion of the surgical instrument should be impelled by the gravity of the surgical instrument rather than by the surgeon's mechanical push. The cotton patties are then removed, which is often followed by some mucosal bleeding.

Mucosal bleeding from the rostrum of the sphenoidal sinus between the middle turbinate and nasal septum is controlled with electrocoagulation using a malleable monopolar suction coagulator. The mucosa at the rostrum of the sphenoidal sinus is completely coagulated before being divided vertically approximately 1.5 cm in length rostrally from the level of the inferior margin of the middle turbinate. The posterior lateral septal artery arises from the sphenopalatine artery and passes at the inferolateral corner of the sphenoethmoidal recess, which is approximately the posteromedial corner of the inferior margin of the middle turbinate. The posterior lateral septal artery must often be coagulated and divided to prevent intraoperative and postoperative nasal bleeding. The site for an anterior sphenoidotomy is again confirmed with reference to the surgical landmarks, which are the inferior margin of the middle turbinate and the nasopharynx.

Anterior sphenoidotomy is made with two different surgical techniques: power drilling or rongeuring with fracture. In the first technique, the use of a power drill creates a clean opening at the anterior wall of the sphenoidal sinus. The endoscope is placed on the endoscope holder, and the power drill is inserted along with a suction cannula next to the endoscope shaft. The vomer is drilled first, and then the nasal septum is pushed to the contralateral side when it loosens. At the contralateral rostrum of the sphenoidal sinus, submucosal dissection is carried out to expose the bilateral rostrum of the sphenoidal sinus. Then the exposure at the rostrum of the sphenoidal sinus is very similar to the exposure through a conventional transseptal approach. Drilling is performed along the lateral gutter at the anterior wall of the sphenoidal sinus, and the sphenoidal mucosa is exposed bilaterally. Using Kurze scissors, an opening is made at the sphenoidal sinus mucosa. Now the posterior wall of the sphenoidal sinus can be directly visualized demonstrating the tuberculum sella, clivus, cavernous sinus, and optic system.

The second technique involves rongeuring after mechanical fracture of the nasal septum and vomer from the rostrum of the sphenoidal sinuses using the septal breaker, which is a special instrument designed for this endoscopic operation. The rostral nasal septum is relatively easy to break; however, the caudally located vomer is often too thick to break without using the specially made septal breaker. The fractured nasal septum is pushed contralaterally, and the contralateral rostrum of the sphenoidal sinus is dissected submucosally. The anterior aspect of the sphenoidal rostrum is exposed bilaterally. With Kerrison rongeurs, the anterior wall of the sphenoidal sinus is first opened along the lateral gutter. Then the bony opening of an anterior sphenoidotomy is completed using Kerrison rongeurs.

The sinus mucosa is opened in the same manner as previously mentioned. Attention is paid not to strip the sphenoidal sinus mucosa because inadvertent stripping can cause unwanted oozing of blood from the bony sinus wall. The anterior wall of the sphenoidal sinus is removed, performing an anterior sphenoidotomy of about 1 to 1.5 cm in size. The sphenoidal sinus septum is trimmed with a power drill or rongeurs. Further rostral extension of the anterior sphenoidotomy is performed accordingly, relative to the sella. Often the sella is exposed from the tuberculum sella to the clival indentation in the vertical dimension and from one cavernous sinus to the other in the transverse dimension. At this point, endoscopic view demonstrates the tuberculum sella rostrally, optic protuberances at the 11 and 1 o'clock positions, the bony wall covering the cavernous sinus and carotid artery laterally, clival indentation caudally, and the internal carotid arteries at the 7 and 5 o'clock locations (see Fig. 27-7D). The endoscope is mounted to the endoscope holder as the endoscope tip is advanced for a close-up view of the sella.

Using a bipolar suction coagulator, the sphenoidal mucosa at the anterior wall of the sella is coagulated and removed. A small hole is made at the inferolateral corner of the anterior bony wall of the sella. The anterior bony wall of the sella is removed with a 1-mm Kerrison punch circumferentially, from one cavernous sinus to the other, and from the sellar floor to the tuberculum sella. Sometimes the anterior bone wall can be opened like a door, with the hinge attached at the sellar floor or tuberculum sella. At the end of operation, the bony door can be closed for sellar reconstruction. The dura mater is coagulated along the periphery circumferentially with a single-bladed bipolar coagulator. The dural opening is made along the inferior margin at the floor of the sella using a Jannetta 45-degree microdissector. The anterior dural wall is incised and removed circumferentially for biopsy. An alternative is an X-shaped incision of the dura mater.

In the case of a microadenoma covered by normal pituitary tissue, the pituitary tissue is sliced or split with a Jannetta 45-degree microdissector to locate the tumor tissue. When the tumor is identified, it is first curetted out. At the tumor resection cavity, a thin layer of the normal pituitary tissue is shaved off to accomplish complete resection of the tumor, because microadenomas that require surgical resection are usually hormonally hyperactive tumors. In the case of a macroadenoma, the adenoma tissue often spills out when the dura mater is opened. Care has to be taken not to lose the tumor specimen by suctioning because the tumor tissue should be sampled for pathologic examination. Once enough of the tumor specimen is collected, the tumor is removed with a suction cannula at the central portion of the sella for debulking. Two No. 5 French or No. 7 French suction cannulas can be used for tumor removal. When the tumor is fibrotic, either from previous medical and surgical treatments or by its intrinsic nature, the tumor tissue is gently curetted with a pituitary ring curette held in one hand, in addition to being suctioned with a suction cannula held in the other hand.

When the tumor resection cavity is created at the central portion of the pituitary fossa, a 45-degree angled curette is used first, followed by a 90-degree angled curette used to remove the lower portion of the tumor from the floor of the sella. An inferiorly angled pituitary ring curette is used in one hand and an inferiorly curved suction cannula is used in the other for removal of the lower portion of the tumor.

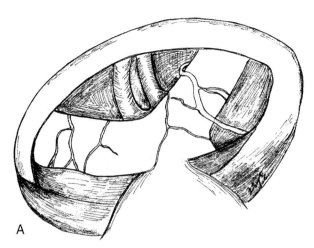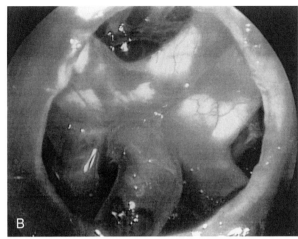

FIGURE 27-8 When the suprasellar portion of the tumor is removed, the optic nerves, chiasm, and anterior cerebral arterial system are under direct 30-degree-lens endoscopic view. *A*, A schematic drawing. *B*, A 30-degree endoscopic view after removal of a suprasellar craniopharyngioma.

The dura mater at the floor of the sella is exposed directly when the lower portion of the tumor is removed. Next the lateral portion of the tumor is removed with a superiorly angled suction cannula and a superiorly angled pituitary ring curette, 45 degrees as well as 90 degrees. The medial wall of the cavernous sinus is directly exposed when the lateral portion of the tumor is removed. The rostral portion of the tumor is removed circumferentially using various superiorly curved and angled suction cannulas and pituitary ring curettes.

When normal pituitary gland tissue is identified, it is preserved as much as possible. The tumor is removed either with suction cannulas in each hand or with a suction cannula in one hand and a pituitary ring curette in the other. When the diaphragma sella is identified along the peripheral edge of the rostral portion of the tumor, the tumor is continuously removed circumferentially. When the tumor is removed along the edge of the diaphragma sella, the suprasellar portion of the tumor progressively descends through the central opening of the diaphragma sella. The suprasellar portion of the tumor that is progressively descending is continuously removed with either two superiorly curved suction cannulas or a suction cannula and a pituitary ring curette, both angled superiorly.

Thinned pituitary tissue is often identifiable rostrally when the suprasellar portion of the tumor has been removed. When the pituitary tissue is severely stretched out, the rostrally located pituitary tissue appears to be a transparent membrane similar to the arachnoid membrane. When this rostral tissue is penetrated, the arachnoid membrane may rupture, resulting in a CSF leak. Sometimes the arachnoid membrane bulges down along the anterior edge of the diaphragma sella in front of the thinned pituitary tissue. The last piece of the pituitary tumor is often located at the insertion point of the pituitary stalk. When this last piece of the tumor is removed at the reversed dimple of the pituitary stalk, the transparent and thinned pituitary tissue descends, looking much like a lily with a dimple at the center. It continuously bulges downward with pulsation toward the floor of the sella. When the tumor resection cavity in the sella is large and the remaining tissue is very thin, the tumor resection cavity may have to be filled and supported with an abdominal fat graft in order to prevent postoperative CSF leak caused by delayed rupture of the membrane. Delayed CSF leak can also occur from a Valsalva maneuver produced by repeated coughs, bearing-down during extubation, or at any time postoperatively.

When the tumor is so solid and fibrotic that the suprasellar portion of the tumor does not descend spontaneously, the suprasellar portion can be exposed directly using a 30-degree lens endoscope or by further removal of the bone at the tuberculum sella or planum sphenoidale. When the arachnoid membrane is ruptured, the optic nerves and chiasm, anterior cerebral artery system, and inferior aspect of the hypothalamus are under direct view with a 30-degree lens endoscope (Fig. 27-8A and B). When CSF leakage does not occur intraoperatively and the tumor is a microadenoma, an abdominal fat graft is unnecessary. After removal of a macroadenoma, the tumor resection cavity is supported with an abdominal fat graft. Occasionally a piece of Gelfoam sponge is used instead of an abdominal fat graft when a sufficient amount of the pituitary tissue still remains rostrally.

An abdominal fat graft is harvested via a 1- to 2-cm transverse skin incision just inferior to the umbilicus. The anterior wall of the sella is reconstructed using autogenous bone saved at the time of the anterior sphenoidotomy (Fig. 27-9A). When autogenous bone is not available, a piece of thin titanium mesh is placed (Fig. 27-9B). No foreign material is placed in the sphenoidal sinus or nasal cavity. The endoscope is removed from the holder to be manipulated by hand again; the nasopharynx and nasal cavity are inspected and cleaned, and any stagnant blood is removed with a suction cannula. The middle turbinate is placed back to its normal position. The abdominal incision is closed in subcuticular fashion and covered with a small bandage to complete the operation.

Surgical Approach to the Anterior Cranial Skull Base

For meningiomas located in the olfactory groove, planum sphenoidale, or tuberculum sella, and for repair of CSF

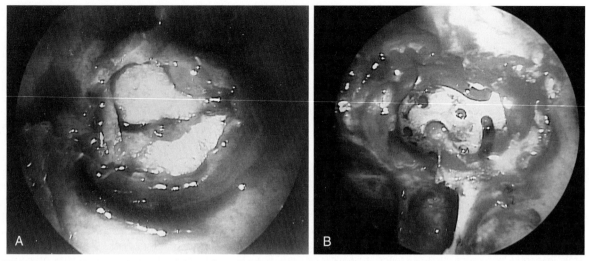

FIGURE 27-9 A small piece of abdominal fat graft is placed at the tumor resection cavity when the tumor resection cavity is too large or cerebrospinal fluid leakage is encountered intraoperatively. The anterior wall of the sella is reconstructed with (*A*) autogenous bone or (*B*) titanium mesh.

leakage at the anterior cranial fossa, the endoscopic endonasal approach to the anterior fossa skull base has been employed (Fig. 27-10A).[25,27] This approach is also useful for suprasellar craniopharyngiomas or for large suprasellar pituitary tumors with fibrotic solid natures. For CSF leak repair, either a paraseptal or a middle meatal approach can be used. For tumor removal, a paraseptal approach is used. As with the approach to the anterior cranial skull base, a fluoroscopic C-arm image is used for intraoperative guidance. Frameless stereotactic guidance can be also used.

The head is positioned in 15-degree extension of the forehead-chin line to maintain the endoscope insertion angle at about 25 degrees, which is naturally comfortable for the surgeon. Otherwise, the patient is prepared in the same manner as described earlier for pituitary surgery. For the middle meatal approach, the middle turbinate is pushed medially, and an ethmoidectomy is performed to reach the anterior skull base. Any CSF leak is often directly visible. The mucosa is dissected around the skull base defect, and an abdominal fat graft is inserted into the cranial cavity. After the entire fat graft is inserted into the cranial cavity, a portion of the fat is grabbed and pulled gently to wedge it into the skull defect. A piece of thin titanium mesh is then placed at the skull defect. The middle turbinate is placed back to its normal position.

For anterior cranial fossa tumor surgery, a paraseptal approach is often used. For tumors located at the tuberculum sella, planum sphenoidale, or olfactory groove, the surgical

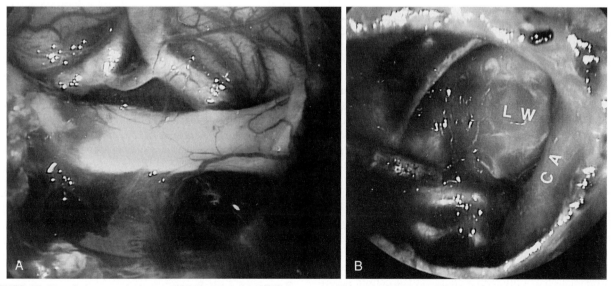

FIGURE 27-10 *A*, As a meningioma at the planum sphenoidale is removed by an endoscopic endonasal anterior skull base approach, the pituitary stalk, optic system, and anterior cerebral artery system are directly visualized in a 0-degree-lens endoscope. *B*, As a pituitary tumor encasing the carotid artery in the cavernous sinus is removed, the carotid artery (CA) and lateral wall of the cavernous sinus (LW) are visualized directly under the 30-degree-lens endoscope.

approach is similar to the aforementioned pituitary operation except that further rostral exposure is required. The middle turbinate is laterally displaced, and the nasal septum is fractured contralaterally. A rostral anterior sphenoidotomy is performed to enter the sphenoidal sinuses, and then the sella and tuberculum sella are identified. Under fluoroscopic guidance, further rostral exposure is made at the anterior skull base, removing the posterior ethmoid sinuses. This approach itself interrupts anterior or posterior ethmoidal arteries during exposure, resulting in complete devascularization of the meningioma.

A portion of the midline anterior skull base approximately 2 cm wide can be exposed with this technique. Bone of the skull base can be removed with a high-speed drill or Kerrison punch. The dura mater is opened, and the tumor is removed with central debulking followed by peripheral dissection. When the central portion of the tumor is excised, peripheral dissection is carried out to inspect the posterior aspect of the tumor. The remaining tumor is gradually flipped, and dissection along the posterior wall of the tumor is carried out until the remaining tumor is excised. The main potential problem related to this surgery is postoperative CSF leak and subsequent meningitis; therefore, adequate skull base reconstruction is essential. When active CSF leak is noted at the time of surgery, a small piece of fat graft is inserted at the various corners intracranially in order to obstruct the active CSF inflow. Then a large dural graft is placed intradurally with enough margin overlapping, dural suture is performed with titanium clips, and another layer of dural graft is laid extradurally. The skull base defect is reconstructed with autogenous bone graft or titanium mesh placement. Abdominal fat grafts are used at the ethmoidectomy site as additional support. When fat graft material is placed at the tumor resection cavity, care must be given not to cause compression to the optic nerve system. The middle turbinate is placed back in its normal position, and the operation is finished.

Surgical Approach to the Cavernous Sinus or Optic Nerve

Although surgical indication for the decompression of the optic nerve is a controversial issue, the optic nerve at the optic canal can be easily exposed using this endoscopic endonasal approach.[22] The surgical approach to the cavernous sinus is similar to that of the optic nerve.[23–25,28] This endoscopic approach to the cavernous sinus is best suited for pituitary adenomas invading the cavernous sinus. Tough fibrotic tumors (e.g., meningiomas) are challenging to remove using an endoscopic technique. Biopsy for the histologic diagnosis of cavernous sinus lesions can be performed with this technique.

The endonasal endoscopic approach to the cavernous sinus is an anteromedial approach, and the fact that cavernous cranial nerves are located at the lateral wall of the cavernous sinus makes this approach advantageous. Pituitary adenomas can involve the cavernous sinus by mechanical compression with lateral tumor bulging, by intrusion into the cavernous sinus through a defect of the medial wall of the cavernous sinus, or by direct extension by dural infiltration. A laterally bulged tumor can be removed by the pituitary approach described previously and does not need any further particular maneuvering. The 30-degree-lens endoscope

discloses the medial wall of the cavernous sinus well when the lateral portion of the tumor is completely removed. Tumors that have intruded into the cavernous sinus by a defect of the medial wall can be removed completely under direct endoscopic visualization. The cavernous carotid artery is exposed during this procedure. Invasive pituitary adenomas of an infiltrating nature may not be completely resectable; however, they can be debulked to reduce the size of the tumor so that focused beam radiation treatment can be performed for the residual portion of the tumor postoperatively.

The optic nerves or cavernous sinuses can be approached via a paraseptal, middle meatal, or middle turbinectomy approach.[24] In the paraseptal approach, the endoscope visualizes the contralateral optic nerve or cavernous sinus better than it does the ipsilateral one, and this technique exposes the anteromedial aspect of the cavernous sinus. The middle meatal approach with a posterior ethmoidectomy provides a straight anterior approach to the cavernous sinus. The middle turbinectomy approach renders a larger corridor that can reach the optic nerve or cavernous sinus, although the paraseptal approach has been sufficient for approaching the optic nerve or cavernous sinus.

The anteromedial exposure of the optic nerve or cavernous sinus through the contralateral nostril, using the paraseptal approach, is similar to that of the previously described endoscopic endonasal pituitary adenoma surgery. When an anterior sphenoidotomy is made, submucosal dissection at the contralateral side of the sphenoidal rostrum is extended further laterally, and the anterior sphenoidotomy can be performed generously at the contralateral side of the sphenoid sinus. This exposes the contralateral cavernous sinus laterally up to the medial anterior temporal fossa. The bone is removed from the anterior aspect of the sella as well as from the cavernous sinus, and unroofing the internal carotid artery may be completed if necessary. The sellar portion of the pituitary tumor is removed first before attacking the tumor portion in the cavernous sinus.

For an isolated cavernous sinus tumor, the tumor is approached directly by opening the dura mater medial to the carotid siphon. The tumor is removed with various pituitary ring curettes and suction cannulas. Attention must be taken not to traumatize the lateral wall of the cavernous sinus, because this can cause ocular cranial nerve dysfunction. The carotid artery pulsation is directly visible, and tumor resection is performed medially and posteriorly to the carotid siphon, which is arced in a reversed C-shape for the right carotid artery or in a C-shape for the left with the convexity directed anterolaterally. When the tumor is completely removed, the lateral wall of the cavernous sinus can be completely visualized (see Fig. 27-10B). The cavernous carotid artery is wrapped with an abdominal fat graft to protect the artery postoperatively. If necessary, the sphenoid sinus can additionally be filled with an abdominal fat graft for protection of the exposed carotid artery. In contrast with pituitary surgery, the sphenoidal sinus mucosa should be removed completely before the fat graft is placed.

Surgical Approach to the Pterygoid Fossa and Petrous Apex

A tumor involving the pterygoid fossa can be approached with a middle meatal or a middle turbinectomy approach.

The posteromedial wall of the maxillary sinus can be removed if necessary, and then the pterygoid fossa is fully exposed. The vidian nerve or sphenopalatine ganglion in the pterygoid fossa can also be approached with this technique. The petrous apex can be approached with a paraseptal approach. This endoscopic endonasal approach is particularly useful for drainage of a cholesterol granuloma. Approach through a contralateral nostril gives a little more lateral angulation to the petrous apex.

When the sphenoidal sinus is entered, the sellar floor and carotid artery protuberance provide anatomic orientation, and a stereotactic image-guidance device may assist anatomic orientation. The carotid artery is exposed at the medial margin, and the petrous apex is approached through the clivus inferior to the sellar floor and medial to the paraclival segment of the cavernous sinus carotid artery. When the cholesterol granuloma is entered, xanthochromic fluid and material will be drained. Unless the carotid artery is fully exposed, placement of fat graft material over the carotid artery for arterial protection is not necessary. Once the cholesterol granuloma is drained, the operation is complete.

Surgical Approach to the Clivus and Posterior Fossa

In the endonasal surgical approach to the clivus and posterior fossa, the endoscopic technique has the advantages of flexibility and a range of endoscopic visualization that spans from the crista galli at the anterior fossa to the foramen magnum.[25,29,30] This endoscopic approach exposes the entire clivus from the floor of the sella to the foramen magnum in a width of approximately 2 cm (Fig. 27-11A), with the internal carotid arteries serving as the lateral limits of this exposure. This technique has been used for radical resection of clival chordomas and midline clival meningiomas. A paraseptal approach is used, but the middle turbinectomy approach can be used when a larger surgical corridor is required.

A fluoroscopic C-arm image or frameless stereotactic technique is used for guidance in the vertical dimension. A high-speed drill is used to remove the clival bone between the internal carotid arteries (in the transverse dimension) and from the floor of the sella to the foramen magnum or to the lower clival level, as needed. The chordoma is then removed with suction cannulas and pituitary rongeurs. Bone is shaved at the tumor resection margin until normal bone is clearly documented. Intradural tumor is then resected, during which the pons and medulla can be visualized. A 30- or 70-degree-lens endoscope visualizes the further rostral aspect of the brain stem or cranial nerves laterally (see Fig. 27-11B and C). Dural defects are repaired with an abdominal fat graft, but once appropriate surgical instruments are fully developed, direct repair by a dural graft will be the ideal method for reconstruction. The dural titanium microclip applicator currently available is too short to be used for this purpose.

POSTOPERATIVE MANAGEMENT

Patients are kept in a regular hospital room overnight. If they do well, they are discharged home the next day. Postoperative discomfort is minimal and often does not require strong analgesics. Postoperative nasal bleeding has also been very minimal since the techniques of meticulous hemostasis and eliminating intraoperative use of vasoconstrictors were adopted. Patients may note a few drops of bloody discharge

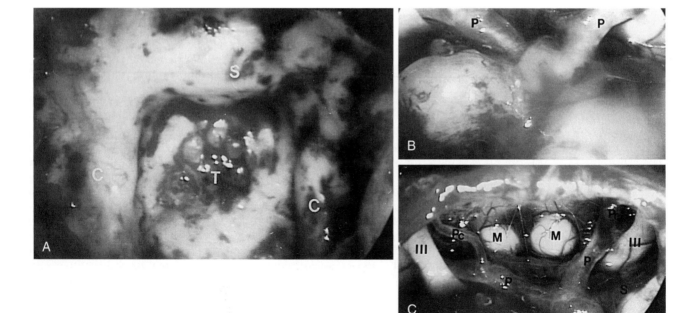

FIGURE 27-11   The clivus is exposed by an endonasal endoscopic approach for removal of the clival and posterior fossa chordoma. *A,* The sella (S), internal carotid arteries (C), and the tumor at the center of the clivus (T) are demonstrated by a 0-degree-lens endoscope. *B,* As a tumor in the posterior fossa encasing the basilar artery is removed, the basilar bifurcation, posterior cerebral arteries (P), posterior communicating arteries (Pc), superior cerebellar arteries (S), mammillary bodies (M), and bilateral oculomotor nerves (III) are demonstrated through a 70-degree-lens endoscope (*C*).

for a day or two when they get up early in the morning or from a prolonged lying position. This minimal nasal drainage is bloody discharge accumulated at the sellar area in the sphenoidal sinus during a recumbent position. Watery nasal discharge may indicate a postoperative CSF leakage, which is a potential complication that can delay hospital discharge. A few drops of CSF leakage are often benign, usually stopping in a day or so.

Although stress doses of corticosteroids were used intraoperatively and postoperatively in the earliest patients, an intraoperative or postoperative corticosteroid is no longer used when the patient's preoperative pituitary-adrenal function is normal. Instead, a morning cortisol level is measured the day after surgery to confirm that it is higher than 15 μg/dL. If the morning cortisol level is less than 15 μg/dL, postoperative treatment is instituted with oral hydrocortisol, 20 mg every morning and 10 mg every night, until the pituitary-adrenal axis is proven to be normal.

Target hormone levels for functioning adenomas (e.g., prolactin for prolactinomas, growth hormone for acromegaly, TSH for TSH-secreting adenomas, and cortisol for Cushing's disease) are measured the first postoperative day. When target hormone levels are not within the expected normal ranges, they are measured again the following day. If the levels do not normalize by the third postoperative day, re-exploration is considered. For patients with Cushing's disease, dexamethasone is administered postoperatively 1 mg orally once or twice a day. Serum cortisol and 24-hour urinary free cortisol levels can be measured to judge the postoperative outcome of Cushing's disease when dexamethasone is used instead of hydrocortisol. Once serum cortisol and 24-hour urinary cortisol levels are confirmed to be normal postoperatively, dexamethasone medications can be changed to hydrocortisol.

Serum electrolytes are measured at the recovery room, on the first postoperative day, and 1 week postoperatively. During the hospital stay, urine specific gravity is measured each time the patient urinates, and fluid intake and output are also measured. In our early patients, postoperative diuresis was an annoying problem that often prolonged hospital stays to more than 1 night. However, we found that excessive intravenous fluid administration was responsible for this postoperative diuresis, which stopped occurring when the intraoperative intravenous fluid volume was judiciously given. Vasopressin (Pitressin) is used immediately when diabetes insipidus is confirmed by exhibition of the classic symptoms of polyuria and polydipsia, diluted urine with low urinary specific gravity, and increased serum osmolarity and sodium concentration. When patients develop diabetes insipidus, 1 μg of DDAVP is given intravenously. Then, if patients experience a breakthrough of diabetes insipidus with increased urine volume, intranasal administration of DDAVP is instituted in the evening. Most often patients who develop diabetes insipidus only require one or two doses of DDAVP because their diabetes insipidus is transient. Development of diabetes insipidus may delay hospital discharge by 1 or 2 nights.

In our early cases, we gave oral antibiotics (clarithromycin, 500 mg twice a day) prophylactically for 5 days postoperatively because the endonasal approach trespasses the putatively semicontaminated sinonasal cavity. However, the use of postoperative antibiotics was found to be unnecessary,

and we have not observed any increased incidence of infection in the absence of prophylactic antibiotics. A single dose of intravenous antibiotics is given intraoperatively in all patients, either as 2 g cefazolin or a combination of 1 g vancomycin and 80 mg gentamycin. Formal endocrine evaluation, visual examination (if necessary), nasal examination, and postoperative MR scans are performed a few weeks postoperatively. Then patient follow-ups are made with interval endocrine evaluations and yearly MR scans.

SURGICAL RESULTS

Among the 200 patients in our early series, 160 had pituitary adenomas, 10 had anterior skull base meningiomas, 8 had clival chordomas, and 22 had other skull base pathologies. Fifty-five patients had previously undergone surgical and/or radiation treatments. Among the 160 patients with pituitary adenomas, 37 patients (23%) had microadenomas, and 123 patients (77%) had macroadenomas. Among the 90 patients with non–hormone-secreting adenomas, 71 patients (79%) had gross total removal. Among the 38 patients with prolactinomas, 25 patients (66%) normalized their postoperative prolactin levels. Thirteen of 18 patients with Cushing's disease (72%) had normal postoperative cortisol levels. Among the 13 patients with acromegaly, 11 (85%) had normalized postoperative IGF-1 levels.

The length of hospital stay was less than 1 day for 75% of the patients. Although same-day surgery has been performed in selective cases on the demand of patients, 1-night stays have been routine for uncomplicated cases. Although our early surgical results are comparable to those reported with microscopic transsphenoidal surgery, our surgical outcome has been continually improving as our experience increases.

POTENTIAL COMPLICATIONS AND THEIR AVOIDANCE

CSF leakage is a major potential complication in endoscopic transsphenoidal surgery; it can occur intraoperatively, or in a delayed fashion and postoperatively. When the tumor resection cavity is large, or if an intraoperative CSF leak is noted, an abdominal fat graft is placed and the anterior sellar wall is reconstructed with autogenous bone or a piece of titanium mesh. Fibrin glue or other adhesives are not used. Earliest postoperative leakage occurs when patients are extubated with excessive coughing, which can rupture the thin membrane.

In our patient series, most CSF leaks occurred in delayed fashion, commonly within the first day of surgery. When patients leak only a drop or two of clear fluid from the nasal cavity, the leak usually stops spontaneously; however, if patients leak clear fluid continually when they sit with the head positioned leaning forward, the leak must be repaired endoscopically without delay in order to prevent meningitis. The challenging case in which to repair a CSF leak is in a patient following tuberculum sellar tumor removal, because too much fat graft can cause compression to the optic system. The optic nerves, located laterally at the tuberculum sella and the optic chiasm posteriorly, can limit the adequate placement of fat graft material to seal the CSF leak.

Reconstruction at the olfactory groove or clivus is much simpler than at the tuberculum sella area. The use of a lumbar drain is reserved for rare occasions (e.g., in patients with CSF leakage despite complete mechanical reconstruction). Although meningitis is an extremely rare occurrence, CSF leakage must be promptly repaired with administration of intravenous antibiotics if meningitis is confirmed, and CSF from a spinal tap can provide bacteriologic information for antibiotics.

Diabetes insipidus is another complication that can prolong hospital stay, but diabetes insipidus can easily be managed using the aforementioned remedies. However, the importance of corticosteroids in the postoperative management of Cushing's patients cannot be overemphasized. When patients with Cushing's disease display the usual hypocortisolism postoperatively, they must take steroid medications until they recover normal pituitary-adrenal axis function, which may take a few weeks to a year. The outcome may be fatal if they fail to comply with their steroid medications. In addition, postoperative hyponatremia can occur several days to a few weeks after surgery. Hyponatremic patients may need to be treated as inpatients because they may become symptomatic with nausea, vomiting, malaise, and altered consciousness.

Delayed massive epistaxis can occur a few days to 2 weeks postoperatively. When patients go to an emergency room, carotid artery rupture is the first diagnosis suspected. However, the most common cause of occasional delayed nasal hemorrhage after transsphenoidal surgery is bleeding from the stump of the posterior septal artery. It can be easily repaired with endoscopic electrocoagulation. Carotid artery injury can potentially occur with any technique of transsphenoidal surgery, and its occurrence requires tamponade with packing followed by endovascular intervention.

ADVANTAGES AND DISADVANTAGES OF THE ENDONASAL ENDOSCOPIC TECHNIQUE

In our description of technique, we already outlined many of the advantages associated with endoscopic transsphenoidal surgery, but we will add a few additional comments. The endoscopic endonasal approach results in minimal postoperative discomfort or pain while obviating the need for postoperative nasal packing. We have also observed that avoidance of nasal packing offers a significant advantage for patient comfort and rapid recovery with early release from the hospital. Despite the naturally narrow nasal passages in pediatric patients (the youngest patient in our series was 13 years old) and in people of East Asian ethnicity, we have yet to encounter a patient who has nostrils too narrow for endoscopic endonasal surgery. This endonasal technique does not require sublabial or nasal transfixion incisions, and it minimizes the chances of dental, gingival, or sinonasal complications. The normal sinonasal physiologic anatomy is also well maintained because the endoscopic endonasal technique is minimally traumatic. In addition, previously described optical advantages of an endoscope may improve overall surgical outcomes.

There are three major disadvantages of endoscopic pituitary surgery in comparison with conventional microscopic surgery: (1) the inferior quality of 2-dimensional monitor-generated flat images, (2) inadequate development of commercially available surgical instruments, and (3) the lack of formalized endoscopic training of pituitary neurosurgeons. Endoscopic 2-dimensional video images are still inferior in resolution to the images generated by 3-dimensional direct microscopic visualization, even though the endoscope allows close-up direct views unachievable by the microscope. A digitally enhanced camera has improved the picture quality to some degree, and high-definition cameras and monitors would further improve the quality of endoscopic views. Secondly, commercially available instruments for endoscopic neurosurgery are still in development and may not be ready for some time. Thirdly, there is a steep learning curve for neurosurgeons who are already well-trained in conventional microscopic surgery. Maneuvering skills involved in endoscopic neurosurgery are quite different from conventional microsurgery techniques and may be likened to using a pair of chopsticks in each hand. Despite a neurosurgeon's painstaking training in microsurgery, most are not used to endoscopic surgical maneuvering and will need to spend considerable time getting accustomed to new endoscopic surgical skills.

In addition, the neurosurgeon must adapt to operating with the endoscope shaft occupying the central portion of the surgical corridor. A major concern expressed by microscopic pituitary surgeons has been regarding the ability to control unexpectedly significant bleeding within a limited exposure. Although tumors involving high vascularity can bleed significantly (e.g., in microscopic pituitary surgery), the endoscopic endonasal technique has not proven to be a handicap for these types of tumors. Venous sinus bleeding may occasionally become cumbersome, but there has not been a single case that had to be aborted. Finally, the operating time for endoscopic surgery may initially be longer than that for microscopic surgery because of the intrinsic learning curve, but the operating time becomes comparable or even shorter once the surgeon masters the technique.

CONCLUSIONS

As described, endoscopic endonasal transsphenoidal surgery is useful for the neurosurgical treatment of pituitary adenomas as well as for other skull base lesions located at the midline anterior cranial skull base, cavernous sinus, optic nerve, pterygoid fossa, petrous apex, and the midline clivus or posterior fossa.

Acknowledgments

The authors thank Mi-Ja Jho, B.E., and Robin A. Coret, B.A., for their assistance in preparation of this manuscript.

REFERENCES

1. Guiot G, Rougerie J, Fourestler A, et al: Une nouvelle technique endoscopique: Exploration endoscopiques intracraniennes. Presse Med 71:1225–1228, 1963.
2. Stammberger H: Endoscopic endonasal surgery-concepts in treatment of recurring rhinosinusitis. II: Surgical technique. Otolaryngol Head Neck Surg 94:147–156, 1986.
3. Jho HD, Carrau RL, Ko Y, Daly M: Endoscopic pituitary surgery: An early experience. Surg Neurol 47:213–223, 1997.
4. Carrau RL, Jho HD, Ko Y: Transnasal transsphenoidal endoscopic surgery of the pituitary gland. Laryngoscope 106:914–918, 1996.
5. Jankowski R, Auque J, Simon C, et al: Endoscopic pituitary tumor surgery. Laryngoscope 102:198–202, 1992.

6. Shikani AH, Kelly JH: Endoscopic debulking of a pituitary tumor. Am J Otolaryngol 14:254–256, 1993.

7. Wurster CF, Smith DE: The endoscopic approach to the pituitary gland (Letter). Arch Otolaryngol Head Neck Surg 120:674, 1994.

8. Gamea A, Fathi M, El-Guindy A: The use of the rigid endoscope in transsphenoidal pituitary surgery. J Laryngol Otol 108:19–22, 1994.

9. Sethi DS, Pillay PK: Endoscopic management of lesions of the sella turcica. J Laryngol Otol 109:956–962, 1995.

10. Helal MZ: Combined micro-endo trans-sphenoid excisions of pituitary macroadenomas. Eur Arch Otorhinolaryngol 252:186–189, 1995.

11. Landolt AM: History of transsphenoidal pituitary surgery. In Landolt AM, Vance ML, Reilly PL (eds): Pituitary Adenomas. New York: Churchill Livingstone, 1996, pp 307–314.

12. Griffith HB, Veerapen R: A direct transnasal approach to the sphenoid sinus: Technical note. J Neurosurg 66:140–142, 1987.

13. Cooke RS, Jones RAC: Experience with the direct transnasal transsphenoidal approach to the pituitary fossa. Br J Neurosurg 8:193–196, 1994.

14. Jho HD: Endoscopic endonasal pituitary surgery: Technical aspects. Contemp Neurosurg 6:1–7, 1997.

15. Jho HD, Carrau RL, Ko Y: Endoscopic pituitary surgery. In Wilkins RH, Rengachary SS (eds): Neurosurgical Operative Atlas, vol 5. Baltimore: Williams & Wilkins, 1996, pp 1–12.

16. Jho HD, Carrau RL: Endoscopy assisted transsphenoidal surgery for pituitary adenoma: Technical note. Acta Neurochir (Wien) 138:1416–1425, 1996.

17. Jho HD, Carrau RL: Endoscopic endonasal transsphenoidal surgery: Experience with 50 patients. J Neurosurg 87:44–51, 1997.

18. Jho HD, Alfieri A: Endoscopic transsphenoidal pituitary surgery: Various surgical techniques and recommended steps for procedural transition. Br J Neurosurg 14(5):424–432, 2000.

19. Jho HD, Park IS, Alfieri A: The future of pituitary surgery. Clin Neurosurg 47:83–98, 2000.

20. Jho HD, Alfieri A: Endoscopic endonasal pituitary surgery: Evolution of surgical technique and equipment in 150 operations. Minim Invasive Neurosurg 44:1–12, 2001.

21. Jho HD: Endoscopic transsphenoidal surgery. J Neurooncol 54:187–195, 2001.

22. Jho HD: Endoscopic endonasal approach to the optic nerve: A technical note. Minim Invasive Neurosurg 44:190–193, 2001.

23. Alfieri A, Jho HD: Endoscopic endonasal approach to the cavernous sinus: An anatomic study. Neurosurgery 48:827–837, 2001.

24. Alfieri A, Jho HD: Endoscopic endonasal approach to the cavernous sinus: Surgical approaches. Neurosurgery 49:354–362, 2001.

25. Jho HD: Expanding role of endoscopy in skull base surgery. Clin Neurosurg 48:287–305, 2001.

26. Alfieri A, Jho HD, Tschabitscher M: Endoscopic endonasal approach to the ventral cranio-cervical juncture: anatomical study. Acta Neurochir (Wien) 144:219–225, 2002.

27. Jho HD, Ha HG: Endoscopic endonasal skull base surgery: Part 1 - The midline anterior fossa skull base. Minim Invasive Neurosurg 47:1–8, 2004.

28. Jho HD, Ha HG: Endoscopic endonasal skull base surgery: Part 2 - The cavernous sinus. Minim Invasive Neurosurg 47:9–15, 2004.

29. Jho HD, Ha HG: Endoscopic endonasal skull base surgery: Part 3 - The clivus and posterior fossa. Minim Invasive Neurosurg 47:16–23, 2004.

30. Jho HD, Carrau RL, Mclaughlin ML, Somaza SC: Endoscopic transsphenoidal resection of a large chordoma in the posterior fossa. Acta Neurochir (Wien) 139:343–348, 1997.

Transcranial Surgery for Pituitary Macroadenomas

CHRIS B. T. ADAMS

INDICATIONS FOR TRANSCRANIAL SURGERY FOR PITUITARY TUMORS

Pituitary tumors are usually treated by the transsphenoidal approach for several reasons. First, it is a less intrusive operation; the surgeon comes straight down onto the tumor and can preserve the normal pituitary tissue. There is also negligible risk of epilepsy, and recovery of vision and the visual fields is quicker because the optic nerves and chiasm are not manipulated. In some circumstances, transsphenoidal surgery is contraindicated or insufficient. The procedure is insufficient when the surgery fails to remove adequate amounts of tumor, particularly enough to decompress the optic chiasm.

The alternative transcranial approach is indicated when transsphenoidal surgery is contraindicated. The usual reason for using the transcranial approach is doubt about the diagnosis. If the lesion may not be a pituitary adenoma, but perhaps is a meningioma or craniopharyngioma, a craniotomy is advisable. Occasionally an entirely intrasellar meningioma or craniopharyngioma can be removed by the transsphenoidal route, but in general these lesions are more safely removed transcranially. A particular clue to a meningioma is seeing a tongue of pathologic tissue extending along the floor of the anterior cranial fossa. A clue to a craniopharyngioma is a presentation with diabetes insipidus. Diabetes insipidus is indicative of a hypothalamic disorder, and pituitary adenomas do not cause diabetes insipidus initially.

Another indication for the transcranial approach is failed transsphenoidal surgery. There may be several reasons for this failure. One is that the pituitary adenoma is too tough: transsphenoidal surgery relies on the surgeon removing the intrasellar component, then the suprasellar component falling into the cavity created. A few adenomas are tough. In those circumstances, it is advisable to take no more than a biopsy specimen and obliterate the sphenoid sinus. The latter action may seem unnecessary with a large tough tumor between the nasal cavity and the cerebrospinal fluid, but the author has regretted not obliterating the sphenoid sinus in these (unusual) circumstances when subsequently performing transcranial surgery. It is the consistency of the tumor, not the size, that limits the effectiveness of transsphenoidal surgery.

Failure of the suprasellar extension to descend is another reason for failed transsphenoidal surgery. The usual cause is that a component of the tumor is extending superiorly, laterally, or anteriorly (Fig. 28-1). If the suprasellar extension has pushed vertically, it usually falls into the tumor cavity created by the transsphenoidal surgeon. If an extension of

tumor hooks around the optic nerve or carotid artery, this extension prevents descent of the tumor, and the tumor extension above the carotid artery or chiasm is inaccessible. The anterior extension is particularly troublesome for the transsphenoidal surgeon, being just at the wrong angle to the line of approach (Fig. 28-2). Finally, recurrent pituitary adenomas may not fall down satisfactorily because of adhesions between the tumor and the surrounding brain. In these circumstances, the combined transcranial/transsphenoidal approach may be the best way of total eradication of the tumor, which may be justified if the tumor has recurred despite previous irradiation. Radical surgery is also indicated for a hormone-secreting adenoma such as acromegaly (or Cushing's syndrome), in which hormonal cure depends on total removal of the tumor.

PREOPERATIVE CONSIDERATIONS

All patients should have a magnetic resonance imaging (MRI) scan. This scan shows the vessels so well that formal

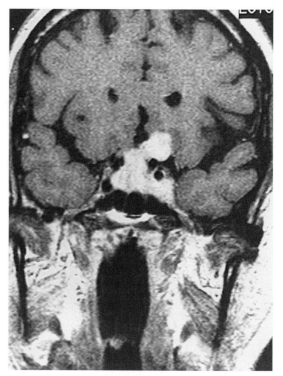

FIGURE 28-1 A magnetic resonance imaging scan showing the suprasellar extension hooking laterally and preventing the descent of the tumor during transsphenoidal surgery.

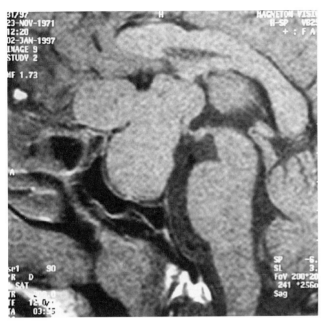

FIGURE 28-2 A magnetic resonance imaging scan showing the suprasellar extension of a growth hormone–secreting tumor that extends anteriorly. A radical removal was achieved by a transcranial approach. Note the position of the anterior communicating artery.

angiography is not usually indicated. The visual fields should be formally recorded, and pituitary function tests should be performed. The transcranial route almost inevitably causes hypopituitarism because the normal pituitary tissue is pushed superiorly under the diaphragma sella, and it is this tissue that is coagulated and cut by the surgeon en route to the tumor (Fig. 28-3). Two pints of blood should be crossmatched. Epilepsy is possible after transcranial surgery, and anticonvulsants such as a hydantoin should be started preoperatively. The patient should be warned of this possibility and the effect this might have on driving, working with machinery, or ascending heights.

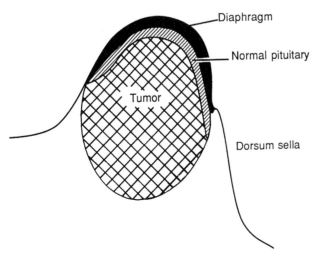

FIGURE 28-3 Diagram showing how the adenoma pushes the normal pituitary superiorly as a thin rind. This makes the normal pituitary tissue particularly vulnerable during transcranial surgery, whereas it is relatively protected with transsphenoidal surgery.

The patient should be warned of the risks of surgery, both general and specific. General risks are those of any operation (e.g., deep vein thrombosis, bleeding into the operative cavity, infection, the anesthetic), and of epilepsy when a craniotomy is carried out. The specific risks are those of damage to the optic nerve or nerves (resulting in impaired vision or visual fields), damage to the blood vessels (i.e., internal carotid artery or anterior cerebral arteries), and damage to the pituitary stalk (resulting in hypopituitarism and diabetes insipidus). Cerebrospinal fluid rhinorrhea occasionally occurs, as does anosmia, especially if excessive retraction of the frontal lobe is needed.

PREFIXED CHIASM

The length of the intracranial optic nerves varies from patient to patient. The tumor extension influences the distance of the optic nerves to the tuberculum sella. If the suprasellar extension thrusts between the optic nerves, it pushes the chiasm upward and backward, allowing good access for the surgeon. Sometimes the suprasellar extension pushes the chiasm upward and forward, however, severely limiting the surgeon's access: this is called prefixed chiasm. The position of a chiasm can be predicted on the sagittal MRI scan by finding the anterior communicating artery (shown in the sagittal MRI section as a black dot; see Fig. 28-3), which denotes the position of the chiasm.

AIMS OF SURGERY

The aims of pituitary surgery are ultimately to cure the patient of the tumor, without damage to the pituitary; to relieve the symptoms and the signs that have been caused by the tumor; and to achieve this relief without damage to the patient. When the tumor is secreting hormone, total extirpation of the tumor is necessary to achieve a cure. A nonfunctioning tumor does not necessarily require total removal, especially if the risks of such an attempt are significant. In these circumstances, the aims should be an adequate debulking of the tumor to produce chiasmal and optic nerve decompression before radiotherapy or radiosurgery.

TECHNIQUE OF TRANSCRANIAL PITUITARY SURGERY

The author advises a pterional craniotomy[2]; in general, it is unnecessary to use a bifrontal approach. In determining which side to operate on, there are two main factors. If one eye is already blind, it is advisable to operate on the side of the blind eye because the ipsilateral optic nerve (to the craniotomy) is most vulnerable to operative manipulation. The other factor is the lateral extension of the tumor: it makes more sense to operate on the side of maximal tumor extension.

The patient is positioned supine with the head turned about 40 degrees to the opposite side and slightly extended. An incision is marked out just behind the hairline from the zygomatic arch to the midline.[2] The author turns a pterional free bone flap and prefers making drill holes with a Gigli saw, believing it is safer. The sphenoid wing is nibbled away, then the dura is opened. If the tumor is large, the anesthetist is asked to administer mannitol or a diuretic to shrink the brain. If the tumor is blocking the third ventricle or the foramen of Monro, causing hydrocephalus, a ventricular drain can be inserted.

The dura is opened in a gentle curve just above the eyebrow and hitched up. The operating microscope is then introduced, and the sylvian fissure is split. This is a key maneuver that allows the main middle cerebral artery, the anterior cerebral artery, and the internal carotid artery to be identified and safeguarded. The exposed frontal lobe is covered with absorbable fabric (Surgicel); this covering protects the brain and allows cotton strips or patties to be placed on and peeled off without damaging the brain surface. A retractor should never be placed on bare brain but always on a pattie. While the sylvian fissure is split, cerebrospinal fluid is gently sucked away, relieving intracranial pressure. Having traced back to the internal carotid artery, the optic nerve is then identified.

The next step is to debulk the tumor. If there is sufficient space, this debulking is done by working between the optic nerves. If a chiasm is prefixed, it may be easier to work between the optic nerve and the chiasm (Fig. 28-4). Early in the operation, the surgeon should avoid working near the ipsilateral optic nerve and concentrate on debulking the tumor. The author uses bipolar coagulation and cuts out the contents with scissors. If soft, the tumor center can be sucked out, which is easier for the surgeon. The author finds the ultrasonic aspirator too bulky and potentially dangerous. Angled curettes (the Bronson Ray type) are helpful. As the debulking proceeds, the opposite optic nerve and internal carotid artery are identified. The author avoids coagulating and cutting vessels running to the chiasm if possible, and also avoids taking vessels when working between the optic nerves and carotid artery because these are often perforating vessels.

As debulking proceeds, the tumor capsule (i.e., the compressed tumor and thinned diaphragma sella) can be gradually drawn down and excised. The sucker, held in the left hand, is a useful instrument to bring the capsule down, especially if the surgeon makes a hole in the capsule and inserts the sucker in the hole. The author starts the capsule removal near the left (if operating on the right) optic nerve and internal carotid artery so that these vital structures become defined. Having done this, the surgeon works superiorly toward the chiasm. If the anterior cerebral artery is surrounded or severely distorted, this needs defining at an early stage. At this point, the right (ipsilateral) anterior cerebral artery is traced from the carotid bifurcation. By working from one side (laterally), then from the other side (medial side), the anterior communicating artery and the chiasm at the summit of the tumor are defined.

Having delivered the summit of the tumor, the surgeon is in a better position to remove the most difficult part of the tumor: the ipsilateral component compressing the optic nerve and internal carotid artery on the side of the exposure. This stage of the operation is the only time the author invariably uses angled bipolar forceps: these forceps are invaluable for coagulating the capsule hidden by the ipsilateral optic nerve.

Once the suprasellar component is delivered, the capsule at the level of the dorsum sellae is coagulated, amputating the suprasellar component from the intrasellar component. The pituitary stalk is almost invariably seen in the angle between the optic nerve and the carotid artery. The stalk is easily recognized by the striated appearance of the long axis of pituitary stalk resulting from the portal venous system.[3]

Using angled curettes, the intrasellar component is removed. Much of this removal is done blindly, with the bleeding controlled by pressure, patience, and Surgicel. If previous transsphenoidal surgery has been carried out, and the sphenoid sinus has not been obliterated, pericranium and temporalis muscle are taken to produce a watertight cerebrospinal fluid closure of the pituitary fossa (Fig. 28-5).

The wound is then closed in a routine fashion, checking hemostasis, replacing the cerebrospinal fluid that was sucked away with Ringer's solution, closing the dura, and replacing the bone flap. Particular care should be taken to inspect the frontal lobe; excessive retraction too easily can occur while the surgeon concentrates on the pituitary tumor down the microscope, not appreciating the degree of fixed retraction on the frontal lobe.

FIGURE 28-4 A diagrammatic view of the usual anatomy. Note the approach between the optic nerve and the internal carotid artery to the pituitary adenoma.

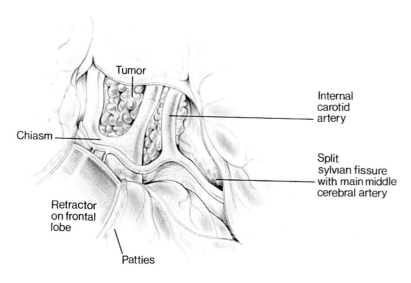

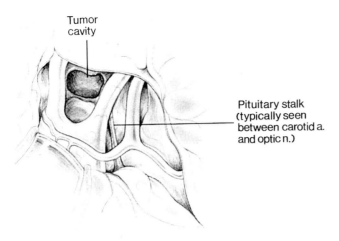

FIGURE 28-5 The anatomy after the removal of the tumor. The pituitary stalk is usually seen between the optic nerve and the internal carotid artery.

RADICAL COMBINED TRANSCRANIAL AND TRANSSPHENOIDAL APPROACH

Occasionally, it is necessary to aim for a complete radical removal of the tumor (e.g., when a tumor has recurred despite radiotherapy). In these circumstances, the author has completed removal of the suprasellar component, then drilled off the tuberculum sella between the optic nerves and the optic foramina (Fig. 28-6). The sphenoid sinus is entered, allowing the mucosa to be displaced and the anterior wall of the pituitary fossa to be removed. Removal of the sellar component can be achieved under direct vision except for the ipsilateral intrasellar tumor, which is less visible. Alternatively, a separate transsphenoidal approach can be carried out; that has the advantage of better bilateral tumor exposure, but it also has the disadvantage of possibly failing to see remaining tumor superiorly. Whichever method the surgeon uses, particular care must be taken to achieve a tight cerebrospinal fluid closure with obliteration of the sphenoid sinus.

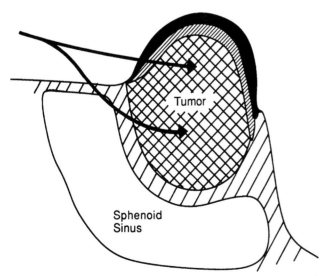

FIGURE 28-6 The combined transcranial, transsphenoidal approach for the radical removal of a pituitary adenoma.

POSTOPERATIVE COMPLICATIONS

General Complications

General complications include infection, bleeding into the operative cavity, epilepsy, and leakage of cerebrospinal fluid. These complications are common to any supratentorial craniotomy and will not be considered further except cerebrospinal fluid leakage. This complication occurs in two circumstances. The first is if a previous transsphenoidal operation has been performed and an inadequate obliteration of the sphenoid sinus has been achieved. Previous sections have alluded to the necessity to obliterate the sphenoid sinus during a transsphenoidal approach when a transcranial procedure is clearly going to be necessary in the future. This necessity exists even when no cerebrospinal fluid is seen. Failure to do so means cerebrospinal fluid rhinorrhea is extremely likely to occur after the transcranial approach, because the dural lining of the pituitary fossa has been penetrated during the transsphenoidal approach. In these circumstances, fascia and fat may be introduced into the pituitary fossa transcranially, but it is not easy to obtain a watertight closure this way. The second circumstance in which cerebrospinal fluid rhinorrhea may be seen is when bone is drilled away from the skull base, thus entering an extension of the sphenoid sinus. If recognized, a fat and fascia repair is necessary. Rhinorrhea usually ensues when such an occurrence has not been recognized.

Frontal Lobe Damage

Frontal lobe damage is perhaps the most common complication, although it is often unappreciated because its manifestations may be subtle. Frontal lobe damage is particularly likely to occur in the elderly, and is caused by excessive frontal lobe retraction. The elderly take longer to recover from this surgery than from transsphenoidal surgery. There may be subtle changes of memory, judgment (on a social or professional level), concentration, and personality. These changes can be minimized by gentle surgical technique and, especially, by minimal brain retraction. A pattie or cotton strip should always be placed between the brain and the retractor. The retractor should be moved often, and should be removed when it is not needed. Splitting the sylvian fissure to separate the frontal and temporal lobes also minimizes the amount of retraction. If there is evidence of an area of soft, blue brain at the end of the operation, the surgeon should beware: this area may represent hemorrhagic infarction, which often causes postoperative bleeding and deterioration. Such areas should be removed surgically before closing the dura.

Frontal Lobe Cyst Formation

Cystic enlargement of an area of frontal lobe damage, sufficient to act as a space-occupying lesion, may occur. The author has described one such case and speculated on the causal mechanism.[2]

Anosmia

Unilateral or bilateral anosmia often reflects the vigor of frontal lobe retraction. If there is a significant subfrontal extension of the pituitary tumor, anosmia is inevitable.

Perioperative Optic Nerve Damage

If an eye is blind preoperatively, it will not recover postoperatively. If vision is severely impaired preoperatively, it is also unlikely to recover. If an already-damaged optic nerve is manipulated at all, vision is likely to be lost altogether postoperatively. The patient should be thus warned.

The most vulnerable nerve is the ipsilateral optic nerve. The rule is not to touch or manipulate it, but this is rarely possible to achieve. Before teasing tumor away, the tumor should be debulked as much as possible; only at the last stage, when space has been created, should the remaining tumor be rolled away from the optic nerve. Meningiomas creep down the optic foramen, but in the author's experience, pituitary tumors do not behave in that fashion.

The blood supply of the optic nerve, nerves, and chiasm varies. The chiasm is supplied by small vessels from the anterior communicating artery, and these must be preserved. The rule is not to coagulate or cut any significant-looking vessel running to the chiasm or optic nerves. In general, however, the author suspects that it is manipulation of these structures, rather than ischemia, that usually causes the damage.

Damage to the Internal Carotid, Anterior Cerebral, or Anterior Communicating Arteries

One of the most unpleasant occasions of the author's neurosurgical career was cutting an internal carotid artery. The patient was elderly, had undergone two previous craniotomies and radiotherapy for the pituitary tumor, and the artery was embedded in scar tissue. Although the artery was not visible, it should have been traced proximally from the middle cerebral artery. This tracing can be extremely difficult. On another occasion, both anterior cerebral arteries were damaged. The tumor was firmly adherent to these vessels, and the author should have stopped the operation, leaving tumor behind around the vessels; this was an error of judgment.

Although the literature describes such vascular damage repaired by fine sutures, the author has been unable to achieve such repairs in these circumstances. Placing aneurysm clips so as to occlude the hole in the vessel without occluding the vessel has occasionally worked; usually, however, the vessel has to be occluded to stop the bleeding.

Occasionally a small vessel is pulled out of the side of a larger vessel. It can be difficult to stop the bleeding, but by placing the finest bipolar forceps on either side of the hole and using low bipolar coagulation, the hole is sealed without occluding the main vessel.

Hypothalamic Damage

Hypothalamic damage is rare after removal of a pituitary adenoma, but it is easily caused by overenthusiastic removal of a craniophyaryngioma. With hypothalamic damage, the patient loses the senses of thirst and hunger. Fluid control can be achieved only by weighing the patient, and excessive weight gain is usual. Hypothalamic wasting or a precocious puberty occurs in the presence of tumors (usually hypothalamic gliomas) and not after surgical trauma. To remove or not to remove a craniopharyngioma intimately involved

in the hypothalamus demands the finest surgical judgment to balance the desire to achieve a total removal with the need to avoid devastating hypothalamic damage. Any publication addressing the results of craniopharyngioma surgery that does not include dispassionate assessment of endocrine and psychological tests (especially for memory) is not worth reading.

Pituitary Damage, Including Diabetes Insipidus

Damage to anterior pituitary function is common after transfrontal surgery because the normal pituitary gland is usually pushed superiorly against the diaphragma sella, rather like a rind around the tumor (see Fig. 28-3). The diaphragma is the first thing to be coagulated and cut when removing such tumor transcranially, hence destroying normal function. Pituitary hormone replacement therapy maintains reasonable health, but the patient never returns to normal. The patient seems sluggish, both physically and mentally, and gains weight. The standard hormone replacement therapy does not include growth hormone or other hormones given in the physiologically pulsatile fashion. Perhaps there are other hormones yet to be discovered.

Fluids should be restricted to 2 L/day for 48 hours postoperatively. A postoperative diuresis is normal, especially in patients cured of acromegaly. If the urinary output is more than 200 mL/hour for 3 hours, plasma and urinary osmolalities are measured. If the former is more (and the latter less) than 295 mOsm/kg, desmopressin should be administered. The osmolality measurements should be repeated in 24 hours.

Salt-Losing Syndrome

Salt-losing syndrome is rare. The syndrome is also alarming, and usually occurs 1 to 2 weeks after the operation.[4–7] One of the author's patients developed a headache, then lapsed rapidly into a coma, and on admission had a low sodium value. The mechanism is unknown, but salt-losing syndrome is assumed to be caused by inappropriate antidiuretic hormone secretion. It is difficult to measure antidiuretic hormone, and so not enough is known about this rare condition. It is advisable to place a central venous line to determine if the problem is primarily low sodium (low venous pressure) or water overload (high venous pressure). The author's patient was treated empirically (successfully) with rapid infusions of fluids and salt, then restricted fluids to increase the serum sodium. Until more is known about this mysterious condition, it can be treated only empirically. Kelly and colleagues[6] recommend using urea for salt-losing syndrome, pointing out that urea enhances sodium reabsorption at the kidney. The author has no experience using urea, but would try it if again faced with this problem.

Postoperative Visual Deterioration

Acute visual deterioration within hours of surgery is usually caused by a postoperative hematoma in the tumor cavity (Table 28-1). The best way to avoid this situation is to be sure to remove the tumor in its entirety. If, however, the tumor invades the clivus, bleeding from the cancellous bone can be

TABLE 28-1 ▪ Cause of Postoperative Visual Failure

Immediately postoperatively	Hematoma Operative damage Acute empty sella syndrome
Subacute (usually 8 days postoperatively)	Unilateral; probably ischemic
Months after operation/irradiation	Recurrent tumor Irradiation damage ?Empty sella syndrome–doubtful ?Scarring of chiasm without displacement—doubtful

TABLE 28-2 ▪ Classification of Results

Type	Size (mm)	% Cure Rate after Transsphenoidal Approach
Microadenoma	<10	80
Mesoadenoma	10–20	80
Macroadenoma	>20	40

difficult to stop, although bone wax, Surgicel, and patience are usually sufficient. Reoperation is necessary.

Olsen and co-workers[8] have described acute deterioration after transsphenoidal surgery resulting from herniation of a chiasm into the pituitary fossa. This condition is amazingly rare, considering how, after transsphenoidal surgery, the diaphragma rapidly descends to the floor of the pituitary fossa on many occasions without visual impairment. The question can be asked if herniation per se (apart from Guiot's unique case) can cause visual deterioration.

Occasionally, a unilateral loss of vision occurs about 8 days after surgery. (The author's experience with this has been just after transsphenoidal surgery, but there is no reason why it should not happen after transcranial surgery.) Morello and Freral[9] describe a similar patient, and the author agrees with their conclusion that ischemic damage is the most likely explanation.

Insidious visual deterioration is almost always caused by recurrent tumor, which usually reproduces the original visual field deficit (i.e., a bitemporal hemianopia). Another possibility is radiation damage to the optic nerves or chiasm after radiotherapy. This visual deterioration usually occurs 9 to 18 months after radiotherapy and is often sudden and unilateral. The mechanism is vascular damage and hence similar to stoke. Some improvement may occur. Guy and colleagues[10] suggest gadolinium-enhanced MRI scanning to confirm the diagnosis of radiation damage.

A third possibility has been suggested: herniation of the chiasm into the pituitary fossa, as described previously, acutely. The author believes that most of these cases have been caused by radiation damage. There is also confusion in much of the literature regarding damage resulting from scarring around the optic nerve and chiasm (without necessarily any significant herniation into the fossa) and actual displacement of the optic nerves and chiasm. The author is not convinced of visual deterioration by the so-called empty sella syndrome. At this time, there are no studies with controls (i.e., MRI studies of chiasmal or optic nerve positions on postoperative patients without visual deterioration). Those interested should consult references 8 through 26.

RESULTS

There are no modern meaningful results for transcranial surgery because such an approach is usually carried out only when the standard transsphenoidal approach fails. The older literature provides the sort of results obtained by transcranial surgery.[27–38] In general, the author's results from transsphenoidal surgery mirror the size of the tumor. A simple classification (Table 28-2) is used. The author recommends the introduction of a group, mesoadenoma, signifying tumors 1 to 2 cm in maximum diameter as measured on MRI. Often, these are classified by other authors as macroadenomas, but the surgical results are similar to microadenomas, and they should be delineated from macroadenomas. Invasive adenomas are usually macroadenomas, and the few exceptions to this rule do not justify more complicated classifications.[1] Dolenc[39] has advocated the direct exploration of a cavernous sinus. The author suspects, however, that gamma knife radiosurgery will be the treatment of choice for extensions within the cavernous sinus, although further evaluation of both of these techniques is required.

REFERENCES

1. Adams CBT: The management of pituitary tumours and postoperative visual deterioration. Acta Neurochir (Wien) 94:103–116, 1988.
2. Adams CBT: A Neurosurgeon's Notebook. Oxford: Blackwell Scientific, 1998.
3. Harris GW: Neural control of the pituitary gland. II: The adenohypothesis. BMJ 2:627–634, 1951.
4. Andrews BT, Fitzgerald PA, Tyrell JB, Wilson CB: Cerebral salt wasting after pituitary exploration and biopsy: Case report. Neurosurgery 18:469–471, 1986.
5. Siva Kumar V, Raj Shekhar V, Chandy MJ: Management of neurosurgical patients with hyponatremia and natriuresis. Neurosurgery 34:269–274, 1994.
6. Kelly DF, Laws ER Jr, Fossett D: Delayed hyponatremia after transsphenoidal surgery for pituitary adenoma: Report of nine cases. J Neurosurg 83:363–367, 1995.
7. Olson BR, Gumowski J, Rubino D, Oldfield EH: Pathophysiology of hyponatremia after transsphenoidal pituitary surgery. J Neurosurg 87:499–507, 1997.
8. Olson DR, Guiot G, Derome P: The symptomatic empty sella: Prevention and correction via the transsphenoidal approach. J Neurosurg 37:533–537, 1972.
9. Morello G, Frera C: Visual damage after removal of hypophyseal adenomas: Possible importance of vascular disturbances of the optic nerve and chiasm. Acta Neurochir (Wien) 15:1–10, 1966.
10. Guy J, Mancuso A, Beck R, et al: Radiation-induced optic neuropathy: A magnetic resonance imaging study. J Neurosurg 74:426–432, 1991.
11. Buys SN, Kerns TC: Irradiation damage to the chiasm. Am J Ophthalmol 44:483–486, 1957.
12. Crompton MR, Layton DD: Delayed radionecrosis of the brain following therapeutic x-radiation of the pituitary. Brain 83:85–101, 1961.
13. Colby MY Jr, Kearns TP: Radiation therapy of pituitary adenomas with associated visual impairment. Mayo Clin Proc 37:15–24, 1962.
14. Lee WM, Adams JE: The empty sella syndrome. J Neurosurg 28:351–356, 1968.
15. Mortara R, Norrell H: Consequences of a deficient sellar diaphragma. J Neurosurg 32:565–573, 1970.
16. Hodgson SF, Randall RV, Holman CB, Maccarthy CS: Empty sella syndrome: Report of 10 cases. Med Clin North Am 56:897–907, 1972.
17. Harris JR, Levene MB: Visual complications following irradiation for pituitary adenomas and craniopharyngiomas. Radiology 120:167–171, 1976.

18. Lee FK, Richter HA, Tsai FY: Secondary empty sella syndrome. Acta Radiol Suppl (Stockh) 347:313–326, 1976.

19. Aristizabal S, Caldwell WL, Avila J: The relationship of time-dose fractionation factors to complications in the treatment of pituitary tumours by irradiation. Int J Radiat Oncol Biol Phys 2:567–573, 1977.

20. Basauri L, Castro M, Garcia JA: The empty sella syndrome: Analysis of 10 cases. Acta Neurochir (Wien) 38:111–120, 1977.

21. Atkinson AB, Allen IV, Gordon DS, et al: Progressive visual failure in acromegaly following external pituitary irradiation. Clin Endocrinol 10:469–479, 1979.

22. Hodgson SF, Randall RV, Laws ER: Empty sella syndrome. In Youmans J (ed): Neurological Surgery, 2nd ed. Philadelphia: WB Saunders, 1982, p 3176.

23. Sheline GE: Radiation therapy of pituitary tumours. In Givens JR (ed): Hormone Secreting Tumours. Chicago: Year Book Medical Publishers, 1982, p 139.

24. McFadzean RM: The empty sella syndrome: A review of 14 cases. Trans Ophthal Soc UK 103:537–541, 1983.

25. Grossman A, Cohen BL, Charlesworth M, et al: Treatment of prolactinomas with megavoltage radiotherapy. BMJ 288:1105–1109, 1984.

26. Jones A: Radiation oncogenesis in relation to the treatment of pituitary tumours. Clin Endocrinol 35:379–397, 1991.

27. Halstead AE: Remarks on the operative treatment of tumours of the hypophysis. Surg Gynecol Obstet 10:494–502, 1910.

28. Cushing H: The Pituitary Body and Its Disorders. Philadelphia: JB Lippincott, 1912.

29. Cairns H: The prognosis of pituitary tumours I. Lancet 2:1310–1311, 1935.

30. Cairns H: The prognosis of pituitary tumours II. Lancet 2:1363–1364, 1935.

31. Henderson WR: The pituitary adenomata: A follow up study of the surgical results in 338 cases (Dr. Harvey Cushing's series). Br J Surg 26:811, 1939.

32. Bakay L: The results of 300 pituitary adenoma operations (professor Herbert Olivecrona's series). J Neurosurg 7:240, 1950.

33. Obrador AS: Adenomas of the pituitary based on a neurosurgical experience of 65 operated patients. Rev Clin Esp 81:396–401, 1961.

34. Jefferson AA: Chromophobe pituitary adenomata: The size of the suprasellar portion in relation to the safety of operation. J Neurol Neurosurg Psychiatry 32:633, 1969.

35. Stern WE, Batzdorf U: Intracranial removal of pituitary adenomas: An evaluation of varying degrees of excision from partial to total. J Neurosurg 33:564, 1970.

36. Ray BS, Patterson RH Jr: Surgical experience with chromophobe adenomas of the pituitary gland. J Neurosurg 34:726, 1971.

37. Symon L, Jakubowski J: Transcranial management of pituitary tumours with suprasellar extension. J Neurol Neurosurg Psychiatry 42:123, 1979.

38. Rand RW: Transfrontal transsphenoidal craniotomy in pituitary and related tumours. In Rand RW (ed): Microneurosurgery, 3rd ed. St. Louis: CV Mosby, 1984.

39. Dolenc VV: Transcranial epidural approach to pituitary tumours extending beyond the sella. Neurosurgery 41:542–552, 1977.

29 Surgical Management of Endocrinologically Silent Pituitary Tumors

ANDRÉ VISOT, PHILIPPE PENCALET, ANNE BOULIN, and STEPHAN GAILLARD

Improvements in the survey of hypophyseal hormones have considerably modified our knowledge of so-called non-functional pituitary adenomas (also called nonfunctioning silent, endocrine-inactive, or nonsecretory adenomas). It is now known that, after immunocytochemical staining, most of these nonfunctioning adenomas are true gonadotrope adenomas secreting one or many hormonal products.[1,2] However, true gonadotrope adenomas and silent tumors have similar clinical and therapeutic features. The secreting character of the tumor is most often established in surgically removed specimens.

In the past, pituitary tumors producing one or more of the glycoproteins (i.e., thyroid-stimulating hormone [TSH], luteinizing hormone [LH], follicle-stimulating hormone [FSH], and the α-glycoprotein subunit) were thought to be rare. However, using modern immunocytochemical and molecular biologic techniques, increasing numbers of these tumors are being detected.[1,3,4] Many of them produce α- and β-glycoprotein subunits in addition to intact glycoprotein. Their hormone production is often low compared with the size of the tumor, and serum hormone levels may not be elevated.[5]

Tumors that produce the gonadotropins LH or FSH, or the α-subunit, account for most clinically nonfunctioning adenomas; they do not cause a specific clinical syndrome, and usually exhibit symptoms of a large mass lesion or hypopituitarism. In surgical series, gonadotrope adenomas account for 12% to 17% of operated pituitary adenomas.[1,5] Table 29-1 shows that in a large series of pituitary adenoma operated at Foch Hospital from 1960 to June 2003 (5134 cases), the rate of endocrinologically silent adenomas was 24.5%. Table 29-2 shows that in 1 year (2002) the prevalence of these pituitary tumors was the same: 24.2%. Table 29-3 demonstrates the current prevalence of gonadotrope adenomas in a series of 145 endocrinologically silent pituitary tumors operated from January 2000 to June 2003.

ANATOMOCLINICAL CONSIDERATIONS

Clinical Features

The most common presenting complaint is the impairment of vision or a peripheral field abnormality (77% in the authors' series).

These complaints are found in all the reported series: in 84% of cases in Taiwan,[3] 74% in Montreal,[6] 72% in the American series reported by Laws and colleagues,[7] 44% in Arafah's series,[8] 60% in a Spanish series,[9] and more than 60% in the report by Black and associates.[1] The visual impairment sometimes is severe, especially in the oldest patients, and may consist of unilateral blindness and visual field cut in the opposite eye. This is caused by the insidious growth of the tumor and concomitant progressive visual deterioration. Occasionally, a distinct ophthalmologic problem (e.g., a cataract or glaucoma) has delayed the correct diagnosis, and some of the authors' patients have been operated on by an ophthalmologist. However, the lack of improvement has led to pituitary imaging and to the correct diagnosis. Bitemporal hemianopsia remains the main criterion for differentiating between an ophthalmologic disease and chiasmal compression. Sometimes, the initial visual symptoms are acute and reach the oculomotor nerves. In these cases, the clinical presentation is similar to that of a subarachnoid hemorrhage, with headache; meningism; and unilateral ophthalmoplegia, with or without visual impairment (9% in

---

TABLE 29-1 ▪ Surgical Series of Pituitary Adenomas: 1960–June 2003, 5134 Cases, Hôpital Foch—Neurosurgical Department

Prolactin adenomas	1866 cases (36.4%)
Endocrinologically silent adenomas	1246 cases (24.3%)
Growth hormone adenomas	1113 cases (21.7%)
Cushing and Nelson's adenomas	875 cases (17%)
Thyreotrop adenomas	34 cases (0.6%)

TABLE 29-2 ▪ Surgical Series of Pituitary Adenomas in 1 Year (2002): 170 Cases, Hôpital Foch—Neurosurgical Department

Prolactinomas	51 cases (30%)
Endocrinologically silent adenomas	41 cases (24.2%)
Growth hormone adenomas	39 cases (22.9%)
Corticotrop adenomas	32 cases (18.9%)
Nelson's disease	4 cases (2.3%)
Thyreotrop adenomas	3 cases (1.7%)

TABLE 29-3 ▪ Endocrinollogically Silent Adenomas from January 2000 to June 2003 (Foch Hospital)

145 Cases

95 gonadotrop adenomas

50 nonsecreting adenomas

the authors' series). These cases result from a sudden necrotic or hemorrhagic transformation of the tumor, which is always identified in surgery.

Endocrinologic symptoms are the second characteristic exhibited by patients with such pituitary adenomas. In the authors' experience, these symptoms are present in 75% of cases, but only 35% exhibit clinical symptoms considered to be caused by hypopituitarism, subsequently confirmed by laboratory tests. These symptoms include amenorrhea; loss of libido; hypothyroidism; hypogonadism; and symptoms of inadequate production of adrenal steroids, sometimes leading to lethargy, fever, and abdominal pain with hyponatremia because of adrenal insufficiency. None of the authors' patients had preoperative diabetes insipidus which, if present, requires careful review of the diagnosis of pituitary adenoma.[10] In the rare cases of proven pediatric nonfunctioning pituitary adenomas, primary amenorrhea and the arrest of growth and sexual development are the initial clinical symptoms.[11–13] The third presenting feature is the incidental discovery of pituitary adenomas on brain imaging, computed tomography (CT), or magnetic resonance imaging (MRI). These events increase with the improvement of neuroimaging procedures. However, screening for hormone overproduction by these tumors must be performed. These cases may constitute a difficult therapeutic challenge.[5,14]

Radiologic Considerations

Magnetic resonance imaging has proven to be the most useful brain imaging technique for the study of a nonfunctioning pituitary adenoma. T1-weighted MRI should be performed in the sagittal and coronal planes, with and without gadolinium. Dynamic sequences are useful, especially in microadenomas, which are rarely nonfunctioning. If MRI is contraindicated because of a pacemaker or intraocular foreign body, CT scanning, with and without contrast material, must be obtained, especially in the coronal section. Most of the pertinent data concerning the characteristics of a pituitary adenoma may be obtained by careful study of MRIs.

Size and Extension of the Adenoma

At diagnosis, most nonfunctioning pituitary adenomas are already macroadenomas.[6,8,14,16] All symptomatic "silent" macroadenomas have extended beyond the confines of an enlarged sella, and the most common form of expansion can be represented as a medial suprasellar expansion filling the suprasellar space. The authors usually distinguish three types of medial suprasellar expansion (Fig. 29-1):

Type a: Constituting 14% in our series, this type is a suprasellar expansion presenting as a bulge in the diaphragma sellae that extends into the suprasellar space and reaches the lower part of the optic tract.

Type b: The expansion of this type fills all the suprasellar space, and chiasmal compression is obvious.

Type c: Expansion of this type reaches the foramen of Monro. Visual symptoms are present, and hydrocephalus is possible.[17] Types b and c together constitute 86% of the authors' series.

Sphenoidal extension is often combined with suprasellar extension, but it may be isolated; it usually takes the form of a bulging of a thin sellar floor into the sphenoid sinus. However, if the sellar floor has been destroyed, the dura may be invaded, and the invasive adenoma can then extend into the sphenoid sinus and posteriorly into the spongy bone of the sphenoid. It is important to recognize the other types of intracranial tumor expansion because they may modify the therapeutic strategy, particularly the operative approach (Fig. 29-2). Subfrontal expansion can occur medially between the optic nerves and extend above the sphenoidal planum, lifting up the frontal lobes. This kind of expansion cannot reasonably be reached by a transsphenoidal approach, except in cases of visual decompression and incomplete removal in an elderly patient who cannot be operated by a cranial approach. Retrochiasmatic expansion is a kind of expansion that occurs in cases of optic nerve shortening. Such expansion extends the tumor into the interpeduncular cistern and upward as far as the foramen of Monro. Occasionally, an adenoma is found behind the dorsum sellae and the clivus, stretching the brain stem.

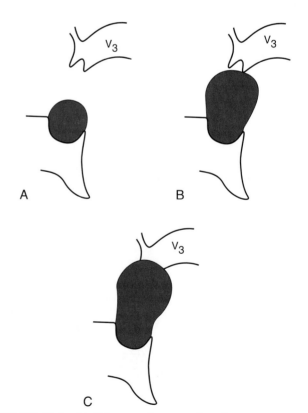

FIGURE 29-1 Medial suprasellar expansion of macroadenomas. *A,* Moderate suprasellar expansion filling (in part) the suprasellar cistern with no chiasmal compression. *B,* Expansion in contact with the anteroinferior part of the third ventricle. Visual symptoms are common. *C,* Amputation of the anterior part of the third ventricle. There is a risk of hydrocephalus; visual symptoms are obvious.

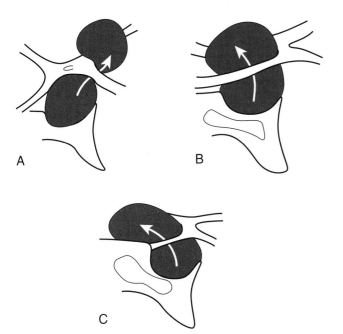

FIGURE 29-2 Different kinds of suprasellar expansions. *A,* Retrochiasmatic. *B,* Prechiasmatic. *C,* Subjugual.

Cavernous involvement by a pituitary adenoma is often questionable. A true invasion is identified as a perforation of the dura of the cavernous sinus with involvement extending into the sinus, around the carotid artery. In these cases, unilateral progressive oculomotor palsies are common. More often, the macroadenoma displaces the intact dural wall of the cavernous sinus laterally over a great distance without invading the dura. Lastly, the most specific signs of cavernous sinus invasion are internal carotid artery encasement and lateral bulging of the external wall of the cavernous sinus.[18,19]

Middle fossa expansion of a macroadenoma consists of a lateral cranial extension of the tumor between the optic nerve and supraclinoid carotid artery, or between the carotid artery and third nerve or ipsilateral optic bundle. Such tumor expansion can be reached only by a pterional cranial approach (Fig. 29-3).

Enclosed or Invasive Macroadenomas

Most nonfunctioning macroadenomas remain enclosed adenomas. In these cases, MRI shows a well-shaped, round

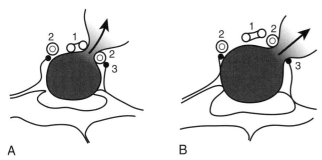

FIGURE 29-3 Pituitary adenomas with lateral suprasellar expansions (*1,* optic chiasma; *2,* internal carotid artery; *3,* third nerve). *A,* Adenoma escape between the optic chiasma and internal carotid artery. *B,* Adenoma escape between internal carotid artery and third nerve.

tumor that stretches the adjacent structures without disrupting the dura or the sellar walls. Total removal is then considered possible. In one third of cases,[6] invasion clearly extends into the cavernous sinus, sphenoid body, or cranial space by perforation of the diaphragma sellae. The tumor is surgically unresectable unless the invasion is local and the surgeon is prepared to repair a cerebrospinal fluid (CSF) leak (Fig. 29-4).

Brain imaging by CT or MRI is also useful for preoperative evaluation of possible intraoperative surgical problems. Potential problems include vascular injury, if the carotid arteries are bulging into the sella; CSF leakage, in cases of extreme distortion of the diaphragma sellae; and an irregularly shaped upper part of the tumor, indicating possible rupture of the arachnoid membrane. Hemorrhage from a fibrous adenoma can be suspected before surgery in patients exhibiting marked contrast enhancement on brain imaging or vascular blush supply on angiography. Routine cerebral angiography is not performed in the authors' institution unless the diagnosis is doubtful. MR angiography is now considered of little value for preoperative evaluation of the consistency of the adenoma. In the authors' series of nonfunctioning pituitary adenomas, 72% were considered by the surgeon to be soft tumors, sometimes fluid or necrotic (Fig. 29-5); and the other 28%, had a fibrous, hemorrhagic (Fig. 29-6), or semifibrous appearance.

ENDOCRINE EVALUATION

For patients with nonfunctioning adenomas, endocrine evaluation should include measurement of the levels of serum prolactin, growth hormone, cortisol, T3, T4, FSH, and LH. In approximately 71% of these adenomas, preoperative partial hypophyseal insufficiency has been demonstrated.[6,9,16]

Moderate hyperprolactinemia (less than 200 ng/mL) is usual (in 50% to 65% of patients). Negative immunocytochemical staining in these cases argues strongly for hypothalamohypophyseal disconnection.[6,8,9,20] α-Subunit and TSH levels should also be tested; even if they are often normal, they might be useful markers for follow-up if their levels are elevated.

Although most nonfunctioning pituitary adenomas are shown by immunocytochemical staining to be gonadotropic adenomas, they are commonly considered silent, with levels of plasma gonadotropins or their subunits that are usually low. Increased basal FSH seems to be more common, especially in men.[21,25] Increased basal LH is rare and is often combined with an excess of α-subunit.[20,22,24,26,27] Overproduction of α-subunit is common, but overproduction of basal LH β-subunit is rare. On the last 95 gonadotropic adenomas, immunocytochemical staining in one third was positive to FSH-β, and in two thirds was positive to a mixed reactivity for FSH-β and LH or FSH-β and α subunit.[22,23]

SURGICAL MANAGEMENT

Goals of Surgery

Visual Prognosis

Because most nonfunctioning pituitary adenomas are macroadenomas, usually accompanied by visual symptoms, the first goal of surgery is the resolution of the visual state.

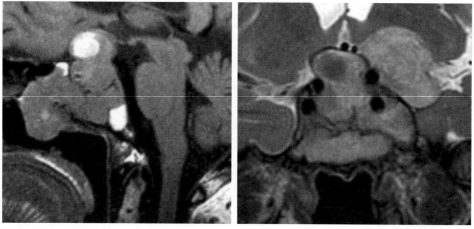

FIGURE 29-4   Invasive partially hemorrhagic pituitary adenoma: coronal (*left*) and sagittal (*right*) sections.

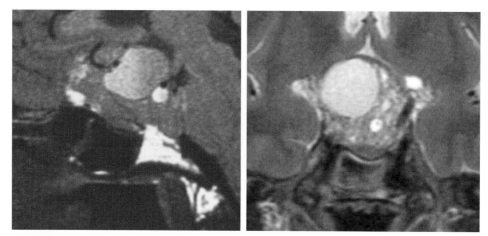

FIGURE 29-5   Partially necrotic pituitary macroadenoma: coronal (*left*) and sagittal (*right*) sections.

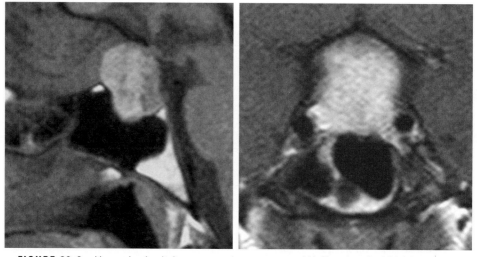

FIGURE 29-6   Hemorrhagic pituitary macroadenoma: coronal (*left*) and sagittal (*right*) sections.

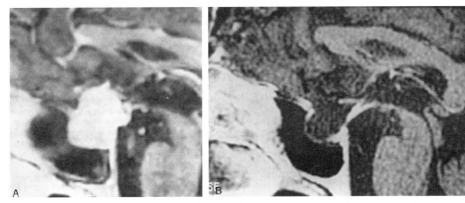

FIGURE 29-7   The goal of surgery is complete removal. *A,* Preoperative magnetic resonance imaging scan of a nonsecreting pituitary adenoma. *B,* Complete removal after transsphenoidal surgery.

Postoperative results are usually good or excellent, especially after transsphenoidal surgery.[6,7,14,28] In the authors' institution, visual results after transsphenoidal surgery for nonfunctioning adenomas are as follows:

Improvement, 80%
No change, 13.8%
Worsening, 6.2%

- 2.8% after first surgery
- 18% after second surgery for recurrence

Improvements in visual symptoms concern visual field and visual acuity, and depend on preoperative visual status, operative approach, and duration of symptoms. Postoperative worsening of visual symptoms is much more predictable in older patients with poor preoperative vision. In macroadenoma extending into the suprasellar space but without pertinent visual deficit, the indication for transsphenoidal surgery to prevent visual symptoms is questionable.

Endocrinologic Prognosis

Preoperative antehypophyseal insufficiency is often present in patients with nonfunctioning pituitary adenomas. After transsphenoidal surgery, the endocrinologic status is often unchanged and requires substitution therapy, but it may also be either worsened or improved.[6,9,14,16]

Pituitary insufficiency can be improved if surgery is not delayed too long and if the insufficiency is caused by compression of normal tissue.[8] The goal of surgery is to preserve pituitary function and, sometimes, to achieve partial restoration.

Total Removal: Goal and Challenge

In patients with nonfunctioning pituitary adenomas, the authors advocate complete tumor removal (Fig. 29-7)[29] because there is no proven effective medical therapy and because radiation therapy is known to be harmful, especially in elderly patients. Total removal must therefore be the goal of surgery, because the tumor is soft, noninvasive, and well delimited by normal tissue (Fig. 29-8). Even in large adenomas, a clean surgical plane can be found at the beginning of the procedure and progressively followed and separated from the adjacent compressed normal structures (see Fig. 29-8). This procedure is valid for the transsphenoidal approach. On the other hand, pituitary adenomas operated through a cranial approach are always invasive tumors and are totally unresectable without major postoperative complications.

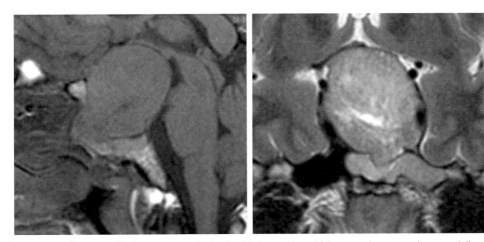

FIGURE 29-8   Huge suprasellar expansion is not a contraindication for transsphenoidal surgery because a large neck lies between intrasellar (*left*) and suprasellar (*right*) components.

The goal of surgery using a cranial approach is subtotal removal and decompression of the optic nerves and chiasm.

Cranial Approaches

Indications for a cranial approach in patients presenting with a nonfunctioning pituitary adenoma are infrequent (2.3% in the authors' series). In fact, craniotomy is indicated only in patients with visual symptoms not improved by medical therapy and an adenoma that is unresectable by the transsphenoidal route. Such cases are mostly encountered when the intracranial part of an extension is separated from the intrasellar part by a narrow neck, or when the intracranial extension is huge and multidirectional (Fig. 29-9). Extensions that are subfrontal, lateral middle fossa, retroclival, or suprasellar with a narrow neck can be indications for a primary cranial approach, but the latter may also be indicated as the second stage of a two-step procedure after transsphenoidal surgery. The choice and side of the cranial approach depend on the location and size of the adenoma as seen on MRI (Fig. 29-10):

- Bifrontal medial craniotomy, such as that used in olfactory groove meningiomas, is recommended for the removal of huge subfrontal tumors.
- The pterional approach is commonly used when the tumor fills the suprasellar medial and lateral cisterns.
- The subtemporal approach is advocated for subtemporal retroclival and infratentorial extensions.
- The transbasal subfrontal approach is not indicated for pituitary tumors, even when extensive, because this approach is entirely extradural, and because the larger part of the adenoma threatening the visual pathways is intradural.

- Approaches to the cavernous sinus, as described by some authors,[30,31] do not, apart from exceptional cases, seem to be of any value for the surgical management of nonfunctioning pituitary adenomas. The main reason is that a pituitary adenoma extending into the cavernous sinus as a space-occupying lesion is an invasive, unresectable tumor (Fig. 29-11).

Complications of the Cranial Approach

Complications of the cranial approach are well known[32]; they are closely related to elevation of the frontal or temporal lobes, dissection of major arteries and perforating vessels, and manipulations of the optic tract and oculomotor nerves. One particular feature of cranial surgery for nonfunctioning pituitary adenomas should be stressed: when such adenomas are operated through a cranial approach, they are usually huge, heterogeneous, fibrous, or hemorrhagic. Therefore, as in meningiomas in the same area, close adhesions to vascular and adjacent brain structures are encountered. Not infrequently, rupture of the arachnoidal plane is noted, so that dissection behind the optic chiasm involving the posterior wall of the carotid artery and optic bundle becomes hazardous and often leads to incomplete tumor removal. After a cranial approach, manipulation of the optic tract or partial devascularization of the optic nerves or chiasm leads to postoperative worsening of visual status more often than after transsphenoidal surgery.

Every attempt should be made to preserve the pituitary stalk, which often adheres closely to the tumor. As in

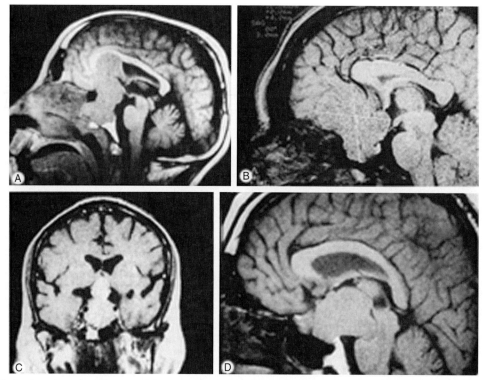

FIGURE 29-9 Indications for a cranial approach in endocrinologically silent pituitary tumors. *A,* Huge suprasellar expansion. *B,* Subfrontal expansion. *C,* Suprasellar expansion with a narrow neck linking with the intrasellar expansion. *D,* Retrochiasmatic expansion.

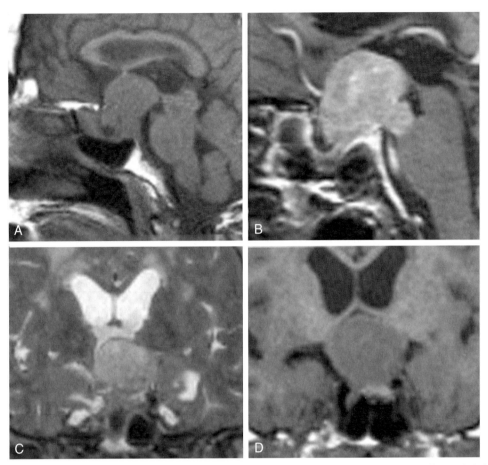

FIGURE 29-10   Indication for cranial approach: a huge pituitary adenoma with suprasellar expansion. *A* and *B*, saggital view. T1-weighted images before (*A*) and after (*B*) gadolinium injection. *C* and *D*, coronal view. T2-weighted (*C*) and T1-weighted (*D*) images.

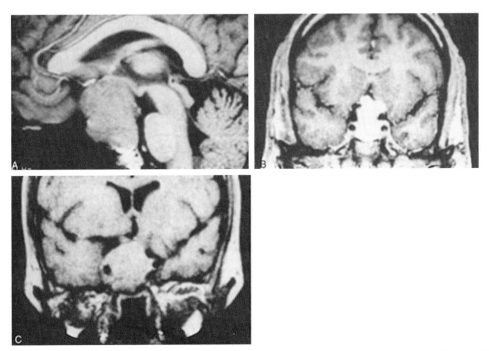

FIGURE 29-11   Invasive endocrinologically silent pituitary adenomas. *A*, Invasive suprasellar sphenoidal tumor. *B*, Suprasellar multilobulated expansion. *C*, Invasive cavernous sinus tumor.

craniopharyngiomas, the choice is then between cutting the stalk or leaving the residual tumor in place.

TRANSSPHENOIDAL APPROACH

The surgical technique for the removal of pituitary adenomas by the transsphenoidal approach has remained almost identical to the one Cushing[33] used initially, with the addition of improvements by Kanavel[34] and Hirsch[35] and as modified by Halstead,[36] who first used the sublabial incision. As he developed the techniques of intracranial surgery, Cushing abandoned the transsphenoidal route, and it was forgotten by most of his students, with the notable exception of Dott.[37] With the technical advances introduced by Guiot[38] and Hardy,[39] the transsphenoidal approach has been commonly used for the surgical treatment of pituitary adenomas and other tumors of the sellar area.[40] The different steps in the procedure are described in detail in Chapter 25, as well as in many well-documented reports.[29,38,40,42] However, the authors wish to stress special aspects of transsphenoidal surgery observed in our institution, where it was initially practiced under the direction of Guiot:

- Preoperative hormonal substitution therapy is routinely used for nonfunctioning pituitary adenomas; it consists of administration of 50 mg of succinate hydrocortisone intramuscularly, 1 hour before surgery, and 25 mg every 6 hours thereafter. Twenty mg of oral hydrocortisone is given 18 hours after the first injection.
- Perioperative antibiotic medication consists of lincomycin, 10 mg/kg every 8 hours; and gentamicin, 1 mg/kg over 24 hours. The choice of these two antibiotics is based on the fact that they do not pass through the brain barrier and are not able to mask an eventful postoperative meningitis.
- Preoperative review of CT and MRI scans is essential to demonstrate the configuration of the sphenoid bone and the position of the carotid arteries, particularly in cases of reoperation.

Careful positioning of the patient is essential. The patient is placed in a semisitting position. The patient's head is fixed to the operative frame to secure the midline parallel to the walls of the room. This landmark is probably the most important, whatever the operative approach (i.e., nasal or sublabial).

Even in macroadenomas, a lumbar drain is not inserted, because surgery is performed under a C-arm fluoroscope so that the progression of instruments can be followed at each step in the procedure. When tumor removal is almost complete, the operative cavity fills up with air, and the position and the prolapse of the diaphragma sellae are controlled using a television screen. Bilateral jugular vein compression is usually enough to debulk a soft suprasellar tumor and make the diaphragma sellae prolapse into the sella. It is thought that raising the intracranial pressure by injection through a lumbar catheter is not a safe procedure for the optic nerves or chiasm, which are already compressed, especially in fibrous adenomas.[43,44]

Except for reoperation, when the endonasal approach may be an effective alternative method to avoid the scar made by previous surgery, the conventional sublabial approach is favored at the authors' institution. For many years, the sublabial has not been sutured at the end of the procedure, without any adverse consequence. The sublabial incision has two main advantages: (1) enlargement of the piriform sinus to avoid fracture of the turbinates as the retractor is opened; and (2) a wide exposure of the sellar floor, an essential condition for exposing the dura as far as possible laterally in relation to the cavernous sinus.

The mucosa inside the sphenoid sinus is usually removed because it may be extensive, and its removal probably reduces the risk of postoperative infection or mucocele.

The dura is not coagulated before opening, because this can induce its shrinkage and extradural bleeding.

The lateral and suprasellar parts of the tumor are usually removed without direct visual inspection, thanks to two anatomic landmarks: (1) the coronaire sinus, running upward; and (2) the cavernous sinus, which lies on each side of the sphenoid bone. These parts of the tumor are removed with "homemade" instruments (i.e., malleable and variously angled curets and suckers). These instruments permit constant but gentle contact with the walls of the sella and the operative cavity.

After tumor removal, normal pituitary tissue can be identified, even with macroadenomas. This tissue is compressed against the wall of the sella as a pink, adhesive tissue. Sometimes, however, the normal pituitary is not visible, and this is always noted in the surgical report as an important item of information for further endocrinologic follow-up. The absence of any residual tumor is confirmed by microscopic examination, flexible fiberoptic endoscopy, and aspiration toward the walls with variously angled instruments.

Hemostasis is ensured with Gelfoam even if bleeding from the intradural venous sinus is significant.

Hemostasis must be obtained carefully, especially in cases of subtotal removal. The authors have had rare but memorable experiences of postoperative rebleeding into the operative cavity from a residual tumor. For a trained pituitary surgeon, this rebleeding is most predictable in cases of huge suprasellar fibrous adenomas without collapse of the diaphragma sellae during surgery (semifibrous or fibrous adenomas constituted 7% of the nonfunctioning pituitary adenomas in the authors' series).

After the adenoma is removed and hemostasis is obtained, a piece of Gelfoam is usually left in the operative cavity.

A piece of bone, extracted from the nasal septum, is inserted below the edges of the opening of the anterior wall of the sella.

In the authors' institution, surgery is performed by the neurosurgeon alone. The mean duration of the procedure is 1 hour.

The patient is discharged on the fifth postoperative day; the removal of the nasal packing takes place on the third postoperative day.

It is noted that there are multiple refinements of the standard transsphenoidal approach; the problem is just a question of experience. The transsphenoidal route, in experienced hands, is secure and effective with most cases of pituitary tumors; however, if the main rules are not strictly applied, this surgery may be troublesome or even stormy.

Postoperative Management

Immediately after surgery, the patient's water balance and urinary output and density should be measured every hour and, for 2 days thereafter, every 3 hours. Serum electrolyte levels should be monitored daily. Diabetes insipidus must be detected quickly to institute medical therapy. In cases of nonfunctioning pituitary adenomas, the patient is always discharged with steroid hormonal substitution therapy until the postoperative endocrinologic evaluation on day 8 after surgery. The patient also must be tested at home for delayed hyponatremia by systematic staining.

Complications

The complications of transsphenoidal surgery observed in the authors' institution are listed in Table 29-4. Many well-documented papers have been published on the subject.[40,41,43–45,47] Here, only some important possible complications are stressed.

A CSF fistula may occur in cases of nonfunctioning pituitary adenoma if the diaphragma sellae is injured or invaded by an invasive tumor; this can be suspected with an irregularly shaped suprasellar extension. This situation also may be predictable in patients who have undergone previous transcranial or transsphenoidal surgery and radiation therapy.[46,48] In such cases, two distinct situations are possible. First, a distorted diaphragma sellae can sustain a minor tear, which can be routinely repaired by clipping the two edges of the tear together with a bayonet clip holder and inserting a piece of fascia lata under the diaphragma. Watertight closure of the sella is completed by introduction of muscle to support the fascia lata, and by a bone graft that closes the sella.

The second possibility, a complete laceration of the diaphragma sellae, requires a more aggressive procedure to close the fistula and avoid resurgery. A piece of fascia lata is sutured to the anterior dura just under the transverse sinus with a long needle holder (used in heart surgery) and then pushed upward to "reconstruct" the diaphragma sellae. This fragment is maintained in position by meticulous packing of the sella with muscle and fat. Closure of the sella is easy if the firm, bony part of the anterior wall remains intact, in which

case a piece of bone (grafted extradurally) ensures permanent closure. On the other hand, if the anterior wall and floor of the sella have already been destroyed by the adenoma because of sphenoidal extension or an invasive sphenoidal adenoma, no osseous structure is available to keep the bone graft in place. In this event, packing of the sphenoidal sinus is mandatory using the same materials as mentioned previously (i.e., muscle, fat, and glue). Spongy bone extracted from the iliac crest can be useful for reconstructing a watertight closure of the sphenoid sinus. The insertion of any foreign material into the sphenoid sinus is prohibited in the authors' department because of the risk of infection. In such cases, postoperative lumbar drainage is used for 6 or 7 days. Despite this meticulous procedure, cases of recurrent CSF rhinorrhea have been described, and in the authors' experience, 1% of patients (in a series of 5000 cases) had to be reoperated for CSF leakage. The authors stress the following:

1. An intraoperative CSF fistula in patients with macroadenoma must be treated and closed in a single operation.
2. Postoperative CSF rhinorrhea after transsphenoidal surgery must be detected and closed as soon as possible, using the same approach.
3. Insertion of a permanent CSF shunt is a rescue procedure.

The secondary empty sella syndrome may occur under three conditions: (1) an enlarged sella, (2) a large suprasellar extension, and (3) adherences between the distended diaphragm sellae and optic tract. This rare syndrome, described in the early period of transsphenoidal surgery, has not been observed for many years because it has been prevented by extradural packing of the sellar floor.[45,46,49]

Suspected postoperative hematoma after transsphenoidal surgery is difficult to manage, particularly in elderly patients with marked impairment of preoperative vision.

Early brain CT or MRI scans are difficult to evaluate because they often reproduce the preoperative size of the tumor. The authors came to the conclusion that postoperative worsening of visual status without improvement after 3 hours of high-dose corticosteroid therapy is an absolute indication for reoperation, which, however, often gives disappointing findings. Such reoperation involves the gentle removal of noncompressive clots until the pulsations of the upper part of the hematoma are obvious. Nevertheless, it must be stated that this reoperation is often successful, with quick improvement of vision. Such reoperations can be prevented by meticulous hemostasis, particularly in cases of fibrous adenoma or proven residual tumor, or in elderly patients with marked impairment of preoperative vision.

RECURRENCES

The mean rate of recurrence for nonfunctioning pituitary adenomas after surgery alone is approximately 30% (range, 10% to 69%).

Because nonfunctioning pituitary adenomas cannot be followed up on the basis of hormonal criteria, CT or MRI criteria must be used. The schedule for postoperative brain imaging is discussed.[50–53] For some neurosurgical teams, MRI is often performed on the day following surgery. It is advocated that this immediate control is useful to detect

---

TABLE 29-4 ▪ Complications of the Transsphenoidal Approach in a Series of 5134 Cases Hôpital Foch—Neurosurgical Department

Surgical mortality
  Before 1985: 1%
  Last decade (1993–2003): 0.2%
Mechanical complications: <2%
Cerebrospinal fluid leak: 2% (1% reoperated)
Secondary empty sella: 0.2% (0% last decade, 1993–2003)
Transient oculomotor palsy: 1.5%

Visual worsening
  In microadenoma: 0%
  In macroadenoma
    First surgery: 2.8%
    Reoperation: 18%
Endocrinologic complications: rare but difficult to summarize because of the usual partial preoperative pituitary insufficiency

immediate hemorrhagic complications, to presize the aspect of the pituitary mass in relation to the optic tract, and to detect residual pathological tissue. A precise operative report is essential for an accurate interpretation at that time. The results of this study included first the pituitary mass: the weight of the mass can be decreased, unchanged, or increased because of excessive packing. The Gelfoam or Surgicel will have a heterogeneous signal in T1- and T2-weighted imaging. This material is blood impregnated, and some air bubbles may be seen. Usually, a peripheric rim is visible around this kind of packing after gadolinium injection. The fat has a typical hypersignal in T1-weighted imaging. The biological glue has an isosignal to the brain. The clear evaluation of a residual tumor at that time is difficult. Normally, the residual tumoral tissue has the same aspect it did preoperatively; however, it presents a nodular enhancement after gadolinium injection. The sphenoid sinus is usually opacified with hemorrhagic fluid, and mucosal thickening is often noted. In the authors' institution, this immediate postoperative control is not use routinely except if a complication is suspected (Fig. 29-12).

On the other hand, the postoperative control MRI 3 months after surgery (Fig. 29-13) is essential because most of the material used for packing (except the fat) has disappeared and the analysis of residual tumor can be more accurate: it has the same signal as the primitive tumor. After gadolinium infusion, the enhancement of residual tissue is less marked than is the normal pituitary gland. At 3 months, except for proven invasive residual tumor (which can be proposed for radiotherapy), a repeat control at 9 months and every year after surgery is proposed, with a better evaluation of a residual tumor, or the presence of an empty sella with homolateral pituitary stalk attraction (Fig. 29-14). After gadolinium injection, the normal tissue enhances homogenously.

The interval after which further morphologic studies are performed has not been clearly defined, but because the largest number of recurrences occur between 4 and 8 years after surgery,[6,54,57] the follow-up period must be extended for many years (Fig. 29-15).

The absence of late recurrences in some follow-up series is surprising and is probably caused by the limitation of the observation period. In the authors' department, 55 recurrent nonfunctioning pituitary adenomas were observed out of 395 cases (14%) with a long-term follow-up of more than 10 years. Summarized data for this series are listed in Table 29-5. From the results, it can be concluded that, as stated previously, radiation therapy does not prevent recurrence but delays it. Ninety percent of the authors' patients experienced new visual symptoms at the time of recurrence, probably either because the morphologic follow-up had not been sufficiently meticulous or because patients had been lost to follow-up because of an uneventful clinical course. Forty-seven of these 55 cases of recurrence concerned macroadenomas, and 8 were known residual tumors that had increased in size.

Table 29-6 summarizes the therapeutic management of these recurrent cases. The authors' experience leads to the following conclusions:

1. Reoperation is highly recommended if visual symptoms are present.
2. The choice of surgical approach is subject to the same rules as the first surgery.
3. Prior radiation therapy and surgery increase the fibrous component of the tumor.
4. Reoperation led to incomplete removal in 40% of the authors' cases.

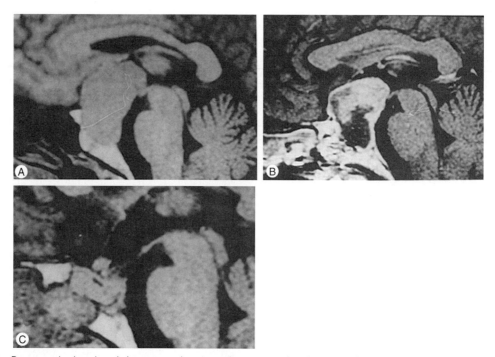

FIGURE 29-12 Postoperative imaging. *A,* A postoperative magnetic resonance imaging seen of a huge adenoma. *B,* The same adenoma 4 days after transsphenoidal surgery. *C,* Same cases 2 months after surgery.

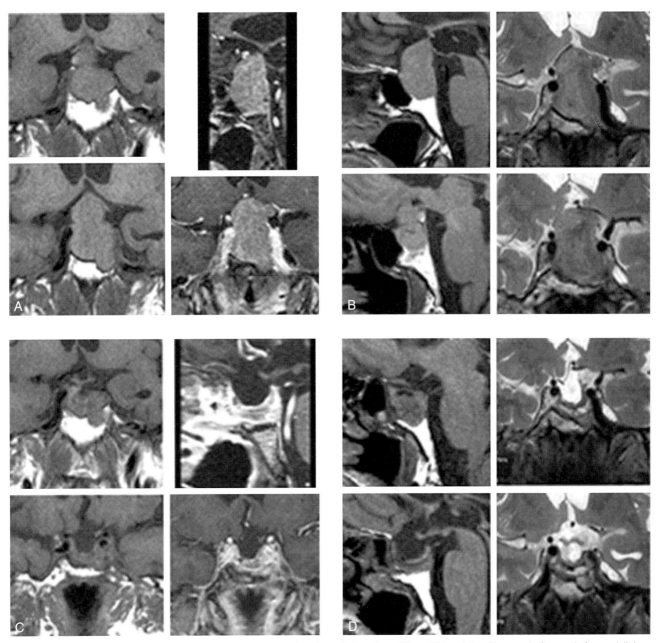

FIGURE 29-13 *A* and *B*, Preoperative macroadenoma coronal and saggital sections: T2- and T1-weighted images before and after gadolinium injection. *C* and *D*, Control MRI at 3 months post-transsphenoidal approach. Subtotal removal with residual tumor in left cavernous sinus.

5. Reoperation by the transsphenoidal approach, in cases of recurrent nonfunctioning pituitary adenomas, leads to more complications: 20% postoperative visual worsening (instead of 3.1% after initial surgery in the authors' department) and 9% CSF fistula (instead of 3.6% at the first surgery) were seen. Table 29-7 gives the results of follow-up after treatment for recurrences.

RADIATION THERAPY

Although the indications for postoperative radiation therapy are not questionable in cases of proven residual tumor, controversy persists between the supporters and opponents of systematic postoperative irradiation, even if there is no obvious residual adenoma.[54] In patients with nonfunctioning pituitary adenomas, systematic postoperative radiation therapy led to a mean rate of recurrence of 11%, whereas in patients who underwent surgery alone, this rate was 27%. These data argue in favor of the value of postoperative irradiation for the prevention of recurrence. On the other hand, all pituitary adenomas do not display the same behavior. The growth of pituitary adenomas, particularly the endocrine inactive type, is usually slow, but it may be faster with more recurrences, especially in young patients.

The final decision regarding radiation therapy would be easier if markers of aggressivity and invasiveness were available. These markers cannot yet be used routinely, but the first results of studies based on the use of genetic molecular markers seem promising.[55–57] Because the goal of radiation therapy is to deliver the maximal dose to the target and the

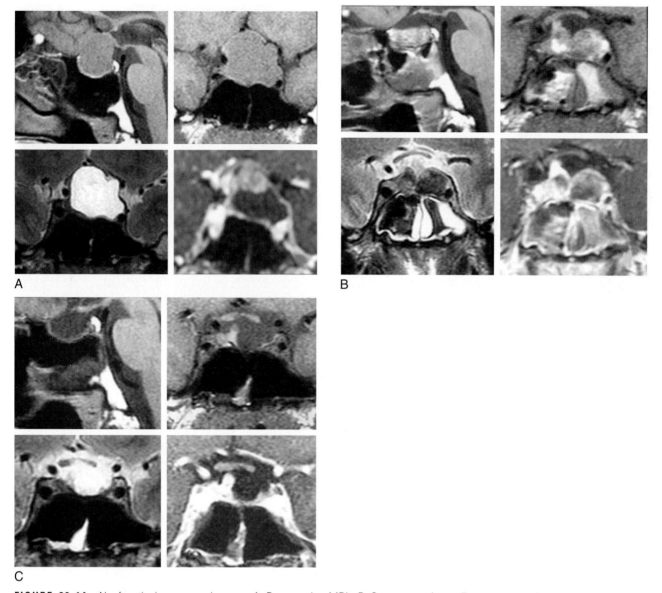

FIGURE 29-14   Nonfunctioning macroadenoma. *A,* Preoperative MRI. *B,* Same case: immediate postoperative control at fourth day. *C,* Same case: 5 months after surgery by transsphenoidal approach.

minimal dose to adjacent structures, different methods of irradiation can be proposed, including heavy particles; gamma knife surgery; or x-ray irradiation, either conventional or delivered by linear accelerator[58–61] (Fig. 29-16).

The control rates for nonfunctioning pituitary adenomas after adjuvant radiation therapy seem to be high, at nearly 85%[60] and 90.3% for 10-year progression-free survival.[61] However, with adjuvant radiation therapy, the mean rate of recurrence is 11%. In the authors' institution, 15 of 104 patients with nonfunctioning pituitary adenomas (14%) who had postoperative radiation therapy with a mean 10-year follow-up had a recurrence. Irradiation does not prevent recurrence, but merely delays it.

Radiation therapy may have pernicious effects, and the progressive onset of hypopituitarism in a few months or years is a well-known complication.[62,63]

The rate of pituitary insufficiency is higher if the radiation dose is 50 Gy or more. Other complications of radiation

therapy have been reported and were observed in the authors' series. These included:

1. Subacute incompletely regressive encephalitis[64,65]
2. Delayed brain radionecrosis[66]
3. Radiation-induced brain tumors, including glioma,[67] astrocytoma,[68] and meningioma[68]

The authors observed one radiation-induced glioblastoma and one skull base sarcoma several years after conventional radiation therapy for nonfunctioning pituitary adenomas. Symptomatic bilateral supraclinoid carotid artery stenosis was also observed in one patient 15 years after conventional radiation therapy for pituitary adenoma.

The pernicious neuropsychological effects of radiation therapy are well known in children, but not in adults.

Because the complications of postoperative radiation therapy are known, its advantages and risks must be carefully weighed (especially in older patients) if pituitary function is

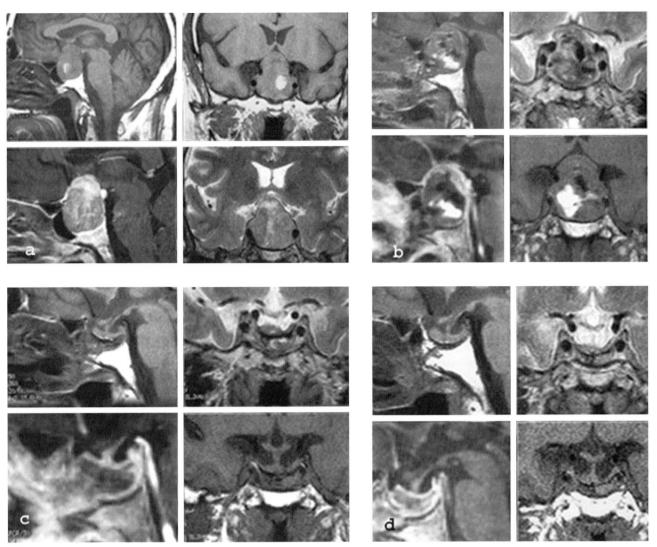

FIGURE 29-15 Nonfunctioning macroadenoma. *A*, Preoperative MRI. *B*, Postoperative MRI second day post-transsphenoidal surgery. *C*, Three months postop. *D*, One year postop: the sella is partially empty. Some normal tissue is visible at the bottom of the sella.

TABLE 29-5 ▪ **Fifty-five (14%) Recurrent Nonfunctioning Pituitary Adenomas of 395 Cases with Long-Term Follow-up, Hôpital Foch—Neurosurgical Department**

Mean age at time of recurrence	60 years
Sex	36 male
	19 female
Mean time to recurrence after surgery	
Less than 5 years	21 cases
5–10 years	17 cases
More than 10 years	17 cases
Mean time to recurrence	
With previous radiation therapy	15 years
Without radiation therapy	6 years

TABLE 29-6 ▪ **Therapeutic Management of 55 Recurrent Nonfunctioning Pituitary Adenomas, Hôpital Foch—Neurosurgical Department**

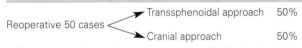

Reoperative 50 cases
Transsphenoidal approach 50%
Cranial approach 50%

Twenty cases incomplete removal -> 16 of radiation therapy
Thirty cases of subtotal or total removal
Radiation therapy: 4 cases
Medical treatment: 1 case

Table 29-7 ▪ Follow-up of 55 recurrent Nonfunctioning Pituitary Adenomas after Treatment of the Recurrence, Hôpital Foch—Neurosurgical Department

Five patients died (two of brain radionecrosis).
Fifty patients are still alive after several procedures and radiation therapy.

normal and if there is no obvious residual tumor. In the past, radiation therapy was always proposed in the authors' department after surgery for nonsecreting pituitary adenomas, even if total removal was visually achieved by the neurosurgeon. However, because of the increasingly common complications reported after radiation therapy, and above all thanks to the development of brain imaging, this policy has gradually changed. The attitude now is to weigh the pros and cons according to the age of the patient and the size of the residual tumor, as follows:

1. If there is no obvious residual tumor on delayed, controlled MRI, radiation therapy is not performed.
2. If a documented residual tumor is present, and if the tumor is less than 10 mm in diameter and separated from the optic tract, gamma knife surgery or linear accelerator radiation is proposed. If the tumor is more than 10 mm in diameter, conventional radiation therapy is proposed, with a lower dose for older patients.

SURGICAL STRATEGY

As stated in this and other documented reports by pituitary surgeons throughout the world, radiation therapy should be considered an adjuvant treatment for endocrinologically silent pituitary adenomas, and medical therapy is not yet routinely effective. The main challenge in treating these adenomas is the surgical strategy. Because, in experienced hands, the transsphenoidal approach is relatively benign, is of short duration, and gives good results, it has for many years been the first choice in the surgical treatment of nonfunctioning pituitary adenomas. The transsphenoidal approach was performed in 95% of the authors' cases regardless of the size of the adenoma. Inferior sphenoidal extension of the tumor is an absolute indication for the transsphenoidal approach. However, for removal by this approach, a suprasellar medial extension has to have widespread connections with the intrasellar part, thus enabling the instruments to reach the uppermost portion of the tumor without risk. The encapsulated adenoma allows the suprasellar portion to descend to the sellar floor after the sella has been evacuated. In general, when there is a narrow neck between an intrasellar and a suprasellar medial or lateral extension, transsphenoidal surgery allows only the removal of the intrasellar part of the tumor.

Therefore, the transsphenoidal approach may constitute the first step in a two-stage procedure comprising the transsphenoidal and cranial approaches. This strategy must be carefully considered when a cranial extension is unresectable by the transsphenoidal route (i.e., in cases of a subfrontal, subtemporal, or suprasellar extension of the tumor with a narrow connection with its intrasellar part) (Fig. 29-17). The transsphenoidal approach should usually be proposed as the first step because:

1. It allows the removal of the intrasellar part of the tumor and the subsequent acquisition of important information on tumor consistency; and because it

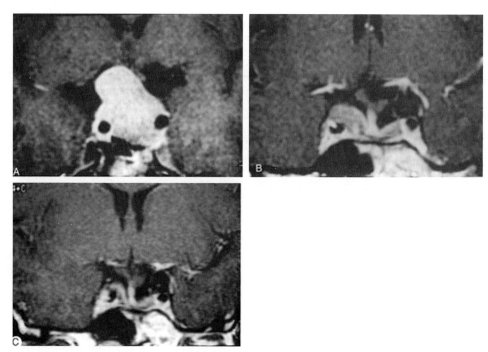

FIGURE 29-16   A nonfunctioning pituitary adenoma: combined transsphenoidal and radiosurgery. *A,* A pituitary adenoma before surgery. *B,* The same case with a magnetic resonance imaging (MRI) scan 4 months after incomplete removal of the paracavernous part of the tumor. *C,* The same case with an MRI scan 1 year after radiosurgery by gamma knife.

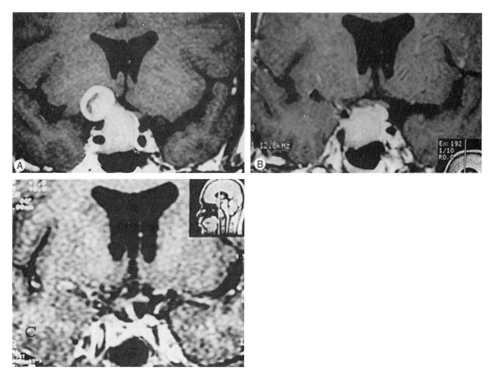

FIGURE 29-17   Nonfunctioning pituitary tumors: cranial and transsphenoidal surgery in two steps. *A,* Lateral expansion with a narrow neck, which is an indication for a cranial approach. *B,* A magnetic resonance imaging (MRI) scan 3 months after the craniotomy. *C,* The same case with an MRI scan 6 months after secondary surgery using a transsphenoidal approach.

confirms the silent, nonfunctionning character of the adenoma by immunocytochemical studies. This information is very important to ensure that no postoperative medical treatment is indicated.

2. Above all, this approach allows meticulous closure of the sella, thus ensuring the absence of CSF leakage after cranial surgery.

The transsphenoidal approach may also be proposed after craniotomy to preserve normal hypophyseal tissue.[16]

Evidence of residual tumor in the cavernous sinus after transsphenoidal surgery is not an indication for secondary cranial surgery because tumor removal might in any case be incomplete. Usually, 1 or 2 months separate the two steps of the combined procedure. This period allows the immunocytochemical results to be obtained, as well as postoperative visual evaluation and watertight closure of the sella.

In some large, nonfunctioning pituitary adenomas, transsphenoidal surgery can be intentionally repeated[69] (Fig. 29-18). This strategy may be considered often, but has proved effective in some of the author's cases. It consists of the following: during the first transsphenoidal surgery, the upper part of the tumor does not prolapse into the sella, either spontaneously or by the artificial means of jugular compression. If its removal is thought to be hazardous, the tumor is left in place after meticulous hemostasis. After this decompressive surgery, visual recovery usually is observed. Some 2 or 3 months after surgery, MRI may show evidence of the descent of the residual upper part of the tumor into the sella, thus making a second transsphenoidal operation a reasonable indication (Fig. 29-19). The goal of this strategy is to achieve complete removal in two stages while preserving,

if possible, the normal hypophyseal tissue and avoiding radiation therapy. The mandatory anatomic condition for the upper part of the tumor to prolapse secondarily into the sella is a wide link between its intrasellar and suprasellar extensions (Fig. 29-20). This technique must not be used for lateral suprasellar extensions, which must be removed by a cranial approach.

PITUITARY INCIDENTALOMA

The finding of pituitary incidentaloma has become more common (by 13%)[15] because brain CT scanning or MRI has become more routinely performed for unrelated reasons.

In such cases, endocrinologic evaluation is recommended. It should indicate hormonal overproduction in cases of secreting but silent adenomas such as prolactinoma, growth hormone adenoma, or corticotropic adenoma. The therapy indicated for each specific tumor type may therefore be necessary. If there is no evidence of hormone overproduction, pituitary function should be evaluated by screening for hypopituitarism. Water deprivation and urinary excretion should be measured to detect diabetes insipidus because if this is present, the pituitary tumor is probably not an adenoma. A microadenoma usually exhibits normal pituitary function. Therefore, when a nonsecreting incidental microadenoma is discovered, first-intention surgery does not seem to be indicated because the risk of significant tumor growth is small.[70,71] However, brain imaging has to be repeated every year and surgery proposed if there is clearly documented enlargement of the adenoma. In cases of nonfunctioning incidental macroadenoma, surgery is

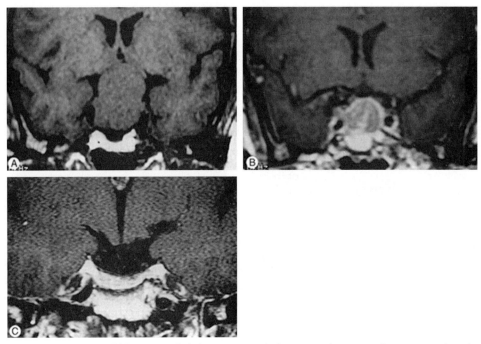

FIGURE 29-18   Two-stage transsphenoidal surgery of pituitary tumors. *A*, A preoperative magnetic resonance imaging (MRI) scan of an expanding pituitary adenoma. *B*, The same case with an MRI scan 3 months after the initial transsphenoidal surgery. *C*, The same case 6 months after the repeat transsphenoidal surgery.

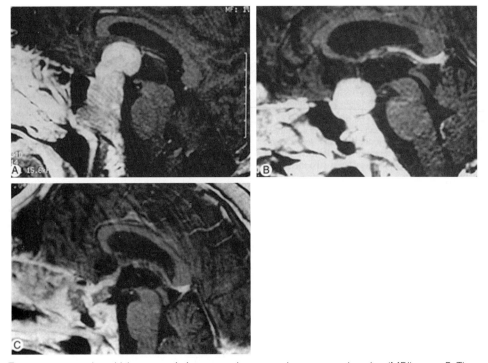

FIGURE 29-19   Two-stage transsphenoidal surgery. *A*, A preoperative magnetic resonance imaging (MRI) scan. *B*, The same case with an MRI scan 3 months after transsphenoidal surgery. The upper part of the tumor has prolapsed into the sella. *C*, The same case with an MRI scan 6 months after the second transsphenoidal approach.

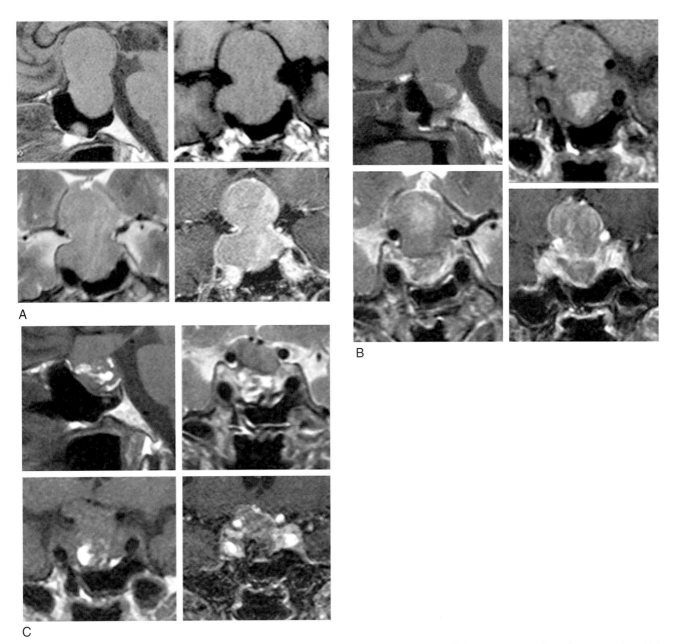

FIGURE 29-20 *A,* Preoperative MRI of a nonfunctioning macroadenoma: two-step surgery. *B,* The same case after a first transsphenoidal surgery. *C,* Postoperative MRI after a second transsphenoidal approach.

highly advisable if there are marked visual symptoms or hypopituitarism. In the absence of these symptoms, it is possible to wait 6 months and then reevaluate the situation, but the patient and his or her family must be aware that surgery may be necessary. Of course, in such cases, the clinical verdict determines the final decision, especially for older patients with a concomitant ophthalmologic disease.

THE FUTURE

Because of the possible occurrence of giant tumors, invasiveness, unusual tumor consistency, a tendency toward recurrence, the risk of radiation therapy, and the absence of effective medical treatment, some nonsecreting pituitary adenomas still constitute a difficult challenge for the neurosurgeon.[72]

What are the reasonable prospects for the future?

- Extensive surgery is thought to be of little use, even in the most experienced hands, and even despite further developments in neuronavigation. Extensive surgery cannot claim to achieve total removal of an invasive macroadenoma without damage to the adjacent structures, vessels, nerves, brain stem, and hypothalamus, and surgery does not avoid the need for subsequent radiation therapy.

- New trends in the field of medical therapy will probably constitute the most significant advances. At present, neither dopaminergic agonists nor somatostatin analogues should be proposed as first therapy if visual symptoms are present, unless surgery is strongly contraindicated. However, drugs can be useful as adjuvant therapy in patients not cured by surgery. More extensive use of new scintigraphic studies of dopaminergic receptors might be promising.[73]
- Radiosurgery is probably underused, especially in Europe, and should replace conventional radiation therapy on the condition that the neurosurgeon leaves residual tumor suitable for radiosurgery (see Fig. 29-16).
- Refinements in operative technology (e.g., neuronavigation or intraoperative MRI) in pituitary surgery are not actually able to supply experienced hands in this field.[74]

REFERENCES

1. Black PM, Hsu DW, Klibanski A, et al: Hormone production in clinically nonfunctioning pituitary adenomas. I Neurosurg 66:244–250, 1987.
2. Jameson JL, Klibanski A, Black PM, et al: Glycoprotein hormone genes are expressed in clinically nonfunctioning pituitary adenomas. Clin Invest 80:1472–1478, 1987.
3. Ming-Tak D, Hsu E, Ting LT, et al: The clinicopathological characteristics of gonadotroph cell adenoma: A study of 118 cases. Hum Pathol 28:905–911, 1997.
4. Thapar K, Kowacs K, Laws ER, et al: Pituitary adenomas: Current concepts in classification, histopathology and molecular biology. Endocrinologist 3:39–56, 1993.
5. Chaidarun SS, Khibawski A: Gonadotropinomas. Semin Reprod Med 20:339–348, 2002.
6. Comtois R, Beauregard M, Somma M, et al: The clinical and endocrine outcome to transsphenoidal microsurgery of nonsecreting pituitary adenomas. Cancer 68:860–866, 1991.
7. Ebersold MI, Quast LM, Laws ER Jr, et al: Long-term results in transsphenoidal removal of nonfunctioning pituitary adenomas. J Neurosurg 64:713–719, 1986.
8. Arafah BM: Reversible hypopituitarism in patients with large nonfunctioning pituitary adenomas. J Clin Endocrinol Metab 62:1173–1179, 1986.
9. Marazuela M, Astiganaga B, Vicente A, et al: Recovery of visual and endocrine function following transsphenoidal surgery of large nonfunctioning pituitary adenomas. J Endocrinol Invest 17:703–707, 1994.
10. Chanson P, Petrossians P: Les Adenomes Hypophysaires Non Fonctionnels. Paris: John Libbey. Eurotext (Eds), pp 5–127, 1998.
11. Dyer H, Civit T, Visot A, et al: Transsphenoidal surgery for pituitary adenomas in children. Neurosurgery 34:207–212, 1994.
12. Minderman T, Wilson GB: Pediatric pituitary adenomas. Neurosurgery 36:259–269, 1995.
13. Abe T, Ludecke DK, Saeger W: Clinically nonsecreting pituitary adenomas in childhood and adolescence. Neurosurg 42(4):744–751, 1998.
14. Harris PE, Afshar F, Goates P, et al: The effects of transsphenoidal surgery on endocrine function and visual fields in patients with functionless pituitary tumors. QJM 71:417–427, 1989.
15. Molitch ME: Evaluation and treatment of the patient with a pituitary incidentaloma. J Clin Endocrinol Metab 80:3–6, 1995.
16. Greenman Y, Tordjman K, Kisch E, et al: Relative sparing of anterior pituitary function in patients with growth hormone secreting macroadenomas: Comparison with nonfunctioning macroadenomas. J Clin Endocrinol Metab 80:1577–1583, 1995.
17. Verhelst J, Berwaerts J, Abo R, et al: Obstructive hydrocephalus as complication of a giant nonfunctioning pituitary adenoma: Therapeutical approach. Acta Clin Belg 53(1):47–52, 1998.
18. Scotti G, Yu G-Y, Dillon WP, et al: MR imaging of cavernous sinus involvement by pituitary adenomas. Am J Roentgenol 151:799–806, 1988.
19. Yokayoma S, Hirano H, Monoki K, et al: Are nonfunctioning pituitary adenomas extending into the cavernous sinus aggressive and/or invasive? Neurosurg 49(4):857–863, 2001.
20. Boute D, Dewailly D, Fossati P: Adénomes gonadotropes. Ann Med Interne (Paris) 69:42–52, 1990.
21. Kwekkeboom DJ, Dejong FH, Lamberts SWJ: Gonadotropin release by clinically nonfunctioning and gonadotroph pituitary adenomas in vivo and vitro: Relation to sex and effects of thyrotropin releasing hormone, gonadotropin releasing hormone and bromocryptine. J Clin Endocrinol Metab 68:1128–1135, 1989.
22. Danesdoost L, Gennarelli TA, Bashey HM, et al: Identification of gonadotroph adenomas in men with clinically nonfunctioning adenomas by the luteinizing hormone beta subunit response to thyrotropin-releasing hormone. J Clin Endocrinol Metab 77:1352–1355, 1993.
23. Snyder PJ: Gonadotroph cell adenomas of the pituitary. Endocr Rev 6:552–563, 1985.
24. Oppenheim DS, Kana AR, Sanghar JS, et al: Prevalence of alpha subunit hypersecretion in patients with pituitary tumors: Clinically nonfunctioning and somatotroph adenomas. J Clin Endocrinol Metab 70:859–864, 1990.
25. Chanson P, Pantel I, Young D, et al: Free luteinizing hormone beta subunit in normal subjects and patients with pituitary adenomas. J Clin Endocrinol Metab 82:1397–1402, 1997.
26. Klibanski A, Deutsch PJ, Dameson JL, et al: Luteinizing hormone secreting pituitary tumor: Biosynthetic characterization and clinical studies. J Clin Endocrinol Metab 64:536–542, 1987.
27. Trouillas I, Girod C, Sassolas G, et al: The human gonadotropic adenoma: Pathologic and hormonal correlations in 26 tumors. Semin Diagn Pathol 3:42–57, 1986.
28. Sassolas G, Trouillas I, Treluyer C, et al: Management of nonfunctioning pituitary adenomas. Acta Endocrinol 129(Suppl l):21–26, 1993.
29. Wilson GB: Surgical management of pituitary tumors: Extensive personal experience. J Clin Endocrinol Metab 82:2381–2385, 1997.
30. Sekhar LN, Chen GN, Jho HD, et al: Surgical treatment of intracavernous neoplasm. Neurosurgery 24:18–30, 1989.
31. Almefty O, Smith RR: Surgery of tumors invading the cavernous sinus. Surg Neurol 30:370–381, 1988.
32. Guiot G, Derome PJ: Surgical problems of pituitary adenomas. Tech Stand Neurosurg 3:3–33, 1976.
33. Cushing H: Surgical experience with pituitary disorders. JAMA 63:1515–1525, 1914.
34. Kanavel AB: Removal of tumors of the pituitary body by an infranasal route. JAMA 53:1704, 1909.
35. Hirsch O: Endonasal method of removal of hypophyseal tumors with a report of two cases. JAMA 55:772, 1910.
36. Halstead AE: Remarks on the operative treatment of tumors of hypophysis: Two cases operated on by an oronasal route. Trans Am Surg Assoc 27:75, 1910.
37. Dott N, Bailey P: A consideration of the hypophyseal adenomata. Br I Surg 13:314–366, 1925.
38. Guiot G: Transsphenoidal approach in surgical treatment of pituitary adenoma: General principles and indications in nonfunctioning adenomas. International Congress Series, vol 303. Amsterdam: Excerpta Medica, pp 159–178, 1973.
39. Hardy J: Transsphenoidal surgery of the normal and pathological pituitary. Glin Neurosurg 16:185–217, 1969.
40. Laws ER Jr: Transsphenoidal approach to pituitary tumors. In Schmidek HH, Sweet WH (eds): Operative Neurosurgical Techniques, 3rd ed. Philadelphia: WB Saunders, pp 283–292, 1995.
41. Landolt AM: Surgical management of recurrent pituitary tumors. In Schmidek HH, Sweet WH (eds): Operative Neurosurgical Techniques, 3rd ed. Philadelphia: WB Saunders, pp 315–326, 1995.
42. Jane JA, Thapar K, Kaptain G, et al: Pituitary surgery: Transsphenoidal approach. Neurosurg 51:435–444, 2002.
43. Barrows DL, Tindall GT: Loss of vision after transsphenoidal surgery. Neurosurgery 27:60–68, 1990.
44. Decker RE, Chalif DJ: Progressive coma after the transsphenoidal decompression of a pituitary adenoma with marked suprasellar extension: Report of two cases. Neurosurgery 28:154–158, 1991.
45. Derome PJ, Visot A, Delalande O, et al: Mechanical complications after transsphenoidal removal of pituitary adenomas. In Derome PJ, Jedynak CP, Peillon F (eds): Pituitary Adenomas. Paris: Ascelpios, pp 233–235, 1980.

46. Spaziante R, de Devitiis E, Cappabianca P: Repair of the sella following transsphenoidal surgery. In Schmidek HH, Sweet WH (eds): Operative Neurosurgical Techniques, 3rd ed. Philadelphia: WB Saunders, pp 327–345, 1995.

47. Laws ER, Fode NC, Redmond MJ: Transsphenoidal surgery following unsuccessful prior therapy. J Neurosurg 63:823–829, 1985.

48. Nicola GC, Tonnarelli G, Griner AC, et al: Surgery for recurrence of pituitary adenomas. In Faglia G, Beck-Peccoz P, Ambroso B, et al (eds): Pituitary Adenomas: New Trends in Basic and Clinical Research. International Congress Series, vol 961. Amsterdam: Excerpts Medica, pp 329–336, 1991.

49. Olson DR, Guiot G, Derome P: The symptomatic empty sella: Prevention and correction via the transsphenoidal approach. J Neurosurg 37:533–537, 1972.

50. Rodriguez O, Mateos B, De La Predaja R: Postoperative follow up of pituitary adenomas after transsphenoidal resection: Mifi and clinical correlation. Neuroradiology 38:747–754, 1996.

51. Dinar TS, Feasier SH, Laws ER Jr, et al: MR of the pituitary gland postsurgery = serial MR studies following transsphenoidal resection. AJNR Am J Neuroradiol 14:763–769, 1993.

52. Bonneville JF, Bonneville F, Schillo F, et al: L'IRM après chirurgie transsphenoidale. J Neuroradiol 30:268–279, 2003.

53. Rodriguez O, Mateos B, De La Pedraja R, et al: Postoperative follow-up of pituitary adenomas after transsphenoidal resection: MRI and clinical correlation. Neuroradiology 38:747–754, 1996.

54. Bradley KM, Adams CBT, Potter CPS, et al: An audit of selected patients with nonfunctioning pituitary adenomas treated by transsphenoidal surgery without irradiation. Clin Endocrinol 41: 655–659, 1994.

55. Bates AS, Farrel WE, Bicknell EI, et al: Allelic deletion in pituitary adenomas reflects aggressive histological activity and has a potential value as a prognostic marker. J Clin Endocrinol Metab 82:818–824, 1997.

56. Tanaka Y, Hongo K, Tada T, et al: Growth pattern and rate in residual nonfunctioning pituitary adenomas: Correlation among tumor volume doubling time, patient age and MBI 1 index. J Neurosurg 98:359–365, 2003.

57. Losa M, Franzin A, Mangili F, et al: Proliferation index of nonfunctioning pituitary adenomas: Correlation with clinical characteristics and long-term follow-up results. Neurosurg 47(6):1313–1319, 2000.

58. Sheehan JP, Kondziolka D, Flickinger J, et al: Radiosurgery for residual or recurrent nonfunctioning pituitary adenomas. J Neurosurg 97(5):408–414, 2002.

59. Petrovitch Z, Chen YU, Gionotta SL, et al: Gamma knife radiosurgery for pituitary adenoma: Early results. Neurosurgery 53(1):51–61, 2003.

60. Tran LM, Blount L, Horton D: Radiation therapy in pituitary tumors: Results in 95 cases. Am J Clin Oncol 14:25–29, 1991.

61. Zangg M, Adaman O, Pescia R, et al: External irradiation of macroinvasive pituitary adenomas with telecobalt: A retrospective study with long-term follow-up in patients irradiated with doses mostly of between 40-45 Gy. Int J Radiat Oncol Biol Phys 32:671–680, 1995.

62. Snyder PJ, Fowble BF, Schatz NJ, et al: Hypopituitarism following radiation therapy of pituitary adenomas. Am J Med 81:457–462, 1986.

63. Shalet SM: Radiation therapy and pituitary dysfunction (Editorial). N Engl J Med 328:131–132, 1993.

64. Delattre JY, Poisson M: Complications neurologiques de la radiothéapie cérébrale: Apport des etudes expérimentales. Bull Cancer 77:715–724, 1990.

65. Creange A, Felten D, Kiesel I, et al: Leucoencephalopathie subaiguë du rhombocéphale après radiothérapie hypophysaire. Rev Neurol 150:704–708, 1994.

66. Al-Mefty O, Kerab JE, Routh A, et al: The long-term side effects of radiation therapy for benign tumors in adults. J Neurosurg 73: 502–512, 1990.

67. Tsang RW, Laperrière NJ, Simpson WJ, et al: Glioma arising after radiation therapy for pituitary adenoma: A report of four patients and estimation of risk. Cancer 72:2227–2233, 1993.

68. Brada M, Ford D, Ashley S, et al: Risk of second brain tumor after conservative surgery and radiotherapy for pituitary adenoma. BMJ 304:1343–1346, 1992.

69. Saito K, Kuwayama A, Yamamoto N, et al: The transsphenoidal removal of nonfunctioning pituitary adenomas with suprasellar extensions: The open sella method and intentionally staged operation. Neurosurgery 36:668–676, 1995.

70. Reincke M, Allolio B, Saeger W, et al: The incidentaloma of the pituitary gland: Is neurosurgery required? JAMA 263:2772–2776, 1990.

71. Donovan LE, Corenblum B: The natural history of the pituitary incidentaloma. Arch Intern Med 155: 181–183, 1995.

72. Kurosaki M, Ludecke DK, Flitsch J, et al: Surgical treatment of clinically nonsecreting pituitary adenomas in elderly patients. Neurosurgery 47(4):843–849, 2000.

73. De Herder WW, Reij AE, Kwekkeboom DJ, et al: In vivo imaging of pituitary tumors using a radiolabeled dopamine D2 receptor radiologland. Clin Endocrinol 45:755–767, 1996.

74. Bohinski RJ, Warwick RE, Gaskill Shiplay M: Intraoperative magnetic resonance imaging to determine the extent of resection of pituitary macroadenomas during transsphenoidal surgery. Neurosurgery 49(5):1333–1344, 2001.

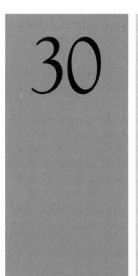

30 Surgical Management of Growth Hormone–Secreting and Prolactin-Secreting Pituitary Adenomas

MARK D. KRIEGER, WILLIAM T. COULDWELL, ARUN P. AMAR, JAMES K. LIU, and MARTIN H. WEISS

MANAGEMENT OF GROWTH HORMONE–SECRETING PITUITARY ADENOMAS

Somatotropes, or growth hormone (GH)–producing cells of the pituitary gland, make up approximately 50% of the normal adenohypophysial cell population; they are located in the lateral wings of the anterior lobe. GH is a 191-amino-acid polypeptide hormone that opposes the effect of insulin, stimulates the uptake of amino acids, and causes a release of free fatty acids from tissue storage sites. In the liver and other tissues, GH also mediates the synthesis of somatomedins (also called insulin-like growth factors), which induce protein synthesis in the skeleton and in muscle, and glucose oxidation in adipose tissue. Somatomedins also stimulate cell replication at these sites. The secretion of GH is stimulated by GH-releasing hormone (GHRH) and inhibited by somatostatin. GH and somatomedin-C (also known as insulin-like growth factor-1 [IGF-1]) stimulate the release of somatostatin, thereby downregulating the secretion of GH. GH is secreted in episodic surges occurring every 3 to 4 hours; in young people, the greatest peaks occur after the onset of deep sleep. Stimuli of GH secretion include insulin-induced hypoglycemia, arginine, exercise, L-dopa, clonidine, propranolol, and GHRH.

Acromegaly and gigantism are the result of oversecretion of GH into the somatic circulation. Collectively, they are second in frequency to hyperprolactinemia as pituitary hypersecretory syndromes. They are almost always caused by a somatotroph (i.e., GH-secreting) adenoma of the pituitary (>99% of cases), as opposed to somatotroph hyperplasia from excess secretion of ectopic GHRH.[1] Although most of these pituitary tumors exhibit a moderate growth rate, they often present relatively early in their growth because of the detection of a hypersecretory syndrome. In the authors' personal series, more than 70% were microadenomas on presentation[2]; however, they can present as macroadenomas with extrasellar extension and focal destruction.[3,4] (In other series, as many as 85% to 90% of patients present with macroadenomas and 10% to 15% present with microadenomas.[1]) Younger patients with acromegaly often harbor larger and more rapidly growing tumors.[5]

Acromegalic tumors may contain and also secrete prolactin (PRL) or the α-subunit (common to all the glycoprotein adenohypophysial hormones); and, rarely, thyroid-stimulating hormone (TSH) in addition to GH.[3] Most patients with large tumors have mixed GH and PRL hypersecretion,[6] which results in concomitant hyperprolactinemia in 20% to 40% of patients.[3,5] PRL is most often secreted from a tumor containing a mixed population of somatotroph and lactotroph cells (e.g., an acidophilic stem cell tumor), but it is occasionally secreted from a bipotential mammosomatotroph adenoma.[4] In patients harboring mammosomatotroph adenomas, the two hormones, by definition, are present within the same cell, or the same secretory granule, or both, and are usually secreted in a similar dynamic pattern.[5]

The total amount of GH secreted in a 24-hour period varies among patients harboring GH-secreting tumors and depends on cell activity, but it roughly correlates with the size of the tumor.[7] GH oversecretion results in elevated plasma IGF-1 levels[3] that are fairly stable and that reflect the integrated pulsatile 24-hour secretion of GH. As GH levels increase, IGF-1 rises linearly until GH reaches approximately 20 ng/mL, after which the IGF-1 level plateaus. As a corollary, to achieve any measure of successful treatment, GH must decrease to a level below 20 ng/mL for IGF-1 levels to drop or for clinical improvement to occur.[1] However, plasma GH levels and clinical manifestations of acromegaly are poorly correlated, presumably because of variable responsiveness of peripheral tissues to GH excess.[3]

Clinical Manifestations and Diagnosis

The clinical manifestations of excess secretion of GH depend on the age of the patient. If the excess secretion occurs in childhood or adolescence, before the epiphyses of long bones have fused, the result is gigantism: people with such a condition may attain great height if the disease progresses unchecked (often more than 7 feet). After fusion of the epiphyses, excess GH produces the syndrome of acromegaly in adults, with soft-tissue and bony enlargement in characteristic locations. Clinical manifestations of these soft-tissue changes include coarsening of facial features, laryngeal enlargement, goiter, thick heel pads, acanthosis nigricans, cardiomegaly, and hepatomegaly. Bony changes are extensive, producing prognathism (enlargement of the mandible with increased spacing between the teeth) and bony enlargements of hands and feet. Soft-tissue and bony changes may produce compressive neuropathies and arthropathies. Metabolic manifestations include associated hypertension; diabetes mellitus; goiter; and, commonly, hyperhidrosis. Deficiencies in corticotropin-releasing hormone and TSH are found in less than 20% of patients.[3] Hypogonadism occurs in 30% to 40% of patients, but it may be attributable to associated hyperprolactinemia[3] and may result in osteoporosis. Acromegaly affects men and women with approximately equal frequency.

The diagnosis is made by assessing GH secretion. A basal fasting GH level greater than 10 ng/mL is present in 90% of acromegalic patients; however, because GH is secreted in several peaks throughout the day, a single fasting level may fail to demonstrate an elevated level in some patients. Therefore, the suspected diagnosis is confirmed by the glucose suppression test. In the acromegalic person, an oral administration of 100 g of glucose fails to suppress the serum GH level to less than 5 ng/mL at 60 minutes. Serum IGF-1 levels are elevated in acromegalic patients, and their measurement proves to be a more reliable measure of the disease and its response to treatment. Radiographic imaging (magnetic resonance imaging [MRI], computed tomography [CT], or both) demonstrates the presence of a pituitary adenoma in greater than 90% of patients with endocrinologically documented acromegaly. High-field, thin-section MRI scans are the most sensitive imaging method for preoperative localization of pituitary adenomas. On unenhanced images, focal glandular hypodensity identified on coronal images is the most sensitive predictor of adenoma location. Radiographic evaluation should consist of coronal, sagittal, and axial MRI, with large tumors usually having signal intensity similar to that of brain on T1-weighted images. The normal pituitary gland, infundibulum, and cavernous sinuses enhance immediately after administration of gadolinium-diethylenetriamine-penta-acetic acid (DTPA), allowing contrast between the enhancing normal glandular tissue and the low-intensity adenomas. A T1-weighted image obtained after the infusion of gadolinium-DTPA is the method of choice for the delineation of intrasellar disease. Shortly after administration, the normal vascular pituitary increases in signal intensity, and a pituitary tumor is visible but remains less intense, being slower to perfuse with the contrast agent.

Indications for Therapy and Goals of Treatment

Excess secretion of GH should be considered a malignant endocrinopathy: it may result in life-threatening medical complications, and thus should be treated aggressively once diagnosed. Left untreated, the mortality rate is double that of healthy age-matched control subjects, from complications that include hypertension, cardiac disease, diabetes, pulmonary infections, and associated malignancies.[8–11] The goals of therapy in management of a GH-secreting pituitary adenoma include: (1) resolution of tumor mass effect; (2) restoration of normal GH physiology (i.e., absolute normalization of GH and somatomedin C [IGF-1] levels); and (3) replacement of any associated hormone deficiencies.

To date, there are no generally accepted criteria for assessment of cure of acromegaly.[9,12–14] Various biochemical tests have been proposed in the postoperative period, including basal GH level, mean GH levels, GH response to the oral glucose tolerance test, GH response to thyrotropin-releasing hormone, and IGF-1 (somatomedin C) levels. Each of these tests has been found limited in determining a cure. Many authors now believe that the criteria for successful therapy (i.e., chemical cure) include a 24-hour integrated GH concentration of no more than 2.5 ng/mL, together with normalization of the circulating IGF-1 level.[4,15]

In the authors' institution, normalization of the IGF-1 level is used as the ultimate determinant of successful therapy. We have found that, in 99% of cases, an early postoperative growth hormone level of 2 ng/mL or less correlates with long-term normalization of the IGF-1 level and thus long-term disease remission. However, higher levels of GH rarely indicate long-term chemical cure.[2]

Microadenomas

If the patient harboring a GH-secreting microadenoma is medically stable enough to undergo a surgical procedure, surgical resection should be considered the optimal first choice for management. Transsphenoidal microsurgical adenomectomy is currently the most accepted and efficient first-line therapy for the GH-secreting tumors of acromegaly.[9,16–27] Some authors indicate that the transnasal dissection in the acromegalic patient with associated soft-tissue and bony changes may present an added challenge for the surgeon. In the authors' experience, however, this has never been a limiting factor in the use of the transsphenoidal approach. Such tumors may be cured by chemical criteria in most cases. A large, combined analysis of 1360 acromegalic patients by Ross and Wilson[24] documented an overall postoperative cure rate of 60.4%. Microadenomas have an even higher rate of cure, exceeding 76% to 84% in large surgical series.[9,16,19–21,26–28] In the authors' series, 78% of patients with microadenomas undergoing transsphenoidal resection achieved normal long-term IGF-1 levels and were considered cured. This rate was determined using very stringent criteria for cure: a postoperative growth hormone level not greater than 2 ng/mL, a normal 5-year IGF-1, and clinical evidence of disease remission at 5 years.[2] Postoperative persistent elevation of GH or IGF-1 levels would be an indication for pharmacotherapy or radiation therapy (see the following).

Macroadenomas

The patient harboring a GH-secreting macroadenoma poses a more difficult management dilemma. Certainly, the likelihood of cure is low in cases of large tumors with frank cavernous sinus invasion; in the authors' series, only 31% of all patients with a macroadenoma achieved chemical cure by surgery alone.[2] Pharmacotherapy or radiation therapy should thus be considered as integral components in the overall management plan. In these cases, initial pharmacotherapy may be indicated; however, surgical resection may be helpful in decreasing the tumor load to effect an absolute normalization of IGF-1 levels by pharmacotherapy.

Pharmacotherapy

Pharmacotherapy should be considered in three groups of patients: (1) patients in whom surgery is contraindicated; (2) patients whose GH and IGF-1 levels are still elevated after surgery, as an alternative to radiation therapy at this stage; and (3) patients with elevated GH and IGF-1 levels after surgery and radiation therapy.[1] Medical therapy may be administered in conjunction with radiation therapy to provide interim GH suppression while awaiting the beneficial effects of the radiation.

Somatostatin Analogues

PHYSIOLOGY

Native somatostatin is believed to control GH secretion by suppression of GH release from the pituitary gland and GHRH release from the hypothalamus.[29] At present, only one Food and Drug Administration (FDA)–approved analogue, octreotide (Sandostatin; Sandoz, East Hanover, NJ; previously designated as SMS 201-995), is appropriate for clinical use.[30] Octreotide contains the active sequence of somatostatin, and it appears to control GH secretion similarly by suppression of GH release from the pituitary gland and by suppression of GHRH from the hypothalamus.[29] Compared with the native hormone, it has both an enhanced binding affinity to the somatostatin receptor and a prolonged half-life of 110 minutes after subcutaneous injection of a 50- to 100-μg dose, providing an overall duration of effect of 6 to 8 hours.[31] A single injection of octreotide produces a decrease in GH levels within 30 to 60 minutes, with maximum suppression of GH levels occurring in 2 to 4 hours.[32] Analogues are under investigation that have greater biologic potency than octreotide and that are more specific for the pituitary gland.[4]

TUMOR SOMATOSTATIN RECEPTOR STATUS

Large numbers of specific somatostatin-binding sites in human GH-secreting pituitary adenomas have been demonstrated.[33–35] The number of somatostatin receptors between tumors and their distribution within a particular tumor appear to be heterogeneous. Most tumors contain somatostatin receptors in densities that are comparable with those in normal somatotrophs,[35] and these respond normally to somatostatin.[36] However, 10% to 30% of GH-secreting tumors have reduced numbers of somatostatin receptors; patients with such tumors exhibit diminished in vivo responses to octreotide.[35]

DOSE AND MODE OF ADMINISTRATION

The usual initial dose of octreotide is 100 μg subcutaneously every 8 hours, and this dose should be increased until adequate suppression is achieved. In acromegalic patients treated with octreotide, a close correlation has been found between the mean 24-hour GH and IGF-1 levels before and during therapy.[37–40] Therefore, regular IGF-1 measurements on an outpatient basis enable optimization of the daily dose and number of octreotide injections needed for each individual patient.[38,39] Most patients achieve control with 300 to 600 μg/day.[32] In a national survey, doses of 750 μg/day resulted in increased frequency of tumor shrinkage without adding any biochemical or clinical benefit.[41] Over a 6-month period, the size of the pituitary tumor was reduced in 34% of patients receiving this latter dose, compared with only 17% of patients receiving 300 μg/day. The maximum recommended dose is 1500 μg/day.[4] As many as 50% of patients can be maintained on a twice-daily regimen,[42] but some patients may achieve better control by receiving the same daily dose every 6 hours instead.[4] In this regard, continuous subcutaneous pump infusion of 100 to 600 μg/day has been shown to provide superior and more stable suppression of mean 24-hour GH levels.[43]

EFFICACY

Seventy-five percent to 90% of acromegalic patients experience some biochemical, clinical, and metabolic improvement with octreotide therapy. Clinical improvement may be heralded by the disappearance or the amelioration of excessive sweating, headaches, paresthesia, soft-tissue swelling, and joint pain improvement of nerve entrapment symptoms, together with a general sense of well-being.[4,41] Immediate and prolonged relief of headaches is experienced in some patients with acromegaly, usually in those with evidence of suprasellar tumor extension.[44] Visual field improvement has been noted, in many cases without demonstrable change in tumor size (see the following).[4] In some patients, dose- and time-related symptoms indicative of drug dependency occur,[45] which may be mediated by the binding of octreotide to opioid receptors.[4]

Effective decreases of GH and IGF-1 levels occur in 30% to 53% and in 40% to 68% of patients, respectively, according to various studies.[4,31,32,41,46,47] In most patients, IGF-1 levels fall within 1 week of the start of treatment and tend to normalize in 37% to 81% of patients with continued therapy.[41,42,48–50] GH and IGF-1 levels have been shown to continue to decrease with long-term treatment of 1.5 to 2 years when compared with levels at 6 to 12 months.[51] Long-term responsiveness can be predicted by the acute GH suppression effect of a single test injection of 50 μg of octreotide. The mean hourly GH level from 2 to 6 hours after drug injection exhibits a high degree of correlation with the 24-hour integrated GH level after long-term (1- to 2-year) therapy.[52] The plasma IGF-1 and GH level responses 2 hours after drug injection, or at any time during subcutaneous infusion, are also useful predictors of efficacy.[4] Plasma PRL levels in patients with mixed GH/PRL-containing tumors have been shown to be suppressed by octreotide in approximately 50% of patients.[51] Elevated concentrations of the α-subunit, which can be found in approximately 35% of acromegalic patients,[53] respond to octreotide in a similar fashion to GH level.[32]

Preoperative treatment with octreotide causes the tumor to become soft and to exhibit a grayish red color at surgery.[54] Several neurosurgical groups have concluded that pretreatment with octreotide to soften the adenoma has facilitated surgical resection.[54,55] Long-term octreotide therapy produces a slight decrease in pituitary tumor size in approximately 20% to 50% of acromegalic patients.[37,38,41,56] Complete tumor shrinkage has been reported in isolated cases.[57] Tumor size may increase soon after the drug is stopped,[58] but in occasional patients, a period off the drug may subsequently permit comparable control to be achieved at a lower dose. This phenomenon is possibly explained by a reversal of somatostatin receptor downregulation.[4]

HISTOLOGIC CHANGES

Shrinkage of adenomas during octreotide therapy might reflect a decrease in the size of individual tumor cells.[32] Electron microscopy of adenomas pretreated with octreotide revealed small necrotic cells and a greater number of macrophages, whereas normal pituitary cells showed an accumulation of lipoprotein and secretory granules.[59] These morphologic findings were primarily consistent with chronic suppression of GH release.

SIDE EFFECTS

Although octreotide is usually well tolerated, several side effects have been reported. Within the first few days of administration, a transient decrease in gastrointestinal motility and slowed absorption occur in most patients. The patient may experience transient abdominal pains and bloating. Steatorrhea, presumably caused by a reduction in pancreatic exocrine secretion,[21] occurs less commonly but may persist with long-term therapy. Treatment using pancreatic enzymes, if necessary, is usually effective.[1]

Nutritional deficiency has not been reported. Toxic hepatitis has occurred very infrequently. Inhibition of insulin secretion can lead to hyperglycemia, although the concomitant improvement in glucose tolerance as a consequence of a decrease in GH secretion is usually sufficient to prevent this. Although somatostatin inhibits TSH secretion, hypothyroidism has not been reported during long-term octreotide therapy.[37,38,50] The side effect of greatest concern is cholelithiasis, which is caused by suppression of cholecystokinin secretion and a resulting decrease in bile flow. The incidence of gallstone formation in patients on long-term octreotide therapy is 40% to 50%[15,60]; thus all patients should be screened regularly for the development of gallstones during treatment.[42] No allergic problems related to octreotide have been reported, although antibodies to octreotide have been detected in one patient.[6] Tachyphylaxis and desensitization have not been observed during long-term treatment.[32] Although the injections are often painful, this may be minimized by slow injection of the drug.[1]

Dopaminergic Analogues

PHYSIOLOGY

Dopamine agonists stimulate GH secretion from normal subjects through a central nervous system–mediated mechanism that increases GHRH secretion,[61] and possibly also through the regulation of somatostatin secretion.[4] In contrast, in at least half of acromegalic patients, dopamine agonists suppress GH secretion[62] through a PRL-dependent D_2 receptor mechanism.[63] Dopamine agonists are primarily effective in GH-secreting tumors that also secrete PRL.[4] Unfortunately, many acromegalic tumors contain few or no D_2 receptors, which is reflected by a poor clinical response to these drugs.

DOSE AND MODE OF ADMINISTRATION

All available agents are members of the ergoline family of compounds. Both bromocriptine (Parlodel; Sandoz) and pergolide (Permax; Lilly, Indianapolis, IN) are available for use in the United States. Newer dopamine agonists do not seem to offer any major advantage over bromocriptine in these patients.[4] Bromocriptine is administered orally every 8 to 12 hours.[4] Up to 20 to 30 mg bromocriptine per day has been used to obtain maximum benefit, a dose that has been commonly associated with side effects.[1,4] To avoid the occurrence of side effects when initiating therapy, a low dose of 1.25 mg should be administered at bedtime. Gradual increases in increments of 1.25 mg should be made every 3 to 4 days until the desired effect is reached.[1] The medication should be taken with meals.[64]

EFFICACY

Amelioration of signs and symptoms of GH excess occurs in 70% of treated acromegalic patients, although GH levels are reduced to 10 ng/mL or less in only 50% and to 5 ng/mL or less in only 20% of these patients.[4] Only 8% of patients achieve normal IGF-1 levels, which is the only reliable parameter for assessing overall normality of pulsatile GH secretion.[1] Less favorable results are seen with larger tumors and if initial GH levels are above 50 ng/mL.[63] Tumor shrinkage is uncommon, occurring in only 10% to 15% of patients.[4,65]

The only known factor predicting responsiveness to dopaminergic agonists is coexistence of PRL hypersecretion. Even in such patients, it is not unusual to achieve total suppression of PRL secretion with only partial or no suppression of GH.[4] A single test dose of bromocriptine (2.5 mg orally) followed by hourly plasma GH levels for 4 to 6 hours may be used to assess therapeutic efficacy. Caution should be observed during this test because side effects may occur after the administration of this dose.

HISTOLOGIC CHANGES

At a morphologic level, bromocriptine produces almost no change in human GH-secreting adenomas, except for an increase in the stromal tissue volume with occasional occurrence of vacuolation and single-cell necrosis.[66]

SIDE EFFECTS

Significant side effects of bromocriptine include malaise, nausea, vomiting, and postural hypotension. Less commonly, headache, abdominal cramps, constipation, nasal congestion, and depression have been described. Hallucinations have been reported in 1.3% of patients[67]; and, rarely, cold-induced vasospasm, most pronounced in the digits, may occur.[1]

Combined Use of Bromocriptine and Octreotide

Few patients who do not respond to either octreotide or bromocriptine alone respond to the combination of octreotide and bromocriptine.[32,51,68,69]

Radiation Therapy

With the advent of a pharmacotherapeutic agent effective in a large percentage of these tumors, it is hoped that the need for radiation therapy in these patients will diminish. At the authors' institution, radiation therapy is considered only for those patients in whom chemical cure through surgery has not been achieved and in those whom medical therapy is contraindicated, not tolerated, or demonstrated to be ineffective.

Radiation therapy has been advocated for the management of pituitary tumors since 1907.[70] Radiation therapy per se, however, should not be considered a completely benign therapy or an equivalent alternative to microsurgical resection.[71] Adverse effects from radiation in this region may range from mild to severe. Radiation carries a significant risk of worsening of preexisting hypopituitarism, with an overt 10% to 15% frequency of panhypopituitarism.[72] Radiation also may increase the rate of atherogenesis in the major vessels in the field, and may cause visual impairment.[71] These complications increase as a function of total treatment dose.[73] The visual impairment may result from one of several mechanisms that include empty sella syndrome, treatment failure, and direct radiation damage to optic pathways. The latter complication is seen with significant frequency with daily fractionation of greater than 220 cGy.[73] Other minor complications from radiation therapy include epilation, scalp swelling, and otitis.[74]

Should radiation therapy be indicated in an acromegalic patient, a dose of 4000 cGy by external beam is considered optimal by most radiation therapists.[73,75] In a reported series of 12 patients treated with radiation therapy alone, Chun and colleagues[71] described a 50% recurrence rate, with a 75% incidence of local control after salvage treatment. Other authors report a local control rate of 50% to 79%, with an adequate salvage in cases of recurrence.[76,77] The rationale for the use of postoperative radiation therapy is to reduce the incidence of recurrence, with several studies suggesting improved tumor control with the combination of surgery plus radiation.[71,72,78,79] This is especially true in large and invasive lesions, which exhibit an increased rate of recurrence. This treatment, however, by no means ensures recurrence-free survival, but the time to recurrence may be prolonged. Valtonen and Myllymaki[80] have reported a surprisingly high 36% recurrence rate in patients with so-called "total removal" after transfrontal craniotomy and postoperative radiation therapy, with recurrences up to 18 years after therapy. Thus published recurrence rates may be misleading in series with short follow-up times.

The development of focal radiation therapy techniques (i.e., stereotactic radiosurgery) offers a potentially improved method of delivering accurate, lethal dosages of radiation to the tumor while limiting toxicity to the surrounding visual and neural structures. Clinical trials are under way.

Follow-up

As noted earlier, most patients with microadenomas experience postoperative amelioration of their endocrinopathy. Overall, 78% of patients with microadenomas and 64% of all patients (microadenomas and macroadenomas) in the authors' personal series attained normal postoperative IGF-1 levels.[2]

Although the surgical experience with microadenomas has been satisfying, cure with restoration of intact pituitary function is rarely achieved with large macroadenomas.[63] In the authors' series, only 31% of patients with macroadenomas achieved a chemical cure from surgery alone.[2] Even when normal postoperative GH levels are achieved, normal pulsatile secretion of GH and glucose suppression often are not restored.[4] Clinically, the physical manifestations of acromegaly are rarely reversed; however, there appears to be little progression of the clinical manifestations of disease when GH levels are below 5 ng/mL.

All acromegalic patients, regardless of initial tumor size, must be followed assiduously for recurrence of their endocrinopathy after surgery. This vigilance is mandated by the increased morbidity and mortality associated with persistent disease. Physical examination for progression of acromegaly and for the development of hypopituitarism is indicated. Whereas GH levels less than 5 ng/mL are not usually associated with persistent clinical disease, levels greater than 2 ng/mL indicate a risk for recrudescent disease and must be monitored closely. After an initial postoperative IGF-1 level obtained at 6 weeks, follow-up measurements of GH or IGF-1 should be performed every 6 months.[3] If octreotide is administered after irradiation, it is withdrawn for 2 weeks every 1 to 2 years, and GH and IGF-1 levels are measured. If they are normal, the drug should be discontinued.[1]

MANAGEMENT OF PROLACTIN-SECRETING PITUITARY ADENOMAS

The mammotropes, also called lactotropes, secrete PRL in the normal pituitary and represent 15% to 25% of the adenohypophysial cells. They are located in the lateral gland, and they accumulate during pregnancy and lactation and after estrogen therapy. PRL is a 198–amino acid polypeptide known to facilitate the development of breast tissue to ensure the production of milk. PRL secretion is stimulated by thyrotropin-releasing hormone, estrogens, stress, and exercise. Dopamine is acknowledged to be the principal PRL-inhibitory factor.

Prolactin-secreting adenomas are the most common type of secretory pituitary tumor and are second in frequency only to null-cell adenomas in overall incidence.[64] In the pediatric population, however, they represent the most common type of adenoma overall.[81]

Clinical Manifestations and Diagnosis

Although these tumors are found pathologically at autopsy with equal frequency in men and women, they are clinically significantly more common in women. They are also more common in girls than in boys.[81] A recent meta-analysis of the literature regarding the prevalence of pituitary adenomas indicates that approximately 17% of patients harbor a microadenoma based on a combination of imaging (MRI) and histological evaluation; one third of these stain positive for prolactin, which indicates the potential for secretion in a large number of incidental adenomas and therefore a gross underdiagnosis of the prolactinomas (W.T.C., unpublished observations). Hyperprolactinemia causes galactorrhea (in women) and hypogonadism, which are exhibited as anovulatory infertility in females and impotence in males.[82,83] Presumed abnormalities in pulsatile secretion of GHRH and gonadotropins precipitate a relative estrogen deficiency.[84,85] This hypogonadal state is associated with osteoporosis in women[86] and with both cortical and trabecular osteopenia in men.[87]

In a series of some 392 PRL-secreting pituitary tumors operated on by one author (M.H.W.), 321 (82%) were in female patients. The most common presenting symptom in this group was the development of secondary amenorrhea (72%); only approximately 50% of those with amenorrhea had associated galactorrhea.[88] Epidemiologically, approximately 5% of women with primary amenorrhea and 25% of women with secondary amenorrhea (other than those who are pregnant) harbor a PRL-secreting pituitary tumor as the cause of their clinical symptoms. Because of this readily identifiable symptom, female patients usually present relatively early in the course of evolution of the tumors; this is unfortunately not true in the male population. Because the primary symptom of a PRL-secreting tumor in the male patient is usually a decrease in libido well before true impotence is observed, this problem is often ascribed to the aging process or functional causes. Approximately two thirds of men with hyperprolactinemia caused by a PRL-secreting tumor have a low serum testosterone level[89]; this condition may be secondary to hyperprolactinemia per se or to mechanical compression of adjacent normal pituitary gland. Thus men often present at a more advanced age and later in the course of their disease with chiasmal compression and visual compromise. In our series, visual loss ranging in duration from 2 to 24 months was the initial complaint in 60% of men but in only 10% of women.[88] For the same reasons, large tumors associated with hypothyroidism and adrenal insufficiency are more common in men.[89] In the pediatric population, boys tend to have much larger tumors and higher preoperative PRL levels than do girls, and they commonly present with focal neurologic deficit or other signs of significant mass effect.[81]

The diagnosis is secured by radiographic evidence of a pituitary lesion with an elevation of serum PRL. As with GH-secreting tumors, high-field, thin-section MRI is the most sensitive imaging method for preoperative localization of pituitary adenomas. A rough correlation exists between the size of the lesion radiographically and pathologically and the serum level of PRL. In addition, local invasion of the tumor into the adjacent venous cavernous sinuses is associated with a marked increase in serum PRL. The diagnosis of pathologic PRL excess should be based on serial blood measurements[63]; PRL levels greater than five times the upper limit of normal are usually associated with a PRL-secreting pituitary tumor.[90] In the endocrinologic evaluation of the patient suspected of harboring a PRL-secreting tumor, it must be appreciated that larger tumors of any endocrine basis may cause a mild-to-moderate hyperprolactinemia resulting from the so-called stalk section effect (i.e., disconnection hyperprolactinemia stalk compression causing loss of dopaminergic inhibition to tonic PRL release),[91] which must be distinguished from a true prolactinoma. Under such circumstances, it is rare to see PRL levels in excess of 100 ng/mL. However, the authors encountered a patient with a preoperative prolactin level above 600 ng/mL confirmed by serial laboratory testing; this was attributed to stalk section effect on the basis of immunohistochemical analysis of the tumor, which failed to stain for prolactin.[92]

In general, large tumors (>2 cm in diameter) associated with PRL levels less than 150 ng/mL (certainly those <100 ng/mL) should be suspected of being nonsecretors when planning management strategies. Such nonsecretors would not be expected to respond to chemical reductions of serum PRL. However, one should be aware of falsely low serum prolactin levels (25 to 150 ng/mL) in the face of giant and invasive prolactinomas (>3 cm), also known as the high-dose "hook effect."[93,94] The hook effect occurs when radioimmunoassays are performed using the two-site

(monoclonal "sandwich") technique. At extremely high levels of serum prolactin, as in the case of giant and invasive prolactinomas, the binding sites of the primary (capture) antibody and secondary (signal) antibody become saturated and the true prolactin level is not accurately measured. The antibody-binding curve is no longer proportional to the amount of serum prolactin, and the measured prolactin declines or hooks downward. This may be resolved by performing serial dilutions of the serum samples in order to overcome the hook effect.

Several reports suggest that neither tumor size nor PRL levels change over a number of years in most women with microprolactinomas.[95,96] In fact, it has been observed that few microprolactinomas progress to macroadenomas.[90] In one of the authors' earlier series, for example, only 3 of 27 women harboring microadenomas demonstrated significant tumor growth over a 6-year interval of observation.[97] In contrast, macroadenomas, which for reasons described earlier often occur in men, may behave in an aggressive manner.[63] They may be associated with invasion of the cavernous sinuses and diffuse invasion of the base of the skull, and they commonly extend to the suprasellar region.[98] Hemorrhage or cyst formation within the tumor may also occur.

The levels of elevated PRL in a diagnosed pituitary adenoma are of great help in determining subsequent management because the ability to successfully extirpate the tumor is reduced with large or invasive lesions (see the following).

Indications for Therapy and Goals of Treatment

Bromocriptine or cabergoline are the first-choice drugs for therapy of PRL-secreting tumors. The efficacy of bromocriptine or cabergoline (dopaminergic agonists) in reducing serum PRL, in addition to reducing tumor size and inhibiting further tumor growth, is well established (see the following). The central considerations related to treating such patients are the ability of the patient to tolerate the medication and the implications for fertility.

With PRL-secreting microadenomas, therapeutic options include medical or surgical management. In the authors' series, 225 of 262 patients (86%) who underwent surgery for tumors less than 1 cm in size had normal (<20 ng/mL) postoperative PRL levels (i.e., chemical cure).[88] The operative mortality rate was zero, and associated morbidity was low. The experience of other centers corroborates this high rate of surgical success.[99–105] Strong consideration should thus be given to surgical intervention in patients harboring smaller tumors without significant hyperprolactinemia.

In patients with larger tumors, however, surgical chemical cures (i.e., postoperative serum PRL <20 ng/mL) are much less common. Those tumors associated with PRL levels greater than 200 ng/mL recur in over 50% of patients after surgery alone[83]; the rate of recurrence of hyperprolactinemia after surgery for macroadenomas (with PRL levels >250 ng/mL) exceeds 70%.[83,106] In the authors' series, only 63 of 130 (49%) of those patients with tumors greater than 1 cm had chemical cure. Although no medical therapy results in cure of a PRL-secreting macroadenoma, only a minority of these patients remain free of their disease after surgery alone. Therefore, medical therapy with bromocriptine or cabergoline should be considered as primary therapy for those patients in whom surgical resection resulting in chemical cure is deemed unlikely.[107]

It is the authors' practice to place all patients who have large or invasive pituitary tumors with endocrinologically documented PRL secretion on a therapeutic trial of dopamine agonist therapy, and then to monitor clinical status and the lesion's radiographic appearance accordingly. All solid primary PRL-secreting tumors should respond to the medication, both by a reduction in tumor size and by a reduction in PRL level. One exception to this management is larger primary cystic tumors, which are less likely to respond with a diminution of size to pharmacotherapy.

The three goals of treatment include: (1) reduction of the tumor mass, (2) correction of the hyperprolactinemic state, and (3) preservation of anterior pituitary function.[83] The tenet of therapy should be absolute normalization of PRL levels, because a prolonged hyperprolactinemic state may be associated with significant osteoporosis and infertility. Surgical resection of these lesions is indicated in patients who are intolerant of the side effects of the medication, who are unable to afford the cost of the medication for a prolonged period, or those in whom sustained tumor reduction is not effected. Furthermore, the FDA recommends discontinuing the medication as soon as pregnancy has been established because of concerns about its safety to the mother and fetus.[108] As will be discussed, expansion of the tumor and compression of the optic structures has been reported in patients while off bromocriptine during gestation.[108] Thus the desire for fertility constitutes another indication for surgical resection, and in the authors' experience, 72 of 96 women (75%) who wanted to achieve pregnancy did so after transsphenoidal surgery.[88] Collectively, these reasons necessitate surgery in approximately 20% to 25% of patients with microadenomas, whereas the remaining patients can be successfully treated with bromocriptine alone.[101,102,109] Among patients with macroadenomas, however, Wilson[105] and others recommend operative removal in most cases.

Subsequent to surgery, if hyperprolactinemia is persistent to some extent, the patient may be able to tolerate greatly reduced doses of dopamine analogues to effect long-term control, or the use of postoperative radiation therapy should be considered to bring the residual tumor under control. In the authors' series, all patients who had endocrinologic recurrence (i.e., relapse of hyperprolactinemia after initial hormonal normalization) or immediate endocrinologic failure (i.e., serum prolactin levels >20 ng/mL on the morning after surgery) were able to resume bromocriptine at much lower doses than they had taken before surgery. All of them tolerated this reduced dose, and although the serum prolactin level was not always restored to normal, no patient has required postoperative radiation therapy.[88]

After radiation therapy for prolactinomas, PRL levels fall slowly over many years, but they rarely reach the normal level[83]; thus these patients may benefit from adjuvant medical therapy.

Pharmacotherapy with Dopaminergic Analogues

Physiology

Bromocriptine is a dopamine agonist that suppresses PRL production and release by the stimulation of dopamine receptors. This orally active dopamine agonist is a semisynthetic ergot alkaloid that was specifically developed as an inhibitor of PRL secretion. Bromocriptine directly stimulates neuronal and pituitary cell membrane dopamine receptors.[110] A single dose of 2.5 mg results in suppression of serum PRL for up to 14 hours.[111] The biologic effect, however, may persist for more than 24 hours in some patients.[64]

The FDA has approved the use of cabergoline (Dostinex), a synthetic ergoline derivative with high specificity and affinity for the D_2 dopaminergic receptor.[112–116] With effects persisting up to 120 days after administration,[117] this long-lasting and potent agonist is typically dosed once or twice a week, thus leading to improved compliance when compared with bromocriptine, which often must be taken up to three times a day. Furthermore, in other comparative studies, cabergoline has been shown to be more effective than bromocriptine in both normalizing serum prolactin and in restoring gonadal function.[114,116] Cabergoline is also better tolerated than other ergot derivatives[114] and may demonstrate efficacy in patients who are refractory to bromocriptine.[116] However, the teratogenic potential of cabergoline has not been extensively investigated.[114] Consequently, the drug is generally not considered first-line therapy for the treatment of infertility associated with hyperprolactinemia, and its current application may be limited to patients who have failed treatment with, or are intolerant of, bromocriptine.[114]

Several other dopamine agonists, including two ergot derivatives (pergolide mesylate and lisuride) and one quinolone (quinagolide), have been shown to suppress serum prolactin and reduce tumor size but have not been approved by the FDA for the treatment of prolactinomas.[2,115,118–127]

Dose and Mode of Bromocriptine Administration

Bromocriptine has proven safe and effective in 27 years of widespread use in the treatment of prolactinomas since its approval in 1978.[64] Initiation of bromocriptine therapy is as described in the previous section for use in GH/PRL-secreting adenomas. Bromocriptine is usually given in a dose of 2.5 mg three times daily. In some patients with large tumors, in whom the tumor size does not decrease or the PRL level is not suppressed by more than 80% of pretreatment levels with the aforementioned dose, much larger doses are required, up to 15 to 20 mg/day.[64,83] However, in certain cases, the dose may be decreased after achievement of adequate suppression.[64] Other authors have reported that if reduction in tumor size has not occurred within a 3-month period after starting bromocriptine, it is unlikely that it will occur and medical therapy should be abandoned.[83] It has been the authors' observation that patients who do not respond by 6 weeks are unlikely to respond by 3 months, so our current practice is to obtain an MRI scan 6 weeks after initiating medical therapy to document tumor reduction.

In the bromocriptine-treated patient who responds to medication but fails to normalize his or her serum PRL levels, and who does not achieve restoration of gonadal function, a combined surgical and medical approach should be considered. After the surgical procedure, hyperprolactinemia is often more responsive to medical therapy, requiring lower doses for control of PRL.[83] As mentioned earlier, reduced doses of bromocriptine have been effective in controlling the authors' patients who were not surgically cured, and adjuvant radiation has not been necessary.[88]

Dopamine agonist therapy must be given chronically. In most patients, withdrawal of the drug results in a return of hyperprolactinemia and reexpansion of the tumor.[128,129] Occasionally, patients with a microadenoma or an unidentifiable tumor do not experience a recurrence after discontinuation of therapy.[64] In a patient with a microadenoma, bromocriptine can be discontinued every 2 years on a trial basis to determine the need for continued therapy.[69]

EFFICACY

After adequate bromocriptine therapy, the PRL levels are usually either lowered by more than 80% or are normalized.[83] The PRL-reducing response to therapy in patients with microadenomas and with macroadenomas is similar with the exception that in the latter group, the time required for effective lowering of PRL is usually longer.[64] In addition, in over 80% of patients, bromocriptine and other dopamine agonists are effective in reversing visual abnormalities and in restoring gonadal and anterior pituitary functions.[83,90] Most female patients begin menstruation within 6 months of initiating therapy. The restoration of fertility in women with bromocriptine has been well documented.[130] However, as stated previously, the continuation of bromocriptine during pregnancy is contraindicated, and patients who wish to become pregnant should undergo surgery.[108]

In addition to reducing PRL secretion, bromocriptine is effective at decreasing tumor size.[131–133] The reduction of the tumor may occur very rapidly (i.e., within days of initiation of therapy) and results in dramatic decompression of the optic chiasm and resolution of headaches and other signs and symptoms of raised intracranial pressure.[83] Some tumors are very responsive to bromocriptine and shrink by more than 80% within 6 weeks of initiation of therapy.[83] Although most patients have a satisfactory biochemical and clinical response to medical therapy, there have been isolated case reports of a lack of response or of progression of disease during bromocriptine therapy.[134–136] Therefore, close monitoring of serum prolactin levels and serial MRI is mandatory. In women, once hyperprolactinemia has been corrected and the menstrual cycle normalized, fertility is usually reestablished and the pregnancy rates are the same as those of normal women in the same age group.[137,138] Although it is tempting intuitively to suggest that pretreatment with bromocriptine may shrink the tumor and facilitate surgical resection, no study has yet reported higher surgical cure rates after such preoperative treatment with bromocriptine.[139,140] Conversely, as discussed later, some surgeons believe that bromocriptine produces adverse effects on the consistency of the adenoma that impede tumor resection,[131] although this has not been the authors' experience.[133]

HISTOLOGIC CHANGES

Bromocriptine therapy of human prolactinomas for a period of 2 weeks has been shown to induce cell shrinkage and degenerative, necrotic, and fibrotic changes in the tumor; the secretory granules within a cell increase in number but not in volume.[66] Others have demonstrated that the cytoplasmic and nuclear volumes are reduced. In the cytoplasm, the amount of rough endoplasmic reticulum and size of the

Golgi apparatus are greatly reduced, and the cell changes from appearing highly active to quiescent. These changes are reversed after bromocriptine withdrawal.[83]

Cabergoline and Other Dopamine Agonists

Cabergoline is a long-lasting, ergot-derivative, selective dopamine D_2-receptor agonist that has been used effectively in the treatment of microprolactinomas and macroprolactinomas.[141–149] Although cabergoline is more expensive than bromocriptine, cabergoline is associated with less common and less severe side effects. Cabergoline appears to be superior to bromocriptine in normalizing prolactin levels, restoring gonadal function, and decreasing the size of the tumor.[143,150,151] It is very useful in patients who become resistant to or who cannot tolerate the adverse effects of bromocriptine. This favorable profile enables escalation of doses to achieve normal serum PRL levels in approximately 85% of patients with microadenomas and, more importantly, in a proportion of bromocriptine-resistant patients.[152] A recent crossover study comparing cabergoline and quinagolide showed similar efficacy of better than 90% biochemical control rates with a slightly better cost effectiveness with cabergoline.[151]

Cabergoline may be administered at doses of 0.5 to 1.5 mg once or twice a week. Because the drug dosing is less frequent and the drug is more tolerable, patient compliance may be higher with cabergoline than with bromocriptine. In a large double-blinded study, cabergoline produced 83% biochemical normalization as compared with 59% in the bromocriptine group.[116]

An important recent study has indicated that the majority of patients who respond to cabergoline with normalization of prolactin levels and reduction in tumor size may manifest remission of hyperprolactinemia following discontinuation of the drug.[141] This indicates a potential for curative treatment of many prolactinomas with this agent (see the following).

Medical Management and Pregnancy

Pregnant women with microprolactinomas rarely experience complications related to tumor expansion, with the reported risk being less than 0.5% to 1%.[64,83] However, in pregnant women with macroprolactinomas, the situation is different: the risk for development of symptoms related to tumor enlargement (e.g., headache, visual field disturbances, and ophthalmoplegia) is approximately 15%, and that for development of asymptomatic tumor enlargement is 9%.[153] These complications appear to occur with equal frequency during all trimesters.[137] Therefore, measures to reduce tumor size such as surgery and radiation are recommended before conception in female patients with macroadenomas who desire to become pregnant. In the event that the tumor enlarges during pregnancy, bromocriptine has been shown to be safe and effective.[154–156] Its administration during pregnancy has not increased the risk of congenital anomalies, spontaneous abortion, or multiple births.[157,158] Motor and psychological development of children born to women treated with bromocriptine during pregnancy were normal.[157]

If pregnancy is a desired goal of the patient with a prolactinoma, bromocriptine should be used whenever possible because of its safety record in pregnancy.[159,160] Although some reports state that cabergoline does not increase the risk of teratogenesis, the experience is limited.[161,162] Cabergoline should not be used as a primary therapy for infertility until there is more evidence supporting its safety during pregnancy. Following dopamine agonist therapy, the subsequent pregnancy rates are the same as those of normal women in the same age group.[137,138] Women should be advised to use a mechanical form of contraception until their menstrual cycle is restored. Normal conception and pregnancy may then follow. Once a menstrual cycle has been missed, bromocriptine should be discontinued immediately.[163] Using bromocriptine in this manner has not been associated with an increased incidence of spontaneous abortion, ectopic pregnancy, or congenital malformation.[153]

Elevation of estrogen levels during pregnancy stimulates pituitary lactotroph DNA synthesis and mitosis, resulting in tumor enlargement.[164,165] These changes are usually transient and resolve after delivery. Nevertheless, the patient should be monitored closely for signs and symptoms of tumor expansion. Formal visual-field testing and serial MR imaging are usually not necessary unless the patient becomes symptomatic. If the tumor becomes symptomatic, these patients may experience visual loss and symptoms of increased intracranial pressure. Women with macroadenomas with suprasellar extension may be offered surgical debulking before conception.[88,166] Patients with asymptomatic macroadenomas should undergo close monitoring with visual field testing once every 3 months. A MRI should be repeated if symptoms of tumor enlargement develop. If the patient develops symptomatic tumor enlargement, bromocriptine therapy can be initiated during pregnancy.[154–156,167] There does not appear to be an increased risk of congenital anomalies or of spontaneous abortions with use of bromocriptine during pregnancy. Alternatively, surgical decompression may also be an option.

If a patient plans to become pregnant while on bromocriptine therapy, a coordinated schedule of follow-up must be observed by the patient, endocrinologist, and neurosurgeon.

Withdrawal of Dopamine Agonist Therapy

After the prolactin level normalizes for a period of at least 2 years, and the size of the tumor has significantly decreased by at least 50% without evidence of optic chiasmal compression, the dopamine agonist can be tapered to lower doses that continue to control hyperprolactinemia and tumor growth. If there is no evidence of cavernous sinus invasion, a trial of cessation may be instituted as long as the patient receives close monitoring for tumor enlargement with serial MR imaging.

The overall success of sustained normoprolactinemia after cessation of bromocriptine has been variable (7% to 38%).[129,168–174] Normoprolactinemia was sustained after cessation of bromocriptine in about 25% of women who were treated for at least 2 years,[170,175] though cessation of bromocriptine in patients with macroprolactinomas usually leads to tumor expansion and recurrence of hyperprolactinemia.[169,176] Tumor enlargement has been noted in about 10% of patients and probably relates to the duration of treatment prior to withdrawal.[168,172] Cessation of bromocriptine within 1 year of treatment appears to have a higher risk of tumor enlargement than does cessation in those who have had longer treatments.[128,176,177] Patients who have

recurrent hyperprolactinemia after cessation of bromocriptine therapy may anticipate tumor recurrence, although the increase in size may be very slow.[168]

Some evidence indicates that cabergoline may have potential for definitive control of hyperprolactinemia and tumor growth. Colao and colleagues[141] reported sustained normalization of serum prolactin levels after withdrawal of cabergoline in 69% of patients with microprolactinomas and 64% of patients with macroprolactinomas without evidence of new tumor growth. The rate of recurrence at 5 years was higher among patients with macroprolactinomas and among those without radiographic evidence of residual tumor. Although there was no evidence of tumor recurrence in the face of recurrent hyperprolactinemia, the follow-up was relatively short and insufficient to determine the true rate of tumor control.

Side Effects and Complications

Commonly occurring side effects of bromocriptine therapy were discussed previously in the section on the GH-secreting pituitary tumor. A rare complication in patients with large prolactinomas is the development of a cerebrospinal fluid leak (caused by shrinkage of the tumor) during treatment.[69] In women, galactorrhea may persist even though the PRL level is lowered to the normal range.[178] It has been reported that if bromocriptine is given for more than 3 months, the tumor may become fibrous in consistency, which may cause difficulty with surgical resection[131]; this has not been the authors' personal experience.[133]

Occasionally, patients who initially respond to bromocriptine with a reduction in tumor size and normalization of serum PRL may subsequently experience recrudescence of the tumor as medical therapy is continued.[134,179,180] In some cases, patient compliance may be responsible, whereas in others, the tumor may undergo a process of dedifferentiation whereby it becomes refractory to dopamine agonist action, as evidenced by the in vitro resistance of cultured lactotrophs to high concentrations of bromocriptine.[134]

Similarly, a discrepancy in the clinical response as judged by tumor size and circulating PRL levels may develop during the course of treatment. Despite marked reduction in serum PRL throughout the duration of bromocriptine therapy, for instance, some patients may experience continued tumor expansion and progressive symptoms from mass effect.[135,181] Conversely, others may simulate the development of bromocriptine resistance, with steady elevations in serum PRL levels after an initial suppression despite serial imaging studies that show continual regression in tumor size.[182] Reports of acquired bromocriptine resistance or dissociation between tumor growth and serum PRL measurements are rare, however, and the true incidence of these phenomena is not known.

Pituitary Apoplexy in Prolactinomas: Medical or Surgical Therapy?

Although most surgeons recommend emergent transsphenoidal decompression and administration of glucocorticoids for patients who present with pituitary apoplexy,[183–188] some have reported excellent results with dopamine agonist therapy in patients with pituitary apoplexy in prolactinomas.[187,189] Brisman and colleagues[189] reported a patient with a macroprolactinoma who presented with pituitary apoplexy and a third nerve palsy who was treated with bromocriptine and glucocorticoids. The third nerve palsy completely resolved within 48 hours. The authors have also successfully managed a patient with bromocriptine who presented with severe headache and right ophthalmoplegia secondary to nonhemorrhagic pituitary apoplexy in a macroprolactinoma.[187] Although the optimal treatment for pituitary apoplexy in prolactinomas remains controversial, the authors recommend an initial trial of dopamine agonist therapy in conjunction with glucocorticoids for patients who have no or minimal visual loss. If patients present with visual loss, or if visual loss progresses despite dopamine agonist therapy, emergency transsphenoidal decompression is indicated.

Surgery for Prolactinomas

The efficacy of pharmacologic therapy has limited the indications of surgical resection of prolactinomas. Surgery is rarely curative in patients with macroprolactinomas, and it therefore is usually reserved for patients who cannot tolerate medical therapy or for whom medical therapy is ineffective.[88,190–192] Because sustained normoprolactinemia following cessation of medical therapy has not been demonstrated in all cases, curative surgery of microprolactinomas may offer an alternative to patients who do not wish to be on long-term medical therapy.[193–196] Surgery may be indicated in patients who are dependent on antipsychotic medications because dopamine agonists can precipitate psychotic episodes.[197] In patients who have persistent hyperprolactinemia, progressive tumor enlargement, or persistent tumor mass effect despite maximal medical therapy, surgery may be indicated. Surgical resection should be considered if restoration of visual function or cranial nerve palsies is not immediately responsive to medical treatment, especially in cases of pituitary apoplexy (as previously mentioned). Even if surgery is not curative, as is the case of most macroprolactinomas (<50% cure rate),[88,191] tumor cytoreduction often increases the responsiveness of dopamine agonists and thereby lowers the dosage.[64,198] Multimodal therapy with surgical debulking and subsequent adjuvant therapy (e.g., stereotactic radiosurgery or medical therapy) may be an effective strategy, especially if there is evidence of cavernous sinus invasion. Although some have reported that prior long-term treatment with dopamine agonists alters tumor consistency and hinders the resection,[131] the authors have not found this to be the case. In cases of giant and invasive prolactinomas, pretreatment with dopamine agonists may improve the safety and success of subsequent surgery.[133]

The transsphenoidal approach is the initial preferred surgical route and is associated with low rates morbidity and mortality.[199–202] The extended transsphenoidal approach may be used in some patients in whom the tumor is located beyond the confines of the sella.[203–206] Even in giant prolactinomas, a transsphenoidal approach should first be considered; however, a pterional approach should be considered if there is extensive tumor extension lateral into the Sylvian fissure.[190,206]

Surgery for Microprolactinomas

In patients with hyperprolactinemia because of a microprolactinoma, transsphenoidal surgery by an experienced pituitary surgeon should be considered a potentially curative procedure.[88,193,196] The realization that medical therapy may require lifelong treatment in some cases (a particularly significant factor in young patients), and consideration of the very low morbidity and mortality rates associated with contemporary transsphenoidal resection in experienced hands, should both factor into the decision-making process. Sustained normoprolactinemia following cessation of medical therapy has been variable. The costs and burden of potentially long-term medical treatment in a young patient with a long life expectancy must be considered, especially in a young female desiring restoration of fertility. In patients with microprolactinomas with serum prolactin levels below 200 ng/mL, transsphenoidal surgery performed by experienced pituitary surgeons at high-volume centers offers a greater than 90% chance of biochemical and oncologic cure[193,207,208] with minimal risks of morbidity and with mortality of less than 1%.[199,205] Furthermore, the continued evolution of endoscopic approaches for tumor resection, which are somewhat less invasive, may reduce the morbidity rate of the surgical approach even further.[209] The financial cost of treatment over a 10-year period is similar in uncomplicated surgical cases to that of long-term dopamine agonist therapy.[210]

In a recent study by Amar and colleagues,[88] a cure rate of 91% was achieved in patients with microprolactinomas. There was a higher correlation with biochemical cure if the preoperative serum prolactin level was less than 200 ng/mL. Similarly, in a study by Tyrrell and colleagues,[191] women with preoperative prolactin levels above 200 ng/mL, and those with larger and more invasive prolactinomas, had worse outcomes (37% to 41% cure rate). In their series, long-term remission was achieved in patients with microadenomas and noninvasive macroadenomas (moderate suprasellar extension and focal sphenoid sinus invasion). Lower postoperative serum prolactin levels are the best predictors of long-term cure. Amar and colleagues[88] demonstrated that fasting morning serum prolactin levels (obtained on the first postoperative day) that were less than 10 ng/mL predicted a 100% cure rate in microprolactinomas and a 93% cure rate in macroprolactinomas. A level between 10 and 20 ng/mL still predicted 100% cure in microadenomas but not for macroadenomas (0% cure rate).

The choice of transsphenoidal surgery for microprolactinomas should take into account the size and location of the tumor, the preoperative serum prolactin level, the age of the patient, the desire for restoration of fertility, the efficacy and tolerability of the dopamine agonists, and the experience of the surgeon. Surgery should not be considered unless a complete removal with chemical cure of the microprolactinoma is an expected outcome. The presence of a symptomatic microprolactinoma, especially in a young patient, should remain an indication for microsurgical or endoscopic transsphenoidal resection.

Radiation Therapy

The reader is referred to the sections on management of GH-secreting pituitary tumors: analogous comments regarding the use of fractionated field radiation therapy in these pituitary tumors can be made.

Stereotactic Radiosurgery

Stereotactic radiosurgery is becoming increasingly popular in the treatment of pituitary adenomas, both functioning and nonfunctioning.[211-218] Current MR imaging enables high resolution and dose planning with excellent accuracy. The preliminary data regarding tumor control and normalization of hypersecretory syndromes after radiosurgery appear favorable. Stereotactic radiosurgery can offer a therapeutic option in patients with prolactinomas as a secondary treatment after failed transsphenoidal surgery or failed medical therapy.[215] Others have proposed stereotactic radiosurgery as a primary treatment for prolactinomas in patients who are reluctant to undergo lifelong medical therapy or surgical resection.[217] The proximity of the pituitary gland to the region of radiosurgical treatment, however, may carry the risk of developing hypopituitarism. Longer follow-up is necessary to assess the likelihood of this complication.

Landolt and Lomax[215] reported 20 patients who underwent gamma knife radiosurgery for residual prolactinomas after unsuccessful transsphenoidal surgery or failed medical therapy. Five patients achieved normoprolactinemia, and medical therapy was discontinued. Eleven patients experienced improvement, which was defined by normalized or decreased (by 20%) prolactin levels with continued requirement of medical therapy at lower doses. The treatment failed in four patients who were receiving dopamine agonist therapy at the time of radiosurgical treatment, suggesting some radioprotective effect of dopamine agonist therapy. Landolt and Lomax have suggested that dopamine agonist therapy be stopped temporarily during radiosurgical treatment.[215]

Pan and colleagues[217] reported 164 patients with prolactinomas who underwent primary treatment with gamma knife radiosurgery. A mean follow-up of 33.2 months was available in 128 patients. Tumor growth was controlled in all but two patients, who eventually underwent transsphenoidal surgery. Biochemical cure was achieved in 52% of patients. Improvement was seen in 28% of patients. Among this group, nine infertile women became pregnant 2 to 13 months after treatment, and all gave birth to normal children. One infertile woman who was unresponsive to bromocriptine became sensitive to the medication after radiosurgery. In 31 (29%) of 108 patients followed for longer than 2 years, persistent hyperprolactinemia could be normalized by bromocriptine after radiosurgery.

Pituitary Transposition (Hypophysopexy)

In cases of macroprolactinomas with cavernous sinus invasion that is refractory to medical therapy, the authors recommend surgical debulking with postoperative stereotactic radiosurgery of residual cavernous sinus tumor. After the tumor is adequately debulked using a transsphenoidal approach, we perform a technique for pituitary gland transposition (hypophysopexy).[219,220] This technique involves transposing the normal pituitary gland away from the cavernous sinus tumor and interposing a fat graft between the normal gland and the tumor in the cavernous sinus. This increases the distance between the normal pituitary gland and residual tumor to facilitate radiosurgical treatment of the tumor, thereby reducing the biologic dose to the normal pituitary gland. This reduction decreases the likelihood of developing hypopituitarism. The details of this technique are described elsewhere in the literature.[219,220]

Follow-up

After surgery in a patient harboring a microprolactinoma, in whom total resection was thought to be achieved, postoperative measurement of PRL levels is the most sensitive measure of completeness of resection and of any recurrence. Because of the short half-life of endogenous PRL, postoperative levels may be checked as early as the morning after surgery. This measurement is repeated at 6 weeks, and it should be performed at regular intervals (every 3 months) in the early postoperative period. Depending on the clinical course, the intervals may be increased accordingly.

The authors have reported the prognostic value of serum PRL levels obtained immediately after transsphenoidal surgery.[88] Our practice is to assess fasting morning PRL levels on postoperative day (POD) 1 and random serum levels sampled at 6 weeks, 12 weeks, and then every 6 months for a minimum of 5 years. Levels less than 10 ng/mL on POD 1 predict long-term endocrinologic cure in patients with microadenomas (100%) as well as in those with macroadenomas (93%). In contrast, patients with "normal" levels of 10 to 20 ng/mL on POD 1 remain at risk for endocrinologic recurrence, especially if preoperative tumor size exceeds 10 mm (100% in the authors' series). However, none of our patients with a microadenoma has had relapse.[88]

In other series, recurrence of hyperprolactinemia after initial hormonal normalization has been reported in 10% to 50% of patients after transsphenoidal resection, depending on the preoperative size of the tumor and the length of follow-up.[100-104] Differences in surgical technique may also underlie this variation. For example, based on the hypothesis that delayed recurrences result in situ from residual tumoral cells at the periphery of an adenoma, Grisoli and colleagues[109] have proposed performing an "enlarged" rather than a selective adenomectomy by removing a layer of normal pituitary gland at the outer edge of the tumor as well as the pituitary capsule in contact with the sellar meninges. Using this technique in 26 patients with tumors less than 20 mm in diameter, they obtained normal serum PRL levels in all cases after an average of 16 months. This length of follow-up is short, however, and it remains to be proven whether this technique results in a lower incidence of delayed recurrence.

Relapses usually occur within the first few years after surgery, although they have been reported after more than 10 years of follow-up.[88,101,103] Often, such recurrences are asymptomatic, but even in patients without overt clinical manifestations, treatment may be indicated to prevent osteoporosis.[101,221] As stated earlier, reduced levels of bromocriptine are usually well tolerated and are often effective in preventing significant enlargement of recurrent tumors.[88,101]

In most cases, however, imaging of the sella turcica fails to reveal residual or recurrent adenoma, and surgical re-exploration is unlikely to achieve chemical cure.[88,100,101,221] This observation may reflect the fact that, with vigilant protocols for sampling postoperative PRL levels, most tumor recurrences are detected early. In the authors' series, for instance, no recurrence was greater than 55 ng/mL.[88] Alternatively, this observation may imply that there are other reasons for recurrent hyperprolactinemia besides regrowth of residual tumor remnants (e.g., a secondary empty sella or a disordered hypothalamic-pituitary axis).[100,101,222]

The clinical response in impotent men with hyperprolactinemia, treated with testosterone, is often unsatisfactory until the PRL levels are lowered.[82] It is presumed that elevated PRL levels interfere with the peripheral effect of testosterone.

REFERENCES

1. Ho P, Barkan A: Acromegaly. In Bardin C (ed): Current Therapy in Endocrinology and Metabolism, 4th ed. Philadelphia: BC Decker, 1991, pp 38–43.
2. Krieger M, Couldwell W, Weiss M: Assessment of surgical long-term remission of acromegaly following surgery cure of acromegaly. J Neurosurg 98:719–724, 2003.
3. Baumann G: Acromegaly. Endocrinol Metab Clin North Am 16:685–702, 1987.
4. Frohman L: Therapeutic options in acromegaly. J Clin Endocrinol Metab 72:1175–1181, 1991.
5. Serri O, Robert F, Comtois R, et al: Distinctive features of prolactin secretion in acromegalic patients with hyperprolactinaemia. Clin Endocrinol 27:429–436, 1987.
6. Wass J: Octreotide treatment of acromegaly. Horm Res 33(Suppl 1): 1–6, 1990.
7. Randall R: Acromegaly and gigantism. In De Groot L (ed): Endocrinology, 2nd ed. Philadelphia: WB Saunders, 1991, pp 330–350.
8. Bengtsson B, Eden S, Ernest I, et al: Epidemiology and long-term survival in acromegaly. Acta Med Scand 223:327–335, 1988.
9. Melmed S: Acromegaly. N Engl J Med 322:966–977, 1990.
10. Nabarro J: Acromegaly. Clin Endocrinol 26:481–512, 1987.
11. Wright A, Hill D, Lowry C, et al: Mortality in acromegaly. QJM 39:1–16, 1970.
12. Arafah B, Rosenzweig J, Fenstermaker R, et al: Value of growth hormone dynamics and somatomedin C (insulin-like growth factor I) levels in predicting the long-term benefit after transsphenoidal surgery for acromegaly. J Lab Clin Med 109:346–354, 1987.
13. Barkan A: Acromegaly. Trends Endocrinol Metab 3:205–210, 1992.
14. Giannella-Neto D, Wajchenberg B, Mendonca B, et al: Criteria for the cure of acromegaly: Comparison between basal growth hormone and somatomedin C plasma concentrations in active and nonactive acromegalic patients. J Endocrinol Invest 11:57–60, 1988.
15. Ho K, Weissberger A, Marbach P, et al: Therapeutic efficacy of the somatostatin analog SMS 201-995 (octreotide) in acromegaly. Ann Intern Med 112:173–181, 1990.
16. Arafah B, Brodkey J, Kaufman B, et al: Transsphenoidal microsurgery in the treatment of acromegaly and gigantism. J Clin Endocrinol Metab 50:578–585, 1980.
17. Aron D, Tyrrell J, Wilson C: Pituitary tumors: Current concepts in diagnosis and management. West J Med 162:340–352, 1995.
18. Baskin D, Boggan J, Wilson C: Transsphenoidal microsurgical removal of growth hormone-secreting pituitary adenomas: A review of 137 cases. J Neurosurg 56:634–641, 1982.
19. Buchfelder M, Brockmeier S, Fahlbusch R, et al: Recurrence following transsphenoidal surgery for acromegaly. Horm Res 35:113–118, 1991.
20. Davis D, Laws E, Ilstrup D, et al: Results of surgical treatment for growth hormone-secreting pituitary adenomas. J Neurosurg 79:70–75, 1993.
21. Fahlbusch R, Honegger J, Buchfelder M: Surgical management of acromegaly. Endocrinol Metab Clin North Am 21:669–692, 1992.
22. Hardy J, Somma M: Acromegaly: Surgical treatment by transsphenoidal microsurgical removal of the pituitary adenoma. In Tindall G, Collins W (eds): Clinical management of pituitary disorders. New York: Raven Press, 1979, pp 209–217.
23. Laws E, Fode N, Redmond M: Transsphenoidal surgery following unsuccessful prior therapy. J Neurosurg 63:823–829, 1985.
24. Ross D, Wilson C: Results of transsphenoidal microsurgery for growth hormone-secreting pituitary adenoma in a series of 214 patients. J Neurosurg 68:854–867, 1988.
25. Serri O, Somma M, Comtoid R, et al: Acromegaly: Biochemical assessment of cure after long term follow-up of transsphenoidal selective adenomectomy. J Clin Endocrinol Metab 61:1185–1189, 1985.
26. Tindall G, Oyesiku N, Watts N, et al: Transsphenoidal adenomectomy for growth hormone–secreting pituitary adenomas in acromegaly: Outcome analysis and determinants of failure. J Neurosurg 78:205–215, 1993.
27. Tucker H, Grubb S, Wigand J, et al: The treatment of acromegaly by transsphenoidal surgery. Arch Intern Med 140:795–802, 1980.
28. Leavens M, Samaan N, Jesse R, et al: Clinical and endocrinological evaluation of 16 acromegalic patients treated by transsphenoidal surgery. J Neurosurg 47:853–860, 1977.
29. Masuda A, Shibasaki T, Kim Y, et al: The somatostatin analog octreotide inhibits the secretion of growth hormone (GH)-release hormone, thyrotropin and GH in man. J Clin Endocrinol Metab 69:906–1000, 1989.
30. Bauer W, Briner U, Doepfner W, et al: SMS 201-995: A very potent selective octapeptide analogue of somatostatin with prolonged action. Life Sci 31:1133–1140, 1982.
31. Barnard L, Grantham W, Lamberton P, et al: Treatment of resistant acromegaly with a long-acting somatostatin analogue (SMS 201-995). Ann Intern Med 105:856–861, 1986.
32. Lamberts S: The role of somatostatin in the regulation of anterior pituitary hormone secretion and the use of its analogs in the treatment of human pituitary tumors. Endocr Rev 9:417–436, 1988.
33. Ikuyama S, Nawata H, Kato K, et al: Specific somatostatin receptors on human pituitary adenoma cell membranes. J Clin Endocrinol Metab 6:666–671, 1985.
34. Moyse E, Le Dafniet M, Epelbaum J, et al: Somatostatin receptors in human growth hormone and prolactin-secreting pituitary adenomas. J Clin Endocrinol Metab 61:98–103, 1985.
35. Reubi J, Landolt A: The growth hormone responses to octreotide in acromegaly correlate with adenoma somatostatin receptor status. J Clin Endocrinol Metab 68:844–850, 1989.
36. Kelijman M, Williams T, Downs T, et al: Comparison of the sensitivity of growth hormone secretion to somatostatin in vivo and in vitro in acromegaly. J Clin Endocrinol Metab 67:958–963, 1988.
37. Barkan A, Kelch R, Hopwood N, et al: Treatment of acromegaly with the long-acting somatostatin analog SMS 201-995. J Clin Endocrinol Metab 66:16–23, 1988.
38. Lamberts S, Uitterlinden P, del Pozo E: SMS 201-995 induces a continuous decline in circulating growth hormone and somatomedin-C levels during therapy of acromegalic patients for over two years. J Clin Endocrinol Metab 65:703–710, 1987.
39. Lamberts S, Uitterlinden P, Verleun T: Relationship between growth hormone and somatomedin-C levels in untreated acromegaly, after surgery and radiotherapy and during medical therapy with Sandostatin (SMS 201-995). Eur J Clin Invest 17:354–359, 1987.
40. Oppizzi G, Petroncini M, Dallabonzana D, et al: Relationship between somatomedin-C and growth hormone levels in acromegaly: Basal and dynamic evaluation. J Clin Endocrinol Metab 63:1348–1353, 1986.
41. Ezzat S, Snyder P, Young W, et al: Octreotide treatment of acromegaly: A randomized, multicenter study. Ann Intern Med 117:711–718, 1992.
42. Page M, Millward M, Hourihan M: Long-term treatment of acromegaly with octreotide (Sandostatin). Horm Res 33(Suppl 1):20–31, 1990.
43. Christensen S, Weeke J, Orskov H: Continuous subcutaneous pump infusion of somatostatin analogue SMS 201-995 versus subcutaneous injection schedule in acromegalic patients. Clin Endocrinol (Oxf) 27:297–306, 1987.
44. Williams G, Ball J, Lawson R: Analgesic effect of somatostatin analogue (octreotide) in headache associated with pituitary tumors. BMJ 295:247–248, 1987.
45. Popovic V, Paunovic V, Micic D: The analgesic effects and development of dependency to somatostatin analogue (octreotide) in headache associated with acromegaly. Horm Metab Res 20:250–251, 1987.
46. Mcknight J, McCance D, Sheridan B: Long-term dose-response study of somatostatin analogue (SMS 201-995, octreotide) in resistant acromegaly. Clin Endocrinol 34:119–125, 1991.
47. Sandler L, Burrin J, Williams G: Effective long-term treatment of acromegaly with a long-acting somatostatin analog (SMS 201-995). Clin Endocrinol (Oxf) 26:85–95, 1987.
48. Barkan A, Lloyd R, Chandler W: Treatment of acromegaly with SMS 201-995 (sandostatin): Clinical, biochemical and morphologic study. In Lamberts S (ed): Sandostatin in the treatment of acromegaly. New York: Springer-Verlag, 1988, pp 103–108.
49. Harris A, Prestele H, Herold K: Long-term efficacy of sandostatin (SMS 201-995, octreotide) in 178 acromegalic patients: Results from the International Multicenter Acromegaly Study Group.

In Lamberts S (ed): Sandostatin in the treatment of acromegaly. New York: Springer-Verlag, 1988, pp 117–125.

50. Lamberts S, Uitterlinden P, Verschoor L: Long-term treatment of acromegaly with the somatostatin analogue SMS 201-995. N Engl J Med 313:1576–1580, 1985.

51. Lamberts S, del Pozo E: Somatostatin analog treatment of acromegaly: New aspects. Horm Res 29:115–117, 1988.

52. Lamberts S, Van Koetsveld P, Hofland L: A close correlation between the inhibitory effects of insulin-like growth factor-1 and SMS 201-995 on growth hormone release by acromegalic pituitary tumours in vitro and in vivo. Clin Endocrinol (Oxf) 31:401–410, 1989.

53. White M, Newland P, Daniels M: Growth hormone secreting pituitary adenomas are heterogeneous in cell culture and commomly secrete glycoprotein hormone alpha-subunit. Clin Endocrinol (Oxf) 25:173–179, 1986.

54. Spinas G, Zaph J, Landolt A: Pre-operative treatment of 5 acromegalics with a somatostatin analogue: Endocrine and clinical observations. Acta Endocrinol (Copenh) 114:249–256, 1987.

55. Landolt A, Osterwalder V, Jantzer R, et al: Pre-operative treatment of acromegaly with SMS 201-995: Surgical and pathological observations. Neuroendocrinol Lett 7:94, 1985.

56. Jackson I, Barnard L, Lamberton P: Role of long-acting somatostatin analogue (SMS 201-995) in the treatment of acromegaly. Am J Med 81(Suppl 6):94–100, 1986.

57. Sadoul J-L, Thyss A, Freychet P: Invasive mixed growth hormone/ prolactin secreting pituitary tumour: Complete shrinking by octreotide and bromocriptine and lack of tumour growth relapse 20 months after octreotide withdrawal. Acta Endocrinol (Copenh) 126:179–183, 1992.

58. Charest L, Comtois R, Beaureguard H, et al: Growth hormone rebound after cessation of SMS 201-995 treatment in acromegaly. Can J Neurol Sci 16:442–445, 1989.

59. George S, Kovacs K, Asa S: Effect of SMS 201-995, a long-acting somatostatin analogue, on the secretion and morphology of a pituitary growth hormone cell adenoma. Clin Endocrinol (Oxf) 26:395–405, 1987.

60. Wass J, Anderson J, Besser G, et al: Gall stones and treatment with octreotide for acromegaly. BMJ 299:1162–1163, 1989.

61. Vance ML, Kaiser DL, Frohman LA, et al: Role of dopamine in the regulation of growth hormone secretion: Dopamine and bromocriptine augment growth hormone (GH)-releasing hormone-stimulated GH secretion in normal man. J Clin Endocrinol Metab 64:1136–1141, 1987.

62. Wass J, Thorner M, Morris D: Long-term treatment of acromegaly with bromocriptine. BMJ 1:875–878, 1977.

63. Alford F, Arnott R: Medical management of pituitary tumors. Med J Austr 157:57–60, 1992.

64. Vance ML, Thorner MO: Prolactinomas. Endocrinol Metab Clin North Am 16:731–753, 1987.

65. Oppizzi G, Liuzzo A, Chiodini P: Dopaminergic treatment of acromegaly: Different effects on hormone secretion and tumor size. J Clin Endocrinol Metab 58:988–992, 1984.

66. Mori H, Maeda T: Changes in prolactinomas and somatotropinomas in humans treated with bromocriptine. Pathol Res Pract 183:580–583, 1988.

67. Turner T, Cookson J, Wass J: Psychotic reactions during treatment of pituitary tumors with dopamine agonists. BMJ 289:1101–1103, 1984.

68. Chiodini P, Cozzi R, Dallabonzana D: Medical treatment of acromegaly with SMS 201-995, a somatostatin analog: A comparison with bromocriptine. J Clin Endocrinol Metab 64:447–453, 1987.

69. Klibanski A, Zervas N: Diagnosis and management of hormone-secreting pituitary adenomas. N Engl J Med 324:822–831, 1991.

70. Gramegna A: Un cas d'acromegalie traité par la radiothérapie. Rev Neurol 17:15, 1909.

71. Chun M, Masko G, Heterlekidis S: Radiotherapy in the treatment of pituitary adenomas. Int J Radiat Oncol Biol Phys 15:305–309, 1988.

72. Noell K: Prolactin and other hormone producing pituitary tumors: Radiation therapy. Clin Obstet Gynecol 23:441–452, 1980.

73. Aristzabal S, Caldwell W, Avila J: The relationship of time-dose fractionation factors to complications in the treatment of pituitary tumors by irradiation. Int J Radiat Oncol Biol Phys 2:667–673, 1977.

74. Baglan R, Marks J: Soft-tissue reactions following irradiation of primary brain and pituitary tumors. Int J Radiat Oncol Biol Phys 7:455–459, 1981.

75. Sheline G: Treatment of non-functioning chromophobe adenomas of the pituitary. AJR Am J Roentgenol 120:553–561, 1974.

76. Kramer S: The value of radiation therapy for pituitary and parapituitary tumors. CMAJ 99:1120–1127, 1968.

77. Urdaneta N, Chessin H, Fisher J: Pituitary adenomas and craniopharyngiomas: Analysis of 99 cases treated with radiation therapy. Int J Radiat Oncol Biol Phys 1:895–902, 1975.

78. Bloom H: Radiotherapy of pituitary tumors. In Jenkins J (ed): Pituitary tumors. London: Butterworth, 1973, pp 165–197.

79. Ciric I, Mikhael M, Stafford T: Transsphenoidal microsurgery of pituitary macroadenomas with long-term follow-up results. J Neurosurg 59:395–401, 1984.

80. Valtonen S, Myllymaki K: Outcome of patients after transcranial operation for pituitary adenoma. Ann Clin Res 18(Suppl 47):43–45, 1986.

81. Mindermann T, Wilson C: Pediatric pituitary adenomas. Neurosurgery 36:259–268, 1995.

82. Evans W, Thorner M: Mechanisms for hypogonadism in hyperprolactinemia. Semin Reprod Endocrinol 2:9–22, 1984.

83. Thorner M: Prolactinoma. In Bardin C (ed): Current therapy in endocrinology and metabolism, 4th ed. Philadelphia: BC Decker, 1991, pp 35–38.

84. Jacobs H, Franks S, Murray M: Clinical and endocrine features of hyperprolactinemic amenorrhea. Clin Endocrinol (Oxf) 5:439–454, 1976.

85. Leyeendecker G, Struve T, Plotz E: Induction of ovulation in chronic intermittent (pulsatile) administration of LH-RH in women with hypothalamic and hyperprolactinemic amenorrhea. Arch Gynecol 229:177–190, 1980.

86. Klibanski A, Greenspan S: Increase in bone mass after treatment of hyperprolactinemic amenorrhea. N Engl J Med 315:542–546, 1986.

87. Greenspan S, Oppenheim D, Klibaski A: Importance of gonadal steroids to bone mass in men with hyperprolactinemic hypogonadism. Ann Intern Med 110:526–531, 1989.

88. Amar AP, Couldwell WT, Chen JC, et al: Predictive value of serum prolactin levels measured immediately after transsphenoidal surgery. J Neurosurg 97:307–314, 2002.

89. Hulting A, Muhr C, Lundberg P, et al: Prolactinoma in men: Clinical characteristics and the effect of bromocriptine treatment. Acta Med Scand 217:101–109, 1985.

90. Cunnah D, Besser M: Management of prolactinomas. Clin Endocrinol (Oxf) 34:231–235, 1991.

91. Lees P, Pickard J: Hyperprolactinemia, intrasellar pituitary tissue pressure, and the pituitary stalk compression syndrome. J Neurosurg 767:192–196, 1987.

92. Albuquerque FC, Hinton DR, Weiss MH: Excessively high prolactin level in a patient with a nonprolactin-secreting adenoma: Case report. J Neurosurg 89:1043–1046, 1998.

93. Chandler WF, Barkan AL, Schteingart DE: Management options for persistent functional tumors. Neurosurg Clin N Am 14:139–145, viii, 2003.

94. Comtois R, Robert F, Hardy J: Immunoradiometric assays may miss high prolactin levels. Ann Intern Med 119:173, 1993.

95. Schlechte J, Dolan K, Sherman B: The natural history of untreated hyperprolactinemia: A prospective analysis. J Clin Endocrinol Metab 68:412–418, 1989.

96. Sisam D, Sheehan J, Sheeler L: The natural history of untreated microprolactinomas. Fertil Steril 48:67–71, 1987.

97. Weiss M, Teal J, Gott P: Natural history of microprolactinomas: Six year follow-up. Neurosurgery 12:180–182, 1983.

98. Lundin P, Nyman R, Burman P: MRI of pituitary macroadenomas with reference to hormonal activity. Neuroradiology 34:43–51, 1992.

99. Giovanelli M, Losa M, Mortini P: Surgical results in microadenomas. Acta Neurochir Suppl (Wien) 65:11–12, 1996.

100. Laws E: Comment on paper by Massoud et al. Surg Neurol 45:344–345, 1996.

101. Massoud F, Serri O, Hardy J: Transsphenoidal adenomectomy for microprolactinomas: 10 to 20 years of follow-up. Surg Neurol 45:341–346, 1996.

102. Molitch M: Pathologic hyperprolactinemia. Endocrinol Metab Clin North Am 21:877–901, 1992.

103. Thomson J, Davies D, McLaren E, et al: Ten-year follow up of microprolactinoma treated by transsphenoidal surgery. BMJ 309:1409–1410, 1994.

104. Webster J, Page M, Bevan J: Low recurrence rate after partial hypophysectomy for prolactinoma: The predictive value of dynamic prolactin function tests. Clin Endocrinol (Oxf) 36:35–44, 1992.

105. Wilson C: A decade of pituitary microsurgery. J Neurosurg 61:814–833, 1984.
106. Adams C: The management of pituitary tumours and post-operative visual deterioration. Acta Neurochir (Wien) 94:103–116, 1988.
107. Serri O, Rasio E, Beauregard H: Recurrence of hyperprolactinemia after selective transsphenoidal adenomectomy in women with prolactinoma. N Engl J Med 309:280–283, 1983.
108. Physicians' Desk Reference, 51st ed. Montvale, NJ: Medical Economics Company, 1997.
109. Grisoli F, Brue T, Graziani N: Enlarged adenomectomy for enclosed prolactinoma: A preliminary study of 26 cases. Acta Neurochir (Wien) 103:92–98, 1990.
110. Corrodi H, Fuxe K, Hokfelt T: Effect of ergot drugs on central cathecolamine neurons: Evidence for stimulation of central dopamine neurons. Pharm Pharmacol 25:409–412, 1973.
111. Thorner M, Schran H, Evans W: A broad spectrum of prolactin suppression by bromocriptine in hyperprolactinemic women: A study of serum prolactin and bromocriptine levels after acute and chronic administration of bromocriptine. J Clin Endocrinol Metab 50:1026–1033, 1980.
112. Bevan J, Davis J: Cabergoline: An advance in dopaminergic therapy. Clin Endocrinol 41:709–712, 1994.
113. Muratori M, Arosio M, Gambino G: Use of cabergoline in the long-term treatment of hyperprolactinemic and acromegalic patients. J Endocrinol Invest 20:537–546, 1997.
114. Rains C, Bryson H, Fitton A: Cabergoline: A review of its pharmacological properties and therapeutic potential in the treatment of hyperprolactinemia and inhibition of lactation. Drugs 49:255–279, 1995.
115. Shimon I, Melmed S: Management of pituitary tumors. Ann Intern Med 129:472–483, 1998.
116. Webster J, Piscitelli G, Polli A: A comparison of cabergoline and bromocriptine in the treatment of hyperprolactinemic amenorrhea. N Engl J Med 331:904–909, 1994.
117. Ciccarelli E, Grottoli S, Razzore P: Long-term treatment with cabergoline, a new long-lasting ergoline derivate, in idiopathic or tumorous hyperprolactinemia and outcome of drug-induced pregnancy. J Endocrinol Invest 20:547–551, 1997.
118. Colao A, Merola B, Sarnacchiaro F, et al: Comparison among different dopamine-agonists of new formulation in the clinical management of macroprolactinomas. Horm Res 44:222–228, 1995.
119. De Luis DA, Becerra A, Lahera M, et al: A randomized cross-over study comparing cabergoline and quinagolide in the treatment of hyperprolactinemic patients. J Endocrinol Invest 23:428–434, 2000.
120. Delgrange E, Donckier J: Prolactinomas apparently resistant to quinagolide respond to cabergoline therapy. J Clin Endocrinol Metab 82:2755–2756, 1997.
121. Ferrari C, Crosignani PG: Medical treatment of hyperprolactinaemic disorders. Hum Reprod 1:507–514, 1986.
122. Morange I, Barlier A, Pellegrini I, et al: Prolactinomas resistant to bromocriptine: Long-term efficacy of quinagolide and outcome of pregnancy. Eur J Endocrinol 135:413–420, 1996.
123. Nickelsen T, Jungmann E, Althoff P, et al: Treatment of macroprolactinoma with the new potent non-ergot D2-dopamine agonist quinagolide and effects on prolactin levels, pituitary function, and the renin-aldosterone system. Results of a clinical long-term study. Arzneimittelforschung 43:421–425, 1993.
124. Orrego JJ, Chandler WF, Barkan AL: Pergolide as primary therapy for macroprolactinomas. Pituitary 3:251–256, 2000.
125. Schultz PN, Ginsberg L, McCutcheon IE, et al: Quinagolide in the management of prolactinoma. Pituitary 3:239–249, 2000.
126. Webster J: Cabergoline and quinagolide therapy for prolactinomas. Clin Endocrinol (Oxf) 53:549–550, 2000.
127. Webster J: A comparative review of the tolerability profiles of dopamine agonists in the treatment of hyperprolactinaemia and inhibition of lactation. Drug Saf 14:228–238, 1996.
128. Thorner M, Perryman R, Rogol A: Rapid changes of prolactinoma volume after withdrawal and reinstitution of bromocriptine. J Clin Endocrinol Metab 53:480–483, 1981.
129. Zarate A, Canales E, Cano C, et al: Follow-up of patients with prolactinomas after discontinuation of long-term therapy with bromocriptine. Acta Endocrinol (Copenh) 104:139–142, 1983.
130. Vance ML, Evans WS, Thorner MO: Drugs five years later. Bromocriptine. Ann Intern Med 100:78–91, 1984.
131. Landolt A: Surgical treatment of pituitary prolactinomas: Postoperative prolactin and fertility in seventy patients. Fertil Steril 35:620–625, 1981.
132. Zervas N: Surgical results for pituitary adenomas: Results of an international survey, in Black P, Zervas N, Ridgeway E (eds): Secretory tumors of the pituitary gland. New York: Raven Press, 1984, pp 377–385.
133. Weiss M, Wycoff R, Yadley R: Bromocriptine treatment of prolactin-secreting tumors: Surgical implications. Neurosurgery 12:640–642, 1983.
134. Breidahl H, Topliss D, Pike J: Failure of bromocriptine to maintain reduction in size of a macroprolactinoma. BMJ 287:451–452, 1983.
135. Crosignani P, Mattei A: Enlargement of a prolactin-secreting pituitary microadenoma during bromocriptine treatment. Br J Obstet Gynaecol 89:169–170, 1982.
136. Martin N, Hales M, Wilson C: Cerebellar metastasis from a prolactinoma during treatment with bromocriptine. J Neurosurg 55:615–619, 1981.
137. Gemzell C, Wang CF: Outcome of pregnancy in women with pituitary adenoma. Fertil Steril 31:363–372, 1979.
138. Skrabanek P, McDonald D, Meagher D, et al: Clinical course and outcome of thirty-five pregnancies in infertile hyperprolactinemic women. Fertil Steril 33:391–395, 1980.
139. Hubbard J, Scheithauer B, Abboud C, et al: Prolactin-secreting adenomas: The preoperative response to bromocriptine treatment and surgical outcome. J Neurosurg 67:816–821, 1987.
140. Fahlbusch R, Buchfelder M, Schrell U: Short-term preoperative treatment of macroprolactinomas by dopamine agonists. J Neurosurg 67:807–815, 1987.
141. Colao A, Di Sarno A, Cappabianca P, et al: Withdrawal of long-term cabergoline therapy for tumoral and nontumoral hyperprolactinemia. N Engl J Med 349:2023–2033, 2003.
142. Colao A, Di Sarno A, Landi ML, et al: Long-term and low-dose treatment with cabergoline induces macroprolactinoma shrinkage. J Clin Endocrinol Metab 82:3574–3579, 1997.
143. Colao A, Di Sarno A, Landi ML, et al: Macroprolactinoma shrinkage during cabergoline treatment is greater in naive patients than in patients pretreated with other dopamine agonists: A prospective study in 110 patients. J Clin Endocrinol Metab 85:2247–2252, 2000.
144. Corsello SM, Ubertini G, Altomare M, et al: Giant prolactinomas in men: Efficacy of cabergoline treatment. Clin Endocrinol (Oxf) 58:662–670, 2003.
145. De Rosa M, Colao A, Di Sarno A, et al: Cabergoline treatment rapidly improves gonadal function in hyperprolactinemic males: A comparison with bromocriptine. Eur J Endocrinol 138:286–293, 1998.
146. Ferrari C, Paracchi A, Mattei AM, et al: Cabergoline in the long-term therapy of hyperprolactinemic disorders. Acta Endocrinol (Copenh) 126:489–494, 1992.
147. Ferrari CI, Abs R, Bevan JS, et al: Treatment of macroprolactinoma with cabergoline: A study of 85 patients. Clin Endocrinol (Oxf) 46:409–413, 1997.
148. Miki N: Cabergoline, a hopeful medicine for prolactinomas and non-tumoral hyperprolactinemia. Intern Med 40:845–846, 2001.
149. Molitch ME: Medical management of prolactin-secreting pituitary adenomas. Pituitary 5:55–65, 2002.
150. Di Sarno A, Landi ML, Cappabianca P, et al: Resistance to cabergoline as compared with bromocriptine in hyperprolactinemia: Prevalence, clinical definition, and therapeutic strategy. J Clin Endocrinol Metab 86:5256–5261, 2001.
151. Di Sarno A, Landi ML, Marzullo P, et al: The effect of quinagolide and cabergoline, two selective dopamine receptor type 2 agonists, in the treatment of prolactinomas. Clin Endocrinol (Oxf) 53:53–60, 2000.
152. Colao A, Di Sarno A, Sarnacchiaro F, et al: Prolactinomas resistant to standard dopamine agonists respond to chronic cabergoline treatment. J Clin Endocrinol Metab 82:876–883, 1997.
153. Molitch ME: Pregnancy and the hyperprolactinemic woman. N Engl J Med 312:1364–1370, 1985.
154. Canales E, Garcia I, Ruiz J: Bromocriptine as prophylactic therapy in prolactinoma during pregnancy. Fertil Steril 36:524–526, 1981.
155. Konopka P, Raymond J, Merceron R: Continuous administration of bromocriptine in the prevention of neurological complications in pregnant women with prolactinomas. Am J Obstet Gynecol 146:935–938, 1983.
156. Van Roon E, Van der Vijver J, Gerretsen G: Rapid regression of a suprasellar extending prolactinoma after bromocriptine treatment during pregnancy. Fertil Steril 36:173–177, 1981.

157. Raymond J, Goldstein E, Konopka P: Follow-up of children born of bromocriptine-treated mothers. Horm Res 22:239–246, 1985.

158. Turkalj I, Braun P, Krupp P: Surveillance of bromocriptine in pregnancy. JAMA 247:1589–1591, 1982.

159. Molitch ME: Management of prolactinomas during pregnancy. J Reprod Med 44:1121–1126, 1999.

160. Rasmussen C, Bergh T, Nillius SJ, et al: Return of menstruation and normalization of prolactin in hyperprolactinemic women with bromocriptine-induced pregnancy. Fertil Steril 44:31–34, 1985.

161. Ricci E, Parazzini F, Motta T, et al: Pregnancy outcome after cabergoline treatment in early weeks of gestation. Reprod Toxicol 16:791–793, 2002.

162. Robert E, Musatti L, Piscitelli G, et al: Pregnancy outcome after treatment with the ergot derivative, cabergoline. Reprod Toxicol 10:333–337, 1996.

163. Schlechte JA: Clinical practice: Prolactinoma. N Engl J Med 349:2035–2041, 2003.

164. Toffle RC, Webb SM, Tagatz GE, et al: Pregnancy-induced changes in prolactinoma as assessed with computed tomography. J Reprod Med 33:821–826, 1988.

165. Vician L, Shupnik MA, Gorski J: Effects of estrogen on primary ovine pituitary cell cultures: Stimulation of prolactin secretion, synthesis, and preprolactin messenger ribonucleic acid activity. Endocrinology 104:736–743, 1979.

166. Weiss M: Pituitary tumors: An endocrinological and neurosurgical challenge. Clin Neurosurg 39:114–122, 1992.

167. Bergh T, Nillius SJ, Enoksson P, et al: Bromocriptine-induced regression of a suprasellar extending prolactinoma during pregnancy. J Endocrinol Invest 7:133–136, 1984.

168. Johnston DG, Hall K, Kendall-Taylor P, et al: Effect of dopamine agonist withdrawal after long-term therapy in prolactinomas: Studies with high-definition computerised tomography. Lancet 2:187–192, 1984.

169. Liuzzi A, Dallabonzana D, Oppizzi G, et al: Low doses of dopamine agonists in the long-term treatment of macroprolactinomas. N Engl J Med 313:656–659, 1985.

170. Passos VQ, Souza JJ, Musolino NR, et al: Long-term follow-up of prolactinomas: Normoprolactinemia after bromocriptine withdrawal. J Clin Endocrinol Metab 87:3578–3582, 2002.

171. Rasmussen C, Bergh T, Wide L: Prolactin secretion and menstrual function after long-term bromocriptine treatment. Fertil Steril 48:550–554, 1987.

172. van't Verlaat JW, Croughs RJ: Withdrawal of bromocriptine after long-term therapy for macroprolactinomas: Effect on plasma prolactin and tumour size. Clin Endocrinol (Oxf) 34:175–178, 1991.

173. Wang C, Lam KS, Ma JT, et al: Long-term treatment of hyperprolactinaemia with bromocriptine: Effect of drug withdrawal. Clin Endocrinol (Oxf) 27:363–371, 1987.

174. Warfield A, Finkel DM, Schatz NJ, et al: Bromocriptine treatment of prolactin-secreting pituitary adenomas may restore pituitary function. Ann Intern Med 101:783–785, 1984.

175. Jeffcoate WJ, Pound N, Sturrock ND, et al: Long-term follow-up of patients with hyperprolactinaemia. Clin Endocrinol (Oxf) 45:299–303, 1996.

176. Orrego JJ, Chandler WF, Barkan AL: Rapid re-expansion of a macroprolactinoma after early discontinuation of bromocriptine. Pituitary 3:189–192, 2000.

177. Molitch ME: Medical treatment of prolactinomas. Endocrinol Metab Clin North Am 28:143–169, vii, 1999.

178. Thorner MO, McNeilly A, Hagen C: Long-term treatment of galactorrhea and hypogonadism with bromocriptine. BMJ 2:419–422, 1974.

179. Bannister P, Sheridan P: Continued growth of a large pituitary prolactinoma despite high dose bromocriptine. Br J Clin Pract 41:712–713, 1987.

180. Bevan J, Webster J, Burke C, et al: Dopamine agonists and pituitary tumor shrinkage. Endocr Rev 13:220–240, 1992.

181. Kupersmith M, Kleinberg D, Warren F: Growth of prolactinoma despite lowering of serum prolactin by bromocriptine. Neurosurgery 24:417–423, 1989.

182. Ahmed S, Shalet S: Discordant responses of prolactinoma to two different dopamine agonists. Clin Endocrinol 24:421–426, 1986.

183. Arnesen M, Scheithauer BW: Aggressive small cell tumor of the skull base. Ultrastruct Pathol 18:191–197, 1994.

184. Bills DC, Meyer FB, Laws ER Jr, et al: A retrospective analysis of pituitary apoplexy. Neurosurgery 33:602–609, 1993.

185. Ebersold MJ, Laws ER Jr, Scheithauer BW, et al: Pituitary apoplexy treated by transsphenoidal surgery: A clinicopathological and immunocytochemical study. J Neurosurg 58:315–320, 1983.

186. Laws ER Jr, Ebersold MJ: Pituitary apoplexy: An endocrine emergency. World J Surg 6:686–688, 1982.

187. Liu JK, Couldwell WT: Pituitary apoplexy: Diagnosis and management. Contemp Neurosurg 25:1–6, 2003.

188. Liu JK, Rovit RL, Couldwell WT: Pituitary apoplexy. Semin Neurosurg 12:315–320, 2001.

189. Brisman MH, Katz G, Post KD: Symptoms of pituitary apoplexy rapidly reversed with bromocriptine: Case report. J Neurosurg 85:1153–1155, 1996.

190. Shrivastava RK, Arginteanu MS, King WA, et al: Giant prolactinomas: Clinical management and long-term follow up. J Neurosurg 97:299–306, 2002.

191. Tyrrell JB, Lamborn KR, Hannegan LT, et al: Transsphenoidal microsurgical therapy of prolactinomas: Initial outcomes and long-term results. Neurosurgery 44:254–263, 1999.

192. Wilson CB: Role of surgery in the management of pituitary tumors. Neurosurg Clin N Am 1:139–159, 1990.

193. Couldwell WT, Rovit RL, Weiss MH: Role of surgery in the treatment of microprolactinomas. Neurosurg Clin N Am 14:89–92, vii, 2003.

194. Liuzzi A, Oppizzi G: Microprolactinomas: Why requiem for surgery? J Endocrinol Invest 19:196–198, 1996.

195. Wang MY, Weiss MH: Is there a role for surgery for microprolactinomas? Semin Neurosurg 12:289–294, 2001.

196. Wolfsberger S, Czech T, Vierhapper H, et al: Microprolactinomas in males treated by transsphenoidal surgery. Acta Neurochir (Wien) 145:935–944, 2003.

197. Peter SA, Autz A, Jean-Simon ML: Bromocriptine-induced schizophrenia. J Natl Med Assoc 85:700–701, 1993.

198. Thorner MO: Prolactinoma. West J Med 139:703–705, 1983.

199. Ciric I, Ragin A, Baumgartner C, et al: Complications of transsphenoidal surgery: Results of a national survey, review of the literature, and personal experience. Neurosurgery 40:225–237, 1997.

200. Couldwell WT: Transsphenoidal and transcranial surgery for pituitary adenomas. J Neurooncol 69:237–256, 2004.

201. Couldwell WT, Weiss MH: Transnasal transsphenoidal approach. In Apuzzo MLJ (ed): Surgery of the third ventricle, 2nd ed. Baltimore: Williams & Wilkins, 1998, pp 553–574.

202. Liu JK, Orlandi RR, Apfelbaum RI, et al: Novel closure technique for the endonasal transsphenoidal approach: Technical note. J Neurosurg 100:161–164, 2004.

203. Jane JA Jr, Thapar K, Kaptain GJ, et al: Pituitary surgery: Transsphenoidal approach. Neurosurgery 51:435–444, 2002.

204. Kaptain GJ, Vincent DA, Sheehan JP, et al: Transsphenoidal approaches for the extracapsular resection of midline suprasellar and anterior cranial base lesions. Neurosurgery 49:94–101, 2001.

205. Liu JK, Das K, Weiss MH, et al: The history and evolution of transsphenoidal surgery. J Neurosurg 95:1083–1096, 2001.

206. Liu JK, Weiss MH, Couldwell WT: Surgical approaches to pituitary tumors. Neurosurg Clin N Am 14:93–107, 2003.

207. Jane JA Jr, Laws ER Jr: The surgical management of pituitary adenomas in a series of 3093 patients. J Am Coll Surg 193:651–659, 2001.

208. Randall RV, Laws ER Jr, Abboud CF, et al: Transsphenoidal microsurgical treatment of prolactin-producing pituitary adenomas: Results in 100 patients. Mayo Clin Proc 58:108–121, 1983.

209. Jho HD, Carrau RL: Endoscopic endonasal transsphenoidal surgery: Experience with 50 patients. J Neurosurg 87:44–51, 1997.

210. Turner HE, Adams CB, Wass JA: Trans-sphenoidal surgery for microprolactinoma: An acceptable alternative to dopamine agonists? Eur J Endocrinol 140:43–47, 1999.

211. Ganz JC: Gamma knife treatment of pituitary adenomas. Stereotact Funct Neurosurg 64(Suppl 1):3–10, 1995.

212. Ganz JC, Backlund EO, Thorsen FA: The effects of Gamma knife surgery of pituitary adenomas on tumor growth and endocrinopathies. Stereotact Funct Neurosurg 61(Suppl 1):30–37, 1993.

213. Kim MS, Lee SI, Sim JH: Gamma knife radiosurgery for functioning pituitary microadenoma. Stereotact Funct Neurosurg 72(Suppl 1):119–124, 1999.

214. Kim SH, Huh R, Chang JW, et al: Gamma knife radiosurgery for functioning pituitary adenomas. Stereotact Funct Neurosurg 72(Suppl 1):101–110, 1999.

215. Landolt AM, Lomax N: Gamma knife radiosurgery for prolactinomas. J Neurosurg 93(Suppl 3):14–18, 2000.
216. Pan L, Zhang N, Wang E, et al: Pituitary adenomas: The effect of gamma knife radiosurgery on tumor growth and endocrinopathies. Stereotact Funct Neurosurg 70(Suppl 1):119–126, 1998.
217. Pan L, Zhang N, Wang EM, et al: Gamma knife radiosurgery as a primary treatment for prolactinomas. J Neurosurg 93(Suppl 3):10–13, 2000.
218. Shin M: Gamma knife radiosurgery for pituitary adenoma. Biomed Pharmacother 56(Suppl 1):178S–181S, 2002.
219. Couldwell WT, Rosenow JM, Rovit RL, et al: Hypophysopexy technique for radiosurgical treatment of cavernous sinus pituitary adenoma. Pituitary 5:169–173, 2002.
220. Liu JK, Schmidt MH, MacDonald JD, et al: Hypophysial transposition (hypophysopexy) for radiosurgical treatment of pituitary tumors involving the cavernous sinus: Technical note. Neurosurg Focus 14(5):Article 11, 2003.
221. Buchfelder M, Fahlbusch R, Schott W, et al: Long-term follow-up results in hormonally active pituitary adenomas after primary successful transsphenoidal surgery. Acta Neurochir Suppl (Wien) 53:72–76, 1991.
222. Maira G, Anile C, DeMarinis L, et al: Prolactin-secreting adenomas: Surgical results and long-term follow-up. Neurosurgery 24:736–743, 1989.

31 Repair of the Sella Turcica after Transsphenoidal Surgery

RENATO SPAZIANTE, ENRICO DE DIVITIIS,
PAOLO CAPPABIANCA, and GIANLUIGI ZONA

SUMMARY

Although at present the microsurgical and the endoscopic endonasal transsphenoidal approaches represent the standard for surgical removal of most pituitary tumors and other sellar lesions,[1-4] little agreement exists concerning reconstruction of the surgical site. Conflicting ideas remain about the usefulness of careful reconstruction and hermetic closure of the sella, which probably should be reserved only to selected cases with elements of high risk. Nevertheless, mechanical complications encountered in this type of surgery should not be underestimated, because, though quite rare, they are very difficult to treat and may be more incapacitating and more severe than the original lesion. Preventing them or treating some specific conditions with appropriate and meticulous surgery remains very important.

The most feared and common complication of transsphenoidal surgery is postoperative hematoma, whereas intrasellar abscess and related infectious complications are quite rare. The possibility of a cerebrospinal fluid (CSF) leak with related dangers of septic meningitis, on the other hand, should be considered more frequently as well.

Risky conditions requiring reconstruction of the sellar region can be summarized as follows:

1. Preoperative or intraoperative CSF leakage
2. A coexisting preoperative or intraoperative empty sella
3. Persistent bleeding after removal of an intrasellar-suprasellar adenoma, even after prolonged compression and irrigation
4. Previous surgery or radiotherapy
5. Ghost sella
6. Age

Natural biologic substances obtained during surgery or common reabsorbable materials used in neurosurgery fulfill the packing requirements in almost every situation. Extradural packing, used on its own or together with intradural packing, constitutes the best method for producing a solid, stable closure of the sella, both immediately and at long-lasting follow-up. Such specific conditions as large or invasive macroadenomas may require no reconstruction at all to favor spontaneous blood drainage as well as progressive intrasellar delivery of the remaining suprasellar tumor to perform a staged transsphenoidal removal (the "open sella" technique). Surgical techniques aimed toward continuous drainage of the cystic fluid into the sphenoidal sinus (cystosphenoidostomy) in case of cystic craniopharyngiomas and to elevation of the sellar contents in the treatment of visual disturbances related to empty sella are described in detail. Personal experiences are discussed in the
last part of this chapter, focusing on the usefulness and indications for sellar repair based on our own experience, which has permitted us to develop more selective criteria for reconstruction.

GENERAL PRINCIPLES

The microsurgical and the endoscopic endonasal transsphenoidal approach to the sella turcica are influenced at each step of their execution by the regional anatomy.[1-3] Specifically, to rebuild the pituitary fossa and nasal and paranasal structures, traditional neurosurgical methods—that is, obtaining hemostasis by coagulation of the operative site under direct visual control, suspending and suturing the dura mater, and fusing the bone flap—cannot be used. In this chapter the alternative methods devised for successfully using the transsphenoidal approach will be discussed, focusing on the specific indications related to different pathologies.

The fundamental goals of reconstruction of the region of the sella follow:

1. Hemostasis
2. Reduction of intrasellar dead space
3. Support for suprasellar structures (the diaphragma sellae, chiasmal cistern, optic structures, and third ventricle)
4. Prevention or arrest of CSF leakage
5. Reconstitution of the integrity of the sellar floor
6. Reconstruction of nasal anatomy

To satisfy these aims, the sellar cavity must be adequately packed and the breech in the bone and dura in its floor sealed.

PACKING OF THE PITUITARY FOSSA AND RECONSTRUCTION OF THE SELLAR FLOOR

An intrasellar tumor causes an increase in the size of the sella turcica, ranging from barely perceptible in the case of a microadenoma to huge in the case of giant adenomas. During its development, an intrasellar lesion first stretches and then causes atrophy or even the disappearance of the diaphragma sellae that normally covers the pituitary fossa, dividing it from the cranial fossa, the chiasmal cistern, and the optic structures.

Removal of a sellar tumor leaves a free space within the pituitary fossa (Fig. 31-1). The walls of this space are potentially hemorrhagic; unless it is obliterated, the space will tend to fill with blood. Therefore, there is the danger of intrasellar hematoma formation with a mass effect.

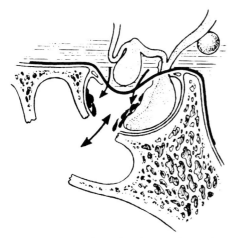

FIGURE 31-1 The conditions that frequently require correction after removal of pituitary fossa lesions. The surgical site is bloody because of many small hemorrhages that arise from the cut surface of the hypophysis and the dura mater covering the sellar floor and the cavernous sinuses. The suprasellar structures tend to be pushed toward the sellar floor because of the ineffectiveness of the sellar diaphragma. Preoperative adhesions, surgical damage, or downward distention of the chiasmal cistern favor the development of cerebrospinal fluid leaks (*upper arrows*). Communication with the septic sphenoidal sinus can lead to contamination of the sellar cavity (*double-faced arrow*).

When the pituitary fossa is not properly separated from the intracranial contents, either because of congenital incompetence of the diaphragma sella or, more commonly, because of its secondary atrophy, the pulsatile action of the brain can force the arachnoid of the chiasmal cistern down toward the sellar floor; it can then involve the optic nerves and cause their downward displacement. In the most serious cases, the third ventricle may herniate into the sellar cavity. The onset or worsening of a CSF fistula can be greatly favored.[5]

No differences exist between the microsurgical and the endoscopic endonasal transsphenoidal approach, because the modifications of sellar anatomy and the indications for sellar reconstruction are similar in both procedures. To avoid the aforementioned problems, the free intrasellar space is obliterated by filling it with substances that will ensure hemostasis and provide both immediate and future support for the suprasellar structures (Fig. 31-2). The substances that best fulfill these requirements are autologous tissues such as subcutaneous fat, fascia, or muscle. The former is preferable to muscle, because it undergoes less necrosis and less scar retraction that would result in a reduction in the volume of the packing. This avoids problems related to insufficient packing or to an excessive amount of material inserted to compensate for later loss in volume.[5] Fragments of cartilage and bone harvested from the nasal septum or the sphenoid bone[5] are easily available after the microsurgical approach, but this is not the case during the endoscopic endonasal approach. In fact, during this procedure, no cartilage is harvested from the nasal septum and only small fragments of bone are achieved from the sphenoid rostrum and the sellar floor, because "en bloc" removal could cause lacerations and bleeding of the nasal mucosa, while passing through an intact nasal cavity. These fragments are insufficient for reconstruction purposes, unless

other tissues are harvested for this purpose from the nasal turbinates[6,7] or from other donor sites of the body.

Autologous tissues are usually harvested from the abdomen or the thigh, requiring additional skin incisions, with prolonged operative time and possible cosmetic and infectious complications. Thus various heterologous or artificial materials can be used instead, mainly in cases of:

- Recurrences of sellar lesions in patients already operated on by means of a transsphenoidal approach, in which there is lack of cartilage or bone from the nasal septum
- A direct microsurgical transnasal transsphenoidal approach in which, as for the endoscopic approach, no incision of the nasal mucosa is necessary and the speculum is introduced into the nasal cavity, passing between the nasal septum and the wall of the nasal turbinates, thus providing insufficient bone or cartilage for sellar repair
- An extended microsurgical transsphenoidal approach to the sphenoid planum or the clivus, in which there is a need for adequate material to reconstruct a large bone defect

Heterologous materials used to fill the sellar cavity should have several properties. They should be absolutely inert, waterproof, and easy to shape in the residual sellar cavity so as not to leave empty spaces through which CSF can pass; have adhesive and coagulative properties so as to favor the seal of the site of CSF leakage and the hemostasis inside the sellar cavity; remain stable in size once positioned inside the sella; be easily recognizable and thus not confound the results of postoperative neuroradiologic studies (especially magnetic resonance [MR] imaging); promote and direct tissue repair so as to reestablish anatomic integrity of the sellar structures. Several heterologous materials such as fibrin or collagen sponge, fibrillar oxidized cellulose hemostat,

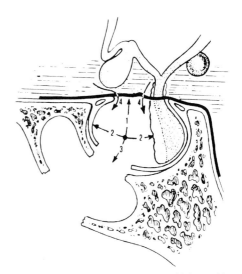

FIGURE 31-2 The basic problems at which packing of the pituitary fossa is directed (in addition to reducing the amount of intrasellar dead space): (1) to support the diaphragma sellae, the chiasmal cistern, and the suprasellar structures; (2) to ensure hemostasis of the surgical bed by contact and light compression; (3) to seal the intrasellar space against external (sphenoidal) agents, and (4) to prevent or arrest cerebrospinal fluid leaks.

Gelfoam, fibrin glue, and lyophilized dura mater[5] fulfill these requirements and have been successfully used alone or in combination for this purpose.[5] The prepared (commercially available) reabsorbable substances and lyophilized dura mater are the most easily and frequently used, with the addition of bone or cartilage fragments when necessary.

We have recently proposed the combined use of fibrin glue and collagen sponge of equine origin to fill the residual sellar cavity during endoscopic transsphenoidal surgery. The efficacy of this combination is demonstrated by the combined effects of hemostasis and stimulation of tissue repair, each of them singularly present on an effective substratum represented by the collagen sponge. This combination of materials has proved to be effective in reducing the risk of postoperative CSF leak and the need for postoperative lumbar drain.[8]

Classically, the pituitary fossa is reached by removing a 1-cm[2] segment of the floor of the sella, opening the dura in a cruciate or H-shaped fashion, and coagulating its edges for hemostasis and to provide wider access to the sella. The resultant bone defect can be repaired so as to support the materials that will eventually be used to fill the pituitary fossa and to create an effective barrier between the intrasellar and infrasellar spaces. Closure of the dura mater is deemed needless and is very difficult to accomplish. Direct closure is possible when dural edges have not been retracted because of coagulation or torn margins and they can be approximated; more often, patch-graft closure can be used.[5] If the opening of the dura of the sellar floor is made in a reversed U shape (as we at present do), a small flap that is hinged downward is obtained that gives a wide, regular, and perfectly sized access to the pituitary fossa. It can be successively replaced, providing a first, highly efficacious component for rebuilding the sellar floor.

The simplest and most effective method of restoring the integrity of the sellar floor is to use a disc of cartilage or bone harvested from the nasal septum or paranasal structures during the initial stages of the surgical exposure.[5] This material is cut to the correct shape and size and is inserted

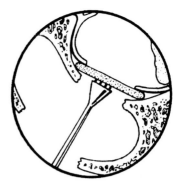

FIGURE 31-3 The sellar floor is usually easily closed by slipping a disc of cartilage or bone (or lyophilized dura mater or synthetic materials) into the extradural space. This disc generously overlaps the breech in the bone and in the dura on all sides.

below the edges of the opening in the bone, in the epidural space, so that pressure from the dura mater will help maintain its position until healing provides a true union (Fig. 31-3). However, this option is not feasible using the unilateral septal technique or the endoscopic endonasal approach, as mentioned before. Hence, in these cases, a substitute for the nasal cartilage is often required to obliterate the bone window. Different materials have been proposed to close the sellar floor instead of autologous material, each one with some advantages and disadvantages (Table 31-1).

Alumina (Al_2O_3) ceramic is a synthetic material that is neither degradable nor osteogenic, but the difficulty of modeling ceramics into the desired shape to seal the sellar floor is a disadvantage limiting its use.[9] The stainless-steel plate used to rebuild the sellar floor is tissue compatible and its position can be checked with radiographs; however, it is not in common use because of its incompatibility with MRI studies.[10] The pure titanium plate is useful and is frequently used in closing large bone defects, mainly for sellar and planum sphenoidale sealing after extended approaches. It has a hard consistency but is easily shaped to

TABLE 31-1 ▪ Summary of the Advantages and Disadvantages of the Various Synthetic Materials Used to Rebuild the Sellar Floor

Material	Advantages	Disadvantages
Alumina (Al_2O_3) ceramic	No infection No rejection	Difficult to shape
Silicone (dimethylpolysiloxene)	Easy to shape and to fit Easy to check on CT and MRI	Possibility of host-tissue reaction
Stainless-steel plate	Easily checked on radiography	Difficult to shape Chemically instable Interference with CT and MRI
Pure titanium	No infection No rejection Chemically stable	Difficult to shape Minimal interference with MRI
Resorbable vicryl patches (polyglactin 910/poly-*p*-dioxanone)	Resorbable	Difficult interpretation on early postop MRI
MacroSorb (polylactide polymers)	Resorbable	Porous Malleable at 70°C (difficult to shape)
Polyester-silicone	Easy to shape and to fit Easy to check on CT and MRI	Possibility of host-tissue reaction

CT, computed tomography; MRI, magnetic resonance imaging.

FIGURE 31-4 *A*, Lines along which the sellar floor can be cut if it has a paper-like consistency. *B*, Two small flaps are reflected to the sides, parallel to the carotid artery grooves.

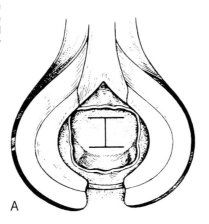 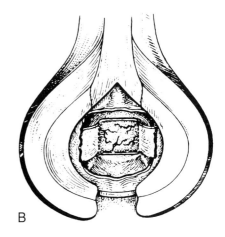

the bone window; its main disadvantages are a minimal ferromagnetic artifact on MRI studies and its cost.[11]

The silicon plate, a synthetic material that possesses a hardness very similar to that of cartilage, has an excellent sealing effectiveness in closing the sellar floor and is easily detected, either intraoperatively or on postoperative MRI. Its only risk is the possibility of a delayed immune response to a foreign body; even though this event is extremely rare, it has been reported in individuals with a predisposition to a strong host-tissue reaction to a foreign body.[12] Prostheses of synthetic histoacrylic resin, and lyophilized bone have also been used.[5] Furthermore, for fusion of the plug (whatever its nature), biologic glues or natural derivatives have been used.[13] Among the resorbable substances, Vicryl (polyglactin 910) patches[14] and plates made from amorphous polymers[15] have been recently proposed with the aim of restoring the anatomic integrity of the sella without leaving a foreign body inside it. Both have proved effective in sealing the bone defect, but the first seems too soft to be used alone and the second is not easy to shape. In our experience with the endoscopic endonasal approach, we have used a polyester-silicone dural substitute (Cousin Biotech, Wervicq-Sud, France) for sellar reconstruction.[16] It is tailored by means of scissors to the adequate size and is introduced in a bent fashion, through the nostril, to be released and spontaneously opened in the chosen site (intradurally and/or extradurally), where a reactive fibrosis occurs thereafter. Its elastic properties allow this material to pass through the nasal cavity without causing lesions to the mucosa. It is compatible and recognizable by diagnostic neuroimaging, and in case of repeat surgery it is easily identified and incised. Analogous results can be obtained with discs of lyophilized dura mater or fascia lata.

In cases in which the floor of the sella is paper thin, it can be opened by cutting two small lateral bone flaps, which can be turned to the side (Fig. 31-4); when the floor is reconstructed, the bone flaps are returned to their original position and secured either by fixing them to each other and to the edges of the breech in the bone or by threading a strip of cartilage beneath the upper and lower margins of the hole in the bone, bridging the medial edge of the two juxtaposed bone flaps (Fig. 31-5). Because the bone edges fit together perfectly and the periosteum has been preserved, the chances for physiologic union of the sella floor are improved.[5]

Methods for Reconstructing the Pituitary Fossa

The underlying lesion and conditions encountered during surgery determine the manner in which the sellar region is reconstructed. Although the needs of each case during surgery are the main guide, general criteria can be formulated for the principal methods.

FIGURE 31-5 To reconstruct the sellar floor after it is opened as noted in Figure 31-4, the bone flaps are returned to their natural position. They can be secured by fitting them into each other and to the edges of the sellar opening (*A*). When this approach proves unreliable, a strip of cartilage can be threaded beneath the edges of the hole in the bone bridging the medial edge of the two juxtaposed bone flaps (*B*).

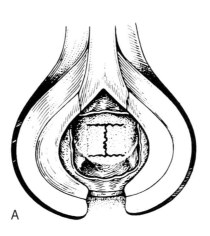 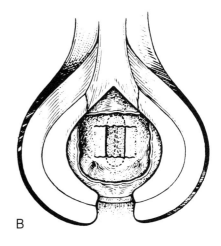

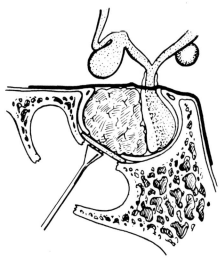

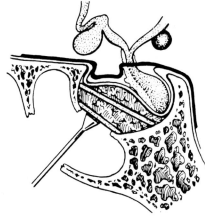

FIGURE 31-6 Simple intradural packing. The packing materials are inserted intradurally, completely filling the intrasellar space. A disc of cartilage or similar material is fitted extradurally close to the sellar floor. (From Spaziante R, de Divitiis E, Cappabianca P: Reconstruction of the pituitary fossa in transsphenoidal surgery: An experience of 140 cases. Neurosurgery 17:453, 1985.)

FIGURE 31-7 Extradural packing. Intradural free space is greatly reduced by detaching the dura mater from the sellar floor. The extradural space is filled with the usual materials interposed between the two cartilage discs, the larger one in contact with the dura mater, the other closing the hole in the sella. (From Spaziante R, de Divitiis E, Cappabianca P: Reconstruction of the pituitary fossa in transsphenoidal surgery: An experience of 140 cases. Neurosurgery 17:453, 1985.)

Simple Intradural Packing

Simple intradural packing is the fundamental method suggested in most classic descriptions of transsphenoidal surgery.[5] Materials for packing the sellar cavity are introduced into the intradural space, and the plug that closes the floor is fixed into the epidural space (Fig. 31-6). This is easily and rapidly performed and is the ideal solution when the empty space left at the end of the operation is no larger than the sella turcica.

This approach has two main limitations: (1) the packing cannot be very tight, even when this is needed, because the pressure developing within the sella is transmitted to suprasellar and parasellar structures, and (2) the packing material is not solidly adherent to the walls of the fossa and can move about.

Extradural Packing

The dura covering the sellar floor can be easily detached from the floor and elevated as far as the insertion to the

cavernous sinus, of which it forms the medial wall, preventing further elevation. The wide space thus obtained can then be packed with the same materials as mentioned earlier (Fig. 31-7), which are interposed between two large bone-cartilage discs, one corresponding with the dural hole, the other with the breech in the bone.[5]

This type of packing can be particularly tight and hermetic, because the elastic forces produced by distending the dura mater make it more compact and stable. Furthermore, there is no risk of introducing an excessive amount of packing material, because the dura cannot be interrupted or elevated beyond the limits imposed by its own elasticity. Thus there is no risk of excessive pressure being transmitted to perisellar structures (Fig. 31-8).

Combined Extradural-Intradural Packing

Extradural packing is advantageous from many points of view; it does not allow complete packing of a particularly large residual cavity, however, because there is a limit to the degree of dural movement at the sellar floor. In this situation,

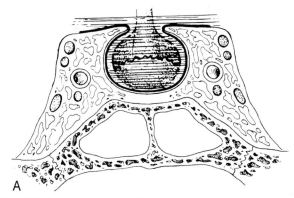

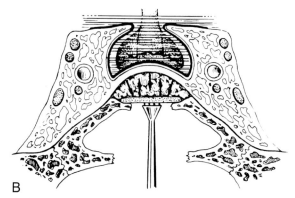

FIGURE 31-8 Cross section of the pituitary fossa along a coronal plane before (A) and after (B) extradural packing. The dura mater of the sellar floor is joined to the walls of the cavernous sinuses. When it is detached from the floor and pushed upward, its distention creates elastic forces that compress the packing materials. The risk of overpacking is avoided, because the dura cannot be elevated to an unlimited degree; increased pressure inside the packed space is not transmitted to suprasellar and perisellar structures. (From Spaziante R, de Divitiis E, Cappabianca P: Reconstruction of the pituitary fossa in transsphenoidal surgery: An experience of 140 cases. Neurosurgery 17:453, 1985.)

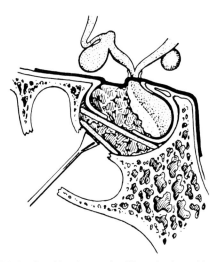

FIGURE 31-9 Combined extradural-intradural packing. The free space within the pituitary fossa is partly filled intradurally; extradural packing, as mentioned earlier, is performed afterward. (From Spaziante R, de Divitiis E, Cappabianca P: Reconstruction of the pituitary fossa in transsphenoidal surgery: An experience of 140 cases. Neurosurgery 17:453, 1985.)

the ideal solution is to make part of the packing intradural (producing volume) and part extradural (providing stability, solidity, and watertight closure) (Fig. 31-9).

The "Open Sella" Technique

Packing of the pituitary fossa and closure of the sellar floor are not mandatory. In patients undergoing subtotal or only partial removal of sellar tumors with suprasellar extension with no evidence of intraoperative CSF leakage, the intrasellar space and the sellar floor may be left unreconstructed.[17] This approach can be helpful in dealing with large macroadenomas that do not descend after the complete removal of the intrasellar tumor either spontaneously or after "provocative" maneuvers (Valsalva maneuver, subarachnoidal injection of saline solution or air, referred to as the "pumping technique"). In this case, intentionally staged removal of the lesion can be planned without aggressively pursuing additional suprasellar tumors. Care must be taken not to produce CSF leakage. Using the open sella method, the remaining suprasellar tumor often delivers into the sellar space within a couple of months, at which time it can be safely removed with a second operation, delaying the need for immediate radiotherapy or reducing the residue volume to a size suitable for radiosurgery (Fig. 31-10). The open sella technique and the intentionally staged operation broaden the indications for the transsphenoidal route also to giant and invasive sellar tumors, whose radical removal by means of more traumatic transcranial approaches is foolishly ambitious in any case.[18]

The choice not to rebuild sellar structures can be advantageous also in case of diffuse bleeding of the suprasellar tumoral residue. In such a case, sellar packing, which should never extend above the interclinoidal plane, is not only useless but also potentially dangerous, because it hinders spontaneous blood drainage with subsequent formation of suprasellar hematomas (Fig. 31-11).

PACKING AND CLOSURE OF THE SPHENOIDAL SINUS

Packing of the sphenoidal sinus is not universally accepted as mechanically useful,[5] but we use this technique to support

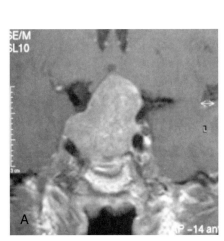
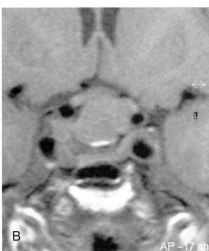
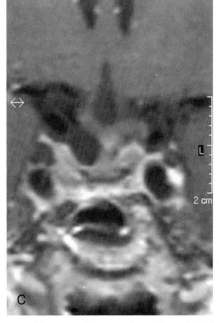

FIGURE 31-10 *A,* A 61-year-old female patient harboring a large nonfunctioning macroadenoma with suprasellar extension. After subtotal transsphenoidal removal, visual field abnormalities rapidly improved. *B,* Magnetic resonance (MR) imaging performed after 5 months showed slight suprasellar extension and the sellar space filled by the tumor residue. Hence, the patient was operated on again by a transsphenoidal approach, with further improvement of visual disturbances. *C,* MR follow-up at 3 months demonstrated gross total removal with complete decompression of optic structures. The patient has been under close follow-up, and radiotherapy has not been performed 6 years after the first operation, because no tumor regrowth has been demonstrated.

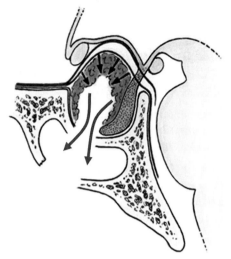

FIGURE 31-11 Schematic drawing illustrating the "open sella" technique. Neither sellar packing nor sellar floor reconstruction is performed so as to allow spontaneous blood drainage into the sphenoid sinus (*bold arrows*) and possible delivery in the sellar space of suprasellar tumor remnants (*small arrows*).

the sellar floor when it is particularly stretched and inconsistent ("ghost" sella) and to create a less septic postoperative environment by using reabsorbable substances soaked in an antibacterial solution.

The same materials are used as for packing the pituitary fossa. The simplest method is to use a fibrin or gelatin sponge soaked in antibiotic solution, together with residual bone-cartilage fragments. The largest fragment can be used to approximately reconstruct the anterior wall of the sphenoidal sinus and separate it from the nasal fossa. Hermetic closure of the sphenoidal sinus by synthetic materials, bone cements, or resins does not prevent the aforementioned mechanical complications or CSF leakage and adds the risks of foreign body reaction and chemical osteitis.[5] Moreover, it prohibits or greatly impedes repeat operation by the transsphenoidal route, which may be necessary either if, despite careful rebuilding of the sellar region, mechanical complications arise, or, later, because of the progression of the pituitary disease.

Filling of the sphenoidal sinus is not indicated if the open sella method has been used, because hemostasis at the operative site is inadequate; a permeable sphenoidal sinus is an excellent route for draining blood that might collect in the pituitary fossa during the first hours after surgery. Likewise, in the case of an intentionally staged operation, a free sphenoidal sinus facilitates the spontaneous descent of the residual tumor.[17,18]

RECONSTRUCTION OF NASAL STRUCTURES

Reconstruction of nasal structures is usually limited to either (nonobligatory) reapposition of the cartilage of the nasal septum, in cases in which this has been removed, or returning the nasal septum to the midline, in the case of a unilateral transseptal approach. The two nostrils are filled with medicated nonadhesive gauze. In the transnasal approach, the columella is held by three or four sutures, of which one transfixes deeply. If a transnasal unilateral approach is

performed, no suture is required, the nasal mucosa being simply replaced on the septum. Nasal packing has been recognized as one of the most common complaints in patients undergoing microsurgical transsphenoidal approach.[19] Hence, to obviate the need for postoperative nasal packing, one recent proposal has been to stitch together the mucosal flaps with a running suture on a short septal needle in a continuous, mattress quilting fashion.[20] When the transoral route is used, the gingival mucosa can be reapposed with a few stitches or can even be left open. Reconstruction of nasal structure and the need for nasal packing is unnecessary during the endoscopic endonasal transsphenoidal approach where submucosal septal dissection is not performed. In fact, the endoscope is inserted in the chosen nostril up to the middle turbinate, which is gently pushed laterally to enlarge the space between itself and the nasal septum. It is subsequently advanced between the inferior turbinate and the nasal septum, up to the choana, where it is angled upward, in the sphenoethmoid recess, for about 1.5 cm, until the natural sphenoid ostium is reached (Fig. 31-12).[21,22]

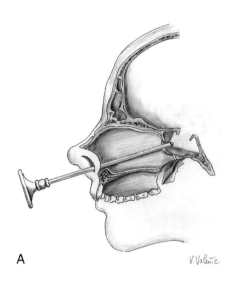

A

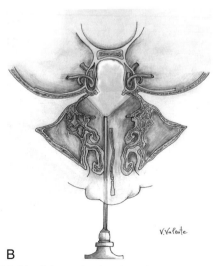

B

FIGURE 31-12 Schematic drawing showing the endoscopic endonasal transsphenoidal approach in sagittal (*A*) and axial (*B*) projection. With this approach the angle of vision is increased from the planum to the clivus (*A*) and from one bony protuberance of the internal carotid artery to the other one (*B*).

INDICATIONS IN RELATION TO THE MOST FREQUENT SELLAR DISEASES

Several variables determine the method used to reconstruct the pituitary fossa. The possibilities range from situations in which no packing or reconstruction of the sellar walls is necessary to those in which they must be performed with obsessive precision.

Pituitary Microadenoma

The size and topographic relationships of pituitary microadenomas mean that there is rarely a need to pack the residual cavity after their removal. Hemostasis usually occurs by the time the lesion has been removed. Suprasellar structures are not involved by the adenoma and are supported naturally (Fig. 31-13). Reconstruction of the sellar floor with a cartilaginous plug fixed in the epidural space is useful for separating the pituitary fossa from the sphenoidal sinus (Fig. 31-14). Two situations, however, may require effective packing: (1) extension of the microadenoma toward the cavernous sinus with persistent hemorrhage after its removal,[5] and (2) a coexisting spontaneous or intraoperatively formed intrasellar arachnoidocele, which rarely occurs. In the event of CSF leakage (which may occur when radical removal is pursued), the provisions outlined later on would have to be implemented.[5]

Intrasellar Adenomas (Mesoadenomas)

In case of intrasellar adenomas (adenomas confined within an enlarged sella or slightly indenting the chiasmal cistern), the sellar cavity is wider than normal and can be very large (e.g., in the case of large adenomas developing downward). The diaphragma sellae is usually atrophied as a result of pressure from the adenoma; nonetheless, suprasellar structures (the cisterns and optic pathways) are virtually unaffected by the growth of the adenoma. Packing the cavity is useful both in ensuring hemostasis of the large cavity and in supporting the suprasellar structures, which could otherwise herniate downward and cause immediate or delayed onset of the empty sella syndrome. Because there is much downward distention of the dura of the sella (Fig. 31-15), extradural packing can be very easy and efficacious and does not carry the risk of overpacking (Fig. 31-16). If intradural packing is used, its upward extent must be checked

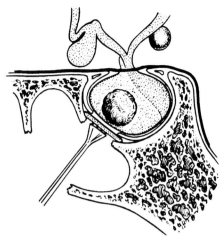

FIGURE 31-13 After removal of a microadenoma, there is usually no need to fill the sellar cavity because of the relationships between the residual cavity and the surrounding anatomic structures. However, plugging the sellar floor with a cartilage disc fitted extradurally may be advisable to restore the sellar wall.

fluoroscopically (Fig. 31-17) to ensure that the packing does not extend above the interclinoid plane.[5]

Adenoma with Large Suprasellar Extension

Large tumors with suprasellar extension present many unfavorable features that influence postoperative complications. The diaphragma sellae is incompetent, and there is compression, stretching, and adherence of the dome of the adenoma to suprasellar and cerebral structures; in some places, adenomatous tissue may reach beyond the capsule. The sella turcica is larger than normal, although its volume is not always proportionate to the overall volume of the adenoma. Following surgical removal, the residual cavity is very large and most of it is out of direct control. These are the most suitable conditions for the development of mechanical complications such as hematomas or empty sella syndrome. CSF leakage can develop because of an interruption in the continuity of the chiasmatic cistern by the adenoma, its accidental rupture during surgery, or as a result of excessive stretching postoperatively.

FIGURE 31-14 An intraoperative fluoroscopic image. *A,* The residual cavity is filled with a sponge soaked in iodinated medium after removal of a microadenoma. *B,* An extradural cartilage disc (*arrowhead*) closes the sellar floor and reduces the intradural free space.

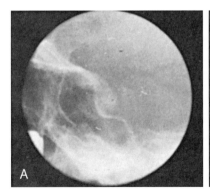
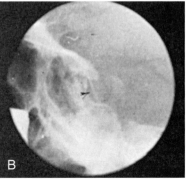

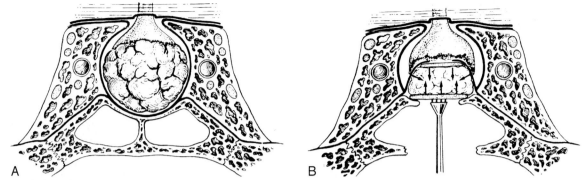

FIGURE 31-15 A cross section of the pituitary fossa along a coronal plane before (*A*) and after (*B*) removal of a large intrasellar adenoma, followed by extradural packing of the residual cavity. Because the dura mater of the sellar floor has been greatly distended, it can be detached very easily and extensively raised before the walls of the cavernous sinus are tightened. Almost the entire intrasellar residual cavity can be filled in this way.

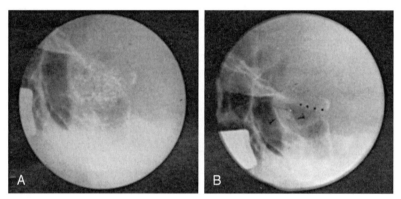

FIGURE 31-16 An intraoperative fluoroscopic image. *A,* The residual cavity after removal of a large intrasellar adenoma is visualized by a radiopaque cottonoid. *B,* The outside and inside limits of extradural packing (*open arrowheads*). The correct position of the diaphragma sellae is outlined by the air bubble remaining within the pituitary fossa (*dotted line*).

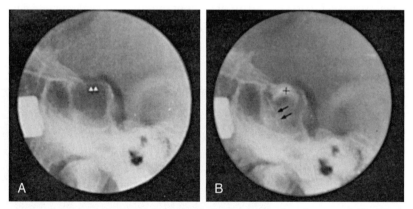

FIGURE 31-17 An intraoperative fluoroscopic image of the removal of a large intrasellar adenoma. *A,* The diaphragma sellae (*white arrowheads*) is outlined by an air bubble within the pituitary fossa, whereas the chiasmal cistern is visualized by means of perioperative pneumoencephalography. *B,* Intradural filling of the defect with reabsorbable materials, the upper limit of which is marked with a sponge soaked in iodinated contrast medium (*cross*). The sellar floor is closed with numerous bone and cartilage fragments that have been inserted extradurally (*arrows*).

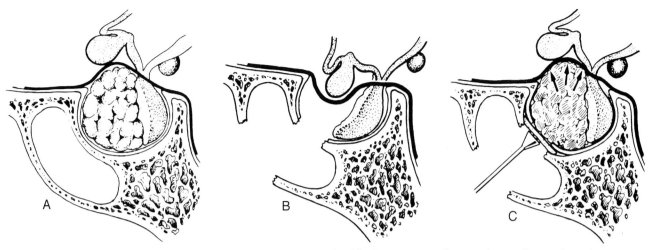

FIGURE 31-18 After removal of an adenoma with suprasellar extension (*A*), there are many features that predispose the patient to post-operative mechanical complications, such as empty sella syndrome, cerebrospinal fluid rhinorrhea, and hemorrhage (*B*). An effective intradural tamponade carries the risk of excessive tightness, causing compression of the suprasellar structures similar to that produced by the growth of the adenoma (*C*). (From Spaziante R, de Divitiis E, Cappabianca P: Reconstruction of the pituitary fossa in transsphenoidal surgery: An experience of 140 cases. Neurosurgery 17:453, 1985.)

Adequately packing this space can be a difficult problem. To fill the cavity completely (Fig. 31-18) would create the same consequences as those caused by the adenoma.[5] To prevent overpacking, filling must be strictly limited to the intrasellar space, its upper limit remaining well beneath the interclinoid plane. Such packing, which is disproportionate to the volume of the residual cavity, risks being mobile and thus ineffective. Furthermore, it may create an obstacle to spontaneous drainage of residual bleeding from surgical bed. These difficulties can be greatly reduced after the adenoma has been removed by returning the chiasmal cistern to its natural position. This can occur spontaneously, or it can be achieved by introducing either a small amount of air or Ringer's solution into the subarachnoid space via a lumbar catheter (perioperative pneumoencephalography) or by compressing the jugular vein in the neck for a few seconds (Fig. 31-19). Greater amounts of air may be injected in more resistant cases (forced cistern air dissection or "pumping" technique).[5] When the capsule of

the adenoma returns to the sellar cavity, the situation becomes analogous to that of an intrasellar adenoma, although it must be remembered that the diaphragma sellae is completely incompetent. Special consideration must be given to cases of giant invasive or hourglass adenoma, in which to achieve intentionally staged surgical removal the "open sella" technique should be used (see section on The "Open Sella" Technique).

Ghost Sella

Ghost sella is particularly problematic, because the large size of the sella and the flimsiness of the floor may prevent efficient performance of any of the methods of repair described. This problem occurs very rarely, but when it is encountered, it may be necessary to resort to intradural packing (Fig. 31-20), combined with packing of the sphenoidal sinus with muscle, fat, and bone-cartilage fragments.[5]

FIGURE 31-19 An intraoperative fluoroscopic image. *A,* Following removal of an adenoma with an extensive suprasellar extension, the dome of the tumor remains raised (*arrowheads*). *B,* Injection of fractionated amounts of air through a lumbar spinal catheter pushed it downward, refilling the chiasmal cistern and dissecting the loose adhesions from surrounding structures.

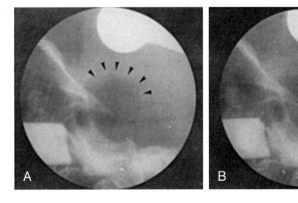

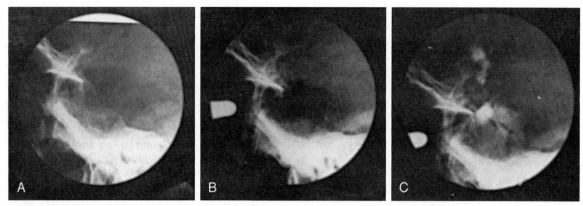

FIGURE 31-20 An intraoperative fluoroscopic image. *A,* A giant pituitary adenoma with extensive suprasellar extension. The sella turcica has completely disappeared. *B,* The residual cavity after removal of the tumor spontaneously filled with air. *C,* Widespread intradural packing with fat lightly soaked in water-soluble nonionic iodinated contrast medium to avoid the risk of overpacking. Some contrast has escaped into the cisternal spaces through an apparently spontaneous disruption of the subarachnoid layer. (Preoperatively, the patient complained of a spontaneous intratumoral hemorrhage.)

Empty Sella

A pituitary adenoma can often be accompanied by an intrasellar arachnoidocele as a consequence of spontaneous necrosis or previous treatment.[23] During removal of the adenomatous tissue, the arachnoid must be protected and elevated and returned to its natural position[5] to avoid risk of CSF leakage and to prevent the serious complications that an empty sella can eventually provoke. Packing must be of sufficient volume, consistency, and stability to avoid recurrence of the empty sella. Extradural mixed packing is probably the best type of repair in this situation, because the arachnoid is protected with a strip of lyophilized dura before being very carefully elevated.[24–26]

Correction of a pure empty sella presents specific problems related to the symptoms to be corrected. The aims of such an operation are to elevate the chiasm and optic structures in cases involving visual disturbances; to prevent progressive stretching and erosion of the sellar floor as a result of transmission by the CSF of the pulsatile action of the brain; to prevent compression and distortion of the pituitary gland and its stalk, and to prevent (or arrest) CSF leakage.[27] The recommended operation in our experience consists of an extradural packing that must be well proportioned, avoiding the risk of overpacking, carried out with minimal trauma, and very stable over time. Elevation of the dura mater greatly reduces the space within the sella, allowing intradural and suprasellar structures to be lifted without the risk of being damaged by direct surgical maneuvers; because they are not directly manipulated, they are protected by the dural and the arachnoidal planes and their upward displacement is self-limited by the insertion of the dura mater of the sellar floor on the medial wall of the cavernous sinuses. Several autologous tissues and prosthetic materials have been suggested for filling the sellar space and for reconstructing the sellar floor, as mentioned earlier. Recently we described a method we have used, aimed at achieving a more stable and simple chiasmapexy and arachnoidopexy,[25] consisting of an extradural sellar packing accomplished by means of a Silastic tube arranged in a

spiral form by means of three transfixed sutures (Fig. 31-21). The resulting "coil" is very easy to create, and it can be quickly tailored to the desired size without the need of complex preoperative measurements. Because the tube is radiopaque and easily recognized on fluoroscopy, the risk of sellar overpacking is reduced (Fig. 31-22). Moreover, it is very elastic (thus minimizing mechanical damage), and it does not present volume changes over time, unlike fat or muscle, both of which bring about necrosis or scar retraction, or deflation as in the case of an inflatable balloon.[28,29] No further skin incisions to harvest autologous tissues (fat or muscle) are necessary, thus lowering the possibility of either cosmetic or infectious complications. Last but not least, this procedure is inexpensive if one considers the low cost of a Silastic catheter for ventricular shunting. We have used this technique to treat primary as well as secondary symptomatic empty sella with excellent results in terms of visual improvement and stable sellar filling (Fig. 31-23).[24–26]

Craniopharyngiomas

The transsphenoidal approach to craniopharyngiomas has limited application, and it is best reserved for patients with preferably cystic extra-arachnoid-infradiaphragmatic tumors with small suprasellar extension, who represent a percentage of 10% to 20% of cases.[30] More recently, its indications have been extended also to lesions with prevalent suprasellar location.[31] Enlargement of the sella turcica and intrasellar development of the tumor are prerequisite for planning a transsphenoidal approach; furthermore, the chiasmal cistern must not lie between the sellar floor and tumor. Relationships with the pituitary gland are less limiting, because it may be split to provide access to the tumor. A transsphenoidal approach is realistically applicable to a greater number of large cystic craniopharyngiomas if the aim is to drain them into the sphenoid sinus. Part of the cystic component, of course, must be intrasellar. Even with a relevant suprasellar portion, in fact, complete emptying of grossly cystic lesions can easily be achieved.

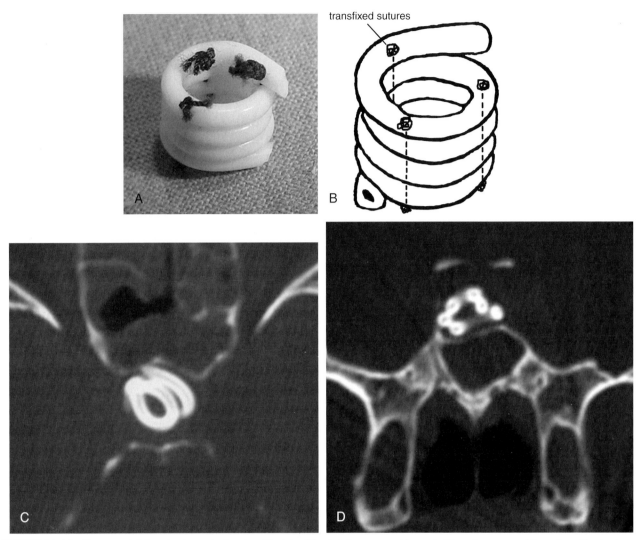

FIGURE 31-21   Photograph (*A*) and schematic drawing (*B*) of the Silastic tube arranged in a spiral form by means of three transfixed sutures. Axial (*C*) and coronal (*D*) computed tomography (CT) scan (bone window) showing the Silastic coil placed within the sella.

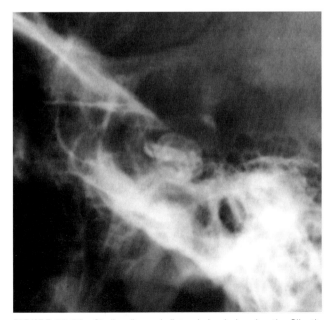

FIGURE 31-22   Skull radiograph (lateral view) showing the Silastic coil in the sellar space.

A wide opening is made in the sellar floor, exposing the cyst wall. The cyst wall is incised, allowing spontaneous outflow of the contents, completed by suction and curettage. The cyst wall is then carefully dissected and removed as far as it is possible. Suitable maneuvers (such as forced air injection of the retrosellar and suprasellar cisterns) are useful to demonstrate the thickness of the solid part of the tumor, to verify an actual cleavage plane with the infundibular area, and to push downward the dome of the tumor. If removal of the cyst wall proves to be critical or even impossible because of a close relationship with surrounding structures, a variation of the described "open sella" technique can be implemented. A permanent transsellar communication between the cyst and the sphenoidal sinus is established—provided the absence of any passage of CSF has been verified—to allow continuous, spontaneous draining of the cyst fluid, thus preventing reexpansion of the tumor (cystosphenoidostomy). Once such a communication has been established, of course, any hazardous maneuver must be avoided that can cause CSF leakage. The permanent fistula is established by means of a Silastic catheter, arranged in a self-securing "X" or bent "H" fashion, placed at the floor

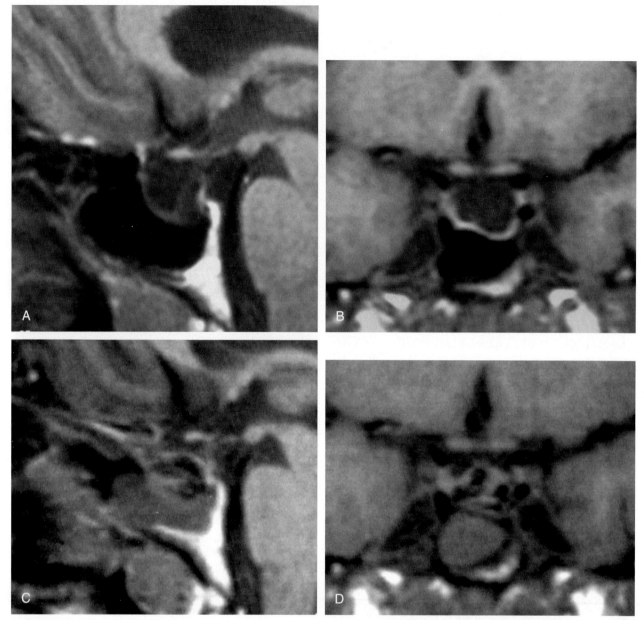

FIGURE 31-23 Primary empty sella: preoperative sagittal (*A*) and coronal (*B*) T1-weighted MR images. Postoperative MRI performed at 1 year (*C* and *D*) shows stable lifting of intrasellar structures. The chiasma and the pituitary stalk are in the normal position; the pituitary gland is raised at the interclinoidal plane, and the sellar cavity is filled by the Silastic coil.

opening so that two arms are within the pituitary fossa and the other two in the sphenoidal sinus (Fig. 31-24). Performed by us for the first time in 1986 as an unplanned expedient (as suggested by Laws[32]) facing unforeseen difficulties of obtaining a radical tumor removal, this method proved to be quite effective and successful, and at present it has been used in more than 25 cases with no mortality or morbidity (Fig. 31-25). Once temporary control of tumor mass has been achieved by such a derivative technique, radiotherapy, with its detrimental effect on visual and pituitary function, especially in younger patients, can be delayed to a more suitable time after surgery, or even suspended with no time limit under careful neuroradiologic follow-up.[33]

Other Sellar Lesions

Other lesions more rarely approached by the transsphenoidal route (e.g., arachnoid cysts, dermoid cysts, meningiomas, chondromas, metastases) involve intraoperative variables similar to those of the more common conditions and can be treated in an analogous manner.[34-36]

Arachnoidal cysts have both intrasellar and suprasellar growth and features similar to those of pituitary adenomas with suprasellar extension (Fig. 31-26); however, their walls do not readily heal solidly postoperatively and they can communicate with the subarachnoid space through a unidirectional valve mechanism, favoring the entry and accumulation of CSF under pressure and the subsequent development

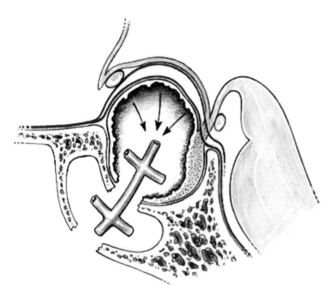

FIGURE 31-24 Schematic drawing of a transsellar permanent communication between the residual cavity of a craniopharyngioma and the sphenoidal sinus by means of a Silastic catheter arranged in an **H** shape.

of CSF rhinorrhea. Postoperative mechanical complications are, therefore, more frequent.

Cerebrospinal Fluid Rhinorrhea

Frequently, but not exclusively, a nontraumatic CSF rhinorrhea occurs as the consequence of the development of an empty sella or a pituitary adenoma.[23] This is perhaps the most difficult condition to treat by the transsphenoidal approach. It can occur as an intraoperative complication in 6% to 20% of cases, depending on the characteristics of the sellar lesion. Furthermore, it can occur as an immediate or delayed postoperative complication in 3% to 6.4% of cases, requiring repeat operation in 1.5% to 2% of cases, although the frequency is decreasing in recent clinical series.[23] The success

rate of an operation or repeat operation for CSF rhinorrhea remains disappointing, with cure rates of approximately 80%, even in patients who have undergone several operations.

The method of sellar reconstruction for repair of a CSF leak must be meticulous, because such a leak can create serious postoperative problems.[23] A strip of fascia lata or lyophilized dura is placed to protect the arachnoid and the diaphragma sellae; the sellar cavity is then partially filled with muscle or subcutaneous fat inserted into the intradural space. A second strip of fascia or lyophilized dura is used on the inner surface of the dura mater to close it.[5] A particularly precise extradural packing is then performed (Figs. 31-27 and 31-28). Continuous CSF lumbar drainage is highly recommended for at least 72 hours to allow the plugging material to consolidate, thus diverting the CSF flow from the fistula and decreasing the CSF pressure. Its working rates must be carefully checked, however, to avoid risk of pneumocephalus, which may even develop into a tension pneumocephalus. To obviate the need for tissue graft, absorbable materials such as Vicryl patches combined with gelatin foam soaked in fibrin glue, a simplified repair using a two-layered collagen sponge technique, or a combination of collagen sponge with fibrin glue have been reported to be effective not only in prevention, but also in the treatment of intraoperative CSF leaks, with or without lumbar drainage.[5,8,14,37]

ERRORS AND COMMON COMPLICATIONS

Reconstruction of the pituitary fossa may be ineffective because either a nonsuitable method was chosen or the volume of packing material inserted was inadequate, either from the outset or because of its subsequent retraction or necrosis (Fig. 31-29) or because it was excessive. The consequences can be: (1) an intrasellar hematoma, (2) contamination of the cavity, (3) postoperative empty sella, or (4) CSF leakage. Care must be taken not to interpret a hyperdense lesion seen on an early postoperative computed tomography (CT) scan as a true postoperative hematoma

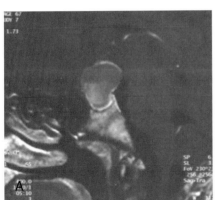
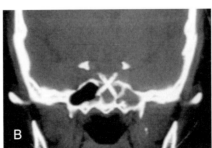
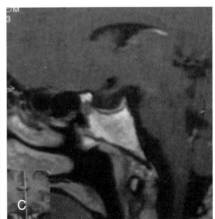

FIGURE 31-25 *A,* Sagittal MR of a huge cystic craniopharyngioma treated by transsphenoidal partial removal with permanent cystosphenoidostomy obtained by means an X-shaped catheter, well recognizable at CT scan (bone window) (*B*). Visual disturbances improved immediately after the operation. *C,* Follow-up at 1 year. The tumor is no longer recognizable, and the patient is free of symptoms. No radiotherapy has been carried out. Annual MR controls up to 7 years showed unmodified findings.

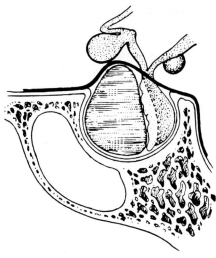

FIGURE 31-26 An intrasellar and suprasellar arachnoid cyst. The anatomic conditions are similar to those of an adenoma with suprasellar extension (see also Fig. 31-18). Even if emptying is surgically more favorable, the structural characteristics of the cyst wall and its relationship with cerebrospinal fluid (CSF) pathways may favor the development of postoperative mechanical complications.

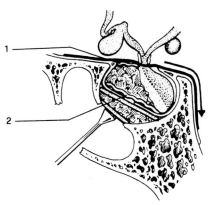

FIGURE 31-27 General rules for packing to treat CSF leakage. The first strip of fascia lata or lyophilized dura mater reinforces the diaphragma sellae and arachnoid of the chiasmal cistern (1). Partial intradural packing is performed, and the dura mater of the sellar floor is closed and reinforced with a second strip of fascia or lyophilized dura (2). Reconstruction of the sella is completed by extradural packing. The *arrow* running along the dorsum sellae demonstrates the usefulness of continuous spinal lumbar drainage during the operation and for the first few postoperative days.

(the actual frequency of which is <1% of cases)[3] (Fig. 31-30), because materials such as oxidized cellulose, Avitene, and fibrin sponge absorb blood and have an appearance on CT scans similar to that of a true blood clot. Also, a certain degree of intrasellar arachnoidocele is a common finding on postoperative radiographic studies and is not a complication unless there are symptoms of an empty sella syndrome, but this is a rare occurrence.[23]

Cerebrospinal fluid rhinorrhea can be transitory or prolonged. Prolonged CSF rhinorrhea persists for days after surgery, and when it does not improve despite suitable provisions, it requires surgical intervention (using the transsphenoidal, transethmoidal, or transcranial routes, a transnasal transseptal endoscopic or even a CSF shunting procedure).[38] Transitory CSF leakage is frequently seen in the early postoperative period but usually stops within a few hours or days, either spontaneously or after continuous CSF drainage. We believe that this measure should be used whenever a CSF leak occurs, whether it is before, during, or immediately after surgery.[5] Therefore, we routinely insert

a lumbar spinal subarachnoid catheter at the outset of the operation in all patients operated on by a microsurgical transsphenoidal approach, except those with a true microadenoma unless problems related to CSF leakage are anticipated.[5] According to this method, in our most recent series (1995–2003), intraoperative CSF leakage was present in 27 cases out of 258 transsphenoidal procedures, but none was followed by postoperative rhinorrhea or required surgical correction. On the contrary, with the endoscopic technique, a lumbar drainage is not usually used; it is adopted only in case of intraoperative CSF leak, when the closure is not judged absolutely watertight, where there are minimal postoperative CSF leaks, or after extended cranial base approaches with removal of the tuberculum sellae and part of the planum sphenoidale.

Excessive packing of the sella is a less frequent event; it is most serious and perhaps most common consequence is extension into the suprasellar cistern (Fig. 31-31), which recreates de novo chiasmal compression and alteration in the visual fields. In addition to the situation where there

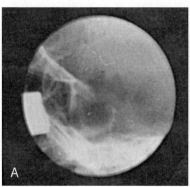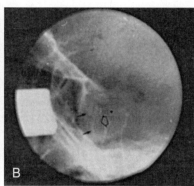

FIGURE 31-28 An intraoperative fluoroscopic image. *A*, Intraoperative CSF leakage after complete removal of a pituitary tumor with intrasellar and suprasellar extensions is clearly demonstrated by spontaneous entrance of air into the suprasellar cistern. *B*, Combined extradural-intradural packing of the sellar cavity. The first strip of lyophilized dura (not visible and indicated by the *asterisk*) reinforces the arachnoid. A second strip of lyophilized dura marked with iodinated contrast medium reinforces the dura mater of the sellar floor (*open arrows*). The packing is completed extradurally (*arrows*).

FIGURE 31-29 A roentgenogram of the sella turcica (lateral view). *A,* Five days and 3 months (*B*) after a transsphenoidal operation. The bone fragment limiting the extradural packing (*arrowheads*) is lowered because of scarring and retraction of the packing material.

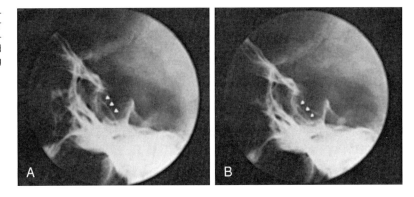

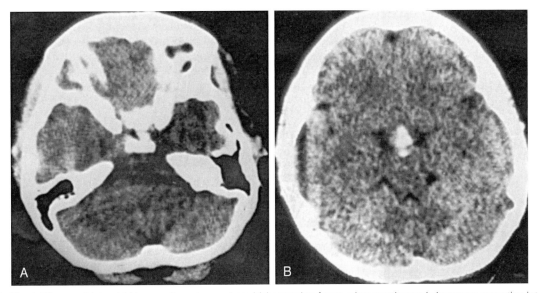

FIGURE 31-30 A CT scan obtained 24 hours after a transsphenoidal operation for an adrenocorticotropic hormone–secreting intrasellar and suprasellar adenoma demonstrating a bloody hyperdensity simulating a hematoma within the tumor bed that appears to be both intrasellar (*A*) and suprasellar (*B*). Because the patient was complaining of worsening vision, she was operated on again. A hemostatic sponge was found.

FIGURE 31-31 An intraoperative fluoroscopic image. *A,* An intrasellar adenoma bulging into the chiasmal cistern. Combined extradural (*arrows*) and intradural packing. There is so much intradural packing material (lightly soaked in iodinated contrast medium) that its upper limit (*arrowheads*) indents the suprasellar cistern demonstrated by means of perioperative pneumoencephalography. *B,* The amount of packing was reduced, freeing the chiasmal cistern. Its upper limit (*open white arrows*) is at the interclinoid plane. The *white arrowheads* outline the extradural packing.

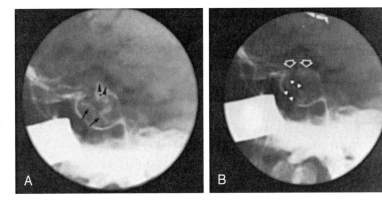

is an unperceived introduction of overabundant filling materials, overpacking is usually a consequence of an attempt to cure intraoperative CSF leakage, a diffuse hemorrhage from a cut surface, or a severe hemorrhage originating from a cavernous sinus. If moderate in amount, the consequences of overpacking may regress because of the expected reduction in the volume of packing materials; otherwise, it is better to operate again and remove this material rather than risk a useless and probably damaging wait. Excessive intrasellar compression, excessive traction, or distortion of the dura mater of the sellar floor and of the wall of the cavernous sinus may cause paresis of the oculomotor nerves, postoperative trigeminal syndrome, or intense and persistent postoperative headaches. More exceptional complications caused by overpacking of the sella include compression or spasm of the carotid artery in its intracavernous segment.[5,23]

Personal Experience

Indications for sellar reconstruction have evolved considerably in our own experience. We do now reconstruct the sellar region only in selected cases at high risk of postoperative complications. In recent years, indeed, two different surgical philosophies are followed in our group. Since 1997 at the Neurosurgical Department of the University of Naples, the endoscopic endonasal approach has replaced the microsurgical approach (Table 31-2), which on the contrary is still used at the Neurosurgical Department of the University of Genoa (Table 31-3). The number of cases in which sellar packing has been necessary has dramatically decreased in recent years in comparison with the microsurgical series jointly performed from 1978 throughout 1992 (73.6% vs. 17.8%) (Table 31-4), even though the postoperative mechanical complication rate requiring surgery has remained almost unchanged (2.8% vs. 2.3%), as well as the type of treated pathologies. Moreover, in the more recent series no mortality has been reported. Such a variation can be explained by the higher number of operations for giant invasive adenomas and macroadenomas, which are ideal candidates for the open sella technique, as well as by an increasing confidence in the surgical technique (i.e., fewer perioperative complications and probably an overassessment of surgical related risks in the ascending part of the learning curve). At present, our indications for sellar repair are summarized in Table 31-5. As a rule, it seems to be realistic to pay careful attention to sellar repair in the following conditions:

- Preoperative or intraoperative CSF leakage
- A coexisting preoperative or intraoperative empty sella
- Persistent bleeding after removal of a large intrasellar-suprasellar adenoma, even after prolonged compression and irrigation
- Previous surgery or radiotherapy
- Ghost sella

Natural biologic substances obtained during surgery or common reabsorbable materials used in neurosurgery fulfill the packing requirements in almost every situation.[39] Extradural packing, used on its own or together with intradural packing, constitutes the best method for producing a solid,

TABLE 31-2 ▪ Synopsis of 280 Transsphenoidal Endoscopic Surgical Procedures Performed from 1997 through 2003 at the Neurosurgical Department of the Università degli Studi di Napoli Federico II

Pathology			Number of Cases
Pituitary adenoma			
NF	Macro	136	136
PRL	Macro	14	20
	Micro	6	
GH	Macro	41	56
	Micro	15	
ACTH	Macro	5	23
	Micro	18	
GH-PRL	Macro	5	5
	Micro		
GH-TSH	Macro	1	1
Craniopharyngioma			8
Rathke's cleft cyst			5
Arachnoid cyst			4
Sellar teratoma			1
Sellar schwannoma			1
Clivus chordoma			3
Olfactory neuroblastoma			1
Sphenoid metastasis			1
Sphenoid mucocele			6
Residual nasal meningocele			1
CSF leak			8
Total			280

ACTH, adrenocorticotropic hormone; GH, growth hormone; NF, nonfunctioning; PRL, prolactin; TSH, thyrotropin.

stable closure of the sella, both immediately and with the passage of time. The consolidation is so effective that patients are often seen in whom all the extradural packing undergoes pronounced ossification (Figs. 31-32 and 31-33). Finally, it is noteworthy that spontaneous ossification of the sellar access often occurs: it would be extremely difficult to conceive of a better result than this (Fig. 31-34).

TABLE 31-3 ▪ Transsphenoidal Microsurgical Procedures Performed from 1995 through 2003 at the Neurosurgical Department of the University of Genoa

Pathology	Number of Cases
Pituitary adenomas:	
Giant invasive	30
Macroadenomas	119
Mesoadenomas	38
Microadenomas	36
Craniopharyngioma + sellar cysts	10
Empty sella	8
Others	10
Complications requiring surgery	
Postoperative hematoma	4
CSF leak	3
Total	258

TABLE 31-4 ▪ Repair of the Sella Turcica following Transsphenoidal Microsurgical Procedures Performed from 1995 through 2003 at the Neurosurgical Department of the University of Genoa

Reconstruction Modality	Number of Cases (%)
Sellar packing	46 (17.8%)
Sellar floor reconstruction	57 (22.1%)
Open sella technique	155 (60.1%)
Total	258 (100%)

TABLE 31-5 ▪ Indications for the Various Techniques in Sellar Repair after Transsphenoidal Surgery

Technique	Condition
Packing of the sella	Prolapse of the suprasellar cistern toward the sellar floor Bleeding from the medial wall of the cavernous sinus Injury of the carotid artery
Packing of the sella with/without packing of the sphenoid sinus	CSF leak Paninvasive macroadenoma
No closure or packing of the sella	Microadenoma Macroadenoma with suprasellar extension incompletely removed or with tumor capsule adherent to the suprasellar cistern

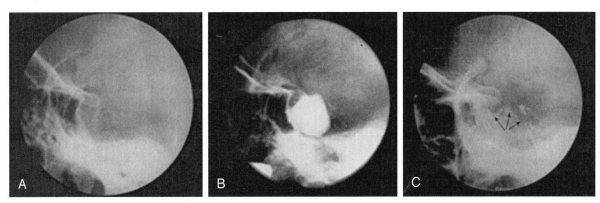

FIGURE 31-32 *A,* A preoperative radiograph of the skull showing an enlarged and eroded sella turcica with disappearance of the dorsum in a case of a growth hormone–secreting intrasellar adenoma. *B,* An intraoperative fluoroscopic image. The dimensions of the adenoma are shown by a sponge soaked in iodinated contrast medium introduced into the residual cavity. *C,* A radiograph of the skull was obtained 3 years later. The sellar boundaries and the dorsum sellae are recalcified. The materials used for intradural and extradural packing (*arrows*) are thinly calcified and ossified, as are the bone fragments lying in the sphenoidal sinus.

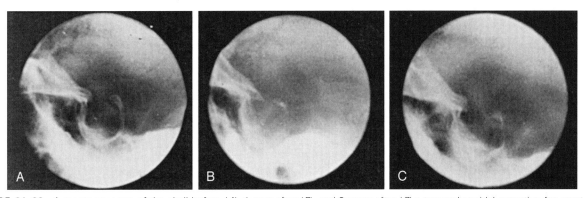

FIGURE 31-33 A roentgenogram of the skull before (*A*), 1 year after (*B*), and 3 years after (*C*) a transsphenoidal operation for empty sella with CSF rhinorrhea that was cured with extradural packing. Progressive ossification of the packing material is clearly visible.

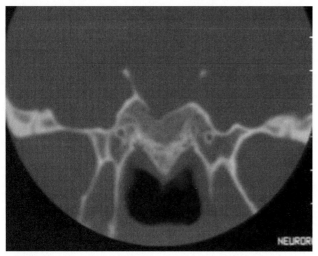

FIGURE 31-34 Sellar CT scan (coronal view) performed 1 year after removal of a large growth hormone–secreting macroadenoma according to the "open sella" technique. Spontaneous ossification of the sellar floor is evident.

REFERENCES

1. Barker FG II, Klibanski A, Swearingen B: Transsphenoidal surgery for pituitary tumors in the United States, 1996–2000: Mortality, morbidity and the effects of hospital and surgeon volume. J Clin Endocrinol Metab 88:4709–4719, 2003.
2. Ciric I, Rosenblatt S, Kerr W Jr, et al: Perspective in pituitary adenomas: An end of the century review of tumorigenesis, diagnosis, and treatment. Clin Neurosurg 47:99–111, 2000.
3. Ciric I, Rosenblatt S, Zhao JC: Transsphenoidal microsurgery. Neurosurgery 51:161–169, 2002.
4. Liu JK, Weiss MH, Couldwell WT: Surgical approaches to pituitary tumors. Neurosurg Clin N Am 14:93–107, 2003.
5. Spaziante R, de Divitiis E, Cappabianca P: Repair of the sella turcica after transsphenoidal surgery. In Schmidek HH, Sweet WH (eds): Operative Neurosurgical Techniques, vol 1. Philadelphia: WB Saunders, 2000, pp 398–416.
6. Citardi MJ, Cox AJ III, Bucholz RD: Acellular dermal allograft for sellar reconstruction after transsphenoidal hypophysectomy. Am J Rhinol 14:69–73, 2000.
7. El-Banhawy OA, Halaka AN, El-Dien AE, Ayad H: Sellar floor reconstruction with nasal turbinate tissue after endoscopic endonasal transsphenoidal surgery for pituitary adenomas. Minim Invasive Neurosurg 46:289–292, 2003.
8. Cappabianca P, Cavallo LM, Valente V, et al: Sellar repair with fibrin sealant and collagen fleece after endoscopic endonasal transphenoidal surgery. Surg Neurol 62:227–233, 2004.
9. Kobayashi S, Sugita K, Matsuo K: Reconstruction of the sellar floor during transsphenoidal operations using alumina ceramic. Surg Neurol 15:196–197, 1981.
10. Freidberg SR, Hybels RL, Bohigian RK: Closure of cerebrospinal leakage after transsphenoidal surgery: Technical note. Neurosurgery 35:159–160, 1994.
11. Arita K, Kurisu K, Tominaga A: Size-adjustable titanium plate for reconstruction of the sella turcica: Technical note. J Neurosurg 91:1055–1057, 1999.
12. Kabuto M, Kubota T, Kobayashi H, et al: Long-term evaluation of reconstruction of the sellar floor with a silicone plate in transsphenoidal surgery. J Neurosurg 88:949–953, 1998.
13. Kumar A, Maartens NF, Kaye AH: Evaluation of the use of BioGlue (R) in neurosurgical procedures. J Clin Neurosci 10:661–664, 2003.
14. Seiler RW, Mariani L: Sellar reconstruction with resorbable Vicryl patches, gelatin foam, and fibrin glue in transsphenoidal surgery: A 10-year experience with 376 patients. J Neurosurg 93:762–765, 2000.
15. Kaptain GJ, Vincent DA, Laws ER, Jr: Cranial base reconstruction after transsphenoidal surgery with bioabsorbable implants. Neurosurgery 48:232–233, 2001.
16. Cappabianca P, Cavallo LM, Mariniello G, et al: Easy sellar reconstruction in endoscopic transsphenoidal surgery with polyester-silicone dural substitute and fibrin glue: Technical note. Neurosurgery 49:473–476, 2001.
17. Saito K, Kuwayama A, Yamamoto N, Sugita K: The transsphenoidal removal of nonfunctioning pituitary adenomas with suprasellar extension: The open sella method and intentionally staged operation. Neurosurgery 36:668–675, 1995.
18. Nishizawa S, Yokoama T, Ohta S, Uemura K: Surgical indications for and limitations of staged transsphenoidal surgery for large pituitary tumors. Neurol Med Chir 38:213–219, 1998.
19. Zada G, Kelly DF, Cohan P, et al: Endonasal transsphenoidal approach for pituitary adenomas and other sellar lesions: An assesment of efficacy, safety, and patient impressions. J Neurosurg 98:350–358, 2003.
20. Liu JK, Orlandi RR, Apfelbaum RI, Couldwell WT: Novel closure technique for the endonasal transsphenoidal approach: Technical note. J Neurosurg 100:161–164, 2004.
21. de Divitiis E, Cappabianca P: Endoscopic endonasal transsphenoidal surgery. In Pickard JD (ed): Advances and Technical Standards in Neurosurgery, vol 27. Wien-New York: Springer Verlag, 2002, pp 137–177.
22. de Divitiis E, Cappabianca P (eds): Endoscopic Endonasal Transsphenoidal Surgery. Wien-New York: Springer Verlag, 2003.
23. Teramoto A: Contemporary transsphenoidal surgery for pituitary adenomas with emphasis on complications. Biomed Pharmacother 56(Suppl 1):154s–157s, 2002.
24. Spaziante R, Zona G, Testa V: Primary empty sella syndrome [letter]. Surg Neurol 60:177–178, 2003.
25. Zona G, Testa V, Sbaffi PF, Spaziante R: Transsphenoidal treatment of empty sella by means of a Silastic coil: Technical note. Neurosurgery 51:1299–1303, 2002.
26. Zona G, Testa V, Sbaffi PF, Spaziante R: Transsphenoidal treatment of empty sella by means of a silastic coil: Technical note [letter]. Neurosurgery 52:1244–1245, 2003.
27. Garcia-Uria J, Ley L, Parajon A, Bravo G: Spontaneous cerebrospinal fluid fistulae associated with empty sellae: Surgical treatment and long-term results. Neurosurgery 45:766–773, 1999.
28. Hudgins WR, Raney LA, Young SW: Failure of intrasellar muscle implants to prevent recurrent downward migration of the optic chiasm. Neurosurgery 8:231–232, 1981.
29. Gazioglu N, Akar Z, Ak H, et al: Extradural ballon obliteration of the empty sella: Report of three cases. Acta Neurochir 141:487–494, 1999.
30. Fahlbusch R, Honegger J, Paulus W, et al: Surgical treatment of craniopharyngiomas: Experience with 168 patients. J Neurosurg 90:237–250, 1999.
31. Maira G, Anile C, Albanese A, et al: The role of transsphenoidal surgery in the treatment of craniopharyngiomas. Neurosurgery 100:445–451, 2004.
32. Laws ER, Jr: Transphenoidal approach to pituitary tumours. In Schmidek HH, Sweet WH (eds): Operative Neurosurgical Techniques, 3rd ed, vol 1. Philadelphia: WB Saunders, 1995, pp 283–292.
33. Spaziante R, de Divitiis E: Drainage techniques for cystic craniopharyngiomas. Neurosurg Quart 7:183–208, 1997.
34. Kato T, Sawamura Y, Abe H, Nagashima M: Transsphenoidal transtuberculum sellae approach for supradiaphragmatic tumors: Technical note. Acta Neurochir 140:715–718, 1998.
35. Kaptain GJ, Vincent DA, Sheehan JP, Laws ER, Jr: Transsphenoidal approaches for the extracapsular resection of midline suprasellar and anterior cranial base lesions. Neurosurgery 49:94–100, 2001.
36. Kouri JG, Chen MY, Watson JC, Oldfield EH: Resection of suprasellar tumors by using a modified transsphenoidal approach. J Neurosurg 92:1028–1035, 2000.
37. Kelly DF, Oskouian RJ, Fineman I: Collagen sponge repair of small cerebrospinal fluid leaks obviates tissue grafts and cerebrospinal fluid diversion after pituitary surgery. Neurosurgery 49:885–889, 2001.
38. Targut S, Ercan I, Pinarci H, Beskonakli E: First experience with transnasal and transseptal endoscopic and microscopic repair of anterior skull base CSF fistulae. Rhinology 38:195–199, 2000.
39. Cappabianca P, Cavallo LM, Valente V, et al: Sella repair in endoscopic endonasal transsphenoidal surgery: Results of 170 cases. Neurosurgery 51:1365–1372, 2002.

32 Management of Cushing's Disease

JOSEPH C. WATSON and EDWARD H. OLDFIELD

Cushing's disease, named for neurosurgery's influential forefather, Harvey Cushing, is best treated by surgery. With proper preoperative evaluation and careful surgical technique, most affected patients can be cured while preserving normal pituitary function. If surgery alone is unsuccessful, almost all patients can be cured of hypercortisolism with irradiation therapy or bilateral adrenalectomy. On the other hand, without treatment or in the case of treatment failure, the patient's quality of life is impaired and his or her life span is shortened.

PATHOPHYSIOLOGY

Cushing's syndrome, the syndrome produced by chronic exposure to excess glucocorticoids, has several etiologies (Table 32-1). The most common cause of Cushing's syndrome is iatrogenic, that is, prescribed glucocorticoids for patients with chronic obstructive pulmonary disease, autoimmune disorders, or transplant recipients requiring chronic immunosuppression. Excluding iatrogenic causes, the most common cause of Cushing's syndrome is an adrenocorticotropic hormone–secreting pituitary adenoma, defined as Cushing's disease, which affects 60% to 80% of patients with spontaneous (noniatrogenic) Cushing's syndrome (see Table 32-1).[1] The other common causes of Cushing's syndrome, which must be distinguished from Cushing's disease, are adrenal tumors and adrenal cortical hyperplasia and ectopic adrenocorticotropic hormone (ACTH) secretion from a nonpituitary tumor, most commonly small cell lung cancer or bronchial carcinoid. Secretion of ACTH by lung carcinoma is not rare, but the ACTH is usually inactive, termed *big ACTH*.[2] A rare cause of Cushing's syndrome is ectopic secretion of corticotropin-releasing hormone (CRH) causing corticotroph hyperplasia.

Pathology

The typical pituitary adenoma causing Cushing's disease is a microadenoma (<1 cm greatest diameter) that stains for ACTH by immunohistochemistry. These tumors are monoclonal.[3] They disrupt the normal acinar pattern of the gland when stained for reticulin. They are typically basophilic by hematoxylin and eosin staining, but this terminology is no longer used because immunohistochemistry for ACTH is more specific. Occasionally Cushing's syndrome is attributed to corticotroph hyperplasia. When no definite tumor is identified at surgery and partial or total hypophysectomy is performed, the specimen must be meticulously and thoroughly examined with serial slices at closely spaced intervals because tumors as small as 1 mm diameter, or less, may cause endocrinopathy from excess ACTH secretion. Corticotroph hyperplasia, which is usually a diagnosis of exclusion (i.e., only after no tumor can be found in the specimen from pituitary surgery), should be considered only after a careful search of the gland has ruled out a discrete adenoma. In the experience at the National Institutes of Health, hyperplasia is exceedingly rare (only two suspected, but unproven, cases from more than 800 operations for Cushing's disease). A unique cytoplasmic staining pattern, known as Crooke's hyaline change, occurs in corticotrophs of the normal pituitary, cells from which ACTH production has been shut down by chronic exposure to hypercortisolemia. The "hyaline" is composed of intracytoplasmic microfilaments that do not stain for ACTH. Crooke's changes may also be found in the cells of the adenoma itself.

Mechanism of Hypercortisolemia in Adrenocorticotropic Hormone–Secreting Pituitary Adenomas

The basic endocrine disorder of the adenomas causing Cushing's disease is that the sensitive negative feedback of cortisol on the production and release of ACTH is impaired (Fig. 32-1). ACTH-secreting pituitary adenomas are well-differentiated tumors derived from pituitary corticotrophs; thus, they typically retain negative feedback to glucocorticoids, it is just set at a higher threshold for suppression, as inhibition of ACTH release is retained in response to high doses of glucocorticoid. These well-differentiated tumor cells also retain their expression of CRH receptors and the cellular machinery necessary to respond to CRH. It is these features that underlie the typical diagnostic responses with provocative endocrine tests used for the differential diagnosis of Cushing's syndrome (see later). Excessive production of ACTH leads to overproduction of cortisol by the adrenal

TABLE 32-1 ▪ Etiology of Cushing's Syndrome	
ACTH-Dependent	**85%**
Cushing's disease	80–85%
Ectopic ACTH-secreting tumor	15–20%
Ectopic CRH-secreting tumor	Rare (<1%)
ACTH-Independent	**15%**
Adrenal adenoma	7%
Adrenocortical carcinoma	7%
Bilateral micronodular adrenocortical hyperplasia	Rare (1%)
Bilateral micronodular adrenocortical hyperplasia	Rare (<1%)

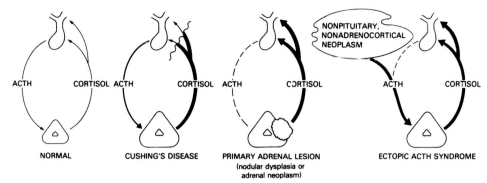

FIGURE 32-1 Normal physiology of the hypothalamic-pituitary-adrenal axis and pathophysiology of hypercortisolism. *Left,* Hypothalamic corticotropin-releasing hormone stimulates production of and secretion of adrenocorticotropic hormone (ACTH) from the corticotrophs of the anterior pituitary. ACTH in turn regulates cortisol production and secretion by the adrenals. Cortisol potently exerts negative feedback on the pituitary and the hypothalamus. (From Loriaux DL, Cutler GB Jr: Diseases of the adrenal glands. In Peter O, Kohler MD (eds): Clinical Endocrinology. New York: John Wiley & Sons, 1986, p 188.)

cortex, loss of normal diurnal plasma cortisol rhythm, and sustained hypercortisolemia. It is the excessive cortisol rather than ACTH per se that causes the clinical manifestations of Cushing's disease.

CLINICAL MANIFESTATIONS

The typical patient with Cushing's syndrome has truncal obesity with associated moon facies, enlarged dorsal fat pads ("buffalo hump"), and abdominal fat deposition with associated purple striae or "stretch marks" (Table 32-2). Hirsutism, especially noticeable on the face of women, is a common component, as are thin skin and easy bruisability, especially of the hands and forearms. Along with the outward appearance, mood or psychiatric disturbances are common, especially depression. A reversible form of brain atrophy is frequently displayed on imaging studies[4] and may be a clue to the presence of Cushing's syndrome in pediatric patients. Other signs include hypertension and hyperglycemia, often with frank diabetes mellitus. A hypercoagulable state has been

described with Cushing's syndrome, so prophylaxis for deep venous thrombosis in high-risk situations has been encouraged.[5] Patients also may have complications related to immunosuppression, such as fungal or opportunistic infections. Spinal epidural lipomatosis may be symptomatic.[6] Osteoporosis is common; related complications include vertebral compression fractures and susceptibility to traumatic long-bone fractures with minor trauma. Pediatric patients with Cushing's disease stop growing linearly and gain weight, often producing morbid obesity.[7] This "crossing of the weight and height curves" is so common in childhood Cushing's syndrome that many consider it diagnostic of the condition. Affected children often appear cherubic. Symptoms caused by tumor growth and pressure on the optic nerves and chiasm are rare with Cushing's disease because the tumors are usually microadenomas.

Life expectancy is greatly shortened by untreated Cushing's disease. If left untreated, most patients succumb to complications of the disease (diabetes, hypertension, myocardial infarction, stroke, or complications associated with immunosuppression) within 5 to 10 years.[8]

Diagnosis

The diagnosis of Cushing's syndrome and its differential diagnosis must be established with a high degree of certainty to avoid unnecessary surgery and treatment failure. Provocative endocrine testing is important in patients with Cushing's syndrome because hypercortisolism may come from causes other than a pituitary tumor, and ectopic ACTH-secreting tumors (typically lung neoplasia) and the pituitary adenomas causing Cushing's disease are often too small to be detected with radiographic techniques.

Establishing Hypercortisolism

Cushing's syndrome, when suspected clinically, is confirmed by demonstrating hypercortisolism or characteristics of its effects on the normal functioning of the hypothalamic-pituitary-adrenal axis. Confirmation of excess cortisol production is made by one or more standard testing procedures. Most commonly today, these tests include one or more of the following: serial 24-hour urine free cortisol measurements,

---

TABLE 32-2 ▪ Symptoms and Signs of Cushing's Syndrome

Fat Distribution	Skin Manifestations
Centripetal obesity	Purple striae
Moon facies	Plethora
"Buffalo hump"	Hirsutism
Supraclavicular fat pads	Acne
Epidural lipomatosis	Bruising
Musculoskeletal	**Fat Distribution**
Osteoporosis, fractures	Hypertension
Proximal muscle weakness	Glucose intolerance
Pituitary Dysfunction	Hypokalemic alkalosis
Amenorrhea	**Mental Changes**
Decreased libido, impotence	Irritability
Hypothyroidism	Psychosis
Dwarfism (children)	

diurnal plasma cortisol levels, evening salivary cortisol levels to detect loss of diurnal rhythm of cortisol secretion, or the overnight dexamethasone suppression test.

Urine free cortisol measurements are assayed using a variety of techniques. The normal upper levels vary with the technique used and with the laboratory performing the assay (Fig. 32-2). Hypercortisolism is associated with loss of normal diurnal variation in cortisol secretion, which is demonstrated by obtaining morning (8 to 9 AM) and evening (11 PM to 12 AM) plasma cortisol levels (Fig. 32-3). Salivary cortisol levels are also reliably used for this and are well suited for outpatient screening of adult and pediatric patients for hypercortisolism.[9] A recent study of more than 140 patients demonstrated a sensitivity of 93% and a specificity of 100% using this test to determine the presence of Cushing's syndrome (Fig. 32-4).[10] Because of its simplicity, the overnight low-dose (1 mg) dexamethasone suppression test is commonly used to detect hypercortisolism (Fig. 32-5). In persons with a normal hypothalamic-pituitary-adrenal axis, morning cortisol levels are suppressed by the overnight low-dose dexamethasone suppression test (1.0 mg given the night before a morning [7 to 8 AM] cortisol measurement). A morning plasma cortisol level greater than 1.8 μg/dL after the bedtime (11 PM) administration of 1 mg dexamethasone

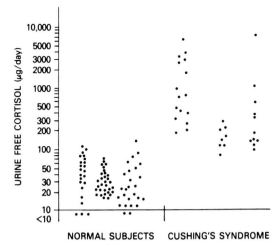

FIGURE 32-2 Twenty-four-hour excretion of urine free cortisol to screen patients for Cushing's syndrome. Comparison of 24-hour excretion of urine free cortisol value in normal subjects and patients with confirmed Cushing's syndrome. (Data from Murphy DEP: Clinical evaluation of urinary cortisol determinations by competitive protein-binding radioassay. J Clin Endocrinol Metab 28:343, 1968; Hsu TH, Bledsoe T: Measurement of urinary free corticoids by competitive protein-binding radioassay in hypoadrenal states. J Clin Endocrinol Metab 30:443, 1970; Beardwell CG, Burke CW, Cope CL: Urinary free cortisol measured by competitive protein binding. J Endocrinol 42:79, 1968.)

FIGURE 32-3 *A,* Diurnal rhythms of adrenocorticotropic hormone (ACTH), β-endorphin, and cortisol in normal subjects. Plasma ACTH, β-endorphin, and cortisol concentrations in each of two normal men who received blood sampling every 10 minutes for 24 hours. (From Veldhuis JD, Iranmanesh A, Johnson ML, Lizarralde G: Amplitude, but not frequency, modulation of adrenocorticotropin secretory bursts gives rise to the nyctohemeral rhythm of the corticotropic axis in man. J Clin Endocrinol Metab 71:452–463, 1990.)

(Continued)

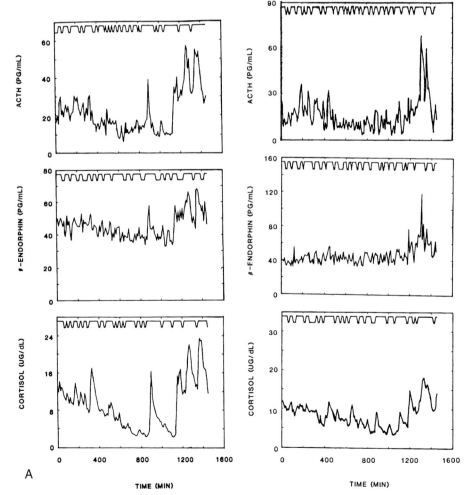

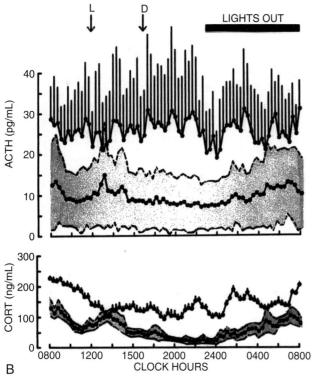

FIGURE 32-3 Cont'd *B,* Diurnal rhythms of plasma ACTH and cortisol levels in nine normal women (*shaded area*; ±95% confidence limits) and in five women with Cushing's disease (mean ± SD). L, lunch; D, dinner. (From Liu JH, Kazer RR, Rasmussen DD: Characterization of the twenty-four hour secretion patterns of adrenocorticotropin and cortisol in normal women and patients with Cushing's disease. J Clin Endocrinol Metab 64:1027–1035, 1987.)

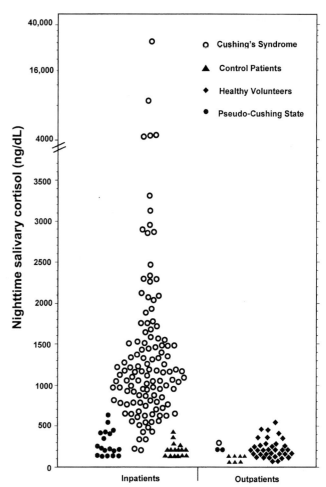

FIGURE 32-4 Salivary cortisols. Nighttime salivary cortisol values in healthy volunteers, control patients, pseudo-Cushing state patients, and patients with Cushing's syndrome. Samples were collected at 12 AM from inpatients and at bedtime (9 PM to 2 AM) from outpatients. To convert salivary cortisol nanograms per deciliter to nanomoles per liter, multiply by 0.0276. (From Papanicolaou DA, Mullen N, Kyrou I, et al: Nighttime salivary cortisol: A useful test for the diagnosis of Cushing's syndrome. J Clin Endocrinol Metab 87:4515–4521, 2002.)

detects most patients with Cushing's syndrome and justifies further diagnostic evaluation.[11]

Differential Diagnosis of Hypercortisolism

Once excess cortisol production has been established, plasma ACTH levels are measured to distinguish between an ACTH-dependent and ACTH-independent etiology (Fig. 32-6; see also Fig. 32-1). With Cushing's disease or ectopic ACTH secretion, the ACTH levels will be normal or elevated relative to the degree of glucocorticoid secretion. For this reason, these two entities are categorized as ACTH-dependent Cushing's syndrome (see Table 32-1), in contrast to adrenal disease, in which plasma ACTH is low (<5 pg/mL) or undetectable (ACTH-independent Cushing's syndrome because the adrenal cortical cortisol secretion is autonomous).

The presence of Cushing's syndrome and the differential diagnosis of Cushing's disease from adrenal disease and ectopic ACTH secretion at one time were examined with the 6-day dexamethasone suppression test, as described by Liddle.[12,13] The first 2 days of the test are used for measurement of basal cortisol secretion. In most patients with Cushing's disease, cortisol secretion, an indirect measure of ACTH secretion by the pituitary gland or the tumor, is not suppressed during the 2 days of low-dose dexamethasone (0.5 mg every 6 hours for 48 hours), but 24-hour urinary cortisol secretion is suppressed to less than 10% of baseline values by 2 days of high-dose

dexamethasone (2 mg every 6 hours for 48 hours). In contrast, high-dose dexamethasone fails to suppress cortisol secretion in most cases of ectopic ACTH secretion. Because of the difficulty in successfully completing this test today, it is now rarely used and has been replaced with the high-dose overnight dexamethasone suppression test. For this test, 8 mg dexamethasone is administered orally at 11 PM, and morning (7 to 8 AM) plasma cortisol measurements are obtained[14]; for greatest diagnostic accuracy, suppression of morning serum cortisol of greater than 68% is required to assign a diagnosis of Cushing's disease (Fig. 32-7).[14,15]

Another test commonly used today to distinguish ectopic ACTH secretion from an ACTH-secreting pituitary tumor is the CRH stimulation test.[16–18] Because they are well-differentiated tumors derived from pituitary corticotrophs, most ACTH-secreting adenomas retain receptors for, and response to, CRH, whereas most ectopic tumors, tumors that are not derived from pituitary tissue, do not express receptors for CRH and do not respond to it (Fig. 32-8). The sensitivity

FIGURE 32-5 Detection of Cushing's syndrome with the low-dose overnight dexamethasone suppression test. Plasma cortisol levels at 8 AM on successive days before and after 1 mg dexamethasone given orally at 11 PM in healthy subjects and patients with Cushing's syndrome. (From Melby JC: Assessment of adrenocortical function. N Engl J Med 285:735–739, 1971.)

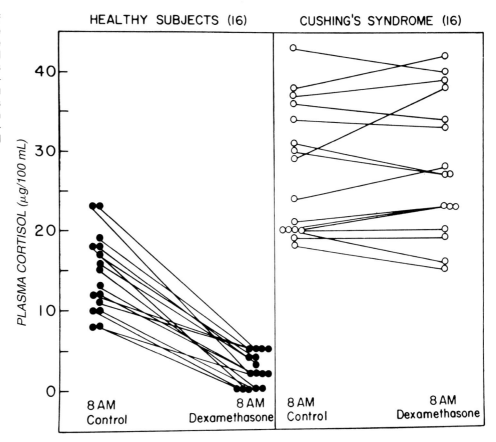

and specificity of the test are optimal using ≥35% for the maximum ACTH response from the 15- or 30-minute samples to indicate Cushing's disease (see Fig. 32-8B).[19]

If ACTH-dependent hypercortisolism is established, sella magnetic resonance imaging (MRI) with and without contrast is performed (see later). In many patients with Cushing's disease, high-resolution sella MRI will demonstrate the presence and location of a pituitary tumor. However, negative sella MRI does not rule out an adenoma because the false-negative rate using the standard T1-weighted spin echo after contrast enhancement in Cushing's disease is as high as 50% at some centers.

If the results of the high-dose dexamethasone suppression test and the CRH stimulation test are consistent with Cushing's disease and the pituitary MRI reveals a definite adenoma, no further diagnostic testing is necessary. However, if either of these provocative endocrine tests is inconsistent with Cushing's disease, inferior petrosal sinus sampling is performed.

The test with the greatest diagnostic accuracy for the differential diagnosis of Cushing's disease versus ectopic ACTH syndrome is bilateral simultaneous inferior petrosal sinus sampling performed with and without intravenous CRH administration.[20] The test is performed by placing catheters with their tips in the inferior petrosal sinuses and in a peripheral vein (Fig. 32-9A) and then obtaining serial, simultaneous samples for central and peripheral plasma ACTH concentrations at 2 and 0 minutes before and at 3, 5, and 10 minutes after intravenous CRH administration (1 µg/kg body weight). Inferior petrosal sinus sampling is only used in patients with

confirmed hypercortisolism because the test cannot discriminate between normal subjects and patients with Cushing's disease. Further, because this is an invasive procedure with rare but serious associated risks,[21] it is generally used in patients in whom the results of provocative endocrine testing to distinguish ectopic ACTH secretion from Cushing's disease are conflicting or equivocal and in instances in which the sella MRI is negative. In this test, the levels of ACTH in the primary venous drainage of the pituitary, the inferior petrosal sinuses, are compared with simultaneous ACTH measurements in the peripheral blood. A peak ratio of 2:1 during baseline (before CRH) or 3:1 before or after CRH indicates a pituitary source of the excess ACTH, Cushing's disease.[20] The sensitivity of the test is increased by sampling after administration of CRH, which, because it stimulates an adenoma to secrete ACTH, enhances the ACTH concentration differential between the central (inferior petrosal sinus) and the peripheral blood (see Fig. 32-9B).[20] It originally seemed that the procedure had a diagnostic accuracy of 100%. However, reports of false-negative and false-positive results have appeared, although in our experience, the diagnostic accuracy approaches 100%. The accuracy of the test also relies on successful placement of the catheter tips in the petrosal sinus bilaterally. Thus venography is performed to ensure correct catheter placement and to evaluate the venous anatomy. A hypoplastic or anomalous inferior petrosal sinus in 0.8% of 501 patients was associated with false-negative results in patients with proven Cushing's disease.[22] It was briefly thought that comparison of petrosal sinus ACTH from the right to left sides would accurately indicate the side

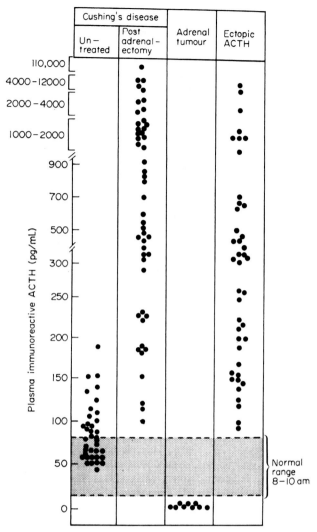

FIGURE 32-6   Plasma adrenocorticotropic hormone (ACTH) levels distinguish patients with ACTH-independent (primary adrenal disease) and ACTH-dependent forms of Cushing's syndrome. Plasma ACTH levels in 137 patients with Cushing's syndrome. (From Besser GM, Edwards CRW: Cushing's syndrome. Clin Endocrinol Metab 1:451–490, 1972.)

of the pituitary in which a small pituitary tumor was located, permitting a more focused search for it at surgery or removal of the half of the pituitary containing an adenoma that was too small to identify despite a thorough search of the gland during surgery.[23] However, more experience with the technique for lateralization indicated that the lateralization accuracy is only approximately 70%, compromising its usefulness as a localizing measure during surgery.[20]

Imaging

Sella MRI is the imaging procedure of choice for detecting and localizing the pituitary adenoma in patients with Cushing's disease. MRI should be performed with and without contrast because the adenomas typically have decreased enhancement compared with the normal gland (Fig. 32-10). The resolution of a 1.5-T magnet may reveal tumors as small as 3 mm in diameter. MRI provides other important anatomic information for the surgeon: aeration of the sphenoid,

parasellar anatomy, location of the carotid arteries, coexisting aneurysms, extent of supra- or parasellar extension of an adenoma, and ectopic parasellar tumors. Recently, the spoiled gradient recalled acquisition technique, used with 1-mm nonoverlapping slices, was shown to be more sensitive than the conventional spin echo approach (sensitivity 80% versus 49%).[24] However, the incidence of false positives was also higher (4% versus 2%). Because the sensitivity of the conventional MRI techniques (spin echo) for Cushing's disease is only 50% to 75%,[25–28] many patients have a negative MRI. Furthermore, MRI is not always available or possible because patients with a cardiac pacemaker or morbidly obese patients cannot be accommodated by the scanner. In these patients, sella computed tomography with and without contrast may demonstrate a tumor, but it is less sensitive than MRI. Furthermore, because the specificity of MRI is not 100% (MRI abnormalities consistent with adenomas occur in the pituitary gland in 10% of normal volunteers[29]) and incidental adenomas are found in the pituitary gland in approximately 5% to 20% of subjects in unselected autopsy studies,[30,31] the results of MRI must be confirmed by endocrinologic testing before surgery. In general, in Cushing's disease, endocrine testing provides the diagnosis and computerized imaging localizes the adenoma within the pituitary and defines the anatomy in its vicinity.

TREATMENT

Surgery

Transsphenoidal microsurgery is the treatment of choice for Cushing's disease. Identification of the adenoma and selective adenomectomy provides remission of hypercortisolism in most patients with an adenoma that is contained within the anterior lobe and that is large enough to be detected by MRI. Surgery for these tumors is similar to the procedures that have been described for pituitary tumors in general.

However, many tumors that cause Cushing's disease are small, frequently so small that they are not identified on preoperative MRI. In these patients, the first task for the surgeon is to locate the adenoma. A wide exposure of the pituitary gland permits visualization of the anterior lobe from one edge to the other. This requires removal of the bone of the anterior face of the sella until the medial portion of the cavernous sinus is visible bilaterally. The pseudocapsule of a microadenoma is almost always a gray-white or gray-yellow color. Because coagulation of the dura will discolor a circumscribed area of the pituitary surface, producing a local white region that can mimic an adenoma just beneath the site of dural coagulation, bipolar cautery of the dura is avoided. A wide cruciate dural opening extending to the lateral corners of the exposure, to the junction of the circular sinus with the cavernous sinus superiorly, and to the medial wall of the cavernous sinus inferiorly, while avoiding entry into the capsule of the pituitary gland, allows visualization of most of the anterior surface of the anterior lobe. In many cases, an adenoma will be seen during careful inspection of the gland's surface while using the operating microscope to look for a focal mass or discoloration on the surface of the gland. Localization of adenomas with intraoperative ultrasonography, using a specially designed probe, has also proven useful in patients with negative MRI scans.[32] When it is used,

FIGURE 32-7 High-dose (8 mg) overnight dexamethasone suppression test for the differential diagnosis of Cushing's syndrome. Comparison of the high-dose overnight dexamethasone suppression test with the high-dose portion of the standard 6-day dexamethasone suppression test. ACTH, adrenocorticotropic hormone. (Graph created using data from Tyrrell JB, Findling JW, Aron DC, et al: An overnight high-dose dexamethasone suppression test for rapid differential diagnosis of Cushing's syndrome. Ann Intern Med 104:180–186, 1986.)

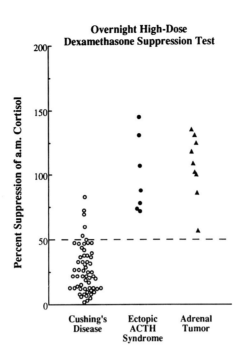

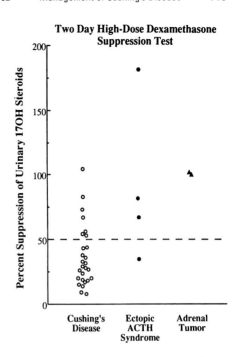

intraoperative ultrasonography is obtained after the bone removal is complete, but before the dura is opened, and with a bloodless field. However, in our experience the most reliable clue to the identification of a microadenoma is visualization of its pseudocapsule. This is especially important for the small tumors that are buried in the gland.

When the location of an adenoma is identified by inspection of the surface of the gland, the pituitary capsule is sharply incised just beyond the visible margin of the tumor pseudocapsule, which is a margin of compressed normal gland surrounding the adenoma. If the adenoma is not identified by examining the pituitary capsule anteriorly and inspecting the lateral surfaces of the anterior lobe, a series of incisions is made vertically in the gland at intervals of 1.5 to 2 mm, each carried deeper in increments until either the pseudocapsule of the tumor is identified or the juncture of the anterior and posterior lobes is reached. By identification of the interface between the pseudocapsule of the adenoma and the surrounding normal gland, the adenoma is discretely dissected from the normal pituitary, ideally without entering the soft body of the adenoma. In this way, total resection is commonly performed. If the tumor breaches the capsule of the pituitary gland, careful inspection of the contiguous dura is performed to ensure that dural invasion by the tumor is not overlooked. This is particularly important laterally along the medial wall of the cavernous sinus, where even small tumors may spread into the adjacent dura and cavernous sinus.

In the rare instance when the ACTH-secreting adenoma is located outside the adenohypophysis, such as in a suprasellar (Fig. 32-11) or parasellar location,[33] special techniques are required. For tumors of the pituitary stalk in the suprasellar cistern, an extended transsphenoidal approach may be used.[34] With this technique, during the standard transseptal approach, bone removal is extended rostrally over the planum sphenoidale. The dura anterior to the gland is opened in the midline to expose the suprasellar cistern (Fig. 32-12).

Bleeding from the opened circular sinus is stopped by packing it with small pieces of Gelfoam or with bipolar coagulation. Direct visual access of the pituitary stalk is thus provided.

Endonasal or endoscopic approaches to the sella are being examined, although their utility for resection of endocrine-active adenomas, such as Cushing's disease, remains to be established.

Postoperative Assessment

The chronic hypercortisolism associated with Cushing's disease suppresses the hypothalamic CRH-producing cells and the secretion of ACTH by the normal corticotrophs but does not fully suppress ACTH secretion by the tumor. In most patients who are cured by surgery, it takes several months for the hypothalamic-pituitary-adrenal axis to recover and the patient has hypocortisolism and requires glucocorticoid replacement therapy for the 6 to 24 months required for recovery of the hypothalamic neuron, the normal pituitary corticotroph, and the adrenal cortex and return of normal endogenous circadian cortisol secretion (Fig. 32-13). Therefore, complete removal of the abnormal source of ACTH should produce hypocortisolism in the immediate postoperative interval and for several months.[35] Thus in almost all instances of successful surgery for Cushing's disease, the patient will be hypocortisolemic (a morning cortisol of <7 μg/dL and 24-hour urine free cortisol secretion of <20 μg). Because of this, postoperative cortisol replacement must be provided. There are several protocols for postoperative cortisol replacement therapy. We use 0.5 mg dexamethasone every 6 hours for 36 hours. The dexamethasone is then discontinued and daily morning cortisol and 24-hour urine cortisol are obtained for three consecutive days. This permits immediate determination as to whether surgery has been successful in eliminating hypercortisolism and provides the potential for immediate early

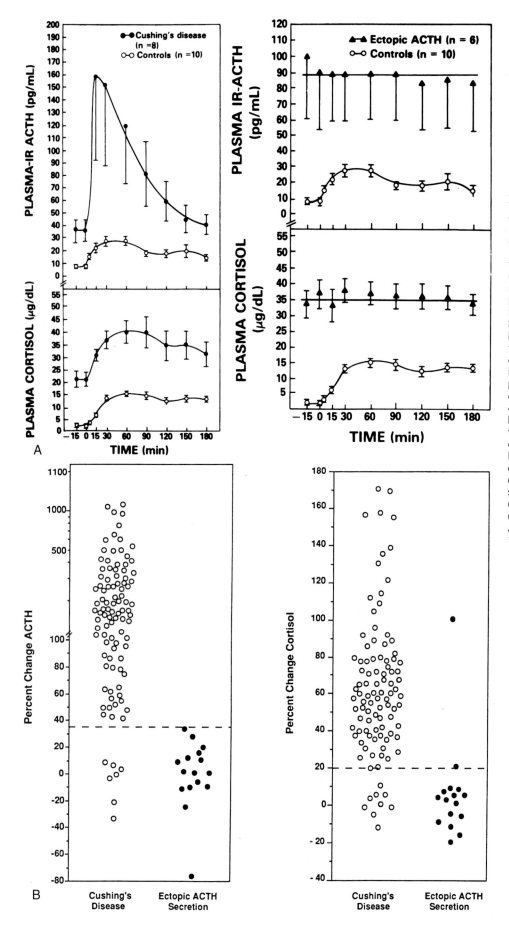

FIGURE 32-8 Corticotropin-releasing hormone (CRH) stimulation test for the differential diagnosis of Cushing's syndrome. *A*, Plasma adrenocorticotropic hormone (ACTH) (*top*) and cortisol (*bottom*) responses to CRH in eight untreated patients with Cushing's disease, six patients with Cushing's syndrome due to ectopic ACTH secretion, and 10 human controls. (From Chrousos GP, Schulte HM, Oldfield EH, et al: The corticotropin-releasing factor stimulation test: An aid in the evaluation of patients with Cushing's syndrome. N Engl J Med 310:622–626, 1984.) *B*, Responses of plasma ACTH and cortisol to intravenous administration of ovine CRH in patients with Cushing's disease and ectopic ACTH secretion. ACTH responses are expressed as the percentage of change in the mean ACTH concentration 15 and 30 minutes after CRH from the basal value 1 and 5 minutes before the injection. *Dashed line* indicates a response of 35%. Cortisol responses are expressed as the percentage of change in mean cortisol concentration 30 and 45 minutes after CRH from the basal value 1 and 5 minutes before the injection. *Dashed line* indicates a response of 20%. (From Nieman LK, Oldfield EH, Wesley R, et al: A simplified morning ovine corticotropin-releasing hormone stimulation test for the differential diagnosis of adrenocorticotropin-dependent Cushing's syndrome. J Clin Endocrinol Metab 77: 1308–1312, 1993.)

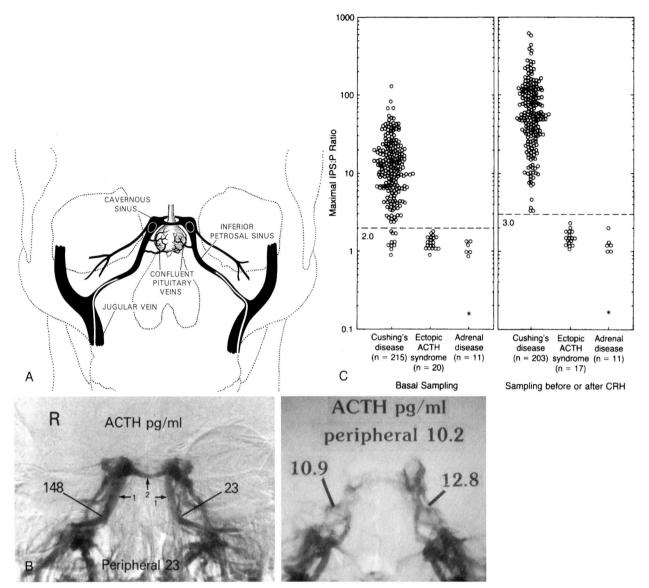

FIGURE 32-9 *A,* Anatomy and catheter placement in bilateral simultaneous blood sampling of the inferior petrosal sinuses. Confluent pituitary veins empty laterally into the cavernous sinuses, which drain into the inferior petrosal sinuses. (From Oldfield EH, Chrousos GP, Schulte HM, et al: Preoperative lateralization of ACTH-secreting microadenomas by bilateral and simultaneous inferior petrosal sinus sampling. N Engl J Med 312:100–103, 1985.) *B,* Venous sampling during inferior petrosal venous sampling with adrenocorticotropic hormone (ACTH) levels from a patient with Cushing's disease (*left*) and a patient with a bronchial carcinoid and ectopic ACTH secretion (*right*). *C,* Bilateral inferior petrosal vein sampling in the differential diagnosis of Cushing's syndrome. Maximal ratio of ACTH concentration from one of the inferior petrosal sinuses to the simultaneous peripheral venous ACTH concentration in patients with Cushing's syndrome in basal samples (*left*) and in basal and corticotropin-releasing hormone (CRH)-stimulated samples (*right*). During basal sampling, the maximal IPS:P (inferior petrosal sinus to peripheral) ACTH ratio was = 2.0 in 205 of 215 patients with confirmed Cushing's disease but was <2.0 in all patients with ectopic ACTH syndrome or primary adrenal disease. All patients with Cushing's disease who received CRH had maximal IPS:P ACTH ratios of ≥3.0, whereas all patients with ectopic ACTH syndrome had IPS:P ratios of = 3.0. The *asterisks* represent five patients with primary adrenal disease in whom ACTH was undetectable in the peripheral blood before and after CRH administration. (From Oldfield EH, Doppman JL, Nieman LK, et al: Bilateral inferior petrosal sinus sampling with and without corticotropin-releasing hormone for the differential diagnosis of Cushing's syndrome. N Engl J Med 325:897–905, 1991.)

reoperation, if indicated, which is successful in many patients.[36] Others use postoperative low-dose dexamethasone suppression testing as follows: on the first postoperative day, the patient receives 50 mg hydrocortisone intravenously in the morning and 25 mg in the evening. On the second day, the patient is given 50 mg hydrocortisone in the morning and 1 mg dexamethasone in the evening at 10 PM. Blood is withdrawn from the patient at 8 AM on the third postoperative morning, and a fasting serum cortisol

level is measured. With this approach, patients with a morning plasma cortisol greater than 2 μg/dL will have a high likelihood of having recurrent disease: 100% of patients in the report by Arnott and colleagues[37] and in the larger experience of Chen and colleagues.[38] Conversely, 93% of patients with a morning cortisol value of 2 μg/dL or less still had sustained remission of Cushing's disease at 5 years (Fig. 32-14).[38] Many authors prefer either or to provide cortisol replacement therapy and to test the patient's

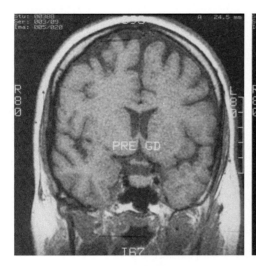
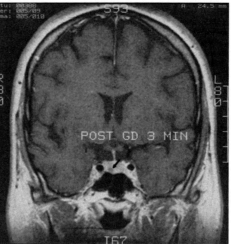

FIGURE 32-10 Magnetic resonance imaging (MRI) of the pituitary in a patient with a 4-mm adenoma in the right half of the anterior lobe. This image was acquired before (*left*) and immediately after (*right*) infusion of gadolinium-diethylene-triamine-pentaacetic acid (T1-weighted MRI, TR 500, TE 20). (From Doppman JL, Frank JA, Dwyer AJ, et al: Gadolinium DTPA enhanced imaging of ACTH-secreting microadenomas of the pituitary gland: Correlation of MR appearance with surgical findings. J Comput Assist Tomogr 12: 728–735, 1988.)

cortisol secretion several weeks after hospital discharge or to provide no cortisol replacement and to measure the immediate postoperative plasma cortisol levels.[39]

Without glucocorticoid replacement, the patient may be symptomatic from an addisonian state and will typically complain of symptoms of lethargy, anorexia, and abdominal discomfort or nausea. As the patient's blood pressure will be normal or even low postoperatively, preoperative medications used to treat hypertension are withheld until it is determined that they are required after surgery. Similarly, because glycemic control may be restored after surgery, preoperative diabetic medications are withheld, and blood glucose is carefully monitored in the immediate postoperative interval. After discharge, twice-daily physiologic cortisol replacement is provided (15 to 20 mg cortisol in the morning and 5 mg in the evening) until normal function of the hypothalamic-pituitary-adrenal axis is reestablished, which usually does not occur until 6 to 24 months after surgery.

With eucortisolism immediately or within a few weeks of surgery, clinical remission is still likely, although Cushing's disease is much more likely to recur than in patients with postoperative hypocortisolism (Fig. 32-15).[40,41]

Early Repeat Surgery

If results of cortisol measurement shortly after surgery indicate persistent hypercortisolism, immediate repeat surgery should be considered in certain circumstances.[42] Early reoperation (within 1 to 6 weeks) can induce remission in the majority of patients, although with a risk of hypopituitarism. Surgical or pathologic confirmation of an ACTH-positive adenoma that is incompletely resected during the initial pituitary exploration is the most significant predictor of success with early re-exploration, in terms of both remission and avoidance of hypopituitarism. Patients who have undergone limited exploration of the pituitary and selective excision of an area that at surgery appears to be, but proves not to have been, a corticotroph adenoma, also are likely to benefit from repeat surgery. Conversely, patients who undergo extensive initial exploration and partial resection of the anterior lobe are unlikely to benefit from a repeat

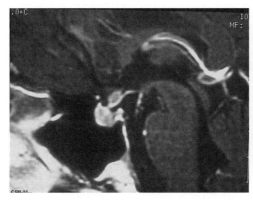
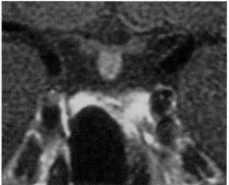

FIGURE 32-11 Adenoma in pituitary stalk. Magnetic resonance T1-weighted images reveal a 7-mm adenoma arising high in the pituitary stalk, just beneath the optic chiasm (*left*, sagittal view; *right*, coronal view) after contrast enhancement with gadolinium-diethylene-triamine-pentaacetic acid. Note the enhancement of the anterior lobe and stalk, but not the tumor. (From Mason RB, Nieman LK, Doppman JL, et al: Selective excision of adenomas originating in or extending into the pituitary stalk with preservation of pituitary function. J Neurosurg 87:343–351, 1997.)

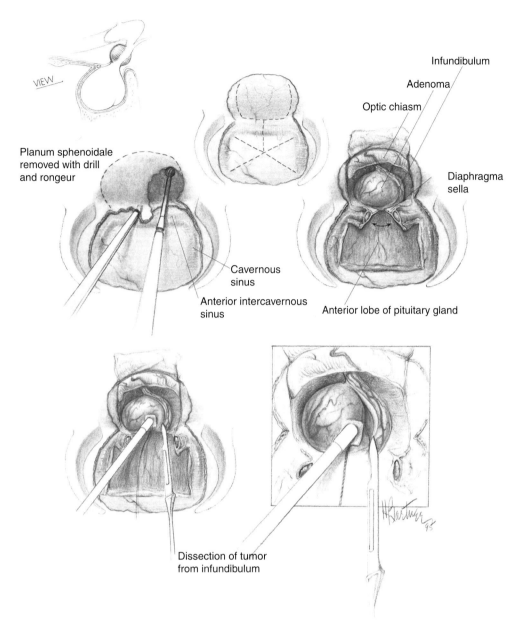

FIGURE 32-12 Extended transsphenoidal technique for removing suprasellar tumor of the pituitary stalk. Drawings depict the routine wide exposure of the anterior surface of the sella and bone removal to expose the medial portion of the cavernous sinus bilaterally. The posterior portion of the planum sphenoidale (the posterior 4 to 6 mm) is removed by first drilling with a rough diamond burr until the plate of bone was paper thin and then using a 2-mm thin footplate cervical Kerrison rongeur. Removal of the planum sphenoidale aids access to the suprasellar cistern, the pituitary stalk, and the superior surface of the gland. The dura mater covering the anterior pituitary surface is opened widely. Bilateral parasagittal incisions are made 8 to 10 mm apart in the dura overlying the planum sphenoidale. A transverse incision just above the anterior portion of the circular sinus is then used to connect the parasagittal incisions. The resulting dural flap is opened posteriorly while, initially, preserving the intact arachnoid. After entering the suprasellar cistern, the superior hypophyseal artery is identified and care is taken not to injure it. The exposed diaphragma sella is incised in the midline, in an anteroposterior direction, to reach the stalk and the supradiaphragmatic tumor. A small piece of Gelfoam or cottonoid is placed superiorly in the subarachnoid space to prevent passage of blood into the cerebrospinal fluid. Characteristic vertical striations produced by the vertical course of the surface blood vessels permit identification of the stalk. A sharp incision is made in the pia with a No. 15 scalpel at the junction of the capsule of the tumor with the pituitary stalk and, when appropriate, in the superior surface of the anterior lobe at the margin of the adenoma. The adenoma is then resected using standard microsurgical technique. (From Mason RB, Nieman LK, Doppman JL, et al: Selective excision of adenomas originating in or extending into the pituitary stalk with preservation of pituitary function. J Neurosurg 87:343–351, 1997.)

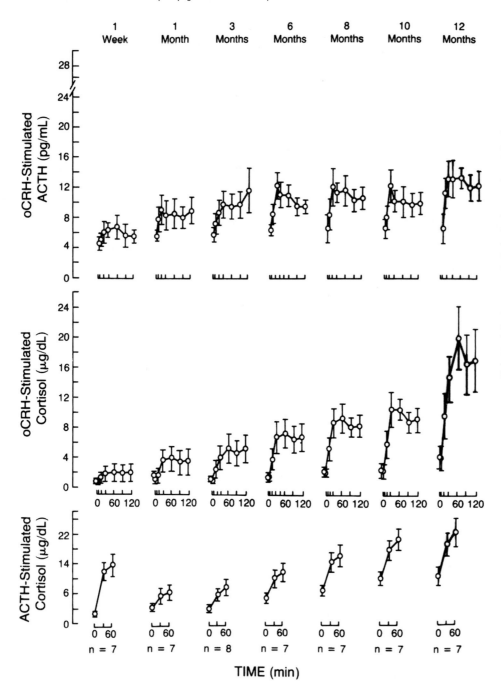

FIGURE 32-13 Recovery of the hypothalamic-pituitary-adrenal axis from chronic hypercortisolism. Nine patients with Cushing's syndrome (six patients with Cushing's disease, two with adrenal adenomas, and one with ectopic adrenocorticotropic hormone [ACTH] syndrome) were tested longitudinally for 12 months after surgical correction of Cushing's syndrome with the 1-hour ACTH test (*bottom*) and the ovine corticotropic-releasing hormone (oCRH) test (*top and middle*). The times at the top of the figure indicate the interval between the testing and surgery, and the number of patients studied at each time point is shown at the bottom. The *shaded areas* represent the mean (± SD) responses in normal subjects. (From Avgerinos PC, Chrousos GP, Nieman LK, et al: The corticotropin-releasing hormone test in the postoperative evaluation of patients with Cushing's syndrome. J Clin Endocrinol Metab 65: 906–913, 1987.)

operation if there is no ACTH-positive adenoma in the excised specimen.[36] With appropriate patient selection, early repeat surgery deserves consideration, especially when prompt control of hypercortisolism is required.

Surgical Management of Recurrent Cushing's Disease

Patients who have remission of hypercortisolism after surgery occasionally develop recurrent Cushing's disease. What should be done for the patient with recurrent Cushing's disease after previous surgery? In a report detailing the results of transsphenoidal surgery in 31 patients who had previously undergone a transsphenoidal operation and

two patients who had had previous pituitary irradiation only, in 24 (73%) of the 33 patients, remission of hypercortisolism was achieved by surgery.[42] Although computerized imaging (computed tomography) identified an adenoma in only three of the 33 patients, in 20 patients a discrete adenoma was identified at pituitary exploration. The incidence of remission of hypercortisolism was greatest if an adenoma was identified at surgery and the patient underwent selective adenomectomy (19 [95%] of 20 patients), if there was evidence at surgery or by preoperative imaging that the previous surgical exposure of the pituitary was incomplete (seven [78%] of nine patients), if an adenoma was seen on preoperative imaging (three of three patients), or if the patient had had previous pituitary irradiation without surgery

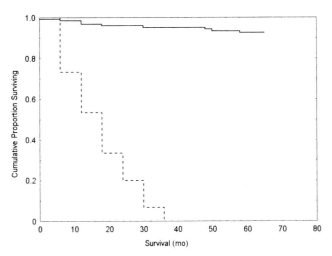

FIGURE 32-14 Postoperative remission of Cushing's disease predicted by the overnight low-dose dexamethasone suppression test. Kaplan-Meier graph compares recurrence-free survival for patients with morning plasma cortisol levels lower than 3 μg/dL (*solid line*) or 3–8 μg/dL (*broken line*) on the third postoperative day after receiving 1 mg dexamethasone at 10 to 11 PM the previous evening. (From Chen JCT, Amar AP, Choi SH, et al: Microsurgical treatment of Cushing's disease: Postoperative assessment of surgical efficacy using overnight low-dose dexamethasone suppression test. J Neurosurg 98:967–973, 2003.)

(two of two patients). In contrast, only five (42%) of 12 patients who underwent subtotal or total hypophysectomy had remission of hypercortisolism. Surgically induced hypopituitarism occurred in six (50%) of these 12 patients, but in only one (5%) of the 20 patients who underwent selective adenomectomy. Three (13%) of the 24 patients who were in remission from hypercortisolism after repeat surgery developed recurrent hypercortisolism 10 to 47 months postoperatively.

More recent reports have established that the recurrent adenoma is always at, or immediately contiguous to, the site of the adenoma at the original surgery.[43,44] Furthermore, the recurrent tumor usually is invading the dura, usually the cavernous sinus wall contiguous to the former location of the adenoma. In the series of Dickerman and Oldfield,[44] repeated surgery (44 ± 35 months after the initial surgery) in all 43 patients in whom tumor had been identified at the initial surgery, the tumor was found at the same site or contiguous to the same site. Dural invasion by an ACTH-producing tumor was identified during repeated surgery in 42 (62%) of the 68 patients re-explored after previous surgery and recurrent or persistent Cushing's disease. In addition, 39 (93%) of the 42 invasive adenomas were located laterally and involved the cavernous sinus. Adenoma invasion of the dura mater was found in 31 (54%) of 57 microadenomas and in all 11 macroadenomas at repeated surgery. The presence of tumor was not detected in 28 of the 59 patients studied with MRI, and in none of these 59 patients was dural invasion evident on MRI. The results of this study thus established that recurrent and persistent Cushing's disease consistently results from residual tumor. At repeated surgery, the residual tumor can be found at, or immediately contiguous to, the site at which the tumor was originally found. Unappreciated dural invasion with growth of residual tumor within the cavernous sinus

dura, which frequently occurs without residual tumor or dural invasion being evident on MRI or to the surgeon during surgery, is the basis of surgical failure in many patients with Cushing's disease.

Thus repeat transsphenoidal exploration of the pituitary and treatment limited to selective adenomectomy should be considered in patients with hypercortisolism despite previous pituitary treatment. If an adenoma is identified during surgery, the chance of remission of Cushing's disease is high and the risk of hypopituitarism is low; however, if no adenoma can be found and partial or complete hypophysectomy is performed, remission of hypercortisolism is less likely and the risk of hypopituitarism is approximately 50%.

Radiation Therapy

Fractionated radiation of the sella after failed transsphenoidal surgery achieves biochemical remission in most patients (80% at 4 years) (Fig. 32-16).[45] Because remission is delayed 6 months to several years after radiation therapy, medical therapy is used to block adrenal[40] production of glucocorticoids, permitting remission of the clinical syndrome of hypercortisolism until the effects of irradiation occur. Hypopituitarism is an expected side effect but usually occurs 5 to 10 years after treatment. Other risks of sellar irradiation include, in decreasing likelihood, optic neuropathy, oculomotor neuropathy, and secondary neoplasia. Stereotactic radiosurgery may produce an earlier response than fractionated conventional radiation therapy, but whether it will reduce or increase the risk of radiation-induced complications has not been established. Radiosurgery of the sella, or of the focus of known residual tumor, also appears to be an effective primary treatment of Cushing's disease, but, as in fractionated therapy remission of hypercortisolism, biochemical remission is delayed and the incidence of permanent hypopituitarism is expected to be high.[46]

Medical Therapy

Chemical adrenalectomy, by medically blocking production of biologically active cortisol by the adrenal cortex, eliminates hypercortisolism and induces remission from the signs and symptoms of Cushing's disease while awaiting transsphenoidal surgery or, more commonly, while awaiting the effects of pituitary irradiation. For this, ketoconazole, which blocks steroidogenesis, is used.[47,48] Its use is limited primarily by hepatic toxicity. Other side effects include reduced androgen production and gynecomastia in men and a disulfiram reaction. Metyrapone inhibits glucocorticoid and mineralocorticoid production, but its clinical usefulness is also limited by toxicity.

Adrenalectomy

Although adrenalectomy was the treatment for Cushing's disease in the midportion of the century, the current use of bilateral adrenalectomy is limited to patients in whom other treatments have failed. Adrenalectomy may be used in lieu of irradiation to avoid hypopituitarism in young patients with Cushing's disease refractory to surgery or it may be

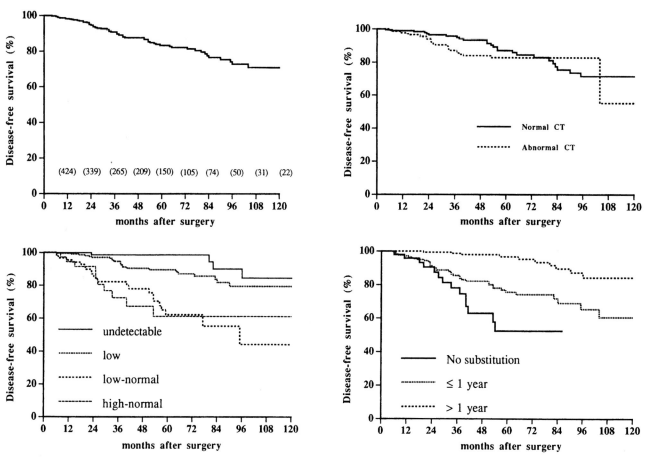

FIGURE 32-15 Analysis of the recurrence of Cushing's disease in patients in remission after transsphenoidal operation. *Top left,* The disease-free survival in the whole group is shown (numbers in parentheses represent patients at risk at the end of each year). *Top right,* The disease-free survival according to the presence of a normal (*n* = 220) or abnormal (*n* = 239) pituitary computed tomography (CT) scan among the 459 patients who were examined before surgery is shown. Patients with an abnormal preoperative CT scan had a higher risk of recurrence, but the difference was of borderline significance (*P* < 0.053). *Bottom left,* The disease-free survival according to the early postoperative morning cortisol level is shown for the 482 patients for whom the result was available. Patients with undetectable (*n* = 94) and low (*n* = 250) cortisol levels had fewer recurrences during follow-up than did patients with low-normal (*n* = 97) and high-normal (*n* = 41) cortisol levels. The overall difference among the four groups was highly significant (*P* < 0.0001). *Bottom right,* The disease-free survival according to the length of glucocorticoid substitution therapy is reported for all 510 patients who had successful operations. Patients who did not need any substitution therapy (*n* = 821) and those who required glucocorticoid replacement for less than 1 year (*n* = 248) showed a higher risk of recurrence than did patients treated for more than 1 year (*n* = 180). The overall difference among the three groups was highly significant (*P* < 0.0001). (From Bochicchio D, Losa M, Buchfelder M: Factors influencing the immediate and late outcome of Cushing's disease treated by transsphenoidal surgery: A retrospective study by the European Cushing's Disease Survey Group. J Clin Endocrinol Metab 80:3114–3120, 1995.)

combined with irradiation to reduce the risk of development of Nelson's syndrome, which occurs in 10% to 20% of patients after adrenalectomy for Cushing's disease.[49]

NELSON'S SYNDROME

As the adenomas of Cushing's disease are under negative feedback, albeit incomplete negative feedback, by high circulating levels of glucocorticoids, plasma ACTH levels increase greatly after adrenalectomy for Cushing's disease and some ACTH-secreting pituitary tumors aggressively enlarge after correction of hypercortisolism. Nelson's syndrome, hyperpigmentation associated with unbridled production of pro-opiomelanocortin and very high levels of plasma ACTH and α-melatonin-stimulating hormone, and the appearance of a rapidly growing pituitary macroadenoma

after bilateral adrenalectomy for Cushing's disease, was identified in the era before microneurosurgery, when bilateral adrenalectomy was the treatment of choice for Cushing's disease. The risk of Nelson's syndrome after adrenalectomy is 10% to 20% in most series but is as high as 30% in others, and it may present 1 to 29 years after adrenalectomy.[50] It is a serious complication that is characterized by uncontrolled tumor growth and parasellar invasion and compression syndromes that are otherwise atypical of Cushing's disease. The success of surgical treatment Nelson's syndrome is limited by the large size and invasiveness of these tumors; the incidence of remission from surgery is the range of 20%[51] but is higher if the tumors are detected before parasellar spread. Surgery followed by irradiation is the preferred treatment,[50] although many of these tumors are refractory to surgical and/or radiation therapy.

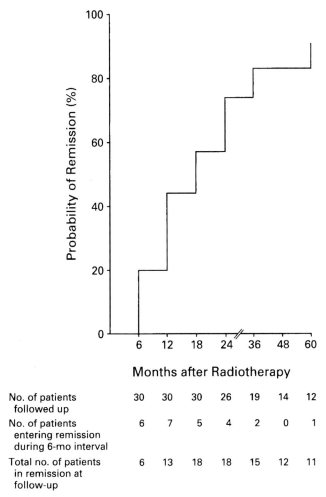

No. of patients followed up	30	30	30	26	19	14	12
No. of patients entering remission during 6-mo interval	6	7	5	4	2	0	1
Total no. of patients in remission at follow-up	6	13	18	18	15	12	11

FIGURE 32-16 Probability of remission of Cushing's disease in 30 patients treated with pituitary irradiation after unsuccessful transsphenoidal surgery. Response to radiotherapy. (From Estrada J, Boronat M, Mielgo M, et al: The long-term outcome of pituitary irradiation after unsuccessful transsphenoidal surgery in Cushing's disease. N Engl J Med 336:172–177, 1997.)

REFERENCES

1. Boscaro M, Barzon L, Fallo F, Sonino N: Cushing's syndrome. Lancet 357:783–791, 2001.
2. Ayvazian LF, Schneider B, Gewirtz G, Yalow RS: Ectopic production of big ACTH in carcinoma of the lung. Its clinical usefulness as a biologic marker. Am Rev Respir Dis 111:279–287, 1975.
3. Schulte HM, Oldfield EH, Allolio B, et al: Clonal composition of pituitary adenomas in patients with Cushing's disease: Determination by X-chromosome inactivation analysis. J Clin Endocrinol Metab 73:1302–1308, 1991.
4. Bourdeau I, Bard C, Noel B, et al: Loss of brain volume in endogenous Cushing's syndrome and its reversibility after correction of hypercortisolism. J Clin Endocrinol Metab 87:1949–1954, 2002.
5. Boscaro M, Sonino N, Scarda A, et al: Anticoagulant prophylaxis markedly reduces thromboembolic complications in Cushing's syndrome. J Clin Endocrinol Metab 87:3662–3666, 2002.
6. Koch CA, Doppman JL, Watson JC, et al: Spinal epidural lipomatosis in a patient with the ectopic corticotropin syndrome. N Engl J Med 341:1399–1400, 1999.
7. Magiakou MA, Mastorakos G, Oldfield EH, et al: Cushing's syndrome in children and adolescents: Presentation, diagnosis, and therapy. N Engl J Med 331:629–636, 1994.
8. Plotz CM, Knowlton AI, Ragan C: The natural history of Cushing's syndrome. Am J Med 13:597–614, 1952.
9. Gafni RI, Papanicolaou DA, Nieman LK: Nighttime salivary cortisol measurement as a simple, noninvasive, outpatient screening test for Cushing's syndrome in children and adolescents. J Pediatr 137:30–35, 2000.
10. Papanicolaou DA, Mullen N, Kyrou I, Nieman LK: Nighttime salivary cortisol: A useful test for the diagnosis of Cushing's syndrome. J Clin Endocrinol Metab 87:4515–4521, 2002.
11. Wood PJ, Barth JH, Freedman DB, et al: Evidence for the low dose dexamethasone suppression test to screen for Cushing's syndrome—recommendations for a protocol for biochemistry laboratories. Ann Clin Biochem 34:222–229, 1997.
12. Liddle GW: Pathogenesis of glucocorticoid disorders. Am J Med 53:638–648, 1972.
13. Liddle GW: Tests of pituitary-adrenal suppressibility in the diagnosis of Cushing's syndrome. J Clin Endocrinol Metab 20:1539–1560, 1960.
14. Tyrrell JB, Findling JW, Aron DC, et al: An overnight high-dose dexamethasone suppression test for rapid differential diagnosis of Cushing's syndrome. Ann Intern Med 104:180–186, 1986.
15. Dichek HL, Nieman LK, Oldfield EH, et al: A comparison of the standard high dose dexamethasone suppression test and the overnight 8-mg dexamethasone suppression test for the differential diagnosis of adrenocorticotropin-dependent Cushing's syndrome. J Clin Endocrinol Metab 78:418–422, 1994.
16. Chrousos GP, Schulte HM, Oldfield EH, et al: The corticotropin-releasing factor stimulation test: An aid in the evaluation of patients with Cushing's syndrome. N Engl J Med 310:622–626, 1984.
17. Nieman LK, Chrousos GP, Oldfield EH, et al: The ovine corticotropin-releasing hormone stimulation test and the dexamethasone suppression test in the differential diagnosis of Cushing's syndrome. Ann Intern Med 105:862–867, 1986.
18. Nieman LK: Diagnostic tests for Cushing's syndrome. Ann N Y Acad Sci 970:112–118, 2002.
19. Nieman LK, Oldfield EH, Wesley R, et al: A simplified morning ovine corticotropin-releasing hormone stimulation test for the differential diagnosis of adrenocorticotropin-dependent Cushing's syndrome. J Clin Endocrinol Metab 77:1308–1312, 1993.
20. Oldfield EH, Doppman JL, Nieman LK, et al: Petrosal sinus sampling with and without corticotropin-releasing hormone for the differential diagnosis of Cushing's syndrome. N Engl J Med 325:897–905, 1991.
21. Miller DL, Doppman JL, Peterman SB, et al: Neurologic complications of petrosal sinus sampling. Radiology 185:143–147, 1992.
22. Doppman JL, Chang R, Oldfield EH, et al: The hypoplastic inferior petrosal sinus: A potential source of false-negative results in petrosal sampling for Cushing's disease. J Clin Endocrinol Metab 84:533–540, 1999.
23. Oldfield EH, Girton ME, Doppman JL: Absence of intercavernous venous mixing: evidence supporting lateralization of pituitary microadenomas by venous sampling. J Clin Endocrinol Metab 61:644–647, 1985.
24. Patronas N, Bulakbasi N, Stratakis CA, et al: Spoiled gradient recalled acquisition in the steady state technique is superior to conventional postcontrast spin echo technique for magnetic resonance imaging detection of adrenocorticotropin-secreting pituitary tumors. J Clin Endocrinol Metab 88:1565–1569, 2003.
25. Colombo N, Loli P, Vignati F, Scialfa G: MR of corticotropin-secreting pituitary microadenomas. AJNR Am J Neuroradiol 15:1591–1595, 1994.
26. Peck WW, Dillon WP, Norman D, et al: High-resolution MR imaging of pituitary microadenomas at 1.5 T: Experience with Cushing disease. AJR Am J Roentgenol 152:145–151, 1989.
27. Doppman JL, Frank JA, Dwyer AJ, et al: Gadolinium DTPA enhanced MR imaging of ACTH-secreting microadenomas of the pituitary gland. J Comput Assist Tomogr 12:728–735, 1988.
28. Tabarin A, Laurent F, Catargi B, et al: Comparative evaluation of conventional and dynamic magnetic resonance imaging of the pituitary gland for the diagnosis of Cushing's disease. Clin Endocrinol (Oxf) 49:293–300, 1998.
29. Hall WA, Luciano MG, Doppman JL, et al: Pituitary magnetic resonance imaging in normal human volunteers: Occult adenomas in the general population. Ann Intern Med 120:817–820, 1994.
30. Camaris C, Balleine R, Little D: Microadenomas of the human pituitary. Pathology 27:8–11, 1995.
31. Teramoto A, Hirakawa K, Sanno N, Osamura Y: Incidental pituitary lesions in 1,000 unselected autopsy specimens. Radiology 193:161–164, 1994.
32. Watson JC, Shawker TH, Nieman LK, et al: Localization of pituitary adenomas by using intraoperative ultrasound in patients with Cushing's disease and no demonstrable pituitary tumor on magnetic resonance imaging. J Neurosurg 89:927–932, 1998.

33. Pluta RM, Nieman L, Doppman JL, et al: Extrapituitary parasellar microadenoma in Cushing's disease. J Clin Endocrinol Metab 84:2912–2923, 1999.
34. Mason RB, Nieman LK, Doppman JL, Oldfield EH: Selective excision of adenomas originating in or extending into the pituitary stalk with preservation of pituitary function. J Neurosurg 87:343–351, 1997.
35. Oldfield EH: Cushing disease. J Neurosurg 98:948–951, 2003.
36. Ram Z, Nieman LK, Cutler GB Jr, et al: Early repeat surgery for persistent Cushing's disease. J Neurosurg 80:37–45, 1994.
37. Arnott RD, Pestell RG, McKelvie PA, et al: A critical evaluation of transsphenoidal pituitary surgery in the treatment of Cushing's disease: Prediction of outcome. Acta Endocrinol (Copenh) 123:423–430, 1990.
38. Chen JCT, Amar AP, Choi SH, et al: Microsurgical treatment of Cushing's disease: Postoperative assessment of surgical efficacy using overnight low-dose dexamethasone suppression test. J Neurosurg 98:967–973, 2003.
39. Simmons NE, Alden TD, Thorner MO, Laws ER Jr: Serum cortisol response to transsphenoidal surgery for Cushing disease. J Neurosurg 95:1–8, 2001.
40. Bochicchio D, Losa M, Buchfelder M: Factors influencing the immediate and late outcome of Cushing's disease treated by transsphenoidal surgery: A retrospective study by the European Cushing's Disease Survey Group. J Clin Endocrinol Metab 80:3114–3120, 1995.
41. Estrada J, Garcia-Uria J, Lamas C, et al: The complete normalization of the adrenocortical function as the criterion of cure after transsphenoidal surgery for Cushing's disease. J Clin Endocrinol Metab 86:5695–5699, 2001.
42. Friedman RB, Oldfield EH, Nieman LK, et al: Repeat transsphenoidal surgery for Cushing's disease. J Neurosurg 71:520–527, 1989.
43. Nakane T, Kuwayama A, Watanabe M, et al: Long term results of transsphenoidal adenomectomy in patients with Cushing's disease. Neurosurgery 21:218–222, 1987.
44. Dickerman RD, Oldfield EH: Basis of persistent and recurrent Cushing's disease: An analysis based on findings at repeat pituitary surgery. J Neurosurg 97:1343–1349, 2003.
45. Estrada J, Boronat M, Mielgo M, et al: The long-term outcome of pituitary irradiation after unsuccessful transsphenoidal surgery in Cushing's disease. N Engl J Med 36:172–177, 1997.
46. Hoybye C, Grenback E, Rahn T, et al: Adrenocorticotropic hormone-producing pituitary tumors: 12- to 22-year follow-up after treatment with stereotactic radiosurgery. Neurosurgery 49:284–292, 2001.
47. Engelhardt D, Weber MM: Therapy of Cushing's syndrome with steroid biosynthesis inhibitors. J Steroid Biochem Mol Biol 49:261–267, 1994.
48. Sonino N, Boscaro M, Paoletta A, et al: Ketoconazole treatment in Cushing's syndrome: Experience in 34 patients. Clin Endocrinol (Oxf) 35:347–352, 1991.
49. Nagesser SK, van Seters AP, Kievit J, et al: Long-term results of total adrenalectomy for Cushing's disease. World J Surg 24:108–113, 2000.
50. Kemink SA, Grotenhuis JA, De Vries J, et al: Management of Nelson's syndrome: Observations in fifteen patients. Clin Endocrinol (Oxf) 54:45–52, 2001.
51. Wilson CB, Tyrrell JB, Fitzgerald PA, Pitts LH: Cushing's disease and Nelson's syndrome. Clin Neurosurg 27:19–30, 1980.

33 Craniopharyngiomas: A Summary of Data

WILLIAM H. SWEET[†]

By far the most comprehensive published account of craniopharyngioma is the major monograph by Choux and colleagues.[1] Although most of the monograph is in French, it includes extensive summaries in English, including the legends to all figures. It is based primarily on data from 474 patients younger than 16 years of age. These data were collected from members of the Société de Neurochirurgie de Langue Française and the International Society for Pediatric Neurosurgery and are described as the ISPC-91 series. Many of the tables include data from all age groups and many nations, as attested by the 579 references cited by the authors. The symposium organized by Epstein and colleagues at New York University and held on December 17 through 19, 1993, in which 24 authors from all over the world presented their findings, will become the most broadly based source of expert information on the subject. Most of the presentations concentrated on the authors' personal data. Its organizers have kindly supplied me with most of the manuscripts so that a supplemental account to Samii's valuable chapter (see Chapter 34) can be included in these volumes.

PATHOLOGY

Agreement has long existed that almost none of the cells in craniopharyngiomas displays malignant features. Peet reported on a case of a child whose tumor, which was mainly "adamantinomatous," had some carcinomatous features.[2] Nelson and colleagues[3] reported on a patient who, 35 years after the first operation, also showed malignant zones in the tumor.[3] The widely ranging types of parenchymal cells need concern us no further because their blood supply of all types is so meager as never to interfere with removal. Differentiation of various types of cells that at times predominate in these tumors led to the terms *adamantinoma* and *ameloblastoma*, which are applied to embryonic cells of the dental enamel organs. Epithelial cells are common; even cholesteatomatous and teratomatous areas occur. Trying to correlate specific histologic features with any other behavioral aspect of interest has proved to be fruitless. The most successful attempt is that of Kahn and co-workers,[4] who in 1973 reported that an oropharyngeal type of squamous epithelial cell without calcification found in 11 of 12 adults and only 1 of 28 children was associated with a much better prognosis than the faster growing type. This cell is said to have distinctive histologic features: groups of radially arranged columnar cells around aggregates of round or polygonal cells. These central masses may become transparent or die. This appearance of dead cells, the authors say, "has reminded some observers of the earliest fetal tooth buds. … The discrete areas of dead cells often underwent slow calcification."[4] Although Adamson and associates[5] have confirmed these findings, other thorough studies, such as those of Miller[6] and Petito and colleagues,[7] have failed to do so. Light microscopic and electron microscopic appraisals conducted by Lisczak and co-workers,[8] even those showing "aggressive growth patterns," failed to agree with what actually occurred.[9] Although Giangaspero and associates[10] described six adults who had tumors and the appearance of a favorable prognosis, three of them actually had a short downhill course to death, and the other three had been followed up for only 8 months or less.[10]

CAPSULE

The detailed structure and extent of the cells often surrounding the actual tumor do not represent the usual kind of capsule. This feature is the surgeon's most commonly unsolved problem. Critchley and Ironside,[11] in one of the earlier comprehensive accounts, describe "the glial tumor reaction in the surrounding structures" as a consistent third element of the lesion along with the epithelial elements and connective tissue stroma. They say that "the glial proliferation forms a sort of capsule," invading extensively in a few cases, even into the central portion of the tumor. They also say that "transection through the capsule reveals a definitely laminated system of connective tissue elements composed externally of neuroglia and internally of fibrous tissue. Within these coverings, there is usually a fine epithelial stratum made up of two or more layers of stratified epithelium." Thus they say that in one of their cases, "The tumor was surrounded by a fibrous capsule except where it was united to the anterior surface of the infundibulum from the upper part of which it seemed to arise." This external glial layer was reported also by Bailey and co-workers[12] to be invaded by epithelial neoplastic streamers, often with the glial layer so substantial and perhaps so tenacious that the plane of cleavage would be more likely to lie in the normal hypothalamus. Ingraham and Scott,[13] however, though describing large cysts as often having a tough fibrous capsule, also say that "the solid masses of the craniopharyngiomas are usually separated from neighboring brain or hypophyseal tissue by only a thin layer of gliosis and possess no well defined capsule." These three descriptions present the problem "in capsule form," so to speak; namely, do these patients have a sufficiently complete glial investment where it is needed against normal brain to permit a delicate and complete removal of tumor plus a normally functioning brain?

Some pathologists,[5] including Miller,[6] described the finger-like epithelial streamers invading the glial layer as invasions of brain. This is not brain any more than solid glioma is brain.

[†]Deceased.

425

I saw the autopsy of a patient in the 1940s who during life had been subjected to repeated cyst aspirations; the firm-walled entire tumor could be gently lifted away from the brain after some tiny avascular strands of tissue had been cut. Bartlett[14] states that "a slow growing tumor usually fell out of its bed at autopsy," whereas "fast growing tumors excited a gliotic or collagenous reaction." By 1948, I had decided that one should explore every resectable-sized craniopharyngioma so as not to leave in situ any readily removable mass. My first such patient was a 14-year-old boy; the cystic portion of his tumor lay lateral to the left optic nerve, compressing it and its blood vessels so that it was white. Aspiration of the cyst permitted the nerve to resume its normal shape and its blood vessels to fill. The solid parts of the tumor were removed from between the left internal carotid artery and the nerve, including a left inferoposterolateral extension into the cerebellopontine angle. The tumor capsule, which had no tenacious adherence to neighboring structures, was sturdy enough to permit a probable total removal. We did not know enough about supplemental corticosteroids to administer any. Probably, no pressure was exerted on the hypothalamus, and the patient recovered smoothly and fully. Forty-five years later, he continued to work full time as a certified nurse's aid.

This lucky result led me to reinvestigate accounts of the pathologic characteristics of the capsule. There was and remains general agreement that a reactive gliosis commonly occurs whenever the tumor is in contact with or invading hypothalamus, and the publications on this issue continue to emanate from several distinguished neuropathologists.[15–18] Those whom I consulted in 1951 gave me no encouragement, however, that this layer might permit innocuous dissection by the neurosurgeon. They emphasized its density and the general toughness of glial scars.

In early 1952, a neurology colleague, Quadfasel, referred to me a close and favorite relative only on the condition that I remove her tumor completely, even if during the operation I estimated the risk of death to be over 90% if I continued the removal. He had arrived at this decision because the relentless downhill course of these patients treated by discouraging successive cyst aspirations, shunts, and partial removals would have been intolerable to this highly intelligent lady. Our endocrinologists were informed about the merits of cortisone, but I also described to him the capsule problem. He nevertheless urged taking the unknown degree of risk involved. Her tumor, which filled most of the third ventricle, had pushed the chiasm forward to be flush with the tuberculum sellae. Removal via the lamina terminalis between the optic tracts required easing some right-sided tumor medially under the right tract, resulting in a partial hemianopia. The tumor in the upper posterior part of the third ventricle crept downward and forward with minimal surgical urging. In my experience, this type of tumor has only minor adhesions to the posterior part of the third ventricle, a view of Matson's (of the Boston Children's Hospital) with which I agree. Because the main adhesions are to brain and vessels anteroinferiorly, the most likely site of the cells of origin, it is safer to deal with these through the lamina terminalis than by a superior transventricular route. The patient had a delightful first postoperative week, so encouraging that our endocrinologist abruptly stopped the cortisone late one day and left the hospital. This action was followed by a precipitous fall in blood pressure. We did not spot the trouble until hours of cerebral ischemia had ruined her higher mental functions. Fortunately, she died 4 months later, having rendered a vitally important service, namely, showing that the capsule can be of surgically useful character, even when it lies against much of the third ventricular wall.

My initial experience, which is encouraging with respect to tumor removal without mortal injury to the brain, is presumably related to a safety feature of the glial layer. The tendency of glial proliferation to occur with these tumors can be so pronounced that the lesion may seem to be a glioma of the visual pathways. I have had two such patients and was saved from leaving the tumor in situ only by the assiduity of the neuropathologist Richardson, who looked through many sections of operative biopsy samples until he found a cluster of epithelial cells. Removal of such a tumor in one patient resulted in complete recovery of her visual fields and acuity from a grossly impaired preoperative level. In another patient, the glial investment appeared grossly to be soft white matter, yet happily turned out microscopically to contain no neurons or nerve fibers.

In one patient, a very thin layer of pseudocapsule was still intact in one area of the surgical specimen, yet he recovered and had no recurrence and no disability in 18 years of follow-up.[19]

Conversely, we treated a patient whose tissue from the posterior edge of his chiasm looked normal. Both with macroscopic techniques and even with the operating microscope, this area was indistinguishable from the rest of the chiasm. Hematoxylin and eosin staining showed mostly astrocytes but with small epithelial rests. The remainder of the largely third ventricular tumor had been removed, but I feared major visual impairment if I removed more chiasm. The patient worked effectively in the family butcher shop for 10 years, when after 2 months of recurrent symptoms we found almost all of his third ventricle to be reoccupied by tumor. At our repeat operation, Crowell and I clearly left a small amount of tumor. His further course was described again in 1980 by Sweet[9]; it was at first satisfactory as a result of careful regulation of his hormonal supplement (as is discussed later) but by 1988 had steadily deteriorated to level "poor."[19]

Confirmation that the glial reactive layer facilitates the surgeon's dissection has been noted by Hoffman and colleagues,[20] Kahn and colleagues,[4] Katz,[19] and Symon.[21] Kobayashi and associates[22] conducted the most extensive pathologic study of the surface of this tumor vis-à-vis the brain in seven patients who went to autopsy without previous surgery. Their serial sections revealed that significant cystic portions of the tumors had a connective tissue membrane between the tumor inside and its smooth attachment to the adjacent glial barrier outside. A distinct layer of gliosis lay between the cyst wall and viable ganglion cells in the hypothalamus and thalamus that ranged in thickness from several hundred micrometers to a few millimeters. Degenerated neurons and demyelinated fibers in this layer were largely replaced by Rosenthal fibers and fibrillary astrocytes (Fig. 33-1). However, the solid portions of the tumors had no connective tissue membrane; protrusions of tumor invaded the gliotic zone. In some areas, tumor cells were only a few micrometers away from viable neurons of hypothalamus or thalamus, and no glial reaction occurred. Prevention of

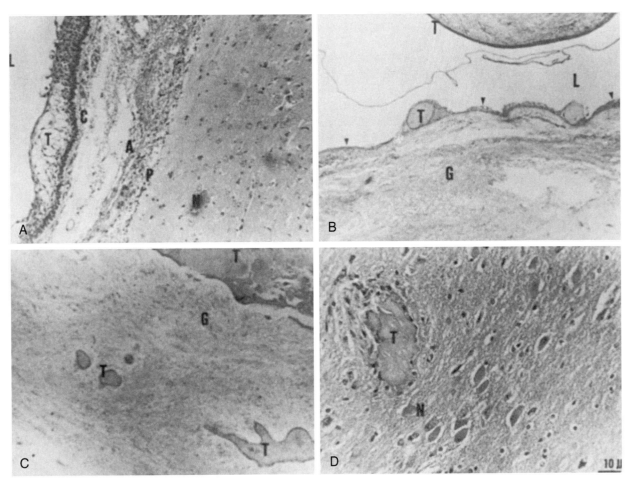

FIGURE 33-1 *A,* The wall of a cystic portion of the tumor's surface showing a connective tissue membrane between the inside of the tumor and its smooth attachment to the adjacent arachnoid and pia. No gliosis appears in the adjoining brain. *B,* Cystic portion of tumor (T); this layer of scattered tumor cells is next to extensive glial reaction between tumor and brain. *C,* The solid portions of the tumor have no outer connective tissue membrane. Papillary protrusions of tumor have invaded the gliotic zone. With and without the connective tissue layer, the layer of gliosis varied in thickness from several hundred micrometers to a few millimeters. *D,* The exceptional situation of a cluster of epithelial cells within viable neurons of hypothalamus with no glial reaction is seen. A, arachnoid; C, connective tissue; F, normal nerve fibers; G, glia; L, lumen; N, normal brain; P, pia; T, tumor. (With thanks to Kobayashi T, Kageyama N, Yoshida J, et al: Pathological and clinical basis of the indications for treatment of craniopharyngiomas. Neurol Med Chir 21:39–47, 1981, who did serial sections on the interface between tumor and brain in seven patients who came to autopsy having had no previous surgery in the tumor area.)

significant hypothalamic injury remains the surgeon's principal problem.

RADIOLOGIC EVALUATION

The ability to determine the precise location and volume of cystic and solid components of the tumor has greatly improved treatment by all modalities, especially those involving stereotaxis.

Magnetic resonance imaging (MRI) and MR angiography are responsible for the discovery of a new syndrome, fusiform dilatation of the carotid artery. Sutton[23] has described an unusual complication resulting from neurosurgeons' attempts to dissect the last bit of tenacious adherences to the supraclinoid internal carotid artery of craniopharyngioma (nine patients) or chiasmatic-hypothalamic glioma (two patients). The complication consists of the delayed appearance of aneurysmal dilatation of the entire circumference of the vessel. Figure 33-2A is a normal digital subtraction angiogram

obtained preoperatively in a patient with a hypothalamic astrocytoma. Figure 33-2B is the right carotid arteriogram of the same patient that was obtained 10 years after right pterional craniectomy and radiation therapy. It shows striking dilatation of the entire supraclinoid internal carotid. None of the nine patients with craniopharyngioma had a hemorrhage or any other symptom referable to the lesion, and no treatment has been given. MRI proton density–weighted spin-echo sequences demonstrate a flow void that depicts the dilated artery (Fig. 33-2C). MR angiography also shows the lesion well and confirms flowing blood within it. The lesion was found 6 to 12 months after operation in the patients with craniopharyngiomas and several years after operation and radiation in those with gliomas. However, of the two patients with fusiform dilatation of the carotid artery that was discovered 8 and 11 years after operation for glioma, one experienced headaches and possibly a hemorrhage. Operation for the lesion yielded a poor result, and no further operations have been performed in the asymptomatic patients.

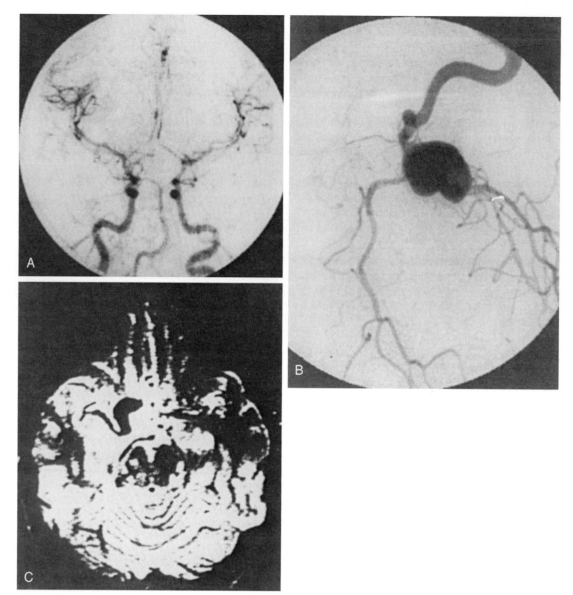

FIGURE 33-2 *A,* Digital subtraction angiogram performed as part of the original preoperative evaluation of a patient with a hypothalamic astrocytoma. No carotid artery abnormality is seen. *B,* Right carotid arteriogram performed on the same patient 10 years after right pterional craniotomy and radiation therapy shows marked aneurysmal dilatation of the entire supraclinoid carotid artery segment. *C,* Proton density-weighted magnetic resonance image, demonstrating a flow void within a dilated supraclinoid carotid artery on the right side.

ENDOCRINE ABNORMALITIES

Sklar[24] describes endocrine abnormalities seen at the first presentation, at which only a few children with craniopharyngiomas complain of symptoms of hormonal deficiency. However, 80% to 90% of them prove to have such inadequacies, along with their common symptoms of headache, vomiting, and visual problems.[24] A summary of laboratory measurements[25–28] is shown in Table 33-1. Almost half of the patients are short in stature, and growth rate is subnormal in most of these patients. Sorva[26] found that the growth records showed impairment in 19 of 22 children with craniopharyngioma and preceded the diagnosis by an average of 4 years. An alert pediatrician spotted this feature

TABLE 33-1 ▪ Craniopharyngioma: Hypothalamic-Pituitary Function before Treatment

Abnormality	Incidence (%)
Growth hormone deficient	75
Luteinizing hormone, follicle-stimulating hormone deficient	40
Adrenocorticotropin deficient	25
Thyroxine-stimulating hormone deficient	25
Increased prolactin	20
Antidiuretic hormone deficient	9–17

Data from references 25–28.

in a 17-year-old young man as the only sign or symptom of his modest-sized third ventricular tumor. This tumor was readily removed by Sweet, and the patient achieved a good record at university and thereafter.

A raised prolactin level suggests damage to hypothalamic areas, which normally inhibit release of prolactin. Although diabetes insipidus is common after a major or radical removal of the tumor, it is found in only a few before the operation. As became apparent in the early 1950s, preoperative testing for corticotropin-adrenal insufficiency and assessment of sodium and water balance are vitally important. Even if these results are normal, any operative trauma to the hypothalamus requires prophylactic administration of large doses of glucocorticosteroids. The necessity of continuing administration of cortisone and regular studies on the entire hormone picture of these patients led our endocrinologists to emphasize to patients and parents the imperative need for frequent monitoring of the endocrine status and immediate supplemental medication, even with such minor stress as a common cold. This approach has resulted in a great reduction in the late postoperative endocrine-related deaths described by Matson and Crigler.[29] The burgeoning understanding of the importance of administering hormonal supplements in the management of surgical and any other form of stress has yielded gratifying results.

One of the many metabolic effects of cortisone is that it decreases polyuria and increases urine osmolality in patients with diabetes insipidus of central origin, thus tending to obscure that diagnosis. Moreover, high-dose glucocorticoids can decrease the secretion of growth hormone, corticotropin, thyroid-stimulating hormone, thyroxine, and prolactin. Also, the commonly used prophylactic anticonvulsants phenytoin and carbamazepine may cause reduced levels of thyroid-stimulating hormone and thyroxine, both total and free.[30,31] Carbamazepine also rarely causes diabetes insipidus. The complexity of these hormonal interactions is evidenced also by the variable changes in growth rate occurring in the first postoperative year. The rate may be increased, normal, or decreased, with about equal numbers in each of the groups. Those with excessive growth in height also gain weight; they had hyperinsulinism, normal immunoreactive insulin-like growth factor-1 level, elevated prolactin level, and delayed thyroid-stimulating hormone response to thyroid-stimulating hormone–releasing hormone, which indicate a hypothalamic lesion. The one-third of patients growing at a normal rate had low insulin levels, with values of the other hormones the same as those in the fast growers. Those growing too slowly had low levels of insulin, insulin-like growth factor-1, prolactin, and thyrotropin.[32] The value of the endocrinologist is illustrated by the case of the patient discussed earlier, who had become less active and heavier on our postoperative discharge regimen of thyroxine, 0.2 mg/day, and hydrocortisone, 25 mg/day. He continued to have visual acuity of J1 and J4 and small inferior temporal field defects. The endocrinologist rightly suspected that we were giving him too much glucocorticosteroid, gradually reduced his prednisone to 3 mg in the morning and 1 mg in the evening, changed his pitressin tannate in oil to desmopressin acetate, increased the dosage of thyroxine from 0.2 mg to 0.3 mg/day, and added 5 mg/day of amphetamine (Dexedrine). The symptoms I was attributing to recurrence vanished. The patient lost 16 kg, dropping to 66 kg; his visual fields and acuity

improved to nearly normal; and he was again earning his living as a meat cutter. I trust that the neurosurgeon will require no further evidence that the collaboration of an exceedingly well-informed endocrinologist is necessary to follow up and treat these patients for a very long time.

VISUAL PROBLEMS

That visual problems deserve special attention is indicated by a 1990 statement of Yasargil and colleagues: "The destructive effects of these tumors on the optic pathways were disastrous in two thirds of the patients in this series and were especially pronounced in the children."[33] Pierre-Kahn and co-workers[34] addressed this problem in 16 children who had severe loss of vision, severe papilledema with hemorrhage, or episodes of transient amaurosis. With the objective of prompt amelioration of pressure against the anterior visual pathways achieved with a minimum of general stress, he sought to puncture a sizable cyst and slowly drain it into a reservoir, which he left in situ for an average of 50 days in 12 children before performing his principal operation. In the other 4 children, he was unable to enter a cyst. In 18 children with less visual loss or cysts too small to identify, he proceeded to immediate tumor removal. Tumor removal was total in 25 of the 30 cases. In the children who had repeated puncture of the cyst through the reservoir, the visual acuity improved in 7 of 17 eyes and worsened or stayed the same in 12 of 20. The authors also point out that the surgeon must take care that the interopticocarotid space is adequately widened by tumor before this area is dissected lest he or she injure tiny arteries from the internal carotid passing superomedially to optic nerve and chiasm.

TREATMENT

Observation

In the ISPC-91 series, 11 children with only endocrine symptoms were at first merely observed. Of these, the symptoms of two progressed, and the patients had operations 2 years later.[1] Follow-up data are provided for only two other patients, who showed no further growth 4 and 10 years later, respectively.

Surgery

Since 1970, a gradual, and more recently, a rapid swing has occurred toward the objective of achieving a total or near-total removal of these tumors at the first operation. The route chosen depends on the principal site of the tumor; the great variability on this score is illustrated and the corresponding variations in approach are discussed by Samii and co-workers in this volume (Chapter 34) and by Yasargil and co-workers,[33] Symon and co-workers,[35,36] and Lapras and co-workers.[37]

Transsphenoidal Approach

We owe our most authoritative information on this tactic to Laws.[38] A summary of his presentation at the Epstein symposium follows: Craniopharyngiomas arising below the sella diaphragm produce progressive enlargement of the sella, giving a radiographic picture seen in 30% to 60% of previously reported series. The diaphragm usually remains as an effective barrier that prevents intimate tumor attachment to any of the important overlying intracranial structures. However, the tumor usually fuses with the diaphragm, which must frequently be removed. The floor of the sella is also removed as widely as possible to create the greatest possible working area. The necessary careful reconstruction of the sella after the tumor has been removed is described by Laws as "a major challenge of this operative approach." Likewise, similar tumor attachments to the medial dural wall of both cavernous sinuses must be stripped away "with bleeding from the sinus, damage of the intracavernous carotid artery or trauma to the cranial nerves in the cavernous sinuses." Laws routinely dissects the tumor from the pituitary stalk "with minimal trauma" and finds that he can remove via the sphenoid route most tumors associated with enlarged sellas. In 65% of these patients, major suprasellar and parasellar extensions were present. He has also approached transsphenoidally some predominantly suprasellar craniopharyngiomas, usually with only a palliative goal.

From 1973 to 1993, Laws performed transsphenoidal removals on 76 such tumors. Of the 29 patients treated primarily by this route and followed up over 5 years, total removal was achieved in 27, with 1 operative death, 1 living disabled patient, 25 well patients, and 2 who had recurrences, one of whom is well and the other disabled. Of the 17 patients in whom only subtotal removal was achieved, 11 were well, 5 disabled, and 1 dead from other causes. Of the 18 such patients treated secondarily by the transsphenoidal route, the results were almost as good as those in the primary subtotal removals. In Laws' 89 operations, only two deaths occurred. Anyone wishing to emulate or improve on the record of this skillful, thoughtful man would do well to begin with some personal tutorial sessions with him.

Stereotactic Methods of Focal Radiation

By far the most successful proponent of stereotactic methods of focal radiation is Backlund,[39,40] who has brought to fruition Leksell's two pioneering concepts. First, the larger cysts are treated by the instillation of pure electron, beta-emitting isotope ^{90}Y or [32]P. The former, which has a 62-hour half-life and 2.3-MeV electrons, is slightly less convenient and penetrates deeper compared with the 14.3-day half-life and 1.74-MeV electrons of [32]P. The electrons at these energies are unlikely to damage visual or hypothalamic structures beyond the fibrous connective tissue and gliotic layers forming the cyst wall. Second, the solid components are treated by photons from ^{60}Co admitted to the target area via air-containing channels in a lead helmet that are directed to a focal target area. This tactic does not have the effective cutoff of radiation beyond the target provided by particle radiation with electrons, protons, or helium atoms.

However, Backlund has included in his standard therapeutic protocol an open microsurgical total removal if "the size and shape of the tumor" indicate that safe surgery with a problem-free postoperative course could be expected. In 1993, he reported the results from his first 43 consecutive patients who had no previous therapy and who were treated between 1964 and 1976.[40] Of the 13 patients selected for tumor removal, the 9 who underwent open operations described earlier and the 4 who underwent focused photon treatment (gamma knife) had a smooth post-treatment course and tumor elimination. Colloidal ^{90}Y was the primary treatment in 18 patients with a large, usually monocystic tumor. In the remaining 12 patients, different combinations of treatment were used. In 4, initial intracystic radiation to reduce bulk was followed by open subtotal removal; in 4 others, focused photons to the solid tumor followed intracystic ^{90}Y administration; in 1 patient, the cystic radiation was followed by linear accelerator radiation. In the 9 patients with very large tumors, linear accelerator radiation was paired with partial surgical removal in only 2.

Follow-up revealed that 6 patients (14%) died of their tumors, and 4 died of autopsy-proven other causes. However, in 1 of these 4, the autopsy revealed a subarachnoid hemorrhage from an erosion of the posterior communicating artery—probably related to the treatment of the tumor. Only 1 patient was lost to follow-up, leaving 32 who were all "alive and well." The thoroughness of the staff of the Karolinska Institute and Sweden's social security system have resulted in an unusually complete appraisal of the status of the survivors. Of 29 patients younger than 65 years of age, 23 (79%) work regularly, and 21 of these work full time. Of the 4 with disability pensions, 2 had cognitive and neurologic deficits related to radiation in childhood, and 1 had poor endocrine follow-up findings. Of those treated in childhood, only 2 were married, and they had no children. Comparison of days off work per year and days of hospitalization per year between the craniopharyngioma survivors and the general Swedish population revealed a slight advantage in terms of lesser disability for the group of 23 tumors.

From these results, we may conclude that when one considers the near-certain improvement from heavy-particle focused radiation and microsurgical removal by the most skilled neurosurgeons, one can hope for improvement in the results.

Although the number of patients in whom the advantages of microsurgical removal is probably higher than the 9 of 43 (21%) recorded here, the place for stereotactically controlled radiation is also firmly established by these carefully assembled data.

Stereotactic Control of Radiation Treatments

Procedures involving *stereotactic radiosurgery* are defined as methods for delivering a single dose to distinct volumes that are determined by precise imaging. *Stereotactic radiotherapy* refers to the same general tactic for the distinction, usually of larger volumes by fractionation. Tarbell and associates[41] gave a full account of methodology for achieving these two closely related objectives. Patients are treated on a prototype linear accelerator that delivers radiation in multiple coplanar arcs through small circular collimators measuring 0.5 to 50 mm. Reproducibility of the precise position of the frame attached to the head is a requirement for treatment in repeated fractions. In over 3300 sets of multiple scalp readings, individual measurements between fittings varied only 0.31 mm. The facility opened June 1, 1992, and had treated 10 craniopharyngiomas by late 1993.

Chemotherapy for Cysts

Umezawa and co-workers[42] found that the antibiotic bleomycin is toxic to squamous cell cancer cells. Because benign squamous epithelial cells often occur in craniopharyngiomas, Kubo and colleagues[43] checked the toxicity of bleomycin in cultures of these cells. The results encouraged Takahashi and colleagues[44] to carry out multiple such injections into the cysts of seven patients; they had three excellent and one poor result in predominantly cystic tumors, and three deaths occurred in solid or mixed tumors. Broggi and co-workers[45] described the disappearance of 13 cysts and the decrease in size of 5 cysts in 18 patients followed up from 3 to 31 months. Fischer and associates,[46] however, having used the agent both in a cyst and systemically, evoked progressive blindness and hemiparesis gradually over 2 years without radiographic evidence of recurrence. Several conferees at the Epstein symposium derived cautious encouragement from their experiences.

Comparison of the Two Customary Methods of Treatment

Intensive efforts to reach well-founded conclusions on this subject are not helped by the mental agility of many of us in presenting the data on our own favored tactic in the most alluring fashion. In the words of Brada and Thomas, "The results are ... often retrospective, not standardized and frequently colored in favor of the treatment modality reported."[47] For example, Table 33-2 (Degree of Disability after Treatment), contains the footnote "Does not include patients dead from disease or complications."[48] No other part of the original article gives this information. Numerous authors emphasize the necessity of long follow-ups with full information on the extent of deficits in all of the visual, endocrine, metabolic, and neuropsychologic areas so likely to be affected. The well-known major problems in the treatment of these tumors lead to referrals at long distances, making intensive follow-up on these aspects the more difficult and proper vigilance in endocrine support less likely. The sketchy definitions of classes of recovery also obscure comparisons between reports. For example, total blindness can usually be compensated for by an otherwise normal person but may lead to total disability in the presence of moderate mental or psychosocial retardation.

Subtotal Surgical Resection Only

Subtotal surgical resection can be dismissed now on the basis of many publications, of which only six are cited here.[49–54] Many early, rapidly growing recurrences are the almost universal experience.

POLL OF NEUROSURGEONS

As a component of the monograph of Choux and colleagues,[1] the philosophy of craniopharyngioma management in children was solicited from 17 prominent neurosurgeons. Microscopic complete removal, when possible, is the first choice of 13 (Basso, Fukushima, Hoffman, Kobayashi, Konovalov, Lapras, Laws, Mori, Samii, Symon, Takahashi, Takakura, Yasargil). Backlund, Lunsford, and Steiner, all pupils of Leksell, follow his pioneering technique of using ^{90}Y or ^{32}P radiation on the cystic component and focused gamma radiation on the solid component. Derome is the most conservative, favoring initial observation in children,[1] "especially if the tumor is calcified." This is a startling statement because most children show calcium in tumor on computed tomography scanning. Derome thinks that radiation should be postponed until after the first decade of life. Although most publications by neurosurgeons agree with the huge majority of 76% recorded in the poll, a few neurosurgeons, including, interestingly, the successors of Matson at the Boston Children's Hospital and the group at the University of California, San Francisco (UCSF), as well as radiation oncologists, are giving radiation therapy a steadily increasing role. After the death of Matson in 1969, the next publication on the subject from the Boston Children's Hospital by Fischer and colleagues[54] reported on 37 children treated between 1972 and 1984. Total removal was thought to be accomplished in 8 of 14 initial attempts to excise the tumor; 23 other patients were initially irradiated. At the Epstein symposium, Scott and colleagues[48] from the Boston Children's Hospital continued the same emphasis on irradiation as the usual initial therapy and reported on 15 patients who had initial extensive surgery and 37 who had lesser surgery plus radiation. The surgeon thought that total removal was achieved in 10, but recurrence took place in 9 of them. Scott and co-workers,[48] in Table 33-2, show the degree of disability in the two groups.

The University of California, San Francisco, group, represented by Wara and associates[55] at the Epstein symposium, summarized their view of the literature as appears in Table 33-3. These figures may be compared with the more detailed data from the ISPC-91 series of 454 patients, in which an operative mortality rate of 3.7% was reported, and with the data from Choux and co-workers' article, which includes individual figures for 17 services from 1975 through 1991.[1] In 5 services that performed 167 operations, the mortality rate was 0%; it varied from 12% to 15% in the 5 services that performed 155 operations and that had the highest mortality rate. Mortality rate averaged 6.7% in the 7 intermediate services. In general, as the surgeon's experience increased, the mortality rate declined: For example, my rate of

---

TABLE 33-2 ▪ Degree of Disability after Treatment of Childhood Craniopharyngioma*

	Surgery (No = 15)		Surgery and Radiotherapy (No = 31)	
	No Recurrence No. (%)	Recurrence No. (%)	No Recurrence No. (%)	Recurrence No. (%)
1. No disability	3 (20)	3 (20)	18 (58)	0 (0)
2. Mild handicap	1 (7)	3 (20)	7 (23)	0 (0)
3. Major disability	2 (15)	3 (20)	2 (6)	4 (13)
4. Incapable of self-care	0 (0)	0 (0)	0 (0)	0 (0)

*Does not include patients dead from disease or complications.
From Scott RM, Hetelekidis S, Barnes P, et al: Surgery, radiation, and combination therapy in the treatment of childhood craniopharyngioma—a 20-year experience. Presented at the Symposium on Craniopharyngioma: The Answer. New York, New York Medical Center, December 17–19,1993. Reprinted with permission from S. Karger, AG, Basel.

**TABLE 33-3 ▪ Radiation Oncologists'
Viewpoint on Craniopharyngioma Outcome**

Outcome Measure	Incidence (%)	
	Total Resection	Subtotal Resection and Radiotherapy
Death	10	1–2
Recurrence	60–70	—
Morbidity	30	10
New tumor or vascular complication	—	1–2

Modified from Brada M, Thomas DG: Craniopharyngioma revisited. Int J Radiat Oncol Biol Phys 27:471–475, 1993. With kind permission from Elsevier Science Ltd, The Boulevard, Langford Lane, Kidlington OX5 1GB, UK.

7.5% for my whole series of radical removals fell from 10% for the first 28% to zero for the last 12.

Again, in the ISPC-91 series, in which follow-ups lasted longer than 3 years, in 53 children who underwent operation plus radiation, 6 (11.3%) died, whereas in the 239 children who had operation only, 14 (5.8%) died. French investigators have emphasized the danger of brain injury from radiation in childhood. Comprehensive appraisals of performance under the general heading of psychosocial adjustment were classified by Pierre-Kahn as indicating normal performance in 81% of patients not irradiated, but in only 22% of patients who had irradiation early or as a complement to surgery.[56] The intelligence quotient averaged 88 after surgical treatment only and was only 75 in the irradiated patients reported by Pierre-Kahn and associates. This discrepancy in the results of the irradiations and the extirpations points to the need for more critically assembled data.

Although the short range of the beta-emitting ^{90}Y and ^{32}P makes radiation of the cysts attractive, focused gamma radiation for the solid tumor is more dangerous because of the vulnerability of the hypothalamic and visual systems, which are usually in direct contact with tumor. However, see the article by Backlund and colleagues[39] for contrary evidence.

The actual completeness of the initial removal varies greatly. In Russia, in Konovalov's far-flung catchment area, which spread through nine time zones, approximately one-third of his more than 500 craniopharyngiomas were of "giant" size (>5 cm in diameter).[57] There is general agreement that the morbidity and mortality rates are significantly higher in this "giant" group; Yasargil's operative mortality rate was seven of eight in tumors larger than 6 cm in diameter. The degree of determination to remove the tumor balanced against eagerness to prevent brain damage is bound to be variably assessed by different surgeons. The risk of external radiation, especially in children in this particular situation, is poorly known. The modes of handling the recurrences involve differing decisions as to: (1) the minimally or asymptomatic lesions demonstrated by surgery, (2) the age of the patient, (3) the variably crucial invaded brain, and (4) the neurologic and general medical status of the patient.

Although drawing conclusions from the entire world literature is difficult, I venture to try to appraise my own experience of 40 patients who underwent a radical removal.

Regarding the three immediate postoperative deaths, I would not repeat the mistake I made of trying to dissect tumor away from an artery in two of them. During operation, I would also send for histologic examination any specimen with an appearance suggestive of neural tissue to be guided on the wisdom of further removal. As the length of observation has increased, the number of deaths relatively unrelated to tumor has increased more than the number of those resulting from recurrence. Thus all deaths in the 6 patients who died of recurrence occurred 112 to 1412 months after their initial operation. Of the 10 patients whose deaths were of causes unrelated to tumor, 5 died in the zero to 15-year survival group, and the remaining 5 lived from 16 to 26.9 years (mean, 22.3 years). The patients in whom recurrences have taken place were in 4 of 6 cases in the good or excellent category at first. However, 6 of the patients who had recurrences have died, and 4 of the 5 still living have deteriorated to the fair-to-poor category. Of the 19 still living, 15 are in the good or excellent category. In the same categories were 8 of the 10 who died of unrelated causes and 4 of 6 before their fatal recurrence. The main good feature of the series is that the status of 23 of the 40 patients was good to excellent in reference to their craniopharyngiomas; the patients died of other causes. The main weak feature of the series is the progression to the failed III and IV groups, or death in 10 of the 11 recurrences. I would now recommend that the primary objective of total removal be maintained but that clinical imaging studies be performed every 6 months for the first several years. Focal proton radiation should be given as soon as clear-cut recurrence develops, unless there is good reason to expect that the tumor can be removed totally at reoperation.

Acknowledgments

The author wishes to express his appreciation to the Neuro-Research Foundation for its support in the preparation of this manuscript and Deborah Wallace for her intelligent assistance.

REFERENCES

1. Choux M, Lena G, Genitori L: Le craniopharyngiome de l'enfant. Neurochirurgie 37(Suppl 1):1–174, 1991.
2. Peet MM: Pituitary adamantinomas: Report of three cases. Arch Surg 15:829–854, 1927.
3. Nelson GA, Bastian FO, Schlitt M, White RL: Malignant transformation in craniopharyngioma. Neurosurgery 22:427–429, 1988.
4. Kahn EA, Gosch HH, Seeger JF, Hicks SP: Forty-five years' experience with the craniopharyngiomas. Surg Neurol 1:5–12, 1973.
5. Adamson TE, Wiestler OD, Kleihues P, Yasargil MG: Correlation of clinical and pathological features in craniopharyngiomas. J Neurosurg 73:12–17, 1990.
6. Miller DC: Pathology of craniopharyngiomas: Clinical import of pathological findings. Presented at the Symposium on Craniopharyngioma: The Answer. New York, New York Medical Center, December 17–19, 1993.
7. Petito CK, DeGirolami E, Earle K: Craniopharyngiomas: A clinical and pathological review. Cancer 37:1944–1952, 1976.
8. Lisczak T, Richardson EP, Phillips JP, et al: Morphological, biochemical, ultrastructural, tissue culture and clinical observations of typical and aggressive craniopharyngiomas. Acta Neuropathol (Berl) 43:191–203, 1978.
9. Sweet WH: Recurrent craniopharyngiomas: Therapeutic alternatives. Clin Neurosurg 27:214–224, 1980.
10. Giangaspero F, Osburne DR, Burger PC, Stein RB: Suprasellar papillary squamous epithelioma ("papillary craniopharyngioma"). Am J Surg Pathol 8:57–64, 1984.

11. Critchley M, Ironside RN: The pituitary adamantinomata. Brain 49:437–481, 1926.
12. Bailey P, Buchanan DN, Bucy PC: Intracranial Tumors of Infancy and Childhood. Chicago: University of Chicago Press, 1939, pp 349–375.
13. Ingraham FD, Scott HW: Craniopharyngiomas in children. J Pediatr 29:95–116, 1946.
14. Bartlett JR: Craniopharyngiomas—a summary of 85 cases. J Neurol Neurosurg Psychiatry 34:37–41, 1971.
15. Van den Bergh R, Brucher JM: L'abord transventriculaire dans les cranio-pharyngiomes du troisième ventricule: Aspects neurochirurgicaux et neuro-pathologiques. Neurochirurgie 16:51–65, 1970.
16. Ghatak NR, Hirano A, Zimmerman HM: Ultrastructure of a craniopharyngioma. Cancer 27:1465–1475, 1971.
17. Grcevic N, Yates PO: Rosenthal fibers in tumors of the central nervous system. J Pathol 73:467–472, 1957.
18. Zülch KJ: Brain Tumors: Their Biology and Pathology, 2nd ed. New York: Springer, 1965.
19. Katz EL: Late results of radical excision of craniopharyngiomas in children. J Neurosurg 42:86–90, 1975.
20. Hoffman HJ, Hendrick EB, Humphreys RP, et al: Management of craniopharyngioma in children. J Neurosurg 47:218–227, 1977.
21. Symon L: Radical excision of craniopharyngioma: Results in 20 patients. J Neurosurg 62:174–181, 1985.
22. Kobayashi T, Kageyama N, Yoshida J, et al: Pathological and clinical basis of the indications for treatment of craniopharyngiomas. Neurol Med Chir 21:39–47, 1981.
23. Sutton LN: Vascular complications of surgery for craniopharyngioma and hypothalamic glioma. Presented at the Symposium on Craniopharyngioma: The Answer. New York Medical Center, New York, December 17–19, 1993.
24. Sklar CA: Craniopharyngioma: Endocrine abnormalities at presentation. Presented at the Symposium on Craniopharyngioma: The Answer. New York, New York Medical Center, December 17–19, 1993.
25. Thomsett MJ, Conte FA, Kaplan SL, Grumbach MM: Endocrine and neurologic outcome in childhood craniopharyngioma. J Pediatr 97:728–735, 1980.
26. Sorva R: Children with craniopharyngioma. Acta Pediatr Scand 77:587–592, 1988.
27. Stahnke N, Grubel G, Lagenstein I, Willig RP: Long-term follow-up of children with craniopharyngioma. Eur J Pediatr 142:179–185, 1984.
28. Blethen SL: Growth in children with a craniopharyngioma. Pediatrician 14:242–245, 1987.
29. Matson DD, Crigler JF, Jr: Management of craniopharyngiomas in childhood. J Neurosurg 30:377–390, 1969.
30. Smith PJ, Surks MI: Multiple effects of 5,5-diphenylhydantoin on the thyroid hormone system. Endocr Rev 5:514–524, 1984.
31. Isojarvi JIT, Pakarinen AJ, Myllyla VV: Thyroid function in epileptic patients treated with carbamazepine. Arch Neurol 46:1175–1178, 1989.
32. Bucher H, Zapf J, Torresani T, et al: Insulin-like growth factors I and II, prolactin and insulin in 19 growth hormone–deficient children with excessive, normal or decreased longitudinal growth after operation for craniopharyngioma. N Engl J Med 309:1142–1146, 1983.
33. Yasargil MG, Curcic M, Kis M, et al: Total removal of craniopharyngiomas. J Neurosurg 73:3–11, 1990.
34. Pierre-Kahn A, Sainte-Rose C, Renier D: Surgical approach to children with craniopharyngiomas and severely impaired vision. Presented at the Symposium on Craniopharyngioma: The Answer. New York, New York Medical Center, December 17–19, 1993.
35. Symon L, Pell MF, Habib AHA: Radical excision of craniopharyngioma by the temporal route: A review of 50 patients. Br J Neurosurg 5:539–549, 1991.
36. Symon L: Adult craniopharyngioma: A different problem? Presented at the Symposium on Craniopharyngioma: The Answer. New York, New York Medical Center, December 17–19, 1993.
37. Lapras C, Patet JD, Mottolese C, et al: Craniopharyngiomas in childhood: Analysis of 42 cases. Prog Exp Tumor Res 30:350–358, 1987.
38. Laws E: Transsphenoidal approach to craniopharyngiomas. Presented at the Symposium on Craniopharyngioma: The Answer. New York Medical Center, New York, December 17–19, 1993.
39. Backlund E, Axelsson B, Bergstrand CG, et al: Treatment of craniopharyngiomas—the stereotactic approach in a ten to twenty-three years' perspective. Acta Neurochir 99:11–19, 1989.
40. Backlund E: Treatment of craniopharyngiomas: The multi-modality approach. Presented at the Symposium on Craniopharyngioma: The Answer. New York, New York Medical Center, December 17–19, 1993.
41. Tarbell NJ, Barnes P, Scott M, et al: Advances in radiation therapy for craniopharyngiomas. Presented at the Symposium on Craniopharyngioma: The Answer. New York, New York Medical Center, December 17–19, 1993.
42. Umezawa H, Maeda K, Takeuchi T, et al: New antibiotics bleomycin A and B. J Antibiot 19:200–209, 1966.
43. Kubo O, Takakura K, Miki Y, et al: Intracystic therapy of bleomycin for craniopharyngioma—effect of bleomycin on cultured craniopharyngioma cells and intracystic concentration of bleomycin. No Shinkei Geka 2:683–688, 1974.
44. Takahashi H, Nakazawa S, Shimura T: Evaluation of postoperative intratumoral injection of bleomycin for craniopharyngioma in children. J Neurosurg 62:120–127, 1985.
45. Broggi G, Giorgi C, Franzini A, et al: Preliminary results of intracavitary treatment of craniopharyngioma with bleomycin. J Neurosurg Sci 33:145–148, 1989.
46. Fischer EG, Welch K, Shillito J, et al: Craniopharyngiomas in children: Long-term effects of conservative surgical procedures combined with radiation therapy. J Neurosurg 73:534–540, 1990.
47. Brada M, Thomas DG: Craniopharyngioma revisited. Int J Radiat Oncol Biol Phys 27:471–475, 1993.
48. Scott RM, Hetelekidis S, Barnes P, et al: Surgery, radiation, and combination therapy in the treatment of childhood craniopharyngioma—a 20-year experience. Presented at the Symposium on Craniopharyngioma: The Answer. New York, New York Medical Center, December 17–19, 1993.
49. Hoogenhout J, Otten B, Kazem I, et al: Surgery and radiation therapy in the management of craniopharyngiomas. Int J Radiat Oncol Biol Phys 10:2293–2297, 1984.
50. Manaka S, Teramoto A, Takakura K: The efficacy of radiotherapy for craniopharyngioma. Br J Radiol 58:480–482, 1985.
51. Sung DI, Chang CC, Harisiadis L, Carmel PW: Treatment results of craniopharyngiomas. Cancer 47:847–852, 1981.
52. Weiss M, Sutton L, Marcia V, et al: The role of radiation therapy in the management of childhood craniopharyngioma. Int J Radiat Oncol Biol Phys 17:1313–1321, 1989.
53. Wen BC, Hussey DH, Staples J, et al: A comparison of the roles of surgery and radiation therapy in the management of craniopharyngiomas. Int J Radiat Oncol Biol Phys 16:17–24, 1989.
54. Fischer EG, Welch K, Belli JA, et al: Treatment of craniopharyngiomas in children: 1972–1981. J Neurosurg 62:496–501, 1985.
55. Wara WM, Sneed PK, Larson DA: The role of radiation therapy in the treatment of craniopharyngioma. Presented at the Symposium on Craniopharyngioma: The Answer. New York, New York Medical Center, December 17–19, 1993.
56. Pierre-Kahn A, Brauner R, Renier D, et al: Traitement des craniopharyngiomes de l'enfant: Analyse retrospective de 50 observations. Arch Fr Pediatr 45:163–167, 1988.
57. Konovalov AN: Techniques and strategies of direct surgical management of craniopharyngiomas. In Apuzzo M (ed): Surgery of the Third Ventricle. Baltimore: Williams & Wilkins, 1987, pp 542–552.

Craniopharyngiomas: A Decade Later

ANN-CHRISTINE DUHAIME

In times of rapid technologic change and in the face of mountains of often contradictory data, pinning down "The Answer" about the optimal management of craniopharyngiomas remains an elusive goal. Since Dr. Sweet's chapter was written, showcasing the symposium on this topic held at New York University in December 1993, much has been written and the pendulum has swung a bit, but no consensus has yet been reached. The proceedings of that symposium were published in *Pediatric Neurosurgery* in September 1994. In the summary article, Dr. Fred Epstein stated that "there was agreement that with a small or moderate sized non-cystic craniopharyngioma a child is best treated surgically, and that there is about a 70% chance of accomplishing a gross total removal".[1] The consensus figure reported for the percentage of tumors that could not be completely removed was 25%, and the morbidity in those treated surgically was placed at 25%. Dr. Sweet notes in his chapter that "since 1970, a gradual, and more recently, a rapid swing has occurred toward the objective of achieving a total or near-total removal of these tumors at the first operation." This commentary will address some of these conclusions in light of more recent series.

As was the case a decade ago, most newly available information comes from retrospective case reviews and is subject to all the limitations inherent in this mode of analysis. Nonetheless, several themes can be appreciated. While studies vary widely, there is an overall increased recognition of a lower rate of "complete" resection than the foregoing figures might suggest, when based on careful postoperative MRI studies and/or surgeon's assessment. Thus recent series suggest that even when the initial intent was to achieve a total resection, this could only be accomplished on average in about 50% (range 19% to 76%).[2–9] This may be in part because in some series patients "underwent an initial resection as extensive as was compatible with subsequent good neurological function" as judged by the surgeon.[7] The availability of adjuvant treatments with the potential for lower morbidity as well as the recognition of the life-altering hypothalamic and behavioral dysfunction that can occur with radical surgery, discussed in more detail later, may be altering the threshold for some surgeons to stop short of total resection in some patients.

In addition, more recent studies suggest a higher long-term recurrence rate for surgical resections considered "complete" when patients have been followed carefully for longer intervals. The long-term recurrence rate for patients in whom a "total" resection was initially thought to have been achieved has been reported to approach or surpass 50% in recent series (range 13% to 53%).[2–4, 6,8–10] Thus the question that the surgeon asks is the age-old one about the relative risks and benefits of available treatment options.

Reports during the past decade have continued to confound the neurosurgeon attempting to make the right choice and to counsel the family of an individual patient presenting with this disorder. One can find support for the idea that even radical surgery results in an excellent cognitive outcome for the majority of patients.[4,9,11,12] One can also find series from excellent centers that report that few patients remain functionally "normal" and that most are plagued with memory dysfunction.[6,13–15] Even in series that report mostly good outcomes, significant behavioral disorders, including "frontal lobe dysfunction," unpredictable anger outbursts, and emotional difficulties, are described in approximately one-quarter to one-half of patients.[6,9,11,12] Family rating scales may elucidate behavioral disturbances that can be missed by conventional measures.[6,14] Whether these cognitive and psychosocial effects result from the tumor itself or the surgical or adjuvant therapy is not entirely clear.

The one aspect of outcome that has been shown to vary with extent of surgery is endocrine status. While most patients

treated with either surgery alone or with surgery plus radiation therapy will show some degree of endocrine dysfunction, the incidence of diabetes insipidus in recent series remains higher with radical surgery, consistent with older studies.[2,4,6,16,17] When this occurs in a very young child, especially when coupled with a deficient thirst mechanism, medical management can be extremely difficult and morbidity and mortality can be high.

Another of the most common associations of craniopharyngioma and its treatment is obesity. One-third to two-thirds of patients develop this complication, which can occur even after subtotal resection.[2,3,9,12,18–21] Despite the wide recognition of the high incidence of obesity as a single outcome measure in these patients, it is difficult to find specific sources of information that help the neurosurgeon avoid what is perhaps the most dreaded complication in craniopharyngioma management—the constellation of symptoms creating the morbidly obese, hypothalamically impaired, behaviorally crippled long-term survivor. Most pediatric neurosurgeons can name their patients who fall into this category, but little is written specifically about the causes of this outcome profile. It is generally assumed that radical surgery with hypothalamic damage is the most likely culprit, but descriptions of these patients are cryptic in the literature. Dr. Chris Adams, in his comment on Dr. Sweet's chapter for the last edition of this text, described such a patient:

"As a young surgeon, I was extremely proud of having totally removed a large craniopharyngioma in a 12-year-old boy. The result was disastrous owing to hypothalamic damage. The boy developed an uncontrolled appetite and lost his ability to feel thirst. His fluid intake could be controlled only by weighing him. I did that boy and his parents no favors."[22]

Other prominent surgeons have described postoperative patients who had such extreme hyperphagia that nearly all waking activity was directed by food-seeking behavior, making the lives of the patient and family unbearable, and serving as an example of why radical surgery may not be worth risking this outcome.[23] The assumption underlying this point of view is that less radical surgery will decrease the incidence of this small but disastrous patient group. The neurosurgeon wrestles with the choice of decreasing the risk of this outcome while possibly increasing the risk of a multiply recurrent, gradually declining patient who resists all attempts to control the tumor, ultimately succumbing from what might have been cured with aggressive surgery.

To weigh the option of radical versus subtotal surgery plus adjuvant therapy, the early and long-term risks of nonsurgical treatments for subtotally resected or recurrent tumors must be understood. Since the last edition of this text, continued advances have been made in radiotherapy in general and that applied to craniopharyngioma specifically. There has been a technologically driven movement toward more focused radiation, which is thought to be better able to target the area of interest while limiting radiation to wider areas of the surrounding brain.[13,24–30] Progression-free survival has been reported at 59% to 100% at 5 years and 56% to 89% at 10 years.[7,13,24,28,29] Late recurrences after 10 years also are reported.[8,27] Complications include radiation damage to endocrine and visual structures, radiation necrosis, cognitive deficits, and second tumors, the last of which so far appear rare.[13,31] Although most authors advocate immediate radiation therapy in the case of subtotal resection, salvage rates for delayed recurrence or growth of known residual tumor are also high, prompting some authors to utilize delayed radiation, especially in young children.[2,3] Intracystic treatment with ^{32}P or bleomycin is another approach designed to reduce toxicity in selected patients.[6,16,25]

Some authors have attempted to predict which patients have a high risk of poor outcome from more radical surgery, but the conclusions are sometimes contradictory.[32] In addition, most of the risk factors for poor outcome from aggressive surgery are also risk factors for tumor recurrence. De Vile and colleagues used a retrospective analysis of cases to show that predictors of poor outcome include severe hydrocephalus, intraoperative adverse events, and age of 5 years or younger. Hypothalamic morbidity was associated with presurgical hypothalamic disturbance, midline vertical height of the tumor of 3.5 cm or more, and adherence of the tumor to the hypothalamus at surgery.[33] Other authors recommend a primary surgical approach specifically in children under 5 years of age, presumably because of the adverse effects of radiation in the very young.[3] Merchant and colleagues recommend surgical excision with an attempt to remove the entire tumor "when an experienced neurosurgeon can reasonably expect to achieve gross total resection with limited adverse effects." They caution that "dissection of tumor from the hypothalamus can cause unpredictable damage and should be avoided."[6] In their comparison of patients treated with radical surgery compared to those treated with more limited surgery plus radiation, the quality of life was better in the latter group, and the long-term survival in both groups was similar.

Thus the recent past has seen the pendulum swing toward more individualized selection of primary treatment options for each patient. Whether the decision to perform limited surgery plus adjuvant therapy is best made in advance of the operation or whether it is decided during surgery based on intraoperative findings also has not been clarified. There is as yet no clear consensus as to which patients are best treated by which modality (Table 33-4), but there is now a more vocal group of surgeons who do not approach all craniopharyngiomas with intent for total removal at the initial surgery—and are not considered cowardly or insufficiently skilled. While it is little mentioned in the medical literature, part of the impetus for this shift may arise because patients and families are better informed and expect to have greater understanding of the options, complications, and likely long-term outcomes, especially from a "benign" tumor in which long-term survival can be expected. In a climate of higher expectations, curing the tumor but leaving the child devastated is increasingly less likely to be considered an acceptable result.

TABLE 33-4 ▪ Selection Criteria Used for Radical Surgery

Radical Surgery Considered Treatment of Choice

Age < 5 years[3]
Small tumors with no hypothalamic symptoms[3]
Intrasellar or pure intraventricular location[3]
"Experienced neurosurgeon can reasonably expect to achieve a gross total resection with limited adverse effects."[6]

Predictors for Poor Outcome from Radical Surgery

Age < 5 years[33]
Preoperative Criteria
   Hydrocephalus[33]
   Hypothalamic symptoms[33]
   Tumor "height" > 3.5 cm[33]
   Large tumors that invade critical structures[6]
   Large tumor with retrochiasmatic location[32]
Intraoperative criteria
   Tumor adherent to hypothalamus[6,33]
   Intraoperative complications (hemorrhage, arterial spasm or damage, frontal bruising, cardiorespiratory problems)[33]

REFERENCES

1. Epstein FJ: Meeting summary. Craniopharyngioma: The Answer. Pediatr Neurosurg 21(Suppl 1):129–130, 1994.
2. Stripp DC, Maity A, Janss AJ, et al: Surgery with or without radiation therapy in the management of craniopharyngiomas in children and young adults. Int J Radiat Oncol Biol Phys 58:714–720, 2004.
3. Kalapurakal JA, Goldman S, Hsieh YC, et al: Clinical outcome in children with craniopharyngioma treated with primary surgery and radiotherapy deferred until relapse. Med Pediatr Oncol 40:214–218, 2003.
4. Van Effenterre R, Boch A. Craniopharyngioma in adults and children: A study of 122 surgical cases. J Neurosurg 97:3–11, 2002.
5. Chen C, Okera S, Davies PE: Craniopharyngioma: A review of long-term visual outcome. Clin Exp Ophthalmol 31:220–228, 2003.
6. Merchant TE, Kiehna EN, Sanford RA, et al: Craniopharyngioma: The St. Jude Children's Research Hospital experience 1984–2001. Int J Radiat Oncol Biol Phys 53:533–542, 2002.
7. Fisher PG, Jenab J, Goldthwaite PT, et al: Outcomes and failure patterns in childhood craniopharyngiomas. Childs Nerv Syst 14:558–563, 1998.
8. Bulow B, Attewell R, Hagmar L, et al: Postoperative prognosis in craniopharyngioma with respect to cardiovascular mortality, survival, and tumor recurrence. J Clin Endocrinol Metab 83:3897–3904, 1998.
9. Villani RM, Tomei G, Bello L, et al: Long-term results of treatment for craniopharyngioma in children. Childs Nerv Syst 13:397–405, 1997.
10. Fahlbusch R, Honegger J, Paulus W, et al: Surgical treatment of craniopharyngiomas: Experience with 168 patients. J Neurosurg 90:237–250, 1999.
11. Donnet A, Schmitt A, Dufour H, Grisoli F: Neuropsychological follow-up of twenty-two adult patients after surgery for craniopharyngioma. Acta Neurochir (Wien) 141:1049–1054, 1999.
12. Riva D, Pantaleoni C, Devoti M, et al: Late neuropsychological and behavioural outcome of children surgically treated for craniopharyngioma. Childs Nerv Syst 14:179–184, 1998.
13. Habrand JL, Ganry O, Couanet D, et al: The role of radiation therapy in the management of craniopharyngioma: A 25-year experience and review of the literature. Int J Radiat Oncol Biol Phys 44:255–263, 1999.
14. Anderson CA, Wilkening GN, Filley CM, et al: Neurobehavioral outcome in pediatric craniopharyngioma. Pediatr Neurosurg 26:255–260, 1997.
15. Carpentieri SC, Waber DP, Scott RM, et al: Memory deficits among children with craniopharyngiomas. Neurosurgery 49:1057–1058, 2001.
16. Hasegawa T, Kondziolka D, Hadjipanayis CG, Lunsford LD: Management of cystic craniopharyngiomas with phosphorus-32 intracavitary irradiation. Neurosurgery 54:813–822, 2004.
17. Honegger J, Buchfelder M, Fahlbusch R: Surgical treatment of craniopharyngiomas: Endocrinological results. J Neurosurg 90:251–257, 1999.
18. Lustig RH, Post SR, Srivannaboon K, et al: Risk factors for the development of obesity in children surviving brain tumors. J Clin Endocrinol Metab 88:611–616, 2003.
19. Anonymous. Long-term outcomes for surgically resected craniopharyngiomas. Neurosurgery 46:291–302, 2000.
20. Srinivasan S, Ogle GD, Garnett SP, et al: Features of the metabolic syndrome after childhood craniopharyngioma. J Clin Endocrinol Metab 89:81–86, 2004.
21. Pinto G, Bussieres L, Recansens C, et al: Hormonal factors influencing weight and growth patterns in craniopharyngioma. Horm Res 53:163–169, 2000.
22. Adams CBT: Management of craniopharyngiomas: Additional comment. In Schmidek H, Sweet WH (eds): Operative Neurosurgical Techniques, 4th ed, Philadelphia, Saunders, pp 487–488.

23. Sanford RA: Craniopharyngioma. Presented at Joint Section for Pediatric Neurosurgery Annual Meeting, American Association of Neurological Surgeons and Congress of Neurological Surgeons Salt Lake City, UT, 2003.

24. Schulz-Ertner D, Frank C, Herfarth KK, et al: Fractionated stereotactic radiotherapy for craniopharyngiomas. Int J Radiat Oncol Biol Phys 54:1114–1120, 2002.

25. Schefter JK, Allen G, Cmelak AJ, et al: The utility of external beam radiation and intracystic ^{32}P radiation in the treatment of craniopharyngiomas. J Neurooncol 56:69–78, 2002.

26. Barajas MA, Ramirez-Guzman G, Rodriguez-Vazquez C, et al: Multimodal management of craniopharyngioma: Neuroendoscopy, microsurgery, and radiosurgery. J Neurosurg 97(Suppl 5):607–609, 2002.

27. Varlotto JM, Flickinger JC, Kondziolka D, et al: External beam irradiation of craniopharyngiomas: Long-term analysis of tumor control and morbidity. Int J Radiat Oncol Biol Phys 54:492–499, 2002.

28. Isaac MA, Hahn SS, Kim JA, et al: Management of craniopharyngioma. Cancer J 7:516–520, 2001.

29. Kalapurakal JA, Goldman S, Hsieh YC, et al: Clinical outcome in children with recurrent craniopharyngioma after primary surgery. Cancer J 6:388–393, 2000.

30. Chung WY, Pan DH, Shiau CY, et al: Gamma knife radiosurgery for craniopharyngiomas. J Neurosurg 93(Suppl 3):47–56, 2000.

31. Rittinger O, Kranzinger M, Jones R, Jones N: Malignant astrocytoma arising 10 years after combined treatment of craniopharyngioma. J Pediatr Endocrinol Metab 16:97–101, 2003.

32. Rutka JR: Craniopharyngioma [Editorial]. J Neurosurg 97:1–2, 2002.

33. De Vile CJ, Grant DB, Kendall BE, Neville BG, et al: Management of childhood craniopharygioma: Can the morbidity of radical surgery be predicted? J Neurosurg 85:73–81, 1996.

34

Surgical Management of Craniopharyngiomas

MADJID SAMII, AMIR SAMII, WOLF LÜDEMANN, and VENELIN GERGANOV

Craniopharyngiomas are benign, slow-growing, well-encapsulated tumors of variable consistency (solid and/or cystic, with or without calcification) that involve primarily the sellar region. These tumors grow by expansion, although glial reaction and small papillary tumor projections into the glial undersurface may falsely lead to the impression of tumor invasion. In general, there are two histologically distinct types of craniopharyngioma: the adamantinous type and the squamous-papillary type.

The overall incidence of craniopharyngioma is 0.13 per 100,000 person-years and does not vary by gender or race. A bimodal distribution by age is determined with peak incidence rates in children (aged 5 to 14 years) and among older adults (aged 50 to 74 years).

Radical microsurgical removal is the treatment of choice to cure the patient. However, the sellar region is a crossroad for major blood vessels supplying the brain, several cranial nerves that govern vision and eye movement, the centers of both the endocrinologic and autonomic system, and those concerned with the emotional sphere of our being. These structures can be affected by the tumor, making the surgical procedure a challenge that requires a skilled and experienced team familiar with this extremely vulnerable region.

Alternative treatment options, such as nonradical surgery followed by radiation therapy, stereotactic cyst puncture with or without intracavitary radioisotope or bleomycin instillation, and stereotactic radiosurgery, are available. In general, these alternatives fail to solve the patient's problems over the long term. However, in combination with conservative surgery, radiotherapy, for instance, appears to significantly prolong the progression/recurrence-free interval when compared with conservative surgery only but not when compared with radical removal, in which tumor-free survival rates of 100% have been reported.[2–4]

CLASSIFICATION

It is of fundamental importance to the surgeon to possess a clear anatomic definition of the tumor and its relationship to the third ventricle.

In 1962, Rougerie[5,6] was the first to propose a surgical classification for craniopharyngiomas. He defined five anatomic forms: prechiasmatic craniopharyngiomas, intrasellar craniopharyngiomas, retrochiasmatic craniopharyngiomas, les formes geantes, and atypical craniopharyngiomas. In 1975, Pertuiset[7] recommended the following classification: intrasellar craniopharyngiomas, suprasellar (prechiasmatic, subchiasmatic, and retrochiasmatic) craniopharyngiomas,

intrasellar and suprasellar craniopharyngiomas, and intraventricular craniopharyngiomas. Konovalov[8] has classified craniopharyngiomas as follows: endosuprasellar craniopharyngiomas, suprasellar-extraventricular craniopharyngiomas, intraventricular craniopharyngiomas, and giant craniopharyngiomas.

Kobayashi[9] singled out four types: type I, anterior; type II, intrasellar; type III, ventricular; and type IV, posterior. Steno[10] considered the following classification: intrasellar and suprasellar, and suprasellar: extraventricular, intraventricular, and mixed. Hoffman[11] described three types of craniopharyngiomas: intrasellar, prechiasmatic, and retrochiasmatic.

However, independent of the numerous historical and present-day classifications, many authors suggest that the axis of tumor growth in craniopharyngiomas, which in the first instance is in a vertical projection, is the essential selection criteria for the various surgical approaches.[12–15] Based on this and considering the different classification proposals and the possible tumor extension to the anterior, middle, and posterior fossa, as well as into the ventricular system and into the sphenoid sinus, we propose the following classification.

The vertical tumor extension can be classified into five grades of severity from grade I to grade V (Fig. 34-1):

- In grade I, the tumor is located purely in the intrasellar or infradiaphragmatic region.
- In grade II, the tumor is localized in the cistern with or without an intrasellar component.
- In grade III, the tumor extends into the lower half of the third ventricle.
- In grade IV, the tumor expands to the upper half of the third ventricle.
- In grade V, the tumor dome reaches the septum pellucidum and/or extends into the lateral ventricle(s).

With regard to the tumor growth on the horizontal plane, lateral and sagittal extensions can be described, respectively. Infrasellar extension into the sphenoid sinus with destructive sellar expansion (S) may be present. A lateral extension (L) would include a temporal skull base invasion, and corpus striatum involvement or the temporal lobe itself in the paraventricular expansion. Finally, sagittal extension would be exhibited as midbrain compression in the posterior protrusion or even as growth into the posterior fossa (P), and interhemispheric fissure or frontal lobe invasion as characteristic of an anterior expansion (A).

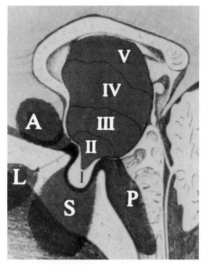

FIGURE 34-1 This drawing represents the grading of cranio-pharyngiomas. The main focus is on the vertical tumor extension. Grade I, intrasellar tumor; grade II, intracisternal tumor, with or without intrasellar component; grade III, intracisternal tumor extending into the lower half of the third ventricle; grade IV, intracisternal tumor extending into the upper half of the third ventricle; grade V, intracisternal tumor extending to the septum pellucidum or into the lateral ventricles. Classification of craniopharyngioma: A: anterior (prechiasmal) expansion; S: infrasellar (sphenoidal sinus) expansion; P: posterior fossa (infratentorial expansion); L: lateral (temporal) expansion.

Atypical craniopharyngiomas may be located within the pharynx, limited entirely to the sphenoid sinus, or even in the pineal region.[16]

CLINICAL FEATURES AND PREOPERATIVE EVALUATION

Craniopharyngiomas, by virtue of their location, can produce a combination of neurologic and endocrine symptoms. The main presenting symptoms are visual disturbances. In 70% of patients, visual field defects are present, whereas in 89.9%, hypoplasia is found.[17,18] In approximately 50%, increased intracranial pressure is clinically evident, and papilledema occurs in 18.5% of patients.[19] Selective hormonal disturbances can precede neuro-ophthalmologic symptoms. The frequency of endocrine manifestations ranges from 24% to 53% in patients from 2 to 15 years of age, and in patients older than 15 years, it increases to approximately 75%. At the time of diagnosis, the signs of hypophyseal-hypothalamic involvement are usually those of growth retardation (33%), obesity (25%), diabetes insipidus (20%), and delayed puberty (50%).[19]

Magnetic resonance imaging, computed tomography, endocrine studies, and neuro-ophthalmologic and neuropsychological evaluation are the standard tools for diagnosis and planning of surgical treatment of craniopharyngiomas. Magnetic resonance imaging, with and without paramagnetic contrast administration (gadolinium), is the prime imaging tool for diagnostic screening, whereas computed tomography is mandatory for evaluating changes in the bony structures of the skull base and determining the presence of tumor calcifications. Large craniopharyngiomas almost always stretch and sometimes engulf the surrounding arteries; therefore,

preoperative angiography can be helpful to establish the surgical strategy. Magnetic resonance imaging/angiography represents a reliable noninvasive procedure that has increasingly replaced conventional angiographic studies.

Typically, 50% of patients with craniopharyngiomas demonstrate intracranial calcifications and 30% have hydrocephalus.[19] The tumor never seems to deform the planum sphenoidale without enlarging the sella turcica. Furthermore, the optic canals generally are not enlarged.[16] In our experience, when we suspected infiltration of the cavernous sinus on the basis of the preoperative neuroradiologic studies, it was not confirmed intraoperatively. Endocrine deficits are reported as follows: growth hormone (60%), luteinizing hormone/follicle-stimulating hormone (LH/FSH) (60%), adrenocorticotropic hormone (30%), and thyroid hormone (30%).[19]

PATIENT SELECTION AND MANAGEMENT DECISIONS

There is abundant controversy among physicians regarding the treatment of choice for craniopharyngioma. Depending on personal specialty and experience, different treatment modalities have been proposed. Most neurosurgeons consider total surgical tumor excision as the treatment of choice. Other neurosurgeons who are experienced with stereotactic methodology advocate stereotactic aspiration and drainage of cystic craniopharyngiomas and, as an additional option, implantation of β-emitting isotopes. Another stereotactic treatment modality is the intracavitary instillation of bleomycin. Others suggest that external fractionated radiation or radiosurgery or subtotal tumor removal combined with radiotherapy should be performed. However, in combination with conservative surgery, radiotherapy, for instance, appears to significantly prolong the progression/recurrence-free interval when compared with conservative surgery only but not when compared with radical removal, for which tumor-free survival rates of 100% have been reported.[2–4] Because radical tumor excision carries a very low rate of morbidity,[10,19,20] we advocate the radical removal of craniopharyngiomas as the method of choice, as well as early surgery after diagnosis. This latter approach may reduce the incidence of irreversible defects at the level of the optic pathway, mesodiencephalon, and frontal lobes.

REGIONAL SURGICAL ANATOMY

Purely intrasellar craniopharyngiomas are uncommon; they expand within the sella and compress the pituitary, producing endocrinopathies before compressing the optic nerve. More frequently, the tumor grows by pushing the diaphragm upward, breaking through it, and extending in any direction. In relation to the optic chiasm, the tumor may extend anteriorly in the direction of the subfrontal space (prechiasmatic craniopharyngioma). These are frequently cystic tumors and achieve large sizes before being diagnosed. When the tumor grows posterior to the chiasm (retrochiasmatic craniopharyngioma), it displaces the pituitary stalk forward and the chiasm forward and upward, making the optic nerve appear falsely prefixed (pseudoprefixity of the optic chiasm). Cystic retrochiasmatic craniopharyngiomas may reach an enormous size by expanding into the posterior fossa into the prepontine cistern.

Tumor extension down to the cervical spine has been described.[21] The tumor may also displace the chiasm upward (subchiasmatic craniopharyngioma) and the pituitary stalk backward. Both retrochiasmatic and subchiasmatic craniopharyngiomas are frequently solid tumors, and they usually press against the third ventricle as they grow, causing compression of the hypothalamus and obstruction of the foramen of Monro. When it is pushed upward by the tumor, the floor of the third ventricle becomes paper thin and tears so that the tumor protrudes directly into it. Craniopharyngiomas may also grow laterally into the subtemporal space, producing compression of the temporal lobe.

Craniopharyngiomas may arise directly from the floor of the third ventricle. This is essentially a retrochiasmatic tumor, but it may extend anteriorly to the prechiasmatic space, superiorly into the lumen of the third ventricle, posteriorly to the interpeduncular and prepontine cisterns, and laterally to the basal ganglia and temporal lobe.

Although large craniopharyngiomas frequently grow into the third ventricle, purely intraventricular craniopharyngiomas are exceptional.[22] A recent review of the literature revealed only 24 cases.[23] The intraventricular craniopharyngiomas have been hypothesized to arise from a pars tuberalis containing squamous epithelial rests or remnants of Rathke's pouch and to then grow along the pituitary stalk, extending to the infundibulum or tuber cinereum in the floor of the third ventricle.[24,25]

Craniopharyngiomas usually adhere to the major arteries at the skull base and to the small perforating arteries arising from the anterior communicating artery, posterior communicating artery, and branches from the anterior choroidal artery and thalamoperforating vessels.[20,25] Vascular adhesions are one of the most important reasons for incomplete tumor removal. Attempts at radical dissection of the tumor capsule from the arterial wall have been associated with weakening of the adventitia by injuring the vasa vasorum, causing fusiform dilatations of the carotid artery.[26]

The anterior part of the tumor is supplied by perforators from the anterior communicating artery and proximal anterior cerebral artery. The lateral part of the tumor receives branches from the posterior communicating artery, and the intrasellar portion is usually supplied from intracavernous meningohypophyseal vessels. Craniopharyngiomas do not usually receive a blood supply from the posterior cerebral arteries or the basilar artery unless the anterior blood supply for the lower hypothalamus and floor of third ventricle is absent (anatomic variant).

CHOICE OF SURGICAL APPROACH

Many different surgical approaches have been used in the treatment of craniopharyngiomas (Fig. 34-2). According to the localization and expansion of the tumor, different approaches have characteristic advantages and disadvantages. Therefore, the best surgical approach can be selected only after careful evaluation of the topography of the tumor, based on detailed neuroradiologic studies.

Some approaches may be superior in specific situations, such as the transsphenoidal approach route for grade I purely intrasellar tumors, whereas purely intraventricular tumors can be excised by a transventricular approach, small retrochiasmatic tumors by the subtemporal route, and large retrochiasmatic tumors with extension along the clivus may best be operated on by a transpetrosal-transtentorial approach.

Based on our experience, we prefer the frontolateral approach to treat grade II, III, and IV tumors. Craniopharyngiomas originate from remnants of Rathke's pouch, which is a midline structure, and a more medial route than that offered by the pterional approach is preferable. The frontolateral is a safe and fast approach that has minimal approach-related morbidity. Conversely, it provides sufficient access to sellar, suprasellar, and parasellar tumor extensions.

In cases of a prefixed chiasm and retrosellar location of the tumor expanding into the interpeduncular-pontine cistern and the third ventricle, the lamina terminalis represents a window through which these extensions can be removed.

Usually the transsphenoidal approach is taken to remove grade I and II tumors.

FIGURE 34-2 Different approach options for the removal of craniopharyngiomas.

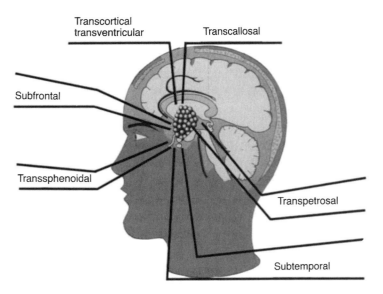

Additional Approaches Described in the Literature

Orbitocranial approaches have been used by some surgeons to achieve a more basal view due to bone removal instead of frontal lobe retraction.[27]

The endoscopic endonasal transsphenoidal approach, endoscopic resection or marsupialization of cystic craniopharyngiomas, endoscopic positioning of the catheter connected to the Ommaya reservoir, and placement of a drainage shunt to the sphenoid sinus to ensure continuous drainage of the cyst contents are all claimed to achieve a high precision rate while limiting approach-related morbidity.[28–30]

The bifrontal basal interhemispheric approach with or without division of the anterior communicating artery has been used successfully by Shibuya and colleagues[31] in 22 patients. The authors conclude that it is appropriate for large lesions because it offers a wide bilateral operative field and better orientation and visualization of important neural and vascular structures. To reduce the morbidity related to such a major approach, Shirane and colleagues[32] use its modification, the so-called frontobasal interhemispheric approach. It requires a smaller bilateral frontobasal craniotomy and, if combined with the translamina terminalis approach, allows removal of lesions of all sizes.

In cases of extremely hard craniopharyngiomas, some authors favor the transfacial approaches, the advantages of which are reduced depth, improved visual and working field, reduced brain retraction, and avoidance of vascular and cranial nerve damage.[33]

SURGICAL TECHNIQUES

Subfrontal Approach

For this approach, the patient is positioned supine, with slight flexion of the trunk and knees. The patient's head is placed in a fixation device, with the head elevated above the heart for venous drainage. The vertex is tilted down with slight extension of the neck to allow the frontal lobes to fall away without excessive retraction. This position provides a comfortable working setting for the surgeon and offers exposure of the entire frontal fossa floor to the basilar apex.

The subfrontal unilateral approach begins with a bitemporal coronal incision. For cosmetic reasons, we prefer this to a circumscribed flap incision on the forehead. Generally, three burr holes are sufficient for the craniotomy (Fig. 34-3). (1) The lateral burr hold is placed at the root of the zygomatic process of the frontal bone, which forms a palpable ridge at its junction with the infratemporal fossa. The hole should be placed approximately 1 to 1.5 cm above the frontozygomatic suture. A small slit can be made in the aponeurosis of the temporal muscle to expose the bony ridge at the temporal fossa. The burr hole is placed directly on that ridge. As the hole is drilled, care is taken not to enter the bony orbit, which would injure Tenon's capsule and so that the hole is as close as possible to the floor of the anterior cranial fossa. This approach will also allow troublesome bony overlapping to be avoided later. (2) The medial burr hole is situated approximately 4 cm from the lateral hole. We try to place the hole as low as possible (at the level of the glabella) and close to the midline. This procedure can be carried out even with a large frontal sinus that extends far superiorly. When the

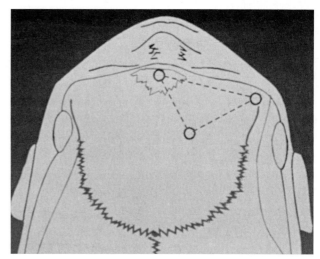

FIGURE 34-3 Placement of the three burr holes for unilateral frontal craniotomy.

frontal sinus is opened, its mucosal lining is stripped downward so that the drill can be advanced through the posterior sinus wall without damaging the mucosa. We mention this detail because it is of importance in preventing the spread of pathogenic organisms from the paranasal sinuses into the cranial cavity and eliminates the need for tube drainage of the frontal sinus into the nasal cavity in case the frontal sinus has been widely opened and a portion of mucosa has been removed. After the frontal sinuses have been exposed, the mucosa is cleaned out, and the sinuses are packed with antibiotic gauze until the end of the operation. (3) The superior burr hole is placed approximately 3 cm above and midway between the lateral and medial perforation. (4) For the bilateral approach (Fig. 34-4), two lateral burr holes are placed as in step 1, a third hole is placed above the glabella, and the fourth one is positioned 3 cm higher.

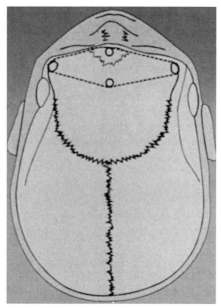

FIGURE 34-4 Placement of the four burr holes for a bifrontal craniotomy.

FIGURE 34-5 Intraoperative findings in a case of a postfixed optic chiasm. After retraction of the right frontal lobe, the suprasellar tumor capsule is identified in the anterior angle of the optic chiasm and is opened. A piecemeal enucleation of the tumor is performed with a curette and suction tip. (From Samii M: Surgery of the Skull Base. Berlin: Springer-Verlag, 1989, p 277.)

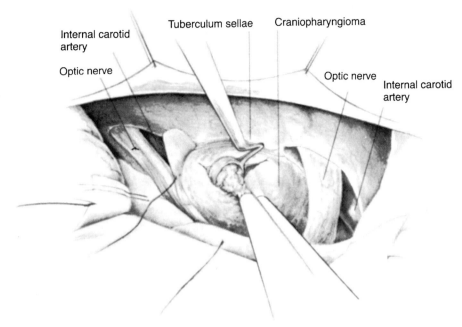

In the unilateral approach, the dura is then opened with a frontobasal incision lateral to the superior sagittal sinus. Intradural exposure is carried out in standard fashion, facilitating frontal lobe retraction by progressively opening the arachnoid and draining cerebrospinal fluid (CSF). It has proved useful and advantageous to expose the anterior skull base from the lateral side, using the lesser sphenoid wing as a landmark. The olfactory nerves are identified, exposed, and preserved in continuity without exerting traction. Microdissection begins until both optic nerves have been exposed. The basal cisterns are then opened to remove more cerebrospinal fluid. For an optimal overview of the suprasellar structures and the tumor, the arachnoidal sheet of both optic nerves and the optic chiasm is dissected (Fig. 34-5).

The condition of the chiasm, which cannot be completely evaluated neuroradiologically, determines whether we proceed subchiasmatically or via the lamina terminalis or by both routes. In cases of a postfixed (Fig. 34-6) chiasm, tumor removal is first performed between the optic nerves; removal of this part of the tumor decompresses the optic pathway, which allows the surgeon to visualize the pituitary stalk. If the pituitary stalk has not been infiltrated, it should be preserved (see Fig. 34-6). If it is cystic, the contents should be drained by puncture. Feeding vessels to the capsule should be coagulated. When the chiasm is prefixed (Fig. 34-7), a situation that occurs in large, predominantly retrochiasmatic tumors, the removal is performed via the lamina terminalis (Figs. 30-8 and 30-9), which offers easy access to the inferior part of the third ventricle. Because this bifrontal approach offers a panoramic multidirectional dissection of the most adherent parts of the tumors, they can be manipulated anterior to the chiasm through the lamina terminalis and also through the opticocarotid space of both sides (Fig. 34-10). A further option is to drill the tuberculum sellae to improve the view into the sella (Fig. 34-11). Here, opened ethmoid cells do not present a problem because they can be covered with free muscle grafts or with the same galea-periosteal flap used to close the frontal sinuses. Fibrin glue is used as sealant.

Transsphenoidal and Extended Transsphenoidal Approaches

The classic transsphenoidal approach (see Chapter 31) is preferred in cases of craniopharyngiomas located completely within an enlarged sella turcica or show symmetrical intra- and suprasellar growth (grades I and II). They comprise approximately 20% to 39% of all cases. Purely intrasellar craniopharyngiomas comprise 10% to 18%.[34,35] The technique is similar to the transsphenoidal approach for pituitary adenomas but requires wider opening of the sphenoid sinus and sellar floor, as far as the internal carotid artery laterally and the tuberculum sellae superiorly.[34] Craniopharyngiomas involving the sella are frequently cystic and friable, making their removal easier, in contrast to infundibular craniopharyngiomas, which are frequently calcified. In a series of

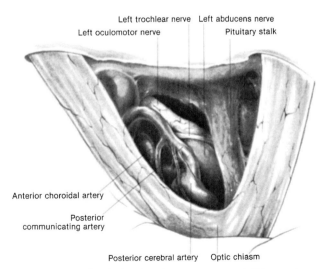

FIGURE 34-6 Surgical cavity after tumor removal. Microanatomy as viewed through the anterior angle of the optic chiasm. The pituitary stalk is intact. (From Samii M: Surgery of the Skull Base. Berlin: Springer-Verlag, 1989, p 277.)

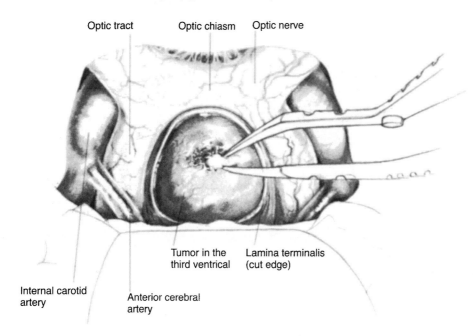

Optic tract   Optic chiasm   Optic nerve

Tumor in the third ventrical   Lamina terminalis (cut edge)

Internal carotid artery   Anterior cerebral artery

FIGURE 34-7 Intraoperative findings after a bifrontal craniotomy in a case of an anteriorly displaced (prefixed) optic chiasm. The lamina terminalis is opened for removal of the interior of the tumor through the retrochiasmal angle. (From Samii M: Surgery of the Skull Base. Berlin: Springer-Verlag, 1989, p 279.)

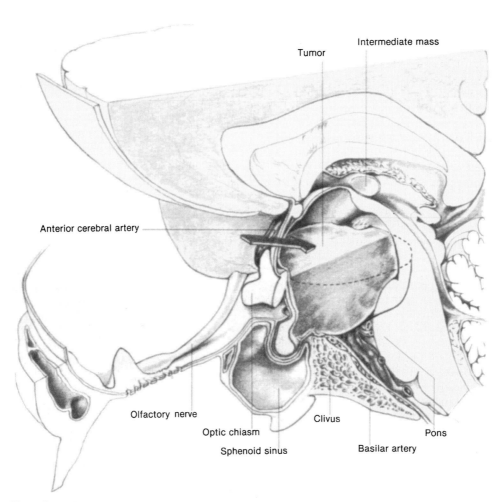

Tumor   Intermediate mass

Anterior cerebral artery

Olfactory nerve   Clivus

Optic chiasm   Pons

Sphenoid sinus   Basilar artery

FIGURE 34-8 Three-dimensional representation of the tumor extent in the transverse and sagittal planes, including the route of surgical access. (From Samii M: Surgery of the Skull Base. Berlin: Springer-Verlag, 1989, p 280.)

FIGURE 34-9 View into the prepontine space shows the microsurgical anatomy after tumor removal through the lamina terminalis. (From Samii M: Surgery of the Skull Base. Berlin: Springer-Verlag, 1989, p 280.)

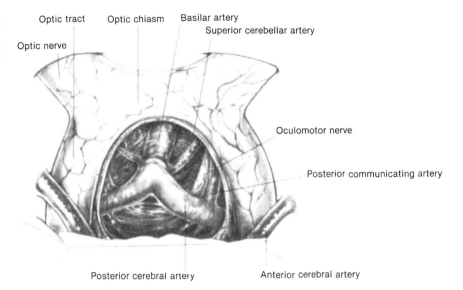

168 patients, total tumor removal is achieved in 86% of the cases operated transsphenoidally and in 46% of those operated via a craniotomy. The morbidity rates are 5.7% and 12.8%, respectively.[36] A normal or slightly enlarged sella does not preclude the transsphenoidal approach. It has been successfully used in a large series of children as well.[37] The disadvantage of the technique is the fact that the pituitary gland is displaced ventrally in 50%, and pituitary splitting is frequently required. The tumor capsule might be attached firmly to the pituitary stalk or diaphragma sellae, precluding its safe dissection. CSF leaks are observed in as many as 80% of the cases.[36]

For craniopharyngiomas with a larger intracranial extension, modified extended transsphenoidal approaches have been proposed. Patients with severe visual impairment or serious general condition precluding craniotomy are

regarded as suitable. In the transsphenoidal presellar approach (presellar transtubercular approach), a wider bone opening and removal of tuberculum sellae is achieved. Part of the planum sphenoidale (4 to 10 mm) is removed, the dura overlying the planum sphenoidale is opened, and the suprasellar cisterns are reached. For lesions requiring wider exposure, the anterosuperior part of the circular sinus can be divided and the diaphragma sellae incised along the midline up to the pituitary stalk. The optic nerves define the lateral limits of the exposure.[38,39] The advantage of this approach is the direct access to supradiaphragmatic lesions, adjacent or anterior to the pituitary stalk. It obviates the need of resecting the pituitary gland. The area provided by the classic transsphenoidal approach can be further extended in lateral and superior directions by performing submucosal posterior ethmoidectomy.[40] The transsellar

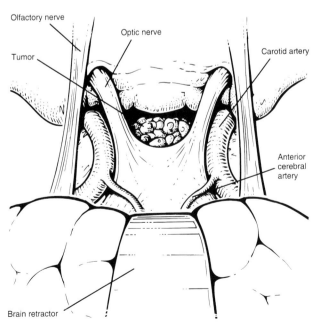

FIGURE 34-10 Intraoperative picture after bifrontal craniotomy and exposure of the sellar region in a patient with a craniopharyngioma.

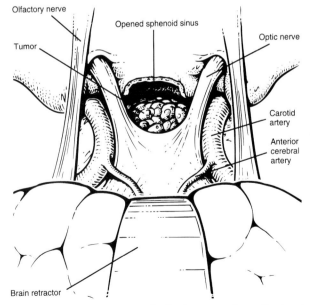

FIGURE 34-11 Intraoperative finding in a case of a prefixed optic chiasm in which the tuberculum sellae is removed and the sphenoid sinus is seen.

transdiaphragmatic approach requires splitting and displacing of the pituitary gland and opening of the diaphragma sellae.[41] It is considered useful in cases of retrochiasmatic craniopharyngiomas with a low-lying chiasm and anterior communicating artery complex. A common disadvantage inherent to all extended transsphenoidal approaches is the high rate of CSF leakage.

Pterional Approach

The frontotemporal or pterional approach may be used alone or in combination with a transsphenoidal or transcallosal approach to remove large craniopharyngiomas.

A frontotemporal craniotomy is performed. The lower margin of the opening has to be positioned well in relation to the floor of the middle cranial fossa. The tumor is dissected in the parachiasmal spaces, such as prechiasmatic, opticocarotid, carotidotentorial, in the triangle superior to the carotid bifurcation and through the opening of the lamina terminalis.[14] The technique of tumor removal is the same as the one employed with the subfrontal approach. Extending the frontal part of the frontotemporal approach, some surgeons use both the subfrontal and transsylvian pathways.[35,42]

The disadvantage of the pterional approach is the narrow corridor in cases of a prefixed optic chiasm. The lateral view through the opticocarotid triangle might be obstructed by perforating arteries. In cases of large retrosellar lesions, the oblique angle through the lamina terminalis does not allow sufficient visualization of the posterior third ventricle and retrosellar space.

Frontolateral Approach

In recent years, the frontolateral approach has been favored by the senior author (M.S.) for all craniopharyngiomas, excluding those with a pure intrasellar location or in cases of large septated lesions extending to the corpus callosum, where the transcallosal approach has certain advantages.[43] The frontolateral approach avoids the approach-related morbidity of the bifrontal or unilateral subfrontal approaches, which are more complex and time consuming, require inevitable opening of the frontal sinus, and endanger the venous structures. It could be regarded as a minimally invasive version of the unilateral subfrontal approach or as a modification of the pterional approach, including its frontal part only.

Technique

The right frontolateral approach is used most commonly. It avoids retraction to the dominant frontal lobe and is easier for right-handed surgeons. The patient is positioned supine, with the head fixed in a Mayfield headholder. The head is slightly extended 35 degrees and rotated 10 to 50 degrees contralaterally. This allows the frontal lobe to fall away from the anterior skull base so that less brain retraction is required.

The skin incision is behind the hair line. It begins 1 cm superior to the zygomatic arch and 1 cm anterior to the tragus and reaches the midline at the anterior edge of the hairline. Scalp elevation is performed in two layers. The galea is elevated from the pericranium by sharp dissection. The pericranium is left intact over the frontal bone. It is used

to create a vascularized pericranial flap later, if needed. The scalp is elevated to the supraorbital rim and the frontozygomatic suture and reflected with the help of fishhook retractors. The pericranial flap is also retracted anteriorly. The anterior part of the temporal muscle is detached from the frontozygomatic region and anterior part of the superior temporal line. Then it is dissected bluntly and retracted posteroinferiorly for 1 to 1.5 cm.

The frontal extent of the craniotomy is just lateral to the supraorbital notch, so that the supraorbital nerve and artery can be preserved. Laterally it extends to the key point. The positioning of the craniotomy in relation to the frontal sinus and the location of the intracranial lesion is further refined by the application of the neuronavigation. With a high-speed bone drill, a single burr hole is made at the key point. Entering the orbital cavity is avoided by adequately directing the drill. An osteoplastic osteotomy positioned just above the supraorbital margin is cut with the craniotome. It is usually 25 to 35 mm in width and 20 to 25 mm in height. Entering the frontal sinus is usually avoided. In the case of a large sinus, it is entered inevitably. If the defect is large, the mucosa should be exenterated to decrease the risk of mucocele formation. The integrity of the sinus is reconstructed at the end with the pericranial flap. The dura is opened in a semicircular manner, with an inferior base and sutured forward.

Under optic magnification, the frontal lobe is retracted slightly using the suction tube and CSF is drained from the basal cisterns. The relaxed frontal lobe is held by a single self-retaining retractor. The arachnoid attachments between the undersurface of the frontal lobe and the optic chiasm are dissected. The olfactory cistern is opened with delicate dissection so that small blood vessels are preserved. The olfactory bulb is exposed, and the olfactory tracts are dissected sharply within the arachnoid plane from the base of the frontal lobe to their origins. No tension on the olfactory tracts should exist at the end, even if the frontal lobes are further elevated. Retraction of the frontal lobe should be kept to a minimum, not more than 1.5 cm, and is directed as needed for each individual case.

The approach gives the surgeon the possibility to work at different angles. Multiple avenues for dissection can be used. Through the preexisting anatomic windows, subchiasmatic, optocarotid, and retrocarotid, craniopharyngiomas extending in the suprasellar and parasellar regions can be accessed. The subchiasmatic approach, directed between the optic nerves and below the chiasm, is used if the tumor elevates the chiasm and opens the space between the optic nerves and chiasm. A prefixed chiasm (15% of the cases) and a prominent tuberculum sellae limit the exposure to the retrochiasmatic and sellar areas. To overcome it, the tuberculum sellae might be drilled with a diamond drill to the level of the superior intercavernous sinus. The sphenoid sinus is then opened, and the anterior wall of the sella turcica is removed. Good exposure of the sella is crucial because approximately 50% of recurrences originate in this region.[36] If the chiasm is prefixed and tumor extension is seen through the stretched wall of the third ventricle, the translamina terminalis approach may be used. It is performed above the chiasm and the anterior communicating artery, medial to the optic tracts. The perforating arteries from the anterior communicating artery that ascend on the lamina terminalis must be preserved because they supply the columns of fornix and damage may result in memory deficit. Therefore, delicate movement of the microinstruments and dissection is required. The more medial subfrontal route provides visualization of the third ventricle behind the lamina terminalis. Tumor parts extending in the retrosellar region, in the interpeduncular and even prepontine cisterns, can be accessed. Endoscopic control ensures that no fragments have been left behind.

During tumor removal, meticulous microsurgical dissection of involved vessels is crucial. Injury to the penetrating vessels supplying the brain stem relates to surgical morbidity. The importance of pituitary stalk preservation is highlighted by the fact that if it is sectioned, the rate of severe endocrinologic deficit is as high as 76%, whereas in cases of preservation, the rate is 48%.[19]

The extent of resection depends on the consistency of the lesion, its location, and invasion of surrounding structures.[35] Invasion of the walls of the ventricle, optic tract, or brain stem is the main limiting factor of total removal. Other factor, found to relate to radicality are tumor size, presence of hydrocephalus, tumor extension in the third ventricle, and more than a 10% rate of calcifications.[36,41]

If the tuberculum sellae has been drilled, muscle or fat tissue is placed over it and fixed with fibrin glue. Final hemostasis is achieved, and the dura is closed in a watertight manner. A large piece of Gelfoam is placed over the dura. The bone flap is fixed with titanium plates. The burr hole is covered by the temporalis muscle so that an optimal cosmetic result is achieved.

The main advantages of the approach are its simplicity and flexibility. It does not require extensive bone removal. Entering the frontal sinus is usually prevented. The risk of injury to the superior sagittal sinus or bridging veins is avoided and their integrity is preserved. The small size of the craniotomy leads to less exposure of the brain, thereby reducing its inadvertent injury or desiccation but provides enough room for surgical manipulations. Retraction of both frontal lobes is avoided. The risk of CSF leakage is very low.

Transcallosal Approach

Transcallosal exposure is possible through a small paramedian frontal craniotomy. Its posterior margin is just behind the coronal suture line. The dura flap is turned over the superior sagittal sinus, and the approach is made along the falx with minimal lateral retraction of the frontal lobe away from the falx. The corpus callosum is exposed; it is usually very thin as a result of obstructive hydrocephalus. A transcallosal incision of approximately 2 cm is made between or just immediately lateral to the pericallosal arteries above the location of the foramen of Monro, 1 cm anterior to the interauricular line. This approach provides access into the lateral ventricles through the dilated foramen of Monro. The tumor capsule is easily visualized. Internal decompression of the tumor by aspiration of cystic contents and piecemeal removal of calcified parts are carried out. The fornix, anterior commissure, choroid plexus, choroidal arteries, and veins of the wall and floor of the third ventricle are key structures to preserve to minimize iatrogenic morbidity.

Case Reports

CASE REPORT 1

A 12-year-old boy was referred to our department after having been operated on 3 years previously. Originally, he presented with deteriorating visual acuity and ataxia. A computed tomography scan of the head revealed a suprasellar cystic tumor that had been partly removed via a right frontal approach. This resulted in an amelioration of his visual acuity. The boy was able to return to bike riding.

Three years later, a physical examination at school detected a renewed deterioration of his visual acuity bilaterally. One month later, hyperphagia, hyperdipsia, drowsiness, headache, nausea, and discrete ataxia were evident. At our department, an endocrine screening confirmed an almost complete breakdown of the adrenotropic and gonadotropic function of the anterior lobe of the pituitary gland. The hormonal dysregulation was treated with compensatory endocrine substitution therapy. A computed tomography scan revealed a large suprasellar cystic tumor occupying the entire third ventricle, with obstructive hydrocephalus (Fig. 34-12A). Shunt placement was performed, which ameliorated the patient's nausea and headaches. One week later, a bifrontal osteoplastic craniotomy was performed with preservation of the left olfactory nerve (the right olfactory nerve having been sacrificed at the first operation) (see Fig. 34-12B and C). A large cystic tumor was completely removed, preserving the pituitary stalk (see Fig. 34-12D and E). After surgery, the patient's hormonal status did not recover, and he was maintained on endocrine substitution therapy. The boy was discharged in good general condition and was able to resume his education.

CASE REPORT 2

A 50-year-old locksmith had complained of severe bifrontal headache for 2 years. He was often tired and lacking in motivation. For 1 year, he was hoarse and ataxic, and his visual acuity deteriorated predominantly in his left eye to the point where he could only detect outlines. Then he developed polydipsia, polyuria, and nocturia. A computed tomography scan revealed a suprasellar tumor, which was then operated on via a subtemporal route. Vegetative abnormalities that occurred intraoperatively prevented the surgeon from removing the tumor. The patient was referred to our department as an emergency case, and he was found to be somnolent and obese with panhypopituitarism. The patient was immediately treated with hormonal substitution and subsequently was operated on (Fig. 34-13A and B). Using a bifrontal approach with preservation of both olfactory nerves, the cystic parts of the tumor were aspirated and the tumor was removed radically leaving the surrounding structures intact (see Fig. 34-13C). The patient's visual acuity did not improve after the operation. His postoperative diabetes insipidus was treated with 1-deamino-(r-D-arginine) vasopressin. Hormonal substitution therapy was continued, and the patient was discharged in a good general condition.

MAJOR INTRAOPERATIVE COMPLICATIONS AND THEIR MANAGEMENT

In the past 15 years, the subfrontal approach is our approach of choice for removing craniopharyngiomas. The following remarks focus on this approach.

Starting with the skin incision, the surgeon must be cautious to avoid damage of the frontal branch of the facial nerve. The scalp incision should be positioned no more than 1 cm anterior to the tragus. In detaching the scalp from the orbital rim, the supraorbital nerve must be identified, the supraorbital foramen should be opened, and the supraorbital nerve should be moved slightly downward to prevent damaging the nerve(s) during the craniotomy.

The frontal sinus, if opened, should be exenterated to prevent formation of a mucocele. If there is a bleeding tendency or oozing into the frontal sinus, the opening to the nasal cavity should be enlarged to provide optimal drainage and reduce the risk of a postoperative hematoma in the frontal sinus area.

After the dura is opened, very careful handling is the absolute requisite for the preservation of the olfactory nerve(s) during microsurgery. The surgeon must refrain from manipulating the nerve(s) directly. He or she should dissect only the arachnoid around the nerve and not coagulate feeding vessels. Extreme caution with the aspiration and suction instrument is advisable because this cranial nerve is particularly vulnerable to injury.

The following aspects will minimize the risk of iatrogenic cerebral contusion:

- A shunt should be placed before surgery if hydrocephalus is present.
- The patient should receive adequate hormonal substitution therapy.
- Neuroanesthesiologic "brain relaxation" techniques are used during the intervention.
- The frontal craniotomy must provide an optimal view to the skull base without shifting and compressing the forebrain unnecessarily.
- Exposure of the anterior fossa should be performed stepwise with increasing CSF drainage so that the frontal lobe can fall back gently with minimal compression.

In the microsurgical era, iatrogenic lesions of the optic nerve and optic pathway are preventable. First, the surgeon must enucleate the tumor through removal of solid parts or through puncture of the cyst before the dissection of the tumor capsule is started along the optic pathway. The same principle is also applicable to the handling of vessels around the tumor, especially small-caliber vessels. An optimal postoperative outcome depends on the preservation of the perforating vessels, particularly the perforators of the thalamus and hypothalamus.

In some cases, the pituitary stalk can be identified and preserved. Hypothalamic disturbances may occur if very large craniopharyngiomas engulf or infiltrate the pituitary stalk so that it cannot be identified early during surgery.

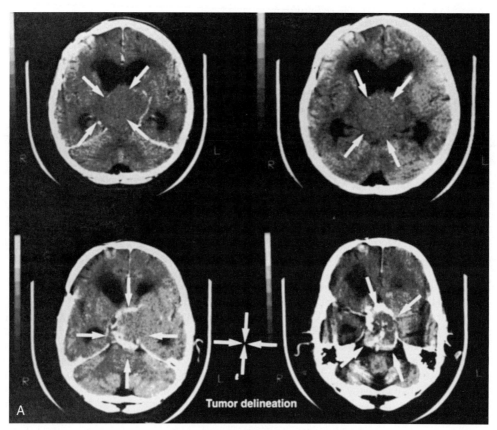

FIGURE 34-12   A 12-year-old boy (case report 1). *A*, Preoperative computed tomography (axial plane) demonstrates a large, solid, cystic, and calcified craniopharyngioma with occlusion hydrocephalus and periventricular edema. Condition after right frontal craniotomy.

(Continued)

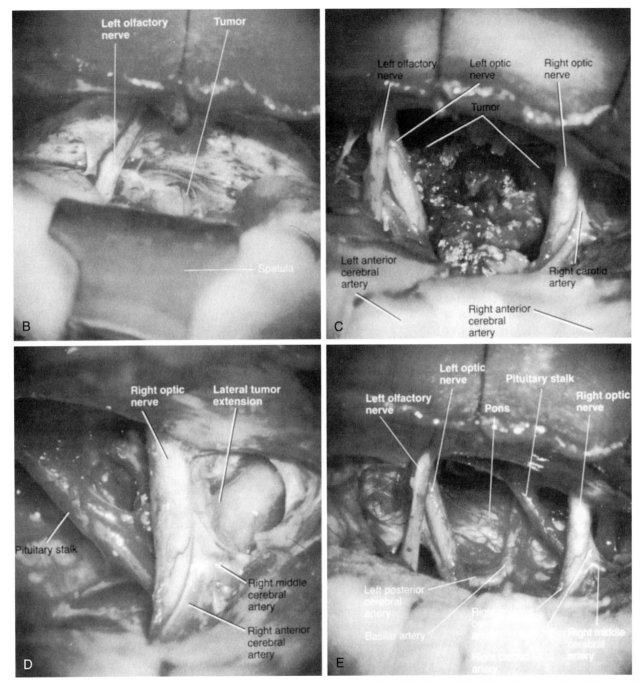

FIGURE 34-12 Cont'd *B*, Intraoperative findings after bifrontal craniotomy opening of the dura and ligation and transection of the superior sagittal sinus. The right olfactory nerve was sacrificed during the first operation; the left olfactory nerve is preserved and exposed. The brain spatula is retracting the frontal lobe; the anterior part of the tumor is visible. *C*, Intraoperative picture after partial tumor removal. Both optic nerves are freed from tumor tissue. The right carotid, middle cerebral, and anterior cerebral arteries are demonstrated. *D*, The parasellar extension of the tumor into the middle fossa as well as the preserved infundibulum are shown. *E*, Surgical site after total tumor removal. All surrounding structures are preserved (optic nerves, carotid artery, basilar artery and its branches, pituitary stalk, left olfactory nerve).

Any pulling or pressure on the pituitary stalk can result in traction to the hypothalamus, which can produce lesions with severe postoperative complications, either through direct damage of the parenchyma or through microvascular rupture. Therefore, it is important that after the basic enucleation, systematic exposure and resection of the tumor capsule are performed with utmost attention paid to the identification of the pituitary stalk.

POSTOPERATIVE MANAGEMENT

The most common postoperative complication in the management of craniopharyngioma is of endocrine origin. The following deficits are often observed: growth hormone (95%), thyroid hormone (90%), adrenocorticotropic hormone (75%), and luteinizing hormone/follicle-stimulating hormone (95%). Diabetes insipidus occurs in 70% of patients.[19]

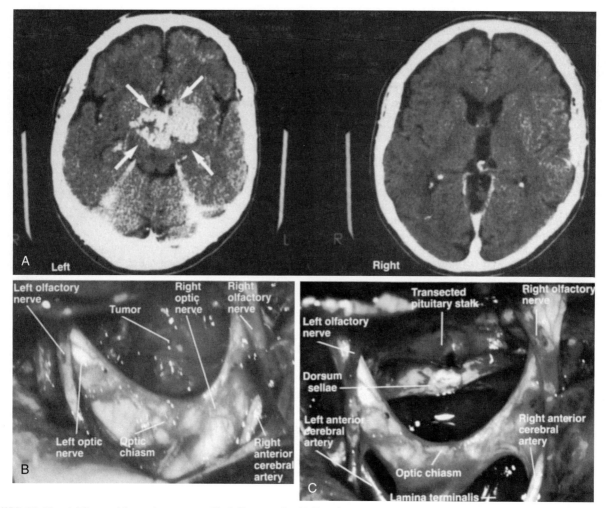

FIGURE 34-13 A 50-year-old man (case report 2). *A,* Preoperative (*left*) and postoperative (*right*) computed tomography (axial plane) of a large suprasellar, intraventricular craniopharyngioma. *Arrows* indicate tumor extension. *B,* Surgical exposure demonstrates both olfactory and optic nerves, the optic chiasm, and the anterior portion of the tumor. *C,* Intraoperative findings after total tumor removal. The retrochiasmal opening of the lamina terminalis, both anterior cerebral arteries, diaphragma sellae with transected pituitary stalk, dorsum sellae, and both preserved olfactory nerves can be seen.

All hormonal deficiencies are treated with replacement medication.

Postoperative hypothalamic syndromes such as hypersomnia, temperature dysregulation, profound amnesia, and disturbances of water, electrolyte, and caloric balance have been tremendously improved by the incorporation of microsurgical techniques. These syndromes do not result primarily from a direct iatrogenic trauma to this region but rather from rupture or coagulation of the small but important peritumoral vessels feeding the thalamus and hypothalamus.

RECURRENT CRANIOPHARYNGIOMAS

Patients with recurrent craniopharyngiomas represent a substantial group who have initially undergone subtotal operations and finally must be operated on again because the tumor has progressed. These patients invariably return with worsening, recurrent, or new symptoms.

Subtotally resected tumors have a 57% recurrence rate, whereas those that have been resected totally have a 19% recurrence rate. A combined therapy of subtotal surgery and postoperative irradiation results in a recurrence rate of 29%. Most of the recurrences appear during the first 3 years after initial treatment.[19]

The recurrence rate, usually in 2 to 5 years, is 7% to 29% after total removal and as high as 80% after subtotal resection.[11,15,35,36] The rate depends on the efficacy of initial surgery and the growth potential of the tumor. Management of recurrences is related to clinical manifestation and size, location, and type (cystic or solid) of lesion. The treatment modalities for recurrences are multiple. Many patients remain asymptomatic for a long time. One of the options is the wait-and-see strategy with regular magnetic resonance imaging follow-up. Surgery is performed in selected cases or in all recurrences. Some surgeons[35,36] propose total removal of all recurrences, provided that the patient's condition is not a contraindication. Radical reoperation in craniopharyngiomas has a higher morbidity rate because the tumor may be more adherent to the surrounding structures.[44] However, recurrent cases should be operated on radically, if possible, by an experienced surgeon to give the patient the best chance for a cure if the general condition of the patient is suitable for surgery. If not, cystic puncture with radionuclide implantation or radiotherapy should be considered in those patients in whom medical or surgical steps (e.g., shunt placement, hormone replacement) cannot achieve a stable and suitable scenario for open microsurgical removal.

Radiotherapy

Radiotherapy is regarded as beneficial for patients with residual or recurrent tumor. It is effective in preventing regrowth of cystic and solid craniopharyngiomas. The well-known side effects, such as radionecrosis, optic neuritis, secondary malignancies, impairment of intellectual functions, and endocrinologic abnormalities, make it an unfavorable option, especially in children. Because surgery after irradiation is far more difficult, radiotherapy is recommended for adults in selected cases who are not suitable for repeated surgery.[36] Varlotto and colleagues[45] suggest that approximately 60 Gy must be delivered in 1.6- to 1.7-Gy fractions for tumors that cannot be totally resected. Radiotherapy of tumor remnants or recurrences is sometimes effective in preventing further tumor progression. Using stereotactic radiosurgery (gamma knife), the tumor control rate was shown to be only 36%.[46] However, the risk of tumor progression in the long term places such patients at particular risk because the possibilities of further surgical treatment are limited.

Intracavitary Irradiation

Intracavitary irradiation with β-emitting radioisotope proved to be beneficial for patients with single cysts larger than 3 cm^3. Some authors suggest it as a first treatment option or as adjuvant therapy in mixed craniopharyngiomas as well. Most beneficial in contemporary series is the application of ^{32}P in colloidal suspension to deliver 250 Gy to the inner wall of the cyst. The limited penetration of its ß particles limits the danger to adjacent structures. The response rate is 71% to 88%, more than 70% of the lesions show a decrease in size, and the recurrence rates after limited follow-up are 9.7% to 33%.[47-49] Five- and 1-year actuarial survival rates are 55% and 45%, respectively.[47] Tumor progression was the cause of death in one third of the cases followed by Voges and colleagues.[47] Some cysts progress rapidly even after repeated radioisotope installation. Several recent studies suggest that combination of intracavitary irradiation and bleomycin administration leads to significantly improved survival rates. Leakage of isotope has been observed in several cases. Its clinical importance is not clear, but anterior or posterior pituitary dysfunction, visual deficits up to amaurosis and cranial nerve palsies have been observed after intracavitary irradiation.[47] Patients remain at risk of the formation of new cysts and require diligent magnetic resonance imaging follow-up.

Chemotherapy

Craniopharyngiomas are composed of benign stratified epithelium, so intratumoral application of bleomycin has been advocated. Bleomycin is an antineoplastic antibiotic medication that inhibits the synthesis of DNA, proteins, and, to a lesser extent, RNA.

Indications for its application are cystic recurrences. Advantages of this treatment mode are the possibility of repeating the cycle of application, while avoiding new surgery.

A universal protocol of treatment with bleomycin has not been accepted. Most authors propose repeated administration for a certain time period through an Ommaya reservoir.[50] The catheter, connecting the reservoir to the cyst, could be positioned by craniotomy, endoscopically or stereotactically.

Bleomycin decreases the secretion of cystic fluid and causes degeneration of tumor cells, which finally leads to reduction of the tumor volume. Lower activity of L4 and L5 isoenzymes of lactate dehydrogenase have been observed. The activity of these enzymes has been shown to correlated with the biologic activity of craniopharyngiomas.[51] Long-term follow-up demonstrates that the rate of tumor control is 42% to 94%.[50,51] Broggi and colleagues[50] observed complete disappearance of the cyst in 50% of their patients. However, the published results are variable, presumably due to the different treatment protocols, cyst sizes, and dose of the drug.

Unfortunately, bleomycin has toxic effect on normal structures as well. The risk of local complications is 10%.[50] Leakage from the cyst or direct action on hypothalamus leads to hypersomnia, thermal dysfunction, memory impairment, bilateral hypacusis, and middle cerebral artery infarction. One case with lethal outcome has been described.[52]

Due to these possible toxic effects, bleomycin cannot be regarded as a primary treatment option. It could be seen as an alternative in patients with cystic recurrences.

RESULTS

The overall 10-year post-treatment survival rate for craniopharyngiomas is 92.5% after total removal and 85.6% after subtotal removal (if radiotherapy is combined with subtotal removal, the survival rate improves to 90%).[19]

Yasargil and colleagues[15] achieved total removal in 90% of 144 patients. In tumors smaller than 2 cm, the outcome was good (improved, totally independent) in 93% of patients. In intermediate-sized tumors (2 to 4 cm), 82.1% of patients were ranked good postoperatively. Sixty-five percent of patients harboring large tumors (4 to 6 cm) had a good outcome. The giant (>6 cm) craniopharyngiomas had a "good" result in only 12.5% of patients.

The following data of the series of Yasargil and colleagues suggest that primary surgery has a significantly better outcome than secondary surgery. In children, the clinical outcome was good in 72.5% after primary surgery, whereas after secondary surgery, only 31.6% of the children were in good condition. In adults, the clinical outcome was good in 80.3% after primary surgery, whereas the results after secondary surgery were good in only 38.5% of the patients.[15]

Similar data have been reported by Fahlbush and colleagues.[36] The mortality rate rises from 1.2% at initial surgery to 10.5% in reoperations and the independent functioning falls from 78% to 58%.

Regarding the ophthalmologic outcome, Cabezudo and colleagues[53] have shown that the prognosis for improvement of preoperative visual deficits is related to the preoperative symptoms. In patients in whom symptoms existed for less than 1 year, 87% of the patients had improved vision, whereas patients in whom symptoms existed for more than 1 year, only 33% experienced visual improvement after surgery.

In cases of repeated surgery, the risk for vision is greater. New visual deficit developed in 13% after first surgery and increased to 75% at reoperation.[19]

After surgical treatment, the endocrine status of these patients is often worse. Thirty-three percent of patients become obese, 70% have diabetes insipidus, and 33% of the pediatric patients undergo paradoxic spontaneous growth during some months. Hormonal deficits are usually observed as follows: growth hormone (95%), thyroid hormone (90%), adrenocorticotropic hormone (75%), and luteinizing hormone/follicle-stimulating hormone (95%).[19]

Postoperative neuropsychological disorders occur in 30% to 60% of children.[19] Pierre-Kahn and colleagues[54] noted that social integration of children after therapy without radiation is normal in 88% of patients, whereas after radiation therapy (either alone or combined with surgery), it is normal in only 22% of patients.

SUMMARY

Radical excision of craniopharyngiomas is considered the method of choice for the treatment of this tumor, delivering the best outcome for the patient without sacrificing functional outcome.[12–14,55–59]

Which hurdles may make total excision impossible? The effectiveness of an attempt for total removal can be evaluated by three factors: morbidity, recurrence, and mortality. These three points are conditioned by three objective and one very individual aspects. The three objective conditioners are size (e.g., which structures are involved?), the consistency of the tumor, and the adhesions between the tumor and the surrounding structures (e.g., calcified adhesion to the carotid artery or optic pathway). Nevertheless, the fundamental variable is the skill and experience of the surgeon. The optimal surgical approach for the removal of craniopharyngiomas is clearly influenced by the experience of the surgeon.[20,60–68] A good approach for tumor removal through real or potential spaces must allow a good overview and control of nearby vital neurovascular structures throughout the procedure.[66,68,69] Conversely, it should not increase the morbidity rate due to its complexity. The frontolateral approach offers sufficiently wide exposure to the region. Through the subchiasmatic, optocarotid, and retrocarotid avenues, craniopharyngiomas extending in the suprasellar and parasellar regions can be accessed. Furthermore, the retrochiasmatic component may be removed by opening the lamina terminalis, by working in the opticocarotid space, or both. The advantage of opening the lamina terminalis is that one may carefully excise that part of the tumor in its retrochiasmatic location at the level of the third ventricle. Even large tumors can be removed through a frontolateral approach with a very low rate of morbidity or postoperative complications. The surgical anatomy encountered allows good visualization of the area. Through the different spaces or portals, complete removal of the tumor is possible.

The other main surgical approaches are the transsphenoidal route, the extended transsphenoidal approaches, the subtemporal or extended pterional approach, the transventricular route and the transpetrosal-transtentorial exposure.

The transsphenoidal route is the approach of choice for grade I and II craniopharyngiomas. Low surgical morbidity and improvement of preoperative visual field deficits and hyperprolactinemia have been reported.[70] If suprasellar calcifications are found, complete tumor removal is unlikely, and a craniotomy will be necessary to accomplish as complete an excision as possible. Special attention must be paid to avoid trauma to the optic nerves and chiasm. Tumors with significant suprasellar extension and attachments to the optic chiasm, hypothalamus, and vascular structures should not be approached by the transsphenoidal route. The extended transsphenoidal approaches offer the possibility of removing lesions with larger suprasellar part, but at the price of a high CSF leak rate.

The pterional, or frontotemporal approach, allows better exposure of the interopticocarotid space, and if it is extended posteriorly and combined with a superior retraction of the temporal lobe, it may expose somewhat better the lateral tumor portion in the space between the third cranial nerve and the posterior communicating artery inferiorly and the optic tract superiorly. However, as regards morbidity, third nerve palsies are not rare; fluctuating hemiparesis resulting from involvement of the intrinsic vascular hemispheric supply and homonymous visual field defects may occur. The transventricular route, which is an approach that descends from above, determines that the surgeon must incise either some cortical tissue or must split a part of the corpus callosum and work at a considerable depth and pass the foramen of Monro.[71] This may constitute a handicap. Therefore, there is greater risk that the neurovascular structures (e.g., the optic nerve, internal carotid artery, and anterior cerebral artery) eventually may be engulfed and iatrogenic lesions may occur, especially during dissection of the tumor capsule.

By means of proper preoperative evaluation, microsurgical technique, and prevention of hormone insufficiency and maintenance of the fluid-electrolyte balance, cure can be achieved in this challenging and "baffling problem to neurosurgeons," as Cushing[72] described craniopharyngioma surgery in 1932.

Total removal of craniopharyngiomas as the method of choice should not be interpreted as "radicality by all means." Unnecessary risks should not be taken if unfavorable situations become evident during surgery. Neurosurgeons should refrain from planning a primary subtotal removal of the tumor with adjuvant irradiation therapy. The overall recurrence rate for this type of combined therapy is approximately 29%, whereas the recurrence rate in totally resected craniopharyngiomas is 19%. Evidence has been provided that reoperation of these recurrent tumors has the worst outcome in terms of morbidity and mortality (20.5%).[19]

Combined therapy of surgery and irradiation should be considered as a method of second choice, strictly reserved for extremely difficult cases in which total removal was attempted but could not be achieved.

REFERENCES

1. Bunin GR, Surawicz TS, Witman PA, et al: The descriptive epidemiology of craniopharyngioma. J Neurosurg 89:547–551, 1998.
2. Crotty TB, Scheithauer BW, Young WF, et al: Papillary craniopharyngioma: A clinicopathological study of 48 cases. J Neurosurg 83:206–214, 1995.

3. Zuccaro G, Jaimovich R, Mantese B, Monges J: Complications in paediatric craniopharyngioma treatment. Childs Nerv Syst 12:385–390, 1996.

4. Rajan B, Ashley S, Thomas DG, et al: Craniopharyngioma: Improving outcome by early recognition and treatment of acute complications. Int J Radiat Oncol Biol Phys 37:517–521, 1997.

5. Rougerie J: What can be expected from the surgical treatment of craniopharyngiomas in children? Report of 92 cases. Childs Brain 5:433–449, 1979.

6. Rougerie J, Raimondi AJ: Craniopharyngiomas. In Amador LV (ed): Brain Tumors in Young, Springfield, IL: Charles C Thomas, 1983, pp 599–618.

7. Pertuiset B: Craniopharyngiomas. In Vinken PJ, Bruyn GW (eds): Handbook of Clinical Neurology. Amsterdam: North Holland, 1975, pp 531–572.

8. Konovalov AN: Microsurgery of tumours of diencephalic region. Neurosurg Rev 6:37–41, 1983.

9. Kobayashi T: Recent progress in the treatment of craniopharyngioma. Neurosurgery 3:101–112, 1984.

10. Steno J: Microsurgical topography of craniopharyngiomas. Acta Neurochir 35(Suppl):94–100, 1985.

11. Hoffman HJ. In Long (ed): Current Therapy in Neurological Surgery. Philadelphia: BC Decker, 1989, pp 82–84.

12. Ammirati M, Samii M, Sephernia A: Surgery of large retrochiasmatic craniopharyngiomas in children. Childs Nerv Syst 6:13–17, 1990.

13. Bhagwati SN, Deopujari CE, Parulekar GD: Lamina terminalis approach for retrochiasmal craniopharyngiomas. Childs Nerv Syst 6:425–429, 1990.

14. Klein HJ, Rath SA: Removal of tumors in the third ventricle using the lamina terminalis approach: Three cases of isolated growth of craniopharyngiomas in the third ventricle. Childs Nerv Syst 5:144–147, 1979.

15. Yasargil MG, Curcic M, Kis M, et al: Total removal of craniopharyngiomas: Approaches and long-term results in 144 patients. J Neurosurg 73:3–11, 1990.

16. Raimondi AJ: Pediatric Neurosurgery. Berlin: Springer-Verlag, 1987, pp 277–291.

17. Symon L: Experiences with radical excision of craniopharyngioma. In Samii M (ed): Surgery of the Sellar Region and Paranasal Sinuses. Berlin: Springer-Verlag, 1991, pp 373–380.

18. Fu X, Wang H: Ocular Symptoms of tumors at sella turcica region. Yen Ko Hsueh Pao Eye Science 12:166–168, 1996.

19. Choux M, Lena G, Genitori L: Le craniopharyngiome de l'enfant. Neurochirurgie 37(Suppl):1–174, 1991.

20. Samii M, Bini W: Surgical treatment of craniopharyngiomas. Zentralbl Neurochir 52:17–23, 1991.

21. Baba M, Iwayama S, Jimbo M, et al: Cystic craniopharyngioma extending down into the upper cervical spinal canal. No Shinkei Geka 6:687–693, 1978.

22. Fukushima T, Hirakawa K, Kimura M, et al: Intraventricular craniopharyngioma: Its characteristics in magnetic resonance imaging and successful total removal. Surg Neurol 33:22–27, 1990.

23. Iwasaki K, Kondo A, Takahashi JB: Intraventricular craniopharyngioma: Report of two cases and review of the literature. Surg Neurol 38:294–301, 1992.

24. Arwell WJ: The development of the hypophysis cerebri in man, with special reference to the pars tuberalis. Am J Anat 37:159–193, 1926.

25. Symon L, Sprich W: Radical excision of craniopharyngioma: Results in 20 patients. J Neurosurg 62:174–181, 1985.

26. Sutton LN, Gusnard D, Bruce DA, et al: Fusiform dilatations of the carotid artery following radical surgery of childhood craniopharyngioma. J Neurosurg 74:695–700, 1991.

27. Shanno G, Maus M, Bilyk J, et al: Image-guided transorbital roof craniotomy via a suprabrow approach: A surgical series of 72 patients. Neurosurgery 48:59–67, 2001.

28. Locatelli D: Endoscopic approach to the cranial base: Perspectives and realities. Childs Nerv Syst 16:686–691, 2000.

29. Cappabianca P, Cavallo LM, Colao A, et al: Endoscopic endonasal transsphenoidal approach: Outcome analysis of 100 consecutive procedures. Minim Invasive Neurosurg 45:193–200, 2002.

30. Joki T, Oi S, Babapour B, et al: Neuroendoscopic placement of Ommaya reservoir into a cystic craniopharyngioma. Childs Nerv Syst 18:629–633, 2002.

31. Shibuya M, Takayasu M, Suzuki Y, et al: Bifrontal basal interhemispheric approach to craniopharyngioma resection with or without division of the anterior communicating artery. J Neurosurg 84:951–956, 1996.

32. Shirane R, Ching-Chan S, Kusaka Y, et al: Surgical outcomes in 31 patients with craniopharyngiomas extending outside the suprasellar cistern: An evaluation of the frontobasal interhemispheric approach. J Neurosurg 96:704–712, 2002.

33. Alvarez-Garijo JA, Cavadas P, Vila M, et al: Craniopharyngiomas in children: Surgical treatment by the transbasal anterior approach. Childs Nerv Syst 14:709–712, 1998.

34. Maira G, Anile C, Albanese A, et al: The role of transsphenoidal surgery in the treatment of craniopharyngiomas. J Neurosurg 100:445–451, 2004.

35. Van Effenterre R, Boch AL: Craniopharyngioma in adults and children: A study of 122 surgical cases. J Neurosurg 97:3–11, 2002.

36. Fahlbusch R, Honneger J, Paulus W, et al: Surgical treatment of craniopharyngiomas: Experience with 168 patients. J Neurosurg 90:237–250, 1999.

37. Abe T, Ludecke DK: Transnasal surgery for infradiaphragmatic craniopharyngiomas in pediatric patients. Neurosurgery 44:957–966, 1999.

38. Kato T, Sawamura Y, Abe H, et al: Transsphenoidal-tuberculum sellae approach for supradiaphragmatic tumors: Technical note. Acta Neurochir (Wien) 140:715–719, 1998.

39. Kouri JG, Chen MY, Watson JC, Oldfield EH: Resection of suprasellar tumors by using a modified transsphenoidal approach: Report of four cases. J Neurosurg 92:1028–1035, 2000.

40. Kitano M, Taneda M: Extended transsphenoidal approach with submucosal posterior ethmoidectomy for parasellar tumors: Technical note. J Neurosurg 94:999–1004, 2001.

41. Kaptain GH, Vincent DA, Sheehan JP, Laws ER: Transsphenoidal Approaches for the extracapsular resection of midline suprasellar and anterior cranial base lesions. Neurosurgery 49:94–101, 2001.

42. Duff GM, Meyer FB, Ilstrup DM, et al: Long-term outcomes for surgically resected craniopharyngiomas. Neurosurgery 46:291–305, 2000.

43. Lüdemann W, Samii M: Comment to Steno et al. Neurosurgery 54:1051–1060, 2004.

44. Konovalov AN: Microsurgery of craniopharyngiomas. In Rand RW (ed): Microneurosurgery, 3rd ed. St. Louis: CV Mosby, 1985, pp 196–213.

45. Varlotto JM, Flickinger JC, Kondziolka D, et al: External beam irradiation of craniopharyngiomas: Long-term analysis of tumor control and morbidity. Int J Radiat Oncol Biol Phys 54:492–499, 2002.

46. Ulfarsson E, Lindquist C, Roberts M, et al: Gamma knife radiosurgery for craniopharyngiomas: Long-term results in the first Swedish patients. J Neurosurg 97(Suppl):613–622, 2002.

47. Voges J, Sturm V, Lehrke R, et al: Cystic craniopharyngiomas: Long-term results after intracavitary irradiation with stereotactically applied colloidal β-emitting radioactive sources. Neurosurgery 40:263–269, 1997.

48. Pollock BE, Natt N, Schomberg PJ: Stereotactic management of craniopharyngiomas. Stereotact Funct Neurosurg 79:25–32, 2002.

49. Blackburn TP, Doughty D, Plowman PN: Stereotactic intracavitary therapy of recurrent cystic craniopharyngioma by instillation of 90yttrium. Br J Neurosurg 13:359–365, 1999.

50. Broggi G, Giorgi C, Franzini A, et al: Therapeutic role of intracavitary bleomycin administration in cystic craniopharyngioma. In Broggi G (ed): Craniopharyngioma: Surgical Treatment. Milan: Springer-Verlag, 1995, pp 113–119.

51. Mottolese C, Stan H, Hermier M, et al: Intracystic chemotherapy with bleomycin in the treatment of craniopharyngiomas. Childs Nerv Syst 17:724–730, 2001.

52. Savas A, Erdem A, Tun K, Kanpolat Y: Fatal toxic effect of bleomycin on brain tissue after intracystic chemotherapy for a craniopharyngioma: Case report. Neurosurgery 46:213–216, 2001.

53. Cabezudo Artero JM, Vaquero Crespo J, Bravo G, et al: Status of vision following surgical treatment of craniopharyngiomas. Acta Neurochir (Wien) 73:165–177, 1984.

54. Pierre-Khan A, Brauner R, Renier D, et al: Traitement des craniopharyngiomes de l'enfant: Analyse retrospective de 50 observation. Arch Fr Pediatr 45:163–167, 1988.

55. Hoffman HJ, Hendrick ZB, Humphreyes RP, et al: Management of craniopharyngioma in children. J Neurosurg 47:218–227, 1977.

56. Sweet WH: Radical surgical treatment of craniopharyngioma. Clin Neurosurg 23:52–70, 1976.

57. Weiner HL, Wishoff JH, Rosenberg ME, et al: Craniopharyngiomas: A clinicopathological analysis of factors predictive of recurrence and functional outcome. Neurosurgery 35:1001–1010, 1994.

58. Anderson CA, Wilkening GN, Filley CM, et al: Neurobehavioral outcome in pediatric craniopharyngioma. Pediatr Neurosurg 26:255–260, 1997.

59. Honegger J, Barocka A, Sadri B, Fahlbusch R: Neuropsychological results of craniopharyngioma surgery in adults: A prospective study. Surg Neurol 50:19–28, 1998.

60. Fujitsu K, Kuwabara T: Zygomatic approach for lesions in the interpeduncular cistern. J Neurosurg 62:340–343, 1985.

61. Hakuba A, Nishimura S, Inove Y: Transpetrosal-transtentorial approach and its application in the therapy of retrochiasmatic craniopharyngiomas. Surg Neurol 24:405–415, 1985.

62. Kobayashi T, Nakane T, Kageyama N: Combined trans-sphenoidal and intracranial surgery for craniopharyngioma. Prog Exp Tumor Res 30:341–349, 1987.

63. Konig A, Lüdecke DK, Hermann HD: Transnasal surgery in the treatment of craniopharyngiomas. Acta Neurochir (Wien) 83:1–7, 1986.

64. Laws ER: Transsphenoidal microsurgery in the management of craniopharyngioma. J Neurosurg 52:661–666, 1980.

65. Long DM, Leibrock L: The transcallosal approach to the anterior ventricular system and its application in the therapy of craniopharyngiomas. Clin Neurosurg 27:160–168, 1980.

66. Mori T, Kodoma N, Takaku A, et al: Bifrontal approach for craniopharyngioma, and postoperative follow-up study. Acta Neurochir (Wien) 51:138–144, 1979.

67. Bini W, Sepehrnia A, Samii M: Some technical considerations regarding craniopharyngioma surgery: The bifrontal approach. In Samii M (ed): Surgery of the Sellar Region and Paranasal Sinuses. Berlin: Springer-Verlag, 1991, pp 373–380.

68. Shillito J: Craniopharyngiomas: The subfrontal approach, or none at all? Clin Neurosurg 27:188–205, 1980.

69. Suzuki J, Katakura R, Mori T: Interhemispheric approach through the lamina terminalis to tumors of the anterior part of the third ventricle. Surg Neurol 22:157–163, 1984.

70. Honegger J, Buchfelder M, Fahlbusch R, et al: Transsphenoidal microsurgery for craniopharyngioma. Surg Neurol 37:189–196, 1992.

71. King TT: Removal of intraventricular craniopharyngiomas through the lamina terminalis. Acta Neurochir (Wien) 45:277–284, 1979.

72. Cushing H: Intracranial Tumors. Notes Upon a Series of Two Thousand Verified Cases with Surgical-Mortality Percentages Pertaining Thereto. Springfield, IL: Charles C Thomas, 1932, pp 93–98.

Intracranial and Intraspinal Cysts

35

Surgical Management of Arachnoid, Suprasellar, and Rathke's Cleft Cysts

DIETER HELLWIG, DIRK MICHAEL SCHULTE, and WUTTIPONG TIRAKOTAI

Most of the intracranial cystic lesions that occur in adults are related to neoplasms, bacterial or parasitic infections, or loss of tissue due to malformation, infarction, or injury, including that resulting from surgical resection of brain tissue. These topics are discussed in other chapters of this book; however, an additional group of cystic intracranial lesions is encountered in neurosurgical practice, and three of these lesions are discussed in this chapter: the arachnoid, suprasellar, and Rathke's cleft cysts. Of particular interest is that the management of these lesions continues to evolve with the development of endoscopic neurosurgical techniques.[1–12]

INTRACRANIAL ARACHNOID CYSTS

Arachnoid cysts are intra-arachnoid benign cystic lesions filled with cerebrospinal fluid (CSF).[13] According to Cohen and Perneczky,[2] in 1831 Bright was the first to describe the intra-arachnoid location of intracranial arachnoid cysts. These lesions are probably developmental in origin and become symptomatic either because of their progressive enlargement or because of hemorrhage into the cyst. The enlargement of arachnoid cysts has been discussed controversially and is at this point in time a matter for discussion. There are various hypotheses to explain the growth of arachnoid cysts:

1. Active fluid secretion from the cyst wall[14,15]
2. Fluid accumulation caused by an osmotic pressure gradient[16]
3. Pumping of CSF through a persistent communication between the cyst and the arachnoid space due to vascular pulsation[17]
4. The so-called slit-valve mechanism, which is described later[1,18,19]

Arachnoid cysts occur throughout the neuraxis, and generally, no communication is demonstrable between the cyst and the subarachnoid space, although occasionally during surgery an arachnoid cyst is observed being filled through an apparent one-way valve.[20,21] Arachnoid cysts may be asymptomatic throughout life, and rarely, they may spontaneously regress[22,23]; however, if they do become symptomatic, the progression results from compression on the underlying brain, overlying bone, or both. There is an ongoing discussion whether space-occupying asymptomatic cysts should be operated on to prevent a hindrance to normal brain development and function.[24–26] If the indication for surgery is questionable,

intracranial pressure (ICP) monitoring should be performed to prove ICP elevation or pathologic pressure waves.[4,27]

CASE REPORT 1
ARACHNOID CYST

A 14-year-old boy was admitted with aggressive attitudes, loss of motivation, headache, and nausea. The neurologic examination was normal. An electroencephalogram showed a left-sided reduction of activity in the frontotemporal region. Magnetic resonance imaging (MRI) demonstrated a large left frontotemporal arachnoid cyst with a slight mass effect (Fig. 35-1). Epidural ICP measurement during a period of 24 hours revealed normal values (Fig. 35-2). We concluded that the cyst was not related to the patient's symptoms, and no further intervention was performed. Long-term follow-up examinations show that the patient is in good neurologic condition with normal age-related capacity.

The clinical symptoms resulting from these arachnoid cysts depend greatly on their location—whether over the Sylvian fissure; over the cerebral convexity; in the interhemispheric region; in the sella and suprasellar region; around the optic nerve, the quadrigeminal plate, or the cerebellopontine angle; in the region of the clivus; over the cerebellar vermis or cerebellar hemisphere; or within the lateral or fourth ventricle.[28–34] Arachnoid cysts have also been described extending across the region of the foramen magnum from the posterior cranial fossa into the upper cervical spine posterolateral to the spinal cord.[35,36] The midline lesions often lead to an obstruction of the CSF flow and result in focal symptoms and raised ICP.[37–40] There is a continuing discussion about whether intracranial arachnoid cysts are related to a specific seizure type and electroencephalographic focus.[41,42]

The arachnoid cyst wall is histologically indistinguishable from normal arachnoidal membrane. Moderate thickening of the arachnoid and an increase in connective tissue are common (Fig. 35-3).[43] Ultrastructural studies confirm the similarity of the cyst membrane with the normal meningeal counterpart, including the cell-cell connections and the occurrence of basal laminal structures. Quantitative differences in the contribution of the single components have

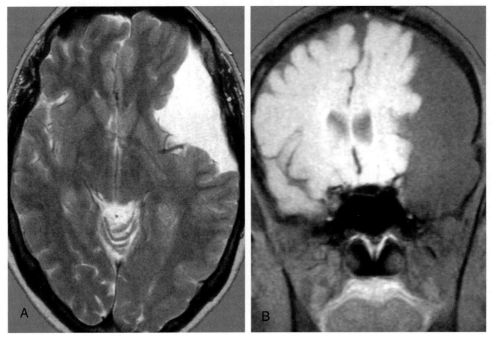

FIGURE 35-1 See Case Report 1, Arachnoid Cyst.

been found both between different cysts and between cysts and normal arachnoid.

A special kind of arachnoid cyst formation consists of a luminal epithelial layer connected with a glial sheet, followed peripherally by a thin connective tissue covering (Fig. 35-4). The glial nature of parts of the cyst lining can be shown by glial fibrillary acidic protein staining. Some authors have called these cysts "glioependymal."[44]

In many cases, arachnoidal cysts are incidental findings noted on CT scanning or MRI of the head performed for a reason unrelated to the cyst. Such patients are informed about the radiographic finding; provided with a copy of the study so they can present it to a physician at a later date, if necessary; and followed up annually. In approximately 15%

of middle fossa arachnoid cysts, an asymptomatic lesion may become symptomatic as a result of bleeding in association with the cyst and raised ICP. This event may occur after minor head trauma.[45–47]

In a report of 6 cases of subdural hematoma occurring in 18 patients with previously asymptomatic middle cranial fossa arachnoid cysts, Rogers and colleagues[48] recommended a cystoperitoneal shunt to treat the cyst after evacuation of the hematoma. Auer and co-workers[49] also recommended evacuation of the hematoma and the cyst's wall in one procedure. Handa and associates[50] reported on the two-stage removal of bilateral cysts and hematomas. They recommend that the hematomas be drained initially through burr holes and that 3 months later the cyst wall be resected and a

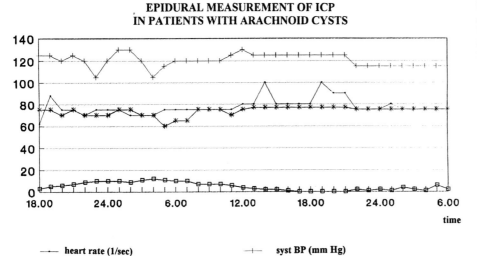

EPIDURAL MEASUREMENT OF ICP IN PATIENTS WITH ARACHNOID CYSTS

FIGURE 35-2 See Case Report 1, Arachnoid Cyst. diast BP, diastolic blood pressure; ICP, intracranial pressure; syst BP, systolic blood pressure.

—•— heart rate (1/sec)

—✳— diast BP (mm Hg)

—+— syst BP (mm Hg)

—□— ICP (mm Hg)

CASE REPORT 2
ARACHNOID CYST

This 72-year-old woman suffered from headache, stupor, and right hemiparesis. A large left hemispheric cystic process with a midline shift was diagnosed by computed tomography (CT) and MRI examination (Fig. 35-5A and B). Using 3-dimensional stereotactic trajectory and target-point calculation, the cyst membrane was approached endoscopically through a right frontal burr hole. The gray membrane was opened by radiofrequency coagulation, and biopsies were taken (Fig. 35-5C). The cyst contained CSF-like fluid. There was no evidence of tumor or other pathology. The histopathologic diagnosis was that of an epithelial cyst. The cyst was opened endoscopically to the left lateral ventricle. After surgery, the CT scan showed that the midline shift was greatly reduced. The left frontal horn was enlarged again (Fig. 35-5D). A few days after the intervention, the patient was alert and she was discharged with only a slight hemiparesis.

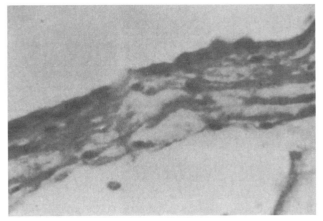

FIGURE 35-3 Lining of subarachnoid cysts consisting of a single layer of arachnoid and adjacent loose subarachnoid network and psammoma body. H&E stain. (From Youmans JR: Neurological Surgery, 2nd ed, vol 3. Philadelphia: WB Saunders, 1982, p 1437.)

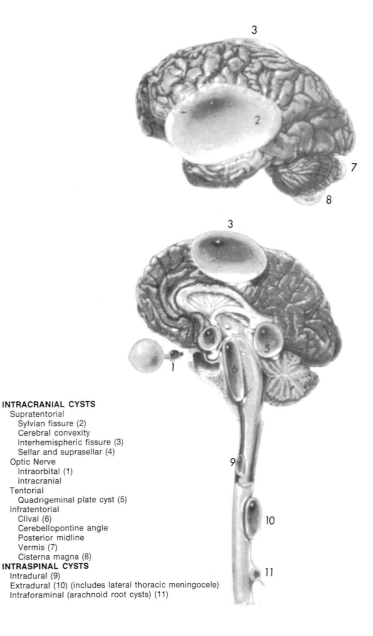

INTRACRANIAL CYSTS
Supratentorial
    Sylvian fissure (2)
    Cerebral convexity
    Interhemispheric fissure (3)
    Sellar and suprasellar (4)
Optic Nerve
    Intraorbital (1)
    Intracranial
Tentorial
    Quadrigeminal plate cyst (5)
Infratentorial
    Clival (6)
    Cerebellopontine angle
    Posterior midline
    Vermis (7)
    Cisterna magna (8)
INTRASPINAL CYSTS
Intradural (9)
Extradural (10) (includes lateral thoracic meningocele)
Intraforaminal (arachnoid root cysts) (11)

FIGURE 35-4 Intracranial and spinal cysts. (From Youmans JR: Neurological Surgery, 2nd ed, vol 3. Philadelphia: WB Saunders, 1982, p 1439.)

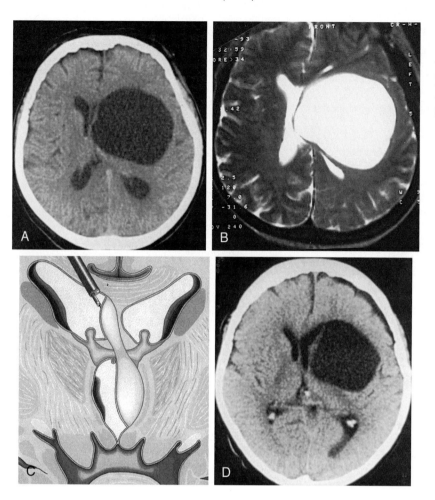

FIGURE 35-5 Electrosurgical technique for cystoventriculostomy. The rigid endoscope is placed into the right frontal horn, 5 mm distant from the cyst's surface. The electrosurgical coagulation and cutting probe is forwarded through the endoscope's working channel. With the tip of the probe, the cystoventriculostomy is performed in a contact mode.

CASE REPORT 3
ARACHNOID CYST AND CHRONIC SUBDURAL HEMATOMA

A 12-year-old boy had been hit on the head by a hockey stick. He suffered from headaches, and 2 weeks later his consciousness was impaired. MRI examination showed a left chronic subdural hematoma (Fig. 35-6A) related to a temporal arachnoid cyst (Fig. 35-6B). The subdural hematoma was drained through a silicone catheter. On CT examination, the subdural hematoma was greatly reduced with no signs of raised ICP or mass effect (Fig. 35-6C). We decided to leave the arachnoid cyst without further operative intervention. The patient did not develop complications during the postoperative course. Over a follow-up period of 9 years, the arachnoid cyst has remained unchanged.

cystoperitoneal shunt inserted. Mori and colleagues as well propose a two-step procedure. Hematoma evacuation is adequate at first operation. If the preoperative symptoms persist, additional arachnoid cyst surgery should be considered.[51] Markakis and colleagues[52] also recommend a two-stage approach to the management of large arachnoidal cysts,

beginning with a shunt procedure, which is followed several weeks later by the resection of the cyst wall and a ventriculostomy. Another treatment option is to evacuate the hematoma through an endoscopic burr hole approach and perform a cystostomy to the CSF space in one procedure.[53]

Cerebral convexity cysts occurring in adults present as seizures, headache, raised ICP, and, sometimes, marked reactive thickening of the overlying skull with erosion of the inner table. These cases can be managed by the wide excision of the membranes and the establishment of communication between the cyst interior and the CSF of the subarachnoid space. The same approach has been used in the treatment of symptomatic interhemispheric arachnoid cysts and cysts in the region of the quadrigeminal plate that produce aqueductal obstruction that leads to hydrocephalus. Before the advent of MRI, arachnoid cysts of the cerebellopontine angle often presented a diagnostic dilemma that required differentiation from other mass lesions located in the cerebellopontine angle.[29] Cysts of the cerebellopontine angle may mimic other lesions in this location and may cause hearing loss and cerebellar signs. These cysts may present as intermittent downbeat nystagmus with an associated hydrocephalus or as vague symptoms, including hearing loss and disequilibrium, contralateral trigeminal neuralgia, or hemifacial spasm.[54–57]

Surgical options for the management of symptomatic arachnoid cysts include the endoscopic resection of the cyst wall with opening of the membranes, which establishes

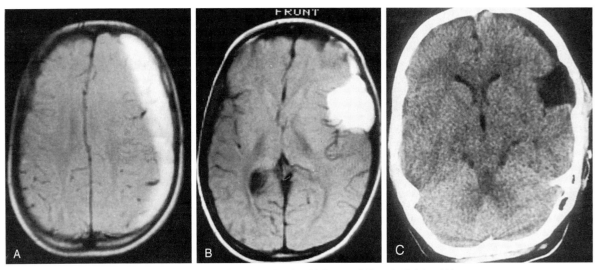

FIGURE 35-6   See Case Report 3, Arachnoid Cyst and Chronic Subdural Hematoma.

communication with the hemispheric or ventricular CSF pathways. Levy and co-workers described their results using the microsurgical keyhole approach for middle fossa arachnoid cysts.[58] This procedure can be performed with a minimal morbidity via a minicraniotomy. Compared with an endoscopic approach, better control of hemostasis can be obtained. The operative time and length of hospital stay were not excessively increased. Other options are stereotactic cyst aspiration,[59-61] shunt drainage or drainage of the lesion through a burr hole,[62] craniotomy with resection or marsupialization of the cyst walls,[63] and craniectomy and ventriculostomy of the cyst.[24,64] In a cooperative European study of the management of arachnoid cysts in children, total excision or marsupialization emerged as the first-choice surgical procedure, and shunting procedures were often applied to cysts located in deeper locations. Among the 285 patients, from birth to 15 years of age, there was a resultant reduction of the size of the cyst in approximately two thirds of the cases, and in 18%, the cyst had disappeared completely on follow-up CT scanning.[65] Another study of the relative merits of different approaches to the management of arachnoid cysts in children is based on an analysis of 40 children treated between 1978 and 1989 at the University of California, San Francisco. Of 15 patients with cysts that were treated initially by fenestration alone, 67% showed no clinical or radiographic improvement and subsequently required cyst-peritoneal or ventriculoperitoneal shunting. All of these patients improved postoperatively, although shunt revision was required in approximately one third of cases as a result of the recurrence of a cyst. These authors concluded that, irrespective of the location of the lesion, cyst-peritoneal or cyst-ventriculoperitoneal shunting is the treatment of choice.[24] Two groups reported about their results in neuroendoscopic treatment of arachnoid cysts. In a prospective study, Schroeder and co-workers[8] treated seven consecutive patients with symptomatic arachnoid cysts in different locations endoscopically. The authors performed cystocisternostomies and ventriculocystostomies

via burr holes with the aid of a universal neuroendoscopic system. Symptoms were relieved in five patients and improved in one patient, whereas the size of the cyst decreased in six patients. Although the follow-up period was short (15–30 months), the authors recommend neuroendoscopic treatment of arachnoid cyst as the first therapy of choice. The second study was conducted by Hopf and co-workers.[7] They evaluated 24 patients with intracranial arachnoid cysts that were treated endoscopically. Their surgical strategy was to create broad communication between the cyst and the subarachnoid space. Various techniques were used: endoscopic fenestration (10 cases), endoscopic controlled microsurgery (5 cases), and endoscopy-assisted microsurgery (9 cases). In all patients sufficient fenestration of the cysts could be achieved, with a favorable outcome in 17 patients. Operative complications included infection (3 patients), bleeding into the cyst (1 patient), and subdural fluid collections (4 patients). The authors conclude that different endoscopic techniques do provide sufficient treatment of selected arachnoid cysts.

CASE REPORT 4

ARACHNOID CYST AND POST-OPERATIVE CHRONIC SUBDURAL HEMATOMA

This female patient suffered from headache, vertigo, and partial oculomotor palsy. CT demonstrated a left-sided temporal arachnoid cyst (Fig. 35-7A). Endoscopic cysto-cisternostomy was performed. Postoperative CT examination showed reduction of the cyst size (Fig. 35-7B), and symptoms improved. However, in the follow-up a subdural fluid collection with mass effect developed (Fig. 35-7C and D). This subdural hematoma was evacuated successfully by a burr hole drainage as seen in control CT examination (Fig. 35-7E).

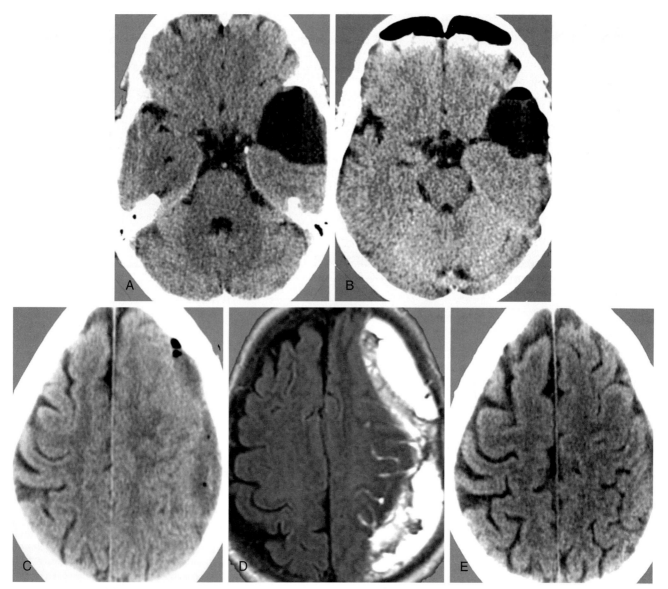

FIGURE 35-7 See Case Report 4, Arachnoid Cyst and Postoperative Chronic Subdural Hematoma.

Neuroendoscopic Instrumentation and Operative Technique in Treatment of Arachnoid Cysts

Endoscopes

Various rigid and flexible endoscopes are available to perform cystostomy, cystoventriculostomy, or cystocisternoventriculostomy. The advantages of rigid-lens scopes are the brilliant and bright pictorial quality and the guidance via a predetermined direct trajectory. Angled rigid scopes are used together with microscopes and neuronavigational devices in endoscopy-assisted microsurgery.[66] They offer the possibility to look around corners. Flexible neuroscopes have the advantages of steerability and maneuverability, which make inspection and interventions on multifocal and multiseptated cystic lesions easier.[67]

Guidance

There are different methods to perform endoscopic interventions on arachnoid cysts. The easiest and most time-sparing technique is the "freehand method." The approach is a single burr hole, and during the intervention the surgeon orients on anatomic landmarks. The advantage is to be free from holding and guiding devices; however, the operative approach and the targeting could be inaccurate.

Frame-based stereotactic guidance provides high accuracy and ensures orientation but could be time consuming and restricts endoscope movements. Newly developed neuronavigation systems provide image guidance, which is interactive and precise. These systems can be applied in a freehand mode or in combination with holding and guiding devices (Fig. 35-8A to C).

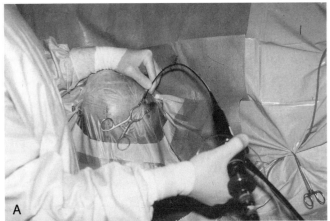

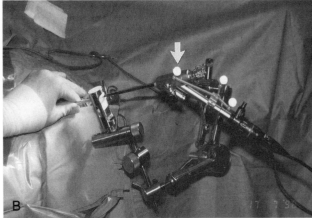

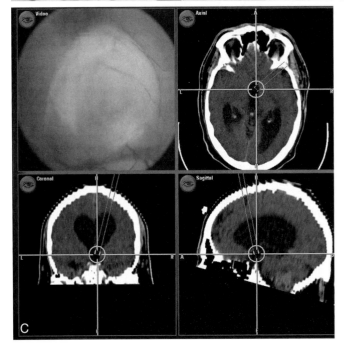

FIGURE 35-8 Various neuroendoscopy guiding techniques. *A*, Freehand technique with the flexible steerable endoscope. *B*, Fixed technique with the rigid endoscope (Zeppelin Co.) adjusted to a stereotaxy holding and guiding device in combination with neuronavigational guidance (see the white star-shaped instrument adapters, *arrow*). *C*, Neuronavigation assembly for 3-dimensional calculation and real-time visualization of the endoscopic approach to a ventricular cystic lesion.

Instruments

Moving neuroendoscopic working instruments within pre-formed or pathologic CNS cavities, as arachnoid cysts are, is not easy and requires training for several reasons: distances might be estimated incorrectly; the instrument may enter the viewing field from the side or is out of view; the surgeon controls the procedure at a video screen, and not directly as in microsurgery.

Various instruments are available for endoscopic interventions on arachnoid cysts. Microforceps and scissors are helpful to open and resect cyst membranes (Fig. 35-9A). In many cases, it is advisable to open the arachnoid cysts using electrosurgical devices. In cooperation with Erbe Company, we have developed a bipolar cutting and coagulation microprobe, which is controlled automatically by an electrosurgical unit. The regulated energy release avoids thermal damage to vulnerable structures. Safe hemostasis is ensured by pinpoint accuracy and effective coagulation of small vessels. The cutting depth is freely adjustable up to 3 mm. The cutting needle can be retracted into the endoscope's working channel. The probes are available for both rigid and flexible endoscopes with diameters of between 0.9 and 1.5 mm (Fig. 35-9B).[68] Balloon catheters (Fogarty, double balloon) are very useful to enlarge the stomas in an atraumatic fashion.

Imaging

Intraoperative digital dynamic subtraction cystography (cystoventriculography) is performed routinely to show the communication of the arachnoid cyst to the adjoining CSF compartments and the restoration of normal CSF flow (Fig. 35-10A and B). After the endoscopic intervention postoperative electrocardiogram-gated dynamic MRI examination demonstrates the normalized CSF flow under real-time conditions. In a recently published study Hoffmann and colleagues[69] could show a 90% accuracy in diagnosis of communication between arachnoid cysts and neighboring CSF spaces using cine-mode MR imaging.

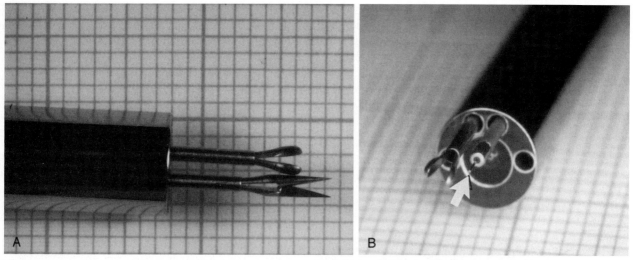

FIGURE 35-9 Supplementary endoscopy working instruments. *A,* Microscissors and grasping forceps guided through the rigid endoscope's working channel. *B,* Biopsy forceps and the tip of the bipolar coagulation and cutting microelectrode, which has a diameter of 0.9 mm (Erbe Co.) *(arrow).*

SUPRASELLAR CYSTS

Suprasellar cysts are arachnoid cysts that occur in the sella region and become symptomatic as locally expanding lesions. Arachnoid cysts in relation to the sella turcica represent 10% of all cases.[70] The term *suprasellar cyst,* formerly a synonym for craniopharyngioma, designates a small group of lesions, usually congenital, with a thin, even transparent wall that is filled with clear, colorless, or light-yellow fluid. The congenital effect from these cysts, which constitute fewer than 1% of all intracranial mass lesions, was severe enough to cause symptoms in the first 2 decades in 46 of the 54 reports collected by Hoffman and co-workers.[71] The lesion evolves as a consequence of prevention of CSF circulation into the chiasmatic cistern or laterally from the interpeduncular cistern beneath the hypothalamus and behind the pituitary stalk and optic chiasm. The presence of CSF from below the pontine cistern then pushes the hypothalamic floor upward and thins it greatly, so that above the arachnoid dome are only at most a few glial and ependymal cells, as described by Harrison[72] in three of four cases. In many of the cases, thin, even transparent, connective tissue is the only lining to the cyst. As do arachnoid cysts in other locations, suprasellar arachnoid cysts may enlarge over time. This change could be effected by active secretion of the membrane[73] or from ectopic choroid-like structures[14] or osmotic pressure gradients.[16] Another theory for the enlargement of

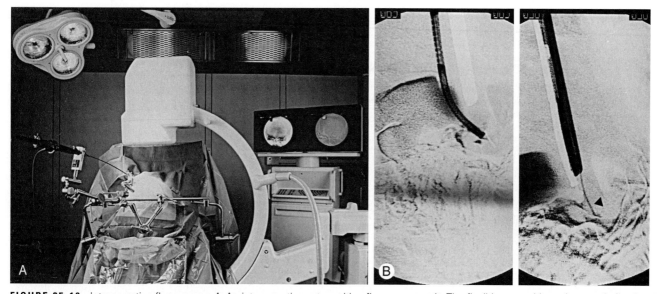

FIGURE 35-10 Intraoperative fluoroscopy. *A,* An intraoperative setup with a fluoroscopy unit. The flexible, steerable endoscope is fixed to the Marburg neuroendoscopy holding and guiding system. *B,* Intraoperative digital dynamic subtraction ventriculography offers a real-time movement control of the endoscope and the working instruments. The flexible, steerable endoscope is guided to the sellar region using a road mapping technique. At the tip of the endoscope, the bipolar electrode is forwarded *(black arrow).*

suprasellar arachnoid cysts is based on the endoscopic and cine-mode evidence of a slit valve,[1,18,19] formed by an arachnoid membrane around the basilar artery. This valve is supposed to open and close with arterial pulsations and lead to an inflow of CSF into the cyst forced by a pressure gradient.

By the time that the diagnosis is made, much or all of the third ventricle is usually filled by the cyst, causing an obstruction of one or both foramina of Monro, lateral ventricular dilatation, and a huge head. Indeed, the dome of the cyst is usually much higher than that shown in Figure 35-11, lying just beneath the corpus callosum. One possible mechanism for this block is excessive development of an arachnoidal curtain that extends from the posterior hypothalamus to the dorsum sellae below, originally described by Key and Retzius.[74] Its presence, confirmed by Lillequist[75] and by Fox and Al-Mefty,[76] becomes a menace when it and the arachnoid lateral to it become imperforate. Another mechanism of pathogenesis, proposed by Starkman and co-workers,[77] is that intra-arachnoidal spaces in the embryo persist and expand exclusively within the arachnoid. This event was demonstrated incidentally at autopsy in a careful dissection of an intact suprasellar cyst by Krawchenko and Collins.[13] Most suprasellar arachnoid cysts occur in children, with a male prevalence.[2] The clinical picture often includes, in addition to hydrocephalus with a big head and ataxia, disturbed visual acuity and fields due to forward and upward displacement of the chiasm, and hypopituitarism due to pressure in the hypothalamus and pituitary stalk. These symptoms caused by a suprasellar cystic lesion had been first described by Pieter Pauw, a Dutch anatomist, in the 16th century.[78]

A constant forward and backward nodding of the head and neck, the bobble-head doll syndrome, is an inconstant sign.[79–82] An unusual symptom is precocious puberty.[83]

Headache may occur in older patients. On CT scans, the cyst has the density of CSF; its wall shows neither enhancement nor calcification and is often mistaken for a dilated third ventricle. According to Cohen and Perneczky,[2] suprasellar arachnoid cysts appear as midline round or oval hypodense lesions adjacent to the dilated frontal horns. They have a typical "Mickey Mouse" configuration on axial CT scans or MRI. Prenatal diagnosis is possible using antenatal ultrasound combined with antenatal MRI.[84] Effective surgical treatment, which would seem to require simply making a big opening between the cyst and a normal CSF compartment, proves to be surprisingly difficult. Various combinations have been tried, including the transfrontal removal of the lower anterior wall of the cyst beneath the chiasm, a transcorticoventricular or transcallosal approach to remove much of the dome, the insertion of catheters between the cyst and ventricle or chiasmatic cistern, and the insertion of shunts from the lateral ventricles. Any one of these operations alone has a poor chance of sustained success. Agreement seems to be converging on the insertion of a combination of shunts from the lateral ventricles to the peritoneal cavity, with either a transcallosal route to remove the cystic dome, which was used with sustained success by Hoffman and co-workers in five cases,[71] or subfrontal removal of the anterior cyst wall. This latter tactic was successful in two cases from Gonzalez and colleagues,[85] three cases from Raimondi and colleagues,[86] and two cases from Murali and Epstein.[87] However, the lower opening closed, and symptoms recurred in one case of each of the last two groups and in one of Hoffman and co-workers' cases. That shunts from the ventricles alone may not suffice was demonstrated in a case from Murali and Epstein, in a child in whom a neonatal shunt kept the ventricles small but who also required opening of a suprasellar cyst to control bilateral visual loss 9 years

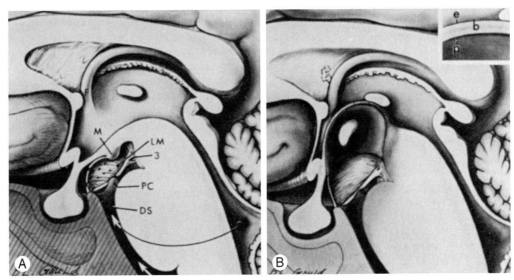

FIGURE 35-11 Anatomy of a suprasellar cyst. *A,* Artist's conception of the sagittal section of a normal brain and the sellar region, looking to the right. *Arrows,* normal flow of cerebrospinal fluid through the prepontine and interpeduncular cisterns. F, fornix; M, mammillary body; LM, Lillequist's membrane; 3, right oculomotor nerve; PC, right posterior clinoid process; DS, dorsum sellae. *B,* The membrane of Lillequist has ballooned forward and backward, compressing the floor of the third ventricle to the level of the massa intermedia. The left base of the nearly 3-dimensional cyst has been cut away to show the right oculomotor nerve. *Inset,* Enlargement of the compressed cyst-ventricular floor junction. e, Ependymal lining of the floor of the third ventricle; b, brain parenchyma of the compressed hypothalamus; p, pia. (From Fox JL, Al-Mefty O: Suprasellar arachnoid cysts: An extension of the membrane of Lillequist. Neurosurgery 7:617, 1980.)

later. Ventriculoperitoneal shunting alone was satisfactory in Raimondi's fourth case. Each of the traditional approaches has been associated with a high rate of recurrence of cysts.[2]

Upcoming neuroendoscopic techniques seem to solve some of the major surgical problems in treatment of suprasellar arachnoid cysts. Pierre-Khan and associates[81] were the first to publish their results after performing endoscopic ventriculocystostomy of suprasellar arachnoid cysts. They used a monopolar electroprobe to create the wide stoma between the cyst and the ventricular cistern (ventriculocystostomy). In contrast to them, Caemaert and associates[1] prefer to use the neodymium:yttrium aluminum garnet (Nd:YAG) laser to open the cyst to the ventricular system and the basal cisterns (ventriculocystcisternostomy). None of the patients had postoperative complications or need for a secondary shunting procedure. Additional authors have published similar successful results.[2,19,88–90]

Neuroendoscopic Technique in Treatment of Suprasellar Arachnoid Cysts

Preoperatively, it is advisable to plan the operative approach whether stereotactically or by neuronavigation. Through a frontal precoronal burr hole approach, the surgeon enters the frontal horn of the lateral ventricle with the endoscope.[67] Usually, the cyst dome is bulging through the foramen of Monro. Ventriculocystostomy is performed using microscissors and microforceps as well as the bipolar coagulation and cutting device. It is advisable to create a large stoma (10–15 mm in diameter). After inspection of the parasellar region, it is absolutely necessary to open the membrane of Lillequist (cystocisternostomy), which forms the inferior wall of the cyst toward the prepontine cistern, using the basilar artery as a landmark. Our bipolar coagulation and cutting electrode proves to be the best instrument to make bloodless openings and avoids thermal effects to the surrounding nerval tissue.[68]

Because many patients are severely impaired by the time of initial diagnosis, prompt aggressive effort and close follow-ups are required. In rare cases prepontine arachnoid cysts can disappear spontaneously as described by Dodd and colleagues.[91]

CASE REPORT 5
SUPRASELLAR ARACHNOID CYST

An 8-year-old girl presented with signs of raised ICP, ataxia, and a cognitive disorder. MRI showed a hydrocephalus caused by a large suprasellar cyst with brain stem compression (Fig. 35-12A). The girl was operated on with the neuroendoscopic technique using the frontal transventricular burr hole approach. The cyst bulged into the foramen of Monro (Fig. 35-12B). After cystocisternostomy the pituitary stalk was clearly seen (Fig. 35-12D). Six days after the intervention, the girl's clinical condition was good and she was discharged. A control MRI, taken 1 year after the intervention, shows that the cystic lesion has reduced greatly in volume, and free CSF communication exists between the ventricular system and

the basal cisterns, which is documented by a postoperative MRI scan with typical flow-void signal in T2-weighted sequences (Fig. 35-12C). The girl still has no neurologic signs.

RATHKE'S CLEFT CYSTS

Rathke's pouch, the superiorly directed evagination from the stomodeum of the 4-week-old human embryo, becomes obliterated at all but its cranial portion by the seventh week of gestation. The anterior wall of the remaining small cavity, "the pituitary pouch," develops into the anterior lobe of the pituitary gland, and its posterior wall proliferates much less to become the pars intermedia of the gland. At autopsy, Shanklin[92] found that a residual lumen between a portion of these two structures persisted in 22 of 100 normal pituitary glands. Small, asymptomatic, fluid-containing cysts were found in 13 of these 22 specimens. Such cysts of Rathke's cleft were recorded in 26% of routine autopsy series in five publications.[93–96] Infrequently, these cysts enlarge enough to produce symptoms. These residual clefts of Rathke's pouch are usually lined with cuboidal or columnar epithelial cells, which are often ciliated and include mucin-secreting goblet cells that stain positively by the periodic acid–Schiff method. Stratified or pseudostratified squamous epithelium may also be present and may rest on a collagenous connective tissue stroma.

By November 1989, Voelker and co-workers[97] had collected a total of 155 histologically confirmed symptomatic cases from the world literature, including their own 8 cases. The increased recognition of the disorder is evident from the total of only 35 cases found in the literature in 1977 by Yoshida and associates.[98] The Rathke's cleft cyst was both intrasellar and suprasellar in 90 patients, intrasellar in 22, suprasellar in 15, and intrasphenoidal in 1. The cyst capsule varies in thickness and can be any color. Common colors of the more watery fluids are yellow, blue, or green, at times with cholesterol crystals. The content of the cyst may vary from watery or serous (in 15 cases) to mucoid, gelatinous, and caseous, like motor oil, to white and creamy. This last appearance may be suggestive of pus. The content of one of the cysts was so tough as to require a rongeur for removal. Although in these series reported with only a few patients a limited range of abnormal appearances may be described in CT scans and MRI, the extreme differences in the cystic content of protein and other chemicals are matched by similar variation in the scans, as pointed out by many authors.[99–106] However, the size and location of the lesion were delineated in approximately 100% of the MRI studies and 90% of the CT scans. Image features such as a sellar epicenter, smooth contour, absence of calcification, absence of internal enhancement, and homogeneous attenuation or signal intensity within the lesion suggest the diagnosis of a Rathke's cleft cyst.[107,108]

Kleinschmidt and associates[109] proposed a new pathognomonic MR feature—the posterior ledge sign—of Rathke's cleft cysts. Ross and colleagues[99] stated that the diagnosis can be made at operation after the cystic cavity is irrigated. The lining of Rathke's cleft cyst is smooth and transparent; that of a craniopharyngiomatous or a pituitary adenomatous cyst is lined at least at some point by tumor.

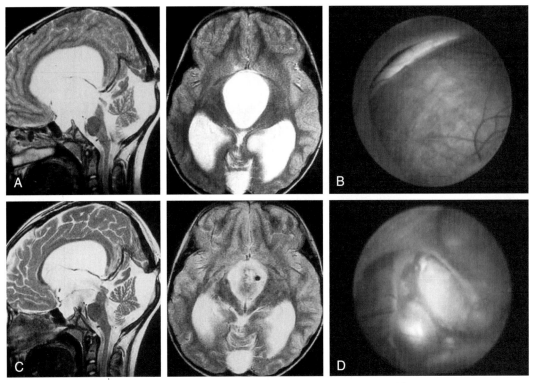

FIGURE 35-12   See Case Report 5, Suprasellar Arachnoid Cyst.

CASE REPORT 6
LOW-GRADE ASTROCYTOMA

This 62-year-old woman was admitted with a progressive bitemporal hemianopia and agitated psychosis (Karnofsky score of 30%). On MRI, a large cystic suprasellar space-occupying lesion with a blockage of foramen of Monro (Fig. 35-13A and B) was noted. Endoscopic stereotactic cyst evacuation was performed as an emergency procedure. The cystic lesion was reached through a right frontal burr hole. The gray membrane that bulged into the foramen of Monro was coagulated and was opened by microscissors. The sticky yellow contents of the cyst were aspirated. The remaining cyst membrane was vaporized using a laser. The histopathologic diagnosis was of a low-grade astrocytoma. Visual loss and the psychologic disturbances of the patient normalized immediately after the procedure. A postoperative MRI showed that the cystic process was totally evacuated (Fig. 35-13C and D). The patient was discharged 12 days after the procedure (Karnofsky score of 90%).

CLINICAL DATA OF RATHKE'S CLEFT CYST

Fager and Carter,[110] who had the earliest reported series of five living patients, found no solid abnormal tissue other than the thin wall in any of them. Visual fields and acuity, grossly abnormal in four of the patients preoperatively, improved greatly after the operation. The authors did not remove the cyst wall completely, but no symptoms recurred in any of the patients, who were followed up for as long as 9 years. They, therefore, regard total excision of the wall as unnecessary, concluding that a less radical approach suffices for these purely cystic intrapituitary or parapituitary lesions containing milky or mucoid fluid.

The following data are taken mainly from the reviews by Voelker and associates.[97] The female-to-male ratio was greater than 2:1, and the patients ranged in age from 4 to 78 years, with a mean age of 38 years and the highest frequency in the sixth decade. The preoperative duration of symptoms was from 3 days to 18 years, with an average of 34.9 months. Clinical presentation of patients is characterized by the triad: pituitary dysfunction, visual impairment, and headache.[104,111] The most common symptoms were those caused by pituitary hypofunction. Dwarfism occurred in more than 70% of those younger than 18 years of age. Of the 37 patients with amenorrhea-galactorrhea, 14 had also a pituitary adenoma. Hyperprolactinemia might have occurred whether or not the amenorrhea-galactorrhea syndrome was present. Half of the patients had visual field defects, and about one fourth had decreased visual acuity. Almost half of the patients had headaches, which were often frontal headaches. Nausea and vomiting were noted in only 18 patients. Bouts of aseptic meningitis, though infrequent, should be recognized and are discussed later. A few patients described vertigo, diplopia, lethargy, or syncope.

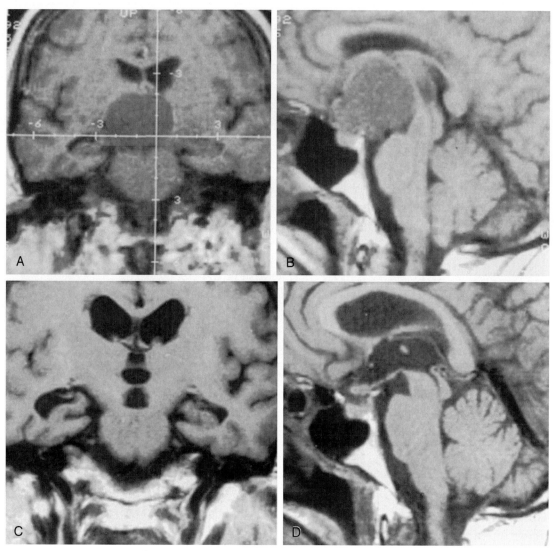

FIGURE 35-13   See Case Report 6, Low-Grade Astrocytoma.

Intermittent episodes of fever in only six cases were, at least in the patient of Van Hilten and colleagues,[112] an unusual symptom of hypothalamic involvement. Attacks of fever at approximately 2-week intervals sometimes woke her at night or occurred randomly. They lasted for 6 hours, during which she had a rectal temperature of 39°C, followed by 3 hours of excessive sweating and a gradual return of temperature to normal. This picture proved to result from a 20 by 20 by 20 mm suprasellar cyst extending up to the foramina of Monro and causing dilatation of both lateral ventricles and increased ICP. After lasting drainage of the cyst (three operations), all symptoms virtually disappeared.

Surgical excision of the cyst (usually partial) was carried out in 137 of the 155 patients, the remaining 18 cysts having been found at necropsy. The approach was by craniotomy in 60 cysts and via the sphenoid sinus in 59 cysts. Ross and co-workers[99] used the transsphenoidal route in 40 of 43 patients. The three patients with suprasellar lesions involving the pituitary stalk had transcranial approaches. The 10 patients of Midha and co-workers[113] were all operated on transsphenoidally, as were the 28 patients of El Mahdy and Powell.[104] This route was selected in only three of Voelker and co-workers' eight patients, all of whom had suprasellar extensions from the main intrasellar mass.[97] Operative mortality was zero in each of these four series. The recurrence rate after a craniotomy is approximately twice as high as that following the transsphenoidal route. Furthermore, if the cyst wall is removed only partially at craniotomy, the material secreted by the remnant may provoke an aseptic meningeal reaction. However, headache is not satisfactorily controlled by the partial removal of cyst wall advocated by the neurosurgeon Ross and colleagues.[99] Of their 32 patients whose preoperative symptoms included headaches, 21 obtained relief. Of 14 patients in whom headache was the only preoperative symptom, the headache persisted after operation in 7 patients. No correlation existed between the size of the lesion and the incidence of headache or the likelihood of disappearance of the headache after operation. The two patients with the largest lesions (23 and 25 mm) did not have a headache. However, of the 17 patients who had preoperative hyperprolactinemia, only 3 have continued to have prolactin levels above normal after operation. No data have been collated on the results on these scores after craniotomies.

Ross and co-workers[99] advocate the extremely conservative simple drainage of the cyst transsphenoidally, "accompanied by biopsy of the cyst wall, when this is possible without entering the subarachnoid space or damaging normal structures." In fact, they took no operative pathologic specimen to confirm the diagnosis in 17 of their 40 patients. El Mahdy and Powell[104] performed a partial excision of the cyst wall and drainage of the contents into the sphenoid sinus. In seven patients with an intraoperative CSF leakage, they used fascia lata or fat grafts.

Midha and associates[113] obtained biopsies of the cyst wall in eight patients and removed all of it in two. The preoperative symptoms and signs in all 10 had disappeared, except those related to pituitary dysfunction and in 3 patients with visual problems. Although Ross and colleagues[99] followed up their patients for a mean of 68 months, with the longest follow-up at 126 months, they have seen only one symptomatic recurrence.

Totally benign behavior is far from invariable, however. One Japanese patient presented with acute adrenal insufficiency, which capped the hypopituitarism secondary to the intrasellar Rathke's cleft cyst.[114] There are two reports of an acute hemorrhage into a Rathke's cleft cyst.[115,116] Another report is of hemosiderin deposits in the calcified epithelium of a Rathke's cleft cyst,[117] which emerged with an abrupt onset of severe headache and gave rise to an enhancing intrasellar and suprasellar mass. The mass was successfully removed transsphenoidally. One of Yoshida and associates' patients had a small nodule on her cyst wall that was scraped out with a curet.[98] Only part of the cyst wall was removed, and a serious recurrence took place within 1 year. Raskind and co-workers' patient, whose cyst contained a clear, colorless fluid, experienced a recurrence requiring repeat surgery 26 years later.[118] The patient reported by Berry and Schlezinger[119] had only a fragment of the cyst wall removed at the first craniotomy. At a major recurrence 37 months later, the cyst was three times the original size but contained the same clear, colorless mucoid fluid. The recurrences described by Yoshida and colleagues,[98] Iraci and colleagues,[120] and Matsushima and colleagues[121] were in patients with solid components to their lesions that contained stratified epithelium. In Matsushima's case, although the cyst was filled with the typical mucinous, puslike material and some of its lining comprised ciliated, mucin-containing columnar cells, most of it consisted of stratified squamous epithelium. This last component determined the outcome, namely death from recurrent tumor 20 months after its subtotal removal. Clearly, the solid portion of the tumor more than the appearance of the cystic fluid determines the prognosis. Two patients of Marcincin and Gennarelli[122] and one of Rout and colleagues[123] experienced recurrences in 4 months to 2 years after transsphenoidal evacuation of the cysts, even though the cyst fluid and wall were typical of pure Rathke's cleft lesions. A permanent visual loss ensued in one of the patients. The lesion was approached intracranially at recurrence in the second patient, and the entire cyst wall was removed. Two more recurrences after craniotomy have been reported by Yamamoto and co-workers[124] and by Leech and Olafson,[125] and four more have been reported after transsphenoidal approaches by

Roux and co-workers,[126] Midha and co-workers,[113] Ross and co-workers,[99] and El Mahdy and Powell.[104] Surprisingly, Mukherjee and associates[127] describe a reexpansion rate of 33% in 12 patients with Rathke's cleft cysts during a follow-up time from 1 to 168 months (median of 30 months). They propose to evaluate the role of radiotherapy for recurrent symptomatic tumors. As the reports have accumulated, it has become clear that many patients have transitional lesions or even highly unusual accompanying lesions. Russell and Rubenstein[128] were among the first to point this out, describing in two patients dumbbell cysts, the intrasellar portion of which was lined by a single layer of ciliated epithelium that changed abruptly at the diaphragma sellae to the squamous epithelium characteristic of a craniopharyngioma for the suprasellar portion. In a case reported by Yoshida and associates,[98] there was a tumor nodule with an inner lining of columnar cells that covered many layers of stratified squamous epithelium. Tajika and co-workers[129] found some areas of stratified epithelium in two of their three patients with Rathke's cleft cysts; in one of the two patients, cholesterol crystals, calcification, and brown fluid were present. Conversely, some ciliated, combined with columnar, cell areas were found in two other patients with histologic findings otherwise typical of a craniopharyngioma. This underlines the assumption that Rathke's cleft cysts may originate from squamous cell rests along the craniopharyngeal canal, resulting in a spectrum of cystic lesions in this area ranging from simple Rathke's cleft cysts to complex craniopharyngiomas.[104,130]

CASE REPORT 7
RATHKE'S CLEFT CYST

A 28-year-old patient suffering from a secondary amenorrhea was admitted to our department. An MRI scan showed a cystic lesion growing up from the sellar region and bulging into the third ventricle (Fig. 35-14A). We decided to perform primarily an endoscopic cyst evacuation using the frontal transventricular burr hole approach. The cyst was totally evacuated, and the cyst membrane was partly resected (Fig. 35-14B). The histopathologic diagnosis of the cyst membrane and its contents was ambiguous; some cells showed characteristics of craniopharyngioma cells, whereas others seemed to be of epithelial origin. Crystalloid and amorphic material was found in the contents of the cyst. The established histopathologic diagnosis was that of Rathke's cleft cyst; the differential diagnosis was a craniopharyngioma.

Goodrich and co-workers[131] described a suprasellar soft necrotic tumor rather than a fluid-containing tumor that contained many ciliated cuboidal or columnar cells typical of the lesion under discussion; however, other parts of the tumor included masses of squamous epithelium. Another Rathke's cleft cyst was reported that had characteristics of an epidermoid cyst.[132] Harrison and associates[133] suggested that Rathke's cleft cysts, epithelial cysts, epidermoid cysts, dermoid cysts, and craniopharyngiomas represent a continuum

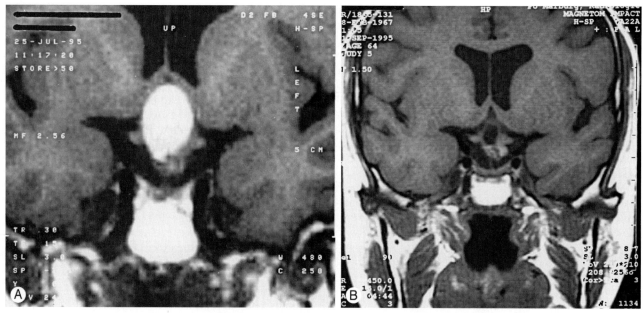

FIGURE 35-14 See Case Report 7, Rathke's Cleft Cyst.

of ectodermally derived epithelial cystic epithelial lesions. Other groups described the association of pituitary adenomas with the typical histologic form of Rathke's cleft cyst.[134-140] The more solid tissue there is associated with the cyst, the more likely it is to include a chronic inflammatory process or the stratified epithelium of a craniopharyngioma or of the glandular tissue of a pituitary adenoma. These tissues are likely to show enhancement in a scan.

These lesions are also more likely to have a major or completely suprasellar portion. Yuge and co-workers[141] have added two more exclusively suprasellar Rathke's cleft cysts to the 15 cysts collected by Voelker and co-workers.[97] In the patients from Miyagi and co-workers,[136] the lesions extended into the third ventricle. The patients in each of two publications[141,142] actually presented with hypothalamic tumors, one as a noncystic hypothalamic mass. This patient had an X, X, Y karyotype in all cells (Klinefelter's syndrome). These larger tumors were not totally removed. In the case from Itoh and Usui,[143] the subepithelial tissue consisted of normal pituitary gland. Wenger and colleagues added in 2001 another case of an entirely suprasellar Rathke's cleft cyst.[144] The Rathke's cleft cyst reported by Onda and colleagues[145] was associated with an arachnoid cyst; the cyst reported by Ikeda and colleagues[146] was associated with an eosinophil (acromegalic) adenoma. Arita and co-workers[147] described a case of Cushing's disease accompanied by Rathke's cleft cyst, and Ersahin and associates[148] presented a case of Rathke's cleft cyst with diabetes insipidus. Rathke's cleft cysts should be kept in mind as a potential cause for the syndrome of inappropriate secretion of antidiuretic hormone and adrenal insuffiency.[149] Two papers have reported chronic (granulomatous) hypophysitis related to Rathke's cleft cyst.[150,151]

Cannova and associates[152] found a granulomatous sarcoidotic lesion of the hypothalamic-pituitary region associated with a Rathke's cleft cyst. More distant accompanying lesions have been described by Koshiyama and colleagues[153] in the form of Hashimoto's thyroiditis with diabetes insipidus

and by Kim and colleagues[154] as a maldevelopmental mass with absence of pituitary gland; a rudimentary prosencephalon; and two other cysts, one a pigmented epithelial cyst (possibly a rudimentary eye) and the other a dorsal ependymal cyst, plus several other congenital abnormalities.

A single case report was published of a large suprasellar tumor extending downward to attach to the anterior wall of the pituitary gland. The cyst wall of the tumor was consistent with Rathke's cleft cyst in many places, but both its immunohistochemical and ultrastructural features were indistinguishable from colloid cysts of the third ventricle.[155] The cyst wall was totally removed via a subfrontal approach, and the authors achieved an excellent clinical result. Graziani and associates[156] assumed a common embryologic origin of suprasellar neurenteric cysts, the Rathke's cleft cyst, and the colloid cyst.

CASE REPORT 8
COLLOID CYST

A 41-year-old woman had chronic headache and gait disturbances, CT and MRI including 3-dimensional reconstructions revealed a cystic lesion in the third ventricle with obstructive hydrocephalus (Fig. 35-15A to C). Through a right frontal burr hole, an endoscopic cyst perforation and evacuation of the colloidal material was performed. The histopathologic diagnosis was a colloid cyst. The cyst wall was shrunk using the bipolar microelectrode. Membranous material adherent to the ventricular ependyma was left in situ. This was confirmed by a postoperative MRI examination (Fig. 35-15D). Seven days after the intervention, the patient was discharged without any new neurologic deficit. Five years after the operation, the patient showed no clinical or radiologic signs of cyst recurrence.

The reports of recurrences after mere evacuation of cysts have provided support for those who, from the first, included readily removable cyst wall as part of the surgical objective. In a 1984 publication (when high-resolution CT scanning was available), Shimoji and co-workers[157] noted enhanced capsules around low-density cysts in all three of their patients. They, therefore, elected to remove "as much as possible of the capsule" in all three and achieved good clinical results. Specimens from all three patients showed a histologic pattern typical of Rathke's cleft cyst, with the addition of squamous epithelium in the third case. Swanson and co-workers[138] also used the presence of capsular enhancement at CT scanning of an intrasellar mass to guide them to a transfrontal excision of the cyst wall.

Nonfunctional pituitary adenomatous cells constituted a part of that wall; therefore, they gave the patient a course of radiation therapy. This patient represented the sole reported case thus treated. The transsphenoidal route has been favored for most cases, especially when the suprasellar portion shows minimal enhancement.

In our experience with nontumorous cystic midline lesions, involving more than 100 patients, it is not necessary to resect the whole cyst membrane to prevent a recurrence. As an example, we have operated on 24 colloid cysts of the third ventricle in neuroendoscopic technique using the frontal burr hole approach. The cysts were evacuated and the membranes were resected subtotally. During a follow-up period from 6 months to 10 years, there was not one recurrence.[158]

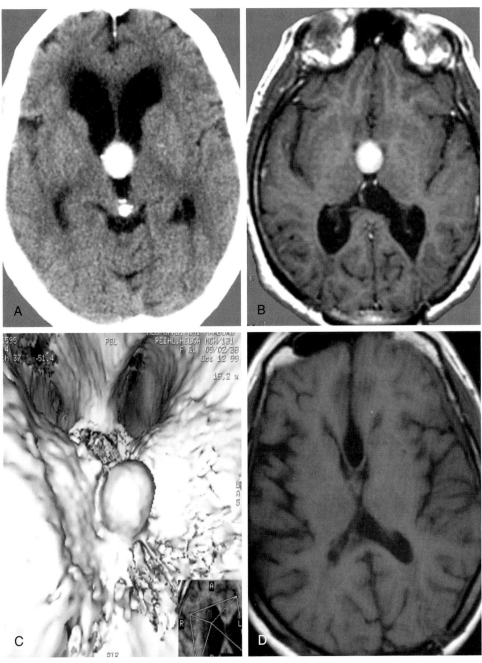

FIGURE 35-15 See Case Report 8, Colloid Cyst.

INTRASELLAR OR SUPRASELLAR ABSCESS

Gomez Perun and associates[159] stated in 1981 that 50 intrasellar abscesses had been reported; usually, the infection was propagated from a neighboring air or vascular sinus. The uninfected content of Rathke's cleft cyst may be a thick, white, or yellowish puslike fluid that was mistaken for pus by the authors. Typically, the cellular reaction in the CSF is predominantly lymphocytic, and culture results of the "pus" and CSF are repeatedly negative. The patient is reacting to a "foreign body" that he himself has secreted, as described in the following section.[160]

BOUTS OF CHEMICAL MENINGITIS: THE SYNDROME OF THE TOXIN-LEAKING CENTRAL NERVOUS SYSTEM CYST

An important point emerges from collation of the data from scattered individual case reports of patients with curious repeated febrile episodes, often with CSF pleocytosis. A culture was obtained from an organism in only one case. Attacks of a recurrent chemical febrile meningitis in a craniopharyngioma, presumably from a leakage of keratin or cholesterol, are a rare but well-authenticated occurrence.[161]

CASE REPORT 9
CYSTIC CRANIOPHARYNGIOMA

The 44-year-old patient had two febrile episodes with headache and opisthotonos 2 years before admission. Repeated CSF punctures revealed a slight pleocytosis. The first MRI scan showed no evidence of an intracranial space-occupying lesion. Later, it was suggested that these symptoms were the result of an aseptic meningitis after spontaneous perforation of a cystic craniopharyngioma. An MRI scan that was performed 3 months after the second febrile attack showed a cystic process in the anterior part of the third ventricle growing up from the suprasellar region (Fig. 35-16A and C). The cyst was approached by 3-dimensional stereotactic calculation under direct endoscopic control. The cyst wall was coagulated using bipolar radiofrequency, and the cyst was opened using microscissors. The cyst contained a thick yellow fluid. The cyst was emptied, and the capsule was coagulated. The postoperative follow-up was uneventful. On MRI, the residual tumor membrane was visible (Fig. 35-16B and D). The patient was discharged 12 days after the intervention without neurologic symptoms or psychologic disorder (Karnofsky score of 100%). The patient decided to undergo gamma knife treatment for the remaining tumor capsule.

In the first such case of Rathke's cleft cyst, reported as an abscess by Obenchain and Becker,[162] the patient had five episodes in 3 years of severe headaches, nausea, vomiting, general malaise, and fever, all leading to hospital admissions but resolving spontaneously a few days later. Finally, blurring of vision in her inferior temporal quadrants led to the diagnosis of her intrasellar and minimally suprasellar mass, from which, via a subfrontal route, 2 mL of "purulent" fluid was aspirated. *Staphylococcus epidermidis* was cultured from this fluid, and the patient was given penicillin, isoniazid, and ethambutol for 1 month. Then, via the transsphenoidal route, 3 mL of "pus" was aspirated, and the capsule was removed. Histologically, the wall was fibrous and lined by columnar epithelium with chronic inflammatory cells. The patient's recovery was excellent and sustained. The absence of acute inflammatory cells and the spontaneously subsiding brief attacks that had occurred for 3 years cast doubt on the role of the staphylococci.

In the next reported case,[163] similar recurrent brief episodes occurred. These episodes each lasted only 2 or 3 days and were characterized by intense supraorbital pain, fever to 39°C or 40°C, and about 50 clear-cut temporal lobe seizures a day. These seizures each lasted for several seconds and occurred mainly during the bouts of fever. These mysterious episodes continued for 10 years, during which time the patient's weight increased from 50 to 72 kg. Although the patient did not develop nuchal rigidity in the attacks, a lumbar puncture finally performed in 1977 revealed a largely lymphocytic pleocytosis and a normal protein level. Demonstration of an infratemporal quadrantanopia was followed by pneumography, which revealed a suprasellar mass. At a subfrontal exposure, thick, puslike fluid was removed from a subchiasmatic cyst, the capsule of which was largely removed. The cyst wall was heavily vascularized and infiltrated with inflammatory cells but lined with the typical ciliated columnar and cuboidal epithelium. The patient had also developed the symptoms and laboratory findings of deficient thyroid-stimulating hormone, adrenocorticotropic hormone, and luteinizing hormone–releasing hormone. The febrile episodes involving a headache stopped at once after operation, and the patient gradually made a full recovery. The seizures continued to require phenobarbital and valproic acid for control.

The following year, Verkijk and Bots[132] described a patient in whom meningeal reactions developed after surgery on a cyst; these reactions resolved spontaneously in 9 months. In the case reported by Steinberg and co-workers,[164] the initial symptoms pointed to a pituitary origin because of defects in visual acuity and fields, but then over the next 2 years, the patient was in the hospital numerous times with bouts of severe headache, nausea, vomiting, confusion, stiff neck, decreased visual acuity, and ataxic gait. On different occasions, the CSF showed pleocytosis, an increased protein level, and elevated pressure. All culture results were always negative. The episodes either resolved spontaneously or disappeared promptly after increases in the dosage of dexamethasone. Decreases in this dosage were followed by a recurrence of the symptoms. The sella was found to be enlarged and to contain a mass without suprasellar extension; the sella was, however, partially empty, with its anterior portion filling with air. These findings were apparently considered to be incidental. The lateral and third ventricles became increasingly dilated, and egress of contrast was delayed through the aqueduct and out of the fourth ventricle. The hydrocephalus was treated by ventriculoatrial shunt in 1972. Intracranial obstruction of the shunt required two revisions; each time, the symptoms promptly resolved. The patient died 1 year later of pneumonia. At autopsy, the

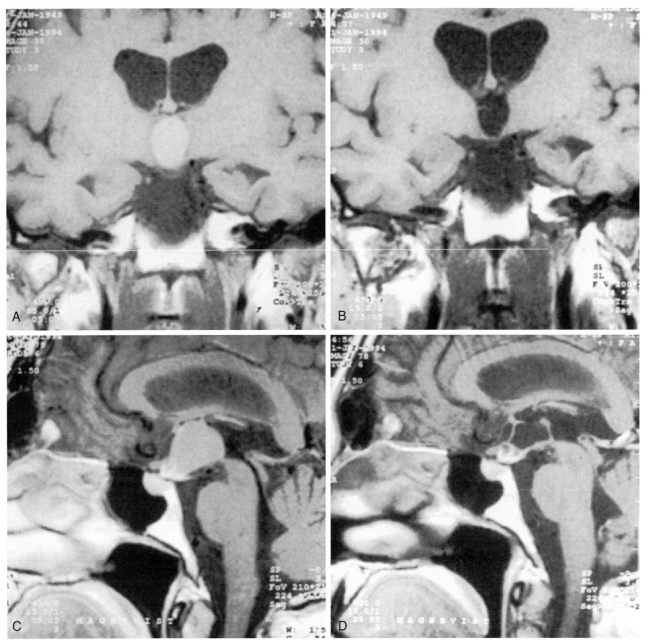

FIGURE 35-16   See Case Report 9, Cystic Craniopharyngioma.

Rathke's cleft cyst occupying the entire sella was filled with thick, yellow-green fluid. The cyst epithelium was largely ciliated and columnar, squamous in one area and keratinized in others. The leptomeninges adjacent to the chiasm and third ventricle were "moderately fibrotic with mild chronic inflammation."

Episodes of severe meningeal symptoms and signs, also with completely negative culture results, characterized a patient reported on by Gomez Perun and co-workers.[159] One episode in May 1977 was especially severe. When a suprasellar lesion was demonstrated and explored 6 months later, the cyst contained a thick, white fluid, which had an intense inflammatory reaction, and numerous vessels in the cyst wall, along with a lining of ciliated columnar epithelium. Also, an extensive frontal basal arachnoiditis

was present that was not noted in the other cases. The "pus" was sterile, and the patient made a prompt recovery but soon regressed, with similar episodes of aseptic meningitis. Despite three more operations, he too died; no organism was ever grown.

The patient reported on by Sonntag and co-workers[165] had only two episodes of a lymphocytic aseptic meningeal reaction before his intrasellar-suprasellar mass was subfrontally exposed. Seven milliliters of "pus" were aspirated, and the cyst wall was subtotally removed. The aspirate was sterile, but rare gram-negative rods were seen, and chloramphenicol was administered for 1 week. The symptoms recurred in 1 month, leading to transsphenoidal drainage of 5 mL of "pus" and "extensive removal of its wall." Culture results from this fluid were also negative.

Therapy with chloramphenicol was continued for 1 month, and the patient had remained well for almost 2 years at this writing.

Shimoji and associates[157] described three clear-cut cases of chemical meningitis. In the first, brief episodes of headache, nausea, vomiting, and fever were accompanied by enough eye signs to point to the sellar region and its cyst. At craniotomy, the "abscess-like viscous fluid" was sterile. As much cyst wall as possible was removed, and an excellent result persisted 2 years later. In the second case, a 52-year-old woman, four episodes of aseptic meningitis were required before a transsphenoidal evacuation of "milky, abscess-like viscous fluid" occurred and "as much as possible" of the cyst wall was removed. She, too, made an excellent recovery, which continued at 2 years. Both patients were also given 3000 cGy of ^{60}Co radiation. In the third case, an intermittent fever to 38°C on hospitalization rose to 39°C after pneumoencephalography; the patient, a 42-year-old woman, had meningeal signs and a CSF pleocytosis of 456 neutrophils and 74 lymphocytes. No growth occurred on culture. A week of antibiotic therapy brought no change, but 30 mg/day of prednisolone given in addition to the antibiotics dropped the temperature to normal the next day. The yellowish white gelatinous cyst fluid and, "as far as possible," its capsule, were removed via craniotomy. The periodic acid–Schiff-positive stratified squamous epithelium was heavily infiltrated with inflammatory cells. Good recovery persisted at 28 months.

Thick, yellow, puslike material and a cyst wall accompanied by squamous epithelium and thick connective tissue infiltrated with inflammatory cells was described in two other reports.[123,166]

One more clear-cut case of a foreign body reaction to the content of Rathke's cleft cyst was reported by Albini and associates.[167] The 19-year-old woman developed headache, galactorrhea, and a few months later, amenorrhea. Bitemporal hemianopia and deficiencies in thyroid-stimulating hormone, adrenocorticotropic hormone, luteinizing hormone, and luteinizing hormone–releasing hormone were identified. There had never been any episodes of fever or other suggestion of an aseptic meningeal reaction. The sella was enlarged, and while in the hospital, the patient developed a partial right third nerve paresis along with polydipsia and polyuria. At right pterional craniotomy, a large cyst seen on CT scan arising from the sella turcica was emptied of its thick, white fluid, and the cyst wall was insofar as possible removed. An excellent clinical result was obtained. The cyst wall was lined by the ciliated columnar and squamous epithelium of a Rathke's cleft cyst. The rest of the specimen was infiltrated with lymphocytes, plasmacytes, and multinucleated giant cells among islands of preserved pituitary tissue. No organisms were ever demonstrated. Apparently, the cystic fluid never seeped into the subarachnoid space. At 3-year follow-up, the patient had had no more headache and no mass observed by CT. From the service of Bognàr and co-workers[168] comes the report of two more patients with symptomatic histologically typical Rathke's cleft cysts and no preoperative episodes, which suggested aseptic meningitis. In both of them, the cyst contents were removed via the sphenoid sinus. Inflammatory cells and bacteria were recognized in the operative specimen, but technical problems were said to have prevented identification of organisms. Antibiotics were used, and one patient recovered uneventfully. In the other patient, transsphenoidal partial removal was followed by worsening in 2 weeks, leading to a frontolateral craniotomy, which likewise did not eliminate all of the abnormal tissue. *Staphylococcus aureus* and *Streptococcus pyogenes* grown from the specimen at the second operation were treated by antibiotics, but they failed to avert death on the ninth postoperative day. This sequence suggests that the cyst content facilitated the bacterial growth seen only after the second operation. Because of the diagnosis of infection, neither of these patients was given large doses of corticosteroids. Both patients may have been reacting primarily to the chemicals in the cyst fluid.

At least four reports have been published of spontaneous rupture of cystic craniopharyngiomas into the subarachnoid space that gave rise to a major but sterile meningeal reaction. This reaction was not different from those associated with Rathke's cleft cyst in that a predominantly neutrophilic, rather than lymphocytic reaction occurred in the severe cases.[157,168–170] Another case with spontaneous intraventricular rupture of a craniopharyngioma cyst was described in 2000 by Kulkarni and colleagues. The rupture resulted in an acute neurologic deterioration with consecutive bilateral optic nerve atrophy due to chemical meningitis. The patient was treated with ventricular drainage, steroids, and anticonvulsants. CSF showed high cholesterol and l-lactate dehydrogenase levels. The diagnosis of craniopharyngioma was subsequently verified histologically.[171]

Intracranial epidermoid tumors[172,173] and dermoid cysts[174,175] also rarely show this behavior as reported by several authors. In conclusion, Rathke's cleft cysts tend to occur mainly within the sella; their precise extent can now be determined by modern CT and MRI scanning. Most of these cysts are best approached transsphenoidally; however, approximately 10% that are wholly suprasellar should be removed via craniotomy. Whether transsphenoidal aspiration of the cyst and biopsy suffice, as urged by Ross and colleagues,[99] the endoscopic transventricular approach with cyst opening and aspiration proposed by Hellwig and colleagues,[67] or whether removal of as much cyst wall as seems safe is preferable is currently unclear. The neurosurgeons who favor a more aggressive stance will need to show that they achieve better relief of symptoms such as significant headache as well as fewer recurrences. The suprasellar component may need to be removed to the full extent dictated by safety because a repeat craniotomy is probably more hazardous than a second transsphenoidal approach.

In patients suffering from Rathke's cleft cysts, recurrent episodes of systemic or usually meningeal febrile illness can occur. This finding suggests that some of these typically thin-walled cysts may contain a peculiar chemical irritant that can leak out enough to contaminate the CSF and possibly the bloodstream at intervals and produce these dangerous responses. In our experience, after endoscopic cyst evacuation (Rathke's cleft cyst, craniopharyngioma, colloid cyst), the contents that contact the CSF compartments lead to a temporary increase in body temperature as a result of aseptic meningitis, which lasts for almost 24 hours and recurs spontaneously.

REFERENCES

1. Caemaert J, Abdulah J, Calliauw L, et al: Endoscopic treatment of suprasellar arachnoid cysts. Acta Neurochir (Wien) 119:68–73, 1992.
2. Cohen A, Perneczky A: Endoscopy and the management of third ventricular lesions. In Apuzzo MLJ (ed): Surgery of the Third Ventricle, 2nd ed. Baltimore: Williams & Wilkins, 1998, pp 922–927.
3. Fitzpatrick MO, Barlow P: Endoscopic treatment of prepontine arachnoid cysts. Br J Neurosurg 15:234–238, 2001.
4. Gaab MR, Schroeder HWS: Arachnoid cysts. In King W, Frazee J, DeSalles A (eds): Endoscopy of the Central and Peripheral Nervous System. New York: Thieme, 1998, pp 136–147.
5. Grotenhuis JA: The use of endoscopes during surgery of the suprasellar region. In Hellwig D, Bauer BL (eds): Minimally Invasive Techniques for Neurosurgery. Heidelberg: Springer-Verlag, 1998, pp 107–110.
6. Hellwig D, Bauer BL, List-Hellwig E: Stereotactic endoscopic interventions in cystic brain lesions. Acta Neurochir Suppl 64:59–63, 1995.
7. Hopf NJ, Resch KDM, Ringel K, Perneczky A: Endoscopic management of intracranial arachnoid cysts. In Hellwig D, Bauer BL (eds): Minimally Invasive Techniques for Neurosurgery. Heidelberg: Springer-Verlag, 1998, pp 111–119.
8. Schroeder HW, Gaab MR, Niendorf WR: Neuroendoscopic approach to arachnoid cysts. J Neurosurg 85:293–298, 1996.
9. Kamikawa S, Inui A, Tamaki N, et al: Application of flexible neuroendoscopes to intracerebroventricular arachnoid cysts in children: Use of videoscopes. Minim Invasive Neurosurg 44:186–189, 2001.
10. Kirollos RW, Javadpour M, May P, et al: Endoscopic treatment of suprasellar and third ventricle–related arachnoid cysts. Childs Nerv Syst 17:713–718, 2001.
11. Nomura S, Akimura T, Imoto H, et al: Endoscopic fenestration of posterior fossa arachnoid cyst for the treatment of presyrinx myelopathy—case report. Neurol Med Chir (Tokyo) 42:452–454, 2002.
12. Tirakotai W, Schulte DM, Hellwig D, et al: Neuroendoscopic surgery of intracranial cysts in adults. Childs Nerv Syst 20:842–851, 2004.
13. Krawchenko J, Collins GH: Pathology of an arachnoid cyst: Case report. J Neurosurg 50:224–228, 1979.
14. Go KG, Houthoff HJ, Blaauw EH, et al: Arachnoid cysts of the Sylvian fissure: Evidence of fluid secretion. J Neurosurg 60:803–813, 1984.
15. Little J, Gomez M, MacCarty C: Infratentorial arachnoid cysts. J Neurosurg 39:380–386, 1973.
16. Hanieh, A, Simpson DA, North JB: Arachnoid cysts: A critical review of 41 cases. Childs Nerv Syst 4:92–96, 1988.
17. Williams D, Gutkelch AN: Why do central arachnoid pouches expand? J Neurol Neurosurg Psychiatry 37:1085–1092, 1974.
18. Santamarta D, Aguas J, Ferrer E: The natural history of arachnoid cysts: Endoscopic and cine-mode MRI evidence of a slit-valve mechanism. Minim Invasive Neurosurg 38:133–137, 1995.
19. Schroeder HW, Gaab MR: Endoscopic observation of a slit-valve mechanism in a suprasellar prepontine arachnoid cyst: Case report. Neurosurgery 40:198–200, 1997.
20. Santamarta D, Morales F, Sierra JM, et al: Arachnoid cysts: Entrapped collections of cerebrospinal fluid variably communicating with subarachnoid space. Minim Invasive Neurosurg 44:128–134, 2001.
21. Hornig GW, Zervas NT: Slit defect of the diaphragma sellae with valve effect: Observation of a "slit valve." Neurosurgery 30:265–267, 1992.
22. Weber R, Voit T, Lumenta C, Lenard HG: Spontaneous regression of a temporal arachnoid cyst. Childs Nerv Syst 7:414–415, 1991.
23. Pandey P, Tripathy M, Chandra PS, et al: Spontaneous decompression of a posterior fossa arachnoid cyst. Pediatr Neurosurg 35:162–163, 2001.
24. Ciricillo SF, Cogen PH, Harsh GR, et al: Intracranial arachnoid cysts in children: A comparison of the effects of fenestration and shunting. J Neurosurg 74:230–235, 1991.
25. Hund-Georgiadis M, Yves Von Cramon D, Kruggel F, et al: Do quiescent arachnoid cysts alter functional organization?: A fMRI and morphometric study. Neurology 59:1935–1939, 2002.
26. Sgouros S, Chapman S: Congenital middle fossa arachnoid cysts may cause global brain ischaemia: A study with ^{99}Tc-hexamethylpropyleneamineoxime single-photon emission computerized tomography scans. Pediatr Neurosurg 35:188–194, 2001.
27. Di Rocco C, Tamburrine G, Caldarelli M, et al: Prolonged ICP monitoring in Sylvian arachnoid cysts. Surg Neurol 60:211–218, 2003.
28. Akor C, Wojno TH, Newman NJ: Arachnoid cyst of the optic nerve: Report of two cases and review of literature. Ophthal Plast Reconstr Surg 19:466–469, 2003.
29. Brooks ML, Mayer DP, Staloff RT, et al: Intracanalicular arachnoid cyst mimicking acoustic neuroma: CT and MRI. Comput Med Imaging Graph 16:283–285, 1992.
30. Floris R, Pastore FS, Silvestrini M, et al: Supracerebellar arachnoid cyst and reversible tonsillar herniation: Magnetic resonance imaging and pathophysiological considerations. Neuroradiology 34:404–406, 1992.
31. O'Reilly RC, Hallinan EK: Posterior fossa arachnoid cysts can mimic Meniere's disease. Am J Otolaryngol 24:420–425, 2003.
32. Ottaviani F, Neglia CB, Scotti A, et al: Arachnoid cyst of the posterior cranial fossa causing sensorineural hearing loss and tinnitus: A case report. Eur Arch Otorhinolaryngol 259:306–308, 2002.
33. Turgut M, Ozcan OE, Onol B: Case report and review of the literature: Arachnoid cyst of the fourth ventricle presenting as a syndrome of normal pressure hydrocephalus. J Neurosurg Sci 36:55–57, 1992.
34. Yamasaki F, Kodama Y, Hotta T, et al: Interhemispheric arachnoid cyst in the elderly: Case report and review of the literature. Surg Neurol 59:68–74, 2003.
35. Bhatia S, Thakur RC, Devi BI, et al: Craniospinal intradural arachnoid cyst. Postgrad Med J 68:829–830, 1992.
36. Price SJ, David KM, O'Donovan DG, et al: Arachnoid cyst of the craniocervical junction: Case report. Neurosurgery 49:212–215, 2001.
37. Arunkumar MJ, Korah I, Chandy MJ: Dynamic CSF flow study in the pathophysiology of syringomyelia associated with arachnoid cysts of the posterior fossa. Br J Neurosurg 12:33–36, 1998.
38. Punzo A, Conforti R, Martiniello D, et al: Surgical indications for intracranial arachnoid cysts. Neurochirurgia 35:35–42, 1992.
39. Pagni CA, Canavero S, Vinci V: Left trochlear nerve palsy, unique symptom of an arachnoid cyst of the quadrigeminal plate: Case report. Acta Neurochir (Wien) 105:147–149, 1990.
40. Kurokawa Y, Sohma T, Tsuchita H, et al: A case of intraventricular arachnoid cyst: How should it be treated? Childs Nerv Syst 6:365–367, 1990.
41. Mazurkiewicz-Beldzinska M, Dilling-Ostrowska E: Presentation of intracranial arachnoid cysts in children: Correlation between localization and clinical symptoms. Med Sci Monit 8:462–465, 2002.
42. Yalcin AD, Oncel C, Kaymaz A, et al: Evidence against association between arachnoid cysts and epilepsy. Epilepsy Res 99:255–260, 2002.
43. Miyagami M, Tsunokawa T: Histological and ultrastructural findings of benign intracranial cysts. Noshuyo Byori 10:151–160, 1993.
44. Friede RL, Yasargil MG: Supratentorial intracerebral epithelial (ependymal) cysts: Review, case reports and fine structure. J Neurol Neurosurg Psychiatry 40:127–137, 1977.
45. Servadei F, Vergoni G, Frattarelli M, et al: Arachnoid cyst of middle cranial fossa and ipsilateral subdural haematoma: Diagnostic and therapeutic implications in three cases. Br J Neurosurg 7:249–253, 1993.
46. Passero S, Filosomi G, Cioni R, et al: Arachnoid cysts of the middle cranial fossa: A clinical, radiological and follow-up study. Acta Neurol Scand 82:94–100, 1990.
47. Gelabert-Gonzalez M, Fernandez-Villa J, Cutrin-Prieto J, et al: Arachnoid cyst rupture with subdural hygroma: Report of three cases and literature review. Childs Nerv Syst 18:609–613, 2002.
48. Rogers MA, Klug GL, Siu KH: Middle fossa arachnoid cysts in association with subdural haematomas: A review and recommendations for management. Br J Neurosurg 4:497–502, 1981.
49. Auer L, Gallhofer B, Ladurner G, et al: Diagnosis and treatment of middle cranial fossa arachnoid cysts and subdural hematoma. J Neurosurg 54:366–369, 1981.
50. Handa J, Okamato K, Sato M: Arachnoid cysts of the middle cranial fossa: Report of bilateral cysts in siblings. Surg Neurol 10:127–130, 1981.
51. Mori K, Yamamoto T, Horinaka N, et al: Arachnoid cyst is a risk factor for chronic subdural hematoma in juveniles: Twelve cases of chronic subdural hematoma associated with arachnoid cyst. J Neurotrauma 19:1017–1027, 2002.
52. Markakis E, Heyer R, Stoeppler L, et al: Die Apoplexie der perisylvischen Region. Neurochirurgia 22:211–220, 1979.
53. Hellwig D, Riegel T: Endoscopic evacuation of intracerebral and septated chronic subdural hematomas. In Jimenez D (ed): Endoscopic Intracranial Neurosurgery. Park Ridge, IL: AANS Publications Committee, 1998, pp 185–197.

54. Chan T, Logan P, Eustace P: Intermittent downbeat nystagmus secondary to vermian arachnoid cyst with associated obstructive hydrocephalus. J Clin Neuroophthalmol 11:293–296, 1991.

55. Haberkamp TJ, Monsell EM, House WF, et al: Diagnosis and treatment of arachnoid cysts of the posterior fossa. Otolaryngol Head Neck Surg 103:610–614, 1990.

56. Babu R, Murali R: Arachnoid cyst of the cerebellopontine angle manifesting as contralateral trigeminal neuralgia: Case report. Neurosurgery 28:886–887, 1991.

57. Higashi S, Yamashita J, Yamamoto Y, et al: Hemifacial spasm associated with a cerebellopontine angle arachnoid cyst. Surg Neurol 37:289–292, 1992.

58. Levy ML, Wang M, Aryan HE, et al: Microsurgical keyhole approach for middle fossa arachnoid cyst fenestration. Neurosurgery 53:1138–1144, 2003.

59. D'Angelo V, Gorgoglione L, Catapano G: Treatment of symptomatic intracranial arachnoid cysts by stereotactic cyst-ventricular shunting. Stereotact Funct Neurosurg 72:62–69, 1999.

60. Iacono RP, Labadie EL, Johnstone SJ, et al: Symptomatic arachnoid cyst at the clivus drained stereotactically through the vertex. Neurosurgery 27:130–133, 1990.

61. Pell MF, Thomas DG: The management of intratentorial arachnoid cysts by CT-directed stereotactic aspiration. Br J Neurosurg 5:399–403, 1991.

62. Germano A, Caruso G, Caffo M, et al: The treatment of large supratentorial arachnoid cysts in infants with cyst-peritoneal shunting and Hakim programmable valve. Childs Nerv Syst 19:166–173, 2003.

63. Tamburrini G, Caldarelli M, Massimi L, et al: Subdural hygroma: An unwanted result of Sylvian arachnoid cyst marsupialization. Childs Nerv Syst 19:159–165, 2003.

64. Lange M, Oeckler R, Beck OJ: Surgical treatment of patients with midline arachnoid cysts. Neurosurg Rev 3:35–39, 1990.

65. Oberbauer RW, Haase J, Pucher R: Arachnoid cysts in children: A European co-operative study. Childs Nerv Syst 8:281–286, 1992.

66. Hellwig D, Benes L, Bertalanffy H, Bauer BL: Endoscopic stereotaxy: An eight years' experience. Stereotact Funct Neurosurg 68:90–97, 1997.

67. Hellwig D, Riegel T, Bertalanffy H: Neuroendoscopic techniques in treatment of intracranial lesions. Minim Invasive Ther Allied Technol 7:123–35, 1998.

68. Hellwig D, Haag R, Bartel V, et al: Application of new electrosurgical devices and probes in endoscopic neurosurgery. Neurol Res 21:67–72, 1999.

69. Hoffmann KT, Hosten N, Meyer BU, et al: CSF flow studies of intracranial cysts and cyst-like lesions achieved using reversed fast imaging with steady-state precession MR sequences. Am J Neuroradiol 21:493–502, 2000.

70. Rengachary SS, Watanabe I: Ultrastructure and pathogenesis of intracranial arachnoid cysts. J Neuropathol Exp Neurol 40:61–83, 1981.

71. Hoffman HJ, Hendrick EB, Humphreys RP, et al: Investigation and management of suprasellar arachnoid cysts. J Neurosurg 57:597–602, 1982.

72. Harrison MJG: Cerebral arachnoid cysts in children. J Neurol Neurosurg Psychiatry 34:316–323, 1971.

73. Dei-Anang K, Voth D: Cerebral arachnoid cysts: A lesion of the child's brain. Neurosurg Rev 12:59–62, 1989.

74. Key A, Retzius G: Studien in der Anatomie des Nervensystems und des Bindegewebes, vol 1, plate III. Stockholm: PA Norsted & Soner, 1875.

75. Liliequist B: The anatomy of the subarachnoid cisterns. Acta Radiol 48:61–71, 1956.

76. Fox JL, Al-Mefty O: Suprasellar arachnoid cysts: An extension of the membrane of Lillequist. Neurosurgery 7:615–618, 1980.

77. Starkman SP, Brown TC, Linell EA: Cerebral arachnoid cysts. J Neuropathol Exp Neurol 17:484–500, 1958.

78. Kivela T, Pelkonen R, Oja M, Heiskanen O: Diabetes insipidus and blindness caused by a suprasellar tumor: Pieter Pauw's observations from the 16th century. JAMA 279:48–50, 1998.

79. Benton J, Nellhaus G, Huttenlocher P, et al: The bobble head doll syndrome: Report of a unique truncal tremor associated with third ventricular cyst and hydrocephalus in children. Neurology 16:725–729, 1966.

80. Albright L: Treatment of bobble-head doll syndrome by transcallosal cystectomy. Neurosurgery 8:593–595, 1981.

81. Pierre-Khan A, Capelle L, Brauner R, et al: Presentation and management of suprasellar arachnoid cysts. J Neurosurg 73:355–359, 1990.

82. Desai KI, Nadkarni TD, Muzumdar D, et al: Suprasellar arachnoid cyst presenting with bobble-head doll movements: A report of 3 cases. Neurol India 51:407–409, 2003.

83. Starzyk J, Kwiatkowski S, Urbanowicz W, et al: Suprasellar arachnoidal cyst as a cause of precocious puberty—report of three patients and literature overview. J Pediatr Endocrinol Metab 16:447–455, 2003.

84. Golash A, Mitchell G, Malllucci C, et al: Prenatal diagnosis of suprasellar arachnoid cyst and postnatal endoscopic treatment. Childs Nerv Syst 17:739–742, 2001.

85. Gonzalez CA, Villarejo FJ, Blazquez MG, et al: Suprasellar arachnoid cysts in children: Report of three cases. Acta Neurochir (Wien) 60: 281–296, 1982.

86. Raimondi AJ, Shimoji T, Gutierrez FA: Suprasellar cysts: Surgical treatment and results. Childs Nerv Syst 7:57–72, 1980.

87. Murali R, Epstein F: Diagnosis and treatment of suprasellar arachnoid cyst. J Neurosurg 50:515–518, 1979.

88. Dhooge C, Govaert P, Martens F, et al: Transventricular endoscopic investigation and treatment of suprasellar arachnoid cysts. Neuropediatrics 23:245–247, 1992.

89. Decq P, Brugieres P, Le Guerinel C, et al: Percutaneous endoscopic treatment of suprasellar arachnoid cysts: Ventriculocystostomy or ventriculocisternostomy? [Technical note]. J Neurosurg 84:696–701, 1996.

90. Nakamura Y, Mizukawa K, Yamamoto K, et al: Endoscopic treatment for a huge neonatal prepontine-suprasellar arachnoid cyst: A case report. Pediatr Neurosurg 35:220–222, 2001.

91. Dodd RL, Barnes PD, Huhn SL: Spontaneous resolution of a prepontine arachnoid cyst: Case report and review of the literature. Pediatr Neurosurg 37:152–157, 2002.

92. Shanklin WM: The incidence and distribution of cilia in the human pituitary with a description of microfollicular cysts derived from Rathke's cleft. Acta Anat (Basel) 11:361–382, 1951.

93. Bayoumi ML: Rathke's cleft and its cysts. Edinb Med J 55:745–749, 1948.

94. Gillman T: The incidence of ciliated epithelium and mucous cells in the normal Bantu pituitary. S Afr Med J 5:30–40, 1940.

95. McGrath P: Cysts of sella and pharyngeal hypophyses. Pathology 3:123–131, 1971.

96. Rasmussen AT: Ciliated epithelium and mucous-secreting cells in the human hypophysis. Anat Rec 41:273–283, 1929.

97. Voelker JL, Campbell RL, Muller J: Clinical, radiographic and pathological features of symptomatic Rathke's cleft cysts. J Neurosurg 74:535–544, 1991.

98. Yoshida J, Kobayashi T, Kageyama N, et al: Symptomatic Rathke's cleft cyst: Morphological study with light and electron microscopy and tissue culture. J Neurosurg 47:451–458, 1977.

99. Ross DA, Norman D, Wilson CB: Radiologic characteristics and results of surgical management of Rathke's cysts in 43 patients. Neurosurgery 30:173–179, 1993.

100. Asari S, Ito T, Tsuchida S, et al: MR appearance and cyst content of Rathke cleft cysts. J Comput Assist Tomogr 14:532–535, 1990.

101. Christophe C, Flamant-Durand J, Hanquinet S, et al: MRI in seven cases of Rathke's cleft cyst in infants and children. Pediatr Radiol 23:79–82, 1993.

102. Ito H, Nishizaka T, Kajiwara K, et al: Pituitary nonadenomatous tumor (Rathke's cleft cyst). Nippon Rinsho 51:2711–2715, 1993.

103. Nakasu Y, Isozumi T, Nakasu S, et al: Rathke's cleft cyst: Computed tomographic scan and magnetic resonance imaging. Acta Neurochir (Wien) 103:99–104, 1990.

104. El Mahdy WE, Powell M: Transsphenoidal management of 28 symptomatic Rathke's cleft cysts, with special reference to visual and hormonal recovery. Neurosurgery 42:7–16, 1998.

105. Israel ZH, Yacoub M, Gomori JM, et al: Rathke's cleft cyst abscess. Pediatr Neurosurg 33:159–161, 2000.

106. Hsu YJ, Chau R, Yang SS, et al: Rathke's cleft cyst presenting with hyponatremia and transient central diabetis insipidus. Acta Neurol Scand 107:382–385, 2003.

107. Oka H, Kawano N, Suwa T, et al: Radiological study of symptomatic Rathke's cleft cysts. Neurosurgery 35:632–636, 1994.

108. Naylor MF, Scheithauer BW, Forbes GS, et al: Rathke cleft cyst: CT, MR, and pathology of 23 cases. J Comput Assist Tomogr 19:853–859, 1995.

109. Kleinschmidt Demasters BK, Lillehei KO, Steaaars JC: The pathologic, surgical, and MR spectrum of Rathke cleft cysts. Surg Neurol 44:19–26, 1995.

110. Fager CA, Carter H: Intrasellar epithelial cysts. J Neurosurg 24:77–81, 1966.
111. Isono M, Kamida T, Kobayashi H, et al: Clinical features of symptomatic Rathke's cleft cyst [Comment]. Clin Neurol Neurosurg 103:96–100, 2001.
112. Van Hilten BJ, Roos RAC, de Bakker HM, et al: Periodic fever: An unusual manifestation of a recurrent Rathke's cleft. J Neurol Neurosurg Psychiatry 43:533, 1990.
113. Midha R, Jay V, Smyth HS: Transsphenoidal management of Rathke's cleft cysts. Surg Neurol 35:441–454, 1991.
114. Tanigawa K, Yamashita S, Namba H, et al: Acute adrenal insufficiency due to symptomatic Rathke's cleft cyst. Intern Med 31:467–469, 1992.
115. Onesti ST, Wisniewski T, Post KD: Pituitary hemorrhage into a Rathke's cleft cyst. Neurosurgery 27:644–646, 1990.
116. Pawar SJ, Sharma RR, Lad SD, et al: Rathke's cleft cyst presenting as pituitary apoplexy. J Clin Neurosci 9:76–79, 2002.
117. Wagle VG: Hemorrhage into Rathke's cleft cyst. Neurosurgery 28:335, 1991.
118. Raskind R, Brown HA, Mathis J: Recurrent cyst of the pituitary: 26-year follow-up from first decompression. J Neurosurg 28:595–599, 1968.
119. Berry RG, Schlezinger NS: Rathke cleft cysts. Arch Neurol 1:48–58, 1959.
120. Iraci G, Girodano R, Gerosa M, et al: Ocular involvement in recurrent cyst of Rathke's cleft: Case report. Ann Ophthalmol 11:94–98, 1979.
121. Matsushima T, Fukui M, Ohta M, et al: Ciliated and goblet cells in craniopharyngioma: Light and electron microscopic studies at surgery and autopsy. Acta Neuropathol (Berl) 50:199–205, 1980.
122. Marcincin RP, Gennarelli TA: Recurrence of symptomatic pituitary cysts following transsphenoidal drainage. Surg Neurol 18:448–451, 1982.
123. Rout DL, Das L, Rao VRK, et al: Symptomatic Rathke's cleft cysts. Surg Neurol 19:42–45, 1983.
124. Yamamoto M, Takara E, Imanaga H, et al: Rathke's cleft cyst: Report of two cases. Neurol Surg 12:609–616, 1984.
125. Leech RW, Olafson RA: Epithelial cysts of the neuraxis: Presentation of three cases and a review of the origins and classification. Arch Pathol Lab Med 101:196–202, 1977.
126. Roux FX, Constans JP, Monsaingeon V, et al: Symptomatic Rathke's cleft cysts: Clinical and therapeutic data. Neurochirurgia (Stuttg) 31: 18–20, 1988.
127. Mukherjee JJ, Islam N, Kaltsas G, et al: Clinical, radiological and pathological features of patients with Rathke's cleft cysts: Tumors that may recur. J Clin Endocrinol Metab 82:2357–2362, 1997.
128. Russell DS, Rubinstein LJ: Pathology of Tumors of the Nervous System, 3rd ed. Baltimore: Williams & Wilkins, 1971.
129. Tajika Y, Kubo O, Kamiya M, et al: Clinicopathological features of 5 cases of pituitary cyst including Rathke's cleft cyst. Neurol Surg 10:1055–1064, 1982.
130. Ikeda H, Yoshimoto T: Clinicopathological study of Rathke's cleft cysts. Clin Neuropathol 21:82–91, 2002.
131. Goodrich JT, Post KD, Duffy P: Ciliated craniopharyngioma. Surg Neurol 24:105–111, 1985.
132. Verkijk A, Bots GT: An intrasellar cyst with both Rathke's cleft and epidermoid characteristics. Acta Neurochir (Wien) 51:203–207, 1980.
133. Harrison MJ, Morgello S, Post KD: Epithelial cystic lesions of the sellar and parasellar region: A continuum of ectodermal derivates? J Neurosurg 80:1018–1025, 1994.
134. Hiyama H, Kubo O, Yato S, et al: A case of pituitary adenoma combined with Rathke's cleft cysts. Neurol Surg 14:435–440, 1986.
135. Matsumori K, Okuda T, Nakayama K, et al: A case of calcified prolactinoma combined with Rathke's cleft cysts. Neurol Surg 12:833–838, 1984.
136. Miyagi A, Iwasaki M, Shibuya T, et al: Pituitary adenoma combined with Rathke's cleft cyst—case report. Neurol Med Chir (Tokyo) 33:643–650, 1993.
137. Nishio S, Mizuno J, Barrow DL, et al: Pituitary tumors composed of adenohypophysial adenoma and Rathke's cleft cyst elements: A clinicopathological study. Neurosurgery 21:371–377, 1987.
138. Swanson SE, Chandler WF, Latack J, et al: Symptomatic Rathke's cleft with pituitary adenoma: Case report. Neurosurgery 17:657–659, 1985.
139. Troukedes KM, Walfish PG, Holgate RC, et al: Sellar enlargement with hyperprolactinemia and a Rathke's pouch cyst. JAMA 240:471–473, 1978.
140. Sumida M, Migita K, Tominaga A, et al: Concomitant pituitary adenoma and Rathke's cleft cyst. Neuroradiology 43:755–759, 2001.
141. Yuge T, Shigemori M, Tokutomi T, et al: Entirely suprasellar symptomatic Rathke's cleft cyst. No Shinkei Geka 19:273–278, 1991.
142. Wenzel M, Salcman M, Kristt DA, et al: Pituitary hyposecretion and hypersecretion produced by a Rathke's cleft cyst presenting as a noncystic hypothalamic mass. Neurosurgery 24:424–428, 1989.
143. Itoh J, Usui K: An entirely suprasellar symptomatic Rathke's cleft cyst: Case report. Neurosurgery 30:581–585, 1992.
144. Wenger M, Simko M, Markwalder R, et al: An entirely suprasellar Rathke's cleft cyst: Case report and review of the literature. J Clin Neurosci 8:564–567, 2001.
145. Onda K, Tanaka R, Takeda N, et al: Symptomatic Rathke cleft cyst simulating arachnoid cyst: Case report. Neurol Med Chir (Tokyo) 29:1039–1043, 1989.
146. Ikeda H, Yoshimoto T, Katakura R: A case of Rathke's cleft cyst within a pituitary adenoma presenting with acromegaly: Do "transitional cell tumors of the pituitary gland" really exist? Acta Neuropathol (Berl) 83:211–215, 1992.
147. Arita K, Uozumi T, Takcchi A, et al: A case of Cushing's disease accompanied by Rathke's cleft cyst: The usefulness of cavernous sinus sampling in the localization of microadenoma. Surg Neurol 42:112–116, 1994.
148. Ersahin Y, Ozdamar N, Demirtas E, Mutluer S: A case of Rathke's cleft cyst presenting with diabetis insipidus. Clin Neurol Neurosurg 97:317–320, 1995.
149. Iwai H, Ohno Y, Hoshiro M, et al: Syndrome of inappropriate secretion of antidiuretic hormone (SIADH) and adrenal insufficiency induced by Rathke's cleft cyst: A case report. Endocr J 47:393–399, 2000.
150. Wearne MJ, Barber PC, Johnson AP: Symptomatic Rathke's cleft cyst with hypophysitis. Br J Neurosurg 9:799–803, 1995.
151. Roncaroli F, Bacci A, Frank G, Calbucci F: Granulomatous hypophysitis caused by a ruptured intrasellar Rathke's cleft cyst: Report of a case and review of the literature. Neurosurgery 43:141–149, 1998.
152. Cannova S, Romano C, Buffa R, Faglia G: Granulomatous sarcoidotic lesion of hypothalamic-pituitary region associated with Rathke's cleft cyst. J Endocrinol Invest 20:77–81, 1997.
153. Koshiyama H, Kato Y, Masutani H, et al: A case of Rathke's cleft cyst associated with diabetes insipidus and Hashimoto's thyroiditis. Jpn J Med Sci Biol 28:406–409, 1989.
154. Kim TS, Cho S, Dickson DW: Aprosencephaly: Review of the literature and a report of a case with cerebellar hypoplasia, pigmented epithelial cyst and Rathke's cleft cyst. Acta Neuropathol (Berl) 79: 424–431, 1990.
155. Wolfsohn AL, Lach B, Benoit BG: Suprasellar xanthomatous Rathke's cleft cyst. Surg Neurol 38:106–109, 1992.
156. Graziani N, Dufour H, Figarella Branger D, et al: Do the suprasellar neurenteric cyst, the Rathke's cleft cyst and the colloid cyst constitute a same entity? Acta Neurochir (Wien) 13:174–180, 1995.
157. Shimoji T, Shinohara A, Shimizu A, et al: Rathke cleft cysts. Surg Neurol 21:295–310, 1984.
158. Hellwig D, Bauer BL, Schulte DM, et al: Neuroendoscopic treatment for colloid cysts of the third ventricle: The experience of a decade. Neurosurgery 52:525–532, 2003.
159. Gomez Perun J, Eiras J, Carcavilla LI: Abcés intrasellaire au sein d'un kyste de la poche de Rathke. Neurochirurgie 27:201–205, 1981.
160. Hellwig D, Riegel T: Stereotactic endoscopic treatment of brain abscess. In Jimenez DF (ed): Intracranial Endoscopic Neurosurgery. Park Ridge, IL: AANS Publications Committee, 1998, pp 199–207.
161. Martin JB: Case records of the Massachusetts General Hospital: Case 17—1980. N Engl J Med 302:1015–1023, 1980.
162. Obenchain TG, Becker DP: Head bobbing associated with a cyst of the third ventricle. J Neurosurg 37:457–459, 1972.
163. Menault F, Sabouraud O, Javalet A, et al: Kyste de la fente de Rathke. Rev Otoneuroophthalmol 51:383–390, 1979.
164. Steinberg GK, Koenig GH, Golden JB: Symptomatic Rathke's cleft cysts. J Neurosurg 56:290–295, 1982.
165. Sonntag VKH, Lenge KL, Balis MS, et al: Surgical treatment of an abscess in a Rathke's cleft cyst. Surg Neurol 20:152–156, 1983.
166. Okamoto S, Handa H, Yamashita J, et al: Computed tomography in intra and suprasellar epithelial cysts (symptomatic Rathke cleft cysts). Am J Neuroradiol 6:515–519, 1985.
167. Albini CH, MacGillivray MH, Fisher JE, et al: Triad of hypopituitarism, granulomatous hypophysitis and ruptured Rathke's cleft cyst. Neurosurgery 22:133–136, 1988.

168. Bognàr L, Szeifert GT, Fedoresàk I, et al: Abscess formation in Rathke's cleft cyst. Acta Neurochir (Wien) 117:70–72, 1992.

169. Russell RWR, Pennybacker JB: Craniopharyngioma in the elderly. J Neurol Neurosurg Psychiatry 24:13, 1978.

170. Patrick BS, Smith RR, Bailey TO: Aseptic meningitis due to spontaneous rupture of craniopharyngioma cyst: Case report. J Neurosurg 41:387–390, 1974.

171. Kulkarni V, Daniel RT, Pranatartiharan R: Spontaneous intraventricular rupture of craniopharyngioma cyst. Surg Neurol 54:249–253, 2000.

172. De Klerk DJJ, Spence J: Chemical meningitis with intracranial tumours. S Afr Med J 48:131–135, 1974.

173. Schwartz JF, Balentine JD: Recurrent meningitis due to an intracranial epidermoid. Neurology 28:124–129, 1978.

174. Cantu RN, Kjellberg RN, Moses JM, et al: Aseptic meningitis due to dermoid tumor: Case report and confirming test. Neurochirurgia (Stuttg) 11:94–98, 1968.

175. Stendel R, Pietila TA, Lehmann K, et al: Ruptured intracranial dermoid cysts. Surg Neurol 57:391–398, 2002.

Intraspinal Cerebrospinal Fluid Cysts

EDWARD C. TARLOV and CARL A. GEYER

Intraspinal cysts are usually asymptomatic. When they are not, the reason is probably an absence of a free communication between the cyst and the subarachnoid space, causing local pressure effects or causing nerve roots or spinal cord to become trapped in cystic spaces.[1]

PERINEURIAL CYSTS

More than 60 years ago, Tarlov[2–4] described fluid-filled cysts of the posterior sacral nerve roots in 5 of 30 dissections within the sacrum during anatomic dissections carried out for study of the nerve roots. Years later, in the course of surgical exploration of the sacrum in patients with sciatica, Tarlov found such cysts. Because there was often evidence in these patients of local pressure effects, including bone erosion, Tarlov believed that these lesions could be symptomatic. He also noted improvement after cyst excision. The imaging techniques available at that time precluded diagnosing the cysts. Subsequently, it has been possible to demonstrate delayed entry of Pantopaque left in the subarachnoid space into cysts. Confusion arose when dilated normal root sleeves came to be referred to as perineurial cysts: these are ectatic root sleeves that freely communicate with the subarachnoid space and should therefore not cause local pressure and symptoms (Table 36-1, Fig. 36-1).

According to Tarlov, true perineurial cysts are probably congenital in most cases and communicate with the subarachnoid space. Schlesinger implicated a relationship with a connective tissue defect such as that found in Marfan's syndrome. Perineurial cysts are often multiple, and their walls may contain neural elements. Perineurial cysts are uncommon in the cervical and thoracic regions and less common in the lumbar region; the majority are found in the sacral spinal canal, most commonly in relation to the S2 root. This may be because the increased hydrostatic pressure in the lower spinal canal contributes to the formation of these cysts. Tarlov recommended surgery only in those rare cases with progressive or disabling symptoms that could clearly be attributable to the cyst.

Symptoms and Signs

Most perineurial cysts are asymptomatic. In most patients with back and sciatic pain who have these cysts, the cause of symptoms is nonspecific. Interestingly, many patients who have bilateral cysts have unilateral complaints, which speaks against the cysts being the cause of symptoms. When these cysts do cause problems, they may produce sciatica and radiculopathy, most often at S2, where they are most commonly found. The pathophysiology of symptoms, when present, may be anatomic distortion of root fibers in the walls of the cyst or pressure by the cyst on adjacent roots.

Imaging Findings

Erosion of the sacrum may be seen on plain radiographs, computed tomography (CT), and magnetic resonance imaging (MRI). The erosion is smooth and the entire sacral

TABLE 36-1 ▪ Cerebrospinal Fluid–Containing Spinal Cysts

	Location	Incidence	Pathology	Imaging	Comments
Perineurial cyst	Lateral sacral	Common	Lining contains neural elements	Appears as nerve root mass; sacral erosion	Can be excised (usually)
Arachnoid diverticulum	Usually lumbar	Common	Lined with arachnoid	Enlarge nerve root sleeve	Asymptomatic, of no clinical significance
Intradural arachnoid cyst	Usually thoracic, dorsal, or ventral	Rare	Lined with arachnoid	May cause spinal cord compression	Can be excised or fenestrated
Extradural arachnoid cyst	Usually thoracic	Uncommon	Lined with arachnoid	Associated kyphosis dorsalis juvenilis	
Intrasacral meningocele	Sacral, midline	Uncommon	Lined with arachnoid; does not contain neural elements	Sacral erosion	Can be excised; usually asymptomatic
Extradural pseudomeningocele	Usually lumbar	Common	Not lined with meninges	Extradural CSF root sleeve	Of no clinical significance
Root avulsion	Usually cervical	Uncommon	Not lined with meninges	Empty root sleeve	Usually not repairable

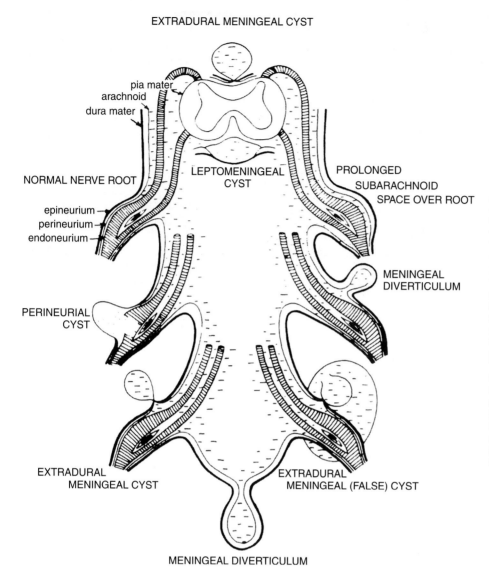

EXTRADURAL MENINGEAL CYST

pia mater
arachnoid
dura mater

NORMAL NERVE ROOT

LEPTOMENINGEAL CYST

PROLONGED SUBARACHNOID SPACE OVER ROOT

epineurium
perineurium
endoneurium

MENINGEAL DIVERTICULUM

PERINEURIAL CYST

EXTRADURAL MENINGEAL CYST

EXTRADURAL MENINGEAL (FALSE) CYST

MENINGEAL DIVERTICULUM

FIGURE 36-1 Illustrations of various cysts and diverticula of nerve roots. Those that do not communicate freely with the subarachnoid space are more likely to cause symptoms. Descriptions of these cysts (*counterclockwise from the top*): An extradural meningeal cyst, usually midline, is either covered by markedly thinned dura or arachnoid herniated through dural defect. A leptomeningeal cyst is seen below the cord, with its wall composed of arachnoid. In the normal nerve root (*upper left*), note that the arachnoid continuation is perineurium, accounting for occasional myelographic filling of perineurial cyst. Note that the perineurial cyst (*left*) lies at the level of the posterior ganglion. The cyst wall contains neural elements. Space within the cyst may have potential communication with the subarachnoid space, as shown, allowing for delayed but not immediate myelographic filling. The extradural meningeal cyst (*lower left*) lies proximal to the posterior root ganglion. The meningeal diverticulum (*bottom*) lies proximal to the posterior root ganglion. This is ordinarily of no pathologic significance, but if communication with the subarachnoid space becomes sealed off, it may form a symptomatic extradural cyst. Prolongation of the subarachnoid space over the nerve root (*upper right*) is a rather common finding of no pathological significance.

lamina can be eroded, with the cyst presenting in the paraspinous musculature. Such erosion is common, even in patients who are asymptomatic.

CT myelography can establish whether the cyst communicates with the subarachnoid space (Figs. 36-2 and 36-3). Modern and less viscous water-soluble nonionic contrast agents (e.g., iopamidol) make entry of contrast material into perineurial cysts more likely than with the use of Pantopaque. Lack of early entry of a water-soluble contrast agent into a cyst indicates that it is a perineurial cyst.

Since the advent of MRI, many perineurial cysts, particularly those that are asymptomatic, have been visualized.[5] On conventional MRI, it is not possible to determine whether a cyst communicates with the subarachnoid space. MRI CSF flow studies have been used to determine whether such communication exists. In one series, five of five asymptomatic cysts communicated with the subarachnoid space on MRI flow studies, whereas seven of seven symptomatic cysts did not communicate. These results correlate well with the earlier observations based on myelography.

Cyst Aspiration

In an effort to clarify if a perineurial cyst was indeed symptomatic, the authors have on occasion carried out CT-guided percutaneous cyst aspiration with a needle placed into these cysts, either through a defect in the sacral lamina or through the thinned sacral lamina itself. Aspiration of the cyst may relieve the symptoms. If the cyst does not communicate with the subarachnoid space, lasting relief can ensue.[6] However, the cyst usually refills, often in a short time. Paulsen and colleagues[6] reported relief of symptoms for 3 weeks to 6 months in five patients in whom cyst aspiration was carried out.

Surgical removal of a perineurial cyst may be indicated when the patient has unilateral pain in a distribution corresponding to the nerve root involved (usually S2), particularly if cyst aspiration has provided some relief.[6–9]

Intradural Arachnoid Cysts

Spinal intradural arachnoid cysts often arise on a congenital basis and may be associated with trauma, vertebral anomalies,

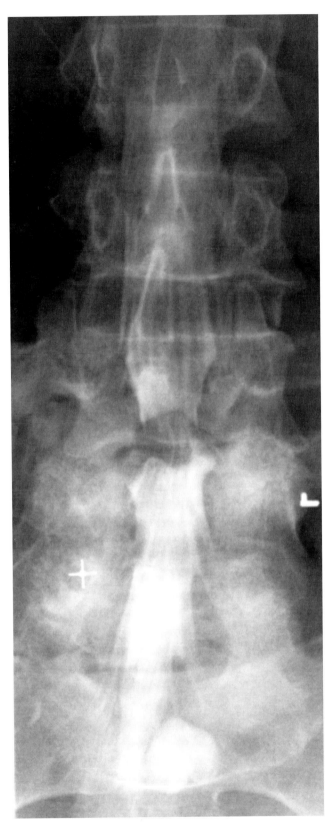

FIGURE 36-2 This lumbar myelogram with Iopamidol enhancement shows a perineurial cyst on the left side at S2. In addition, this image demonstrates a blockage at L3–L4 caused by spinal stenosis, the origin of the patient's symptoms. The cyst is asymptomatic.

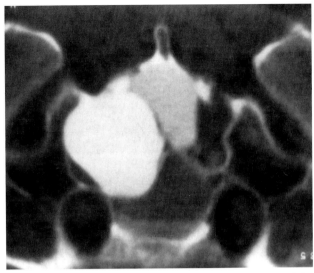

FIGURE 36-3 An axial CT scan with contrast enhancement of the subarachnoid space demonstrates a large perineural cyst on the left; the cyst is eroding the sacrum and is poorly communicating with the subarachnoid space. The contrast material in the cyst is denser than is the contrast material in the subarachnoid space.

neural tube defects, and syringomyelia.[10–13] Infection and arachnoiditis have also been implicated but without convincing proof. These cysts are commonly thoracic, but they can arise in other areas of the spinal canal (see Table 36-1). Intradural arachnoid cysts are depicted as leptomeningeal cysts in Figure 36-1.

If intradural arachnoid cysts do not freely communicate with the subarachnoid space, they may be symptomatic, presenting with myelopathy, nerve root compression, cauda equina syndrome, or a myelopathy.[14–16] MRI or CT myelography will demonstrate a CSF-containing mass that does not communicate with the subarachnoid space (Figs. 36-4, 36-5, and 36-6).

Surgical decompression of such a cyst may result in significant neurologic improvement. If the cyst lies dorsally or in the cauda equina, it can be excised via a laminectomy. If it lies ventrally, it may be fenestrated through a posterolateral laminectomy, with section of the dentate ligaments in the cervical and thoracic area to aid in exposure.

Intraspinal Meningeal Cysts

Nabors and colleagues in 1988 suggested a simplified categorization of intraspinal meningeal cysts.[17,18] They categorized extradural meningeal cysts without spinal nerve root fibers in their walls as type I, extradural spinal cysts with nerve root fibers as type II, and intradural meningeal cysts as type III. They also described successful surgical treatment of each type.

The surgical treatment of intradural arachnoid cysts (type III) requires little comment. Removal of the cyst membranes can ordinarily be done with little difficulty. If the cyst is not in free communication with the subarachnoid space and is causing symptoms, there is often significant improvement after surgery. The surgical treatment of extradural arachnoid cysts not related to nerve roots (type I) is also quite straightforward. Excision of the cyst and closure of any

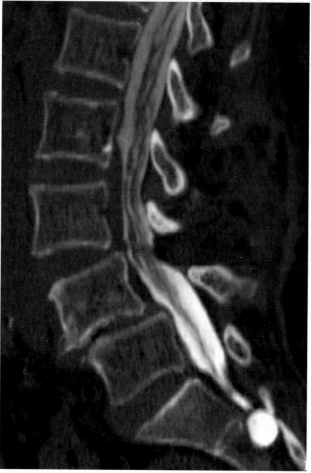

FIGURE 36-4 This sagittal reformat of a CT/myelogram demonstrates stenosis at L3–L4, degenerative changes with spondylolisthesis at L4–L5, and a sacral perineurial cyst (also asymptomatic) in the sacral canal at S2.

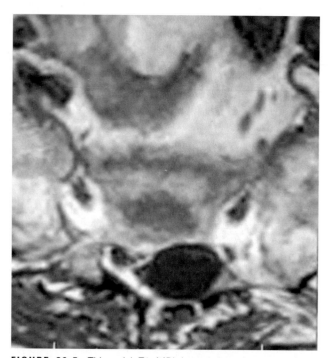

FIGURE 36-5 This axial T1 MRI image demonstrates a large perineal cyst at S2 that is eroding the sacral canal.

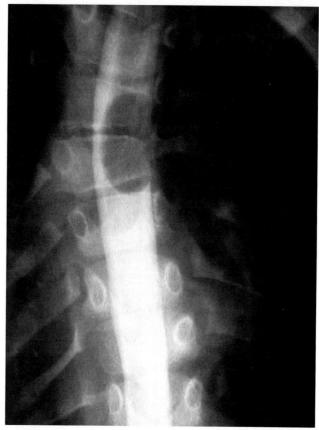

FIGURE 36-6 This metrizamide-enhanced myelogram demonstrates an arachnoid cyst compressing the thoracic spinal cord.

communication with the subarachnoid space by suture (with or without the use of muscle, fat, or fibrin glue reinforcement) also often helps if the lesion is truly symptomatic.

Gentle reduction of any nerve root or spinal cord hernia is carried out as part of such an operation.

The cyst walls of perineurial cysts, as described by Tarlov (the type II cysts of Nabors), contain nerve root elements and require careful handling. Preservation of nerve root function is of paramount importance, but patients must be made aware that manipulation of nerve roots, no matter how gentle, may cause new neurologic symptoms or deficit, although the overlapping cutaneous distribution of adjacent sensory nerve roots usually minimizes the deficit.

The operation is carried out via sacral laminectomy. The lamina overlying the cyst is usually markedly thinned. With magnified vision, the neural elements in the wall of the cyst are obvious and should (and usually can) be preserved. If the cyst communicates at all with the subarachnoid space, it is necessary to obliterate the connection. Surgery to excise a perineurial cyst in toto is likely to result in perineal sensory loss. If the cyst wall is sufficiently strong, it can be imbricated and sutured to reconstruct the dural root sleeve. In recent years, the authors have performed duraplasty, suturing the nerve root sheath after excising the nonneural part of its wall (Fig. 36-7). Marsupialization of cysts can be carried out when there are multiple cysts (Fig. 36-8). A graft of fat can be used to obliterate any dead space. The authors have used this technique on several occasions on noncommunicating cysts with success; however, they have

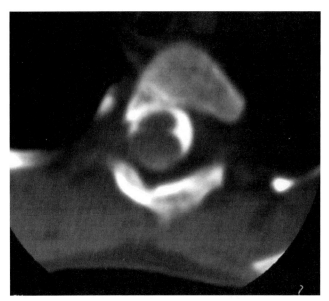

FIGURE 36-7 This CT myelogram shows an arachnoid cyst compressing the spinal cord. Removal of such a laterally placed cyst is surgically feasible, whereas as a more ventrally placed cyst should be fenestrated.

not attempted to reconstruct multiple nerve roots out of concern for causing a neurologic deficit (e.g., bladder impairment). Even in cases in which the cyst appears situated so as to cause pressure on adjacent nerve roots and to be symptomatic, removal of the cyst may not relieve symptoms. For this reason, it is necessary to exercise great caution in selecting patients for operation.

Pressure Dynamics

Whether a cystic space is in free communication with the rest of the subarachnoid space seems to be the most reliable determinant of whether the cyst is exerting pressure on the adjacent neural elements. Thus failure of subarachnoid contrast material to enter a cyst freely is probably the best indicator of whether the cyst is exerting local pressure effects. This logic breaks down, however, in attempting to explain the erosion of the sacrum that occurs in cases of communicating perineurial cysts. The physics of pressure phenomena are not well understood, and the pulsatile component of CSF pressure may be a factor in explaining sacral erosion and bony remodeling in such cases. Sophisticated MRI techniques, such as those previously alluded to, may in the future help clarify this aspect of CSF pressure dynamics.

Extradural Arachnoid Cysts

Elsberg and colleagues described extradural arachnoid cysts as composed of spontaneous herniations of arachnoid through dural defects.[19] (They are depicted in Fig. 36-1 as extradural meningeal cysts.) Occasionally, these cysts accompany vertebral epiphysitis or kyphosis dorsalis juvenilis (Scheuermann's disease). They are very rare and usually present in the thoracic spine.[20] A ball-valve mechanism of formation was described in a patient in whom the cyst formed in relation to a spontaneous dural CSF fistula. These cysts may be symptomatic.

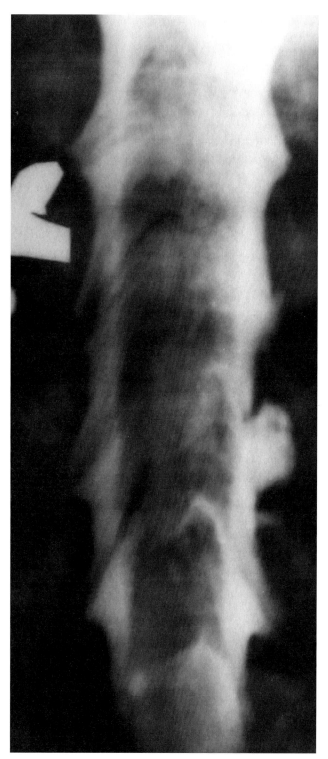

FIGURE 36-8 This cervical myelogram demonstrates cervical nerve root avulsion with pseudomeningocele at the site of an avulsed nerve root.

Intrasacral Meningoceles

Intrasacral meningoceles lie in the midline, are lined with arachnoid, and their walls do not contain neural elements (see Fig. 36-1); they are usually asymptomatic. These lesions may erode the sacrum. These lesions contain CSF, and ordinarily communicate with the subarachnoid space.

Surgery involves closure of the fistula and marsupialization of the lesion; however, because surgery usually does not relieve symptoms, the authors do not surgically treat them.

Arachnoiditis

Loculations of CSF in the subarachnoid space can occur as a consequence of arachnoiditis. Arachnoiditis may be caused by a reaction to Pantopaque; by a mixture of blood and Pantopaque; or by blood at surgery, which can lead to thickening of the arachnoid and scarring in the subarachnoid space. In most cases, this is of no clinical significance because the loculated spaces are in full communication with the rest of the subarachnoid space. In the usual scenario, a painful condition or neurologic disorder leads to investigation by myelography, and subsequently the preexisting symptoms are inappropriately attributed to the myelography.

Extradural Pseudomeningoceles

Pseudomeningoceles are CSF collections outside the dura and are not lined by arachnoid. They commonly result from trauma at surgery. Compared with a true meningocele, in which the arachnoid is intact, in the pseudomeningocele an arachnoid injury results in the leakage of CSF and the subsequent development of a smooth membrane lining the CSF-filled space. This is noted in Figure 36-1 as an extradural meningeal false cyst. Unless neural structures, nerve roots, or the spinal cord herniates and becomes distorted or entrapped, extradural meningoceles and pseudomeningoceles are usually asymptomatic. Local pain related to the swelling can often be treated conservatively, because spontaneous healing of dura and arachnoid can occur. Spinal drainage has occasionally been helpful.

An extradural pseudomeningocele should be considered if continued radicular pain after lumbar surgery is accompanied by evidence of an extradural CSF collection. In such cases, relief can follow surgical reduction of herniated neural elements and dural repair. When dura defects are ventral, conservative management is more often advisable.

Traumatic Pseudocysts in Nerve Root Avulsion

Traction injuries with sufficient force to avulse nerve roots from the spinal cord can also result in tearing of the dural root sleeve and arachnoid; this, in turn, results in extradural arachnoid pseudocysts (see Fig. 36-8). These pseudocysts are seen in brachial plexus injuries, as well as in lumbar root avulsions, and they usually do not require repair. Symptomatic CSF leakage is very rare.

Neurenteric Cysts

Figures 36-9 and 36-10 illustrate neurenteric cysts that presented with myelopathy. These are rare lesions.[21]

CONCLUSIONS

Anomalies of the spinal subarachnoid space and the meningeal membranes are common (Fig. 36-11): many are congenital.[22] In most instances, these anomalies are

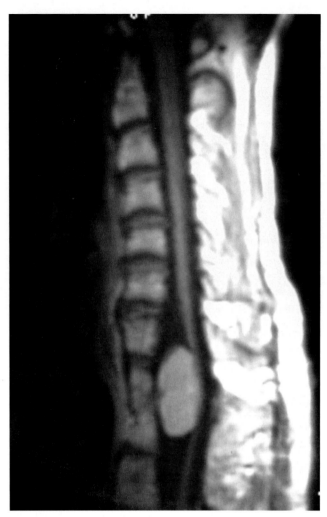

FIGURE 36-9 This sagittal T1 MRI image demonstrates embryologic failure of segmentation of the T1 and T2 vertebrae. A large, ventrally placed neurenteric cyst is posteriorly displacing the spinal cord, which is somewhat atrophic.

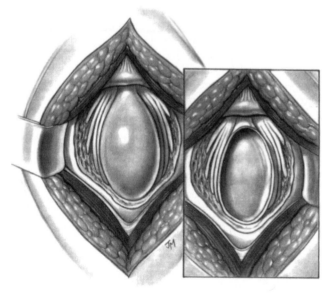

FIGURE 36-10 This diagram shows a sacral laminectomy exposure of a large intrasacral cyst (*left*). The cyst has been marsupialized (*right*) because there was no communication with the subarachnoid space. The sacral roots are displaced laterally.

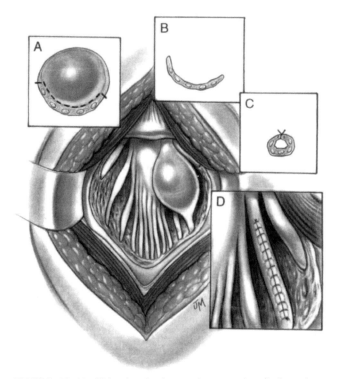

FIGURE 36-11 This sketch shows the operative findings in a typical perineurial cyst. Illustrations *A* to *D* depict the incision of the nonneural portion of the wall and the surgical repair.

innocuous and do not require surgical treatment. When symptomatic, either through herniation of neural elements or because of local pressure effects, the appropriate surgery may be helpful. The major challenge for the clinician is to recognize the small proportion of such cysts that are truly symptomatic. Even when a cyst appears to correlate with a patient's symptoms, relief of pain may not occur after surgery.

REFERENCES

1. Tarlov E, Geyer C: Intraspinal cerebrospinal fluid cysts. In Kaufman H (ed): Cerespinal Fluid Collections. Park Ridge, IL: American Association of Neurological Surgeons, 1998, pp 167–175.
2. Tarlov IM: Perineurial cysts of the spinal nerve roots. Arch Neurol Psychiatry 40:1067–1074, 1938.
3. Tarlov IM: Sacral Nerve Root Cysts: Another Cause of the Sciatic or Cauda Equina Syndrome. Springfield, IL: Charles C Thomas, 1953.
4. Tarlov IM: Spinal perineurial and meningeal cysts. J Neurol Neurosurg Psychiatry 33:833–843, 1970.
5. Davis SW, Levy LM, LeBriham DJ, et al: Sacral meningocele cysts: Evaluation with MR imaging. Radiology 187:445–448, 1993.
6. Paulsen RD, Call GD, Murtagh FR: Prevalence and percutaneous drainage of cysts of the sacral nerve root sheaths (Tarlov cysts). AJNR Am J Neuroradiol 15:293–297, 1994.
7. Casper W, Papavero L, Nabhan A, et al: Microsurgical excision of symptomatic sacral perineurial cysts: A study of 15 cases. Surg Neurol 59(2):101–106, 2003.
8. Andrews BT, Weinstein PR, Rosenblum ML, et al: Intradural arachnoid cysts of the spinal canal associated with intramedullary cysts. Neurosurg 68:544–549, 1988.
9. Voyadzis JM, Bhargava P, Henderson FC: Tarlov cysts: A study of 10 cases with review of the literature. J Neurosurg Spine 97(2):271, author reply 271–272, 2002.
10. Chen HJ, Chen L: Traumatic intradural arachnoid cyst in the upper cervical spine: Case report. J Neurosurg 85:351–353, 1996.
11. Osenbach RK, Godersky JC, Traynelis VC, et al: Intradural extramedullary cysts of the spinal canal: Clinical presentation, radiographic diagnosis and surgical management. Neurosurgery 30:35–42, 1992.
12. Quinones-Hinojosa A, Sanai N, Fischbein NJ, Rosenberg WS: Extensive intradural arachnoid cyst of the lumbar spinal canal: Case report. Sur Neurol 60(1):57–59, 2003.
13. Wang MY, Levi AD, Green BA: Intradural spinal arachnoid cysts in adults. Surg Neurol 60(1):49–56, 2003.
14. Rohrer DC, Burchiel KJ, Gruber DJ: Intraspinal extradural meningeal cyst demonstrating ballvalve mechanism of formation: Case report. J Neurosurg 78:122–125, 1993.
15. Rabb CH, McComb JG, Raffel C, et al: Spinal arachnoid cysts in the pediatric age group: An association with neural tube defects. J Neurosurg 77:369–372, 1992.
16. Siontos P, Arbor E, Tsaris P, et al: Spontaneous thoracic spinal cord herniation. Spine 21:1710–1713, 1996.
17. Nabors MW, Pait TG, Byrd EB, et al: Updated assessment and current classification of spinal meningeal cysts. J Neurosurg 68:366–377, 1988.
18. Abou-Fakhr FS, Kanaan SV, Youness FM, et al: Thoracicspinal intradural arachnoid cyst: Report of two cases and review of literature. Eur Radiol 12(4):877–882, 2002.
19. Elsberg CA, Dyke CG, Brewer ED: Symptoms and diagnosis of extradural cysts. Bull Neurol Inst New York 3:395–417, 1934.
20. Martin G: Spinal cord herniation into an extradural arachnoid cyst. J Clin Neurosci 7(4):330–331, 2002.
21. Martin AJ, Penney CC: Spinal neurenteric cyst. Arch Neurol 58(1):126–127, 2001.
22. Schlesinger EB: The significance of genetic contributions and markers in disorders of spinal structure. Neurosurgery 26:944–951, 1990.

Section VII

Management of Hydrocephalus

37

Cerebrospinal Fluid Shunting and Management of Pediatric Hydrocephalus

JAMES M. DRAKE and MARK R. IANTOSCA

CLINICAL PRESENTATION OF HYDROCEPHALUS

Hydrocephalus is one of the most common complications of virtually any insult to the neonatal, infant, or child's nervous system. It occurs in approximately 1 in 2000 births and is associated with approximately one third of all congenital malformations of the nervous system.[1] It is also a common complication of intraventricular hemorrhage, brain tumors, infections, and head injury.[2] The causes of hydrocephalus in 344 children undergoing a first shunt insertion in the randomized shunt design trial[3] are listed in Table 37-1. The median corrected age of the patients was 55 days, indicating that this is a problem seen most commonly in infancy. An estimated 33,000 shunts are placed in patients of all ages annually in the United States, with an estimated shunt prevalence of more than 56,000 in children younger than 18 years old.[1]

The diagnosis of hydrocephalus is based on clinical and radiologic features. As seen in Table 37-1, children most commonly present with symptoms of irritability, delayed development, vomiting, and headache, and on examination have increasing head circumference and a bulging fontanelle. Magnetic resonance imaging (MRI) has the best diagnostic utility in terms of establishing the cause and defining the site of obstruction but may be combined with computed tomography (CT), particularly if looking for evidence of intracranial calcification. Ultrasound is quite practical in critically ill premature infants with intraventricular hemorrhage or in patients with myelomeningocele in whom the cause is not in doubt. In patients with mild ventricular enlargement, evidence of transependymal flow of cerebrospinal fluid (CSF) usually suggests that the process is more acute. Other signs of progressive hydrocephalus—enlargement of the temporal horns, dilation of the third ventricle, and effacement of the sulci—are not absolutely specific. In cases in which there is doubt, careful observation with serial images, rather than subjecting the patient to the known risks of shunt failure, is prudent.

TREATMENT WITH CEREBROSPINAL FLUID SHUNTS

History of Shunts

The history of hydrocephalus is a fascinating one and dates back to the dawn of civilization. Early attempts at management failed because of ignorance about the pathogenesis, primitive surgical techniques, and lack of appropriate equipment and biocompatible materials. Early 20th-century attempts at achieving closed ventricular drainage included gold, glass, silver, and rubber tubes, as well as catgut and linen threads passed from the ventricle to the subdural space.[4–7] Similar techniques were used to connect the lumbar thecal sac to the peritoneum or renal pelvis.[8–10] After attempts at third ventriculostomy[11,12] and choroid plexectomy,[13] shunts from the lateral ventricle to cisterna magna, Torkildsen shunts,[14] and shunts from the lumbar spine to the ureter came into more widespread use.

The treatment of hydrocephalus was revolutionized when Nulsen and Spitz[15] reported in 1952 the successful use of a ventriculojugular shunt using a spring and stainless-steel ball valve. The two valves were housed in rubber intravenous tubing, which acted as a flushing device, and connected to polyethylene tubing at either end. Occlusion of the venous catheter by blood clot was a frequent problem.

Holter's shunt was the first to use silicone, and he designed a multiple-slit valve out of silicone for use in his son who developed hydrocephalus.[16] Almost at the same time, Pudenz[17] also concluded that silicone was the best material and designed two valves to use as ventriculoauricular shunts.

Mechanical Principles and Available Shunt Components

Cerebrospinal fluid shunts regulate flow by means of one-way valves. The standard valves that have been in use for decades simply open or close depending on the pressure across them (Fig. 37-1A).[17–21] They can be grouped into four general design categories: silicone rubber slit valves, silicone rubber diaphragm valves, silicone rubber miter valves, and metallic spring ball valves.[20] The pressure at which they open is termed the opening pressure, and typically there are low, medium, and high designations, which generally correspond to 5, 10, and 15 mm H_2O pressure, but there are no universal standards. Once open, the valves have little resistance to flow and let large quantities of CSF through the shunt. When patients stand up, this situation

TABLE 37-1 ▪ Cause and Clinical Presentation of Hydrocephalus in 344 Pediatric Patients

Corrected age (median)	55 days
Hydrocephalus causes	
Intraventricular hemorrhage	24.1%
Myelomeningocele	21.2%
Tumor	9.0%
Aqueduct stenosis	7.0%
CSF infection	5.2%
Head injury	1.5%
Other	11.3%
Unknown	11.0%
Two or more causes	8.7%
Presenting symptoms	
Irritability	26.6%
Delayed developmental milestone	19.8%
Nausea or vomiting	19.0%
Headache	17.5%
Lethargy	17.5%
New seizures or change in seizure pattern	6.6%
Diplopia	5.8%
Worsening school performance	4.2%
Fever	2.6%
Presenting signs	
Increase head circumference	81.3%
Bulging frontanelle	70.6%
Delayed developmental milestones	20.9%
Loss of upward gaze	15.8%
Decreased level of consciousness	12.6%
Other focal neurologic deficit	12.4%
Papilledema	12.0%
Sixth nerve palsy	4.6%
Hemiparesis	3.8%
Nuchal rigidity	1.8%

CSF, cerebrospinal fluid.

can lead to siphoning as CSF drains out of the head under the effect of gravity into the abdomen. Large negative intracranial pressures and low-pressure headache and subdural hematomas can result.[18,19,22]

Other valve designs have tried to limit this siphoning effect and include siphon-reducing devices. These have a mobile membrane that moves to narrow an orifice in response to a negative pressure inside the shunt system (see Fig. 37-1B).[23,24] Examples are the antisiphon device and the Delta valve (Medtronic PS Medical, Goletta, CA). A flow-limiting valve has a flexible diaphragm that moves along a piston of increasing diameter (see Fig. 37-1C). This flexible diaphragm reduces the flow orifice, dramatically increasing the resistance to flow. This increase in resistance results in little increase in flow rate despite progressive rise in pressure—essentially a flow limit. The Orbis Sigma NMT (Boston, MA) is an example of this valve.[25]

Other valves try to reduce the effects of gravity by changing their configuration according to how they are positioned (see Fig. 37-1D). In some designs, metallic balls rest on top of a standard spring ball valve to increase the opening pressure when the valve (and patient) are vertical. In another, a single metallic ball rests in an asymmetric valve seat in upright position, increasing the resistance.

There are also several externally adjustable valves. The simplest involves moving metallic balls along Silastic sleeves, to open or occlude two parallel valve systems (see Fig. 37-1E). This leads to four settings: low, medium, high,

and off. Other designs use a magnetized rotor to adjust the tension on a spring ball valve. The rotor may have 3 to 18 pressure settings and be controlled by an external bar magnet or electromagnet. The magnetized systems are susceptible to external magnetic fields, including those of MRI. Verification of the pressure setting by means of a radiographic study is usually required.

Although several different ventricular and peritoneal catheters exist, there is little to choose among them. There are a number of ways of connecting the ventricular catheter to the distal system, including burr hole reservoirs, right-angle connectors, right-angled guides, and preshaped catheters, and some systems come in a completely unitized fashion. In closed-ended peritoneal catheters, the adjacent slits act as a valve.

Shunt Selection

Currently, no data recommend one particular shunt over another. In fact, a randomized trial on CSF shunt design that compared a standard valve to the Delta valve and the Orbis-Sigma valve failed to show any difference in terms of overall shunt failure.[3] There are important considerations to be taken into account, however, when considering the individual patient, including age, weight, skin thickness, head size, size of the ventricles, pathogenesis of hydrocephalus, acuteness of the illness, presence of internal lines or gastrostomy, tracheotomy openings, status of the distal drainage site, and plans for further surgery.

For example, a premature infant with thin skin stretched further by a rapidly expanded head cannot handle adult-size equipment without the risk of skin erosion. If the same infant has blood in the ventricles, immediate implantation of a valve with a narrow flow-limiting orifice might increase the risk of early obstruction. If one ventricle is significantly larger than the other, placing the ventricular catheter on that side is easier. In patients with large ventricles and large skulls with fused sutures, placing a flow-limiting or siphon-reducing device might decrease the risk of subdural hemorrhage.

If there are loculations within the ventricular system, fenestrating them endoscopically at the time of shunt insertion would at least attempt to keep the number of shunts to one. If a patient is expected to have a number of subsequent and important MRI studies, metallic shunt components or magnetic programmable valves might interfere with the interpretation of these images. Finally, if a patient is scheduled to have further intra-abdominal surgery—for example, to close a colostomy or to reconstruct the bladder—this might influence the choice of site of distal drainage.

For most routine cases, it is probably better to use a shunt system with which one is quite familiar. In this setting, we prefer a two-piece system, with a nonflanged ventricular catheter, connected to a flat-bottomed valve with a reservoir, with open-ended distal tubing.

Surgical Technique—Initial Shunt Insertion

Although shunt surgery is often regarded with some disdain by staff and trainee neurosurgeons alike—as "plumbing"—it

Standard Differential Pressure Valve

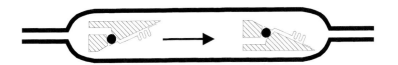

Mechanism

Spring-ball valve

Pressure Flow Characteristics

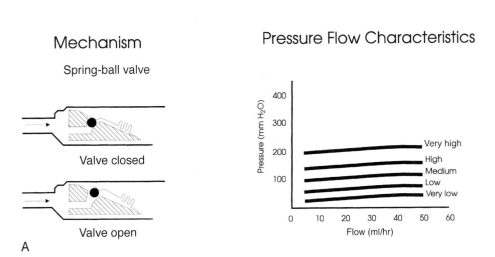

A

PS Medical Delta Valve

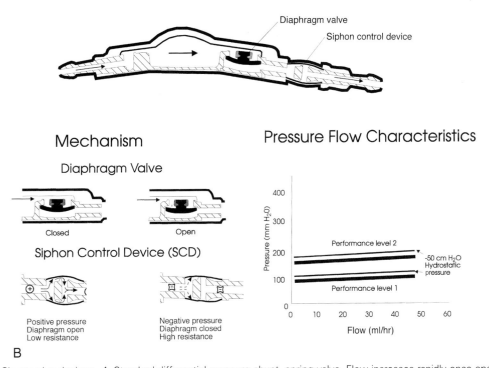

Mechanism

Pressure Flow Characteristics

B

FIGURE 37-1 Shunt valve designs. *A,* Standard differential pressure shunt, spring valve. Flow increases rapidly once opening pressure is exceeded. *B,* Siphon-reducing device distal to a standard differential pressure valve, diaphragm type. The effects of gravity are reduced in the upright position.

(Continued)

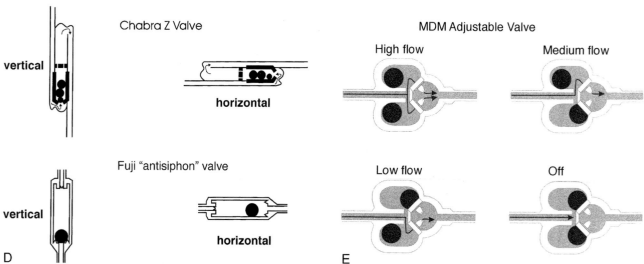

Cordis Orbis Sigma

Diaphragm valve portion

Flow control orifice

Mechanism

Variable Resistance Valve

Diaphragm valve closed

Low pressure
Low resistance

Medium pressure
High resistance
(flow limiting)

High pressure
Low resistance
(safety pressure release)

C

Pressure Flow Characteristics

Low resistance
(Safety valve)

High resistance

Low resistance

Pressure (mm H$_2$0)

Flow (ml/hr)

Chabra Z Valve

vertical

horizontal

Fuji "antisiphon" valve

vertical

horizontal

D

MDM Adjustable Valve

High flow

Medium flow

Low flow

Off

E

FIGURE 37-1 Cont'd   *C,* A flow-limiting valve with a variable-resistance orifice leading to flow limit as seen in flow pressure curve. *D,* Two gravity-actuated devices that increase the opening pressure (*above*), or the resistance (*below*) in the vertical position. *E,* A percutaneous adjustable valve that can be completely occluded. (*A–C,* From Drake JM, Kestle J: Determining the best cerebrospinal fluid shunt valve design: The pediatric valve design trial. Neurosurgery 38:604–607, 1996. *D* and *E,* From Drake JM, Sainte-Rose C: The Shunt Book. New York: Blackwell Scientific, 1995, p 1.)

has the highest failure rate of any neurosurgical procedure, and nothing is less forgiving of any technical errors than a shunt operation. Shunts often fail from tissue occluding the upper or lower end. Parenchymal ventricular catheters, extraperitoneal distal catheters, and spontaneously disconnected or migrated shunts have happened in virtually every neurosurgery service. These complications are avoidable.

We believe that shunt surgery should command great respect, require meticulous attention to detail, and be carried out in a skilled and expeditious fashion.

Body wash and shampoo the night before and again before surgery with an antiseptic solution (e.g., chlorhexidine) is recommended. In the operating room, the patient is positioned under general endotracheal anesthesia, with the head rotated to the side opposite the shunt and the neck extended so that there is almost a straight line between the scalp and abdominal incisions. A number of meta-analyses have shown that prophylactic antibiotics are effective,[26] and they are strongly recommended. Cloxicillin, 50 mg/kg administered 30 minutes before surgery, is often used. For patients in whom an abdominal trochar is being used, the bladder should be emptied either by a Credé maneuver or by urinary catheter. Hair is clipped (not shaved) in the operating room if desired to assist with skin closure and bandage application. Hair removal has never been shown to decrease the risk of infection, however.[27]

The patient should be positioned so that there is a flat plane between the upper and lower incision sites, so that the shunt can be passed easily. For an occipital burr hole, this means rotating the head to the opposite side and extending the neck, usually with a rolled towel (Fig. 37-2A). The site of the burr hole and abdominal incisions should be selected and marked before draping, before the surface landmarks are obscured. Occipital burr holes are usually on the flat part of the occiput 3 to 4 cm from the midline along the course of the lambdoid suture. In patients with Dandy-Walker malformation or huge arachnoid cysts of the posterior fossa, the transverse sinus can be placed much higher than in normal subjects. In these patients, the position of the transverse sinus should be identified preoperatively by MRI, and the placement of the burr hole should be modified according to the results of this examination. Frontal burr holes are along the coronal suture 2 to 3 cm from the midline. The issue of frontal versus occipital burr hole has never been resolved.[28]

The skin is meticulously prepared with a slow-release iodine solution. Disposable, adhesive drapes are used to cover the patient and the operating table entirely except for a small band of skin from the burr hole site to the abdomen (see Fig. 37-2B). The drapes may need to be stapled to the hair-bearing areas of the scalp. Small skin incisions are adequate (see Fig. 37-2C). It is better to position the incision so that the hardware is not afterward directly underneath. The burr hole need not be a standard size, and a twist drill is adequate unless using a burr hole reservoir or intraoperative ultrasound. In infants, particularly if premature, an opening between the splayed sutures at either frontal or occipital sites is all that is required. The dura does not need to be opened widely, and in patients with thinned cortical mantles, a wide dural opening may allow CSF to escape around the ventricular catheter into the subcutaneous tissues, promoting a CSF leak. The brain pia is cauterized and nicked.

The abdominal incision is simultaneously opened by an assistant. The method and site are unimportant. Paraumbilical and upper midline sites are common. One needs to be sure that the peritoneum has truly been opened and not just the preperitoneal space. Passing a blunt dissector easily well into the abdominal cavity verifies this (see Fig. 37-2D). A purse-string suture around the peritoneum tends to prevent omentum from herniating but is not absolutely necessary. We prefer to use abdominal trochars in virgin abdomens from a paraumbilical location. Opening the rectus sheath through a tiny incision and visualizing the posterior wall of the sheath facilitates placement. The posterior sheath is then picked up by the tip of the trochar; then the tip is angled inferiorly and off the midline to avoid hitting the great vessels (see Fig. 37-2E). A gentle pop is felt

as the peritoneum is penetrated. A blunt instrument can also be passed along the trochar sheath to verify peritoneal entry.

Care must be taken when tunneling. If the metal tube is too deep, either the chest or the posterior fossa can be entered. One has to be particularly careful in patients who have had an occipital craniectomy, because it is possible to pass the device into the bone opening by mistake. If the tunneling device is too superficial, a skin laceration, which may be initially unrecognized, can occur. A gentle curve to the tunneling instrument allows one to direct the tip posteriorly when coming over the anterior chest into the neck, then by rotating 180 degrees, the tip anteriorly toward the occiput (see Fig. 37-2F). Significant resistance is usually felt at the posterior nuchal line. Firm pressure, making sure that the pointed central stylet has not backed out, and guarding against plunging usually allow this fascia to be penetrated. If one is using excessive force, a separate incision should be made in the neck.

If passing to a frontal burr hole, an intervening incision is needed over the occiput. There appears to be no logical reason to tunnel down the back of the patient. Not only is it awkward, but also with time a fibrous cord similar to a bow string forms, which is unsightly and can even affect neck mobility. The cord also remains if the shunt hardware is removed. The tunneling device is rigid enough when in place to compress the chest of small children so that the anesthetist typically notes an increase in airway pressure. It should not be left in place too long. The device can also tear the scalp, particularly in small infants, in whom one is trying to bring the straight tunneling tube around the curved skull.

The peritoneal tubing, with or without the attached valve, is then passed along the tube, attaching suction to the distal end and irrigating. The valve should then be attached and irrigated to fill it with fluid, usually the antibiotic solution soaking the shunt equipment. It is not necessary to test the opening pressure of the shunt in the operating room. Merely handling the valve changes its performance characteristics for days, and air bubbles can also affect these measurements. It is important to connect the valve in the right direction.

The ventricular catheter trajectory is then determined according to external landmarks (see Fig. 37-2G). From a frontal burr hole, traditional landmarks for the foramen of Monro or the intersection of the planes through the pupil and the external auditory meatus (or simply being perpendicular to the skull) are used. From the occipital location, a target at the midpoint of the forehead just at the normal hairline ensures that the catheter proceeds into the frontal horn instead of the temporal horn. There is no proven ideal location for the ventricular catheter. Evidence from the pediatric shunt design trial suggests that frontal or occipital locations are better than in the body of the ventricle or in the third ventricle.[29] Hitting small ventricles is easier from a frontal location. In these patients, ultrasound or even stereotaxis may assist with successful ventricular cannulation. We routinely use ultrasound either through the shunt burr hole or, in infants, through the open fontanelle (see Fig. 37-2H). An endoscopic stylet can also be used to place the shunt (see Fig. 37-2I). Whether assisted placement results in improved outcome is the subject of an ongoing

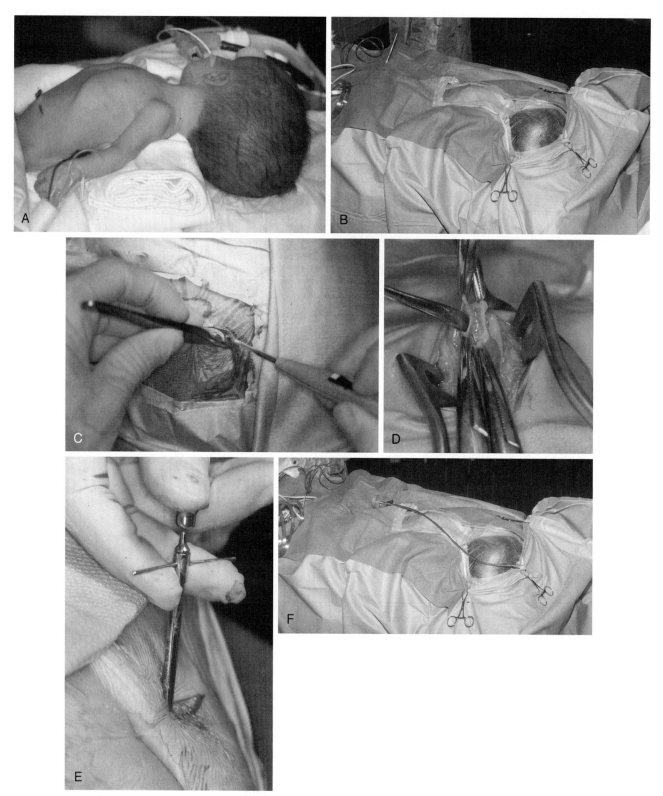

FIGURE 37-2   Sequential steps on shunt insertion. *A*, Patient positioning and marking of incisions. *B*, Draping. *C*, Making a small incision that will not cross over shunt equipment. *D*, Passing a blunt dissector into the peritoneal cavity. *E*, Using an abdominal trochar. *F*, A tunneling device.

clinical trial. With these techniques, the surgeon is as certain as possible that the catheter is in good position at the end of the case and not in one of the unusual sites, such as the sylvian fissure or quadrigeminal cistern.

The ventricular catheter can usually be felt to pop once the ependyma is breached with a concomitant gush of CSF.

Gently irrigating the catheter may show pulsatile CSF flow into and out of the catheter. Withdrawing vigorously simply draws brain tissue into the catheter and plugs the shunt if one is in the parenchyma. Although there is no official limit on the number of passes, after two, we use ultrasound. A little fresh blood that clears is not unusual and is one reason to

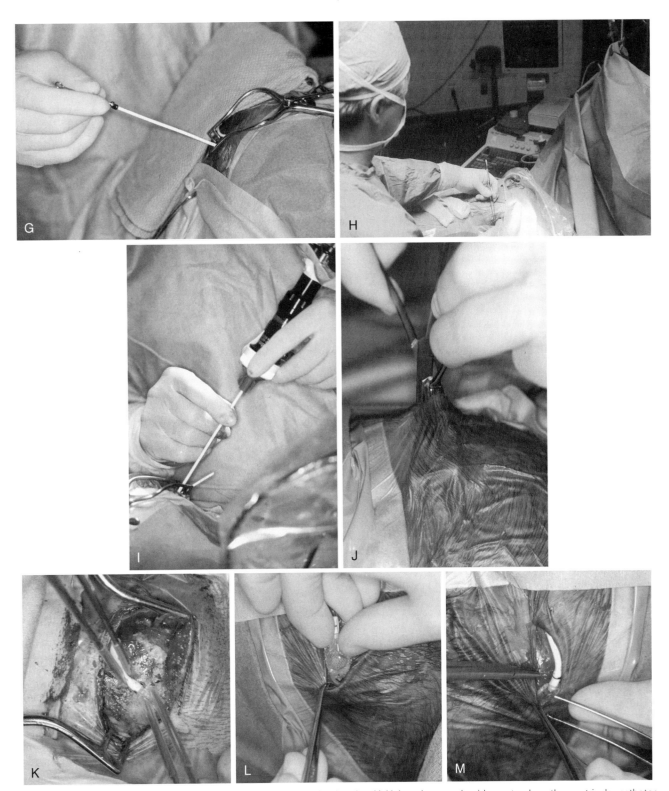

FIGURE 37-2 Cont'd   *G*, Cannulating the ventricle according to landmarks. *H*, Using ultrasound guidance to place the ventricular catheter. *I*, Using a shunt scope to place the ventricular catheter. *J*, Making the subcutaneous pocket for the valve. *K*, Silastic-sleeved forceps coaxing the tubing onto the connector. *L*, Placing the valve into its pocket. *M*, Suturing the valve to the pericranium.

recommend a separate ventricular catheter, so that blood and debris can be cleared before attaching to the valve. Extensive hemorrhage should prompt extensive irrigation until it clears. Installing a narrow-orifice, high-resistance valve is this setting is likely to result in rapid occlusion.

There are a number of ways of getting the ventricular catheter around the burr hole corner; all are somewhat awkward. Simply bending the catheter, using the forces of the brain, burr hole, and dura, is fine, but the inherent stiffness of the catheter tends to move the tip in the opposite direction. In patients with large ventricles and thin cortical mantles, the catheter can take an almost vertical trajectory. Right-angled guides avoid this. When attaching burr hole reservoirs (usually with contained valves), the ventricular catheter must be withdrawn, then readvanced. The attachment site is usually below the cortical surface, where it becomes adherent, and losing the catheter at a subsequent revision is possible.

When using a flat-bottomed valve, a pocket must be created along the distal path. This pocket must be exactly along the course of the catheter or the valve binds when attempting to slide it along (see Fig. 37-2J). This binding can be an enormous nuisance, particularly if the ventricular catheter is already connected. When attaching the ventricular catheter to the valve, one should avoid using metal instruments directly on the tubing forcefully because they can lacerate it, and the tubing can subsequently leak or break. We put Silastic sleeves over forceps and snaps (see Fig. 37-2K) or use a clean gauze sponge. Similarly, when tying the catheter over the connector, having the tie directly over the neck of the connector, tight enough not to allow spontaneous disconnection or, alternatively, not too tight to lacerate the tubing, is vital. The valve system is then placed into its pocket by gently tugging on the peritoneal catheter from below (see Fig. 37-2L). The shunt system should then be secured to the pericranium (see Fig. 37-2M). It is incredible how unsecured systems can migrate. Postfossa catheters are particularly difficult to secure and have a high tendency to move. A three-way connector in this site also seems to come under excessive stress with neck motion and be prone to fracture.

Once in place, the system should be checked that it is flowing, either spontaneously or with gentle pumping of the reservoir. If there is any doubt, the system should be disconnected to verify that both ends are patent. This verification avoids having to return the patient directly from the recovery room back to the operating room. The distal catheter is then inserted, making sure that it enters easily. If the catheter keeps backing out of the abdomen, it may be coiling up in the preperitoneal space. The surgeon needs to ensure that the catheter is truly intraperitoneal. The purse-string suture is then tied snugly, and the abdominal layers are reapproximated.

Skin closure is critical. Any CSF leak predisposes to wound breakdown or infection. Normally the skin is closed in two layers, with careful apposition of the skin edges. The fragile skin of premature infants may fray and leak CSF through large needle holes. An occlusive dressing, which also resists attempts by small children to remove it, is also recommended for 48 hours. Positioning in the postoperative period is important. In patients with large ventricles, early mobilization may risk a subdural hemorrhage. In patients with high-resistance valves, placing them in an upright posture may promote CSF drainage and prevent accumulation under the skin.

The postoperative hospital stay is typically 2 to 3 days. Prophylactic antibiotics are normally given intravenously preoperatively and sometimes postoperatively for a few doses only. Prolonged antibiotic treatment in the postoperative period in an uncomplicated shunt patient is unwarranted. Shunted patients typically have immediate resolution of acute symptoms. In infants, a sunken fontanelle with standard valves is typical. Low-pressure headache can occur in older patients, particularly if the hydrocephalus is long-standing. An initial postoperative CT or MRI study, unless there was some particular problem intraoperatively, is unlikely to be helpful. Normally, patients are seen in follow-up at approximately 3 months postoperatively with a CT or MRI scan at this time and at 1 year with repeat imaging because the ventricles do not reach their final size on average until 1 year of age.[29]

Ventriculopleural Shunts

Pleural shunts are a second choice to peritoneal shunts. Contraindications include previous chest surgery and adhesions, active pulmonary disease including infection, or borderline pulmonary function in patients in whom a significant pleural effusion might push them into respiratory failure. Infants are more likely to develop a significant effusion temporarily. The pleural space can be entered at a variety of sites. Along the anterior axillary line, in the fourth to sixth interspace, is often convenient. A muscle-splitting approach along the upper border of the rib (to avoid the neurovascular bundle) reveals the translucent pleura and the lung moving with ventilation.

The pleura is opened sharply, as with the peritoneum. There is no need to ask the anesthetist to collapse the lung because it moves away slightly as atmospheric pressure enters the chest cavity. The distal catheter is then introduced gently, being careful to guide it along the chest wall, not into the lung parenchyma. The catheter may need to be cut to length to avoid putting excess tubing, even allowing for growth, into the chest. There is no need to place a purse-string suture, and a Valsalva maneuver by the anesthetist inflates the lung adequately. Rapidly closing the muscles with a few sutures avoids further air entry into the chest.

A small pneumothorax is seen on the mandatory postoperative film. It resolves over the next few days, whereas the CSF usually accumulates as a small pleural effusion, especially in infants. These patients must be monitored for any evidence of respiratory distress and with serial chest films.[30,31] Usually the intrapleural fluid disappears over the next several weeks. In patients in whom the pleural fluid progressively accumulates, leading to respiratory distress with significant shift of the mediastinum, percutaneous drainage of the fluid and moving the distal tubing to another site are required.

Ventriculocardiac Shunts

Cardiac shunts are the third choice among the distal sites because of the serious complications of cor pulmonale and shunt nephritis.[32,33] Catheter embolization is also a possibility. With growth, the shunts tend to block as they pull out of the right atrium, so that a small child might need several revisions for growth-related failure. The shunt tip should lie in the superior vena cava just above the triscuspid valve. There are a number of ways of achieving this position. Entrance to the jugular vein is usually achieved via the common facial vein, which is tied proximally and held with a stay suture distal to the venotomy site. The catheter is then advanced down the jugular vein into the superior vena cava, which is much easier to do on the right side. Percutaneous methods into the jugular and subclavian vein have also been described.[34] Positioning the tip can be done under fluoroscopy or even ultrasound.[35,36] Fluoroscopy is useful because occasionally the catheter can be seen traveling out the subclavian vein.

Alternatively, one can use the tip of the catheter as an electrocardiogram lead and look for a change in P-wave polarity.

MANAGEMENT OF SHUNT FAILURE

In most centers, the frequency ratio of shunt revision to initial shunt insertion surgery is 2:1. Having a sound grasp of the nuances of managing patients with failing CSF shunts is extremely important, and shunt revision surgery can be at times quite challenging.

Clinical Presentation and Diagnosis

Mechanical Failure

Shunt mechanical complications may occur at any time, from in the recovery room immediately after the shunt operation to years later; at this time the patient and the family may have all but forgotten about the shunt or falsely believed that the shunt is no longer necessary. The most common time for a shunt to fail is in the first 6 months after insertion (Fig. 37-3).[37] In the shunt design trial, the overall 1-year failure rate was 39%, including an 8% infection rate.[3]

Common to most mechanical complications is the obstruction of CSF shunt flow and the accompanying rise in intracranial pressure. This rise leads most commonly to headache, nausea and vomiting, and lethargy. The clinical signs and symptoms of 150 patients presenting with shunt failure are listed in Table 37-2. The onset of symptoms may be quite variable, ranging from sudden and severe to slow and insidious. A rapid and severe rise in intracranial pressure leads ultimately to unconsciousness. Less obvious signs of shunt mechanical malfunction include irritability, deterioration in school performance, or delay in achievement of developmental milestones. Occasionally, new or increased seizure frequency may be a symptom of mechanical shunt dysfunction.

Patients may also complain of double vision, or families may notice loss of conjugate gaze with sixth nerve palsies. Loss of vision from chronic papilledema may be insidious, particularly in small children. The only sign may be the child moving closer and closer to the television and subsequently "bumping into things."

Signs of mechanical dysfunction relate to the clinical manifestations of raised intracranial pressure as well as abnormalities of the performance of the shunt hardware. Examination of the mental status of the patient may show variation from subtle intellectual deterioration to coma. On physical examination infants often present with a bulging fontanelle, split sutures, and abnormally increased head circumference. Despite the absence of infection, nuchal rigidity may be present from herniation of the tonsils through the foramen magnum. Papilledema appears in patients with closed sutures. Sixth nerve palsy, which may be bilateral, often accompanies papilledema. Loss of vertical gaze is also common. With impending brain herniation, decerebrate posturing, apnea, bradycardia, and pupillary dilatation ensue.

Examination of the site of the shunt equipment implantation may provide confirmatory evidence of shunt dysfunction. Although pumping of the shunt reservoir is a time-honored

TABLE 37-2 ▪ Shunt Failure Presentation

	Mechanical (No. = 122) (%)	Infection (No. = 28) (%)
Symptoms		
Headache	16.2	11.5
Nausea or vomiting	39.3	30.8
Irritability	35.9	34.6
New seizure or change in seizure pattern	1.7	3.8
Loss of development milestones	8.5	3.8
Worsening school performance	1.7	0.0
Abdominal pain		19.2
Signs		
Papilledema	2.6	3.8
Bulging fontanelle	42.7	23.1
Increased head circumference	38.5	19.2
Decreased level of consciousness	18.8	7.7
Nuchal rigidity	0.0	3.8
Sixth nerve palsy	2.6	3.8
Loss of upward gaze	6.0	0.0
Fluid tracking along shunt	23.1	15.4
CSF leak that necessitates shunt revision	3.4	15.4
Shunt reservoir cannot be depressed	5.1	3.8
Shunt reservoir does not refill	12.0	0.0
Fever	2.6	69.2
Meningismus		8.0
Wound erythema		26.9
Skin erosion		23.1
Purulent wound discharge		7.7
Abdominal mass (pseudocyst)		3.8
Peritonitis		15.4
Test result		
Enlarging ventricles	70.9	30.8
Disruption/migration on x-ray study	13.7	0.0
Shunt flow study showing obstruction	2.6	0.0
Positive bacterial culture CSF and/or shunt material		92.3

CSF, cerebrospinal fluid.

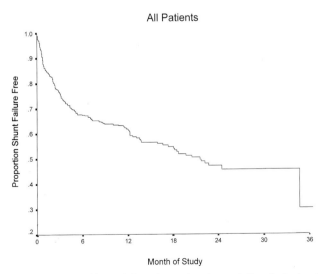

All Patients

FIGURE 37-3 Shunt failure from the time of the first shunt insertion. Most failures occur within 6 months. The 2-year failure rate is 50%. (From Drake JM, Kestle J, Milner R, et al: Randomized trial of cerebrospinal fluid shunt valve design in pediatric hydrocephalus. *Neurosurgery* 43:294–305, 1998.)

technique, in fact, this is often misleading.[38] A patient in whom a reservoir fills slowly may simply have small ventricles. Shunts whose reservoirs remain umbilicated for prolonged periods of time or even permanently, however, are often blocked proximally. A reservoir that is difficult to depress or refills apparently instantaneously frequently indicates a distal obstruction. Some shunt reservoirs contain proximal and distal occluders (or, less satisfactory, two valveless reservoirs). By occluding the distal reservoir and depressing and allowing the reservoir to refill, one can infer that the proximal catheter is patent. Similarly, by occluding the proximal reservoir and flushing distally, one can confirm patency of the distal catheter. In this situation, the reservoir should remain umbilicated if the occluder is working properly.

Fluid collecting around the shunt, particularly if it firmly distends the skin, is progressive, and tracks along the distal catheter are often a sign of shunt occlusion. When shunts fracture, CSF often continues to track along the fibrous sheath. In this scenario, one can often feel a small amount of fluid and a space where the shunt has come apart. It may be difficult, however, to distinguish an empty sheath from a sheath containing shunt tubing, particularly if the shunt has been implanted for some years or the tract is calcified. A fluid thrill can sometimes be felt at the site of a distal catheter disruption, with pumping of the proximal reservoir.

Patients with shunt overdrainage may complain of postural headache—that is, headache that begins with the assumption of the upright posture and disappears with recumbency. Patients with subdural hematoma may present with signs of raised intracranial pressure, but there may be some true localizing signs, such as hemiparesis. Patients with loculated CSF compartments also tend to present with signs of increased pressure. Patients with loculated fourth ventricles may present specifically with bulbar paralysis and apnea. Sometimes, symptoms and signs of syringomyelia, particularly in shunted myelomeningocele patients, may be a manifestation of shunt obstruction. The clinical features of shunt mechanical dysfunction may also be intermittent. This occurs not only in the slit-ventricle syndrome but also with partially occluded proximal or distal catheters.

Diagnostic Tests

Imaging studies are normally the first investigation undertaken. CT, MRI, or ultrasound scanning can determine the size and shape of the ventricles as well as any other collections or loculated compartments. The position and course of the ventricular catheter can also be seen best on CT. Dilatation of the ventricles compared with a previous image when the shunted patient was well is the simplest and clearest evidence of shunt dysfunction. Some patients, however, may have small ventricles or demonstrate minimal enlargement in the presence of shunt obstruction, and the ventricular size alone, in the absence of previous images, may be quite misleading in terms of shunt function (Fig. 37-4A, B). This situation is true particularly in children, in whom growth and development of the brain and congenital malformations alter one's notions of what normal ventricular size is.

Plain anteroposterior and lateral films of the skull, chest, and abdomen demonstrate whether the shunt is in continuity or has come apart or fractured (see Fig. 37-4C). For this reason, all shunt apparatus should be easily seen on radiographic studies. These radiographic studies may also demonstrate a peritoneal catheter that has migrated out of the abdomen with growth or obvious misplacement of the ventricular or peritoneal catheter. The films must often be scrutinized quite closely to detect small separations at connectors or along tubing. Calcification along the tubing is common in old shunts, which are prone to fracture. Common sites of shunt fracture are at connectors between the valve and the peritoneal catheter, where the hard connector repeatedly stresses the soft tubing, and in the neck, where fracture is presumably related to movement.

Uncertainty about the status of the shunt in a patient with symptoms compatible with shunt obstruction often leads to other diagnostic tests. The simplest test is the shunt tap. Under sterile conditions, the reservoir can be punctured with a 25-gauge butterfly needle catheter. Free flow of fluid indicates patency of the proximal catheter. The tubing can be used as a manometer to measure the pressure in the ventricle system. If the reservoir is distal to the proximal valve, flow of CSF back into the shunt gives an indication of the patency of the distal catheter. A shunt tap can also be therapeutic and lifesaving in critically ill shunted patients. Aspiration of 5 to 10 mL of fluid frequently dramatically improves a deteriorating shunted patient while preparations for surgery are made. In life-threatening situations, when the proximal catheter is blocked and no CSF can be aspirated, passing a lumbar puncture needle through the shunt, burr hole, and brain into the ventricle may be lifesaving. Although this needle often destroys the proximal portion of the shunt, this is of little consequence given the gravity of the situation and the forthcoming shunt revision. Other measurements of shunt patency include the use of radionuclide injections[39] or contrast agents.

Surgical Technique—Shunt Revision

The surgery for shunt revision is not very different from an initial shunt insertion, but there are a few important points. Unless one is planning on removing the shunt for an infection, the patient should be prepped and draped as for a shunt insertion, including upper and lower incisions. This prep is necessary even if one strongly suspects one or the other end of the shunt, because these suspicions can turn out to be wrong.

We normally explore the upper end of the shunt first, because one can test both ends from the same location, and piecemeal replacement of the lower end from an abdominal site using connectors is to be discouraged. Once the skin has been incised, cutting cautery can be used to expose the shunt hardware easily with minimal bleeding (Fig. 37-5A). Care must be taken with burr hole reservoir systems, particularly when there is a tie on the ventricular catheter that resides below the pial surface. This tie becomes stuck, and it is easy to lose the catheter when it separates. These lost catheters are extremely difficult to find, and one should probably introduce a ventriculoscope into the ventricle, rather than searching blindly in the parenchyma. For this reason, we rarely recommend burr hole systems. The equipment should then be inspected carefully for signs of damage, CSF egress, or infection.

Disconnecting the ventricular catheter from the valve allows determination of the patency of the upper end as well as the opportunity to take a CSF sample. Slow dripping from the upper end often indicates an incomplete but clinically

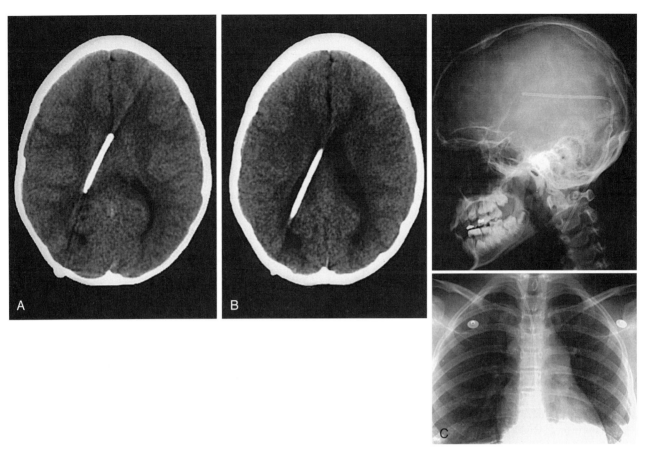

FIGURE 37-4 Diagnosis of shunt failure. A CT scan before (*A*) and after (*B*) shunt obstruction from a disconnection. The size of the ventricles in the scan in *B* appears normal, indicating the importance of a control CT scan when the patient is well. *C,* Plain films of the same patient showing a disconnection in the neck, which is a common site for this occurrence.

significant ventricular catheter obstruction, as evidenced by the gush of high-pressure CSF when the catheter is replaced. If there is doubt, the catheter can be gently manipulated, or a manometer using clear Silastic tubing and a straight connector can be attached to demonstrate free to-and-fro flow.

The lower end is then tested by connecting the clear Silastic tubing manometer to the valve and watching for spontaneous drainage. The distal system may need to be irrigated, but if flow is poor, the lower end should probably be explored. It is possible to reopen the same lower end

incision and, using the cutting cautery, expose the tubing as well as its fibrous tract. Stay sutures on the tract allow the tubing to be removed from the abdomen; then the same catheter or a new one can be passed down the same tract, avoiding a separate laparotomy.

If the upper end of the shunt is the culprit, the ventricular catheter should be gently removed and a new catheter introduced in rapid sequence, being careful not to lose too much CSF, because the ventricles collapse. The standard landmarks are again used, but as with an initial shunt insertion,

FIGURE 37-5 *A,* Dissecting the shunt apparatus during a shunt revision with a cutting cautery, which will not harm the Silastic material. *B,* Applying cautery to the ventricular catheter stylet to free a stuck ventricular catheter.

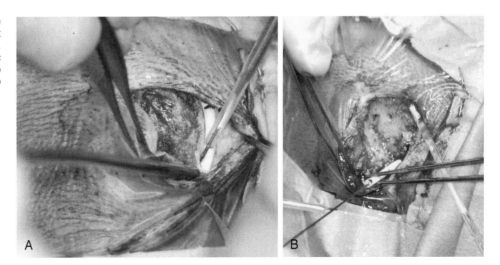

ultrasound, endoscopy, or stereotaxis can be used as aids. Preferably, one uses the metal stylet to direct the catheter, although with small ventricles, sliding the limp catheter down the old tract may suffice. One has no control over the trajectory of the catheter without the stylet, and astonishing catheter positions can result.

If the ventricular catheter is stuck, gently rotating the catheter may free it. Otherwise the metal stylet can be advanced down the lumen to the tip and cautery applied to the metal stylet while rotating the ventricular catheter (see Fig. 37-5B).[40] Badly stuck catheters should probably be left in place rather than produce a serious intraventricular hemorrhage. If hemorrhage does occur, manifested as frankly bloody CSF, the ventricle should be copiously irrigated with warm irrigation fluid. Failure of the CSF to clear should prompt placement of an external ventricular drain and abandonment of the shunt revision.

Lower end obstruction is less common, and its cause should be always be sought. Distal slit valves may accumulate debris, which forms a column inside the shunt eventually blocking the slits. Unclogging the tip or just cutting it off may suffice. If the peritoneal catheter has fractured or is too short, we recommend replacing the entire aging system rather than piecing it together. The latter may result in further disruption in short order. Connectors should not be placed anywhere along the path of the peritoneal catheter below the skull in growing children. They become adherent to the surrounding tissues, and the catheter breaks with growth. If there appears to be an outflow problem into the peritoneum, the catheter should be removed to another site, rather than placing it down the same tract. If the problem is the valve or if one is changing a valve onto the same peritoneal catheter, care should be taken when pulling the peritoneal catheter up into the wound, then again passing it back down from above. It is possible for the catheter to kink or coil out of sight, impeding shunt flow. It is preferable to expose the valve rather than extract and reinsert blindly.

Shunt Infection

Shunt infection remains an important, distressing cause of shunt failure.[41,42] Shunt infection puts the patient at increased risk of intellectual impairment, the development of loculated CSF compartments, and even death. Despite intensive efforts to prevent shunt infection for decades, most centers report infection rates on the order of 5% to 10%. Although the mechanism of shunt contamination seems relatively straightforward, the exact intervention that has led to lower rates in some centers remains elusive.[42–44]

Shunt infection remains in some cases remarkably difficult to establish, even in retrospect. A simple working definition is unequivocal evidence of infection of the shunt equipment, the overlying wound, the CSF, or distal drainage site related to the shunt. Unequivocal evidence requires demonstration of the organism on Gram stain or culture from material in, on, or around the shunt or from fluid withdrawn from the shunt.

Shunt infection is probably best classified in terms of site:

1. Wound infection: An incision or shunt tract with signs of inflammation, purulent discharge, and organisms seen on gram stain or culture.
2. Meningitis: Fever, meningismus, CSF leukocytosis, and organisms seen on Gram stain or culture.

3. Peritonitis: Fever, abdominal tenderness (abdominal pseudocyst and abdominal abscess may present with mass with or without fever), and organisms seen on Gram stain or culture. For vascular shunts, findings are fever, leukocytosis, positive blood culture, with or without evidence of shunt nephritis or cor pulmonale.
4. Infected shunt apparatus: Minimal signs of CSF contamination with bacteria recovered from purulent exudate in or on shunt material, Gram stain of CSF withdrawn from the shunt, or positive culture on fluid aspirated from the shunt under sterile conditions.[45] Organisms that grow only from the shunt equipment or CSF on broth culture are probably contaminants.

Most shunt infections appear within 2 months of surgery. Delayed infections with skin commensal organisms are possible.[46] Contamination of the shunt can occur from other surgical procedures that expose it, such as bladder augmentation with peritoneal shunts; however, it is unusual for remote sepsis to contaminate the shunt.

The most common organisms infecting CSF shunts are staphylococci; approximately 40% of shunt infections are caused by *Staphylococcus epidermidis* infections and 20% by *S. aureus*.[41,47,48] Other species isolated from infected shunts include the coryneforms, streptococci, enterococci, aerobic gram-negative rods, and yeasts. Because these organisms are commonly part of the normal skin flora, and shunt infection usually occurs within 2 months of surgery, endogenous spread from the patient or surgical staff is the logical route of infection.

Bacteria colonize the shunt in the form of a continuous biofilm. This biofilm is composed of bacterial cells, either singly or in microcolonies, all embedded in an anionic matrix of bacterial exopolymers and trapped macromolecules.[49] The biofilm offers protection against many common antibacterial agents, including antibodies, white blood cells, surfactants, and antibiotics. For this reason, treatment of shunt infections by the exclusive use of systemic or intraventricular antibiotics[41,50] has been ineffective.

Clinical Presentation

Most shunt infections present within 2 months of shunt insertion.[3] The clinical features depend on the site of infection. Wound infections are usually manifested as fever, reddening of the incision site or shunt tract; and, with progression, discharge of pus from the incision. In chronic wound infections, the shunt may become exposed as the wound breaks down. Table 37-2 indicates the clinical presentation of shunt infection in 28 patients from the shunt design trial.[3] Erosion of the thin skin in infants, particularly premature infants, from pressure also results in a wound infection. Any leak of CSF from the incision because of a high-resistance valve or poor distal flow also often results in contamination of the shunt and subsequent infection.

Patients with meningitis or ventriculitis usually present with fever, headache, or irritability, and often with some neck stiffness if not nuchal rigidity. Peritonitis is less common. Patients typically present with fever, anorexia or vomiting, and abdominal tenderness. The severity of the symptoms depends to some extent on the infecting organism. Patients infected with *S. epidermidis* may look remarkably well and may have intermittent fever and irritability only.

They may also present with signs of a typical shunt obstruction without fever or leukocytosis. Patients with abdominal pseudocysts (which are invariably infected) may present with a mass only. Small pseudocysts may be difficult to detect on abdominal examination. Historically, patients with ventriculoatrial shunts, in addition to presenting with signs of a septicemia, could manifest shunt nephritis or cor pulmonale.

The infection often involves more than one compartment or progresses to multiple compartments, as in a patient who develops a wound infection that progresses to meningitis. Shunts have been demonstrated to be impervious to bacterial migration across the shunt wall, so that spread occurs along the inside or outside the shunt. Although the possibility of retrograde bacterial movement up the lumen of the shunt has been disputed, clear evidence of spread of infection from the peritoneal cavity to the brain has been reported.

In terms of differential diagnosis, all patients with suspected shunt infection should have a thorough history and physical examination to rule out other possible infections or identify possible sources of infection. This differential diagnosis is particularly important in children, in whom any of the common childhood febrile illnesses can resemble a shunt infection, such as otitis media and, particularly in myelomeningocele patients, urinary tract infection. Patients with an uninfected shunt obstruction can have nuchal rigidity resulting from tonsillar herniation and occasionally a low-grade fever.

Diagnostic Tests

Routine blood tests frequently reveal a polymorphonuclear leukocytosis. Blood culture is perhaps less important in patients with ventriculoperitoneal shunts but should be performed in febrile patients. Culture of the urine or other obvious sites of infections, for example, the wound, should also be taken. Plain film examination of the shunt system reveals whether the shunt system is still intact, whether an abdominal viscus may have been perforated, and whether or not there are any extraneous pieces of shunt equipment from previous revisions that may also be contaminated. A CT or MRI scan of the head is also important to display the size of the ventricles not only as part of determining whether or not the shunt is obstructed, but also how the size and configuration of the ventricles may influence decisions to remove the shunt and insert an external ventricular drain (EVD). Placing an EVD in a patient with a functioning but infected shunt with slit ventricles may be quite difficult. Rarely, evidence of ventriculitis or, even more uncommonly, brain abscess may be revealed on cerebral images.[51,52] Abdominal ultrasound should be performed in any patient with abdominal pain or tenderness or a mass or in patients suspected of having a distal obstruction.

All patients without obvious wound infection or cutaneously extruded hardware should have the shunt system aspirated through an existing reservoir. Examination of the CSF for cell count, Gram stain, and culture confirms the diagnosis of shunt infection and quickly gives an index of the probable infecting organism. Shunt aspiration should be done with meticulous aseptic technique so as not to contaminate a shunt system that is, in fact, sterile or to introduce a second organism in shunts that are already infected. Shunt aspiration provides a high diagnostic yield of shunt infection of approximately 95% and is quite safe. Lumbar puncture or ventricular puncture gives a much lower yield (7% to 26%). Although CSF leukocytosis of 50 to 200 cells/mL is common, a normal CSF count may not rule out a colonized shunt, and CSF protein and glucose are often normal. In patients with a wound infection, care should be taken not to contaminate the interior of the shunt when aspirating the collection surrounding the shunt system.

Because about 30% of patients who prove to be infected also have a shunt obstruction, at the time of surgery, ventricular CSF should be resampled. Sending all the hardware to the microbiology laboratory results in overdiagnosis of shunt infections, because skin commensals contaminating the shunt during removal show up on broth culture. It is recommended that any purulent material on the shunt be swabbed for microscopy and culture. Subsequently, a local area of the shunt should be swabbed with alcohol and fluid aspirated from the lumen of the shunt with a sterile syringe and needle. If no aspirate is obtained, the shunt component should be irrigated with sterile saline.

Treatment

Shunt removal with interval antibiotic treatment (usually with EVD) carries the highest shunt infection cure rate and the lowest mortality rate.[50] CSF shunt removal with immediate replacement carries an almost equal shunt infection cure rate with a higher morbidity and mortality rate. Antibiotic treatment alone has the lowest cure rate and the highest mortality rate. These findings seem sensible given what is now known about bacterial biofilms. Every attempt should be made to remove all existing hardware, even lost ventricular and peritoneal catheters. These can act as a nidus for a repeat infection after treatment.

Normally the EVD is left in place for approximately 1 week. This time provides an opportunity to examine the CSF daily, to verify that the CSF has become sterile, and to verify that the antibiotics in use are appropriate given the organism's antibiotic sensitivity. Intraventricular antibiotic injection and antibiotic level measurement can also be performed with an EVD. At the time of shunt reinsertion after an interval EVD, the EVD is usually clamped for 8 to 12 hours (provided that the patient can tolerate it) to allow the ventricles to expand and facilitate ventricular cannulation with the new shunt.

Organisms that cause meningitis in the general population and that infect patients with shunts or cause hydrocephalus and are discovered at time of shunt insertion can usually be treated with antibiotics alone. This includes *Haemophilus influenzae* and *Streptococcus pneumoniae*.[53,54] It is essential in this form of treatment that the CSF be resampled to verify sterilization. Failure to clear the CSF within 48 to 72 hours should prompt removal of the shunt equipment.

Given the considerable morbidity, let alone financial cost, of shunt infections, prevention is the leading consideration for the future. Several studies have instituted procedures aimed at risk reduction (such as restricting operating room personnel, operating early in the day, soaking the shunt in antibiotics, and using prophylactic antibiotics) and reported a reduction in shunt infection from 7.75% to 0.17% (see reference 43) in one series and from 12.9% to 3.8% (see reference 55) in another, using historical controls from the same institution. These studies leave doubt as to which of the deliberately altered variables is important.

Management of the Difficult Shunt Patient

Difficult shunt patients seem to fall into two general categories. One category is patients with intractable symptoms, usually headache, in whom doubt about the functional status of the shunt exists.[56-58] The other is patients who present repeatedly with shunt malfunction for no apparent reason. Both sets of patients can be difficult to manage. The patients often otherwise lead normal lives and are completely disabled or continuously in the hospital with their shunt problem.

A detailed history, including all the previous shunt surgeries, is mandatory. Previous operating room notes from the hospital where the surgery was done should be sought. The relevant imaging, which should be related to the patient's clinical status at the time the images were obtained, should also be carefully studied. This whole process often requires creating a spreadsheet or log to keep track of the multiple interventions. All culture reports should also be sought, looking for an unrecognized or partially treated infection. A thorough physical examination, including the shunt equipment, follows. Current imaging should be complete, including plain x-ray films of the shunt equipment.

In patients with chronic headache, an idea of whether the headache is postural can often be obtained by the history. Other exacerbating and relieving symptoms as well as concomitant features should be sought. Determining the functional status of the shunt by pumping the reservoir is notoriously unreliable.[38] If the shunt's functional status by standard imaging is still uncertain, a flow study using a radioisotope or other contrast agent should be done. If the reservoir is above the valve, reflux into the ventricles confirms that the upper end is patent. Otherwise, it may be more difficult to decide which end is blocked. Sitting the patient up or pumping the reservoir helps to determine what effect these manipulations have on the shunt system. Collection of contrast material in a localized cyst in the abdomen can also be seen with this technique and confirmed with ultrasound. These flow studies are not infallible, and both false-positive and false-negative results are possible.

If all information suggests that the shunt is working, intracranial pressure monitoring is usually the next step. Using a separate intraparenchymal probe is warranted because it provides the most accurate information. The patient should be monitored for 48 to 72 hours to ensure that prolonged periods of sleep and wakefulness, in various postural positions, are recorded. The patient or family should also keep a timed log to record any headaches, so that they can be related to the pressure recordings. Slightly negative intracranial pressure when upright is normal. In patients with symptomatic postural hypotension, large negative pressures associated with the headache are sought. Patients with slit-ventricle syndrome usually have plateau waves of 20 or 30 minutes with pressures frequently greater than 20 mm Hg and usually when asleep at night.

Patients with postural hypotension usually respond to placement of either a siphon-reducing device or a flow-limiting valve. Verification that both ends of the shunt are functioning properly at surgery is mandatory before replacing the valve. Leaving the pressure monitor in place for a few days ensures that the new valve is functioning as expected. If the patient continues to experience headache, the relationship to the new pressure profile can help to sort this out.

Patients with slit-ventricle syndrome are more difficult to manage.[59-63] We replace any standard differential valve with a flow-limiting valve, provided that the system is shown to be completely patent at surgery. This action often dilates the ventricles slightly and, more importantly, demonstrates progressive decline in plateau waves during sleep.[25] If that fails, one is usually faced with expanding the intracranial compartment. Subtemporal decompression has not stood the test of time for this condition, and though much more extensive, a cranial vault expansion is usually required. One can temporize before embarking on this extensive surgical procedure with antimigrainous drugs (which can be tried before any of these interventions) while the patient and surgeon reconsider the wisdom of this operation.

In patients in whom the pressure monitoring is normal or bears no relationship to headache, surgical restraint is wise. These patients are unlikely to be helped by further shunt surgery, and each attempt increases the risk that they will suffer a surgical complication that will only exacerbate the situation. Assessment by a chronic pain or headache specialist team consisting of physicians and psychiatrists or psychologists is important, particularly if the patient is dependent on narcotic analgesics. Various forms of psychotherapy may dramatically improve the patient's condition. As a last resort, particularly if the opinion of the team is that the headache is organic, the shunt can be explored or changed, but patients have to realize that probably nothing will be found.

In patients with repetitive obstruction for no apparent reason, every search for a possible indolent infection should be made, including anaerobic cultures. Encysted fluid collections in the abdominal cavity, even in the absence of positive cultures, strongly point to an infection. If there is any doubt, the whole shunt system, including any retained hardware (the exception being fragments in the chest wall not in communication with the abdomen) should be removed and an external drain placed. A new system should be placed at new sites in the head and abdomen.

If there are repetitive proximal obstructions, the ventricular catheter may be traveling down a sheath of gliotic tissue to the same site, only to be replugged. Placing the ventricular catheter under ultrasound or endoscopic guidance into a completely different site (even the opposite ventricle) obviates this problem. If the patients have slit ventricles when the shunt is functioning, changing the valve to a flow-limiting one may slightly expand the ventricles and possibly lead to a reduced rate of obstruction. Another possibility is to place a programmable shunt, so that the opening pressure can be changed once implanted.[64] Finally, particularly if the patient has a history of aqueduct stenosis, an endoscopic third ventriculostomy (ETV) may render the patient shunt-free entirely, as discussed in the next section.[65] Dissatisfaction with the long-term outcome and significant failure rates of conventional CSF shunting systems has resulted in a resurgence of interest in the earliest form of treatment for hydrocephalus, ventriculostomy.[66,67]

ENDOSCOPIC THIRD VENTRICULOSTOMY

History

The earliest endoscopic treatment for hydrocephalus was choroid plexus fulguration performed by Lespinasse in

1910 (see reference 68). Dandy[69] subsequently described an open technique for third ventriculostomy for the treatment of noncommunicating hydrocephalus. A percutaneous ventriculostomy technique using an endoscope was first described by Mixter in 1923 (see reference 70). Fay and Grant[71] published the first intraventricular photographs that same year, providing the first visual record of endoscopic anatomy. Because of the limited illumination and large size of early endoscopes, open ventriculostomy procedures as well as percutaneous fluoroscopic and later CT-guided techniques remained popular for many years. Hopkins provided the technical advances necessary for the revival of neuroendoscopy.[72] Hopkins' innovative solid-rod lens and coherent quartz fiber lens systems underlie the basic design of all modern rigid and flexible endoscopic systems. The improved optics and illumination and reduced size of modern endoscopes have greatly increased their utility and reduced associated morbidity and mortality.

Patient Selection

Third ventriculostomy is intended to treat noncommunicating hydrocephalus with patent subarachnoid spaces and adequate CSF absorption. Results of ETV are related to the cause of hydrocephalus encountered as well as clinical and radiographic features of the individual patient. Table 37-3 lists causes of obstructive hydrocephalus classified according to reported success rates of ETV (see later section on Outcome). Patients with acquired aqueductal stenosis or tumors obstructing third or fourth ventricular outflow have demonstrated the highest success rates, exceeding 75% in carefully selected series of patients.[73–76] Previously shunted patients with or without myelomeningocele and patients with congenital aqueductal stenosis or cystic abnormalities leading to obstruction (i.e., arachnoid cyst, Dandy-Walker malformations) have shown intermediate response.[74,75,77–79] Further study of this intermediate group is likely to identify subgroups with higher success rates. Infants presenting with hydrocephalus associated with myelomeningocele, hemorrhage, or infection have demonstrated poor response to ventriculostomy,[73,80,81] and despite limited reports of success in such patients,[75,77,78,82–85] they are more controversial candidates for this procedure. The procedure is not advisable in patients who have undergone prior radiation therapy because of the extremely poor response rates, altered anatomy (i.e., thickened third ventricular floor), and increased risk of bleeding.[75,77,81]

Several clinical features may influence the outcome of third ventriculostomy (Table 37-4). There appears to be a significant association between increasing patient age and a more favorable outcome.[74,75,77,86] Evidence suggests that this association applies to the age at which hydrocephalus initially developed as well as age at the time of ventriculostomy.[75,86] Several studies show success rates of approximately 50% in patients younger that 2 years old, regardless of cause.[74,75,78] Results are even poorer in patients younger than 6 months old.[86]

Many studies have demonstrated a trend toward more successful ventriculostomy outcome in patients with existing shunt systems.[74,78,86] In fact, third ventriculostomy has been found to be useful in the treatment of intractable shunt infections and malfunctions and even slit-ventricle syndrome refractory to other treatments.[65,73,77,87–90] Other series of

ventriculostomy in previously shunted patients have been less promising.[79,91] These contradictory results may reflect the mix of patients in small series. The improved outcome in previously shunted patients is commonly attributed to increased CSF absorptive capacity; however, the effect of

---

TABLE 37-3 ▪ Ventriculostomy Success Rates by Hydrocephalus Cause

High Success Rates (≥75%)

Acquired aqueductal stenosis
Tumor obstructing ventricular outflow
 Tectal
 Pineal
 Thalamic
 Intraventricular

Intermediate Success Rates (50% to 70%)

Myelomeningocele (previously shunted, older patients)
Congenital aqueductal stenosis
Cystic abnormalities obstructing CSF flow
 Arachnoid cysts
 Dandy-Walker malformation
Previously shunted patients with difficulties
 Slit-ventricle syndrome
 Recurrent or intractable shunt infections
 Recurrent or intractable shunt malfunctions

Low Success Rates (<50%)

Myelomeningocele (previously unshunted, neonatal patients)
Posthemorrhagic hydrocephalus
Postinfectious hydrocephalus (excluding aqueductal stenosis of infectious origin)

TABLE 37-4 ▪ Favorable Clinical and Radiographic Features for Endoscopic Third Ventriculostomy

Clinical

Cause of hydrocephalus in high or intermediate success group (see Table 37–3)
Age >6 months at time of hydrocephalus diagnosis
Age >6 months at time of procedure
No prior radiation therapy
No history of hemorrhage or meningitis
Patient previously shunted

Radiographic

Clear evidence of ventricular noncommunication
 Obstructive pattern of HCP
 Aqueductal anatomic obstruction
 Lack of aqueductal flow void on T2–weighted MRI
Favorable third ventricular anatomy
 Width and foramen of Monro sufficient to accommodate endoscope
  Rigid >7 mm
  Flexible >4 mm
  Thinned floor of third ventricle
 Downward bulging floor, draped over clivus
 Basilar posterior to mammillary bodies
Absence of structural anomalies impeding procedure
 AVM or tumor obscuring third ventricular floor
 Enlarged massa intermedia
 Insufficient space between mamillary bodies and basilar and the clivus
 Basilar artery ectasia

AVM, arteriovenous malformation; HCP, hydrocephalus; MRI, magnetic resonance imaging.

the shunt itself on CSF absorption is difficult to distinguish from the effect of increased age in these patients.

Preoperative assessment of CSF absorptive capacity has been advocated by some authors,[92,93] but these techniques have not been widely accepted.[75,86] Because the patency of CSF pathways is one of the assumptions on which the procedure is based, a preoperative CSF absorption study would be invaluable in identifying patients who would likely benefit from ventriculostomy. The observed delay between operation and decrease in ventricular size (see later section on Outcome), however, suggests that CSF absorption may increase slowly after ventriculostomy. Therefore, preoperative assessment of CSF-absorptive capacity may fail to identify all appropriate patients.[75] Until an accurate functional predictor of this capacity is practical, radiographic assessment of the obstructive pattern of hydrocephalus by MRI will probably remain the preoperative diagnostic procedure of choice.

Table 37-4 depicts preoperative radiographic criteria frequently cited for improving outcome and limiting morbidity of ETV. Preoperative MRI optimally demonstrates all relevant anatomic features and should be obtained for all proposed third ventriculostomy patients. Initially, confirmation of noncommunicating hydrocephalus of favorable cause should be established by the pattern of ventricular dilatation. Anatomic obstruction of CSF pathways between the aqueduct and the fourth ventricular outflow foramina may be visible on T2- or T1-weighted contrast images. Additionally, T2-weighted images should reveal absence of the aqueductal CSF flow void frequently present in normal individuals.

Once the patient's suitability for the procedure has been established, the neurosurgeon must clarify the details of third ventricular anatomy that are likely to affect morbidity. First, the width of the third ventricle and diameter of the foramen of Monro must be sufficient to accommodate the endoscope of choice (see later section on Technique). Additionally, the thickness of the third ventricular floor and the anatomy of the proposed puncture site in relationship to vital structures, particularly the basilar artery and its branches, must be assessed. A downward-bulging third ventricular floor draped over the clivus has been cited as a prerequisite for this procedure in the past, but others have not found this to be necessary.[75,81] Ultimately, the surgeon must be satisfied that there is no structural lesion (i.e., tumor or arteriovenous malformation) or anatomic variation that would render the procedure unduly difficult or hazardous. In cases of doubt, it is reasonable to visualize the floor of the third ventricle and abandon the procedure if the floor is unsuitable.

Technique

An ever-increasing variety of endoscopic equipment is currently available for neuroendoscopic procedures. For uncomplicated third ventriculostomy, a 0- or 30-degree rigid scope offers superior optics and anatomic orientation. The Gaab endoscope (Johnson & Johnson, Randolph, MA), inserted through a 7-mm rigid cannula, provides the advantage of two working ports with a third for continuous irrigation. A 4-mm flexible steerable endoscope (Johnson & Johnson, Randolph, MA) introduced through a No. 12 French peel-away sheath allows for improved maneuverability

within the ventricular system, at the expense of some image quality. Flexible scopes are useful for accessing more remote portions of the ventricular system (i.e., pineal recess, aqueduct). Several miniature fiberoptic endoscopes are also now available. These scopes can be inserted through a standard ventricular catheter; however, their inferior optics and lack of an irrigating or working channel limit their potential applications (i.e., ventricular catheter placement).

A miniature video camera is attached to the endoscope, and orientation is adjusted before insertion. The monitor should be placed at a comfortable distance and height for viewing throughout the case. Use of the camera allows the senior surgeon, trainee, and operating room staff to view the entire procedure, greatly enhancing the opportunities for learning without added morbidity.

Adequate continuous irrigation is imperative for proper visualization, particularly if bleeding is encountered. This irrigation is provided by running Ringer's lactate through blood-warming apparatus, with a shut-off valve on the scope. An uninterrupted release pathway for irrigation fluid is equally essential to avoid dangerous elevations of intracranial pressure. A separate channel for fluid release can be intermittently or partially blocked to provide transient pressure tamponade for control of bleeding. Direct pressure using the scope cannula itself can also be useful for homeostasis.

Endoscopic third ventriculostomy can be performed with either a flexible or a rigid endoscope. The patient is positioned supine in a horseshoe headrest with the neck flexed 15 to 20 degrees. A burr hole is made over the right coronal suture, 2 to 2.5 cm lateral to the midline. Optimal positioning of the burr hole varies slightly depending on the proposed trajectory as determined from preoperative MRI. The burr hole is placed more anteriorly to provide access to the posterior third ventricle if desired. The dura is opened in cruciate fashion, and the pial surface is coagulated and incised. A 3-mm-diameter, blunt-tipped brain needle is inserted into the right frontal horn, directed toward the foramen of Monro. After CSF sampling and intracranial pressure assessment, the needle is withdrawn, and the same tract is used for insertion of the endoscope sheath or cannula. This technique allows for blunt separation of the ependymal layer and progressive enlargement of this opening, minimizing ependymal bleeding, a common cause of poor intraventricular visualization.

Once insertion of the endoscope into the lateral ventricle has been achieved, the foramen of Monro is located by identification of the choroid plexus and septal and thalamostriate veins (Figs 37-6A, B and 37-7A). After passage of the endoscope through the foramen of Monro, the optic chiasm, infundibulum, mammillary bodies, massa intermedia, and aqueduct can all be observed along the floor of the third ventricle from anterior to posterior, depending on trajectory (see Figs 37-6C, D and 37-7B, G). A flexible scope is generally necessary to view the lamina terminalis, suprapineal recess, or third ventricular roof. In cases of obstructive hydrocephalus, a diamond-shaped transparent membrane is commonly seen between the mammillary bodies and infundibulum. The dorsum sellae, clivus, and basilar artery are often visible through this membrane (see Fig. 37-7B). This area of the third ventricular floor between the clivus and the basilar artery is the ideal site for third ventriculostomy.

Numerous methods of perforating the third ventricular floor have been described that use the scope itself, a cautery unit, laser, or endoscopic instrument.[74,77,81,94–96] We use a closed blunt biopsy forceps for initial fenestration and a No. 4 French Fogarty balloon catheter for enlargement of the ventriculostomy (see Fig. 37-7C through E). Care is taken to inflate the balloon only under direct vision within the opening, because blindly withdrawing an inflated balloon from the basal cisterns carries a significant risk of injury to perforating vessels. After adequate enlargement of the ventriculostomy, the scope can be advanced to inspect the prepontine and interpeduncular cisterns (see Fig. 37-7F).

Postoperative management of patients after ETV must be individualized to address the unique preoperative and intraoperative details of each case. Patients with subacute hydrocephalus presentations and uneventful procedures may require only short-term postoperative observation, whereas patients with acute presentations or significant intraoperative bleeding often require an external ventricular drain with continuous intracranial pressure monitoring in an intensive care unit setting. Patients undergoing a simultaneous endoscopic tumor biopsy or removal of a prior existing shunt system require particularly close observation and monitoring.

In the past, postoperative CSF shunting has been recommended to promote expansion of pericerebral CSF spaces and to improve absorption.[82,84,91] Compelling evidence suggests, however, that CSF flow through the ventriculostomy maintains its patency, and shunts can lead to closure of the opening.[73,91] We do not recommend a coexisting CSF shunt and ETV.

Outcome

The goal of ETV and, to date, the best objectively quantifiable measure of a successful outcome, is shunt independence. ETV has yielded a higher success rate with lower morbidity and mortality than earlier methods of third ventriculostomy. Mortality rates for open ventriculostomy procedures varied between 5% and 27% with success rates of 37% to 75%.[11,73,81,83,91,97] Percutaneous radiographic and later CT-guided techniques reduced this mortality rate to 2% to 7%, with a 44% to 75% rate of shunt independence.[73,80,81,84,91,98] Studies using modern endoscopic techniques and equipment, with or without stereotactic CT or MRI guidance, have reported low morbidity (3% to 12%) and essentially no mortality, with success rates greater than 75% for carefully selected patient groups. Table 37-5 depicts the results of ETV studies with success rates by cause where this information is available. The current challenge is to

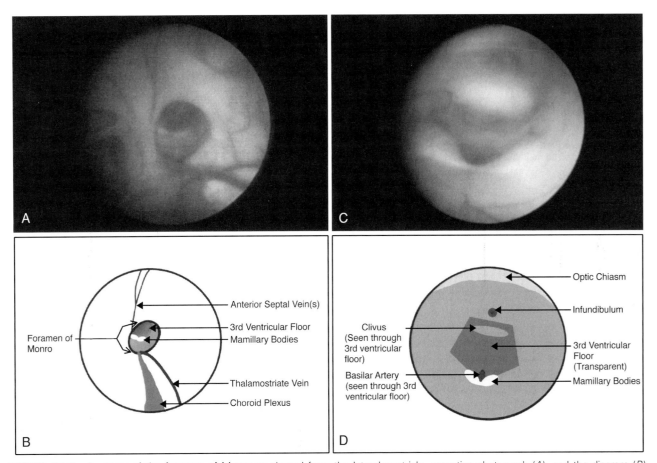

FIGURE 37-6 Anatomy of the foramen of Monro as viewed from the lateral ventricle, operative photograph (*A*), and the diagram (*B*). A close-up view of anatomy of the third ventricular floor, an operative photograph (*C*), and a schematic diagram (*D*).

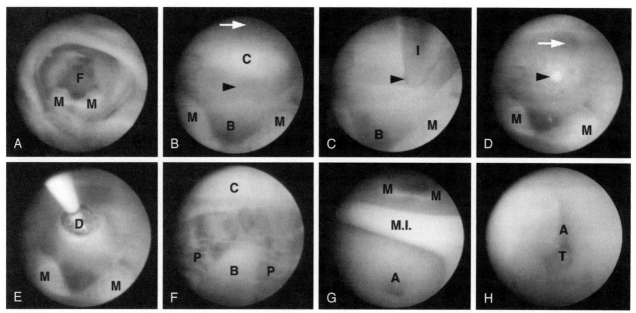

FIGURE 37-7   A series of operative photographs demonstrating the endoscopic third ventriculostomy procedure. *A,* Entrance is through the foramen of Monro from the right lateral ventricle. *B,* A close-up of the third ventricular floor; an *arrowhead* depicts the proposed ventriculostomy site. *C,* Blunt forceps piercing the third ventricular floor. *D,* View of the initial ventriculostomy opening. *E,* Dilatation of the ventriculostomy using a Fogarty balloon catheter. *F,* View of basal cisterns through the ventriculostomy opening. *G,* View of the middle third ventricular floor. *H,* View of the aqueduct demonstrating an obstruction by a tectal tumor (*black arrowhead*). Ventriculostomy site; (*white arrow*) infundibular recess. A, aqueduct; B, basilar artery; C, clivus; D, Fogarty balloon; F, floor of third ventricle; I, blunt forceps; M, mammillary bodies; M.I., massa intermedia; P, basilar perforators; T, tectal tumor.

define appropriate indications and devise objective measures for preoperative and postoperative assessment of these patients.

One of the most confusing aspects of outcome evaluation in ETV patients is the failure of the ventricles to return to normal size. Most studies report a gradual decrease in the ventricular size over months to years postoperatively, with resolution of periventricular edema and increased extracerebral spaces, coinciding with clinical improvement.[73–76,91,95] One series of patients treated with either CSF shunts or ETV showed no difference in intellectual outcome despite enlarged ventricles in the ETV group.[95] Multiple authors have reported late failures, in which the ventriculostomy closes sometimes years postoperatively.[75,87] Radiographic evaluation of suspected closure is confounded by the presence of persistently enlarged ventricles, and closure must often be suspected solely on the basis of clinical evidence.

Studies detailing the serial measurements of multiple radiographic indices of ventricular size postoperatively show that the third ventricular size responds more quickly (usually within 3 months) than the lateral ventricular size (2 years).[99,100] Additionally, third ventricular size appears to correlate most closely with outcome in these patients.[76,99,100]

Several newer modalities appear promising as potential objective measures of ventriculostomy function. MRI detection of T2-weighted flow void around the ventriculostomy has been correlated with clinical outcome in ETV.[101–103] This observation has proven most helpful in confirming ventriculostomy patency postoperatively, particularly in patients with persistent ventriculomegaly.[102,103] Actual quantification of flow velocity through ventriculostomies has also been demonstrated by phase-contrast MRI and

Doppler ultrasonography.[104,105] Intraventricular pressure has been observed to return to normal over 3 months in a patient after third ventriculostomy who underwent concurrent implantation of a telemetric intracranial pressure monitor.[106] It is hoped that methods of quantifying ventriculostomy function will allow neurosurgeons to refine further the techniques necessary to improve outcome. Radiographic confirmation may also help define indications with more subjective outcomes, for example, the observation of less fulminant shunt malfunctions in patients after ventriculostomy.[77]

Complications

Several series of ETV report no mortality and low morbidity (see Table 37-5).[65,73–79,102,107–109] The most common serious complications are related to structures in and around the floor of the third ventricle. In patients with aqueductal obstruction, the third ventricular floor is usually thinned out and transparent, with the hypothalamic nuclei displaced laterally. When the floor is not thinned or the ventriculostomy is not performed at the preferred midline site, injury to the hypothalamus or bleeding can result. These complications have been attributed to direct pressure from the perforating instrument, elevated CSF temperature from cautery or the light source, or distention of the third ventricle from continuous irrigation without adequate drainage.[76] Reported complications from injury to this area include the syndrome of inappropriate secretion of antidiuretic hormone, diabetes insipidus, loss of thirst, amenorrhea, and trancelike states.[107,110] These complications are usually transient. Bradycardia is also observed on occasion when perforating a thickened third ventricular floor, and a near-fatal cardiac arrest has been reported.[111]

TABLE 37-5 ■ Summary of Endoscopic Third Ventriculostomy Trials

Author (Year)	Procedure	Patients (n)	Overall Success (%)	Morbidity (%)	Procedure Abort Rate (%)	Follow-up (mean)	% Success (Shunt Independence) by Cause (n)						
							AS	MMC	Tumor	SVS	Shunt	PHH	Other
Hirsch et al (1986)[107]	ETV	114	70	—	—	—	70 (114)	—	—	—	—	—	—
Jones et al (1990)[77]	ETV	24	50	8	16	NS	57 (14)	40 (5)	67 (3)	—	—	—	0 (2)
Kelly (1991)[73]	SETV	16	94	0	0	1–5 yr (3.5 yr)	94 (16)	—	—	—	—	—	—
Dalrymple and Kelly (1992)[108]	SETV	85	87	—	—	1–66 mo	—	—	—	—	—	—	—
Jones et al (1992)[74]	ETV	54	60	7	9	3 mo–7 yr (27 mo)	65 (31)	40 (10)	86 (7)	—	75 (4)	0 (2)	—
Goodman (1993)[109]	MRETV	3	100	0	0	6–14 mo (10 mo)	100 (3)	—	—	—	—	—	—
Jones et al (1994)[75]	ETV	101	61	5	6	NS	78 (9)	52 (21)	81 (16)	—	—	—	—
Sainte-Rose and Chumas (1996)[76]	ETV	82	81	NS	NS	(1.8 yr)	67 (111)	—	>80 (53)	—	—	—	—
	RTV and STV	104	68	—	—	(5.7 yr)	—	—	—	—	—	—	—
Teo and Jones (1996)[78]	ETV	69	72	3	9	1–17 yr (32 mo)	—	72 (69)	—	—	—	—	—
Goumnerova and Frim (1997)[102]	ETV	23	73	9	—	7–44 mo (17 mo)	69 (13)	—	71 (7)	—	—	0 (1)	100 (2)
Baskin et al (1998)[65]	ETV	16	63	12	—	(18.8 mo)	—	—	—	63 (16)	—	—	—
Brockmeyer et al (1998)[79]	ETV	97	49	6	26	15–69 mo (24.2 mo)	56 (16)	50 (16)	61 (18)	50 (4)	—	0 (4)	38 (13)

As, aqueductal sinus, ETV, endoscopic third ventriculostomy; MMC, myelomeningocele; MRETV, stereotactic (MR-guided) endoscopic third ventriculostomy; NS, not significant; PHH, posthemorrhegic hydrocephalus; RTV, radiography-guided thrid ventriculostomy; SETV, stereotactic (CT-guided) endoscopic third ventriculostomy; shunt, intractable shunt infection or malfunction; STV, stereotactic (CT-guided) thrid ventriculostomy; SVS, slit-ventricle syndrome.

Transient postoperative fevers, which frequently occur in these patients, are commonly attributed to irritation of the ependyma from blood or manipulation of the hypothalamus.[95]

Other structures at risk in this area include the third and sixth cranial nerves, fornix, and caudate. Injuries to all of these structures, usually transient or clinically silent, have been reported.[107,110] The major life-threatening risk during the procedure is injury to the basilar artery and its branches. The basilar bifurcation is usually visible through the thinned third ventricular floor. Extreme caution should be taken to avoid injuring these vessels, particularly when preoperative imaging suggests a thickened ventricular floor or aberrant location (i.e., anterior to the mammillary bodies) of these vessels. We perform the initial fenestration with a blunt instrument rather than the cautery or laser to minimize the risk of arterial damage. Injury to these vessels can result in catastrophic hemorrhage, stroke, or pseudoaneurysm formation.[112]

Other routine complications, associated with most neurosurgical procedures, have also been observed. Superficial wound infections as well as meningitis and ventriculitis, subdural hematomas, and CSF leaks have all been described.[76,107,110]

OTHER ENDOSCOPIC APPLICATIONS

Endoscopic techniques, with and without the addition of stereotactic assistance, are increasingly used for treating a variety of conditions and complications related to hydrocephalus. In stereotactic-guided techniques, the scope target can be selected and intervening structures (i.e., the foramen of Monro) chosen as part of the trajectory.[73,113] CT-based or MRI-based frame systems or the newer frameless stereotactic systems can be easily adapted for use with a rigid endoscope. These systems are particularly useful when planning the trajectory in patients with small ventricles, distorted anatomy as a result of prior shunting procedures or infection, or approaching intraventricular lesions. They are also helpful when operating in large ventricles where the light is diffused, in loculated ventricles where there is essentially no recognizable anatomy, and in CSF turbid from debris or blood when scope image is poor. Collapse of the ventricular system or cystic cavities can rapidly render the preoperative imaging data useless.

Intracranial cysts and loculated regions of the ventricular system have been successfully treated with these techniques.[94,114,115] Endoscopic procedures for colloid cysts and suprasellar arachnoid cysts have been particularly successful.[116–118] Several studies have examined the role of ventriculoscopic shunt catheter placement[119,120]; however, prospective, randomized study of the usefulness of this procedure is under way. Likewise, treatment of intraventricular tumors and their associated hydrocephalus with endoscopic techniques requires further study, particularly in midline posterior fossa tumors.[76] Ventriculoscopic procedures for pineal, suprasellar, and tectal lesions have proven most useful to date.[121–124] Further study and technical refinements will lead to many more potential uses for these procedures in the treatment of hydrocephalus and its associated causes. The challenge for neurosurgeons is to define the indications and outcomes and refine the techniques for safely performing these useful procedures.

REFERENCES

1. Bondurant CP, Jimenez DF: Epidemiology of cerebrospinal fluid shunting. Pediatr Neurosurg 23:254–259, 1995.
2. Aronyk KE: The history and classification of hydrocephalus. Neurosurg Clin N Am 4:599–609, 1993.
3. Drake JM, Kestle J, Milner R, et al: Randomized trial of cerebrospinal fluid shunt valve design in pediatric hydrocephalus. Neurosurgery 43:294–305, 1998.
4. McCullough DC: A history of the treatment of hydrocephalus. Concepts Neurosurg 3:1–10, 1990.
5. Fisher RG: Surgery of the Congenital Anomalies. Baltimore: Williams & Wilkins, 1951.
6. Davidoff LE: Treatment of hydrocephalus. Arch Surg 18:1737–1762, 1929.
7. Sharpe W: The operative treatment of hydrocephalus: A preliminary report of forty-one patients. Am J Med Sci 153:563–571, 1917.
8. Cushing H: The special field of neurological surgery. Cleveland Med J 4:1–25, 1905.
9. Ferguson AH: Intraperitoneal diversion of the cerebrospinal fluid in cases of hydrocephalus. N Y Med 67:902, 1898.
10. Nicholl JH: Case of hydrocephalus in which peritoneo-meningeal drainage has been carried out. Glasgow Med J 63:187–191, 1905.
11. Dandy WE: Diagnosis and treatment of strictures of the aqueduct of Sylvius (causing hydrocephalus). Arch Surg 51:1–14, 1945.
12. Mixter WJ: Ventriculoscopy and puncture of the floor of the third ventricle. Boston Med Surg J 188:277–278, 1923.
13. Dandy WE: Extirpation of the choroid plexus of the lateral ventricles in communicating hydrocephalus. Ann Surg 68:569–579, 1918.
14. Torkildsen A: A new palliative operation in cases of inoperable occlusion of the sylvian aqueduct. Acta Chir Scand 82:117–124, 1939.
15. Nulsen FE, Spitz EB: Treatment of hydrocephalus by direct shunt from ventricle to jugular vein. Surg Forum 2:399–403, 1952.
16. Wallman LJ: Shunting for hydrocephalus: An oral history. Neurosurgery 11:308–313, 1982.
17. Pudenz RH: The surgical treatment of hydrocephalus—an historical review. Surg Neurol 15:15–26, 1981.
18. Fox JL, McCullough DC, Green RC: Effect of cerebrospinal fluid shunts on intracranial pressure and on cerebrospinal fluid dynamics. 2: A new technique of pressure measurements: Results and concepts. 3: A concept of hydrocephalus. J Neurol Neurosurg Psychiatry 36: 302–312, 1973.
19. Fox JL, Portnoy HD, Shulte RR: Cerebrospinal fluid shunts: An experimental evaluation of flow rates and pressure values in the anti-siphon valve. Surg Neurol 1:299–302, 1973.
20. Drake JM, Sainte-Rose C: The Shunt Book. New York: Blackwell Scientific, 1995.
21. Watts C, Keith HD: Testing the hydrocephalus shunt valve. Childs Brain 10:217–228, 1983.
22. Chapman PH, Cosman ER, Arnold MA: The relationship between ventricular fluid pressure and body position in normal subjects and subjects with shunts: A telemetric study. Neurosurgery 26:181–189, 1990.
23. Horton D, Pollay M: Fluid flow performance of a new siphon-control device for ventricular shunts. J Neurosurg 72:926–932, 1990.
24. Portnoy HD, Schulte RR, Fox JL, et al: Anti-siphon and reversible occlusion valves for shunting in hydrocephalus and preventing post-shunt subdural hematomas. J Neurosurg 38:729–738, 1973.
25. Sainte-Rose C, Hooven MD, Hirsch JF: A new approach to the treatment of hydrocephalus. J Neurosurg 66:213–226, 1987.
26. Langley JM, LeBlanc JC, Drake J, Milner R: Efficacy of antimicrobial prophylaxis in placement of cerebrospinal fluid shunts: Meta-analysis. Clin Infect Dis 17:98–103, 1993.
27. Horgan MA, Piatt JH, Jr: Shaving of the scalp may increase the rate of infection in CSF shunt surgery. Pediatr Neurosurg 26:180–184, 1997.
28. Bierbauer KS, Storrs BB, McLone DG, et al: A prospective, randomized study of shunt function and infections as a function of shunt placement. Pediatr Neurosurg 16:287–291, 1990.
29. Tuli S, O'Hayon B, Drake J, et al: Change in ventricular size and effect of ventricular catheter placement in pediatric patients with shunted hydrocephalus. Neurosurgery 45:1329–1333, 1999.
30. Sanders DY, Summers R, DeRouen L: Symptomatic pleural collection of cerebrospinal fluid caused by a ventriculopleural shunt. South Med J 90:345–346, 1997.
31. Beach C, Manthey DE: Tension hydrothorax due to ventriculopleural shunting. J Emerg Med 16:33–36, 1998.

32. Lam CH, Villemure JG: Comparison between ventriculoatrial and ventriculoperitoneal shunting in the adult population. Br J Neurosurg 11:43–48, 1997.

33. Lundar T, Langmoen IA, Hovind KH: Fatal cardiopulmonary complications in children treated with ventriculoatrial shunts. Childs Nerv Syst 7:215–217, 1991.

34. Decq P, Blanquet A, Yepes C: Percutaneous jugular placement of ventriculo-atrial shunts using a split sheath: Technical note. Acta Neurochir (Wien) 136:92–94, 1995.

35. McGrail KM, Muzzi DA, Losasso TJ, Meyer FB: Ventriculoatrial shunt distal catheter placement using transesophageal echocardiography: Technical note [see Comment in Neurosurgery 31:1136, 1992]. Neurosurgery 30:747–749, 1992.

36. Szczerbicki MR, Michalak M: Echocardiographic placement of cardiac tube in ventriculoatrial shunt: Technical note. J Neurosurg 85:723–724, 1996.

37. Drake JM, Kestle J: Determining the best cerebrospinal fluid shunt valve design: The pediatric valve design trial. Neurosurgery 38:604–607, 1996.

38. Piatt JH, Jr: Pumping the shunt revisited: A longitudinal study. Pediatr Neurosurg 25:73–76, 1996.

39. Vernet O, Farmer JP, Lambert R, Montes JL: Radionuclide shuntogram: Adjunct to manage hydrocephalic patients. J Nucl Med 37:406–410, 1996.

40. Steinbok P, Cochrane DD: Shunt removal by choroid plexus coagulation (Letter; Comment). J Neurosurg 85:981, 1996.

41. Drake JM, Kulkarni AV: Cerebrospinal fluid shunt infections. Neurosurg Q 3:283–294, 1993.

42. Borgbjerg BM, Gjerris F, Albeck MJ, Borgesen SE: Risk of infection after cerebrospinal fluid shunt: An analysis of 884 first-time shunts. Acta Neurochir (Wien) 136:1–7, 1995.

43. Choux M, Genitori L, Lang D, Lena G: Shunt implantation: Reducing the incidence of shunt infection. J Neurosurg 77:875–880, 1992.

44. Renier D, Lacombe J, Pierre-Kahn A, et al: Factors causing acute shunt infection: Computer analysis of 1174 operations. J Neurosurg 61:1072–1078, 1984.

45. Bayston R, Hart CA, Barnicoat M: Intraventricular vancomycin in the treatment of ventriculitis associated with cerebrospinal fluid shunting and drainage. J Neurol Neurosurg Psychiatry 50:1419–1423, 1987.

46. Schiff SJ, Oakes WJ: Delayed cerebrospinal-fluid shunt infection in children. Pediatr Neurosci 15:131–135, 1989.

47. Langley JM: Design for a Study of the Risk Factors for Cerebrospinal Fluid Shunt Infection. Master's thesis, McMaster University, Hamilton, Ontario, 1989.

48. Meirovitch J, Kitai-Cohen Y, Keren G, et al: Cerebrospinal fluid shunt infections in children. Pediatr Infect Dis J 6:921–924, 1987.

49. Brydon HL, Bayston R, Hayward R, Harkness W: Reduced bacterial adhesion to hydrocephalus shunt catheters mediated by cerebrospinal fluid proteins. J Neurol Neurosurg Psychiatry 60:671–675, 1996.

50. James HE, Walsh JW, Wilson HD, et al: Prospective randomized study of therapy in cerebrospinal fluid shunt infection. Neurosurgery 7:459–463, 1980.

51. Fischer G, Goebel H, Latta E: Penetration of the colon by a ventriculoperitoneal drain resulting in an intra-cerebral abscess. Zentralbl Neurochir 44:155–160, 1983.

52. Nadvi SS, Parboosing R, van Dellen JR: Cerebellar abscess: The significance of cerebrospinal fluid diversion. Neurosurgery 41:61–66, 1997.

53. Petrak RM, Pottage JC, Jr, Harris AA, Levin S: *Haemophilus influenzae* meningitis in the presence of a cerebrospinal fluid shunt. Neurosurgery 18:79–81, 1986.

54. Klein DM: Shunt infections. In Scott RM (ed): Hydrocephalus. Baltimore: Williams & Wilkins, 1990, p 88.

55. Kestle JRW, Hoffman HJ, Soloniuk D, et al: A concerted effort to prevent shunt infection. Childs Nerv Syst 9:163–165, 1993.

56. James HE, Nowak TP: Clinical course and diagnosis of migraine headaches in hydrocephalic children. Pediatr Neurosurg 17:310–316, 1991.

57. Dahlerup B, Gjerris F, Harmsen A, Sorensen PS: Severe headache as the only symptom of long-standing shunt dysfunction in hydrocephalic children with normal or slit ventricles revealed by computed tomography. Childs Nerv Syst 1:49–52, 1985.

58. Stellman-Ward GR, Bannister CM, Lewis MA, Shaw J: The incidence of chronic headache in children with shunted hydrocephalus. Eur J Pediatr Surg 7:12–14, 1997.

59. Di Rocco C: Is the slit ventricle syndrome always a slit ventricle syndrome? Childs Nerv Syst 10:49–58, 1994.

60. Coker SB: Cyclic vomiting and the slit ventricle syndrome. Pediatr Neurol 3:297–299, 1987.

61. Epstein F, Lapras C, Wisoff JH: 'Slit-ventricle syndrome': Etiology and treatment. Pediatr Neurosci 14:5–10, 1988.

62. Sgouros S, Malluci C, Walsh AR, Hockley AD: Long-term complications of hydrocephalus. Pediatr Neurosurg 23:127–132, 1995.

63. Walker ML, Fried A, Petronio J: Diagnosis and treatment of the slit ventricle syndrome. Neurosurg Clin N Am 4:707–714, 1993.

64. Reinprecht A, Dietrich W, Bertalanffy A, Czech T: The Medos Hakim programmable valve in the treatment of pediatric hydrocephalus. Childs Nerv Syst 13:588–593, 1997.

65. Baskin JJ, Manwaring KH, Rekate HL: Ventricular shunt removal: The ultimate treatment of the slit ventricle syndrome. J Neurosurg 88:478–484, 1998.

66. Sainte-Rose C, Hoffman HJ, Hirsch JF: Shunt failure. Concepts Pediatr Neurosurg 9:7–20, 1989.

67. Hoppe-Hirsch E, Laroussinie F, Brunet L, et al: Late outcome of the surgical treatment of hydrocephalus. Childs Nerv Syst 14:97–99, 1998.

68. Grant JA: Victor Darwin Lespinasse: A biographical sketch. Neurosurgery 39:1232–1237, 1996.

69. Dandy WE: An operative procedure for hydrocephalus. Bull Johns Hopkins Hosp 33:189–190, 1922.

70. Mixter W: Ventriculoscopy and puncture of the floor of the third ventricle. Boston Med Surg J 188:277–278, 1923.

71. Fay T, Grant FC: Ventriculoscopy and intraventricular photography in internal hydrocephalus. JAMA 80:461–463, 1966.

72. Griffith HB: Technique of fontanel and persutural ventriculoscopy in infants. Childs Brain 1:359–363, 1975.

73. Kelly PJ: Stereotactic third ventriculostomy in patients with nontumoral adolescent/adult onset aqueductal stenosis and symptomatic hydrocephalus [see Comment in J Neurosurg 76:890–891, 1992]. J Neurosurg 75:865–873, 1991.

74. Jones RF, Teo C, Stening WA, Kwok CT: Neuroendoscopic third ventriculostomy. In Manwaring KH, Crone KR (eds): Neuroendoscopy. New York: Mary Ann Liebert, 1992, pp 63–77.

75. Jones RF, Kwok BC, Stening WA, Vonau M: The current status of endoscopic third ventriculostomy in the management of noncommunicating hydrocephalus. Minim Invasive Neurosurg 37:28–36, 1994.

76. Sainte-Rose C, Chumas P: Endoscopic third ventriculostomy. Tech Neurosurg 1:176–184, 1996.

77. Jones RF, Stening WA, Brydon M: Endoscopic third ventriculostomy. Neurosurgery 26:86–91, 1990.

78. Teo C, Jones R: Management of hydrocephalus by endoscopic third ventriculostomy in patients with myelomeningocele. Pediatr Neurosurg 25:57–63, 1996.

79. Brockmeyer D, Abtin K, Carey L, Walker ML: Endoscopic third ventriculostomy: An outcome analysis. Pediatr Neurosurg 28:236–240, 1998.

80. Jaksche H, Loew F: Burr hole third ventriculo-cisternostomy: An unpopular but effective procedure for treatment of certain forms of occlusive hydrocephalus. Acta Neurochir (Wien) 79:48–51, 1986.

81. Drake JM: Ventriculostomy for treatment of hydrocephalus. Neurosurg Clin N Am 4:657–666, 1993.

82. Natelson SE: Early third ventriculostomy in meningomyelocele infants—shunt independence? Childs Brain 8:321–325, 1981.

83. Patterson RH, Jr, Bergland RM: The selection of patients for third ventriculostomy based on experience with 33 operations. J Neurosurg 29:252–254, 1968.

84. Sayers MP, Kosnik EJ: Percutaneous third ventriculostomy: Experience and technique. Childs Brain 2:24–30, 1976.

85. Vries JK, Friedman WA: Postoperative evaluation of third ventriculostomy patients using ^{111}In-DTPA. Childs Brain 6:200–205, 1980.

86. Jones RF, Kwok BC, Stening WA, Vonau M: Neuroendoscopic third ventriculostomy: A practical alternative to extracranial shunts in noncommunicating hydrocephalus. Acta Neurochir Suppl 61:79–83, 1994.

87. Jones RF, Stening WA, Kwok BC, Sands TM: Third ventriculostomy for shunt infections in children. Neurosurgery 32:855–859, 1993.

88. Yamamoto M, Oka K, Ikeda K, Tomonaga M: Percutaneous flexible neuroendoscopic ventriculostomy in patients with shunt malfunction as an alternative procedure to shunt revision. Surg Neurol 42:218–223, 1994.

89. Perlman BB: Percutaneous third ventriculostomy in the treatment of a hydrocephalic infant with aqueduct stenosis. Int Surg 49:443–448, 1968.

90. Reddy K, Fewer HD, West M, Hill NC: Slit ventricle syndrome with aqueduct stenosis: Third ventriculostomy as definitive treatment [see Comment in Neurosurgery 25:317–318, 1989]. Neurosurgery 23:756–759, 1988.

91. Hoffman HJ, Harwood-Nash D, Gilday DL: Percutaneous third ventriculostomy in the management of noncommunicating hydrocephalus. Neurosurgery 7:313–321, 1980.
92. Foltz EL: Treatment of hydrocephalus by ventricular shunts (Letter). Childs Nerv Syst 12:289–290, 1996.
93. Pudenz R, Foltz E: Hydrocephalus: Overdrainage by ventricular shunts—a review and recommendations. Surg Neurol 35:200–212, 1991.
94. Heilman CB, Cohen AR: Endoscopic ventricular fenestration using a "saline torch." J Neurosurg 74:224–229, 1991.
95. Sainte-Rose C: Third ventriculostomy. In Manwaring KH, Crone KR (eds): Neuroendoscopy. New York: Mary Ann Liebert, 1992, pp 47–62.
96. Crone KR: Endoscopic technique for removal of adherent ventricular catheters. In Manwaring KH, Crone KR (eds): Neuroendoscopy. New York: Mary Ann Liebert, 1992, pp 41–46.
97. Scarff JE: Evaluation of treatment of hydrocephalus: Results of third ventriculostomy and endoscopic cauterization of choroid plexuses compared with mechanical shunts. Arch Neurol 14:382–391, 1966.
98. Forjaz S, Martelli N, Latuf N: Hypothalamic ventriculostomy with catheter: Technical note. J Neurosurg 29:655–659, 1968.
99. Oka K, Go Y, Kin Y, et al: The radiographic restoration of the ventricular system after third ventriculostomy. Minim Invasive Neurosurg 38:158–162, 1995.
100. Schwartz TH, Yoon SS, Cutruzzola FW, Goodman RR: Third ventriculostomy: Post-operative ventricular size and outcome. Minim Invasive Neurosurg 39:122–129, 1996.
101. Jack CR, Jr, Kelly PJ: Stereotactic third ventriculostomy: Assessment of patency with MR imaging. AJNR Am J Neuroradiol 10:515–522, 1989.
102. Goumnerova LC, Frim DM: Treatment of hydrocephalus with third ventriculocisternostomy: Outcome and CSF flow patterns. Pediatr Neurosurg 27:149–152, 1997.
103. Wilcock DJ, Jaspan T, Worthington BS, Punt J: Neuro-endoscopic third ventriculostomy: Evaluation with magnetic resonance imaging. Clin Radiol 52:50–54, 1997.
104. Lev S, Bhadelia RA, Estin D, et al: Functional analysis of third ventriculostomy patency with phase-contrast MRI velocity measurements. Neuroradiology 39:175–179, 1997.
105. Wilcock DJ, Jaspan T, Punt J: CSF flow through third ventriculostomy demonstrated with colour Doppler ultrasonography. Clin Radiol 51:127–129, 1996.
106. Frim DM, Goumnerova LC: Telemetric intraventricular pressure measurements after third ventriculocisternostomy in a patient with noncommunicating hydrocephalus. Neurosurgery 41:1425–1428, 1997.
107. Hirsch JF, Hirsch E, Sainte-Rose C, et al: Stenosis of the aqueduct of Sylvius: Etiology and treatment. J Neurosurg Sci 30:29–39, 1986.
108. Dalrymple SJ, Kelly PJ: Computer-assisted stereotactic third ventriculostomy in the management of noncommunicating hydrocephalus. Stereotact Funct Neurosurg 59:105–110, 1992.
109. Goodman RR: Magnetic resonance imaging-directed stereotactic endoscopic third ventriculostomy. Neurosurgery 32:1043–1047, 1993.
110. Teo C, Rahman S, Boop FA, Cherny B: Complications of endoscopic neurosurgery. Childs Nerv Syst 12:248–253, 1996.
111. Handler MH, Abbott R, Lee M: A near-fatal complication of endoscopic third ventriculostomy: Case report. Neurosurgery 35:525–527, 1994.
112. McLaughlin MR, Wahlig JB, Kaufmann AM, Albright AL: Traumatic basilar aneurysm after endoscopic third ventriculostomy: Case report. Neurosurgery 41:1400–1403, 1997.
113. Zamorano L, Chavantes C, Moure F: Endoscopic stereotactic interventions in the treatment of brain lesions. Acta Neurochir Suppl 61:92–97, 1994.
114. Lewis AI, Keiper GL, Jr, Crone KR: Endoscopic treatment of loculated hydrocephalus. J Neurosurg 82:780–785, 1995.
115. Cohen AR: Endoscopic ventricular surgery. Pediatr Neurosurg 19:127–134, 1993.
116. Rappaport ZH: Suprasellar arachnoid cysts: Options in operative management. Acta Neurochir (Wien) 122:71–75, 1993.
117. Decq P, Brugieres P, Le Guerinel C, et al: Percutaneous endoscopic treatment of suprasellar arachnoid cysts: Ventriculocystostomy or ventriculocystocisternostomy? Technical note. J Neurosurg 84:696–701, 1996.
118. Lewis AI, Crone KR, Taha J, et al: Surgical resection of third ventricle colloid cysts. Preliminary results comparing transcallosal microsurgery with endoscopy [see Comment in J Neurosurg 81:174–178, 1994]. J Neurosurg 81:174–178, 1994.
119. Ure BM, Holschneider AM: Ventriculoscopic implantation of ventricular shunts in children with hydrocephalus. Eur J Pediatr Surg 7:299–300, 1997.
120. Kellnar S, Boehm R, Ring E: Ventriculoscopy-aided implantation of ventricular shunts in patients with hydrocephalus. J Pediatr Surg 30:1450–1451, 1995.
121. Ellenbogen RG, Moores LE: Endoscopic management of a pineal and suprasellar germinoma with associated hydrocephalus: Technical case report. Minim Invasive Neurosurg 40:13–15, 1997.
122. Drake J: Neuroendoscopy Tumour Biopsy. New York: Mary Ann Leibert, 1992.
123. Ferrer E, Santamarta D, Garcia-Fructuoso G, et al: Neuroendoscopic management of pineal region tumours. Acta Neurochir (Wien) 139:12–20, 1997.
124. Oka K, Yamamoto M, Nagasaka S, Tomonaga M: Endoneurosurgical treatment for hydrocephalus caused by intraventricular tumors. Childs Nerv Syst 10:162–166, 1994.

38 Surgical Management of Adult Hydrocephalus

DAVID M. FRIM, RICHARD PENN, and MAUREEN LACY

INTRODUCTION

Hydrocephalus, from the Greek meaning "water in the head," is a general term used to describe many conditions of fluid collected in the intracranial space. For the purposes of this chapter, we define hydrocephalus as an inappropriate amount of cerebrospinal fluid (CSF) within the intracranial space at an inappropriate pressure. In this way, we can include a variety of both childhood and adult syndromes of abnormal CSF flow and absorption patterns and the sequelae of their treatments. This definition excludes syndromes such as the pseudotumor cerebri syndrome[1,2] whose etiology and treatment may be somewhat different from that of hydrocephalus. It would, however, include low-pressure hydrocephalus syndromes in which the ventricles stay enlarged with relatively normal pressures despite our lack of understanding of these syndromes.[3,4]

From a practical standpoint, the treatment of hydrocephalus in the adult can be divided into two broad categories: childhood onset and adult onset. The first situation revolves mostly around upkeep of shunting devices and monitoring of a care strategy already implemented to prevent or treat complications. The latter situation necessitates a standard approach of evaluation of a clinical entity, choice of intervention strategy, and then implementation of that intervention. We deal with these two situations separately.

MANAGEMENT OF THE ADULT TREATED FOR HYDROCEPHALUS AS A CHILD

As much as 40% of pediatric neurosurgical practice in most large centers involves the treatment of hydrocephalus. The most common etiologic factor is premature birth and intraventricular hemorrhage. The presumption is that blood in the CSF causes either scarring in the subarachnoid space or sclerosis from inflammation at the absorptive surface of the arachnoid villi. This situation decreases the absorption rate of fluid and causes hydrocephalus with four-ventricular dilatation. This condition has been referred to as communicating or absorptive hydrocephalus. Other etiologies for an absorptive defect in children can be a congenital incontinence of the arachnoid villi for a variety of etiologic reasons or an obstruction within the CSF pathways that will cause ventricular dilatation upstream from the obstruction. The most common situation that presents in this fashion is aqueductal stenosis from either scarring or a benign tectal tumor. In children, obstructive hydrocephalus is first approached with the question of whether the obstruction

can be removed or bypassed. Endoscopic third ventriculocisternostomy can be performed to bypass aqueductal obstruction with a high rate of success. At this stage in our ability to treat hydrocephalus, absorptive hydrocephalus causing dilatation of all four ventricles is almost always treated by an extracranial shunting device.

Children who have been treated with a third ventriculocisternostomy bypass need to be monitored into adulthood because there is a risk of the ostomy stenosing many years after its initial placement. The true incidence of this is not yet known but is believed to be relatively low if the ostomy has survived several years. The adult who presents with a third ventriculocisternostomy bypass from childhood can be periodically evaluated by an imaging study such as magnetic resonance imaging with a cinematic gated flow study through the ostomy.[5] If symptoms imply that the ostomy has begun to occlude, the lateral and third ventricles may slowly begin to enlarge. Options for treatment at this time include endoscopic re-exploration for reconstruction of the ostomy or placement of a shunting device.

The management of the majority of adult hydrocephalus that was first treated in childhood revolves around the upkeep of extracranial CSF shunting devices. The utility of yearly or every other year shunt checks for pediatric and adult patients is controversial. Our practice is to maintain a regimen of more or less yearly shunt check evaluations in all our adult patients with shunts to maintain contact with the patient and his or her family as well as to continually review the presentation and dangers of shunt malfunction. Where the upkeep of a shunting device in a child may concern issues of growth, such as ascertaining whether the extracranial portion of the shunt tubing is of adequate length during periods of growth or the ventricular catheter does not extrude from the ventricular system due to head growth, upkeep and management of shunting devices in adults are much more straightforward. In fact, shunt longevity is much longer in older children and adults than in infants,[6] presumably due to issues of growth. In the adult, as in the child, the most common overall complication of shunt placement will be a malfunction due to catheter or valve occlusion or fracture.[7,8] The next most common complication will be shunt infection, which is generally seen in an early phase after implantation.[9] Beyond that, issues of overdrainage and underdrainage may also need to be confronted.

Shunt malfunction in the adult, as generally seen in a child, will present with stereotypic symptoms more or less similar to past shunt malfunctions with the initial presentation of hydrocephalus. In adulthood in patients who are high functioning cognitively, the patient him- or herself may often be able to make the diagnosis on clinical grounds. The evaluation consists of the usual radiographic studies such as plain shunt radiographs and a head computed tomography scan after adequate patient history is taken and physical examination is performed. Oftentimes, the diagnosis of shunt malfunction will be made due to either mechanical obstruction of the shunt tubing or enlargement of the ventricular system. In that situation, the shunt is explored operatively in the usual fashion.

We have generally opened the scalp incision first to determine the ventricular catheter patency versus malfunction of the components from the valve to the distal tubing. We then replace one portion of the shunt, either that in the brain or the extracranial components in their entirety. Our experience, like that of others, has shown no benefit to replacing the entire shunt versus revision of the affected component.[6] Usually we replace a nonfunctioning valve with a valve of similar type if the patient had done well for some time with that same valve. This may be different from the situation in the infant or child in which, as the child grows, drainage needs may require a change to a valve type with other characteristics.

The advent of percutaneously programmable differential pressure valves and programmable valves with fused antisiphoning components (Table 38-1) allows some flexibility in installing a valve that can provide dynamics similar to those of the one being replaced and also retains the option of changing the shunting dynamics without operative intervention. With regard to shunt revision in the adult patient, generally we recommend replacing those components that are nonfunctional but not disturbing other components that appear to be functioning adequately.

Shunt infection in the adult patient presents almost always with some sign of systemic infection, either a fever, elevated serum leukocyte count, or frank meningitis, although the risk factors for infection as well as many commonly used approaches to reduce infection remain insufficiently studied to determine significance.[10] The severity of symptoms depends on the infectious agent and may range from headache with minimal other signs of infection (for relatively benign organisms such as *Staphylococcus epidermidis* or *Corynebacterium*) to a much more virulent picture of

life-threatening meningitis if the etiologic agent is *Staphylococcus aureus* or a gram-negative organism. A shunt infection needs to be treated as any foreign body infection would be in an adult with removal of all the infected foreign body material, which in general means removal of the entire shunt. Depending on the etiology of the hydrocephalus and the need for daily drainage, the shunt can be replaced with an external draining ventricular catheter or a lumbar drainage catheter for the period of the antibiotic treatment. Although the length of this period of temporary external drainage and antibiotic treatment can vary, most recommendations include at least several days of external drainage with negative CSF cultures before replacement of the shunting device in a new location, if possible.[10] Depending on the terminus of the shunt, whether it is in the peritoneum, the pleura, or the cardiac atrium, the infection may spread or become loculated in those areas and require separate treatment. One other late complication of infection in the adult population that is more common than in the pediatric population is sclerosis of an absorbing surface from acute or chronic infection. In the peritoneum, this presents as a CSF pseudocyst or ascites, and in the pleural space this may present as CSF pleural effusion. In that situation, once recurrent infection is ruled out, the distal CSF catheter may be moved to another location or placed in the vascular tree through the cardiac atrium where reabsorptive sclerosis is not present.

Shunt overdrainage and underdrainage in the adult can become a problem with age in which presumably the brain may require lower pressure analogous to the normal-pressure hydrocephalus syndrome, which is described below. In that situation, the approach to the shunting dynamics are similar to the normal- or low-pressure hydrocephalus situation in that a trial of drainage at a low pressure may be tried or a programmable valve can be placed to allow percutaneous programming to lower pressures.

Our impression is that in patients whom we have followed from childhood into adulthood, complications seem to be reduced as children reach adulthood. The etiologic basis for this is unclear but may have to do with cessation of growth and reduced physical activity. Upkeep and care of the adult who was treated for hydrocephalus as a child is quite rewarding and relatively straightforward.

TABLE 38-1 ▪ Example of Currently Available Shunting Valves

Differential pressure (siphoning): Contour valve (Medtronic Neurosurgery, Minneapolis, MN), Hakim valve (Integra Lifesciences, Plainsboro, NJ), Medos (Nonprogrammable) valve (Codman/J&J, Randolf, MA)

Nonsiphoning combination differential pressure valves: Delta valve (Medtronic Neurosurgery, Minneapolis, MN), Equiflow valve (Radionics/Integra Lifesciences, Plainsboro, NJ), Novus valve (Integra)

Percutaneously programmable variable pressure differential valves: Codman-Hakim programmable valve (Codman/J&J, Randolf, MA), Sophy valve (Sophysa, Orsay, France), Strata-NSC valve (Medtronic Neurosurgery, Minneapolis, MN)

Percutaneously programmable variable pressure nonsiphoning valve: Strata (Medtronic Neurosurgery, Minneapolis, MN)

Flow-dependent valves: Orbis-Sigma Valve (Integra Lifesciences, Plainsboro, NJ), Diamond Valve (Phoenix Biomedical, Mississauga, Ontario)

EVALUATION AND MANAGEMENT OF HYDROCEPHALUS PRESENTING IN ADULTHOOD

Introduction

The causes of hydrocephalus presenting in adulthood are the same and yet different from hydrocephalus presenting in childhood. Intraventricular and subarachnoid blood from aneurysmal subarachnoid hemorrhage or hemorrhage from intraparenchymal vascular malformations can cause chronic hydrocephalus via a mechanism believed to be similar to that seen in the absorptive hydrocephalus of prematurity. Similarly, bacterial meningitis can also cause inflammation and presumably scarring in the subarachnoid space or at the arachnoid villi that will cause an absorptive hydrocephalus. These entities will present with four-ventricle enlargement as in childhood. Obstructive lesions such as tectal tumors or even congenital scarring at the Sylvian aqueduct can cause triventricular enlargement and obstructive hydrocephalus, which will present in adulthood.[11] The treatment of aqueductal stenosis in an adult, similar to that in a child, will be third ventriculocisternostomy to bypass the obstruction.[12] Also, intraventricular tumors or large tumors abutting the ventricles can sometimes cause hydrocephalus from what is believed to be a CSF hyperprotein state that may perhaps reduce villus absorption of CSF. These causes of hydrocephalus and its presentation will mirror similar situations in childhood and will, of course, present with symptoms and signs of elevated intracranial pressure.

Normal Pressure Hydrocephalus (Adult-Onset Chronic Hydrocephalus)

Unique to adults is the normal- or low-pressure hydrocephalus seen with advanced age. This syndrome, first described by Hakim and Adams[13] 40 years ago, has been undergoing continual reevaluation over the years. Classically, this syndrome presents as a triad of gait disorder, incontinence, and cognitive dysfunction, usually attention and short-term memory loss that can mimic a dementia.[14] The patient will have CSF pressures measured in the normal range on lumbar puncture and symptoms may often be reduced by large volume removal of CSF. The diagnosis of normal-pressure hydrocephalus syndrome is a subject of considerable controversy, as is the decision to treat the syndrome by CSF shunting.[3] A variety of diagnostic approaches have been described. These include imaging by computed tomography or magnetic resonance imaging, which will show a characteristic pattern of ventricular enlargement with widening of the sylvian fissures and some of the cortical sulci.[15-17] If one or several large-volume lumbar taps reducing CSF pressure and volume relieves or reduces the symptomatology, this has been advocated as an indication for treatment. An infusion test of fluid into either the lumbar or ventricular CSF space while monitoring pressure response to a given volume has also been advocated as a test to predict outcome from shunting for this syndrome.[18] Bolus or continuous infusion can be used to measure compliance and outflow resistance. Long-term intracranial pressure measurements combined with magnetic resonance imaging to detect abnormal brain pressure waves have also been suggested.[19] Better results for shunting may be possible by using a high threshold for selection, but this may miss some patients who would benefit from, but are not selected for, surgery. Protocols of temporary lumbar[20] or ventricular drainage[21] to tonically reduce CSF pressures to even less than what would be the normal range combined with cognitive testing before and after several days of CSF drainage as well as daily physical therapy evaluations to assess gait function have also been used as predictors of outcome from shunting in this syndrome.[22] In our hands, such a protocol has had a 100% positive predictive value in 23 consecutive patients for a good outcome with shunting when clear improvement in neurocognition or gait function is observed after temporary lumbar drainage. However, the false-negative rate in our cohort has not been investigated by shunt placement when no improvement with temporary drainage is seen. The neuropsychology testing protocol used at the University of Chicago is presented in Table 38-2.

TABLE 38-2 ▪ Testing Protocol Used to Assess Neurocongnitive Responses to Long-Term Lumbar Drainage in the Patient with Normal-Pressure Hydrocephalus

Mini-Mental Status Examination
Repeatable Battery for the Assessment of Neuropsychological
  Status
Stroop Color Word Test
Delis-Kaplan Executive Functioning Scale-Card Sorting Test
Trail Making Test
Phoenemic Fluency
Clock Drawing
Grooved Pegboard
Geriatric Depression Inventory-15

Unfortunately, there are not yet universally accepted diagnostic criteria for normal-pressure hydrocephalus or an agreed-on set of predictors of outcome after shunt placement.

THE DECISION OF WHEN TO TREAT HYDROCEPHALUS IN THE ADULT

In adult hydrocephalus, symptoms are primarily due to inappropriate pressure within the ventricular system. Compression of brain tissue by ventricular enlargement may produce problems in gait due to stretching of subcortical white matter tracts. The rate of development of hydrocephalus differs significantly and affects which symptoms occur. Slow progression may lead to subtle changes in cognition; rapid progression will lead to headache and loss of consciousness. These symptoms can include headache, vomiting, mental status change, gait changes, extraocular movement deficit, visual changes, or cognitive changes. Obviously, hydrocephalus presenting after aneurysmal subarachnoid hemorrhage will be diagnosed in the ongoing evaluation and treatment of the lesion that has caused the bleeding. Similarly, hydrocephalus developing after meningitis will be recognized as the meningitis is treated. However, the exact threshold for treatment of hydrocephalus in the adult can sometimes be difficult to define. Clearly, symptoms such as headache or cognitive changes, which are interfering with life or lifestyle, would constitute indications for initiating treatment whether the hydrocephalus is from a process reducing absorption or one of obstruction. Radiographic evidence of enlarging ventricles in the absence of overt symptoms may also constitute indications for intervention, although in many cases, it is difficult to discern whether a process, such as an infection, has begun to cause global brain atrophy as opposed to inappropriate pressure within the ventricular system causing ventricular enlargement.

Using our definition of hydrocephalus as an inappropriate amount of CSF under an inappropriate pressure, a measurement of CSF pressure either by lumbar puncture (in the situation of communicating hydrocephalus) or by direct ventricular access in the setting of triventricular enlargement from obstruction is diagnostic when combined with imaging. A secondary criteria when CSF pressure is measured by lumbar puncture or ventricular tap is to observe a reduction in presenting symptoms by a reduction in CSF pressure. This is the analogous situation to the large-volume CSF removal that is often performed for the diagnosis of normal-pressure hydrocephalus syndrome. The exact limits of what is considered normal CSF pressure in adults is unclear. Many would consider pressures as high as 20 cm H_2O in the lumbar space with the patient in a supine position to be within the normal range. However, sometimes symptoms of elevated intracranial pressure can be witnessed when pressure is measured to be as low as 15 to 18 cm H_2O, and those symptoms can be ameliorated by reduction in the CSF pressure to less than 10 or even less than 5 cm H_2O. This situation begins to establish a continuum of inappropriate CSF pressures in the adult that begins in the clearly abnormal range above 20 or 25 cm H_2O but can end quite squarely in the middle of what most would consider a normal pressure value. In a similar fashion, pressures as high as the mid-20s can be asymptomatic with no change in ventricular size. Whether this defines compensated hydrocephalus or simply a variant of normal is unclear.

In any case, symptoms that are referable to elevated intracranial pressure in the presence of an enlarged ventricular space that can be ameliorated or reduced by drainage of CSF constitutes a clear indication for treatment of hydrocephalus. In the absence of a pressure measurement, symptoms referable to elevated intracranial pressure that coincide with enlarged or enlarging ventricles also call for treatment. Precise indications for intervention are sometimes not possible, even considering ventricular size, CSF pressure, and the effect of drainage of CSF. Each case must be individually evaluated by the treating neurosurgeon. The goal of treatment is to restore a CSF pressure and dynamic that maximally reduces symptoms while maintaining the pressures within a range appropriate for cerebral profusion and also reduction in ventricular size to a normal range.

CHOICES OF TECHNIQUES FOR TREATING HYDROCEPHALUS AND OF SHUNTING STRATEGY AND SHUNTING HARDWARE

The general approach to an individual presenting with symptomatic hydrocephalus or radiographic enlargement of ventricles will depend on the etiology of the hydrocephalus. In practical terms, obstructive hydrocephalus should generally be considered for a bypass procedure or removal of obstruction before resorting to extracranial shunting. Hydrocephalus due to absorption or obstruction of the subarachnoid space with four-ventricle enlargement should be approached with extracranial shunting primarily. Aqueductal stenosis in a center where expertise is available should be treated by a third ventriculocisternostomy, which may avoid the need for permanently implanted hardware.[23] However, extracranial shunting is certainly an option that will also adequately treat this type of hydrocephalus. Extracranial shunting for obstruction or for four-ventricle hydrocephalus does, however, provide the additional possibility of fine-tuning CSF drainage dynamics and pressures that a bypass procedure cannot accomplish.

Shunting Strategy and Shunting Hardware

Adults may be more sensitive to CSF dynamic pressure changes than children. This may be due to the decreased plasticity of the adult brain. Certainly, the existence of normal-pressure hydrocephalus syndrome in adults suggests

that shunting in the adult may require a specific low CSF pressure or high flow rather than simply restoring elevated pressure to a normal range and allowing the brain to accommodate. Therefore, different shunting strategies may be of use in adult hydrocephalus.

The standard extracranial shunt operation now performed in this country is a ventricular catheter placed either frontally or occipitally and subcutaneously tunneled to an entry into the peritoneum. An intervening valve and often a tapping reservoir allow control of shunting pressure and access to the CSF space. The peritoneum provides little pressure of its own and allows drainage and reabsorption of a large volume of fluid. Alternative shunting strategies can rest on a different absorptive surface than the peritoneum. The cardiac atrium provides an egress for a very large volume of CSF. It can also handle high protein content that could cause malabsorption of spinal fluid in the peritoneal space. The pleural space also provides an alternative extracranial absorptive surface, but the pleural space generates its own negative pressure. This can be used to advantage in constructing a shunting system that will provide less than normal pressure or even negative pressure if the valve is chosen appropriately.[24] Antisiphoning components, which prevent negative pressure in the shunt tubing, can be used to counteract the negative pressure "sink" of the pleural space. The gallbladder can also be used as an absorptive surface, and it provides a positive pressure postprandially that prevents overdrainage.[25] In addition, recipient sites such as the internal jugular vein in reverse orientation may also be used in the adult more so than in a child because of easier access and a larger anatomy in which to place the distal shunting tube.[26]

Concerning placement of the catheter into the ventricular system, the larger head and larger ventricles of the adult provide better landmarks than those of the child. We have generally advocated a frontal approach in adults with small ventricles because of ease of ventricular access. An occipital approach is reasonable when the ventricles are large because it allows more catheter length to be placed within the ventricle and, particularly under endoscopic guidance, can allow the catheter tip to be placed as far as possible away from the choroid plexus at the foramen of Monro.

A variety of shunting components are now available for use in constructing a shunting system. Although ventricular catheters and burr hole reservoirs are similar, shunt valves can be divided into three general groupings: differential pressure valves that siphon, differential pressure valves plus an antisiphoning chamber that reduces siphoning, and valves designed to maintain constant flow of CSF called flow control or flow-dependent valves (see Table 38-1). The differential pressure valves will siphon when an adult stands upright and may cause low-pressure symptoms. However, this is a strategy that may be useful in a shunting system that will drain CSF to a less than normal pressure. The antisiphoning shunt valves will provide a more normal postural pressure dynamic but may underdrain in patients with normal-pressure hydrocephalus.[27] The flow control valves are not free of complications of overdrainage in normal-pressure hydrocephalus[28] but are of value in patients who may require constant flow or flow that is more robust than that seen in the nonsiphoning combination valves. In any case, a thoughtful choice of an initial shunt system may prevent valve revision if the shunting system does not match individual patient's needs. However, there are times when two or even all three of the valve types will need to be tried if a patient remains symptomatic from initial valve placement.

There are currently three percutaneously programmable differential pressure valves available for purchase. The valve setting mechanisms range in pressure from 3 and 20 cm H_2O by various increments. Only one of these valves, the Strata valve (Medtronic Neurosurgery) is manufactured with a fused antisiphoning chamber. To make the other two programmable valves (Hakim-Codman valve, Codman/Johnson & Johnson; Sophy valve; Sophysa) into nonsiphoning valves, antisiphoning chambers need to be spliced inline distal to the valve mechanism. The programmable valve can be of great use in the adult shunting system because adults may be less able to adapt to a fixed pressure than children whose brains are more plastic.[29,30] Therefore, variable pressure settings may allow fine-tuning of shunting pressures to symptoms. In addition, there is the theoretical benefit in the situation of normal-pressure hydrocephalus or hydrocephalus with large ventricles and a small cortical mantel in initially placing a shunt in a patient with a high differential pressure setting on the valve and then slowly decreasing that pressure to a more normal or even lower than normal one. This may allow better accommodation and prevent ventricular collapse from sudden overdrainage, with the attendant risk of subdural hematoma due to rupture of bridging subdural veins. In the future, hardware cost may dictate much of the decision making in shunt system construction. For now, the many choices of shunt valves and other accompanying hardware makes selecting shunting hardware difficult, particularly because no randomized studies show any system to be clearly superior.[12] Matching the shunt system to the patient's individual needs is an art.

TECHNICAL ASPECTS IN THE TREATMENT OF ADULT HYDROCEPHALUS

Technique of Endoscopic Third Ventriculocisternostomy

Endoscopic third ventriculocisternostomy is performed in an identical fashion in adults and children. We recommend a coronal burr hole at the mid-pupillary line and dural opening to allow a 12.5- or 14-French introducer with trocar. Once the ventricular space is entered, an endoscope, either rigid or flexible, is placed within the ventricular system and navigated through the foramen of Monro.

The landmarks for this navigation[31] are the choroid plexus in the choroidal fissure, which dives into the foramen, and the septal and thalamostriate veins, which enter medially and anterolaterally into foramen of Monro. Once the foramen is traversed, navigation through the third ventricle is based on identification of the paired mammillary bodies from which one can discern the midline and anteriorly the retrochiasmatic space. Frequently, behind the retrochiasmatic space, a small red stripe that corresponds to the infundibulum is seen. In the space between the retrochiasmatic recess and the mammillary bodies is the flat and often thinned anterior floor of the third ventricle. We use a point

one third of the way back from the retrochiasmatic recess for our ostomy hole. This minimizes the risk of injury to the basilar artery, which is generally positioned beneath the anterior floor in the posterior half. A blunt 1-mm probe is used to gently traverse through the floor of the third ventricle. The probe is left in place for a moment to potentially tamponade bleeding in the floor. Then a Fogerty balloon dilator of either 3 or 4 mm in size is introduced. This can be placed through a working channel of the endoscope either with or without concurrent irrigation. The ostomy is gently dilated by inflating the balloon within it. An alternative technique of inflating the balloon on the inferior side of the ostomy and pulling it through the hole to tear the tissue can be successful though may cause bleeding. Bleeding is controlled either with warm saline irrigation or with unipolar or bipolar cautery devices available for work through the endoscope. Once the bleeding is controlled, the endoscope can be navigated through the ostomy to inspect the prepontine cistern where it is used to fenestrate leaflets of arachnoid if that can be safely done without injury to the basilar artery. Once there is free flow of CSF throughout the prepontine cistern and through the ostomy hole, the ventriculoscope is withdrawn from the third ventricle, inspected for bleeding, and then withdrawn into the lateral ventricle.

In adults, we leave a ventricular catheter placed under endoscopic guidance by withdrawing the endoscope into the introducer sheath and then placing the sheath approximately 1 cm away from Monro's foramen. The ventriculoscope is then removed, and a ventricular catheter is placed so that it will be (by measured length) at the tip of the introducer, which is then peeled away out of the hole. The catheter is cut and connected to a blunt-ended burr hole reservoir. This catheter and tapping reservoir provide emergency access to CSF should there be sudden catastrophic occlusion of the ostomy. The patency of a third ventriculocisternostomy after several months to years is between 60% and 80%. If the ostomy provides egress of CSF for several years, even if it occludes at that time, the procedure can be repeated safely. Early failure of the ostomy generally requires extracranial CSF shunting for a permanent solution.

Techniques for the Placement of an Extracranial Shunting Device in Adults

Ventriculoperitoneal shunts are placed in an identical fashion in adults and children. As a general rule of thumb, connections in the shunt devices should be minimized and whenever possible connections should be against the direction of tube movement such as a right angle connection from a burr hole reservoir device into the proximal end of a ventricular catheter. Ample tubing must be placed into the peritoneal or pleural space for catheter movement; however, issues of selecting a shunt catheter of adequate length for growth no longer apply in adulthood.

The procedures for placement of a ventriculoperitoneal shunt begins with the patient placed in the supine position with the head turned away from the side of the ventricular access. Usually, we place the head in the lateral position with the falx parallel to the floor and a roll under the shoulder ipsilateral to the shunt placement. Hair can be shaved or not per the surgeon's preference.[32] The entry site is chosen to be either at the coronal suture in the mid-pupillary line for frontal access to the ventricle or approximately 5 or 6 cm above the inion and 4 to 5 cm lateral from the midline for occipital access. The surgical prep is continuous from the frontal or occipital region and down along a track to the neck, chest, and belly. The shunting device is tested to make sure that it closes at an appropriate pressure and that all connections are secured. The abdominal incision is either in the upper midline or subcostal. Care is taken to cover all skin surfaces with iodine-impregnated adhesive drapery and to minimize the exposed skin surfaces. We have infused intravenous antibiotics within 45 minutes of placement of the skin incision.

An incision is made and then layers are divided through fascia in the midline or through fascia and muscles in a sub-costal incision until the peritoneum is identified below the linea alba in the midline or below the posterior rectus fascia in the subcostal position. The peritoneum is grasped and then opened. The scalp incision is made over the selected burr hole entry site. A skin flap is then elevated and retracted. A burr hole is made with a perforator using either a power or hand drill. Before the dura is opened, a pocket is made inferior to the burr hole and then a shunt-tunneling device is used to tunnel from the burr hole to the peritoneum. In the case of a frontal entry site, an intermediate incision behind the ear is usually required to "turn the corner" with the tunneling device. Either a tunneling sheath or a long silk tie is then used to pull the shunting components from the head to the abdominal incision. Once in place with a burr hole reservoir or other connector over the burr hole, the dura is opened with unipolar cautery and the pia with bipolar cautery. The trajectory into the ventricular system can be determined either by preoperative computed tomography scanning or by estimate using the contralateral medial canthus at a level in the midforehead for an occipital approach and for a frontal approach using lines from the frontal burr hole to the medial canthus and from the burr hole to halfway between the lateral canthus and tragus. Once the catheter is placed and CSF egress is seen, the con-nection is made to the connector at the burr hole and is secured. All incisions are closed in layers. For ventriculo-pleural access, we make an incision at the third or fourth rib off the midline in the same line that one would use for passage of the peritoneal catheter for a ventriculoperitoneal shunt. We then dissect down to the pleura through the muscles of the anterior chest wall and the intercostal muscles. Once the pleura is identified, it is not opened until the shunt is entirely connected. Analogous to the peritoneal catheter, which is placed in the peritoneum after the ventricular catheter is connected to the shunt, we also connect the ventricular catheter to the shunting device, visualize distal run off of CSF and then under direct vision we have made a pleural egress with a long hemostat and then placed approx-imately 20 cm of tubing into the pleural space. Alternatively, a trocar may be used for the catheter to be placed blindly. We recommend placement of a positive end-expiratory pressure valve in the anesthesia circuit to maintain lung inflation during placement of the pleural catheter and thus avoid a pneumothorax.

For ventriculoatrial shunt placement, the procedure can be done with fluoroscopic assistance. After the shunting device is connected either frontally or occipitally and a valve

and distal tubing are in place, a tunnel is made from either the distal nipple of the valve (if placed occipitally) or from a cut in the tubing at an intermediate incision behind the ear (if placed frontally) to a point over the internal jugular vein. This point is selected by placement of a "finding" needle and then a larger needle and J wire into the internal jugular vein on the neck lateral to the shunt. The incision is enlarged with a stab wound and adequate tubing is tunneled from the exposed distal valve nipple (or intermediate inci-sion behind the ear) to the neck incision to allow the blunt-end catheter tubing into the cardiac atrium with an additional several centimeters for positioning. Once the wire is visual-ized in the cardiac atrium by fluoroscopy, a 9- or 10-French introducer sheath is placed over the wire and the wire removed and the tubing threaded directly through the introducer sheath into the cardiac atrium under fluoroscopic guidance. If there is some kink in the venous system, the wire can be guided into the cardiac atrium and the atrial tubing threaded over the wire into the atrium. The tubing is then pulled back until it makes a straight connection to the shunt with the tip at the right atrium–superior vena cava junction. Before connection, the atrial catheter is flushed with heparinized saline. Incisions are then closed in layers.

In our practice, other places for reabsorption of CSF, such as the gallbladder, are approached with the assistance of a general surgeon. Laparoscopic placement of peritoneal tubes also usually requires the assistance of a general surgeon until comfort is attained with that technique.

Complications of Treatment of Adult Hydrocephalus

Complications of a third ventriculostomy or other bypass procedures, whether they be fenestration of ventricular walls, cyst walls, or removal of obstructing tumors, are specific to the surgery for the bypass procedure. If the surgery proceeds without any immediate complications, the major long-term problem is whether the bypass ostomy occludes with time. This occurrence recapitulates the presenting symptoms of the hydrocephalus. If the ostomy fails, a decision will need to be made as to whether the ostomy can be reconstructed or whether the patient should proceed to placement of an extracranial shunting device.

Complications of extracranial shunting include shunt malfunction, shunt infection, overdrainage and under-drainage of CSF, and complications relating to injury to the absorptive site by the distal shunting catheter.

Shunt malfunction is caused by occlusion or impedance to flow along the shunting device. The most common place for shunt malfunction occurs near the ventricular catheter from ingrowth of choroid plexus or other debris into the catheter, and this is true for both children and adults in our experience. Valve function can be degraded by particulate matter or protein within the CSF and necessitate valve replacement. Distal catheter occlusion in the peritoneal space can be precipitated by tissue ingrowth into the distal shunt tube. In all these situations, surgery must be performed to test the shunt components and to replace that which is malfunctioning.

The patient's history and physical findings most often suggest elevated intracranial pressure. The symptoms often recapitulate those that occurred at the time of initial presentation with hydrocephalus. The elevation in CSF pressure can be tested by lumbar puncture in absorptive hydrocephalus or by direct shunt tap if the shunt does not communicate with the lumbar CSF space. Once the diagnosis of shunt malfunction is established, the patient will need to be brought to the operating room for exploration.

We always "prep" the entire length of the shunt. The incision overlying the ventricular burr hole is first opened, and then the proximal and distal components of the shunt are disconnected and tested individually. The component that is occluded or malfunctioning is replaced. Proximally, the ventricular catheter is frequently occluded and will need replacement. If distal function is compromised, the valve or tubing is occluded and will need to be removed. Sometimes the manipulation of the shunting components during exploration will release a site of impedance of CSF flow. In those situations, the ventricular catheter is the most likely culprit based on clinical experience. In some cases, if shunt function was demonstrated preoperatively to be nonoptimal, the entire shunting system may need to be replaced if no specific malfunction is found at the time of surgery.

Shunt Infection

Shunt infection is treated identically in the adult and the child. Suspicion for shunt infection is based on clinical presentation and CSF cultures. There is a higher yield for positive culture in the setting of infection from fluid obtained directly from the shunt by shunt tap than by a lumbar puncture in our hands. Once laboratory investigation data support infection either by Gram stain or culture results, the entire shunt is removed and replaced by a temporary draining ventriculostomy or, in some cases, a lumbar drainage catheter. In some cases of normal-pressure hydrocephalus in which the patient has no overt or dangerous symptoms of hydrocephalus causing intracranial hypertension, the shunt may be removed in its entirety to have a period with no foreign body in the CSF space. Cultures are monitored daily from the external draining device when present. After several days of negative cultures, a new shunting device can be replaced at a site separate from the infected one. Few data provide a guideline for the length of temporary drainage before a new shunt is placed. Considerable variability in treatment of shunt infections is quite evident from the literature.[9,10] It seems that the standard of care encompasses both direct replacement of shunts under antibiotic coverage with no intermediate phase of external drainage or external drainage that can be anything from a few days to several weeks under antibiotic coverage.

Other Complications

The shunting complication of overdrainage or underdrainage is one that is very difficult to treat. In general, overdrainage from shunting is diagnosed by a postural headache that improves with lying down. This can be approached by insertion of an antisiphoning device if that is not yet in the shunting system or by changing the valve to a higher pressure. The percutaneous programmable valves are particularly useful for finding a pressure that is appropriate. In some cases, the distal shunt tubing will need to be moved to a different location that decreases drainage such as the gallbladder or the internal jugular vein in reverse orientation. Changes of valve type from differential pressure or differential pressure with an antisiphoning component to a flow-dependent valve sometimes will also alleviate symptoms. It should be noted however, that overdrainage is generally a problem that will cause symptoms but as yet has not been described as having long-term effects on neurologic function beyond the symptoms. Underdrainage of extracranial CSF shunting devices is a problem encountered more often in adults than in children. In particular, normal-pressure hydrocephalus, which by definition calls for CSF drainage to a less than normal pressure, can be inadequately treated by underdrainage. Valve changes by removing an antisiphoning component or by replacing a differential pressure valve with a flow-regulated valve may sometimes provide additional drainage. Also, revising the terminus of the shunting device from the peritoneal space to the pleural space, which generates negative pressure, can improve drainage characteristics. One particular caveat of normal-pressure hydrocephalus syndrome is that in several of our patients, we have observed that, with time, the syndrome requires lower and lower pressure drainage to achieve therapeutic results. The etiology of this change is not known, nor is the reason why it only seems to affect a subset of the population. However, eventually manipulations to provide lower and lower pressure can be exhausted.

The one acute potential complication of overdrainage, particularly in the elderly, is ventricular collapse and disruption of the subdural bridging veins causing subdural hematoma. This is a potentially catastrophic complication in individuals who have compromised brain function. In general, when the subdural collection is small, we have advocated placing an antisiphoning device, if one is not yet in the system, and also increasing the valve pressure. Although this will usually resolve a small subdural collection in the situation of normal-pressure hydrocephalus, it results in bringing back the original symptoms. Usually, patients can tolerate several weeks of no symptomatic relief to resolve the subdural hematoma before readjusting valve pressure gradually lower. The use of a percutaneous programmable valve has greatly simplified this process.[33] Another complication of overdrainage is the slit-ventricle syndrome. Thankfully, this is relatively rare in the adult population, but a variety of approaches to this problem have been advocated. They range from changes in valve pressure or the addition of an antisiphoning device to decompression of the intracranial space by craniectomy. Recently, we have found that addition of a lumboperitoneal shunting system to the functioning ventricular shunting system can also alleviate symptoms.[34] The slit-ventricle syndrome can be diagnosed by high CSF pressures in the presence of slitlike ventricles and functioning ventriculoperitoneal shunt. Several more detailed discussions of its manifestations and treatment have been published.[35,36]

CONCLUSIONS

The treatment of the adult with hydrocephalus is similar and yet distinct from that of a child in many respects. Much of the treatment of adult hydrocephalus will be the ongoing maintenance of shunting devices placed during childhood.

Diagnosis of adult-onset hydrocephalus of any type is made based on evidence of an inappropriate amount of CSF at an inappropriate pressure in the intracranial space. However, the normal-pressure hydrocephalus syndrome in the adult population makes the determination of what is an appropriate pressure confusing. Hydrocephalus from an obstructive source can be bypassed or the obstruction can be attacked directly, thereby resolving the symptomatology. For hydrocephalus due to abnormal absorption, shunting of CSF to an extracranial absorptive surface is needed. Various shunting systems with different valve types exist, and several potential absorptive surfaces are available. Choosing the best valve and the optimal absorptive surface must be individualized. Bypassing an obstruction and extracranial shunting can result in several types of surgical complications. However, shunt malfunction, shunt infection, overshunting, and undershunting can be treated successfully if approached in a thoughtful manner. The treatment of hydrocephalus in the adult can be a rewarding exercise in the diagnosis of the syndrome and in the use of current technology to treat it.

REFERENCES

1. Kosmorsky G: Pseudotumor cerebri. Neurosurg Clin N Am 12:775–797, 2001.
2. Johnston I, Paterson A: Benign intracranial hypertension. I: Diagnosis and prognosis. Brain 97:289–300, 1974.
3. Hebb AO, Cusimano MD: Idiopathic normal pressure hydrocephalus: A systematic review of diagnosis and outcome. Neurosurgery 49:1166–1184, 2001.
4. Lamas E, Esparza J, Diez Lobato R: Intracranial pressure in adult non-tumoral hydrocephalus. J Neurosurg Sci 19:226–233, 1975.
5. Goumnerova LC, Frim DM: Treatment of hydrocephalus with third ventriculocisternostomy: Outcome and CSF flow patterns. Pediatr Neurosurg 27:149–152, 1997.
6. Piatt JH Jr, Carlson CV: A search for determinants of cerebrospinal fluid shunt survival: Retrospective analysis of a 14-year institutional experience. Pediatr Neurosurg 19:233–242, 1993.
7. Kast J, Duong D, Nowzari F, et al: Time-related patterns of ventricular shunt failure. Childs Ner Syst 10:524–528, 1994.
8. Puca A, Anile C, Maira G, Rossi G: Cerebrospinal fluid shunting for hydrocephalus in the adult: Factors related to shunt revision. Neurosurgery 29:822–826, 1991.
9. Piatt JH Jr: Cerebrospinal fluid shunt failure: Late is different from early. Pediatr Neurosurg 23:133–139, 1995.
10. Borgbjerg BM, Gjerris F, Albeck MJ, Borgesen SE: Risk of infection after cerebrospinal fluid shunt: An analysis of 884 first-time shunts. Acta Neurochir 136:1–7, 1995.
11. Fukuhara T, Luciano MG: Clinical features of late-onset idiopathic aqueductal stenosis. Surg Neurol 55:132–137, 2001.
12. Aschoff A, Kremer P, Hashemi B, Kunze S: The scientific history of hydrocephalus and its treatment. Neurosurg Rev 22:67–95, 1999.
13. Bret P, Guyotat J, Chazal J: Is normal pressure hydrocephalus a valid concept in 2002? A reappraisal in five questions and proposal for a new designation of the syndrome as "chronic hydrocephalus" [see comment]. J Neurol Neurosurg Psychiatry 73:9–12, 2002.
14. Meier U, Zeilinger FS, Kintzel D: Signs, symptoms and course of normal pressure hydrocephalus in comparison with cerebral atrophy. Acta Neurochir 141:1039–1048, 1999.
15. Raftopoulos C, Massager N, Baleriaux D, et al: Prospective analysis by computed tomography and long-term outcome of 23 adult patients with chronic idiopathic hydrocephalus. Neurosurgery 38:51–59, 1996.
16. Hurley RA, Bradley WG Jr, Latifi HT, Taber KH: Normal pressure hydrocephalus: Significance of MRI in a potentially treatable dementia. J Neuropsychiatry Clin Neurosci 11:297–300, 1999.
17. Mase M, Yamada K, Banno T, et al: Quantitative analysis of CSF flow dynamics using MRI in normal pressure hydrocephalus. Acta Neurochir Suppl 71:350–353, 1998.
18. Meier U, Bartels P: The importance of the intrathecal infusion test in the diagnosis of normal pressure hydrocephalus. J Clin Neurosci 9:260–267, 2002.
19. Qureshi AI, Williams MA, Razumovsky AY, Hanley DF: Magnetic resonance imaging, unstable intracranial pressure and clinical outcome in patients with normal pressure hydrocephalus. Acta Neurochir Suppl 71:354–356, 1998.
20. Walchenbach R, Geiger E, Thomeer RT, Vanneste JA: The value of temporary external lumbar CSF drainage in predicting the outcome of shunting on normal pressure hydrocephalus. J Neurol Neurosurg Psychiatry 72:503–506, 2002.
21. Krauss JK, Regel JP: The predictive value of ventricular CSF removal in normal pressure hydrocephalus. Neurol Res 19:357–360, 1997.
22. Savolainen S, Hurskainen H, Paljarvi L, et al: Five-year outcome of normal pressure hydrocephalus with or without a shunt: Predictive value of the clinical signs, neuropsychological evaluation and infusion test. Acta Neurochir 144:515–523, 2002.
23. Tisell M, Almstrom O, Stephensen H, et al: How effective is endoscopic third ventriculostomy in treating adult hydrocephalus caused by primary aqueductal stenosis? Neurosurgery 46:104–111, 2000.
24. Munshi I, Lathrop D, Madsen JR, Frim DM: Intraventricular pressure dynamics in patients with ventriculopleural shunts: A telemetric study. Pediatr Neurosurg 28:67–69, 1998.
25. Frim DM, Lathrop D, Chwals WJ: Intraventricular pressure dynamics in ventriculocholecystic shunting: A telemetric study. Pediatr Neurosurg 33:237–242, 2000.
26. el-Shafei IL: Ventriculojugular shunt against the direction of blood flow. III. Operative technique and results. Childs Nerv Syst 3:342–349, 1987.
27. Bergsneider M, Peacock WJ, Mazziotta JC, Becker DP: Beneficial effect of siphoning in treatment of adult hydrocephalus [see comment]. Arch Neurol 56:1224–1229, 1999.
28. Weiner HL, Constantini S, Cohen H, Wisoff JH: Current treatment of normal-pressure hydrocephalus: Comparison of flow-regulated and differential-pressure shunt valves. Neurosurgery 37:877–884, 1995.
29. Black PM, Hakim R, Bailey NO: The use of the Codman-Medos programmable Hakim valve in the management of patients with hydrocephalus: Illustrative cases. Neurosurgery 34:1110–1113, 1994.
30. Zemack G, Romner B: Adjustable valves in normal-pressure hydrocephalus: A retrospective study of 218 patients. Neurosurgery 51:1392–1402, 2002.
31. Vinas FC, Dujovny N, Dujovny M: Microanatomical basis for the third ventriculostomy. Minim Invasive Neurosurg 39:116–221, 1996.
32. Horgan MA, Piatt JH Jr: Shaving of the scalp may increase the rate of infection in CSF shunt surgery. Pediatr Neurosurg 26:180–184, 1997.
33. Kamano S, Nakano Y, Imanishi T, Hattori M: Management with a programmable pressure valve of subdural hematomas caused by a ventriculoperitoneal shunt: Case report. Surg Neurol 35:381–383, 1991.
34. Le H, Yamini B, Frim DM: Lumboperitoneal shunting as a treatment for slit ventricle syndrome. Pediatr Neurosurg 36:178–182, 2002.
35. Bruce DA, Weprin B: The slit ventricle syndrome. Neurosurg Clin N Am 12:709–717, 2001.
36. Walker ML, Fried A, Petronio J: Diagnosis and treatment of the slit ventricle syndrome. Neurosurg Clin N Am 4:707–714, 1993.

Section VIII

New Technologies
in Neurosurgery

39 Neuronavigation in Neuroendoscopic Surgery

WUTTIPONG TIRAKOTAI, DIRK MICHAEL SCHULTE, and DIETER HELLWIG

INTRODUCTION

The utilization and further development of novel endoscopic approaches are impeded by the fundamental limitation of direct visualization[1–3] and by intraoperative spatial disorientation (especially encountered by less experienced neurosurgeons).[4] Over the last decade, the rapid advances in computer and software technology have significantly impacted the development of neuronavigation and the techniques of different perspectives of imaging. Because modern optical neuronavigation systems routinely find application in neurosurgical procedures, image guidance has contributed to the safety and proficiency of contemporary neuroendoscopy.[5–8] This means that selected neurosurgical procedures and the safest route of approach can be planned and performed less invasively with better patient outcome.[4,9–11]

Frameless stereotaxy is found to be useful for preoperative planning (of both the entry point of the instrument and the endoscopic trajectory) and for intracavitary orientation, especially in a pathologically altered setting.[6,7,12] The authors of this article describe the stereotactic method, some related principles, and their contributions in this field. At the same time, advantages and pitfalls of the promising techniques are discussed. Consideration of future trends (e.g., 3-dimensional visualization, virtual endoscopy, and robotic-assisted neuroendoscopy), the integration of these newly evolved technologies, and the development of endoscopic tools may remove restrictions on neuroendoscopic procedures in the near future.

STEREOTACTIC METHODS

Neuroendoscopy, combined with frame-based stereotaxy, offers the possibility of performing biopsies of intracranial space-occupying lesions under direct visual control, and also a way to handle previously inaccessible lesions with various endoscopic interventions.[13,14] These frame-based techniques, however, have several limitations. The stereotactic frames themselves are bulky and sometimes interfere with the endoscopic procedures. Patients also complain about the weight of the frame and the pain associated with its application. Most important, these frame-based stereotactic systems do not provide ongoing intraoperative feedback to the surgeon about anatomical structures encountered in the surgical field.[9] As a consequence, frameless stereotactic systems were developed.[15–19]

Similar to traditional frame-based systems, image-guided neuronavigation also requires a surgical reference to be firmly fixed to the patient. For example, the VectorVision[17,20] and the Stealth Station[21] use an array of reflecting spheres or light-emitting diodes fixed to a Mayfield head clamp as a surgical reference. Each sphere or light-emitting diode (LED) is detected by a camera array, and its position is computed. After performing the patient registration, the computer will calculate the correlation between the coordinate system of the imaging data and the fiducial marker positions on the actual patient. By attaching LEDs or reflectors to surgical instruments such as endoscope, ultrasound probe, or ventricular catheter with stylet, their position relative to the reference array can be tracked.

Several other systems that came on the market in the early 1990s use different technologies. The Picker ViStar Medical Imaging System uses ultrasonic emitters sensed by microphones,[15] and the CANS navigator uses magnetic fields.[22] The Neuronavigator, Operating Arm System, and Viewing Wand all use the similar technology, determining surgical coordinates by means of of an articulated arm with sensors in its joints.[19,23]

Computerized neuronavigation was introduced to intracranial microsurgical procedures to minimize craniotomies; to localize small lesions; and to offer the chance of radical tumor resection with minimal morbidity, especially in the eloquent area.[15,24–32] Recently, image guidance has been also increasingly used in neuroendoscopic surgery.[4,7,17,33–37] Since 1998, the authors' group has used the frameless stereotactic method for neuroendoscopic procedures operating on more than 100 patients using endoscopic techniques and image guidance. We use the BrainLab VectorVision system. VectorVision2, which is similar to the first version, consists of a mobile computer workstation and two incorporated infrared cameras. Because of the extension arm, the touch screen is accessible in the operative field, enabling the surgeon to choose the desired features. Before surgery, a 3-dimensional computed tomography (CT) or magnetic resonance imaging (MRI) dataset was obtained. Prior to scanning, MRI-compatible fiducial markers were spherically distributed around the zone of interest. The lesion could be outlined and reconstructed in any plane or in a 3-dimensional mode. Afterwards, the imaging data were transferred to the neuronavigation system either by intranet or by a Zip disk.

STEPS OF NAVIGATED ENDOSCOPY

Position and Patient Registration

After the induction of general anesthesia, the head is fixed by using either a Mayfield clamp or a vacuum headrest.

Most frameless systems fix the system reference to a head clamp, and the surgical coordinate system remains valid as long as there is no relative motion between the surgical reference and the head. The authors' group has proposed the vacuum headrest for navigated endoscopic procedures. After testing a vacuum headrest with dummies and then applying it to endoscopically treated colloid cyst patients,[38,39] the vacuum headrest was found to be safe and appropriate, especially for single burr hole approach use.[8] In selected patients, we use the vacuum pillow and strapping tape to hold the head in place. After fitting the patient with an appropriately sized headrest, the air in the headrest is removed to create a vacuum, and simultaneously the headrest is reshaped according to the individual head contour of the patient (Fig. 39-1A). In cases where an occipital or suboccipital approach is used, we apply a Mayfield clamp to keep the head immobile.

The patient's registration (fiducial registration) is performed using a nonsterile pointer to locate the adhesive skin fiducials, which are detected by the system's infrared cameras and used as the patient's reference point. During registration, the acquired data are matched to the patient's head position. After registration, the computer calculates the correlation between the coordinate system of the imaging data and the fiducial marker positions on the actual patient, and then reports any registration errors in the system. In all cases, the accuracy of the system is checked before and after performing a burr hole by testing the positions of the palpable anatomic landmarks such as nasion and orbital rims. The authors would like to recommend this performance as the significant step in verifying the accuracy of the data before introducing the endoscope.

The following are technical innovations that our group has introduced into the field of computer-aided surgery.

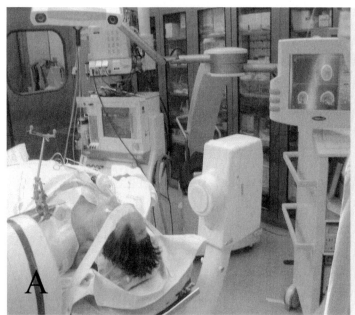
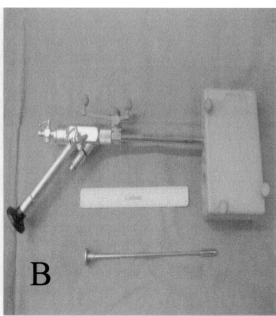
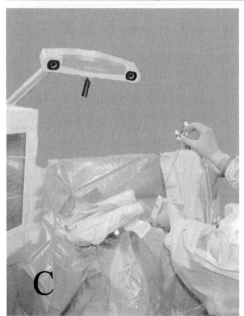

FIGURE 39-1 Instruments. *A,* A vacuum headrest for the minimally invasive surgical procedure. *B,* An instrument calibration matrix (ICM) with size-varied holes. *C,* The ICM is brought into the camera field.

Instrument Calibration and Instrument Calibration Matrix

Because of the different lengths of instruments, and because of the altered correspondence of angle between the instrument axis and instrument adapter, inaccurate data of navigation can occur. The instrument calibration matrix (ICM) was developed to solve this problem. The full registration of any instrument consists of two steps, depending on the correspondence of angle between the instrument axis and instrument adapter. (Nonendoscopic instruments require only one step of registration.) The length of the surgical instrument is registered by touching the calibration cone of the system reference rod. The software automatically detects the universal adapter and calibrates the tip of the instrument. In cases where an instrument's axis does not correspond to the instrument adapter (e.g., in an endoscope), a virtual elongation problem will occur, followed by an error distance from the desired target. Therefore, the correct diameter and exact vector of the instrument must be calibrated in the second step. The instrument is inserted into the appropriate "burr hole" of a special instrument calibration matrix. Later, both instrument and ICM are brought into the camera field (see Fig. 39-1B and C). The system automatically detects the calibration hole and adjusts the parameters to the appropriate diameter and vector of the instrument used. The complete registration procedure is performed in less than 1 minute. A more detailed description of this procedure has been published elsewhere.[40] After this registration, tracking of stereotactic instruments allows visualization of the anatomy at the tip of the instrument in any plane.

Catheter Placement Software (Autopilot Program)

This software, which was developed by our group in collaboration with BrainLab, the surgeon can navigate within 3-dimensional CT images or MR images. The program provides possible routes for ventricular catheter placements or other reservoir catheter placements, and it also guides freehand endoscopic placement. First, a preplanned vector with entry and target point is determined. After selecting the Autopilot mode, two arrows are seen on the screen. The upper arrow, using degree data, indicates at which angle and in which direction the surgeon should move the instrument in order to align it with the preplanned trajectory. The movement of the instrument can be seen and controlled in accordance with the interactive data from the axial, coronal, or sagittal images. The lower arrow indicates the distance between the entry point and the tip of the instrument. Concentric circles represent the funnel effect: when the tip of the instrument closely approaches the target, the circles' color will change from green to red.[8]

Source of Data for Neuronavigation

Imaging coordinate systems for CT or magnetic resonance images are based on a field of view with known dimensions. A voxel can be visualized as pixel that is expanded to a box with a height equal to the slice thickness. The voxel size reflects the resolution of a scan and is a factor in determining the accuracy of surgical procedures. Because of the spatial error of field distortion in MR imaging,[41] and because of the smaller

voxel size of CT when compared with MRI,[42] the CT-guided frameless stereotaxy was found to be either minimally[42] or significantly more accurate than MR image–directed stereotaxy.[41] Hence, we would prefer MR imaging as a data source in a midline lesion procedure and CT imaging as a data source in the endoscopic intervention of peripheral lesion.

Frameless stereotactic systems have proved to be helpful in a variety of neurosurgical procedures, and especially in neuroendoscopic surgery. The system is indispensable for the neurosurgeon in planning an exact approach to avoid the eloquent regions.

APPLICATION OF NEURONAVIGATION IN NEUROENDOSCOPIC SURGERY

Image guidance is helpful for endoscopic neurosurgery in terms of determining the optimal entry point and in planning the exact trajectory to the lesion to avoid injury to vital structures, especially in patients with arachnoid cyst (Fig. 39-2). Cystocisternostomy or ventriculocystostomy can be planned using navigation.[43] Although the individual's anatomy serves as orientation to the lesion (after introduction of the endoscope into the lateral ventricle[44]), the navigation is still useful for intraoperative orientation, especially in cases with impaired visualization, distorted anatomy, or narrowed ventricles.[6] Neuronavigation is beneficial in intraparenchymal cyst or in multiloculated hydrocephalus surgery, because the system orientates the surgeon within the cystic compartment and indicates the appropriate fenestration site. In endoscopic third ventriculostomy, the use of neuronavigation may not be necessary[7]; however, in cases with thickened, nontranslucent third ventricular floors, the authors have found that neuronavigation is useful for anatomic orientation.[10,38,45] The integration of an actual endoscopic image into the navigation system allows the surgeon to check the accuracy of the navigation system and to perform a safe endoscopic operation (including a transventricular biopsy) because of the safe and correct target localization (Fig. 39-3).[8]

Case Reports

CASE REPORT 1

ARACHNOID CYST

This female patient suffered from persisting headaches and a feeling of pressure behind the eyes. During the course of disease she developed daily headaches and uneasiness, together with blurred vision because of a right paresis of the sixth cranial nerve. Subsequent MRI revealed a cystic formation in the rear part of the third ventricle (presumably an arachnoid cyst) leading to obstructive hydrocephalus (see Fig. 39-2B). Considering the clinical symptoms, a neuroendoscopic cystoventriculostomy and a third ventriculocisternostomy were carried out. Image-guided neuronavigation proved to be useful in finding the optimal trajectory for the rigid endoscope to perform the ventriculocisternostomy and to access the arachnoid cyst with the flexible endoscope afterwards (see Fig. 39-2A). After successful cystic evacuation, the cyst collapsed and the reestablishment of cerebrospinal fluid (CSF) flow through the aqueduct was documented by intraoperative ventriculography.

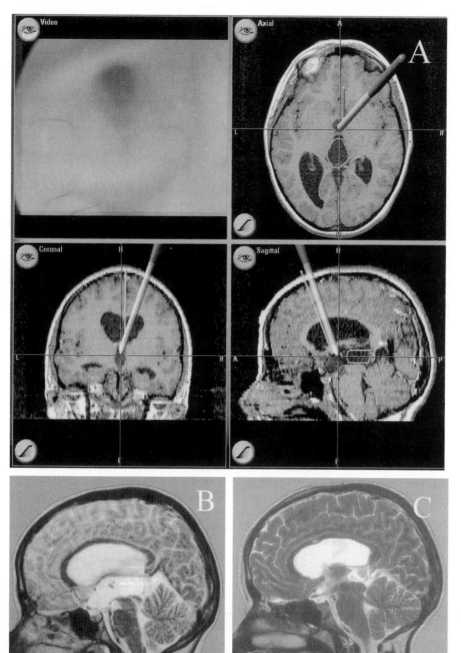

FIGURE 39-2 Cystoventriculostomy of an arachnoid cyst. *A,* Images from the navigation workstation showing the tip of endoscope and the arachnoid cyst; the outer wall of the cyst is demonstrated *(upper left)*. *B* and *C,* Preoperative and postoperative MR sagittal views of the same patient.

CASE REPORT 2
HYPOTHALAMIC LESION

A 40-year-old woman suffered from acute generalized seizures with postictal somnolence. Imaging shows a space-occupying lesion of the hypothalamus without contrast media enhancement (see Fig. 39-3A and B). A transventricular biopsy was selected for obtaining the histopathology of the tumor. After positioning the patient's head in the vacuum headrest, the approach was planned through an image-guidance system. With the aid of the navigation system, the biopsy could be precisely performed and a low-grade astrocytoma was diagnosed. The endoscopic view reveals the ependymal layer above the tumor mass (see Fig. 39-3C). No further treatment was necessary; yearly MRI controls show no change of tumor size and no hydrocephalus.

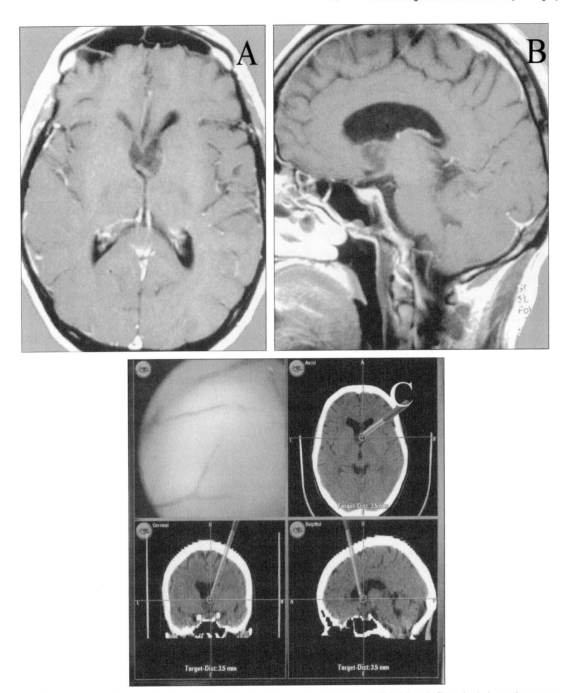

FIGURE 39-3 Transventricular biopsy of a hypothalamic lesion. Preoperative MRI with (*A*) axial and (*B*) sagittal views demonstrate a hypothalamic lesion. *C*, An endoscopic view shows the ependymal layer above the tumor mass (*upper left*), and triplanar CT scan reconstructions measure the distance between the tip of the endoscope and the target lesion as 3.5 mm.

CASE REPORT 3
COLLOID CYST

The patient complained of severe headaches for several days before the admission, and the family reported impaired mental abilities and memory deficits. MRI scans showed an occlusive hydrocephalus caused by a colloid cyst at the level of the foramina of Monro (Fig. 39-4B). An endoscopic evacuation of the cyst was performed under the guidance of neuronavigation. After targeting and

performing a trepanation (4 cm in front of the coronal suture and 3.5 cm right paramedian), the endoscope emerged in front of the foramen of Monro, which was occluded by the cyst. Subsequently, the cyst wall was coagulated and the liquid colloid could be extracted; then the membranes were partially resected and coagulated (see Fig. 39-4A). The CSF route through the foramen was reopened and was documented by ventriculography. An external ventricular drainage was placed to prevent potential aseptic meningitis caused by remnants of the colloid (see Fig. 39-4C).

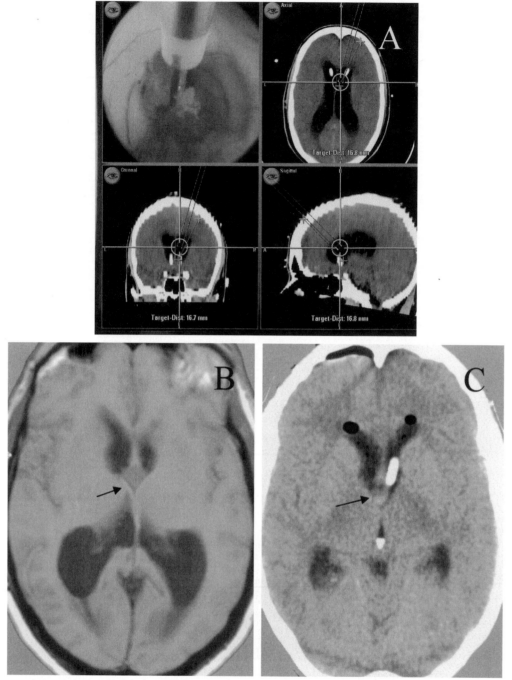

FIGURE 39-4 Colloid cyst evacuation. *A,* After introduction of the rigid endoscope to the region of interest under the control of navigation system and endoscopic view, the cyst wall is opened and the content is removed. Preoperative MRI with (*B*) axial view and (*C*) postoperative CT scan demonstrate an evacuated colloid cyst (*arrow*).

SOURCE OF ERRORS AND PITFALLS

Steinmeier and colleagues proposed that the accuracy of neuronavigation systems may be influenced by (1) imaging (e.g., voxel size, geometric distortion, and compatibility), (2) registration or coordinate transformation (e.g., mapping image space to physical space), (3) the precision and (mechanical) accuracy of the navigation system itself (i.e., technical accuracy), and (4) intraoperative events (e.g., positional shift or brain shift). The application accuracy is determined by the first three factors, whereas application accuracy plus intraoperative events should be defined as clinical accuracy.[42]

Similar to the study of Steinmeier and colleagues, Grunert classified the error of the navigation into three categories: (1) the technical error of the device calculating its own position in space, (2) the registration error caused by inaccuracies in the calculation of the transformation matrix between the navigation and the image space, and (3) the application error caused additionally by anatomic shift of brain structures during operation.[46] Attention should be paid to the details of image acquisition and the source of image. The effect of slice thickness on accuracy has been evaluated systematically in frame-based systems.[47,48]

According to the imaging principle, the pixel size determines the resolution of the image, and structures smaller than a voxel cannot be distinguished by imaging modality. Therefore, voxels should be as small as possible. Because the slice thickness of imaging plots the voxel size, slice thickness of CT and MRI should be thin in order to increase the application accuracy. Because the patient must be moved during acquisition of CT slices, error in the distance between slices potentially can occur and lead to the incorrect reconstruction of the 3-dimensional image. Therefore, the accuracy of table movement should be proved periodically.[49] Although errors from inaccurate table motion are not an issue during MRI, the problem of geometric distortion of MRI compared with CT should be considered.[50–54] This distortion is assumed to be caused by specific physical properties of the scanner (e.g., the magnetic field inhomogeneity) and/or the chemical properties of the scanned tissue (i.e., chemical shift).[55]

The other potential source of error is the registration between image space and physical space (patient registration). Scalp fiducials, especially those near the head pins, may have the tendency to move after head fixation. Therefore, it is necessary to carefully inspect these and avoid displacement of fiducials. Scalp fiducials on the dependent side are sometimes not stable enough to include as registration points and should be excluded from registration.

Intraoperative brain displacement and deformation of the brain have long been observed,[56] and various techniques have been used to decrease these errors.[57,58] Roberts and colleagues found a weak correlation between cortical surface motion and operative time, whereby displacement increased with increasing operative time. They suggested that critical navigational decisions should be made early in a procedure, whenever possible.[56] The surgeon ought to rely on stereotactic guidance only early in the procedure, before extensive CSF drainage. The problem of brain shift will be lessened if precautions are taken to prevent the abrupt change of either the cystic lesion or the lateral ventricle. For example, position the patient with the lesion at the highest point in order to minimize the escape of fluid from the lesion after the introduction of the endoscopic sheath. From the report of Dorward and co-workers in 1998,[59] brain distortion rarely occurs in the midline structures, and most procedures handled by endoscope use the midline structure as an anatomic landmark. Regardless of the perioperative accuracy of the navigation system, it is prudent to intermittently verify the accuracy of the system by cross-checking the location of a known anatomic structure (e.g., the foramen of Monro) from the endoscopic view and its corresponding view on the navigation monitor. In cases where the authors are uncertain about an instrument's position (or even the surgical result), the intraoperative fluoroscopic cysto- or ventriculography may provide additional information and some solutions to these questions. After entering the cyst or ventricle, the surgeon should try to orient the scope as quickly as possible.

Intraoperative sonography provides a workable alternative that is convenient to use and that requires a less time-consuming procedure.[60,61] The surgeon may update the 2-dimensional or 3-dimensional images in seconds during surgery, navigating directly on the monitor screen.[62] The displayed image reflects the patient's true anatomy without a requirement for patient registration. The capabilities of real time 3-dimensional imaging and the relatively less expensive equipment (in comparison with other intraoperative imaging alternatives) may establish ultrasound as a popular tool (in combination with neuronavigation) and as a practical image modality for hospitals with limited financial resources. This combined system may function as an ultrasound scanner and a conventional neuronavigation system; or as an integrated, ultrasound-based neuronavigation system, which is in development. Although both navigation tools present 3-dimensional image volumes, the ultrasound reveals the updated imaging. Duplex scan and Doppler modes of ultrasound are also useful for the detection of vascular structures or malformations because of its capacity to demonstrate the flow and direction of related vessels. This technology will be able to provide real-time navigation at an affordable cost.

FUTURE TRENDS

As the optical digitizing systems that compare images from different perspectives become more sophisticated, and as tracking mechanisms continue to be developed, the capabilities of the neuroendoscope will increase. Frameless stereotaxy and its integration with other technologies (e.g., real time ultrasound, intraoperative imaging, virtual reality, and robot-assisted neuroendoscopy) will undoubtedly lead to some innovative applications.[63] One new development is a robot arm, controlled by the neurosurgeon via a special joystick, that can perform with a very smooth, slow motion. This device can steer the endoscope (with the assistance of navigation) precisely and accurately to the preplanned target, but it is limited to 30 degrees of motion, ruling out endoscopic procedures that require a larger range of motion.[64] In the future, this robot might evolve to move in a wider range of motion or to be controlled via satellite signal (telemedicine) in order to operate on patients in remote areas where specialists are in short supply.

Both intraoperative MRI (including functional MRI, magnetoencephalography) and intraoperative CT offer the advantage of repeated scans of a patient during surgery by transporting the patient in and out of the scanner.[65–72] An updated, high-quality, 3-dimensional image obtained from these sophisticated imaging modalities may be used for further guidance and accurate control of navigation, as well as for functional brain mapping.[73,74] Nevertheless, two important drawbacks of intraoperative images are the relatively long image acquisition procedure (typically a total of 20–60 min) and the financial resources needed for these intraoperative systems.[75] The up-and-coming nanotechnology may simplify the intraoperative procedure and shorten the time consumed by these intraoperative imaging modalities. Before image-guided surgery using intraoperative CT or MRI becomes more practical and economical, the application of intraoperative ultrasound may find use in periodically updating the computer data as brain shift occurs.

Careful planning of neuroendoscopic procedures (based on the patient's individual anatomy) is always essential because the endoscope, once introduced into the ventricles, should not be moved tangentially or repositioned.[2,76] Therefore, examination of the patient's ventricular system using virtual reality methods prior to surgery may help the surgeon comprehend structures and improve the performance of intervention.[77]

Virtual Reality Neuroendoscopic Simulations

The endoscopic view of intraventricular anatomy is different from microsurgery, which is familiar to neurosurgeons.[44] Three-dimensional image software, in combination with modern computer technology, is helpful for preoperative virtual planning and in the simulation of endoscopic approaches. In 2000, the authors published our first results of the relationship of virtual reality neuroendoscopic simulations to actual imaging. Individual anatomic details obtained from the virtual endoscopic system are sufficient to plan intraventricular neuroendoscopic procedures because

of the understanding of spatial relationships between lesions and adjacent structures.[78] Furthermore, the virtual system can also be a valuable tool for training not only neuro-endoscopically inexperienced surgeons but also medical students.[79]

Although virtual reality was used to combine with intraoperative neuronavigation for planning of endoscopic surgery,[80] at present there are some technical problems related to virtual neuroendoscopy. The sensitivity of virtual endoscopy to anatomic variants is lower than that of conventional images.[81] A major drawback is that a clear texture or coloring of the anatomic structures is not possible[78,80] (Fig. 39-5). In particular, specific anatomic structures

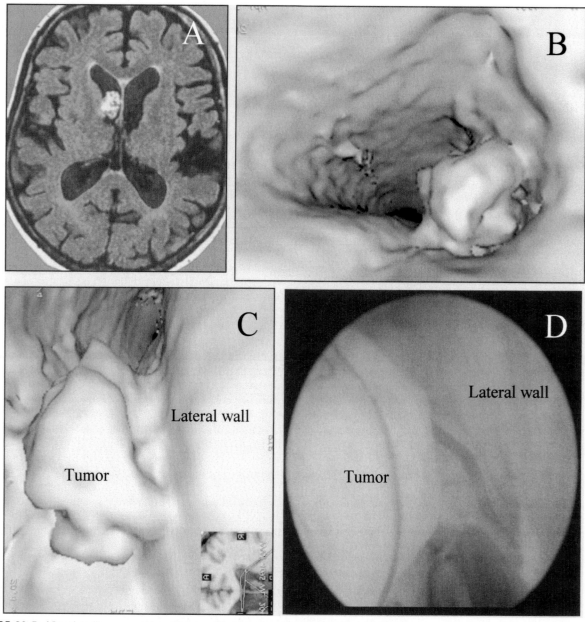

FIGURE 39-5 Virtual reality neuroendoscopic simulations to actual imaging. *A,* Axial MRI shows the right intraventricular tumor. *B* and *C,* Virtual endoscopic image reveals partial occlusion of the foramen of Monro, and the tumor origin can be seen on the lateral wall. A small tumor-supplying blood vessel is not visible. The choroids plexus and thalamostriate vein cannot be demonstrated clearly. *D,* Intraoperative endoscopic view demonstrates a tumor that is partially occluding the foramen of Monro, and the endoscopic dissection of the tumor at the lateral ventricular wall. Histopathologic findings yielded a subependymoma.

(e.g., blood vessels) cannot be identified properly[78,80] (Fig. 39-6). However, the administration of contrast medium, as proposed by Burtscher and colleagues,[82] seems to enhance the identification of both intra- and paraventricular vessels (e.g., the thalamocaudate vein and the basilar artery with all its branches) on the virtual endoscopic image.

Although clinical application of virtual neuroendoscopy is still in its developmental stage, improvements in image processing will transform this technology into a useful tool for rehearsal of the operative procedure in simulated situation and for preoperative approach planning, as well as for intraoperative orientation in the future.

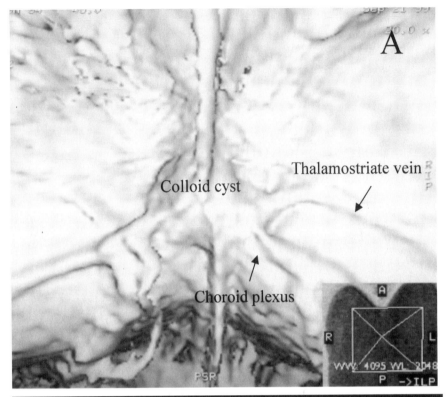

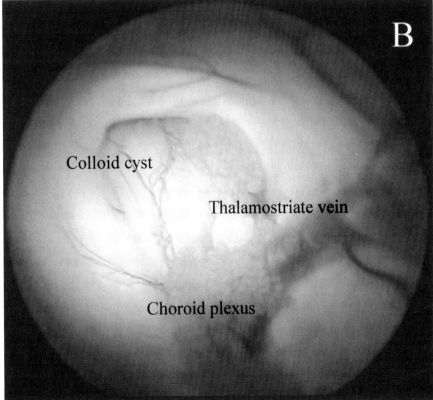

FIGURE 39-6 Virtual reality of colloid cyst. Comparing the virtual image (*A*) with the endoscopic view (*B*), the anteriomedial aspect of the colloid cyst is seen to totally occlude both foramina of Monro. Parts of the septum pellucidum are absent. From the virtual image, the thalamostriate vein and choroids plexus can be identified to some extent. The fornix is not visible.

REFERENCES

1. Fukushima T: Endoscopic biopsy of intraventricular tumors with the use of a ventriculofiberscope. Neurosurgery 2:110–113, 1978.
2. Hellwig D, Bauer BL, List-Hellwig E, et al: Stereotactic endoscopic procedures on processes of the cranial midline. Acta Neurochir Suppl (Wien) 53:23–32, 1991.
3. Walker ML, MacDonald J, Wright LC: The history of ventriculoscopy: Where do we go from here? Pediatr Neurosurg 18:218–223, 1992.
4. Dorward NL, Alberti O, Zhao J, et al: Interactive image-guided neuroendoscopy: Development and early clinical experience. Minim Invasive Neurosurg 41:31–34, 1998.
5. Grunert P, Müller-Forell W, Darabi K, et al: Basic principles and clinical applications of neuronavigation and intraoperative computed tomography. Comput Aided Surg 3:166–173, 1998.
6. Hopf NJ, Grunert P, Darabi K, et al: Frameless neuronavigation applied to endoscopic neurosurgery. Minim Invasive Neurosurg 42:187–193, 1999.
7. Schroeder HWS, Wagner W, Tschiltschke W, et al: Frameless neuronavigation in intracranial endoscopic neurosurgery. J Neurosurg 94:72–79, 2001.
8. Tirakotai W, Riegel T, Sure U, et al: Clinical application of neuronavigation in a series of single burr-hole procedures. Zentralbl Neurochir 65:1–8, 2004.
9. Golfinos JG, Fitzpatrick BC, Smith LR, et al: Clinical use of a frameless stereotactic arm: Results of 325 cases. J Neurosurg 83:197–205, 1995.
10. Riegel T, Alberti O, Hellwig D, et al: Operative management of third ventriculostomy in cases of thickened, non-translucent third ventricular floor: Technical note. Minim Invasive Neurosurg 44:65–69, 2001.
11. Rohde V, Reinges MH, Krombach GA, et al: The combined use of image guided frameless stereotaxy and neuroendoscopy for the surgical management of occlusive hydrocephalus and intracranial cysts. Br J Neurosurg 12:531–538, 1998.
12. Muacevic A, Muller A: Imaged-guided endoscopic ventriculostomy with a new frameless armless neuronavigation system. Comput Aided Surg 4:887–892, 1999.
13. Hellwig D, Bauer BL: Endoscopic procedures in stereotactic neurosurgery. Acta Neurochir Suppl (Wien) 52:30–32, 1991.
14. Hellwig D, Benes L, Bertalanffy H, et al: Endoscopic stereotaxy: An eight-year experience. Stereotact Funct Neurosurg 68:90–97, 1997.
15. Barnett GH, Kormos DW, Steiner CP, et al: Intraoperative localization using an armless, frameless stereotactic wand. J Neurosurg 78:510–514, 1993.
16. Buxton N, Cartmill M: Neuroendoscopy combined with frameless neuronavigation. Br J Neurosurg 14:600–601, 2000.
17. Gumprecht HK, Widenka DC, Lumenta CB: BrainLab VectorVision neuronavigation system: Technology and clinical experiences in 131 cases. Neurosurgery 44:97–104, 1999.
18. Tan KK, Grzeszczuk R, Levin DN, et al: A frameless stereotactic approach to neurosurgical planning based on retrospective patient-image registration. J Neurosurg 79:296–303, 1993.
19. Watanabe E, Mayangi Y, Kosugi Y, et al: Open surgery assisted by the neuronavigator, a stereotactic, articulated, sensitive arm. Neurosurgery 28:792–799, 1991.
20. Gumprecht H, Trost HA, Lumenta CB: Neuroendoscopy combined with frameless Neuronavigation. Br J Neurosurg 14:129–131, 2000.
21. Smith KR, Frank KJ, Bucholz RD: The neurostation: A highly accurate, minimally invasive solution to frameless stereotactic neurosurgery. Comput Med Imaging Graph 18:247–256, 1994.
22. Kato A, Yoshimine T, Hayakawa T, et al: A frameless, armless navigation system for computer-assisted neurosurgery. J Neurosurg 74:845–849, 1991.
23. Guthrie BL: Graphic-interactive cranial surgery. Clin Neurosurg 41:489–516, 1994.
24. Doshi PK, Lemmieux L, Fish DR, et al: Frameless stereotaxy and interactive neurosurgery with the ISG viewing wand. Acta Neurochir Suppl (Wien) 64:49–53, 1995.
25. Drake JM, Prudencio J, Holowaka S, et al: Frameless stereotaxy in children. Pediatr Neurosurg 20:152–159, 1994.
26. Hata N, Dohi T, Iseki H, et al: Development of a frameless and armless stereotactic neuronavigation system with ultrasonographic registration. Neurosurgery 41:608–614, 1997.
27. Olivier A, Germano IM, Cukiert A, et al: Frameless stereotaxy for surgery of the epilepsies: Preliminary experience: Technical note. J Neurosurg 81:629–633, 1994.
28. Olson JJ, Shepherd S, Bakay RAE: The EasyGuide Neuroimage-guided surgery. Neurosurgery 40:1092–1096, 1997.
29. Saenz A, Zamorano L, Matter A, et al: Interactive image guided surgery of the pineal region. Minim Invasive Neurosurg 41:27–30, 1998.
30. Stapleton SR, Kiriakopoulos E, Mikulis D, et al: Combined utility of functional MRI, cortical mapping, and frameless stereotaxy in the resection of lesions in eloquent areas of brain in children. Pediatr Neurosurg 26:68–82, 1997.
31. Tirakotai W, Sure U, Benes L, et al: Image-guided transsylvian, transinsular approach for insular cavernous angiomas. Neurosurgery 53:1299–1304, 2003.
32. Wagner W, Tschiltschke W, Niendorf WR, et al: Infrared-based neuronavigation and cortical motor stimulation in the management of central-region tumors. Stereotact Funct Neurosurg 68:112–116, 1997.
33. Grunert P, Hopf N, Perneczky A: Frame-based and frameless endoscopic procedures in the ventricle. Stereotact Funct Neurosurg 68:80–89, 1997.
34. Iseki H, Kawamura H, Tanikawa T, et al: An image-guided stereotactic system for neurosurgical operations. Stereotact Funct Neurosurg 63:130–138, 1994.
35. Manwaring KH, Manwaring ML, Moss SD: Magnetic field guided endoscopic dissection through a burr hole may avoid more invasive craniotomies. A preliminary report. Acta Neurochir Suppl (Wien) 61:34–39, 1994.
36. McCallum J: Combined frameless stereotaxy and neuroendoscopy in placement of intracranial shunt catheters. Pediatr Neurosurg 26:127–129, 1997.
37. Rhoten RL, Luciano MG, Barnett GH: Computer-assisted endoscopy for neurosurgical procedures: Technical note. Neurosurgery 40:632–638, 1997.
38. Alberti O, Riegel T, Hellwig D, et al: Frameless navigation and endoscopy. J Neurosurg 95:541–543, 2001.
39. Hellwig D, Bauer BL, Schulte M, et al: Neuroendoscopic treatment for colloid cysts of the third ventricle: The experience of a decade. Neurosurgery 52:525–532, 2003.
40. Sure U, Hellwig D, Bertalanffy H: Incorrect vector after calibration of surgical instrument for image-guidance: The problem and the solution: Technical note. Minim Invasive Neurosurg 44:88–91, 2001.
41. Dorward NL, Alberti O, Palmer JD, et al: Accuracy of true frameless stereotaxy: In vivo measurement and laboratory phantom studies: Technical note. J Neurosurg 90:160–168, 1999.
42. Steinmeier R, Rachinger J, Kaus M, et al: Factors influencing the application accuracy of neuronavigation systems. Stereotact Funct Neurosurg 75:188–202, 2000.
43. Wagner W, Gaab MR, Schroeder HW, et al: Cranial neuronavigation in neurosurgery: Assessment of usefulness in relation to type and site of pathology in 284 patients. Minim Invasive Neurosurg 43:124–131, 2000.
44. Riegel T, Hellwig D, Bauer BL, et al: Endoscopic anatomy of the third ventricle. Acta Neurochir Suppl (Wien) 61:54–56, 1994.
45. Broggi G, Dones I, Ferroli P, et al: Image guided neuroendoscopy for third ventriculostomy. Acta Neurochir (Wien) 142:893–898, 2000.
46. Grunert P, Darabi K, Espinosa J, et al: Computer-aided navigation in neurosurgery. Neurosurg Rev 26:73–99, 2003.
47. Galloway RJ Jr, Maciunas RJ, Latimer JW: The accuracies of four stereotactic frame systems: An independent assessment. Biomed Instrum Technol 25:457–460, 1991.
48. Maciunas RJ, Galloway RL Jr, Latimer JW: The application accuracy of stereotactic frames. Neurosurgery 35:682–695, 1994.
49. Kitchen NK, Lemieux L, Thomas DGT: Accuracy in frame-based and frameless stereotaxy. Stereotact Funct Neurosurg 61:195–206, 1993.
50. Go KG, Kamman RL, Mooyaart EL: Interaction of metallic neurosurgical implants with magnetic resonance imaging at 1.5 tesla as a cause of image distortion and of hazardous movement of the implant. Clin Neurol Neurosurg 91:109–115, 1989.
51. Kondzioka D, Dempsey RK, Lunsford LD, et al: A comparison between magnetic resonance imaging and computed tomography of stereotactic coordinate determination. Neurosurgery 30:402–407, 1992.
52. Schad LR, Lott S, Schmitt F, et al: Correction of spatial distortion in MR imaging: A prerequisite for accurate stereotaxy. J Comput Assist Tomogr 11:499–505, 1987.
53. Sumanaweera TS, Adler JR, Napel S, et al: Characterization of spatial distortion in magnetic resonance imaging and its implications for stereotactic surgery. Neurosurgery 35:696–704, 1994.
54. Wyper DJ, Turner JW, Patterson J, et al: Accuracy of stereotactic localization using MRI and CT. J Neurol Neurosurg Psychiatry 49:1444–1448, 1986.
55. Lunsford LD, Albright L: Intraoperative imaging with a therapeutic computed tomographic scanner. Neurosurgery 15:559–561, 1984.
56. Roberts DW, Hartov A, Kennedy FE, et al: Intraoperative brain shift and deformation: A quantitative analysis of cortical displacement in 28 cases. Neurosurgery 43:749–758, 1998.

57. Hartkens T, Hill DL, Castellano-Smith AD, et al: Measurement and analysis of brain deformation during neurosurgery. IEEE Trans Med Imaging 22:82–92, 2003.
58. Paulsen KD, Miga MI, Kennedy FE, et al: A computational model for tracking subsurface tissue deformation during stereotactic neurosurgery. IEEE Trans Biomed Eng 46:213–225, 1999.
59. Dorward NL, Alberti O, Velani B, et al: Postimaging brain distortion: Magnitude, correlates, and impact on neuronavigation. J Neurosurg 88:656–662, 1998.
60. Balasubramaniam C, Seshardi S, Suresh I: Intraoperative sonography in neurosurgery. Ann Acad Med Singapore 22:513–515, 1993.
61. Chandler WF, Knake JE, McGillicuddy JE, et al: Intraoperative use of real-time ultrasonography in neurosurgery. J Neurosurg 57:157–163, 1982.
62. Gronningsaeter A, Kleven A, Ommedal S, et al: SonoWand, an ultrasound-based neuronavigation system. Neurosurgery 47:1373–1379, 2000.
63. Hellwig D: Computer-aided navigation in neurosurgery: Commentary. Neurosurg Rev 26:101, 2003.
64. Zimmerman M, Krishnan R, Raabe A, et al: Robot-assisted navigated neuroendoscopy. Neurosurgery 51:1446–1452, 2002.
65. Balmer B, Bernays RL, Kollias SS, et al: Interventional MR-guided neuroendoscopy: A new therapeutic option for children. J Pediatr Surg 37:668–672, 2002.
66. Black PM, Moriarty T, Alexander E 3rd, et al: Development and implementation of intraoperative magnetic resonance imaging and its neurosurgical applications. Neurosurgery 41:831–845, 1997.
67. Ganslandt O, Fahlbusch R, Nimsky C, et al: Functional neuronavigation with magnetoencephalography: Outcome in 50 patients with lesions around the motor cortex. J Neurosurg 91:73–79, 1999.
68. Kaibara T, Saunders JK, Sutherland GR: Advances in mobile intraoperative magnetic resonance imaging. Neurosurgery 47:131–138, 2000.
69. Nimsky C, Ganslandt O, Kober H, et al: Integration of functional magnetic resonance imaging supported by magnetoencephalography in functional neuronavigation. Neurosurgery 44:1249–1256, 1999.
70. Seifert V, Zimmermann M, Trantakis C, et al: Open MRI-guided neurosurgery. Acta Neurochir (Wien) 141:455–464, 1999.
71. Steinmeier S, Fahlbusch R, Ganslandt O, et al: Intraoperative magnetic resonance imaging with the Magnetom open scanner: Concepts, neurosurgical indications and procedures: A preliminary report. Neurosurgery 43:739–748, 1998.
72. Tronnier VM, Wirtz CR, Knauth M, et al: Intraoperative diagnostic and interventional magnetic resonance imaging in neurosurgery. Neurosurgery 40:891–902, 1997.
73. Rubino GJ, Farahani K, McGill D, et al: Magnetic resonance imaging-guided neurosurgery in the magnetic fringe fields: The next step in neuronavigation. Neurosurgery 46:643–654, 2000.
74. Wirtz CR, Bonsantano MM, Knauth M, et al: Intraoperative magnetic resonance imaging to update interactive navigation in neurosurgery: Method and preliminary experience. Comput Aided Surg 2:172–179, 1997.
75. Unsgaard G, Omnedal S, Muller T, et al: Neuronavigation by intraoperative three-dimensional ultrasound: Initial experience during brain tumor resection. Neurosurgery 50:804–812, 2002.
76. Grunert P, Perneczky A, Resch KDM: Endoscopic procedures through the foramen interventriculare of Monro under stereotactical conditions. Minim Invasive Neurosurg 37:2–8, 1994.
77. Burtscher J, Dessl A, Maurer H, et al: Virtual neuroendoscopy, a comparative magnetic resonance and anatomical study. Minim Invasive Neurosurg 42:113–117, 1999.
78. Riegel T, Alberti O, Retsch R, et al: Relationships of virtual reality neuroendoscopic simulations to actual imaging. Minim Invasive Neurosurg 43:176–180, 2000.
79. Freudenstein D, Bartz D, Skalej M, et al: New virtual system for planning of neuroendoscopic interventions. Comput Aided Surg 6:77–84, 2001.
80. Krombach GA, Rohde V, Haage P, et al: Virtual endoscopy combined with intraoperative neuronavigation for planning of endoscopic surgery in patients with occlusive hydrocephalus and intracranial cysts. Neuroradiology 44:279–285, 2002.
81. Shigematsu Y, Korogi Y, Hirai T, et al: Virtual MRI endoscopy of the intracranial cerebrospinal fluid spaces. Neuroradiology 40:644–650, 1998.
82. Burtscher J, Bale R, Dessl A, et al: Virtual endoscopy for planning neuro-endoscopic intraventricular surgery. Minim Invasive Neurosurg 45:24–31, 2002.

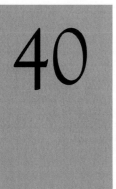

40

Gamma Knife Surgery for Cerebral Vascular Malformations, Tumors, and Functional Disorders

LADISLAU STEINER, JASON SHEEHAN,
CHRISTER LINDQUIST, MATEI STROILA, and
MELITA STEINER

INTRODUCTION

The gamma knife is a neurosurgical tool used either as a primary or as an adjuvant procedure for intracranial pathologies. It was devised in the late 1960s as an alternative to open stereotactic lesioning for functional disorders. Both variations in anatomy and the need for physiologic confirmation of the target limited its usefulness for these indications at that time. However, the technology was found to be efficacious in the management of structural disorders as well. The limited scope of the pathology treated with the gamma knife (i.e., intracranial) and its unique technology make the gamma knife an extension of the neurosurgeon's therapeutic armamentarium and not a separate specialty. It should not be mistaken for a form of radiation therapy because it differs in concept from the radiation oncologist's idea of tumor treatment, which is based on variable tissue response to fractionated radiation. Gamma surgery is a single session, stereotactically guided procedure for various neurosurgical pathologic processes that limits exposure to radiation as much as possible to the lesion only.

Recently it has been shown that the gamma knife can palliate some ocular tumors. In a more limited application of the concept, the treatment of extracranial tumors in spinal, abdominal, and thoracic locations has evolved with the use of the Cyberknife by Stanford and Pittsburgh groups, the LINAC by the University of Arizona group, and by a medical physics group at the Karolinska Hospital.[1-4] Obviously, those lesions that lie outside the central nervous system will not be treated by a neurosurgeon; however, when the gamma knife is used for neurosurgical pathology, no one is more qualified to apply it. It is the operator and the pathology that define the use of a technology. When Walter Dandy placed a cystoscope in a ventricle for the first time, he was not performing a urologic procedure.[5] The microscope, when used by the neurosurgeon, ophthalmologist, or otolaryngologist, is a neurosurgical, ophthalmological, or otolaryngological instrument, respectively.

It is remarkable how difficult it was (and still is) for some neurosurgeons to accept as a neurosurgical tool a physical agent with which they are not accustomed. Some of the causes of this reticence can be identified:

1. Lack of historic perspective makes it difficult for some neurosurgeons to realize that Leksell's concept was rooted in the philosophy of the founders of neurosurgery, as far as recognition of technologic advances and their application to neurosurgical practice. The early adoption by Cushing of the x-ray machine, his use of the "radium bomb" in glioma treatment,[6] and his introduction of the use of radiofrequency lesions are just a few examples of "technology transfer."
2. The difficulty of accepting a neurosurgical procedure without opening the skull, despite the fact that every neurosurgeon knows that trephination is itself a minor part of the neurosurgical act. The laser beam, the bipolar coagulator, and the ultrasound probe are accepted without resistance because they are used after trephining the skull. The recently introduced "photon radiosurgery," with its limited scope as compared with gamma surgery, is widely accepted as "neurosurgery" because it reaches the target through a small burr hole.
3. The loss of the thrill and glamor provided by the open surgical act.
4. The deeply rooted acceptance of the dogma that where ionizing beams are involved, a radiotherapist is needed. The last 20 years have demonstrated that a neurosurgeon can acquire the necessary knowledge of radiophysics and radiobiology to handle ionizing beams. This is much easier than for a radiation oncologist to master neuroanatomy and management of neurosurgical lesions, and thus to exclude bias when deciding whether to use the microscope or the gamma knife in each particular case.

The trend in cranial as well as spinal neurosurgery has been toward minimally invasive approaches. These may be achieved with the increasing skill of the operators and by new technology. If, as a result of these changes in the procedure, aspects are modified or even eliminated, the procedure is still neurosurgical. To relegate less invasive procedures to nonsurgeons is to argue that the only aspect of a patient's care that is unique to a surgeon is purely technical. This is patently untrue; it is the surgeon's responsibility to maintain the standard of surgical care by adapting to new technologies.

There is no substitute at this time for the physical extirpation of a mass lesion in terms of cure or control of either vascular or oncologic pathologies. The attractiveness of radiosurgery is not that it supplants open neurosurgical procedures but that it allows treatment of pathologies only treated earlier with unacceptable morbidity or mortality. There is, and likely always will be, a gray area where the benefits of various modalities are debated. It will only be through evaluation of the long-term results of these various therapies (as well as their availabilities, cost, requirements for experience of the operators, and individual patient preferences) that the "best" therapy in any given case is decided.

This chapter describes the results of the authors' experience with the gamma knife as well as the published results of other centers, where required.

Table 40-1 lists all the cases treated with the gamma knife worldwide through 1997. It should be kept in mind that many of the indications listed are not universally accepted as appropriate for gamma surgery. The authors' version of the facts for each indication are given in the text.

HISTORY

Clarke and Horsley developed the first stereotactic system,[7] and the method was first applied clinically by Spiegel and co-workers.[8] This allowed for the localization of intracranial structures by their spatial relationship to Cartesian coordinates relative to a ring rigidly affixed to the skull. This was a prerequisite to the development of radiosurgery by Lars Leksell: his ambition was to develop a method of destroying localized structures deep within the brain without the degree of coincident brain trauma associated with open procedures. The convergence of multiple beams of ionizing radiation at one stereotactically defined point was the result. A nominal dose is delivered to the paths of each incident beam. However, at the point of intersection of the beams, a dose proportional to the number of individual beams is delivered. The physical specifications of the device would be designed to ensure a sharp drop-off of delivered radiation at the edge of the intersection point. This would allow precise selection of the targeted lesion and minimization of trauma to surrounding tissue. He termed this concept radiosurgery in 1951.

Various sources of ionizing radiation were tried. Leksell first used an orthovoltage x-ray tube coupled to a stereotactic frame in the treatment of trigeminal neuralgia and for cingulotomy in obsessive compulsive disorders.[9] A cyclotron was used as an accelerated proton source and used to treat various pathologies.[10,11] The cyclotron was too cumbersome and expensive for widespread application. A linear accelerator was evaluated but was found at that time to lack the inherent precision necessary for this work. Fixed gamma sources of Co^{60} and a fixed stereotactic target fulfilled

TABLE 40-1 • **Number of Cases Treated with the Gamma Knife Worldwide through June 2003**		
Diagnosis	**No.**	**Percentage**
Vascular	36233	15.78
Arteriovenous malformation	33540	14.60
Aneurysm	127	0.06
Other vascular	2566	1.12
Tumor	177151	77.13
Benign	80517	35.06
Acoustic neuroma	21272	9.26
Meningioma	28421	12.37
Pituitary	19561	8.52
Pineal	2215	0.96
Craniopharyngioma	2294	1.00
Hemangioblastoma	1042	0.45
Chordoma	1134	0.49
Trigeminal neuroma	1450	0.63
Schwannoma	1383	0.60
Other benign tumors	1745	0.76
Malignant	96634	42.08
Metastasis	72749	31.68
Glial tumors	17677	7.70
Chondrosarcoma	234	0.10
Glomus tumor	657	0.29
Ocular melanoma	874	0.38
NPH carcinoma	949	0.41
Hemangiopericytoma	631	0.27
Other malignant tumors	2863	1.25
Functional	16281	7.09
Intractable pain targets	447	0.19
Trigeminal neuralgia	12560	5.47
Parkinson's disease	1058	0.46
Psychoneurosis	109	0.05
Epilepsy	1534	0.67
Other functional targets	573	0.25
Total Indications	229665	100

From Elekta Radiosurgery Inc, 2003. These figures represent cases treated at gamma knife sites throughout the world from 1968 through June 2003.

the requirements of precision and compactness. The first gamma knife was built between 1965 and 1968.

The use of a single high dose of ionizing beams to treat neurosurgical problems was a novel and creative concept 30 years ago, and it changed the direction of development in many fields of neurosurgery. However, a creative innovation is not perfect in its inception, and the gamma knife was not an exception. Contributions of excellence by numerous neurosurgeons and physicists, together with advances in computer technology to improve the software used in planning, have over the years defined the present use of the tool. For instance, improvements in the planning system now allow for systematic shielding of the optic apparatus from exposure during treatment of parasellar masses. In lesions only 2 to 5 mm away, the dose to sensitive structures can be limited to less than 2% to 7% of the maximum dose. However, in spite of all the changes in application of gamma surgery, the underlying concepts behind it have not changed since its inception. This speaks for the sagacity of Lars Leksell and his invention.

Doses delivered and indications for the various pathologies treated were all empiric, initially. In the subsequent discussions this should be considered when doses (both minimal and maximal) and results are discussed.

PATHOPHYSIOLOGY

The effects of single high dose of gamma radiation on pathologic and normal tissue have been studied on clinical human and on experimental animal tissue. These studies are incomplete because the human material tends to come from treatment failures and the experimental material is taken from normal animals. However, some conclusions as to the method of effectiveness and about tissue tolerances can be drawn.

Normal Tissue

The relative radioresistance of normal brain relates to its low mitotic activity. Also, the rate at which a total dose of radiation is applied affects the damage caused by the dose. This is caused by the ability of the cell to effect repairs during the actual time of irradiation. A higher dose rate (i.e., the same total dose applied over a shorter period) consequently increases the lethality of the dose. The normal tissue surrounding the stereotactically targeted pathologic tissue receives a markedly lower dose but over the same period. Therefore, not only is the total dose lower, but the dose rate is lower as well. This effect is seen most clearly at doses above and below 1 Gy/min.[12] This radiobiological phenomenon explains part of the relative safety of single-dose radiation with steep gradients at the edge of targeted tissue. There are likely additional mechanisms of such sparing.

The steep gradient of dose and consequent dose rate described above does not exist in conventional radiotherapy. When treating tumors, the radiation oncologist uses "fractionation" or dividing the total dose into smaller portions, which allows repair of normal tissue as well as transition of dormant cells within the target to cells in division (at which time they are more sensitive to radiation). Creating a dose gradient at the lesion's margin not only eliminates the need for fractionation but also improves the effectiveness of the delivered dose within the target (high-dose rate zone) to 2.5 to 3 times that of the same dose delivered in a fractionated manner. The gamma knife stereotactically excludes normal tissue from the high-dose rate zone area as much as possible. It may also take advantage of the natural difference in susceptibility of pathologic versus normal tissue.

In order to understand the radiobiology of a single high dose of radiation on normal brain, the parietal lobe of rats treated by a gamma knife was studied at the authors' center. It was found that a dose of 50 Gy caused astrocytic swelling without changes in neuronal morphology or breakdown of the blood-brain barrier at 12 months. There was fibrin deposition in the walls of capillaries. At 75 Gy, necrosis was seen at 4 months, as was breakdown of the blood-brain barrier. More vigorous morphologic changes were seen in astrocytes, and hemispheric swelling coincident with the necrosis occurred at 4 months. With the dose increased to 120 Gy, necrosis was seen at 4 weeks but was not associated with hemispheric swelling. Astrocytic swelling occurred

at only 1 week postirradiation.[13] These findings are consistent with earlier reports on the effective dose to produce well-defined lesions in the thalamus in patients treated with the gamma knife.[14,15]

Tumor Response

Little is known about the pathophysiologic changes induced by gamma surgery at the cellular level in tumors. Division of tumor cells is presumably inhibited by radiation-induced damage to DNA. Also, it has been shown that the microvascular supply to tumors is inhibited by changes resulting from gamma surgery. In meningiomas studied after this treatment, there was reduction of blood flow over time.[16] Tumors responding early showed the greatest reduction in blood flow. Other authors have proposed that the induction of apoptosis by gamma radiation to proliferating cells may be responsible for at least a portion of the effect of gamma surgery on tumors.[17,18] Although such contentions may be premature, they may point the direction to future research.

Thus the pathophysiologic effect of gamma surgery seems not to be tumor necrosis. For this, higher doses than typically used would be required. Rarely, necrotic doses are used for gamma surgery (e.g., in functional cases). Ideally, following gamma surgery, tumors begin to shrink without changes in the normal tissue. In general, the rate of shrinkage is slower in more benign tumors.

The effectiveness of the therapy is most dependent on the ability to define and treat the entire lesion. However, the same result can also be obtained at times by treating the nutrient or feeding vessels of tumors (e.g., meningiomas). Malignant gliomas do poorly with any surgical technique, including gamma surgery, because of the inability to include all of the microscopic disease within the treated area. Individual metastatic deposits and small benign tumors are well handled with both open resection and with the gamma knife because the tumor margin can be defined well intraoperatively or on neuroimaging studies.

In order to conformally cover the target, more than one isocenter is nearly always utilized. When multiple radiation fields are made to overlap in this manner, the radiation dose distribution becomes inhomogeneous. The resulting areas of local maxima are called "hot spots." Controversy exists as to whether the presence of hot spots in gamma surgery is beneficial or detrimental. An even dose distribution is an essential and basic concept in radiotherapy. There is some evidence that these hot spot areas may be of benefit in gamma surgery. The factors to keep in mind to understand this line of reasoning are as follows: because of radiation geometry, hot spots are usually located in the deep portions of the target. In tumors, this is usually the areas that receive the poorest blood supply and that are therefore relatively hypoxic. Furthermore, the ability of a cell to respond to otherwise sublethal dosages of radiation can be affected by its own condition, as well as the state of the cells near it. Cells that are sublethally injured and that are in the vicinity of similar cells recover more often than cells that are in the vicinity of lethally injured cells. The hot spots, therefore, create islands of lethally injured cells that will enhance the cell kill in the sublethal injury zone.[19] Oxygen is a radiosensitizer, and the relatively high dose rate of the hot spots will act to offset any loss of efficacy in the hypoxic core of the target. This position is supported by the work of other authors.[20]

Cranial Nerves

The susceptibility of cranial nerves to injury from gamma surgery is of great interest. Tolerance is dependent on the particular nerve and the individual nerve's involvement by the pathologic process requiring treatment. Because of these factors, it is difficult to extrapolate exact numbers in many instances. Some statements can be made with some certainty.

The optic and acoustic nerves are the most sensitive to radiation of the cranial nerves. Being central nervous system tracts, containing oligodendrocytes, and carrying complex information are the reasons thought to be behind their vulnerability. These tracts are unable to regenerate following injury. Optic neuropathy has been reported as a complication following single doses greater than 8 Gy.[21] The tolerable level of radiation to the optic apparatus is still a subject of debate. Some advocate that the optic apparatus can tolerate doses as high as 12 to 14.1 Gy[22–24]; others recommend an upper limit of 8 Gy.[25,26] Small volumes of the optic apparatus exposed to doses of 10 Gy or less may be acceptable in some cases.[27,28] Both the tolerable absolute dose and tolerable volume undoubtedly vary from patient to patient. This degree of variability likely depends on the extent of damage to the optic apparatus by pituitary adenoma compression, ischemic changes, type and timing of previous interventions (e.g., fractionated radiation therapy and surgery), the patient's age, and the presence or absence of other comorbidities (e.g., diabetes).[28,29]

On the other hand, the trigeminal and facial nerves are significantly more resilient. In the treatment of trigeminal neuralgia with radiosurgery, with 50 to 100 mm^3 of the trigeminal roots at the entry zone treated with 60 to 80 Gy, out of 139 patients only 1 had a facial hypoesthesia. The authors have observed 9 mild to profound hypoesthesias in trigeminal neuralgia patients treated with gamma knife doses of 50 to 90 Gy. In a larger group of small acoustic neuromas (not stretching the trigeminal nerve) treated with radiosurgery with periphery doses of 10 to 25 Gy, the incidence of facial hyposthesia was 19%.[30] This seems to indicate that it is the length of nerve exposed that is the critical determinant in injury. In the same 254 patients, the incidence of facial paresis was 17%, although this was in all instances transitory.

The cranial nerves in the cavernous sinus are relatively robust; neuropathies have not been seen with doses up to 40 Gy.[21] The authors have not observed any neuropathies of cranial nerves IX through XII in the treatment of glomus jugulare tumors.

Normal Cerebral Vasculature

There are both clinical and experimental data regarding the effect of single high-dose gamma irradiation of normal cerebral vasculature. In treating 1917 arteriovenous malformations, the authors have seen only 2 incidences of clinical syndromes that were possibly associated with the stenosis of normal vessels. This low incidence has occurred even though occasionally normal vessels are included in the treatment field. One case was reported after treating a glioma with 90 Gy gamma surgery followed by 40 Gy of fractionated

whole brain irradiation of a middle cerebral artery occlusion.[31] Steiner and colleagues described two cases in which disproportionate white matter changes might have been ascribed to venous stenosis and occlusion.[32] Another case, that of a patient with a diencephalic arteriovenous malformation, demonstrated marked edema associated with venous outflow occlusion. This patient suffered visual and cognitive deficits, but over the course of months his neurologic status returned to baseline. Because veins in this region can obliterate spontaneously, it is difficult to assess what was the contribution of the gamma surgery in this process (Fig. 40-1).

In the authors' treatment of pituitary adenomas with cavernous sinus extension or medial sphenoid wing vicinity meningiomas, no occlusion of normal vasculature has been observed. This absence of stenosis is noted even though the internal carotid artery or portions of the circle of Willis, or its proximal branches, are often included in the treatment field. The only incidence of treating an intracranial aneurysm with a gamma knife did lead to narrowing and eventual occlusion of the adjacent small posterior communicating artery segment. Whether this was associated with the obliteration of the aneurysm neck or with primary changes in the artery is unknown. It is possible that the incidence of occlusion of smaller vessels is more common than recognized because the occlusion would occur slowly and compensatory changes could take place, preventing clinical syndromes from occurring. Regardless, the clinical impact is minimal. Others have noted injury to the cavernous segment of the carotid artery following radiosurgery for pituitary adenomas. A total of 4 cases have been reported, and in only 2 of these cases were the patients symptomatic from carotid artery stenosis.[33–35] Pollock and colleagues have recommended that the prescription dose should be limited to less than 50% of the intracavernous carotid artery vessel diameter.[34] Shin and colleagues recommended restricting the dose to the internal carotid artery to less than 30 Gy.[36]

Experimental studies done on normal vasculature in the brains of rats[37] and cats[38] showed similar findings. The primary injury was endothelial necrosis and desquamation, muscular coat hypertrophy, and fibrosis at lower doses (25 to 100 Gy). At doses up to 300 Gy, necrosis of the muscular layer was seen in cats. In only 1 instance (i.e., a rat anterior cerebral artery treated with 100 Gy) was occlusion of a vessel seen. Follow-up of 2 to 20 months was allowed. Similar studies on hypercholesterolemic rabbits treated with 10 to 100 Gy showed no histologic changes in the basilar arteries and no instances of occlusion after 2 to 24 months.[39]

Arteriovenous Malformations

Whereas minimal clinical and only moderate changes are seen in the normal cerebral vasculature after high doses of gamma radiation, this is in sharp contrast to the response of the vessels of an arteriovenous malformation (AVM). Complete radiographic obliteration can be achieved after appropriate gamma surgery. The effects of ionizing radiation, and their role in the management of AVMs, was first reported in 1928 by Cushing and Bailey.[40] During craniotomy for an AVM, he had to interrupt surgery because of a major hemorrhage from the lesion. He then treated the patient with fractionated radiation. At reoperation 5 years later, only an obliterated avascular mass was discovered. This early

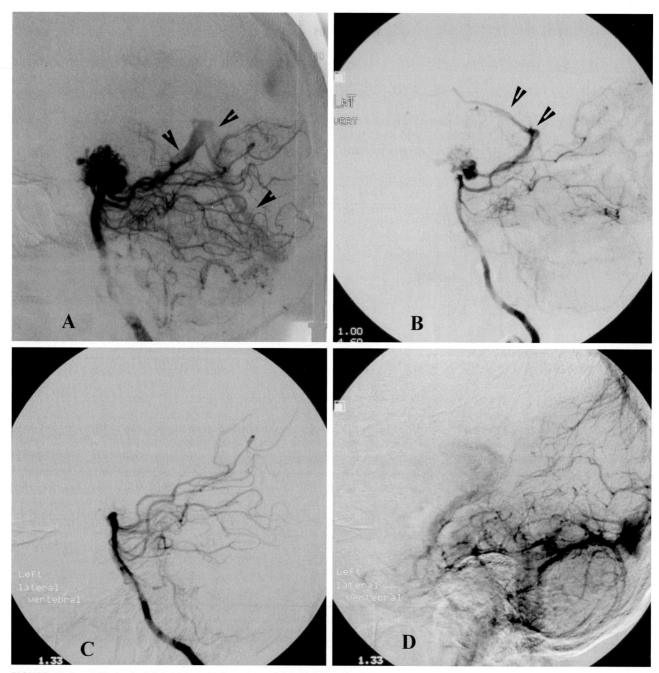

FIGURE 40-1   *A,* Thalamic AVM shown with lateral vertebral arteriography. *B,* Similar view obtained 17 months after gamma surgery shows partial obliteration of the nidus. The basal vein of Rosenthal, the vein of Galen, and the straight sinus were not visualized. Venous drainage of the residual AVM appears to be through ascending choroidal veins and the internal cerebral veins. *C,* Early and (*D*) late-filling vertebral arteriograms obtained 37 months after gamma surgery show obliteration of the AVM and complete absence of the deep venous system.

success was overshadowed by numerous series of failures.[41–57] In this early period, Johnson[48] was the only one to report reasonable results with a 45% angiographic obliteration. The introduction of the gamma knife rekindled interest in the treatment of AVMs with radiation.[49]

The pathologic changes in AVMs treated with the gamma knife have been described by several authors.[50–52] The earliest change is damage to the endothelium, with swelling of the endothelial cells and subsequent denution or separation of the endothelium from the underlying vessel wall. The most important changes are seen later in the intima, with the appearance of loosely organized spindle cells (myofibroblasts) and an extracellular matrix containing collagen type IV, not seen in the intima of untreated vessels. Expansion of the extracellular matrix and cellular degeneration define the final stage prior to luminal obliteration. The occlusion of the vessels is not a thrombotic process but rather the culmination of concentric narrowing of the vessel by an expanding vessel wall. Subsequent recanalization of an angiographically proven obliterated AVM has not occurred in the authors' experience.

INDICATIONS

Vascular Malformations

Arteriovenous Malformations

The indications for gamma surgery of AVMs versus other treatment options is, in many cases, unclear at best. Small, asymptomatic, inoperable AVMs are clearly best treated with the gamma knife, whereas AVMs with a large, symptomatic hemorrhage in noneloquent superficial brain are best treated with open surgery. The reason for this is that the risk-benefit value is clear in both of these situations. In other situations, the risk-benefit value is more ambiguous. A knowledge of the capabilities of various treatments to effect cure, the associated morbidity and mortality associated with the treatment, and the natural history of the disease following various treatments must be known to accurately prescribe the most efficacious treatment plan.

Unfortunately, in most instances, these are not known. The natural history of AVMs is not fully understood. Some authors believe that size matters, with smaller AVMs bleeding at a higher rate than larger ones[53–56] or at a lower rate.[57,58] There is also evidence that size is independent of the hemorrhage rate.[59–63] Similarly, the rate of hemorrhage of an AVM following a previous hemorrhage is thought to be higher than the rate in unruptured AVMs by some authors[54,60,62,64] but not by others.[55,65,66] The effects of age, gender, pregnancy, and AVM location also confound the question of risk of rupture.[53–55,59–62,65,67,68]

The results of microsurgery published in the literature tend to come from centers of excellence, and the patients they treat with open surgery are, by definition, more amenable to this treatment. The effectiveness of the treatment by this manner and its comorbid results are known shortly after surgery. The short-term morbidity of treatment with the gamma knife approaches zero, but because the benefit and potential complications require time to become apparent, follow-up of these patients is problematic. The quality of the AVMs treated with the gamma knife also varies in a large series of those treated by microsurgery. All of these factors make comparison of the modalities difficult. Add to that the additional risks and benefits of preoperative embolization and the matter is much less clear. It is paramount to the physician treating a patient harboring an AVM to be aware, as much as possible, of the options that are available and of the magnitude of the risks and benefits associated with each.

Methods

PERIOPERATIVE MANAGEMENT

Patients are routinely evaluated the day prior to radiosurgery. Preoperative consults are obtained as necessary, including evaluation by the neuroradiology service. The patients are loaded with antiseizure medications, and levels are drawn prior to therapy. Patients already on medication for seizures also have their levels evaluated. Although the authors have never had a patient have a seizure during therapy, the small but serious risk of a generalized seizure while the patient is secured within the gamma unit makes every precaution reasonable. Patients are also started on systemic dexamethasone the evening prior to therapy and this is continued until the following evening. The use of high-dose perioperative dexamethasone is empiric. Although the authors have used steroids in all experiences with the gamma knife, their original purpose (i.e., to minimize vasogenic edema at the time of therapy) has never been documented as a problem. Hence, the prophylactic use of steroids is debatable.

FRAME PLACEMENT

The placement of the head frame is done in the operating room. The patient is given intravenous sedation, usually short-acting narcotics (e.g., fentanyl) and propofol, until he or she is no longer responsive to verbal or moderate physical stimuli. The anesthesia service monitors the patient throughout the procedure. The authors have found this far superior to the previous practice of applying the frame using only local anesthesia. Patients that were treated both before and since the frame is applied in this way have provided clear feedback preferring frame placement under anesthesia.

A simple strap, fashioned with Velcro ends, is placed across the patient's head and then fastened above the frame after it has been lowered into position. This holds the frame in position while the pins are secured. The frame eliminates the need for the earplugs in the auditory canal, which can be painful.

The space available within the gamma knife is limited, as is the 3-dimensional coordinate system within the frame itself. For these reasons, care must be taken to skew the placement of the frame in the direction of the pathology if it is far off the center of the brain. This includes having the frame base at the level of the zygomatic arch, for skull base and posterior fossa lesions; and to the side of the head for lesions that are more than a short distance off the midline. Care must be taken to not compress the ear against the frame.

IMAGING AND DOSE PLANNING
(Figs. 40-2 and 40-3)

In planning the treatment of an AVM, both stereotactic arteriography and stereotactic MRI are used. This requires cooperation between the treating neurosurgeon and the radiologist performing the examination. With the angiogram, the only views that are applicable to the planning of treatment are standardized views relative to the frame. These are A-P and lateral views exactly orthogonal to the frame. The frame is placed in a fixed holder, and a perspex box carrying fiducial markers is applied to it. The relevant digital images are electronically transferred to the planning station or scanned, if necessary. The relative positions of the fiducials and AVM allow localization of the AVM relative to the frame. If evaluation of previous films indicates that any other view is necessary to visualize the AVM, then adjustments must be made in the placement of the frame.

The use of digital subtraction angiography may be helpful in understanding the anatomy of an AVM, but at this time it cannot be used in the planning of treatment. Distortion of the radiograph by the image intensifier is too great to allow for the precision necessary for radiosurgery.

The stereotactic MRI allows better visualization of the dimensions of nonspherically shaped targets in the axial plane. The MRI also helps to define the shape of the AVM and confirms angiographically obtained information. It is difficult to differentiate the nidus from the draining veins, so the MRI tends to overestimate the size of the AVM. The capability to incorporate computerized tomography angiography (CTA) and magnetic resonance angiography (MRA) data into the planning process is expected to be available in future releases of gamma planning software.

THE GAMMA KNIFE

The gamma knife is composed of a body that contains the radiation sources and a treatment couch that delivers the patient into the unit. Within the body are 201 Co^{60} source capsules that are aligned with two internal collimators that direct the gamma radiation toward the center of the unit. A third, external collimator helmet is attached to the

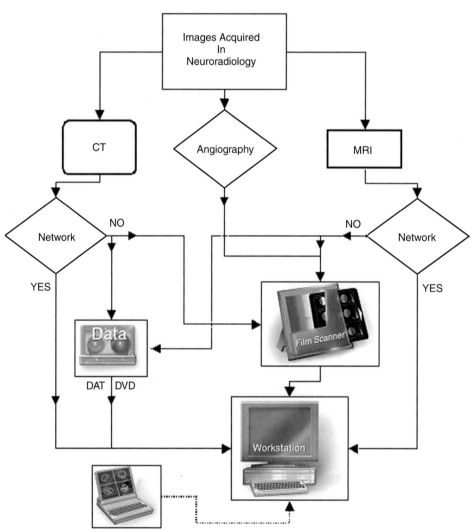

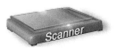

FIGURE 40-2 This diagram depicts the process for obtaining and transferring radiologic information to the Gamma Suite planning workstation.

Flowchart of the Planning Process

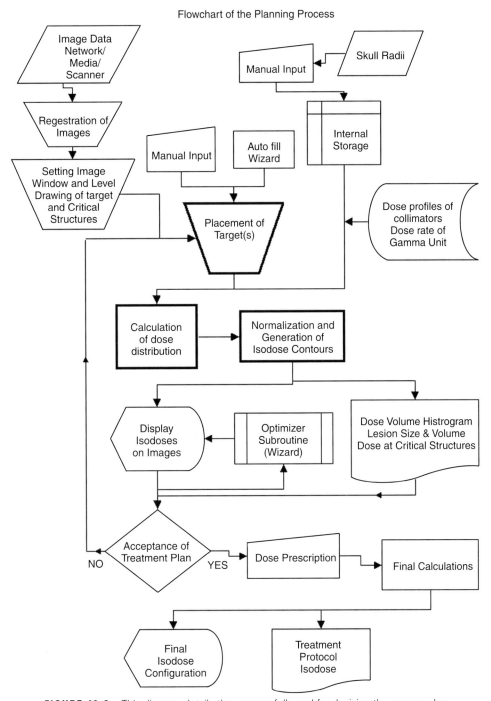

FIGURE 40-3   This diagram details the process followed for devising the gamma plan.

treatment couch. Four external collimator helmets are provided, and they have fixed-diameter apertures that create an isocenter of 4-, 8-, 14-, or 18-mm diameters. By changing external collimator helmets, the diameter of the roughly spherical isocenter can be varied. The 201 individual collimators within the helmet are machined to exact standards to direct the 201 beams of gamma radiation to a common point where they intersect, creating the isocenter. The frame attached to the patient's head is adjusted within the

collimator helmet so that the area to be treated is at that point of intersection.

TREATMENT

After the treatment plan has been made, the patient is moved onto the gamma knife couch and the y and z coordinates for the first exposure are set on the frame attached to the patient's head. The patient's head is placed within the collimator helmet and secured on either side by trunions, and the x coordinate is set. Visual confirmation of correct settings must be made by the operator, in addition to the person who sets the coordinates.

The head, at this point, is suspended by the frame within the helmet, and for comfort the neck should be supported with towels or an equivalent material. The exposure time of the corresponding isocenter is entered at the control panel twice for confirmation, and the session then commences with the entire couch being mechanically pulled into the body of the unit. The external collimator helmet locks into place with the internal collimators. After each exposure, the patient is withdrawn from the collimator helmet and the process is repeated. Necessary changes of the collimator helmet are made as needed according to the plan. The relatively recent introduction of the Automatic Positioning System, a system that sets the coordinates by six independent motors just outside the irradiation field, has led to shorter treatment times, enhanced selectivity, and better physician workflow.[69–71] Improved ergonomics, automatic shielding, and an integrated collimator helmet changer are also planned. Obviously, these changes will not affect the efficacy of the treatment but will make the process simpler for the operator.

At the end of the treatment, the frame is removed from the head within the suite. The patient usually reports a sensation of tightening and discomfort during removal. At least two pairs of hands should be available to steady the frame and prevent injury by the pins as they are removed. Venous bleeding, when it occurs, can be controlled with hand-held pressure for several minutes. The occasional arterial bleeder usually requires a hemostatic suture, and an absorbable one (which obviates the need for later removal) should be readily available. After frame removal the pin sites are dressed in a sterile fashion, steristrips are used to oppose the skin edges for optimal cosmesis, and a modest head wrap is applied.

RESULTS

The authors have treated 2155 vascular malformations (of which 1917 were AVMs with the gamma knife) since 1970. As experience with this tool grows, the capabilities and limitations of the gamma knife are being defined. Serendipitously, the first AVMs were treated by prescribing a 25-Gy periphery dose. That means the edge of the AVM received this dose, and that this was the minimum dose received by the entire AVM. Subsequent changes in protocol showed a significant decrease in success with doses less than 23 Gy, and small improvements in obliteration rates (but with significantly more radiation-associated complications) with higher doses. Optimally, therefore, the authors treat most AVMs with 23 to 25 Gy at the margin. With doses higher than 25 Gy, no added benefit has been observed.

As in microsurgery, feeding arteries or draining veins should be left alone when performing gamma surgery, and only the nidus should be treated. In very large AVMs, only partially treated because of the excessive dose necessary to treat optimally, occasional cures have been achieved. This is thought to be caused by fortuitous inclusion of all the pathologic shunts within the higher dose treatment field. Targeting only the feeding vessels to the AVM has had very limited success because of recruitment of small angiographically occult feeding arteries. Interestingly, the first patient ever treated had only the feeding vessels targeted and a cure

was obtained. The early success with this strategy has not been reproduced.

The results of gamma surgery on AVMs are affected by the minimum dose applied to the AVM and the size of the AVM: these two factors are interdependent. It has been shown that the limitation of the allowed margin dose by the size of the malformation decreases the rate of obliteration. There are reports contending that low-dose gamma surgery with large malformations results in obliteration rates that are comparable to smaller lesions treated with a larger margin dose. It is doubtful that these results will hold up with larger series. Thus far, at the authors' center, larger AVMs have had a lower obliteration rate.

Between 1970 and 1990, 880 patients were optimally treated. (Optimally is defined as at least 25 Gy at the margin of the entire nidus of the AVM.) Of these patients, the age range was 3 to 76 years; approximately 15% were pediatric patients (<17 years old).

The presenting symptoms were hemorrhage (70%), seizures (16%), headache (5%), neurologic deficits not associated with acute hemorrhage (4%), and other symptoms (2%).

The majority of referrals were for AVMs deemed operable only with unacceptable morbidity, explaining the fact that 73% of the AVMs were located in deep areas of the brain (20% in the basal ganglia or thalamus, 16% around or within the ventricular system, and 11% within the brain stem) or within eloquent cortex. Eighty-five percent were supratentorial, and among these 62% were located on the right side, 37% on the left side, and 1% were centrally located.

In this series, the patients treated earlier were subjected to a vigorous protocol of repeated angiograms. Later, with the introduction of computerized tomography and then magnetic resonance imaging, angiography was not performed until nidus was no longer evident on these screening examinations.

Imaging Outcome (Tables 40-2 and 40-3)

Of the 880 patients treated, 461 had adequate angiographic follow-up. Of these 461 patients, 80% were found to be cured within 2 years. In patients with MRI examinations that showed no residual nidus, roughly one third were found on subsequent follow-up angiography to be cured; one third were found to be subtotally obliterated (no residual nidus but early filling vein present on angiography); and

---

TABLE 40-2 ▪ Outcome of Radiosurgery for Arteriovenous Malformations

Series	No. of Cases	Angiographic Obliteration (%)
Bunge et al[†]	374	82
Sutcliffe et al (1992)[272]	160	76
Kawamoto et al[‡]	144	70
Kondziolka et al (1993)[273]	402	71
Steiner et al (1979)	461	80
Chang et al (2000)[274]	277	79
Karlsson, Lindquist, and Steiner (1997)[275]	1319	85
Flickinger et al (1996)[276]	197	72

[†]H. Bunge, personal communication, 1993.
[‡]S. Kawamoto, personal communication, 1994.

TABLE 40-3 ▪ Permanent Neurologic Deficits Following Gamma Knife Radiosurgery of Arteriovenous Malformation

Series	Radiation-Induced Complications	Rebleeding
Bunge et al*	4	5
Sutcliffe et al (1992)[272]	3.8	3.8
Kawamoto et al[†]	3.7	4.2
Steiner et al (1992)[79]	3.1	2.3
Kondziolka et al (1993)[273]	3.1	5.2

*H. Bunge, personal communication, 1993.
[†]S. Kawamoto, personal communication, 1994.

one third were found to be partially obliterated (nidus smaller but still present). Rarely, delayed formation of a cyst on MRI occurs at the site of an obliterated AVM; this infrequent occurrence has been reported by others.[72–74]

Angiographic changes precede obliteration.[75–78] The diameter of the nidus becomes smaller, as do the diameters of the feeding arteries and, occasionally, those of the draining veins. The nidus decreases in size, and the shunt is reduced. We have classified angiographic changes as either no change, partial obliteration (decrease in the size of the nidus) (Fig. 40-4), subtotal obliteration (no evidence of nidus but with a persistent early draining vein) (Fig. 40-5), and total obliteration (Figs. 40-6 through 40-8).

At the time of the last evaluation of our results, only 5% of patients who had had follow-up angiograms had no change in the status of their AVMs. Eighty percent were cured, 10% had subtotal obliteration, and 5% were partially obliterated. The angiogram should be complete, of high quality, and should be reviewed by an experienced and interested neuroradiologist or neurosurgeon. No patient that was harboring an angiographically proven obliterated AVM has ever hemorrhaged, in our experience, nor has a patient with a subtotally obliterated AVM sustained a postradiosurgery hemorrhage. Regardless of this, the authors do not consider a patient cured until he or she has total obliteration of the AVM. The early draining vein represents persistence of the shunt.

In this group of patients, obliteration rates were affected by the size of the nidus. The rate for AVMs less than 1 mL in volume was 88%. For 1 to 3 mL, it was 78%, and for greater than 3 mL, it was 50%.

Evaluation of patients treated suboptimally (i.e., periphery dose less than 23 to 25 Gy) shows a sharp decline in obliteration rates (Fig. 40-9). Doses greater than 25 Gy were associated with little improvement in obliteration rate.

Of the 2500 patients we have treated, 277 had embolization of the AVM prior to gamma surgery. Only 53 had follow-up angiograms. Of these, 43 (81%) were cured. The low rate of follow-up angiograms in this subset is caused disproportionately by evidence of flow voids on follow-up MRI scans. The authors are now undertaking a study of this subgroup, including patients treated up to 2 years ago. It is clear, however, that the ability of the embolization procedure to improve obliteration rates with gamma surgery depends on shrinking the size of the nidus. If the embolization only decreases flow or splits the AVM into multiple portions, it is unlikely to alter the outcome of gamma surgery.

Gamma surgery was performed on 218 patients to treat residual nidus following microsurgery. Of these patients, 182 had an angiogram at 2 years after gamma surgery, and 153 (85%) were cured. Volume appears to be directly related to higher long-term complication rates.

Recently, there has been much discussion of prospective, staged treatment of large AVMs (volume > 15 mL) with gamma surgery. Staging is typically designed to separate out 50% of the volume. Our results for large AVMs indicate an obliteration rate of approximately 16%. At the University of Vienna, Kitz and his team have reported angiographically proven obliteration in 13 out of 14 patients with large AVMs. If there is residual AVM, retreatment is possible. However, complication rates for retreatment are higher than for initial treatment; rates range from 14% reported by Karlsson to 2% in our series.[275] The wide variation in retreatment complication rates likely depends on differences in the initial and residual AVM treatment volumes in each center's experience.

There has been criticism leveled against radiosurgery series for AVMs reported in the literature that the results are biased because angiography is only performed after there is no evidence of nidus residual on MRI. And because the reported obliteration rate is of the patients who had follow-up angiograms, the reported numbers are biased toward a favorable group. To a limited extent, this is true. Evaluation of the group of 880 patients showed that assuming the worst-case scenario, in which every patient with an MRI but not an angiogram was considered not cured, the final percentages of obliteration dropped less than 1%.

Clinical Outcome (see Table 40-3)

A review of the long-term clinical outcome following gamma surgery was carried out on 247 patients the authors treated between 1970 and 1983.[79] The presenting symptoms varied widely, and 94% of the patients had hemorrhaged prior to therapy. Ninety-eight of these patients had chronic headaches, and 66% had complete relief following gamma surgery; an additional 9% improved. Twenty-six percent had seizures prior to therapy, and 19% of these became seizure-free and 51% improved. Eleven patients (5% of patients without a prior seizures) had at least one seizure following therapy. Resolution or significant improvements were also seen in 53 of 74 patients (72%) with motor deficits, 19 of 46 (41%) with a sensory deficit, 23 of 44 (52%) with memory disturbance, and 26 of 35 (74%) with language dysfunction.

The authors have recently, by questionnaires, analyzed in detail the outcome of seizures in our patients. Of 1200 respondents, there were 178 patients with seizures as a preoperative symptom. At the time of analysis, 62% were seizure-free, with almost half of these off medication. An additional 24% were improved.

The cause for clinical improvement following gamma surgery in such a large number of patients is unknown. The natural history of neurologic deficits to improve over time must be presumed to play a major role. The improvement in regional blood flow following AVM obliteration may also be responsible for a portion of the gains made by the patients. Whatever the reason, significant improvement is seen in many patients.

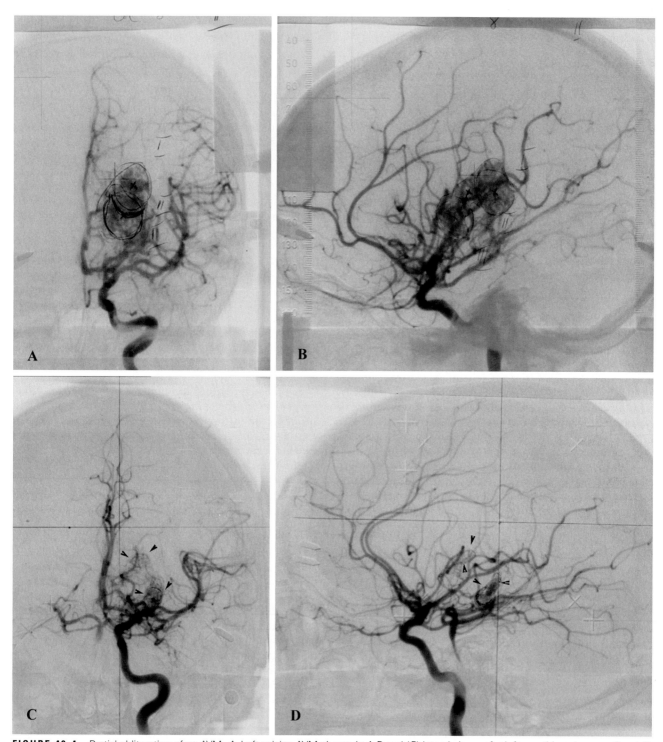

FIGURE 40-4 Partial obliteration of an AVM. *A*, Left sylvian AVM shown in A-P and (*B*) lateral views of a left carotid angiogram. *C* and *D*, Same views 4 years later show a decrease in the size of the nidus but persistent shunting of blood through the partially obliterated malformation (*arrowheads*). The residual AVM was recently retreated.

Hemorrhage Risk in the Treatment-Response Interval

The annual incidence of hemorrhage in untreated AVMs is reported by various authors as between 2% and 5%. From research based on our own material, the authors recently reached several other conclusions. The risk of hemorrhage increases with age, and is also higher in females during the fertile years.[63]

Whether gamma surgery without obliteration of the nidus provides partial protection from hemorrhage is still controversial. It has been demonstrated by some authors that there may be some degree of protective effect.[79–81] Because the incidence of hemorrhage in a matched group of untreated patients will likely never be known, and because the timing of obliteration is not known except as being between diagnostic scans, it is a difficult position to support.

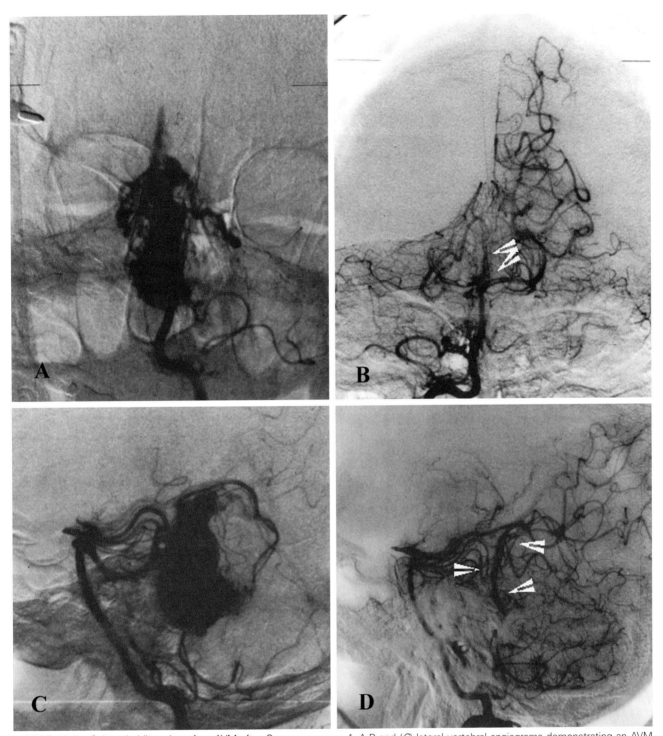

FIGURE 40-5 Subtotal obliteration of an AVM after Gamma surgery. *A*, A-P and (*C*) lateral vertebral angiograms demonstrating an AVM located within the vermis of the cerebellum. *B* and *D*, Control angiography with the same views obtained 3 years after gamma surgery shows no demonstrable nidus but the presence of an early filling vein (*arrowheads*).

The incidence of hemorrhage following gamma surgery during the first 2 years was studied in 1604 of our patients and reported by Karlsson and colleagues.[82] There were 49 hemorrhages, for an annual incidence of 1.4%. This is significantly lower than the generally accepted rate of 3% to 4% per year, but it includes all 1604 patients, including those known and not known to have obliterated AVMs. Of these hemorrhages,

14 were fatal (annual rate of 0.4%) and 9 had permanent neurologic deficits (annual rate of 0.3%).

In 113 patients with subtotal obliteration of the AVM, we observed no hemorrhages. No hemorrhage occurred during 948 risk years (average, 8.5 years). Assuming a natural risk of hemorrhage of 4%, there should have been 34 hemorrhages in this interval. These observations should be

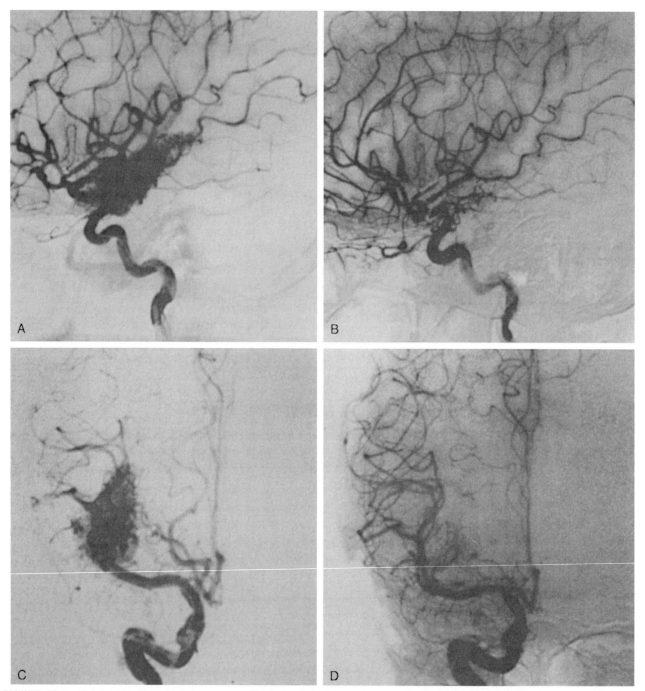

FIGURE 40-6   Total obliteration of arteriovenous malformation following gamma surgery. Arteriovenous malformation in the right sylvian region shown after partial embolization in the (A) lateral and (B) frontal projections and 2 years following gamma surgery, showing complete obliteration of the malformation in the (C) lateral and (D) frontal projections.

tested on larger patient material before final conclusions are made. Moreover, others have noted AVM reappearance after apparent gamma knife surgery obliteration.[83] In the authors' histopathologic analysis, gamma surgery of AVMs caused endothelial damage, proliferation of smooth-muscle cells, and the elaboration of extracellular collagen by these cells; this led to progressive stenosis and obliteration of the AVM nidus.[84] In this same report, there was evidence of small trapped vessels, which would have very little blood flow.[84] It is unclear what histopathologic process would

permit the formation of new vessels following radiosurgical-induced obliteration of the AVM nidus. However, it is clear that the infrequent and small trapped vessels observed by Schneider and colleagues[84] could not explain the angiographic findings reported by Lindqvist and colleagues.[83] Such inconsistent findings following radiosurgical treatment of AVMs suggest the need for further clinical and histopathologic investigation and the continued follow-up of patients, particularly pediatric ones, following gamma surgery.

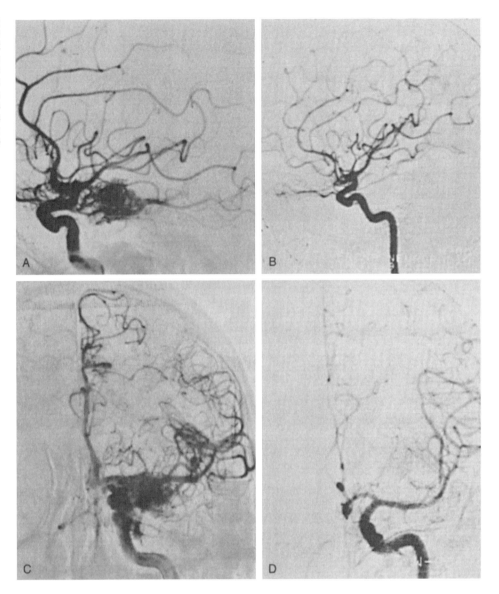

FIGURE 40-7 Early obliteration of an arteriovenous malformation following gamma surgery. Left internal carotid angiogram showing the (A) lateral and (B) frontal views of the malformation before gamma surgery and (C and D) 6 months following gamma surgery. In this case, early angiography was prompted by an MRI, which showed no flow voids in the region of the treated AVM.

Complications

Acute post-treatment nausea and vomiting occurs occasionally and is not associated with any lasting effects; these may be treated symptomatically.

Rare seizures have occurred in the authors' experience, all in the post-treatment period and in patients with a previous seizure disorder. None of our patients experienced a seizure while the head was secured within the gamma unit. However, this possibility should not be discounted because of the risk of cervical spine injury associated with the head being fixed within the unit.

The results of a series of 816 patients treated for AVMs with gamma surgery with follow-up CT (630 patients) and/or MRI (239 patients) showed white matter changes in a significant number of cases.[85–86] CT showed hypointensity changes in 11% of cases, and increased signal on the T2-weighted images on MRI in 37%. The higher percentage in MRI scans represents the higher sensitivity of this imaging modality. The earliest onset of these changes was 3 months, and 92% occurred within 15 months. Resolution of these changes was the usual course, on average

within 5 months (range, 1 to 17 months) (Fig. 40-10). Clinical symptoms were associated with these changes in 6% of the entire group, and resolved completely in one half. Therefore, 3% of patients suffered a fixed neurologic deficit following gamma surgery for AVM (see Table 40-3).

A rare occurrence following gamma surgery for AVMs is the development of an expansive cyst at or adjacent to an obliterated AVM. First reported in 1992[50] in 2 patients out of a series of 40, the authors have seen this event twice in our material. These occurred 5 to 10 years following treatment, and occasionally are symptomatic because of mass effect requiring extirpation. The etiology of these cysts is unclear. There have been 7 cases that we know of worldwide, 5 of which were operated on, usually because of mass effect. There was no evidence of malignancy or tumor noted in any of these cases. All those reported cases were in patients imaged solely with angiograms at the time of treatment, and the condition of the surrounding brain at the time of gamma surgery was not documented by CT or MRI (Fig. 40-11). The authors have preliminary data concerning the occurrence of this adverse effect in 1203 consecutive patients

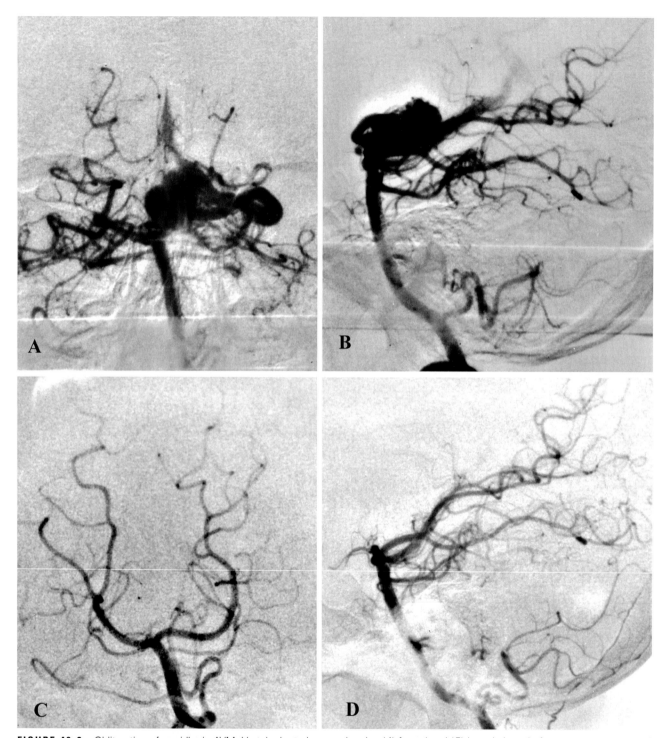

FIGURE 40-8   Obliteration of a midbrain AVM. Vertebral arteriogram showing (*A*) frontal and (*B*) lateral views before gamma surgery and (*C* and *D*) 2 years after gamma surgery. There was no neurologic deficit.

from a study in progress, including 2500 cases of AVMs treated between 1970 and 2002 with gamma surgery. The incidence of cyst formation in the entire 1203 patients was 1.6%; in those with more than 5 years of follow-up, the incidence of cyst formation was 3.6%. Radiation induced tissue change following gamma surgery and embolization were statistically related to the cyst formation.

Dural Malformations

Dural malformations, with or without associated AVMs, are uncommon lesions. Optimal treatment is unknown at this time; however, reasonable cure rates can be achieved with smaller lesions, using gamma surgery. Larger lesions, unless wholly inoperable, should be managed with at least partial open surgical or endovascular treatment prior to radiosurgery.

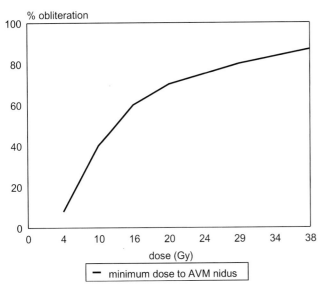

FIGURE 40-9 Dose-response curve of arteriovenous malformations.

The authors have treated 58 dural malformations with gamma surgery. The incidence of cure decreased with increasing length of the fistula. Of the 19 fistulas under 15 mm in length, 10 had angiographic follow-up and 7 of these (70%) were cured (Fig. 40-12) Of those between 15 and 25 mm in length, 6 had adequate follow-up and 3 were obliterated. There were 14 patients with lesions greater than 25 mm in length; and 7 had angiograms, of which 5 were cured. Three patients hemorrhaged after treatment (none with neurologic deficit); the fistulas of 2 of these patients are still patent.

Gamma surgery has been demonstrated to produce excellent results for selected AVMs. However, there have been scattered instances of delayed cyst formation years after treatment of an AVM with the gamma knife. The authors have recently reviewed 2 cases of dural AVMs treated with gamma surgery, and observed cyst formation at 153 and 157 months after radiosurgery. In these 2 cases, the doses to the margin were 20 and 23 Gy, and the maximal doses were 30 and 32 Gy. Both patients were neurologically asymptomatic from the cyst formation.

Spontaneous Carotid-Cavernous Sinus Fistulas

Large symptomatic fistulas require prompt intervention; presently, endovascular treatment is often employed. Ideally, treatment would obliterate the fistula while maintaining patency of the carotid artery. This is often not possible with endovascular techniques, and is certainly not possible with open surgical therapy.

The authors have treated 9 patients with carotid cavernous sinus fistulas using gamma surgery. The age range was 20 to 62 years. There was no acute reversible symptomatology in these cases. Six of these patients have follow-up angiography, and 5 were found to be cured while maintaining the patency of the carotid artery. Gamma surgery should be considered in the treatment of this entity when acute ablation of the fistula is not mandated by the clinical syndrome and when the eye is not threatened with excessive intraocular pressures.

Vein of Galen Malformations

The authors have treated 9 patients with vein of Galen malformations. The patients ranged in age from 4 to 72 years of age. Among these patients, there were 3 with Yasargil type I, 1 with type II, 2 with type III, and 3 with type IV malformations. Prior embolization had failed in 4 of the cases. Three of the vein of Galen malformations were treated twice with radiosurgery. Follow-up angiograms were obtained in 8 of the patients treated.[85] Four malformations were completed obliterated (Fig. 40-13). Another one seems to be obliterated, but definitive confirmation could not be obtained because the patient refused a final angiogram. Another patient has some residual fistula not in the initial radiosurgical treatment field and has been retreated. Two other patients had marked reduction of flow through their malformations.

Cavernous Hemangiomas

The success of treating AVMs prompted the treatment of cavernous hemangiomas (angiographically occult vascular malformations [AOVM]) with the gamma knife. Their tendency to be small, with the lack of intervening normal brain tissue and relatively low rate of clinically significant hemorrhage, made cavernomas a natural target for the gamma knife. The rate of hemorrhage for cavernomas is widely disparate in the neurosurgical literature reported as between 0.1% and 32%.[87–91] This is largely because of semantic differences in defining a hemorrhage, with some authors counting the presence of a haemosiderin ring on MRI as evidence of a hemorrhage and others only recognizing hemorrhages brought to attention by neurologic changes.

Gamma surgery of cavernous malformations appears to have a histologic effect on them that is not evident on imaging studies. In a case reported earlier,[92] a gamma surgery–treated cavernous hemangioma followed for 5 years showed no change on MRI studies. Histologic examination following surgical removal of the lesion showed it to be partially obliterated (Fig. 40-14).

A total of 23 patients have been treated by the authors for cavernous hemangiomas, all between 1985 and 1996; 22 of these are available for follow-up evaluation.[93] The patients either presented with epilepsy[6] or hemorrhage.[16] Maximum treatment dose varied from 11 to 60 Gy (mean, 33 Gy). Minimum, or periphery dose, varied from 9 to 35 Gy (mean, 18 Gy).

Nine symptomatic hemorrhages occurred in this group after therapy, for an annual incidence of 8%. Four of these patients were subsequently operated on. There was a statistical trend ($p = 0.17$) for higher peripheral dose to be associated with greater likelihood of post-treatment hemorrhage. There was no relationship between lesion location and occurrence of hemorrhage.

Six patients suffered neurologic decline secondary to radiation-induced changes, 5 of which were permanent. Two also suffered from a post-treatment hemorrhage. Radiation-induced changes were defined as radionecrosis or radiation-induced transitory changes seen on CT or MRI associated with clinical decline. Two patients subsequently underwent surgery. Thus the radiation-induced complication rate is 22%, nearly eight times higher than expected for

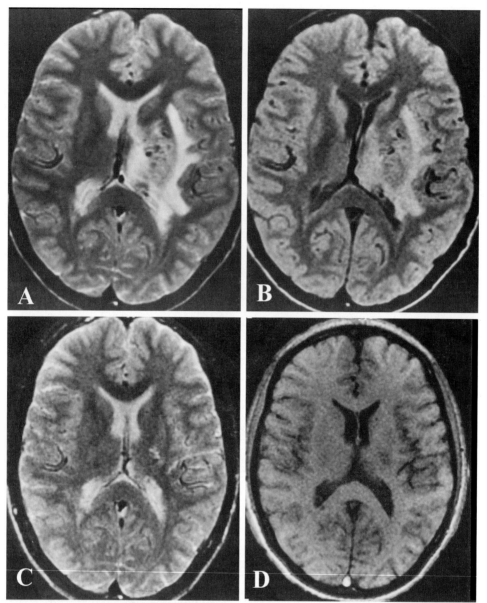

FIGURE 40-10 Onset and resolution of radiation-induced changes of normal brain tissue. Radiation-induced changes 6 months following radiosurgical treatment of a left basal ganglia arteriovenous malformation with a margin dose of 20 Gy. Appearance on (*A*) T2- and (*B*) T1-weighted MRI. These changes showed progressive regression and a complete disappearance at 2 years following the onset (*C* and *D*). Angiography documented total obliteration of the arteriovenous malformation.

a similarly treated group of AVM patients. As expected, there was a significant (*p* = 0.005) relationship between periphery dose of radiation and the occurrence of radiation-associated complications.

The high incidence of post-treatment hemorrhage and radiation-induced complications is greater than the expected morbidity from an untreated group. For this reason, the routine use of the gamma knife in the treatment of cavernous hemangiomas cannot be supported at this time.

There have been observations in literature that demonstrate a protective effect of gamma surgery on the rate of hemorrhage in these lesions. Based on 38 cases with AOVMs, Kondziolka and colleagues[94] maintain that radiosurgery offers benefit to these patients. They report that 6 patients

(15%) had significant reduction in AOVM size, with a 13% hemorrhage rate; 10 of the patients (26%) developed neurologic deficit, and 2 of these underwent surgery and succumbed to the illness. The rate of complications reported by them in the face of the fact that only 15% of the patients in this series had any reduction in the size of the lesion does not, in the authors' opinion, constitute grounds for justifying radiosurgery for an AOVM. Furthermore, their contention that the complications reported by us[95] may in part be caused by the high doses used in treatment does not get support from their statistics with a lower dose.

These 38 patients were a part of a later report on 47 patients from the same authors detailing the outcome. They found a postradiosurgery annual hemorrhage rate

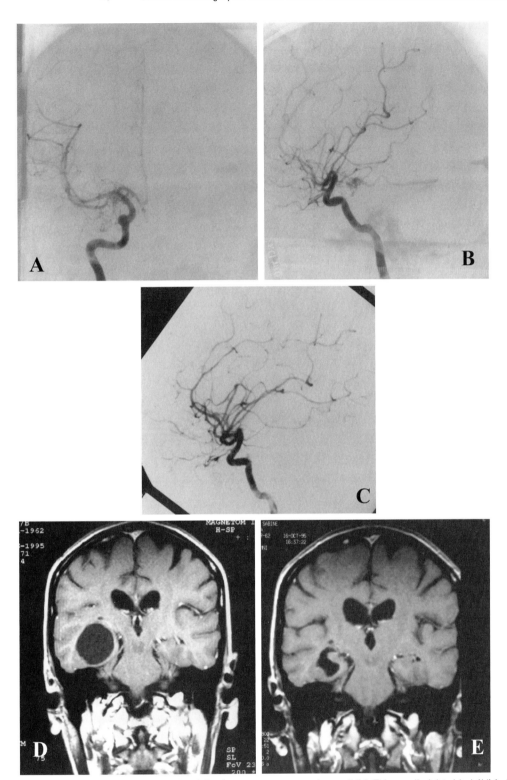

FIGURE 40-11 Delayed occurrence of cyst formation following gamma surgery for an AVM. This small, right-sided AVM visualized (A) on A-P and (B) lateral carotid arteriography was cured, as shown on a control angiogram (C) obtained 2 years after gamma surgery. The development of headaches and personality changes prompted an MRI examination 7 years after gamma surgery (D and E). This cyst was surgically decompressed. Biopsy of the cyst wall did not reveal any evidence of tumor. (Follow-up MRI courtesy of Professor J. Camaert, Chairman, Department of Neurosurgery, Gent, Belgium.)

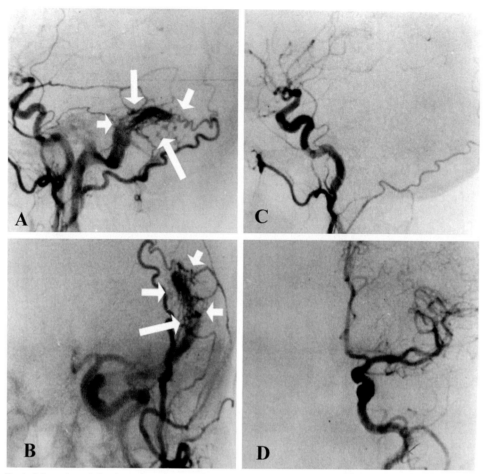

FIGURE 40-12 Total obliteration of dural arteriovenous malformation following gamma surgery. *A,* Left common carotid angiogram lateral and (*B*) frontal projections of a dural arteriovenous malformation in the region of the left transverse sinus. Complete obliteration is demonstrated at 2 years following gamma surgery in the (*C*) lateral and (*D*) frontal projections.

of 8.8%, which if compared to the risk reported by the same authors at 0.6% to 4.5% is high, even if the difference is not statistically significant. They chose, however, to compare their postradiosurgery hemorrhage rates with the preradiosurgery rate in the same subjects, making the assumption that the rate could be based on an epoch starting from first observation or first hemorrhage. This is fallacious because the malformation was present before the presenting hemorrhage and most likely was present from birth. Recomputed on this basis, the preradiosurgery annual bleed rate comes to 5.9%, which is more congruent with the expected natural history. Once again, the incidence of hemorrhages postradiosurgery seems spuriously higher.

A more recent report from this same group on a larger cohort purports a reduction in hemorrhage rate following radiosurgery, and a radiation-induced complication rate of 13.4%.[96] Other respected groups have not observed the same protective effect following radiosurgery for cavernous malformations.[97–99] It is certainly unlikely that radiosurgery would increase the propensity or frequency of hemorrhage. It certainly seems to offer minimal to no protection from hemorrhage, and is associated with a high risk of side effects. We advocate that cavernous malformations should only be treated if patients are suffering from repeated seizures,

hemorrhages, or progressive neurologic deficits; and, if treatment is needed, surgical resection is the best option at present. The future will reveal the ultimate usefulness of gamma surgery for cavernous malformations.

Developmental Venous Anomalies

The natural history of developmental venous anomalies (previously named venous angiomas) is benign[100] and is clearly not a surgical lesion. Prior to clear elucidation of this prognosis, 19 patients were treated for this entity by the authors. One patient was cured and 3 had their anomalies partially obliterated. Three patients suffered radionecrosis, and 1 had symptomatic edema. One patient with radionecrosis underwent subsequent débridement. A 5% cure incidence with a 30% complication incidence for a benign entity is unacceptable.

Tumors

Treatment of tumors with gamma surgery introduces a new approach to the evaluation of the end point of the treatment. Unlike microsurgery, no actual debulking of tissue occurs, and in the short term, there are no visible changes. However, over the long term, the tumors often shrink, and some even disappear entirely on follow-up neuroimaging studies.

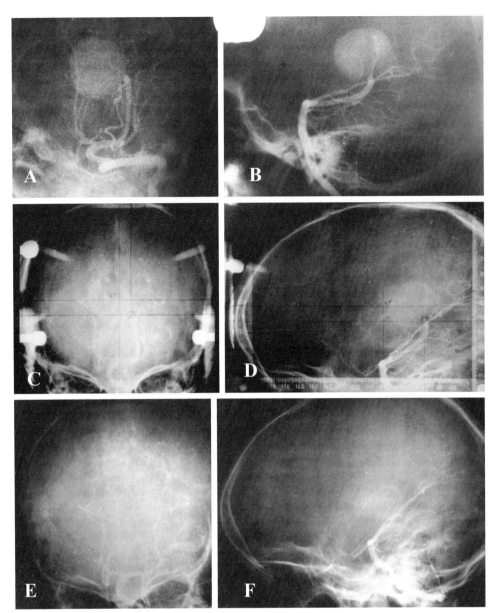

FIGURE 40-13   Gamma surgery for a vein of Galen malformation. *A*, A-P and (*B*) lateral vertebral angiograms show direct shunting of blood into the primitive precursor (promesencephalic vein) of the vein of Galen. *C* and *D*, Stereotactic angiogram obtained at the time of treatment. *E* and *F*, Control angiography obtained 1 year later demonstrates cure of the malformation. (Courtesy of Hernan Bunge, MD, Clinica del Sol, Buenos Aires, Argentina.)

Success is therefore established by a pattern of reducing tumor size over serial follow-up studies or by the lack of growth. With benign tumors, the natural history may be one of no growth for many years. As such, longer follow-up is necessary to ascertain whether gamma knife surgery affords true tumor volume control in slow-growing tumors.

In an attempt to eliminate some of the subjectivity of naked eye observations, and the obvious fallacy resulting from the estimation of a 3-dimensional object on the basis of three linear measurements in orthogonal planes, the authors have developed software that allows estimation of lesion volume based on MR or CT images. The procedure involves scanning the study into a computer program and outlining the pathology in each slice. The computer then measures the area within the contour and calculates a volume based on slice thickness. This process is repeated for each slice, and the total volume is calculated by integrating the individual slice volumes. The error of this method was determined by comparing various hand-partitioned volumes with volumes estimated using polyhedrons to approximate the regions of interest on each slice. The average relative error is strongly dependent on the number of axial slices obtained through the object of interest, and it is fairly independent of the size of the object itself. For objects varying in volume from 0.1 to 10 mL, the average relative errors per number of slices through the object have been computed as follows: 3% for 7 slices; 4% for 6 slices; 6% for 5 slices; 11% for 4 slices; and 21% for 3 slices. Volumetric estimation

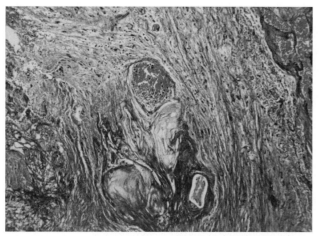

FIGURE 40-14   Hematoxylin- and eosin-stained histologic section of a cavernous malformation that was treated with gamma surgery. Because no change was observed on serial MRI examinations over 5 years, the lesion was excised. Except for a single persistent capillary channel (*arrow*), the malformation was obliterated.

based on 1 or 2 slices through the region of interest produces unacceptable average relative errors of more than 40%. The authors now require all follow-up studies to be performed with a slice thickness of 3 mm with zero overlap or gap between adjacent slices. Such a protocol generally helps ensure the acquisition of 3 or more slices through the region of interest. Even though the technique of volume estimation has an acceptable level of accuracy, we prefer to ignore changes of less than 15%.

Pituitary Adenomas (Tables 40-4 and 40-5)

The efficacy of radiation in the treatment of pituitary adenomas was well documented before gamma surgery was used for this disease.[101,102] Reduced fractionation techniques had been shown to have effectiveness in the treatment of Cushing's disease and was the impetus for the use of radiosurgery. MRI has replaced less exact invasive localization procedures (cisternography) and CT in the planning of gamma surgery in patients with pituitary adenomas. There still remain difficulties with the use of gamma surgery. The periphery dose that can be delivered for macroadenomas is limited if the optic nerve apparatus is in contact with the tumor. Localization of microadenomas can be difficult with even the best MRI examinations (e.g., a fat suppression MRI protocol) and amelioration of hypersecretory syndromes is delayed.

One of the best indications for gamma surgery of secretory or nonsecretory pituitary adenomas is residual tumor that is not removable with microsurgical techniques (i.e., within the cavernous sinus). If it is known before microsurgery that the cavernous sinus is involved and a debulking procedure is considered, then every effort to clear the tumor away from the optic nerves and chiasm should be made in order to make gamma surgery postoperatively more effective. A suprasellar approach should be considered if there is doubt that this can be accomplished through a transsphenoidal approach. There is some difficulty in differentiating residual tumor from postoperative changes on MRI even with fat saturation protocols. A thorough operative note

concerning any foreign material or grafts left behind is important, as well as a high-quality preoperative scan for comparison.

Another indication for gamma surgery is persistence or recurrence of elevated hormone levels after microsurgery. In the presence of residual or recurrent tumor that is not readily amenable to further extirpation, either because of its location or the inability to localize the tumor within the sella, gamma surgery can be applied. Tumor within the cavernous sinus can be treated as with other macroadenomas. Difficulty in localizing the tumor usually requires radiosurgical targeting of all the contents within the sella, and such an approach carries a fair risk of postradiosurgical hormonal insufficiency.[103–105] If the patient has a secretory microadenoma, but the symptomatology is not urgent and microsurgery is for some reason not considered, then gamma surgery can be used as the primary therapy.

In preparation for treatment with high-dose, narrow-beam radiation, many centers have recommended a temporary cessation of antisecretory medications in the peritreatment time period. In 2000, Landolt and colleagues first reported a significantly lower hormone normalization rate in acromegalic patients who were receiving antisecretory medications at the time of radiosurgery.[106] Since then, this same group as well as others has documented a counterproductive effect of antisecretory medications on the rate of hormonal normalization following gamma knife surgery.[34,107] The degree to which and the mechanism by which antisecretory medications lower hormonal normalization rates is unknown, but Landolt and colleagues have hypothesized that these drugs lower the tumor's metabolic rate and decrease its radiosensitivity.[106,107] Moreover, the optimal time to hold antisecretory medications in conjunction with gamma surgery is not clear. Landolt and Lomax recommend that dopamine agonists be withheld 2 months prior to the procedure.[107] For acromegalics, they recommend altering antisecretory medication administration as early as 4 months prior to radiosurgery, and completely halting all antisecretory medications 2 weeks prior to radiosurgery.[107] Although many centers have incorporated such methodology into their treatment regimens, the potential risk and benefits of altering antisecretory medication administration should be weighed. The functional adenoma may be more likely to respond to gamma knife surgery; however, in the absence of antisecretory medication control, it may also enlarge, thereby risking adjacent structures (e.g., the optic apparatus), necessitating a lower prescription dose, and making effective treatment more difficult.

Most centers have observed effective growth control of pituitary adenomas following gamma knife surgery (see Table 40-4)[108–135]; however, there have been a wide range of outcomes with regard to hormonal normalization of secretory adenomas. The varied outcome results for hormonal normalization may arising from the following reasons: (1) early studies utilized CT rather than more precise MR imaging for dose planning; (2) different criteria for defining an endocrinologic cure have been applied in various studies, and there is little consensus even within the neuro-endocrinological community for precise defining criteria; and (3) many studies had short or intermediate follow-up periods and may not have been long enough to observe patients with an endocrinologic recurrence following an initial remission.[125]

TABLE 40-4 ▪ **Results of Gamma Knife Surgery for Pituitary Adenomas**

Type of Pituitary Adenoma	Author (Year)	No. of Patients	Mean or Median Follow-up (Months)	Margin Dose (Gy)	Endocrine Cure Rate (%)	Growth Control (%)
GH secreting	Ganz et al (1993)[108]	4	18	19.5	25	100
	Martinez et al (1998)[109]	7	36	25	71	100
	Landolt et al (1998)[110]	16	NR	25	81	NR
	Lim et al (1998)[111]	20	26	25	38	92
	Morange-Ramos et al (1998)[112]	15	20	28	20	NR
	Witt et al (1998)[113]	20	32	19	20	94
	Hayashi et al (1999)[114]	22	16	24	41	92
	Inoue et al (1999)[115]	12	>24	20	58	94
	Kim et al (1999)[116]	2	12	22	0	100
	Kim et al (1999)[117]	11	27	29	46	68
	Laws et al (1999)[118]	56	NR	NR	25	NR
	Mokry et al (1999)[119]	16	46	16	31	98
	Izawa et al (2000)[120]	29	28	22	41	94
	Shin et al (2000)[121]	6	43	34	67	100
	Zhang et al (2000)[122]	68	34	31	96	100
	Fukuoka et al (2001)[123]	9	42	20	50	100
	Ikeda et al (2001)[124]	17	48	25	82	100
	Feigl et al (2002)[125]	9	55	15	NR	94
	Pollock et al (2002)[126]	26	42	20	42	100
	Attanasio et al (2003)[127]	30	46	20	37	100
	Petrovich et al (2003)[128]	6	41	15	100	NR
ACTH secreting	Ganz et al (1993)[108]	4	18	25	50	100
	Martinez et al (1998)[109]	3	36	24	100	100
	Lim et al (1998)[111]	4	26	25	25	92
	Morange-Ramos et al (1998)[112]	6	20	28	67	NR
	Witt et al (1998)[113]	25	32	19	28	94
	Hayashi et al (1999)[114]	10	16	24	10	92
	Inoue et al (1999)[115]	3	>24	20	100	94
	Kim et al (1999)[116]	8	27	29	62	68
	Laws et al (1999)[118]	50	NR	NR	58	NR
	Mokry et al (1999)[119]	5	56	17	33	98
	Izawa et al (2000)[120]	12	28	22	17	94
	Sheehan et al (2000)[103]	43	44	20	63	100
	Shin et al (2000)[121]	7	88	32	50	100
	Hoybye et al (2001)[129]	18	204	NR	83	83
	Feigl et al (2002)[125]	4	55	15	NR	94
	Kobayashi et al (2002)[130]	20	64	29	35	100
	Pollock et al (2002)[126]	9	42	20	78	100
	Petrovich et al (2003)[128]	4	41	15	50	NR
Prolactin secreting	Ganz et al (1993)[108]	3	18	13.3	0	100
	Martinez et al (1998)[109]	5	36	33	0	100
	Lim et al (1998)[111]	19	26	25	56	92
	Witt et al (1998)[113]	12	32	19	0	94
	Hayashi et al (1999)[114]	13	16	24	15	92
	Inoue et al (1999)[115]	2	>24	20	50	94
	Kim et al (1999)[116]	20	12	22	19	100
	Kim et al (1999)[117]	18	27	29	17	68
	Laws et al (1999)[118]	19	NR	NR	7	NR
	Morky et al (1999)[119]	21	31	14	21	98
	Morange-Ramos et al (1999)[112]	4	20	28	0	NR
	Izawa et al (2000)[120]	15	28	22	20	94
	Landolt et al (2000)[110]	20	29	25	25	NR
	Pan et al (2000)[133]	128	33	32	15	98
	Feigl et al (2002)[125]	18	55	15	NR	94
	Pollock et al (2002)[126]	7	42	20	29	100
	Petrovich et al (2003)[128]	12	41	15	83	NR
Nonsecreting	Martinez et al (1998)[109]	14	36	16		100
	Lim et al (1998)[111]	22	26	25		92
	Witt et al (1998)[113]	24	32	19		94
	Hayahsi et al (1999)[114]	18	16	20		92
	Inoue et al (1999)[115]	18	>24	20		94
	Mokry et al (1999)[119]	31	21	14		98
	Izawa et al (2000)[120]	23	28	22		94
	Shin et al (2000)[121]	3	19	16		100
	Feigl et al (2002)[125]	61	55	15		94
	Sheehan et al (2002)[134]	42	31	16		98
	Wowra and Stummer (2002)[135]	30	58	16		93
	Petrovich et al (2003)[128]	56	41	15		100

NR, information not reported in that particular series.

TABLE 40-5 ▪ Outcome at the University of Virginia for Gamma Surgery for Pituitary Adenomas

Tumor Type	No.	Size Decreased	Size Unchanged	Size Increased	Endocrine Remission
Nonsecretory	92	55	21	6	—
Secretory	178	140	20	18	—
Growth hormone	70	56	6	8	43%
Prolactin	16	11	3	2	44%
ACTH	74	61	7	6	64%
Pleurihormonal	4	2	2	0	—
Nelson's	14	10	2	2	31%
Total	270	195	41	24	—

RESULTS

The authors have treated 270 pituitary tumors, all macroadenomas and locally invasive (see Table 40-5); there were 5 malignant tumors. All had been previously treated one or more times by some other modality. Microsurgery alone was used in 90.3%, radiation therapy and micro-surgery in 8.2%, and radiation therapy alone in 1.5%. Tumor volume ranged from 0.9 to 32 mL, with an average volume of 11 mL.

Tumors were treated with a maximum dose of 6 to 60 Gy (average, 37.5 Gy). Periphery dose ranged from 3 to 28 Gy (average, 15 Gy). This discrepancy is caused by variations in patient profile. Patients that had received previous radiation therapy or that had a tumor close to the optic apparatus in general received lower doses. Currently, Gamma Plan, the planning software for the gamma knife, allows for very specific shielding of the optic nerves and chiasm, and this has allowed for higher doses to be administered when these structures are nearby.

Nonsecretory Tumors

The authors have treated 92 nonsecretory pituitary tumors, 82 of which have radiographic and endocrinologic follow-up of a minimum of 6 months and an average of 34 months. Of these, 55 (67%) had a decrease in the volume of their tumors; 21 (26%) had no change in the size; and 6 (7%) increased in size. New hypopituitarism occurred in 12 patients (15%). The only indication we have to date for treating these tumors is for postoperative residual tumors, in order to lower the incidence of tumor progression or pro-gression in spite of previous radiation therapy (Fig. 40-15).

ACTH-Secreting Tumors

Seventy-four patients with ACTH-secreting tumors under-went 80 gamma knife procedures. These tumors had all been treated with microsurgery before radiosurgical consul-tation. Imaging follow-up demonstrated a decrease in the size of the tumor in 61 cases (76%), no change in 13 (16%), and an increase in size in 6 (8%). However, because the hypercortisolism defines the dangerous character of the ACTH-secreting tumor, the control of endocrine abnor-malities is the true measure of tumor control. Normal 24-UFC levels were achieved in 46 patients (64%), at an average time of 10.6 months post-treatment (range, 1 to 40 months). Six of these patients had repeat gamma knife

procedures, with 4 patients achieving another remission. New endocrine deficiencies developed in 18 patients (24%), with growth hormone deficiency being the most commonly found new endocrinopathy. Four patients developed new-onset visual acuity deficits, 2 of whom had received prior conventional fractionated radiation therapy. Evidence of radiation-induced changes was seen in 3 patients, but only 1 had symptoms attributable to these changes. These find-ings are notably different from the authors' earlier published results in that more patients went on to develop a recur-rence after an initial period of hormonal remission.[103]

The results of 35 patients treated at the Karolinska Institute have been reported.[136] Of the 29 patients that had follow-up of up to 9 years, 22 (76%) had normalization of their endocrine abnormalities, 10 within 1 year and the remainder within 3 years.

Growth Hormone–Secreting Tumors

The authors have performed 74 gamma knife procedures on 70 patients with growth hormone–secreting adenomas. Reliable endocrine follow-up is available for 38 of these patients. There was normalization of IGF-1 in 43% of cases. No patient had an elevation in growth hormone level after gamma surgery. Five patients developed recurrence of their acromegaly after initial remission, with a mean time to recurrence of 47 months. New endocrinologic deficiencies developed in 31% of patients, with hypothyroidism and low testosterone levels being the most common new endocrinopathies.

A decrease in tumor size was seen after 60 gamma knife procedures (79%). Tumor growth was seen after 8 proce-dures. No change in tumor volume was seen after 6 proce-dures. Four patients developed the new-onset of visual acuity deficits; 2 of these patients had received prior conventional fractionated radiation therapy. Three patients developed deterioration in visual fields, likely secondary to tumor growth. Evidence of radiographic changes on postra-diosurgical neuroimaging was seen in only 2 patients, nei-ther of whom developed clinical symptomatology.

Prolactin-Secreting Tumors

Of the 22 prolactin-secreting tumors treated by the authors at Virginia, 16 have radiographic follow-up of 6 months or more. Eleven of these (69%) had a decrease in the size of their tumors, 3 were unchanged (19%), and

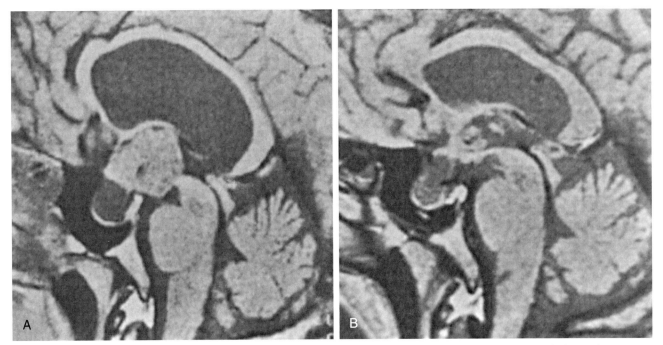

FIGURE 40-15 Nonsecretory pituitary adenoma treated wth gamma surgery following four failed microsurgical resections.

2 were increased (12%). Endocrine follow-up was available for all 22 patients. There was remission in 44% of cases and no change in the remaining 56%.

Nelson's Syndrome

At the University of Virginia, the authors have performed gamma surgery on 14 Nelson's syndrome patients. All patients had documented tumor growth and hyperpigmentation as well as elevated ACTH levels (mean of 840 ng/mL) at the time of radiosurgery. One patient had previously received conventional fractionated radiation therapy, and 2 patients had received prior gamma surgery for Cushing's disease. Mean endocrine follow-up was 33 months (range, 6 to 78 months), and mean radiologic follow-up was 31 months (range, 5 to 72 months). Median dose to the tumor margin was 25 Gy (range, 4 to 30 Gy). Tumor growth control was achieved in 12 of 14 patients (86%). ACTH levels decreased in 14 patients (81%), with a median decrease of 59% (range, –93% to +33%). Five patients (31%) achieved normal ACTH levels, with a mean time to remission of 9.4 months postradiosurgery. New endocrinopathies were seen after 5 gamma knife procedures (31%), with low growth hormone levels being the most common new hormonal deficit. No patients exhibited radiographic or clinical evidence of damage to the optic apparatus or surrounding brain.

It is worth noting that there is a wide variation in both the rates of endocrinologic cure and hypopituitarism following gamma surgery. The difference in cure rates between modern radiosurgical series is likely caused by the definition of cure employed and the length of follow-up. However, the discrepancy in the reported rates of hypopituitarism is more likely a function of the degree to which there is rigorous endocrinologic follow-up testing.

Craniopharyngiomas

Craniopharyngiomas are very difficult tumors to treat. Their benign histology is misleading. Their near impossibility to resect completely, and their usual location in and about the hypothalamus make them difficult to cure. Various medical therapies have been used in the treatment of craniopharyngiomas. Microsurgery; intracystic instillation of radioisotopes; radiation therapy; and, now, radiosurgery have all been used. Long-term evaluation of patients with craniopharyngiomas is available[137,138] after various treatment protocols. The consensus is that the most complete surgical resection possible, without creating significant morbidity, should be performed; this is followed by radiation therapy, and gives reasonable long-term survival. The ill effects on children after receiving fractionated brain irradiation are well known.[139–143] Good results with resection alone have been achieved but only in the hands of a few neurosurgeons. Even so, long-term results of children with subtotal resection followed by radiation therapy has been shown to be superior to complete resection alone,[137] and the deficits incurred with aggressive surgery can be considerable.

Gamma surgery as an adjunct to microsurgical resection has been used in lieu of radiation therapy, or in addition to it, at several centers. The instillation of radioisotopes (e.g., P[32]) into large, nonloculated cystic components of the tumor, and gamma surgery for the solid portion, is the treatment policy for craniopharyngiomas at the authors' center (Fig. 40-16).

The authors have treated 31 craniopharyngiomas in Virginia with gamma surgery, some of whom were reported on earlier.[144] Maximum dose was 25 to 50 Gy (average, 34.2 Gy) with a periphery dose of 9 to 16.7 Gy (average, 13 Gy). Since the introduction of more advanced software for planning, the treatment of all lesions in this region

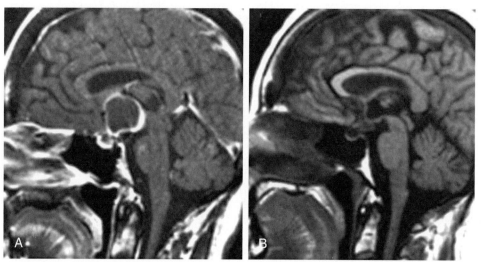

FIGURE 40-16 *A*, Craniopharyngioma shown by postcontrast T1-weighted saggital MRI 12 months after gamma surgery and (*B*) stereotactic instillation of P^{32}. The most recent follow-up MRI, after 5 years, showed the tumor decreased 73% in size.

incorporated shielding to protect the optic apparatus and uninvolved hypothalamus. This has become more refined with the introduction of more sophisticated planning systems (Gamma Plan), but the maximum dose in all cases was kept below 8 Gy.

Of the 31 patients, 2 died at 6 and 15 months after gamma surgery. Three of the tumors increased in size, and one is unchanged. Five (16%) radiographically disappeared, and 19 (61%) decreased in size. One patient was lost to follow-up (Fig. 40-17).

Several other series have reported on the use of gamma surgery in the treatment of craniopharyngiomas[145,146] with results similar to those of the authors. As larger series with longer follow-up become available, it is likely that gamma surgery will either take the place of less discriminate radiation therapy, or be a useful adjunct to it.

Meningiomas (Table 40-6)

Meningiomas are usually benign, circumscribed tumors that arise from the coverings of the central nervous system and therefore tend to be superficial. Because of these attributes, microsurgical extirpation of the entire tumor (and of any involved meninges) is the treatment of choice. Unfortunately, many meningiomas do not have one or more of the mentioned attributes. Aggressive, locally invasive tumors, especially those invading or involving critical or difficult-to-control neural or vascular structures, and those at the skull base can be problematic in their complete removal. The use of radiation to lower the recurrence rate following microsurgical removal of meningiomas was shown to be beneficial.[147–149] Recurrence rates were found to be dramatically decreased, and for patients with residual tumor following surgery, the progression of tumor growth was significantly decreased.

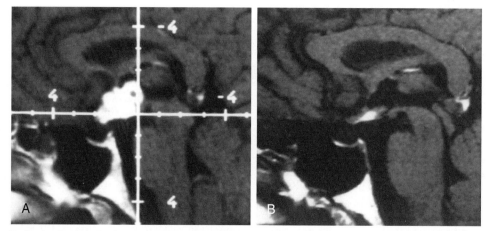

FIGURE 40-17 Reduction in size of craniopharyngioma treated with gamma surgery. Residual craniopharyngioma following microsurgery treated with the gamma knife. Contrast-enhanced T1-weighted images (*A*) before and (*B*) 4 months after treatment show marked reduction in the tumor size. Patient has a normal neurologic examination and endocrine profile.

TABLE 40-6 ▪ **Outcome of Radiosurgery for Meningiomas**

Series	No.	Size			Follow-up (Months)	Complications	Improved
		Decrease	Increase	Unchanged			
Bunge*	16	0	1	7	6–36	—	—
Forster[†]	3	0	1	0	Up to 24	—	—
Kondziolka et al (1993)[151]	81	—	5	27	6–48	3	9
Rähn[‡]	82	1	3	8	3–120	—	12
Steiner[‖]	151	94	17	40	6–252	0	12
Liscak et al (1999)[153]	67	34	0	33	2–60	3	24
Roche et al (2000)[154]	80	25	4	51	12–79	3	21
Lee et al (2002)[160]	159	54	9	96	2–145	11	46
Nicolato et al (2002)[157]	122	75	3	44	>12	4	—
Roche et al (2003)[155]	32	4	0	28	28–118	2	13
Flickinger et al (2003)[156]	219	—	7	—	2–164	12	—

*H. Bunge, personal communication, 1993.
[†]D.M.C. Forster, personal communication, 1993.
[‡]T. Rähn, personal communication, 1993.
[‖]L. Steiner, refers to information in this chapter and relects current data.

The authors have treated 329 meningiomas at the University of Virginia since 1989. The most recent evaluation of our material was for 206 patients with a follow-up of 1 to 6 years. Tumor volume ranged from 1 to 32 mL. These patients received an average of 38 Gy maximum dose (range, 20 to 60 Gy) and an average periphery dose of 14 Gy (range, 10 to 20 Gy). There were 142 patients treated for residual tumor and 64 treated with gamma surgery primarily. Radiographic follow-up was available for 151 patients. Of the evaluated patients, 94 (63%) showed a decrease in the volume of their tumor greater than 15%. No change in size was seen in 40 (26%) and an increase in size in 17 (11%). The results of other centers reported in the literature are similar[150–157] (see Table 40-6).

Tumors within the parasellar compartment, which is a part of the extradural neural axis compartment, can be difficult to remove with microsurgery without significant morbidity.[158,159] Residual tumor that is attached to patent vascular or neural structures can be targeted with gamma surgery; this allows less radical microsurgical resection and a lower incidence of morbidity.

In the group of meningiomas that the authors treated, there were 112 within the cavernous sinus. In 68%, the tumor either disappeared (Fig. 40-18) or shrank; in 30%, they remained the same size; and in 2%, they have grown larger. Petroclinoid meningiomas involving the cavernous sinus were not included in this series and are to be evaluated in the future. The results of cavernous sinus meningiomas treatments from the University of Pittsburgh group are similar in that they reported a 94% long-term tumor control rate.[160] At the Karolinska Hospital between 1987 and 1993, a group of 40 patients were treated for skull-based meningiomas with gamma knife surgery. These 40 patients received a median prescription dose of 16 Gy and have been followed for a median time of 9 years. Tumor control was achieved in 87%, and a reduction in tumor volume was documented in 33%. Neurologic complications were observed in 11% of patients and tended to occur in those patients who received more than 20 Gy to the optic apparatus. Few complications were noted when more modern threshold doses for sensitive structures were administered. Distant tumor recurrences outside of the radiation field were noted in 6%.

The authors now have long-term follow-up of 10 to 21 years in 31 meningiomas treated with the gamma knife. Two thirds of these tumors have either shrunk significantly or remained stable, and among these were cases where only the vascular supply for the tumor was targeted (Fig. 40-19). This has resulted in significant tumor shrinkage and lasting effect, even in the long term.

The authors' practice has been to obtain a stereotactic angiogram prior to gamma surgery for large tumors. This allows treatment to include the vascular supply when ideal treatment is not possible because of radiation dose constraints imposed by the treatment volume. Using MRI, the group from Heidelberg proved that radiation occluded small nutrient vessels of meningiomas, providing the rationale for the treatment we have used since 1976.

No clinical complications were experienced in treating meningiomas; however, a tumor without histologic diagnosis and with equivocal imaging characteristics in the pineal region was treated as a presumed meningioma, and bilateral edema of the basal ganglia occurred. This resulted in cognitive disturbances with incomplete recovery.

The primary therapy for meningiomas is microsurgery. The advantage of histologic diagnosis, debulking, and reasonable chance of cure secures surgical extirpation as the procedure of choice for this tumor. The tumors most amenable to gamma surgery treatment are less than 10 to 15 mL in volume. The ability of gamma surgery to effectively treat small tumors with low morbidity argues strongly, however, for minimizing morbidity during open procedures. The option to treat residual tumor in critical or hard-to-reach locations should temper the ambition of total surgical removal. This is especially true in locations where complete meningeal resection is impossible, and thus the chance of recurrence is high.

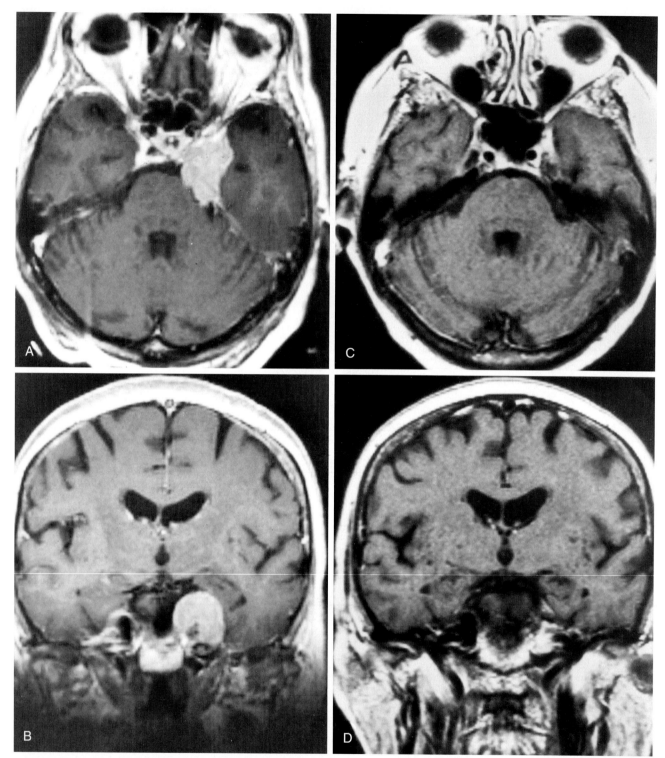

FIGURE 40-18   Large left parasellar meningioma residual following microsurgery visualized on postcontrast T1-weighted (*A*) axial and (*B*) coronal MRI images. *C* and *D*, MRI obtained 6 months following gamma surgery shows that the tumor has disappeared. Repeated control MRI examinations for 5 years show no recurrence of the tumor.

Vestibular Schwannomas (Table 40-7)

Historically and incorrectly referred to as an acoustic neuroma, the authors prefer the designation of vestibular schwannoma, which recognizes the anatomic and histologic origins of these tumors.[161] There may be no other intracranial neuropathology about which the proper treatment arouses as much controversy as the vestibular schwannoma. Neurosurgeons cite the series of surgeons with enormous experience removing these tumors to justify suboccipital removal, whereas otolaryngologists sacrifice the inner ear during the translabarynthine approach in an attempt to better expose and preserve the facial nerve.

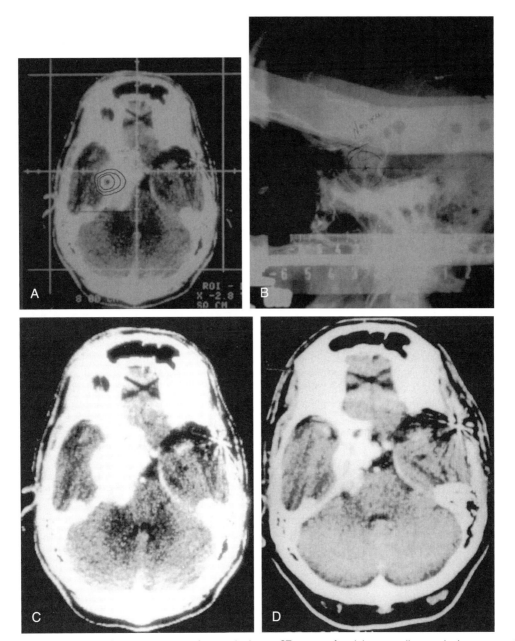

FIGURE 40-19 Long-term result of gamma surgery for meningioma. CT scans of a right parasellar meningioma treated treated with radiation to the nutrient vessel as defined by (A) CT and (B) angiogram. The original size of the tumor is depicted in the pregamma surgery axial CT (C), and the last follow-up at 18 years after gamma surgery is shown (D). The tumor has substantially decreased in size.

TABLE 40-7 ▪ Outcome of Radiosurgery for Acoustic Neuromas

Series	No. of patients with Follow-up Imaging Studies	Mean Follow-up (Months)	Tumor Increased (%)	Tumor Unchanged or Decreased (%)
Noren et al (1993)[30]	209	Minimum of 12	16	84
Flickinger et al (1993)[165]	134	24	11	89
Foote et al (1995)	35	16	0	100
Kwon et al (1998)[169]	63	52	5	95
Prasad et al (2000)[164]	153	51	7	93
Flickinger et al (2001)[168]	190	30	3	97
Bertalanffy et al (2001)[167]	40	36	9	91
Iwai et al (2003)[166]	51	60	4	96

Radiosurgery's proponents cite excellent tumor control and low morbidity but must acknowledge that although the tumor often shrinks, it is still there. Therefore, it is in the best interest of our patients that long-term outcomes in patients treated with these three modalities be thoroughly evaluated, and that small series, anecdotal evidence, and personal beliefs not weigh too heavily in our minds.

The first vestibular schwannomas treated with the gamma knife were by Leksell and Steiner in 1969.[162] However, Dr. Steiner refused to be an author of the initial paper; at the time he had reservations about the treatment of tumors with the gamma knife and was concequently only acknowledged in a footnote by Leksell. Since then, more than 21,272 have been treated around the world as of June 2003. The indications for gamma knife surgery for this tumor vary. Some physicians advocate gamma knife surgery in medically high-risk patients, patients who refuse microsurgery, and in patients with postoperative residual tumor. However, others advocate gamma knife surgery as the treatment of choice in nearly all cases of vestibular schwannomas. The usefulness of irradiation in the postoperative period was shown by Wallner and co-workers in 1987, where external beam irradiation lowered the recurrence rate from 46% to 6% in Boldrey's surgical series at the University of California at San Francisco.[163] By then, gamma surgery was already being widely applied to this disease under many circumstances. The fact is that for a number of reasons few neurosurgeons acquire the necessary competency to satisfactorily extirpate these tumors. This situation may change if a method is found to improve the acquisition of skills required for extirpation of these lesions.

The advent of MRI has made planning for this procedure much more exact. With a high-quality MRI scan and a relatively small tumor, the seventh cranial nerve can occasionally be visualized and carefully excluded from the treatment field. The trigeminal nerve can nearly always be identified except with the largest tumors, which in most cases should not be treated primarily with gamma surgery.

Small collimators are used to better match the isodose configuration to the size and shape of the tumor. The authors have had no brain stem–related complications. Previously, we used minimum periphery doses up to 20 Gy and maximum doses up to 70 Gy. Presently, we use a margin dose of 11 to 15 Gy at the 30% to 50% isodose curve. The incidence of cranial nerve palsies rose considerably at the higher doses without significant improvement in the degree of tumor control.

At the University of Virginia, we have treated 400 patients with vestibular schwannomas. Some 153 of these patients with greater than 12 months' follow-up have been reported.[164] Of these, radiosurgery was the primary treatment for 96 and was adjutant (following microsurgery) in 57. The volume of the treated tumors ranged from 0.02 to 18.3 mL.

Of the patients treated primarily with gamma surgery, a decrease in tumor size was seen in 81% (78 patients), no change in 12%, and an increase in size in 6%. Among those 78 patients with a decrease in the size of their tumors, the decrease was greater than 50% in 20 patients (Fig. 40-20). It is our policy to not consider as significant decreases in volume of less than 15%. This is true of all tumors and vascular malformations that we treat. Radiologic follow-up for these patients ranged from 1 to 10 years.

Of the 57 patients treated with gamma surgery after microsurgery, a decrease in tumor size was seen in 65%, no change was seen in 25%, and an increase in size was seen in 10%. Among the 37 patients with a decrease in the size of their tumors, the decrease was greater than 50% in 12 patients. The outcome, in terms of postradiosurgical volume reduction in patients who had prior microsurgery, is worse than in those who were primarily treated with gamma surgery. This difference is likely a result of the increased difficulty with accurate targeting in those who have undergone prior microsurgery. Of note, although our experience with treating large vestibular schwannomas is small ($n = 19$), we have observed a 95% tumor control rate in those following gamma surgery.

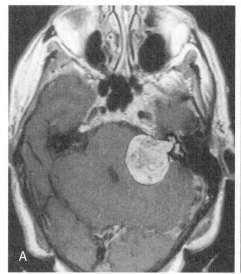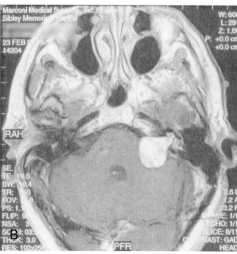

FIGURE 40-20   Reduction in the size of a vestibular schwannoma following gamma surgery. *A,* Contrast-enhanced T1-weighted MRI of a left vestibular schwannoma; *B,* reduction in size 24 months after radiosurgery with a margin dose of 10.8 Gy. The tumor measured 11.2 mL at the time of gamma treatment and decreased to a volume of 4.4 mL. Of note, this patient had a small postradiosurgery change in the pons on an interim MRI scan (not shown). However, this radiologic change resolved, and the patient remains in excellent neurologic condition.

In our patients, there were 5 with transient changes in trigeminal sensation and 3 with facial paresis. One of the patients with facial weakness was operated on shortly after gamma surgery and was lost to follow-up. Another patient recovered completely in 6 weeks, and the third has nearly completely recovered at 10 months. Of the patients with useful hearing prior to gamma surgery, 58% retained their hearing following radiosurgery, 42% experienced some degree of deterioration, and 31% lost useful hearing. The majority of hearing changes were observed at the 2-year checkup, and additional auditory changes were observed as late as 8 years postradiosurgery.

Other centers report similar rates of tumor control (i.e., with no change or decrease in the size of the tumor) in 89% to 100% of patients.[30,165–170]

Evaluation of the material from the Karolinska group included evaluation of radiographic changes other than size.[30] The most common change was loss of central enhancement within the tumor on either contrasted MRI or CT studies. This occurred in 70% of patients, and typically was observed within 6 to 12 months of treatment. However, these changes were reversible. Another change that was observed (and that we have often seen) is a transient increase in the size of the tumor during the first 6 months after gamma surgery. This is commonly seen in tumors that then regress to their original size or smaller (Fig. 40-21).

Previously published incidence of cranial neuropathies at other centers was 17% at Karolinska and 29% at Pittsburgh for facial paresis, which in the vast majority of cases was transient or mild. The trigeminal nerve was affected in a variety of ways in 33% of the time at Pittsburgh, most commonly a mild hypoesthesia. Recent complication rates at these institutions are comparable to those at our center.

The authors have not seen an instance of cerebellar edema or hydrocephalus requiring spinal fluid diversion following gamma surgery for vestibular schwannomas, but both of these have been reported elsewhere.[30,165]

Astrocytomas

The treatment of astrocytomas, whether low or high grade, is largely defined by the ability to effectively reduce the tumor burden as much as possible and to lessen the rate of recurrence. Except in the case of pilocytic astrocytoma, cure is rare. Classically, the goal of reducing tumor burden is obtained by gross total resection with a margin of "normal" brain when possible, and postoperative radiation in the case of more malignant tumors. The indication for radiation therapy for intermediate grade tumors, chemotherapy, repeat surgical debulking, and other therapies is dependent on several factors, many of which are not clearly defined. Into this cornucopia of choices, gamma surgery has been introduced. Intellectually, we have difficulty accepting the application of a focused technique for an infiltrative process. Nevertheless, recent results showing improved survival indicate that this negative attitude may be inappropriate.

In the case of low-grade tumors, gamma surgery can be used in the place of surgical resection when the tumor is in an inaccessible location (e.g., brain stem) or when the patient opts for this alternative. Their small size and relative circumscription makes planning straightforward, and fairly good results have been obtained.

For high-grade tumors, gamma surgery may be employed in several ways. If the tumor is small and in an inaccessible location (e.g., thalamus), gamma surgery is used to treat the tumor primarily. Focal or whole brain irradiation is also used as an adjunct therapy. The incidence of radionecrosis is relatively high when aggressive protocols are used, and differentiating recurrence from this phenomenon can be problematic. Gamma surgery can also be used as an adjunct to surgical resection. The incidence of residual postoperative tumor is unfortunately not uncommon after "total" surgical resections, and care is often taken when the tumor abuts eloquent brain so as not to leave neurologic deficit even at the expense of incomplete gross tumor resection. In these cases, gamma surgery can be used to treat the residual tumor. Whole or focal radiation therapy has been used to lower the recurrence rate after these surgical therapies have been undertaken.

Results

Low-Grade Astrocytomas

The authors have treated 56 benign astrocytomas. The general indication was a deep-seated tumor not amenable to

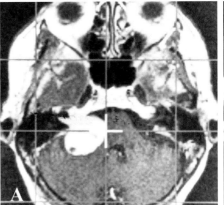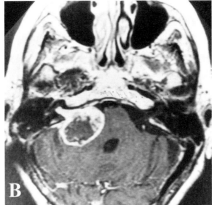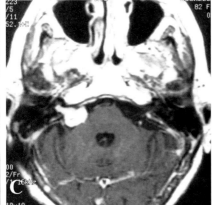

FIGURE 40-21 *A,* A right vestibular schwannoma with a volume of 9.3 mL shown on a postcontrast T1-weighted axial MRI prior to gamma surgery. *B,* The same lesion 6 months after treatment shows central nonenhancement and no change in the size of the lesion. *C,* Thirty-six months after treatment, the lesion is again homogeneously enhancing and is significantly smaller (69%). Control MRI examinations for 6 years show the lesion has remained stable.

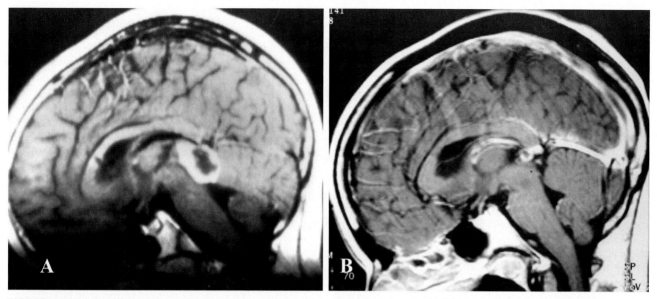

FIGURE 40-22   *A,* A pilocytic astrocytoma shown on a postcontrast T1-weighted sagittal MRI image. Annual control MRI examinations were obtained, and the latest (*B*) was made 9 years following gamma surgery.

surgical resection, or a case in which the patient insisted on gamma surgery.

We have treated 15 patients with grade I astrocytomas with greater than 1 year follow-up. Tumor size was found to be important, with best results found in patients with a tumor volume less than 3 mL. Of these patients, the tumor disappeared in 1 case (7%), shrank in 8 (53%), and increased in 6 (40%) (Fig. 40-22). Two patients were subsequently operated on, 1 for increase in tumor size and 1 for a hemorrhage and radiation-induced changes. In two patients, a cyst associated with the tumor enlarged whereas the solid portion became smaller. One of these patients is the only patient to have a decline in neurologic function following gamma surgery.[171]

We have follow-up of more than 1 year for 17 grade II astrocytomas available. Three (18%) disappeared, 7 (41%) shrank, 2 (12%) remained unchanged, and 5 (31%) increased in size. One patient died from progression of his disease at 46 months after treatment. No relationship was found between pretreatment tumor size and outcome. These results are similar to other reported series.[172]

High-Grade Astrocytomas

From an intellectual standpoint, it is difficult to understand how a patient with a highly invasive and diffuse tumor like a high-grade glioma can benefit from such a focused treatment as gamma surgery. However, when coupled with chemotherapy and fractionated radiation therapy, the gamma knife can be used to treat the largest concentration of the residual tumor based on the neuroimaging studies. It seems clear that no single treatment modality in the neuro-oncology armamentarium is a magic bullet for such tumors, and, as such, this multimodality approach to high-grade gliomas is prudent.

The authors have treated 56 malignant astrocytomas. Our experience has been similar to other reported series,[173–175] with the majority of patients showing initial decrease in size

or remaining stable for a time (Fig. 40-23); however, recurrence and progression is the rule with these tumors, and no therapy is curative. Because of the differences in histology and the variety of therapies and protocols available for these tumors, it is difficult to judge the benefit of gamma surgery. Although our group and Nwokedi and colleagues[176] have observed a statistically significant (sic) prolongation of life expectancy in the group of patients undergoing aggressive multimodality treatment (e.g., including some or all of the following: radical tumor debulking, radiation therapy, chemotherapy, and gamma surgery), it remains to be seen if these findings will be borne out in larger, better-controlled studies.[177] The limit of the benefit that radiation can contribute to the treatment of these lesions seems to have been reached, hence it may be stated that the dose escalation with the gamma knife in the treatment protocol of this disease will change only marginally the clinical outcome. It is also conceivable that targeting tumor angiogenesis and finding ways to induce apoptosis will have some impact on the management of these cases.

Chordoma

Chordomas at the level of the clivus or elsewhere in the skull base are difficult to remove surgically and have a high recurrence rate. The use of postoperative radiation with heavy particles was shown to be associated with a significant long-term survival but with only modest reduction in tumor size.[177–178]

The authors treated 10 patients with a chordoma; follow-up greater than 2 years is available for 6 of these. Two tumors shrank (Fig. 40-24), 2 increased in size, and the remaining 2 are unchanged.

Linear accelerator–based radiosurgery results for chordomas have been published. Thirteen patients followed for an average of 32 months (range, 4 to 80 months) were evaluated. All but 1 patient, who died at 4 months of tumor progression, were alive. Local control of the tumor was

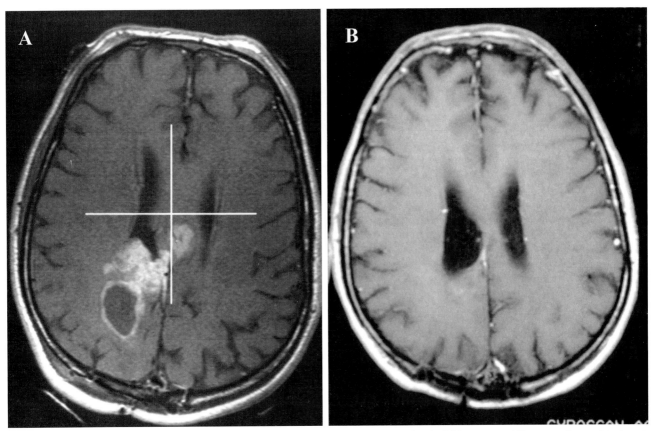

FIGURE 40-23   *A*, A postcontrast T1-weighted axial MRI demonstrating a right parietal glioblastoma multiforme and associated cyst. *B*, The same patient 11 months after gamma surgery shows complete radiographic disappearance of the lesion.

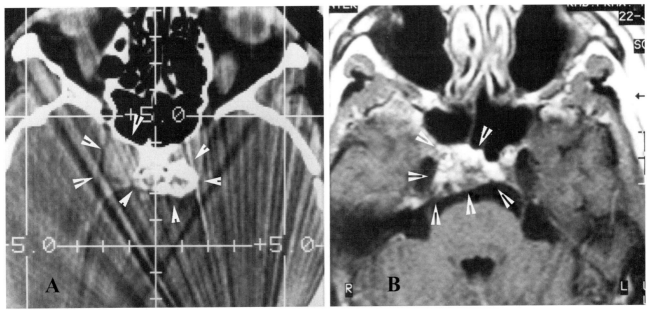

FIGURE 40-24   Gamma surgery for residual chordoma. *A*, Postcontrast axial CT image at the time of treatment. *B*, Postcontrast T1-weighted axial MRI image obtained 7 years after gamma surgery demonstrates a 35% reduction in tumor volume.

69% (tumor unchanged or smaller), and there was 1 significant complication (pituitary dysfunction requiring replacement therapy).[179]

Chondromas and Chondrosarcomas

These are rare tumors in the skull base. The authors have treated 4 chondromas and 7 chondrosarcomas with gamma surgery. Response in some cases was very good (greater than 50% reduction in size), and none have progressed as shown by a follow-up of 1 to 5 years (Fig. 40-25).

Muthukumar and colleagues treated 15 patients (9 with chordomas and 6 with chondrosarcomas) with gamma surgery, and reported their results with an average follow-up of 4 years. Four of their patients had died; only 2 deaths were related to progression of disease, and both of these had progression outside of the treated area. Only 1 of the surviving 11 had tumor progression, and 5 had shrunk.[180] Gamma surgery seems to be a reasonable treatment alternative for these tumors, but longer follow-up and larger series are required before definitive statements can be made.

Metastatic Tumors

Except for solitary lesions causing mass effect, the treatment of metastatic brain tumors is primarily palliative. In the instance of solitary metastasis, the occurrence of long-term survival is not unheard of; however, in general the guiding philosophy is generally palliation, reversal of neurologic deficits, and maintenance of quality in life. There has been some disagreement regarding the total number and volume of tumors that can be treated with gamma surgery in the instance of multiple metastases. The authors' general guideline is not to treat more than three if that is known to be the case. We have treated more, but usually only when additional lesions were discovered on the treatment MRI.

The integral dose that the remainder of the brain receives is difficult to determine when making more than one treatment plan. Studies indicate that treating more than three lesions at the same time will increase the integral dose to the brain to levels requiring lowering of the prescription dose to the individual lesions, reducing the efficacy of the treatment.[101] However, considering the limited survival expectation in these patients, the pertinence of rigid consideration of integral dose is debatable.

If metastatic deposits are located very far from one another in space, the ability to treat them all with the same frame placement may be difficult because of the limitation of the space within the treatment helmet. Such consideration makes frame placement for widely separated metastases a challenge at times.

Surgical extirpation of a solitary brain metastasis has been shown to significantly prolong survival if the primary disease is controlled. Likewise, whole-brain irradiation has been show to be of benefit for some tumor types. These conclusions, and the well-defined limits on neuroimaging studies of most metastatic lesions, make them very amenable to gamma surgery. Because of this, as well as the high incidence of these lesions, the treatment of metastatic tumors is presently a common indication for gamma surgery worldwide.[181]

Most reports regarding gamma surgery for metastatic tumors report a 7- to 15- month survival following treatment[182–204] (Table 40-8). Local tumor control rates range from 71% to 98.5%. The histology, dosages, and previous treatments vary considerably through the literature. Most centers are using a periphery dose of 12 to 20 Gy and a maximum dose of 40 Gy. These doses are adjusted down if whole brain irradiation has been given previously. The reduction of dose in the instance of tumors that appear after

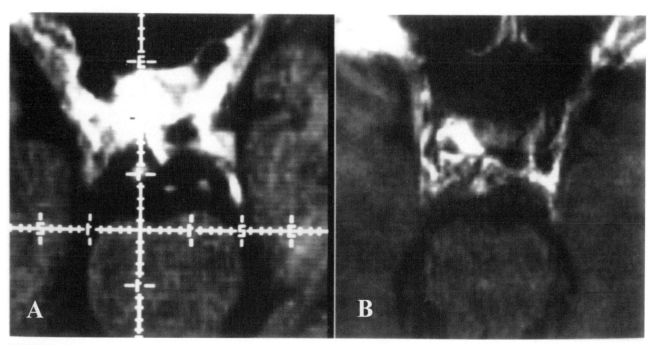

FIGURE 40-25 Gamma surgery for residual chondrosarcoma. CT scans of a 32-year-old man with a postoperative residual chondrosarcoma in the sellar region (*A*) before and (*B*) 18 months after gamma surgery. Note regression in the size of the residual. The patient has no neurologic deficits.

TABLE 40-8 • Outcome of Gamma Surgery for Metastatic Tumors

Type of Brain Metastasis	No. of Patients	Local Tumor Control Rate (%)	Median Survival (Months)	Series
Melanoma	26	96	10.1	Gerosa et al (2002)[186]
Melanoma	45	82	10.4	Mingione et al (2002)[187]
Melanoma	23	97	9	Somaza et al (1993)[188]
Melanoma	60	90	7	Mori et al (1998)[192]
Melanoma	45	97	8	Lavine et al (1999)[191]
Renal	22	98.5	8	Amendola et al (2000)[190]
Renal	35	90	11	Mori et al (1998)[192]
Renal	74	86	14.6	Gerosa et al (2002)[186]
Renal	42	80	12.5	Hoshi et al (2002)[193]
Renal	69	96	15	Sheehan et al (2003)[194]
Lung	30	71	7.9	Williams et al (1998)[195]
Non–small cell lung	273	84	7	Sheehan et al (2002)[196]
Non–small cell lung	211	98	8.6	Serizawa et al (2002)[197]
Small cell lung	34	94.5	9.1	Serizawa et al (2002)[197]
Breast	30	93	13	Firlik et al (2000)[198]
Breast	68	94	7.8	Amendola et al (2000)[199]
Unknown primary	15	93	15	Maesawa et al (2000)

whole-brain irradiation is possibly not necessary or desirable. In a study comparing the efficacy of surgery plus whole-brain radiotherapy with radiosurgery alone in the treatment of solitary brain metastases less than or equal to 3.5 cm in diameter, local tumor control and 1-year death rates did not statistically differ between the two groups.[200] In a large, multi-institutional study, the omission of up-front fractionated radiation therapy did not compromise the overall length of survival in brain metastasis patients who had undergone radiosurgery.[201] Radiosurgery even appears to be efficacious for treating traditionally relatively "radioresistant" brain metastases such as melanoma and renal carcinoma.

The authors have treated 911 patients for metastatic tumors to the brain. Only in some instances has individual histologic type been analyzed. Evaluation of our series demonstrated an 83% control rate of treated lesions (i.e., disappeared, shrank, or did not change) and a median survival of 7 months. Some 11% disappeared, 63% shrank, and 10% were unchanged (Figs. 40-26 and 40-27); the other 16% increased in size. The usual cause of death was systemic disease.

The various primary tumor types have been evaluated separately in some instances. A series of 21 patients with 37 renal cell carcinoma brain metastases was evaluated and treated by the authors at Virginia.[202] There was an average survival of 8 months following radiosurgery. Of the 23 tumors with post-treatment neuroimaging, 1 remained unchanged in volume, 16 decreased in volume, and 6 disappeared; no renal metastasis progressed following gamma surgery. An unmatched control group of 119 patients that

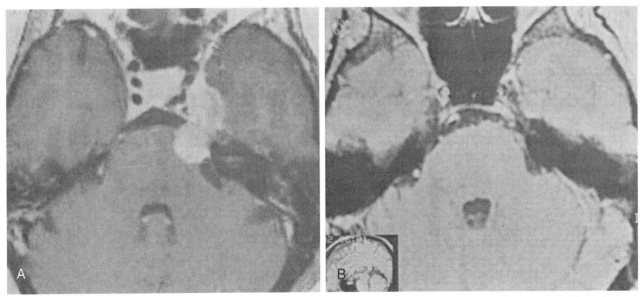

FIGURE 40-26   Patient with metastasis from breast carcinoma to the region of Meckel's cave and the Gasserian ganglion. Contrast-enhanced T1-weighted MRI (A) before and (B) 6 months after gamma surgery. Total regression of the tumor occurred, and 4 years following the treatment the latest MRI reveals no tumor.

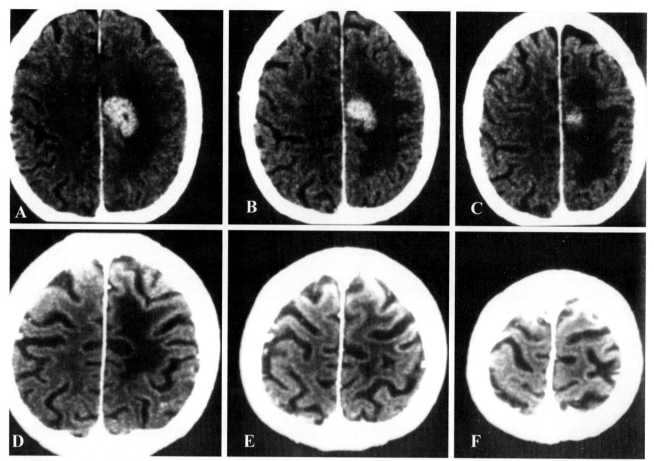

FIGURE 40-27 Gamma surgery for cerebral metastasis from systemic lymphoma. *A* through *C*, This 66-year-old man has cerebral lymphoma metastasis; (*D* through *F*), the same patient 2½ months after gamma surgery. The tumor disappeared completely.

received external brain radiation therapy had an average survival of 4.4 months.[203] Factors associated with longer survival in the group treated with gamma surgery included a higher Karnofsky performance status, absence of extracranial metastases, adjutant whole-brain radiation therapy, and prior surgical resection. Surprisingly, size and the number of metastases did not have a significant effect on survival, although in cases of single metastasis with controlled local disease, long-term survival could be achieved (Fig. 40-28).

A large series of patients with metastatic disease to the brain was reported by Shiau and colleagues.[205] They showed that melanomas had shorter freedom from progression intervals than other histologies (e.g., adenocarcinoma and

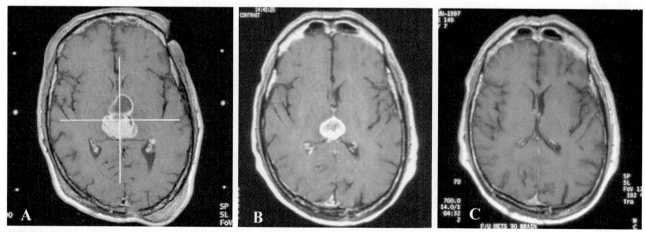

FIGURE 40-28 Gamma surgery for renal cell carcinoma. Postcontrast axial T1-weighted MRI (*A*) at the time of treatment; (*B*) at 3 months; and (*C*) at 1 year following gamma surgery. This patient developed two additional metastases that were subsequently successfully treated with gamma surgery. The patient survived 17 months before succumbing to metastatic deposits outside the brain.

renal cell carcinoma), and that certain imaging characteristics were associated with survival. Multivariate analysis showed that longer control of treated lesions was significantly associated with higher prescribed dose, a homogeneous pattern of contrast enhancement, and a longer interval between primary diagnosis and gamma surgery.[205]

Of 32 metastatic melanomas treated by Somaza and colleagues,[188] 97% disappeared, shrank, or remained unchanged. Average survival in their series was 9 months, with systemic disease being the cause of death in nearly all cases. Three patients remained alive at 13 to 38 months following gamma surgery. Seung and colleagues[204] treated 55 patients with 140 metastatic melanomas and had an average survival just short of 8 months. Freedom from progression was seen in 89% of tumors at 6 months and 77% of tumors at 1 year. Survival was related inversely to total tumor burden and less related to the number of metastases.

In another analysis of 45 patients treated for 92 melanoma metastasis at Virginia, the median survival was 10.4 months following radiosurgery, and local tumor control was 82%.[187] A single metastasis and absence of extracranial disease correlated with improved prognosis. The authors' radiosurgical experience with other histologic subtypes of metastases besides melanoma, lung carcinoma, and renal carcinoma has generally been comparable in terms of survival and local tumor control.

The authors have also treated 191 patients with 425 brain metastases from lung carcinoma. The median survival in those treated with gamma knife alone was 15 months, whereas the median survival in those treated with gamma knife and whole brain irradiation was 14 months ($p = 0.587$). In an analysis of 281 of these brain metastases on follow-up neuroimaging studies, tumor control rates varied according to the tumor size and were as follows: 84.4% (<0.5 mL),

94% (0.5 to 2 mL), 89.1% (2 to 4 mL), 93.4% (4 to 8 mL), 85.7% (8 to 14 mL), and 87.5% (>14 mL). In multivariate analysis, age less than 65 years old, a Karnofsky performance score greater than 70, well-controlled extracranial disease, and more than one gamma surgery were all associated with increased survival.

For brain metastases from breast carcinoma, the authors have treated 43 patients with a total of 84 lesions. Overall median survival was 13 months after gamma knife surgery. Univariate analysis revealed that a high Karnofsky performance score and a single lesion correlated with increased survival, whereas multivariate analysis revealed Karnofsky score and age as related to survival. Overall median time to local tumor control failure was 10 months. Higher Karnosky score and prior chemotherapy led to improved local tumor control.

Hemangioblastomas

The gold standard treatment for hemangioblastomas is the surgical resection of the solid component of the tumor. It is not necessary to resect the cystic portion of the tumor, if present. Similarly, with gamma surgery, the authors have treated only the solid portion of these tumors. The results of 11 of our patients with hemangioblastomas have been reported.[206] Four of these patients had von Hippel-Lindau disease. These patients were followed for an average of 27 months and were treated with a maximum dose of 28 to 60 Gy and a peripheral dose of 11 to 20 Gy. The usual course was either a decrease in the size of the solid component of the tumor (7 of 10 patients) or no change (3 of 10 patients). One patient with a history of multiple hemangioblastomas and extirpations had dramatic tumor shrinkage of a pineal region hemangioblastoma and continues to do well more than 9 years after her gamma surgery (Fig. 40-29). It was not uncommon, however, for the cystic portion of the tumor to

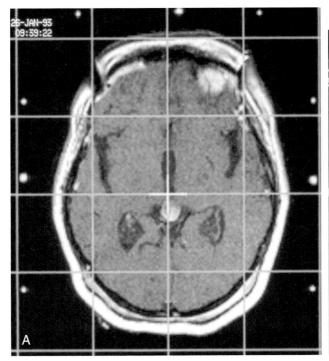
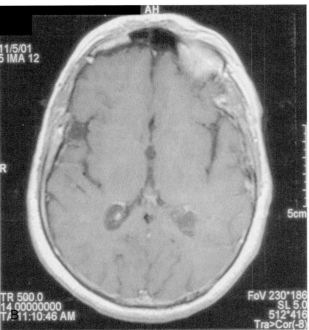

FIGURE 40-29 Gamma surgery for a hemangioblastoma. Postcontrast axial T1-weighted MRI (*A*) at the time of treatment and (*B*) nearly 9 years following gamma surgery. Note the marked reduction in tumor size and loss of enhancement of the pineal region hemangioblastoma. This patient was treated with 21 Gy to the tumor margin and continues to do well.

grow larger regardless of the behavior of the solid portion. During the follow-up of these patients, 4 patients required open surgery for relief of expanding cysts, and 2 required surgery for unresponding solid tumors.

Although several patients responded well, the high incidence of second, open procedures indicates that the microsurgical removal of hemangioblastomas is, in most cases, the initial procedure of choice.

Hemangiopericytomas

Intracranial hemangiopericytomas are richly vascular, rapidly growing mesenchymal neoplasms. They have a predilection for both local and distant central nervous system recurrence and an increased tendency to metastasize. Although surgical resection is the gold standard for these tumors, their high recurrence rate and operative mortality make gamma surgery an attractive option for treatment of hemangiopericytomas.

A retrospective analysis of 12 patients with 15 separate intracranial hemangiopericytomas treated at the University of Virginia revealed reasonable short-term, local tumor control, with 9 tumors decreasing in volume and 3 remaining stable.[207] However, 4 of the 9 tumors that initially shrank later progressed at a mean of 22 months postradiosurgery. In a similar fashion, the University of Pittsburgh group found a local tumor control rate of 76% at a mean follow-up of 31 months postradiosurgery; the 5-year survival rate was 100%.[208] However, radiosurgery did not seem to offer protection against the development of intra- or extracranial metastases. Gamma knife surgery appears to offer effective, acceptable short-term local tumor control for these otherwise untreatable tumors.

Uveal Melanomas

The most common surgical treatment for uveal melanomas is enucleation, but several centers have relatively large series in the treatment of these tumors with gamma surgery.[209–213] Other therapeutic options include radium plaque therapy and proton beam therapy. The first uveal melanoma treated with gamma surgery was in Buenos Aires,[214] and this has become a more commonly used procedure for this unusual pathology. The use of gamma surgery and its stereotactic technique requires that the eyeball be fixated relative to the stereotactic frame. This is accomplished with retrobulbar blocks and external fixative sutures that are attached to the frame. At the University of Vienna, a specially designed suction device that is attached to the frame is utilized.[215]

The Sheffield group reported a series of 29 patients treated and followed for an average of 14 months.[210] The average periphery dose was 73 Gy corresponding to the 50% isodose line. The dose was delivered in two sessions not more than 8 days apart. All but 2 patients had good local control; the two failures required later enucleation. Three patients died of metastatic disease.[210] More recent work suggests that a lower margin dose of 41.5 Gy may be just as effective in terms of tumor control but also may be associated with a lower risk of neovascular glaucoma.[216] In a series of 75 patients with uveal melanoma followed for a minimum of 10 months, Simonova and colleagues reported 84% local tumor control and secondary glaucoma in 25%.[217]

Of the 3 patients treated at the University of Virginia, there has either been no change or a slight decrease in the size of the tumor, with at least 2 years of follow-up. When required, we placed a spacer to elevate the eyelid to prevent radiation injury to the lid. One of the 3 patients was treated with two sessions in order to protect the eyeball from acute increased intraocular pressure, which can be a problem following radiation exposure. The experience treating uveal melanomas with gamma surgery has been shown to be effective for short-term local control. Longer follow-up is required to determine if this procedure is superior to other therapies.

Functional Surgery

Pain

The lack of anatomic and pathophysiologic background knowledge of the mechanisms of pain makes management of pain by open or closed stereotactic techniques largely unsatisfactory.

Early results using gamma surgery to produce thalamotomies for pain control were published by Steiner and colleagues.[15] All of the 52 patients treated suffered from terminal cancer and were treated prior to the advent of CT or MRI. Pneumoencephalography was used to target the thalamic centrum medianum-parafasciculus (CM-Pf complex). Good pain relief was obtained in 8 patients, and moderate pain relief was obtained in 18. The patients had, in general, only temporary relief of pain. Of those with good pain relief, 5 died without recurrence of pain between 1 and 13 months after the procedure, and 3 had recurrence of pain at 3, 6, and 9 months. Doses between 100 and 250 Gy were tested. Observation of an actual lesion was only possible in 21 of 36 patients that had a postmortem examination. Not surprisingly, the presence of a lesion was associated with relief. Lesions were only reliably created with doses greater than 160 Gy. The collimators used were 3 by 5 and 3 by 7 mm. The most effective lesions were more medially located near the wall of the third ventricle, and the greatest relief was for face or arm pain.

These results were not very encouraging; however, with improvements in neuroimaging and alternate target selection, it is possible that more effective lesions can be produced. Recent reports seem to support this expectation.[216] Hayashi and colleagues reported significant pain reduction in patients with severe cancer pain and poststroke thalamic pain after gamma knife lesioning of the hypophysis.[219] Using the 4-mm collimator and doses of 140 to 180 Gy, Young and colleagues have reported effective pain relief in patients with chronic, intractable pain following medial thalamotomy with the gamma knife.[220–222] In a series of 15 patients followed for more than 3 months after a radiosurgical induced medial thalamotomy, 4 (27%) were pain free and 5 others (33%) had greater than 50% pain relief.[222] Additional investigation must be conducted before the role of the gamma knife for pain treatment can be fully defined.

Trigeminal Neuralgia

The first time radiosurgery was used to treat trigeminal neuralgia, Leksell treated 3 patients with an orthovoltage stereotactic technique with long-term relief of symptoms.

With the introduction of the gamma knife, a series of 46 patients were treated at Stockholm with less encouraging results (S. Hakansson, personal communication, 1993). The target in these cases was the gasserian ganglion, and targeting was by bony landmarks or cisternography. With advances in neuroimaging (most notably, MRI), gamma surgery for trigeminal neuralgia was revisited. However, the focus of treatment shifted from the ganglion to the nerve root entry zone. A number of centers have since shown the safety and demonstrated at least short-term pain relief with this approach.

A multicenter trial with 50 patients showed good to excellent relief of pain in 88% of patients (54% pain free and 34% with significant relief) at 2 years. Complete relief was found in 72% of patients treated with 70 Gy or greater.[223] The authors failed to reproduce the reported long-term results.

The majority of 53 patients in a series by Regis and colleagues were pain free at a median follow-up of 55 months after gamma surgery.[224] In a review of 220 patients treated at the University of Pittsburgh with a median radiosurgery dose of 80 Gy, complete pain relief was achieved in 64.9% of patients at 6 months, 70.3% at 1 year, and 75.4% at 33 months.[225,226] At 5 years, only 55.8% had either complete or partial pain relief. The results for patients with atypical facial pain were worse. Following radiosurgery, 10.2% developed new or increased facial paresthesias or numbness. With those who experienced recurrence of their trigeminal neuralgia, repeat gamma surgery afforded complete pain relief in only 48% and, despite a dose reduction to 50 to 60 Gy, carried an increased risk of new sensory deficits.[227] In a series of 54 patients with a median follow-up of 12 months, the results from the Barrow Neurological Institute were less favorable, with only 35% achieving complete pain relief.[228]

Six cases of refractory cluster headache (5 chronic and 1 episodic) were treated by gamma surgery directed at the trigeminal nerve root entry zone. Excellent results were reported in 4 cases (off medication), good in 1 case, and fair in the other cases with an 8 to 14 month follow-up.[229]

At the University of Virginia, the authors have recently reviewed our treatment of 146 cases of trigeminal neuralgia (TN) with gamma knife surgery. In this group, radiosurgery was performed once in 131 patients, twice in 14 patients, and three times in 1 patient. The types of trigeminal neuralgia were as follows: 126 patients with typical TN, 3 with atypical TN, 4 with multiple sclerosis–associated TN, and 10 patients with TN and a history of a cavernous sinus tumor. In each case, the radiosurgical target chosen was 2 to 4 mm anterior to the entry zone of the trigeminal nerve into the pons. The maximal doses varied from 50 to 90 Gy. The median follow-up was 18 months (range, 2 to 96 months). The mean time to pain relief was 24 days (range, 1 to 180 days). The percentage of patients who were pain-free at 1, 2, and 3 years postradiosurgery was 48%, 46%, and 39%, respectively. The percentage of patients who experienced some degree of improvement in their pain was 90%, 77%, and 70% at 1, 2, and 3 years follow-up, respectively. Eleven patients (8%) developed the onset of facial numbness postradiosurgery. Although less effective than microvascular decompression, stereotactic radiosurgery remains a reasonable treatment option for those patients who are unwilling or unable to undergo more invasive surgical approaches, and it offers a low risk of side effects.

Movement Disorders

Thalamotomy for tremor in Parkinson's disease remains one of the most gratifying procedures in functional neurosurgery, defending its place in the therapeutic armory for those common cases in which drugs fail to stop the tremor. However, to avoid the potential risks of open thalamotomies, the prototype of the gamma knife was used by Leksell for the production of thalamic lesions in 5 cases of tremor between 1968 and 1970. At that time, the intended target could not be visualized but was indirectly determined by using derived coordinates relative to the anterior and posterior commisures visualized by pneumoencephalography. Verification that a lesion had been produced could not be obtained because neither CT nor MRI was available. The fixation of the head of the patient for the radiosurgical procedure was also unsatisfactory because the stereotactic frame used for target localization was too large to fit into the collimator helmet. Instead, fixation devices were applied onto a plaster-of-Paris helmet previously molded on the patient's head. It is therefore not surprising that beneficial results were lacking. In 1986, MRI was introduced at Karolinska Hospital, and better anatomic visualization of the target volume became possible. A new stereotactic frame compatible with MRI that also served as the fixation device in the gamma knife was introduced.[230]

These improvements paved the way for new attempts to relieve Parkinsonian tremor by gammathalamotomy, and the first 2 cases were treated using this improved methodology.[231,232] The procedure was performed using an 8-mm collimator, and the volume of the resulting lesion was much larger than intended (1.5 mL). The tremor began to dwindle after 2 months, but a transient hemiparesis and mild speech disturbance ensued secondary to edema. The eventual outcome was, however, satisfactory, and 4 years after the treatment the patient returned free of tremor contralateral to the side of the thalamic lesion, asking for a second procedure to stop the tremor that had developed on the other side.

The second patient was treated using a 4-mm collimator, which gave a smaller volume to the thalamic lesion. In this case, the clinical result was not satisfactory. The patient was treated a second time without relief of tremor. It is not clear whether the lack of effect was caused by the atypical clinical picture in this patient or by the lack of physiologic corroboration of the target. In spite of experience from centers active in this field indicating that modern imaging techniques (especially MRI) may obviate the need for physiologic target definition, this remains controversial. Lim and colleagues showed a high incidence of delayed internal capsule stroke in patients with a previous history of vascular disease who were treated with stereotactic radiofrequency lesioning. If these results are reproduced, then gamma surgery may be the primary treatment of choice, at least for the subgroup most at risk for stroke.[233]

Pioneering works in neuroanatomy and neurophysiology by Hirai and colleagues have shed much light on the position, anatomic organization, and physiologic significance of the thalamus as it pertains to tremor, rigidity, and dyskinesia.[234–239] MRI guidance for selective thalamotomy in the treatment of Parkinsonian or essential tremors has been well established. The correlations between neuroanatomic and electrophysiologic findings in the human ventrolateral thalamic nuclei (e.g., VLa, VLp, VPLa, and VPLc) are better understood. For gamma knife surgery, the difficulty arises in identifying the VLp and VLa nuclei in the human thalamus purely by radiologic methods. As such, thin-slice MRI, Surgiplan, and a neuroanatomic atlas may be required to treat these nuclei with the gamma knife.

Rand has treated 18 cases of movement disorder with radiosurgery (R. Rand, personal communication, 1994). Of the 7 patients with resting tremor, 4 responded to a nucleus ventralis lateralis (NVL) lesion with marked improvement in the tremor, and in 2 patients, rigidity improved as well. Eight other patients underwent radiosurgical pallidotomy for rigidity, and 4 had significant improvement. Two of 3 patients treated with an NVL lesion for intention tremor showed dramatic improvement. Results termed good, excellent, or complete relief of tremor by the authors were accomplished in 63% of patients treated with thalamic lesioning in 34 patients treated by Duma and colleagues.[240] Similar results were obtained by Young and colleagues,[241] Ohye and colleagues,[242–244] and Niranjan and colleagues.[245]

Ohye (C. Ohye, personal communications, 2004) has performed gamma thalamotomies on 56 patients for Parkinson's disease, 21 with essential tremor, and 6 with intention tremor. Thalamotomies were performed using a single 4-mm shot and 130-Gy dose. Follow-up MR imaging revealed two different types of thalamic changes. One type was a round, punched-out lesion with a volume of less than 100 mm[3]; the other was an irregular, high-signal zone (volume up to 800 mm[3]) that may extend into the internal capsule and streak along the border of the thalamus. The efficacy of the procedure did not seem to correlate with the type of postoperative imaging observed. Ohye noted improvements in tremor and/or rigidity in 85% of patients. Hirai (T. Hirai, personal communications, 2004) has treated 14 patients with gamma surgery for involuntary movement disorders. Of these 14 patients, 8 had tremor dominant Parkinson's, 4 had rigidity and dyskinesia-dominant Parkinson's, and 2 had essential tremors. Hirai's target points were the VLp nucleus for control of tremor and the VLa nucleus for control of rigidity and dyskinesia. The maximum dose varied from 130 to 150 Gy; a single 4-mm isocenter was used to make each lesion. At last follow-up, 13 out of 14 patients noted subjective improvement in their symptomatology. In nine of these patients who had at least 1-year follow-up, Hirai noted symptomatic improvement by 50% to 90% in the patients' Unified Parkinson's Disease Rating Scale for tremor, rigidity, and dyskinesia scores. On follow-up MR imaging, Hirai observed T2-weighted changes 3 months after gamma surgery, and these lesions gradually increased to 5 to 8 mm in diameter. In another series, Young and colleagues reported significant improvements in Unified Parkinson's Disease Rating Scale tremor and rigidity scores in 74 out of 102 patients (73%) at 4 years post–gamma knife thalamotomy; in those with essential tremor, 88.2% remained tremor-free at 4 years postoperatively.[246] The gamma knife may even be able to lesion the subthalamic nucleus.[247]

A pertinent change in the surgical management of movement disorders, particularly of Parkinsonian tremor, was the introduction of deep brain stimulation (DBS), which allows the amelioration of symptoms without a destructive lesion.

Good results have been obtained with this technique, and at present deep brain stimulation has supplanted destructive lesions as the surgical procedure of choice in most patients.[248,249] The enthusiasm for deep brain stimulation may be lessened by the high rate of complications and the cost.[250–253] As the benefits and risks for DBS become better defined, neurosurgeons will be able to counsel patients and select the more appropriate neurosurgical tool (i.e., gamma knife or DBS).[250] It is difficult to predict the extent to which these two competing neurosurgical tools will be used in the future for treatment of movement disorders.

Obsessive-Compulsive Neurosis

Despite therapeutic progress in recent years, conventional treatment of anxiety disorders fails or has only a temporary effect in 20% of patients. These disorders are often severely disabling and are associated with rates of suicide comparable to those of depression. First described by Leksell,[254] psychosurgery targeting the frontolimbic connections in both anterior internal capsules (capsulotomy) is a valuable therapeutic method for selected severe cases. The first cases using the gamma knife to create the lesions were also performed by Leksell.

Mindus at the Karolinska Institute[255] reported the effects of such procedures on the anxiety symptoms and personality characteristics presented in conjunction with results of imaging studies performed by MRI and PET. The patient material comprised two series of patients with a 15-year mean duration of psychiatric illness, in all of whom various extensive treatment trials had previously been made. One series consisted of 24 patients subjected to capsulotomy by a conventional thermocoagulation technique and followed for 1 year. The other series comprised 7 patients treated by gamma surgery and followed for 7 years. The clinical effects of these treatments were evaluated subjectively by two independent observers and were also rated on the Comprehensive Psychopathological Rating Scale (CPRS). Ratings were performed 10 days before and 2, 6, and 12 months after surgery. The effects on the personality were evaluated by the Karolinska Scales of Personality (KSP). These scales have been developed to measure traits related to frontal lobe dysfunction and to reflect different dimensions of anxiety proneness.

At the 12-month follow-up, statistically and clinically significant improvement was noted in all assessments of symptomatic and psychosocial function. Freedom from symptoms or considerable improvement was noted in 79% of patients, and none were worse after the operation. Negative effects on the personality were not noted. Behind these numbers are numerous examples of dramatic improvements in individual lifestyles. A number of patients were preoperatively unable to work or function socially owing to such problems as preoccupation with personal cleanliness and the inability to use public transportation, with resulting domestic confinement, aggravated psychological problems, deterioration of family relationships, and devastation of personal economy. Postoperatively, these patients could return to their previous occupation and to a normal social function. The results of gamma capsulotomy were found to be comparable to those of capsulotomy performed by the thermocoagulation technique. Only in 5 of the 7 patients could a lesion be demonstrated by MRI, and those were the patients who benefited from the procedure. The lowest effective target dose was 160 Gy, whereas 100, 120, and 152 Gy failed to produce lesions.

Treatment of a new series of 10 patients was started in 1988, using stereotactic MRI for more accurate anatomic target localization and the new gamma knife model B to produce the lesions. In this series, the lesions were produced by using a 4-mm collimator and three isocenters on each side for overlapping fields, thereby creating a cylindrical lesion. The maximum dose within the target volume was 200 Gy. Although it is too early to evaluate the long-term psychological effects in this series of patients, important radiologic information, which will serve to plan future treatments, is already available. The development of the lesions has been followed by MRI and CT scans every 3 months. Magnetic resonance imaging has, not unexpectedly, been found to be particularly valuable for these follow-up studies. On T2-weighted images, a high signal appears in the target area after approximately 3 months. This signal is most likely produced by local edema. The edema extends to a maximal volume at around 9 months and then slowly subsides. The edema is directly related to the dose and to the volume radiated. The preliminary impression is that the results equal those obtained in the earlier series.

A comparison of the radiobiologic effects between these two series is unfortunately not possible, because neither MRI nor CT was available when the lesions developed in the first series of patients. In the second series, the edema was extensive in a few patients, and it may therefore be wise to adjust the dose or decrease the volume exposed to necrotizing doses in the future. It may be sufficient to use only one isocenter and the 4-mm collimator. With these treatment parameters and a maximal dose of 180 Gy, a lesion measuring approximately 50 mm^3 can be expected within several weeks with only minimal transient edema.

Gammacapsulotomy offers several important clinical as well as scientific advantages over capsulotomy via an open technique.[256] The most important advantage is patient tolerance. It is the authors' experience that this psychologically vulnerable group of patients is much more willing to undergo a closed stereotactic procedure, which in contrast to open surgery, leaves no external marks. Theoretically, the gradual development of the radiolesion may also allow the patient better psychological adjustment to his or her new situation. The psychological rehabilitation phase is an important part of any psychosurgical procedure.

If it would be ethically acceptable, a control group of patients could be subjected to spending time in the collimator helmet without radiation. In a later stage, if this sham procedure is proven to give no result in comparison with the real procedure, the control group would receive the appropriate treatment. Such a controlled study is probably necessary before the capsulotomy procedure is generally accepted. Further efforts should also be made to study the biology of the developing lesions. Important questions to answer include when does the functional effect of the radiation start and what are the characteristics of the MRI and CT images at that time. Even the issue of dose-volume relationships needs to be addressed further. PET or SPECT imaging may help to answer some of these questions, and pre- and post-treatment evaluation is planned for further series of patients. The experience from multiple centers

suggests a degree of optimism for the use of radiosurgery in the treatment of intractable obsessive-compulsive disorder, and future research in psychiatric neurosurgery is proceeding in a cautious fashion.[257] Any such work necessitates the coordination and effort of a multidisciplinary team.[257]

Epilepsy

Seizure was the presenting symptom in 59 of the 247 patients with AVMs of the brain treated by Steiner with Gamma surgery between 1970 and 1984.[79] The treatment resulted in the relief of some or all seizures in 52 of these patients. Eleven were successfully taken off anticonvulsant medication. Interestingly, in 3 patients the seizure disorder stopped although the AVM itself was unaffected by the radiation.[79] These observations and the observations made by others[258–260] prompted the idea of testing focal irradiation as a treatment modality for focal epilepsy.

At the neurosurgery department at the University of Virginia, basic science research was done on changes in neuroexcitability after irradiation. The hippocampal slices from rats treated with the gamma knife were found to have a higher seizure threshold than those of controls when placed in solutions of varying concentrations of penicillin. This effect was lost at high concentrations (Henson and colleagues, personal communication, 2001). Using single doses of either 20 or 40 Gy to the hippocampus in a rat model of chronic spontaneous limbic epilepsy, a reduction in both the frequency and duration of spontaneous seizures was observed.[261] Histologic evaluation of the targeted region revealed no signs of necrosis, and hippocampal slice recordings revealed intact synaptically driven neuronal firing.[261] Subsequent work by the University of Pittsburgh group using a kainic acid–induced hippocampal epilepsy rat model revealed similarly efficacious results in terms of seizure control and the absence of behavioral impairment with subnecrotic doses of radiosurgery.[262,263]

Biochemical analysis of changes in rats brains after gamma surgery, performed by Regis and colleagues, showed changes in the concentrations of excitatory and inhibitory amino acids (particularly gamma-aminobutyric acid [GABA]).[264] Warnke and colleagues showed that patients with low-grade astrocytomas and associated epilepsy had significant relief from seizures following interstitial radiosurgery. SPECT scanning showed a reduced number of GABA receptors prior to treatment in both the tumors and surrounding brain. Levels of these receptors increased following therapy.[265] These early studies show that functional changes may occur at the cellular level without gross structural damage. The implications of this for functional neurosurgery are intriguing.

Epilepsy has been treated with the gamma knife at many centers, but there have been few published long-term results. The authors have treated 6 patients, 3 of whom had structural lesions. The early results for the first 3 patients were encouraging, with significant reduction in seizure activity; however, these results were not durable in the long term.

Barcia-Salorio and colleagues treated 11 patients with idiopathic epilepsy.[266] Preoperative invasive electrodiagnostic confirmation of the epileptogenic focus was performed, and treatment was with low dose (10- to 20-Gy) radiosurgery. Complete relief from seizures was obtained in 4 patients, and significant reduction in seizure activity was seen in 5 patients. The effect of the treatment was not seen for several months in most instances. Regis and colleagues reported a case of mesial temporal lobe epilepsy treated with gamma surgery.[267] They used 25 Gy given to the 50% isodose line. The patient was seizure-free after the treatment. At 10 months a lesion that conformed to the 50% isodose line (amygdala and hippocampus) was evident on both CT and MRI. Whether actual gross structural lesioning with this method is associated with either better results or more complications is unknown. Further results of 25 patients with medically intractable mesial temporal lobe epilepsy treated by Regis and colleagues showed that of the 16 patients with more than 2 years follow-up, 13 are seizure-free and 2 are improved.[268] In addition, they noted minimal morbidity (only 3 cases of nonsymptomatic visual field deficit) and no mortality associated with the gamma surgery.[268]

The potential of a less invasive, nondestructive therapy to treat epilepsy prompted the creation of prospective European- and a National Institutes of Health (NIH) sponsored multicenter studies of gamma surgery for temporal lobe epilepsy. In the European study, three centers enrolled 21 patients with mesial temporal lobe epilepsy. The anterior parahippocampal cortex, the basal and lateral portions of the amygdala, and the anterior hippocampus were targeted, and patients received a mean dose of 24 Gy. At 2 years postradiosurgery, 65% of the patients were seizure-free. However, 9 patients developed visual field deficits, and 5 suffered transient side effects including depression, headache, nausea, vomiting, and imbalance.[269] The NIH-sponsored study, which began in the fall of 2000, randomized 40 patients into two dosage groups and monitored several clinical and radiologic characteristics over 3 years following radiosurgical treatment. These evaluation points include the effect on seizure frequency and severity, MR imaging (including diffusion- and perfusion-weighted studies), MR spectroscopy, and neuropsychological outcomes. Of the patients in the NIH study treated at the University of Virginia, improvements in their epilepsy have been observed. However, 1 of the patients treated at another center as part of the NIH study experienced a serious adverse event that included persistent headaches, visual changes, and cerebral edema, and these consequences necessitated a standard temporal lobectomy.

The safety and demonstrated short-term efficacy of gamma knife surgery for the treatment of epilepsies arising from space-occupying lesions (e.g., low-grade gliomas), hippocampal sclerosis, or hypothalamic hamartomas make it an attractive option.[270] However, gamma knife's long-term feasibility and effectiveness for epilepsy needs to be proved. Also, it is unclear what underlying mechanisms are responsible for amelioration of seizures following radiosurgery. Some have suggested a "neuromodulation" phenomenon following gamma surgery with accompanying glial cell reduction, stem cell migration, neuronal plasticity and sprouting, and biochemical changes.[271] Rigorous scientific studies evaluating the cellular and subcellular mechanisms responsible for improvements in epilepsy post-gamma surgery are thus far lacking. Furthermore, the need for physiologic monitoring (e.g., depth electrodes or cortical grids) to determine conclusively the epileptogenic focus cannot be entirely discarded. Future developments of noninvasive physiologic monitoring will influence the development of gamma surgery for epilepsy. When everything is considered, one may

contend that although gamma knife surgery may be used for functional diseases of the brain, the current efficacy of alternative methods dramatically limits the role of gamma surgery in the management of these diseases.

CONCLUSIONS

The indications and usefulness of gamma surgery are being defined more carefully with the passage of time. The advances of the past several decades have paralleled improvements in neuroimaging. The identification of discrete thalamic, hypothalamic, and basal ganglia nuclei with acceptable confidence may allow the use of gamma surgery in a wider range of functional disorders. This will require a better understanding of the relationship of anatomy and function as well as improved spatial definition of these nuclei. With existing technology the treatment of some functional disorders (e.g., Parkinson's disease, obsessive-compulsive disorder, and chronic pain) are being evaluated now.

Technical advances and improvements of the gamma unit will increase the ease of use of the machine, and better-defined protocols should improve the clinical results obtained with its use. Other advances in fields such as pharmacology may allow the selective sensitization of tumors or provide protective effect to normal tissue, increasing the efficacy and safety in tumor treatment. In the first stage of development of gamma surgery, it is mandatory to define its usefulness in various pathologies. The elimination of its use when not clinically indicated, and to expand its use into new areas when it has been shown to have efficacy, are important goals. The rapidly accumulating material from patients that have been treated will define the place of the gamma knife in the armory of neurosurgery.

REFERENCES

1. Gerszten PC, Ozhasoglu C, Burton SA, et al: Cyberknife frameless real-time image-guided stereotactic radiosurgery for the treatment of spinal lesions. Int J Radiat Oncol Biol Phys 57(2 Suppl):S370–S371, 2003.
2. Hamilton AJ, Lulu BA, Fosmire H, et al: LINAC-based spinal stereotactic radiosurgery. Stereotact Funct Neurosurg 66(1–3):1–9, 1996.
3. Lax I, Blomgren H, Naslund I, et al: Stereotactic radiotherapy of malignancies in the abdomen: Methodological aspects. Acta Oncol 33(6):677–683, 1994.
4. Chang SD, Adler JR: Robotics and radiosurgery: The cyberknife. Stereotact Funct Neurosurg 76(3–4):204–208, 2001.
5. Dandy WE: Cerebral Ventriculoscopy. Bull Johns Hopkins Hosp 33:1922.
6. Schulder M, Loeffler JS, Howes AE, et al: Historical vignette: The radium bomb: Harvey Cushing and the interstitial irradiation of gliomas. J Neurosurg 84:530–532, 1996.
7. Clarke R, Horsley V: One method of investigating the deep ganglia and tracts of the central nervous system (cerebellum). BMJ ii: 1799–1800, 1906.
8. Spiegel E, Wycis H, Marks M, et al: Stereotaxic apparatus for operations on the human brain. Science 106:349–350, 1947.
9. Leksell L: The stereotaxic method and radiosurgery of the brain. Acta Chir Scand 102:316, 1951.
10. Larsson B, Leksell L, Rexed B: The use of high-energy protons for cerebral surgery in man. Acta Chir Scand 125:1, 1963.
11. Leksell L, Larsson B, Andersson B: Lesions in the depth of the brain produced by a beam of high-energy protons. Acta Radiol 54:251–264, 1960.
12. Hall EJ, Marchese M, Hei TK, et al: Radiation response characteristics of human cells in vitro. Radiat Res 114:415–424, 1988.
13. Kamiryo T, Kassell NF, Thai QA, et al: Histological changes in the normal rat brain after gamma irradiation. Acta Neurochir (Wien) 138:451–459, 1996.

14. Flickinger JC, Lunsford LD, Kondziolka D: Dose-volume considerations in radiosurgery. Stereotact Funct Neurosurg 57:99–105, 1991.
15. Steiner L, Forster D, Leksell L, et al: Gammathalamotomy in intractable pain. Acta Neurochir (Wien) 52:173–184, 1980.
16. Hawighorst H, Engenhart R, Knopp MV, et al: Intracranial meningeomas: time- and dose-dependent effects of irradiation on tumor microcirculation monitored by dynamic MR imaging. Magn Reson Imaging 15:423–432, 1997.
17. Tsuzuki T, Tsunoda S, Sakaki T, et al: Tumor cell proliferation and apoptosis associated with the gamma knife effect. Stereotact Funct Neurosurg 66:39–48, 1996.
18. Marekova M, Cap J, Vokurkova D, et al: Effect of therapeutic doses of ionising radiation on the somatomammotroph pituitary cell line, GH3. Endocr J 50(5):621–628, 2003.
19. Hopewell JW, Wright EA: The nature of latent cerebral irradiation damage and its modification by hypertension. Br J Radiol 43:161–167, 1970.
20. Verhey LJ, Smith V, Serago CF: Comparison of radiosurgery treatment modalities based on physical dose distributions. Int J Radiat Oncol Biol Phys 40:497–505, 1998.
21. Tishler RB, Loeffler JS, Lunsford LD, et al: Tolerance of cranial nerves of the cavernous sinus to radiosurgery (see comments). Int J Radiat Oncol Biol Phys 27:215–221, 1993.
22. Stafford SL, Pollock BE, Leavitt JA, et al: A study on the radiation tolerance of the optic nerves and chiasm after stereotactic radiosurgery. Int J Radiat Oncol Biol Phys 55(5):1177–1181, 2003.
23. Chen JC, Giannotta SL, Yu C, et al: Radiosurgical management of benign cavernous sinus tumors: Dose profiles and acute complications. Neurosurgery 48:1022–1032, 2001.
24. Ove R, Kelman S, Amin PP, et al: Preservation of visual fields after peri-sellar gamma knife radiosurgery. Int J Cancer 90:343–350, 2000.
25. Tishler RB, Loeffler JS, Lunsford LD, et al: Tolerance of cranial nerves of the cavernous sinus to radiosurgery. Int J Radiat Oncol Biol Phys 27:215–221, 1993.
26. Girkin CA, Comey CH, Lunsford LD, et al: Radiation optic neuropathy after stereotactic radiosurgery. Ophthalmology 104(10):1634–1643, 1997.
27. Leber KA, Bergloff J, Pendl G: Dose-response tolerance of the visual pathways and cranial nerves of the cavernous sinus to stereotactic radiosurgery. J Neurosurg 88:43–50, 1998.
28. Lundstrom M, Frisen L: Atrophy of optic nerve fibres in compression of the chiasm: Degree and distribution of ophthalmoscopic changes. Acta Ophthalmol (Copenh) 54(5):623–640, 1976.
29. Rodriguez O, Mateos B, de la Pedraja R, et al: Postoperative follow-up of pituitary adenomas after trans-sphenoidal resection: MRI and clinical correlation. Neuroradiology 38(8):747–754, 1996.
30. Noren G, Greitz D, Hirsch A, et al: gamma knife surgery in acoustic tumours. Acta Neurochir Suppl (Wien) 58:104–107, 1993.
31. G. Szikla OB, S. Blond: Data of late reactions following stereotactic irradiation of gliomas. In INSERM Symposium on Stereotactic Irradiations. Paris: Elsevier, North Holland Biomedical Press, 1979.
32. Steiner L, Greitz T, Backlund E, et al: radiosurgery in arterio-venous malformations of the brain undue effects. In INSERM Symposium on Stereotactic Irradiations. Paris: Elsevier, North Holland Biomedical Press, 1979.
33. Lim YL, Leem W, Kim TS, et al: Four years' experiences in the treatment of pituitary adenomas with gamma knife radiosurgery. Stereotact Funct Neurosurg 70(Suppl 1):95–109, 1998.
34. Pollock BE, Nippoldt TB, Stafford SL, et al: Results of stereotactic radiosurgery in patients with hormone-producing pituitary adenomas: Factors associated with endocrine normalization. J Neurosurg 97(3):525–530, 2002.
35. Muramatsu J, Yoshida M, Shioura H, et al: Clinical results of LINAC-based stereotactic radiosurgery for pituitary adenoma. Nippon Igaku Hoshasen Gakkai Zasshi 63(5):225–230, 2003.
36. Shin M, Kurita H, Sasaki T, et al: Stereotactic radiosurgery for pituitary adenoma invading the cavernous sinus. J Neurosurg 93(Suppl 3):2–5, 2000.
37. Kamiryo T, Lopes MBS, Berr SS, et al: Occlusion of the anterior cerebral artery after gamma knife irradiation in a rat. Acta Neurochir (Wien) 138:983–990, 1996.
38. Nilsson A, Wennerstrand J, Leksell D, et al: Stereotactic gamma irradiation of basilar artery in cat: Preliminary experiences. Acta Radiol Oncol Radiat Phys Biol 17:150–160, 1978.
39. Kihlström L, Lindquist C, Adler J, et al (eds): Histological studies of gamma knife lesions in normal and hypercholesterolemic rabbits.
40. Radiosurgery: Baseline and Trends. New York: Steiner L. Raven Press, 1992, pp 111–119.
40. Cushing H, Bailey P: Tumors Arising from the Blood Vessels of the Brain. Springfield, IL: Charles C Thomas, 1928, p 46.
41. Wegemann H-J: Das Schicksal Operierter Patienten mit Arteriovenösem Aneurysma des Gehrins. Zurich: Juris Druck and Verlag, 1969.
42. Krayenbühl H: Discussion des rapports sur "les angiomes supratentoriels." In Congrès International de Neurochirurgie, Bruxelles, 1957.
43. Olivecrona H, Ladenheim J: Congenital arteriovenous aneurysms of the carotid and vertebral systems. Berlin Göttingen Heidelberg: Springer, 1957, p 91.
44. McKissock W, Hankinson J: The surgical treatment of supratentorial angiomas. Congrès International de Neurochirurgie, Bruxelles, 1957.
45. Pool J: Aneurysms and arteriovenous anomalies of the brain: Diagnosis and treatment. New York: Hoeber Medical Division, Harper & Row, 1965.
46. Jefferson G: Les hemorrhagies sous-arachnoidiennes par angiomes et aneurysms chez le jeune. Rev Neurol (Paris) 80:413–432, 1948.
47. Ray B: Cerebral arteriovenous aneurysms. Surg Gynec Obstet 73:614–648, 1941.
48. Johnson J: Cerebral Angiomas: Advances in Diagnosis and Therapy. Berlin: Springer-Verlag, 1975, pp 256–258.
49. Steiner L, Leksell L, Greitz T, et al: Stereotaxic radiosurgery for cerebral arteriovenous malformations: Report of a case. Acta Chir Scand 138:459–464, 1972.
50. Yamamoto M, Jimbo M, Kobayashi M, et al: Long-term results of radiosurgery for arteriovenous malformation: Neurodiagnostic imaging and histological studies of angiographically confirmed nidus obliteration. Surg Neurol 37:219–230, 1992.
51. Schneider BF, Eberhard DA, Steiner L: Histopathology of arteriovenous malformations after gamma knife radiosurgery. J Neurosurg 87:352–357, 1997.
52. Szeifert GT, Kemeny AA, Timperley WR, et al: The potential role of myofibroblasts in the obliteration of arteriovenous malformations after radiosurgery. Neurosurgery 40:61–65, 1997.
53. Albert P, Salgado H, Polaina M, et al: A study on the venous drainage of 150 cerebral arteriovenous malformations as related to haemorrhagic risks and the size of the lesion. Acta Neurochir (Wein) 103:30–34, 1990.
54. Graf CJ, Perret GE, Torner JC: Bleeding from cerebral arteriovenous malformations as part of their natural history. J Neurosurg 58:331–337, 1983.
55. Itoyama Y, Uemura S, Ushio Y, et al: Natural course of unoperated intracranial arteriovenous malformations: Study of 50 cases. J Neurosurg 71:805–809, 1989.
56. Spetzler RF, Hargraves RW, McCormick PW, et al: Relationship of perfusion pressure and size to risk of hemorrhage from arteriovenous malformations (see comments). J Neurosurg 76:918–923, 1992.
57. Jomin M, Lesoin F, Lozes G: Prognosis for arteriovenous malformations of the brain in adults based on 150 cases. Surg Neurol 23:362–366, 1985.
58. Steiner L, Linquist C, Karlsson B, et al: Gamma knife radiosurgery in cerebral vascular malformations. In Pasqualin A, Pian RD (eds): New trends in management of cerebro-vascular malformations. New York: Springer-Verlag, 1994, pp 473–485.
59. Brown RD Jr, Wiebers DO, Forbes G, et al: The natural history of unruptured intracranial arteriovenous malformations. J Neurosurg 68:352–357, 1988.
60. Crawford PM, West CR, Shaw MD, et al: Cerebral arteriovenous malformations and epilepsy: Factors in the development of epilepsy. Epilepsia 27:270–275, 1986.
61. Forster DM, Kunkler IH, Hartland P: Risk of cerebral bleeding from arteriovenous malformations in pregnancy: The Sheffield experience. Stereotact Funct Neurosurg 61:20–22, 1993.
62. Fults D, Kelly DL Jr: Natural history of arteriovenous malformations of the brain: A clinical study. Neurosurgery 15:658–662, 1984.
63. Karlsson B: Gamma Knife Surgery of Arteriovenous Malformations in Neurosurgery. Stochholm: Karolinska Institute, 1996.
64. Forster DM, Steiner L, Hakanson S: Arteriovenous malformations of the brain: A long-term clinical study. J Neurosurg 37:562–570, 1972.
65. Ondra SL, Troupp H, George ED, et al: The natural history of symptomatic arteriovenous malformations of the brain: A 24-year follow-up assessment. J Neurosurg 73:387–391, 1990.
66. Sadasivan B, Malik GM, Lee C, et al: Vascular malformations and pregnancy. Surg Neurol 33:305–313, 1990.

67. Harbaugh KS, Harbaugh RE: Arteriovenous malformations in elderly patients. Neurosurgery 35:579–584, 1994.

68. Robinson JL, Hall CS, Sedzimir CB: Arteriovenous malformations, aneurysms, and pregnancy. J Neurosurg 41:63–70, 1974.

69. Horstmann GA, Van Eck AT: Gamma knife model C with the automatic positioning system and its impact on the treatment of vestibular schwannomas. J Neurosurg 97(5 Suppl):450–455, 2002.

70. Regis J, Hayashi M, Porcheron D, et al: Impact of the model C and automatic positioning system on gamma knife radiosurgery: An evaluation in vestibular schwannomas. J Neurosurg 97(5 Suppl):588–591, 2002.

71. Kondziolka D, Maitz AH, Niranjan A, et al: An evaluation of the Model C gamma knife with automatic patient positioning. Neurosurgery 50(2):429–431, 2002.

72. Yamamoto M, Jimbo M, Hara M, et al: gamma knife radiosurgery for arteriovenous malformations: Long-term follow-up results focusing on complications occurring more than 5 years after irradiation. Neurosurgery 38(5):906–914, 1996.

73. Kihlstrom L, Guo WY, Karlsson B, et al: Magnetic resonance imaging of obliterated arteriovenous malformations up to 23 years after radiosurgery. J Neurosurg 86(4):589–593, 1997.

74. Yamamoto M, Ide M, Jimbo M, et al: Late cyst convolution after gamma knife radiosurgery for cerebral arteriovenous malformations. Stereotact Funct Neurosurg 70(Suppl 1):166–167, 1998.

75. Sutcliffe JC, Forster DM, Walton L, et al: Untoward clinical effects after stereotactic radiosurgery for intracranial arteriovenous malformations. Br J Neurosurg 6(3):177–185, 1992.

76. Karlsson B, Lindquist C, Steiner L: Prediction of obliteration after gamma knife surgery for cerebral arteriovenous malformations. Neurosurgery 40(3):425–430, 1997.

77. Flickinger JC, Pollock BE, Kondziolka D, et al: A dose-response analysis of arteriovenous malformation obliteration after radiosurgery. Int J Radiat Oncol Biol Phys 36(4):873–879, 1996.

78. Chang JH, Chang JW, Park YG, et al: Factors related to complete occlusion of arteriovenous malformations after gamma knife radiosurgery. J Neurosurg 93(Suppl 3):96–101, 2000.

79. Steiner L, Lindquist C, Adler JR, et al: Clinical outcome of radiosurgery for cerebral arteriovenous malformations. J Neurosurg 77:1–8, 1992.

80. Kjellberg RN, Davis KR, Lyons S, et al: Bragg peak proton beam therapy for arteriovenous malformation of the brain. Clin Neurosurg 31:248–290, 1983.

81. Steiner L, Lindquist C, Adler JR, et al: Outcome of radiosurgery for cerebral AVM. J Neurosurg 77:823, 1992.

82. Karlsson B, Lindquist C, Steiner L: The effect of gamma knife surgery on the risk of rupture prior to AVM obliteration, in gamma knife surgery in cerebral arteriovenous malformations (PhD Thesis). Stockholm: Karolinska Institute, 1996, pp 34–52.

83. Lindqvist M, Karlsson B, Guo WY, et al: Angiographic long-term follow-up data for arteriovenous malformations previously proven to be obliterated after gamma knife radiosurgery. Neurosurgery 46(4):803–808, 2000.

84. Schneider BF, Eberhard DA, Steiner LE: Histopathology of arteriovenous malformations after gamma knife radiosurgery. J Neurosurg 87(3):352–357, 1997.

85. Payne BR, Prasad D, Steiner M, et al: Gamma surgery for vein of Galen malformations. J Neurosurg 93(2):229–236, 2000.

86. Guo WY: Radiological aspects of gamma knife radiosurgery for arteriovenous malformations and other non-tumoral disorders of the brain. Acta Radiol Suppl 388:1–34, 1993.

87. Aiba T, Tanaka R, Koike T, et al: Natural history of intracranial cavernous malformations. J Neurosurg 83:56–59, 1995.

88. Curling OD, Kelly DL, Elster AD, et al: An analysis of the natural history of cavernous angiomas. J Neurosurg 75:702–708, 1991.

89. Garner TB, Del Curling O Jr, Kelly DL Jr, et al: The natural history of intracranial venous angiomas. J Neurosurg 75:715–722, 1991.

90. Kondziolka D, Lunsford L, Kestle J: The natural history of cavernous malformations. J Neurosurg 83:820–824, 1995.

91. Robinson JR, Awad IA, Little JR: Natural history of the cavernous angioma. J Neurosurg 75:709–714, 1991.

92. Steiner L, Prassad D, Lindquist C, et al: Clinical aspects of gamma knife stereotactic radiosurgery. In Gildenberg P, Tasker R, Franklin P (eds): Textbook of Stereotactic and Functional Neurosurgery, 1st ed. New York: McGraw-Hill, 1998, pp 763–803.

93. Karlsson B, Kihlstrom L, Lindquist C, et al: Radiosurgery for cavernous malformations. J Neurosurg 88:293–297, 1998.

94. Kondziolka D, Lunsford LD, Flickinger JC, et al: Reduction of hemorrhage risk after stereotactic radiosurgery for cavernous malformations. J Neurosurg 83:825–831, 1995.

95. Weil S Jr, Tew JM, Steiner L: Comparison of radiosurgery and microsurgery for treatment of cavernous malformations of brain stem. J Neurosurg 72:336A, 1990.

96. Hasegawa T, McInerney J, Kondziolka D, et al: Long-term results after stereotactic radiosurgery for patients with cavernous malformations. Neurosurgery 50(6):1190–1197, 2002.

97. Pollock BE, Garces YI, Stafford SL, et al: Stereotactic radiosurgery for cavernous malformations. J Neurosurg 93(6):987–991, 2000.

98. Coffey RJ: Brain stem cavernomas. J Neurosurg 99:1116–1117, 2003.

99. Tathiesen Tiit, Edner G, Kihlstrom L: Brain stem cavernomas. J Neurosurg 99:1117, 2003.

100. Garner TB, Curling JOD, Kelly DL, et al: The natural history of intracranial venous angiomas. J Neurosurg 75:715–722, 1991.

101. Kjellberg RN, Shintani A, Frantz AG, et al: Proton beam therapy in acromegaly. N Engl J Med 278:689–695, 1968.

102. Levy RP, Fabrikant JI, Frankel KA, et al: Charged-particle radiosurgery of the brain. Neurosurg Clin N Am 1:955–990, 1990.

103. Sheehan JM, Vance ML, Sheehan JP, et al: Radiosurgery for Cushing's disease after failed transsphenoidal surgery. J Neurosurg 93:738–742, 2000.

104. Shimon I, Ram Z, Cohen ZR, et al: Transsphenoidal surgery for Cushing's disease: Endocrinological follow-up monitoring of 82 patients. Neurosurgery 51:57–62, 2002.

105. Semple PL, Laws ER Jr: Complications in a contemporary series of patients who underwent transsphenoidal surgery for Cushing's disease. J Neurosurg 91(2):175–179, 1999.

106. Landolt AM, Haller D, Lomax N, et al: Octreotide may act as a radioprotective agent in acromegaly. J Clin Endocrinol Metab 85:1287–1289, 2000.

107. Landolt AM, Lomax N: Gamma knife radiosurgery for prolactinomas. J Neurosurg 93(Suppl 3):14–18, 2000.

108. Ganz JC, Backlund EO, Thorsen FA: The effects of gamma knife surgery of pituitary adenomas on tumor growth and endocrinopathies. Stereotact Funct Neurourg 61(Suppl 1):30–37, 1993.

109. Martinez R, Bravo G, Burzaco J, et al: Pituitary tumors and gamma knife surgery: Clinical experience with more than two years of follow-up. Stereotact Funct Neurosurg 70(Suppl 1):110–118, 1998.

110. Landolt AM, Haller D, Lomax N, et al: Stereotactic radiosurgery for recurrent surgically treated acromegaly: Comparison with fractionated radiotherapy. J Neurosurg 88:1002–1008, 1998.

111. Lim YL, Leem W, Kim TS, et al: Four years' experiences in the treatment of pituitary adenomas with gamma knife radiosurgery. Stereotact Funct Neurosurg 70(Suppl 1):95–109, 1998.

112. Morange-Ramos I, Regis J, et al: Gamma-knife surgery for secreting pituitary adenomas. Acta Neurochir (Wien) 140(5):437–443, 1998.

113. Witt TC, Kondziolka D, Flickinger JC, et al: Gamma knife radiosurgery for pituitary tumors. In Lunsford LD, Kondziolka D, Flickinger JC (eds): Gamma Knife Brain Surgery. Progress in Neurological Surgery, vol 14. Basel: Karger, 1998, pp 114–127.

114. Hayashi M, Izawa M, Hiyama H, et al: Gamma knife radiosurgery for pituitary adenomas. Stereotact Funct Neurosurg 72(Suppl 1): 111–118, 1999.

115. Inoue HK, Kohga H, Hirato M, et al: Pituitary adenomas treated by microsurgery with or without gamma knife surgery: Experience in 122 cases. Stereotact Funct Neurosurg 72(Suppl 1):125–131, 1999

116. Kim MS, Lee SI, Sim JH: Gamma knife radiosurgery for functioning pituitary microadenoma. Stereotact Funct Neurosurg 72(Suppl 1): 119–124, 1999.

117. Kim SH, Huh R, Chang JW, et al: Gamma knife radiosurgery for functioning pituitary adenomas. Stereotact Funct Neurosurg 72(Suppl 1):101–110, 1999.

118. Laws ER, Vance ML: Radiosurgery for pituitary tumors and craniopharyngiomas. Neurosurg Clin N Am 10:327–336, 1999.

119. Mokry M, Ramschak-Schwarzer S, Simbrunner J, et al: A six-year experience with the postoperative radiosurgical management of pituitary adenomas. Stereotact Funct Neurosurg 72(Suppl 1):88–100, 1999.

120. Izawa M, Hayashi M, Nakaya K, et al: Gamma knife radiosurgery for pituitary adenomas. J Neurosurg 93(Suppl 3):19–22, 2000.

121. Shin M, Kurita H, Sasaki T, et al: Stereotactic radiosurgery for pituitary adenoma invading the cavernous sinus. J Neurosurg 93(Suppl 3):2–5, 2000.

122. Zhang N, Pan L, Wang EM, et al: Radiosurgery for growth hormone-producing pituitary adenomas. J Neurosurg 93(Suppl 3):6–9, 2000.

123. Fukuoka S, Ito T, Takanashi M, et al: Gamma knife radiosurgery for growth hormone-secreting pituitary adenomas invading the cavernous sinus. Stereotact Funct Neurosurg 76(3–4):213–217, 2001.

124. Ikeda H, Jokura H, Yoshimoto T: Transsphenoidal surgery and adjuvant gamma knife treatment for growth hormone-secreting pituitary adenoma. J Neurosurg 95(2):285–291, 2001.

125. Feigl GC, Bonelli CM, Berghold A, et al: Effects of gamma knife radiosurgery of pituitary adenomas on pituitary function. J Neurosurg 97(Suppl 5):415–421, 2002.

126. Pollock BE, Young WF Jr: Stereotactic radiosurgery for patients with ACTH-producing pituitary adenomas after prior adrenalectomy. Int J Radiat Oncol Biol Phys 54:839–841, 2002.

127. Attanasio R, Epaminonda P, Motti E, et al: Gamma-knife radiosurgery in acromegaly: A 4–year follow-up study. J Clin Endocrinol Metab 88(7):3105–3112, 2003.

128. Petrovich Z, Yu C, Giannotta SL, et al: Gamma knife radiosurgery for pituitary adenoma: Early results. Neurosurgery 53(1):51–59, 2003.

129. Hoybye C, Grenback E, Rahn T, et al: Adrenocortcotrophic hormone-producing pituitary tumors: 12- to 22-year follow up after treatment with stereotactic radiosurgery. Neurosurgery 49:284–292, 2001.

130. Kobayashi T, Kida Y, Mori Y: Gamma knife radiosurgery in the treatment of Cushing disease: Long-term results. J Neurosurg 97(Suppl 5):422–428, 2002.

131. Pollock BE, Nippoldt TB, Stafford SL, et al: Results of stereotactic radiosurgery in patients with hormone-producing pituitary adenomas: Factors associated with endocrine normalization. J Neurosurg 97(3):525–530, 2002.

132. Pollock BE, Carpenter PC: Stereotactic radiosurgery as an alternative to fractionated radiotherapy for patients with recurrent or residual nonfunctioning pituitary adenomas. Neurosurgery 53(5):1086–1094, 2003.

133. Pan L, Zhang N, Wang EM, et al: Gamma knife radiosurgery as a primary treatment for prolactinomas. J Neurosurg 93(Suppl 3):10–13, 2000.

134. Sheehan JP, Kondziolka D, Flickinger J, et al: Radiosurgery for residual or recurrent nonfunctioning pituitary adenoma. J Neurosurg 97(Suppl 5):408–414, 2002.

135. Wowra B, Stummer W: Efficacy of gamma knife radiosurgery for non-functioning pituitary adenomas: A quantitative follow-up with magnetic resonance imaging-based volumetric analysis. J Neurosurg 97(5 Suppl):429–432, 2002.

136. Rahn T, Thorén M, Hall K: Stereotactic radiosurgery in the treatment of MB Cushing. In INSERM Symposium. Amsterdam: Elsevier, 1979.

137. Hetelekidis S, Barnes PD, Tao ML, et al: 20–Year experience in childhood craniopharyngioma. Int J Radiat Oncol Biol Phys 27:189–195, 1993.

138. Rajan B, Ashley S, Gorman C, et al: Craniopharyngioma: Long-term results following limited surgery and radiotherapy. Radiother Oncol 26:1–10, 1993.

139. Mulhern RK, Kepner JL, Thomas PR, et al: Neuropsychologic functioning of survivors of childhood medulloblastoma randomized to receive conventional or reduced-dose craniospinal irradiation: A Pediatric Oncology Group study. J Clin Oncol 16:1723–1728, 1998.

140. Chadderton RD, West CG, Schuller S, et al: Radiotherapy in the treatment of low-grade astrocytomas. II: The physical and cognitive sequelae. Childs Nerv Syst 11:443–448, 1995.

141. Yang TF, Wong TT, Cheng LY, et al: Neuropsychological sequelae after treatment for medulloblastoma in childhood: The Taiwan experience. Childs Nerv Syst 13:77–80, 1997.

142. Ilveskoski I, Pihko H, Wiklund T, et al: Neuropsychologic late effects in children with malignant brain tumors treated with surgery, radiotherapy and "8 in 1" chemotherapy. Neuropediatrics 27:124–129, 1996.

143. Chapman CA, Waber DP, Bernstein JH, et al: Neurobehavioral and neurologic outcome in long-term survivors of posterior fossa brain tumors: Role of age and perioperative factors. J Child Neurol 10:209–212, 1995.

144. Prasad D, Steiner M, Steiner L: Gamma knife surgery for craniopharyngioma. Acta Neurochirurgica 134:167–176, 1995.

145. Coffey RJ, Lunsford LD: The role of stereotactic techniques in the management of craniopharyngiomas. Neurosurg Clin N Am 1:161–172, 1990.

146. Backlund E-O: Solid craniopharyngiomas treated by stereotactic radiosurgery. In INSERM Symposium No 12 on Stereotactic Irradiations. Paris: Elsevier, North Holland Biomedical Press, Amsterdam, 1979.

147. Barbaro NM, Gutin PH, Wilson CB, et al: Radiation therapy in the treatment of partially resected meningiomas. J Neurosurg 20:525–528, 1987.

148. Taylor BW, Marcus RBJ, Friedman WA, et al: The meningioma controversy: Postoperative radiation therapy. Int J Radiat Oncol Biol Phys 15:299–234, 1988.

149. Goldsmith BJ, Wara WM, Wilson CB, et al: Postoperative irradiation for subtotally resected meningiomas: A retrospective analysis of 140 patients treated from 1967 to 1990. J Neurosurg 80:195–201, 1994.

150. Steiner L, Lindquist C, Steiner M: Meningiomas and gamma knife radiosurgery. In Al-Mefty O (ed): Meningiomas. New York: Raven Press, 1991, pp 263–272.

151. Kondziolka D, Lundsford L, Linskey M, et al: Skull base radiosurgery. In Alexander E III, Lundsford LD (eds): Stereotactic Radiosurgery. New York: McGraw-Hill, 1993, pp 175–188.

152. Kondziolka D, Lunsford LD, Coffey RJ, et al: Stereotactic radiosurgery of meningiomas. J Neurosurg 74:552–559, 1991.

153. Liscak R, Simonova G, Vymazal J, et al: Gamma knife radiosurgery of meningiomas in the cavernous sinus region. Acta Neurochir (Wien) 141(5):473–480, 1999.

154. Roche PH, Regis J, Dufour H, et al: Gamma knife radiosurgery in the management of cavernous sinus meningiomas. J Neurosurg 93(Suppl 3):68–73, 2000.

155. Roche PH, Pellet W, Fuentes S, et al: Gamma knife radiosurgical management of petroclival meningiomas results and indications. Acta Neurochir (Wien) 145(10):883–888, 2003.

156. Flickinger JC, Kondziolka D, Maitz AH, et al: Gamma knife radiosurgery of imaging-diagnosed intracranial meningioma. Int J Radiat Oncol Biol Phys 56(3):801–806, 2003.

157. Nicolato A, Foroni R, Alessandrini F, et al: Radiosurgical treatment of cavernous sinus meningiomas: Experience with 122 treated patients. Neurosurgery 51(5):1153–1159, 2002.

158. Parkinson D: Extradural neural axis compartment. J Neurosurg 92(4):585–588, 2000.

159. Parkinson D: Lateral sellar compartment O.T. (cavernous sinus): History, anatomy, terminology. Anat Rec 251(4):486–490, 1998.

160. Lee JY, Niranjan A, McInerney J, et al: Stereotactic radiosurgery providing long-term tumor control of cavernous sinus meningiomas. J Neurosurg 97(1):65–72, 2002.

161. Henshen F: Über Geschwülste der hinteren Schädelgrube insbesondere des Kleinhirnbrückenwinkels, in Pathologisch-anatomischen. Stockholm: Karolinishen Institut, 1910, p 283.

162. Leksell L: A note on the treatment of acoustic tumours. Acta Chir Scand 136:763–765, 1971.

163. Wallner K, Sheline GE, Pitts LH, et al: Efficacy of irradiation for incompletely excised acoustic neurilemomas. J Neurosurg 67:858–863, 1987.

164. Prasad D, Steiner M, Steiner L: Gamma surgery for vestibular schwannoma. J Neurosurg 92(5):745–759, 2000.

165. Flickinger JC, Lunsford LD, Linskey ME, et al: Gamma knife radiosurgery for acoustic tumors: Multivariate analysis of four year results. Radiother Oncol 27:91–98, 1993.

166. Iwai Y, Yamanaka K, Shiotani M, et al: Radiosurgery for acoustic neuromas: Results of low-dose treatment. Neurosurgery 53(2):282–287, 2003.

167. Bertalanffy A, Dietrich W, Aichholzer M, et al: Gamma knife radiosurgery of acoustic neurinomas. Acta Neurochir (Wien) 143(7):689–695, 2001.

168. Flickinger JC, Kondziolka D, Niranjan A, et al: Results of acoustic neuroma radiosurgery: An analysis of 5 years' experience using current methods. J Neurosurg 94(1):1–6, 2001.

169. Kwon Y, Kim JH, Lee DJ, et al: Gamma knife treatment of acoustic neurinoma. Stereotact Funct Neurosurg 70(Suppl 1):57–64, 1998.

170. Coffey RJ, Swanson JW, Harner SG, et al: Stereotactic radiosurgery using the gamma knife for acoustic neuromas. Int J Radiat Oncol Biol Phys 32(4):1153–1160, 1995.

171. Szeifert GT, Prasad D, Kamiryo T, et al: The role of the gamma knife in the therapy of intracranial astrocytomas. In 2nd Annual Meeting of the Japanese Society for Brain Tumor Surgery, Nagasaki, Japan, 1997.

172. Pozza F, Colombo F, Chierego G, et al: Low-grade astrocytomas: Treatment with unconventionally fractionated external beam stereotactic radiation therapy. Radiology 171:565–569, 1989.

173. Gutin PH, Wilson CB: Radiosurgery for malignant brain tumors. J Clin Oncol 8:571–573, 1990.

174. Loeffler JS, Alexander ED, Shea WM, et al: Radiosurgery as part of the initial management of patients with malignant gliomas. J Clin Oncol 10:1379–1385, 1992.

175. Larson DA, Prados M, Lamborn KR, et al: Phase II study of high central dose gamma knife radiosurgery and marimastat in patients with recurrent malignant glioma. Int J Radiat Oncol Biol Phys 54(5):1397–1404, 2002.

176. Nwokedi EC, DiBiase SJ, Jabbour S, et al: Gamma knife stereotactic radiosurgery for patients with glioblastoma multiforme. Neurosurgery 50(1):41–46, 2002.

177. Suit HD, Goitein M, Munzenrider J, et al: Increased efficacy of radiation therapy by use of proton beam. Strahlenther Onkol 166:40-44, 1990.

178. Austin-Seymour M, Munzenrider J, Goitein M, et al: Fractionated proton radiation therapy of chordoma and low-grade chondrosarcoma of the base of the skull. J Neurosurg 70:13–17, 1989.

179. Latz D, Gademann G, Hawighorst H, et al: The initial results in the fractionated 3-dimensional stereotactic irradiation of clivus chordomas. Strahlenther Onkol 171:348–355, 1995.

180. Muthukumar N, Kondziolka D, Lunsford LD, et al: Stereotactic radiosurgery for chordoma and chondrosarcoma: Further experiences. Int J Radiat Oncol Biol Phys 41:387–392, 1998.

181. Davey P, O'Brien P: Disposition of cerebral metastases from malignant melanoma: Implications for radiosurgery. Neurosurgery 28:8–14, 1991.

182. Coffey RJ, Lunsford LD: Stereotactic radiosurgery using the 201 cobalt-60 source gamma knife. Neurosurg Clin N Am 1:933–954, 1990.

183. Coffey RJ, Flickinger JC, Bissonette DJ, et al: Radiosurgery for solitary brain metastases using the cobalt-60 gamma unit: Methods and results in 24 patients. Int J Radiat Oncol Biol Phys 20:1287–1295, 1991.

184. Flickinger JC, Kondziolka D, Lunsford LD, et al: A multi-institutional experience with stereotactic radiosurgery for solitary brain metastasis. Int J Radiat Oncol Biol Phys 28:797–802, 1994.

185. Kihlstrom L, Karlsson B, Lindquist C: Gamma knife surgery for cerebral metastases: Implications for survival based on 16 years experience. Stereotact Funct Neurosurg 61:45–50, 1993.

186. Gerosa M, Nicolato A, Foroni R, et al: Gamma knife radiosurgery for brain metastases: A primary therapeutic option. J Neurosurg 97 (5 Suppl):515–524, 2002.

187. Mingione V, Oliveira M, Prasad D, et al: Gamma surgery for melanoma metastases in the brain. J Neurosurg 96(3):544–551, 2002.

188. Somaza S, Kondziolka D, Lunsford LD, et al: Stereotactic radiosurgery for cerebral metastatic melanoma. J Neurosurg 79(5):661–666, 1993.

189. Mori Y, Kondziolka D, Flickinger JC, et al: Stereotactic radiosurgery for cerebral metastatic melanoma: Factors affecting local disease control and survival. Int J Radiat Oncol Biol Phys 42(3):581–589, 1998.

190. Amendola BE, Wolf AL, Coy SR, et al: Brain metastases in renal cell carcinoma: Management with gamma knife radiosurgery. Cancer J 6(6):372–376, 2000.

191. Lavine SD, Petrovich Z, Cohen-Gadol AA, et al: Gamma knife radiosurgery for metastatic melanoma: An analysis of survival, outcome, and complications. Neurosurgery 44(1):59–64, 1999.

192. Mori Y, Kondziolka D, Flickinger JC, et al: Stereotactic radiosurgery for brain metastasis from renal cell carcinoma. Cancer 83(2):344–353, 1998.

193. Hoshi S, Jokura H, Nakamura H, et al: Gamma knife radiosurgery for brain metastasis of renal cell carcinoma: Results in 42 patients. Int J Urol 9(11):618–625, 2002.

194. Sheehan JP, Sun MH, Kondziolka D, et al: Radiosurgery in patients with renal cell carcinoma metastasis to the brain: Long-term outcomes and prognostic factors influencing survival and local tumor control. J Neurosurg 98(2):342–349, 2003.

195. Williams J, Enger C, Wharam M, et al: Stereotactic radiosurgery for brain metastases: Comparison of lung carcinoma vs. non-lung tumors. J Neurooncol 37(1):79–85, 1998.

196. Sheehan JP, Sun MH, Kondziolka D, et al: Radiosurgery for non-small cell lung carcinoma metastatic to the brain: Long-term outcomes and prognostic factors influencing patient survival time and local tumor control. J Neurosurg 97(6):1276–1281, 2002.

197. Serizawa T, Ono J, Iichi T, et al: Gamma knife radiosurgery for metastatic brain tumors from lung cancer: A comparison between small cell and non-small cell carcinoma. J Neurosurg 97(5 Suppl): 484–488, 2002.

198. Firlik KS, Kondziolka D, Flickinger JC, et al: Stereotactic radiosurgery for brain metastases from breast cancer. Ann Surg Oncol 7(5): 333–338, 2000.

199. Amendola BE, Wolf AL, Coy SR, et al: Gamma knife radiosurgery in the treatment of patients with single and multiple brain metastases from carcinoma of the breast. Cancer J 6(2):88–92, 2000.

200. Muacevic A, Kreth FW, Horstmann GA, et al: Surgery and radiotherapy compared with gamma knife radiosurgery in the treatment of solitary cerebral metastases of small diameter. J Neurosurg 91(1):35–43, 1999.

201. Sneed PK, Suh JH, Goetsch SJ, et al: A multi-institutional review of radiosurgery alone vs. radiosurgery with whole brain radiotherapy as the initial management of brain metastases. Int J Radiat Oncol Biol Phys 53(3):519–526, 2002.

202. Payne BR, Prasad D, Szeifert G, et al: Gamma surgery for intracranial metastases from renal cell carcinoma. J Neurosurg 92(5):760–765, 2000.

203. Wronski M, Maor MH, Davis BJ, et al: External radiation of brain metastases from renal carcinoma: A retrospective study of 119 patients from the M.D. Anderson Cancer Center. Int J Radiat Oncol Biol Phys 37(4):753–759, 1997.

204. Seung SK, Sneed PK, McDermott MW, et al: Gamma knife radiosurgery for malignant melanoma brain metastases. Cancer J Sci Am 4:103–109, 1998.

205. Shiau CY, Sneed PK, Shu HK, et al: Radiosurgery for brain metastases: Relationship of dose and pattern of enhancement to local control. Int J Radiat Oncol Biol Phys 37:375–383, 1997.

206. Niemela M, Young J, Jääskeläinen J, et al: Gamma knife radiosurgery in 11 haemangioblastomas. In 7th International Meeting of the Leksell Gamma Knife Society. Lanai, Hawaii, 1995.

207. Payne BR, Prasad D, Steiner M, et al: Gamma surgery for hemangiopericytomas. Acta Neurochir (Wien) 142(5):527–536, 2000.

208. Sheehan J, Kondziolka D, Flickinger J, et al: Radiosurgery for treatment of recurrent intracranial hemangiopericytomas. Neurosurgery 51(4):905–910, 2002.

209. Marchini G, Gerosa M, Piovan E, et al: gamma knife stereotactic radiosurgery for uveal melanoma: Clinical results after 2 years. Stereotact Funct Neurosurg 66:208–213, 1996.

210. Rennie I, Forster D, Kemeny A, et al: The use of single fraction Leksell stereotactic radiosurgery in the treatment of uveal melanoma. Acta Ophthal Scand 74:558–562, 1996.

211. Langmann G, Pendl G, Klaus-Mullner, et al: Gamma knife radiosurgery for uveal melanomas: An 8-year experience. J Neurosurg 93(Suppl 3):184–188, 2000.

212. Mueller AJ, Talies S, Schaller UC, et al: Stereotactic radiosurgery of large uveal melanomas with the gamma knife. Ophthalmology 107(7):1381–1387, 2000.

213. Marchini G, Gerosa M, Piovan E, et al: Gamma knife stereotactic radiosurgery for uveal melanoma: Clinical results after 2 years. Stereotact Funct Neurosurg 66(Suppl 1):208–213, 1996.

214. Chinela A, Zambrano A, Bunge H, et al: Gamma knife surgery in uveal melanomas. In Steiner L (ed): Radiosurgery Baselines and Trends. New York: Raven Press, 1992, pp 161–169.

215. Zehetmayer M, Menapace R, Kitz K, et al: Suction attachment for stereotactic radiosurgery of intraocular malignancies. Ophthalmologica 208:119–121, 1994.

216. Langmann G, Pendl G, Mullner K, et al: High-compared with low-dose radiosurgery for uveal melanomas. J Neurosurg 97(5 Suppl): 640-643, 2002.

217. Simonova G, Novotny J Jr, Liscak R, et al: Leksell gamma knife treatment of uveal melanoma. J Neurosurg 97(Suppl 5):635–639, 2002.

218. Young RF: Functional neurosurgery with the Leksell gamma knife. Stereotact Funct Neurosurg 66:19–23, 1996.

219. Hayashi M, Taira T, Chernov M, et al: Role of pituitary radiosurgery for the management of intractable pain and potential future applications. Stereotact Funct Neurosurg 81(1–4):75–83, 2003.

220. Young RF, Jacques DS, Rand RW, et al: Technique of stereotactic medial thalamotomy with the Leksell gamma knife for treatment of chronic pain. Neurol Res 17(1):59–65, 1995.

221. Young RF, Vermeulen SS, Grimm P, et al: Gamma knife thalamotomy for the treatment of persistent pain. Stereotact Funct Neurosurg 64(Suppl 1):172–181, 1995.

222. Young RF, Jacques DS, Rand RW, et al: Medial thalamotomy with the Leksell gamma knife for treatment of chronic pain. Acta Neurochir Suppl (Wien) 62:105–110, 1994.

223. Kondziolka D, Lunsford LD, Flickinger JC, et al: Stereotactic radiosurgery for trigeminal neuralgia: A multiinstitutional study using the gamma unit. J Neurosurg 84:940-945, 1996.

224. Regis J, Metellus P, Dufour H, et al: Long-term outcome after gamma knife surgery for secondary trigeminal neuralgia. J Neurosurg 95(2):199–205, 2001.

225. Kondziolka D, Lunsford LD, Flickinger JC: Stereotactic radiosurgery for the treatment of trigeminal neuralgia. Clin J Pain 18(1):42–47, 2002.

226. Maesawa S, Salame C, Flickinger JC, et al: Clinical outcomes after stereotactic radiosurgery for idiopathic trigeminal neuralgia. J Neurosurg 94(1):14–20, 2001.

227. Hasegawa T, Kondziolka D, Spiro R, et al: Repeat radiosurgery for refractory trigeminal neuralgia. Neurosurgery 50(3):494–500, 2002.

228. Rogers CL, Shetter AG, Fiedler JA, et al: Gamma knife radiosurgery for trigeminal neuralgia: The initial experience of The Barrow Neurological Institute. Int J Radiat Oncol Biol Phys 47(4):1013–1019, 2000.

229. Ford RG, Ford KT, Swaid S, et al: Gamma knife treatment of refractory cluster headache. Headache 38:3–9, 1998.

230. Leksell L, Lindquist C, Adler JR, et al: A new fixation device for the Leksell stereotaxic system: Technical note. J Neurosurg 66:626–629, 1987.

231. Lindquist C, Steiner L, Hindmarsh T: Gamma knife thalamotomy for tremor: Report of two cases. In Steiner L, Lindquist C, Forster D, Backlund E-O (eds): Radiosurgery Baseline and Trends. New York: Raven Press, 1992, pp 237–243.

232. Lindquist C, Kihlstrom L, Hellstrand E: Functional neurosurgery: A future for the gamma knife? Stereotact Funct Neurosurg 57:72–81, 1991.

233. Lim JY, De Salles AA, Bronstein J, et al: Delayed internal capsule infarctions following radiofrequency pallidotomy: Report of three cases. J Neurosurg 87:955–960, 1997.

234. Hirai T, Ohye C, Yoshishige N, et al: Cytometric analysis of the thalamic ventralis intermedius nucleus in humans. J Neurophysiol 61(3):478–487, 1989.

235. Ohye C, Shibazaki T, Hirai T, et al: Further physiological observations on the ventralis intermedius neurons in the human thalamus. J Neurophysiol 61(3):488–500, 1989.

236. Hirai T, Miyazaki M, Nakajima H, et al: The correlation between tremor characteristics and the predicted volume of effective lesions in stereotaxic nucleus ventralis intermedius thalamotomy. Brain 106:1001–1018, 1983.

237. Hirai T, Jones EG: A new parcellation of the human thalamus on the basis of histochemical staining. Brain Research Reviews 14:1–34, 1989.

238. Hirai T, Schwark HD, Yen CT, et al: Morphology of physiologically characterized medial lemniscal axons terminating in cat ventral posterior thalamic nucleus. J Neurophysiol 60(4):1439–1459, 1988.

239. Hirai T, Jones EG: Segregation of leminiscal inputs and motor cortex outputs in cat ventral thalamic nuclei: Application of a novel technique. Exp Brain Res 71:329–344, 1988.

240. Duma CM, Jacques DB, Kopyov OV, et al: Gamma knife radiosurgery for thalamotomy in parkinsonian tremor: A five-year experience. J Neurosurg 88:1044–1049, 1998.

241. Young RF, Vermeulen SS, Grimm P, et al: Electrophysiological target localization is not required for the treatment of functional disorders. Stereotact Funct Neurosurg 66:309–319, 1996.

242. Ohye C, Shibazaki T, Hirato M, et al: Gamma thalamotomy for parkinsonian and other kinds of tremor. Stereotact Funct Neurosurg 66:333–342, 1996.

243. Ohye C, Shibazaki T, Zhang J, et al: Thalamic lesions produced by gamma thalamotomy for movement disorders. J Neurosurg 97(Suppl 5):600–606, 2002.

244. Ohye C, Shibazaki T, Ishihara J, et al: Evaluation of gamma thalamotomy for parkinsonian and other tremors: Survival of neurons adjacent to the thalamic lesion after gamma thalamotomy. J Neurosurg 93(Suppl 3):120–127, 2000.

245. Niranjan A, Jawahar A, Kondziolka D, et al: A comparison of surgical approaches for the management of tremor: Radiofrequency thalamotomy, gamma knife thalamotomy and thalamic stimulation. Stereotact Funct Neurosurg 72(2–4):178–184, 1999.

246. Young RF, Jacques S, Mark R, et al: Gamma knife thalamotomy for treatment of tremor: Long-term results. J Neurosurg 93(Suppl 3):128–135, 2000.

247. Keep MF, Mastrofrancesco L, Erdman D, et al: Gamma knife subthalamotomy for Parkinson disease: The subthalamic nucleus as a new radiosurgical target: Case report. J Neurosurg 97(Suppl 5):592–599, 2002.

248. Tasker RR: Deep brain stimulation is preferable to thalamotomy for tremor suppression. Surg Neurol 49:145–153, 1998.

249. Duff J, Sime E: Surgical interventions in the treatment of Parkinson's disease (PD) and essential tremor (ET): Medial pallidotomy in PD and chronic deep brain stimulation (DBS) in PD and ET. Axone 18:85–89, 1997.

250. Eskandar EN, Flaherty A, Cosgrove GR, et al: Surgery for Parkinson disease in the United States, 1996 to 2000: Practice patterns, short-term outcomes, and hospital charges in a nationwide sample. J Neurosurg 99(5):863–871, 2003.

251. Umemura A, Jaggi JL, Hurtig HI, et al: Deep brain stimulation for movement disorders: Morbidity and mortality in 109 patients. J Neurosurg 98(4):779–784, 2003.

252. Kondziolka D, Whiting D, Germanwala A, et al: Hardware-related complications after placement of thalamic deep brain stimulator systems. Stereotact Funct Neurosurg 79(3–4):228–233, 2002.

253. Beric A, Kelly PJ, Rezai A, et al: Complications of deep brain stimulation surgery. Stereotact Funct Neurosurg 77(1–4):73–78, 2001.

254. Bingley T, Leksell L, Meyerson BA, et al: Long-term results of stereotactic anterior capsulotomy in chronic obsessive-compulsive neurosis. In Sweet WH, et al (eds): Neurosurgical Treatment in Psychiatry, Pain, and Epilepsy. Baltimore: University Park Press, 1977, pp 287–299.

255. Mindus P: Capsulotomy in anxiety disorders: A multidisciplinary study (PhD Thesis). Stockholm: Karolinska Institute, 1991.

256. Lippitz BE, Mindus P, Meyerson BA, et al: Lesion topography and outcome after thermocapsulotomy or gamma knife capsulotomy for obsessive-compulsive disorder: Relevance of the right hemisphere. Neurosurgery 44(3):452–458, 1999.

257. Greenberg BD, Price LH, Rauch SL, et al: Neurosurgery for intractable obsessive-compulsive disorder and depression: Critical issues. Neurosurg Clin N Am 14(2):199–212, 2003.

258. Elomaa E: Focal irradiation of the brain: An alternative to temporal lobe resection in intractable focal epilepsy? Med Hypotheses 6:501–503, 1980.

259. Barcia Salorio JL, Roldan P, Hernandez G, et al: Radiosurgical treatment of epilepsy. Appl Neurophysiol 48:400–403, 1985.

260. Rossi GF, Scerrati M, Roselli R: Epileptogenic cerebral low-grade tumors: Effect of interstitial stereotactic irradiation on seizures. Appl Neurophysiol 48:127–132, 1985.

261. Chen ZF, Kamiryo T, Henson SL, et al: Anticonvulsant effects of gamma surgery in a model of chronic spontaneous limbic epilepsy in rats. J Neurosurg 94(2):270–280, 2001.

262. Maesawa S, Kondziolka D, Dixon CE, et al: Subnecrotic stereotactic radiosurgery controlling epilepsy produced by kainic acid injection in rats. J Neurosurg 93(6):1033–1040, 2000.

263. Mori Y, Kondziolka D, Balzer J, et al: Effects of stereotactic radiosurgery on an animal model of hippocampal epilepsy. Neurosurgery 46(1):157–165, 2000.

264. Regis J, Kerkerian-Legoff L, Rey M, et al: First biochemical evidence of differential functional effects following gamma knife surgery. Stereotact Funct Neurosurg 66:29–38, 1996.

265. Warnke PC, Berlis A, Weyerbrock A, Ostertag CB: Significant reduction of seizure incidence and increase of benzodiazepine receptor density after interstitial radiosurgery in low-grade gliomas. Acta Neurochir Suppl 68:90–92, 1997.

266. Barcia-Salorio JL, Barcia JA, Hernandez G, et al: Radiosurgery of epilepsy. Long-term results. Acta Neurochir Suppl (Wien) 62:111–113, 1994.

267. Regis J, Peragui JC, Rey M, et al: First selective amygdalohippocampal radiosurgery for mesial temporal lobe epilepsy. Stereotact Funct Neurosurg 64:193–201, 1995.

268. Regis J, Bartolomei F, Rey M, et al: Gamma knife surgery for mesial temporal lobe epilepsy. J Neurosurg 93(Suppl 3):141–146, 2000.

269. Regis J, Rey M, Bartolomei F, et al: Gamma knife surgery in mesial temporal lobe epilepsy: A prospective multicenter study. Epilepsia 45(5):504–515, 2004.

270. Regis J, Bartolomei F, Hayashi M, et al: What role for radiosurgery in mesial temporal lobe epilepsy? Zentralbl Neurochir 63(3):101–105, 2002.

271. Regis J, Bartolomei F, Hayashi M, et al: Gamma knife surgery, a neuromodulation therapy in epilepsy surgery. Acta Neurochir Suppl 84:37–47, 2002.

272. Sutcliffe JC, Forster DM, Walton L, et al: Untoward clinical effects after stereotactic radiosurgery for intracranial arteriovenous malformations. British J Neurosurg 6:177–185, 1992.

273. Kondziolka D, Lundsford L, Flickinger J: Gamma knife stereotactic radiosurgery for cerebral vascular malformations. In Alexander E III, Lundsford LD (eds): Stereotactic Radiosurgery. New York: McGraw-Hill, 1993, pp 136–146.

274. Chang JH, Chang JW, Park YG, et al: Factors related to complete occlusion of arteriovenous malformations after gamma knife radiosurgery. J Neurosurg 93(Suppl 3):96–101, 2000.

275. Karlsson B, Lindquist C, Steiner L: Prediction of obliteration after gamma knife surgery for cerebral arteriovenous malformations. Neurosurgery 40(3):425–430, 1997.

276. Flickinger JC, Pollock BE, Kondziolka D, et al: A dose-response analysis of arteriovenous malformation obliteration after radiosurgery. Int J Radiat Oncol Biol Phys 36(4):873–879, 1996.

41

CT/MRI-Based Computer-Assisted Volumetric Stereotactic Resection of Intracranial Lesions

ROGER LICHTENBAUM, HOWARD L. WEINER, and
PATRICK J. KELLY

Before the era of modern neuroimaging, neurosurgical approaches for resection or biopsy of intra-axial brain tumors typically employed large craniotomy flaps, which would be of sufficient size so as to ensure adequate exposure of the lesion in question. Such openings were often imprecise and frequently led to the exposure and potential damage of normal structures. Tumor stereotaxis developed partially as a result of modern neuroradiographic techniques, which provided very precise anatomic localization of the location and volumetric extent of such neoplasms. Furthermore, the explosion of modern computer technology over the past 20 years facilitated the transfer of this information into a database that could be used not only for surgical planning but also for the execution of the actual surgical procedure. As a result, operative procedures could be more precise, minimizing potential morbidity, duration of hospital stay, and, ultimately, cost. Minimally invasive computer-assisted stereotactic tumor surgery, therefore, developed as a method of precise image-guided intracranial navigation for the safe removal of intra-axial brain tumors. It became a technique for gathering, storing, and reformatting image-derived 3-dimensional volumetric information that defined a lesion with respect to the surgical field. It enabled the neurosurgeon to plan and simulate the operative procedure ahead of time (the "virtual" craniotomy) such that the safest and least invasive approach could be used. Moreover, this technology allowed the surgeon to visualize exactly the border between the tumor and the surrounding brain. The necessity for stereotactic volumetric approaches became even more critical with the advent of truly minimally invasive "keyhole" approaches, in which surgeons could no longer rely on visualized intracranial landmarks. The advantages of this technology to the surgeon, the patient, and third-party payers became apparent.

With the original advent of computed tomography (CT) scanning, many neurosurgeons began to rethink classic approaches to common intracranial tumors.[1–4] Compared with projection radiography and ventriculography, which were used in functional stereotactic procedures, CT was a natural data source for tumor stereotaxis. It provided a precise 3-dimensional database that could easily be incorporated into a stereotactic coordinate system. In addition, for the first time surgeons could actually see the intracranial tumor target volume directly. Magnetic resonance imaging (MRI) also became a most valuable addition to the stereotactic preoperative database.

CT-based, and later MRI-based, point-in-space stereotactic biopsy procedures for the diagnosis of intracranial tumors became commonplace.[1,5–7] In addition, point stereotaxis could also be used to drain a tumor cyst, to place multiple radionuclide catheters within a CT-/MRI-defined tumor, and to center a craniotomy precisely over a superficial lesion or to locate a deep one. However, point-in-space stereotactic techniques could not be used to identify tumor margins, which were clearly visible on the imaging studies. The volumetric stereotactic method, in which a tumor volume is represented in stereotactic space by computer reconstruction of planar tumor boundaries defined by stereotactic CT and MRI, was developed to facilitate the intraoperative identification of CT- and MRI-defined tumor borders and to maintain a surgeon's 3-dimensional orientation during the resection of an irregularly shaped neoplasm.[8–10]

We began performing CT-/MRI-based stereotactic volumetric resections of deep-seated intracranial lesions in January 1980.[4] This procedure has been very useful in the resection of superficial and deep-seated intra-axial lesions. As clinical experience was developed, technical innovations increased the facility and accuracy with which these operations were performed. In particular, the operating room computer system and appropriate software replaced cumbersome manual methods used in the early procedures. The computer was used for the transposition of volumetric information derived from axial stereotactic CT scans and MR images into 3-dimensional space and to monitor and display the position of stereotactically directed instruments in relation to computer-generated reconstructions of the tumor volume. In this chapter, we discuss the state-of-the-art aspects of this approach as well as newer developments made possible by the recent revolution in imaging and computer technology.

INSTRUMENTATION

Stereotactic Frame

Although other stereotactic frames could be modified for volumetric stereotactic procedures, the COMPASS stereotactic system (COMPASS International, Rochester, MN) was designed specifically for volumetric tumor stereotaxis. It evolved from modifications made to a standard Todd-Wells stereotactic frame. These modifications were then incorporated into an intermediate system (the so-called Kelly-Goerss frame), which, after some clinical experience, was further modified into the COMPASS system.[11] In addition, basic software for data acquisition, surgical planning, and interactive surgery evolved over an 8-year period and was rewritten for functionality on evolutionary computer and image-processing platforms. The sole purpose of the computer hardware and software was to render volumetric stereotactic procedures more convenient and time efficient.

The contemporary version of the COMPASS stereotactic frame consists of a fixed arc-quadrant 3-dimensional slide and removable headholder (Fig. 41-1). It can be fixed onto a semipermanent base unit or mounted onto the lateral support rails of a standard operating table. In addition, data acquisition hardware (localization systems for CT, MRI, and digital subtraction angiography) and computer support hardware and software are also considered to be part of the system.

Headholder

The headholder (Fig. 41-2) consists of a round base ring, four vertical supports, and a skull fixation system. The headholder attaches to the patient's skull by means of flanged carbon fiber pins that are inserted into four holes drilled in the outer table of the patient's skull into the diploë.

Detachable micrometers are used to measure the distance between the end of the carbon fiber pins and the outer face of the vertical supports. These measurements and the fact that the pins are replaced in previously drilled holes in the skull provide a method for accurate replacement of the stereotactic headholder. Thus, data acquisition and surgery do not need to be performed on the same day, and additional procedures can be performed later using the same database.

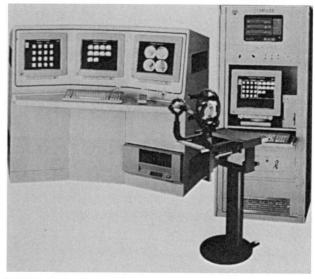

FIGURE 41-1 Modern COMPASS stereotactic system includes a three-screen workstation console (*left*), electronic control panel with digital readout for stereotactic coordinates (*right*), and an arc-quadrant stereotactic frame with cartesian robotic slide mechanism and optical encoder position sensors.

Arc-Quadrant

The 160-mm radius arc-quadrant attaches to horizontal arms that extend from the base plate of the 3-dimensional slide. Probes and retractors are directed by an attachment on the upper face of the arc. The arc-quadrant provides two angular degrees of freedom for approach trajectories: a collar angle (from the horizontal plane) and an arc angle (from the vertical plane).

3-Dimensional Positioning Slide

The headholder fits into a support yoke of a 3-dimensional slide that moves the patient's head within the fixed arc-quadrant (Fig. 41-3). Each axis of the 3-dimensional slide is moved by worm gear and a computer-controlled stepper motor that is activated at a remote control console located

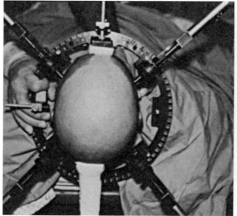
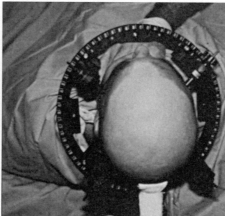

FIGURE 41-2 The COMPASS stereotactic head frame with (*left*) and without (*right*) attached micrometers. Note the indexing marks on the base ring of the headholder. The headholder fixes to the patient's skull by means of four fixed-length flanged carbon fiber pins that insert into twist drill holes made in the outer table of the skull. Micrometers measure the extension of the carbon fiber pin beyond the plane of the vertical support and provide a mechanism for precise frame reapplication.

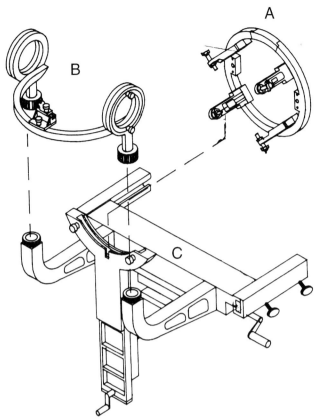

FIGURE 41-3 This schematic of a simplified COMPASS stereotactic frame demonstrates the circular headholder (A), the 160-mm radius arc-quadrant (B), and the slide mechanism containing three axes (C), which attaches to a semipermanent floor stand or to a standard operating room table. Hand cranks, which provide mechanical backups to three-axis computer-controlled stepper motors, are shown.

outside the surgical field. Hand cranks are provided on each of the three axes for manual backup.

Stereotactic coordinates on the slide are detected by optical encoders on the x, y, and z axes that transmit the coordinates to digital readout scales and to the computer. In addition, vernier scales on each axis for direct reading of stereotactic coordinates are provided as a backup to the optical encoders.

Computer System

The computer, although not absolutely necessary, saves a great deal of time when calculating target points, interpolating imaging-defined tumor volumes, cross-registering points and volumes between CT, MR images, and digital angiography (DA) and in real-time interactive image displays during the surgical procedure. The computer makes volumetric stereotactic procedures practical and time efficient.

Hardware

The COMPASS stereotactic frame is supported by a SUN SPARC 10 (SUN Microsystems, Mountainview, CA) with three X terminal display monitors mounted in a custom-designed ergometrically efficient workstation-style console (COMPASS International, Rochester, MN).

Software

Data acquisition, surgical planning, and interactive display software run by mouse/cursor and menu interactive devices and voice recognition systems allows user-friendly interaction with the operating room computer system before and during surgery. Stereotactic tumor resections are possible using manual methods for calculation of stereotactic coordinates and cross-correlation of target points between the different imaging modalities.

Laser

The carbon dioxide (CO_2) laser has been found to have very limited application in the resection of superficial lesions but has several advantages in the stereotactic resection of deep tumors. First, the laser is convenient for removing tissue from a deep cavity and is relatively hemostatic. Second, the laser removes tissue by means of a narrow beam of light; thus, one less instrument that must be inserted into a narrow surgical field. At present, a Sharplan 1100 CO_2 Laser System (Medical Industries, Tel Aviv, Israel) is used in stereotactic resections.

Stereotactic Retractors

An arc-mounted stereotactic retractor system comprises cylindrical retractors, dilators, and an arc-quadrant adapter. The retractor is a thin-walled hollow cylinder that is 140 mm in length and 2 cm in diameter. The retractor cylinder is directed toward the focal point of the stereotactic arc-quadrant. Dilators that fit inside the retractor cylinder are 1 cm longer than the retractor. The distal end of the dilator is wedge shaped and spreads an incision to the diameter of the retractor so that the retractor cylinder can be advanced. The retractor is used not only to maintain exposure but also to provide a fixed stereotactic reference structure within the stereotactic surgical field.

Accessory Instruments

Extra-long bipolar forceps with a shaft length of 150 mm are required to control bleeding in the surgical field when working through the stereotactic retractors. In addition, 150- to 160-mm long suction tips, dissectors, and alligator scissors are also used.

Heads-up Display for the Operating Microscope

In a specially designed heads-up display unit (similar to that used in jet fighter aircraft), the image output of a small video monitor mounted on the operating microscope is optically superimposed on the surgical field viewed through the microscope. The computer-generated image displayed on the video monitor is scaled by a system of lenses to the desired size. Thus the surgeon sees the actual surgical field with the computer-generated rendition of that field based on CT and MRI, which are superimposed.

MATERIALS AND METHODS

Computer-assisted volumetric stereotactic resections are performed in three phases: (1) database acquisition, (2) treatment planning, and (3) interactive procedure.

Data Acquisition

A CT-/MRI-compatible stereotactic head frame is placed on the patient's head and secured by carbon fiber pins inserted into 18-inch twist drill holes through the outer table of the skull into the diploë. For frame replacement, detachable micrometers are used to measure the carbon fiber fixation pins with respect to the fixed vertical support elements of the headholder. This provides a mechanism for accurately replacing the frame for subsequent data acquisition or surgical procedures.

After frame application, the stereotactic CT scan, MRI scan, and angiographic examinations as shown in Figure 41-4 follow.

A CT table adaptation plate receives the stereotactic headholder CT localization system, which consists of nine carbon fiber localization rods that are arranged in the shape of the letter N on either side of the head and anteriorly to create nine reference marks on each CT slice. Stereotactic CT scanning is done on a General Electric 9800 CT scanning unit, which gathers 5-mm slices through the lesion and uses a medium body format. In some patients, a stereotactic MRI examination is also done.

The MRI localization system consists of capillary tubes filled with copper sulfate solution, which also create nine reference marks on each MR image.

Digital substraction angiography is used for the localization of important blood volumes that must be preserved in the surgical approach and tumor resection. An adaptation plate receives the stereotactic headholder on the General Electric DF 5000 DA unit. The localization system consists of four Lucite plates, each of which contains nine radiopaque reference marks located on either side of the

head anteriorly and posteriorly. This creates 18 reference marks on each anteroposterior and lateral DA image. The mathematical relationships between the fiducial marks and their locations on the DA images are the basis from which stereotactic coordinates for intracranial vessels can be calculated and stereotactic target points derived from CT and MRI can be displayed on angiographic images. DA is performed using a femoral catheterization technique. Angiography is carried out under the direction of New York University, Division of Interventional Neuroradiology.

Surgical Planning

After data acquisition, the archived computer data tapes from the CT, MRI, and DA examinations are entered into the operating room computer system. The nine reference marks on each CT slice and MRI scan are detected automatically by an intensity detection algorithm. This suspends the position of each slice in a 3-dimensional computer image storage matrix.

Volume Reconstruction

Volumes defined by CT contrast enhancement, CT low attenuation, and T1 and T2 signal abnormalities on MRI scans are each established in the computer matrix as follows. First, the surgeon, who is seated at the computer console, digitizes the tumor by tracing around the outline of the lesion defined by CT contrast enhancement; sometimes, the surgeon traces around that defined by CT hypodensity, by the T1- and T2-weighted signal abnormalities of the MRI scan. Then each of these digitized contours is suspended in a separate computer image matrix. Finally, a computer program interpolates intermediate slices at 1-mm intervals between the digitized contours and creates separate volumes in space by filling in each of these slices with 1-mm cubic voxels.[6]

Surgical Trajectory

The actual surgical approach (or view line) is expressed in stereotactic frame adjustments (collar angle, the angle from the horizontal plane; arc angle, the angle from the

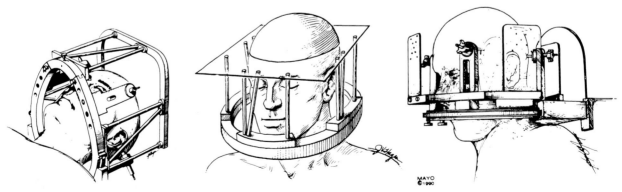

FIGURE 41-4 Stereotactic localization device for computed tomography (CT) and magnetic resonance imaging (MRI) (*left*) contains nine rods arranged in the shape of the letter N. These produce nine reference marks on each CT slice from which stereotactic coordinates are calculated (*middle*). Stereotactic digital angiography fiducial reference plates fix the base ring of the COMPASS stereotactic frame bilaterally, anteriorly, and posteriorly (*right*). These create a set of 18 reference marks for the calculation of stereotactic coordinates from angiograms and the cross-registration of CT and MRI data onto the angiographic images. (Reprinted with permission of the Mayo Clinic, © 1990.)

vertical plane) that access a selected point with the interpolated tumor volumes from an entry point on the surface of the brain. In general, the surgical approach selected takes into account the 3-dimensional shape of the lesion, important overlying cortical regions, subcortical white matter pathways, and vascular structures that must be preserved. In most cases, the stereotactic surgical approach to the lesion is selected on anteroposterior and lateral digital subtraction angiography images on which the digitized tumor volume has been displayed.

Patient Rotation

The COMPASS stereotactic headholder has indexing marks inscribed around its circumference that align to an indexing mark in the headholder receiving yoke of the 3-dimensional slide system. Thus the patient's head can be rotated to any position that will provide a comfortable working position for the surgeon. In addition, to avoid possible spatial shifts of the intracranial contents, the surgeon must rotate the patient's head in the stereotactic headholder so that the trephine opening will be at the least dependent position in the surgical field (i.e., on top). This places the proposed trephine in the most superior position within the surgical field, and the spatial integrity of the brain is maintained by the intact skull that encases it. This is similar to opening a jar of liquid. The top is directed in the least dependent position, and the liquid within the jar does not move.

To illustrate this point, the following example is provided. An approach is planned to a posterior dorsal thalamic tumor through the superior parietal lobule (Fig. 41-5). Here, a patient rotation of 180 degrees is selected with appropriate collar and arc angles (approximately 35 degrees on the collar and 0 degrees on the arc) (Fig. 41-6). The patient's body is placed in the park bench position. The head in the COMPASS stereotactic headholder is turned to 180 degrees, and the operating room table is elevated to approximately 35 degrees in a reverse Trendelenburg position.

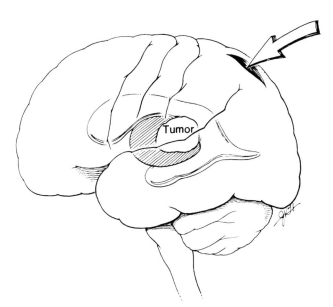

FIGURE 41-5 Dorsal thalamic tumor is approached through the superior parietal lobule and the atrial region of the lateral ventricle.

Surgical Procedures

The technical aspects of the surgical procedure depend on whether the lesion is superficial or deep. In the approach to superficial lesions, the stereotactic instrument is used to center a circular trephine of known diameter over the tumor. The relationship between the computer display of the circular trephine superimposed by the heads-up display onto the actual trephine in the surgical field and slices from the CT- or MRI-defined tumor volumes will orient the surgeon during dissection around and removal of the neoplasm with the CO_2 laser. Deep tumors are removed through a cylindrically shaped stereotactically directed retractor using a CO_2 laser.

Superficial Lesions

Procedural Aspects

The patient is anesthetized with general endotracheal anesthesia. The stereotactic head frame is replaced using the same pinholes in the skull, pin placements, and frame micrometer settings used during the data acquisition phase. The patient is then positioned in the stereotactic frame. In the COMPASS system, the patient's head in the stereotactic headholder may be rotated to any position that will provide not only a comfortable working situation for the surgeon but will also minimize brain shifts as described in the previous section. The headholder rotation angle has usually been determined during the surgical planning phase, but if this has been modified for some reason (e.g., when encountering a previously made surgical incision), the new rotation is entered into the computer program, and the computer calculates new stereotactic frame adjustments that place the center of the tumor into the focal point of the stereotactic arc-quadrant and accounts for the modified patient rotation. The head of the operating room table is raised to place the position of the intended trephine in the least dependent portion of the surgical field (usually equivalent to the collar angle).

After preparing and draping the head, the stereotactic arc-quadrant is positioned. The selected arc and collar approach angles are set on the instrument. Through an incision in the scalp, a pilot hole is drilled in the outer table of the skull by a stereotactically directed 18-inch drill. The scalp is then opened with a linear incision. A craniotomy is performed using a power trephine centered on the pilot hole. The size of the trephine selected is equal to or slightly larger than the largest cross-sectional area of the tumor as viewed from the selected surgical approach angles that were determined during the planning phase.

The computer displays the configuration of the trephine in relationship to the reformatted tumor outlines into the heads-up display unit of the operating microscope (Fig. 41-7). The surgeon then superimposes the graphic image of the trephine over the actual trephine in the surgical field using the most superficial computer-generated tumor slice as a template. A section of cortex that has the same size and configuration as a superficial computer-generated slice image is removed with bipolar forceps and scissors. We have found that cortex is nonviable when tumors extend to within 1 cm of the surface. A plane is then developed around the tumor using suction and bipolar forceps.

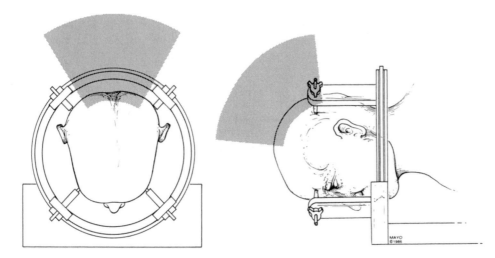

FIGURE 41-6 Patient rotation of 180 degrees is used for parasagittal approaches in which collar angles of 0 to 80 degrees and arc angles from 15 to 15 can be used (*shaded area*). A three-fourths prone body position is employed. (By permission of the Mayo Foundation.)

During tumor resection, the computer displays 1-mm thick slice configurations of the lesion at successively deeper levels in the correct spatial relationship to a circle, which represents in size and position the location of the stereotactically placed trephine within the surgical field. It is best to first isolate the lesion from surrounding brain tissue and keep the specimen intact. Computer displays of deep tumor slices along the view line provide information on the expected configuration of the tumor as it is encountered during the procedure. Measurements may be taken from the edges of the trephine opening and compared with the tumor-generated slice images. Slice depth can be determined by measuring from the level of the cranium at the edge of the trephine to the depth in the brain at which the surgeon is working. This is simply measured on the bipolar forceps with a millimeter ruler. This measurement, added to the distance from the outer surface of the probe carrier assembly on the stereotactic arc-quadrant, is subtracted from 135 mm (the distance from the outer surface of the probe carrier assembly to the focus of the arc-quadrant) and will provide

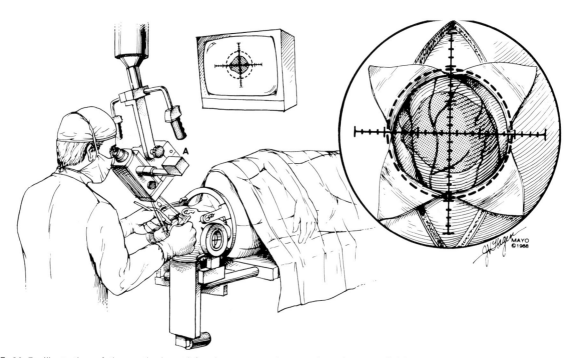

FIGURE 41-7 Illustration of the method used for the stereotactic resection of a superficial tumor. A trephine opening of the skull is performed centered on a pilot hole drilled by means of the stereotactic frame. The computer displays the position of a tumor slice in proper position with respect to the location of the trephine at a specified distance along the view line on the display monitor and into the heads-up display unit of the operating microscope (A). The image is scaled in the heads-up display, and the microscope is moved until the configuration of the trephine in the image display is exactly the same size as the actual trephine in the surgical field and aligns with the trephine. The surgeon then uses the tumor slice image as a template that will aid in identification of the surgical plane between the computed tomography– and magnetic resonance imaging–defined tumor and surrounding brain tissue. This facilitates isolation of the tumor from the surrounding brain tissue. (From Kelly PJ: Volumetric stereotactic surgical resection of intra-axial brain mass lesions. Mayo Clin Proc 63:1186–1198, 1988.)

the distance in millimeters from the plane of the surgical field to the focal point plane of the stereotactic arc-quadrant. The computer-generated tumor slice image corresponding to this plane may then be displayed. If the surgeon notes that hyperventilation, mannitol given by the anesthesiologist, or loss of subarachnoid fluid has resulted in the brain collapsing away from the dura and inner table of the skull, this amount of collapse can be measured and the depth of the slice images can be updated accordingly.

Compared with classic neurosurgical internal tumor decompressions, volumetric resection mandates that the interior of the lesion should not be entered until late in the procedure because the walls of the lesion may collapse and render subsequent computer-generated slice images no longer accurate. Employing this method, we have found that intermediate- and high-grade gliomas can be totally removed as intact specimens with negligible bleeding. In addition, infiltrated areas of brain parenchyma in low-grade gliomas located in nonessential brain tissue can also be resected in this way. In fact, we have found that the intraoperative heads-up display of the reconstructed tumor volume has enhanced the surgeon's technical ability to develop a surgical plane around a specified lesion.

DEEP TUMORS

Volumetric stereotactic resection of periventricular, basal ganglia, or thalamic tumors requires stereotactic retractors, extra-long bipolar forceps, and dissecting instruments.

The stereotactic retractors are mounted on the stereotactic arc-quadrant. The position of these retractors is also indicated on the computer display terminal in the operating room and in the heads-up display unit of the operating microscope (Fig. 41-8). The position of the cylindrical retractor is shown as a circle in the computer display in relationship to the tumor slice. During surgery, the computer-generated image of the retractor is superimposed on the actual view of the retractor in the operating microscope.

Various surgical approaches have been developed for various deep tumor locations. These approaches include transcortical, transsulcal, transsylvian, and interhemispheric exposure. The actual approach selected depends on the proximity of the tumor to deep sulci that can be split microsurgically and spread wide enough to provide adequate exposure. The approach to thalamic tumors depends on whether they are located anteriorly (and thus approached from the anterosuperior position), posterodorsally (and exposed through the lateral ventricle by way of the superior parietal lobule), or posteroventrally (and approached from posterior laterally). The issue is the preservation of normal thalamic tissue. Multiplanar MRI is invaluable in defining the anatomic relationships between a tumor and normal structures to select the best surgical approach trajectory for stereotactic craniotomy.

The stereotactic resection of deep tumors is performed under general anesthesia. The patient is placed in the stereotactic headholder and positioned in the stereotactic frame. The selected target point within the tumor volume is positioned into the focal point of the stereotactic arc-quadrant.

In cystic tumors, intraventricular tumors, or tumors near the ventricular system, the monitoring of possible movements of the tumor during the procedure may be necessary.

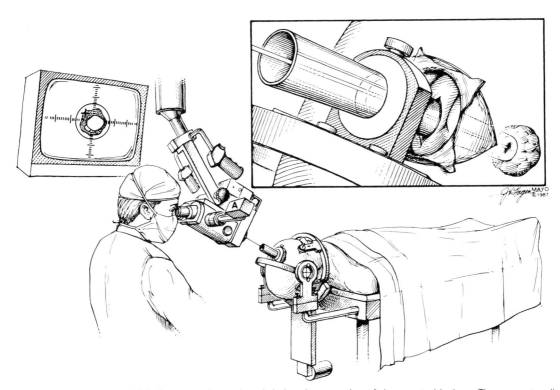

FIGURE 41-8 The stereotactic cylindrical retractor is employed during the resection of deep-seated lesions. The computer displays the configuration of a cross-section of the retractor (*circle*) with respect to a selected slice through the tumor volume cut perpendicular to the surgical view line. This information is displayed on a computer monitor in the operating room as well as in the heads-up display unit of the operating microscope (A). (From Kelly PJ: Volumetric stereotactic surgical resection of intra-axial brain mass lesions. Mayo Clin Proc 63:1186–1198, 1988.)

This is accomplished by means of a series of 0.5-mm stainless steel reference balls that are deposited at 5-mm intervals along the surgical view line in the tumor by a stereotactically directed biopsy cannula inserted through an 18-inch drill hole in the skull. Anteroposterior and lateral radiographs are obtained. The position of these steel balls on subsequent radiographs after exposure of the lesion may indicate shifts in the position of the tumor that can be adjusted in the computer software for updated accurate tumor slice images.

The scalp is opened with a linear or slightly curved incision. A 1.5-inch trephine craniotomy is performed, and a cruciate opening of the dura is accomplished. A linear incision is made in the cortex, and then the subcortical white matter incision is progressively deepened with the stereotactically directed CO_2 laser. Alternatively, a convenient sulcus can be split microsurgically, and the cortical incision can be made in the depths of this sulcus.

The direction of the subcortical incision should be through nonessential brain tissue and in a direction parallel to major white matter fibers. As the incision is deepened, the stereotactic retractor is advanced to maintain the developing exposure.

The computer has calculated the range of the tumor along the surgical view line. At the outer border of the tumor, the laser beam is deflected laterally, a dilator is placed through the retractor, and the retractor is advanced. This creates a shaft from the surface to the outer border of the tumor. Using the computer display, which demonstrates the relationship of the computer-generated tumor slice images to the edges of the retractor as a guide, the surgeon creates

a plane of dissection around the lesion with the laser or with suction and bipolar forceps. The length of the suction and bipolar forceps is 10 to 15 mm longer than the stereotactic retractor; thus, the plane between tumor and brain tissue can be developed for 10 to 15 mm beyond the end of the retractor using the computer-generated slice images as a guide, which helps the surgeon to identify and develop that plane. Once the plane has been developed entirely around the tumor to a uniform depth, tumor tissue within the retractor is then removed with 65 to 85 W of defocused laser power. In general, a tumor is removed slice by slice, extending from the most superficial slices to the deepest ones. Hemostasis is secured using the extra-long bipolar forceps.

When stainless steel reference balls have been placed (because of concern over spatial shifting of the tumor), anteroposterior and lateral teleradiographs are obtained and compared with the initial pictures to record possible movements of the reference balls. In our experience, shifting of a deep tumor occurs rarely unless it is associated with a tumor cyst that is entered early in the procedure or adherent to the walls of the lateral or third ventricle, which are opened with the loss of ventricular fluid.

Tumors that are larger than the retractor opening can be removed as follows. First, one side of the tumor is positioned under the retractor, and the surgeon creates a plane between this side of the tumor and brain tissue with the laser. The display image is then translated on the computer display terminal to position the other side of the lesion under the retractor (Fig. 41-9). The computer calculates new stereotactic frame adjustments, which are duplicated on the servomotor-driven slide mechanism of the frame

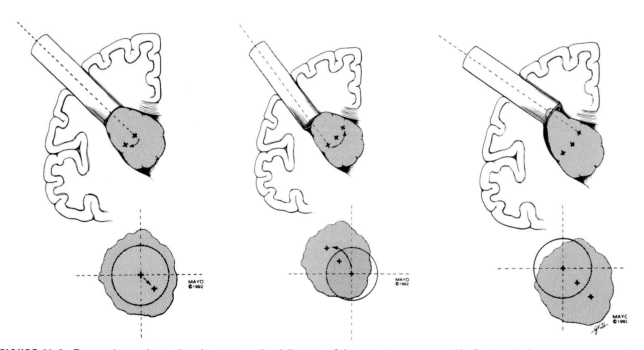

FIGURE 41-9 Tumors that are larger than the cross-sectional diameter of the retractor are removed by first translating to a new target point within the tumor volume to place a new target point beneath the retractor opening (*left*). In principle, the surgeon first isolates the tumor from surrounding brain tissue before removing it. The computer indicates the computed tomography–/magnetic resonance imaging–defined edge of the tumor with respect to the edge of the cylindrically shaped retractor (*middle*). A plane between the tumor and the surrounding brain tissue is established using the computer-generated slice images as a guide. Then another part of the tumor is translated under the retractor, and the computer image is correspondingly updated (*right*). (By permission of the Mayo Foundation.)

by remote control. This side of the tumor is then separated from brain tissue with the laser. After isolating the lesion from surrounding brain tissue, it may then be vaporized by a laser or removed by biopsy forceps and suction as previously described.

Tumors of the Posterior Parahippocampal Gyrus

We have described a novel, computer-assisted volumetric stereotactic approach for resecting tumors of the posterior parahippocampal gyrus.[12] This approach illustrates the novel ways in which volumetric stereotaxis can be exploited for removal of lesions in difficult locations. Earlier attempts to resect lesions in this location were limited by a significant risk of injury to lateral temporal lobe cortical (language, visual) and vascular (vein of Labbé) structures. To avoid these problems, we designed a lateral occipital-subtemporal trajectory, which is essentially under this region of the brain. Originally described in seven patients,[12] this technique has now been used in 40 such operations for various intra-axial neoplasms of the brain.[13] We found that it was advantageous to avoid unnecessary brain resection or retraction, thus reducing the risk of injury to lateral temporal lobe structures and helping to maintain precise spatial and anatomic orientation for the surgeon. Furthermore, like all computer-assisted volumetric approaches, we delineated the margin between the tumor and the surrounding neural tissue.[12,13]

Patient Selection for Stereotactic Resection

In general, the techniques outlined can be used to resect any intracranial tumor. However, in some regions, there is little need to employ the volumetric method; for example, in the resection of skull base lesions where one can easily find the tumor and discern its boundaries. In addition, the volumetric stereotactic technique is not appropriate for lesions located in frontal, temporal, or occipital poles because these can be managed with a standard lobectomy. For most other locations, however, the volumetric stereotactic method can be useful. However, because glial neoplasms represent the most common tumor type for which these procedures are indicated, the selection of appropriate surgical coordinates is imperative. Metastatic tumors, intraventricular lesions, vascular malformations, and many others can be performed by employing this minimally invasive surgical approach.

Spatial Types of Glial Tumors

Glial neoplasms can be classified into three types based on the growth patterns and presence or absence of tumor tissue, with or without surrounding tumor cell–infiltrated parenchyma.

Type I

Tumor tissue only with no surrounding parenchymal isolated tumor cell infiltration (Fig. 41-10). In general, type I tumors include gangliogliomas, most juvenile pilocytic astrocytomas, many xanthoastrocytomas, rare protoplasmic astrocytomas, and some oligodendrogliomas in young patients. Complete surgical resection can, in theory, cure these patients (Fig. 41-11).

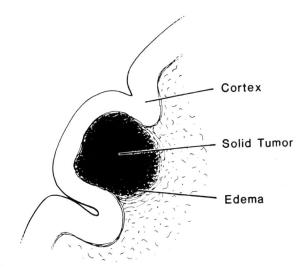

FIGURE 41-10 Type I glial neoplasm comprises solid tumor tissue only, usually presents as a contrast-enhancing mass, and can be completely resected.

Type II

Tumor tissue parenchyma is surrounded by isolated infiltrating tumor cells (Fig. 41-12). These cells are frequently high-grade gliomas. Low-grade tumors can also have a mass of tumor tissue that is hypodense within a field of infiltrated parenchyma. Surgical resection of the tumor tissue mass will benefit the patient in direct relationship to the proportion of the lesional volume that the tumor tissue proper comprises (Fig. 41-13). Resection of a small mass of tumor tissue within a large field of infiltrated parenchyma is of questionable benefit.

Type III

Parenchyma is infiltrated with isolated tumor cells only and no tumor tissue (Fig. 41-14). Type III tumors are more frequently low-grade gliomas. However, rare grade IV astrocytomas can present as type III tumors. However, these are usually hypodense or isodense on CT scanning. Resection of these lesions essentially involves resection of viable, albeit infiltrated, brain tissue.

Surgical Patient Selection in Glial Neoplasms

Precision removal by means of computer-assisted volumetric stereotaxis of the imaging-defined intracranial tumor is dependent on the ability to recognize tumor boundaries on imaging studies. The technique is not appropriate for all glial neoplasms. Patient selection for computer-assisted volumetric resection in glial neoplasms, as in all surgeries, is based on a risk:benefit ratio and the following guidelines.

Contrast-Enhanced Lesions

If the tumor volume defined by contrast enhancement on CT scanning (or gadolinium enhancement on MRI) is approximately equal to the volume defined by the T2-weighted image of the MRI (or the volume of perilesional hypodensity on a CT scan), the lesion is frequently a type I tumor. This, in most cases, can (and should) be resected. The postoperative results will be good, and the morbidity will be low.

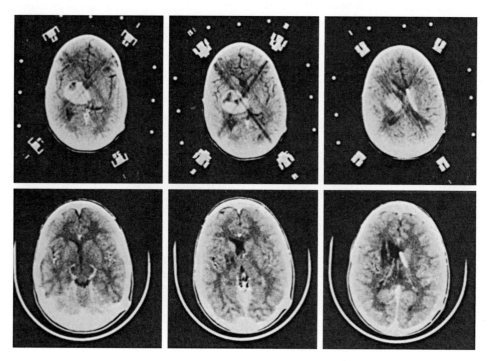

FIGURE 41-11 Preoperative (*top*) and postoperative (*bottom*) computed tomography scans of a 7-year-old girl with a pilocytic astrocytoma involving the right thalamus, internal capsule, and basal ganglia. The patient had a mild hemiparesis preoperatively that was essentially unchanged postoperatively.

However, in a type II lesion, the volume defined by gadolinium enhancement on MRI or CT contrast enhancement is less than the volume defined by T2 prolongation on MRI. An important exception can be noted in type I lesions in patients with seizures: the perilesional hypodensity or surrounding regions of T2 prolongation in these cases may represent edema and not infiltrated parenchyma. A stereotactic serial biopsy can be performed to exclude the presence of infiltrating tumor cells before consideration for definitive surgery. One study indicates that patients harboring type IV gliomas undergoing computer-assisted volumetric resection followed by radiation therapy have a better chance of survival than do those who have radiation therapy after a biopsy alone.[14] Resection provides not only internal decompression but also significant tumor cell reduction and sets the stage for more effective radiation therapy and chemotherapy.

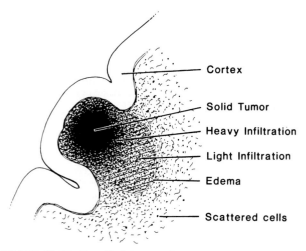

FIGURE 41-12 Type II glial tumor featuring a solid tumor tissue mass surrounded by parenchyma infiltrated by isolated tumor cells.

In nonessential brain regions, volumetric stereotactic resection of the entire volume of tumor tissue as well as infiltrated brain tissue can provide very significant cytoreduction and should theoretically prolong survival in high- and low-grade glial tumors.[15]

Nonenhancing Tumors

No imaging method can prospectively differentiate solid tumor tissue from parenchyma infiltrated by isolated tumor cells in tumors that do not exhibit contrast enhancement. In most cases, the absence of contrast enhancement usually indicates that the lesion comprises isolated tumor cells within parenchyma only. Resection of the imaging-defined lesional volume is, in fact, resection of intact and usually functional brain parenchyma, and a neurologic deficit is usually the result. Therefore, in many of these cases, stereotactic biopsy and (when appropriate) radiation therapy may represent the only surgical and therapeutic options.

In some low-grade glial tumors, tumor tissue is present and hypodense. A serial stereotactic biopsy procedure can establish whether the lesion comprises tumor tissue, infiltrated parenchyma, or both. Some CT hypodense nonenhancing tumor tissue lesions can be resected from essential brain regions with low morbidity (Fig. 41-15).

In particular, low-grade oligodendrogliomas, dysembryoplastic neuroepithelial tumors, and some gangliogliomas in young patients (usually presenting with seizures) will manifest a solid tumor tissue mass that is hypodense and nonenhancing on CT scanning. Serial biopsies in these lesions will show only tumor tissue with minimal or no surrounding infiltrated parenchyma (type I tumor).

Tumors located in eloquent brain, which on biopsy are found to comprise isolated tumor cells within parenchyma with or without tumor tissue (type II or III, respectively), should not be resected unless careful cortical mapping techniques establish that the involved parenchyma is "silent" (Fig. 41-16).

FIGURE 41-13 In essential brain regions, resection of the only tumor tissue mass in a type II glioma is possible as in this 43-year-old man with a left posterodorsal thalamic grade 4 astrocytoma. Preoperative (*left*) and postoperative (*right*) contrast-enhanced computed tomography scans are shown.

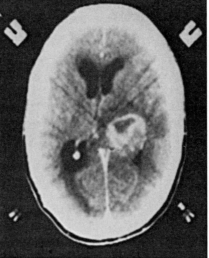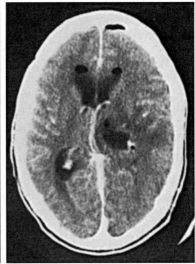

Hypodense type II or III tumors, which are located in nonessential brain tissue, can be completely resected. Low-grade oligodendrogliomas, mixed gliomas, and astrocytomas located in frontal or anterior or mediotemporal lobes or superoparietal lobules can be selectively resected by imaging-based volumetric stereotactic methods with rewarding postoperative results.

RESULTS

A total of 1165 patients underwent computer-assisted, volumetric stereotactic resection procedures at the Mayo Clinic (from August 1984 to September 1993) and at New York University Medical Center (from September 1993 to December 1994) over a 10-year period between August 1984 and December 1994. Overall surgical morbidity was 6.5%, and mortality was less than 1%. Postoperative imaging

studies confirmed complete resection of the radiographically defined target volume in more than 90% of cases. Postoperative and follow-up results have been published previously in a series of publications.[4,7,8,10–12,16–27] Moreover, the average global charges (physician related plus hospital related) for tumor resection by volumetric, minimally invasive stereotaxis was 67% of the charges for patients undergoing classic craniotomy for similar lesions.

Morbidity and Mortality

Forty-three patients were neurologically worse after the operation: 14 patients were neurologically normal before and had deficits afterward, and 29 additional patients experienced worsening of a deficit noted on the preoperative neurologic examination. Postoperative deficits resulted from the surgical approach or from local perilesional trauma. In 18 of 43 patients, postoperative neurologic deficits were consistent with neuronal injury along the surgical approach. For instance, 14 patients with mediotemporal or posteroventral thalamic lesions sustained a permanent contralateral superior quadrantanopsia, and two others had a homonymous hemianopsia after the temporo-occipital approach that was necessary to resect their lesions. The transsylvian exposure of a left subinsular metastatic tumor produced a contralateral arm dyspraxia in another patient. Finally, a transvermian exposure of a midline cerebellar thrombosed arteriovenous malformation resulted in increased gait apraxia.

The remaining 25 patients who were worse after surgery sustained deficits consistent with local trauma inflicted while resecting the neoplasm or disruption of the parenchymal blood supply. Most often, this occurred in high-grade glial neoplasms with peritumoral tumor cell infiltration. However, deficit followed resection in some low-grade, apparently circumscribed lesions. For example, a 27-year-old woman noted worsening of a postoperative hemiparesis after resection of a 3-cm thrombosed arteriovenous malformation that was located in the left lateral basal ganglia. Six patients with thalamic pilocytic astrocytomas noted worsened preoperative hemiparesis postoperatively, which was slight in four patients and moderate in two patients. Recently, we reported a 26% overall incidence of postoperative deficit and supplementary

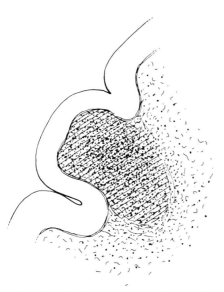

FIGURE 41-14 Type III gliomas consist of isolated tumor cells, which reside in and infiltrate a volume of intact brain tissue. Resection of these lesions is, in fact, resection of functioning (albeit diseased) brain parenchyma.

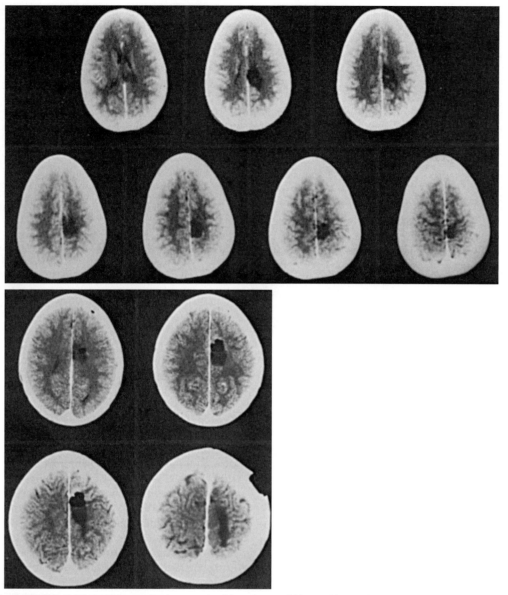

FIGURE 41-15 Preoperative computed tomography scan (*top*) in a 3-year-old boy with a subcortical oligodendroglioma located beneath the postcentral convolution. The tumor comprises solid tumor tissue only and was completely resected (*bottom*) with no postoperative neurologic deficit.

motor area (SMA) syndrome after stereotactic resection of glial neoplasms involving the posterior one third of the superofrontal convolution.[28] In this study, seven of a total of 27 patients had SMA-related deficits, with three having a complete SMA syndrome and four having a partial SMA syndrome. Low-grade gliomas were associated with a higher incidence of SMA syndrome, likely indicating the removal of more functional SMA cortex in these patients.

In a series of 657 patients, operated on between August 1984 and December 1991 (Table 41-1), six deaths occurred within 1 month of surgery. One death was the result of massive brain stem edema after removal of a ventral thalamic mixed pilocytic/fibrillary astrocytoma with brain stem infiltration apparent on the MRI and two from massive pulmonary embolization (one 2 weeks after resection of a large left lateral ventricle meningioma and the other 6 days after resection of a thalamic glioblastoma). Another patient had a herniation syndrome and died owing to a subdural

hygroma, which had developed 2½ weeks after resection of a larger intraventricular neurocytoma. Two additional patients with grade 4 astrocytomas continued to deteriorate neurologically owing to tumor progression despite tumor resection; these patients died within 30 days of the surgical procedure.

High-Grade Glial Tumors

Computer-assisted stereotactic resection can remove all CT-defined, contrast-enhancing portions of high-grade glial neoplasms from neurologically important subcortical areas with acceptable levels of mortality and morbidity.[2,8,9,18,23] Postoperative CT studies usually demonstrate an absence of contrast enhancement around the surgical defect. Nevertheless, the mean postoperative survival time for our patients harboring grade 4 astrocytomas treated with postoperative external beam radiation therapy (50–65 Gy)

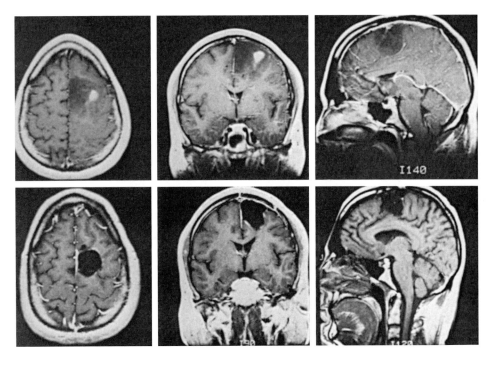

FIGURE 41-16 Preoperative (*top*) and postoperative (*bottom*) results in a 39-year-old man presenting with intractable seizures and an infiltrating grade 2 oligodendroglioma in the posterior third of the left superofrontal convolution, which was resected using a stereotactically placed trephine and the volumetric resection technique. The patient's neurologic examination was normal before and after surgery.

was 50.6 weeks. This survival rate compares favorably with a consecutive series of patients harboring grade 4 gliomas who underwent radiation therapy after a biopsy alone (mean survival of 33 weeks).[29] However, after resection, new areas of contrast enhancement on CT scanning developed within low-density areas surrounding the surgical defect within 6 to 9 months of the procedure.

Computer-assisted volumetric stereotactic resection allows safe and complete resection of the contrast-enhancing

mass lesion in high-grade gliomas. However, preoperative stereotactic MRI (especially the T2-weighted image) in high-grade glial tumors always demonstrates much larger areas of abnormality than those indicated by contrast enhancement on CT scanning.[6,7] An examination of stereotactic serial biopsy specimens obtained in patients with high-grade gliomas from these MRI-defined abnormalities outside the contrast-enhancing tumor mass reveals a larger area of intact edematous brain parenchyma infiltrated by aggressive isolated tumor cells.[5–7,17,30] In fact, this edematous infiltrated parenchyma usually extends as far as (and in some cases beyond) the area of signal prolongation abnormality on the T2-weighted MRI.[6,7] It would be technically possible using volumetric stereotaxis to resect the volume defined by the MRI abnormality, and this, in theory, would substantially prolong postoperative survival.[31,32] However, unacceptable neurologic deficits would result from removal of the intact albeit infiltrated parenchyma.

A similar problem exists for patients with grade 3 astrocytomas, mixed gliomas, and oligodendrogliomas. Although the cellular elements within these tumors are not as mitotically active as in the grade 4 tumor, isolated tumor cells also infiltrate intact and surrounding edematous parenchyma[6,7] and defy surgical attempts to cure them. In addition, grade 3 gliomas, particularly astrocytomas, tend to have larger infiltrative components with respect to tumor tissue components than do grade 4 lesions. Thus, the benefit of resecting a relatively small tumor tissue mass in the face of a large volume of infiltrated parenchyma is questionable.

Low-Grade Astrocytomas

The resectability of these tumors depends on the degree of histologic circumscription. In adults, low-grade astrocytomas are usually manifest by an area of low density on CT scanning and prolongation of signal on MRI.[7] Stereotactic serial biopsy studies of these so-called fibrillary

TABLE 41-1 ▪ Location of Tumors in 657 Patients Undergoing Stereotactic Resection (August 1984–December 1991)

Location	Total	Right	Left
Supratentorial			
Central	63	32	31
Basal ganglia	31	19	12
Thalamus	55	19	36
Third ventricle	37	—	—
Posterior/deep frontal	142	66	76
Parietal	108	51	57
Occipital	26	10	16
Temporal	67	33	34
Temporo-occipital	15	6	9
Temporoparietal	20	7	13
Parieto-occipital	11	7	4
Corpus callosum	3	—	—
Lateral ventricle	25	17	8
Total	603		
Infratentorial			
Deep cerebellar hemisphere	23		
Vermis	7		
Mesencephalon	8		
Pons	11		
Medulla	5		
Total	54		

astrocytomas reveal that the tumor consists almost entirely of infiltrated intact parenchyma with little tumor tissue proper.[6,7] Therefore, resection of the tumor by stereotactic craniotomy involves resection of intact but infiltrated parenchyma defined by the low-density areas on CT scanning and signal prolongation on MRI. However, in important brain areas, this results in a postoperative neurologic deficit, and stereotactic resection is therefore rejected as an option.[8,33] In some cases, the lesion is confined to expendable brain tissue, such as the posterior portion of the superofrontal convolution.

Juvenile pilocytic astrocytomas, conversely, which tend to occur in children and young adults, are histologically circumscribed. Despite the fact that many are located in the thalamus and other important subcortical locations, they can be completely resected by computer-assisted stereotactic technique with excellent postoperative results.[8,34] These lesions exhibit prominent contrast enhancement on CT or on MRI with gadolinium, and the histologic borders are defined accurately by the contrast enhancement.

Metastatic Tumors

Many surgeons have had the unsettling experience of trying unsuccessfully to locate deep subcortical metastatic lesions during a conventional craniotomy. In fact, reported surgical series of metastatic tumors removed at nonstereotactic craniotomies report a percentage of patients with incomplete resections.[34–37] Metastatic tumors are usually located at the gray-white junction subcortically. They can be located superficially near the crown of a gyrus. They can also be located at the gray-white junction in the depths of a deep sulcus, and they can be difficult to find at conventional craniotomy. Other tumors may be deep to the insular cortex, deep to the mesial occipital cortex, or under the cortex of the interhemispheric fissure.

Stereotactic techniques can be advantageous in the resection of the superficial metastases as well as the deeply situated lesions.[24] First, stereotactic point localization helps to center small cranial trephines directly over superficial lesions (the trephine need be no larger than the cross-sectional

area of the neoplasm). The approach is, therefore, selective and direct, and no more brain need be exposed than is absolutely necessary. With volumetric stereotaxis and intraoperative image displays, identification of the plane between the tumor and the brain is straightforward and, in fact, simple. These lesions can be completely resected by the computer-assisted stereotactic craniotomy.

Our postoperative morbidity for stereotactic resection of centrally located and deep-seated metastatic tumors (0% mortality rate, 4.3% morbidity rate) compares favorably with that associated with conventional craniotomy for these lesions in the past (11% mortality rate).[34–38]

Vascular Malformations

Angiographically, occult arteriovenous malformations (AVMs) and cavernous hemangiomas are well-circumscribed lesions that can be completely removed stereotactically with relatively low risk. A byproduct of establishing the histology is that cessation or significant reduction of seizures, when present, usually results.

Small, deep-seated, active arteriovenous malformations may also be resected using similar techniques (Fig. 41-17). At our institution, we have successfully used the frame-based stereotaxis for resection of deep-seated AVMs. In a series of 44 consecutive patients, we reported that the use of stereotaxis decreased operative time and intraoperative blood loss without any increase in morbidity.[39] Stereotaxis is of particular value in these lesions because the position of the feeding vessels is established in the 3-dimensional surgical planning matrix and is approached and clipped or coagulated before the remainder of the lesion is dissected away from the surrounding parenchyma.

Intraventricular Lesions

A more limited but direct approach to intraventricular lesions can be made stereotactically. Brain and ventricular incisions need to be only large enough to remove the lesion. Thus intraventricular lesions are removed through a 1.5-inch trephine and 2-cm cylindrical retractor (Fig. 41-18).

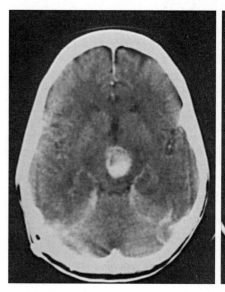 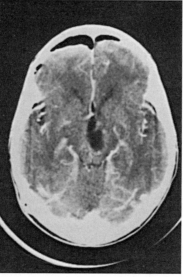

FIGURE 41-17 Preoperative (*left*) and postoperative (*right*) computed tomography scans in a 29-year-old woman with a mesencephalic arteriovenous malformation (AVM) with a hemorrhage. The hematoma and AVM were resected using the 2-cm-diameter stereotactic retractor. The patient was lethargic and had Weber's syndrome preoperatively. She made an excellent neurologic recovery after evacuation of the hematoma and resection of the AVM.

FIGURE 41-18 Preoperative (*A*) and postoperative (*B*) magnetic resonance imaging studies in a 58-year-old woman with a large intraventricular subependymal astrocytoma and associated hydrocephalus. The lesion was totally resected using a 2-cm stereotactic retractor and multiple translations. A gross total excision of the lesion was accomplished. The patient did not require a shunt.

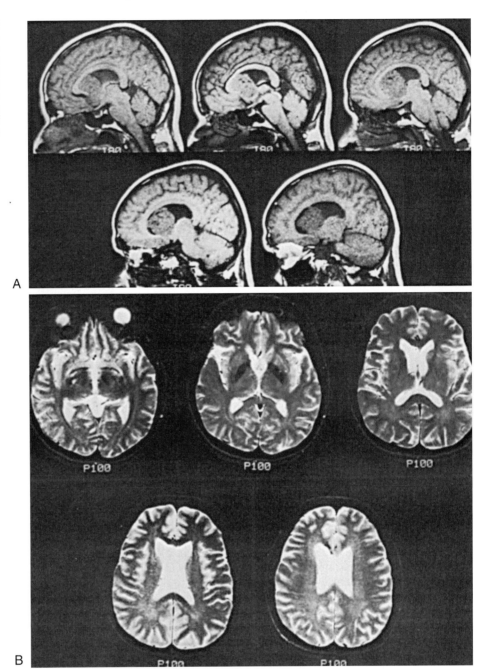

Colloid cysts are approached through the lateral ventricle and foramen of Monro into which the cyst extends. The approach features an anterior trephine craniotomy (about at the frontal hairline), splitting of the superior frontal sulcus, and exposure of the cyst in the foramen of Monro by means of the 2-cm diameter stereotactic retractor (Fig. 41-19). This approach does not violate epileptogenic brain tissue and provides an anterior vantage point for dealing with the attachment of the cyst. We have resected 28 colloid cysts in this manner without permanent complications.[16]

Large third ventricular lesions are usually approached through the right lateral ventricle, unless the lesion has a significantly enlarged foramen of Monro on the left side. In the latter instance, the lesion would be approached from the left side (Fig. 41-20). One fornix can be incised to extend the stereotactic retractor into the third ventricular lesion, where an internal decompression of the lesion is performed with a CO_2 laser until only a thin rim of the capsule remains. The computer display of the cross-sections of the digitized CT-/MRI-defined tumor volume is extremely useful in this step because the surgeon, knowing where the tumor stops and the third ventricular wall begins, can be aggressive within the tumor with no risk of extending through the capsule and damaging the walls of the third ventricle. After this internal decompression, the retractor is withdrawn to the level of the roof of the third ventricle, and the capsule is carefully dissected from the walls of the third ventricle. The tumor capsule can be contracted using the defocused laser, which facilitates the dissection of the capsule from the wall of the third ventricle.[25]

R:23   L:7

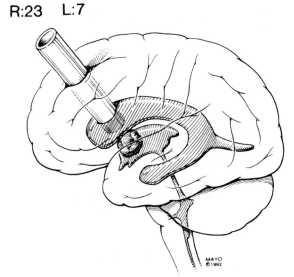

FIGURE 41-19 Exposure of the anterior third ventricular lesion. A stereotactic retractor is placed through a microsurgically opened superofrontal sulcus and subcortical incision into the lateral ventricle. The ipsilateral fornix can be sacrificed if foramen of Monro must be enlarged to extend the retractor into the third ventricle itself. (By permission of the Mayo Foundation.)

FRAMELESS STEREOTAXIS

The advantages of computer-assisted stereotactic neurosurgery have become evident over the past several years, as have the ease and applicability of computer technology. These developments have enabled us to embark on several new projects that have rapidly become incorporated into our neurosurgical armamentarium. It has become clear that computers can be used to monitor and display to the surgeon the position of surgical instruments within a stereotactically defined work environment. This makes possible a trend toward even more minimally invasive as well as endoscopic surgery, not only in subarachnoid and intraventricular spaces but also for intra-axial target volumes.

Computers make possible instrumentation for online registration of surgical instrument position within the surgical work envelope by transmitting the position of a surgical tool to an operating room computer system. Several frameless systems are currently available and in use at our institution. These include multiple-jointed, articulated arm digitizers. These may be cumbersome and require frequent repositioning during the operative procedure. In addition, image-guided, stereotactic navigational microscopes, based on optical digitizing methods using a system of light-emitting diodes, have also been introduced. These, however, are limited by "line-of-sight" considerations, which often only become apparent during real-time operations, when the patient is positioned on the operating table and the entire team of surgeons, anesthesiologists, and nurses are at work. Alternatively, we have developed magnetic field digitizers to cross-register points from the imaging database to the actual surgical field (Fig. 41-21). Sensors on this device are connected to a wire similar to that attached to bipolar forceps. With tuning of the magnetic field and computer-generated distortion corrections, we have reliable and reasonable accuracy with this instrument as a pointing device. We have also incorporated a suction device and a heads-up display

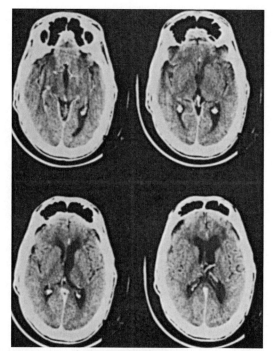

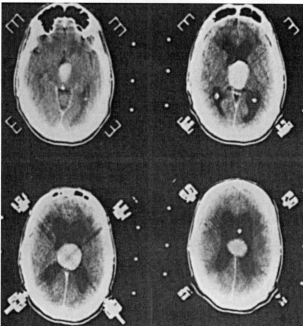

FIGURE 41-20 Preoperative (*top*) and postoperative (*bottom*) contrast-enhanced computed tomography scans in a 56-year-old man who presented with a recent memory deficit and hydrocephalus due to a giant, partially calcified colloid cyst of the third ventricle. He was neurologically intact postoperatively; his recent memory had improved to better than preoperative levels by 3 months after surgery.

to this unit to increase its utility in the operating room. The REGULUS and, more recently, the CYGNUS systems (COMPASS International) have been developed to give surgeons more freehand efficiency. The latter system is the first portable image-guided surgery system that is operated from a laptop computer with a network image-acquisition interface, thus reducing the costs of this technology significantly (Fig. 41-22). At our institution, this system is actually shared between affiliated hospitals.

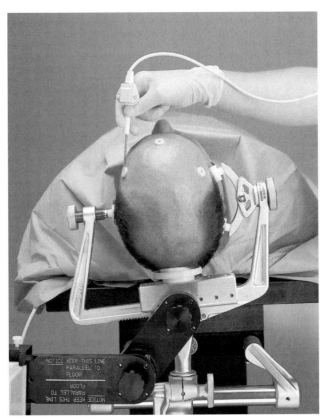

FIGURE 41-21 Intraoperative registration of the CYGNUS frameless stereotactic system (COMPASS International, Rochester, MN) to cross-register points from the imaging database to the actual surgical field.

We recently mathematically compared all three prototypical image-guided navigational systems that are in use at our institution for actual precision and accuracy.[27] Using a stereotactic "phantom," we calculated the mean accuracy and precision of localization for three frameless stereotactic systems. The Cygnus system attained a mean accuracy of

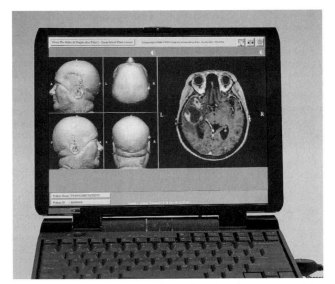

FIGURE 41-22 Intraoperative view of the laptop computer of the CYGNUS frameless stereotactic system. Note the ability to view the 3-dimensional representation and the axial images of the preoperative magnetic resonance imaging concurrently.

1.90 ± 0.7 mm, the ISG viewing wand system a mean accuracy of 1.67 ± 0.43 mm, and the SMN microscope a mean accuracy of 2.61 ± 0.99 mm. The precision was not significantly different between systems. With accuracy and precision being similar among the three systems, at our institution now we use predominantly the CYGNUS system because of its ease of use, low cost, and easy portability.

Integration of Stereotaxis and Endoscopy

We have incorporated computer-assisted, frameless stereotaxis into our freehand endoscopic procedures over the past several years. In one author's (H.W.) experience in pediatric neurosurgery, intraventricular anatomy may frequently be distorted and devoid of normal anatomic landmarks, rendering such surgical procedures unacceptably risky. With the integration of the visual information obtained endoscopically and the navigational information provided by stereotaxis, we and others have been able to successfully place ventricular catheters in complex hydrocephalus, fenestrate irregular cysts and loculated ventricles, retrieve retained catheters, and perform endoscopic septostomy and third ventriculostomy.[40,41]

The combination of frameless stereotaxy and endoscopy has proven useful in the biopsy and/or resection of numerous intraventricular lesions, such as tumors and colloid cysts,[42] with improved accuracy, confidence, and safety.

Transphenoidal Lesions

Frame-based stereotaxis has historically been of little use in the treatment of skull-based lesions. The more recent acquisition of frameless systems has allowed most major institutions to use stereotaxis for accurate localization of skull-based lesions. Frameless stereotaxy now has been used both as an adjunct to and as a replacement for fluoroscopy in transsphenoidal resection of pituitary tumors.[43,44] It is most helpful in establishing 3-dimensional intraoperative localization of important midline structures, especially in cases of recurrent surgery in which the anatomy is distorted. Both fiducial-based and headset-based systems are now in use for registration of selected anatomic points.

Integration of Functional Brain Mapping in Image-Guided Neurosurgery

Magnetoencephalography is a noninvasive, accurate, and reproducible method for the preoperative assessment of patients with lesions associated with eloquent sensory and motor cortex.[19,26,45] We have incorporated the interactive use of magnetoencephalography functional mapping in our stereotactic, volumetric resections, allowing for safer approaches for resection of eloquent cortex lesions. We have, therefore, developed magnetoencephalography mapping–derived functional risk profiles that are used as powerful tools for both presurgical planing and intraoperative guidance. We have developed a process for transforming the magnetoencephalography-derived sensorimotor localization coordinates into the COMPASS stereotactic coordinate system. This, in turn, is incorporated into the stereotactic database, enabling the simultaneous visualization of functional and anatomic data. The results of this technique have appeared in several publications.[19,26,45]

Frameless Stereotaxis and Epilepsy Surgery

Intracranial operations for placement of subdural recording electrodes and resection of epileptogenic foci have benefited greatly from frameless stereotaxis. The accurate localization of each subdural electrode series is now greatly enhanced, and the 3-dimensional navigational information provided by stereotaxis allows the placement of depth electrodes in the medial temporal lobe for direct sampling of that area.[46] Once the seizure focus is identified, stereotaxis also allows the subsequent targeting and resection of abnormal tissue with excellent results for seizure control.[47] Other epilepsy surgeries, including partial or complete corpus callosotomy for atonic seizure control, have also used frameless stereotaxis for enhanced anatomic localization of midline structures, including the sagittal sinus and draining cerebral veins.[48]

Pediatric Neurosurgery

The use of frameless stereotaxis is an obvious advantage in children who are generally unlikely to tolerate frame-based procedures. In addition to its use in epilepsy surgery, frameless stereotaxis has proven to be useful in almost every kind of pediatric neurosurgical procedure, including shunting of the ventricular system,[49] endoscopic third ventriculostomy,[50] and resection of tumors.[51]

NEW DIRECTIONS IN MINIMALLY INVASIVE COMPUTER-ASSISTED STEREOTACTIC NEUROSURGERY

Stereotaxis and Molecular Neurosurgery

With new molecular biologic advances in the field of neuro-oncology, stereotactic methods combined with modern computing power and imaging databases provide powerful options for molecular neurosurgery. Point-in-space and volumetric computer-assisted, imaging-based tumor stereotactic procedures can be easily modified for the preplanned and precise delivery of genetic and chemotherapeutic agents to an imaging-defined anatomic target volume. These techniques could provide more uniform coverage and dose levels of the therapeutic material within the defined target structure.[20] As the molecular basis for each disease process is uncovered, specific targets can be chosen and strategies employed via stereotactic delivery systems to enhance our ability to treat neurologic disease.

CONCLUSION

With the computer-assisted volumetric stereotactic method described, it is theoretically possible to resect all tumors detected by CT or MRI. The procedure has been found to be most effective for the resection of well-circumscribed lesions in deep-seated intra-axial locations. For instance, juvenile pilocytic astrocytomas can be totally removed with minimal morbidity from any subcortical location, such as the thalamus, by this method. Furthermore, patients with

other circumscribed glial tumors, metastatic tumors, and thrombosed vascular malformations can derive significant benefit from this procedure.

Without volumetric stereotaxis, the surgeon may become lost, resulting in unnecessary tissue damage. This may lead to neurologic deficits and a prolonged and expensive recovery period. Furthermore, the border between tumor and surrounding normal brain may not be obvious, possibly leading to the resection of normal tissue in eloquent brain regions. The neurosurgeon benefits from this technology by being able to localize the lesion, visualize the border between the lesion and surrounding tissue, conceptualize the 3-dimensional character of the neoplasm, and plan the safest approach preoperatively, based on the neural and vascular anatomy. The patient benefits from a smaller skin incision, craniotomy flap, and brain exposure, resulting in reduced operative morbidity, shorter hospitalization, and reduced cost.

In conclusion, computer-assisted volumetric stereotactic craniotomy provides several advantages over conventional freehand neurosurgical techniques in the management of intra-axial mass lesions. First, the stereotactic method maintains surgical orientation as the procedure extends below the cortical surface, and the approach is preplanned to disrupt as little important brain tissue as possible. Beyond the gross appearance of a tumor at surgery and its apparent margins on visual inspection, the computer display images provide additional information to the surgeon regarding where tumor boundaries lie in relationship to surrounding brain tissue. The method allows us to resect as much of a lesion as we choose to remove. However, limitations in malignant glial neoplasms lie in the biology of the disease process itself, unresectable intact parenchyma that is infiltrated by isolated tumor cells. The best candidates for computer-assisted stereotactic volumetric resection, therefore, are patients with histologically circumscribed glial and nonglial tumors and nonneoplastic lesions.

REFERENCES

1. Apuzzo ML, Chandrasoma PT, Zelman V, et al: Computed tomographic guidance stereotaxis in the management of lesions of the third ventricular region. Neurosurgery 15:502–508, 1984.
2. Brown RA: A computerized tomography-computer graphics approach to stereotaxic localization. J Neurosurg 50:715–720, 1979.
3. Goerss S, Kelly PF, Kall B, Alker GJ Jr: A computed tomographic stereotactic adaptation system. Neurosurgery 10:375–379, 1982.
4. Kelly PJ, Alker GJ Jr: A stereotactic approach to deep-seated central nervous system neoplasms using the carbon dioxide laser. Surg Neurol 15:331–334, 1981.
5. Daumas-Duport C, Monsaingeon V, Szenthe L, Szikla G: Serial stereotactic biopsies: A double histological code of gliomas according to malignancy and 3-D configuration, as an aid to therapeutic decision and assessment of results. Appl Neurophysiol 45:431–437, 1982.
6. Kelly PJ, Daumas-Duport C, Scheithauer BW, et al: Stereotactic histologic correlations of computed tomography- and magnetic resonance imaging-defined abnormalities in patients with glial neoplasms. Mayo Clin Proc 62:450–459, 1987.
7. Kelly PJ, Daumas-Duport C, Kispert DB, et al: Imaging-based stereotaxic serial biopsies in untreated intracranial glial neoplasms. J Neurosurg 66:865–874, 1987.
8. Kelly PJ: Volumetric stereotactic surgical resection of intra-axial brain mass lesions. Mayo Clin Proc 63:1186–1198, 1988.
9. Kelly PJ, Kall BA, Goerss S, Alker GJ Jr: Precision resection of intra-axial CNS lesions by CT-based stereotactic craniotomy and computer monitored CO_2 laser. Acta Neurochir (Wien) 68:1–9, 1983.

10. Kelly PJ, Kall BA, Goerss S: Transposition of volumetric information derived from computed tomography scanning into stereotactic space. Surg Neurol 21:465–471, 1984.

11. Kelly PJ, Goerss SJ, Kall BA: Evolution of contemporary instrumentation for computer-assisted stereotactic surgery. Surg Neurol 30:204–215, 1988.

12. Weiner HL, Kelly PJ: A novel computer-assisted volumetric stereotactic approach for resecting tumors of the posterior parahippocampal gyrus. J Neurosurg 85:272–277, 1996.

13. Russell SM, Kelly PJ: Volumetric stereotaxy and the supratentorial occipitosubtemporal approach in the resection of posterior hippocampus and parahippocampal gyrus lesions. Neurosurgery 50:978–988, 2002.

14. Frankel SA, German WJ: Glioblastoma multiforme; review of 219 cases with regard to natural history, pathology, diagnostic methods, and treatment. J Neurosurg 15:489–503, 1958.

15. Jelsma R, Bucy PC: The treatment of glioblastoma multiforme of the brain. J Neurosurg 27:388–400, 1967.

16. Abernathey CD, Davis DH, Kelly PJ: Treatment of colloid cysts of the third ventricle by stereotaxic microsurgical laser craniotomy. J Neurosurg 70:525–529, 1989.

17. Daumas-Duport C, Scheithauer BW, Kelly PJ: A histologic and cytologic method for the spatial definition of gliomas. Mayo Clin Proc 62:435–449, 1987.

18. Devaux BC, O'Fallon JR, Kelly PJ: Resection, biopsy, and survival in malignant glial neoplasms: A retrospective study of clinical parameters, therapy, and outcome. J Neurosurg 78:767–775, 1993.

19. Hund M, Rezai AR, Kronberg E, et al: Magnetoencephalographic mapping: Basic of a new functional risk profile in the selection of patients with cortical brain lesions. Neurosurgery 40:936–943, 1997.

20. Kelly PJ: Stereotactic procedures for molecular neurosurgery. Exp Neurol 144:157–159, 1997.

21. Kelly PJ, Alker GJ Jr, Goerss S: Computer-assisted stereotactic microsurgery for the treatment of intracranial neoplasms. Neurosurgery 10:324–331, 1982.

22. Kelly PJ, Kall B, Goerss S: Stereotactic CT scanning for the biopsy of intracranial lesions and functional neurosurgery. Appl Neurophysiol 46:193–199, 1983.

23. Kelly PJ: Computer-assisted stereotaxis: New approaches for the management of intracranial intra-axial tumors. Neurology 36:535–541, 1986.

24. Kelly PJ, Kall BA, Goerss SJ: Results of computed tomography-based computer-assisted stereotactic resection of metastatic intracranial tumors. Neurosurgery 22:7–17, 1988.

25. Morita A, Kelly PJ: Resection of intraventricular tumors via a computer-assisted volumetric stereotactic approach. Neurosurgery 32:920–927, 1993.

26. Rezai AR, Hund M, Kronberg E, et al: The interactive use of magnetoencephalography in stereotactic image-guided neurosurgery. Neurosurgery 39:92–102, 1996.

27. Benardete EA, Leonard MA, Weiner HL: Comparison of frameless stereotactic systems: Accuracy, precision, and applications. Neurosurgery 49:1409–1416, 2001.

28. Russell SM, Kelly PJ: Incidence and clinical evolution of postoperative deficits after volumetric stereotactic resection of glial neoplasms involving the supplementary motor area. Neurosurgery 52:506–516, 2003.

29. Kelly PJ, Hunt C: The limited value of cytoreductive surgery in elderly patients with malignant gliomas. Neurosurgery 34:62–67, 1994.

30. Burger PC, Dubois PJ, Schold SC Jr, et al: Computerized tomographic and pathologic studies of the untreated, quiescent, and recurrent glioblastoma multiforme. J Neurosurg 58:159–169, 1983.

31. Hoshino T: A commentary on the biology and growth kinetics of low-grade and high-grade gliomas. J Neurosurg 61:895–900, 1984.

32. Hoshino T, Barker M, Wilson CB, et al: Cell kinetics of human gliomas. J Neurosurg 37:15–26, 1972.

33. Kelly PJ, Kall BA, Goerss S, Earnest F 4th: Computer-assisted stereotaxic laser resection of intra-axial brain neoplasms. J Neurosurg 64:427–439, 1986.

34. McGirr SJ, Kelly PJ, Scheithauer BW: Stereotactic resection of juvenile pilocytic astrocytomas of the thalamus and basal ganglia. Neurosurgery 20:447–452, 1987.

35. MacGee EE: Surgical treatment of cerebral metastases from lung cancer: The effect on quality and duration of survival. J Neurosurg 35:416–420, 1971.

36. Haar F, Patterson RH Jr: Surgical for metastatic intracranial neoplasm. Cancer 30:1241–1245, 1972.

37. Yardeni D, Reichenthal E, Zucker G, et al: Neurosurgical management of single brain metastasis. Surg Neurol 21:377–384, 1984.

38. van Eck JH, Ebels EJ, Go KG: Metastatic tumours of the brain. Psychiatr Neurol Neurochir 68:443–462, 1965.

39. Russell SM, Woo HH, Joseffer SS, Jaraf JJ: Role of frameless stereotaxy in the surgical treatment of cerebral arteriovenous malformations: Technique and outcomes in a controlled study of 44 consecutive patients. Neurosurgery 51:1108–1118, 2002.

40. Alberti O, Reigel T, Hellwig D, Bertalanffy H: Frameless navigation and endoscopy. J Neurosurg 95:541–543, 2001.

41. Fratzoglou M, Grunert P, Leite dos Santos A, et al: Symptomatic cysts of the cavum septi pellucidi and cavum vergae: The role of endoscopic neurosurgery in the treatment of four consecutive cases. Minim Invasive Neurosurg 46:243–249, 2003.

42. Kumar K, Kelly M, Toth C: Stereotactic cyst wall disruption and aspiration of colloid cysts of the third ventricle. Stereotact Funct Neurosurg 71:145–152, 1998.

43. Walker DG, Ohaegbulam C, Black PM: Frameless stereotaxy as an alternative to fluoroscopy for transsphenoidal surgery: Use of the InstaTrak-3000 and a novel headset. J Clin Neurosci 9:294–297, 2002.

44. Jane JA Jr, Thapar K, Alden TD, Laws ER Jr: Fluoroscopic frameless stereotaxy for transsphenoidal surgery. Neurosurgery 48:1302–1308, 2001.

45. Rezai AR, Mogiler AY, Cappell J, et al: Integration of functional brain mapping in image-guided neurosurgery. Acta Neurochir Suppl (Wien) 68:85–89, 1997.

46. Murphy MA, O'Brien TJ, Cook MJ: Insertion of depth electrodes with or without subdural grids using frameless stereotactic guidance systems—Technique and outcome. Br J Neurosurg 16:119–125, 2002.

47. Rosenfeld JV, Harvey AS, Wrennall J, et al: Transcallosal resection of hypothalamic hamartomas, with control of seizures, in children with gelastic epilepsy. Neurosurgery 48:108–118, 2001.

48. Hodaie M, Musherbash A, Otsubo H, et al: Image-guided, frameless stereotactic sectioning of the corpus callosum in children with intractable epilepsy. Pediatr Neurosurg 34:286–294, 2001.

49. Gil Z, Siomin V, Beni-Adani L, et al: Ventricular catheter placement in children with hydrocephalus and small ventricles: The use of a frameless neuronavigation system. Childs Nerv Syst 18:26–29, 2002.

50. Muacevic A, Muller A: Image-guided endoscopic ventriculostomy with a new frameless armless neuronavigation system. Comput Aided Surg 4:87–92, 1999.

51. Herrera EJ, Caceres M, Viano JC, et al: Stereotactic neurosurgery in children and adolescents. Childs Nerv Syst 15:256–261, 1999.

42 Intraoperative Neurophysiology: A Tool to Prevent and/or Document Intraoperative Injury to the Nervous System

VEDRAN DELETIS and FRANCESCO SALA

INTRODUCTION

To detect and/or prevent intraoperatively induced neurologic injuries, intraoperative neurophysiology (ION) has established itself as a clinical discipline that uses neurophysiologic methods especially developed or modified from existing methods of clinical neurophysiology. Developments in ION over the past 25 years, especially its most recent achievements, have solidified its role in neurosurgery and other surgical disciplines. The ideal goal of ION is to prevent intraoperatively induced injury to the nervous system. Furthermore, ION can be used to document the exact moment when the injury occurred. As a result, it can be used for both educational and medicolegal purposes.

Generally, ION techniques can be divided in two groups: mapping and monitoring.

Neurophysiologic mapping is a technique that, when applied intraoperatively, enables us to identify anatomically indistinct neural structures by their neurophysiologic function. This allows the surgeon to avoid lesioning critical structures in the course of the surgical procedure. In essence, the information gained from neurophysiologic mapping allows the surgeon to operate more safely.

The following procedures use a neurophysiologic mapping technique: mapping of the sensory motor cortex with phase reversal median nerve somatosensory evoked potentials (SEPs), mapping of the cranial nerve motor nuclei on the surgically exposed floor of the fourth ventricle, mapping of the corticospinal tract (CT) subcortically (i.e., at the level of the cerebral peduncle or at the spinal cord), mapping of the pudendal afferents in the sacral roots, before selective dorsal rhizotomy, and so on.

Neurophysiologic monitoring is a technique that continuously evaluates the functional integrity of nervous tissue and gives feedback to the (neuro)surgeon. This feedback can be instantaneous, as in a recently developed technique of monitoring motor-evoked potentials (MEPs) from the epidural space of the spinal cord or limb muscles. If the surgical procedure allows us to combine monitoring with mapping techniques, then optimal protection of nervous tissue can be achieved during neurosurgery.

Furthermore, ION uses provocative tests to examine their influence on neurophysiologic signals before the surgical procedure. The typical example of a provocative test is the temporary placement of a clip on the feeding vessel of a cerebral or spinal arteriovenous malformation. Before permanent occlusion takes place, observation of changes in neurophysiologic signals are used as an indicator of an ischemic event. A temporary clamping of the carotid artery during endarterectomy with monitoring of SEPs or electroencephalography is another example of a provocative test that measures the ability of the collateral cerebral circulation to supply a potentially ischemic hemisphere. Endovascular injection of a short-acting barbiturate or Xylocaine into a vascular malformation of the spinal cord, before embolization, and observation of its influence on the neurophysiologic signals is another kind of provocative test.

USE OF INTRAOPERATIVE NEUROPHYSIOLOGIC TECHNIQUES

Supratentorial Surgery

Surgery for brain gliomas has become more and more aggressive. This is based on clinical data that support better patient survival and quality of life after gross total removal of both low- and high-grade lesions.[1,2]

However, the resection of tumors located in eloquent brain areas, such as the rolandic region and frontotemporal speech areas, requires the identification of functional cortical and subcortical areas that must be respected during surgery. Moreover, the dogmatic assumption that tumoral tissue could not retain function has been repeatedly questioned by neurophysiologic and functional magnetic resonance imaging studies.[3–5] In response to the need for a safe surgery in eloquent brain areas, the past decade has seen the development of a number of techniques to map brain functions, including, but not limited to, functional magnetic resonance imaging, magnetoencephalography, and positron emission tomography.[6–11]

The neurophysiologic contribution to brain mapping has been evident since the late 19th century with the pioneering work of Fritsch and Hitzig[12] and Bartholow.[13] In the 20th century, Penfield and colleagues[14,15] made invaluable contributions through intraoperative mapping of the sensorimotor cortex, the findings of which have been substantiated by a number of recent studies.[16–18]

Somatosensory Evoked Potential Phase Reversal Technique

To indirectly identify the central sulcus, SEPs can be recorded from the exposed cerebral cortex by using the phase reversal technique.

SEPs are elicited by stimulation of the median nerve at the wrist and the posterior tibial nerve at the ankle (40-mA intensity, 0.2-msec duration, 4.3-Hz repetition rate). Recordings are performed from the scalp at CZ'-FZ (for legs) and C3'/C4'-CZ' (for arms) according to the 10-20 International Electroencephalography System. After craniotomy, a strip electrode is placed across the exposed motor cortex and primary somatosensory cortex, transversing the central sulcus. This technique is based on the principle that an SEP, elicited by median nerve stimulation at the wrist, can be recorded from the primary sensory cortex.[19] Its mirror-image waveform can be identified if some of the contacts of the strip electrode are placed on the opposite side of the central sulcus, over the motor cortex[20,21] (Fig. 42-1). For phase reversal, a strip electrode with four to eight stainless steel contacts with an intercontact distance of 1 cm is used. In the literature, the success rate of the phase reversal technique to indirectly localize the primary motor cortex ranges between 91%[20,21] and 97%.[18] Interestingly, identification of the central sulcus by magnetic resonance imaging provided contradictory results when compared with intraoperative phase reversal.[20] Although it is expected that ongoing progress in the field of functional magnetic resonance imaging will eventually replace the need for neurophysiologic tests, ION still retains the highest reliability in mapping of the motor cortex and language areas when compared with functional neuroimaging.[23–26]

Direct Cortical Stimulation (60-Hz Penfield Technique)

Once the motor strip has indirectly been identified by the phase reversal technique, direct cortical stimulation is needed to confirm the localization of the motor cortex.

Most current methods are based on the original Penfield technique. This calls for continuous direct cortical stimulation over a period of a few seconds with a frequency of stimulation of 50 to 60 Hz and observation of muscle movements.[14,16,27] An initial current intensity of 4 mA is used and, if no movements are elicited in contralateral muscles of the limbs and face, stimulation is increased in steps of 2 mA to the point at which movements are elicited.[16] Muscle responses can either be observed visually or documented by multichannel electromyography, which appears to be more sensitive.[28] If no response is elicited with an intensity as high as approximately 16 mA, that area of cortex is considered not functional and can therefore be removed.[29] It should be emphasized that a negative mapping does not always ensure safety. To increase the chances of obtaining a positive mapping result, technical and anesthesiologic drawbacks have to be carefully ruled out and cortical exposure should be generous.

Spreading of the current using the 60-Hz stimulation technique is limited to 2 to 3 mm as detected by optical imaging in monkeys.[30] Accordingly, one can assume that using this technique is safe for removal of tumors very close to the motor and sensory pathways as long as stimulation is repeated whenever a 2- to 3-mm section of tumoral tissue is removed.[29] Similarly, this technique allows us to map motor pathways subcortically while removing tumors that arise or extend to the insular, subinsular, or thalamic areas.[27,31] At the subcortical level, the stimulation intensity required to elicit a motor response is usually lower than that required for cortical mapping. When performing subcortical mapping, however, we have to keep in mind that a distal muscle response after stimulation of subcortical motor pathways can be misleading. Although this stimulation activates axons distal to the stimulation point, the possibility of damage to the pathways proximal to that point cannot be ruled out. This is a concern, especially when dealing with an insular tumor where there is a risk of cortical or subcortical ischemia induction secondary to manipulation of perforating vessels (Fig. 42-2).

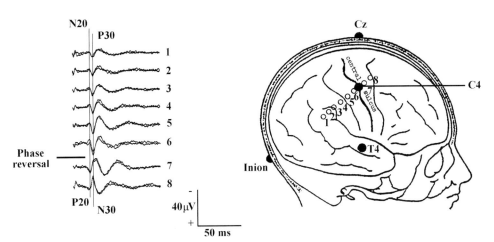

FIGURE 42-1 Identification of the central sulcus by phase reversal of median nerve cortical somatosensory evoked potentials. To the right is schematic drawing of the exposed brain surface with a grid electrode position orthogonally to the central sulcus. On the left are the recorded evoked potentials phase reversed between electrode 6 and 7, showing a mirror image of the evoked potential between the motor and sensory cortices, depicting the central sulcus lying between electrodes 6 and 7. (Reproduced from Deletis V: Intraoperative neurophysiological monitoring. In McLone D (ed): Pediatric neurosurgery: Surgery of the developing nervous system, 4th ed. Philadelphia: WB Saunders, 1999, pp 1204–1213.)

Despite the large consent and popularity acquired in the past, this 60-Hz Penfield technique has some disadvantages. With the exception of speech mapping, it is our opinion that these disadvantages should prevent its use as a motor cortex/pathways mapping technique. First, this technique can induce seizures in as many as 20% of patients, despite therapeutic levels of anticonvulsants and regardless of whether there is a preoperative history of intractable epilepsy.[32,33] Second, in children who are younger than 5 years old, direct stimulation of the motor cortex for mapping purposes may not yield localizing information because of the relative unexcitability of the motor cortex.[19,34] Third, because this is a mapping and not a monitoring technique, no matter how often cortical or subcortical stimulation is repeated, the functional integrity of the motor pathways cannot be assessed continuously during surgery.

In the illustrative case presented in Figure 42-2,[35] an impairment of muscle MEPs occurred at the end of tumor removal when opening and closing mapping procedures had already been done and confirmed the integrity of motor pathways distal to the stimulation point at the level of the internal capsule. However, ischemia of the pyramidal tracts secondary to severe vasospasm of the main perforating branches of the middle cerebral artery occurred during hemostasis and were detected by muscle MEP monitoring. If not detected in time, this event would have likely resulted in an irreversible loss of muscle MEPs and, consequently, a permanent motor deficit. Mapping techniques are unlikely to detect these events because they do not allow a continuous "online" assessment of the functional integrity of neural pathways.

Direct Cortical Stimulation and Motor Evoked Potential Monitoring (Short Train of Stimuli Technique)

Recently, mapping techniques have integrated monitoring techniques to continuously assess the functional integrity of the motor pathways and therefore increase the safety of these procedures.[20,35-37]

The following is a description of the technique that we use at our institutions and have found suitable for both mapping and monitoring.

Muscle MEPs are initially elicited by multipulse transcranial electrical stimulation (TES). Short trains of five to seven square-wave stimuli of 500-μsec duration with an interstimulus interval of 4 msec are applied at a repetition rate of as high as 2 Hz through electrodes placed at C1 and C2 scalp sites, according to the 10-20 International Electroencephalography System. The maximum stimulation intensity should be as high as 200 mA, which is strong enough for most cases. Muscle responses are recorded via needle electrodes inserted into the contralateral upper and

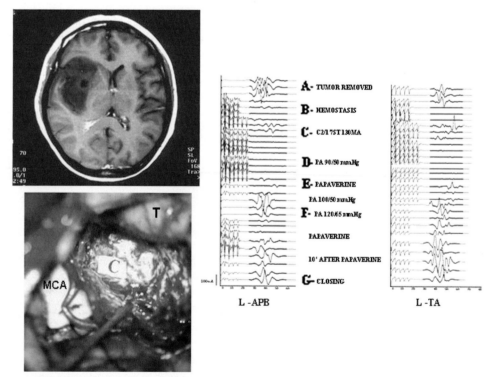

FIGURE 42-2 *Upper left:* Preoperative axial contrast-enhanced magnetic resonance T1-weighted image of a right frontotemporoinsular anaplastic astrocytoma that was removed with the assistance of intraoperative neurophysiologic monitoring. *Lower left:* Intraoperative view at the end of tumor resection. The internal capsule (C) has been identified using mapping of the subcortical motor pathways with the short train of stimuli technique. The temporal lobe (T) and branches of the middle cerebral artery (MCA) are on view. *Right:* Motor-evoked potentials (MEPs) recorded intraoperatively from the left abductor brevis pollicis (L-APB) and tibialis anterior (L-TA) muscles. A, MEP recordings at the end of tumor removal; B, MEP loss during hemostasis; C, transitory MEP reappearance by increasing stimulation to seven stimuli and 130-mA intensity; D, new disappearance of MEPs despite increased stimulation; E, F, progressive MEP reappearance after papaverine infusion and increased systemic blood pressure; G, MEPs at the end of the procedure. (Modified from Sala F, Lanteri P: Brain surgery in motor areas: The invaluable assistance of intraoperative neurophysiological monitoring. J Neurosurg Sci 47:79–88, 2003.)

lower extremity muscles. We usually monitored the abductor pollicis brevis and the extensor digitorum longus for the upper extremities and the tibialis anterior and the abductor hallucis for the lower extremities. For the face area, the orbicularis oculi and orbicularis oris muscles are typically used.

After exposure of the cortex and once phase reversal has been performed, direct cortical stimulation of the motor cortex can be achieved by using a monopolar-stimulating probe to identify the cortical representation of contralateral facial and limb muscles. The same parameters of stimulation used for TES, except for a much lower intensity (≤20 mA), can be used.[29] Sometimes the short train of stimuli technique requires slightly higher current intensities than those required by the bipolar Penfield technique. However, by using a very short train, the charge applied to the brain is significantly reduced[38] and, consequently, the risk of inducing seizures. The number of pulses in the short-train technique is five to seven pulses per second, whereas in the Penfield technique, there are 60 pulses per second. The effect of stimulation on the cerebral cortex, from a neurophysiologic point of view, differs between the Penfield technique and the short train of stimuli technique. The Penfield technique delivers one stimulus every 15 to 20 msec continuously for a couple of seconds. The short train of stimuli technique delivers five to seven stimuli in a period of approximately 30 msec with a long pause between trains (470 to 970 msec, which depends on train repetition rate; 1 or 2 Hz). Therefore, the Penfield technique is more prone to produce seizures, activating the cortical circuitry more easily than short-train stimuli do. Furthermore, compared with the Penfield technique, the short-train technique does not induce strong muscle twitches that may interfere with the surgical procedure. Responses are usually recorded from needle electrodes used to record muscle MEPs elicited by TES. However, any combination of recording muscles can be used, according to the tumor location. The larger the number of monitored muscles, the lower the chance of a false-negative mapping result. We suggest that stimulation of the tumoral area should always be performed to rule out the presence of some functional cortex. As already described, this is especially true in the case of low-grade gliomas.[3-5]

In our experience with using the short-train technique, a threshold lower than 5 to 10 mA for eliciting muscle MEPs usually indicated proximity to the motor cortex. When muscle responses are elicited through higher stimulation intensities, activation of the CT is of less localizing value because of the possibility of spreading of the current to adjacent areas.[35]

Once mapping of the cortex has clarified the relationship between eloquent motor areas and the lesion, continuous MEP monitoring of the contralateral muscles can be sustained throughout the procedure to assist during the surgical manipulation. To do so, one of the same contacts of the strip electrode can be used as an anode for stimulation while the cathode is at Fz. The stimulation point on the motor cortex with the lowest threshold used to elicit muscle MEPs from contralateral limbs or face usually corresponds with the contact from which the largest amplitude of the mirror-image SEPs was obtained. The same stimulation parameters as those used for the short-train mapping technique can be used.

When removing a tumor that extends subcortically, preservation of muscle MEPs during monitoring from the strip electrode will guarantee the functional integrity of motor pathways and avoid the need for periodic remapping of the cortex at known functional sites.[35]

For insular tumors where the motor cortex is not exposed by the craniotomy, a strip electrode can still be gently inserted into the subdural space to overlap the motor cortex. Phase reversal and/or direct cortical stimulation can be used to identify the electrode with the lowest threshold to elicit muscle MEPs.

Warning Criteria and Correlation with Postoperative Outcome

Still debated are the warning criteria for changes in muscle MEPs that are used to inform the surgeon about an impending injury to the motor system. It should be stressed that although for spinal cord surgery, a "presence/absence" of muscle MEPs criterion has proved to be reliable and strictly correlates with postoperative results,[39,40] there are not definite MEP parameters indicative of significant impairment during supratentorial surgery.[41] We believe that the predictive value of muscle MEPs is different for supratentorial and spinal cord surgeries. As such, different warning criteria must be employed. This judgment is based on the difference in types of CT fibers in supratentorial portion of the CT as compared with the spinal cord. Different groups with established experience in this field have proposed similar criteria,[30,41] suggesting that a shift in latency between 10% and 15% and a decrease in amplitude of more than 50% to 80% correlate with some degree of postoperative motor deficit. However, a permanent new motor deficit has consistently correlated only with irreversible complete loss of muscle MEPs.[41]

A persistent increase in the threshold to elicit muscle MEPs or a persistent drop in muscle MEP amplitude, despite stable systemic blood pressure, anesthesia, and body temperature, represents a warning sign. However, it should be noted that muscle MEPs are easily affected by muscle relaxants and high concentrations of volatile (and other) anesthetics such that wide variation in muscle MEP amplitude and latency can be observed.[42] Due to this variability, the multisynaptic nature of the pathways involved in the generation of muscle MEPs, and the nonlinear relationship between stimulus intensity and the amplitude of muscle MEPs, the correlation between intraoperative changes in muscle MEPs (amplitude and/or latency) and the motor outcome are not linear. Further clinical investigation is needed to clarify sensitive and specific neurophysiologic warning criteria for brain surgery.

Brain Stem Surgery

The human brain stem is a small and highly complex structure containing a variety of critical neural structures. These include sensory and motor pathways; sensory and motor cranial nerve nuclei; cardiovascular and respiratory centers; neural networks supporting swallowing, coughing, articulation, and oculomotor reflexes; and the reticular activating system. In such a complex neural structure, even small lesions can produce severe and life-threatening neurologic deficits.

The neurosurgeon faces two major problems when attempting to remove brain stem tumors. First, if the tumor is intrinsic and does not project on the brain stem surface, approaching the tumor implies a violation of the anatomic integrity of the brain stem. Knowledge of the location of critical neural pathways and nuclei is mandatory when considering a safe entry into the brain stem[43,44] but may not suffice when anatomy is distorted. Morota and colleagues[45] reported that visual identification of the facial colliculus based on anatomic landmarks was possible in only three of seven medullary tumors and was not possible in five pontine tumors. The striae medullares were visible in four of five patients with pontine tumors and in five of nine patients with medullary tumors.

Therefore, functional rather than anatomic localization of brain stem nuclei and pathways should be used to identify safe entry zones.

Mapping Techniques

Neurophysiologic mapping techniques have been increasingly used to localize CT and cranial nerve motor nuclei on the lateral aspect of the midbrain and on the floor of the fourth ventricle.[45-49]

Mapping of the Corticospinal Tract at the Level of the Cerebral Peduncle

This is a recently described technique used to map the CT tract within the brain stem at the level of the cerebral peduncle.[49] To identify the CT, we use a hand-held monopolar-stimulating probe (0.75-mm tip diameter) as a cathode, with a needle electrode inserted in a nearby muscle as an anode. If the response (D wave) is recorded from an epidural electrode, a single stimulus is used. Conversely, if the response is recorded as a compound muscle action potential from one or more muscles of contralateral limbs, a short train of stimuli should be used.

We usually increase stimulation intensity to 2 mA. When a motor response is recorded, the probe is then moved in small increments of 1 mm to find the lowest threshold to elicit that response.

This technique is particularly useful for midbrain tumors that have displaced the CT tract from its original position. Usually, the so-called midbrain lateral vein described by Rhoton[50] represents a useful anatomic landmark because it allows an indirect identification of the CT tract, located anterior to the vein. However, when an expansive lesion distorts anatomy, only neurophysiologic mapping allows the identification of the CT and, consequently, a safe entry zone to the lateral midbrain.

In the case of a cystic midbrain lesion, sometimes mapping of the CT is negative at the beginning of the procedure, but a positive response can be recorded when mapping from within the cystic cavity toward the anterolateral cystic wall.[51]

Mapping of Motor Nuclei of Cranial Nerves on the Floor of the Fourth Ventricle

This technique is based on intraoperative electrical stimulation of the motor nuclei of the cranial nerves on the floor of the fourth ventricle, using a hand-held monopolar-stimulating probe. Compound muscle action potentials are then elicited in the muscles innervated by the cranial motor nerves. A single stimulus of 0.2-msec duration is delivered at a repetitive rate of 2.0 Hz. Stimulation intensity starts at approximately 1 mA and is then reduced to determine the point with the lowest threshold that elicits muscle responses corresponding with the mapped nucleus (Fig. 42-3). No stimulation intensity higher than 2 mA should be used.[45,46] To record the responses from cranial motor nerves VII, IX/X, and XII, wire electrodes are inserted into the orbicularis oculi and orbicularis oris muscles, the posterior wall of the pharynx, and the lateral aspect of the tongue muscles, respectively. Based on mapping studies, characteristic patterns of motor cranial nerve displacement, secondary to tumor growth, have been described[52] (Fig. 42-4). The case described in Figure 42-5 is consistent with this observation.

A similar methodology can be applied to identify the motor nuclei of cranial nerves innervating ocular muscles (nerves III, IV, and VI) during a dorsal approach to midbrain lesions as well as quadrigeminal plate, tectal, and pineal region tumors.[53,54]

Despite the relative straightforwardness of the fourth ventricle mapping technique and its indisputable usefulness in planning the most appropriate surgical strategy to enter the brain stem, postoperative functional outcome is not always predicted by postresection responses.[45] In the case of mapping of the motor nuclei of the seventh cranial nerve, brain stem mapping cannot detect injury to the supranuclear tracts originating in the motor cortex and ending on the cranial nerve motor nuclei. Consequently, a supranuclear paralysis would not be detected, although lower motoneuron integrity has been preserved. Similarly, the possibility of stimulating the intramedullary root more than the nuclei itself exists. This could result in a false-negative peripheral response still being recorded despite an injury to the motor nuclei.[45]

Mapping of the glossopharyngeal nuclei is also of limited benefit. Recording activity from the muscles of the posterior pharyngeal wall after stimulation of the ninth cranial nerve motor nuclei on the floor of the fourth ventricle assesses the functional integrity of the efferent arc of the swallowing reflex. This technique, however, does not provide information on the integrity of afferent pathways and afferent/efferent connections within brain stem, which are indeed necessary to provide functions involving reflexive swallowing, coughing, and the complex act of articulation. Recently, however, Sakuma and colleagues[55] succeeded in monitoring glossopharyngeal nerve compound action potentials after stimulation of the tongue in dogs, opening the possibility of a new field of investigation in humans. Functional magnetic resonance imaging of the brain stem has also provided a new, yet experimental, tool to localize cranial nerve nuclei in humans.[56]

An intrinsic limitation of all mapping techniques, however, is that these do not allow the continuous evaluation of the functional integrity of a neural pathway. The identification of the safe entry zone for approaching a pontine astrocytoma, as in Figure 42-5, does not provide any information on the well-being of the adjacent corticospinal, corticobulbar, sensory, and auditory pathways during the surgical manipulation aimed to remove the tumor. Therefore, it is essential to combine mapping with monitoring techniques.

Monitoring Techniques

SEPs and brain stem auditory evoked potentials have been extensively used to assess the functional integrity of the

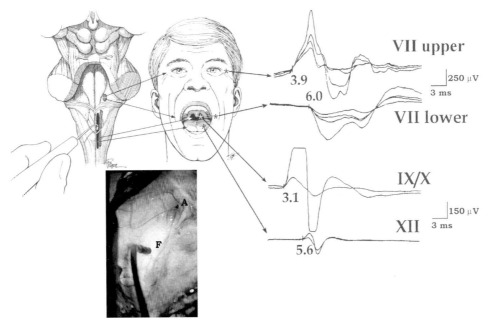

FIGURE 42-3 Mapping of the brain stem cranial nerve motor nuclei. *Upper left:* Drawing of the exposed floor of the fourth ventricle with the surgeon's hand-held stimulating probe in view. *Upper middle:* The sites of insertion of wire hook electrodes for recording the muscle responses are depicted. *Far upper right:* Compound muscle action potentials recorded from the orbicularis oculi and oris muscles after stimulation of the upper and lower facial nuclei (*upper two traces*) and from the pharyngeal wall and tongue muscles after stimulation of the motor nuclei of cranial nerves IX/X and XII (*lower two traces*). *Lower left:* Photograph obtained from the operating microscope shows the hand-held stimulating probe placed on the floor of the fourth ventricle (F). A, aqueduct. (Reproduced from Deletis V, Sala F, Morota N: Intraoperative neurophysiological monitoring and mapping during brain stem surgery: A modern approach. Oper Tech Neurosurg 3:109–113, 2000.)

brain stem, and we refer the reader to the related literature for a review of these classic techniques. Unfortunately, SEPs and brain stem auditory evoked potentials can evaluate only approximately 20% of brain stem pathways.[57] As a result, their use is of limited valued when the major concern is related to corticospinal and cranial nerve motor function. Still, brain stem auditory evoked potentials can provide useful information on the general well-being of the brain stem, especially during those procedures in which a significant surgical manipulation of the brain stem and/or of the cerebellum is expected. When interpreting brain stem auditory evoked potential recordings, a thoughtful analysis of the waveform and of their correlation with neural generators provides useful information about the localization of the changes.

When an initial myelotomy is performed at the region of dorsal column nuclei of the medulla, further monitoring with SEPs is compromised due to limitations similar to those related to intramedullary spinal cord tumor surgery after myelotomy.[49] For pontine and midbrain tumors, SEPs have little localizing value but can still be used to provide nonspecific information about the general functional integrity of the brain stem (because it is expected that a major impending brain stem failure will be detected by changes in SEP parameters).

Similar to what has occurred for brain and spinal cord surgery, the major breakthrough in modern ION of the brain stem has been the advent of MEP-related techniques.

With regard to motor function within the brain stem, standard techniques for continuously assessing the functional integrity of motor cranial nerves relies on the recording of spontaneous electromyographic activity in the muscles innervated by motor cranial nerves.[54,58,59] Several criteria have been proposed to identify electromyographic activity patterns that may anticipate transitory or permanent nerve injury, but these patterns are not always easily recognizable and criteria remain vague or at least subjective. Overall, convincing data regarding a clinical correlation between electromyographic activity and clinical outcomes is still lacking.[54,58]

Seeking more reliable techniques in the neurophysiologic monitoring of motor cranial nerve integrity, the possibility of extending the principles of CT monitoring to the corticobulbar tracts is currently under investigation.[51]

Monitoring of Corticobulbar (Corticonuclear) Pathways

For this purpose, TES with a train of four stimuli, with an interstimulus interval of 4 msec, and a train-stimulating rate of 1 to 2 Hz, intensity between 60 and 100 mA can be used. The stimulating electrode montage is usually C3/Cz for right side muscles and C4/Cz for left side muscles. For recording muscle MEPs, electromyographic wire electrodes are inserted in the orbicularis oris and orbicularis oculi muscles for nerve VII, in the posterior pharyngeal wall for the cranial motor nerves IX and X, and in the tongue muscles for the hypoglossal nerve (i.e., in the same manner as described for mapping of motor nuclei of the cranial nerves). Reproducible muscle MEPs can be continuously recorded from the facial, pharyngeal, and tongue muscles

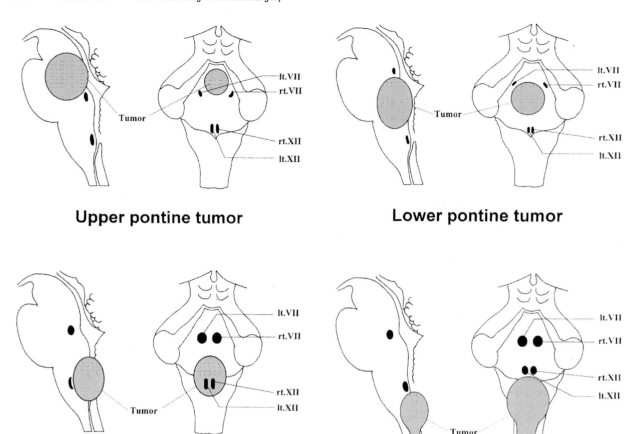

Upper pontine tumor

Lower pontine tumor

Medullary tumor

Cervicomedullary junction spinal cord tumor

FIGURE 42-4 Typical patterns of cranial nerve motor nuclei displacement by brain stem tumors in different locations. Upper and lower pontine tumors: Pontine tumors typically grow to push the facial nuclei around the edge of the tumor, suggesting that precise localization of the facial nuclei before tumor resection is necessary to avoid their damage during surgery. Medullary tumors: Medullary tumors typically grow more exophytically and compress the lower cranial nerve motor nuclei ventrally; these nuclei may be located on the ventral edge of the tumor cavity. Because of the interposed tumor, in these cases mapping before tumor resection usually does not allow identification of cranial nerve IX/X and XII motor nuclei. Responses, however, could be obtained close to the end of the tumor resection when most of the tumoral tissue between the stimulating probe and the motor nuclei has been removed. At this point, repeat mapping is recommended because the risk of damaging motor nuclei is significantly higher than at the beginning of tumor debulking. Cervicomedullary junction spinal cord tumors: These tumors simply push the lower cranial nerve motor nuclei rostrally when extending into the fourth ventricle. (Reproduced from Morota N, Deletis V, Lee M, et al: Functional anatomic relationship between brain stem tumors and cranial motor nuclei. Neurosurgery 39:787–794, 1996.)

while the brain stem is surgically manipulated (see Fig. 42-5). This technique allows one to monitor the entire pathway, from the motor cortex down to the neuromuscular junction so that a supranuclear injury can be detected. However, the corticobulbar tract monitoring technique is still far from becoming standardized due to some theoretical and practical drawbacks. First, from a neurophysiologic perspective, use of the lateral montage as an anodal stimulating electrode (C3 or C4) increases the risk that strong TES may not activate the corticobulbar pathways but the cranial nerve directly. Accordingly, an injury to the corticobulbar pathway rostral to the point of activation may be masked by a misleading preservation of the muscle MEP. To minimize this risk, stimulation intensity should be kept as low as possible. Furthermore, given the continuous fluctuations in the threshold required to elicit muscle MEPs intraoperatively (i.e., due to variability in room temperature, anesthesiologic regimen, and physiologic variability in muscle MEP

threshold, and so on), the appropriate threshold for monitoring corticobulbar pathways should be rechecked throughout the surgical procedure. Another limitation of this technique is that spontaneous electromyographic activity can sometimes hinder the recording of reliable muscle MEPs from the same muscles. In our experience, this spontaneous activity appears to be more common in the pharyngeal muscles as compared with the facial and tongue muscles. Further experience with this technique will indicate the extent to which monitoring of the corticobulbar tract predicts postoperative function and allows an impending injury to the motor cranial nerves to be recognized in time to be corrected (see Fig. 42-5).

Due to the complexity of the brain stem's functional anatomy, the more neurophysiologic techniques that can be rationally integrated, the better the chances are for successful monitoring.[60] The battery of techniques to be used should be tailored to each individual patient according to tumor

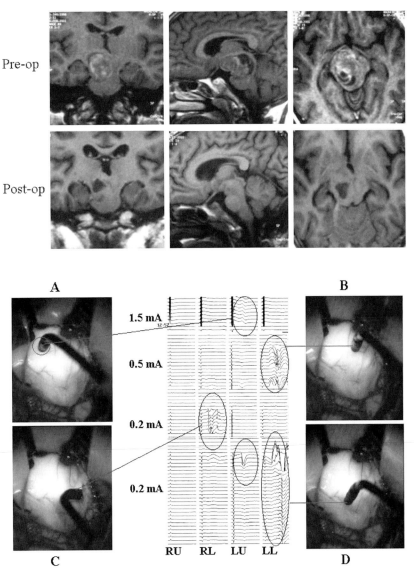

FIGURE 42-5 *Upper panel:* Preoperative contrast-enhanced T1-weighted magnetic resonance images of a right midbrain pilocytic astrocytoma in a 4-year-old child. Postoperative magnetic resonance imaging (MRI): Total removal of the tumor is documented at a 4-month follow-up MRI study. *Middle panel:* Direct mapping of the facial nerve motor nuclei on the floor of the fourth ventricle in a patient with a left pontine low-grade astrocytoma. The tumor was approached through a median suboccipital craniectomy. When the floor of the fourth ventricle was exposed, the median sulcus appeared dislocated to the right and the left median eminence was expanded. Electromyographic wire electrodes were inserted bilaterally in the left (LU) and right (RU) orbicularis oculi and left (LL) and right (RL) orbicularis oris muscles for mapping and monitoring of the seventh nerve, and in the abductor pollicis brevis (LA and RA) for continuous monitoring of the corticospinal tract integrity. We initially stimulated on the left side, approximately 1.5 cm rostral to the striae medullares, where the motor nuclei were expected to be according to normal brain stem functional anatomy. A response was obtained from the left orbicularis oculi (LU) at a stimulation intensity of 1.5 mA (*A*). By moving the stimulating probe caudally and to the right, a consistent response from the left orbicularis oris (LL) was recorded at a stimulation intensity of 0.5 mA (*B*). At this point, we moved the stimulation probe more laterally to the right side, approximately 1 cm above the striae medullares, and a clear response was recorded from the right orbicularis oris (RL) at the lowest threshold intensity of 0.2 mA (*C*). Finally, by moving the stimulating probe paramedially to the left side, a few millimeters above the striae medullares, a consistent response was recorded from both the left orbicularis oris (LL) and orbicularis oculi (LU), using the same low threshold (0.2 mA) (*D*). The conclusion was drawn that the tumor displaced caudally the facial nerve motor nuclei, especially on the left side. Based on mapping results, the surgeon decided to enter the brain stem on the left side in correspondence with the higher threshold stimulating point (*A*).

(Continued)

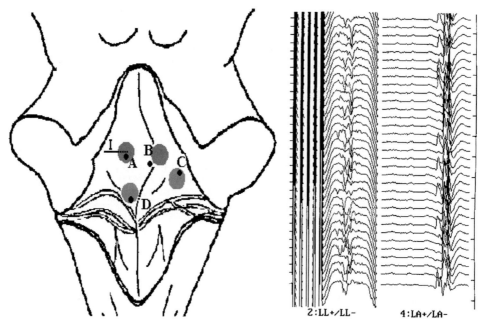

FIGURE 42-5 Cont'd   *Lower left:* Schematic summary of mapping results. A and B represent the original position of the left and right facial colliculi, as expected according to brain stem anatomy. A, B, C, and D correspond to the stimulating point illustrated in the upper panel. C and D also correspond to the lower threshold to elicit a consistent response from, respectively, the right and left muscles innervated by the facial nerve. The conclusion was made that real location of facial nerve motor nuclei (C and D) was more caudal than expected, especially on the left side, due to the tumor mass effect. Accordingly, initial incision (I) was carried on transversely in correspondence with stimulating point A. *Lower right:* Continuous neurophysiologic monitoring of muscle motor-evoked potentials during tumor removal. Electromyographic wire electrodes were inserted in the left orbicularis oris (LL) and abductor pollicis brevis (LA) muscles for continuous monitoring of, respectively, the corticobulbar and corticospinal tract integrity, after transcranial electrical stimulation (electrode montage C4/Cz; short train of four stimuli; intensity 50 mA). (Modified from Sala F, Lanteri P, Bricolo A: Intraoperative neurophysiological monitoring of motor evoked potentials during brain stem and spinal cord surgery. Adv Tech Stand Neurosurg 29, 2004, pp 133–169.)

location and clinical status. Keeping this in mind, SEPs and brain stem auditory evoked potentials should always be considered. However, unlike in the past decade when these classic monitoring methods allowed only a very limited assessment of the brain stem functional integrity, current techniques of MEP monitoring and motor nuclei mapping are receiving increasing credit in assisting the neurosurgeon during brain stem surgery.

Spinal and Spinal Cord Surgery

These surgeries are potentially burdened with serious neurologic deficits such as para- or quadriplegia (paresis). As a rule, the closer to the spinal cord that the neurosurgeon operates, the higher is the risk of injury. Of course, there is always the possibility that surgeries on the bony structures of the spinal cord can result in paraplegia.[61] Furthermore, long-lasting intraoperative hypotension can be disastrous for the spinal cord if neurophysiologic monitoring has not been used because no other routine methods are available to evaluate the functional integrity of the spinal cord during hypotension.

It has been shown that the use of SEPs to monitor the functional integrity of the spinal cord is inadequate and can result in false-negative results (i.e., no changes in SEP parameters intraoperatively, but the patient wakes up paraplegic after surgery[61,62]). Therefore, it is mandatory that during spinal and spinal cord surgeries, monitoring of both sensory and motor modalities of evoked potentials is conducted. Each of these methods evaluates different long tracts; SEPs evaluate

the dorsal columns, whereas MEPs evaluate CT. If a lesion to the spinal cord is diffuse in nature, affecting both long tracts, monitoring one of them may suffice. Unfortunately, this is not always the case. A typical example is anterior spinal cord artery syndrome with preservation of SEPs and disappearance of MEPs.

Surgery for intramedullary spinal cord tumors requires a special approach concerning monitoring with MEPs. During this type of surgery, very precise surgical instruments are used, such as the Contact Laser System (SLT, Montgomeryville, PA),[63] and a very selective lesion within the spinal cord can occur. Therefore, monitoring this type of surgery using only MEPs recorded from limb muscles can be insufficient. Monitoring the D wave (i.e., recording descending activity of the CT using catheter electrodes placed over the exposed spinal cord) should be combined with MEP recording from limb muscles. Combining both of these techniques proved highly effective in preventing paraplegia/quadriplegia. This gives the neurosurgeon the opportunity to be more radical in tumor resection. This combined type of monitoring can precisely predict transient postoperative motor deficits[40,64] and clearly distinguish them from permanent ones.

Neurophysiologic Monitoring of the Spinal Cord and Spinal Surgeries with Motor-Evoked Potentials

A schematic drawing of techniques for eliciting MEPs by TES or direct electrical stimulation of the exposed motor cortex while recording them from the spinal cord (D wave) or limb muscles (muscle MEPs) is presented in Figure 42-6.

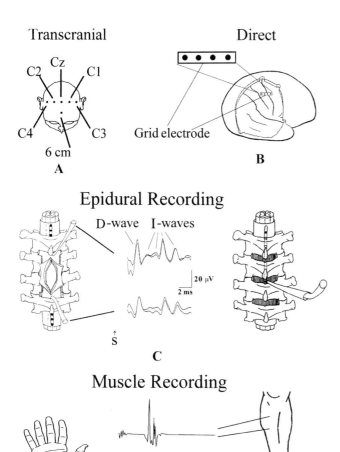

Transcranial

Cz
C2   C1
C4   C3
6 cm
A

Direct

Grid electrode

B

Epidural Recording

D-wave   I-waves

20 µV
2 ms

Ŝ

C

Muscle Recording

D

FIGURE 42-6 *A*, Schematic illustration of electrode positions for transcranial electrical stimulation of the motor cortex according to the 10-20 International Electroencephalography System. The site labeled 6 cm is 6 cm anterior to Cz. *B*, Illustration of grid electrode overlying the motor and sensory cortexes. *C*, Schematic diagram of the positions of the catheter electrodes (each with three recording cylinders) placed cranial to the tumor (control electrode) and caudal to the tumor to monitor the descending signal after passing through the site of surgery (*left*). In the middle are D and I waves recorded rostral and caudal to the tumor site. On the right is depicted the placement of an epidural electrode through a flavectomy/flavotomy when the spinal cord is not exposed. *D*, Recording of muscle motor-evoked potentials from the thenar and tibial anterior muscles after eliciting them with short train of stimuli applied either transcranially or over the exposed motor cortex. (Modified from Deletis V, Rodi Z, Amassian VE: Neurophysiological mechanisms underlying motor evoked potentials in anesthetized humans. Part 2: Relationship between epidurally and muscle recorded MEPs in man. Clin Neurophysiol 112:445–452, 2001.)

TABLE 42-1 ▪ Principles of Motor-Evoked Potential Interpretation

D Wave	Muscle MEP*	Motor Status
Unchanged or 30%–50% decrease	Preserved	Unchanged
Unchanged or 30%–50% decrease	Lost uni- or bilaterally	Transient motor deficit
>50% decrease	Lost bilaterally	Long-term motor deficit

*In the tibial anterior muscle(s).

Reproduced from Deletis V: Intraoperative neurophysiological monitoring. In McLone D (ed): Pediatric Neurosurgery: Surgery of the Developing Nervous System, 4th ed. Philadelphia: WB Saunders, 1999, pp 1204–1213.

achieve a good postoperative motor outcome, it is imperative that the critical decrement in D wave amplitude not be permitted. The neurophysiologic explanation for transient paraplegia is that the D wave is generated exclusively by the descending activity of the transcranially activated fast neurons of the CT, whereas muscle MEPs are generated by the combined action of the fast neurons of the CT and propriospinal and other descending tracts within the spinal cord (of course with consecutive activation of alpha motoneurons, peripheral nerves, and muscles). The selective lesion to the propriospinal and other descending tracts can occur with the use of precise neurosurgical instruments (e.g., contact laser with a tip of 200 µm, producing minimal collateral damage).[63] Lesioning of the propriospinal system and other descending tracts can be functionally compensated postoperatively, whereas a lesion to the fast neurons of the CT cannot. Empirically, we have discovered that decrements in the amplitude of the D wave occur in a stepwise fashion (except in the case of anterior spinal artery lesion). Therefore, the neurosurgeon has enough time to make a decision and can immediately stop the surgery when a critical decrement in D wave amplitude occurs. The previous statement has been tested in 100 surgeries for intramedullary spinal cord tumors performed by one neurosurgeon and using a combined monitoring method. This approach showed a sensitivity of 100% and a specificity of 91%.[40] Based on these results, Table 42-1 was produced to explain the meaning and predictive features of combined monitoring of the spinal cord surgery using muscle MEPs and D wave.

Combined monitoring of MEPs in one typical patient with an intramedullary spinal cord tumor showed a disappearance of muscle MEPs and a sustained D wave. This resulted in a transient postoperative paraplegia, with a complete recovery from paraplegia, as presented in Figure 42-7.

Mapping of the Corticospinal Tract within the Surgically Exposed Spinal Cord

Further improvement in the prevention of lesioning of the CT during spinal cord surgery has been achieved by introducing a neurophysiologic method of mapping the CT by using a D wave collision technique. This technique has recently been developed by our group and has allowed us to precisely map the anatomic location of the CT when the anatomy of the spinal cord has been distorted.[65] The anatomic position of the CT is difficult to determine by visual inspection alone.

Table 42-1 summarizes the results from the combined use of D wave and muscle MEP recordings during surgery for intramedullary spinal cord tumors. The neurosurgeon can proceed with the surgery aggressively, without jeopardizing the patient's motor status despite the complete disappearance of the muscle MEPs during surgery. This is only allowed when the D wave amplitude does not decrease more than 50% from the baseline amplitude. After disappearance of muscle MEPs, patients will have only transient postoperative motor deficits, with a full recovery of muscle strength later on. Therefore, to

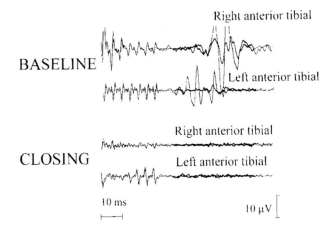

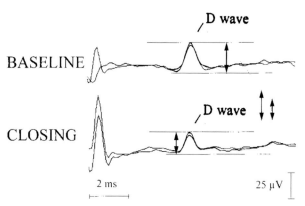

FIGURE 42-7 A 9-year-old boy underwent gross total resection of a pilocytic astrocytoma of the thoracic spinal cord that spanned four spinal segments. Preoperatively, there were no motor deficits. During surgery, the muscle motor-evoked potentials from the left and right tibial anterior muscles were lost (*upper*) and the D wave decreased, although not less than 50% of baseline value (*lower*). Postoperatively, the patient was paraplegic. Within 1 week, he regained antigravity force in both legs, and by 2 weeks he walked again. (Reproduced from Kothbauer K, Deletis V, Epstein FJ: Intraoperative spinal cord monitoring for intramedullary surgery: An essential adjunct. Pediatr Neurosurg 26:247–254, 1997.)

D wave collision is accomplished by simultaneously stimulating the exposed spinal cord (with a small hand-held probe delivering a 2-mA intensity stimulus), with TES to elicit a D wave. Because the resulting signals are transmitted along the same axons, the descending D wave collides with the ascending signal carried antidromically along the CT (Fig. 42-8). This results in a decrease in the D wave amplitude recorded cranially to the collision site. This phenomenon indicates that the spinal cord–stimulating probe is in close proximity to the CT. This could potentially guide surgeons to stay away from the "hot spot." Mapping of the CT is now in the process of a technical refinement. Its initial use indicates an impressive ability to selectively map the spinal cord for the CT's anatomic location. Using this method, the CT can be localized within 1 mm. This is in concordance with the other CT mapping techniques used within the brain stem that show the same degree of selectivity.[45]

Mapping of the Dorsal Columns of the Spinal Cord

To protect the dorsal columns from lesioning during myelotomy, a novel neurophysiologic technique has been developed. To approach an intramedullary tumor, accepted neurosurgical techniques require a midline dorsal myelotomy. Distorted anatomy, however, often does not allow a precise determination of the anatomic midline by visual inspection and anatomic landmarks. Therefore, to facilitate the precise determination of the medial border between the left and right dorsal columns of the spinal cord, a technique for dorsal column mapping has been developed.[66] Dorsal column mapping is based on two basic principles: First, after stimulation of the peripheral nerves, evoked potentials traveling through the dorsal columns can be recorded. Second, the area over the dorsal columns of the spinal cord where the maximal amplitude of the SEPs is recorded represents the point on the recording electrode in closest proximity to the dorsal columns. For recording these traveling waves, a miniature multielectrode is placed over the surgically exposed dorsal columns of the spinal cord. This electrode consists of eight parallel wires, 76 μm in diameter and 2 mm in length, placed 1 mm apart and embedded in a 1-cm² (approximately) silicone plate (Fig. 42-9). An extremely precise amplitude gradient of the SEPs is recorded as the conducted potentials pass beneath the electrodes after alternating stimulation of the tibial nerves.

The amplitude gradient of the conducted potentials indicates the precise location of the functional midline corresponding to the dorsal fissure of the spinal cord (i.e., the optimal site for myelotomy). These data can be used by the neurosurgeon to prevent injury to the dorsal columns that could occur through an imprecise midline myelotomy. This is especially useful during surgery for intramedullary spinal cord tumors or during the placement of a shunt to drain syringomyelic cysts (see Fig. 42-9).

Neurophysiologic Monitoring during Spinal Endovascular Procedures

Endovascular procedures for the embolization of spinal and spinal cord vascular lesions carry the risk of spinal cord ischemia.[67] Whenever these procedures are performed under general anesthesia, only neurophysiologic monitoring can provide an "online" assessment of the functional integrity of sensory and motor pathways. Monitoring of SEPs and muscle MEPs is performed in the same fashion as described for monitoring of intramedullary spinal cord tumor surgery.[68,69] The D wave, in contrast, is usually not monitored during these procedures because these patients receive a considerable amount of heparin in the perioperative period and the percutaneous placement of the recording epidural electrode would expose the patient to the risk of an epidural bleed. Besides safety issues, there is also no evidence that monitoring the D wave is an essential adjunct to muscle MEPs during these endovascular procedures. Both peripheral and myogenic MEPs have, in fact, been proven to be more sensitive than the D wave in detecting spinal cord ischemia. Similar results have been consistently reported both in experimental and clinical studies, supporting the hypothesis that whenever the mechanism of spinal cord injury is purely ischemic, muscle MEPs may suffice.[70–73]

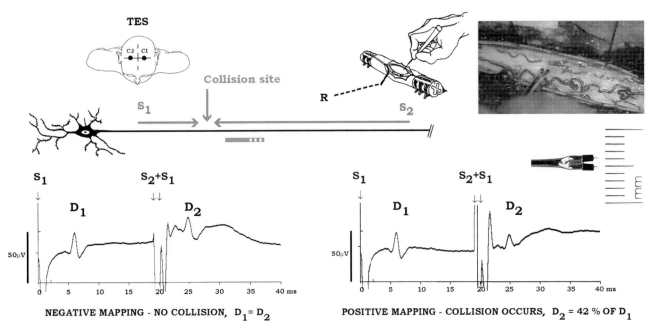

FIGURE 42-8 The neurophysiologic basis for intraoperative mapping of the corticospinal tract (CT). Mapping of the CT by the D wave collision technique (see text for details). S_1, transcranial electrical stimulation (TES); S_2, spinal cord electrical stimulation; D_1, control D wave (TES only); D_2, D wave after combined stimulation of the brain and spinal cord; R, the cranial electrode for recording D wave in the spinal epidural space. *Lower left:* Negative mapping results ($D_1 = D_2$). *Lower right:* Positive mapping results (D_2-wave amplitude significantly diminished after collision). *Inset:* Hand-held stimulating probe over the exposed spinal cord. (Modified from Deletis V, Camargo AB: Interventional neurophysiological mapping during spinal cord procedures. Stereotact Funct Neurosurg 77:25–28, 2001.)

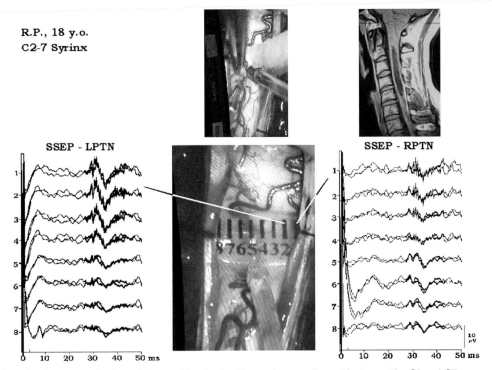

FIGURE 42-9 Dorsal column mapping in an 18-year-old patient with a syringomyelic cyst between the C2 and C7 segments of the spinal cord. *Upper right:* Magnetic resonance imaging shows the syrinx. *Lower middle:* Placement of miniature electrode over surgically exposed dorsal column; vertical bars on the electrode represent the location of the underlying exposed electrode surfaces. Sensory evoked potentials after stimulation of the left and right tibial nerves showing maximal amplitude between electrodes 1 and 2 (*lower left and right*). These data strongly indicate that both dorsal columns from the left and right lower extremities have been pushed to the extreme right side of the spinal cord. Using these data as a guideline, the surgeon performed the myelotomy using a YAG laser through the left side of the spinal cord and inserted the shunt to drain the cyst (*upper middle*). The patient did not experience a postoperative sensory deficit. (Reproduced from Kržan MJ: Intraoperative neurophysiological mapping of the spinal cord's dorsal column. In Deletis V, Shils JL (eds): Neurophysiology in Neurosurgery. A Modern Intraoperative Approach. San Diego, CA: Academic Press, 2002, pp 153–164.)

Given the complexity of spinal cord hemodynamics, which is even more unpredictable in the presence of a spinal cord hypervascularized lesion, it is mandatory to perform both SEP and MEP monitoring to enhance the safety of these risky procedures.[69]

A critical step regarding neurophysiologic monitoring during these procedures consists of the provocative tests.[69,74,75] These tests rely on the properties of two drugs, lidocaine and amobarbital, to selectively block axonal and neuronal conduction (respectively) when injected intra-arterially in the spinal cord.[76] Provocative tests are usually performed once the endovascular catheter has reached the embolizing position, before any embolizing material is injected. If that specific vessel not only feeds the target of the embolization (e.g., spinal cord arteriovenous malformation, hemangioblastoma, arteriovenous fistula) but also perfuses normal spinal cord, it is expected that the provocative drug will block the white and/or gray matter conduction, and this will be reflected in neurophysiologic tests. Criteria for positive provocative tests are the disappearance of the MEPs and/or a 50% decrease in SEP amplitude. If the test is positive, embolization from that specific catheter position is not performed and embolization from a different feeder or from a more selectively advanced catheter position is attempted. Provocative tests mimic the effect of the embolization and select those patients amenable to a safe embolization. Although the specificity of provocative tests has not been tested (because the procedure is abandoned whenever provocative tests are consistently positive), their sensitivity has proven to be very high and no false-negative results (i.e., new postoperative neurologic deficit despite embolization performed after a negative provocative test) have so far been reported.[69]

Surgery of the Lumbosacral Nervous System

Intraoperative monitoring during surgery of the lumbosacral nervous system is a very demanding task and is still not developed in comparison with monitoring of the surgeries for other parts of the central and peripheral nervous systems. The neurophysiologic techniques used to monitor the lumbosacral nervous system are dependent on the pathology and structures involved. Generally, monitoring of the lumbosacral system involves the epiconus, conus, and cauda equina. These structures are essential in both voluntary and reflexive control of micturition, defecation, and sexual function as well as somatosensory and motor innervation of the pelvis and lower extremities. So far, only methodologies for monitoring and mapping of the somatomotor and somatosensory components of the lumbosacral nervous system have been developed. Intraoperative monitoring of the vegetative component of the lumbosacral nervous system is still in the embryonic stage.

One of the most widely used applications of intraoperative monitoring of the lumbosacral nervous system, at least in the pediatric population, is for patients undergoing surgery for a tethered spinal cord. During these procedures, the surgeon cuts the filum terminale or removes the tethering tissue that envelopes the conus and/or the cauda equina roots. In a large series of patients operated on for tethered spinal cords, permanent neurologic complications have been described

in as many as 4.5%.[77,78] The rate increased to 10.9% when transient complications were considered. Due to the tethering, the lumbosacral nerve roots leave the spinal cord in different directions than in a healthy spinal cord. Furthermore, the cord may be skewed and sometimes a nerve root may pass through a lipoma. Nerve roots may also be involved in the thickened filum terminale that is cut during untethering. Direct electric stimulation of these structures in the surgical field or direct recording from them after peripheral nerve stimulation has proven helpful. Using mapping techniques, functional neural structures of the lumbosacral region can be correctly identified and thus possibly preserved. In Figure 42-10, schematic drawings of the most important neurophysiologic techniques for monitoring afferent and efferent events (i.e., recording and monitoring neurophysiologic signals from sensory or motor parts of the lumbosacral system) are presented. During intraoperative testing with these techniques, it has been found that some of them are more important than others, from pragmatic point of view. Only these are described.

Pudendal Dorsal Root Action Potentials

In the treatment of spasticity (e.g., in cerebral palsy), sacral roots are increasingly being included during rhizotomy procedures.[79] Children who underwent L2–S2 rhizotomies had an 81% greater reduction in plantar/flexor spasticity compared with children who underwent only L2–S1 rhizotomies. However, as more sacral dorsal roots have been included in rhizotomies, neurosurgeons have experienced an increased rate of postoperative complications, especially with regards to bowel and bladder functions.

To spare sacral function, we have attempted to identify those sacral dorsal roots carrying afferents from pudendal nerves using recordings of dorsal root action potentials after stimulation of dorsal penile or clitoral nerves. Patients were anesthetized with isoflurane, nitrous oxide, fentanyl, and a short-acting muscle relaxant introduced only at the time of intubation. The cauda equina was exposed through a T12–S2 laminotomy/laminectomy, and the sacral roots were identified using bony anatomy. The dorsal roots were separated from the ventral ones, and dorsal root action potentials were recorded by a hand-held sterile bipolar hooked electrode (the root being lifted outside the spinal canal) (Fig. 42-11). The dorsal root action potentials were evoked by electrical stimulation of the penile or clitoral nerves. One hundred responses were averaged together and filtered between 1.5 and 2100 Hz. Each average response was repeated to assess its reliability. Afferent activity from the right and left dorsal roots of S1, S2, and S3 were always recorded, along with occasional recordings from the S4–5 dorsal roots. Of special relevance was the finding that in 7.6% of these children, all afferent activity was carried by only one S2 root (see Fig. 42-11C and F). These findings were confirmed by a later analysis of results of mapping in 114 children (72 male, 42 female; mean age, 3.8 years).[80] Mapping was successful in 105 of 114 patients. S1 roots contributed 4%, S2 roots 60.5%, and S3 roots 35.5% of the overall pudendal afferent activity. The distribution of responses was asymmetrical in 56% of the patients (see Fig. 42-11B, C, and F). Pudendal afferent distribution was confined to a single level in 18% (see Fig. 42-11A) and even to a single root in 7.6% of patients (see Fig. 42-11C and F).

FIGURE 42-10 Neurophysiologic events used to intraoperatively monitor the sacral nervous system. *Left:* Afferent events after stimulation of the dorsal penile/clitoral nerves and recording over the spinal cord: 1, pudendal somatosensory evoked potentials (SEPs), traveling waves; 2, pudendal dorsal root action potential; and 3, pudendal SEPs, stationary waves recorded over the conus. *Right:* Efferent events: 4, anal M wave recorded from the anal sphincter after stimulation of the S1–3 ventral roots; 5, anal motor-evoked potentials recorded from the anal sphincter after transcranial electrical stimulation of the motor cortex; 6, bulbocavernosus reflex obtained from the anal sphincter muscle after electrical stimulation of the dorsal penile/clitoral nerves. BCR, bulbocavernosus reflex; DRAP, dorsal root action potentials; MEP, motor-evoked potential. (Reproduced from Deletis V: Intraoperative neurophysiological monitoring. In McLone D (ed): Pediatric Neurosurgery: Surgery of the Developing Nervous System, 4th ed. Philadelphia: WB Saunders, 1999, pp 1204–1213.)

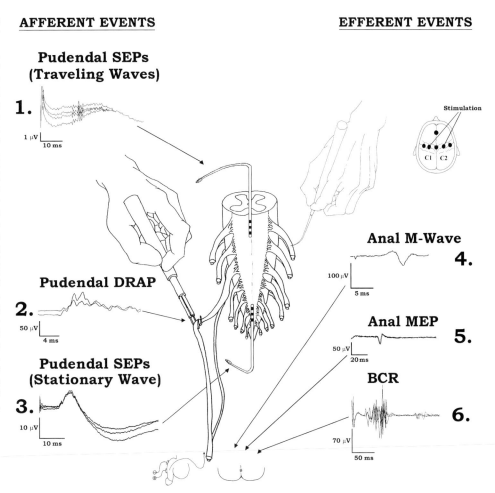

AFFERENT EVENTS

Pudendal SEPs (Traveling Waves)

1.

1 μV | 10 ms

Pudendal DRAP

2.

50 μV | 4 ms

Pudendal SEPs (Stationary Wave)

3.

10 μV | 10 ms

EFFERENT EVENTS

Stimulation

C1 C2

Anal M-Wave

4.

100 μV | 5 ms

Anal MEP

5.

50 μV | 20 ms

BCR

6.

70 μV | 50 ms

Fifty-six percent of the pathologically responding S2 roots during rhizotomy testing (using electrical stimulation of dorsal roots with spreading activity in adjacent myotomes) were preserved because of the significant afferent activity (as demonstrated during pudendal mapping). None of the 105 patients developed long-term bowel or bladder complications.

All our results in the early series of dorsal root mapping with 19 patients have been confirmed by analysis of the larger series of 105 patients.[80] With this series, we showed that selective S2 rhizotomy can be performed safely without an associated increase in residual spasticity while preserving bowel and bladder function by performing pudendal afferent mapping.[79] Therefore, we suggest that the mapping of pudendal afferents in the dorsal roots should be employed whenever these roots are considered for rhizotomy in children with cerebral palsy without urinary retention. In children with cerebral palsy with hyperreflexive detrusor dysfunction, in whom sacral rhizotomy may be considered to alleviate the problem, preoperative neurourologic investigation of the child should help in making appropriate decisions. In any case, intraoperative mapping of sacral afferents should make selective surgical approaches possible and provide the maximal benefit for children with cerebral palsy. Mapping of pudendal afferents has been further expanded by introducing methodology that maps afferents

from the anal mucosa by stimulating them using anal plug electrodes and recording them in the same way as penile/clitoral afferents.[81]

Mapping and Monitoring of Motor Responses from the Anal Sphincter

These responses can be elicited by direct stimulation of the S2 to S5 motor roots and recording from the anal sphincters, after surgical exposure of the cauda equina, or by TES of the motor cortex. The first method of cauda equina stimulation, using a small hand-held monopolar probe, is easy to perform with recording of responses from each anal hemisphincter with intramuscular wire electrodes identical to the ones used to record the bulbocavernosus reflex.[82] This mapping method is very useful when it becomes necessary to identify roots within the cauda equina during tethered cord or tumor surgeries in which the normal anatomy is distorted. To perform mapping, the surgeon must stop surgery and map the roots with a monopolar probe. To continuously monitor the functional integrity of parapyramidal motor fibers (for volitional control of the anal sphincters) and the motor aspects of the pudendal nerves from the anterior horns to the anal sphincters, the method of TES and recording of anal responses was introduced. Because the response recorded from the anal sphincter after TES has to pass multiple synapses at the level of the spinal

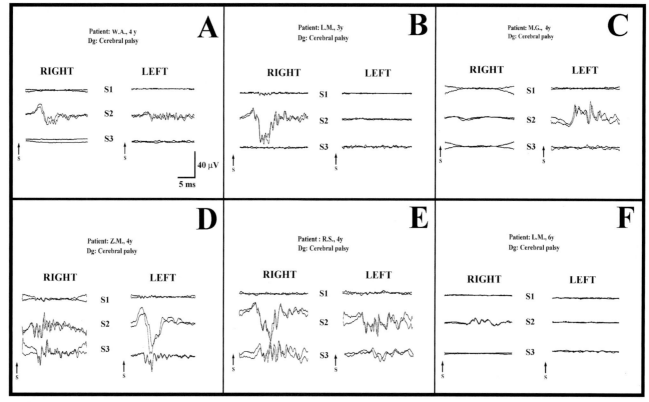

FIGURE 42-11   Six characteristic examples of dorsal root action potentials showing the entry of a variety of pudendal nerve fibers to the spinal cord via S1–3 sacral roots. *A,* Symmetrical distribution of dorsal root action potentials confined to one level (S2) or three levels (*D*). Asymmetrical distribution of dorsal root action potentials confined to the one side (*B*), only one root (*C* or *F*), or all roots except right S1 (*E*). Recordings were obtained after electrical stimulation of bilateral penile/clitoral nerves. (Reproduced from Vodusek VB, Deletis V: Intraoperative neurophysiological monitoring of the sacral nervous system. In Deletis V, Shils J (eds): Neurophysiology in Neurosurgery. A Modern Intraoperative Approach. San Diego: Academic Press, 2002, pp 197–217.)

cord, this method is moderately sensitive to anesthetics and rather light anesthesia should be maintained. So far no clinical correlation using this method has been published.

Monitoring of the Bulbocavernosus Reflex

The bulbocavernosus reflex is an oligosynaptic reflex mediated through the S2–4 spinal cord segments that is elicited by electrical stimulation of the dorsal penis/clitoris nerves with the reflex response recorded from any pelvic floor muscles. The afferent paths of the bulbocavernosus reflex are the sensory fibers of the pudendal nerves and the reflex center in the S2–4 spinal segment. The efferent paths are the motor fibers of the pudendal nerves and anal sphincter muscles. In neurophysiologic laboratories, the bulbocavernosus reflex is usually recorded from the bulbocavernosus muscles, and this is where it gets its name. We have described an intraoperative method for recording the bulbocavernosus reflex from the anal sphincter muscle, with improvement in methodology reported by others.[82,84] The advantage of bulbocavernosus reflex monitoring is that it tests the functional integrity of the three different anatomic structures: the sensory and motor fibers of the pudendal nerves and the gray matter of the S2–4 sacral segments (see Fig. 42-10).

Because of a lack of published statistical data collected for large groups of patients, the reliability of monitoring for conus and cauda equina surgeries remains unclear.

REFERENCES

1. Nitta T, Sato K: Prognostic implications of the extent of surgical resection in patients with intracranial malignant gliomas. Cancer 75:2727–2731, 1995.
2. Hentschel SJ, Sawaya R: Optimizing outcomes with maximal surgical resection of malignant gliomas. Cancer Control 10:109–114, 2003.
3. Skirboll SS, Ojemann GA, Berger MS, et al: Functional cortex and subcortical white matter located within gliomas. Neurosurgery 38:678–685, 1996.
4. Ojemann JG, Miller JW, Silbergeld DL: Preserved function in brain invaded by tumor. Neurosurgery 39:253–259, 1996.
5. Schiffbauer H, Ferrari P, Rowley HA, et al: Functional activity within brain tumors: A magnetic source imaging study. Neurosurgery 49:1313–1321, 2001.
6. George JS, Aine CJ, Mosher JC, et al: Mapping function in the human brain with magnetoencephalography, anatomical magnetic resonance imaging, and functional magnetic resonance imaging. J Clin Neurophysiol 12:406–431, 1995.
7. Kober H, Nimsky C, Moller M, et al: Correlation of sensorimotor activation with functional magnetic resonance imaging and magnetoencephalography in presurgical functional imaging: A spatial analysis. Neuroimage 14:1214–1228, 2001.
8. Kaplan AM, Bandy DJ, Manwaring KH, et al: Functional brain mapping using positron emission tomography scanning in preoperative neurosurgical planning for pediatric brain tumors. J Neurosurg 91:797–803, 1999.
9. Meyer PT, Sturz L, Sabri O, et al: Preoperative motor system brain mapping using positron emission tomography and statistical parametric mapping: hints on cortical reorganisation. J Neurol Neurosurg Psychiatry 74:471–478, 2003.

10. Sobottka SB, Bredow J, Beuthien-Baumann B, et al: Comparison of functional brain PET images and intraoperative brain-mapping data using image-guided surgery. Comput Aided Surg 7:317–325, 2002.

11. Schulder M, Maldjian JA, Liu WC, et al: Functional image-guided surgery of intracranial tumors located in or near the sensorimotor cortex. J Neurosurg 89:412–418, 1998.

12. Fritsch G, Hitzig E: Uber die elektrische Errgebarkeit des Grosshirns. Arch Anat Physiol Wiss Med 37:300–332, 1870.

13. Bartholow R: Experimental investigations into the functions of the human brain. Am J Med Sci 67:305–313, 1874.

14. Penfield W, Boldrey E: Somatic motor and sensory representation in the cerebral cortex of man as studied by electrical stimulation. Brain 60:389–443, 1937.

15. Penfield W, Rasmussen T: The cerebral cortex of man: A clinical study of localization and function. New York: Macmillan, 1950.

16. Berger MS, Ojemann GA, et al: Techniques for functional brain mapping during glioma surgery. In Berger MS, Wilson CB (eds): The Gliomas. Philadelphia: WB Saunders, 1999, pp 421–435.

17. Duffau HL, Capelle J, Sichez P, et al: Intéret des stimulations électriques corticales et sous-corticales directes peropératoires dans la chirurgie cérébrale en zone fonctionnelle. Rev Neurol 155:553–568, 1999.

18. Kombos T, Suess O, Funk T, et al: Intra-operative mapping of the motor cortex during surgery in and around the motor cortex. Acta Neurochir 142:263–268, 2000.

19. Goldring S, Gregorie EM: Surgical management of epilepsy using epidural recordings to localize the seizure focus: Review of 100 cases. J Neurosurg 60:457–466, 1984.

20. Cedzich C, Taniguchi M, Schafer S, et al: Somatosensory evoked potential phase reversal and direct motor cortex stimulation during surgery in and around the central region. Neurosurgery 38:962–970, 1996.

21. Wood CC, Spencer DD, Allison T, et al: Localization of human sensorimotor cortex during surgery by cortical surface recording of somatosensory evoked potentials. J Neurosurg 68:99–111, 1988.

22. King RB, Schell GR: Cortical localization and monitoring during cerebral operations. J Neurosurg 67:210–219, 1987.

23. Lehericy S, Duffau H, Cornu P, et al: Correspondence between functional magnetic resonance imaging somatotopy and individual brain anatomy of the central region: Comparison with intraoperative stimulation in patients with brain tumors. J Neurosurg 92:589–598, 2000.

24. Puce AR, Constable T, Luby ML, et al: Functional magnetic resonance imaging of sensory and motor cortex: Comparison with electrophysiological localization. J Neurosurg 83:262–270, 1995.

25. Fandino J, Kollias SS, Weiser HG, et al: Intraoperative validation of functional magnetic resonance imaging and cortical reorganization patterns in patients with brain tumors involving the primary motor cortex. J Neurosurg 91:238–250, 1999.

26. Roux FE, Boulanouar K, Lotterie JA, et al: Language functional magnetic resonance imaging in preoperative assessment of language areas: Correlation with direct cortical stimulation. Neurosurgery 52:1335–1347, 2003.

27. Duffau H, Capelle L, Sichez JP, et al: Intra-operative direct electrical stimulations of the central nervous system: The Salpetrière experience with 60 patients. Acta Neurochir (Wien) 141:1157–1167, 1999.

28. Yingling CD, Ojemann S, Dodson B, et al: Identification of motor pathways during tumor surgery facilitated by multichannel electromyographic recording. J Neurosurg 91:922–927, 1999.

29. Berger MS: Functional mapping-guided resection of low-grade gliomas. Clin Neurosurg 42:437–452, 1995.

30. Haglund MM, Ojemann GA, Blasdel GG: Optical imaging of bipolar cortical stimulation. J Neurosurg 78:785–793, 1993.

31. Berger MS: Lesions in functional ("eloquent") cortex and subcortical white matter. Clin Neurosurg 41:444–463, 1994.

32. Sartorius CJ, Wright G: Intraoperative brain mapping in a community setting: Technical considerations. Surg Neurol 47:380–388, 1997.

33. Sartorius CJ, Berger MS: Rapid termination of intraoperative stimulation-evoked seizures with application of cold Ringer's lactate to the cortex: Technical note. J Neurosurg 88:349–351, 1998.

34. Hines M, Boynton EP: The maturation of "excitability" in the precentral gyrus of the young monkey (Macaca mulatta). Contrib Embryol 178:313–451, 1940.

35. Sala F, Lanteri P: Brain surgery in motor areas: The invaluable assistance of intraoperative neurophysiological monitoring. J Neurosurg Sci 47:79–88, 2003.

36. Kombos T, Suess O, Ciklatekerlio O, et al: Monitoring of intraoperative motor evoked potentials to increase the safety of surgery in and around the motor cortex. J Neurosurg 95:608–614, 2001.

37. Zhou HH, Kelly PJ: Transcranial electrical motor evoked potential monitoring for brain tumor resection. Neurosurgery 48:1075–1081, 2001.

38. Riviello JJ, Kull L, Troup C, et al: Cortical stimulation in children: Techniques and precautions. Tech Neurosurg 7:12–18, 2001.

39. Kothbauer K, Deletis V, Epstein FJ: Intraoperative spinal cord monitoring for intramedullary surgery: An essential adjunct. Pediatr Neurosurg 26:247–254, 1997.

40. Kothbauer K, Deletis V, Epstein FJ: Motor evoked potential monitoring for intramedullary spinal cord tumor surgery: Correlation of clinical and neurophysiological data in a series of 100 consecutive procedures. Neurosurg Focus 4:1–9, 1998.

41. Neuloh G, Schramm J: Mapping and monitoring of supratentorial procedures. In Deletis V, Shils JL (eds): Neurophysiology in Neurosurgery: A Modern Intraoperative Approach. San Diego, CA: Academic Press, 2002, pp 339–401.

42. Deletis V, Camargo AB: Transcranial electrical motor evoked potential monitoring for brain tumor resection. Neurosurgery 49:1488–1489, 2001.

43. Bricolo A, Turazzi S: Surgery for gliomas and other mass lesions of the brainstem. In Symon L (ed): Advances and Technical Standards in Neurosurgery, vol.22. Vienna: Springer-Verlag, 1995, pp 261–341.

44. Kyoshima K, Kobayashi S, Gibo H, et al: A study of safe entry zones via the floor of the fourth ventricle for brain-stem lesions. J Neurosurg 78:987–993, 1993.

45. Morota N, Deletis V, Epstein FJ, et al: Brain stem mapping: Neurophysiological localization of motor nuclei on the floor of the fourth ventricle. Neurosurgery 37:922–930, 1995.

46. Suzuki K, Matsumoto M, Ohta M, et al: Experimental study for identification of the facial colliculus using electromyography and antidromic evoked potentials. Neurosurgery 41:1130–1136, 1997.

47. Strauss C, Romstock J, Fahlbusch R: Intraoperative mapping of the floor of the fourth ventricle. In Loftus CM, Traynelis VC (eds): Intraoperative Monitoring Techniques in Neurosurgery. New York: McGraw-Hill, 1994, pp 213–218.

48. Strauss C, Romstock J, Fahlbusch R: Pericollicular approaches to the rhomboid fossa. Part II: Neurophysiological basis. J Neurosurg 91:768–775, 1999.

49. Deletis V, Sala F, Morota N: Intraoperative neurophysiological monitoring and mapping during brain stem surgery: A modern approach. Oper Tech Neurosurg 3:109–113, 2000.

50. Rhoton AL: The posterior fossa veins. Neurosurgery 47:S69–S92, 2000.

51. Sala F, Lanteri P, Bricolo A: Intraoperative neurophysiological monitoring of motor evoked potentials during brain stem and spinal cord surgery. Adv Tech Stand Neurosurg 29:133–169, 2004.

52. Morota N, Deletis V, Lee M, et al: Functional anatomic relationship between brain stem tumors and cranial motor nuclei. Neurosurgery 39:787–794, 1996.

53. Sekiya T, Hatayama T, Shimamura N, et al: Intraoperative electrophysiological monitoring of oculomotor nuclei and their intramedullary tracts during midbrain tumor surgery. Neurosurgery 47:1170–1177, 2000.

54. Schlake HP, Goldbrunner R, Siebert M, et al: Intra-operative electromyographic monitoring of extra-ocular motor nerves (Nn. III, VI) in skull base surgery. Acta Neurochir (Wien) 143:251–261, 2001.

55. Sakuma J, Matsumoto M, Ohta M, et al: Glossopharyngeal nerve evoked potentials after stimulation of the posterior part of the tongue in dogs. Neurosurgery 51:1026–1033, 2002.

56. Komisaruk BR, Mosier KM, Liu WC, et al: Functional localization of brainstem and cervical spinal cord nuclei in humans with fMRI. AJNR Am J Neuroradiol 23:609–617, 2002.

57. Fahlbusch R, Strauss C: The surgical significance of brain stem cavernous hemangiomas. Zentralbl Neurochir 52:25–32, 1991.

58. Grabb PA, Albright L, Sclabassi RJ, et al: Continuous intraoperative electromyographic monitoring of cranial nerves during resection of fourth ventricular tumors in children. J Neurosurg 86:1–4, 1997.

59. Romstock J, Strauss C, Fahlbusch R: Continuous electromyography monitoring of motor cranial nerves during cerebellopontine angle surgery. J Neurosurg 93:586–593, 2000.

60. Sala F, Kržan MJ, Deletis V: Intraoperative neurophysiological monitoring in pediatric neurosurgery: Why, when, how? Childs Nerv Syst 18:264–287, 2002.

61. Jones SJ, Buonamassa S, Crockard HA: Two cases of quadriparesis following anterior cervical discectomy, with normal perioperative

somatosensory evoked potentials. J Neurol Neurosurg Psychiatry 44:273–276, 2003.

62. Minahan RE, Sepkuty JP, Lesser RP, et al: Anterior spinal cord injury with preserved neurogenic 'motor' evoked potentials. Clin Neurophysiol 112:1442–1450, 2001.

63. Jallo G, Kothbauer K, Epstein F: Contact laser microsurgery. Childs Nerv Syst 18:333–336, 2002.

64. Deletis V: Intraoperative neurophysiology and methodology used to monitor the functional integrity of the motor system. In Deletis V, Shils JL (eds): Neurophysiology in Neurosurgery: A Modern Intraoperative Approach. San Diego: Academic Press, 2002, pp 25–51.

65. Deletis V, Camargo AB: Interventional neurophysiological mapping during spinal cord procedures. Stereotact Funct Neurosurg 77:25–28, 2001.

66. Kržan MJ: Intraoperative neurophysiological mapping of the spinal cord's dorsal column. In Deletis V, Shils JL (eds): Neurophysiology in Neurosurgery: A Modern Intraoperative Approach. San Diego, CA: Academic Press, 2002, pp 153–164.

67. Berenstein A, Lasjaunias P: Spine and spinal cord vascular lesions. In Berenstein A, Lasjaunias P (eds): Surgical Neuroangiography: Endovascular Treatment of Spine and Spinal Cord Lesions. Berlin, Heidelberg: Springer, 1992, pp 1–109.

68. Berenstein A, Young W, Benjamin V, Merkin H: Somatosensory evoked potentials during spinal angiography and therapeutic transvascular embolization. J Neurosurg 60:777–785, 1984.

69. Sala F, Niimi Y: Neurophysiological monitoring during endovascular procedures on the spine and the spinal cord. In Deletis V, Shils JL (eds): Neurophysiology in Neurosurgery: A Modern Intraoperative Approach. San Diego, CA: Academic Press, 2002, pp 119–151.

70. de Haan P, Kalkman CJ, de Mol BA: Efficacy of transcranial motor-evoked myogenic potentials to detect spinal cord ischemia during operations for thoracoabdominal aneurysms. J Thorac Cardiovasc Surg 113:87–101, 1997.

71. de Haan P, Kalkman CJ, Jacobs MJ: Spinal cord monitoring with myogenic motor evoked potentials: Early detection of spinal cord ischemia as an integral part of spinal cord protective strategies during thoracoabdominal aneurysm surgery. Semin Thorac Cardiovasc Surg 10:19–24, 1998.

72. Konrad PE, Tacker WA Jr, Levy WJ, et al: Motor evoked potentials in the dog: Effects of global ischemia on spinal cord and peripheral nerve signals. Neurosurgery 20:117–124, 1987.

73. Kai Y, Owen JH, Allen BT, et al: Relationship between evoked potentials and clinical status in spinal cord ischemia. Spine 19:1162–1168, 1994.

74. Sadato A, Taki W, Nakamura I, et al: Improved provocative tests for the embolization of arteriovenous malformations: Technical note. Neurol Med Chir (Tokyo) 34:187–190, 1994.

75. Touho H, Karasawa J, Ohnishi H, et al: Intravascular treatment of spinal arteriovenous malformations using a microcatheter: With special reference to serial Xylocaine tests and intravascular pressure monitoring. Surg Neurol 42:148–156, 1994.

76. Tanaka K, Yamasaki M: Blocking of cortical inhibitory synapses by intravenous lidocaine. Nature 209:207–208, 1966.

77. Choux M, Lena G, Genitori L, et al: The surgery of occult spinal dysraphism. Adv Tech Stand Neurosurg 21:183–238, 1994.

78. Piere-Kahn A, Zerah M, Renier D, et al: Congenital lumbosacral lipomas. Childs Nerv Syst 13:298–335, 1997.

79. Lang FF, Deletis V, Valasquez L, et al: Inclusion the S2 dorsal rootlets in functional posterior rhizotomy for spasticity in children with cerebral palsy. Neurosurgery 34:847–853, 1994.

80. Huang JC, Deletis V, Vodušek DB, et al: Preservation of pudendal afferents in sacral rhizotomies. Neurosurgery 41:411–415, 1997.

81. Deletis V, Kržan MJ, Bueno de Camargo A, Abbott R: Functional anatomical asymmetry of pudendal nerve sensory fibers. In Bruch HP, Kocherling F, Bouchard R, Schug-Pass C (eds): New Aspects of High Technology in Medicine. Bologna, Italy: Monduzzi, 2001, pp 153–158.

82. Deletis V, Vodušek DB: Intraoperative recording of the bulbocavernosus reflex. Neurosurgery 40:88–92, 1997.

83. Deletis V: Intraoperative neurophysiological monitoring. In McLone D (ed): Pediatric Neurosurgery: Surgery of the Developing Nervous System, 4th ed. Philadelphia: WB Saunders, 1999, pp 1204–1213.

84. Rodi Z, Vodušek DB: Intraoperative monitoring of bulbocavernous reflex—The method and its problems. Clin Neurophysiol 112:879–883, 2001.

43

Ultrasound in Neurosurgery

MICHAEL WOYDT

HISTORY

In the early 1950s, French and colleagues[1] reported on the experimental use of A mode (amplitude modulated) ultrasound (US) in an experimental setting to scan a brain tumor. This was confirmed 2 years later by Wild and Reid[2] in a clinical setting. During the following 20 years, different applications of A mode were used intraoperatively and transcranially.[3] With the invention of real-time sector scanning (B mode) intraoperative US (IOUS) in neurosurgery has become a widely used intraoperative diagnostic tool since the early 1980s,[4,5] until other methods of intraoperative navigation (frameless neuronavigation, intraoperative MRI) became available. US imaging during the past 10 years was characterized by a multitude of technical inventions and new methods, some of which are explained in this chapter.

OVERVIEW OF TECHNICAL DETAILS

Physical Principles

Successful application of IOUS requires an understanding of the basic principles of US imaging. First, US pictures are the result of reflection, absorption, and scattering. For image buildup, reflection is the most important part; absorption and scattering require an intricate interpretation of the resulting artifacts.

Many surgeons are not satisfied with US imaging because of bad image quality. Provided that the US machine is not older than 5 years, it is in the hands of the surgeon (or the radiologist) him- or herself to optimize image quality and to achieve maximal resolution (25 μm at 50 MHz); therefore, the three most important characteristics of image buildup in IOUS, which could be chosen at the US machine, are explained:

Frequency: High frequencies (e.g., 10 MHz) will yield a high resolution but result in a high degree of absorption, whereas low frequencies (e.g., 5 MHz) show less absorption (will travel deeper in tissue) but also provide less resolution.

Focus: Electronic focusing can narrow the US beam, which will result in a high resolution in the focal zone but also dramatically lower resolution beyond the focal zone.

Depth: The deeper the chosen depth, the more overview of brain tissue is possible. However, details at the surface will become very small and sometimes invisible.

In summary, scanning a small lesion at the surface (e.g., ≤15 mm subcortically, for instance, a sulcus), one has to choose a high frequency, set the focus at 20 mm, and switch the depth to a maximum of 40 mm. Conversely, to gain an overview of a deep-seated lesion (e.g., a ventricular tumor), the frequency has to be downregulated (e.g., 5 to 6 MHz),

the focus should be in the region of the tumor (e.g., 50 mm), and the depth has to be open to 70 mm (Fig. 43-1).

Hardware

US platforms can be differentiated into different subcategories depending on the incorporated modes, storing features, transducers, and financial considerations. The possible modes (see the following) and transducers are important for the neurosurgeon. Intraoperative scanning is best performed with a small-phased array, which should have a small rectangular acoustic lens (area with contact to the brain surface; maximum, 20 to 25 mm) with a radial scanning field. Convex and linear arrays are less well suited due to artifacts with transducer-brain coupling (convexity of brain and transducer, size of transducer). Today, only electronic arrays are used in IOUS (except in endosonography). For burr hole scanning (e.g., ventricular puncture), specially designed probes fitting into standard 12-mm burr holes are available (Fig. 43-2). New crystals and focus technology as larger bandwidth and increased sensitivity of the transducers now generate images not comparable with those of 10 or 15 years ago.

Modes

The standard application is the B mode (brightness mode). All structures are displayed in different shades of gray in a real-time fashion (>18 frames per second). To interpret the images, it is helpful to use a dedicated US language terminology (corresponding to intensity in magnetic resonance imaging, density in computed tomography imaging), especially addressing the following:

Echogenicity: Depending on the reflections of tissue (cell density, calcifications), there are grades from no echogenicity/ anechogenicity (e.g., ventricles), to low echogenicity (normal white matter), to high echogenicity (gliomas) until hyperechogenicity is reached (nearly total reflection as with bone or calcified plexus).

Homogenicity: Structures with uniform echogenicity (e.g., low-grade gliomas) are homogeneous, whereas structures with different echogenic parts inside (e.g., high-grade gliomas) are termed inhomogeneous (Fig. 43-3).

Demarcation: Depending on the level of reflections at the tissue borders, some structures, such as ventricles, are well demarcated from brain tissue. Conversely, invasive brain tumors are less well delineated due to the infiltrated brain tissue.

When scanning vascular structures, one has to add the C mode (color mode). All moving particles (e.g., erythrocytes) become encoded with different shades of red and blue, depending on the velocity and direction (in general, structures

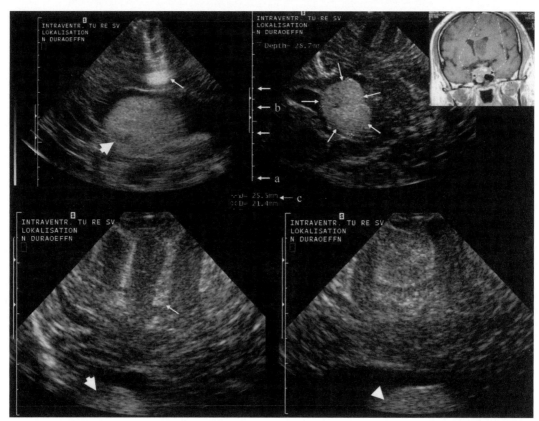

FIGURE 43-1 Left intraventricular tumor (subependymoma). *Upper right:* To get an overview of anatomic structures and tumor localization, the depth is at 7.7 cm (a), focus zone is from 3.5 to 5.5 cm (b), and frequency is at 6 MHz. The size of the high echogenic tumor (c) (*small arrows*) fits well with corresponding magnetic resonance image (*inset*). *Lower left and right:* To display the sulcus (transsulcal dissection planned), the setting for depth (4 cm), focus zone (0.5–2.5 cm), and frequency (9 MHz) are corrected; the tumor is only partially displayed (*arrowhead*); the echogenic sulcus in the coronal plane (*lower left*) and sagittal plane (*lower right*) is shown. *Upper left:* After preparation (bottom of the sulcus), intraoperative ultrasound is performed with a hemostypticum as an artificial landmark (*small arrow*).

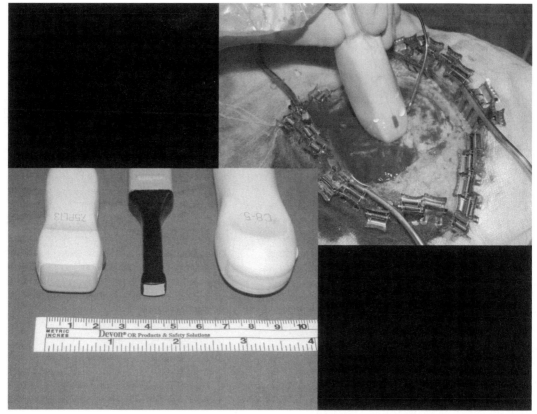

FIGURE 43-2 Intraoperative ultrasound probes. *Upper right:* Phased array probe covered with a sterile sheath placed on the durol surface. *Lower left:* Intraoperative transducers with phased array, burr hole transducer, and curved array (from left to right).

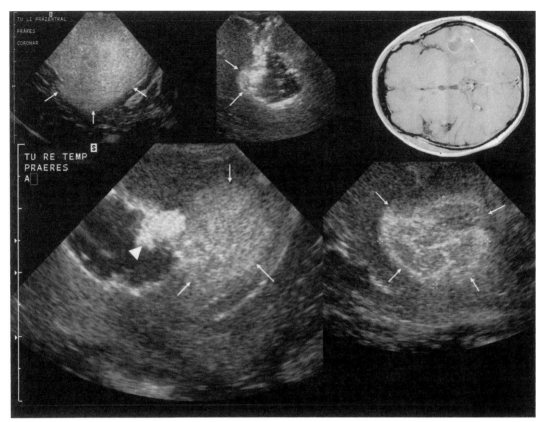

FIGURE 43-3 Different types of tumors and resection control. *Upper left:* Low-grade tumor with homogeneous echotexture. *Lower right:* Preresection intraoperative ultrasound (IOUS) of a heterogeneous high-grade tumor (with corresponding magnetic resonance image). *Upper middle:* Small echogenic area adjacent to the frontal part of the resection cavity (*arrows,* corresponding echogenicity to tumor tissue in preresection IOUS), histopathologically solid tumor. *Lower left:* Localization of satellite tumor dorsally located (*small arrows;* see magnetic resonance image). Navigation with small hemostypticum (*arrowhead*) after resection of the frontal part of the tumor (hypoechoic resection cavity).

moving toward the probe are encoded in red). The color bar indicates the different velocities. A more sensitive method (e.g., for small and slow-flow arteries) of displaying flow is the power or angio mode (color Doppler energy) because it rather depends on the amplitude of moving structures and not on the velocity. New US platforms incorporate this feature also as a direction-encoded mode. Adding the D mode (Doppler mode) in real-time fashion results in the so-called triplex mode (or color duplex sonography, color flow sonography), which offers information on angle-corrected flow velocities in vessels deep in the brain and therefore comparable information between different measurements.

For a better display of large tumors or spinal lesions, extended field of view techniques can help the visualization of these structures.

Preparation and Artifacts

For IOUS, the probe has to be covered with a sterile sheath because most of the modern probes are not suited for sterilization. Therefore, great care has to be taken that the sheath is not damaged, and this ought to be checked every time before the probe comes in contact with tissue. To avoid damage of the gloving, storing the probe in an extra pouch during surgery is recommended. In our clinic (with experience with more than 1500 IOUS examinations), we are not aware of higher infection rates using US intraoperatively. Most problems with blurred images are due to air bubbles

trapped between contact surfaces (brain/sheath and probe/contact gel/sheath), which should be checked. Best images are generated before or after dural opening, and artifacts during the surgical procedure may result from air bubbles, hemostyptics, and fresh blood. Other types of artifacts are reverberations (e.g., from spatulas), shadowing (e.g., distally from calcifications), and increased echogenicity of structures lying beyond water-like structures (e.g., cysts).

Flow Chart

Figure 43-4 provides a short checklist for application of IOUS.

CRANIAL APPLICATIONS (WITH SPECIAL METHODS)

Tumors (Resection Control)

Meningiomas are in most cases highly echogenic lesions sharply demarcated from surrounding brain tissue. Calcifications within the meningioma may result in a shadowing of structures lying behind the tumor. IOUS may be helpful in localizing tumors at the lower edge of the falx that are not visible at the brain surface, so one might choose a different dissection route, respecting bridging veins at the surface. Adding C or power mode, pathoanatomic relations between tumor and main arteries and their branches become visible[6] and (as a quality control) hemodynamic control

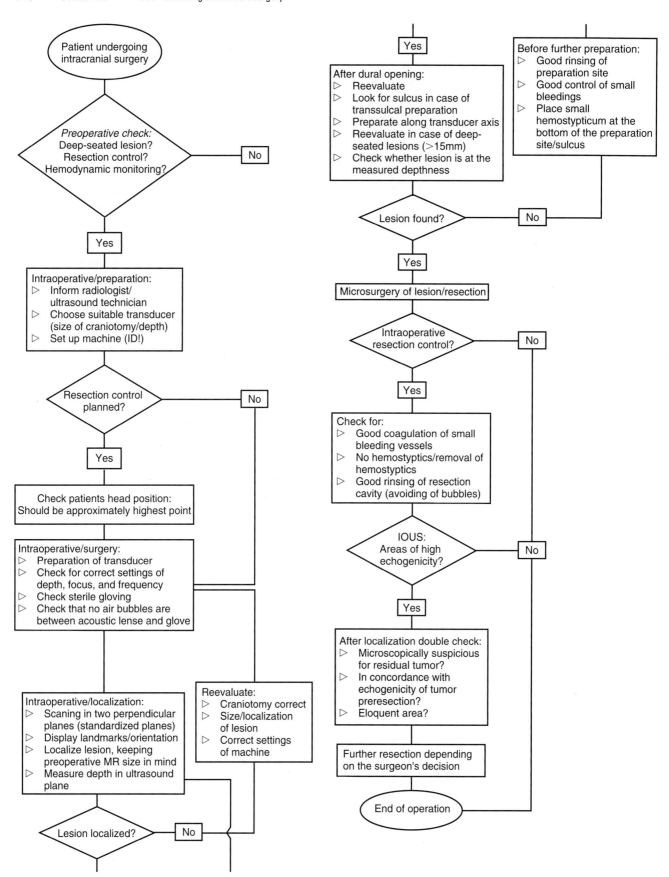

FIGURE 43-4 Flow chart for use of intraoperative ultrasound.

before and after resection can be verified in combination with angle-corrected D mode (color Doppler sonography). IOUS is not useful for bone-invading tumors (e.g., spheno-orbital meningiomas) because bone reflects the US beam resulting in a very high echogenic imaging of the skull base.

Metastases are highly echogenic and mostly well demarcated. Depending on their histopathology, they may appear inhomogeneous: cystic metastases may have only a small echogenic rim surrounding the anechogenic cyst (no reflections). The surrounding brain with edema is slightly more echogenic than normal brain (Fig. 43-5).

Gliomas show a higher echogenicity than normal brain tissue, irrespective of whether they are contrast-enhancing tumors. This once again shows the physical difference between imaging with computed tomography (radiograph), magnetic resonance imaging (electron relaxation), and IOUS (US wave propagation). To differentiate between solid tumor tissue and infiltration zone and surrounding brain tissue, using frequencies as high as possible (e.g., 7 to 10 MHz), depending on the depth of the lesion, is recommended.

Low-grade gliomas are homogeneous and have a moderate echogenicity,[7] whereas high-grade gliomas, due to their histopathologic composition, mostly appear inhomogeneous (bleeding residuals, necrosis, cysts) and more echogenic than low-grade gliomas[8] (see Fig. 43-3). Furthermore, most gliomas are sonographically characterized by a spherical manifestation and small calcifications in oligodendrogliomas

can be identified reliably due to their hyperechogenic appearance. By adding C or power mode, it is possible to obtain an impression of the vascularization of the tumor. Typically, a homogeneous distribution of the intratumoral vessels is seen in low-grade gliomas and a more peripheral vascularization is found in high-grade gliomas.

Intraoperative resection control with US can be performed if the following points are accounted for. First, only when IOUS is used before tumor resection, can it be used after resection because it is vital to compare the degree of echogenicity of suspected tumor remnants with the echogenicity of the tumor before resection (as is the rule with all other imaging techniques). Second, the site of the craniotomy should be optimally the highest point of the head, so that the tumor cavity can be sufficiently filled with saline after resection. Most important, the resection cavity should be free of blood coagels and hemostyptics, and H_2O_2 should not be used. During the scanning process of the rim of the resection cavity, solid echogenic areas with echogenicity comparable with that of the tumor before resection are suspicious of solid tumor remnants (see Fig. 43-3). Specificity is nearly 90%[9,10] when verifying the echogenic area in two perpendicular US planes. An alternative method (especially suited for deep-seated tumors) is to enlarge the craniotomy or to make a second craniotomy large enough for the US probe and scan through normal brain tissue to the resection cavity.[11]

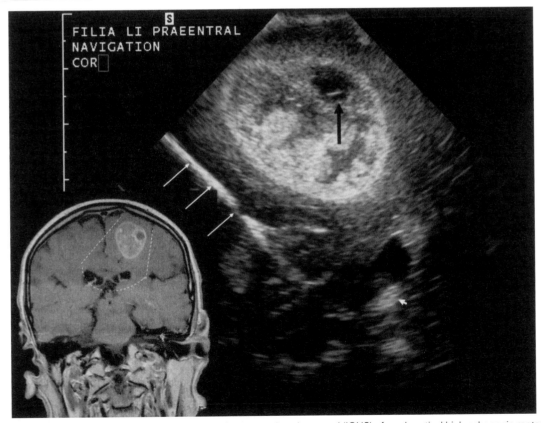

FIGURE 43-5   Subcortical metastases (colon carcinoma). Intraoperative ultrasound (IOUS) of a subcortical high echogenic metastases (with corresponding magnetic resonance image). Landmarks: Falx (*small arrows*) and anechoic ventricle (with hyperechoic plexus, *arrowhead*). Hypoechoic cyst within the metastases (*black arrow*).

Vascular Malformations (Sononavigation)

Cavernomas are lesions with low to high hyperechogenicity and are easy to localize with IOUS in B mode. Their appearance can be inhomogeneous due to microcalcifications, very small cysts, and microthromboses (Fig. 43-6). In approximately one fourth of cases, the demarcation of the cavernoma from brain tissue is not sharp because of iron deposits in the surrounding brain tissue. It is practically not possible to identify vessels in the cavernomas (without use of echo contrast enhancers) with conventional C or power mode due to the very low flow. Associated deep venous anomalies can be identified using color duplex sonography. Criteria are venous signal (slow flow, <5 cm/second) and flow away from the lesion. Vessel patency can be verified after the resection.[12]

Sononavigation can be used alone or in combination with frameless neuronavigation devices (see later) to localize and navigate to deep-seated cavernomas or other subcortically located lesions (metastases, hematomas, deep-seated gliomas). In superficially located lesions (≤10 to 15 mm), the US probe has to be moved in two perpendicular planes on the dura to safely identify the lesion. After dural opening, the angioarchitecture of the cortex may show that the direct dissection plane to the lesion would result in a destruction of small vessels at the cortex. In these cases, another point for the corticotomy has to be chosen and the US probe has to be placed at that point. The angulation of the probe (while displaying the lesion) defines the dissection path (along the long axis of the probe). Before dissection, the depth from surface to the lesion should be measured on the frozen screen of the US device. In deep-seated lesions with a transgyral/transfissural dissection, the lesion is located in the first step, and in the second step, the best fitting sulcus is identified (e.g., comparing preoperative magnetic resonance imaging or depending on cortical vessel anatomy) by the typical high echogenicity of a sulcus (small line in one plane and broad band in the perpendicular plane). After dissection of the sulcus/fissure, a small hemostypticum can be placed (as an artificial hyperechoic landmark) at the bottom of the sulcus and a reevaluation done (see Fig. 43-1). Then the dissection plane can be adjusted and the distance between the artificial landmark and the lesion should be measured. Whenever the lesion is not encountered at the measured distance, a reevaluation should be done. With this technique of sononavigation, the preparation could be double-checked at every stage of dissection in a real-time fashion.[12]

Arteriovenous malformations (AVMs) should be identified first with C or power mode because of their high vascularization. The perfused parts of the AVM will be

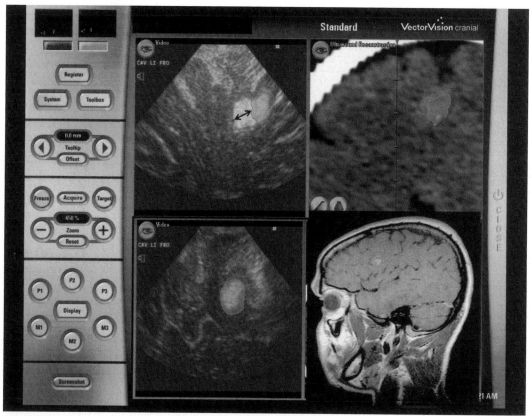

FIGURE 43-6   Left frontal subcortical cavernoma. Screen shot from a frameless neuronavigation system (FLNN). *Upper left:* Intraoperative ultrasound (IOUS) with high echogenic subcortical cavernoma (green: localization of cavernoma with FLNN) in coronal plane. *Upper right:* Reconstructed computed tomography image from ultrasound plane. *Lower left:* IOUS in sagittal plane. *Lower right:* Corresponding magnetic resonance image. Due to difference of 5 mm between FLNN and IOUS, localization of the cavernoma (*upper left, black arrow*) object was shifted in FLNN and navigation was successful. (See Color Plate.)

displayed in C mode as a mixture of red and blue pixels encoding the convolute of vessels in the nidus. Power mode is very sensitive for displaying small vessels, and the angiography-like picture helps in understanding the angioarchitecture of the AVM. Switching to the B mode, perfused parts of the nidus will be displayed as anechoic, and interventionally embolized parts will appear moderate to highly echogenic due to the thrombosed vessels. B mode is also very suitable for identifying associated hematomas (see later).[13] For the differentiation of feeder, draining, and transit vessels, triplex mode must be chosen. Feeder vessels can be separated from transit vessels by placing the Doppler sample volume to the vessel of interest: flow direction of feeder vessels is toward the nidus (color and direction of Doppler spectrum) and the Doppler spectral curve shows very high systolic (up to 300 cm/second) and diastolic flows with a low resistance index (<0.6) (Fig. 43-7). Transit vessels have normal Doppler spectral curves. Draining vessels show flow away from the nidus with high systolic and diastolic velocities in D mode. IOUS is very helpful for resection control in AVM surgery: corresponding to glioma surgery, the resection cavity must be filled with saline solution. To identify perfused residual AVM parts, one must pay attention to areas close to the cavity with the characteristic red and blue pixels (like preresection).[14]

Aneurysms (Hemodynamic Monitoring)

The easiest way to identify aneurysms is to use power mode and to begin with displaying all the basal arteries. After gaining the anatomic overview, the site of the aneurysm (e.g., internal cerebral artery) must be focused and zoomed to optimally display the aneurysm and adjacent arteries (Fig. 43-8). A perfused aneurysm is characterized by anechoic presentation in B mode (because perfused structures are nonreflective), bichromatic display in C mode (because of the flow inversion within the aneurysm), and a typical bidirectional flow signal with a "sloshing" noise in D mode.[15] Using this technique, even small peripheral aneurysms can be identified and sononavigated.[16]

Hemodynamic monitoring is the main advantage of IOUS in aneurysm surgery. Qualitative and quantitative comparison of blood flow velocities in the adjacent arteries before and after clipping is possible by the angle correction modality (Doppler sample volume) in the triplex mode. Before dural opening, the vessels of interest are visualized in C or power mode and measured (e.g., middle and anterior cerebral arteries in the case of an internal carotid artery aneurysm) by recording peak systolic flow, end-diastolic flow, and resistance index. After clipping and removal of the spatulas, a second measurement is performed following

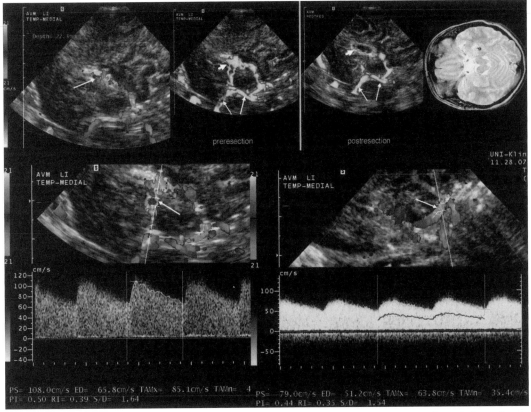

FIGURE 43-7   Left temporobasal arteriovenous angioma. *Upper left:* Localization of the AVM nidus in C mode (*arrow*); measurement of depth from the cortical surface (22.3 mm). *Upper middle and right:* Display of the angioarchitecture pre- and postresection in power mode and corresponding magnetic resonance image. Nidus and resection cavity, respectively (*arrowheads*) and posterior cerebral artery (P2 and P3 segment) with feeder vessels (*small arrows*). *Lower left:* Measurement of flow velocity in feeder vessel with triplex mode (angle corrected Doppler sample volume marked with *arrow*); at the bottom, spectral curve with elevated peak systolic flow of 108.0 cm/second and low resistance index of 0.39 are shown. *Lower right:* Triplex mode of draining vessel (sample volume, *arrow*) with flow away from nidus. (See Color Plate.)

the identical protocol. Inspecting the vessel anatomy in C or power mode allows a qualitative assessment of whether all vessels are still visible after clipping. Quantitative assessment is possible comparing the peak systolic flow and resistance index before and after clipping (see Fig. 43-8). An increase of peak systolic flow and resistance index can be detected when vessels are narrowed by the clip.[17]

Hematomas/Cysts (Biopsy)

Fresh intracerebral hematomas are highly echogenic in B mode. In case of emergency surgery with an atypical location of the hemorrhage, a repeat IOUS examination after partial hematoma evacuation with C/power mode can serve to detect an AVM or aneurysm.[13] Two weeks after hemorrhage, the central parts of the hematoma become iso- to hypoechoic and 6 to 8 weeks later, the hematoma is more or less isoechoic.[18]

Cysts (associated with gliomas, metastases, or other lesions) appear hypoechoic like the ventricles. Therefore, they are normally very well demarcated from surrounding brain tissue.

US-guided biopsy of intracerebral lesions can be performed in two ways: freehand and with a needle-guided adapter.

For ventricular tapping through a burr hole or in case of swelling of brain (e.g., during aneurysm surgery), the freehand method can be used. It can be done in a real-time fashion by placing the probe at the surface and advancing the ventricular catheter in the US plane toward the ventricle under real-time control. Another way is to visualize the ventricle in two perpendicular planes and place the catheter in the same angulation as the US probe. A safer approach is to use a biopsy guide attached to the probe. This fixation guarantees that the biopsy needle is always in the plane of the US beam and the angulation of the needle guide can be chosen according to the guideline on the US screen.[19] It must be kept in mind that the so-called burr hole US probes have (due to the miniaturization of the scan head and therefore limited space for crystals) a limited resolution and a lower signal-to-noise ratio compared with other modern scan heads. However, US-guided biopsies are diagnostic in 85% to 100% of cases, depending on histology and mainly the depth of the lesion.[19]

SPINAL APPLICATIONS

Generally, the statements for intracranial US imaging are also valid for intraspinal application. There are some differences concerning the practical use of IOUS during

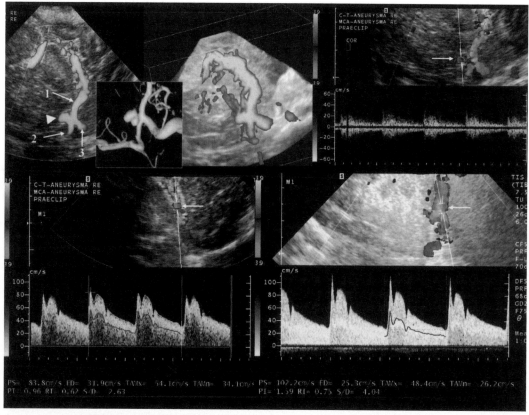

FIGURE 43-8 Aneurysm of the left carotid bifurcation. *Upper left:* Aneurysm (*arrowhead*) and bifurcation (1 = middle cerebral artery, 2 = anterior cerebral artery, 3 = carotid artery) in power mode (coronal plane, with corresponding 3-dimensional angiography). *Upper middle:* Intraoperative 3-dimensional ultrasound image of the aneurysm. *Upper right:* Triplex mode of the aneurysm with bichromatic display (*arrow*) and bidirectional Doppler signal (*bottom line*). *Lower left* (preclipping) and *lower right* (postclipping): Hemodynamic monitoring of middle cerebral artery with quantitative assessment of velocities due to angle-corrected Doppler sample volume (*arrows*). Postclipping there is only slight elevation of peak systolic flow (83.3 to 102.2 cm/second) and resistance index (0.67 to 0.73). (See Color Plate.)

spinal procedures. Through the saline solution–filled (hemi-) laminectomy site and due to the limited depth of the intraspinal space, high frequencies (7 to 10 MHz) should always be used to achieve a detailed display. In our experience, the borders of intramedullary tumors are much more difficult to ascertain (e.g., in astrocytomas) than in intracranial gliomas; therefore, IOUS for the purpose of resection control in intramedullary tumors is advisable only with limitations.[20] In these cases, intratumoral cysts can prove helpful because they are easy to identify and compare with preoperative magnetic resonance imaging. To minimize exposure and dural opening, spinal IOUS can be very valuable and, due to the high echogenicity of two of the most frequent intraspinal extramedullary tumors (meningiomas and neurinomas, Fig. 43-9), IOUS offers maximal information in a short time.

SPECIAL APPLICATIONS AND NEW TECHNIQUES

Transcranial Applications

Although transcranial US imaging in neurology is gaining more interest, its application in neurosurgery is of low importance because of the limited imaging quality.[22] However, in craniectomized patients the size of the ventricles and midline shift can be monitored because image quality improves dramatically without absorption and scattering by the skull.

Combination with Other Navigation Techniques

The combination of IOUS with frameless neuronavigation systems is one way to overcome the problem of brain shift and the resulting inaccuracy of navigation and localization tools that rely on preoperative data (as in frameless neuronavigation; see Fig. 43-6). Further advantages are the combination of three or more different image acquisition methods (computed tomography, magnetic resonance imaging, US) and the advantages of every image modality. Displaying the corresponding computed tomography/ magnetic resonance imaging parallel to the IOUS image plane makes it easier to interpret the IOUS image, especially for the surgeon not accustomed to US images.[23] There are two ways to implement this. One way is to add the frameless neuronavigation system to an already existing US platform, which has the advantage of excellent image quality due to digital data transfer and an all-in-one machine solution.[24] The other is to combine already existing frameless neuronavigation systems with any available US platform via an analogue signal, which offers the advantage of a high flexibility in the fast-growing US market.[25]

Another possible combination is IOUS and neuroendoscopy. Mechanical rotating or electronic probes (10 to 15 MHz) small enough to fit into endoscopes can produce radial US images at the tip of the endoscope and enable one to see "behind" structures seen in the endoscope.[26]

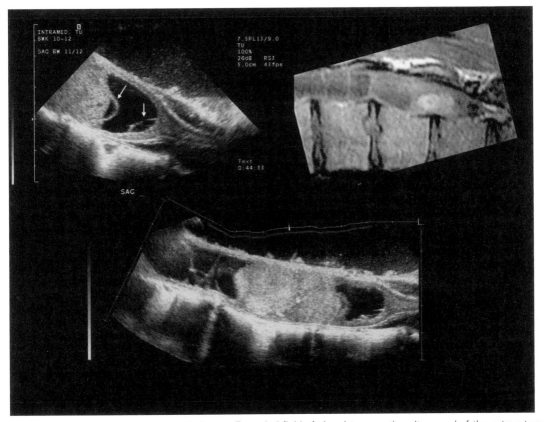

FIGURE 43-9 Intramedullary tumor (astrocytoma). *Lower:* Extended field of view intraoperative ultrasound of the astrocytoma to get an overview. *Upper left:* Detail of the distal end of the tumor with extension into conus (very small septa within the cyst, *arrow*).

Three-Dimensional Intraoperative Ultrasound

Three-dimensional IOUS is realized with different techniques. First, one has to differentiate whether IOUS is used in combination with a frameless neuronavigation system or as a stand-alone tool. In the first case, the frameless neuronavigation system reconstructs the IOUS data set as 3-dimensional images.[27] In the second case, there are two main techniques for 3-dimensional IOUS: sensor and processor based. While the first procedure is somewhat cumbersome (although measurements are highly reliable with this technique), the second is integrated in most high-end US machines today.[28] The latter is possible to do at any stage of the operation because it generates 3-dimensional images instantaneously. Postprocessing is possible with segmentation and choosing different display modes (volume/surface mode). In vascular neurosurgery, power mode can display aneurysms effectively as in 3-dimensional angiography (see Fig. 43-8).

Echo Contrast Enhancers and Other Applications

Echo contrast enhancers are small (~5 μm) air- or gas-filled bubbles with a more or less firm capsule (e.g., galactose, albumin). They can be administered intravenously, and very small vessels (capillaries) can be visualized due to their high acoustic impedance. Although echo contrast enhancers vibrate nonlinearly, they reflect harmonic frequencies to the transducer that can be received selectively, resulting in what is called harmonic imaging.[6] This technique can also be applied without echo contrast enhancers, dramatically improving signal-to-noise ratio (tissue harmonic imaging).[23] Using echo contrast enhancers, many new techniques (e.g., acoustic densitometry, transient response imaging, stimulated acoustic emission) are possible, and during the past years, perfusion measurement is one of the fields of growing interest using echo contrast enhancers and harmonic imaging. Other experimental intraoperative and intracranial applications are elastography and interventional US.

SUMMARY

IOUS is an intraoperative imaging modality that offers a multitude of possibilities. A sound knowledge of the physical principles of US and the willingness to acquaint oneself with the US image are both requisites for effective use of IOUS. It can be used in emergency cases, is not based on preoperative data, and is a real-time method. Continued practice will help the operator to judge artifacts and will in time increase the rate of yield. The technical possibilities and image quality are growing rapidly.

REFERENCES

1. French LA, Wild JJ, Neal D: The experimental application of ultrasonics to the localization of brain tumors. J Neurosurg 8:198–203, 1951.
2. Wild JJ, Reid JM: The effects of biological tissues on 15-m pulsed ultrasound. J Acoust Soc Am 270–280, 1953.
3. Leksell L: Echoencephalography. II: Midline echo from the pineal body as an index of pineal displacement. Acta Chir Scand 115:255–259, 1958.
4. Rubin JM, Mirfakhraee M, Duda EE, et al: Intraoperative ultrasound examination of the brain. Radiology 137:831–832, 1980.
5. Chandler WF, Knake JE, McGillicuddy JE, et al: Intraoperative use of real-time ultrasonography in neurosurgery. J Neurosurg 57:157–163, 1982.
6. Otsuki H, Nakatani S, Yamadaki M, et al: Intraoperative ultrasound arteriography with the "coded harmonic angio" technique. J Neurosurg 94:992–995, 2001.
7. LeRoux PD, Berger MS, Wang K, et al: Low-grade gliomas: Comparison of ultrasound characteristics with preoperative imaging studies. J Neurooncol 13:189–198, 1992.
8. McGahan JP, Ellis WEG, Budenz RW, et al: Brain gliomas: Sonographic characterization. Radiology 159:485–492, 1986.
9. Hammoud MA, Ligon BL, El Souki R, et al: Use of intraoperative ultrasound for localizing tumors and determining the extent of resection: A comparative study with magnetic resonance imaging. J Neurosurg 84:737–741, 1996.
10. Woydt M, Krone A, Becker G, et al: Correlation of intra-operative ultrasound with histopathologic findings after tumor resection in supratentorial gliomas. Acta Neurochir (Wien) 138:1391–1398, 1996.
11. Unsgaard G, Gronningsaeter A, Ommedal S, et al: Brain operations guided by real-time two-dimensional ultrasound: New possibilities as a result of improved image quality. Neurosurgery 51:402–412, 2002.
12. Woydt M, Krone A, Soerensen N, et al: Ultrasound-guided neuronavigation of deep-seated cavernous haemangiomas: Clinical results and navigation techniques. Br J Neurosurg 15:485–495, 2001.
13. Kitazawa K, Nitta J, Okudera H, et al: Color Doppler ultrasound imaging in the emergency management of an intracerebral hematoma caused by cerebral arteriovenous malformations: Technical case report. Neurosurgery 42:405–407, 1998.
14. Woydt M, Perez J, Meixensberger J, et al: Intraoperative color Duplex sonography in the surgical management of cerebral AV-malformations. Acta Neurochir (Wien) 140:689–698, 1998.
15. Woydt M, Greiner K, Perez J, et al: Intraoperative color Duplex sonography of basal arteries during aneurysm surgery. J Neuroimaging 7:203–207, 1997.
16. Payer M, Kaku Y, Bernays R, et al: Intraoperative color-coded duplex sonography for localization of a distal middle cerebral artery aneurysm: Technical case report. Neurosurgery 42:941–943, 1998.
17. Woydt M, Horowski A, Krone A, et al: Guiding and hemodynamic monitoring in aneurysm surgery with intraoperative color-duplex-sonography. J Neurosurg 90:411A, 1999.
18. Enzmann DR, Britt RH, Lyons B, et al: Natural history of experimental intracerebral hemorrhage. Am J Neuroradiol 2:517–526, 1981.
19. Strowitzki M, Moringlane JR, Steudel WI, et al: Ultrasound-based navigation during intracranial burr hole procedures: Experience in a series of 100 cases. Surg Neurol 54:134–144, 2000.
20. Epstein FJ, Farmer J-P, Schneider SJ: Intraoperative ultrasonography: An important surgical adjunct for intramedullary tumors. J Neurosurg 74:729–733, 1991.
21. Maiuri F, Iaconetta G, de Divitiis O: The role of intraoperative sonography in reducing invasiveness during surgery for spinal tumors. Minim Invasive Neurosurg 40:8–12, 1997.
22. Mursch K, Vogelsang JP, Zimmerer B, et al: Bedside measurement of the third ventricle's diameter during episodes of arising intracranial pressure after head trauma. Acta Neurochir (Wien) 137:19–24, 1995.
23. Woydt M, Vince GH, Krauss J, et al: New ultrasound techniques and their application in neurosurgical intraoperative sonography. Neurol Res 23:97–705, 2001.
24. Gronningsaeter A, Kleven A, Ommedal S, et al: Sono-Wand, an ultrasound-based neuronavigation system. Neurosurgery 47:1373–1380, 2000.
25. Trobaugh JW, Richard WD, Smith KR, et al: Frameless ultrasonography: Method and applications. Comput Med Imaging Graph 18:235–246, 1994.
26. Resch KDM, Perneczky A, Schwarz M, et al: Endo-neuro-sonography principles and 3-D technique. Childs Nerv Syst 13:616–621, 1997.
27. Jödicke A, Deinsberger W, Erbe H, et al: Intraoperative three-dimensional ultrasonography: An approach to register brain shift using multidimensional image processing. Minim Invasive Neurosurg 41:13–19, 1998.
28. Woydt M, Horowski A, Krauss J, et al: Three-dimensional intraoperative ultrasound of vascular malformations and supratentorial tumors. J Neuroimaging 12:1–7, 2002.

Section IX

Brain Tumors

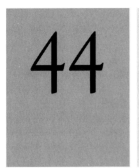

Frame-Based Stereotactic Brain Biopsy

KENDALL H. LEE, BRENT T. HARRIS, and DAVID W. ROBERTS

INTRODUCTION

Stereotactic brain biopsy is used increasingly to aid in the diagnosis and management of intracranial lesions.[1-3] When lesions are judged not suitable for radical excision because of their location (such as the brain stem), histology, or number, the goal of this procedure in nearly all cases is to obtain tissue for accurate pathologic diagnosis so that a final management strategy can be instituted. It is a technique widely used with minimal morbidity in the management of lesions such as pineal region tumors, primary cerebral lymphomas, acquired immunodeficiency syndrome–related brain masses, and deep-seated and eloquent region inflammatory masses,[4] offering a high diagnostic yield. Therefore, it is essential that the clinical teams that are caring for the neurosurgical patient including neurosurgeons, oncologists, neurologists, and pathologists be well aware of the choice of established and emerging techniques as well as diagnostic utility and limitations of this important neurosurgical procedure.

HISTORICAL ASPECTS OF STEREOTAXIS

In the 17th century, Pierre de Fermat and René Descartes independently recognized that a system composed of two perpendicular lines can be used to identify any point within a plane.[5] The distances along each of these lines (the *x*- and *y*-axes) from the origin to a given point provide an ordered pair of numbers that is unique to that point. Such a rectangular coordinate system is called Cartesian, in honor of Descartes. In such a manner, each location in a given space can be uniquely and quantitatively defined.

In 1873, Dittmar[6] was the first to report the use of guided probes into the medulla oblongata of animals. In 1890, Zernov, a Russian anatomist, developed an instrument called the encephalometer, which used the polar coordinates and an arc-based guiding mechanism[7,8] to guide a probe to a location. In 1908, Horsley and Clarke[9] reported the instrumentation and method for producing lesions at specific locations within the cerebellum. However, it was not until 1947 when Spiegel, a neurologist, and Wycis, a neurosurgeon, introduced a new stereotactic system and techniques that allowed the use in humans.[10] Their technique used a frame and 3-dimensional coordinate system related to intracranial landmarks defined by pneumoencephalography. These first human devices were used to lesion particular brain regions for the treatment of movement disorders. However, to identify specific intracranial

targets required the stereotactic coordinates of each target, and in 1952, Spiegel and Wycis[11] published a human stereotactic brain atlas.

Conway[12] reported the first series on stereotactic biopsy of 31 deep-seated intracranial tumors in 1973. In the ensuing decades, there have been tremendous improvements in the ability to identify specific neuroanatomic targets with the introduction of computed tomography (CT)–guided neurosurgery in 1976[13] and of magnetic resonance imaging (MRI) in the mid-1980s.[14]

STEREOTACTIC INSTRUMENTATION

All stereotactic instrument systems are based on some mathematical system of 3-dimensional spatial coordinates and some system of achieving controlled movement along defined geometric axes. The mathematical systems of special coordinates that are often used are the Cartesian and Polar coordinate systems, in which the location of a point in *n*-dimensional space may be uniquely defined by the assignment of *n* coordinates to that point. The Cartesian system is composed of perpendicular lines (what may be called *x*-, *y*-, *z*-axes) from the origin (the axes' intersection, in which each axis is usually assigned a value of 0). The Polar system localizes a point in space by specifying its distance and direction from an origin, that is, a radius and one or more angles (perpendicular with respect to each other). Indeed, these systems are mathematically equivalent, and one may convert the coordinates of one system to those of another by the following the formulas: $x = r \sin\theta \cos\varphi$, $y = r \sin\theta \sin\varphi$, $z = r \cos\theta$.

There are several designs for a stereotactic apparatus and these include (1) translational systems, (2) arc-centered systems, (3) focal point systems, (4) Polar coordinate systems, (5) burr hole–mounted devices, (6) phantom target systems, (7) a system of interlocking arcs, (8) computer-based systems, and (9) the so-called frameless systems.

The translational system (also called rectilinear system), used by Horsley and Clarke in 1906, allows maneuverability of the biopsy needle or probe in longitudinal or vertical directions by linear displacement of the electrode carrier.[15] Interestingly, circa 1918, Aubrey Mussen also had made a frame-based on a translational system intended for human use, but it was never used.[16]

Arc-centered systems, such as that introduced by Leksell[17] in 1949, work on the principle that a probe whose length is equal to the radius of an arc will reach the center of the arc when introduced perpendicular to a tangent anywhere along the arc. By linear adjustments of the arc

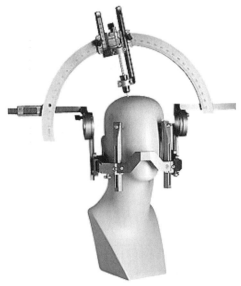

FIGURE 44-1   The Leksell Model G stereotactic frame. (Courtesy of Elekta AB. www.elekta.com/healthcareus.nsf.)

support system in three dimensions, the probe is brought to the target. The system is based on the center-of-arc principle and the basic components are the Cartesian coordinate frame and a semicircular arc (Fig. 44-1). The Cosman-Roberts-Wells is another arc radius system (Radionics; Fig. 44-2). Couldwell and Apuzzo[18] reported in 1990 their initial experience with a new arc radius design of stereotactic frame that interfaced with the existing components of the Brown-Roberts-Wells instrument.

Focal point systems, such as the Todd-Wells system, are similar to arc-radius systems except that the patient's head is moved within the arc, bringing the target to the center of the arc.

Polar coordinate systems use a combination of angles and a probe depth measurement to specify a trajectory and a target point. A minimum of two angles in planes perpendicular to each other plus the probe length are required to specify a unique trajectory in 3-dimensional space. The Cooper[19] device involves a polar coordinate system that includes calibrated protractors used with a ventriculogram. A line is marked from entry point to target while the desired trajectory is compared with the actual trajectory, and angular corrections are made.

In burr hole systems, the device is mounted to the margins of a hole in the skull, allowing guidance of a probe to different lengths at various angles. Examples of such a system is the plastic ball-and-socket system reported by Austin and Lee[20] in 1958 and that reported by McCaul[21] in 1959. These burr hole–mounted systems are limited by the inherent inaccuracy of a single-point fixation so that the fractional adjustments of the angular device are translated via the fulcrum, which may lead to inaccurate targeting.

Phantom target systems, such as the Riechert-Mundinger,[22] Gillingham-modified Guiot,[23] and Brown-Roberts-Wells[24] designs, use a phantom frame and target to allow a mechanical setting of the probe impact point. The phantom target principle can be used with any coordinate system but is most commonly used in combination with polar coordinate systems. An advantage of the phantom target system is that procedures can be rehearsed before performing surgery on the patient.

Newer systems have been developed that use advances in computer technology. One of these is the microtargeting platform for the microtargeting drive system.[25] This system for surgical targeting attaches directly to a skull-based fiducial system and aligns the microtargeting microdrive with a selected target (Fig. 44-3). The technology behind the

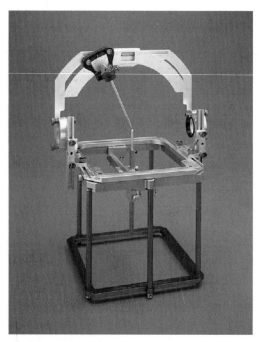

FIGURE 44-2   Cosman-Roberts-Wells frame with phantom base. (Courtesy of Radionics.)

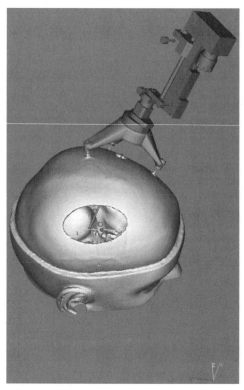

FIGURE 44-3   Computer image of microtargeting system. (Courtesy of F.H.C., Inc.)

microtargeting platform is based on a computer-generated virtual custom mounting interface for a particular patient that allows precise localization of the target, entry point, and a fixed reference. A data file is generated that allows the platform to be fabricated. The microtargeting platform can then be attached to the fixed reference points and will provide a known location relative to the patient anatomy from which the microtargeting drive can be guided by direct attachment.

Frameless stereotactic systems provide the surgeon with navigational information relating the location of instruments in the operative field to preoperative imaging data. The first application of a frameless system was developed by Roberts and colleagues[26,27] in 1986. Such information minimizes invasiveness by more accurately selecting the best trajectory to the target.[28] To achieve these goals, these systems use the stereotactic principle of coregistration of the patient with an imaging study.[27,29] Using such systems, even neurosurgical units with a limited number of procedures, can successfully implement neuronavigation in daily routines.[30]

INDICATIONS AND CONTRAINDICATIONS FOR STEREOTACTIC BRAIN BIOPSY

Given the ease, safety, and accuracy of stereotactic techniques, the indications for open biopsy is rare. Stereotactic biopsy is optimal in patients with (1) deep, intrinsic lesions that have a high risk of significant neurologic deficit such as in the brain stem; (2) lesions poorly defined on imaging that may be considered for further surgical or medical therapy, depending on the lesion's pathology, which is usually neoplastic, infectious, or inflammatory[31]; (3) those who appear to have a lesion in which the value of open surgery is questionable; and (4) patients in poor medical condition precluding general anesthesia.[32–34]

The presence of an extensively vascular lesion or a lesion that is near a major vascular structure (i.e., near the sylvian region or the area adjacent to the cavernous sinus/carotid artery complex) represent a relative contraindication to stereotactic biopsy. In the series of Apuzzo and colleagues,[1] 5% of patients evaluated for stereotactic biopsy under these circumstances were managed by alternative strategies such as observation or conventional craniotomy.

IMPACT ON TREATMENT PLANNING

Friedman and colleagues[35] reported that the rate of discrepancy between the clinical impression and histologic diagnosis was 13%, in which the management was changed after the stereotactic biopsy. Lunsford and Martinez[36] reported an even higher rate of 26% (26 of 102 patients). Kim and colleagues[37] reported that the disagreement rate between the preoperative clinical and subsequent histologic diagnosis that led to a change of treatment was 27%. Plunkett and colleagues[31] reported that management was altered in 57 of 141 patients (40%) due to histology after stereotactic biopsy. Given these relatively high rates in which the stereotactic biopsy result changed the management plan, histologic confirmation of intracranial lesions is warranted.

NEURORADIOLOGY FOR IMAGING-DIRECTED BIOPSY

CT, MRI, positron-emission tomography (PET), and angiography are each used in planning brain biopsies. Fontaine and colleagues[38] present the results of 100 consecutive MRI-guided biopsies in cases in which CT guiding was considered dangerous or impossible. MRI guidance was preferred to CT guidance for cases in which lesions were located in the central area or were not clearly visible on CT scan or where the visualization of vessels was considered necessary. MRI guiding for stereotactic biopsies was effective for CT-invisible or ill-defined lesions, lesions located in functional or densely vascularized areas, and in the brain stem.

Vindlacheruvu and colleagues[39] audited their experience of MRI-guided biopsy and demonstrated that it is feasible and comparable with CT-guided biopsy in terms of diagnostic accuracy with a low procedural morbidity. Hall and colleagues[40] reported on 35 brain biopsies performed in a high-field strength interventional MRI unit. Diagnostic tissue was obtained in all 35 brain biopsies, and in all cases magnetic resonance spectroscopy was accurate in distinguishing recurrent tumors (five cases) from radiation necrosis (one case). Hall and colleagues concluded that interventional 1.5-T MRI is a safe and effective method for evaluating lesions of brain. Magnetic resonance spectroscopic targeting is likely to augment the diagnostic yield of brain biopsies. The interrelationships between MRI, CT, angiography, and stereotactic biopsy and their respective roles in the establishment of a definitive diagnosis were discussed by Baleriaux and colleagues.[32]

Recently, dynamic susceptibility contrast MRI technique has been used in determining the stereotactic biopsy site. Dynamic susceptibility contrast MRI can provide relative cerebral blood volume and is one of the most reliable methods to evaluate in vivo tumor vascularity. Tumor vessel size is extremely variable, and the gradient-echo echo-planar imaging technique, being sensitive to the total vascular bed, is well suited for the purpose of visualizing tumor vasculature in vivo. Dynamic susceptibility contrast MRI is especially useful for grading glioma, and Sugahara and colleagues[41] found that this technique can also provide information to differentiate between malignant lymphoma and glioma because the absence of tumor neovascularization of malignant lymphoma leads to low regional cerebral blood volume, in contrast to those of malignant gliomas.

Although not necessary to do routinely, in cases in which the lesion may be vascular (e.g., aneurysm, arteriovenous malformation) or may have displaced major vascular structures (e.g., pineal tumor's relationship to the deep veins), it is advisable to obtain an angiogram before performing a biopsy.

Positron-Emission Tomography

In an effort to optimize yield and decrease sampling error, PET is used to guide the biopsy needle trajectory. Levivier and colleagues[42] reported 100% diagnostic yield in 90 stereotactic trajectories planned in 43 patients using PET with fluorodeoxyglucose F18 (FDG). In 36 patients, an area of abnormal FDG uptake is used to guide at least one biopsy trajectory. A total of 90 stereotactic trajectories were performed; among them, 55 based on PET-defined targets and 35 based on CT-defined targets. Histologic diagnosis was obtained in all patients, but six of the 90 trajectories were nondiagnostic; all six were based on targets defined by CT alone. Differences between the diagnostic yield of trajectories based on PET-defined targets and those based on CT-defined targets were statistically significant in patients with contrast-enhanced lesions but not in patients with nonenhancing lesions.[42] These results support the view that PET may contribute to the successful management of patients with brain tumor requiring stereotactic biopsy. Because there is no increase in discomfort or morbidity related to the technique, it is suggested that the development of similar techniques integrating PET data in the planning of stereotactic biopsy be considered by centers performing stereotactic surgery and having access to PET technology.[42] Thompson and colleagues[43] evaluated the utility of PET to distinguish radiation necrosis from recurrent tumor in a retrospective review of patients with primary glial neoplasms. Fifteen patients had preoperative contrast-enhanced MRI and PET images followed by stereotactic biopsy or craniotomy and histologic confirmation. The sensitivity of PET was 43% (six of 14) and the specificity was 100% (one of one). The authors conclude that, given the clinical significance of distinguishing tumor progression from radiation necrosis, PET is insufficient to resolve the issue of radiation necrosis versus tumor progression.[43]

Pirotte and colleagues[44] report their results in a consecutive series of 38 patients who underwent combined PET and CT-guided stereotactic biopsy. In 31 patients, at least one trajectory was defined using an abnormality visualized on PET. A histologic diagnosis was obtained in all cases. The diagnostic yield of each trajectory according to the FDG uptake of PET and contrast enhancement on CT showed that most low-grade tumors were found in hypometabolic/hypodense areas and glioblastomas were all diagnosed in areas with increased FDG uptake and contrast enhancement on CT, whereas data for anaplastic astrocytomas are heterogeneously distributed. In their series, six targets defined on CT were nondiagnostic; however, this never occurred when targets were defined on PET.[44]

Pirotte and colleagues[45] combined PET and MRI in the planning of stereotactic brain biopsy in nine children (five boys and four girls, aged 2 to 14 years) with infiltrative, ill-defined brain lesions. The tracers used for PET are ^{18}F-fluoro-2-deoxy-D-glucose in four cases, ^{11}C-methionine in two cases, and both tracers in three cases. Biopsy targets were selected in hypermetabolic areas. PET-guided stereotactic brain biopsy provided accurate histologic diagnosis in all patients and allowed a reduction in the number of trajectories in lesions located in functional areas. This preliminary series also suggests that combining PET and MRI in the planning of stereotactic biopsy in children improves the diagnostic yield in infiltrative, ill-defined brain lesions and makes it possible to reduce the sampling in high-risk/functional areas, thereby improving the quality of therapeutic management of pediatric brain tumors.[45]

SURGICAL TECHNIQUE

There are many acceptable surgical techniques and stereotactic frames that are currently being used for stereotactic

brain biopsy. No one technique is universally accepted, nor is there one that is better than another in all situations. However, based on our experience, we describe here the technique used at Dartmouth-Hitchcock Medical Center neurosurgical service.

After informed consent is obtained, the patient is taken to the anesthesia holding area, where the Leksell Model G frame is placed. The patient is placed in the sitting position, and the forehead and occipital scalp are cleaned with iodine solution. The base is secured during placement by tape extending from the nose part to the occiput, while an observer standing at the front of the patient visually monitors the base position. After the desired position is achieved, the scalp is infiltrated at the four fixation points with 1% lidocaine with 1:200,000 units of epinephrine. Frame fixation to the patient's head is achieved with adjustable fixation posts and self-tapping screws. A variety of exchangeable front pieces allows flexibility, both with regard to access to the patient's nose and mouth and frame positioning. The localizing unit is attached to the base ring and CT or MRI is then performed. CT, MRI, radiography, angiography, or PET localization may be performed with the same frame in any sequence (Fig. 44-4). The adapter ensures that the patient's head is supported throughout the scanning procedure. CT and MR scans are made parallel to the frame providing reproducibility. This feature allows scans to be compared with each other or with an atlas. The localizing unit is then removed from the base ring, and the patient taken to the operating room. Localization and target coordinate determination may be performed with an entirely manual method, standard scanner software, or dedicated computer software systems.

For the manual method for calculating x, y, and z coordinates, the (0, 0, 0) coordinate has been arbitrarily define at right, superior, posterior, for the Leksell Model G system. The x coordinate is obtained by measuring the distance from midpoint (100, 100, z) to target in the horizontal direction, then adding to 100 if the lesion is to the left of midpoint or subtracting from 100 if the lesion is to the right of midpoint. Thus right-sided lesions will have a value

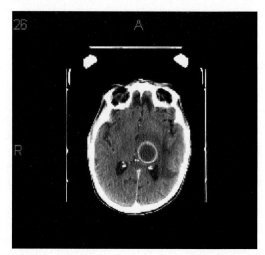

FIGURE 44-4 Axial head computed tomography scan of a patient undergoing stereotactic brain biopsy with Leksell Model G frame in place.

less than 100, and left-sided lesions will have a value greater than 100. The y coordinate is obtained by measuring the distance from midpoint (100, 100, z) to target in the perpendicular direction, adding to 100 if the lesion is anterior to the midpoint or subtracting from 100 if the lesion is posterior to the midpoint. Thus anterior lesions will have a value greater than 100, and posterior lesions will have a value less than 100. The z coordinate is obtained by measuring the distance from posterior set point to the variable side bar mark, then adding to 40, to get the z value.

A target point is selected that is most representative of the mass. The exact point within a mass lesion that is most representative varies with the type of lesion, so that with a cystic lesion, the wall provides the most diagnostic material, whereas the central part is usually the most representative area in a solid neoplasm, with exception of glioblastoma multiforme, in which the center may be necrotic. Multiple biopsies may be taken from different points along a single trajectory. Entry areas along a major arterial watershed zones are also deemed preferable as they are relatively safer.

Once localization is completed, the stereotactic arc is attached to the frame. The arc is positioned according to the calculated x, y, and z coordinates of the target so its center coincides with the selected target. Because of the complete freedom of choice for the entry point, the target can be reached from any direction without further computer calculations or phantom simulations. The frame is secured to the operating table with a Leksell clamp adaptor for use with the Mayfield headrest. In general, the semisitting position with local anesthesia (monitored anesthesia care) is used. This positioning is more comfortable for the surgeon and the patient.

For most biopsies, a burr hole is made near the coronal suture, although a parietal or occipital approach may also be used. The skull hole is made with the $^{3}/_{16}$-inch bit that is able to fit within the drill guide attached to the Leksell frame. This allows the Sedan needle (Fig. 44-5) to be placed at the target. Using a syringe, 2 mL are withdrawn from the target site. Additional specimens are obtained at this site by rotating the biopsy needle in 90-degree increments. The needle is withdrawn progressively, and additional specimens may be taken along the biopsy trajectory. With the inner canula removed, the outer canula is examined for bleeding, after which the inner canula is replaced and the needle removed. The skin incision is closed with 4-0 Prolene suture, the wound is cleaned, and then bacitracin, Xeroform, dry sterile gauze, and tape are applied.

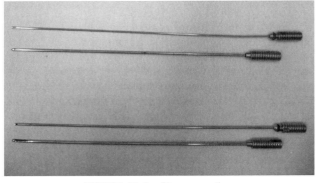

FIGURE 44-5 Biopsy needles.

The Leksell Model G stereotactic frame is removed, and the patient transferred to the post anesthesia care unit for observation.

NEUROPATHOLOGY

Clear communication and coordination between the surgical and pathology teams are critical. It may be helpful for the pathologist to enter the operating room suite during the procedure. Providing the pathologist with the patient's age, presentation of illness, previous relevant diagnoses and treatment, location of lesion, and pertinent imaging findings is basic to helping the pathologist generate a differential diagnosis. Because most patients undergoing stereotactic procedures are sedated but awake, discussions should be kept quiet, especially when the pathologist returns to the room with the diagnosis. Some pathologists will be unaware of the patient's level of consciousness. Less desirable are pass-through tube specimen systems with communication between the pathologist and surgeon via an intercom or telephone. Such tube systems have been known to malfunction or cause small specimens to be damaged in their containers.

Slide Preparation

Preserving the integrity of the specimen occurs immediately on removal. Optimally, two to four cores at least 0.5 cm in length should be obtained. These are placed on saline-moistened gauze or Telfa pad material and positioned in a Petri dish or specimen container; they should be neither too dry nor submerged in saline. If infection is in the differential diagnosis, the specimens should be obtained for microorganism studies in the OR rather than the nonsterile frozen section room. Often abnormal tissue can be differentiated grossly from normal based on coloration, texture, and consistency. Necrotic tissue may not form solid cores and often has a yellow-tan or hemorrhagic appearance. Once passed on to the pathologist, it is his or her responsibility to efficiently generate a rapid preliminary report (or at least indicate whether the tissue is sufficient for a diagnosis after full processing and examination) and notify the surgical team.

Depending on the amount of material submitted for intraoperative consultation and the preferences of the pathologist, cytologic smears and/or frozen sections are prepared. Ideally, both should be prepared because the findings are often complementary in forming the intraoperative consult diagnosis. With less than 1 mm of tissue, a smear preparation can yield useful results. Also called squash or touch preparation by some, the minute piece of abnormal tissue is cut from the core with a clean scalpel and placed delicately on a glass slide.[46] While this slide is being held, another slide is positioned above and squashed down, sandwiching the tissue. Then the slides are rapidly pulled apart lengthwise to smear the tissue out along both slides. The slides can be air dried and stained or, more often, quickly placed in methanol to fix the tissue and then taken through staining steps with hematoxylin and eosin. The advantages of the smear preparation are better cytologic detail, no freeze artifact, and speed. The primary disadvantage is loss of cytoarchitecture and relational orientation of the lesion with normal central nervous system structure.

Frozen sections are prepared by choosing a likely abnormal portion of the core(s) by color/texture/consistency and placing the tissue piece on a platform "chuck" in a semifrozen medium. Some tissue from the core (we generally take half for the intraoperative consult and leave the other half for permanent sections) should not be frozen or smeared but preserved in formalin for permanent sections. The tissue/ medium is then fully frozen within a cryostat to approximately −20°C. Several sections of the tissue are cut within the cryostat at low temperature, placed on slides, and processed similarly to the smear preparations. The major advantage of frozen sections is that most pathologists are more familiar with sections of tissue that retains normal and lesion cytoarchitectural landmarks as compared with neurocytologic smears. However, cutting frozen sections can be quite challenging with the small amounts of tissue available from these biopsies, and artifacts are largely unavoidable. These artifacts can include freezing vacuoles usually within neuropil or chatter artifact that leaves the tissue looking like venetian blinds.

Final diagnosis resides with examination of the permanent sections after full processing of the tissues. Tumor typing is aided by the use of immunohistochemistry and ultrastructural examination, and the examination of serial sections is of value in grading.[47]

POSTOPERATIVE MANAGEMENT

Given that currently there is little consensus on the postoperative care of patients undergoing stereotactic biopsy,[48] a survey of active members of the American Association of Neurological Surgeons/Central Nervous System Section on Tumors was performed by Warnick and colleagues.[48] They found that most surgeons (59%) routinely ordered postoperative CT scans, and the remainder ordered scans based on specific indications. Furthermore, patients were transferred from the recovery room to a special care unit in 47%, a regular room in 47%, or home in 6%.[48] Warnick and colleagues also retrospectively reviewed 84 consecutive stereotactic biopsy procedures at their institution to assess the potential benefit of routine CT scanning and intensive care unit monitoring.[48] In this retrospective review, 81 patients underwent 84 stereotactic biopsy procedures; 79 underwent postoperative CT scanning, and all 81 were monitored overnight in the intensive care unit. Among five (6%) patients who experienced intraoperative hemorrhage, two (2%) underwent craniotomy to control arterial bleeding. Three (4%) patients developed new neurologic deficits, which occurred within 2 hours of surgery. In both groups, CT scans were helpful in excluding hemorrhage that would require reoperation. In the remaining patients (90%), findings on routine postoperative CT did not alter patient management, and intensive care unit monitoring appeared unnecessary because neurologic complications occurred within 2 hours postoperatively. They confirmed these results in the prospective study of 54 patients undergoing stereotactic biopsy without routine postoperative CT scanning or intensive care unit monitoring. In contrast with national practice patterns reported, based on their study, Warnick and colleagues recommended that CT scanning and intensive care unit monitoring be reserved for patients who have intraoperative hemorrhage or new deficits after surgery. All other patients are recommended to be monitored for 2 hours in the recovery room and transferred to a regular hospital room without a postoperative CT scan.[48]

Linhares and colleagues[49] evaluated the efficacy of postoperative CT to diagnose intracerebral damage and to determine the existence of postbiopsy hemorrhage. They evaluated 80 consecutive cases of patients who underwent a stereotactic brain biopsy; 63 of them had a control CT scan from 4 to 6 hours after the procedure. There were inconclusive results in five patients (6.25%), significant morbidity in four cases (5%), and no mortality. Control CT scanning revealed no alterations in 25 patients and vestigial hemorrhage in 27. In the remaining 11 patients, the hemorrhage was of little significance. The authors concluded that the realization of a control CT scan within few hours after biopsy allows the identification of a subgroup of patients without intracerebral hemorrhage who may be discharged from the hospital on the same day.

DIAGNOSTIC YIELD

Over the past decade, a number of studies have investigated the efficacy of stereotactic brain biopsy. Many of these have been summarized by Hall[50] who found in some 17 different studies on a total of almost 7500 patients undergoing stereotactic brain biopsy that the average diagnostic yield was 91% (range, 80% to 96%). Some of the reasons given for diagnostic failure include small sample size, inaccurate tissue targeting and sampling error, target choice in areas of high signal on T2-weighted MRI, and small target size. In Hall's own series, he describes an increase in diagnostic yield from 80% to 96% after instituting intraoperative review by pathologists. Most of the pathology literature is in agreement that intraoperative consultation improves the diagnostic efficacy of the procedure by providing feedback to the surgeon regarding the adequacy of the tissue and indicating when additional biopsies might be required.[51,52]

The efficacy of combining cytologic and histologic techniques has also been advocated to assist in improving the accuracy of grading gliomas,[53] although in some cases it remains difficult to distinguish gliosis from low-grade astrocytomas with either method. In a large series of 650 central nervous system lesions, cytologic smears were prepared alone at intraoperative consult and provided an accurate diagnosis in 97.3% (concordance with paraffin sections).[54] Review of eight other large series show similar diagnostic yields of cytopathologic preparations averaging greater than 90%. In summary, the diagnostic yield for stereotactic brain biopsy is quite high with low morbidity and mortality and is improved with the implementation of intraoperative pathology consultation and cytologic smear preparation.

There is general agreement that stereotactic biopsy provides a definitive diagnosis in 91% to 98.1% of patients.[1,46,49,50] Fratkin and colleagues[46] reported that in their series of 29 patients with CT-guided stereotactic biopsy, 7% were nondiagnostic due to sampling error. Reasons for diagnostic failure include lesion location adjacent to the ventricular system, inaccurate targeting, and the inability to penetrate the tumor.[50] In addition, diagnostic difficulties in interpreting the biopsy specimen include accurate tumor typing and grading and the distinction between reactive and neoplastic astrocytic proliferations.[47] Ryken and colleagues,[34] reviewing 12 infratentorial stereotactic biopsies in 11 patients, concluded that stereotactic biopsy of infratentorial lesions can be performed safely with a high probability of obtaining a diagnosis. In an attempt to ascertain the incidence of unexpected pathologic findings, 100 consecutive stereotactic biopsies were reviewed by Friedman et al,[35] who found that 12 patients were found to have diagnoses of pathologic conditions that preoperatively were considered unlikely or not considered at all.

Chadrasoma and colleagues[33] reported the pathologic accuracy of image-directed stereotactic brain biopsy in 30 patients who had mass lesions of the brain and subsequently underwent resection of the mass. The histologic diagnosis at stereotactic biopsy was appropriate for direction of clinical management in 28 of 30 patients. Correlation between the stereotactic and resection diagnoses was exact in 19 of 30 cases. These included 11 of 12 nonastrocytic neoplasms and eight of 13 astrocytic neoplasms. Correlation was imperfect in nine of 30 cases, which included two cases of anaplastic astrocytoma that were upgraded to glioblastoma multiforme, two cases of astrocytoma that had a significant oligodendroglial component, and five nonneoplastic lesions that were reported on biopsy as showing nonspecific reactive changes. In two of 30 patients, the stereotactic biopsy was not accurate, which included one patient who had glioblastoma multiforme whose stereotactic biopsy specimen showed only necrotic tissue. Thus Chandrasoma and colleagues concluded that, with careful target placement, stereotactic biopsy can provide biopsy material that represents the entire lesion with an accuracy that is sufficient for clinical management. Serious diagnostic error that resulted in clinical mismanagement occurred in one patient who had a pineal germinoma that had large areas of granulomatous inflammation at which the stereotactic biopsy was directed.[33]

In addition, Feiden and colleagues[55] reported the concordance rate to be 89% between stereotactic biopsy and subsequent craniotomy or autopsy, whereas Voges and colleagues[56] reported it to be 88%. Kim and colleagues[37] found the concordance rate was 96.6% between stereotactic biopsy and the biopsy at craniotomy (29 of 30 cases).

SAFETY/COMPLICATIONS

Complications arising from stereotactic biopsy are infrequent, with mortality being reported in less than 1% and significant morbidity occurring in 5%.[1,57,58] The four most common complications are hemorrhage, new neurologic deficit, seizures, and infections. Thus preoperative identification of high-risk characteristics may permit modification of either operative technique, patient selection, or both to reduce the risk of these adverse outcomes. For example, Sawin and colleagues[58] studied factors that may confer an increased risk of morbidity from stereotactic brain biopsy by evaluating 225 consecutive stereotactic brain biopsy procedures and noting that the demographic, anatomic, surgical, and histologic data were compiled and putative risk factors for morbidity identified. They performed univariate and logistic regression analyses to determine the significance as independent predictors of operative risk. Twelve patients had complications as a consequence of the biopsy procedure, eight from hemorrhage and four from direct trauma. Major morbidity (hemiparesis, aphasia, obtundation) occurred 3.6%, and 1.3% had minor morbidity (transient, mild neurologic deficits); there was one operative fatality (0.4%). An increased risk of morbidity was associated with the preoperative use of antiplatelet agents, long-term

corticosteroid therapy, deep-seated lesions, malignant gliomas, and a greater number of biopsy attempts.[58] Factors not conferring increased morbidity included gender, age, preexisting illness, extracranial malignancy, cardiac disease, hypertension, diabetes, human immunodeficiency virus status, and instrument used to procure the specimen.[58] These results suggests that the morbidity of stereotactic brain biopsy may be minimized by risk factor modification.

Investigations into the incidence and timing of complications after stereotactic biopsy revealed that most occurred within hours of the procedure, although there have been reports of complications arising 1 to 2 days later. Bernstein and colleagues[57] documented neurologic complications in 19 (6.3%) patients, including 3 who deteriorated more than 8 hours after surgery. Interestingly, Bhardwaj and Bernstein[59] reported the results of a prospective trial of 76 patients who underwent outpatient stereotactic biopsy and found that only 2 patients were not discharged on the same day (97.4% success rate). The two patients underwent inpatient admission because one required intravenous antibiotic treatment of a brain abscess and the other had a hard lesion in the brain stem that precluded biopsy needle penetration; admission for further investigation of the lesion was elected. Two patients experienced complications (2.6%), that is, one small area of intraventricular hemorrhage that produced only a mild headache and one case of mild worsening of preexisting leg weakness, with negative CT results. Thus Bhardwaj and Bernstein[59] concluded that discharging patients home after 4 hours of observation after stereotactic biopsies seems to be a safe, well-tolerated practice.

The influence of lesion location on morbidity is not a new or particularly novel concept. Operative manipulation of eloquent brain regions, whether by open craniotomy or by a stereotactic approach, carries with it an increased risk of neurologic impairment. Direct operative trauma, perilesional edema, or intraparenchymal hemorrhage is less well tolerated within the confines of the thalamus, basal ganglia, or brain stem than within the expanses of the nondominant lobar white matter and is much more likely to manifest itself as neurologic dysfunction. Bouvier and colleagues[60] noted a 26% incidence of neurologic decline after stereotactic biopsy of perirolandic lesions. Bernstein and Parrent[57] postulated that malignant lesions such as lymphoma and malignant glioma would be more prone to hemorrhage and/or produce edema after manipulation because of the anomalous neovascularity of these lesions; experience with malignant gliomas confirms a trend toward poorer operative outcome in patients with this histology. Furthermore, Favre and colleagues[61] showed that there was no statistically significant difference in the risk of hematoma formation between morphologic (139 biopsies, 18 lesion evacuations [cysts, abscesses, and hematomas], and 18 drain implantations) and 186 functional procedures (137 lesions [thalamotomy or pallidotomy], 47 deep brain electrode implantations, and 2 physiologic explorations without lesions or implantations), suggesting that the risk of bleeding for stereotactic procedures is related more to the patient than to the type of procedure performed.[61]

Bernstein and Parrent[57] reviewed a series of 300 consecutive stereotactic biopsies for intra-axial brain lesions performed by one neurosurgeon and critically analyzed the complications of the procedure. There were complications in a total of 19 patients (6.3%). Five patients (1.7%) died after the procedure, all due to intracranial hypertension: one from subarachnoid hemorrhage, one from intracerebral hemorrhage, and three from increased edema without hemorrhage. The three patients who died without hemorrhage all had marked intracranial hypertension at the time of biopsy. All five patients who died harbored a glioblastoma multiforme. The surviving 14 patients (4.7%) with complications had increased neurologic deficit due to hemorrhage. In 10 patients (3.3%), the deficit was mild and/or transient; in the other four (1.3%), there was a major deficit that markedly affected the remainder of the patients' life. Therefore, mortality or major morbidity was seen in 3.0% of patients and minor morbidity in 3.3%. Stereotactic biopsy is a very effective procedure with a complication rate significantly lower than that of craniotomy, but in a small number of patients, the outcome is devastating.[57]

Hemorrhage

Interestingly, Kulkarni and colleagues[62] found that of 102 patients who underwent stereotactic biopsy, 61 patients (59.8%) exhibited hemorrhages, mostly intracerebral (54.9%), on the immediate postoperative scan. However, only six of these patients were clinically suspected to have had a hemorrhage based on immediate postoperative neurologic deficit: In the remaining 55 (53.9%) of 102 patients, the hemorrhage was clinically silent and unsuspected. Of the 55 patients with clinically silent hemorrhages, only three demonstrated a delayed neurologic deficit (one patient with seizure and two with progressive loss of consciousness), and these complications all occurred within the first 2 postoperative days. Thus clinically silent hemorrhage after stereotactic biopsy is very common. However, the authors did not find that knowledge of its existence ultimately affected individual patient management or outcome. The authors, therefore, suggest that the most important role of postoperative CT scanning is to screen for those neurologically well patients with no hemorrhage. These patients could safely be discharged on the same day that they underwent the biopsy.

Kaakaji and colleagues[63] showed that of 130 biopsies performed, there were five serious complications (3.8%), of which four were transient, and one death (0.8%). The death and any sustained deficit occurred in patients in whom a clot had been demonstrated on postoperative CT scans. All complications were detected within 6 hours after surgery. Guidelines for early discharge (<8 hours) after stereotactic biopsy were developed and stipulated the absence of the following: (1) intraoperative hemorrhage, (2) new postoperative deficit, and (3) clot on a postoperative CT scan. In this report, all complications were detected within 6 hours after surgery, with no deaths. These authors concluded that early discharge of patients after stereotactic biopsy of supratentorial lesions is safe in the absence of excessive intraoperative bleeding, new postoperative deficit, and clot on a postoperative CT scan.[63]

In another study of hemorrhage rate, 500 consecutive patients undergoing stereotactic brain biopsy underwent immediate postbiopsy intraoperative CT scanning to prospectively determine the acute hemorrhage rate.[64] In 40 patients (8%), hemorrhage was detected using immediate postbiopsy intraoperative CT scanning. Neurologic deficits developed in six patients (1.2%), and one patient (0.2%) died. Symptomatic delayed neurologic deficits developed in two patients (0.4%), despite the fact that the initial postbiopsy CT scans in these patients did not show acute hemorrhage. Both patients had large intracerebral hemorrhages that were confirmed at the time of repeated imaging. The results of a multivariate logistic regression analysis of the risk of postbiopsy hemorrhage of any size showed a significant correlation only with the degree to which the platelet count was less than 150,000/mm^3. The results of a multivariate analysis of a hemorrhage measuring greater than 5 mm in diameter also showed a correlation between the risk of hemorrhage and a lesion location in the pineal region.[64] The rate at which a nondiagnostic biopsy specimen was obtained increased as the number of biopsy samples increased and in accordance with younger patient age.[64] Stereotactic brain biopsy was associated with a low likelihood of postbiopsy hemorrhage. The risk of hemorrhage increased steadily as the platelet count decreased to 150,000/mm^3. The authors found a small but definable risk of delayed hemorrhage, despite unremarkable findings on an immediate postbiopsy head CT scan.[64] This risk justifies an overnight hospital observation stay for all patients after having undergone stereotactic brain biopsy.[64]

Management of intraoperative hemorrhage resulting from stereotactic biopsy has been outlined by Kelly,[65] in which the most important step is not to move the cannula. The blood will flow out of the cannula because it is the point of least resistance, thereby avoiding an intraparenchymal clot. Irrigation of the cannula is important to keep it open. If the bleeding is venous, it will stop with gentle irrigation and patience. However, if the bleeding is arterial, it has been suggested to use 0.5 mL of thrombin to stop the bleeding.[66] If a large intraparenchymal hemorrhage requiring craniotomy is suspected, an emergent CT may be performed.

New Neurologic deficit

New neurological deficits may occur that may be transient or permanent, even without an accompanying hematoma, particularly those trajectories that pass through eloquent brain areas such as motor cortex, internal capsule, Broca/Wernike areas. Thus choosing the safest and most direct route to the lesion is warranted. Often, we use dexamethasone (4 mg PO/IV every 6 hours for 24 hours) to decrease the cerebral edema after stereotactic biopsy.

Seizures

Seizures have been reported to occur during a stereotactic biopsy, especially if the projected trajectory is in the rolandic, perirolandic, or temporal lobe regions. Some authors have routinely loaded their patients with anticonvulsants at the therapeutic level (usually phenytoin [Dilantin]), whereas others have preferred to perform the surgery under general anesthesia.[65,67]

Infection

The reported infection rate after stereotactic biopsy is relatively low, on the order of 0.2% to 0.8%,[1,68,69] most being localized to the scalp and subgaleal space, which are easily treated with oral antibiotics. However, more serious infection such as abscesses secondary to stereotactic biopsies have been reported.[70] Thus to avoid the potential for an infectious complication, we generally give perioperative antibiotics (Kefzol 1 g IV every 8 hours for three doses), except in cases in which infection is in the differential diagnosis of the target lesion.

CASE EXAMPLES

Oligodendroglioma

Patient 1

The patient is a 39-year-old woman with a history of a grade II astrocytoma resected 6 years previously who now presents with increased headache, nausea and vomiting, and drowsiness. She had been relatively symptom free until 2 months before admission when she started developing these symptoms that have steadily increased. Brain MRI demonstrated a recurrence of her left frontal tumor, now with bilateral spread and mass effect (Fig. 44-6). She denied chest pain, shortness of breath, coughing, changes in her vision or hearing, ability to speak and eat, fevers/chills/sweats, dizziness, seizures, loss of consciousness, focal weakness or numbness, changes in bowel or bladder, or decreased memory. The patient underwent stereotactic brain biopsy.

In contrast to the patient's biopsy specimen from 6 years ago that suggested a WHO grade II diffuse astrocytoma, her current stereotactic biopsy sample displays a low-grade oligodendroglioma (WHO grade II). A representative pathology slide showed predominantly neoplastic oligodendroglial cells diffusely spread throughout the neural tissue. The tumor cells have the characteristic uniform, round nuclei surrounded by an artifact-produced clear cytoplasm giving a "halo" or "fried-egg" appearance.

FIGURE 44-6 Oligodendroglioma.

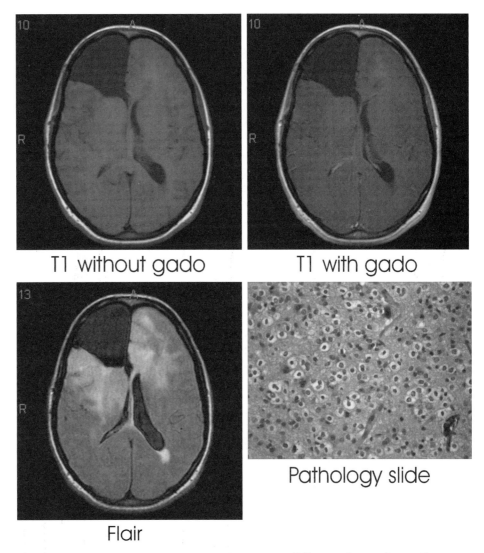

T1 without gado

T1 with gado

Flair

Pathology slide

Oligodendroglioma

It should be noted, however, that not all oligodendrogliomas will display this clearing effect or necessarily have uniform, round nuclei. Microcalcifications are also often seen in oligodendrogliomas, as in this case, but are not specific to this neoplasm. No mitotic figures, areas of necrosis, or endothelial proliferation were identified in the biopsy sample. An immunohistochemical stain against the antigen Ki-67 (MIB1), a marker of cells within the cell cycle, indicated a low proliferation rate.

Unstained sections were sent to a reference laboratory to perform fluorescence in situ hybridization (FISH) to look for genetic alterations, especially in chromosomes 1 and 19. Recent clinical studies have suggested that the combined loss of chromosome 1p and 19q in oligodendroglial neoplasms is associated with prolonged survival and increased sensitivity to chemotherapy. In this particular case, there were deletions of both 1p and 19q, consistent with the "genetically favorable" variant of oligodendroglioma. The associations between genetic phenotype and clinical behavior have not been absolute, and at present, the data should be considered preliminary and experimental. It is not uncommon within larger glial neoplasms to have variability of tumor grade as well as even cellular phenotype and possibly genotype arguing for multiple sampling at the time of biopsy from different regions. Mixed oligodendroglioma/astrocytomas are a distinct entity under the WHO classification system, and distinguishing between oligodendrogliomas and astrocytomas or mixed neoplasms can, on occasion, be challenging for the pathologist, especially in small biopsy specimens.

Brain Abscess

Patient 2

The patient is 53-year-old man with emphysema and alcoholism who was brought to the emergency department by his roommate because he was disoriented to time, place,

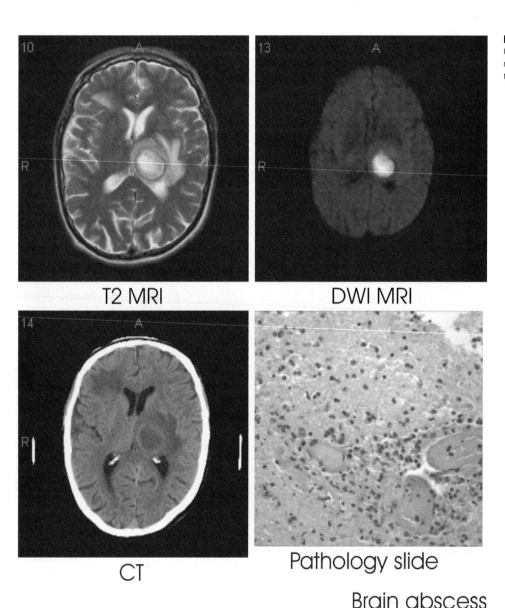

FIGURE 44-7 Brain abscess. CT, computed tomography; DWI, diffusion-weighted imaging; MRI, magnetic resonance imaging.

T2 MRI

DWI MRI

CT

Pathology slide

Brain abscess

and age and incontinent of urine and stool for 2 days. His roommate suspected that he was under the influence of some drug but offered no more information. In the emergency department, results of a breathalyzer test were negative for alcohol, and a fingerstick showed a blood glucose of 125. His vital signs were stable, and he was afebrile and found to be disoriented to time and place. A head CT done in the emergency department displayed three ringlike lesions showing low attenuation with associated edema in the right frontal, left thalamus, and left temporal regions and no midline shift. A chest radiograph revealed a left lower lobe infiltrate versus a mass. Laboratory studied were significant for a white blood cell count of 16.9 and a mild hypoxemia. A subsequent MRI of the brain with and without gadolinium confirmed the CT findings and highlighted vasogenic edema around fairly thin walled, uniformly enhancing rims (Fig. 44-7). The impression was that of multiple abscesses versus cavitating metastatic neoplasms. The patient underwent stereotactic brain biopsy. Cultures taken intraoperatively were positive for a few *Fusibacterium* and *Peptostreptococcus* species, but no acid-fast bacillus–positive organism or fungal species. The biopsy displayed fragments of acutely inflamed neural parenchyma with reactive blood vessels and infiltrates of lymphocytes and neutrophils. Necrotic fragments were also present, but organisms were not identified. No neoplastic cells were identified, and the diagnosis was brain abscess.

CT-guided stereotaxic aspiration is useful in the management of brain abscesses.[71] Leuthardt and colleagues[72] reported their experience with diffusion-weighted imaging in five patients with lesions on MRI to assess the usefulness of this technique in the preoperative evaluation of cerebral abscess. All lesions were markedly hyperintense on diffusion-weighted imaging and had a diminished apparent diffusion coefficient. Of 165 nonpyogenic lesions with diffusion-weighted imaging findings, 87 were hypointense or isointense, 78 lesions had variable hyperintensities, and a few manifested the degree of hyperintensity observed with abscesses.[72] Thus restricted water diffusion, as indicated by the hyperintensity on diffusion-weighted imaging and low apparent diffusion coefficient, in ring-enhancing lesions assists in differentiating brain abscess from necrotic tumor. This information facilitates stereotactic surgical planning: abscesses should be preferentially centrally aspirated, whereas necrotic brain tumors should have diagnostic tissue biopsied from cavity walls. Although not definitive for brain abscess, restricted water diffusion is an important MRI sign and is useful in neurosurgical treatment strategies for ring-enhancing lesions.[72] The importance of early diagnosis and treatment of infection cannot be overemphasized. Because it is relatively noninvasive, stereotactic neurosurgery has been used increasingly to diagnose brain masses in patients with acquired immunodeficiency syndrome, establishing diagnoses in all suspected cases of cerebral infection.[73]

FIGURE 44-8 Brain metastasis. MRI, magnetic resonance imaging.

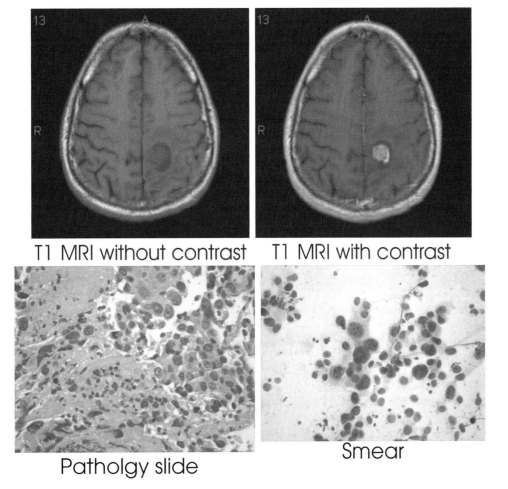

T1 MRI without contrast   T1 MRI with contrast

Patholgy slide   Smear

Brain Metastasis

Patient 3

The patient is 43-year-old man transferred from another hospital for a workup of a 1.4-cm brain mass. He presented to the emergency department of the referring hospital after passing out while driving and hitting a stone wall. He regained consciousness and reported to the emergency department that he had had 2 months of right flank and upper back pain as well as progressing numbness in his right leg to the point recently that he "couldn't make it work." A head CT revealed a 1.4-cm lesion in the left temporal lobe without mass effect. His social history was significant for alcoholism and 50-pack per year history of smoking. After transfer, his admitting neurologic examination was grossly normal. MRI revealed three intracranial, round, enhancing lesions in the right frontal, left parietal, and left temporal lobes (Fig. 44-8). A stereotactic biopsy of the left parietal lesion was performed. Sections from the biopsy specimen and cytologic smears prepared intraoperatively showed

tumor cells infiltrating within a background of inflammation and necrosis. The neoplastic cells had large, pleomorphic nuclei with prominent nucleoli and nonfibrillar cytoplasm. They immunostained with several keratin markers. The patient was also found to have non–small cell lung cancer. Thus he was diagnosed with a metastatic brain tumor with primary lung cancer.

Glioblastoma Multiforme

Patient 4

The patient is an 85-year-old, right-handed woman who was well until she experienced several episodes of "sick feeling" in her abdomen followed by shivering that ascended to the upper neck and sometimes sweating and shortness of breath, lasting 1 minute. On examination, she had subtle left upper extremity drift. Otherwise, the patient was neurologically intact. CT followed by MRI was performed that revealed a right temporal mass (Fig. 44-9), for which she underwent

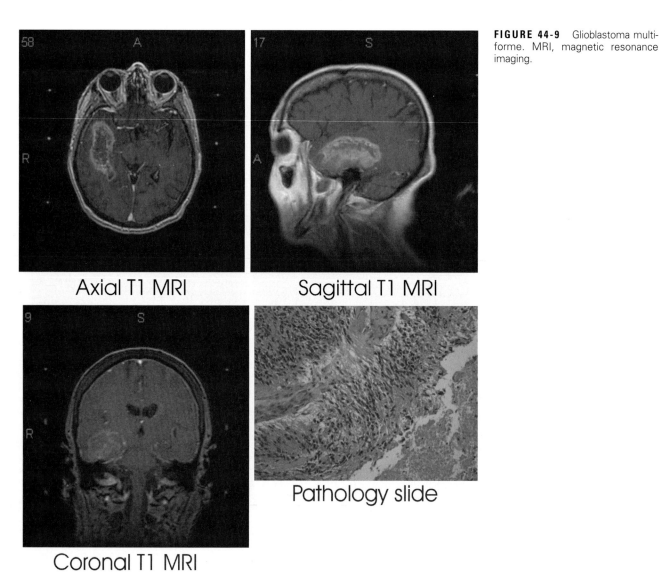

Axial T1 MRI

Sagittal T1 MRI

Coronal T1 MRI

Pathology slide

FIGURE 44-9 Glioblastoma multiforme. MRI, magnetic resonance imaging.

stereotactic brain biopsy. Sections of the biopsy specimen displayed a high-grade glial neoplasm with extensive areas of necrosis and tumor cells pseudopalisading. The tumor cells were fibrillar and showed hyperchromatic, pleomorphic nuclei and many mitotic figures. Vascular endothelial proliferation was also evident. These were the diagnostic architectural and cytologic features of a glioblastoma, the most malignant variety of astrocytic neoplasms (WHO grade IV of IV).

CONCLUSIONS

The indication for stereotactic biopsy to obtain a diagnosis that enables rational treatment has increased with progressively more sophisticated neuroimaging. At the same time, stereotactic methodology has been refined to incorporate these imaging modalities, effect accurate and reliable coregistration, and accomplish tissue acquisition in a safe and efficient manner. Understanding the appropriate application of this methodology to the management of specific patients and conditions requires continual reappraisal of the sensitivity and specificity of less invasive diagnostic tests (such as neuroimaging) and the implications of that diagnostic information on potential therapeutic interventions. Currently, we are at a point where neuroimaging is generating indications for but not yet supplanting stereotactic biopsy in the majority of neoplastic and infectious disease processes. Thus there remains an important role for tissue diagnosis by stereotactic brain biopsy.

REFERENCES

1. Apuzzo ML, Chandrasoma PT, Cohen D, et al: Computed imaging stereotaxy: Experience and perspective related to 500 procedures applied to brain masses. Neurosurgery 20:930–937, 1987.
2. Apuzzo ML, Chandrasoma PT, Zelman V, et al: Computed tomographic guidance stereotaxis in the management of lesions of the third ventricular region. Neurosurgery 15:502–508, 1984.
3. Apuzzo ML, Sabshin JK: Computed tomographic guidance stereotaxis in the management of intracranial mass lesions. Neurosurgery 12:277–285, 1983.
4. Rajshekhar V: Current status of stereotactic biopsy. Stereotact Funct Neurosurg 76:137–139, 2001.
5. West B, Griesbach E, Taylor J, et al: The Prentice-Hall Encyclopedia of Mathematics. Englewood Cliffs, NJ: Prentice-Hall, 1982, pp 119–126.
6. Dittmar C: Uber die Lage des sogenamnten Gefafsszentrums in der Medulla oblongata. Ber Saechs Ges Wiss Lepizig Math Phys 25: 449–469, 1873.
7. Kandel E, Schavinsky Y: Stereotaxic apparatus and operations in Russia in the 19th century. J Neurosurg 37:407–411, 1972.
8. Zernov D: L'encepalometre. Rev Gen Clin Ther 19:302, 1890.
9. Horsley V, Clarke R: The structure and functions of the cerebellum examined by a new method. Brain 31:45–124, 1908.
10. Spiegel E, Wycis H, Marks M, et al: Stereotaxic apparatus for operations on the human brain. Science 106:349–350, 1947.
11. Spiegel E, Wycis H: Stereoencephalotomy, Part 1. Orlando, FL: Grune & Stratton, 1952.
12. Conway LW: Stereotaxic diagnosis and treatment of intracranial tumors including an initial experience with cryosurgery for pinealomas. J Neurosurg 38:453–460, 1973.
13. Bergstrom M, Greitz T: Stereotaxic computed tomography. Am J Roentgenol 127:167–170, 1976.
14. Leksell L, Leksell D, Schwebel J: Stereotaxis and nuclear magnetic resonance. J Neurol Neurosurg Psychiatry 48:14–18, 1985.
15. Bullard DE, Nashold BS Jr: Evolution of principles of stereotactic neurosurgery. Neurosurg Clin N Am 6:27–41, 1995.
16. Picard C, Olivier A, Bertrand G: The first human stereotaxic apparatus. The contribution of Aubrey Mussen to the field of stereotaxis. J Neurosurg 59:673–676, 1983.
17. Leksell L: A stereotaxic apparatus for intracerebral surgery. Acta Chir Scand 99:229–233, 1950.
18. Couldwell WT, Apuzzo ML: Initial experience related to the use of the Cosman-Roberts-Wells stereotactic instrument: Technical note. J Neurosurg 72:145–148, 1990.
19. Cooper I: Cryogenic surgery: a new method of destruction or extirpation of benign or malignant tissue. N Engl J Med 268:743–749, 1963.
20. Austin G, Lee A: A plastic ball-and-socket type of stereotaxic director. J Neurosurg 15:264–268, 1958.
21. McCaul I: A method for the localization and production of discrete destructive lesions in brain. J Neurol Neurosurg Psychiatry 22: 109–112, 1959.
22. Riechert T: Stereotactic brain operations. Methods, clinical aspects, indications. In Huber H (ed). Bern: Jack Burgess, 1980.
23. Gillingham F: Surgical management of the dyskinesias. J Neurol Neurosurg Psychiatry 23:347–348, 1960.
24. Brown R, Roberts T, Osborn A: Stereotaxic frame and computer software for CT-directed neurosurgical localization. Invest Radiol 15:308–312, 1980.
25. Dawant BM, Li R, Cetinkaya E, et al: Computerized atlas-based positioning of deep brain stimulators: A feasibility study. In Second Workshop on Biomedical Image Registration (WBIR'03): New York: Springer-Verlag, 2003, pp 1–10.
26. Roberts DW, Strohbehn JW, Friets EM, et al: The stereotactic operating microscope: Accuracy refinement and clinical experience. Acta Neurochir Suppl (Wien) 46:112–114, 1989.
27. Roberts DW, Strohbehn JW, Hatch JF, et al: A frameless stereotaxic integration of computerized tomographic imaging and the operating microscope. J Neurosurg 65:545–549, 1986.
28. Roberts DW, Nakajima T, Brodwater B, et al: Further development and clinical application of the stereotactic operating microscope. Stereotact Funct Neurosurg 58:114–117, 1992.
29. McInerney J, Roberts DW: Frameless stereotaxy of the brain. Mt Sinai J Med 67:300–310, 2000.
30. Brommeland T, Kloster R, Ingebrigtsen T: A four-year experience with a stereotactic computer in a small neurosurgical department. Surg Neurol 57:190–194, 2002.
31. Plunkett R, Allison RR, Grand W: Stereotactic neurosurgical biopsy is an underutilized modality. Neurosurg Rev 22:117–120, 1999.
32. Baleriaux D, Parizel PM, Matos C, et al: Stereotactic indications for neuroradiological differential diagnosis. Acta Neurochir (Wien) 124:31–33, 1993.
33. Chandrasoma PT, Smith MM, Apuzzo ML: Stereotactic biopsy in the diagnosis of brain masses: Comparison of results of biopsy and resected surgical specimen. Neurosurgery 24:160–165, 1989.
34. Ryken TC, Hitchon PW, Roach RM, et al: Infratentorial stereotactic biopsy: A review of 11 cases. Stereotact Funct Neurosurg 59:111–114, 1992.
35. Friedman WA, Sceats DJ Jr, Nestok BR, et al: The incidence of unexpected pathological findings in an image-guided biopsy series: A review of 100 consecutive cases. Neurosurgery 25:180–184, 1989.
36. Lunsford LD, Martinez AJ: Stereotactic exploration of the brain in the era of computed tomography. Surg Neurol 22:222–230, 1984.
37. Kim JE, Kim DG, Paek SH, et al: Stereotactic biopsy for intracranial lesions: Reliability and its impact on the planning of treatment. Acta Neurochir (Wien) 145:547–555, 2003.
38. Fontaine D, Dormont D, Hasboun D, et al: Magnetic resonance-guided stereotactic biopsies: Results in 100 consecutive cases. Acta Neurochir (Wien) 142:249–256, 2000.
39. Vindlacheruvu RR, Casey AT, Thomas DG: MRI-guided stereotactic brain biopsy: A review of 33 cases. Br J Neurosurg 13:143–147, 1999.
40. Hall WA, Martin AJ, Liu H, et al: Brain biopsy using high-field strength interventional magnetic resonance imaging. Neurosurgery 44:807–813, 1999.
41. Sugahara T, Korogi Y, Shigematsu Y, et al: Value of dynamic susceptibility contrast magnetic resonance imaging in the evaluation of intracranial tumors. Top Magn Reson Imaging 10:114–124, 1999.
42. Levivier M, Goldman S, Pirotte B, et al: Diagnostic yield of stereotactic brain biopsy guided by positron emission tomography with [18F] fluorodeoxyglucose. J Neurosurg 82:445–452, 1995.
43. Thompson TP, Lunsford LD, Kondziolka D: Distinguishing recurrent tumor and radiation necrosis with positron emission tomography versus stereotactic biopsy. Stereotact Funct Neurosurg 73:9–14, 1999.
44. Pirotte B, Goldman S, Brucher JM, et al: PET in stereotactic conditions increases the diagnostic yield of brain biopsy. Stereotact Funct Neurosurg 63:144–149, 1994.

45. Pirotte B, Goldman S, Salzberg S, et al: Combined positron emission tomography and magnetic resonance imaging for the planning of stereotactic brain biopsies in children: Experience in 9 cases. Pediatr Neurosurg 38:146–155, 2003.

46. Fratkin JD, Ward MM, Roberts DW, et al: CT-guided stereotactic biopsy of intracranial lesions: Correlation between core biopsy and aspiration smear. Diagn Cytopathol 2:126–132, 1986.

47. Robbins PD, Yu LL, Lee M, et al: Stereotactic biopsy of 100 intracerebral lesions at Sir Charles Gairdner Hospital. Pathology 26:410–413, 1994.

48. Warnick RE, Longmore LM, Paul CA, et al: Postoperative management of patients after stereotactic biopsy: Results of a survey of the AANS/CNS section on tumors and a single institution study. J Neurooncol 62:289–296, 2003.

49. Linhares P, Aran E, Goncalves JM, et al: [Stereotactic brain biopsy: Review of 80 cases: The need of CT-scan in the first hours]. Neurocirugia (Astur) 13:299–304, 2002.

50. Hall WA: The safety and efficacy of stereotactic biopsy for intracranial lesions. Cancer 82:1749–1755, 1998.

51. Burger PC, Nelson JS: Stereotactic brain biopsies: Specimen preparation and evaluation. Arch Pathol Lab Med 121:477–480, 1997.

52. Vinters HV, Mischel PS, Ranchod M: Central nervous system. Pathology (Phila) 3:513–534, 1996.

53. Gaudin PB, Sherman ME, Brat DJ, et al: Accuracy of grading gliomas on CT-guided stereotactic biopsies: A survival analysis. Diagn Cytopathol 17:461–466, 1997.

54. Bleggi-Torres LF, de Noronha L, Schneider Gugelmin E, et al: Accuracy of the smear technique in the cytological diagnosis of 650 lesions of the central nervous system. Diagn Cytopathol 24:293–295, 2001.

55. Feiden W, Steude U, Bise K, et al: Accuracy of stereotactic brain tumor biopsy: Comparison of the histologic findings in biopsy cylinders and resected tumor tissue. Neurosurg Rev 14:51–56, 1991.

56. Voges J, Schroder R, Treuer H, et al: CT-guided and computer assisted stereotactic biopsy: Technique, results, indications. Acta Neurochir (Wien) 125:142–149, 1993.

57. Bernstein M, Parrent AG: Complications of CT-guided stereotactic biopsy of intra-axial brain lesions. J Neurosurg 81:165–168, 1994.

58. Sawin PD, Hitchon PW, Follett KA, et al: Computed imaging-assisted stereotactic brain biopsy: A risk analysis of 225 consecutive cases. Surg Neurol 49:640–649, 1998.

59. Bhardwaj RD, Bernstein M: Prospective feasibility study of outpatient stereotactic brain lesion biopsy. Neurosurgery 51:358–364, 2002.

60. Bouvier G, Couillard P, Leger SL, et al: Stereotactic biopsy of cerebral space-occupying lesions. Appl Neurophysiol 46:227–230, 1983.

61. Favre J, Taha JM, Burchiel KJ: An analysis of the respective risks of hematoma formation in 361 consecutive morphological and functional stereotactic procedures. Neurosurgery 50:48–57, 2002.

62. Kulkarni AV, Guha A, Lozano A, et al: Incidence of silent hemorrhage and delayed deterioration after stereotactic brain biopsy. J Neurosurg 89:31–35, 1998.

63. Kaakaji W, Barnett GH, Bernhard D, et al: Clinical and economic consequences of early discharge of patients following supratentorial stereotactic brain biopsy. J Neurosurg 94:892–898, 2001.

64. Field M, Witham TF, Flickinger JC, et al: Comprehensive assessment of hemorrhage risks and outcomes after stereotactic brain biopsy. J Neurosurg 94:545–551, 2001.

65. Kelly PJ: Stereotactic biopsy procedures. In Kelly PJ (ed): Tumor Stereotaxis. Philadelphia: WB Saunders, 1992, pp 183–222.

66. Chimowitz M, Barnett GH, Palmer J: Treatment of intractable arterial hemorrhage during stereotactic brain biopsy with thrombin. J Neurosurg 74:301–303, 1991.

67. Kitchen N, Bradford R, Thomas D: Stereotactic surgery: Methods of CT and MRI directed biopsy. In Thomas DG (ed): Stereotactic and Image Directed Surgery of Brain Tumors. Edinburgh: Churchill Livingstone, 1993.

68. Lunsford LD, Coffey DJ, Cojocaru T, et al: Image-guided stereotactic surgery: A 10-year evolutionary experience. Stereotact Funct Neurosurg 54/55:375–387, 1989.

69. Wild A, Xuereb J, Marks PV, et al: Computerized tomographic stereotaxy in the management of 200 consecutive intracranial mass lesions: Analysis of indications, benefits and outcome. Br J Neurosurg 4:407–415, 1990.

70. De la Porte C: Technical possibilities and limitations of stereotaxy. Acta Neurochir (Wien) 124:3–6, 1993.

71. Cordoliani YS, Hor F, Derosier C, et al: [Emergency stereotaxic cerebral punctures]. J Radiol 70:465–470, 1989.

72. Leuthardt EC, Wippold FJ 2nd, Oswood MC, et al: Diffusion-weighted MR imaging in the preoperative assessment of brain abscesses. Surg Neurol 58:395–402, 2002.

73. Duma CM, Kondziolka D, Lunsford LD: Image-guided stereotactic management of non-AIDS-related cerebral infection. Neurosurg Clin N Am 3:291–302, 1992.

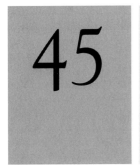

45 Surgical Management of Cerebral Metastases

STEPHEN J. HENTSCHEL and FREDERICK F. LANG

INTRODUCTION

Cerebral metastases are a significant source of morbidity and mortality for patients with systemic cancer and are a common problem encountered by neurosurgeons. In the modern era, neurosurgical management of brain metastases has become progressively more complex for several reasons. Most importantly, treatment options have increased. In the past, therapy was limited to corticosteroids and whole-brain radiation therapy (WBRT). In the more modern era, surgical resection and stereotactic radiosurgery have become integral parts of the management armamentarium; thus the appropriate application of surgery vis-à-vis other therapies must be clearly understood. Because operative techniques have improved, there is an increasing potential for resecting lesions that in the past were considered unresectable. This has expanded the indications for surgical resection. Furthermore, whereas in the past brain metastases were usually detected when they were large and symptomatic, screening by magnetic resonance (MR) imaging has resulted in the detection of brain metastases when they are asymptomatic and small. This early detection allows for "elective" and highly controlled surgical resections, but has also raised questions of whether less invasive interventions (e.g., radiosurgery) should be undertaken. Finally, there is an increasing trend toward aggressive systemic therapy that has led to the expectation that treatment of the brain should not excessively delay or interfere with treatment of the systemic disease. Modern neurosurgeons therefore must be familiar with the complexities of brain metastasis management in order to integrate surgical options into the overall treatment plan of the cancer patient.

This chapter provides an overview of the surgical management of brain metastases in order to define the role of neurosurgery in the management of the cancer patient. Particular attention is given to patient selection and surgical techniques, as well as emphasizing surgical outcomes and potential complications.

MAGNITUDE OF THE PROBLEM

Cerebral metastases are the most common brain tumor in adults.[1] Approximately 20% to 40% of patients with cancer develop brain metastases during the course of their illness.[2-5] It has been estimated that of the more than 560,000 patients in the United States dying each year of cancer, approximately 19%, or more than 100,000 patients, will have brain metastases.[6-8] Most brain metastases arise from lung, breast, and kidney primaries; however, melanoma, lung carcinoma, breast carcinoma, and renal cell carcinoma have the greatest propensity to develop brain metastases (Table 45-1). Whereas breast and renal cell carcinomas tend to present as single metastases within the brain, melanoma and lung cancers have an increased incidence of multiplicity.[3,9,10] In addition, the interval between the diagnosis of the primary cancer and the brain metastasis depends on the histology of the primary cancer. Breast cancer tends to have the longest interval to present as brain metastases (mean, 3 years), whereas lung cancer tends to have the shortest interval (mean, 4 to 10 months).[11] The highest incidence of brain metastases is seen in the fifth to seventh decades of life and is equally common among males and females. However, lung carcinoma is the source of most brain metastases in males, and breast carcinoma are the most common source of metastases in females. Males with melanoma are more likely to develop brain metastases than are females.[10]

TREATMENT GOALS: ADVANTAGES OF SURGICAL RESECTION

The goals of treating brain metastases are to establish a histologic diagnosis, relieve symptoms, and provide long-term local control. Compared with the other treatment options (i.e., corticosteroids, WBRT, and stereotactic radiosurgery), surgical resection has several advantages for achieving these aims.

Surgery is the only treatment modality that can provide a histologic diagnosis. Although in the future, imaging techniques such as spectroscopy may allow for determinations of tumor pathology, surgery is the only currently available method for documenting the histologic diagnosis. Thus surgery is a critical part of the management of any patient in whom the diagnosis of brain metastasis is in question. This occurs most commonly for patients without a known

TABLE 45-1 ■ Proportion of Brain Metastases and Propensity to Metastasize to Brain According to Primary Tumor

Overall Incidence		Propensity to Metastasize*	
Lung carcinoma	45%	Melanoma	50%
Breast carcinoma	20%	Lung carcinoma	25%
Melanoma	15%	Breast carcinoma	25%
Renal cell carcinoma	10%	Renal cell carcinoma	15%
Colon carcinoma	5%	Colon carcinoma	5%
Other	5%		

*Proportion of patients with primary cancer developing brain metastases.

primary cancer but may also occur in the rare situation where a patient has two known cancers or where the brain lesion may be of a noncancerous etiology. For patients with known systemic cancer, it must be remembered that failure to obtain histologic confirmation may lead to erroneous diagnosis in 5% to 11% of cases.[12,13]

Compared with other modalities, surgery is capable of most rapidly relieving symptoms by eradicating the lesion and thereby reducing intracranial pressure, eliminating local compression, and abolishing the source of edema. Although corticosteroids reduce the effects of vasogenic edema, they do not alter the direct mass effect of the lesion itself, and their side effects preclude long-term use. Conventional radiation may reduce the tumor mass, but the effect is not immediate and many metastases are radio-resistant. Stereotactic radiosurgery is limited to small lesions (<3 cm) that are less likely to cause symptoms.

Ultimately, local cure is the most important goal of surgery. Although WBRT and radiosurgery may provide local control, eradication of the lesion (defined as no visible lesion on radiographic studies) is less predictable for these modalities when compared with surgery. With modern techniques, complete resection can be achieved in nearly all cases (see the following). The ability to predict such an outcome is a major advantage over radiation-based modalities, for which tumor response depends on unpredictable, intrinsic, biologic properties of a given tumor.

PATIENT SELECTION

Patient selection is the cornerstone of surgical management. Not all patients with brain metastases are candidates for resection, and decisions to operate should be based on a firm understanding of the variables influencing surgical outcomes. Determining whether surgical resection is best for a particular patient requires that the physician consider the number, location, and size of the lesion(s) in the context of the clinical features of the patient, as well as the histology of the primary tumor. The value of surgery must be weighed against the role of other treatment options, including corticosteroids, WBRT, and stereotactic radiosurgery.

Radiographic Assessment

Preoperative studies, particularly MR imaging, are used to determine the number, location, size, and resectability of intracranial metastases. These tumor features are critical aspects of selecting patients for surgery.

Number of Lesions

A primary consideration in deciding to operate is the number of lesions. MR imaging is more sensitive than computed tomography (CT) for the detection of small metastases or those within the posterior fossa.[14–16] and is thus recommended for definitively establishing the number of intracranial metastases. A single cerebral metastasis is defined as one metastasis to the brain in the face of other systemic metastases, whereas "solitary" cerebral metastases indicates that the brain is the only site of metastatic disease within the body.[17] It has been found that single and solitary cerebral metastases constitute approximately 50% to 65% of all

cases of patients with brain metastases.[18] Patients should be divided into those with single/solitary metastases or those with multiple brain metastases.

Single and Solitary Brain Metastasis

Patients with single/solitary brain metastases are the best candidates for surgery. It has been demonstrated by class I evidence that surgical resection of single or solitary brain metastases is superior to treatment with WBRT alone. Although Mintz and colleagues[19] reported a randomized trial in which there were no differences between surgery and WBRT, two prospective randomized trials have shown that surgical resection followed by WBRT is superior to WBRT alone for patients with single brain metastases.[12,20]

In a prospective randomized trial of patients with single cerebral metastases, Patchell and colleagues compared surgical resection plus WBRT ($n = 25$) with needle biopsy and WBRT ($n = 23$).[12] These authors found that the overall length of survival was significantly longer ($p < 0.01$) in the surgically resected group (median, 40 weeks) than in the WBRT group (median, 15 weeks). The predictors of prolonged survival from a multivariate analysis were surgical resection ($p < 0.04$), increased interval between diagnosis of primary tumor and brain metastasis ($p < 0.04$), absence of disseminated disease ($p < 0.02$), and younger patient age ($p < 0.01$). Importantly, functional independence was maintained longer in the surgical group (median, 38 weeks) than in the radiation group (median, 8 weeks; $p < 0.005$). A statistically significant difference in the incidence of local recurrence was also seen between the two groups, with surgical patients having a much lower incidence of local recurrence (20%) than the radiation group (52%; $p < 0.02$). In addition, the time to recurrence was significantly shorter in the radiation group (median, 21 weeks) than the surgery group (median, 59 weeks; $p < 0.0001$). The development of new metastases remote from the original site was no different between the two groups, indicating that surgical resection does not promote the development of new metastases. A multivariate analysis found that surgical resection ($p < 0.0001$) and the absence of disseminated disease ($p < 0.0004$) were predictors of a lower risk of recurrence.

In a similar trial, Vecht and colleagues also compared the outcome of patients with single brain metastases who were randomized to surgical resection plus WBRT or to WBRT alone.[20] A major difference from the trial of Patchell and colleagues was that these authors stratified the patients by site (lung cancer vs. non-lung cancer) and by status of extracranial disease (progressive vs. stable). Patients with stable extracranial disease had a more prolonged survival when treated with surgical resection and WBRT (median, 12 months) than when treated with WBRT alone (median, 7 months). The difference in survival between the two groups was statistically significant ($p = 0.04$). Patients with progressive extracranial disease did worse than those with stable disease. Patients with progressive disease had overall survival times of 5 months after surgical resection plus WBRT, compared with less than 3 months survival after WBRT alone. The tumor type, lung versus nonlung histology, was not a strong predictor of survival.

Based on the results of these studies, it is generally accepted that the standard of treatment of patients with single brain metastases is surgical resection. Although other treatment modalities, particularly radiosurgery, are becoming increasingly popular, it must be remembered that to date there has been no randomized trial comparing radiosurgery with surgery for single brain metastases (see the following). Thus choosing radiosurgery instead of surgery as the primary treatment of a single brain metastasis is a decision based on conflicting retrospective studies (see the following).

Multiple Brain Metastases

Traditionally, the presence of multiple metastases has been considered a contraindication to surgery, even when the tumors are surgically accessible.[21–24] However, a report from The University of Texas M.D. Anderson Cancer Center has suggested that there may be a role for surgery in the treatment of patients with multiple metastases.[25] This study reported the outcome of 56 patients who underwent resection for multiple brain metastases. Patients were divided into those who had one or more lesions left unresected (Group A, $n = 30$), and those who had undergone resection of all lesions (Group B, $n = 26$). These patients were compared with a group of matched controls who had single metastases that were surgically resected (Group C, $n = 26$). There was no difference in surgical mortality (3%, 4%, and 0% for groups A, B, and C, respectively) or morbidity (8%, 9%, and 8% for Groups A, B, and C, respectively) regardless of treatment group. Patients with multiple metastases who had all the lesions resected (Group B) had a significantly longer survival (median, 14 months) than patients who had some lesions left unresected (Group A; median, 6 months; $p = 0.003$). The survival time of patients who had all lesions removed (Group B) was similar to that of patients with resected single metastases (Group C; median, 14 months). Bindal and colleagues concluded that removal of multiple metastatic lesions is as effective as resection of single metastases, so long as all lesions are removed.[25]

In support of the above findings, Iwadate and colleagues reported a median survival of 9.2 months following resection of multiple brain metastases; this was similar to the survival following resection of a single brain metastasis (8.7 months).[26] Predictors of shorter survival were age greater than 60 years, Karnofsky performance score (KPS) less than 70, incomplete surgical resection, and the presence of extensive systemic cancer. Thus the presence of multiple brain lesions was not a significant predictor of shorter survival, suggesting that surgical resection is potentially worthwhile.

Based on these studies, patients with multiple metastases should not be excluded from surgery. It should be remembered, however, that the surgical definition of "multiple" in the reported studies was three or fewer lesions. In this context, the authors generally recommend surgery only if all lesions can be resected. However, surgery may also be used as part of a multitreatment approach that will result in the eradication of all the tumors. For example, resection of a large symptomatic lesion and treatment of several smaller lesions with radiosurgery may be a reasonable approach. Of course, all patients with multiple metastases should receive adjunctive WBRT.

Location

Resectability (i.e., whether a tumor can be removed without morbidity) is dictated primarily by tumor location.

With modern microneurosurgical techniques there are very few, if any, regions within the brain that are inaccessible to the neurosurgeon. However, accessibility and resectability are not the same. The most important features that determine resectability are whether the tumor is deep or superficial and whether the tumor is within or near eloquent brain. Stereotactic image-guided surgical techniques and skull base exposures have made previously unreachable tumors resectable. A variety of techniques help preserve functionally important brain regions during resection. Nevertheless, lesions that are deep and within eloquent areas are associated with slightly higher surgical morbidity than are those within silent, superficial areas (see the following). Sawaya and colleagues studied 400 consecutive patients undergoing craniotomies for brain tumor resection.[27] They found that major neurologic complications occurred in 13% of patients undergoing resection of tumors from eloquent brain regions, whereas the incidence was 5% and 3%, respectively, for patients undergoing resection of tumors located within "near-eloquent" and "noneloquent" brain regions. Ultimately, the potential morbidity (hence, recovery time) associated with surgical removal must be weighed against the limited survival expectancy of this patient population. Patients with metastases to the brain stem, thalamus, and basal ganglia are generally not considered surgical candidates, except in rare circumstances. Treatment of lesions in these locations with alternatives such as radiosurgery may be warranted. However, it must be remembered that there is no good study demonstrating that the morbidity of surgery is more than that of radiosurgery when the lesion is located in eloquent brain.

Lesion Size

The size of the lesion is another factor that must be considered when choosing therapy. For lesions that are greater than 3 cm in maximum diameter, surgical resection is the primary option because surgery rapidly relieves the mass effect that commonly occurs with larger, often symptomatic lesions, and because the large size precludes radiosurgery.[28,29] For lesions less than 1 cm in maximum diameter, radiosurgery may be more appropriate because localizing small lesions at surgery, even with MR imaging guidance, may be difficult, especially when deep in the brain. The most difficult lesions with regard to surgical decision making are those between 1 and 3 cm in maximum diameter. For these lesions, the decision is complex because either surgery or radiosurgery can be applied and because no prospective randomized study has demonstrated the superiority of one treatment over the other. The authors believe that surgical resection, based on current evidence supporting it (see the following) and its predictability, is the primary option for these patients and that radiosurgery should be reserved for patients with extensive systemic disease, poor performance status, or medical problems that increase the risk of surgical intervention.

Clinical Assessment

The status of the patient's systemic disease (i.e., the extent of the primary tumor and of noncerebral metastases) is a critical consideration in the decision to resect a brain metastasis because advanced systemic disease is a major predictor of short-term survival, whereas limited systemic disease is associated with long survival in patients undergoing surgery for cerebral metastases.[12,20,25,30–32] Indeed, after resection of a single brain metastasis, up to 70% of patients will succumb to their systemic disease and not to their brain disease.[12] In this context, most patients with absent systemic disease are surgical candidates, whereas most patients with widely disseminated cancer are not. Decision making in patients with "controlled" or "limited" systemic disease is usually more difficult. Patients with a significant systemic cancer burden that is responding to therapy may be an even greater decision-making challenge. One practical approach is to determine the expected survival time for the patient, excluding the presence of cerebral metastases. At M.D. Anderson, patients who are expected to survive for more than 3 to 4 months are usually candidates for surgical resection.

In addition, the patient's general medical status must be evaluated prior to surgery. Patients who have major cardiac, pulmonary, renal, or hematologic diseases may be better suited for nonsurgical therapies. Finally, the preoperative neurologic status should be considered, because patients with marked neurologic deficits have been shown to have a shorter median survival than patients who are neurologically intact.[32,33] However, it is important not to exclude patients from surgery on this basis alone, because there are many patients whose neurologic deficits improve following resection of the offending lesion. One way to determine the potential for recovery is to assess the response of the deficit to corticosteroid administration. Patients whose neurologic deficits are likely to improve after resection usually demonstrate an improvement after treatment with corticosteroids, whereas patients who will not improve postoperatively do not have such a response to corticosteroids. In general, a surgical patient should have an expected survival of at least 4 months, be able to withstand anesthesia, and have a KPS greater than or equal to 70 (Table 45-2).

Several investigators have advocated dividing patients into prognostic categories based on several clinical features determined in retrospective analyses of patient outcome. However, this method of prognostication should not necessarily be used for surgical decision making. Gaspar and colleagues identified three prognostic groups of patients with brain metastases by applying recursive partitioning analysis (RPA) to patients enrolled in three consecutive Radiation Therapy Oncology Group (RTOG) trials.[34] The analysis consisted of 1200 patients from studies conducted between 1979 and 1993 that were originally designed to evaluate radiation fractionation paradigms and radiation sensitizers. RPA, a sophisticated statistical technique, identified three variables (i.e., age, KPS, and systemic cancer status) that were significant predictors of survival. Based on these results, the patients with brain metastases were divided into three groups: class I (KPS >70, age <65 years, controlled primary cancer, no extracranial metastases); class III (KPS <70); and class II (all other patients). Class I patients survived a median of 7.1 months, whereas class II and III patients survived only 4.2 months and 2.3 months, respectively. Based on this analysis it has been suggested that class III patients (KPS <70) are not good candidates for aggressive treatment (including surgery) because their expected survival is short. However, a subsequent study has identified a subgroup of class III patients with a more favorable prognosis; these patients are less than 65 years old, have a controlled primary cancer, and harbor a single metastasis.[35] These RPA classes may not be applicable to surgical decision making because patients with a KPS of less than 70 owing to mass effect from the tumor may dramatically improve postoperatively after resection of the lesion and thus may actually be good surgical candidates.

Histologic Assessment

The type of primary cancer is of importance, mainly because of differences in radiosensitivity (Table 45-3). The most common tumors to metastasize to the brain, breast and non–small cell lung cancer, are intermediately sensitive to conventional fractionated radiotherapy, and surgery will have a role in many cases. Primary treatment with radiotherapy should be strongly considered for patients with tumors having highly radiosensitive histologies (e.g., lymphoma, germ cell tumors, and small cell lung cancer), whereas resection should be strongly considered for patients with radioinsensitive tumors (e.g., melanoma, renal cell carcinoma, and sarcomas). Although these categories of radiation sensitivity apply to conventional fractionated radiotherapy, the same does not hold true for stereotactic radiosurgery, to which melanoma, renal cell, and sarcomas may respond well.[36]

SURGICAL TECHNIQUE

Successful extirpation of cerebral metastases is based on good basic neurosurgical techniques in conjunction with technologies for tumor localization and functional brain mapping. A clear understanding of the surgical anatomy of these lesions results in safe and effective tumor removal.

TABLE 45-2 ▪ Considerations in Patient Selection for Surgical Removal of Brain Metastases

Factor	Requirement for Surgery
Status of Systemic Disease	
Control of primary cancer	Expected survival > 4 months
General medical condition	Able to withstand surgery/anesthesia
Neurologic status	KPS ≥ 70
Resectability	
Accessibility	Not brain stem, basal gangila, thalamus
Number of lesions	≤3 lesions
Histology	
Radiosensitivity	See Table 45-3

TABLE 45-3 ▪ Radiosensitivity of Brain Metastases to Conventional Fractionated Radiotherapy

Highly Sensitive	Intermediately Sensitive	Poorly Sensitive
Lymphoma	Breast	Melanoma
Germinoma	Lung (non–small cell)	Renal
Lung (small cell)	Colon	Sarcoma

Data from references 2 and 39.

Surgical Anatomy

Cerebral metastases consist of solid tumor material without intervening brain tissue between the cells. Although there may be some infiltration of tumor cells into the surrounding brain, this is usually less than 5 mm deep.[8] Typically, the mass of tumor cells is surrounded by a gliotic rim that separates the tumor from the surrounding edematous brain. The lesions commonly arise at the gray-white junction, where a reduction in blood vessel diameter causes the embolic tumor to become trapped.[37]

In the supratentorial space, metastases may be classified based on their relationship to adjacent sulci and gyri.[37,38] Metastases may occur just under the cortex and fill a gyrus (subcortical), deep within a gyrus adjacent to a sulcus (subgyral), deep to a sulcus (subsulcal), deep within the hemispheric white matter (lobar), or within the ventricle (intraventricular).[39] In the posterior fossa, cerebellar metastases can be categorized as occurring in either deep or hemispheric locations; hemispheric lesions can be considered as lateral or medial. A subset arises directly within the vermis. Knowledge of the relationship to the sulcus is particularly important because this may determine the appropriate surgical path to the tumor (see the following).

Another important aspect of the surgical anatomy is the location of blood vessels. "Arterialized" veins that drain the lesion are often evident on the brain surface, and surgeons must carefully consider the venous drainage when resecting the lesion. More importantly, the arterial supply to most metastases comes from vessels parasitized from branches of larger vessels that arise within the sulci.

Resection Methods

Careful planning and meticulous attention to detail are necessary to minimize surgical complications. The surgeon must devote appropriate attention to each stage of the operative procedure including positioning, opening, tumor resection, and closure. The technique must result in complete removal of the lesion, with preservation of neurologic function and minimal disruption of the surrounding brain.

Positioning

After careful review of the preoperative imaging and correlation with known anatomic landmarks, it should be possible to identify and mark the location of the tumor as it projects onto the scalp and to tentatively define the incision prior to immobilization of the head and final positioning of the patient. This is a useful exercise not only as a check of the neuronavigation system (see the following) and to decrease total reliance on such devices but also to aid in proper placement of the head immobilizer and to determine the most appropriate position for the patient. Typically, patients are positioned with the guiding principle that the lesion should be at the top of the operative field. After selection of the most appropriate position for the patient, the head is rigidly fixed in a neurosurgical headholder (e.g., the Mayfield 3-pin clamp) and then secured to the operating table. Now, the tumor can be marked out on the scalp using the neuronavigation system, if available. After the location of the tumor has been determined, a final appropriate skin incision is planned. The authors generally prefer linear skin incisions, where possible, because the risk of compromising the vascular supply to the scalp is decreased compared with flaps.

Exposure and Operative Approach

Standard neurosurgical principles of preservation of blood supply and minimal injury to tissues guide the operation. Frameless stereotaxy is preferred because it allows for smaller cranial and dural openings with minimal exposure of normal brain and because it assists in determining the optimal trajectory to the tumor. However, unless intraoperative imaging with CT or MR (and, in some cases, ultrasound) is available, the system cannot be updated during the operative procedure.

Surgical approaches to a brain metastasis are based on its anatomic location.[37] Supratentorial subcortical lesions are best resected by an incision in the apex of the sulcus and circumferential dissection of the tumor (transcortical approach) (Fig. 45-1). Removal of a cortical plug above the lesion improves exposure; this may be problematic when the lesion arises within eloquent cortex. In such a situation, a longitudinal incision dictated by local functional mapping performed with direct brain stimulation (see the following) may minimize injury to the surrounding brain.

Lesions in subgyral or subsulcal locations are best approached by splitting the sulcus leading to the lesion. Subgyral tumors are removed by making an incision in the side of the split sulcus, whereas subsulcal lesions are entered at the sulcal base (transsulcal approach) (see Fig. 45-1). Metastases located deep within the white matter, independent of a single sulcus or gyrus (lobar), may be approached either transcortically or transsulcally (see Fig. 45-1). Tumors in the subinsular cortex may be approached by splitting the sylvian fissure. Midline metastases are best approached by

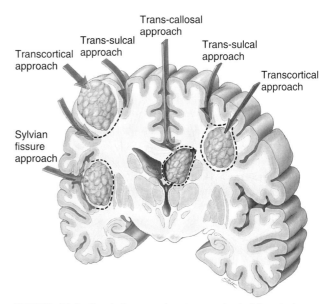

FIGURE 45-1 Surgical approaches to supratentorial metastases: transsylvian approach to a metastasis of the external capsule; transcortical and transsulcal approaches to a subcortical metastasis, which is shown filling the gyrus; transcallosal approach to an intraventricular tumor. (From Lang FF, Chang EL, Suki D, et al: Metastatic brain tumors. In Winn HR (ed): Youmans Neurologic Surgery, 5th ed. Philadelphia: WB Saunders, 2004.)

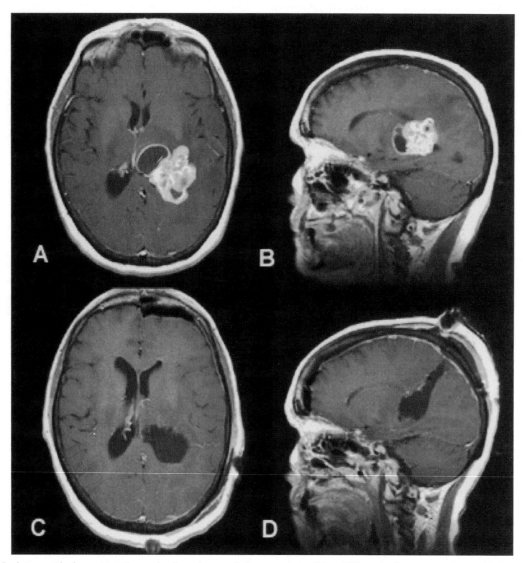

FIGURE 45-2 Intraventricular metastatic renal cell carcinoma. *A,* Preoperative axial and (*B*) sagittal contrast-enhanced MR images showing a metastasis in the atrium of the left lateral ventricle. The lesion was completely resected utilizing a transcortical approach through the superior parietal lobule (*C* and *D*). (From Vecil GG, Lang FF: Surgical resection of metastatic intraventricular tumors. Neurosur Clin N Am 14:593–606, 2003.)

splitting the interhemispheric fissure; tumors may then be resected by further splitting or entering a deep gyrus (see Fig. 45-1). Intraventricular lesions may be approached transcallosally or transcortically (Fig. 45-2; see Fig. 45-1).

Cerebellar tumors are best approached along the shortest transparenchymal route to the lesion. Superior hemispheric lesions are approached via the supracerebellar cistern and then incising the cerebellum at the closest point to the tumor. This requires a high suboccipital craniotomy with exposure of the transverse sinus. Lateral hemispheric lesions are approached directly from a posterior trajectory. Inferior cerebellar tumors require opening of the foramen magnum. Midline tumors can be resected after splitting the vermis.

Lesion Extirpation

Once the lesion is reached, resection is usually performed in a circumferential, en bloc fashion by dissection in the gliotic pseudocapsule surrounding the lesion (Fig. 45-3).

Circumferential dissection is carried out in this gliotic plane without violating the wall of the tumor. Such an approach ensures gross-total resection (because tumor cells rarely infiltrate beyond the gliotic plane) and also reduces spillage of cells into the surrounding area. For lesions located directly in eloquent brain (e.g., motor strip or speech centers), a longitudinal incision parallel to the orientation of the gyrus can be made and the tumor resected in an "inside-out," piecemeal fashion, rather than en bloc. Piecemeal removal may also be preferred for very large lesions in difficult areas (e.g., within the ventricle).

When resecting cerebral metastases, care must be taken to preserve the main arteries that lie within sulci. Most tumors receive their blood supply from several small branches arising from the main vessel. It is critical to identify these branches and to individually coagulate and cut them. This step reduces bleeding during resection and ensures that the main artery is not damaged. Likewise, significant care

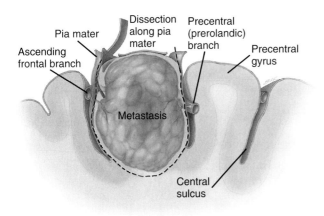

FIGURE 45-3 En bloc technique of metastasis resection. A metastasis filling a gyrus is pictured. The tumor is removed en bloc after dissection in the adjacent sulci and deep to the lesion through the base of the sulci. All but those vessels directly supplying the tumor are preserved. (Modified from Hentschel SH, Lang FF: Current surgical management of glioblastoma. Cancer J 9:113–126, 2003.)

should be taken to preserve all surface veins so that the drainage of the normal brain is not disrupted.

Technical Issues in Resecting Multiple Metastases

When resecting multiple brain metastases, special attention must be given to planning the operation. Resection of multiple metastases can be performed via one craniotomy that encompasses all the lesions or via multiple, separate craniotomies. The decision to perform multiple craniotomies is determined by the proximity of the lesions to each other: lesions that are some distance apart generally require separate craniotomies. When multiple craniotomies are required, it is usually possible to perform all the craniotomies simultaneously without having to redrape the patient. The patient

may be placed in a neutral position and turned from side to side on the operating table so that the lesion that is being operated on is positioned at the top of the operative field. Linear skin incisions are particularly effective when performing multiple craniotomies, and they also reduce the risk of compromising the vascular supply to the scalp. To maximize efficiency, each step of the operation (i.e., skin incision, bone flap elevation, dural opening, tumor removal, hemostasis, and closure) is performed at each location before the next step is performed. This approach is preferred to removing one lesion at one site and closing that wound and then removing one lesion at another site, not only because it is more efficient, but also because it minimizes the time between hemostasis and patient awakening. Thus any untoward events (e.g., hematoma formation) do not go undetected while the patient is under anesthesia.

Surgical Adjuncts

Safe and effective resection of cerebral metastases requires accurate identification of the location of each lesion and the surgical corridor through which it can be resected. The ability to identify the lesion is enhanced by the use of computer-assisted image-guided stereotaxis, intraoperative ultrasonography, and (in some centers) intraoperative MR imaging. Other useful adjuncts include somatosensory evoked potentials (SSEPs) and intraoperative direct brain stimulation, both of which allow for identification of functional (eloquent) brain regions.

Ultrasound

Intraoperative ultrasound is a valuable adjunct available to the surgeon that provides a relatively low-cost method for visualizing tumors below the surface of the brain. Most brain metastases appear homogeneously hyperechogenic, although those with necrotic centers or cysts may be hypoechoic centrally (Fig. 45-4). Compared with other methods of localization, ultrasound has the advantage of real-time imaging; therefore, changes in the tumor, as well as brain shift,

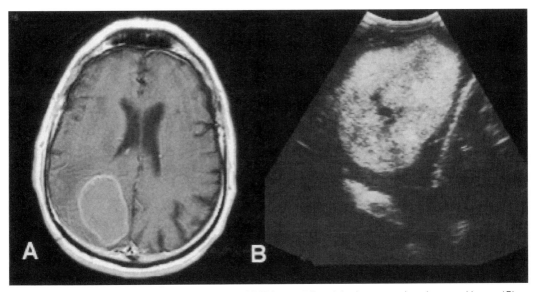

FIGURE 45-4 Occipital lobe metastasis. The contrast-enhanced MR image (*A*) and the intraoperative ultrasound image (*B*) are shown. The central hypodensity on the ultrasound image represents necrosis within the tumor.

are readily identifiable as the resection proceeds. Ultrasound also allows for visualization of the adjacent sulci and other intracranial landmarks (e.g., the ventricle), thus assisting in selection of a corridor of approach to the tumor. Ultrasound can assist in the determination of the extent of tumor resection because gross-total resection corresponds to complete removal of the echogenic mass, in most cases. However, in cases of recurrent tumors after radiotherapy, radiation necrosis may obscure the boundaries of the lesion, making determination of the extent of resection more difficult.[40]

Stereotaxis

Advances in localization technology have allowed for the evolution of rigid frame-based stereotaxy into frameless systems. These "neuronavigation" devices allow neurosurgeons to navigate the brain based on the preoperative images. These systems are particularly useful for planning the skin incision and craniotomy and the initial trajectory to the lesion. However, they suffer from the inability to compensate for intraoperative changes such as brain shift unless they can be updated with intraoperative imaging (usually MR images or even ultrasonography).[41] Thus the authors generally rely on ultrasound as the resection proceeds.

Intraoperative MR Imaging

The inability of neuronavigation systems to track intraoperative changes in real time has led to the development of intraoperative MR imaging systems. Surgery may be performed within the magnet itself or outside of it, necessitating that the patient be brought into the unit or that the unit be brought to the patient. The main uses of these systems are to update the neuronavigation system during the operation, to confirm the extent of tumor resection, and to rule out intracranial complications prior to leaving the operating room. The cost of current systems has precluded widespread application, particularly for well-demarcated lesions such as brain metastases.

Functional Mapping

When resecting metastases within eloquent areas of the brain, mapping the location of the critical functions is vital to safe tumor resection. Preoperative identification of sensory, motor, and language cortices is possible with functional MR imaging,[42] and diffusion-tensor imaging allows for identification of important white matter tracts (e.g., internal capsule).[43] These preoperative studies, however, are only a general guide, and precise localization of function usually requires verification during the surgical resection. Consequently, functional mapping methods have been used to precisely define eloquent brain regions intraoperatively.

Neurophysiologic techniques, such as SSEPs, can be utilized to identify the reversal of phase that occurs between the motor and sensory cortices. A strip electrode is placed on the cortical surface, and stimulation of median, ulnar, or posterior tibial nerves results in cortical potentials that are detected by the electrodes. A "reversal of phase" is seen when the electrode covers both the motor and the sensory cortex because the motor potentials are typically positive and sensory potentials are typically negative. This permits an intraoperative indirect identification of motor and sensory cortices. The technique has also been used to continuously monitor the

potentials throughout the operative procedure to guide resections adjacent to the primary somatosensory cortex.[44]

Direct cortical electrical stimulation can be used to identify eloquent cortex and is particularly useful in the localization of language areas. The technique involves stimulation of the cerebral cortex at a frequency of 60 Hz for 1 millisecond with biphasic square wave pulses and a current of 1 to 15 mA (Fig. 45-5).[45-47] Stimulation of the motor cortex elicits a motor response in the patient, thus resulting in an objective response, which is an advantage over the SSEP technique. Stimulation of subcortical motor pathways can also be performed in a similar manner; however, the results are somewhat less reliable than cortical stimulation.[48]

Although motor mapping can be performed with patients under general anesthesia, language mapping requires an awake patient. The authors' current method of awake craniotomy employs intubation with a laryngeal mask and short duration anesthetics, along with a local anesthetic scalp block prior to placement of the three-point head fixator.[49] The muscle (if exposed) and dura are carefully infiltrated with local anesthetic. Once the craniotomy is completed, the patient is awakened and the laryngeal mask is removed. Cortical stimulation with mapping of speech may then commence. Speech areas are usually defined as sites where electrical stimulation elicits speech arrest. In addition, patients can freely converse during the resection of the tumor in order to avoid loss of function as the resection proceeds. Once the resection is completed, the laryngeal mask may be replaced and the patient anesthetized, if required; or a short-acting sedative, along with a narcotic, may be given during the closure. This awake method allows for the safe removal of the tumor from eloquent brain and provides the patient with maximal comfort.

OUTCOMES AFTER SURGICAL RESECTION

Surgical Mortality

Most studies define surgical mortality as death that occurs within 30 days of operation, although some of the earlier surgeons used shorter intervals.[50-52] Other series include deaths after 30 days if the patient did not leave the hospital.[31,53] Surgical mortality has decreased dramatically since the earliest reports. For example, Cushing found that the mortality after resection of brain metastases was quite high (38%).[53] In contrast, in the 1990s, using modern techniques, surgical mortalities of 3% or less have often been reported (Table 45-4). In fact, some of the more recent series report no mortality after surgery for brain metastases.[30,40,54,55] In the randomized trial of Patchell and colleagues,[12] the 30-day operative mortality and the 30-day postradiotherapy mortality were both 4%. In a very comprehensive analysis of 400 craniotomies from M.D. Anderson (1992–1994), 194 craniotomies were performed for resection of brain metastases.[27] The overall mortality for these patients was 2% (4/194), with the cause of death being sepsis in two patients and progressive leptomeningeal carcinomatosis in two others.

Surgical Morbidity

Postoperative morbidity after surgery for brain metastases includes those related to neurologic changes and those related

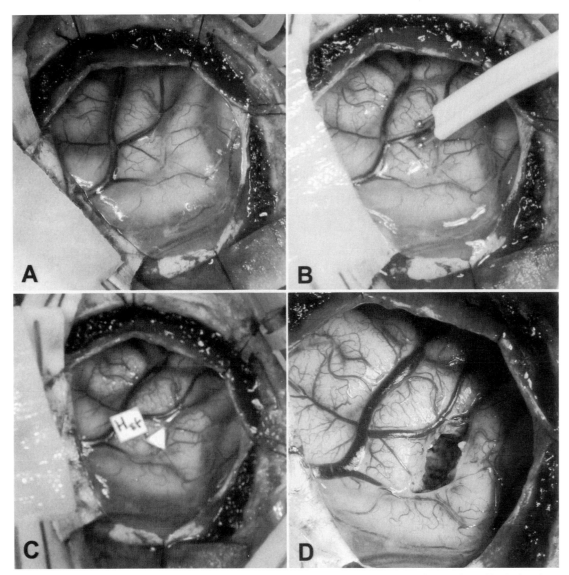

FIGURE 45-5 Intraoperative photographs depicting removal of a metastasis from the motor area of the brain. *A,* The brain prior to resection demonstrating slightly clouded leptomeninges along with an enlarged gyrus. *B,* A bipolar cortical stimulator was used to electrically stimulate the cerebral cortex, and a motor response was elicited. *C,* The cortical stimulation resulted in hand movement in the area marked by the white label (Hst). The white arrowhead marks a sulcus overlying the tumor. *D,* The tumor has been completely resected and all vascular structures preserved utilizing a transsulcal approach through the sulcus identified in *C.* The patient experienced no permanent alteration of neurologic function.

TABLE 45-4 ▪ Results of Surgical Resection of Single Brain Metastases, Including Mortality and Morbidity

Study	No.	Histology	WBRT	Mortality	Morbidity	Survival Median (Months)	1-Year
Ferrara et al[56]	100	Mixed	71%	6%	N/A	13	N/A
Patchell et al[12]	25	Mixed	100%	4%	8%	10	45%
Bindal et al[25]	26	Mixed	54%	0%	8% (0% neuro)	14	50%
Vecht et al[20]	32	Mixed	100%	9%	41% total 13% (major)	10	41%
Wronski et al[73]	231	Lung	84%	3%	17% (neuro)	11	46%
Bindal et al[54]	62	Mixed	66%	0%	5%	16.4	58%
Pieper et al[75]	63	Breast	86%	5%	N/A	16	62%
Muacevic et al[76]	52	Mixed	100%	1.6%	7.7%	17	53%
Wronski and Arbit[77]	73	Colon	43.8%	4%	N/A	8.3	31.5%
Schoggl et al[65]	66	Mixed	100%	0%	4.5%	9	83%
O'Neill et al[68]	74	Mixed	82%	N/A	13.5% (neuro) 9.5% (systemic)	N/A	62%
Overall	804		80%	3%	12%	12	53%

N/A, not available.

to nonneurologic problems (e.g., postoperative hematoma, wound infection, deep venous thrombosis, pneumonia, and pulmonary embolism). Some studies separate these two aspects of morbidity,[25,30,32] others consider them together,[12,20,22] a few report only neurologic morbidity,[33,50,56–58] and many do not report morbidity at all (see Table 45-4).[24,31,51,52,59,60]

One of the most comprehensive recent analyses of postoperative complications for brain metastases was conducted by Sawaya and colleagues.[27] This series from M.D. Anderson reviewed the complications that occurred after 194 craniotomies for brain metastases performed using all the modern technologies described above. Importantly, complications were categorized as either neurologic (directly producing neurologic compromise), regional (at the surgical site), or systemic (more generalized medical problems). Complications were considered to be minor (not life-threatening and not prolonging the length of the hospital stay) when they resolved within a few days to 30 days without surgical intervention. They were considered to be major when they persisted for more than 30 days (reducing the quality of life) or required aggressive treatment because of their life-threatening nature. The rates of major neurologic, regional, and systemic complications were 6%, 3%, and 6%, respectively. In a critical analysis of factors contributing to complications, the authors reported that the most important variable affecting the frequency of neurologic complications was the relationship of the tumor to functional (eloquent) brain. Specifically, tumors located within or near eloquent brain had more neurologic complications than did those in noneloquent areas. Nevertheless, the risk of major neurologic complications, even when the lesion was within eloquent areas, was low (13%). Based on their extensive data, the authors used a statistical model to predict the risk of major complications from any source. They found that patients who were relatively young (age 40 years), with a KPS score of 100 and a metastasis in noneloquent brain, had a 5% risk of a major complication; whereas, at the opposite extreme, for a relatively old patient (age 65 years) with a low KPS score (of 50) and a tumor in eloquent brain, this risk was 23%.

Recurrence

Recurrence is fairly easily measured after resection because surgery typically removes the entire gadolinium contrast-enhancing tumor mass (as visualized by MR imaging) and causes regression of the secondary brain edema. Thus reappearance of a contrast-enhancing mass and edema on an MR image can be determined, although minimal postoperative contrast enhancement may be present for up to 3 months after surgery. In addition, one must distinguish between recurrence at the surgical site (i.e., local recurrence) and the development of new lesions in the brain at sites outside the initial resection site (i.e., distant recurrence). These events represent two distinct biologic processes. Local recurrence represents regrowth of microscopic residual disease after surgery, whereas distant recurrence is believed to arise from hematogenous dissemination of tumor cells to the brain from the primary site. When evaluating rates of local and distant tumor recurrence, it is important to know whether the patients received adjunctive WBRT. In the prospective study by Patchell and colleagues of patients with single brain metastases who were then randomized either to receive or not to receive WBRT after surgery,[61] the local recurrence rate after surgery alone was 46% (21 of 46 patients), whereas the distant recurrence rate was 37% (17 of 46 patients). This high rate of local recurrence is not consistent with the results of other studies, which suggest recurrence rates of 10% to 15%.[62] Table 45-5 lists the local and distant recurrence rates in recent surgical series of brain metastases.

Survival

Most series from the modern neurosurgical era that include metastases with different tumor histologies indicate a median patient survival time of 11 months (range, 6 to 16 months) and a 1-year survival rate of 42% (range, 22% to 63%) (see Table 45-4). Kelly and colleagues[37] reported a 1-year survival rate of 63% using computer-assisted stereotactic craniotomy. Studies from M.D. Anderson report a median survival time of 14 months, with a 1-year survival rate of 50% for patients with single brain metastases.[25,30] Similar median (14 months) and 1-year (55%) survival values were observed in patients with multiple metastases in whom all the lesions were removed.[25] In most studies, variables associated with poor survival are the presence of multiple metastases, extensive and progressive systemic cancer, and a poor KPS.

TABLE 45-5 ▪ Local and Distant Recurrence following Resection of a Single Brain Metastases

Study	No.	Local Recurrence	Distant Recurrence	Both	Latency (Median)
Patchell et al[12]	25	20%	20%	12%	15 months (l)
Bindal et al[25]	26	16%	27%	8%	25% at 6 months
Wronski et al[73]	231	23.8%	36.6%	3%	N/A
Bindal et al[54]	62	13%	26%	5%	N/A
Pieper et al[75]	63	17%	16%	N/A	15 months
Muacevic et al[76]	52	25% at 1 year	10% at 1 year	N/A	N/A
Wronski and Arbit[77]	73	49.3%	Overall		3.6 months
Schoggle et al[65]	66	16.7%	15.2%	N/A	3.9 months (l)
					3.7 months (d)
O'Neill et al[68]	74	18%	18%	5.4%	N/A
Overall	672	20%	25%	5%	8.1 months

l, local; d, distant recurrence; N/A, not available.

ROLE OF STEREOTACTIC RADIOSURGERY

Stereotactic radiosurgery via the gamma knife or linear accelerator uses small, multiple, well-collimated beams of ionizing radiation to destroy lesions localized by stereotaxy. An advantage of this technique over conventional surgery is that it lends itself to treatment of brain metastases that might be considered surgically inaccessible, especially where eloquent brain would be transgressed to reach the lesion. It is also less costly, less invasive (no incisions; requires placement of stereotactic headframe under local anesthesia), and necessitates shorter hospital stays, because only a single-fraction radiation dose is given. Moreover, multiple reports suggest that stereotactic radiosurgery controls the growth of the tumor in approximately 85% to 95% of patients.[63–65] A recent review of 21 reports, including 1700 patients undergoing radiosurgery for brain metastases, found that the median survival was 9.6 months and the local control rate was 83%.[66] Yet radiosurgery is limited to treatment of small lesions, usually to those not exceeding 3 cm in maximum diameter (volume < 10 to 12 cm^3).[28,29] In addition, no histologic verification of the metastatic nature of the lesion can be obtained with radiosurgery, which is important considering that 5% to 11% of patients with systemic cancer are found to have nonmetastatic brain lesions (e.g., primary brain tumors or abscesses).[8,12,13] Furthermore, because radiosurgery does not have the immediate effect of conventional surgery, patients may have to remain on high steroid doses for longer intervals, and compression effects of tumors (e.g., neurologic deficits and intracranial pressure elevation) are not quickly relieved.

Primarily because radiosurgery is easy to perform and has a presumed lower cost, it has been suggested that conventional surgery should be replaced by radiosurgery for eradication of all small metastases (<3 cm in greatest diameter). To date, no prospective randomized trial has been performed comparing treatment of brain metastases by craniotomy to treatment by radiosurgery. There have, however, been several retrospective studies attempting to evaluate the efficacy of these modalities.[54,63,67] Nevertheless, because the conclusions of these retrospective reports are completely divergent, the controversy has not been resolved. For example, the authors' group at M.D. Anderson conducted a retrospective study comparing surgery and radiosurgery. A group of 31 consecutive radiosurgically treated patients was matched to 62 patients treated by surgery during the same time interval (using sex, age, extent of systemic disease, primary tumor histology, pretreatment KPS, number of brain metastases, and time to occurrence of brain metastases).[54] The median survival time was 16.4 months for the group undergoing surgery versus 7.5 months for the radiosurgery group; the difference was significant using both multivariate ($p = 0.0009$) and univariate ($p = 0.0041$) analyses. These findings are in direct contrast to the results recently reported by O'Neill and colleagues, who compared the outcome of 74 patients treated with surgery to that of 23 patients treated with radiosurgery.[68] All of these patients were eligible for either radiosurgery or surgical resection. The 1-year survival rates for surgery and radiosurgery were 67% and 56%, respectively ($p = 0.18$). These survival rates were not statistically different. However, the local recurrence rate was 58% in the surgical group and 0% in the radiosurgical group ($p=0.02$).

Resolution of the current controversy will require completion of a prospective randomized trial comparing surgery with radiosurgery. Until such a trial is completed, however, it is probably best to view surgery and radiosurgery as complementary rather than as competing therapies. In particular, the potential ability of radiosurgery to treat small, deep lesions with minimal morbidity is quite distinct from the ability of surgery to rapidly reverse neurologic deficits from larger symptomatic lesions. Currently at M.D. Anderson, surgery is the treatment of choice for single brain metastases. Radiosurgery is used primarily as an alternative to surgery. Radiosurgery is typically recommended in three situations: (1) for single lesions that are surgically inaccessible, (2) in patients who are not surgical candidates because of advanced systemic disease or medical conditions that preclude surgery, and (3) as part of a multimodal attack on multiple brain lesions. For example, in patients with a single, large, symptomatic lesion and one small lesion (<3 cm in maximum diameter), surgical resection of the large lesion is often followed by radiosurgery on the smaller, less accessible lesion.

ROLE OF WHOLE-BRAIN RADIATION THERAPY AS A POSTOPERATIVE ADJUVANT

After resection of a single brain metastasis, patients are often given adjuvant WBRT on a routine basis in an effort to eradicate residual cancer cells at the resection site as well as microscopic foci at other sites. Although some retrospective studies have shown this to benefit patients,[69–71] others have not.[32,72,73] Moreover, irreversible neurotoxicities (e.g., dementia) often occur in long-term surviving patients given WBRT.[74]

Recently, Patchell and colleagues[61] reported the results of a randomized prospective trial examining the benefits of adjunctive WBRT in the surgical treatment of single brain metastases. After surgery, patients were randomly assigned either to treatment with 50.4 Gy over 5.5 weeks or to observation (median follow-up, 43 weeks), and the patients were classified according to extent of disease and primary tumor type. The patients who received WBRT showed a striking reduction in tumor recurrence (distant and local) relative to the observation group (18% versus 70%, respectively; $p < 0.001$). The local recurrence rate was 46% in the surgery alone group and 10% in the surgery plus WBRT group, and patients in the radiotherapy group were less likely than those in the observation group to die of neurologic causes (14% vs. 44%, respectively; $p = 0.003$). Nevertheless, overall patient survival was not improved by adjunctive WBRT. Moreover, the KPS scores for the patients undergoing WBRT declined at the same rate as for those in the surgery only (observation) group, raising the possibility that the toxicity of WBRT offset its beneficial effect. An unexplained result was that among patients who died from systemic disease, those not receiving WBRT survived longer than those in the observation group. Although the authors concluded WBRT to be a valuable adjunct to surgical resection (partly on the basis of preventing deaths from neurologic causes), the lack of overall survival improvement, their use of higher-than-standard radiation doses (50 Gy rather than the more common 30 Gy), and the potential for radiation toxicity leave some unresolved concerns as to the best recommendations for treatment of patients with single brain metastases. Confirmation of the findings of Patchell and colleagues with more careful assessments of cognitive function would be helpful. Moreover, in this study,[61] it is difficult to draw conclusions for patients with renal cell carcinoma (RCC) or melanoma (tumors that are considered radioresistant) because each arm of the study contained only one melanoma patient and an unspecified number of RCC patients. Thus for patients having tumors with so-called radioresistant histologies (e.g., metastatic melanoma and RCC), the need for adjunctive postoperative WBRT remains unclear. A randomized trial of postoperative WBRT exclusively for RCC or melanoma patients will be needed to help resolve the controversy.

REFERENCES

1. Wingo PA, Tong T, Bolden S: Cancer statistics, 1995. CA Cancer J Clin 45:8–30, 1995.
2. Cairncross JG, Kim JH, Posner JB: Radiation therapy for brain metastases. Ann Neurol 7:529–541, 1980.
3. Delattre JY, Krol G, Thaler HT, et al: Distribution of brain metastases. Arch Neurol 45:741–744, 1988.
4. Patchell RA: Brain metastases. Neurol Clin 9:817–824, 1991.
5. Posner JB, Chernik NL: Intracranial metastases from systemic cancer. Adv Neurol 19:579–592, 1978.
6. Jemal A, Tiwari RC, Murray T, et al: Cancer statistics, 2004. CA Cancer J Clin 54:8–29, 2004.
7. Landis SH, Murray T, Bolden S, et al: Cancer statistics, 1998. CA Cancer J Clin 48:6–29, 1998.
8. Sawaya R, Bindal RK, Lang FF, et al: Metastatic brain tumors. In Kaye AH, Laws ER (eds): Brain Tumors: An Encyclopedic Approach. Edinburgh: Churchill Livingstone, 2001, pp 999–1026.
9. Byrne TN, Cascino TL, Posner JB: Brain metastasis from melanoma. J Neurooncol 1:313–317, 1983.
10. Madajewicz S, Karakousis C, West CR, et al: Malignant melanoma brain metastases: Review of Roswell Park Memorial Institute experience. Cancer 53:2550–2552, 1984.
11. Black P: Surgical and radiotherapeutic management of brain metastasis. In Schmidek HH (ed): Operative Neurosurgical Techniques: Indications, Methods, and Results. Philadelphia: WB Saunders, 2000, pp 717–732.
12. Patchell RA, Tibbs PA, Walsh JW, et al: A randomized trial of surgery in the treatment of single metastases to the brain. N Engl J Med 322:494–500, 1990.
13. Voorhies R, Sundaresan N, Thaler H: The single supratentorial lesion: An evaluation of preoperative diagnostic tests. J Neurosurg 53:338–344, 1980.
14. Kuhn MJ, Hammer GM, Swenson LC, et al: MRI evaluation of "solitary" brain metastases with triple-dose gadoteridol: Comparison with contrast-enhanced CT and conventional-dose gadopentetate dimeglumine MRI studies in the same patients. Comput Med Imaging Graph 18:391–399, 1994.
15. Nomoto Y, Miyamoto T, Yamaguchi Y: Brain metastasis of small cell lung carcinoma: Comparison of Gd-DTPA enhanced magnetic resonance imaging and enhanced computerized tomography. Jpn J Clin Oncol 24:258–262, 1994.
16. Sze G, Milano E, Johnson C, et al: Detection of brain metastases: Comparison of contrast-enhanced MR with unenhanced MR and enhanced CT. Am J Neuroradiol 11:785–791, 1990.
17. Macchiarini P, Buonaguidi R, Hardin M, et al: Results and prognostic factors of surgery in the management of non-small cell lung cancer with solitary brain metastasis. Cancer 68:300–304, 1991.
18. Johnson JD, Young B: Demographics of brain metastasis. Neurosurg Clin N Am 7:337–344, 1996.
19. Mintz AH, Kestle J, Rathbone MP, et al: A randomized trial to assess the efficacy of surgery in addition to radiotherapy in patients with a single cerebral metastasis. Cancer 78:1470–1476, 1996.
20. Vecht CJ, Haaxma-Reiche H, Noordijk EM, et al: Treatment of single brain metastasis: Radiotherapy alone or combined with neurosurgery? Ann Neurol 33:583–590, 1993.
21. Elvidge AR, Baldwin M: Clinical analysis of 88 cases of metastatic carcinoma involving the central nervous system. J Neurosurg 6:495–502, 1949.
22. Haar F, Patterson R: Surgery for metastatic intracranial neoplasm. Cancer 30:1241–1245, 1972.
23. Oldberg E: Surgical considerations of carcinomatous metastases to the brain. JAMA 101:1458–1461, 1933.
24. Ransohoff J: Surgical management of metastatic tumors. Semin Oncol 2:21–27, 1975.
25. Bindal RK, Sawaya R, Leavens ME, et al: Surgical treatment of multiple brain metastases. J Neurosurg 79:210–216, 1993.
26. Iwadate Y, Namba H, Yamaura A: Significance of surgical resection for the treatment of multiple brain metastases. Anticancer Res 20:573–577, 2000.
27. Sawaya R, Hammoud M, Schoppa D, et al: Neurosurgical outcomes in a modern series of 400 craniotomies for treatment of parenchymal tumors. Neurosurgery 42:1044–1055, 1998.
28. Kondziolka D, Lunsford LD: Brain metastases. In Apuzzo MLJ (ed): Brain Surgery: Complication Avoidance and Management. New York: Churchill Livingstone, 1993, pp 615–641.
29. Sturm V, Kimmig B, Engenhardt R, et al: Radiosurgical treatment of cerebral metastases. Method, indications and results. Stereotact Funct Neurosurg 57:7–10, 1991.
30. Bindal RK, Sawaya R, Leavens ME, et al: Reoperation for recurrent metastatic brain tumors. J Neurosurg 83:600–604, 1995.
31. Galicich JH, Sundaresan N, Arbit E, et al: Surgical treatment of single brain metastasis: Factors associated with survival. Cancer 45:381–386, 1980.
32. Sundaresan N, Galicich JH: Surgical treatment of brain metastases: Clinical and computerized tomography evaluation of the results of treatment. Cancer 55:1382–1388, 1985.
33. Winston KR, Walsh JW, Fischer EG: Results of operative treatment of intracranial metastatic tumors. Cancer 45:2639–2645, 1980.
34. Gaspar L, Scott C, Rotman M, et al: Recursive partitioning analysis (RPA) of prognostic factors in three Radiation Therapy Oncology Group (RTOG) brain metastases trials. Int J Radiat Oncol Biol Phys 37:745–751, 1997.
35. Lutterbach J, Bartelt S, Stancu E, et al: Patients with brain metastases: Hope for recursive partitioning analysis (RPA) class 3. Radiother Oncol 63:339–345, 2002.
36. Brown PD, Brown CA, Pollock BE, et al: Stereotactic radiosurgery for patients with "radioresistant" brain metastases. Neurosurgery 51:656–665, 2002.
37. Kelly PJ, Kall BA, Goerss SJ: Results of computed tomography-based computer-assisted stereotactic resection of metastatic intracranial tumors. Neurosurgery 22:7–17, 1988.
38. Yasargil MG: Topographic anatomy for microsurgical approaches to intrinsic brain tumors. In Microneurosurgery, vol IVA. New York: Thieme Medical Publishing Inc., 1994, pp 2–114.
39. Lang FF, Sawaya R: Surgical management of cerebral metastases. Neurosurg Clin N Am 7:459–484, 1996.
40. Hammoud M, Ligon BL, elSouki R, et al: Use of intraoperative ultrasound for localizing tumors and determining the extent of resection: A comparative study with magnetic resonance imaging. J Neurosurg 84:737–741, 1996.
41. Unsgaard G, Ommedal S, Muller T, et al: Neuronavigation by intraoperative 3-dimensional ultrasound: Initial experience during brain tumor resection. Neurosurgery 50:804–812, 2002.
42. Heilbrun M, Lee J, Alvord L: Practical application of fMRI for surgical planning. Stereotact Funct Neurosurg 76:168–174, 2001.
43. Witwer B, Moftakhar R, Hasan K, et al: Diffusion-tensor imaging of white matter tracts in patients with cerebral neoplasm. J Neurosurg 97:568–575, 2002.
44. Grant G, Farrell D, Silbergeld D: Continuous somatosensory evoked potential monitoring during brain tumor resection. J Neurosurg 97:709–713, 2002.
45. Berger MS, Ojemann GA: Intraoperative brain mapping techniques in neuro-oncology. Stereotact Funct Neurosurg 58:153–161, 1992.
46. Matz P, Cobbs C, Berger M: Intraoperative cortical mapping as a guide to the surgical resection of gliomas. J Neurooncol 42:233–245, 1999.
47. Taylor M, Bernstein M: Awake craniotomy with brain mapping as the routine surgical approach to treating patients with supratentorial

intraaxial tumors: A prospective trial of 200 cases. J Neurosurg 90:35–41, 1999.

48. Skirboll S, Ojemann G, Berger M, et al: Functional cortex and subcortical white matter located within gliomas. Neurosurgery 38:678–685, 1996.

49. Toms S, Ferson D, Sawaya R: Basic surgical techniques in the resection of malignant gliomas. J Neurooncol 42:215–226, 1999.

50. Raskind R, Weiss SR, Manning JJ, et al: Survival after surgical excision of single metastatic brain tumors. AJR Am J Roentgenol 111:323–328, 1971.

51. Stortebecker TP: Metastatic tumors of the brain from a neurosurgical point of view: A follow-up study of 158 cases. J Neurosurg 11:84–111, 1954.

52. Vieth RG, Odom GL: Intracranial metastases and their neurosurgical treatment. J Neurosurg 23:375–383, 1965.

53. Cushing H: Notes upon a series of 2000 verified cases with surgical-mortality percentages pertaining thereto. Springfield, IL: Charles C Thomas, 1932, p 105.

54. Bindal AK, Bindal RK, Hess KR, et al: Surgery versus radiosurgery in the treatment of brain metastasis. J Neurosurg 84:748–754, 1996.

55. Brega K, Robinson WA, Winston K, et al: Surgical treatment of brain metastases in malignant melanoma. Cancer 66:2105–2110, 1990.

56. Ferrara M, Bizzozzero L, Talamonti G, et al: Surgical treatment of 100 single brain metastases: Analysis of the results. J Neurosurg Sci 34:303–308, 1990.

57. Lang EF, Slater J: Metastatic brain tumors: Results of surgical and non-surgical treatment. Surg Clin North Am 44:865–872, 1964.

58. Sause WT, Crowley JJ, Morantz R, et al: Solitary brain metastasis: Results of an RTOG/SWOG protocol evaluation surgery + RT versus RT alone. Am J Clin Oncol 13:427–432, 1990.

59. Simionescu MD: Metastatic tumors of the brain: A follow-up study of 195 patients with neurosurgical considerations. Ann Surg 84:635–646, 1960.

60. White KT, Fleming TR, Laws ER Jr: Single metastasis to the brain: Surgical treatment in 122 consecutive patients. Mayo Clin Proc 56:424–428, 1981.

61. Patchell RA, Tibbs PA, Regine WF, et al: Postoperative radiotherapy in the treatment of single metastases to the brain: A randomized trial. JAMA 280:1485–1489, 1998.

62. Sawaya R: Surgical treatment of brain metastases. Clin Neurosurg 45:41–47, 1999.

63. Auchter RM, Lamond JP, Alexander E, et al: A multiinstitutional outcome and prognostic factor analysis of radiosurgery for resectable single brain metastasis. Int J Radiat Oncol Biol Phys 35:27–35, 1996.

64. Fuller BG, Kaplan ID, Adler J, et al: Stereotaxic radiosurgery for brain metastases: The importance of adjuvant whole brain irradiation. Int J Radiat Oncol Biol Phys 23:413–418, 1992.

65. Schoggl A, Kitz K, Reddy M, et al: Defining the role of stereotactic radiosurgery versus microsurgery in the treatment of single brain metastases. Acta Neurochir (Wien) 142:621–626, 2000.

66. Boyd TS, Mehta MP: Stereotactic radiosurgery for brain metastases. Oncology 13:1397–1409, 1999.

67. Cho KH, Hall WA, Lee AK, et al: Stereotactic radiosurgery for patients with single brain metastasis. J Radiosurg 1:79–85, 1998.

68. O'Neill BP, Iturria NJ, Link MJ, et al: A comparison of surgical resection and stereotactic radiosurgery in the treatment of solitary brain metastases. Int J Radiat Oncol Biol Phys 55:1169–1176, 2003.

69. DeAngelis LM, Mandell LR, Thaler HT, et al: The role of postoperative radiotherapy after resection of single brain metastases. Neurosurgery 24:798–805, 1989.

70. Hagen NA, Cirrincione C, Thaler HT, et al: The role of radiation therapy following resection of single brain metastasis from melanoma. Neurology 40:158–160, 1990.

71. Smalley SR, Schray MF, Laws ER Jr, et al: Adjuvant radiation therapy after surgical resection of solitary brain metastasis: association with pattern of failure and survival. Int J Radiat Oncol Biol Phys 13:1611–1616, 1987.

72. Dosoretz DE, Blitzer PH, Russell AH, et al: Management of solitary metastasis to the brain: The role of elective brain irradiation following complete surgical resection. Int J Radiat Oncol Biol Phys 6:1727–1730, 1980.

73. Wronski M, Arbit E, Burt M, et al: Survival after surgical treatment of brain metastases from lung cancer: A follow-up study of 231 patients treated between 1976 and 1991. J Neurosurg 83:605–616, 1995.

74. Sundaresan N, Galicich JH, Deck MD, et al: Radiation necrosis after treatment of solitary intracranial metastases. Neurosurgery 8:329–333, 1981.

75. Pieper DR, Hess KR, Sawaya RE: Role of surgery in the treatment of brain metastases in patients with breast cancer. Ann Surg Oncol 4:481–490, 1997.

76. Muacevic A, Kreth FW, Horstmann GA, et al: Surgery and radiotherapy compared with gamma knife radiosurgery in the treatment of solitary cerebral metastases of small diameter. J Neurosurg 91:35–43, 1999.

77. Wronski M, Arbit E: Resection of brain metastases from colorectal carcinoma in 73 patients. Cancer 85:1677–1685, 1999.

46 Management of Primary Central Nervous System Lymphomas

CAMILO E. FADUL and PAMELA ELY

INTRODUCTION

The phrase primary central nervous system lymphoma (PCNSL) is used to designate an extranodal lymphoma restricted to the nervous system; these constitute about 3% of all brain tumors. Most are large B-cell lymphomas but a few cases of T-cell lymphomas have been reported. A common location is the brain parenchyma surrounding the ventricular system, but any craniospinal structure, in addition to the eye, can be involved. Although not as common, isolated spinal cord, meningeal, or ocular PCNSL can also occur. On the other hand, brain lesions can be accompanied by lepto meningeal and ocular dissemination. This chapter does not cover nervous system involvement as the first manifestation of systemic lymphoma, which can masquerade as PCNSL.

Among the brain tumors, PCNSL has gained notoriety because, though still rare, it has recently increased in incidence and, unlike other brain tumors, has a high response rate to chemotherapy and radiation therapy. Before 1980, PCNSL would occur in a few individuals who were immune suppressed, usually after kidney transplant. The advent of the acquired immunodeficiency syndrome (AIDS) epidemic brought a steep increase in the frequency of this entity. Nevertheless, the increased incidence was also seen in individuals without AIDS or other known immuno-suppressive states, except for older age. Pathogenesis, diag-nostic approach, treatment, and prognosis differ according to the patient's immune state; thus when there is a suspicion of PCNSL, establishing an individual's immunocompetency is of fundamental importance in deciding the most appropriate management.

At some point in his or her career, the neurosurgeon will be required to decide about surgery for a lesion sus-pected of being PCNSL by imaging studies. Unfortunately, the appearance is not specific, making it necessary to have this entity in mind as part of the differential diagnosis of any mass lesion. Because this tumor is highly responsive to nonsurgical forms of therapy, the role of surgery has to be tempered accordingly. In some cases, it will entail the defer-ral of surgical resection of a mass until the pathologic result of a diagnostic biopsy is available for review. In others, it involves refraining from the use of steroids until after the biopsy is performed to ensure the best diagnostic yield from the specimen. Moreover, in many cases, placement of a reservoir with intraventricular catheter for chemotherapy administration is required as part of the treatment. Therefore, it is important for the neurosurgeon to be aware of the clinical and diagnostic characteristics suggestive of PCNSL while actively participating in the subsequent therapeutic antineoplastic phase.

This chapter describes concepts pertaining to PCNSL of relevance for the neurosurgical practice taking into account, where appropriate, differences according to the patient's immune state. Initial consideration will be given to the pathogenesis, etiology, and epidemiology of this type of lymphoma. Clinical presentation and diagnostic approach when the suspicion of PCNSL arises will be reviewed. Finally, therapeutic interventions, its complications, and prognostic factors will be described in detail, insofar as they are important to understanding the surgical role in the overall interdisciplinary treatment approach of PCNSL.

PATHOGENESIS AND MOLECULAR PATHOLOGY

As previously mentioned, PCNSLs are uncommon lym-phomas arising in the CNS without evidence of extracerebral or intravascular involvement. These lymphomas are almost exclusively of B cell origin with only 2% of T cell origin. Histologically, T-cell lymphomas may be indistinguishable from other entities such as inflammatory processes, but molecular genetic verification of clonal T cell receptor (TCR) gene rearrangements help to establish the diagnosis.[1] The most common histologic subtype is the diffuse large B cell non-Hodgkin's lymphoma by the WHO classification, with a smattering of other more indolent B cell lymphomas reported. The disease is more common in the immuno-compromised than in the immunocompetent, but the pathogenesis of these disorders is uncertain regardless of the immunocompetency of the patient.[2,3] Indeed, how does a B-cell lymphoma arise in a setting that has been considered, under normal circumstances, to be immunologically privi-leged, and what is the origin of these cells?

Normal B cells arise from the hematopoietic stem cell and initially undergo antigen-independent differentiation, with immunoglobulin rearrangement in the bone marrow prior to emerging from the marrow as mature but virgin B cells. These B cells may move to secondary lymphoid organs where, upon encountering antigen, they undergo somatic hypermutation of the immunoglobulin variable region in the germinal center microenvironment. The presence of T cells and the appropriate cytokine milieu is generally considered a requirement for somatic hypermutation.[4] Those B cells displaying the highest affinity for antigen are rescued from apoptosis and become either a memory cell or the terminally differentiated plasma cell.

Malignant B cells can be viewed as B cells arrested at a certain stage of differentiation. The developmental state, and thus the origin, of the cell, will be reflected in its morphologic attributes, the degree of immunoglobulin rearrangement, the expression of BCL-6 (which serves as a marker of the B cell's transition through the germinal center), and the presence of intraclonal heterogeneity. There is good evidence that the B cell of origin in PCNSL has undergone somatic hypermutation, suggesting that the malignant cell is a postgerminal center B cell.[5] Because there are no germinal centers in the brain, the malignant cell has, in all likelihood, migrated from a node to the CNS, probably in response to antigen.[6]

A rat model has been developed by Knopf and colleagues[7] to show that nonmalignant B lymphocytes do, in fact, enter the normal brain with an intact blood-brain barrier (BBB) in response to antigen localized to the CNS. Their data supports the hypothesis that there is first an efflux of antigen from the brain into draining secondary lymphoid organs. This is followed by antigen-specific recruitment of naive lymphocytes with clonal expansion in the germinal center. Finally, there is trafficking of these lymphocytes back to the brain via the blood, with production of antibody in the CNS.[7] Applying this model to PCNSL, it would be postulated that PCNSL arises in response to an antigenic stimulus, an infection perhaps, where the antigen has moved into a draining lymph node and serves to recruit naive B cells. Presumably, antigen is retained in the CNS that prompts trafficking of cells back into the CNS. Although this hypothetical scenario is compatible with the pathologic stage of development and differentiation of the malignant cell, several questions remain unanswered, including identification of the site of malignant transformation, the complete lack of involved lymph nodes, and the identification of the intracerebral antigen driving the process. Furthermore, there is uncertainty about ongoing hypermutation in the CNS despite the lack of secondary follicles and their accompanying T cells and antigen presenting cells.

Intraclonal heterogeneity suggests that there is ongoing hypermutation in the CNS, but the details of the necessary accessory cells remain unclear.[6] Two studies have found a preferential usage of V_H gene, V4-34, which raises yet another issue, that being whether the CNS promotes expansion of B lymphocytes whose antibody production uses that particular gene segment. Of note, polyomaviruses, herpes viruses (e.g., cytomegalovirus [CMV] and Epstein-Barr virus [EBV], and mycoplasma give rise to increased serum levels of V4-34 encoded antibody; some of these entities are known to persist in the CNS, making them possible candidates as the antigenic stimulus for the malignant lymphocyte.[6,8] Certainly, there is abundant data that EBV is involved in the pathogenesis of PCNSL in the HIV-positive patient, perhaps through EBV-encoded LMP1-induced up-regulation of the antiapoptotic gene BCL-2.[5,9,10] There are, however, equally compelling data that EBV positivity is a rarity in PCNSL occurring in the immunocompetent individual.[5,10,11] Thus it is quite possible that the underlying pathogenesis differs, depending on the immunocompetency of the patient.

Chromosomal alterations and oncogene expression that commonly characterize many of the histologic subtypes of lymphoma have been sought in PCNSL. With respect to immunophenotypic and molecular characteristics, primary CNS, large-cell, B-cell lymphomas, which constitute the vast majority of PCNSL, are quite similar to systemic diffuse, large-cell, B-cell lymphomas.[12] Several studies have shown expression of BCL-6, BCL-2, p53, and C-MYC in PCNSL.[5,11,13] BCL-6 expression (though not mutations involving BCL-6 rearrangement) has been associated with improved overall survival in both systemic as well as primary CNS, diffuse, large-cell lymphomas.[14,15] Braaten and colleagues found that the median survival for patients with BCL-6 positive tumors was 101 months but was 14.7 months for those patients with BCL-6 negative tumors.[15] Furthermore, like its systemic counterpart, there is no evidence of recurring translocations characterizing diffuse, large-cell PCNSL, unlike extracerebral Burkitt's, anaplastic large-cell, follicular, and mantle cell lymphomas, in which t(8;14), t(2;5), t(14;18), and t(11;14) characterize the respective histologic subtypes. Recurring chromosomal abnormalities of number, however, have been found for the diffuse large-cell subtype, whether limited to the CNS or systemic. Using a comparative genomic hybridization technique to identify DNA copy number imbalances in the genome of 22 primary CNS lymphomas, Rickert and colleagues found gains on chromosomes 1, 9, 11, 12, 16, 17, 18, and 22 and losses on chromosomes 6, 18, and 20.[16] However, the loss of 6q was correlated with reduced survival and may be of prognostic relevance. Further, 6q loss has subsequently been shown to have a disproportionately high frequency in PCNSL as opposed to systemic lymphoma.[17] This is of note because of the increased incidence of 6q deletions in testicular lymphoma, a lymphoproliferative disorder of another sanctuary site.[17] Three sites of potential tumor suppressor genes have been identified on 6q and may play a role in the pathogenesis of lymphomas of immunologically privileged sites.[18]

EPIDEMIOLOGY

PCNSL was considered a rare tumor occurring in a few immune-suppressed organ transplant recipients, until the early 1980s when, coinciding with the AIDS epidemic, there was a marked increase in its frequency. The increase in incidence was seen in all age groups but was more evident in men than in women.[19] Although the increase is more pronounced in HIV-infected individuals, there is also a definite, but less dramatic, rise in incidence in the immunocompetent population. Patients without immune suppression are usually older, and the male-to-female ratio is 1.2 to 1.7:1.[19] Most studies corroborate that this change in the incidence of PCNSL is independent of trends in the incidence of brain tumors and in non-Hodgkin's lymphoma (NHL).[20]

Approximately 3% of AIDS patients will develop this tumor, either as the first manifestation of the AIDS diagnosis or during the subsequent course of the illness.[21] A similar percentage of organ transplant recipients develop PCNSL. Epidemiologic studies that exclude data obtained from cancer registries, where AIDS is highly prevalent, and from individuals whose marital status was single, never married, or unknown, support the concept that the incidence of PCNSL has increased in immunocompetent individuals of all ages and both genders. There are several other factors, however, independent of immune suppression that could have resulted in an artificial rise in the incidence of PCNSL. When comparing data before and after the availability of modern imaging studies like computed tomography (CT) scan and magnetic resonance imaging (MRI), there is a threefold increase in PCNSL, whereas no change was noted in the frequency of gliomas. This suggests that improved diagnostic tools alone cannot explain the increase[20] and, therefore, the increased incidence of this neoplasm in the immunocompetent population appears to be real, although still low compared with other brain tumors or NHL.

Recently, the incidence seems to have decreased (or at least plateaued) for all groups except those older than 60 years.[22] In the AIDS population, the leveling has been attributed to the availability of highly active antiretroviral therapy (HAART) and increased awareness of the condition; however, there is no apparent explanation for this phenomenon in the immunocompetent population. Despite being an uncommon tumor, this entity should be considered in the differential diagnosis of any patient presenting with a brain mass, and there should be a heightened awareness in the patient who has an underlying immunodeficiency.

CLINICAL MANIFESTATIONS

The clinical effects of PCNSL are indistinguishable from those associated with other brain tumors, but a thorough medical history and physical examination might provide clues to the diagnosis. In addition to the routine medical history, special care should be taken to elicit information about the possibility of immune suppression, especially secondary to HIV infection. PCNSL usually occurs several years after the diagnosis of HIV infection has been made.[23] Even when the diagnosis of AIDS has been established, these patients present great difficulty in diagnosis because of their increased risk of diverse types of infections. Because PCNSL only occurs in about 3% of all AIDS patients, infections like toxoplasmosis are a more likely diagnosis in this setting.

Approximately 8% of immunocompetent patients will have a history of successful treatment of a non–nervous system malignancy many years before the diagnosis of PCNSL.[24] In these cases, the diagnosis is even more challenging and might be delayed because of the concern of secondary nervous system involvement from the previous malignancy. When the previous malignancy is an NHL, absence of systemic disease on diagnostic workup and comparison of gene rearrangement studies on the biopsy specimens of both lymphomas can demonstrate that they are separate entities. Whether these patients have an increased predisposition to multiple neoplastic processes, or the PCNSL is the result of the antineoplastic treatment for the first tumor, is unknown.[24]

The relative frequency of clinical manifestations of PCNSL does not differ greatly between immunosuppressed and immunocompetent individuals. Nevertheless, there are some differences that might be of clinical relevance when considering the diagnosis (Table 46-1). In immunocompetent patients, the median age at presentation is in the sixth decade of life, whereas the median age for AIDS patients is in the fourth decade of life. Patients with AIDS more often have multiple lesions than do immunocompetent individuals, making the clinical topographic diagnosis difficult, and the latency between the onset of symptoms and diagnosis seems to be shorter.[21]

TABLE 46-1 ▪ Characteristics According to Immune State

	Immunocompetent	Immunocompromised
Mean age	Sixth decade	Fourth decade
Lesions	Single	Multiple
Symptoms	Nonfocal	Focal
Past medical history	Malignancy	Risk factor (HIV infection, transplant)
CSF-EBV PCR	Negative	Positive
Contrast enhancement	Homogenous	Ringlike

The clinical course is usually subacute, with a few months elapsing between the onset of symptoms and the diagnosis of a mass lesion by imaging studies. There are several reports of spontaneous transient remission of symptoms associated with PCNSL.[25] In addition, the clinician has to bear in mind that signs and symptoms associated with PCNSL can rapidly improve with steroids. The most common symptoms associated with PCNSL are focal neurologic deficit, increased intracranial pressure, alteration of mental function, or a combination of these manifestations. At the time of initial presentation, approximately one third will have symptoms of increased intracranial pressure, about 50% will have behavioral changes, and approximately 10% will have seizures.[21] Between 30% and 42% of patients will experience a combination of focal and nonfocal symptoms at the time of diagnosis. Although they can locate anywhere, PCNSL lesions have a predilection for the periventricular region, and therefore alteration in mental function and behavioral changes are prominent symptoms.

The neurologic examination will yield a variety of signs that can be focal or nonlocalizing (e.g., increased intracranial pressure or alteration in the mental function). Hemiparesis and ataxia are the most common focal neurologic signs,[21] but aphasia, acalculia, visual field defects, and cranial nerve palsies are also common.[21] Cranial-spinal nerve palsies and hydrocephalus might be secondary to lymphomatous meningeal infiltration, which is present in up to 42% of all patients with PCNSL.[21]

Visual symptoms might precede or follow the diagnosis of PCNSL and will depend on the ocular structure affected by the tumor. The vitreous, the retina, and the optic nerve/chiasm are the areas most commonly compromised. However, 50% of the patients with PCNSL and ocular involvement detected by slit-lamp examination are asymptomatic.[26] Clinically there is ocular involvement in about 8% to 10% of these patients,[21] but vitreous involvement of the eye occurring prior to and during the course of CNS lymphoma has been noted in up to 25% of patients.[27] In about half of the cases with ocular involvement, visual symptoms can be the first manifestation of PCNSL, preceding neurologic symptoms by several months. Decreased visual acuity or floaters may prompt the patient to seek medical attention, and any nonspecific uveitis refractory to topical or systemic steroids should bring ocular PCNSL to mind.[26]

Rare clinical syndromes that sometimes can be associated with PCNSL include those where the tumor location is restricted to the spinal cord, the leptomeninges, and the hypothalamus. These are especially challenging cases because, in addition to other neoplastic diseases, benign inflammatory entities can have a similar clinical and radiologic presentation. Isolated spinal cord involvement occurs in 1% to 2% of all PCNSL[21] and can be associated with syringomyelia.[28] The level and extent of myelopathic involvement will guide the clinical presentation. Secondary involvement of the spinal cord in patients with cerebral lesions is not a rare occurrence.[29] There have been case reports where the lymphoma is limited to the leptomeninges without evidence of brain, spinal cord, or extraneural tumor. PCNSL presenting as hypothalamic dysfunction causing diabetes insipidus has also been described.[21]

DIAGNOSIS

A definitive diagnosis of PCNSL cannot be made on clinical or imaging grounds, and histologic confirmation is essential. CT scan or MRI will initially establish the presence of a mass lesion with characteristics that, although suggestive of PCNSL, are not specific for this entity (Fig. 46-1). CSF analysis helps in the differential diagnosis and in some cases makes the diagnosis by the demonstration of malignant B lymphocytes.[21] Because immunosuppression is a predisposing factor, HIV testing is required in all patients suspected of having PCNSL. In spite of the information obtained from these studies, tissue diagnosis is required in most circumstances.

Imaging Studies

There are some characteristics on imaging studies that, although not pathognomonic, would strongly suggest that the mass lesion identified might be of lymphomatous origin. In the immunocompetent host a higher level of suspicion is required. Head CT scan shows a hyperdense or isodense mass, solitary in 86% of the cases,[30] that usually exhibits homogenous enhancement after the administration of iodinated contrast as a consequence of local blood-brain barrier disruption.[31] Lesions are usually supratentorial and localized in the deep periventricular areas.[30] Because of their infiltrative nature, the lesions might have indistinct borders and result in minimal surrounding edema or compressive effect (see Fig. 46-1). Occasionally it can appear as

a ring-enhancing lesion with a hypodense, necrotic core, indistinguishable from a high-grade glioma. Lesions can be multiple, suggestive of metastatic disease or infection, but the scarce perilesional edema should raise the suspicion of PCNSL. In about 10% of the cases the lesions are localized in the posterior fossa. On MRI, most of the lesions are hypointense or isointense on T1-weighted images, and only about 40% are hyperintense on T2-weighted images.[31] Nearly all the lesions enhance after the administration of gadolinium except in cases when the study follows the administration of steroids. The appearance of PCNSL is of such heterogeneity that it should be considered in the differential diagnosis of any mass lesions detected on imaging studies (Fig. 46-2).

PCNSL in the immunocompromised patient may have a more variable appearance on imaging studies.[32] The increased incidence of infection is another difficulty in this population, where infection is more likely to be responsible for a mass or enhancing lesion on imaging studies than PCNSL. No specific pattern has been established that can be used to distinguish between CNS lymphoma, toxoplasmosis, or other CNS diseases that occur in patients with AIDS.[21] Unlike immunocompetent patients, AIDS-associated PCNSL has been reported to present with multiple lesions in 71% to 80% of cases, to show ringlike enhancement in 50% of cases, and to lack enhancement in about 10% to 27% of the lesions.[32] Spontaneous hemorrhage, a nonenhancing lesion, or diffuse white matter changes do not exclude lymphoma in an immunocompromised patient.[32]

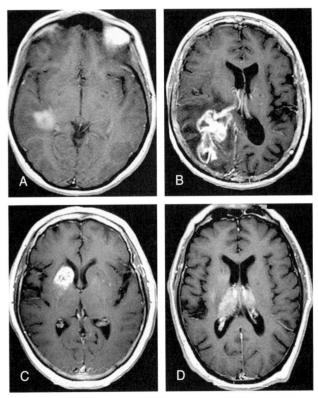

FIGURE 46-2 T1-enhanced MRI of entities mimicking PCNSL on imaging studies: (*A*) multiple sclerosis, (*B*) toxoplasmosis in a patient with a history of renal transplant, (*C*) stroke, and (*D*) arteriovenous malformation.

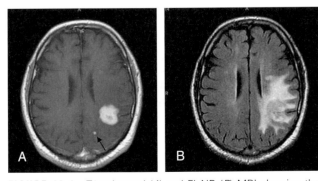

FIGURE 46-1 T1-enhanced (*A*) and FLAIR (*B*) MRI showing the infiltrative character of PCNSL. *Arrow* shows small satellite area of enhancement that on the FLAIR seems to be connected to the larger lesion.

Diverse techniques have been considered in an attempt to improve the specificity of the diagnosis of PCNSL by imaging studies. Magnetic resonance spectroscopy (MRS) has been proposed as a useful modality to differentiate PCNSL from solid astrocytomas. PCNSL may have massively elevated lipid resonances that may also be present in glioblastoma, but in combination with a markedly elevated choline/creatine ratio, MRS provides metabolic information that may improve the preoperative differentiation of PCNSL and glioma.[33]

Nuclear medicine has also been suggested as a possible method to discriminate between PCNSL and other types of malignant as well as nonmalignant pathologies without resorting to histologic diagnosis. In one study, 10 patients with PCNSL, 14 with malignant gliomas, and 7 with meningioma underwent N-isopropyl-p-(^{123}I)-iodoamphetamine (^{123}I-IMP) single photon emission computerized tomography (SPECT). The ^{123}I-IMP retention uptake in delayed (6 hours) to extradelayed (24 hours) SPECT images was significantly higher in PCNSL than in those of both malignant gliomas and meningioma.[34] In patients with AIDS, the Thallium[201]-SPECT delayed retention index may be useful to discriminate PCNSL from infectious lesions with high sensitivity and specificity.[35] The diagnostic utility of these techniques has yet to be determined in larger series, and histologic confirmation is still considered the gold standard for diagnosis of PCNSL.

Tumor infiltration of the nervous system can be more diffuse than is appreciated on imaging studies. Correlation of autopsy and MRI findings in 10 patients who died with PCNSL showed that all had tumor infiltration in CNS regions that were normal radiographically, including T2 sequences.[36] Therefore, the infiltrative microscopic tumor burden of PCNSL renders futile any attempt to resect these lesions. The surgical role is restricted to a tissue biopsy for histologic diagnosis.

On rare occasions when the intra-axial spinal cord is the only location of PCNSL, the diagnosis is even more challenging. MRI might be initially normal or reveal diffuse T2 abnormality with patchy areas of enhancement. In some cases, syringomyelia is present in association with the neoplastic mass.

Tissue Diagnosis and Staging

As noted previously, the diagnosis of PCNSL is usually suggested by the appearance of a focal lesion on CT or MRI; confirmation of the diagnosis of PCNSL in the immunocompetent requires tissue to definitively differentiate PCNSL from metastatic disease, glioma, sarcoidosis, and inflammatory lesions. Because the CSF is involved at diagnosis 20% of the time, a brain biopsy can be avoided if malignant cells can be obtained from the CSF.[37] Similarly, malignant (though often asymptomatic) uveitis is apparent in 10% to 20% of patients with PCNSL at presentation and may serve as the source of cells on which the diagnosis may be based.[38,39] Cytologic examination of cells, as the sole parameter by which the diagnosis is made, is not optimal because it cannot determine monoclonality, a condition that is necessary though not sufficient for the diagnosis of lymphoma. In the case of B-cell lymphoma, monoclonality can be determined by flow cytometric detection of light-chain

restriction if there are sufficient cells available. In T-cell disease, and when there are inadequate numbers of malignant B cells for flow cytometry, the diagnosis can be established by polymerase chain reaction (PCR) studies on the basis of T-cell receptor or immunoglobulin rearrangement, respectively. This technique is susceptible to false positives if there are too few cells present, and to false negatives if the DNA is highly degraded. In one recent multicenter study,[40] CSF was examined from 76 immunocompetent patients with PCNSL by a nested complementary determining region (CDR) III PCR technique to detect immunoglobulin rearrangement in conjunction with cytologic examination. DNA could be obtained from 52 patients, and monoclonality was detected by PCR in 8 of them, which is within the range of the published incidence. However, in 10 patients, the PCR result did not correlate with the CSF cytologic examination.[40] It is important to underscore the fact that most lymphomas, including PCNSL, are quite sensitive to steroids. Cell death and tumor regression may occur as early as 24 hours after initiation of therapy. If tissue or a specimen for cytology is obtained following initiation of steroids, the result may be nondiagnostic because of cell death and tissue necrosis. Unless the patient is showing evidence of rapid neurologic deterioration or impending herniation, tissue should be obtained prior to starting any steroid therapy.[41,42]

Once the diagnosis is made, patients generally undergo staging to determine the extent of involvement. PCNSL usually presents as a single or sometimes multifocal process in the brain, but it can also involve other nervous system compartments including the meninges, eye, and the spinal cord.[29,37] Because systemic involvement tends to occur more commonly at relapse, and because evidence of systemic disease is found in less than 5% at diagnosis, the necessity for a full lymphoma staging has been called into question.[43] There is general agreement that, besides a complete history and physical, a CBC, standard chemistries with an LDH, HIV status, chest x-ray, CSF examination, and slit-lamp examination are absolutely required. A full staging would include imaging with CT of the chest, abdomen, and pelvis, as well as bilateral bone marrow biopsies; this is usually required for any patient enrolled in a study.

The approach to a focal brain lesion in the HIV population is slightly different. The detection of Epstein-Barr virus DNA (EBV-DNA) by PCR in the CSF is a sensitive (80% to 84%) and highly specific (100%) diagnostic marker of AIDS-related PCNSL, and it has a positive predictive value of 100%.[44,45] Therefore, a CSF sample positive for malignant lymphoma cells or EBV-DNA obviates the need for further tissue. The recommended algorithm for the workup of a focal brain lesion with nondiagnostic CSF starts with presumptive antitoxoplasmosis therapy and proceeds to brain biopsy if there is no response after a full course of treatment for toxoplasmosis[23] (Fig. 46-3). In one recent study of focal brain lesions in AIDS patients, a diagnosis was successfully established on the biopsy specimen in 88%; but the morbidity and mortality of the procedure was 8.4% and 2.9%, respectively.[46] As expected, *Toxoplasmosis gondii*, PCNSL, and progressive multifocal leukoencephalopathy accounted for the vast majority of diagnoses in this population. A disconcerting retrospective study of 2500 HIV-positive patients identified 38 with the presumed or confirmed diagnosis of PCNSL between 1986 and 1998. Twenty-six patients were

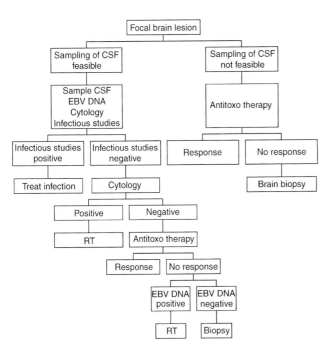

FIGURE 46-3 Algorithm for the management of HIV-infected individuals with focal brain lesions. CSF, cerebrospinal fluid; antitoxo, antitoxoplasmosis; RT, radiotherapy. (From Sparano JA: Clinical aspects and management of AIDS-related lymphoma. Eur J Cancer 37(10):1296–1305, 2001, Figure 1, page 1299.)

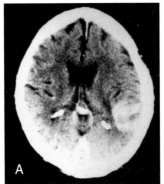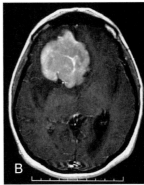

FIGURE 46-4 *A,* Head CT scan with contrast demonstrating left temporal-parietal enhancing mass. Biopsy revealed PCNSL. *B,* T1-enhanced MRI showing a right frontal PCNSL. The lesion was dural-based, infiltrating brain parenchyma, and malignant meningioma was considered in the differential diagnosis before surgery.

presumed to have PCNSL following the failure of antitoxoplasmosis therapy, and 12 had the diagnosis confirmed with tissue or CSF. Sixteen patients received therapy for PCNSL; 10 of these patients were from the 26 with presumed disease, and 6 were from the biopsy-confirmed cohort. The overall survival for the entire group was 1.2 months with no difference in survival between the presumptive and confirmed group.[47] Bower and colleagues conclude that there may be little benefit in subjecting the patient to the diagnostic procedure when the outcome is so dismal. The use of HAART and its impact on the CD4 count has allowed the use of more aggressive chemotherapeutic regimens without undue toxicity, and resulted in improved life expectancy for these patients. These changes will undoubtedly influence the algorithm, and they suggest that earlier diagnostic procedures may be in order for this patient population.

Differential Diagnosis

Clinically, PCNSL may present with a variety of signs and symptoms and has a capacity to mimic many other neurologic conditions.[48] PCNSL can be confused with multiple sclerosis (MS) in patients who present with neurologic dysfunction, a nonenhancing periventricular lesion, and CSF pleocytosis. Administration of corticosteroid causes clinical improvement and regression of PCNSL in some patients; this may be interpreted as a steroid-induced remission from an exacerbation of MS. Sustained clinical dependence on corticosteroid is unusual in MS, and should lead to consideration of PCNSL. Repeat CSF examination and gadolinium-enhanced MRI scan obtained off corticosteroid should differentiate between the two diagnostic possibilities.[49] PCNSL cortical lesions may be difficult to distinguish from

extra-axial masses such as meningioma on imaging studies (Fig. 46-4). In the case of immunocompromised individuals, infections such as *Toxoplasma gondii* should always be included in the differential diagnosis (Table 46-2).

TREATMENT

In spite of its infiltrative nature, PCNSL is one of the few brain tumors in which a durable remission can be achieved with appropriate treatment. Unfortunately, this sometimes is at the expense of significant treatment-related toxicity. Because PCNSL is rare, and because the disease behaves in an aggressive manner (with a life expectancy of less than 5 months if left untreated), the design of and accrual to large clinical trials has been limited. These hindrances to progress not withstanding, there are now several interventions with varying toxicities available that can result in an increased disease-free period as well as overall survival. An interdisciplinary, multimodality therapeutic strategy can, therefore, be designed to accommodate specific patient characteristics such as age, comorbid conditions, and immune status.

Steroids

Steroids induce apoptosis of lymphoid cells and can result in complete disappearance of the clinical and imaging

---

TABLE 46-2 ▪ Differential Diagnosis of PCNSL

Differential Diagnosis	
Disease	**Diagnostic Studies**
Multiple sclerosis	Past medical history-CSF
High grade glioma	SPECT-MRS
Infection	HIV infection-CSF
Sarcoidosis	ACE level, calcium
Meningioma	MRS
Vascular	Cerebral angiogram-MRI DWI

CSF, cerebrospinal fluid; MRS, magnetic resonance spectroscopy; HIV, human immunodeficiency virus; ACE, angiotensin-converting enzyme; SPECT, single photon emission computerized tomography; DWI, diffusion-weighted images.

manifestations associated with PCNSL.[50] Although decrease in edema plays a role, most of the rapid and dramatic responsiveness to glucocorticoids is mediated by their cytotoxic activity. Because of the exquisite sensitivity of lymphoma cells to steroids, their administration to the patient with PCNSL carries important diagnostic and therapeutic implications.

Steroids given before a biopsy is performed may preclude the correct pathologic diagnosis from the specimen obtained, mandating that steroids be withheld until the biopsy has been performed when PCNSL is considered in the differential diagnosis. Further, there can be a complete response after steroids in about 15% of the cases, resulting in the complete disappearance of the target for the biopsy.[50] A dramatic clinical and MRI improvement would make the diagnosis of PCNSL very likely, although as previously mentioned there are other entities (e.g., multiple sclerosis and sarcoidosis) that exhibit similar steroid-responsiveness.

In 40% of patients, a rapid and dramatic regression of PCNSL follows the administration of steroids.[51] There are several reports of complete long-term responses of the disease following only steroid therapy, but eventually the disease will recur either at the same or a remote site within the nervous system. It is likely, however, that some tumors develop glucocorticoid resistance, because the second response is often shorter or even absent. The use of steroids as monotherapy for PCNSL, therefore, is not recommended though they are usually used in combination with chemotherapy as part of the therapeutic regimen. In a study to determine the feasibility and efficacy of single-agent high-dose methotrexate therapy without concomitant radiotherapy, the application of corticosteroids during the first methotrexate course was associated with a higher rate of complete responses.[52]

The possible benefit has to be weighed against the multiple serious side effects associated with long-term use of steroids. Steroids are known immune suppressants that, in combination with chemotherapy or in patients already immunocompromised, may lead to opportunistic infections such as *Pneumocystis carinii* pneumonia (PCP), listeriosis, and fungal infections. PCP prophylaxis is routinely used while patients are on steroids and chemotherapy.

Surgery

PCNSL is an infiltrative tumor, usually localized in the deep periventricular regions, and is highly responsive to radiation and chemotherapy. Therefore, surgical resection is of limited benefit and can carry significant morbidity. In a retrospective study including 248 immunocompetent patients with PCNSL, 132 underwent stereotactic biopsy for diagnosis of PCNSL, resulting in a procedure-related morbidity of 3.7% and no mortality. The remainder 116 underwent surgical resection (because imaging studies were not suggestive of lymphoma) with a mortality rate of 3.4%. Multivariate analysis revealed that surgical resection was an unfavorable prognostic factor[30] and may increase functional deficit.[21] When there is the suspicion of PCNSL, the role of surgery is restricted to a stereotactic biopsy to provide tissue for diagnostic purposes. As previously mentioned, when PCNSL is suspected, steroids should be avoided before the biopsy to increase the diagnostic yield of the procedure.

In AIDS patients, a diagnostic stereotactic biopsy may be avoided using thallium-201 (201Tl) SPECT combined with EBV-DNA in CSF. The diagnosis of PCNSL is extremely likely in patients with hyperactive lesions and positive EBV-DNA. If the lesion is hypoactive on SPECT, with negative CSF EBV-DNA, the recommendation is empiric antitoxoplasma therapy. If there is disagreement between the SPECT and CSF PCR results, a brain biopsy is advisable.[45]

Despite common contiguity with the ventricular system, only 7% of the patients have hydrocephalus requiring shunting.[30] When leptomeningeal lymphomatous spread is documented, intraventricular chemotherapy is often recommended. An intraventricular catheter with a subgaleal reservoir for ease of administration is usually placed. Before therapeutic use of the reservoir, a nuclear medicine flow study is performed to ensure correct catheter placement as well as good distribution of the chemotherapy agent.

Reservoirs have been associated with complications necessitating removal of the device. Infection is the most common complication, occurring in about 15% of patients with PCNSL. A rare complication is the development of a porencephalic cyst around the catheter that improves after the catheter is surgically removed (Fig. 46-5).

Radiation Therapy

Radiotherapy was the first intervention to have a significant impact on PCNSL survival, with an increased median survival of 12 to 18 months.[30,42,53] Systemic lymphomas are considered to be extremely radiosensitive. This is equally true of PCNSL, as was exemplified in a Radiation Therapy Oncology Group study using 40 Gy to the whole brain and a 20-Gy boost to the lesion(s) with a 2-cm margin. An 83%

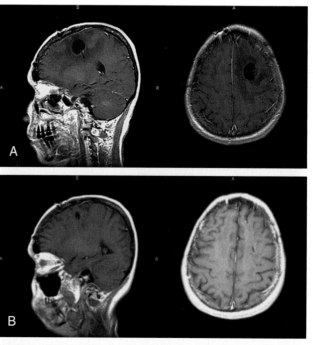

FIGURE 46-5 T1-enhanced sagittal and axial MRI of a patient with PCNSL who developed a porencephalic cyst surrounding a reservoir catheter (*A*) and that decreased in size after removal of the device (*B*).

complete remission rate was obtained in this study, but unfortunately the remissions were not durable; the median survival from the start of radiation therapy was only 11.6 months. Because the disease is multifocal, the target for treatment is the whole brain, and the benefit obtained from using a boost is questionable. For the same reason, although there are some case reports to the contrary, radiosurgery is not considered a suitable alternative. Finally, unlike other tumors, there is no classic dose response curve for radiation in PCNSL, but there does appear to be a threshold dose of 50 Gy. A review of the literature, including patients receiving only radiation therapy (RT), found a 42.3% 5-year survival for 54 patients receiving greater than 50 Gy, as compared with a 12.8% 5-year survival for 154 patients receiving less than 50 Gy.[53]

Because of the potential for neurotoxicity, especially in the elderly and in long-term survivors, deferred RT or the use of low-dose RT consolidation after chemotherapy has been considered in several small, noncontrolled clinical trials. Deferring RT even when a complete response has been achieved with chemotherapy may result in a higher recurrence rate.[51] Reduced-dose RT (40 to 45 Gy) in patients younger than 60 years who achieve a complete response with aggressive chemotherapy may decrease the occurrence of severe cognitive impairment, but the cost is an extremely high incidence of chemotherapy-related toxicity and lower response rates.[54] For patients who are 60 years or older, radiotherapy is often eliminated or deferred because of the high risk of severe cognitive impairment and neurotoxicity-related mortality.

Methotrexate-Based Chemotherapy

At present, the use of combined modality chemoradiation therapy is generally considered to yield improved outcomes over radiation therapy alone, although this consensus has not been confirmed by a randomized controlled trial[51] (Fig. 46-6). A large retrospective study of 226 patients was undertaken by Blay and colleagues[55] to identify treatment modalities associated with improved outcome, including prolonged remission duration as well as decreased late toxicity. As expected, extent of surgical resection did not influence survival. In univariate analysis, the use of chemotherapy in addition to radiation therapy, and the use of either high-dose methotrexate or high-dose cytarabine was associated with improved survival. These two chemotherapeutic agents are commonly used in lymphoma therapy and have excellent penetration into the CNS, even in the presence of an intact blood-brain barrier. However, only treatment regimens including high-dose methotrexate (defined as more than 1.5 gm/m² per cycle), remained an independent, favorable prognostic factor after adjustment for age, performance status, CSF protein, and the patient's International Prognostic Index score.[55] Equally important, Blay studied the incidence of late neurotoxicity, evaluating 208 patients by clinical symptomatology and imaging studies. The projected incidence at 1 year, 2 years, and at just under 6 years was 4%, 8%, and 26%, respectively. In this study, neither age nor treatment with chemotherapy, regardless of route (e.g., intrathecal versus intravenous) or agent, correlated with increased neurotoxicity by either univariate or multivariate analysis. The sequence of radiation followed by

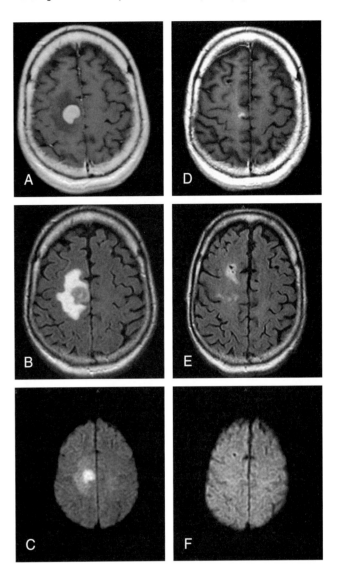

FIGURE 46-6 T1-enhanced (A), FLAIR (B), and DWI (C) MRI of patient with PCNSL at the time of diagnosis (A, B, C) and after five cycles of chemotherapy (D, E, F).

chemotherapy, as opposed to the reverse, was found by both univariate and multivariate analysis to increase the risk of late neurotoxicity, whereas the total dose of radiation (greater than 50 Gy) was associated with an increased risk of neurotoxicity by univariate analysis alone.[55] Multiple studies have confirmed these findings over the past decade, with median survivals ranging from 33 months to 60 months when a high-dose methotrexate regimen was used with or without subsequent WBRT (Table 46-3).[56–66]

A single study devoted to PCNSL in the elderly, using single-agent, high-dose methotrexate without radiation therapy, revealed that response rates and durability of remission remain lower in the elderly than in younger patients with PCNSL. The relatively low dose of methotrexate (1 gm/M²) used in this study may have contributed to both the low complete response (CR) rate of 42% and the short overall survival of 14.3 months.[61] Nevertheless, DeAngelis has also found that patients older than 60 years enjoy a significantly shortened overall (11.1 months versus 38.8 months) and progression-free (21.8 months versus 50.4 months) survival when compared

TABLE 46-3 ▪ Results of Recent Clinical Trials for PCNSL

Study	Number	WBRT	Therapy	Response	OS	Delayed Neurotoxicity	TTF Median
Sandor et al (1998)[65]	14	No	MTX 8.4 g/M²	79% CR 21% PR	57 months 68.8%	2/7 severe impairment	16.5 months
Guha-Thakurta et al (1999)[64]	31	No	MTX 8 g/M²	65% CR 35% PR	All pts: 2 yr 63% CR pts: 2 yr 90% 3 yr 72%	No leukoencephalopathy	14.3 months
Abrey et al (2000) Pilot data[57]	52	34: 45 Gy 22: No	MTX 3.5 g/M² IT MTX	87% CR 7% PR 94% ORR	Median 60 months	All pts 13/52 10/12 >60 yr with XRT 1/22 >60 yr no XRT	
O'Brien et al (2000)[56]	46	Yes 45 Gy with 5.4 Gy boost	MTX 1 g/M² IT MTX if +CSF	32% CR 13% PR 45% ORR	2 yr 62% Median 33 months	6/44 dementia median 16 months	17 months
Schlegel et al (2001)[59]	20	No	Bonn therapy MTX 5 g/M² IT MTX	55% CR 5% CR 70% ORR	Median 54 months 10% PR	1/20 showed cognitive impairment median	20.5 months 21 months
Bessell et al (2002)[60]	57	Yes Reg I: 45 Gy Reg II: 30.6 Gy	MTX 1.5 g/M²	I 64% CR I 13% PR 77% ORR II 62% CR II 8% PR 70% ORR	All pts: 3 yr 55% 5 yr 36% Median 40 months	30 Gy 0/13 45 Gy 7/22	
DeAngelis et al (2002)[58]	102	Yes 45 Gy	MTX 2.5 g/M² IT MTX	58% CR 36% PR 94% ORR	<60 50.4 months >60 21.8 months	12/82 neurotoxicity median 16 months	24 months
Batchelor et al (2003)[62]	25	No	MTX 8 g/M²	52% CR 22% PR 74% ORR	Median not reached 22.8+ months		12.8 months
Hoang-Xuan et al (2003)[61]	50 all >60 yr	No	MTX 1 g/M² IT MTX	42% CR 6% PR 48% ORR	1 yr 52% Median 14.3 months	7% pts with CR >2 yr	10.6 months
Pels et al (2003)[66]	65	No	MTX 5 g/M² IT MTX	61% CR 10% PR	<60: median OS not reached 2 yr 80% >60: median 34 months 2 yr 59%	3% severe cognitive dysfunction	<60: median not reached, 26 months f/u >60: 15 months
Poortmans et al (2003)[63]	52	Yes 39-40 Gy	MTX 3 g/M² IT MTX	69% CR 12% PR 81% ORR	2 yr 69% 4 yr 58% Median 46 months		

CSF, cerebrospinal fluid; MTX, methotrexate; WBRT, whole brain radiation therapy; Gy, gray; CR, complete response; PR, partial response; ORR, overall response rate; OS, overall survival; IT, intrathecal; TTF, time to treatment failure.

with younger patients in her treatment regimen, which included higher doses of methotrexate as well as high-dose cytarabine.[58]

The questions of optimal chemotherapeutic combination and the role of postchemotherapeutic radiation remain unanswered. Both of these issues turn on the balance of increased toxicity (both acute and delayed) versus increased remission durability. High-dose methotrexate and high-dose cytarabine carry extensive toxicity profiles that include significant bone marrow suppression, orointestinal mucositis, dermatitis, and neurotoxicity. For both drugs, the extent and severity of toxicity depends on rapid and reliable renal excretion and, in the case of methotrexate, restoration of the intracellular stores of reduced folate in normal cells by the administration of leucovorin (5-formyl-tetradyrofolic acid). Thus aggressive hydration, alkalinization of the urine, initiation of leucovorin rescue within 24 to 48 hours following the methotrexate infusion, and close monitoring of renal function and methotrexate level are imperative when giving methotrexate. Infection caused by marrow

suppression will remain a significant problem, particularly as more aggressive chemotherapeutic regimens are used. Counts must be monitored closely and broad-spectrum antibiotics administered prospectively in the event that the patient develops a neutropenic fever. The addition of steroids to high-dose methotrexate renders these patients increasingly susceptible to opportunistic infections, specifically PCP. Current recommendations include the use of PCP prophylaxis in patients undergoing therapy for PCNSL.

Intrathecal Therapy

High-dose methotrexate, which penetrates an intact blood-brain barrier and results in therapeutic levels of drug in the CSF, has brought into question the routine use of intrathecal (IT) therapy for patients with PCNSL. There has been no prospective study performed to determine if IT methotrexate improves the outcome when used in conjunction with systemic high-dose methotrexate in patients with PCNSL, regardless of CSF involvement at diagnosis.

A case-controlled retrospective study has been done, however, in which all patients received the same high-dose methotrexate and high-dose cytarabine systemic chemotherapy.[67] Patients were matched for age, performance status, CSF cytology, and use of WBRT in a two-to-one ratio IT-MTX: no IT-MTX. There was no significant difference in overall survival, in event-free survival, in CSF relapse, or in delayed neurotoxicity between the two groups.[67] There is, therefore, a growing consensus that outside of a clinical trial, IT therapy is used only in the setting of a positive CSF cytology, if at all, in up-front treatment. In addition, it is used at relapse or if leptomeningeal disease persists after initiation of systemic high-dose methotrexate therapy.[67,68] Should IT therapy be required, methotrexate, cytarabine, and hydrocortisone have all been used singly or in combination. A sustained released, liposomal form of cytarabine is available that can be administered on an every 2-week basis, as opposed to the more common twice-weekly injections when the standard drug formulations are used. This has been shown to improve the response rate but not the time to neurologic progression or survival in an open-label, randomized trial comparing liposomal cytarabine to free cytarabine in patients with lymphomatous meningitis.[69]

Other Therapeutic Options

Although improvements in the overall and progression-free survival rates have been made in patients with PCNSL, durable remissions and cure rates are distinctly lower in diffuse large-cell lymphoma of the CNS than in systemic diffuse large-cell, B-cell NHL. This is, in part, because of the difficulty in obtaining adequate drug levels when given systemically across an intact blood-brain barrier. The chemotherapeutic regimens for systemic diffuse large-cell lymphoma that result in durable remissions generally contain an alkylator, an anthracycline, a vinca alkaloid, and a steroid. Of these agents, only the alkylator class has been shown to penetrate the CNS. Within this class, penetration varies from drug to drug (Box 46-1).

In a recent review of strategies to increase the uptake of drugs given intravenously, Siegel and Zylber-Katz list the use of a lipid-soluble prodrug (i.e., temozolomide), increased plasma concentrations, intra-arterial drug injection, and osmotic disruption of the blood-brain barrier. Intra-arterial delivery and osmotic disruption of the blood-brain barrier

| BOX 46-1 | *Systemic Antineoplastic Agents Used in Lymphoma Therapy That Penetrate the BBB* |

Methotrexate
Cytosine arabinoside
Procarbazine
BCNU
CCNU
Tiotepa
Temozolomide
Mercaptopurine (low concentrations)
Melphalan (low concentrations)
Cyclophosphamide (low concentrations)

have been used, though these are invasive techniques with significant toxicity.[70] High-dose IV therapy, which results in better penetration, is limited by systemic toxicity. However, if the dose-limiting toxicity of the agents is bone marrow suppression or ablation, stem cell rescue can be used to overcome that particular toxicity. Indeed, it has been found that patients with systemic, diffuse, large-cell NHL, relapsing after standard chemotherapy, or patients presenting with poor prognosis, high-risk disease can still be cured using high chemotherapy with hematopoietic stem cell rescue.[71,72] Applying the lessons learned from systemic disease, high-dose chemotherapy with hematopoietic stem cell rescue is now being tried in young PCNSL patients who have particularly poor prognostic indicators or relapsed/refractory disease.[73-75] Soussain and colleagues have reported a 3-year overall and event-free survival probability of 63.7% and 53%, respectively, for 22 relapsed or refractory patients who underwent high-dose chemotherapy with stem cell rescue.[74]

In patients who are older, have significant comorbid disease, refuse to undergo toxic therapy, or have become resistant to first line therapies, options are somewhat limited. Early reports and case studies using the immunotherapeutic rituximab (which is directed against the CD20 antigen found on most mature B cells) are now appearing in the literature.[76] Temozolomide, an oral alkylating agent with excellent CNS penetration and a modest toxicity profile, has produced complete remissions in two patients reported by Herrlinger and another elderly patient reported by Lerro.[77,78] More standard chemotherapeutic regimens have resulted in good response in patients who have failed high-dose methotrexate regimens; these include the use of PCV (procarbazine, CCNU, and vincristine), which contains two agents known to cross the blood-brain barrier well.[79,80]

Therapy for Intraocular Lymphoma

The therapy for intraocular lymphoma, whether it occurs in isolation or in the presence of other CNS lesions, deserves separate mention. In a recent review by Ferreri, neither involved field irradiation nor chemotherapy (including agents with good CNS penetration) alone resulted in durable remissions in the eye. The addition of orbital radiation to a high-dose, methotrexate-based regimen has been associated with both a higher response rate and decreased intraocular relapse rate. Radiation of both orbits is recommended, because bilateral eye involvement occurs in close to 80% of cases.[26] This carries with it substantial ocular morbidity, including radiation retinitis, dry eye syndrome with corneal erosions, glaucoma, and cataracts. Intravitreal methotrexate, given in a dose of 400 micrograms on a once- or twice-weekly basis, has been used with success.[81,82] In one case report, serial vitreous sampling allowed pharmacokinetic studies to be performed, and a first-order kinetic rate of elimination was observed. Presuming 1 micromol/liter is tumoricidal, the 400-microgram dose would remain effective for 5 days.[81] The optimal therapy for PCNSL with intraocular involvement remains to be defined. At present, combined chemotherapy followed by ocular irradiation appears to give the best results. Identification of chemotherapeutic agents that penetrate the vitreous humor well when given systemically, or infusion of chemotherapeutic agents directly into the vitreous humor may provide another option without invoking the toxicity associated with ocular irradiation, although this possibility will require further study.

Treatment for AIDS-Related PCNSL

Treatment of AIDS-related lymphomas in general has been discouraging until the recent advent of HAART. Full-dose chemotherapy in the immunocompromised host results in an unacceptable morbidity and mortality, whereas dose reduction results in inadequate therapy, with tumor progression and drug resistance. Standard therapy had been palliative, using corticosteroids and WBRT, with only 10% of patients surviving more than 1 year. As expected, CHOP (cyclophosphamide, hydroxyl daunorubicin, oncovin, prednisone)–like regimens, which contain agents incapable of adequately penetrating an intact blood-brain barrier, have not improved median survivals.[23] Combination radio-chemotherapy has been given to patients with AIDS-related PCNSL using a PCV regimen. Although numbers are small, this appears to increase the survival from a median of 4 months with radiation alone to 13 months.[83] The benefit of combined modality therapy over radiotherapy has been confirmed in other studies.[47] The decision to treat with combined modality, as opposed to radiation alone, should be based on the patient's performance status, extent of disease, comorbid conditions, projected prognosis, and the patient's desire for aggressive therapy.[83] Because AIDS-related PCNSLs are essentially 100% EBV driven, interventions targeting the virus have been considered; this includes the use of hydroxyurea, which at a low dose can deplete deoxyribonucleotide reserves, exerting an antiviral effect.[84] As with systemic AIDS-related lymphomas, the hope for both decreased incidence and improved survival in AIDS-related PCNSL resides in restoration of the immune system through HAART. To date there are only case reports of regression of PCNSL following initiation of HAART and improvement in the CD4+ cell count.[85] Further study will be needed to establish a causal link between disease remission and restoration of immunocompetency.

PROGNOSIS

At present, regardless of immunocompetency, the primary cause of death for patients with PCNSL is their disease. For the patient with AIDS-related PCNSL, until immunocompetency can be restored, the prognosis will remain grim. The best survival results obtained with current therapeutic strategies are no more than 1 year. In the immunocompetent population, if PCNSL is untreated, the median survival is less than 5 months. Treated with radiation alone, median survival is approximately 1 year. However, median survival has improved dramatically as combination modality therapies have been introduced, and median survivals of 2 to 5 years are routinely being reported using high-dose methotrexate regimens. Given that systemic, diffuse, large-cell lymphoma is a curable disease in a significant percentage of patients, there is no theoretical reason why some patients with PCNSL of the diffuse, large-cell subtype cannot be cured. The features unique to the CNS, however, need to be incorporated into the lessons learned about the treatment of systemic aggressive lymphomas.

As oncologists have learned from the International Prognostic Index developed for systemic, diffuse large-cell lymphoma,[86] the ability to determine which patients will likely do well would be of great benefit and aid in the ability to tailor therapy to the patient. There is general agreement that age and performance status are the most important predictors of outcome.[58,61,87] In a multicenter retrospective study of 378 immunocompetent patients, Ferreri and colleagues have attempted to identify other factors that may predict response. Besides age and performance status, serum LDH, CSF protein concentration, and involvement of the deep structures of the brain were independent predictors of survival. Survival curves, generated according to a prognostic score based on these five parameters, reveal a significant survival difference between groups having 0 or 1, 2 or 3, and 4 or 5 unfavorable features, with a 2-year overall survival (OS) of 80%, 48%, and 15%, respectively.[88] Survival, of course, is not the only end point worthy of measure, and chronic toxicity to the CNS, resulting in an unacceptable quality of life, must be factored into the equation. In a recent update of a German PCNSL study using a high-dose methotrexate- and cytarabine-based regimen without radiotherapy, neither a median overall survival nor a time-to-treatment failure has been reached, with an estimated 5-year survival of 75% in patients younger than 60 years.[66] In this younger population, there appears to be a plateau in the survival curve after 30 months without further relapses, suggesting the possibility of cure. As expected, those older than 60 years experienced a shorter OS and time to treatment failure (34 months and 15 months, respectively). Most impressive, however, is the fact that of the 61 patients, only 2 patients (3%) manifested severe cognitive dysfunction.[66] Although the optimal therapy for PCNSL has not yet been determined, it does appear that PCNSL may, like its systemic counterpart, be a potentially curable malignancy. Current therapies hold out the hope that the price of cure will not include unacceptable cognitive dysfunction.

REFERENCES

1. Harder A, Dudel C, Anagnostopoulos I, et al: Molecular genetic diagnosis of a primary central nervous system T cell lymphoma. Acta Neuropathol (Berl) 105:65–68, 2003.
2. Schlegel U, Schmidt-Wolf IG, Deckert M: Primary CNS lymphoma: Clinical presentation, pathological classification, molecular pathogenesis and treatment. J Neurologic Sci 181:1–12, 2000.
3. Paulus W: Classification, pathogenesis and molecular pathology of primary CNS lymphomas. J Neurooncol 43:203–208, 1999.
4. MacLennan IC: Germinal centers. Annu Rev Immunol 12:117–139, 1994.
5. Larocca LM, Capello D, Rinelli A, et al: The molecular and phenotypic profile of primary central nervous system lymphoma identifies distinct categories of the disease and is consistent with histogenetic derivation from germinal center-related B cells. Blood 92:1011–1019, 1998.
6. Thompsett AR, Ellison DW, Stevenson FK, et al: V(H) gene sequences from primary central nervous system lymphomas indicate derivation from highly mutated germinal center B cells with ongoing mutational activity. Blood 94:1738–1746, 1999.
7. Knopf PM, Harling-Berg CJ, Cserr HF, et al: Antigen-dependent intrathecal antibody synthesis in the normal rat brain: Tissue entry and local retention of antigen-specific B cells. J Immunol 161:692–701, 1998.
8. Montesinos-Rongen M, Kuppers R, Schluter D, et al: Primary central nervous system lymphomas are derived from germinal-center B cells and show a preferential usage of the V4-34 gene segment. Am J Pathol 155:2077–2086, 1999.
9. Camilleri-Broet S, Davi F, Feuillard J, et al: High expression of latent membrane protein 1 of Epstein-Barr virus and BCL-2 oncoprotein in acquired immunodeficiency syndrome-related primary brain lymphomas. Blood 86:432–435, 1995.

10. Anthony IC, Crawford DH, Bell JE: B lymphocytes in the normal brain: Contrasts with HIV-associated lymphoid infiltrates and lymphomas. Brain 126:1058–1067, 2003.

11. Krogh-Jensen M, Johansen P, D'Amore F: Primary central nervous system lymphomas in immunocompetent individuals: Histology, Epstein-Barr virus genome, Ki-67 proliferation index, p53 and bcl-2 gene expression. Leuk Lymphoma 30:131–142, 1998.

12. Camilleri-Broet S, Martin A, Moreau A, et al: Primary central nervous system lymphomas in 72 immunocompetent patients: Pathologic findings and clinical correlations. Groupe Ouest Est d'etude des Leucenies et Autres Maladies du Sang (GOELAMS). Am J Clin Pathol 110:607–612, 1998.

13. Korfel A, Finke J, Schmidt-Wolf I, et al: Report on workshop: Primary CNS lymphoma. Ann Hematol 80:B20–B23, 2001.

14. Lossos IS, Jones CD, Warnke R, et al: Expression of a single gene, BCL-6, strongly predicts survival in patients with diffuse large B-cell lymphoma. Blood 98:945–951, 2001.

15. Braaten KM, Betensky RA, de Leval L, et al: BCL-6 expression predicts improved survival in patients with primary central nervous system lymphoma. Clin Cancer Res 9:1063–1069, 2003.

16. Rickert CH, Dockhorn-Dworniczak B, Simon R, et al: Chromosomal imbalances in primary lymphomas of the central nervous system. Am J Pathol 155:1445–1451, 1999.

17. Boonstra R, Koning A, Mastik M, et al: Analysis of chromosomal copy number changes and oncoprotein expression in primary central nervous system lymphomas: Frequent loss of chromosome arm 6q. Virchows Arch 443:164–169, 2003.

18. Offit K, Parsa NZ, Gaidano G, et al: 6q Deletions define distinct clinico-pathologic subsets of non-Hodgkin's lymphoma. Blood 82:2157–2162, 1993.

19. Schabet M: Epidemiology of primary CNS lymphoma. J Neurooncol 43:199–201, 1999.

20. Olson JE, Janney CA, Rao RD, et al: The continuing increase in the incidence of primary central nervous system non-Hodgkin lymphoma: A surveillance, epidemiology, and end results analysis. Cancer 95:1504–1510, 2002.

21. Herrlinger U, Schabet M, Bitzer M, et al: Primary central nervous system lymphoma: From clinical presentation to diagnosis. J Neurooncol 43:219–226, 1999.

22. Kadan-Lottick NS, Skluzacek MC, Gurney JG: Decreasing incidence rates of primary central nervous system lymphoma. Cancer 95: 193–202, 2002.

23. Sparano JA: Clinical aspects and management of AIDS-related lymphoma. Eur J Cancer 37:1296–1305, 2001.

24. Reni M, Ferreri AJ, Zoldan MC, et al: Primary brain lymphomas in patients with a prior or concomitant malignancy. J Neurooncol 32:135–142, 1997.

25. Al-Yamany M, Lozano A, Nag S, et al: Spontaneous remission of primary central nervous system lymphoma: Report of 3 cases and discussion of pathophysiology. J Neurooncol 42:151–159, 1999.

26. Ferreri AJ, Blay JY, Reni M, et al: Relevance of intraocular involvement in the management of primary central nervous system lymphomas. Ann Oncol 13:531–538, 2002.

27. Hochberg FH, Miller DC: Primary central nervous system lymphoma. J Neurosurg 68:835–853, 1988.

28. Landan I, Gilroy J, Wolfe DE: Syringomyelia affecting the entire spinal cord secondary to primary spinal intramedullary central nervous system lymphoma. J Neurol Neurosurg Psych 50:1533–1535, 1987.

29. Kawasaki K, Wakabayashi K, Koizumi T, et al: Spinal cord involvement of primary central nervous system lymphomas: Histopathological examination of 14 autopsy cases. Neuropathology 22:13–18, 2002.

30. Bataille B, Delwail V, Menet E, et al: Primary intracerebral malignant lymphoma: Report of 248 cases. J Neurosurg 92:261–266, 2000.

31. Coulon A, Lafitte F, Hoang-Xuan K, et al: Radiographic findings in 37 cases of primary CNS lymphoma in immunocompetent patients. European Radiology 12:329–340, 2002.

32. Thurnher MM, Rieger A, Kleibl-Popov C, et al: Primary central nervous system lymphoma in AIDS: A wider spectrum of CT and MRI findings. Neuroradiology 43:29–35, 2001.

33. Harting I, Hartmann M, Jost G, et al: Differentiating primary central nervous system lymphoma from glioma in humans using localised proton magnetic resonance spectroscopy. Neurosci Lett 342:163–166, 2003.

34. Shinoda J, Yano H, Murase S, et al: High 123I-IMP retention on SPECT image in primary central nervous system lymphoma. J Neurooncol 61:261–265, 2003.

35. Lorberboym M, Estok L, Machac J, et al: Rapid differential diagnosis of cerebral toxoplasmosis and primary central nervous system lymphoma by thallium-201 SPECT. J Nucl Med 37:1150–1154, 1996.

36. Lai R, Rosenblum MK, DeAngelis LM: Primary CNS lymphoma: A whole-brain disease? Neurology 59:1557–1562, 2002.

37. Behin A, Hoang-Xuan K, Carpentier AF, et al: Primary brain tumours in adults. Lancet 361:323–331, 2003.

38. Verbraeken HE, Hanssens M, Priem H, et al: Ocular non-Hodgkin's lymphoma: A clinical study of nine cases. Br J Ophthalmol 81:31–36, 1997.

39. Merchant A, Foster CS: Primary intraocular lymphoma. Int Ophthalmol Clin 37:101–115, 1997.

40. Gleissner B, Siehl J, Korfel A, et al: CSF evaluation in primary CNS lymphoma patients by PCR of the CDR III IgH genes (comment). Neurology 58:390–396, 2002.

41. Nasir S, DeAngelis LM: Update on the management of primary CNS lymphoma. Oncology 14:228–234, 2000.

42. Plasswilm L, Herrlinger U, Korfel A, et al: Primary central nervous system (CNS) lymphoma in immunocompetent patients. Ann Hematol 81:415–423, 2002.

43. Herrlinger U: Primary CNS lymphoma: Findings outside the brain. J Neurooncol 43:227–230, 1999.

44. Cingolani A, De Luca A, Larocca LM, et al: Minimally invasive diagnosis of acquired immunodeficiency syndrome-related primary central nervous system lymphoma. J Natl Cancer Inst 90:364–369, 1998.

45. Antinori A, De Rossi G, Ammassari A, et al: Value of combined approach with thallium-201 single-photon emission computed tomography and Epstein-Barr virus DNA polymerase chain reaction in CSF for the diagnosis of AIDS-related primary CNS lymphoma. J Clin Oncol 17:554–560, 1999.

46. Skolasky RL, Dal Pan GJ, Olivi A, et al: HIV-associated primary CNS lymorbidity and utility of brain biopsy. J Neurol Sci 163:32–38, 1999.

47. Bower M, Fife K, Sullivan A, et al: Treatment outcome in presumed and confirmed AIDS-related primary cerebral lymphoma. Eur J Cancer 35:601–604, 1999.

48. Grant JW, Isaacson PG: Primary central nervous system lymphoma. Brain Pathol 2:97–109, 1992.

49. DeAngelis LM: Primary central nervous system lymphoma imitates multiple sclerosis. J Neurooncol 9:177–181, 1990.

50. Weller M: Glucocorticoid treatment of primary CNS lymphoma. J Neurooncol 43:237–239, 1999.

51. Ferreri AJ, Abrey LE, Blay JY, et al: Summary statement on primary central nervous system lymphomas from the Eighth International Conference on Malignant Lymphoma, Lugano, Switzerland, June 12 to 15, 2002. J Clin Oncol 21:2407–2414, 2003.

52. Herrlinger U, Schabet M, Brugger W, et al: German Cancer Society Neuro-Oncology Working Group NOA-03 multicenter trial of single-agent high-dose methotrexate for primary central nervous system lymphoma. Ann Neurol 51:247–252, 2002.

53. Nelson DF: Radiotherapy in the treatment of primary central nervous system lymphoma (PCNSL). J Neurooncol 43:241–247, 1999.

54. DeAngelis LM: Primary central nervous system lymphoma: A curable brain tumor. J Clin Oncol 21:4471–4473, 2003.

55. Blay JY, Conroy T, Chevreau C, et al: High-dose methotrexate for the treatment of primary cerebral lymphomas: Analysis of survival and late neurologic toxicity in a retrospective series. J Clin Oncol 16:864–871, 1998.

56. O'Brien P, Roos D, Pratt G, et al: Phase II multicenter study of brief single-agent methotrexate followed by irradiation in primary CNS lymphoma. J Clin Oncol 18:519–526, 2000.

57. Abrey LE, Yahalom J, DeAngelis LM: Treatment for primary CNS lymphoma: The next step. J Clin Oncol 18:3144–3150, 2000.

58. DeAngelis LM, Seiferheld W, Schold SC, et al: Combination chemotherapy and radiotherapy for primary central nervous system lymphoma: Radiation Therapy Oncology Group Study 93-10. J Clin Oncol 20:4643–4648, 2002.

59. Schlegel U, Pels H, Glasmacher A, et al: Combined systemic and intraventricular chemotherapy in primary CNS lymphoma: A pilot study. J Neurol Neurosurg Psych 71:118–122, 2001.

60. Bessell EM, Lopez-Guillermo A, Villa S, et al: Importance of radiotherapy in the outcome of patients with primary CNS lymphoma: An analysis of the CHOD/BVAM regimen followed by two different radiotherapy treatments. J Clin Oncol 20:231–236, 2002.

61. Hoang-Xuan K, Taillandier L, Chinot O, et al: Chemotherapy alone as initial treatment for primary CNS lymphoma in patients older than 60 years: A multicenter phase II study (26952) of the European Organization for Research and Treatment of Cancer Brain Tumor Group. J Clin Oncol 21:2726–2731, 2003.

62. Batchelor T, Carson K, O'Neill A, et al: Treatment of primary CNS lymphoma with methotrexate and deferred radiotherapy: A report of NABTT 96-07. J Clin Oncol 21:1044–1049, 2003.

63. Poortmans PM, Kluin-Nelemans HC, Haaxma-Reiche H, et al: High-dose methotrexate-based chemotherapy followed by consolidating radiotherapy in non-AIDS-related primary central nervous system lymphoma: European Organization for Research and Treatment of Cancer Lymphoma Group Phase II Trial 20962. J Clin Oncol 21:4483–4488, 2003.

64. Guha-Thakurta N, Damek D, Pollack C, et al: Intravenous methotrexate as initial treatment for primary central nervous system lymphoma: Response to therapy and quality of life of patients. J Neurooncol 43:259–268, 1999.

65. Sandor V, Stark-Vancs V, Pearson D, et al: Phase II trial of chemotherapy alone for primary CNS and intraocular lymphoma. J Clin Oncol 16:3000–3006, 1998.

66. Pels H, Schmidt-Wolf IG, Glasmacher A, et al: Primary central nervous system lymphoma: Results of a pilot and phase ii study of systemic and intraventricular chemotherapy with deferred radiotherapy. J Clin Oncol 21:4489–4495, 2003.

67. Khan RB, Shi W, Thaler HT, et al: Is intrathecal methotrexate necessary in the treatment of primary CNS lymphoma? J Neurooncol 58:175–178, 2002.

68. Plotkin SR, Batchelor TT: Advances in the therapy of primary central nervous system lymphoma. Clin Lymphoma 1:263–277, 2001.

69. Glantz MJ, LaFollette S, Jaeckle KA, et al: Randomized trial of a slow-release versus a standard formulation of cytarabine for the intrathecal treatment of lymphomatous meningitis. J Clin Oncol 17:3110–3116, 1999.

70. Siegal T, Zylber-Katz E: Strategies for increasing drug delivery to the brain: Focus on brain lymphoma. Clin Pharmacokinet 41:171–186, 2002.

71. Perry AR, Goldstone AH: High-dose therapy for diffuse large-cell lymphoma in first remission. Ann Oncol 9(Suppl 1):S9–S14, 1998.

72. Shipp MA, Abeloff MD, Antman KH, et al: International Consensus Conference on High-Dose Therapy with Hematopoietic Stem Cell Transplantation in Aggressive Non-Hodgkin's Lymphomas: Report of the jury. J Clin Oncol 17:423–429, 1999.

73. Cheng T, Forsyth P, Chaudhry A, et al: High-dose thiotepa, busulfan, cyclophosphamide and ASCT without whole-brain radiotherapy for poor prognosis primary CNS lymphoma. Bone Marrow Transplantation 31:679–685, 2003.

74. Soussain C, Suzan F, Hoang-Xuan K, et al: Results of intensive chemotherapy followed by hematopoietic stem-cell rescue in 22 patients with refractory or recurrent primary CNS lymphoma or intraocular lymphoma. J Clin Oncol 19:742–749, 2001.

75. Abrey LE, Moskowitz CH, Mason WP, et al: Intensive methotrexate and cytarabine followed by high-dose chemotherapy with autologous stem-cell rescue in patients with newly diagnosed primary CNS lymphoma: An intent-to-treat analysis. J Clin Oncol 21:4151–4156, 2003.

76. Pels H, Schulz H, Manzke O, et al: Intraventricular and intravenous treatment of a patient with refractory primary CNS lymphoma using rituximab. J Neurooncol 59:213–216, 2002.

77. Herrlinger U, Kuker W, Platten M, et al: First-line therapy with temozolomide induces regression of primary CNS lymphoma. Neurology 58:1573–1574, 2002.

78. Lerro KA, Lacy J: Case report: a patient with primary CNS lymphoma treated with temozolomide to complete response. J Neurooncol 59:165–168, 2002.

79. Herrlinger U, Brugger W, Bamberg M, et al: PCV salvage chemotherapy for recurrent primary CNS lymphoma. Neurology 54:1707–1708, 2000.

80. Reni M, Ferreri AJ: Therapeutic management of refractory or relapsed primary central nervous system lymphomas. Ann Hematol 80 (Suppl 3):B113–B117, 2001.

81. de Smet MD, Vancs VS, Kohler D, et al: Intravitreal chemotherapy for the treatment of recurrent intraocular lymphoma. Br J Ophthalmol 83:448–451, 1999.

82. Fishburne BC, Wilson DJ, Rosenbaum JT, et al: Intravitreal methotrexate as an adjunctive treatment of intraocular lymphoma. Arch Ophthalmol 115:1152–1156, 1997.

83. Chamberlain MC, Kormanik PA: AIDS-related central nervous system lymphomas. J Neurooncol 43:269–276, 1999.

84. Slobod KS, Taylor GH, Sandlund JT, et al: Epstein-Barr virus-targeted therapy for AIDS-related primary lymphoma of the central nervous system. Lancet 356:1493–1494, 2000.

85. Taiwo BO: AIDS-related primary CNS lymphoma: A brief review. AIDS Reader 10:486–491, 2000.

86. A predictive model for aggressive non-Hodgkin's lymphoma. The International Non-Hodgkin's Lymphoma Prognostic Factors Project. N Engl J Med 329:987–994, 1993.

87. Corry J, Smith JG, Wirth A, et al: Primary central nervous system lymphoma: Age and performance status are more important than treatment modality. Int J Radiat Oncol Biol Phys 41:615–620, 1998.

88. Ferreri AJ, Blay JY, Reni M, et al: Prognostic scoring system for primary CNS lymphomas: The International Extranodal Lymphoma Study Group experience. J Clin Oncol 21:266–272, 2003.

Current Surgical Management of High-Grade Gliomas

RAY M. CHU and KEITH L. BLACK

INTRODUCTION

The malignant glioma has been the neurosurgeon's hydra, continually growing despite attempts to defeat it. High-grade gliomas (HGGs) are heterogeneous and include anaplastic astrocytoma (AA), glioblastoma multiforme (GBM), gliosarcoma, and anaplastic oligodendroglioma (AO). The annual incidence of new primary brain tumors in the United States is estimated to be 14 per 100,000, resulting in approximately 40,000 new primary brain tumors per year, of which 22,000 are high grade.[1] Some 13,100 deaths in 2002 were attributed to primary malignant brain tumors.[2] Despite continually renewed efforts at treating HGGs, the odds of significant long-term survival has remained poor and stable for the past three decades, with 2% to 4% of patients with GBM surviving to the 5-year point.[3]

PREOPERATIVE WORKUP

MRI with and without gadolinium is essential for preliminary differential diagnosis, for the decision for surgery, and for operative planning. For selected patients who cannot undergo MRI (e.g., the patient with a cardiac pacemaker), CT with and without contrast provides similar although less detailed information. Thallium SPECT scan, PET scan, or MR spectroscopy may help in determination of high-grade versus low-grade tumor, although none of these studies is definitive, and the differentiation between HGGs and metastases is difficult.[4] These studies are more useful in patients with previous surgery and radiation, in helping determine recurrent tumor versus radiation effect.

A Wada (intracarotid amobarbital) test is the definitive (albeit invasive) method to establish cerebral hemispheric dominance for language and memory. It is required for procedures in patients with a seizure disorder with tumor in whom a formal temporal lobectomy is planned. A Wada may be useful in selected other patients, such as the patient with a dominant hemisphere temporal lobe tumor in whom tumor resection without temporal lobectomy is planned. Although both functional MRI and a Wada test offer similar information about cerebral dominance,[5,6] a Wada test does not offer anatomic localization of critical areas for language because MRI does not truly investigate the potential bilaterality of language.[7,8] Functional MRI is more useful than a Wada test for lesions of the dominant hemisphere near the motor cortex, frontal lobe pars triangularis and opercularis (Broca's area), or Wernicke's area. With changes in metabolic activity and blood flow demand, an active area of the brain during a silent speech or motor task becomes infused with more oxygenated blood; this change can be detected, because oxygenated blood

carries a different paramagnetic signal than does deoxygenated blood (the blood oxygen level-dependent or BOLD signal) (Fig. 47-1A and B).[9,10] One limitation of functional MRI is that it becomes less useful in patients with recurrent tumor because of altered vascular patterns and MR artifact from the previous surgery.

CYTOREDUCTION

Although decompression of mass effect is a surgical goal and influences symptomatic survival, controversy exists over whether the extent of resection influences survival or time to progression for HGGs. Dandy originally proposed hemispherectomy for selected patients with malignant tumors, but there was no significant effect on mortality.[11] Next there were data suggesting that for GBMs, biopsy and resection were equivalent in terms of survival, and that it was really postoperative radiation that had a meaningful effect on survival. More recently, the Glioma Outcomes Project reported a statistically significant extension of survival for patients with HGGs who undergo resection over biopsy (median survival 51.6 weeks versus 27.1 weeks, respectively).[12] This study was limited by lack of central pathologic review, lack of quantification of amount of resection, sampling error from a biopsy, and selection bias in biopsy versus resection. Other surgeons have also reported extension of survival for patients with 90% or better resection; resection better than 98% was associated with a median survival of 13 months versus 8.8 months with less than 98% in one study.[13] Additionally, the volume of residual tumor at the time of first recurrence may negatively influence the response to chemotherapy in terms of time to progression and overall survival.[14] However, even gross total resection does not truly address the diffuse nature of malignant gliomas.

INTRAOPERATIVE IMAGING

Even with the continual improvements being seen in operating microscopes, some form of intraoperative imaging or navigation is useful. A high-quality intraoperative ultrasound assists in many types of surgeries but cannot aid in incision and craniotomy planning. Also, many tumors, especially lower grade tumors, may not be dense enough, compared with the normal brain, to be visualized adequately by this method. Ultrasound is more helpful when the density difference is greater (e.g., if there is a hematoma to evacuate in addition to tumor, if there is a cystic component, or if it is used to obtain ventricular access).

Frameless stereotactic navigation is becoming more common. This technology incorporates a preoperatively

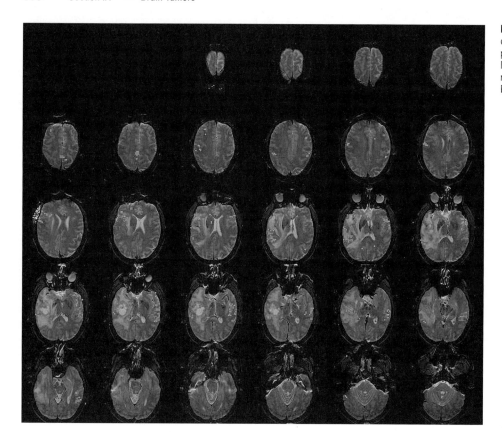

FIGURE 47-1 Functional MRI during a silent speech task in a patient with a glioblastoma of the left temporal glioblastoma (left and right are reversed). (See Color Plate.)

obtained MRI or CT with fiducial markers that are left in place on the scalp. In the operating room, these markers or contours of the face can be registered in reference to a frame, which is visualized by a computer via an optical apparatus, electromagnetic waves, or mechanical arms. This technology allows the surgeon to visualize points on the scalp and skull and compare them with the MRI, aiding in planning of a small, localized incision and craniotomy as well as ensuring that the exposure of the lesion is adequate. Surgical navigation can be performed intracranially with a localizing probe or with image fusion into the operating microscope based on focus depth. Because frameless navigation is based on a preoperative set of images without updating in the operating room, the surgeon needs to account for brain shift during the procedure. Brain shift up to 2 centimeters can occur and is more common with increased patient age, cortical rather than subcortical structures, larger tumor volume, and lesions far from some point of tethering (e.g., the skull base or falx).[15] Once brain shift is taken into account, resection to the imaging abnormality borders (when safe) assists in the goal of cytoreduction.

Intraoperative MRI systems are available as well. Low-field (less than 0.5-T) systems allow most normal operating room equipment to be used throughout the surgery except right at the point of imaging.[16,17] Because the imaging can be updated, the surgeon does not need to account for brain shift. For craniotomies, once resection is deemed complete by the surgeon, an MRI can be performed to assess whether there is occult residual tumor, thereby aiding in the aim of cytoreduction. These systems offer a smaller field of view, less detailed images, longer acquisition time, and less types of imaging options than conventional diagnostic MRIs.

High-field (1.5-T) systems exist which offer all the imaging capabilities of a standard, diagnostic MRI.[18] A biopsy needle can be watched in near-real time as it is passed to target and verified at target before samples are taken. With craniotomies, intraoperative imaging can confirm completeness of tumor resection, which is especially helpful in cases of low-grade gliomas where the distinction between tumor and normal brain is less apparent. At closure, an MRI can be performed to exclude hemorrhage; for patients with a biopsy or simple craniotomy, excluding hemorrhage may allow a patient to be transferred to a step-down unit instead of the ICU. These systems, however, require construction of an operating room suite specifically designed for an intraoperative MRI to provide adequate shielding and safety measures. The high-field strength requires a larger magnet than the low-field systems, limiting access to the patient. Normal operating room equipment can be used outside the 5-gauss line (several feet from the center of the bore of the magnet); inside that line, only MRI-compatible (i.e., titanium or surgical-grade stainless steel) instruments can be used.

MOTOR STRIP MAPPING

Surgery in the parietal lobe or the posterior frontal lobe may require motor strip mapping. Short-acting muscle relaxants are used during induction, and anesthetics are lightened for the mapping, but the patient does not need to emerge from anesthesia fully. Rather than identification of the motor cortex itself, this technique relies on identification of the sensory cortex by looking for somatosensory evoked potentials (SEPs). A 1 × 8 or other-sized subdural electrode is used.

By noting the electrodes with a positive (precentral) as opposed to a negative (postcentral) amplitude, and electrodes between which there is phase reversal, the primary motor cortex can be identified and protected. This technique has good correlation to magnetoencephalography when integrated into the surgical navigation system.[19]

AWAKE CRANIOTOMY

Awake craniotomy with cortical mapping affords the ultimate protection for surgery in or near language areas. Patients are nasotracheally intubated so that the endotracheal tube can later be withdrawn out of the vocal cords and language tasks can be performed. In addition to local anesthetic to the incision, a field block is performed with a long-acting anesthetic such as bupivacaine to the scalp in the area of the incision and the Mayfield pins. Muscle relaxants may be used at induction, but they must be short-acting. Draping is per routine except that the face needs to have an unobstructed view so visual naming and interaction with the neuropsychologist are possible. Once the craniotomy is created, anesthetics are lightened, the endotracheal tube is withdrawn out of the vocal cords, and a hand-held bipolar stimulator is used to stimulate areas likely to have language function or areas of planned resection to determine the effect. Continuous language testing can be performed during resection to reconfirm safety. Once resection is complete, the endotracheal tube is replaced and general anesthesia is reinstated for closure.

FRONTAL LOBE

HGGs are most common in the frontal lobe because it occupies one third of the surface of the brain and is the largest lobe.[20] The frontal lobe tolerates unilateral surgical resection very well as long as the motor cortex and Broca's area are respected. Frontal lobe tumors are often amenable to image-complete resection. For tumors with significant growth into the corpus callosum and across the midline, surgical resection is unlikely to provide significant cytoreduction, and therefore a biopsy may be the more prudent choice.

Motor Cortex

For lesions in the posterior frontal lobe, operative anatomy and imaging are not always sufficient to make adequate surgical plans. Functional MRI can reliably identify the motor strip, but even with modern neuronavigation systems, surgical resection is safer with some type of functional evaluation. Two current ways to identify motor cortex include intraoperative cortical stimulation mapping and placement of a subdural grid for mapping out of the operating room.

Proponents of subdural grid placement argue that electrocorticography while out of the operating room and without sedation is superior. Time is not limited, and residual effects of anesthetics and narcotics can be minimized. Operating room time is minimized. The additional risks of the second surgery for grid removal and surgical resection are minimal; however, some surgeons prefer intraoperative testing to subdural grid placement. Intraoperative mapping

may gain an extra margin of safety from continuous testing during surgical resection.

Broca's Area

Approximately 95% of right-handed, 85% of ambidextrous, and 75% of left-handed persons will have left-sided cerebral dominance for language.[21] Broca's area encompasses the middle and posterior parts of the inferior frontal gyrus (i.e., the pars opercularis and the pars triangularis). Protection of language area via awake craniotomy and intraoperative corticography or subdural electrode placement for cortical mapping is essential for tumors adjacent to Broca's area (Fig. 47-2A and B).

Premotor Area

Deficits from surgical resection in the premotor area generally recover over a period of weeks to months through reorganization. Premotor weakness generally shows a better response to stimulation than to voluntary initiation.

Supplementary Motor Area

The supplementary motor area (SMA) occupies the posterior one third of the superior frontal gyrus and is responsible for planning of complex movements of ipsilateral and contralateral extremities.[22] SMA syndrome involves speech arrest, contralateral weakness, and near-total recovery in weeks to months. For tumors involving the SMA, functional MRI shows ipsilateral decreased SMA activity compensated by increased contralateral activity.[23] After resection in the SMA, the motor deficit is further compensated by recruitment of activity in the contralateral SMA and premotor cortex.

TEMPORAL LOBE

Anterior temporal lobe lesions are amenable to surgical resection. Decompression of mass effect in this area is especially important because of proximity to the brain stem. Resection is generally safe to 4 centimeters back from the temporal tip on the dominant hemisphere and 6 centimeters back on the nondominant side. Removal of temporal lobe back to 6 centimeters is often associated with at least a rim of visual defect in the contralateral superior quadrant, but this deficit is generally well tolerated. Resection at or behind 4 centimeters back from the tip of the middle cranial fossa on the left requires either intraoperative electrocorticography or subdural grid placement for identification of Wernicke's area (Fig. 47-3A and B). When a lesion involves the hippocampus, it is possible that the contralateral hippocampus is compensating for function; for the dominant hemisphere, this is best proven with a Wada test before surgery.

PARIETAL LOBE

Complete lesions of the dominant parietal lobe can be characterized by Gerstmann's syndrome, which consists of left/right confusion, digit agnosia, acalculia, and agraphia.[24] Clinically, even with a large parietal lobe neoplasm, the

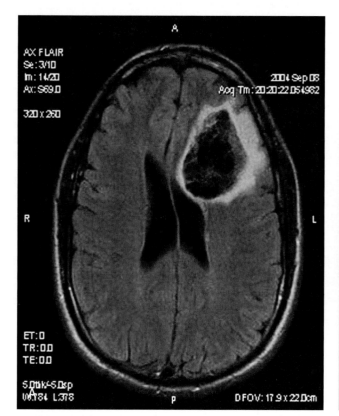
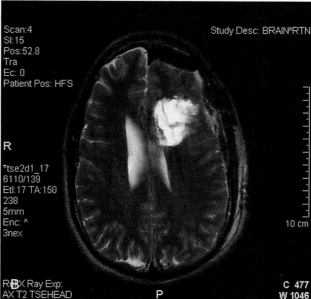

FIGURE 47-2 Preoperative (*A*) and postoperative (*B*) brain MRI in a patient with seizures, revealing a heterogeneous lesion of mixed signal on FLAIR which was nonenhancing (not shown). Surgery with awake craniotomy was performed, and an image-complete resection was achieved. Pathology revealed an anaplastic oligodendroglioma, and the patient was referred for chemotherapy.

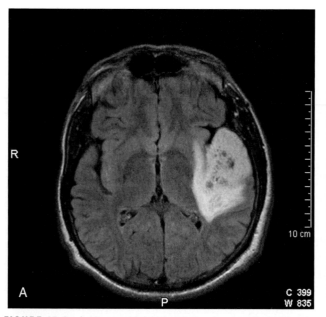
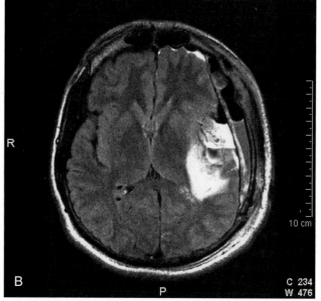

FIGURE 47-3 A 40-year-old right-handed male presented with seizures. Preoperative brain MRI (*A*) was remarkable for a nonenhancing left temporal lesion. Functional imaging revealed language posterior to the lesion (not shown). Craniotomy for gross total resection was performed. Postoperative imaging (*B*) showed resection of the lesion with residual FLAIR abnormality posteriorly. Pathology showed mixed oligoastrocytoma.

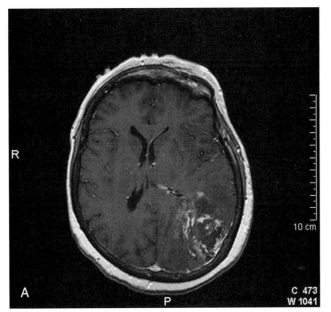
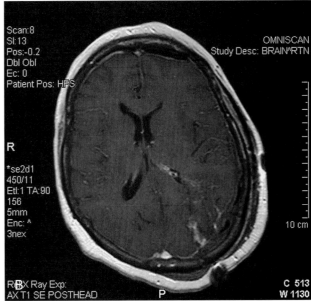

FIGURE 47-4 A 60-year-old right-handed woman presented with increasing word-finding difficulty and right-sided hemiparesis. A brain MRI (*A*) revealed an enhancing left parietal mass with edema. At awake craniotomy, there was no involvement of the language area by tumor, and an image-complete resection was achieved (*B*). Pathology demonstrated glioblastoma, and the patient is undergoing radiation therapy and chemotherapy. Her speech improved after surgery, possibly because of resolution of mass effect and little direct involvement of the speech area by tumor.

deficit is usually incomplete. Lesions of the dominant superior parietal lobule alone rarely cause the full syndrome; the angular gyrus has to be involved.[25] Low-grade gliomas are more likely than HGGs to have infiltration into still functioning cortical areas; HGGs tend more to displace and destroy function. Restoration of a preoperative dominant parietal deficit is unlikely unless there is a cystic component, a hematoma to evacuate, or significant mass effect from edema that resolves with surgery and radiation (Fig. 47-4A and B). Surgery within the nondominant parietal lobe is generally tolerated well. Motor strip mapping adds an extra layer of safety as described above.

OCCIPITAL LOBE

Occipital lobe surgery almost invariably results in some form of visual field cut, although most high-grade tumors that present in this location have already caused a visual defect. Some tumors that present more laterally may leave less visual field disturbance but may cause occipital association symptoms such as visual auras, color agnosia, or episodic blindness.

PROGNOSIS

Outcome from diagnosis for a HGG depends on several factors. Precise pathologic diagnosis contributes a significant impact because approximately 30% of patients with GBM survive to the 1-year point versus 60% of patients with anaplastic astrocytoma in one study.[26] However, glioblastoma and the rare gliosarcoma do not differ significantly in behavior, response to therapy, or cytogenetics.[27] According to recently published data from the Glioma Outcomes Project, resection instead of biopsy, age less than or equal to 60 years, and a Karnofsky Performance

Scale of 70 or greater were all significantly correlated with outcome.[12]

NEW DIRECTIONS

Certainly, surgery alone for HGGs will not provide a cure; surgeons also have impact on radiation and chemotherapy delivery to the brain. Besides local chemotherapy with BCNU-impregnated wafers,[28] other avenues proposed to effect change in the local tumor environment include convection-enhanced delivery (CED) of chemotherapy or targeted toxins.[29] This concept is currently being tested in a randomized trial. An option for increasing the local dose of radiation is an implantable balloon system for radioactive iodine,[30] but it is unclear if this method of radiation delivery is clearly better than focused conventional radiation to the area. Overall, these local delivery approaches to HGGs raise interesting questions but also battle with the notion over whether malignant glioma is a focal or diffuse disease.

An approach that attacks the diffuse nature of gliomas is immunotherapy. One option involves creation of a subcutaneous vaccine specific to the patient's resected tumor using tumor lysate-pulsed dendritic cells.[31,32] Vaccinated patients demonstrate an antigen-specific T-cell response and survival benefit as well as increased responsiveness to chemotherapy.[33] Other potential strategies include interleukin gene introduction via viral vectors,[34] vaccination with dendritic-glioma cell fusions using interleukin-12,[35] or scores of other targets to immunotherapy.

CONCLUSIONS

Craniotomy for tumor resection is a mainstay of current treatment for high-grade gliomas when it can be done safely.

Neuroanatomy is the foundation that allows safe surgical resection. Newer technologies allow ever-improving levels of surgical safety. Overall, surgical resection alone will not cure malignant brain tumors unless coupled with other strategies that address the diffuse nature of the disease (e.g., novel chemotherapy delivery options or immunotherapy), but these possibilities are on the horizon.

REFERENCES

1. CBTRUS 2002-3: Primary Brain Tumors in the United States Statistical Report 1995–1999. Central Brain Tumor Registry of the United States.
2. Cancer Facts and Figures 2002: Atlanta: American Cancer Society, Inc. Surveillance Research, 2002.
3. McLendon RE, Halperin EC: Is the long-term survival of patients with intracranial glioblastoma multiforme overstated? Cancer 98:1745–1748, 2003.
4. Majos C, Alonso J, Aguilera C, et al: Proton magnetic resonance spectroscopy (^{1}H MRS) of human tumours: assessment of differences between tumour types and its applicability in brain tumour categorization. Eur Radiol 13(3):582–591, 2003.
5. Desmond JE, Sum JM, Wagner AD, et al: Functional MRI measurement of language lateralization in Wada-tested patients. Brain 118:1411–1419, 1995.
6. Binder JR, Swanson SJ, Hammeke TA, et al: Determination of language dominance using functional MRI: A comparison with the Wada test. Neurology 46:978–984, 1996.
7. Benbadis SR, Binder JR, Swanson SJ, et al: Is speech arrest during wada testing a valid method for determining hemispheric representation of language? Brain Lang 65(3):441–446, 1998.
8. Sabsevitz DS, Swanson SJ, Hammeke TA, et al: Use of preoperative functional neuroimaging to predict language deficits from epilepsy surgery. Neurology 60:1788–1792, 2003.
9. Bandettini PA, Wong EC, Hinks RS, et al: Time course EPI of human brain function during task activation. Magn Reson Med 25:390–397, 1992.
10. Logothetis NK, Pauls J, Augath M, et al: Neurophysiological investigation of the basis of the fMRI signal. Nature 412:150–157, 2001.
11. Dandy WE: Removal of right cerebral hemisphere for certain tumors with hemiplegia: Preliminary case report. JAMA 90:823–825, 1928.
12. Laws ER, Parney IF, Huang W, et al: Survival following surgery and prognostic factors for recently diagnosed malignant glioma: Data from the Glioma Outcomes Project. J Neurosurg 99(3):467–473, 2003.
13. Lacroix M, Abi-Said D, Fourney DR, et al: A multivariate analysis of 416 patients with glioblastoma multiforme: Prognosis, extent of resection, and survival. J Neurosurg 95:190–198, 2001.
14. Keles GE, Lamborn KL, Chang SM, et al: Volume of residual disease as a predictor of outcome in adult patients with recurrent supratentorial glioblastomas multiforme who are undergoing chemotherapy. J Neurosurg 100:41–46, 2004.
15. Reinges MH, Nguyen HH, Krings T, et al: Course of brain shift during microsurgical resection of supratentorial cerebral lesions: Limits of conventional neuronavigation. Acta Neurochir (Wien) 146(4):369–377, 2004.
16. Tronnier VM, Wirtz CR, Knauth M, et al: Intraoperative diagnostic and interventional magnetic resonance imaging in neurosurgery. Neurosurgery 40:891–902, 1997.
17. Steinmeier R, Fahlbusch R, Ganslandt O, et al: Intraoperative magnetic resonance imaging with the Magnetom open scanner: Concepts, neurosurgical indications, and procedures: A preliminary report. Neurosurgery 43:739–748, 1998.
18. Chu RM, Tummala RP, Hall WA: Intraoperative magnetic resonance imaging-guided neurosurgery. Neurosurg Q 13:234–250, 2003.
19. Romstock J, Fahlbusch R, Ganslandt O, et al: Localisation of the sensorimotor cortex during surgery for brain tumors: Feasibility and waveform patterns of somatosensory evoked potentials. J Neurol Neurosurg Psychiatry 72:221–229, 2002.
20. Carpenter MB: Core Text of Neuroanatomy, 4th ed. Baltimore, MD: Williams & Wilkins, 1991.
21. Knecht S, Drager B, Deppe M: Handedness and hemispheric language dominance in healthy humans. Brain 123:2512–2518, 2000.
22. Russell SM, Kelly PJ: Incidence and clinical evolution of postoperative deficits after volumetric stereotactic resection of glial neoplasms involving the supplementary motor area. Neurosurgery 52:506–516, 2003.
23. Krainik A, Duffau H, Capelle L, et al: Role of the healthy hemisphere in recovery after resection of the supplementary motor area. Neurology 62:1323–1332, 2004.
24. Gerstmann J: Syndrome of finger agnosia, disorientation for right and left, agraphia, and acalculia. Arch Neurol Psychiatry 44:398–408, 1940.
25. Roux F, Boetto S, Sacko O, et al: Writing, calculating, and finger recognition in the region of the angular gyrus: A cortical stimulation study of Gerstmann syndrome. J Neurosurg 99:716–727, 2003.
26. Barnholtz-Sloan JS, Sloan AE, Schwartz AG: Relative survival rates and patterns of diagnosis analyzed by time period for individuals with primary malignant brain tumor, 1972–1997. J Neurosurg 99:458–466, 2003.
27. Galanis E, Buckner JC, Dinapoli RP, et al: Clinical outcome of gliosarcoma compared with glioblastoma multiforme: North Central Cancer Treatment Group results. J Neurosurg 89:425–430, 1998.
28. Westphal M, Hilt DC, Bortey E, et al: A phase 3 trial of local chemotherapy with biodegradable carmustine (BCNU) wafers (Gliadel wafers) in patients with primary malignant glioma. Neuro-Oncology 5(2):79–88, 2003.
29. Kunwar S: Convection-enhanced delivery of IL13-PE38QQR for treatment of malignant glioma: Presentation of interim findings from ongoing phase 1 studies. Acta Neurochir Suppl 88:105–111, 2003.
30. Tatter SB, Shaw EG, Rosenblum ML, et al: An inflatable balloon catheter and liquid ^{125}I radiation source (GliaSite Radiation Therapy System) for treatment of recurrent malignant glioma: Multicenter safety and feasibility trial. J Neurosurg 99:297–303, 2003.
31. Yamanaka R, Abe T, Yajima N, et al: Vaccination of recurrent glioma patients with tumour lysate-pulsed dendritic cells elicits immune responses: results of a clinical phase I/II trial. Br J Cancer 89(7):1172–1179, 2003.
32. Yu JS, Liu G, Yong WH, et al: Vaccination with tumor lysate-pulsed dendritic cells elicits antigen-specific, cytotoxic T-cells in patients with malignant glioma. Cancer Res 64:4973–4979, 2004.
33. Wheeler CJ, Das A, Liu G, et al: Clinical responsiveness of glioblastoma multiforme to chemotherapy after vaccination. Clin Cancer Res 10:5316–5326, 2004.
34. Ren H, Boulikas T, Lundstrom K, et al: Immunogene therapy of recurrent glioblastoma multiforme with liposomally encapsulated replication-incompetent Semliki forest virus vector carrying the human interleukin-12 gene-a phase I/II clinical protocol. J Neurooncol 64(1–2):147–154, 2003.
35. Kikuchi T, Akasaki Y, Abe T: Vaccination of glioma patients with fusions of dendritic and glioma cells and recombinant human interleukin 12. J Immunother 27(6):452–459, 2004.

48 Surgical Management of Low-Grade Gliomas

RENATO GIUFFRÈ[†] and FRANCESCO S. PASTORE

CLASSIFICATION—PATHOLOGY

Astrocytomas, oligodendrogliomas, and mixed (oligoastrocytic) gliomas are low grade, that is, Grade I gliomas according to the classification of the World Health Organization (WHO). "The Yale Neuro-Oncology Tumor Data Bank reported an incidence of these oncotypes of 60%, 23.3%, and 16.7%, respectively, among all low-grade gliomas."[1]

Fibrillary, gemistocytic, protoplasmic, or mixed astrocytomas present different surgical problems according to whether they are solid or cystic. A solid astrocytoma has a hard or rubbery consistency, is sometimes cartilaginous, and is whitish in the fibrillary form; it is softer, gelatinous, and translucent in the gemistocytic and protoplasmic varieties. On the surface, the growth is either diffuse or apparently circumscribed. Under the surface, it usually has less consistency and tends to form either several small cysts or a single large one; a single large cyst is most often found in the fibrillary and gemistocytic varieties.[2] The pilocytic variety is rare among astrocytomas of the cerebral hemispheres and is found more often in the posterior fossa (cerebellum and brain stem), diencephalon, and anterior optic pathways. In most cases, cerebral pilocytic astrocytoma consists of a large unilocular cyst with a mural nodule; it differs from other forms of astrocytoma in biologic behavior and in a marked responsiveness to therapy.[3–5]

Oligodendroglioma is often very hard and gritty on section, because it contains palpable calcifications: it is grayish pink and has clear-cut limits on the surface (where it infiltrates the gyri, giving them a hypertrophied, "scalloped or garlanded" appearance) to become indistinct in depth, where small mucinous cysts may be found. Small nodules as hard as warts are found in the cortex and are detected by the surgeon on inspection or on palpation. When the tumor spreads through the leptomeninges, it forms large lumps that project beyond the surface like bluish red fungi. In such cases, the tumor may adhere to the dura mater and may be mistaken at first sight for a meningioma.[2]

Mixed oligoastrocytomas do not differ in gross appearance from true oligodendrogliomas and constitute a purely histologic variety. Tumors such as pleomorphic xanthoastrocytomas and gangliogliomas are low grade, usually resectable tumors with a very low incidence and will not be considered here.

Both oncotypes (astrocytoma and oligodendroglioma) occur preferentially in the frontal lobes, after which come the temporal, parietal, and occipital lobes, in this order. These diffusely infiltrative tumors do not respect boundaries, however, and most low-grade gliomas straddle the fissures to involve contiguous lobes.

There are no typical sites by oncotype, except perhaps the frontolateral region for oligodendroglioma. Both of these gliomas may be parasagittal, affecting the frontal and parietal lobes. Hard gliomas "of the edge," bordering on the sagittal fissure, develop along the medial gyri and may infiltrate the corpus callosum or spread contralaterally through the corpus callosum ("butterfly gliomas").

Whether these tumors emerge on the surface or are subcortical, they infiltrate the white substance diffusely and may spread in depth toward the ventricular system or basal nuclei. Gliomas arising from the diencephalon, which are distinguished by certain histologic and clinical features (occurrence of pilocytic astrocytomas, preference for youth) and which present peculiar biologic behavior and peculiar problems of treatment, are discussed in Chapter 61.

Any centrencephalic spread of a hemispheric glioma limits surgical resection, a point that is addressed in the section on Surgical Technique. Such spread occurs along the projection fibers (Fig. 48-1). Seeger[6] recognized two other possible routes of tumor spread: (1) along the associative fibers (intrahemispheric spread) and (2) along the commissural fibers (interhemispheric spread). An example of the latter is the contralateral spread via the corpus callosum, as already mentioned. An example of intrahemispheric spread is the subcortical migration of neoplastic cells via the short associative U-shaped fibers between two adjacent gyri.

However, tumor progression is a process of dislocation or infiltration of the surrounding neural tissue, and these two patterns of growth may explain the neurophysiologic data showing "in toto" displacement of eloquent areas but also the occasional presence of neural activity in the tumor core.[7]

The WHO classification criteria are purely histopathologic, and their limitations were highlighted in the 1980s and 1990s by the advances of immunohistochemistry, molecular biology, and neuroimaging. When classifying gliomas today, one must take account of specific markers of different cell types, parameters of cellular kinetics, and metabolic data relating to neoplastic tissue in vivo. Thus, tumor grading based solely on morphology is supplemented by neurodiagnostic grading (the presence or absence of contrast enhancement on computed tomograpy [CT] and magnetic resonance imaging [MRI]),[8] metabolic grading (increased glucose consumption on positron-emission tomography [PET]), and grading based on parameters of cellular molecular biology and kinetics.

[†]Deceased.

671

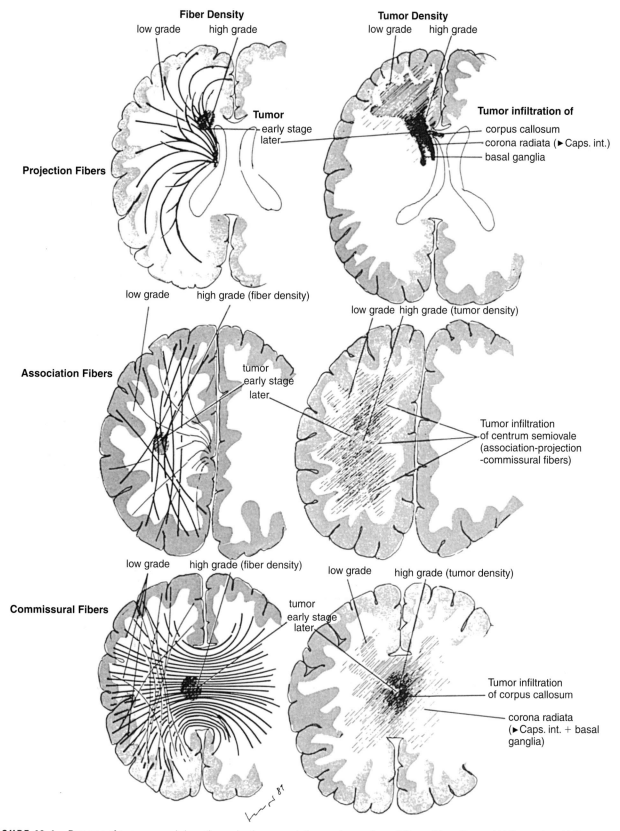

FIGURE 48-1 Patterns of tumor spread along the projection, association, and commissural fibers. (From Seeger W: Strategies of Microsurgery in Problematic Brain Areas. Vienna: Springer-Verlag, 1990, p 25.)

On the last point, histologically similar tumors may exhibit differing proliferative potential. Subgroups of low-grade astrocytomas exist that have different proportions of cells in the S phase of DNA synthesis, expressed by different values of the labeling index (LI). One subgroup with a low LI (<1%) is characterized by slow growth, and another with the same or higher LI is biologically more aggressive, which partially explains the very different clinical behavior often seen in histologically similar tumors.[9] The proliferative potential of a given tumor (expressed in the LI) correlates with necrosis and tissue hypervascularization rather than with the number of mitoses and cellular anomalies (or monstrosities).[10,11] This fact confirms the undue importance that was formerly attached to the mitotic count in gliomas as an index of growth rate. It is now known that mitoses may be lacking in a glioblastoma multiforme and may be present in a slow-growing oligodendroglioma.[12]

The PET tumor grading based on glucose consumption by area is also a better predictor of the long-term prognosis of gliomas than is histologic grading.[13]

The data on the biology of gliomas have been, in the last decade, increasing exponentially. These data will eventually form the basis of a new classification of the far from homogeneous group of low-grade gliomas.

Because low-grade gliomas do not constitute a homogeneous group, treatment clearly cannot be uniform in all cases, and the results are not easily comparable.

CLINICAL AND BIOLOGIC FEATURES OF LOW-GRADE GLIOMAS

Low-grade gliomas of the cerebral hemispheres occur less frequently than malignant gliomas (glioblastomas, primitive neuroectodermal tumors), affect a younger population, and have a better prognosis. Perhaps because these tumors occur less frequently and patients may remain well for a long time, few formal clinical trials have been mounted; therefore, the natural history of low-grade gliomas is less well known than is that of the high-grade varieties. In addition, the preoperative clinical history has changed substantially in recent years as a result of neuroimaging techniques, which have ensured much earlier diagnosis. In the pre-CT era, patients with low-grade hemispheric glioma often presented with headache, papilledema, and focal deficits, whereas today they undergo surgery after only a few episodes of convulsions and are absolutely normal neurologically. For example, in the series of Laws and co-workers,[14] consisting of patients treated between 1915 and 1975, 40% had papilledema at the time of presentation, almost half complained of headache, and 51% exhibited motor deficits. In the series of Gol,[15] composed of patients treated before 1960, 72% had a headache at the time of diagnosis, 59% papilledema, 56% hemiparesis, and 56% seizures. By contrast, in Piepmeier's series,[16] in which all the patients were diagnosed by CT, 5% initially had a headache 15%, motor weakness, and more than 90% seizure activity (the frequency of papilledema was not stated). In addition, in the series of Vertosick and associates,[17] 16% had headache, 8% papilledema, 16% motor deficits, and 92% seizures.

Epileptic activity in patients with low-grade cerebral gliomas is important not only clinically, because it is the earliest symptom, but also surgically. Electrocorticographic recordings in patients with a slow-growing glioma have revealed epileptogenic foci separate from the tumor.[18] This nontumoral cortex, though not marked by neuronal loss, nonetheless shows a change in neuronal subpopulations, that is, a reduction of neurons immunoreactive to γ-aminobutyric acid and to somatostatin,[19] which is an expression of local hyperexcitability. Hence, the seizures in these patients, which are often refractory to drugs, can be controlled only if the epileptogenic foci are removed along with the tumor. A patient with chronic epilepsy may thus have a glioma. Among 51 patients with epilepsy of 1 to 27 years' duration (mean duration of 11 years), Goldring and colleagues[20] found 40 gliomas, including 25 low-grade astrocytomas and 1 oligodendroglioma. In one patient with a 22-year history of epilepsy, they found a glioblastoma, evidently the outcome of secondary degeneration, as is discussed later. CT and, even better, MRI define the lesion, but these modalities have limitations: the lack of increase in lesion volume on serial CT scans does not exclude a tumor. The clinical features, warn Goldring and co-workers, may be very deceptive; a history typical of essential epilepsy does not exclude a tumor as the cause. For instance, generalized febrile convulsions in infancy followed by complex partial seizures—a history typical of temporal mesial sclerosis—was the history of some subjects with temporal glioma.

The biology (cellular kinetics and metabolism) of these nonsymptomatic tumors that have a long natural history (remaining silent or nonsymptomatic for years and then exploding dramatically) cannot be considered benign and certainly arouse scientific interest. Low-grade gliomas (astrocytomas, mixed gliomas, and ependymomas) have a lower percentage of cells in the S phase (LI = 2% to 6.7%) than do malignant gliomas (LI = 9.1% to 46.5%).[21] The growth fraction (GF) (i.e., the total number of cells involved in cellular proliferation as a proportion of the entire cell population of the tumor) is correspondingly low: GF = 0 to 4.5% in low-grade astrocytomas, and GF = 1.7% to 32.2% in glioblastomas.[22] Flow cytometry of nuclear DNA in well-differentiated gliomas shows that most of the cells have the same ploidy (as a rule, they are diploid), with little variation from one area of the tumor to another. Malignant gliomas, by contrast, display hyperploidy (up to octaploid cells) or aneuploidy, and the ploidy varies from one area of the tumor to another.[12] The disordered distribution of nuclear DNA evidently betrays the disordered reproduction of cells in malignant gliomas. As PET shows, low-grade gliomas are quantitatively comparable in blood flow, oxygen utilization, and glucose consumption to the adjacent normal brain tissue. Although no difference exists in blood flow between low-grade and high-grade gliomas,[23] glucose consumption is much higher in the latter.[24] PET also shows, through the uptake of [^{11}C]L-methionine, a much higher rate of protein synthesis in high- than in low-grade gliomas.[25]

A mature glioma takes much longer to grow than does a glioblastoma. Noninvasive estimates have been made on serial CT scans, but few data exist on mature gliomas. Tsuboi and associates[26] evaluated the doubling time in four Grade II astrocytomas and mixed gliomas at 937.3 ± 66.5 days and compared this with 48.1 ± 20.9 days on 11 glioblastomas. In mature gliomas, the production of daughter cells must be almost exactly equal to cell loss and inactivation. Hoshino[27] supplied a theoretical basis for this clinical intuition.

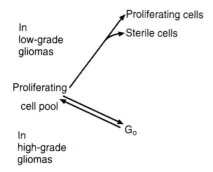

FIGURE 48-2 Cytodynamic of low-grade gliomas.

Determining the LI at necropsy in patients in whom it had been determined before operation, he found that, unlike immature gliomas, the well-differentiated varieties conserved the labeled cells for a long time. He, therefore, called this mode of cell proliferation of low-grade gliomas "conservative." In malignant gliomas, all the daughter cells proliferate, whereas in low-grade gliomas, one of two appears to retain the capacity for mitosis, whereas the other loses it. As a result, the proliferating pool grows moderately while sterile nonproliferating cells are continually being added to the cell population; therefore, the GF progressively slackens (Fig. 48-2).

However, the most worrying aspect of the biology of low-grade gliomas is the possibility alluded to earlier of malignant degeneration over time. In a study of 137 recurrent low-grade gliomas, Müller and co-workers[28] found that only 14% of Grade I astrocytomas had not changed grade by the time of the recurrence, whereas 55.5% had become Grade II, and 30.5% had become glioblastomas. Similarly, of 23 Grade I oligodendrogliomas, 15 (65.1%) had recurred as Grade II oligodendrogliomas and 2 (8.6%) as glioblastomas.[29] Laws and associates[14] found that at least half of the 79 low-grade astrocytomas in their series that recurred after treatment had advanced to Grade III or Grade IV. Zülch,[2] in a series of 104 supratentorial astrocytomas, found malignant degeneration in 23%. Rubinstein,[30] who studied 129 glioblastomas at necropsy, estimated that about 20% may have derived from the malignant degeneration of low-grade astrocytomas. Piepmeier found that over a median follow-up of 8 years, 50% of the astrocytomas and 10% of the oligodendrogliomas recurred as higher grade.[1] In the series of Wallner and co-workers,[31] 10 of the 29 patients with oligodendroglioma had a recurrence: at reoperation or at necropsy, only four had undergone no change, two had become glioblastomas, three had become Grade III mixed gliomas, and one had become a Grade II astrocytoma.

During the last 10 years, it has become evident that classification systems that are morphologically based are inadequate to describe either the biologic identity of these lesions or their biologic potential (malignant transformation).[32] The relevance of these features in the choice of therapeutic options and for determining a reliable prognosis has produced an overwhelming amount of studies on gliomas genetics and molecular biology, almost 75% of all the literature articles on the subject in recent years. A slow-growing tumor as the low-grade astrocytoma is expected to have a low proliferative activity. Many studies have identified as a measure of

this activity the percentage of astrocytoma cells expressing the proliferation antigen Ki-67 MIB-1 (expressed during the entire cell cycle) and the proliferating nuclear antigen (PCNA) (only expressed during S_1 phase). For a low-grade glioma the MIB-1 Labeling Index should not exceed 4%.[33,34] MIB-1 expression reflects differences in biologic behavior, such as the rapid progression of a residual tumor or stable remaining tumor. MIB-1 LI is reported to be lower in "quiescent" tumors.[35]

However, it is a common experience that a variable percentage (50% to 85%) of low-grade gliomas undergo malignant transformation. The molecular neuropathologic basis of this process is the summation of significant genetic alterations.

These mutations concern two categories of genes: (1) oncosuppressors and (2) oncogenes. As a consequence, the former will lose function in two stages. At the beginning, a copy of the gene is lost through an inactivating mutation, often a deletion. This situation may establish a predisposition to tumor formation. A second genetic event, however, is necessary for the complete inactivation of a suppressor gene. For oncogenes, mutations have an activating effect, and only one could be enough to induce a neoplastic phenotype.[36]

Cytogenetic analysis identified several alterations in pilocytic astrocytomas, but none is specific. In only few cases, a modification of oncosuppressor gene p53 has been described. Through a comparative genome hybridization technique, detecting losses and gains of DNA copy number across the entire genome, a constantly increased copy number of 8q emerged as the most frequent change in low-grade gliomas.[37]

Conversely, in diffuse astrocytomas, the p53 mutation is more frequent and may represent an indicator of malignant transformation. In fact, astrocytomas with a significant gemistocytic fraction, typically carrying a p53 mutation, seem to progress more rapidly.[38] Protoplasmic astrocytomas have low MIB-1 indices, and p53 reactivity is observed in a few of these tumors.[39]

p53 genes regulate the G_1 phase of the cell cycle that activates p21, and its inactivation seems to play a relevant role in neoplastic progression, determining further genomic instability.[40] However, the function of p53 appears also to prevent DNA rupture, duplication errors, and anomalous regional genomic amplification, therefore deserving the appellative of DNA caretaker. In fact, the cell cycle is normally stopped by p53 to allow repair; if the latter is not possible, the cell undergoes apoptosis. Moreover, p53 is claimed to function as genomic gatekeeper (i.e., regulate the expression of many genes).[41] There is evidence that the loss of only one allele for p53 increases the risk of tumorigenesis, suggesting that a decreased genic dosage is sufficient to compromise the surveillance function.[42] The implications for therapy of these data are evident. For instance, adenoviral vectors may carry a normal p53 gene in mutated tumoral cell nuclei.[43]

The cell kinetics of a low-grade glioma should differ only slightly from normal adult astrocytes, and the inactivation of p53 is a consequence not only of mutation or allelic loss but also of "transcriptional silencing."[44] The overexpression of Mdm2, establishing a linkage to mutant or wild-type p53, inhibits transcription.[45]

The overexpression of *PDGFRB* (encoding for a growth factor) and the mutations of *TP53*, inactivating the p53, have often been indicated as responsible for the proliferative stimulus, with the contemporary inhibition of apoptosis. *Bcl2* is a proto-oncogene that also blocks apoptosis.[46] Apoptosis is a sequence of morphologic and biochemical changes that lead to cell death. Tumorigenesis is the consequence not only of cell proliferation but also of the loss of the ability to undergo apoptosis. These events provide the necessary genomic instability for further phenotype changes, cell cycle deregulation, and the selection of malignant cell clones. Although in slow-growing gliomas the cell cycle is not deregulated, Grade II astrocytomas must have an imbalance between proliferative activity and apoptosis. Grade II astrocytomas have been divided in two groups with significantly different survival (1062 versus 1686 days), related to the value over or under 8% of the MIB-1 LI. The presence of well-differentiated astrocytes with a high MIB-1 LI suggests that cell cycle deregulation precedes further alterations with phenotypic transformation and that MIB-1 LI might be used as a prognostic indicator.[33]

There is still debate on the clonality of the resultant malignant tumors. The tumor originates from confluent clones of multiple transformed cells or from a single cell clone. Polymerase chain reaction assay studies through amplification of a high polymorphic microsatellite marker locus suggested that low-grade and malignant gliomas are usually monoclonal and that tumor cell migration represents the basis for extensively infiltrating tumors.[47] Different populations of cells with diverse genetic alterations may coexist in the same tumor, but this appears to be a transitional state, because the cell clone with the more efficient features of growth will rapidly prevail.

Loss of heterozygosity on chromosomes 19q and 1p are the most common reported alterations in oligodendrogliomas. The loss of a chromosome region carrying the residual copy of an oncosuppressor gene is revealed by a contiguous marker absence, using DNA amplification.[48]

Many factors that are intrinsic or extrinsic to the cell microenvironment keep under control the replication and differentiation of the neuroepithelial cell. Growth and trophic factors are small proteinic molecules identified in molecular biology studies that may represent potential pharmacologic agents to regulate neuroepithelial pathologic proliferation and differentiation. A peculiarity of this regulatory system is that the same factor may exert different and also opposite effects on neuroepithelial cells in different stages of differentiation or to neuroepithelial cells that belong to different parts of the nervous system.[49] This is probably the consequence of differences in number and type of growth factors receptors or of a fine modulatory intracellular process regarding transcription pathways of the signal generated after receptor–growth factor linkage. Therefore, tumors that are morphologically alike may differ substantially in their biologic behavior, as a result only of different receptor expression, thus disclosing further identification methods.

The transcriptional factors induce specific gene transcription, possibly modifying the cell phenotype. There are suggestions that activation of protein STAT 1 and STAT 2 by transcriptional factors allows differentiation toward an astrocytic phenotype of the neoplastic cells of the low-grade gliomas. Conversely, a differentiation to a high grade implies an inhibition of the pathway, determining lower levels of STAT proteins.[50] In view of future therapeutic application, this is evidence in favor of preservation of differentiation mechanisms also during oncogenesis.

Growth factors have been proved to determine the angiogenic potential of glioma cells, and angiogenesis has been used as a biologic marker for low-grade gliomas at risk of malignant transformation. Patients with more than seven microvessels counted on a 400-μm microscopic field of tumor tissue are reported to have a shorter survival time and a greater chance of tumor progression. Higher staining for vascular endothelial growth factor (VEGF) seems related to a worse prognosis.[51] Fibrillary astrocytomas, studied with determination of microvessel density and VEGF levels, appear not as a single pathologic entity but as a wide spectrum of tumors with differing tendencies toward malignant transformation. VEGF secretion may also represent the common pathway of microvascularization and progression to glioblastomas.[52] The p53 gene is thought to regulate VEGF and, consequently, tumor neovascularization.[53]

The recent progress in molecular neuropathology helped to discover anomalies of oncogenes and tumor suppressor genes, new sites for putative tumor suppressor genes (through microsatellite analysis), and peculiar molecular pathways for each tumor type. The presence of alterations in cell cycle regulatory genes of anaplastic gliomas may explain their amazing growth potential. Autocrine and paracrine growth factors and their respective protein receptors appear to contribute to glial and endothelial cell proliferation. The pattern of genetic alterations will help to further differentiate histopathologic entities into genetic distinct groups and to better define the mechanisms of angiogenesis. The common target is to establish a correlation between histopathologic, molecular, and clinical data.

NEURODIAGNOSTIC IMAGING

The "typical" imaging features for the diagnosis of a low-grade glioma in an adult patient were considered: CT scan hypodensity, without contrast enhancement; lack of contrast enhancement on a CT scan; hypointensity on short TR (repetition time) T1-weighted and hyperintensity on long TR T2-weighted MRI scans; no contrast enhancement on MRI.[54] Nevertheless, further experience has demonstrated the unreliability of these parameters also in high-standard radiodiagnostics. Forty-eight biopsies performed by Bernstein contradicted the radiologic diagnosis in 31.3% of cases, and a refutation of neuroimaging-based hypotheses followed the 20 bioptic procedures of Kondziolka in 50% of cases. Unrecognized pathologies included higher grade gliomas, oligodendrogliomas, mixed astrocytomas, and inflammatory lesions. However, the opinions of these authors are not convergent when the treatment of these patients has to be considered: histologic diagnostic confirmation with biopsy is imperative for Kondziolka, whereas Bernstein reserves biopsy for lesions that are very likely to be treated surgically. Bernstein recommends observation for others.[54,55]

Berger analyzed different MRI aspects of low-grade tumors while looking for a correlation with the histologic type. He concluded that no predictive value for histology exists in the presence of a cyst, the degree of mass effect, the cortical or subcortical location, the ratio of tumor volume T1-weighted versus T2-weighted, the diameter of the tumor, the presence of hemorrhage, or vascular flow voids. Only T1 hypointensity seems to correlate well with the softness of a tumor at surgery. This could be explained by the loose structure of astrocytoma presenting with a microcystic mesh with some degree of mucinous degeneration. Less hypointense lesions express a firmer architecture as typically seen in oligodendrogliomas and mixed astrocytomas.[56]

Further steps in characterization of low-grade gliomas with a propensity to malignant transformation and in tumor boundary definition are represented by PET and high-resolution magic angle spinning proton (HRMAS 1H) magnetic resonance.

[^{11}C]Methionine PET has been reported to be useful to detect changes in the endothelium and blood-brain barrier related to malignant low-grade glioma transformation.[57,58] It proved to be better than fluorodeoxyglucose in delineating the borders of low-grade gliomas, but methionine uptake cannot differentiate anaplastic gliomas.[59]

Some researchers have claimed that a thallium-201 single photon emission CT (^{201}Tl SPECT) scan can permit differential diagnosis between low-grade and high-grade gliomas.[60,61] Though less expensive than PET, it may give false-positive results in low-grade gliomas. It demonstrates high sensitivity for tumors with a bromodeoxyuridine LI equal or inferior to 5%.[62]

HRMAS 1H magnetic resonance spectroscopy produces well-resolved spectra of metabolites from an intact tissue specimen. The metabolic ratio presented the highest sensitivity in differentiating normal tissue from a tumor as well as in distinguishing between tumor groups. For instance, the resonance ratio of inositol to creatine may help to differentiate the tumor type.[63]

HRMAS 1H for choline showed that all progressive astrocytomas had elevated choline levels of more than 45%, whereas stable cases showed an elevation of less than 35%, no change, or even a decreased signal.[64-68]

1H nuclear magnetic resonance spectra of human brain tumor homogenates revealed a broad resonance at 5.3 to 5.4 ppm in glioblastomas and is not detectable in low-grade gliomas. This resonance has been identified as ceramide, a sphingosine–fatty acid combination portion of ganglioside (with an immunosuppressive activity), indicating an abundance of monounsaturated fatty acids. It is suggested a role for aberrant ganglioside and ceramide precursors in the grade of malignancy and invasiveness.[69]

There is evidence that no major difference exists between the PET investigation of glucose metabolism and the less expensive SPECT measurement of amino acid uptake(^{123}I-α-methyl tyrosine [[123]IMT]).[70-72]

MANAGEMENT DECISIONS

With the advances in neurodiagnostics, the pathology that confronts the clinician today is different from what it was 20 years ago, and this development requires new and more demanding decisions. In the days of angiography, encephalography, and radionuclide scanning, low-grade cerebral gliomas reached the surgeon after years of history, when they had grown large, with mass effect and signs of hypertension. These gliomas sometimes already contained foci of dedifferentiation inside. Today, at the first convulsive seizures, CT and MRI reveal small, less malignant tumors in patients who are neurologically intact. When it is considered that this pathology arises in young individuals on the convexity of a cerebral hemisphere, frequently beside "eloquent" cortical and subcortical areas, the magnitude of the dilemma facing the surgeon becomes clear.[73]

Although oncologic surgery should generally be performed as early and as radically as possible, some contend that an operation should be postponed when serial scanning shows no change in the volume or structure of the lesion. Others argue that biopsy plus radiotherapy is just as effective as surgical resection. Yet others[17] question the use of radiotherapy because of its long-term detrimental effects, asserting that because these patients never die as a result of a progression of the low-grade tumor but instead of its malignant degeneration, a management strategy designed to prevent dedifferentiation would be just as effective as eradication of the original tumor. The point is highly controversial and must be examined from several perspectives (Table 48-1).

Surgery is questioned first because of the risk of postoperative deficits in a young, neurologically sound patient with a long life expectancy. This situation requires the utmost precision in the diagnosis of the anatomic limits of the tumor and the functional status of the most important adjacent nervous structures.

Second, early surgery has yet to be proved to improve survival. As is discussed later in the section on Results, one of the issues in long-term survival is a long preoperative history. The follow-up study of Laws and co-workers,[74] which is one of the most important studies in terms of numbers and time span, makes this point.

Third, no proof exists that more generous resection correlates significantly with longer survival. A correlation of this kind, generally valid for any tumor, is argued by Salcman,[75] who cites Laws and associates.[14] However, although Laws and associates found a significantly higher 5-year survival rate among patients who had undergone total removal than among those who had undergone biopsy and subtotal removal or radical subtotal removal, statistical significance was not maintained at 15 years, total removal excluded. Furthermore, as these authors state, the most

TABLE 48-1 ■ Surgery in Low-Grade Gliomas

Indications	Reasons That Surgery Is Questionable
Diagnosis and classification	Risk of postoperative deficits in a young, neurologically sound patient with a long life expectancy
Debulking the mass and alleviating symptoms	
Reducing the proliferating cell pool	Early surgery has not been proved to lengthen survival
Decreasing the number of cells inherently resistant to radiation therapy	There is no significant correlation between the extent of surgical resection and the length of survival
Preventing or reducing the risk of increase in malignancy	
Cytoreduction makes subsequent radiotherapy more effective	
Chemotherapy has proved ineffective in all cases	

favorable lesions tend to be treated more radically, and the least favorable (deep-seated, infiltrative, noncystic) more sparingly. Weir and Grace,[76] Piepmeier,[16] and Vertosick and colleagues[17] deny any significant correlation between the extent of surgical resection and the length of survival.

All these points, which tend to undermine the importance of surgery in low-grade cerebral gliomas, are counterbalanced by the following considerations, according to which surgery is indicated: (1) for diagnosis and classification, (2) for debulking the mass and relieving symptoms, (3) for reducing the proliferating cell pool, (4) for preventing or reducing the risk of degeneration, (5) for decreasing the number of cells inherently refractory to radiotherapy, (6) because cell reduction makes subsequent radiotherapy more effective, and (7) because chemotherapy has proved ineffective.

Each of these assertions calls for comment. First, surgery is valuable as a diagnostic check on a patch of low density on a CT scan and on one of low intensity in the T1 sequences and of increased intensity in the T2 sequences of MRI. A tumor must be differentiated from an infective or vascular lesion, and the borders of the tumor must be demarcated from the surrounding edema. The tumor must be typed not only histologically but also, if possible, for proliferative potential by immunochemistry (monoclonal antibodies to bromodeoxyuridine for the LI and antigen to Ki-67 for the GF). For these purposes, stereotactic surgery may be preferred to open surgery, a point that is discussed in Chapter 52. Surgical resection is needed for debulking the mass and palliating symptoms when a glioma is discovered at a late stage and has already grown large. In any case, surgical resection reduces the proliferating pool and delays the growth of the tumor. As Hoshino[27] pointed out, low-grade gliomas differ from more malignant gliomas in the lack of cellular traffic between the nonproliferating pool and the proliferating pool (see Fig. 48-2). In low-grade gliomas, the conservative mode of proliferation ensures the continual addition to the cell population of sterile, permanently nonproliferating cells (for which there is no return to the reproductive cycle). In glioblastoma, by contrast, frequent reciprocal traffic exists between nonproliferating and proliferating cells: its growth may be depressed by cell bunching; partial surgical resection may stimulate the cells in G_0 to return to the proliferating pool and thus end, paradoxically, by accelerating tumor growth. Nonetheless, surgical resection, however satisfactory, is always limited. As Sano[77] reminded us, 99% removal of a tumor corresponds with only a 2-log reduction of the number of cells that constitute a neoplastic population (10^7 to 10^8).

As we have seen, at the time of a recurrence, low-grade gliomas exhibit increased malignancy and resistance to treatment. Because it is not known which cells will be subject to dedifferentiation or what factors contribute to the process, the risk is presumably proportional to the number of neoplastic cells. Therefore, the most extensive cytoreduction possible should be advantageous. In addition, no one has ever suggested that surgical resection may favor dedifferentiation. On the evidence of Vertosick and associates,[17] two points emerge: (1) Patients who present dedifferentiation tended to be diagnosed at a younger age than did those who did not (mean of 33 vs. 43 years), and (2) those who received radiotherapy underwent dedifferentiation an average of 5.4 years later than did those who did not

(3.7 years later). However, these data are preliminary and have not been statistically validated.

When does a low-grade glioma degenerate—that is, at what stage in its natural history? How can the change be detected in time? Clinical experience shows that dedifferentiation occurs several years after the initial symptoms of the tumor—on average 5 years after in the 12 cases of Francavilla and co-workers,[78] with a range of 1.5 to 10 years. PET with [^{18}F]-deoxyglucose is currently the most sensitive tool for detecting incipient malignant transformation, which manifests increased metabolism (increased glucose consumption), is focal (in agreement with the histologic data), and is similar to the hypermetabolic state observed in de novo malignant gliomas. One PET scan at one point in the natural history may not have predictive value, any more than does a histologic examination performed at that time. Serial PET scans are needed to identify variations in the biologic behavior of a tumor.

Apart from all the foregoing reasons, surgical resection is indicated in low-grade gliomas because no concrete alternative exists, given their biologic resistance to chemotherapy and scant sensitivity to radiotherapy. The cellular kinetics and metabolism of these oncotypes, which differ little from those of healthy nervous tissue, and the integrity of the blood-brain barrier prevent cytostatic agents from entering the tumor with a higher concentration gradient than that of the surrounding healthy tissue.[75] Radiotherapy is recommended in only a few cases, as is discussed later.

In conclusion, we can share in part the statements of Bernstein[79] regarding the presumed absence of negative prognostic indicators in a patient younger than 40 years of age, with epilepsy but without neurologic deficits, harboring a low-density intrinsic lesion, without enhancement and without mass effect. As mentioned, molecular markers may enhance the predictive accuracy. For a patient older than 40 years, with or without neurologic deficits, mass effect, or enhancement, we think that more aggressive treatment should be considered. For lobar lesions, we recommend the most radical surgery followed by radiotherapy; for deeper or "diffuse" lesions (particularly if located in "eloquent" areas), stereotactic biopsy and radiotherapy should be the treatment of choice.

PATIENT SELECTION AND CHOICE OF SURGICAL APPROACH

The conditions in favor of surgical treatment for slow-growing gliomas outweigh those in favor of waiting or abstaining both in number and in importance.

The surgical choice is between open resection and stereotactic surgery followed by other treatment (irradiation or interstitial radiotherapy). The criteria for the stereotactic option depend, according to Salcman,[80] on the characteristics of: (1) the tumor (centrally sited, poorly demarcated, extremely small, containing a large cyst or changing character), (2) the patient (either too ill for a craniotomy or neurologically intact), and (3) subsequent treatment (catheter-based, requires repeated sampling). "In essence, the same criteria employed in the selection of open versus closed techniques can be applied to low-grade tumors, but with more stringent emphasis on neurologic condition and radiographic definition."[75] In summary, in the case of low-grade cerebral glioma, as for almost all other central nervous system diseases, surgical treatment must be tailored to the neurologic status and social needs of the patient, to the site and size of the lesion, to the ability of the surgeon, and to the facilities available to him or her. General directives can come only from randomized prospective studies conducted over a sufficiently long time by several institutions on series matched for pathology, patient selection, and management.

PREOPERATIVE EVALUATION

The brain is a singular organ in that many of its main functions are represented on its surface. Areas of the cortex both near and distant are connected subcortically by short and long associative fibers. A surgeon preparing to approach a subcortical hemispheric glioma traditionally has the problem of tumor projection to the surface in relation to the functionally most important cortex and its principal projections. Neuroimaging now solves this problem noninvasively. The rolandic fissure, which delineates the sensorimotor cortex, has always been the pole star of the topography of the cerebral cortex, something that Giacomini intuited in Turin in 1878.[81] That the rolandic fissure is the pole star does not, of course, apply to polar so much as to "central" sites: it is no accident that in the English-speaking world, the rolandic fissure is the central sulcus and the rolandic convolutions, the precentral and postcentral gyri. On the basis of careful studies on cadavers, Giacomini found a way of projecting the central sulcus onto the skull surface by means of an ingenious pair of cardboard compasses. The transverse line from ear to ear, intercepted at the vertex by the sagittal midline, is divided into segments, one on either side. When the vertical leg of the compasses is centered on the central

point of one segment, the other leg, inclined at 30 degrees, identifies the sulcus (Fig. 48-3). Constant in site, unlikely to be displaced, especially in its medial portion, the pararolandic cortex is now detectable in the highest axial CT cuts (Fig. 48-4). Parasagittal MRI sections locate the central sulcus through the cingulate and marginal sulci. Less accurately, the lower half of the rolandic cortex is shown adjacent to the lateral sulcus: lateral sagittal MRI sections identify it with the perpendicular to the posterior roof of the insula (Fig. 48-5).[82] To identify the whole length of the central sulcus, 3-dimensional MRI is needed.[83] Imaged on the lateral surface of the hemisphere are also the inferior frontal gyrus and the superior temporal gyrus, which in the left hemisphere comprise Broca's area and the auditory area, respectively. Thus, a large part of the cortex, which is known traditionally as being "eloquent," is located via the rolandic area.

This precise anatomic definition supplied by neuroimaging may not be sufficient for planning and performing the operation for several reasons. First, the anatomic structures may be displaced or distorted, especially by slow-growing space-occupying lesions such as the ones that we are considering; therefore, the anatomic landmarks may be unreliable. The surgical damage feared by surgeons on the basis of the standard anatomic landmarks is, surprisingly and fortunately, not usually found in the postoperative course. Second, major centers and nervous pathways may or may not be infiltrated, damaged, or interrupted by the neoplastic process; the surgeon should know their functional status. Third, although the sensorimotor cortex is more constant in its anatomy, the cortex related to language and cognitive functions has a much more variable and complex organization, hence the need to see the functional data for the various cortical areas alongside

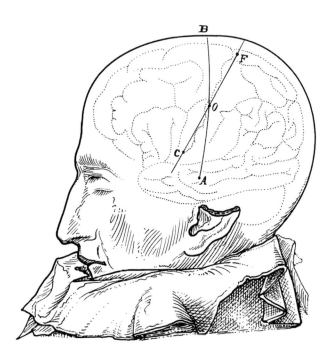
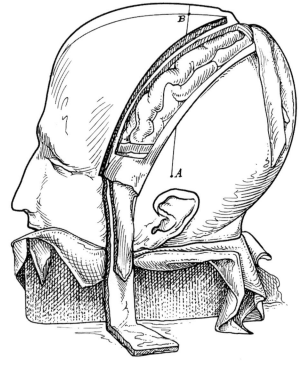

FIGURE 48-3 Goniometric identification of the central sulcus. (From Giacomini C: Guida allo studio delle circonvoluzioni cerebrali dell'uomo, 2nd ed. Torino: E Loescher, 1884.)

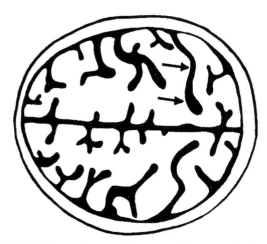

FIGURE 48-4   Tomographic aspect of the central sulcus.

or superimposed on the anatomic images. PET and single photon emission CT, which supply quantitative maps of physiologic, biochemical, and biophysical parameters but have poor spatial anatomic resolution, are superimposed on CT and MRI in the "computerized brain atlas."[84–87] The performance of various motor, verbal, and cognitive tasks or sensory stimulation is known to show a constant focal increase on PET, both in the glucose metabolism and in regional cerebral blood flow in certain areas of the cerebral cortex. For practical reasons, the regional blood flow has been investigated by use of $H_2{}^{15}O$. Once again, the rolandic cortex has proved to be the easiest to study, both on the motor side and on the sensory side: images are altered during either the performance of simple motor tasks involving a single limb or during sensory stimulation of it. Language, being a more complex function, still defies precise localization: numerous areas of the cortex and circuits are involved in the act of repeating words heard or of generating new ones; the nervous pathways activated in the production of new words and in getting used to them (repeating a list of names) are numerous. PET performed on volunteers and the speech map obtained by Ojemann and co-workers[88] by intraoperative

stimulation (arrest or error in naming known objects presented) agree on the following: (1) extreme individual variation, (2) language cannot be located reliably on purely anatomic criteria, and (3) the traditional area of Broca needs to be revised.

Nariai and colleagues[89] pointed out that a glioma may be located within a single gyrus without altering its external morphology. Alternatively, a tumor may cause swelling or distortion of the cortical surface of the gyrus. In the latter situation, 3-dimensional MRI may not warrant the identification of "eloquent" areas, and the functional mapping with PET [^{11}C]methionine seems to offer the necessary accuracy. Localization of speech, motor, and memory function is now achieved with good accuracy by functional MRI (fMRI), but it still represents only a surrogate guide to neurophysiologic intraoperative methods.[90,91]

ANESTHETIC CONSIDERATIONS AND AIDS TO SURGERY

Craniotomy for cerebral glioma is almost always performed with the patient under general anesthesia and with monitoring of various parameters (e.g., electrocardiographic reading, arterial pressure, central venous pressure, and blood gas analysis) and checking of the fluid balance. Black and Ronner[92] and Walsh and associates[93] have mapped the sensorimotor and language cortex in a few cooperative patients by use of electrical stimulation while the patients were under local anesthesia. Systemic anesthetic agents were used occasionally on completion of the mapping studies. Ebeling and colleagues[94] localized the motor cortex intraoperatively with patients under general anesthesia and with temporary decurarization. However, these are all isolated experiments. Somatosensory evoked potentials are more widely used for illustrating the rolandic cortex when tumors are adjacent to it. They require appropriate screening of the operating room to reduce artifacts. For cortical mapping, Berger and colleagues[95] operate on patients who are awake with mild fentanyl sedation, using a local anesthetic for the scalp. Alternatively, during bone flap removal, propofol provides a deep sedative effect that can be reversed in 10 minutes.

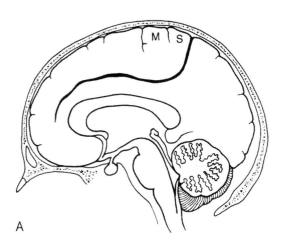

A

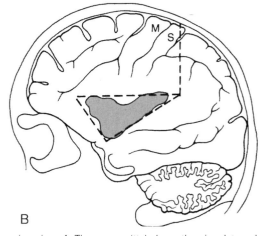

B

FIGURE 48-5   Geometric identification of central sulcus on magnetic resonance imaging. *A,* The parasagittal plane: the cingulate sulcus ends superiorly as the marginal sulcus (MS). *B,* The far lateral sagittal plane (*dashed line*).

Obviously, the operating microscope and microsurgical instruments, bipolar cautery, ultrasonic aspirators, and laser equipment are now part of routine neurosurgical practice. B-mode ultrasound with surface ultrasound probes is also useful in cases of subcortical glioma, as is explained later.

Last, the previous spatial incompatibility—recently resolved by "portable" CT and "in-built" MRI—between cumbersome neurodiagnostic machines and operating room demands, and also between stereotactic frames and freehand surgery, prompted few leading centers to develop sophisticated and complex equipment. The precision of stereotactic methods is often needed in the surgery for gliomas.

SURGICAL TECHNIQUE

Craniotomy

The importance of neuroimaging, especially with 3-dimensional MRI, in highlighting simultaneously the tumor and the layout of the cortex of the entire cerebral hemisphere concerned with its main sulci and gyri has already been discussed. The cerebral hemisphere can, furthermore, be sectioned according to various planes on the computer display to illustrate the relations between the tumor and the deep-seated structures (e.g., internal capsule, basal nuclei, and ventricular cavities). MR angiography relies on "angiographic" pulse sequences that potentiate the signal from the blood flow at the expense of that from the static tissues. Thus, the relations between the tumor and the cerebral vascular network are studied on the 3-dimensional model both on the surface of the hemisphere and in sections. The structural features of the tumor (e.g., cysts, calcifications, or necrosis) are also illustrated. As mentioned, functional data from eloquent structures may also be integrated by fMRI.

Knowing the volume and spatial disposition of the neoplastic mass in relation to the eloquent cortex and to no less eloquent deep structures can permit simulation of a test flap on the computer screen. This image is then projected onto the image of the skull surface and transferred to the patient's head either by means of external points of reference (e.g., eye, ear, previous operation scar) or stereotactically. It is not transferred by a conventional stereotactic procedure, because the frame or ring would obstruct the operative field and is unsuitable for freehand surgery, such as that required for gliomas.

Frameless stereotactic surgery is performed by means of a localizing arm.[96] The five-part jointed arm operated by the surgeon is connected to a graphic-oriented computer (Fig. 48-6). Its tip, which runs along the surface of the skull, records the coordinates of each point on it in relation to reference points consisting of three metal pins, which are lodged noncolinearly in sterile conditions (under local anesthesia) in the patient's scalp. These skull markers, which appear on the two CT scout scans (anteroposterior and lateral), likewise constitute the points of reference of the CT coordinates. Because the arm coordinates and CT coordinates are correlated in the same computer, after appropriate calibration the tip of the localizing arm that runs along the skull surface is shown on the CT scan by a cursor. The optimal approach to the underlying tumor, even if it is small, can easily be centered. The craniotomy is thus targeted and personalized. It may consist of a trephine hole 4 to 5 cm in diameter. The chosen approach need not be the most direct, but it must be the safest for the neurologic integrity of the patient.

Cortical Approach

In surgeries for subcortical lesions that do not emerge on the surface, the following procedure is used. After the dura mater is opened, the surgeon has to recognize the tumor, size up its spatial relations with the adjacent structures, and decide where to incise the cortex. B-mode ultrasound[97,98] now replaces manual palpation: it localizes the tumor in relation to the cortex, to the underlying ventricle, to the falx, to the tentorium, or to the bony base; it also characterizes the tumor structure (calcifications or secluded cysts), specifies its volume,[99] and demarcates its margins.

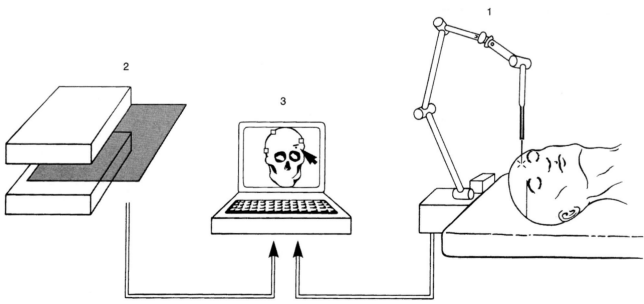

FIGURE 48-6 Frameless stereotactic surgery system. See text for details.

Although CT shows low-grade gliomas as hypodense, ultrasonography shows them as hyperechogenic.[98] The surrounding edema appears as hypoechogenic or very faintly echogenic against the healthy parenchyma.[99]

Even when the dura mater has been opened, recognition of the eloquent cortex and its relations with paracentral tumors is not necessarily straightforward. The smallness of the craniotomy opening, the extreme variability of the morphology of the cortical sulci even in normal individuals, and the asymmetry of a given sulcus in the two hemispheres may make recognition of the areas of reference difficult,[100] the more so because of the adjacent pathology. Once again, neurophysiologic methods are helpful, mainly in the topography of the rolandic cortex. Easiest to obtain and most constant (reproducible) is the cortical representation of the hand by somatosensory evoked potentials on stimulation of the contralateral median nerve. With the patient under general anesthesia, the topography of the hand is clear on both gyri separated by the central sulcus. The potentials are approximately mirrored in form on the two sides, the P_{20}–N_{30} waves being of greater amplitude in the precentral area and the N_{20}–P_{30} waves in the postcentral area (Fig. 48-7).[101] Focal somatosensory evoked potentials of great amplitude have also been obtained from the posterosuperior bank of the Sylvian fissure. Could this be a secondary somatosensory area?[102] Unfortunately, evoked potentials are not as helpful in identifying the visual and auditory cortex intraoperatively.

The cortex involved in the expression of language can only be demarcated by stimulation with the patient under local anesthesia. Electrostimulation of the cortex, pioneered by Bartholow[103] and Horsley[104] and later systematized by Penfield and Boldrey,[105] still has applications for delineation of speech areas,[88] as already discussed. Whatever the means used, the neurophysiologic and/or neuroradiologic identification of the eloquent cortex are an aid not only in the planning of an operation but also in its execution.[106,107] Because of possible displacement by the tumor, the surgeon is freer to be more aggressive than if he or she is working only from anatomic landmarks.

However, is there really a "silent" cortex? Brodmann's areas 1 through 7, 17 through 19, 27 through 28, and (in the dominant hemisphere) 40 through 45 are considered to be eloquent (Fig. 48-8). The problem with the remainder of the cortex is that it gives no elementary responses to stimulation; rather it is involved in complex mechanisms of neurophysiologic and neuropsychologic integration, and it does not give signals in laboratory animals that are easily applied to humans. Furthermore, although projection fibers (motor, special, or general sensory) underlie the eloquent cortex, short and long intrahemispheric associative fibers underlie the rest.

Desire to spare the lobar cortex and underlying fibers as far as possible has led to the proposal of the transsulcal surgical approach[108,109]: by using these natural corridors, the surgeon can go down 2 to 3 cm in pseudo depth without incising tissue, thus remaining outside the brain. Furthermore, because the sulci, especially the major ones, are full of fluid, their opening ensures decompressive depletion, hence the renewed interest in the anatomy of the cerebral sulci.[100,110] Several varieties of sulci are recognized: axial, limiting, opercular, and complete (Fig. 48-9). Their extreme variation from one individual to another and between hemispheres in a single individual is confirmed, and efforts are being made to define the numerous ways in which one sulcus continues with another (full, partial, or simulated communication). The depth of some sulci has been measured on several specimens: the superior frontal sulcus is 17 to 24 mm deep; the superior temporal, 15 to 25 mm; and the junction of the interparietal with the postcentral sulcus, 20 to 27 mm.[111] The course of the blood vessels in the sulci is not uniform: some descend to the bottom of the sulcus before penetrating the brain substance, whereas others only cross the sulcus to rise to the top of the adjacent gyrus.[69] In either case, they are easily dissected between the arachnoid trabeculations of the sulcus or retracted toward one or the other gyrus with a spatula. An advantage of a transsulcal over a transgyral incision is that the cortex is less thick at the bottom of a sulcus than at the summit of a gyrus. A disadvantage is that an incision at the bottom of a sulcus interrupts the subcortical associative U-shaped fibers that connect two neighboring gyri.

On superficial inspection, deciding which sulcus to approach is not always easy. The arachnoid must be incised at several points to distinguish first the deep from the shallow sulci and from a sulcus-like impression of an artery on the cortex (Fig. 48-10).[6] Rarely, minute blood vessels obstruct

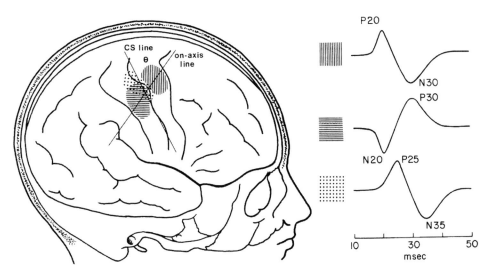

FIGURE 48-7 Somatosensory evoked potential–guided mapping of the cortical sensory (CS) motor area. (From Wood CC, Spencer DD, Allison T, et al: Localization of human sensory motor cortex during surgery by cortical surface recording of somatosensory evoked potentials. J Neurosurg 68:99–111, 1988.)

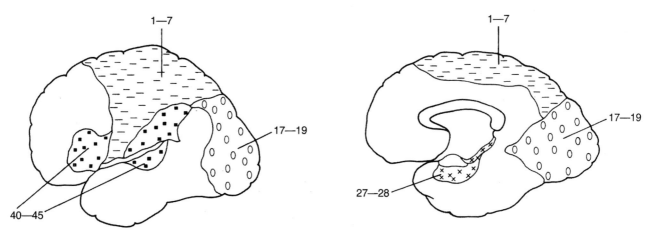

FIGURE 48-8 Schematic topography of eloquent cortical regions of the brain.

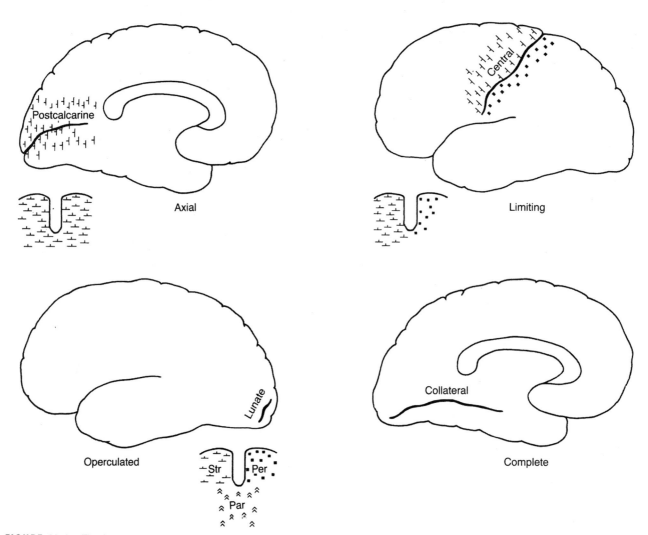

FIGURE 48-9 The four types of cortical sulci: Axial: an infolding in homogeneous areas. Limiting: separates the cortex into two areas different in both morphology and function. Operculated: separates distinct functional areas at its entrance, and often a third area of function is present in its floor—for example, the lunate sulcus separating with its walls the striate (Str), peristriate (Per), and parastriate (Par) areas. Complete: that which is so deep that it produces an elevation in the ventricular walls.

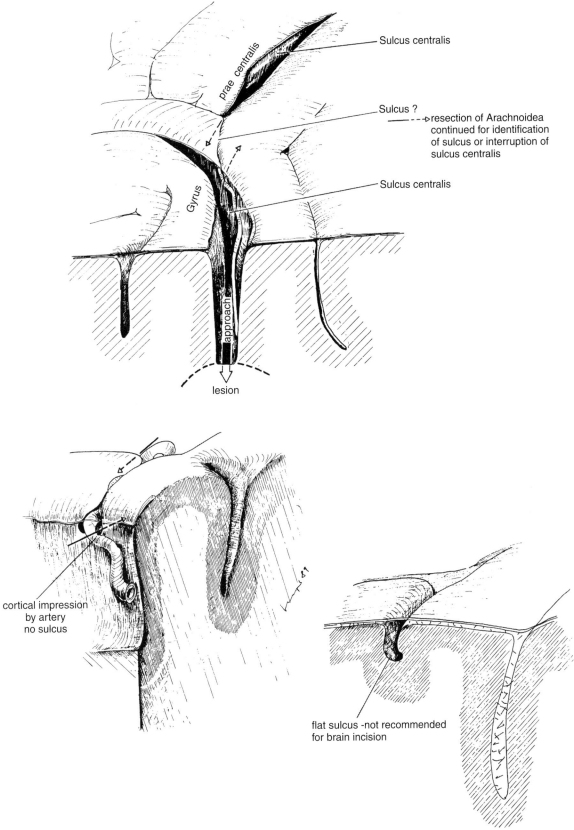

FIGURE 48-10 The arachnoid has to be incised at several points in order to distinguish the deep sulci from a sulcus-like impression of an artery on the cortex. (From Seeger W: Strategies of Microsurgery in Problematic Brain Areas. Vienna: Springer-Verlag, 1990, p 13.)

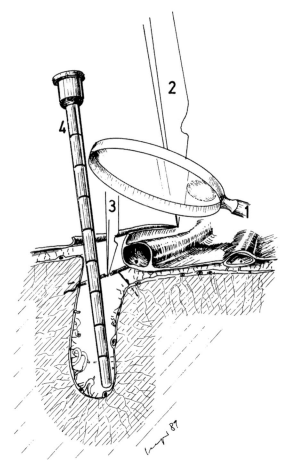

FIGURE 48-11 Sulcal approach strategies. 1, Lens; 2 and 3, scalpel; 4, Cushing needle. (From Seeger W: Strategies of Microsurgery in Problematic Brain Areas. Vienna: Springer-Verlag, 1990, p 11.)

access to a sulcus; if they do, they must be cauterized and cut (Fig. 48-11). Not only must the depth of the sulcus be noted but also its orientation with respect to the cortical plane. In normal brains, the sulci are almost perpendicular to the surface. A subcortical tumor diverts their course (Fig. 48-12). The tumor, therefore, must be sought via the compressed and oblique deep sulci. The incision does not have to be made at the bottom of the sulcus; it can be made in a lateral wall if the latter is closer to the tumor (Fig. 48-13).[6] Both in the transsulcal approach and in the transgyral approach, the primary branches of the superficial arteries can still be dissected fairly comfortably because they remain outside the parenchyma in the perivascular spaces.

Because the operating microscope is an optic instrument, it is Yasargil's impression that the divergence of the light beams allows the surgeon to work at a depth of 10 to 12 cm through an opening 1.5 cm long and 0.5 cm wide (Fig. 48-14).[109] However small the cortical incision is, it nonetheless interrupts an enormous number of neurons and their connections and fibers. A wedge of cortex with a section that is 1 mm² and 2.5 mm deep contains up to 60,000 neurons. Neuronal density varies, of course, from one area of the cortex to another, being greatest in the striate area and lowest, perhaps, in the precentral gyrus.

Tumor Resection

Microsurgical debulking of the tumor proceeds piecemeal from its center to its periphery. The resultant cavity is cleared with a spatula only when it allows gentle, nontraumatic retraction of the adjacent tissue. Last comes resection of the peripheral zone of tumor infiltration, which is biologically the most active because it consists of the largest number of neoplastic cells proliferating and migrating into the adjacent tissue.

The operative plane is established according to the objective conditions of the tumor and subjective variables relating to the surgeon and the patient.[80] The following situations cover most cases (Fig. 48-15)[6]:

1. Superficial tumor infiltrating only one gyrus: Tumor resection must spare the long fibers projecting to neighboring gyri and converging deep to the tumor margins. Preservation of vessels is the main problem.
2. Tumor infiltrating more than one gyrus on the surface: A larger number of long projection fibers is sacrificed, but other long fibers converging from the healthy cortex must be spared in depth.
3. Diffuse subcortical tumor: Resection deafferents the underlying intact cortex and intercepts a certain number of intact fibers.

For solid gliomas diffusely infiltrating the centrum ovale, a lobectomy is not indicated, because it does not prolong life and results in psychologic deficits. This type of tumor develops deeper than the cortex. Under the cortex, the limits to resection are the allocortical areas, the basal nuclei, and the internal capsule. A selective tumorectomy, whether centrotumoral or including as much as possible of the marginal zone, affords the same survival and better health. The rare cystic astrocytomas of the cerebral hemispheres are much less of a surgical problem. The pilocytic variety is particularly favorable, because simple resection of the mural nodule yields a good short and long-term result, whether the cyst wall is completely removed or not. There are suggestions that contrast enhancement of the cyst wall at CT or MR requires its complete removal to ensure radicality.[112] Brachytherapy has been used for small tumors and restricted to selected areas of the brain. Sealed radioactive isotopes, such as ¹⁹²Ir or ¹²⁵I, are stereotactically positioned usually in cases of a recurrence of a postsurgical glioma.[113]

Ultrasonic aspiration[114] has several advantages over the former combined use of aspirating cannula and electric loop in the debulking of a solid tumor. A single instrument leaves the operating field more free of instruments, minimizes mechanical damage to nervous tissue (traction), and eliminates damage resulting from heating. Observed in slow motion, the ultrasonic aspirator works in three stages: (1) fragmentation of the tissue adjacent to the vibrating tip within a radius of not more than 2 mm, (2) suspension of the fragmented tissue in irrigating fluid supplied by the instrument, and (3) aspiration of the aqueous emulsion. The power of the vibrating tip and of aspiration is adjustable. The speed of action depends on the consistency of the tissue to be removed. However, the lower the power of fragmentation, the less damage will occur to the vascular framework. Fragmentation is selective for a tissue with a large aqueous component and spares the vessel walls, which

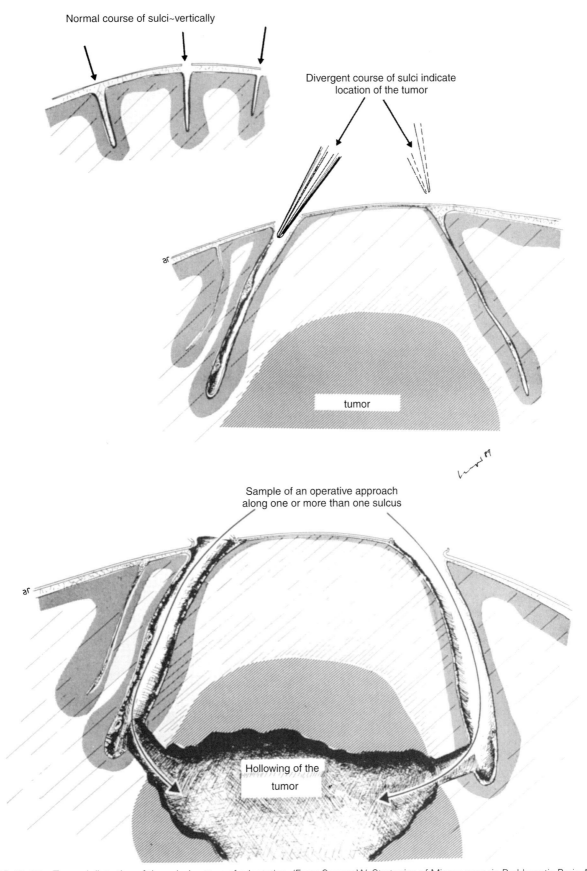

Normal course of sulci~vertically

Divergent course of sulci indicate location of the tumor

tumor

Sample of an operative approach along one or more than one sulcus

Hollowing of the tumor

FIGURE 48-12 Tumoral distortion of the sulcal pattern of orientation. (From Seeger W: Strategies of Microsurgery in Problematic Brain Areas. Vienna: Springer-Verlag, 1990, p 15.)

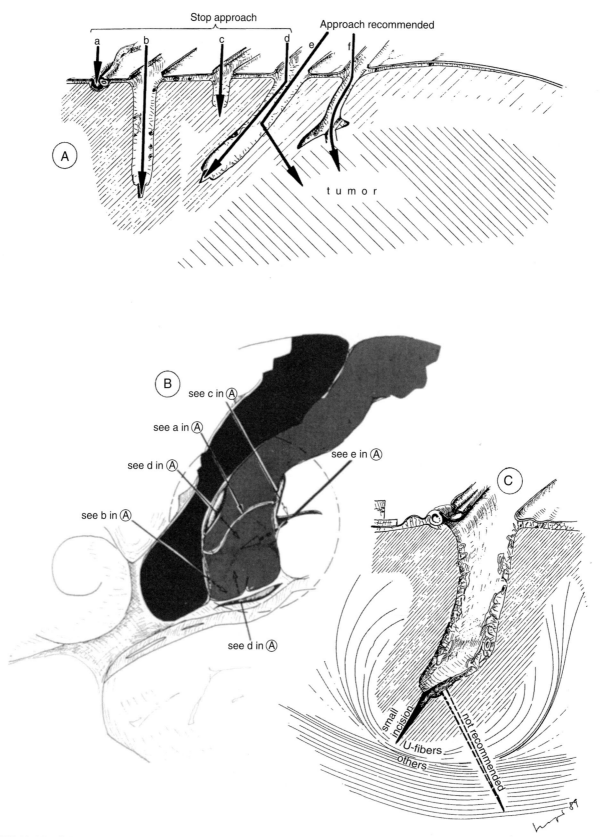

FIGURE 48-13 Sulcal approach strategies. (From Seeger W: Strategies of Microsurgery in Problematic Brain Areas. Vienna: Springer-Verlag, 1990, p 17.)

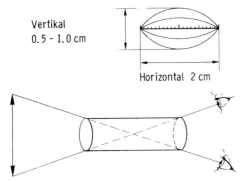

Vertikal
0.5 - 1.0 cm

Horizontal 2 cm

FIGURE 48-14 Optic effect in the operating microscope. (From Yasargil MG, Cravens GF, Roth P: Surgical approaches to "inaccessible" brain tumors. Clin Neurosurg 34:42–110, 1988. Copyright © Williams & Wilkins.)

have collagenous and elastic components. The tiny vessels are freed from the surrounding parenchyma and are easily cauterized without being torn. Hard or moderately calcified, poorly vascularized, low-grade gliomas are an elective indication for the ultrasonic aspirator. Because the instrument does not provide for hemostasis, this is handled by bipolar coagulation. An aspirator with an ultrasonic vibrating tip is useful not only in the debulking of the central mass of a glioma but also in the dissection of its peripheral margins, which are very indistinct. The instrument gives the operator some tactile feedback on the tissue encountered and thus warns him or her of variations in resistance in the transition from the tumor to the surrounding edema or healthy tissue.

The 1970s brought another very useful aid to tumor resection: the laser beam. The carbon dioxide laser is preferred both for incising the cortex and for debulking the tumor.[115–117] Introduced by Patel in 1965, it operates at a wavelength of 10.6 m. It emits an invisible beam in the far infrared zone, which is absorbed by water and thus may be applied to all tissues. It vaporizes the water content of tissues; when appropriate, the penetration depth is only 0.2 mm into soft tissue. The advantages of this immaterial knife include: (1) precise dissection of the tumor mass, (2) speed, (3) vaporization of deep tumor processes with a nontouch technique, and (4) less risk of surgical infection because the laser knife not only has sterilizing effects but also does not touch the tissues. In addition, because it has no electromagnetic field, it does not stimulate the nervous structures or interfere with the electrophysiologic monitoring equipment (e.g., electrocardiogram, electroencephalogram, and pulse rate). The disadvantages are the cumbersomeness of the equipment, the risk of explosion of anesthetic gases because of the high temperatures that the laser beam may reach (1700 °C to 1800 °C), and the restriction of hemostasis to vessels with a diameter of less than 0.5 mm. Because of the last feature, the carbon dioxide laser beamis indicated for low-grade gliomas. In more vascularized tumors (glioblastomas or angioblastic meningiomas), which require greater capacity for hemostasis, the neodymium:yttrium aluminum garnet laser is more suitable.

When a tumor is massive and superficial, it is best to use a focusing laser beam to shorten the vaporization time; in deep regions of the brain, the tumor should be vaporized

with a defocused beam with continuous movement to avoid injury to the normal deep structures.

Last, laser technology has rekindled the recurrent interest in the possibility of inducing fluorescence by tissue photosensitizers to discover the tumor margins in the course of surgery. New generations of photosensitizing agents (phthalocyanine) have been proposed.[118]

Haglund and co-workers[119] developed a technique of optic image enhancement with intravenous injection of indocyanine green. This method allows the surgeon to differentiate normal brain, low-grade gliomas, and high-grade gliomas as an effect of different dynamics of optic signals. The technique also provides a clear image of the resection margins in malignant tumors during surgical removal. An analogous method developed by Allen and Maciunias at Vanderbilt University[56] involves the use of implanted fiducial markers combined with an infrared tracking system relating fiducial-based images to the position of the tip of an infrared probe, with an estimated error of less than 1 mm. Both the techniques are based on the different light penetration coefficient of tissues, due to the optic characteristics of the tissue and to the wavelength of the light.

It has always been the surgeon's dream to have visual control of his or her work during the surgery. Some information is supplied by intraoperative ultrasound: tumor residues are shown to be hyperechogenic. A close correspondence was demonstrated between low-grade glioma volumes evaluated with neuroimaging techniques and the volumes found intraoperatively using ultrasound-based methods.[99] However, previous radiation therapy may generate hyperechogenic false-positive images due to gliosis.

Intraoperative neurophysiologic methods are likely to make a contribution that is of theoretical rather than practical interest. King and Schell[102] noted that somatosensory evoked potentials increase in amplitude as tumor debulking proceeds. Whether the phenomenon depends on improved cerebral perfusion (general effect) or on decompression of fibers of the internal capsule that project to the cortex lying against the tumor mass (local effect) is unknown.

Since 1985, the problem has been moving to a more brilliant solution, based on sophisticated imaging techniques.[120] The principle is similar to that of the Guthrie-Adler localizing arm. A jointed sensor arm tells a computer the position of its tip in the cranial cavity (Fig. 48-16). The preoperative CT (or MRI or angiographic) findings are projected on the computer display. The fiducial points are three metal markers (for CT) or three fat-filled capsules (for MRI) affixed to the nasion and the two tragi with adhesive tape (Fig. 48-17). After calibration, the machine gives the surgeon the spatial position of the tip of the sensor arm as it is moved over the neuroimages. The arm, fixed to the Mayfield headrest, is introduced into the operative field only when the surgeon wants to know the exact position of the tip. The margin of error is around 2 mm, negligible in open surgery, in which the target inevitably moves during the procedure (respiratory movements or vascular pulsations). Watanabe and associates[120,121] called the instrument a "neuronavigator."

In recent years, although the routine use of this apparatus spread diffusely and many different models have been released by the industry, few reports appeared in the literature specifically addressing the surgical treatment of low-grade gliomas.

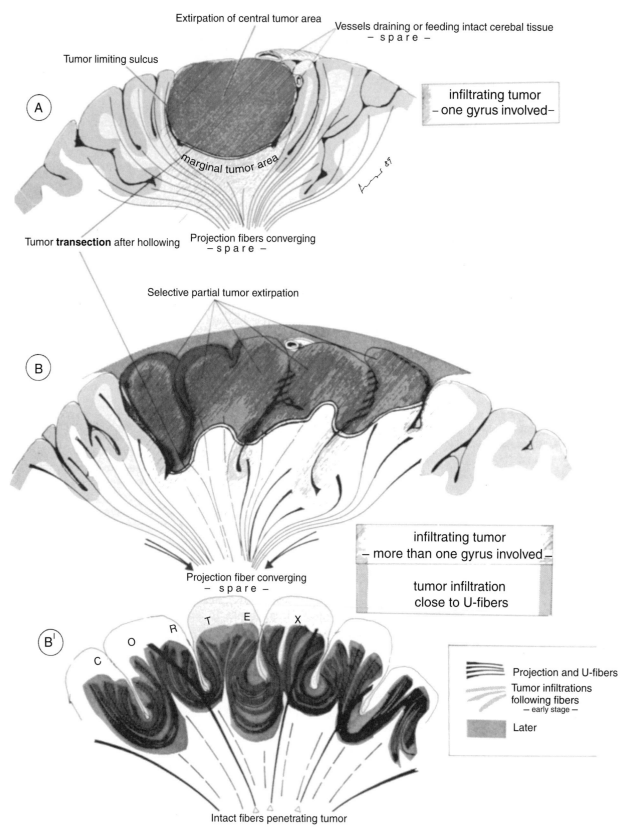

FIGURE 48-15   Different patterns of glioma infiltration. (From Seeger W: Strategies of Microsurgery in Problematic Brain Areas. Vienna: Springer-Verlag, 1990, p 21.)

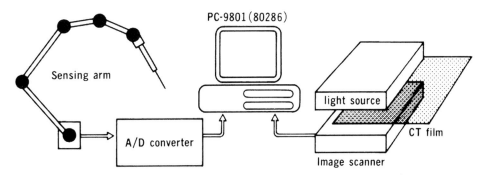

FIGURE 48-16 Neuronavigator. (From Watanabe E, Mayanagy Y, Kasugi Y, et al: Open surgery assisted by the neuronavigator: A stereotactic, articulated, sensitive arm. Neurosurgery 28:792–800, 1991.)

The spatial incompatibility between neurodiagnostic apparatus (CT, MRI, digital angiography) and the requirements of the operating room has been overcome by Kelly[122] by a complex organization centering on a heads-up display system, similar to that used on fighter aircraft, which projects the tumor sections obtained by the computer from CT or MRI data into the operating microscope. A detailed account is provided in Chapter 41. The introduction of portable CT and, moreover, high-field intraoperative MRI—the latter at this point available in a limited number of neurosurgical units—should provide more information about eloquent areas, allow adequate control over the surgical "work in progress," and consequently ensure better results. However, we are not as yet aware of reports detailing morbidity and recurrence figures in low-grade gliomas series using these intraoperative aids.[123–125]

Another method is that proposed by Hassenbusch and colleagues.[126] Craniotomy is performed under a stereotactic frame; when the dura mater has been opened, two or three stereomarkers are introduced at the tumor margins (the ones most difficult to distinguish or situated in the most critical areas) according to the coordinates supplied by CT or MRI (Fig. 48-18). They are "micropatties" (0.6 × 0.6 cm), each with a string tail or silicone sheeting microtubes, either of which are introduced through a microbiopsy forceps

with the ends left emerging from the cortex. The stereotactic frame is then removed, and the surgeon proceeds to free-hand tumor resection. The advantage of this method is that the markers remain lodged at the edges of the tumor (in the brain adjacent to it) despite shifts in the tumor or in the cerebral hemispheres resulting from cyst drainage or tumor debulking.

Berger[56] also reports the use of ultrasonic guidance to introduce catheters at the tumor boundaries as a "fence" to mark the limit of surgical resection. The proposed method of ultrasonic neuronavigation includes a program to calculate the shift of intracranial content occurring with tumor progressive debulking and cerebrospinal fluid (CSF) removal, performing a continuous correction of the initial spatial parameters.

Associated Intractable Epilepsy

Often epileptic foci are associated to low-grade gliomas. Berger and co-workers[95] have registered intraoperatively this pathologic activity, establishing relevant correlations with the clinical status. Only in 6 of 45 patients studied did electrocorticography fail to demonstrate epileptic activity. Twenty-one patients harbored one epileptic focus, and 18 patients harbored at least two foci. Some of these foci

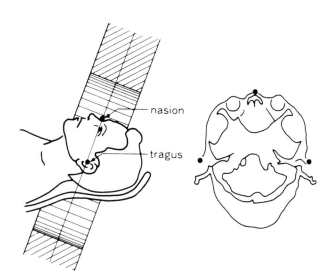

FIGURE 48-17 Artificial coordinates method(s): fiducial points. (From Watanabe E, Mayanagy Y, Kasugi Y, et al: Open surgery assisted by the neuronavigator: A stereotactic, articulated, sensitive arm. Neurosurgery 28:792–800, 1991.)

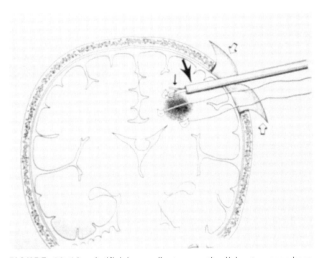

FIGURE 48-18 Artificial coordinates method(s): stereomarkers. (From Hassenbusch SJ, Anderson JS, Pillay PK: Brain tumor resection aided with markers placed using stereotaxis guided by magnetic resonance imaging and computed tomography. Neurosurgery 28:801–806, 1991.)

were adjacent; others were far from the tumor. The latter were mainly associated with temporal lobe gliomas. Epileptiform discharges rose from temporal mesial structures even in tumors of the lateral cortex. The neural tissue of 90% of the identified foci were histologically free of tumor infiltration, which was usually normal and resulted only in a few cases with mild gliosis. Multiple epileptogenic foci were associated with a longer history of seizures. The authors stress the importance of tumor and epileptic focus resection under the guide of electrocorticography, particularly in children and for long-lasting epilepsy, with the goal to optimize seizure control and allow possible interruption or reduction of drug therapy.

Hemostasis and Closure

Hemostasis is ensured in the usual way under the operating microscope by means of bipolar cautery, discontinuous irrigation with lukewarm isotonic saline solution, and dabbing of the walls with cottonoids. Even the smallest nontumoral vessels are spared. As little use as possible is made of foreign materials (e.g., fibrin sponge, oxidized cellulose net) for lining the cavity, which is then filled with physiologic saline.

An extended internal decompressive operation impinging on sound nervous tissue is now viewed with great circumspection, because any sacrifice of nervous tissue always involves neurologic or behavioral deficits, even if they are not detectable with the tests currently available. No such rule applies to the resection of epileptogenic cortical foci separate from the neoplastic mass, which is recommended by Ghatan and associates.[18]

Once the dural margins have been secured to the periosteum by interrupted sutures along the perimeter of the craniotomy, the dural flap is made watertight. The bone is replaced; because the craniotomy is small and its site is at the convexity, there is no point in removing the bone flap for decompression (the classic decompressive operation is to be performed at the base). If the surgeon desires, an epidural probe for prolonged intracranial pressure (ICP) recording is positioned by tunneling the cable beneath the scalp for a few centimeters and bringing it to the surface through a tiny incision in the scalp at a distance from the main wound.

In conclusion, although neurosurgery is not rejecting its origins (the foundations of surgical technique laid down by Cushing and Dandy), this specialty is preparing to take a qualitative leap with the aid of image digitalization techniques. The firm establishment of neuroimaging technologies (which now form part of the operating room setup), the first clinical applications of robotics, and the computerized management of neurophysiologic monitoring systems (e.g., evoked potentials, PET, SPECT) have set the stage for a revision of technique. The main advantages are: (1) personalized instead of standardized craniotomy, (2) prior simulation and not just planning of the operation, and (3) intraoperative verification of the extent of resection so that no surprises occur postoperatively. Genuine tumorectomy replaces the former lobectomy, lobulectomy, and polectomy. In addition, tumorectomy does not have to be total. The surgeon's aim is to remove the tumor, but he or she will later decide between grossly total resection and subtotal resection according to the requirements of the case.

Stereotactic and open biopsies are addressed in other chapters.

MAJOR INTRAOPERATIVE COMPLICATIONS AND THEIR MANAGEMENT

Improved anesthetic technique, the prophylactic use of corticosteroids, and the intraoperative use of a mannitol bolus before the dural incision if the dura mater is tense are the means whereby the operative field is made fit for surgical manipulation. The surgeon takes great care not to damage veins and to prevent the leakage of blood into the CSF compartment (ventricles, cisterns, and sulci of the convexity). A spatula is used only if it does not traumatize the surrounding nervous tissue; scooping with retractors fixed to the Mayfield headrest is preferable to manual scooping, which is always discontinuous.

These conditions minimize the risk of intraoperative and postoperative complications. The intraoperative risks are lobar or hemispheric swelling, episodic or subcontinuous bleeding, and incarceration of CSF in the operative cavity or in a ventricular pole or, less likely, in a cistern. Swelling of the operative field may be the result of hyperemia (increased cerebral blood volume) or edema; either may be local or diffuse. Hydrostatic edema may be caused by congestion of a vessel that results from a rise in capillary and venous pressure after distention of the walls of resistance vessels. Hyperemia may be associated with normal, decreased, or increased blood flow.

Determination of the cerebral blood flow still presents technical problems and furnishes only an overall picture of the blood perfusion of each cerebral hemisphere. Particularly useful are regional blood flow data, which PET and SPECT can supply, but not in the course of an operation (except when high-field intraoperative MRI is available). Thus, we still do not know how the blood flow and cerebral metabolism are regulated in single areas of the brain adjacent to space-occupying lesions or after they have been evacuated surgically, nor do we know what the regional response will be to drugs or to variations in pressure of the respiratory gases. An intravenous mannitol bolus (which increases the blood flow irrespective of the ICP), hyperventilation, and, on occasion, cautious withdrawal of CSF are options if intraoperative congestion of the brain occurs. Initially, the surgeon must ensure that the swelling is not a result of anesthesia or a large tumor residue, of a clot deep in the operative cavity, or of incarcerated CSF.

POSTOPERATIVE MANAGEMENT

An operation on a cerebral glioma is not high-risk surgery; therefore, the immediate postoperative management is the same as that required for any other neurosurgical operation of average complexity. It has now been standardized after decades of experience.

The patient is kept in intensive care for the first 48 to 72 hours under close neurologic supervision and monitoring of autonomic parameters. Drainage, if applied, is removed after 24 hours. The ICP recording probe is removed on postoperative day 3. Antiedema osmotic treatment is discontinued on day 4, and corticosteroid therapy is titrated down a few days later. Prophylactic antibiotics are discontinued between days 4 and 6. CT scanning is performed on day 7 of an uneventful course, and a neurophysiologic (evoked potentials) and neuropsychologic assessment is performed on day 10. Antiepileptic therapy or prophylaxis is given for years.

The immediate postoperative period may be marked by the same complications as those that may arise during the operation (e.g., brain swelling, bleeding, engorgement of CSF), as well as infarction adjacent to the operative field or distant from it, resulting from the interruption of arteries or veins. Neuroimaging and continuous ICP recording are diagnostic. To differentiate swelling resulting from congestion from that resulting from edema, CT scanning is essential after contrast injection. The hypodensity found in the standard images increases by a few Hounsfield units if the blood volume is increased, an increase that is too small, however, to be appreciable on the CT scan. Even minimal bleeding in the operative cavity, either subdural or extradural, shows up clearly on CT and MRI. Regarding ICP, whether a given cerebral perfusion pressure is sufficient in a particular individual to ensure perfusion to all parts of the brain is unknown. Particularly vulnerable are those areas adjacent to the operative focus, whose vascular autoregulation is presumably altered. It has been decided arbitrarily that an ICP of over 20 mm Hg must be corrected by hyperventilation and antiedema osmotic agents. These measures are adopted only in severe neurologic conditions, which are rarely found in patients with low-grade cerebral glioma. If infiltration of deep structures occurs, the surgeon will choose a biopsy rather than extensive resection. Indeed, if surgical series since the introduction of CT are evaluated, the following situation is illustrative. Of the 25 patients that Vertosick and associates[17] operated on between 1978 and 1988, 5 underwent debulking, 4 had an open biopsy, and 16 had stereotactic biopsy, with zero operative mortality and zero morbidity. Of Piepmeier's[16] 50 patients operated on between 1975 and 1985, 19 underwent total resection, 17 subtotal resection, and 14 biopsy, with only one postoperative death. In the series of McCormack and co-workers,[127] of 53 patients (10 gross total resections, 34 subtotal resections, and 9 biopsies) operated on between 1977 and 1988, only 1 died of myocardial infarction in the postoperative period, and 5 died after the 30-day period but while the patients were still in hospital. Three patients who had been neurologically intact before surgery had mild deficits thereafter. In the series of McCormack and colleagues, 15 reoperations were necessary: 3 for shunts, 3 for cyst aspiration, 2 for infection, and 7 for further tumor resection.

The role of radiotherapy in the management of low-grade gliomas is discussed in several excellent review articles.[128–132] Unfortunately, no uniform or systematic studies have been performed that would allow a firm judgment, but the number of patients receiving radiotherapy in the past few years has increased.[133,134] Retrospective analysis of past series, with all their limitations, seems to show that as far as astrocytomas are concerned, (1) patients who undergo surgery for pilocytic astrocytoma (even if incompletely) should not be irradiated; (2) patients with fibrillary or protoplasmic astrocytoma who have undergone gross total resection should not be irradiated but should be followed up closely with neuroimaging; (3) patients with these tumors who have undergone incomplete resection should receive conventional

fractionated radiotherapy at doses of 4500 to 5500 cGy in a limited volume (dose to be reduced and commencement of radiotherapy deferred for patients younger than 2 to 3 years of age); and (4) patients with gemistocytic astrocytoma should receive postoperative radiotherapy regardless of the extent of resection.[135,136] With regard to oligodendrogliomas[137] and the rarer mixed gliomas, the published data are still more fragmentary and discordant. It does seem, however, that radiotherapy slows tumor regrowth.[133]

GROWTH RESUMPTION

It is more appropriate to speak of growth resumption long after treatment than of recurrence, because an infiltrating tumor is never completely eradicated. The literature supplies data on the rates of recurrence, on the length of the interval since operation, and on the histologic differences on the second appraisal (at surgery or at necropsy) compared with the first. Very few opinions on the treatment of a recurrence have been published. Among the series explicitly discussing this topic, one refers to a long period and the other to the CT era: Laws and colleagues[74] reported on 151 recurrences of Grade I and Grade II astrocytomas that were treated surgically between 1915 and 1976. Of the recurrences, 105 were treated surgically (alone or associated with other therapy), 36 nonsurgically, and 10 were not treated. The 12-month survival rates were 45.7%, 46.1%, and 47.6%, which is virtually the same for the three groups. McCormack and associates[127] reported on 24 recurrences among 41 patients who survived total or subtotal removal: 7 had a second operation, and 12 received chemotherapy. The mean survival of those who had a second operation was 12 months from the recurrence. The authors stated that neither reoperation nor chemotherapy prolonged postrecurrence survival. Such data increase the importance of the first management decision; at the time of recurrence, the tumors exhibit increased malignancy and resistance to treatment.

RESULTS

The largest series (461 cases) and the one covering the longest time span (1915–1975) is that of the Mayo Clinic.[14,74] Although the long-term results are obviously better in patients treated since 1950 as a result of improved surgical and anesthetic techniques and antiedema agents, the variables that correlate with longer survival are age under 20 years, good neurologic status before and after operation, epileptic seizures as the onset symptom, preoperative history of symptoms for not less than 6 months, grossly total surgical resection, and parietal or occipital tumor site. Sex, astrocytoma histologic Grade I or II, the presence of an intratumoral cyst, the side affected, and surgical lobectomy (which in malignant astrocytoma improves the prognosis) had little or no impact on survival. Laws and co-workers[14] combined patient age with six of the most important prognostic indicators to score the probability of survival (Table 48-2). Operative mortality excluded, survival varies widely (Fig. 48-19): the 5-year survival rate ranges from 69% to 35%. At 15 years, the rate is over 50% in low-risk patients, versus 16% for the mean. The effectiveness of postoperative radiotherapy could not be assessed per se but only in relation to other parameters. Its value is proved only

TABLE 48-2 ▪ Scoring System for Low-Grade Hemispheric Gliomas

Score = Age at Diagnosis × 0.072

+ 0	+ 1
Surgery after 1949	Surgery before 1949
No personality change	Personality change
Normal consciousness	Altered consciousness
Total resection	Partial resection
Site other than the frontal or temporal lobe	Frontal or temporal lobe
Mild postoperative neurologic deficit	Moderate-to-severe post-operative neurologic deficit

Scoring system based on the data by Laws ER, Taylor WF, Clifton MB, Okazaki H: Neurological management of low-grade astrocytoma of the cerebral hemispheres. J Neurosurg 61:665–673, 1984.

in patients older than 40 years of age with high scores (i.e., with several risk factors). Patient age proved to be by far the most important factor in prognosis, more important than all the other clinical variables and forms of treatment combined, and this aspect is confirmed by the experience of many authors.[79,138,139] The reason for this result is unclear, but what is clear is a difference in biologic behavior of these oncotypes between the young and the adult host.

We dealt with the subject of different low-grade astrocytomas of the cerebral hemispheres as a whole, but we also mentioned that this pathologic entity includes three oncotypes: (1) the astrocytomas representing about 60%, (2) oligodendrogliomas approximately 23%, and (3) mixed oligoastrocytomas about 17%. Actually, the biologic and clinical features of these oncotypes are comparable if we consider the age at presentation, symptomatology, possibility of tumor progression to a higher grade, and absence of spinal diffusion or metastases. With respect to long-term survival, however, pure oligodendrogliomas emerge more favorably, pure astrocytoma appear worse, and mixed oligoastrocytomas display intermediate behavior.[140,141] The series of Shaw and colleagues[142] of the Mayo Clinic, which was drawn from a 20-year period, compares the survival of patients with pure and mixed oligodendrogliomas using

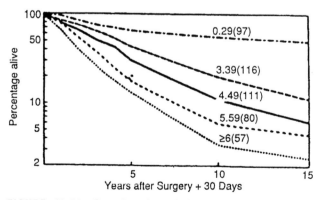

FIGURE 48-19 Score-based survival curves of patients with low-grade hemispheric glioma. See Table 48-2 for basis of scoring system. (From Laws ER, Taylor WF, Clifton MB, Okazaki H: Neurosurgical management of low-grade astrocytoma of the cerebral hemispheres. J Neurosurg 61:665-673, 1984.)

univariate and multivariate analysis and examining 14 prognostic indicators. The tumor grade emerged as the variable that was most significantly related to survival. Less significant was the extent of surgical resection. Younger age was also significantly related with a more favorable prognosis for both oncotypes so that, after gross total surgical resection, radiotherapy may not be required. Conversely, radiotherapy with doses of 5000 cGy is advocated in older patients and for partially resected tumors.

Reports confirm the importance of the length of clinical history among the clinical factors considered relevant for long-term prognosis. Tumors with a longer duration of symptoms and chronic epilepsy seem much less likely to progress toward malignancy over time.[143,144]

The routine use of CT since the time of the series by Laws and colleagues has added a new variable to be evaluated in the long-term prognosis of low-grade cerebral gliomas: the absence of contrast enhancement (i.e., the integrity of the blood-brain barrier) is associated with a better prognosis.[143]

The 1975 to 1985 experience of Yale University[16] shows that the only variables relevant to a better prognosis are age under 40 years and no contrast enhancement on the CT scan. The results of the 1977 to 1988 series at New York University[127] agree: multivariate regression analysis demonstrates that the most important prognosticators for improved survival are young age, absence of contrast enhancement of the original tumor on CT, and the performance status of the patient. The CT contrast enhancement of the original tumor is associated with a 6.8-fold increase in risk for a late recurrence. However, the prognostic significance of contrast enhancement is questioned by some authors,[1] whose further experience contradicts the results obtained in the series covering the decade 1975 to 1985. Bernstein[79] still ascribes some value to the presence of contrast enhancement as related to malignant progression, but Philippon and co-workers[145] deny these findings.

The value of aggressive surgical behavior has also been questioned.[144,146] The likelihood of malignant transformation has been demonstrated to be proportional to the preoperative tumor volume or to residual volume and the latter result inversely related to the time of recurrence.[147] On the other hand, Bernstein[79] emphasizes the unreliability of retrospective studies regarding tumors with different locations being treated differently: these limitations explain the dichotomy existing in the literature between supporters of aggressive surgery and supporters of "wait and see" behavior.

CONCLUSIONS

There has been a revival of scientific and clinical interest in low-grade gliomas, which were neglected for many years in the literature. Within this group of tumors, extraganglionic gliomas have attracted even less attention, and many surgical series group them together with those of the cerebellum, hypothalamus, brain stem, and anterior optic pathways. This grouping is inadvisable, because both histologically and biologically as well as from the diagnostic and therapeutic viewpoints, the latter gliomas are altogether different from those of the cerebral hemispheres.

One reason for this revival of interest is that in the neuroimaging age, the clinician is confronted with pathology different from that seen 20 years ago. The clinician now sees a small lesion in a young, neurologically intact subject whose only complaint is a short history of epileptic seizures. The lesion is of the cerebral convexity, is diffusely infiltrative, and may have connections with the higher functions of the hemisphere: eloquent cortex, its projections, and associative fibers.

For tumors that are indolent for years, one may legitimately wonder whether aggressive treatment—surgery or radiotherapy—is appropriate in all cases and whether the potential benefits of treatment may not be counterbalanced by its risks and adverse effects.[73,148,149] Retrospective studies are of little help in shaping judgment, for the reasons given already (unselected series of tumors much larger than those that are treated now), to which must be added: nonuniformity of pathologic classification criteria, the question of sampling errors, nonuniformity in classifying preoperative neurologic status (Karnofsky's performance scale), nonuniformity of the extent of surgical resection or of a dose of radiotherapy, and the lack of a contemporary group of matched control subjects who did not receive treatment. The final and fundamental reason that retrospective studies are not helpful is the nonuniformity of biologic behavior of the tumor through time; it is subject to dedifferentiation in a high percentage of cases in the course of its natural history. We have no sure data on which to form a judgment regarding the optimal treatment for low-grade cerebral gliomas. These data can come only from prospective, randomized studies of large series. Meanwhile, surgery has both a diagnostic and a therapeutic role. Its diagnostic role may well diminish with advances in neuroimaging procedures, like PET and SPECT, and the chemical quantification in vivo of metabolites in selected regions of the brain, such as can be obtained with proton MR spectroscopy.[150] On the therapeutic front, surgery may well maintain its hold, unless valid alternatives are developed. Although surgery has so far been limited by the risks of damage that it induces, the progress of technology will reduce the risk of undesired side effects and allow surgery to be more aggressive and safer.

REFERENCES

1. Piepmeier JH: Criteria for patient selection: Low-grade gliomas. Clin Neurosurg 44:51–62, 1997.
2. Zülch KJ: Brain Tumors, 3rd ed. Berlin: Springer-Verlag, 1986.
3. Schisano G, Tovi D, Nordenstam H: Spongioblastoma polare of the cerebral hemisphere. J Neurosurg 20:241–251, 1963.
4. Palma L, Guidetti B: Cystic pilocytic astrocytomas of the cerebral hemispheres: Surgical experience with 51 cases and long-term results. J Neurosurg 62:811–815, 1985.
5. Afra D, Müller W, Slowik F, Firsching R: Supratentorial lobar pilocytic astrocytomas: Report of 45 operated cases, including 9 recurrences. Acta Neurochir (Wien) 81:90–93, 1986.
6. Seeger W: Strategies of Microsurgery in Problematic Brain Areas, with Special Reference to NMR. New York: Springer-Verlag, 1990.
7. Skirboll SL, Ojemann GA, Berger MS, et al: Functional cortex and subcortical white matter located within gliomas. Neurosurgery 38:678–685, 1996.
8. Silverman C, Marks JE: Prognostic significance of contrast enhancement in low-grade astrocytomas of the adult cerebrum. Radiology 139:211–213, 1981.
9. Hoshino T, Rodriguez LA, Cho KG, et al: Prognostic implications of the proliferative potential of low-grade astrocytomas. J Neurosurg 69:839–842, 1988.
10. Germano IM, Ito M, Cho KG, et al: Correlation of histopathological features and proliferative potential of gliomas. J Neurosurg 70:701–706, 1989.
11. Labrousse F, Daumas-Duport C, Batorski L, Hoshino T: Histological grading and bromodeoxyuridine labeling index of astrocytomas: Comparative study in a series of 60 cases. J Neurosurg 75:202–205, 1991.
12. Hoshino T: Cell kinetics of brain tumors. In Salcman M (ed): Neurobiology of Brain Tumors, vol 4: Concepts in Neurosurgery. Baltimore: Williams & Wilkins, 1991, pp 145–159.
13. Patronas NJ, Di Chiro G, Kufta C, et al: Prediction of survival in glioma patients by means of positron emission tomography. J Neurosurg 62:816–822, 1985.
14. Laws ER, Taylor WF, Clifton MB, Okazaki H: Neurosurgical management of low-grade astrocytoma of the cerebral hemispheres. J Neurosurg 61:665–673, 1984.
15. Gol A: The relatively benign astrocytomas of the cerebrum: A clinical study of 194 verified cases. J Neurosurg 18:501–506, 1961.
16. Piepmeier JM: Observations on the current treatment of low-grade astrocytic tumors of the cerebral hemispheres. J Neurosurg 67:177–181, 1987.
17. Vertosick FT, Selker RG, Arena VC: Survival of patients with well-differentiated astrocytomas diagnosed in the era of computed tomography. Neurosurgery 28:496–501, 1991.
18. Ghatan S, Berger MS, Ojemann GA, Dobbins J: Seizure control in patients with low-grade gliomas: Resection of the tumor and separate seizure foci. J Neurosurg 74:355A, 1991.
19. Haglund MM, Berger MS, Kunkel DD, et al: Changes in gamma-aminobutyric acid and somatostatin in epileptic cortex associated with low-grade gliomas. J Neurosurg 77:209–216, 1992.
20. Goldring S, Rich KM, Picker S: Experience with gliomas in patients presenting with a chronic seizure disorder. Clin Neurosurg 33:15–42, 1986.
21. Yoshii Y, Maki Y, Tsuboi K, et al: Estimation of growth fraction with bromodeoxyuridine in human central nervous system tumors. J Neurosurg 65:659–663, 1986.
22. Zuber P, Hamou MF, De Tribolet N: Identification of proliferating cells in human gliomas using the monoclonal antibody Ki-67. Neurosurgery 22:364–368, 1988.
23. Tachibana H, Meyer JS, Rose JE, Kandula P: Local cerebral blood flow and partition coefficients measured in cerebral astrocytomas of different grades of malignancy. Surg Neurol 21:125–131, 1984.
24. Di Chiro G, De La Paz RL, Brooks RA, et al: Glucose utilization of cerebral gliomas measured by [18F]fluorodeoxyglucose and positron emission tomography. Neurology 32:1323–1329, 1982.
25. Bustany P, Chatel M, Derlon JM, et al: Brain tumor protein synthesis and histological grades: A study by positron emission tomography (PET) with 11C-L-methionine. J Neurooncol 3:397–404, 1986.
26. Tsuboi K, Yoshii Y, Nakagawa K, Maki Y: Regrowth patterns of supratentorial gliomas: Estimation from computed tomographic scans. Neurosurgery 19:946–951, 1986.
27. Hoshino T: A commentary on the biology and growth kinetics of low-grade and high-grade gliomas. J Neurosurg 61:895–900, 1984.
28. Müller W, Afra D, Schröder R: Supratentorial recurrences of gliomas: Morphological studies in relation to time intervals with astrocytomas. Acta Neurochir (Wien) 37:75–91, 1977.
29. Müller W, Afra D, Schröder R: Supratentorial recurrence of gliomas: Morphological studies in relation to time intervals with oligodendrogliomas. Acta Neurochir (Wien) 39:15–25, 1977.
30. Rubinstein LJ: The correlation of neoplastic vulnerability with central neuroepithelial cytogeny and glioma differentiation. J Neurooncol 5:11–27, 1987.
31. Wallner KE, Gonzales M, Sheline GE: Treatment of oligodendrogliomas with or without postoperative irradiation. J Neurosurg 68:684–688, 1988.
32. Piepmeier JM, Christopher S: Low-grade gliomas: Introduction and overview. J Neurooncol 34:1–3, 1997.
33. Schiffer D, Cavalla P, Chio A, et al: Proliferative activity and prognosis of low-grade astrocytomas. J Neurooncol 34:31–35, 1997.
34. Fisher BJ, Naumova E, Leighton CC, et al: Ki 67: A prognostic factor for low-grade glioma? Int J Radiat Oncol Biol Phys 52:996–1001, 2002.
35. Dirven CM, Koudstall J, Mooij JJ, Molenaar WM: The proliferative potential of the pilocytic astrocytoma: The relation between MIB-1 labeling and clinical and neuro-radiological follow-up. J Neurooncol 37:9–16, 1998.
36. Knudson AG, Jr: Mutations and cancer: Statistical study of retinoblastoma. Proc Natl Acad Sci U S A 68:820–823, 1971.
37. Nishizaki T, Ozaki S, Harada K, et al: Investigation of genetic alterations associated with the grade of astrocytic tumor by comparative genomic hybridization. Genes Chromosomes Cancer 21:340–346, 1998.

38. Watanabe K, Tachibana O, Yonekawa Y, et al: Role of gemistocytes in astrocytoma progression. Lab Invest 76:277–284, 1997.

39. Prayson RA, Estes ML: MIB1 and p53 immunoreactivity in protoplasmic astrocytomas. Pathol Int 46:862–866, 1996.

40. Bogler O, Huang HJ, Cavenee WK: Loss of wild-type p53 bestows a growth advantage on primary cortical astrocytes and facilitates their in vitro transformation. Cancer Res 55:2746–2751, 1995.

41. Chernova OB, Chernov MV, Agarwal ML, et al: The role of p53 in regulating genomic stability when DNA and RNA synthesis are inhibited. Trends Biochem Sci 20:431–434, 1995.

42. Venkatachalam S, Shi YP, Jones SN, et al: Retention of wild-type p53 in tumors from heterozygous p53+/- mice: Reduction of p53 dosage can promote cancer transformation. EMBO J 17:4657–4667, 1998.

43. Gomez Manzano C, Fueyo J, Kyritsis AP, et al: Adenovirus-mediated transfer of the p53 gene produces rapid and generalized death of human glioma cells via apoptosis. Cancer Res 56:694–699, 1996.

44. Fueyo J, Gomez-Manzano C, Bruner JM, et al: Hypermethylation of the CpG island of p16/CDKN2 correlates with gene inactivation in gliomas. Oncogene 13:1615–1619, 1996.

45. Ehrmann J, Jr., Kolar Z, Vojtesek B, et al: Prognostic factors in astrocytomas: Relationship of p53, MDM-2, BCL-2 and PCNA immunohistochemical expression to tumor grade and overall patient survival. Neoplasma 44:299–304, 1997.

46. Carroll RS, Zhang J, Chauncey BW, et al: Apoptosis in astrocytic neoplasms. Acta Neurochir (Wien) 139:845–850, 1997.

47. Kattar MM, Kupsky WJ, Shimoyama RK, et al: Clonal analysis of gliomas. Hum Pathol 28:1166–1179, 1997.

48. Reifenberger J, Ring GU, Gies U, et al: Analysis of p53 mutation and epidermal growth factor amplification in recurrent gliomas with malignant progression. J Neuropathol Exp Neurol 55:822–831, 1996.

49. Noble M, Mayer-Prochel M: Molecular growth factors, glia and gliomas. J Neurooncol 35:193–209, 1997.

50. Bonnie A, Sun Y, Nadal-Vicens M, et al: Regulation of gliogenesis in the central nervous system by the JAK-STAT signaling pathway. Science 278:477–483, 1997.

51. Abdulrauf SI, Edvardsen K, Ho KL, et al: Vascular endothelial growth factor expression and vascular density as prognostic markers of survival in patients with low-grade astrocytoma. J Neurosurg 88:513–520, 1998.

52. Jensen RL: Growth factor–mediated angiogenesis in the malignant progression of glial tumors: A review. Surg Neurol 49:189–195, 1998.

53. Takekawa Y, Sawada T: Vascular endothelial growth factor and neovascularization in astrocytic tumors. Pathol Int 48:109–114, 1998.

54. Kondziolka D, Lunsford LD, Martinez AJ: Unreliability of contemporary neurodiagnostic imaging in evaluating suspected adult supratentorial (low-grade) astrocytoma. J Neurosurg 79:533–536, 1993.

55. Bernstein M, Guha A: Biopsy of low-grade astrocytomas. J Neurosurg 80:776–777, 1994.

56. Berger MS: Surgery of low-grade gliomas: Technical aspects. Clin Neurosurg 44:161–180, 1997.

57. Herholz K, Holzer T, Bauer B, et al: 11C-methionine PET for differential diagnosis of low-grade gliomas. Neurology 50:1316–1322, 1998.

58. Nuutinen J, Sonninen P, Lehikoinen P, et al: Radiotherapy treatment planning and long-term follow-up with [11C]methionine PET in patients with low-grade astrocytoma. Int J Radiat Oncol Biol Phys 48:43–52, 2000.

59. Kaschten B, Stevenaert A, Sadzot B, et al: Preoperative evaluation of 54 gliomas by PET with fluorine-18-fluorodeoxyglucose and/or carbon-11-methionine. J Nucl Med 39:778–785, 1998.

60. Gungor F, Bezircioglu H, Guvenc G, et al: Correlation of thallium-201 uptake with proliferating cell nuclear antigen in brain tumors. Nucl Med Commun 21:803–810, 2000.

61. Terada H, Kamata N: Contribution of the combination of (201) Tl SPECT and (99m)T(c)O(4)(−) SPECT to the differential diagnosis of brain tumors and tumor-like lesions: A preliminary report. J Neuroradiol 30:91–94, 2003.

62. Tamura M, Shibasaki T, Zama A, et al: Assessment of malignancy of glioma by positron emission tomography with [18F]fluorodeoxyglucose and single photon emission computed tomography with thallium-201 chloride. Neuroradiology 40:210–215, 1998.

63. Cheng LL, Chang IW, Louis DN, Gonzalez RG: Correlation of high resolution magic angle spinning proton magnetic resonance spectroscopy with histopathology of intact brain tumor specimens. Cancer Res 58:1825–1832, 1998.

64. Tedeschi G, Lundbom N, Raman R, et al: Increased choline signal coinciding with malignant degeneration of cerebral gliomas: A serial proton magnetic resonance spectroscopy imaging study. J Neurosurg 87:516–524, 1997.

65. Tzika AA, Cheng LL, Goumnerova L, et al: Biochemical characterization of pediatric brain tumors by using in vivo and ex vivo magnetic resonance spectroscopy. J Neurosurg 96:1023–1031, 2002.

66. Galanaud D, Chinot O, Nicoli F, et al: Use of proton magnetic resonance spectroscopy of the brain to differentiate gliomatosis cerebri from low-grade glioma. J Neurosurg 98:269–276, 2003.

67. Wu WC, Chen CY, Chung HW, et al: Discrepant MR spectroscopic and perfusion imaging results in a case of malignant transformation of cerebral glioma. AJNR Am J Neuroradiol 23:1775–1778, 2002.

68. Isobe T, Matsumura A, Anno I, et al: Quantification of cerebral metabolites in glioma patients with proton MR spectroscopy using T2 relaxation time correction. Magn Reson Imaging 20:343–349, 2002.

69. Lombardi V, Valko L, Valko M, et al: 1H NMR ganglioside ceramide resonance region on the differential diagnosis of low and high malignancy of brain gliomas. Cell Mol Biol 17:521–535, 1997.

70. Woesler B, Kuwert T, Morgenroth C, et al: Non-invasive grading of primary brain tumors: Results of a comparative study between SPECT with 123I-alpha-methyltyrosine and PET with 18F-deoxyglucose. Eur J Nucl Med 24:428–434, 1997.

71. Molenkamp G, Riemann B, Kuwert T, et al: Monitoring tumor activity of low-grade glioma of childhood. Klin Padiatr 210:239–242, 1998.

72. Weber WA, Dick S, Reidl G, et al: Correlation between postoperative 3-[123I]iodo-alpha-methyltyrosine uptake and survival in patients with gliomas. J Nucl Med 42:1144–1150, 2001.

73. Morantz RA: Controversial issues in the management of low-grade astrocytomas. In Wilkins RH, Rengachary SS (eds): Neurosurgery Update I. New York: McGraw-Hill, 1990, pp 245–251.

74. Laws ER, Taylor WF, Bergstralh EJ, et al: The neurosurgical management of low-grade astrocytoma. Clin Neurosurg 33:575–588, 1986.

75. Salcman M: Radical surgery for low-grade glioma. Clin Neurosurg 36:353–366, 1990.

76. Weir B, Grace M: The relative significance of factors affecting postoperative survival in astrocytomas, grades one and two. Can J Neurol Sci 3:47–50, 1976.

77. Sano K: Integrative treatment of gliomas. Clin Neurosurg 30:93–124, 1983.

78. Francavilla TL, Miletich RS, Di Chiro G, et al: Positron emission tomography in the detection of malignant degeneration of low-grade gliomas. Neurosurgery 24:1–5, 1989.

79. Bernstein M: Low-grade gliomas: In search of evidence-based treatment. Clin Neurosurg 44:315–330, 1997.

80. Salcman M: Surgical decision-making for malignant brain tumors. Clin Neurosurg 35:285–311, 1989.

81. Giacomini C: Topografia della scissura di Rolando. Torino: Vercellino Tip, 1878.

82. Berger MS, Cohen WA, Ojemann GA: Correlation of motor cortex brain mapping data with magnetic resonance imaging. J Neurosurg 72:383–387, 1990.

83. Hu X, Tan KK, Levin DN, et al: Three-dimensional magnetic resonance images of the brain: Application to neurosurgical planning. J Neurosurg 72:433–440, 1990.

84. Fox PT, Burton H, Raichle ME: Mapping human somatosensory cortex with positron emission tomography. J Neurosurg 67:34–43, 1987.

85. Levin DN, Hu X, Tann KK, et al: The brain: Integrated three-dimensional display of MR and PET images. Radiology 172:783–789, 1989.

86. Evans AC, Marrett S, Torrescorzo J, et al: MRI-PET correlation in three dimensions using a volume-of-interest (VOI) atlas. J Cereb Blood Flow Metab 11:A69–A78, 1991.

87. Martin N, Grafton S, Vinuela F, et al: Imaging techniques for cortical functional localization. Clin Neurosurg 38:132–165, 1992.

88. Ojemann G, Ojemann J, Lettich E, Berger M: Cortical language localization in left dominant hemisphere: An electrical stimulation mapping investigation in 117 patients. J Neurosurg 71:316–326, 1989.

89. Nariai T, Senda M, Ishii K, Maehara T, et al: Three-dimensional imaging of cortical structure, function and glioma for tumor resection. J Nucl Med 38:1563–1568, 1997.

90. Rees J: Advances in magnetic resonance imaging of brain tumors. Curr Opin Neurol 16:643–650, 2003.

91. Nimsky C, Ganslandt O, von Keller B, Fahlbusch R: Preliminary experience in glioma surgery with intraoperative high-field MRI. Acta Neurochir Suppl 88:21–29, 2003.

92. Black PMCL, Ronner SF: Cortical mapping for defining the limits of tumor resection. Neurosurgery 20:914–919, 1987.

93. Walsh AR, Schmidt RH, Marsh HT: Cortical mapping and resection under local anaesthetic as an aid to surgery of low and intermediate grade gliomas. Br J Neurosurg 4:485–491, 1990.

94. Ebeling U, Schmid UD, Reulen HJ: Tumour-surgery within the central motor strip: Surgical results with the aid of electrical motor cortex stimulation. Acta Neurochir (Wien) 101:100–107, 1989.

95. Berger MS, Saadi Ghatan BS, Haglund MM, et al: Low-grade gliomas associated with intractable epilepsy: Seizure outcome utilizing electrocorticography during tumor resection. J Neurosurg 79:62–69, 1993.

96. Guthrie BL, Adler JR: Computer-assisted preoperative planning, interactive surgery, and frameless stereotaxy. Clin Neurosurg 38:112–131, 1992.

97. Auer LM, Van Velthonen V: Intraoperative ultrasound imaging: Comparison of pathomorphological findings in US and CT. Acta Neurochir (Wien) 104:84–95, 1990.

98. Rubin JM, Chandler WF: Ultrasound in Neurosurgery. New York: Raven Press, 1990.

99. Leroux PD, Berger MS, Ojemann GA, et al: Correlation of intraoperative ultrasound tumor volumes and margins with preoperative computerized tomography scans: An intraoperative method to enhance tumor resection. J Neurosurg 71:691–698, 1989.

100. Ono M, Kubik S, Abernathey CD: Atlas of the Cerebral Sulci. New York: G Thieme Verlag, 1990.

101. Wood CC, Spencer DD, Allison T, et al: Localization of human sensorimotor cortex during surgery by cortical surface recording of somatosensory evoked potentials. J Neurosurg 68:99–111, 1988.

102. King RB, Schell GR: Cortical localization and monitoring during cerebral operations. J Neurosurg 67:210–219, 1987.

103. Bartholow R: Experimental investigations into the functions of the human brain. Am J Med Sci 67:305–313, 1874.

104. Northfield DWC: Sir Victor Horsley: His contributions to neurological surgery. Surg Neurol 1:131–134, 1973.

105. Penfield WG, Boldrey E: Somatic motor and sensory representation in the cerebral cortex of man as studied by electrical stimulation. Brain 60:389–443, 1937.

106. Duffau H, Capelle L, Sichez N, et al: Intraoperative mapping of the subcortical language pathways using direct stimulations: An anatomo-functional study. Brain 125:199–214, 2002.

107. Duffau H, Capelle L, Denvil D, et al: Usefulness of intraoperative electrical subcortical mapping during surgery for low-grade gliomas located within eloquent brain regions: Functional results in a consecutive series of 103 patients. J Neurosurg 98:764–768, 2003.

108. Pia HW: Microsurgery of gliomas. Acta Neurochir (Wien) 80:1–11, 1986.

109. Yasargil MG, Cravens GF, Roth P: Surgical approaches to "inaccessible" brain tumors. Clin Neurosurg 34:42–110, 1988.

110. Harkey HL, Al-Mefty O, Haines DE, Smith RR: The surgical anatomy of the cerebral sulci. Neurosurgery 24:651–654, 1989.

111. Szikla G, Bouvier G, Hori T, Petrov V: Angiography of the human brain cortex: Atlas of vascular patterns and stereotactic cortical localization. Berlin: Springer-Verlag, 1977.

112. Berger MS, Ojemann GA, Lettich E: Cerebral hemispheric tumors of childhood. Neurosurg Clin N Am 34:839–852, 1992.

113. Hellwig D, Bauer BL, List-Hellwig E, et al: Stereotactic-endoscopic procedures on processes of the cranial midline. Acta Neurochir Suppl 53:23–32, 1991.

114. Epstein F: The Cavitron ultrasonic aspirator in tissue surgery. Clin Neurosurg 31:497–505, 1984.

115. Gonghai C, Qiwu X: Carbon dioxide laser vaporization of brain tumors. Neurosurgery 12:123–126, 1983.

116. Ascher PW, Heppner F: CO_2 laser in neurosurgery. Neurosurg Rev 7:123–133, 1984.

117. Koivukangas J, Koivukangas P: Treatment of low-grade cerebral astrocytoma: New methods and evaluation of results. Am Clin Res 47(Suppl):115–124, 1986.

118. Poon WS, Schomacker KT, Deutsch TF, Martuza RL: Laser-induced fluorescence: Experimental intraoperative delineation of tumor resection margins. J Neurosurg 76:679–686, 1992.

119. Haglund MM, Berger MS, Hockman DW: Enhanced optical imaging of human gliomas and tumor margins. Neurosurgery 38:308–317, 1996.

120. Watanabe E, Mayanagy Y, Kosugi Y, et al: Open surgery assisted by the neuronavigator, a stereotactic, articulated, sensitive arm. Neurosurgery 28:792–800, 1991.

121. Watanabe E, Watanabe T, Manaka S, et al: Three-dimensional digitizer (neuronavigator): New equipment for computed tomography-guided stereotaxic surgery. Surg Neurol 27:543–547, 1987.

122. Kelly PJ: Stereotactic imaging, surgical planning and computer-assisted resection of intracranial lesions: Methods and results. In Symon L (ed.): Advances and Technical Standards in Neurosurgery. New York: Springer-Verlag, 1990, pp 77–118.

123. Schneider JP, Schulz T, Schmidt F, et al: Gross-total surgery of supratentorial low-grade gliomas under intraoperative MR guidance. AJNR Am J Neuroradiol 22:89–98, 2001.

124. Tummala RP, Chu RM, Liu H, et al: Optimizing brain tumor resection. High-field interventional MR imaging. Neuroimaging Clin North Am 11:673–683, 2001.

125. Hall WA, Liu H, Maxwell RE, Truwit CL: Influence of 1,5-Tesla intraoperative MR imaging on surgical decision making. Acta Neurochir Suppl 85:29–37, 2003.

126. Hassenbusch SJ, Anderson JS, Pillay PK: Brain tumor resection aided with markers placed using stereotaxis guided by magnetic resonance imaging and computed tomography. Neurosurgery 28:801–806, 1991.

127. McCormack BM, Miller DC, Budzilovich GN, et al: Treatment and survival of low-grade astrocytoma in adults 1977–1988. Neurosurgery 31:636–642, 1992.

128. Garcia D, Fulling K, Marks JE: The value of radiation therapy in addition to surgery for astrocytomas of the adult cerebrum. Cancer 55:917–919, 1985.

129. Shaw EG, Wisoff JH: Prospective clinical trials of intracranial low-grade glioma in adults and children. Neurooncol 5:153–160, 2003.

130. Sheline GE: The role of radiation therapy in treatment of low-grade gliomas. Clin Neurosurg 33:563–574, 1986.

131. Morantz RA: Radiation therapy in the treatment of cerebral astrocytoma. Neurosurgery 20:975–982, 1987.

132. Jeremic B, Bamberg M: Radiation therapy for incompletely resected supratentorial low-grade gliomas in adults. J Neurooncol 55:101–112, 2001.

133. Marks JE: Ionizing radiation. In Salcman M (ed): Neurobiology of Brain Tumors, vol 4: Concepts in Neurosurgery. Baltimore: Williams & Wilkins, 1991, pp 299–320.

134. Karim AB, Afra D, Cornu P, et al: Randomized trial on the efficacy of radiotherapy for cerebral low-grade glioma in the adult: European Organization for Research and Treatment of Cancer Study 22845 with the Medical Research Council study BRO4: An interim analysis. Int J Radiat Oncol Biol Phys 52:316–324, 2002.

135. Weingart J, Olivi A, Brem H: Supratentorial low-grade astrocytomas in adults. Neurosurg Q 1:141–159, 1991.

136. Brandes AA, Vastola F, Basso U: Controversies in the therapy of low-grade glioma: when and how to treat. Expert Rev Anticancer Ther 2:529–536, 2002.

137. Bullard D, Rawlings CE, Phillips B, et al: Oligodendroglioma: An analysis of the value of radiation therapy. Cancer 60:2179–2188, 1987.

138. Piepmeier J, Christopher S, Spencer D, et al: Variations in the natural history and survival of patients with supratentorial low-grade astrocytomas. Neurosurgery 38:872–879, 1996.

139. Vecht CJ: Effect of age on treatment decisions in low-grade glioma. J Neurol Neurosurg Psychiatry 56:1259–1264, 1993.

140. Cillekens JM, Belien JA, van der Valk P, et al: A histopathological contribution to supratentorial glioma grading, definition of mixed gliomas and recognition of low-grade glioma with Rosenthal fibers. J Neurooncol 46:23–43, 2000.

141. Feigenberg SJ, Amdur RJ, Morris CG, et al: Oligodendroglioma: Does deferring treatment compromise outcome? Am J Clin Oncol 26:E60–E66, 2003.

142. Shaw EG, Scheithauer BW, O'Fallon JR, Davis DH: Mixed oligoastrocytomas: A survival and prognostic factors analysis. Neurosurgery 34:577–582, 1994.

143. Bauman G, Lote K, Larson D, et al: Pretreatment factors predict overall survival for patients with low-grade glioma: A recursive partitioning analysis. Int J Radiat Oncol Biol Phys 45:923–929, 1999.

144. Van Veelen ML, Avezaat CJ, Kros JM, et al: Supratentorial low-grade astrocytoma:prognostic factors, dedifferentiation, and the issue of early versus late surgery. J Neurol Neurosurg Psychiatry 64:581–587, 1998.

145. Philippon JH, Clemenceau SH, Fauchon FH, Foncin JF: Supratentorial low-grade astrocytomas in adults. Neurosurgery 32:554–559, 1993.

146. Bampoe J, Bernstein M: The role of surgery in low grade gliomas. J Neurooncol 42:259–269, 1999.

147. Berger MS, Deliganis AV, Dobbins J, Evren Keles G: The effect of the extent of resection on recurrence in patients with low-grade cerebral hemisphere gliomas. Cancer 74:1784–1791, 1994.

148. Cairncross JG, Laperriere NJ: Low-grade glioma: To treat or not to treat? Arch Neurol 46:1238–1239, 1989.

149. Laws ER: The conservative management of primary gliomas of the brain. Clin Neurosurg 36:367–374, 1990.

150. Sutton LN, Wang Z, Gusnard D, et al: Proton magnetic resonance spectroscopy of pediatric brain tumors. Neurosurgery 31:195–202, 1992.

49 Surgical Management of Lesions in Eloquent Areas of Brain

MARK A. PICHELMANN and FREDRIC B. MEYER

Lesions presenting themselves in close proximity to eloquent cortex and underlying white matter tracts provide a challenging subset of disorders for the neurosurgeon. Advances over the last 40 years in the ability to localize functional parenchyma by a variety of means has facilitated a more aggressive approach to the management of these lesions from a surgical standpoint. Neuronavigational systems in combination with anatomic and functional imaging advances as well as electrophysiologic study have greatly advanced the neurosurgeon's ability to effectively and safely treat these lesions. The goals of surgery for tumors located in eloquent areas of the brain are to maximize the extent of resection, minimize neurologic morbidity, and treat intractable tumor-related epilepsy.

This chapter will focus on lesions juxtaposed or involving eloquent areas of the brain. Any number of pathologic entities can potentially manifest in functionally eloquent regions; however, gliomas will be a particular focus because of their more invasive nature compared with more focal lesions. The techniques described can be applied to any lesion located in potentially eloquent cortex or subcortical white matter.

RATIONALE FOR AGGRESSIVE RESECTION

Resection of focal tumors in theory involves resection of the tumor mass without disruption of adjacent "normal" brain, since these tend to displace rather than invade. In the absence of the tumor presenting to the cortical surface, however, identifying eloquent cortex in an effort to minimize trauma to adjacent functioning brain during resection is of prime importance. Circumscribed lesions such as gangliogliomas, metastases, cavernomas, and arteriovenous malformations (AVMs) are examples of more focal masses that are usually more amenable to complete resection with less risk to adjacent cortex and white matter when compared with infiltrating gliomas. The exception to this may be epileptogenic zones that are separate from the tumor mass or gliotic tissue that is not easily distinguishable from tumor-involved brain.

Surgery for diffuse tumor masses such as oligodendrogliomas and astrocytomas involves consideration of another dimension, that being resection of tumor infiltrating functional brain. It is well recognized that these diffuse tumors extend into otherwise grossly normal-appearing or slightly gliotic and potentially eloquent areas.[1,2] The identification of this functional brain within the tumor margin

is important for ensuring continued neurologic function. The topic concerning the benefits of extent of resection with respect to high- and low-grade gliomas is controversial. Unfortunately, there are no prospective, randomized controlled trials to specifically address the benefits of radical resection. We are thus restricted to considering non-randomized, retrospective data in an effort to guide clinical therapy. It cannot be overemphasized that decision making must be individualized and is best undertaken with a multi-disciplinary approach to each patient considering the risks and benefits of each specific treatment option. Any benefit of surgery will come only by way of minimizing operative and neurologic morbidity related to the treatment.

The literature, overall, supports a positive effect of surgery on the natural history of low-grade gliomas. In a number of studies, gross or near-gross total resection of low-grade astrocytomas was correlated with lower recurrence rates and longer times to progression as compared with subtotal resection.[3–9] Fewer studies have correlated extent of resection with a survival advantage.[10] The rationale for aggressive resection is based on the assumption that small tumors will with time progress to larger tumors and become potentially either more difficult to resect or nonresectable. There is also good evidence to suggest that the potential for malignant degeneration is related to the tumor size and length of time the mass has been present.[3,11] Malignant degeneration has been variously reported, and probably occurs in about 50% of patients harboring these lesions.[12,13] An exhaustive review of this literature is beyond the scope of this chapter, and the reader is referred to a recent review by Keles and colleagues.[14] Surgery for high-grade gliomas is less controversial. Several studies not only indicate a benefit for time to progression and improved neurologic performance, but also improved survival.[15–22]

Therefore, the advantages to utilizing a maximal tumor resection strategy include less likelihood of tissue sampling error, an immediate reduction in signs and symptoms of mass effect, improved control of intractable seizures with dedicated seizure monitoring, and the potential positive effects in decreasing the risk of malignant dedifferentiation through cytoreduction and influencing outcome as it pertains to delaying progression.

DEFINITIONS OF ELOQUENT CORTEX

The concept of cortical localization with respect to language dates back to Broca's seminal report of two patients with nonfluent aphasia after having suffered autopsy-proven left inferior frontal strokes.[23] Wernicke subsequently added the description of another form of aphasia, variously termed *fluent aphasia*, in 1874 under similar circumstances.[24] These experiments of nature have opened the door to extensive research efforts at anatomically localizing various aspects of language and motor function to specific regions of the cerebral cortex. Numerous types of language deficit can result from injury both to cortical and subcortical regions. The focus here will be directed toward those regions essential for language and motor function as it applies to neurosurgical procedures and practice.

Harvey Cushing is credited for the first stimulation mapping of the cerebral cortex in a patient when he stimulated the motor and somatosensory cortex producing contralateral limb movement and paresthesias.[25] Almost 30 years later, Penfield and Boldrey detailed their results in stimulation of the precentral and postcentral gyri and noted that primary motor and sensory function is reliably located in these regions, although they may be displaced from their usual anatomic location as a result of mass effect from adjacent tissue.[26] They found these areas to be indispensable for movement and emphasized that during surgery every effort to preserve their structural integrity should be made. An exception to this general rule may be the face region, which is represented bilaterally, and resection of lesions in the nondominant motor cortex have been described.[27] This is not advocated in the dominant hemisphere because of the close proximity of language areas and the greater role the face motor region may play as association cortex with the language areas.

The most extensive work done on mapping primary essential language areas up to recent years was done by Penfield and colleagues as well.[28,29] Penfield tested naming, counting, spelling, and reading in patients during awake craniotomy and documented these areas on maps of the lateral and superior cortical surface. Three main areas were identified as being essential for language function. These were the inferior frontal opercular area (corresponding to Broca's area), the posterior temporal area (corresponding to Wernicke's area), and a third area located on the medial and superior surfaces of the superior frontal gyrus (the supplementary motor area). They also noted that these sites had relative importance in subserving language function, with the posterior temporal and inferior frontal regions being unresectable if language function was to be preserved. They also noted that the mesial frontal region was associated with severe expressive deficits postoperatively but that these deficits gradually disappeared in the weeks following surgery. Numerous others have confirmed this observation, indicating that resection of the supplementary motor area does not generally lead to permanent deficits as long as the more posterior primary motor cortex is spared.[30,31]

The standard technique for intraoperative stimulation mapping was also developed by Penfield to a large extent and later refined by Ojemann.[32] Of note in Penfield's stimulation maps is that errors in naming and object recognition were indeed clustered in the classical Broca's and Wernicke's areas, but a significant number of sites occurred outside of these traditional boundaries. In mapping studies done by Ojemann and colleagues on 117 patients, 67% had more than one distinct essential language area and 24% had

three or more distinct areas subserving language function in the dominant hemisphere peri-Sylvian region. There was also greater variability in the temporal language area as compared with the frontal region. Additionally, essential language sites were found to be confined to an area of 2.5 cm^2 or less in about 50% of people, with only 16% of patients having an area equal to or larger than 6 cm^2.[32] Seldom are the entire extents of classical language areas essential for language function.

To summarize, motor and sensory cortex are reliably localized to the precentral and postcentral gyri, respectively, in both hemispheres and are often readily identified on magnetic resonance imaging (MRI). The majority of essential motor neurons are located in the posterior portion of the precentral gyrus adjacent to the central sulcus. Compartmentalization of language functions is imprecise. In contrast to classic views of motor and sensory localization, language does not provide the surgeon with the same degree of certainty based on anatomic landmarks. There is wide variability in both the number and location of essential language sites within individual patients. Language sites cannot be accurately defined with anatomic imaging only, and other means, such as functional imaging and/or direct stimulation mapping, must be used to minimize patient morbidity when considering resection of lesions in the peri-Sylvian region of the dominant hemisphere. It must be kept in mind that language functions as a network of interconnected areas involved in parallel processing to accomplish a task, although it is convenient to think of these areas as having discrete anatomic boundaries for the purposes of surgical planning and resection.

TESTING OF CEREBRAL DOMINANCE

The evaluation of cerebral dominance has interested scientists since the time of Broca. It is well established that the vast majority of right-handed individuals are left brain dominant for speech and language function, while fewer left-handed individuals are left brain dominant, but still a majority. Efforts at finding out which patients may have atypical language localization (i.e., bilateral or right sided) is of great importance to the neurosurgeon particularly when operating in the peri-Sylvian region of the right hemisphere. Strauss and Wada evaluated patients for various lateralized preferences including hand, foot, eye, and ear and found that taken together, these had a higher correlation with cerebral dominance than any one did alone. Perhaps more revealing in this study was that only 3% of patients with all left-sided preferences were left hemisphere dominant, indicating a high-risk group for undergoing right-sided surgical procedures.[33] Noninvasive means of testing for dominance offer clues about the lateralization of cerebral dominance, but application to a broad population base is problematic. These evaluations alone cannot be used to predict cerebral dominance reliably in individual patients, especially those with any left-sided preference. The intracarotid amobarbital procedure is the method of choice for the determination of dominance in this setting.

The intracarotid amobarbital procedure was initially developed by Wada in 1949[34] and later applied to a larger number of patients in reports by Wada and Rasmussen[35] and Branch and colleagues[36] for determining cerebral dominance with respect to language function. Milner and colleagues applied the technique to study the dominance of memory in patients undergoing resection of mesial temporal lobe structures for epilepsy.[37] There have been numerous other applications of this technique, but the focus of this chapter will be on testing for language and memory dominance as it applies to lesions in eloquent cortex.

Tumors involving peri-Sylvian and mesial temporal structures are often in close proximity to potentially essential language cortex and the hippocampus, which has been shown to be of prime importance in memory processing. It is also well established that memory in addition to language tends to lateralize in individuals. It is important for the surgeon to know to which hemisphere language is dominant and in certain circumstances, as with medial temporal lobe lesions, to know potential memory lateralization before embarking on aggressive resection. Wada testing can add light to the decision about whether or not more detailed preoperative or intraoperative study is necessary in individual patients. At a minimum, patients with planned peri-Sylvian or medial temporal resections without strict right-sided preferences should be considered for Wada testing because these individuals will often have atypical language representation. Currently, Wada testing, with certain limitations, as will be briefly discussed in the following, can localize dominant language and memory function with a single testing procedure.

Procedure for Wada Test

Performance of the Wada test requires a multidisciplinary approach involving the neurosurgeon, neurologist, neuropsychologist, and interventional radiologist. Testing consists of a limited angiogram of the internal carotid artery to document the presence of anomalous circulation or significant cross filling that may alter interpretation of the results. Language and memory testing must be presented in an efficient and coordinated fashion, because the time to administer such testing may be relatively short depending on the side tested and whether it is dominant for language. Typically, the patient is tested before the injection of amobarbital to get a baseline assessment of language and memory function to compare to postinjection results. This consists of naming objects, reading words aloud, counting, spelling, following simple commands, and memory items such as remembering drawings or short sentences. Amobarbital, typically at a dose between 100 and 175 mg, is injected, and the effect of the drug is initially assessed by weakness of the contralateral upper extremity. It is important to assess both speech-language function and memory function during the procedure, as documented by Dodrill and Ojemann and others later.[38] In general, it is advisable to administer lower doses of amobarbital to minimize side effects and carryover of the drug's effects when planning to evaluate the contralateral hemisphere. The vast majority of the drug clears within 30 minutes, permitting injection and evaluation of the opposite side.

Selective amobarbital testing has been described and may, in limited circumstances, offer additional information not provided by a carotid injection, although this is not routinely done and may pose an additional risk.[39] Selective injection of the posterior circulation has been described in an effort to isolate the mesial temporal structures[40,41] but is usually not necessary because the function of the hippocampus with respect to memory is affected by the carotid injection. If doubt arises, the amobarbital test may be combined with single photon emission computed tomography imaging to help with interpretation of nonlateralizing studies.[42]

The information obtained from Wada testing should be interpreted with knowledge of the assumptions and limitations that go with the procedure. The main assumptions are that amobarbital will functionally and completely deactivate the regions through which it flows, the carotid injection reaches all areas of the hemisphere that are involved in language function, and there is no substitution of these language functions by areas ipsilateral or contralateral to the injection. Regional blood flow, collateral circulation, and anomalous arterial supply may all contribute to false-negative testing, although typically a limited angiogram prior to the procedure can assess for these before the test is begun.

ANATOMIC IMAGING

Several methods have been described for localizing the central sulcus based on external (skull) landmarks. This gives the surgeon a general idea of where the precentral and postcentral gyri are located preoperatively and can help in planning the craniotomy in the absence of neuronavigational aids. These techniques are based on Taylor-Haughton lines.[43] The motor strip is typically located 4 to 5 cm posterior to the coronal suture in the midsagittal plane.[44]

The central sulcus is often readily identified on preoperative imaging. Berger and colleagues correlated intraoperative stimulation mapping of motor cortex with preoperative MRI scans and found that the central sulcus is reliably identified on high-vertex axial T2-weighted imaging as transverse sulci with the motor cortex located immediately anterior (Fig. 49-1). Additionally, it was found less reliably on slightly

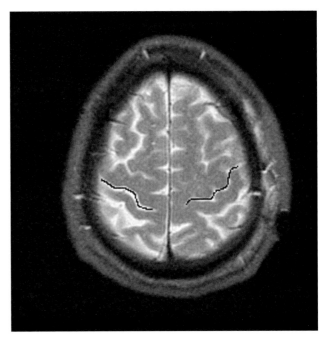

FIGURE 49-1 High vertex axial imaging can be used to locate the central sulcus (*black line*) on most patients as a transversely oriented sulcus posterior to the end of the superior frontal sulcus.

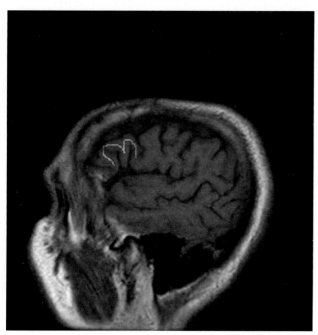

FIGURE 49-2 The frontal operculum can often be identified as an M-shaped gyrus (*gray line*) on lateral sagittal imaging just superior to the Sylvian fissure.

parasagittal images using the termination of the cingulate sulcus in the marginal sulcus with the sensorimotor cortex anterior to this.[45] Efforts at localizing language areas have been less certain, although for Broca's area, which is more constant in location, Quiñones-Hinojosa and colleagues have demonstrated 87% to 89% accuracy when the frontal opercular area is categorized in specific anatomic subtypes when compared to intraoperative stimulation mapping.[46] This may be readily identified on sagittal imaging as an "M-shaped" gyrus representing the pars orbitalis, triangularis, and opercularis (Fig. 49-2).

Though attractive, this method may be most useful for identifying lesions that are in proximity to the rolandic sulcus and thus require more invasive testing either preoperatively with functional imaging and/or with intraoperative mapping.

INTRAOPERATIVE STIMULATION MAPPING

Localization of eloquent areas of the brain during surgery is of paramount importance both in preserving function and in ensuring the most radical resection possible when lesions are in close proximity to them. Furthermore, tumors may abut eloquent cortex, displacing it and making landmarks more difficult to identify, or they may invade critical structures. Intraoperative cortical stimulation is widely used and has been validated in numerous studies. It is currently the "gold standard" in the identification and preservation of eloquent areas to which all other modalities such as functional imaging should be compared.

Localization of Rolandic Cortex

The method of using somatosensory evoked potentials to identify the sensorimotor cortex was introduced by

Goldring in treating pediatric epilepsy patients.[47] It has since broadened to include use in patients having tumors in the rolandic region.[48,49] Somatosensory evoked potential mapping is quick and reliable in identifying the somatosensory region. Typically, an eight–contact strip electrode array is placed over the region of interest in a transverse orientation, and stimulation of the median or tibial nerve, depending on the lesion location, is done with recording of the contralateral cortical surface, either epidurally or subdurally. The somatosensory cortex is located at the point of phase reversal between two adjacent contacts. The array of electrodes may then be repositioned to confirm the location of the central sulcus superiorly or inferiorly.

The advantages of this procedure over stimulation mapping are that the risk for inducing seizures is significantly less, and it may be performed epidurally, thus potentially limiting exposure of eloquent cortex through a tailored dural opening suitable for the needs at hand. Additionally, electrodes may be placed beneath the adjacent bone not involved in the craniotomy flap to localize sensorimotor cortex. Tibial or median nerve stimulation may be used depending on the location of the craniotomy with respect to sensorimotor cortex—that is, tibial for lesions located near the vertex and median for those located over the lateral convexity.

Motor-evoked potentials have more recently been used to identify motor cortex specifically and allow direct stimulation monitoring of motor cortex and subcortical pathways with a high-frequency stimulator in patients under general anesthetic.[48,50,51]

Cortical stimulation mapping can be used to map the rolandic cortex with great precision (Figs. 49-3 to 49-5). Mapping of the motor cortex can be done with the patient either awake or under general anesthesia. Somatosensory stimulation can only be done with the patient awake.

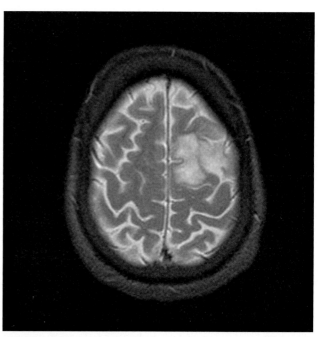

FIGURE 49-3 Preoperative T2-weighted magnetic resonance imaging revealing a low-grade glial tumor adjacent to the motor cortex in the supplementary motor area.

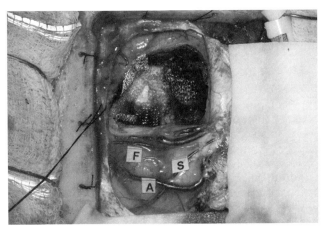

FIGURE 49-4 Intraoperative photograph of the patient in Figure 49-3 showing stimulation mapping of the right upper arm and leg region done before tumor removal. The resection was done with stereotactic guidance and ongoing neurologic examinations, both motor and speech, to protect the radiating white matter tracts during the resection of the deeper components of the tumor. A, arm; F, face; S, shoulder.

Stimulation may involve the cortex or subcortical white matter, which may be especially advantageous for tumors that extend deeply into the hemisphere or in the region of the internal capsule in the case of insular masses. Notably, children may have relatively inexcitable cortex as compared to adults, making stimulation mapping more difficult.[52]

Localization of Language Cortex

Permanent language dysfunction, even relatively minor, can be of considerable distress to the patient and family. Identification of essential language sites is of great importance during lesion resection in the peri-Sylvian region of

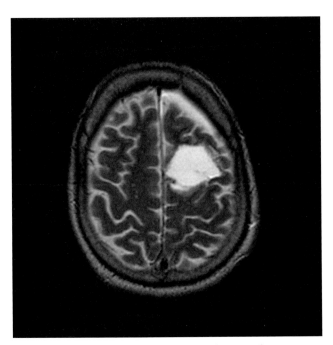

FIGURE 49-5 Postoperative T2-weighted magnetic resonance imaging of the patient in Figure 49-3 revealing complete removal of all T2 signal abnormality.

the dominant hemisphere. Language mapping, in contrast to mapping motor cortex, must be done with the patient awake and cooperative. If speech function, reading, or comprehension is impaired because of the location of the mass, intraoperative stimulation mapping for language function will not usually be helpful. Additionally, adults with neurologic, psychiatric, or significant medical comorbidities such as obesity or pulmonary problems may not be able to tolerate an awake procedure. Prior to surgery, the patient is counseled by the surgeon, anesthesiologist, and speech pathologist or neurologist about the nature of the procedure, the environment, and their expected duties. It is crucial to assess a patient's language function prior to surgery to obtain a baseline against which to compare intraoperative testing. It is often more labor intensive and time consuming for the surgical team and requires perseverance in identifying essential language regions.

Stimulation Mapping Technique

Patient positioning is of great importance to balance the requirements of a multidisciplinary team during the surgical procedure. The patient must be comfortable enough with respect to head position and padding of pressure points to allow cooperation for often extended periods of time. He or she must have an unobstructed view of the examiner so as to participate fully in testing during the procedure. The anesthesiologist must also have ready access to the airway for emergency intubation as well as monitoring during pin placement and craniotomy, when the patient is under more sedation. In our practice, frameless stereotaxis is often used and, therefore, patient positioning must also consider line-of-sight issues of the infrared camera and stereotactic equipment.[53] With these issues in mind, the surgeon must often determine if there will be adequate access to the lesion. Often, optimal positioning from the surgical standpoint is somewhat compromised, and judgment must be exercised about the feasibility of doing an awake procedure as opposed to using alternative methods such as extraoperative mapping. Usually, however, a satisfactory solution can be found, facilitating safe tumor resection.

The patient is given fentanyl and propofol for conscious sedation for placement of the pinion, scalp incision, and craniotomy, then awakened for the cortical and/or subcortical mapping. A mixture of bupivacaine (0.25%) and lidocaine (0.5%) that is pH adjusted is used to infiltrate the pin sites and subsequently the scalp incision when the head has been positioned. Intraoperative stereotactic neuronavigation is useful to plan the craniotomy and scalp incision as well as to allow necessary exposure of the tumor and for mapping of adjacent language or sensorimotor cortices. This will also allow for feedback intraoperatively with respect to tumor volume excision, as discussed further later. Preoperatively, the maximum volume of local anesthetic that can be safely used throughout the procedure is calculated based on the patient's weight (2–3 mg/kg of bupivacaine or 4–6 mg/kg of lidocaine). A reserve of 10 to 15 mL is kept on hand for application to the dura after the craniotomy as well as for additional discomfort the patient may have during the stimulation mapping portion of the procedure. After the mapping has been completed, the patient may again be sedated to finish the necessary resection and closure.

The stereotactic navigation system can be used to outline the tumor and identify possible motor and sensory cortex to minimize the amount of time spent mapping as well as serving as a useful guide about the extent of tumor resection. Intraoperatively, the main concern with stereotaxis and the use of preoperative imaging is brain shift. As the operation progresses, this distortion increases as cerebrospinal fluid is lost and the tumor is resected. This distortion is accentuated when the tumor is large or when the ventricle is entered. Intraoperative ultrasound is an alternative method to ensure maximal resection after mapping has been done to localize the tumor boundaries. Small tickets or catheters may be used to outline the depth of the tumor around the periphery in a "picket fence" arrangement, with resection proceeding up the edge of each catheter. This minimizes the chance that brain shift will have an adverse effect on tumor resection. Ultrasound has shown good correlation to T2 signal abnormality on MRI.[54]

Standard cortical mapping is then done with the Ojemann stimulator, as has been described previously.[52] An established anesthesia protocol should be in place in anticipation of the rare instance that stimulation induces a seizure, especially if the patient's head is fixed in a pinion. To minimize induction of intraoperative seizure activity, a surface electrocorticography strip is placed outside the resection field on the cortical surface to monitor for afterdischarges. Stimulation current is selected to be less than that which results in 1 or 2 afterdischarges. If there is evidence of cortical irritability following a stimulation, the brain's surface is irrigated with ice-cooled saline. A low-setting (2–5 mA) constant current, 60-Hz biphasic square wave stimulus with a 1-msec duration is used to stimulate various regions of interest. Motor stimulation may have to be higher than sensory stimulation. If no response is elicited at 16 mA, then no functional cortex is located in the stimulated area. A quick test of the temporalis muscle reflected from the craniotomy site can confirm that the equipment is functional in sleeping patients. Electromyography can be used when performing mapping of the motor cortex to provide greater sensitivity and lessen the chances of stimulation-induced seizure activity.[55] Contact of the bipolar stimulator, parallel to the adjacent sulci, should last 1 to 2 seconds, and no two stimulation trials should be attempted in succession in one area. Current may need to be increased to identify certain areas such as the face motor region and depends on the anesthesia used if the patient is asleep. Pediatric patients also may require higher stimulation current to elicit a response, as noted earlier. The patient is assessed for motor or sensory findings with each stimulus when mapping the perirolandic areas. The cortex is stimulated in stepwise fashion at 1.5-cm intervals, with two to three positive stimulations defining functional cortex.[53] A numbered tag is then placed on the brain surface at these sites. Subcortical tracts may also be stimulated similarly during tumor resection with the same or slightly higher current parameters.[56-58] This may be particularly useful for insular gliomas adjacent to the internal capsule or medial temporal tumors growing over the tentorial edge to identify the cerebral peduncle at the medial extent of the resection.

Language mapping is done similarly, with a speech pathologist examining the patient with confrontational naming, spelling, counting, reading, or other site-specific test.

The patient is shown objects or assessed every 4 seconds with any errors, anomia, dysnomia, hesitation, or speech arrest being noted. After each stimulation trial, the patient is allowed to name an object without stimulation to ensure recovery of function. Afterdischarges are allowed to dissipate prior to the next stimulation. It is important to note when stimulating the posterior inferior frontal lobe that speech arrest is not caused by oropharyngeal motor arrest, as occurs when stimulating the precentral gyrus, by observing the patient as well as listening. Stimulation of the postcentral gyrus may aid in this distinction, because the patient is able to note oropharyngeal sensory stimuli. Cortical sites essential for language function have been found to be located on the crests of gyri and not generally in sulci unless continuous with an adjacent gyrus, according to Ojemann and co-workers.[32]

Most stimulation-induced seizures last only 10 to 30 seconds, and cold saline can be applied to the cortical surface to abort the majority of these. Seizures lasting longer than this should be treated more aggressively with benzodiazepines, because generalization of a focal seizure can lead to an unsafe situation with a patient in pinions and limited access to the airway. Again, every effort should be made to use low stimulation current as well as meticulous monitoring of afterdischarges to prevent this complication.

A limitation of intraoperative cortical mapping is that high-intensity stimulation may inhibit or activate functional areas whereas low-intensity stimulation may not identify intended target areas.[59] Other pitfalls to be aware of are that more than two language areas can exist, and thus the inability to identify any eloquent cortex should raise caution that the stimulation is not working rather than lead to the conclusion that none exists in a given area. Also, preservation of cortex with disruption of subcortical tracts by undercutting gyri may lead to permanent morbidity.

It is often straightforward to identify by MRI the central sulcus or to map eloquent motor and language cortex as just described. However, it is far more difficult to map the subcortical white matter tracts. One technique to minimize the risk of injury to radiating white matter tracts is to conduct repetitive neurologic and speech examinations during the ongoing tumor resection. This obviously requires a coordinated team approach, which includes having both a neurologist and speech pathologist, possibly with interpreters for mapping multiple language regions available in the operating room. With ongoing examinations, the surgeon is able to be more aggressive and proceeds with resection until the onset of neurologic deficits. In this circumstance, a maximum neurologically permissible resection of infiltrative tumors can be performed with a risk of significant neurologic injury that approximates 15%.[53]

There is evidence that epilepsy associated with slow-growing low-grade neoplasms resides in adjacent tumor-free cortex.[60] Epilepsy associated with AVMs may be similar.[61] With respect to lesions in eloquent cortex, this epileptogenic zone may also reside in functional cortex, hence the need to perform either extraoperative mapping as described later, or intraoperative electrocorticography to define this area. Multiple studies have shown that resection of adjacent electrocorticography-active foci results in improved seizure control as compared with resection of the tumor mass alone.[60] Children may fare better in this regard than adults.[62] Combining an epilepsy operation with an oncologic operation may provide the best chance at tumor and seizure control. It is also important to monitor for epileptic discharges after resection to ensure that additional seizure foci are not left behind.

Intraoperative cortical mapping combined with appropriate functional imaging and stereotactic neuronavigation should theoretically protect the patient from iatrogenic neurologic morbidity. This, however, is not always the case, and there are several possible reasons for this. First, patients with lesions in eloquent areas already have some degree of neurologic impairment, and manipulation or close resection to critical areas may worsen the neurologic condition. Additionally, maximizing resection by removing tumor until a deficit becomes apparent is a strategy sometimes used.[7,52] Second, regional ischemia and peritumoral edema may become manifest after an apparently uneventful resection.[63] Third, a lack of specificity of the testing paradigm to the area of resection may miss potentially eloquent areas. This is minimized by using naming as a part of language evaluation, as the majority of aphasias have anomia as a component of the syndrome. More specific tests, however, can be done when there is concern about important association cortex or functions such as calculation.[64] Complex language functions may in time be better identified with more specific testing paradigms used after assessment with functional MRI (fMRI), evaluating the specific functional modalities at risk during lesion resection.[65]

Resection of gliomas to within 2 cm of eloquent tissue used in naming carries a risk of persistent postoperative deficit, as noted by Ojemann and Dodrill.[66] Haglund and colleagues later reported in a study of patients undergoing temporal glioma resection that a margin of greater than 8 mm was associated with no postoperative deficits lasting more than 30 days.[67] In general, it is best to keep a margin of about 1 cm between resection and eloquent cortex. Subcortical pathways from sensorimotor and language areas are thought to descend perpendicular to gyri; therefore, undercutting identified eloquent cortex is not recommended.

The majority of the deficits induced during awake craniotomy are temporary in nature and lasting major neurologic morbidity relatively rare. Patients must be counseled preoperatively of this risk and the expected temporary nature of the postoperative deficits.

EXTRAOPERATIVE STIMULATION MAPPING

Epileptic monitoring is by far the most widely cited indication for intracranial monitoring with grid placement. This allows both monitoring for epileptic discharges for a prolonged period, as well as stimulation mapping of functional cortex. It is analogous to intraoperative stimulation mapping, but there are important differences and indications for using one or the other procedure. It is often used in the surgical treatment of extratemporal nonlesional intractable epilepsy.

In lesional epilepsy, it is important to know whether the structural abnormality in question is responsible for the patient's seizure and to ensure that any resection being planned also accounts for adjacent epileptic foci if possible. This is particularly evident in patients with multiple lesions, for example cavernomas, or patients with medially placed temporal lesions and hippocampal atrophy, with respect to

which lesion or how extensive a surgery should be planned. Typically, patients with a dominant lesion and concordant preoperative data supporting the supposition that the lesion in question is responsible for seizures, do not need extraoperative electrocorticography or mapping and can have it done intraoperatively. However, patients who have more than one lesion or infrequent disabling seizures, or who have discordant data may be good candidates for grid placement and monitoring, because the duration of monitoring can be extended up to 2 weeks if necessary. The grid placement and subsequent resection can sometimes be enhanced with awake mapping.[68] Additionally, patients who do not meet the criteria for intraoperative stimulation mapping, such as children or adults who are unable to cooperate as a result of neurologic or psychiatric disease or medical comorbidities such as severe obesity or pulmonary problems, are good candidates for this technique.

The disadvantages to grid placement are that it requires at least two operations, or sometimes three if the grids have to be repositioned after a period of monitoring, and an increased risk of infection due to having a foreign body in place. Furthermore, in patients with large mass lesions, adding the additional mass of grid electrodes, however small, to a condition in which intracranial pressure is already increased may be problematic. Methods to minimize the mass effect include leaving the bone flap out during monitoring and using various medical modalities to reduce intracranial pressure such as steroids or diuretics. Additionally, the resolution of grid electrodes is typically 1 cm, as compared with standard bipolar electrodes, which are 5 mm apart. Usually this has little consequence, however.

The decision whether to resect the hippocampus for patients who have intractable epilepsy related to tumors located in the medial temporal lobe can be addressed with the evaluation of memory during Wada testing. For patients with dominant memory functions on the side of the tumor, it may be reasonable to spare the hippocampus if it is not directly involved with the tumor mass. More commonly, however, the hippocampus will be atrophic and dominant memory function will be represented in the contralateral hippocampus, allowing for resection of mesial temporal structures along with the tumor mass to maximize seizure control.

FUNCTIONAL IMAGING

There has been an explosion in recent years in the research and application of functional imaging to neurosurgery. These techniques are based on identifying regions of the brain that are "active" relative to other regions of the brain during a specific testing algorithm. This technology is extremely helpful in that it offers the possibility of localizing eloquent areas of cortex with respect to a mass lesion preoperatively, determining the best surgical approach, and potentially guiding the decision to use intraoperative mapping in a given patient.

Functional MRI (fMRI) and positron emission tomography (PET) scanning are being used more frequently in the preoperative assessment of eloquent areas of the brain. Functional MR signal changes are believed to be a result of local blood oxygenation differences between activated and, therefore, more metabolically active, brain and relatively

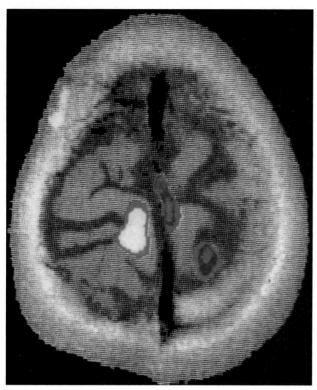

FIGURE 49-6 Functional magnetic resonance image using the BOLD technique for identifying motor cortex preoperatively.

silent areas. This has been termed the blood oxygen level–dependent (BOLD) contrast method and requires no contrast agent[69] (Fig. 49-6). Various paradigms exist for testing certain areas of the brain. All are dependent on a comparison with the performance of a task and a resting state or alternate task. fMRI studies and their interpretation, therefore, are extremely dependent on the tasks and comparisons used. While fMRI measures the changes in deoxyhemoglobin levels reflecting oxygen consumption, PET measures regional differences in cerebral blood flow through use of an injected radioisotope, most commonly [15O]H2O or 2-[18F]-2-desoxy-D-glucose (FDG). Despite the inherent differences in the physiologic basis for the imaging modalities, concordance between them when compared to intraoperative stimulation mapping has been good.[70,71] In the future, fMRI may have more efficacy in comparison with PET because of its noninvasive nature and more widespread availability.

Maps of eloquent areas identified on fMRI or PET can be coregistered or "fused" to standard MRI scans, slice by slice manually or with fusion software, to give better anatomic detail in most neuronavigational systems.[72,73] This coregistration can in turn be applied in planning the surgical procedure, as well as during the formal operation. The potential benefit to using fMRI data is that it preoperatively determines the general location of eloquent cortex with respect to the lesion in question, allowing for preprocedural planning of the craniotomy and the approach to the tumor, as well as aiding in the decision whether to apply intraoperative stimulation. It may further reduce the size of the craniotomy,

thus minimizing both surgical morbidity and the amount of time spent performing intraoperative mapping.[74]

More recently there has been interest in combining fMRI with diffusion-weighted MR images to identify the motor cortex and pyramidal tracts with respect to space-occupying lesions.[75] This may also add additional insight into the preoperative planning and again reduce the time needed for intraoperative stimulation of subcortical tracts, which can be tedious and time consuming. The major disadvantage at this point is the spatial resolution of the diffusion-weighted sequences. More studies evaluating this potential application and direct comparison to intraoperative subcortical mapping must be done to validate this technique.

Several potential pitfalls should be taken into account when relying on fMRI or PET data. There can be significant technical issues in integrating functional scans with a neuronavigational system with respect to echo-planar image distortion and complementary slice integration. This may lead to functional mislocalization of eloquent tissue.[76] The areas identified by fMRI or PET utilized for a specific task are often much larger than those identified at surgery with electrical mapping. This poses a problem in deciphering on fMRI the areas that are essential for a given task and the areas that simply participate in a task but are nonessential. This has been more problematic in mapping language areas than in mapping sensorimotor regions.[77,78] Additionally, local vasoreactivity in peritumoral brain may distort results that rely on vasoreactivity and oxygen consumption for producing data maps.[79]

Intraoperative stimulation mapping remains the gold standard for identifying and preserving functional cortex and subcortical white matter; however, noninvasive methods such as fMRI are desirable, and further research and paradigm validation may improve the usefulness of this technique in the future.

CONCLUSIONS

Surgery of lesions or epileptic foci located in eloquent areas of the brain provides a unique challenge to the neurosurgeon. The goals are to maximize resection and minimize neurologic morbidity. Several techniques for achieving these goals have been presented. A multidisciplinary approach to treating these patients is the standard, and it should be kept in mind that these techniques should be viewed as complementary to each other, with no one approach serving as a stand-alone method of ensuring safe removal of lesions in eloquent brain.

REFERENCES

1. Kelly PJ, Daumas-Duport C, Kispert DB, et al: Imaging-based stereotaxic serial biopsies in untreated intracranial glial neoplasms. J Neurosurg 66:865–874, 1987.
2. Skirboll SS, Ojemann GA, Berger MS, et al: Functional cortex and subcortical white matter located within gliomas. Neurosurgery 38:678–684, 1996.
3. Berger MS, Deliganis AV, Dobbins J, et al: The effect of extent of resection on recurrence in patients with low grade cerebral hemisphere gliomas. Cancer 74:1784–1791, 1994.
4. Hirsch JF, Rose CS, Pierre-Kahn A, et al: Benign astrocytic and oligodendrocytic tumors of the cerebral hemispheres in children. J Neurosurg 70:568–572, 1989.
5. Berger MS, Rostomily RC: Low grade gliomas: Functional mapping resection strategies, extent of resection, and outcome. J Neurooncol 34:85–101, 1997.

6. Nakamura M, Konishi N, Tsundoda S, et al: Analysis of prognostic and survival factors related to treatment of low-grade astrocytoma in adult. Oncology 58:108–116, 2000.
7. Peraud A, Meschede M, Eisner W, et al: Surgical resection of grade II astrocytomas in the superior frontal gyrus. Neurosurgery 50:966–977, 2002.
8. Piepmeier J, Christopher S, Spencer D, et al: Variations in the natural history and survival of patients with supratentorial low-grade astrocytomas. Neurosurgery 38:872–878, 1996.
9. Vives KP, Piepmeier JM: Complications and expected outcome of glioma surgery. J Neurooncol 42:289–302, 1999.
10. Soffietti R, Chio A, Giordana MT, et al: Prognostic factors in well-differentiated cerebral astrocytomas in the adult. Neurosurgery 24:686–692, 1989.
11. Shafqat S, Hedley-White ET, Henson JW: Age-dependent rate of anaplastic transformation in low-grade astrocytoma. Neurology 52:867–869, 1999.
12. Laws ER Jr, Taylor WF, Clifton MB, et al: Neurosurgical management of low-grade astrocytoma of the cerebral hemispheres. J Neurosurg 61:665–673, 1984.
13. Schmidt MH, Berger MS, Lamborn KR, et al: Repeated operations for infiltrative low-grade gliomas without intervening therapy. J Neurosurg 98:1165–1169, 2003.
14. Keles GE, Lamborn KR, Berger MS: Low-grade hemispheric gliomas in adults: A critical review of extent of resection as a factor influencing outcome. J Neurosurg 95:735–745, 2001.
15. Ammirati M, Vick N, Liao Y, et al: Effect of the extent of surgical resection on survival and quality of life in patients with supratentorial glioblastomas and anaplastic astrocytomas. Neurosurgery 21:201–205, 1987.
16. Ciric I, Ammirati M, Vick N, et al: Supratentorial gliomas: Surgical considerations and immediate postoperative results. Neurosurgery 21:21–26, 1987.
17. DeVaux BC, O'Fallon JR, Kelly PJ: Resection, biopsy and survival in malignant glial neoplasma: A retrospective study of clinical parameters, therapy, and outcome. J Neurosurg 78:767–775, 1993.
18. Lacroix M, Abi-Said D, Fourney DR, et al: A multivariate analysis of 416 patients with glioblastoma multiforme: Prognosis, extent of resection, and survival. J Neurosurg 95:190–198, 2001.
19. Nitta T, Sato K: Prognostic implications of the extent of surgical resection in patients with intracranial malignant gliomas. Cancer 75:2727–2731, 1995.
20. Sawaya R: Extent of resection in malignant gliomas: A critical summary. J Neurooncol 42:303–305, 1999.
21. Laws ER, Parney IF, Huang W, et al: Survival following surgery and prognostic factors for recently diagnosed malignant glioma: Data from the glioma outcomes project. J Neurosurg 99:467–473, 2003.
22. Jeremic B, Grujicic D, Antunovic V, et al: Influence of extent surgery and tumor location on treatment outcome of patients with glioblastoma multiforme treated with combined modality approach. J Neurooncol 21:177–185, 1994.
23. Broca P: Remarques sur le siège de la faculté du language articulé, suivies d'une observation d'aphémie (perte de la parole). Bull Soc Anat 36:330–357, 1861.
24. Wernicke C: Der Aphasische Symptomen Komplex. Breslau: Cohn & Weigart, 1874.
25. Cushing H: A note upon the faradic stimulation of the postcentral gyrus in conscious patients. Brain 32:44–54, 1909.
26. Penfield W, Boldrey E: Somatic motor and sensory representation in the cerebral cortex of man as studied by electrical stimulation. Brain 60:389–443, 1937.
27. LeRoux PD, Berger MS, Haglund MM, et al: Resection of intrinsic tumors from nondominant face motor cortex using stimulation mapping: Report of two cases. Surg Neurol 36:44–48, 1991.
28. Penfield W, Jasper H: Epilepsy and the Functional Anatomy of the Human Brain. Boston: Little, Brown & Co., 1954.
29. Penfield W, Roberts L: Speech and Brian Mechanisms. Princeton, NJ: Princeton University Press, 1959.
30. Rostomily R, Berger M, Ojemann G, et al: Postoperative deficits and functional recovery following removal of tumors involving the dominant hemisphere supplementing motor area. J Neurosurg 75:62–68, 1991.
31. Zentner J, Hufnagel A, Pechstein U, et al: Functional results after resective procedures involving the supplementary motor area. J Neurosurg 85:542–549, 1996.
32. Ojemann G, Ojemann J, Lettich E, et al: Cortical language localization in left, dominant hemisphere. J Neurosurg 71:316–326, 1989.
33. Strauss E, Wada J: Lateral preferences and cerebral speech dominance. Cortex 19:165–177, 1983.
34. Wada J: A new method for the determination of the side of cerebral speech dominance: A preliminary report of the intracarotid injection of sodium amytal in man. Igaku Seibutsugaki (Medicine and Biology) 14:221–222, 1949.
35. Wada J, Rasmussen T: Intracranial injection of amytal for the lateralization of cerebral speech dominance. J Neurosurg 17:266–282, 1960.
36. Branch C, Milner B, Rasmussen T: Intracarotid sodium amytal for the lateralization of cerebral speech dominance: Observations in 123 patients. J Neurosurg 21:399–405, 1964.
37. Milner B, Branch C, Rasmussen T: Study of short-term memory after intracarotid injection of sodium amytal. Trans Am Neurol Assoc 87:224–226, 1962.
38. Dodrill CB, Ojemann GA: An exploratory comparison of three methods of memory assessment with the intracarotid amobarbital procedure. Brain Cogn 33:210–223, 1997.
39. Wieser HG, Muller S, Schiess R, et al: The anterior and posterior selective temporal lobe amobarbital tests: Angiographic, clinical, electroencephalographic, PET, SPECT findings, and memory performance. Brain Cogn 33:71–97, 1997.
40. Morton N, Polkey CE, Cox T, et al: Episodic memory dysfunction during sodium amytal testing of epileptic patients in relation to posterior cerebral artery perfusion. J Clin Exp Neuropsychol 18:24–37, 1996.
41. Urbach H, Klemm E, Linke DB, et al: Posterior cerebral artery Wada test: Sodium amytal distribution and functional deficits. Neuroradiology 43:290–294, 2001.
42. Kim BG, Lee SK, Kim JY, et al: Interpretation of Wada memory test for lateralization of seizure focus by use of (99m) technetium-HMPAO SPECT. Epilepsia 41:65–70, 2000.
43. Taylor AJ, Haughton VM, Syvertsen A, et al: Taylor-Haughton line revisited AJNR Am J Neuroradiol 1:55–56, 1980.
44. Kido DK, LeMay M, Levinson AW, et al: Computed tomographic localization of the precentral gyrus. Radiology 135:373–377, 1980.
45. Berger MS, Cohen WA, Ojemann GA: Correlation of motor cortex brain mapping data with magnetic resonance imaging. J Neurosurg 72:383–387, 1990.
46. Quiñones-Hinojosa A, Ojemann SG, Sanai N, et al: Preoperative correlation of intraoperative cortical mapping with magnetic resonance imaging landmarks to predict localization of the Broca area. J Neurosurg 99:311–318, 2003.
47. Goldring S: A method for surgical management of focal epilepsy, especially as it relates to children. J Neurosurg 49:344–356, 1978.
48. Cedzich C, Taniguchi M, Schafer S, et al: Somatosensory evoked potential phase reversal and direct motor cortex stimulation during surgery in and around the central region. Neurosurgery 38:962–970, 1996.
49. Romstock J, Fahlbusch R, Ganslandt, et al: Localization of the sensorimotor cortex during surgery for brain tumours: Feasibility and waveform patterns of somatosensory evoked potentials. J Neurol Neurosurg Psychiatry 72:221–229, 2002.
50. Kombos T, Suess O, Funk T, et al: Intra-operative mapping of the motor cortex during surgery in and around the motor cortex. Acta Neurochir (Wien) 142:263–268, 2000.
51. Cedzich C, Pechstein U, Schramm J, et al: Electrophysiological considerations regarding electrical stimulation of motor cortex and brain stem in humans. Neurosurgery 42:527–532, 1998.
52. Berger MS, Kincaid J, Ojemann GA, et al: Brain mapping techniques to maximize resection, safety, and seizure control in children with brain tumors. Neurosurgery 25:786–792, 1989.
53. Meyer FB, Bates LM, Goerss SJ, et al: Awake craniotomy for aggressive resection of primary gliomas located in eloquent brain. Mayo Clin Proc 76:677–687, 2001.
54. LeRoux P, Berger MS, Wang K, et al: Low grade gliomas: Comparison of intraoperative ultrasound characteristics with preoperative imaging studies. J Neurosurg 13:189–198, 1992.
55. Yingling CD, Ojemann S, Dodson B, et al: Identification of motor pathways during tumor surgery facilitated by multichannel electromyographic recording. J Neurosurg 91:922–927, 1999.
56. Berger MS, Ojemann GA: Intraoperative brain mapping techniques in neuro-oncology. Stereotact Funct Neurosurg 58:153–161, 1992.

57. Berger MS, Ojemann GA, Lettich E: Neurophysiological monitoring during astrocytoma surgery. Neurosurg Clin N Am 1:65–79, 1990.

58. Duffau H, Capelle L, Denvil D, et al: Usefulness of intraoperative electrical subcortical mapping during surgery for low-grade gliomas located within eloquent brain regions: functional results in a consecutive series of 103 patients. J Neurosurg 98:764–778, 2003.

59. Carpentier A, Pugh KR, Westerveld M, et al: Functional MRI of language processing: dependence on input modality and temporal lobe epilepsy. Epilepsia 42:1241–1254, 2001.

60. Berger MS, Ghatan S, Geyer JR, et al: Seizure outcome in children with hemispheric tumors and associated intractable epilepsy: The role of tumor removal combined with seizure foci resection. Pediatr Neurosurg 17:185–191, 1991.

61. Yeh HS, Kashiwagi S, Tew JM Jr, et al: Surgical management of epilepsy associated with cerebral arteriovenous malformations. J Neurosurg 72:216–223, 1990.

62. Berger MS, Ghatan S, Haglund MM, et al: Low-grade gliomas associated with intractable epilepsy: Seizure outcome utilizing electrocorticography during tumor resection. J Neurosurg 79:62–69, 1993.

63. Duffau H, Lopes M, Denvil D, et al: Delayed onset of the SMA syndrome after surgical resection of the mesial frontal lobe: A time course study using intraoperative mapping in an awake patient. Stereotact Funct Neurosurg 76:74–82, 2001.

64. Duffau H, Denvil D, Lopes M, et al: Intraoperative mapping of the cortical areas involved in multiplication and subtraction: An electrostimulation study in a patient with a left parietal glioma. J Neurol Neurosurg Psychiatry 73:733–820, 2002.

65. Whittle IR, Borthwick S, Haq N: Brain dysfunction following 'awake' craniotomy, brain mapping and resection of glioma. Br J Neurosurg 17:130–137, 2003.

66. Ojemann GA, Dodrill CG: Intraoperative techniques for reducing language and memory deficits with left temporal lobe lobectomy. In Wolf P, Dam M, Janz D, Dreifuss F (eds): Advances in epileptology. New York: Raven Press, 1987, pp 327–330.

67. Haglund MM, Berger MS, Shamseldin M, et al: Cortical localization of temporal lobe language sites in patients with gliomas. Neurosurgery 34:567–576, 1994.

68. Cohen-Gadol AA, Britton JW, Collignon FP, et al: Nonlesional central lobule seizures: Use of awake cortical mapping and subdural grid monitoring for resection of seizure focus. J Neurosurg 98:1255–1262, 2003.

69. Ogawa S, Lee TM, Kay AR, et al: Brain magnetic resonance imaging with contrast dependent on blood oxygenation. Proc Natl Acad Sci U S A 87:9868–9872, 1990.

70. Bittar RG, Olivier A, Sadikot AF, et al: Presurgical motor and somatosensory cortex mapping with functional magnetic resonance imaging and positron emission tomography. J Neurosurg 91:915–921, 1999.

71. Ramsey NF, Kirkby BS, Van Gelderen P, et al: Functional mapping of human sensorimotor cortex with 3D BOLD fMRI correlates highly with H2[15]O PET rCBF. J Cereb Blood Flow Metab 16:755–764, 1996.

72. McDonald JD, Chong BW, Lewine JD, et al: Integration of preoperative and intraoperative functional brain mapping in a frameless stereotactic environment for lesions near eloquent cortex. J Neurosurg 90:591–598, 1999.

73. Schulder M, Maldjian JA, Liu WC, et al: Functional image-guided surgery of intracranial tumors located in or near the sensorimotor cortex. J Neurosurg 89:412–418, 1998.

74. Rutten GJ, Ramsey NF, van Rijen PC, et al: Development of a functional magnetic resonance imaging protocol for intraoperative localization of critical temporoparietal language areas. Ann Neurol 51:350–360, 2002.

75. Krings T, Reinges MH, Thiex R, et al: Functional and diffusion-weighted magnetic resonance images of space-occupying lesions affecting the motor system: Imaging the motor cortex and pyramidal tracts. J Neurosurg 95:816–824, 2001.

76. Roux FE, Ibarrola D, Tremoulet M, et al: Methodological and technical issues for integrating functional magnetic resonance imaging data in a neuronavigational system. Neurosurgery 49:1145–1156, 2001.

77. Roux FE, Boulanouar K, Lotterie JA, et al: Language functional magnetic resonance imaging in preoperative assessment of language areas: Correlation with direct cortical stimulation. Neurosurgery 52:1335–1347, 2003.

78. Lehericy S, Duffau H, Cornu P, et al: Correspondence between functional magnetic resonance imaging somatotopy and individual brain anatomy of the central region: Comparison with intraoperative stimulation in patients with brain tumors. J Neurosurg 92:589–598, 2000.

79. Roux FE, Boulanouar K, Ranjeva JP, et al: Usefulness of motor functional MRI correlated to cortical mapping in rolandic low-grade astrocytoma. Acta Neurochir (Wien) 141:71–79, 1999

50

Surgical Management of Recurrent Gliomas

GRIFFITH R. HARSH IV

Renewed growth of a mass at the site of a previously treated brain glioma raises issues pertaining to the indications for and choices of treatment. Important considerations include the following: (1) Is the mass a recurrence of the original tumor, (2) why did the tumor regrow, (3) does this regrowth pose a threat to the patient's neurologic function and survival, and (4) what additional therapy is appropriate?

CONFIRMATION OF RECURRENCE

When recurrent growth of a glioma is suspected either clinically or radiographically, the full set of imaging studies should be reviewed with careful attention directed toward detecting any change of imaging signals and documenting the size of the lesion. The original pathologic specimen should be reviewed.

Differential Diagnosis

An enlarging lesion at the site of a previously treated glioma probably represents renewed growth of an incompletely eradicated initial tumor rather than the development of a new pathologic entity. Exceptions are infrequent, but they do occur, as is noted in the following list:

- A tumor of related histology may supplant the original tumor; for example, the astrocytic component may replace the oligodendrocytic component as the predominant subtype of a mixed glioma, or a gliosarcoma may arise from a previously treated glioblastoma.
- A distinctly new tumor may arise near the site of an eradicated tumor. This is more likely to occur if there is a genetic predisposition to tumor development shared by cells in the area; for example, multiple gliomas may occur in a patient with tuberous sclerosis or neurofibromatosis.
- Nonneoplastic lesions induced by treatment of the original tumor may mimic tumor growth; for example, an abscess may be found at the site of tumor resection, or radiation necrosis may follow focal high-dose irradiation.

These differential diagnoses must be excluded before prognosis is addressed and therapy chosen. Neurodiagnostic imaging usually permits accurate prediction of the diagnosis. The first sign of recurrent tumor on a magnetic resonance imaging (MRI) scan is often an increase in T2 hyperintensity about the tumor bed. An original consistently thin contrast-enhancing rim will develop focal thickening and nodularity.[1] From this nodularity develops a mass that often has imaging features similar to those of the original lesion. A recurrent malignant glioma will probably have central low-density rim enhancement, and hypodense surrounding components on computed tomographic (CT) scans. On MRI scans, the center and surrounding area will be T1-hypointense and T2-hyperintense, and the rim will enhance.[2] In some cases, however, attention to subtle differences may be required: A more spherical, sharply demarcated, highly enhanced rim may suggest an abscess rather than recurrent malignant glioma, while a more diffuse, irregularly marginated pattern of surrounding edema may indicate radionecrosis rather than recurrent tumor. Two scenarios, malignant progression and radiation effects, often pose particular diagnostic difficulty. In each case, alternative diagnoses often cannot be distinguished by imaging criteria alone.

Malignant Progression

The first scenario is the renewed growth of a low-grade tumor. When low-grade gliomas regrow after therapy, approximately half remain nonanaplastic, but the other 50% progress to a more malignant form.[3-6] Molecular analyses have delineated genetic correlates of this progression.[7] Enlarging low-grade tumors usually resemble the original tumor on imaging studies. When a progression in grade has occurred, the new tumor may also resemble the old one, especially if the original tumor enhanced with contrast. Enhancement is highly predictive of recurrence; low-grade enhancing tumors are six to eight times as likely to recur as nonenhancing tumors.[8] Most commonly, new malignant growth enhances in a previously nonenhancing glioma and thus is readily identified. In one study, only 30% (16 of 42) of low-grade tumors enhanced initially, but 92% (22 of 24) enhanced at recurrence.[8] Occasionally, however, an enlarging malignant focus may not enhance. However, it might be apparent as a region of hypermetabolism on a 2-deoxyglucose positron-emission tomography (PET) study, increased activity on a thallium or iodine single photon emission CT (SPECT) scan, or increased cerebral blood volume on a functional MRI (fMRI) scan.[9,10] Proton MR spectroscopy (MRS) may show increase of choline relative to creatine and N-acetyl aspartate (NAA).[11,12] The sensitivity of these modalities for detecting tumor recurrence is approximately 80%.[13,14] Usually, however, histologic analysis after biopsy or resection is warranted to verify malignant transformation.

Radiation Effects

The second scenario that causes diagnostic difficulty is renewed enlargement of a tumor mass following radiation. Usually only large, very malignant tumors grow sufficiently fast to show significant enlargement during, or within

3 months of completing, a course of radiation. When this does occur, the prognosis is particularly poor.[15] Radiation can cause tumor enlargement in three ways: (1) through an early reaction, which is likely to be edema occurring during or shortly after irradiation; (2) through an early delayed reaction that involves edema and demyelination arising a few weeks to a few months after radiation; and (3) through a late delayed reaction that occurs 6 to 24 months after radiation and reflects radiation-induced necrosis.[16]

Regional teletherapy at a dose of 60 Gy is the current standard radiation treatment for most gliomas.[17] Although this dose has a low risk of inducing radiation necrosis, regional early and early delayed effects are relatively common. In most cases tissue swelling represents edema and is transient. Acute symptoms from early or early delayed effects of radiation usually respond quickly to a short course of corticosteroids. The low-density, T1-hypointense, T2-hyperintense regions of edema correspond to the area irradiated. Chronically, these volumes of brain will demonstrate parenchymal atrophy, enlargement of subarachnoid spaces, and ex vacuo ventricular dilatation. Dementia with apathy, inanition, and memory loss, as well as decline in fine motor control are the clinical correlates. In the absence of new tumor growth, enhancement on CT and MRI beyond the initial tumor resection margin is infrequent; when it does occur, it is patchy, diffuse, irregularly margined, and easily distinguished from the more focal, nodular appearance of recurrent tumor.

In contrast, the late delayed effect of radiation-induced necrosis appears at about the time malignant tumors might be expected to recur.[18] The risk of radiation necrosis increases with the volume of tissue treated, the dose delivered, and the fraction size.[19] Radiation necrosis following fractionated treatment to doses of less than 70 Gy is rare; its incidence rises steadily with higher doses, however.[20] Radiation necrosis is much more common following brachytherapy and radiosurgery. These methods deliver high doses of radiation to relatively small volumes over a short time period.[18,21] A common protocol for brachytherapy is a 50- to 60-Gy boost (to 60 Gy of regional external beam radiotherapy) to a 0- to 5-cm tumor delivered over approximately 1 week. The radiosurgical equivalent is a 10- to 20-Gy boost to a 0- to 3-cm tumor delivered in less than 1 hour. Necrosis is radiographically and pathologically evident in almost all cases and symptomatic in as many as half.

Whether arising from higher doses of fractionated radiotherapy, brachytherapy, or radiosurgery, radiation necrosis is often difficult to distinguish radiographically from recurrent tumor. It forms a ringlike contrast-enhancing mass that resembles a malignant tumor. It has these characteristics: a CT-hypodense, T1-hypointense, T2-hyperintense center; an enhancing annular region; and a hypodense, T1-hypointense, T2-hyperintense surrounding area. The surrounding area corresponds to edema that conforms strikingly to the patterns of white matter tract radiations. The similarity of this appearance to that of recurrent tumors and the time course of its occurrence frequently necessitate additional measures to differentiate radiation-induced necrosis from recurrent tumor. A variety of functional neurodiagnostic imaging techniques help to distinguish between these two possibilities. Regions of high activity on PET scans, SPECT scans, dynamic MRI, and MRI cerebral blood volume mapping are thought to distinguish recurrent tumor from relatively metabolically inactive and hypovascular radiation necrosis.[9,10] An increase in the ratio of choline to creatine and of choline to NAA of a mass on MRS is suggestive of tumor recurrence (present in >80% of 34 recurrent tumors); the ratio of NAA to creatine and levels of lipid and lactate did not help differentiate recurrent tumor from radiation necrosis after radiosurgery.[11,12,22]

Although specificity for differentiation of tumor recurrence from radiation necrosis of up to 100% has been claimed for these techniques, in many cases, the data from these studies are inconclusive and the diagnosis is revealed by either the clinical course or analysis of a pathologic specimen.[9,14] The prognostic importance in making this distinction and the utility of MRI-directed stereotactic biopsy was defined in a study that showed that a diagnosis of radiation effect rather than recurrent tumor portended significantly longer survival only if the abnormal signal warranting diagnosis appeared at least 5 months after initial radiotherapy. When biopsy performed within 5 months of radiation therapy showed radiation effect but no tumor, 86% of cases developed recurrent tumor (at a mean interval of 11 months from biopsy). When biopsy was not needed for at least 5 months, only 25% of cases developed recurrent tumor (at a mean interval of 12 months).[23]

When an enlarging mass that is recurrent tumor, radiation necrosis, or both becomes symptomatic, corticosteroid therapy is required. Up to half of the patients receiving high-dose-rate brachytherapy and radiosurgery develop symptoms that either prove refractory to corticosteroids or require debilitating long-term steroid use.[18,21] In early studies, surgery for resection of an enlarging, symptomatic mass was needed in 20% to 40% of patients following such brachytherapy or radiosurgery of a malignant glioma.[18,21] At reoperation for presumed radiation necrosis following focal radiation treatment of a malignant glioma, necrosis was found in 5% of cases, tumor alone in 29%, and a mixture of radiation necrosis and tumor in 66%.[18] In almost all cases, the tumor that is seen is of reduced viability.[24,25]

CAUSES OF RECURRENCE

Renewed growth of a brain glioma following surgery and possibly radiation and chemotherapy indicates failure of these therapies to reduce the tumor to a size that would permit its eradication by the patient's immune system (Fig. 50-1). Failure arises from a number of conditions that limit the efficacy of each modality.

Recurrence after Surgery

Surgery may fail because of anatomic considerations, pathologic features, or errors in judgment or technique. The involvement of critical structures may limit the initial resection. Tumor investment of the anterior or middle cerebral arteries; involvement of the optic pathway, the diencephalon, the internal capsule, or brain stem; or proximity to eloquent cortex all warrant incomplete removal. Tumor recurrence, despite removal of all macroscopically evident tumor, can occur if there is microscopic infiltration of adjacent structures. All but Grade I cerebral gliomas are infiltrative, and microscopic foci of neoplastic cells are

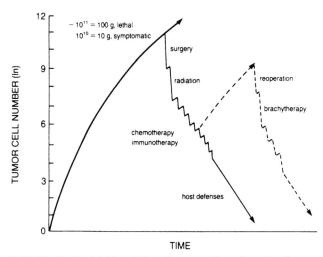

FIGURE 50-1 Multimodality therapy of malignant gliomas. Various therapeutic methods, including reoperation, are used in an attempt to reduce the number of tumor cells.

frequently found several centimeters from the densely cellular tumor. Anaplastic astrocytomas and glioblastomas characteristically are widely invasive. Finally, errors in judgment, such as preoperatively underestimating the amount of tumor that can be safely removed or intraoperatively failing to remove tumor that was targeted, result in leaving potentially resectable tumor as a nidus of regrowth.

Recurrence after Radiation

Radiation therapy may fail because of inadequate targeting, underutilization of tolerable dose, or radiation resistance of the tumor cells. The correlations between imaging abnormality and tumor extent are incomplete. Pathologic studies have shown that individual tumor cells can be found throughout and even beyond CT-hypodense and MRI T2-hyperintense areas of malignant glioma.[2] The value of functional imaging techniques, such as PET and MRS, as guides to targeting of radiation is being studied.[26] The choice of field size for irradiation of such a lesion nonetheless remains difficult and relies as much on the trade-off between target volume and tolerable dose as on the accurate delineation of tumor boundaries. Failure to include an adequate annulus of tissue about the tumor to accommodate imaging uncertainty and technical error may leave tumor cells incompletely irradiated. Even if the maximal dose tolerated by infiltrative surrounding brain is delivered, tumor cells may remain viable. Hypoxic, nonproliferating cells are particularly radioresistant; with time or change in the physiologic conditions following therapy, reentry of cells into the cell cycle permits the proliferation that results in clinically apparent tumor recurrence. One study of high-dose fractionated proton irradiation following radical resection of glioblastomas showed the following: (1) a dose between 80 and 90 Gy is sufficient to prevent tumor regrowth; (2) outside this high-dose volume, tumor regrows, usually in areas receiving between 60 and 70 Gy; and (3) enlargement of the high-dose volume to include more peripheral areas is likely to be accompanied by unacceptably high levels of symptomatic radiation-induced necrosis.[20]

Recurrence after Chemotherapy

Chemotherapy fails as a result of inadequate drug delivery, toxicity, or cell resistance. The blood-brain barrier is deficient in the contrast-enhancing region of the tumor, but it is usually intact in surrounding brain; thus, lipid-insoluble drugs have limited access to tumor cells infiltrating peripheral regions. The margin between drug efficacy and neurotoxicity, bone marrow suppression, pulmonary injury, and intestinal side effects is often narrow. Noncycling cells are resistant to cell cycle–specific drugs, and potentially vulnerable cells often rapidly develop biochemical means of resistance to chemotherapeutic agents. Specific targeting of molecular mechanisms of cellular proliferation and apoptosis or of tumor invasion and neovascularization may be inefficacious because of the many pathways governing tumor cell cycling and death as well as tumor growth and angiogenesis.

Even if these therapies significantly reduce the tumor burden, the patient's immune response may be rendered ineffective by chemotherapy and by the tumor's secretion of factors that are antagonistic to mechanisms of immune response. Each of these limitations of each component of multimodality therapy may contribute to failure to prevent tumor regrowth. At the time of tumor recurrence, consideration of these reasons for failure is essential to the assessment of prognosis and to the choice of subsequent therapy.

PROGNOSTIC IMPLICATIONS OF RESIDUAL AND RECURRENT TUMOR

In the management of a recurrent glioma, consideration of the prognostic implications of regrowth is essential. The presence of residual tumor and the occurrence of tumor regrowth probably have different prognostic implications.

Residual Tumor

Radiologic demonstration of residual tumor after initial treatment may be consistent with preoperative goals and expectations; the prognosis would be that which was originally formulated. If, however, residual tumor is identified unexpectedly, the prognosis may have to be altered. The prognostic import of residual tumor is best seen in the relationship between the extent of resection and the probability of tumor recurrence.

Cytoreductive surgery is a fundamental part of the treatment of most systemic malignancies. In most cases, there is a strong relationship between the extent of resection and outcome. For gliomas, the relationship is less clear between the extent of resection or, more significantly, the size of residual tumor, and outcome measures, such as interval to tumor progression and survival.

Correlation of survival with the extent of resection for low-grade gliomas has been suggested by retrospective uncontrolled reviews and comparisons with historical reports.[4,8] The median survival following resection and radiation compared favorably (10 years vs. 8 years) with that following biopsy and radiation.

For high-grade gliomas, the correlations between the extent of resection at the initial operation and both the time to tumor recurrence and the duration of patient survival are disputed.[27,28] Historical reports and reviews of large series have noted the association of survival and the extent of resection for both astrocytomas and oligodendrogliomas. Extensive reviews of the literature, however, have failed to locate randomized, controlled clinical trials comparing survival after biopsy with that after radical resection of malignant gliomas. Nevertheless, the benefit of surgical cytoreduction has been strongly suggested.

1. Multivariate regression analysis of multicentered trials has shown that the extent of resection is an important prognostic factor ($p < 0.0001$) for survival.[29]
2. Single-center studies have confirmed this relationship: in one study containing 21 patients with glioblastomas and 10 patients with anaplastic astrocytomas, median survival time after gross total resection was 90 weeks versus only 43 weeks following subtotal resection, and the 2-year survival rates were 19% and 0%, respectively, even though the two groups were well matched for other prognostically significant variables.[30] In another study, patients with a gross total resection of their malignant glioma lived longer (76 weeks vs. 19 weeks) than those who underwent only a biopsy, even after correction for tumor accessibility and all other prognostically significant variables.[31]
3. In two larger series, patients with resected cortical and subcortical Grade IV gliomas lived longer (50.6 weeks vs. 33 weeks[32] and 39.5 weeks vs. 32 weeks[33]) after surgery and radiation than those who underwent biopsy and radiation.
4. Small postoperative tumor volume correlates with time to tumor progression after surgery and longer patient survival.[15]

The data that exist for gliomas and experience with tumors outside the central nervous system suggest that cytoreduction, though less than ideal, does have a benefit when a near-total removal (1 to 2 log reduction of tumor cell number) of a glial tumor can be achieved. Therefore, failure to identify and remove a readily accessible tumor mass at an initial operation might warrant reoperation before regrowth occurs.

Recurrent Tumor

Regrowth of tumors after an initial response (diminution or stability) to surgery and radiation therapy is ominous. This is particularly true if the growth is more rapid, better supported by neovasculature, and more infiltrative than that of the original tumor. Such changes usually reflect additional genetic abnormalities that also make the tumor less responsive to subsequent therapy. A short interval between initial treatment and the recurrence of symptoms often indicates rapid regrowth and a poor prognosis. Variables to be considered in estimating prognosis include the biology of the tumor (its pathology, growth rate, vascularity, and invasiveness), its resectability, its prior response to radiation and chemotherapy, and the age and performance status of the patient. Estimates of the recurrent tumor's size, growth rate, invasiveness, and location must be made in assessing its potential for causing both neurologic deficit and death. Reappearance of a slowly growing, well-demarcated frontal oligodendroglioma in a young patient in good neurologic condition after a 10-year interval of postsurgical quiescence clearly carries a much different prognosis from that of diffuse diencephalic spread of a glioblastoma multiforme in an elderly patient with a poor performance status 3 months after treatment with surgery, radiation, and chemotherapy.

THERAPY OF RECURRENT TUMORS

The choice of therapy of a recurrent glioma is based on a comparison of the natural history of the regrowing tumor with the benefits and risks of potential therapies. Gliomas that recur warrant aggressive multimodality therapy if the patient is in good neurologic and general medical condition and therapeutic options offer a realistic chance for significant improvement in neurologic status or extension of survival.[34]

Patterns of Recurrence

When gliomas recur, most do so locally. Secondary lesions that appear distinct on imaging studies are usually connected to the original tumor site by microscopic trails of invasive tumor evident histologically. Truly metastatic dissemination of malignant gliomas within the central nervous system, such as drop metastases to the spine, is uncommon. Almost all recurrent glioblastomas arise within 2 cm of the original margin of contrast-enhancing tumor (Fig. 50-2). In one series, 97% of glioblastomas recurred within the 90% isodose volume of the original radiation.[35] This tendency to recur locally is a function of tumor cell distribution. There is a gradient of tumor cell density in which tumor cell number decreases rapidly at increasing distances from the contrast-enhancing rim of solid tumor. Thus, although individual tumor cells are spread throughout the brain at great distances from the primary site, there are so many more cells locally that the odds favor local reaccumulation of tumor mass.[2] Conditions contributing to the likelihood of local recurrence include the following: (1) the relative predominance of tumor cell mass in the region, (2) the statistical probability that a local cell will be the cell that first develops a competitive proliferative advantage, and (3) the possibility that the physiologic milieu (hypervascularity, disrupted tissue architecture, and paracrine growth factor stimuli) at the site is particularly conducive to regrowth.

As tumor cell proliferation resumes at the initial tumor site, cells again spread rapidly and diffusely. Tumor cell proliferation resumes at distant sites as a result of the influx of these new, mitotically active cells or the renewed growth of cells that spread before the initial treatment. Consequently, treatments targeting local recurrence alone are, at best, briefly palliative. Treatment of tumor recurrence thus usually involves a combination of modalities aimed at both local and distant disease.

Multimodality Therapy

An enlarging lesion that was originally a low-grade glioma should undergo biopsy (stereotactically or, if resection is anatomically feasible, by open craniotomy) to confirm its histology (Fig. 50-3). If the tumor remains low grade and a large part of the lesion can be resected without inflicting significant neurologic deficit, it should be removed.[36] For recurrent pilocytic astrocytomas in children, reoperation

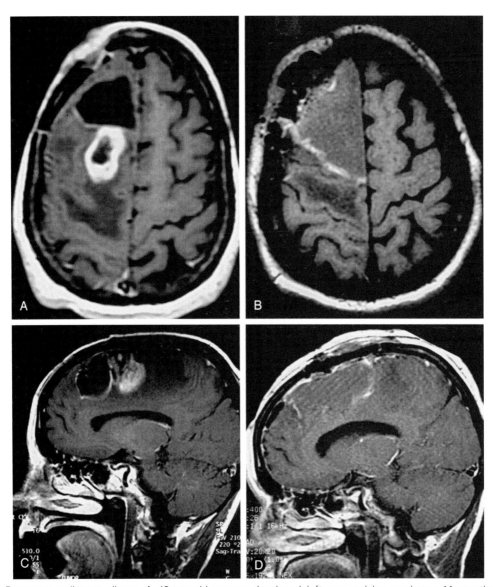

FIGURE 50-2 Recurrent malignant glioma. A 43-year-old woman developed left arm and leg weakness 11 months after complete resection and irradiation (60 Gy) of a right frontal glioblastoma. Preoperative axial (*A*) and sagittal (*C*) magnetic resonance imaging scans show ring contrast enhancement just posterior to the resection cavity. Reoperation, guided by intraoperative electrocorticographic mapping of the right primary motor area, accomplished gross total removal of the tumor and surrounding frontal lobe back to the prefrontal sulcus, as seen on postoperative axial (*B*) and sagittal (*D*) images. After the perioperative edema resolved, full strength returned to the patient's extremities.

accomplishing gross total resection may prove curative; in one series, only 2 of 12 tumors with near-total or gross total resection recurred after a mean follow-up of more than 3 years.[37] With other histologies, reoperation should usually be followed by radiation, chemotherapy, or both.

If the tumor is inaccessible to surgery and has not been irradiated, fractionated radiotherapy should be prescribed. If the tumor is surgically inaccessible and has been irradiated previously, reirradiation at doses reduced in inverse proportion to the time elapsed since initial treatment may be possible.[38] Stereotactic radiosurgery is an option for surgically inaccessible recurrent low-grade tumors whether they have been previously irradiated or not.

If the low-grade tumor recurs as a high-grade tumor, or if a high-grade tumor recurs, reoperation should be attempted if the patient has a Karnofsky score of at least 70 and removal of all or almost all of the contrast-enhancing tumor is potentially attainable, or if the tumor mass is causing neurologic symptoms that might be palliated by its reduction.[39] If the tumor was not irradiated previously, the tumor bed and its annular margin should receive regional radiotherapy. Even when radiotherapy has been used initially, it is an option at recurrence.[40,41] Hypofractionated stereotactic radiotherapy (SRT, 5 Gy per fraction to doses ranging from 20 to 50 Gy) given to 29 patients with recurrent high-grade astrocytomas resulted in a median survival time after retreatment of 11 months.[42] Steroid-dependent toxicity occurred in 36% of patients, reoperation was required in 6%, and a total dose in excess of 40 Gy predicted radiation damage ($p < 0.005$). A different study showed a 79% response rate,

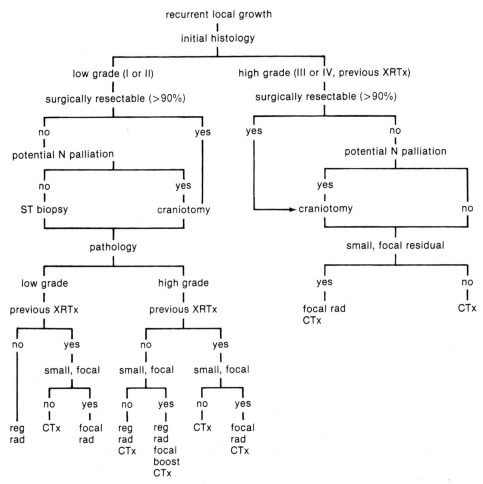

FIGURE 50-3 Management of recurrent gliomas. Decisions regarding the management of a recurrent tumor should consider grade, resectability, and prior therapy. CTx, chemotherapy; focal rad/boost, stereotactic radiosurgery, brachytherapy, or radiotherapy; N, neurologic; reg rad, regional fractionated radiation therapy; small, focal, less than 10 cm³, radiographically demarcated; ST, stereotactic; XRT, radiotherapy.

no Grade 3 toxicity, and no need for reoperation for radiation necrosis in 19 recurrent glioblastomas treated for 10 days with 3.0 or 3.5 Gy daily fractions (30–35 Gy total dose) at a median interval from completion of initial radiotherapy of 3.1 months. Neurologic improvement occurred in 45% of patients and steroid requirements declined in 60%.[40]

Others advocate that a stereotactically delivered focal boost of interstitial brachytherapy or radiosurgery should be given to any contrast-enhancing residual of acceptably small size, particularly if the recurrent tumor is a glioblastoma. Brachytherapy has proved valuable in treating glioblastomas, both initially and at the time of recurrence.[41,42] The median survival following brachytherapy using temporary implantation of high-activity ¹²⁵I sources was 49 weeks for recurrent glioblastomas but only 52 weeks for anaplastic astrocytomas.[18] Patients receiving brachytherapy were highly selected; only about 20% of recurrent tumors met the criteria of appropriate size and focality. Almost 10% of patients suffered severe acute toxicity, and approximately 40% required reoperation for delayed medically refractory neurologic deterioration and intracranial mass effect. Although tumor was identified in 95% of the specimens harvested at reoperation, reoperation was associated with longer survival time after brachytherapy (90 weeks vs. 37 weeks for those not undergoing reoperation).

The authors suggested that this rate of morbidity was justified by the prolongation of survival achieved in patients with glioblastomas but not by that for those with anaplastic astrocytomas.[18] Subsequent studies using low-activity ¹²⁵I sources implanted permanently at open operation have shown similar survival outcomes but lower rates of necrosis and reoperation after brachytherapy.[5,43] In one subset of 18 recurrent glioblastomas, median survival after reoperation and implantation was 64 weeks; only one patient had symptomatic radiation injury, and this did not require surgery.[43] A liquid ¹²⁵I radiation source injected into an inflatable balloon placed into a tumor resection cavity provides a more homogeneous distribution of dose to surrounding brain. This may reduce the incidence of symptomatic radiation necrosis. A preliminary study in 21 patients with high-grade recurrent gliomas treated with 40 to 60 Gy found no symptomatic radiation necrosis during 21.8 patient-years of follow-up.[44]

Stereotactic radiosurgery is a less invasive way of stopping tumor growth. In a retrospective comparison of interstitial brachytherapy and radiosurgery, the median durations of survival times of the two groups were similar (11.5 months and 10.2 months, respectively). The actuarial risks of reoperation for necrosis at 12 and 24 months were 33% and 48%, respectively, after radiosurgery and 54% and 65%, respectively, after brachytherapy, with the caveat that the brachytherapy group had larger tumors and longer follow-up.[45] Fractionation may reduce the risk of symptomatic radionecrosis. One study comparing single-fraction (median dose of 17 Gy of stereotactic radiosurgery at the 50% isodose line) and multiple-fraction (median dose of 37.5 Gy in 15 fractions of SRT to the 85% isodose line) irradiation of recurrent malignant gliomas found a lower complication rate (2/25 vs. 14/46) and equal efficacy (despite poorer pretreatment prognostic factors) in the fractionated group.[46] The ability of radiation sensitizers, such as arsenic trioxide, to improve the therapeutic ratio for radiosurgery is currently being studied.[47] Other forms of focal radiation therapy such as photodynamic therapy (PDT), boron neutron capture therapy (BNCT), avidin-biotin targeting of ^{90}Y, ^{131}I-labeled tenascin-specific monoclonal antibody, and intraoperative radiation (IORT) have been used sparingly for recurrent glioma.[6,48–50]

Chemotherapy of recurrent gliomas is often valuable. Low-grade tumors will generally not have been treated by chemotherapy at their initial presentation unless a predominant oligodendrocytic component warranted temozolamide or PCV (procarbazine, lomustine, and vincristine).[51] If not previously used, these agents may produce sustained response, particularly in oligodendrogliomas with prognostically favorable 1p and 19q deletions.[52] In one series, 62% of recurrent oligodendrogliomas and oligoastrocytomas responded to PCV for a median time of 24 months (32 months for oligodendrogliomas and 12 months for oligoastrocytomas).[53] Adjuvant chemotherapy of malignant gliomas, in combination with radiation and surgery, increases the percentage of patients surviving at 1 year by 10% (a relative increase of 23.4%) and at 2 years by 8.6% (a 52.4% relative increase).[54] A systematic review of 32 chemotherapy studies involving 1031 patients with recurrent malignant gliomas treated with chemotherapy identified nitrosoureas as the sole class of agents capable of significantly extending time to tumor progression.[54] At the time of renewed growth of a high-grade tumor, if the tumor has not been exposed previously to a nitrosourea, then carmustine (also called BCNU), the PCV combination, or temozolamide should be tried.[51] For Grade IV tumors, BCNU and PCV provide similar results, but the PCV combination is superior for Grade III tumors.[54,55] Novel methods of delivery of nitrosourea to surgically inaccessible recurrent malignant gliomas include stereotactic infusion of BCNU in ethanol solvent (DTI-015) into the tumor.[56] If nitrosourea therapy is unsuccessful, alternatives such as carboplatin, cisplatin, or tamoxifen might be tried.[57] The response rates (partial response or stable disease) to such chemotherapy at the time of recurrence range from 20% to 50%.[58]

Multivariate statistical analysis of multimodality therapy for recurrent gliomas has been used to identify variables affecting response.[41] Fifty-one patients with recurrent malignant gliomas were treated in a phase II trial of multidrug chemotherapy. Of the 51 patients, 31 (61%) patients underwent reoperation consisting of radical tumor debulking before chemotherapy was begun. Disease stabilization or partial response occurred in 29 of the 51 (57%) patients. Median time to tumor progression was 19 weeks for all pathologies, ranging from 32 weeks for patients with anaplastic astrocytomas to 13 weeks for those with glioblastoma multiforme. Median survival time was 40 weeks for all pathologies,

79 weeks for patients with anaplastic astrocytoma, and 33 weeks for those with glioblastoma multiforme. Thirty-five percent of patients had a serious chemotoxicity, but none had permanent morbidity or mortality. Variables associated with a longer mean time to tumor progression included a higher Karnofsky score, lower initial histologic grade, lack of prior chemotherapy, greater degree of myelotoxicity, smaller postoperative tumor volume, greater extent of resection, and a local rather than diffuse pattern of recurrence. Variables associated with a longer mean survival time were a higher Karnofsky score, anaplastic astrocytoma rather than glioblastoma at recurrence, greater degree of myelotoxicity, and lobar rather than central location of the tumor.[41]

Alternative approaches have involved intracavitary or interstitial immunotherapy, chemotherapy, or gene therapy following reoperation for recurrent malignant gliomas.[59–63] One study using lymphokine-activated killer cells and interleukin-2 (IL-2) described a median survival time of 53 weeks after reoperation and immunotherapy compared with 26 weeks following reoperation and chemotherapy.[59] Another showed survival in excess of 4 years for two of nine patients with recurrent malignant gliomas following immunization with autologous tumor cells and bacille Calmette-Guérin (BCG) and harvest, activation (with antibody to CD-3), expansion (with IL-2), and intravenous reinfusion of T cells.[64] The initial randomized, double-blind clinical trial with intracavitary BCNU wafers showed improved survival rates in the BCNU arm relative to the placebo arm at 6 months after treatment, but the survival curves converged at longer follow-up.[65] An independent, retrospective, cohort-matched study showed no statistically significant difference in survival (median survival after reoperation and implantation of 14 weeks vs. 50 weeks for reoperation alone) and a higher risk of postoperative complications (13 among 17 patients vs. 8 among 45 patients) after wafer implantation.[66] Subsequent study has identified a maximum tolerated dose of 20% BCNU that might be more effective.[63] Intracavitary injection of bleomycin and mitoxantrone following resection of recurrent glioblastomas resulted in a median total survival time of 27.6 months, significantly longer than that achieved by patients who lacked either reoperation or intracavitary chemotherapy.[67] Preliminary gene therapy studies using modified herpes virus or ganciclovir activated by a thymidine kinase gene delivered by a retrovirus produced by a modified mouse fibroblast packaging cell line have proved feasible and safe but have not yet demonstrated efficacy.[60–62]

Rationale for Reoperation

Early reoperation, within months of the initial procedure, might be indicated for complications such as intracerebral, subdural, or epidural hematoma; wound dehiscence and infection; or hydrocephalus and cerebrospinal fluid leakage. Failure to identify and remove an accessible tumor at a first operation might warrant reoperation; in the Royal Melbourne Hospital experience, 5 of 200 patients underwent early reoperation.[3] More frequently, true tumor recurrence after an interval of response to the initial therapy is the reason for considering reoperation. Reoperation is justified if it produces sustained improvement of neurologic condition and quality of life, as well as significant enhancement of response rates to adjuvant therapy, which might prolong survival. Palliation of neurologic symptoms by surgery results from reduction of the local mass effect produced by the tumor and tumor-induced edema.

Multiple studies have shown that primary surgical cytoreduction of malignant gliomas can both improve neurologic deficits and promote maintenance of high-performance status. One study showed that patients undergoing gross total resection of their malignant gliomas were likely to have improved neurologic outcome (97% of 36 patients had either improved or stable neurologic conditions), improved functional status (mean Karnofsky score improvement of 6.8%), and extended maintenance of good functional status (mean of 185 weeks).[68] Another study confirmed that the extent of surgery correlated with better immediate postoperative performance, lower 1-month mortality rate, and longer survival: 43% of patients with malignant gliomas improved, 50% remained unchanged, and 7% suffered deterioration in their neurologic condition following resection of at least 75% of their tumor, as opposed to the outcomes of a more limited resection (28% improved, 51% were unchanged, and 21% were worse).[29]

Similar results can be achieved by reoperation. Forty-five percent of the patients had an improved Karnofsky score following reoperation in one series.[68] In another series of 46 patients undergoing reoperation for glioblastoma, Karnofsky scores improved after surgery in 28%, were unchanged in 49%, and decreased (between 10 and 30 points) in 23%; there was no perioperative mortality.[15] In a third series focusing on reoperation, when gross tumor resection was achieved, 82% (32 of 39) of patients showed improvement or stability in Karnofsky score.[69] In a fourth, patients with Karnofsky scores of 50 or less also underwent reoperation. Two thirds improved from a dependent to an independent state, and the median survival of patients with an initially low Karnofsky score was similar to that for all patients undergoing reoperation.[70]

The doubling rate of malignant gliomas is so high, however, that the benefits gained by reoperation will be very brief unless adjuvant therapies are used to induce remission of tumor growth. Surgical resection is especially beneficial when reduction of tumor burden improves the response rate to such therapies. Studies from the University of California at

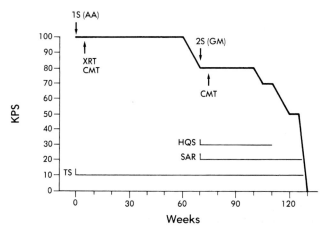

FIGURE 50-4 Quality-of-life considerations in the management of patients with malignant gliomas. Maintenance of high-performance status is a critical feature of outcome. The Karnofsky score (KPS) as a function of time indicates the quality of the survival time that follows each intervention. AA, anaplastic astrocytoma; CMT, chemotherapy; GM, glioblastoma multiforme; HQS, high-quality survival ($K = 70$); 1S, initial surgery; 2S, reoperation; SAR, survival after reoperation; TS, total survival; XRT, radiation therapy.

San Francisco (UCSF), Memorial Sloan-Kettering, and the University of Washington at Seattle have shown that reoperation followed by chemotherapy leads to stabilization of the performance score for significant intervals (Fig. 50-4).[71-73] At UCSF, 44% of patients with a glioblastoma maintained a performance level of at least 70—a level consistent with self-care and judged to be survival of high quality[74] (Table 50-1)—for at least 6 months after reoperation; 18% maintained this level for at least a year; and three patients did so for longer than 3 years. Most patients (52% of 31) with an anaplastic astrocytoma maintained this performance level for at least 12 months after reoperation; 13% had more than 4 years of high-quality survival. Approximately 90% of the survival after reoperation for anaplastic astrocytoma was of high quality.[73] In the Memorial Sloan-Kettering group, the median duration of maintenance of independent status (a Karnofsky score of at least 80) was 34 weeks.[71] In the University of Washington series, patients

TABLE 50-1 ■ Karnofsky Performance Status

Definition	%	Criteria
Able to carry on normal activity and to work; no special care is needed	100	Normal; no complaints; no evidence of disease
	90	Able to carry on normal activity; minor signs or symptoms of disease
	80	Normal activity with effort; some signs or symptoms of disease
Unable to work; able to live at home, care for most personal needs; a varying amount of assistance is needed	70	Cares for self; unable to carry on normal activity or to do active work
	60	Requires occasional assistance, but is able to care for most needs
	50	Requires considerable assistance and frequent medical care
Unable to care for self; requires equivalent of institutional or hospital care; disease may be progressing rapidly	40	Disabled; requires special care and assistance
	30	Severely disabled, hospitalization is indicated although death is not imminent
	20	Very sick; hospitalization necessary; active supportive treatment necessary
	10	Moribund; fatal processes progressing rapidly
	0	Dead

From Karnofsky D, Burchenal JH, Armistead GC Jr, et al: Triethylene melamine in the treatment of meoplastic disease. Arch Intern Med 87:477–516, 1951.

with a Karnofsky score of at least 70 maintained this high level of function for an average of 37 weeks after reoperation for glioblastoma and for 70 weeks after reoperation for anaplastic astrocytoma.[72]

Aggressive surgical cytoreduction at the time of recurrence may increase the duration as well as the quality of patient survival. Support for reoperation is found in comparisons of the outcomes in cases in which different degrees of tumor removal were accomplished and in comparisons of the survival of patients following reoperation with that of control patients not undergoing reoperation.[75,76] Patients in whom gross total resection of a glioblastoma is achieved survive longer (45.6 weeks vs. 25.6 weeks) than do those receiving near-total or subtotal resections; for anaplastic astrocytomas, the effect of the extent of resection is similar (87.5 weeks vs. 55.7 weeks).[72] In the Sloan-Kettering series that grouped glioblastomas and anaplastic astrocytomas together, a similar difference was found (51.2 weeks vs. 23.3 weeks).[71] In the UCSF series, survival of patients undergoing reoperation and chemotherapy for either anaplastic astrocytoma or glioblastoma was longer than that of patients receiving chemotherapy alone at the time of tumor recurrence.[73]

The benefit of reoperative surgery is also suggested by experience with brachytherapy. Patients undergoing reoperation for tumor recurrence, radiation necrosis, or both following brachytherapy for a glioblastoma either initially or at first recurrence survived longer than those not receiving reoperation: The median duration of total survival was 120 weeks versus 62 weeks for patients with primarily treated tumors, and 90 weeks versus 37 weeks for patients treated with brachytherapy at the time of first recurrence.[18] In another study of 40 patients with recurrent glioblastoma, maximal surgical resection accompanied by implantation of permanent ^{125}I seeds delivering 120 to 160 Gy yielded an actuarial duration of survival of 47 weeks. No patient developed symptomatic radiation necrosis. Multivariate analysis showed both a definite effect of gross total resection on time to tumor progression and a trend toward its effect on duration of survival.[77]

Reoperation as a part of the multimodality treatment of recurrent gliomas is further supported by study of long-term survivors of glioblastoma multiforme. A review of the UCSF experience identified 22 of 449 (5%) patients with glioblastomas who survived at least 5 years after diagnosis. Sixteen of 22 patients had tumor recurrence that was treated; 9 underwent between one and three reoperations. For 8 of the 16 patients with treated recurrence, survival time after treatment of recurrence (median of 4.5 years) was longer than the remission produced by the initial treatment.[78]

The benefit to survival from reoperation is not above dispute. As noted, multivariate analyses of chemotherapy studies have found that greater extent of resection and smaller postoperative volume are associated with prolongation of time to tumor progression but not of survival.[79] A similar study of survival after progression of malignant gliomas identified high Karnofsky score and age less than 50 years as independent prognostic factors for longer survival.[80] Those who underwent reoperation (58 of 143 patients) lived longer (median of 35 weeks vs. 16 weeks, $p < 0.005$ in univariate analysis) after tumor recurrence than those treated without reoperation, but multivariate analysis identified only a trend toward reduction of risk of death (relative risk = 0.74; 95%

confidence interval = 0.50 – 1.11; $p = 0.014$) following reoperation. Randomized controlled trials using MRC brain tumor prognostic indices for analysis of outcomes are needed to evaluate definitively the benefits of reoperation.[81]

Selection of Patients for Reoperation

Case selection is critical to outcome. The patient's profile of prognostic factors, his or her predicted tolerance of the procedure, and the feasibility of extensive tumor resection without undue risk of new neurologic morbidity must all be considered.[82] Multiple characteristics have been identified as predictive of a good response to reoperation (Table 50-2). Foremost among these are tumor histologic type, patient age, performance status, interoperative interval, and extent of resection.[15,39,76]

The prognostic significance of tumor grade is evident in most series. Median survival after reoperation was 88 weeks for patients with an anaplastic astrocytoma but only 36 weeks for those with a glioblastoma at UCSF and was 61 weeks and 29 weeks, respectively, at Sloan-Kettering.[71,73]

Age may be more significant than tumor grade. In one series, survival after reoperation was 57 weeks for those younger than 40 years but only 36 weeks for older patients.[34] Other authors found an association between youth and total survival after diagnosis and between youth and quality of survival after reoperation, but not between youth and duration of survival after reoperation.[15,71,73]

The patient's preoperative performance score significantly affects the outcome of reoperation.[15,72,73,76] In the University of Washington series, for glioblastomas, survival after reoperation was almost twice as long (71 weeks vs. 36 weeks) for patients with Karnofsky scores of at least 70.[72]

The prognostic importance of the duration of the interval between initial treatment and recurrence is disputed. At the University of Washington, a threefold difference (150 weeks vs. 48 weeks for glioblastoma and 164 weeks vs. 52 weeks for anaplastic astrocytomas) was noted when the time to progression exceeded 3 years.[6] Others, however, have found either no relation or an inverse relation between the interoperative interval and the survival time after reoperation.[15,34,71,73]

A more complete resection of recurrent tumor portends longer survival. At Sloan-Kettering, gross total resection afforded a median survival of 51.2 weeks versus 23.3 weeks for a more limited resection.[69,71] Others have noted a strong trend in the correlation between a more complete removal of tumor and survival duration.[83] The ability to remove sufficient tumor mass to be of oncologic benefit depends on the location of the tumor and its physical characteristics. Removal is facilitated by a more superficial location in noneloquent areas; a discrete pseudoencapsulated mass is more easily removed than a less well-marginated, diffuse one; drainage of a cystic component often provides immediate reduction of mass, as well as an avenue for further resection of tumor.

During the interval between initial surgery and tumor recurrence, the patient usually undergoes therapy that might affect his or her tolerance of further surgery. The decision to reoperate must consider the patient's overall physical condition, tissue viability, blood coagulability, hematologic reserve, and immune function following surgery, radiation,

TABLE 50-2 ▪ Reoperation for Recurrent Gliomas

Author	No.of Patients	Pathology	SAR	HQS	Morb	Mort	⁻K	Px Relations	Weeks
Young et al[89]	24	GM	14		52%	17%	25%	K⁻³ 60 → SAR	22 vs. 9
								II > 12 m → SAR	16.5 vs. 8.5
Salcman et al[34]	40	MG	37			0%		Age < 40 → SAR	57 vs. 36
Ammirati et al[68]	55	64% GM	36	34	16%	64%	45%	K > 70 → SAR	48.5 vs. 19
								Grade → SAR	61 vs. 29
								Ext resect → SAR	51.2 vs. 23.3
Harsh et al[73]	49	GM	36	10	8%	5%	5%	Age → SAR	
								K⁻³ 70 → HQS	
Harsh et al[73]	21	AA	88	83	3%	3%	10%	Age → HQS	
								Grade → SAR	
Berger et al[72]	56	GM						K⁻³ 70 → SAR	70.7 vs. 36.5
								K⁻³ 70 → SQE	36.6 vs. 8.4
								Age² 60 → SQE	mo 35.1 vs. 9.4
								II > 12 m → SAR	150 vs. 48
Berger et al[72]	14	AA						II > 12 m → SQE	mo 99.5 vs.22.4
Kaye[3]	50	GM				16%	0%	Age → SAR	
								Grade → SAR	
								II → SAR	
								Age → HQS	
								Grade → HQS	
								II → HQS	
Barker et al[15]	46	GM	36	18	23%	0%	28%	K → SAR	

AA, anaplastic astrocytoma; Cx, complications; Ext resect, extent of resection; HQS, high-quality survival; K ≥70; II, intraoperative interval; ⁻K, increased performance score; Morb, morbidity; Mort, mortality; Px, prognostic relations; SAR, survival after reoperation; SQE, same-quality existence.

corticosteroids, and chemotherapy. A high risk of multisystem failure, failure to thrive, intracranial hemorrhage, anemia, wound infection, pneumonia, or neurologic damage may exist. This risk should be assessed for each patient by obtaining preoperative chemical, hematologic, and radiographic studies.

In choosing patients for reoperation, careful consideration of the individual patient's profile of these prognostically significant factors permits a reasonable estimate of the likelihood that he or she will benefit from the procedure.

Preparation for Reoperation

Before surgery, the patient usually receives corticosteroids; they should be continued. At the time of induction of anesthesia, the patient is fitted with thigh-high intermittent compression air boots. He or she is first given additional steroids, prophylactic antibiotics, an anticonvulsant, and osmotic and loop diuretics, and is then hyperventilated. In positioning the patient, the likelihood of elevated intracranial pressure makes elevation of the head above the level of the heart particularly important.

Reoperative Exposure

In planning the needed exposure, the location of the tumor should be identified by noting its relationship to the margins of the craniotomy plate, to specific cortical gyri and sulci, and to deeper structures. Close study of a preoperative MRI, computer stereotactic-assisted navigation, or intraoperative MRI may be used.[83–86] The procedure should be planned in advance to ensure adequate skin opening, craniotomy, and durotomy to expose the recurrent mass. All may have to be shifted or enlarged relative to the original procedure because of the increased extent of the tumor or

a desire to perform corticography for mapping of motor or speech function, or both.

The skin incision from the previous operation is usually used. The skin opening can be increased by introducing additional incisions. They should be external to the previous flap, avoid its base and other vascular pedicles, and intersect the previous incision at right angles. The margins of the prior craniotomy flap should be defined. Generally, this is best accomplished with a curet beginning at a prior trephination. Only rarely does the prior curf need to be recut. Dissection in the epidural plane can be begun with a curet followed by a no. 3 and then a no. 2 Penfield dissector. The craniotomy plate is further elevated as the dura is stripped from its inner surface with a periosteal elevator. Unless the craniotomy has to be enlarged, epidural adhesions affixing dura to the craniotomy margin should be preserved as prophylaxis against postoperative extension of an epidural fluid collection. If required, these adhesions are dissected with a curet and trimmed. After the dura has been stripped from the undersurface of the cranial plate, an additional segment of bone can be removed with a craniotome.

The durotomy may have to be enlarged, but often it can be limited to part of the dural exposure. It should be planned to minimize traverse of cortical adhesions. For instance, in re-exposing a temporal lesion, the durotomy can be placed over the cyst remaining from the prior resection. Flapping the dura superiorly then allows adhesions to be put on traction such that they may be dissected from cortex, coagulated, and sharply divided. Extending a durotomy along an old incision line should be avoided. The prior incision line should be traversed perpendicularly and as infrequently as possible, because it is often the site of the densest adhesions. Microdissection of larger vessels from dural attachments may be necessary.

Once the dura has been opened and retracted, the exposed cortex is inspected for the surface presentation of the tumor; its abnormal color, consistency, and vascularity should be apparent.

Localization of the subcortical extent of the tumor is then undertaken. Again, preoperative imaging studies including diffusion tensor imaging of white matter tracts, computer-assisted stereotactic navigation, and intraoperative imaging can be highly valuable (Fig. 50-5).[83–86] Electrophysiologic mapping of motor, sensory, and speech cortical areas and deeper white matter tracts may reduce the chance of inflicting a neurologic deficit. By revealing the relationship of the site of cortical traverse and of the subsequent subcortical dissection to eloquent brain, it may also encourage a more extensive resection (see Figs. 50-2 and 50-5).[86,87]

This technique is often more difficult at the time of reoperation because of cortical disruption by the tumor and prior surgery. An intraoperative photograph from cortical mapping at the time of the initial craniotomy may also be helpful.

Transcortical ultrasonography also has its advocates, although this technique tends to overestimate the volume of recurrent tumor.[88] Tumor may also be found by locating a cystic resection cavity or encephalomalacic brain left after the previous operation. In that almost all tumors recur within 2 cm of the original tumor's margin, exposure and careful inspection of the initial tumor's surgical bed usually reveals at least part of the recurrent mass.

Generally, the appearance of the tumor itself is the best guide to its extent. Tumor-infiltrated cortex is likely to have increased vascular markings, a pink to gray color, and a firm consistency. Its central core may vary from yellow cystic fluid of low viscosity to high-viscosity, soupy, white necrosis that resembles pus to a yellow-gray, granular, honeycomb-like material. Generally, the center is relatively avascular, although it may be traversed by thrombosed blood vessels.

Some authors advocate incision into the tumor mass and internal debulking with an ultrasonic aspirator or large sucker as an initial step. However, this often induces significant hemorrhage. Enucleation of the mass by circumferential dissection in the pseudoplane about the rim of solid tumor is usually more satisfactory. Arteries supplying the tumor and veins draining it can be coagulated and divided as they enter the tumor mass, much as the vascular supply of an arteriovenous malformation is handled. Softened, necrotic, highly edematous white matter around the tumor provides an excellent plane of dissection. The use of bipolar cautery forceps and suction together accomplishes this dissection while reducing local mass. In areas of noneloquent brain, the dissection can extend more widely into surrounding brain tissue that is likely infiltrated by tumor. In potentially eloquent areas, the dissection should adhere more closely to the tumor surface, since adjacent normal brain, though edematous and possibly injured by prior retraction and radiation therapy, is often functional and should be preserved.

Often, the tumor can be removed as a single specimen without the need for significant retraction of surrounding brain. In general, gentle, temporary displacement of a cottonoid patty lying on the margin of resection provides sufficient exposure of the dissection plane so that fixed, self-retaining retractors are unnecessary. Retraction of the tumor mass is preferable to retraction of surrounding brain. Often, identification of the appropriate plane for the circumferential dissection is facilitated by this retraction on the tumor; coherence of the tumor mass helps delineate the plane between solid tumor and tumor-infiltrated brain.

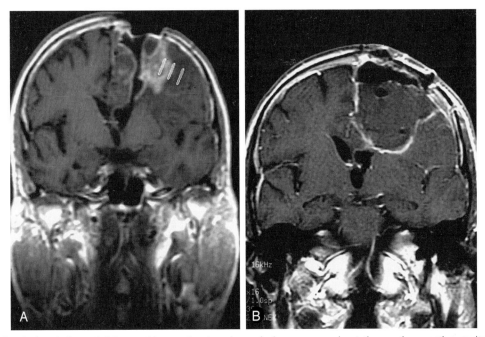

FIGURE 50-5 Surgical technique. A 39-year-old man developed marginal recurrence about the cystic resection cavity remaining after removal and irradiation of an anaplastic astrocytoma 3 years earlier. As part of a gene therapy trial, three columns of vector-producing cells were infused within the tumor, at the tumor margin, and in surrounding infiltrated brain. A, Coronal MRI. Five days later, the tumor and the infused tissue were removed to be analyzed. Care was taken to extend the resection to the margin of eloquent areas and to achieve watertight closure. B, Coronal, immediately postoperative magnetic resonance imaging scan.

Once the tumor mass has been removed, the margins of resection should be inspected to verify that the excision is complete. The margins should be free of tumor, which is usually more firm, glassy, opaque, and hypervascular than surrounding brain. Computer-assisted navigation and intra-operative MRI can also be used to verify the extent of resection.[83,86]

Biopsy specimens of the surrounding edematous brain should be sent for frozen-section analysis to verify absence of tumor. If solid tumor or tumor infiltrating into noneloquent areas remains, it should be removed. In some cases, extension of tumor into eloquent areas or diencephalic structures precludes resection of the entire mass. In such cases, the tumor should be divided. This process often entails coagulation of numerous strands of small, thin-walled blood vessels, particularly if the extension is in the direction of the vascular supply, such as occurs with medial extension of a temporal lobe tumor toward the posterior aspect of the Sylvian fissure. Care should be taken to coagulate and sharply divide these vessels. Tearing them without prior coagulation will leave a loose end that will retract and continue to bleed. Such loose ends should be directly coagulated rather than tamponaded with hemostatic packing, which may encourage deeper dissection of a hematoma.

After the resection has been completed, hemostasis should be confirmed by filling the tumor cavity with saline and, during a Valsalva maneuver, observing for wisps of continuing hemorrhage. This check should be performed with the patient's blood pressure at least as high as his or her normal level. The cavity is then aspirated, lined with a single layer of Surgicel, and filled again with irrigation fluid. Hyperventilation is then reversed to permit expansion of the brain during closure.

Watertight dural closure is essential (see Fig. 50-5B). Often, this can be attained by primary suturing, given the decompression achieved by tumor removal. If the dura is incompetent, it may be supplemented by a pericranial graft. Peripheral dural tacking sutures are placed where needed. Any craniotomy plate fragments are fastened together, and then the entire plate is fastened to the cranium with nonabsorbable monofilament suture, stainless-steel wire, or titanium miniplates. Any craniectomy defect is covered by titanium mesh to prevent cosmetically unacceptable scalp concavities. The wound is irrigated several times with antibiotic solution and then closed in layers with 2-0 absorbable suture in muscle, fascia, and galea. The galeal sutures should be inverted and the knots should be cut short to avoid superficial erosion. They should be placed in sufficient proximity so that tension-free closure of the skin is possible. Simple running 4-0 nylon skin sutures or staples provide adequate skin closure except at sites of attenuation, where horizontal mattress sutures may be less likely to compromise blood supply.

Postoperatively, the patient should be monitored closely for at least 24 hours for signs of increased intracranial pressure from hematoma or edema. Fluid restriction, dehydration, and corticosteroids should be continued throughout this period. The patient should be mobilized as soon as possible, and a gadolinium-enhanced MRI scan should be obtained as soon as he or she is able to tolerate it.[1]

Key Points

Renewed growth of a mass at the site of a previously treated brain glioma raises the following issues: (1) is the mass a recurrence of the original tumor, (2) why did the tumor regrow, and (3) what additional therapy is appropriate?

An enlarging lesion at the site of a previously treated glioma probably represents renewed growth of an incompletely eradicated initial tumor or a more malignant variant rather than a distinctly new tumor, abscess, or radiation necrosis.

Functional imaging is usually helpful to assess malignant progression and radiation effects, but biopsy is often necessary.

Gliomas that recur warrant aggressive multimodality therapy if the patient is in good neurologic and general medical condition and therapeutic options offer a realistic chance for significant improvement in neurologic status or extension of survival.

When gliomas recur, most do so locally, but cells often spread rapidly and diffusely. Treatment thus usually involves a combination of modalities aimed at both local and distant disease.

An enlarging lesion that was originally a low-grade glioma should undergo biopsy to confirm its histology. If the tumor remains low grade and a large part of the lesion can be resected without inflicting significant neurologic deficit, it should be removed. Reoperation should usually be followed by radiation, chemotherapy, or both.

If the tumor is inaccessible to surgery and has not been irradiated, fractionated radiotherapy should be prescribed. If the tumor is surgically inaccessible and has been irradiated previously, reirradiation at doses reduced in inverse proportion to the time elapsed since initial treatment may be possible. Stereotactic radiosurgery is an option for surgically inaccessible recurrent low-grade tumors whether they have been previously irradiated or not.

If the low-grade tumor recurs as a high-grade tumor, or if a high-grade tumor recurs, reoperation should be attempted if the patient has a Karnofsky score of at least 70 and removal of all or almost all of the contrast-enhancing tumor is potentially attainable or if the tumor mass is causing neurologic symptoms that might be palliated by its reduction. If the tumor was not irradiated previously, the tumor bed and its annular margin should receive regional radiotherapy. Even when radiotherapy has been used initially, hypofractionated SRT, interstitial brachytherapy, and radiosurgery are options at recurrence. Chemotherapy of recurrent gliomas is often valuable. Alternative approaches include intracavitary or interstitial immunotherapy, chemotherapy, or gene therapy following reoperation for recurrent malignant gliomas.

Aggressive surgical cytoreduction of recurrent tumor may increase the duration as well as the quality of patient survival. Case selection is critical to outcome. Predictors of a good response include tumor histology, patient age, patient performance status, interoperative interval, and extent of resection.

In planning the surgical exposure, the location of the tumor should be identified by noting its relationship to the margins of the craniotomy plate, to specific cortical gyri and sulci, and to deeper structures using preoperative imaging studies including diffusion tensor imaging of white matter tracts, computer-assisted stereotactic navigation, and/or intraoperative imaging. Electrophysiologic mapping of motor, sensory, and speech cortical areas and deeper white matter tracts may reduce the chance of inflicting a neurologic deficit. Generally, the appearance of the tumor itself is the best guide to its extent. Enucleation of the mass by circumferential dissection in the pseudoplane about the rim of solid tumor can usually be accomplished without significant retraction of surrounding brain.

REFERENCES

1. Ekinci G, Akpinar IN, Baltacioglu F, et al: Early postoperative magnetic resonance imaging in glial tumors: Prediction of tumor regrowth and recurrence. Eur J Radiol 45:99–107, 2003.
2. Kelly PJ, Daumas-Duport C, Scheithauer B, et al: Stereotactic histologic correlation of computed tomography and magnetic resonance imaging defined abnormalities in patients with glial neoplasma. Mayo Clin Proc 62:450–459, 1987.
3. Kaye AH: Malignant brain tumors. In Rothenberg RE (ed): Reoperative Surgery. New York: McGraw-Hill, 1992, pp 51–76.
4. Laws ER, Taylor WF, Clifton MB, Okazaki H: Neurosurgical management of low-grade astrocytoma of the cerebral hemispheres. J Neurosurg 61:665–673, 1984.
5. McDermott MW, Sneed PK, Gutin PH: Interstitial brachytherapy for malignant brain tumors. Semin Surg Oncol 14:79–87, 1998.
6. Muller PJ, Wilson BC: Photodynamic therapy for recurrent supratentorial gliomas. Semin Surg Oncol 11:346–354, 1995.
7. Von Diemling A, Louis DM, Von Ammon K, et al: Subsets of glioblastoma multiforme defined by molecular genetic analysis. Brain Pathol 3:19–26, 1993.
8. McCormich BM, Miller DC, Budzilovich GN, et al: Treatment and survival of low grade astrocytoma in adults, 1977–1988. Neurosurgery 31:636–642, 1992.
9. Alavi JB, Alavi A, Chawluk J, et al: Positron emission tomography in patients with gliomas: A predictor of prognosis. Cancer 62:1074–1078, 1988.
10. Le Bihan D, Douek M, Argyropoulou M, et al: Diffusion and perfusion magnetic resonance imaging in brain tumors. Top Magn Reson Imaging 5:25–31, 1993.
11. Graves EE, Nelson SJ, Vigernon DB, et al: Serial proton MR spectroscopic imaging of recurrent malignant gliomas after gamma knife radiosurgery. AJNR Am J Neuroradiol 22:613–624, 2001.
12. Rabinov JD, Lee PL, Barker FG, et al: In vivo MRS at 3 Tesla predicts recurrent glioma vs. radiation effects. Radiology 225:871–879, 2002.
13. Kuwert T, Woesler B, Morgenroth C: Diagnosis of recurrent glioma with SPECT and iodine-123-alpha-methyl tyrosine. J Nucl Med 39:23–27, 1998.
14. Carvalho PA, Schwartz RB, Alexander E III, et al: Detection of recurrent gliomas with quantitative thallium-201/technetium-99m HMPAO single-photon emission computerized tomography. J Neurosurg 77:565–570, 1992.
15. Barker FG, Chang SM, Gutin PH, et al: Survival and functional status after resection of recurrent glioblastoma multiforme. Neurosurgery 42:709–723, 1998.
16. Leibel SA, Sheline GE: Radiation therapy for neoplasms of the brain. J Neurosurg 66:1–22, 1987.
17. Vick NA, Coric IS, Eller TW, et al: Reoperation for malignant astrocytoma. Neurology 39:430–432, 1989.
18. Scharfen CD, Sneed PK, Wara WM, et al: High activity iodine-125 interstitial implant for gliomas. Int J Radiat Oncol Biol Phys 24:583–591, 1992.
19. Marks JE, Boylan RJ, Prossal SC, et al: Cerebral radionecrosis; incidence and risk in relation to dose, time, fractionation, and volume. Int J Radiat Oncol Biol Phys 7:243–252, 1981.
20. Fitzek M, Thornton A, Lev M, et al: Accelerated fractionated proton/photon irradiation to 90 cobalt gray equivalent for glioblastoma multiforme: Results of a phase II prospective trial. J Neurosurg 91:251–260, 1999.
21. Loeffler JS, Alexander E III, Shea WM, et al: Radiosurgery as part of the initial management of patients with malignant glioma. J Clin Oncol 10:1379–1385, 1992.
22. Schlemmer HP, Bachert P, Herfarth KK, et al: Proton MR spectroscopic evaluation of suspicious brain lesions after stereotactic radiotherapy. AJNR Am J Neuroradiol 22:1316–1324, 2001.
23. McGirt MJ, Bulsara KR, Cummings TJ, et al: Prognostic value of magnetic resonance imaging-guided stereotactic biopsy in the evaluation of recurrent malignant astrocytoma compared with a lesion due to radiation effect. J Neurosurg 98:14–20, 2003.
24. Daumas-Duport C, Blond S, Vedrenee C, Szikla G: Radiolesion versus recurrence: Bioptic data in 30 gliomas after interstitial implant or combined interstitial and external radiation treatment. Acta Neurochir (Wien) 33(Suppl):291–299, 1984.
25. Rosenblum ML, Chiu-Liu H, Davis RL, Gutin PH: Radiation necrosis versus tumor recurrence following interstitial brachytherapy: Utility of tissue culture studies. Proc Am Assoc Neurol Surgeons 53:264, 1985.
26. Levivier M, Wikier D, Goldman S, et al: Integration of the metabolic data of positron emission tomography in the dosimetry planning of radiosurgery with the gamma knife: Early experience with brain tumors. J Neurosurg 93:233–238, 2000.
27. Nazzaro J, Neuwelt E: The role of surgery in the management of supratentorial intermediate and high-grade astrocytomas in adults. J Neurosurg 73:331–344, 1990.
28. Quigley MR, Maroon JC: The relationship between survival and the extent of the resection in patients with supratentorial malignant gliomas. Neurosurgery 29:385–389, 1991.
29. Vecht CJ, Avezaat CJ, van Patten WL, et al: The influence of the extent of surgery on the neurological function and survival in malignant glioma: A retro-operation analysis in 243 patients. J Neurol Neurosurg Psychiatry 53:466–471, 1990.
30. Ciric I, Ammirati M, Vick N, et al: Supratentorial gliomas: Surgical considerations and immediate postoperative results: Gross total resection versus partial resection. Neurosurgery 21:21–26, 1989.
31. Winger MJ, MacDonald DR, Cairncross JG: Supratentorial anaplastic gliomas in adults: The prognostic importance of extent of resection and prior low grade glioma. J Neurosurg 71:487–493, 1989.
32. Devaux BC, O'Fallon JR, Kelly PJ: Resection, biopsy, and survival in malignant gliomas: A retrospective study of clinical parameters, therapy, and outcome. J Neurosurg 78:767–775, 1993.
33. Kreth FW, Warnke PC, Scheremet R, Ostertag CB: Surgical resection and radiation therapy in the treatment of glioblastoma multiforme. J Neurosurg 78:762–766, 1993.
34. Salcman M, Kaplan RS, Durken TB, et al: Effect of age and reoperation on survival in the combined modality treatment of malignant astrocytomas. Neurosurgery 10:454–463, 1982.
35. Oppitz U, Maessen D, Zunterer H, et al: 3D recurrence patterns of glioblastomas after CT planned postoperative irradiation. Radiother Oncol 53:53–57, 1999.
36. Schmidt MH, Berger MS, Lamborn KR, et al: Repeated operations for infiltrative low-grade gliomas without intervening therapy. J Neurosurg 98:1165–1169, 2003.
37. Bowers DC, Krause TP, Aronson LJ, et al: Second surgery for recurrent pilocytic astrocytoma in children. Pediatr Neurosurg 34:229–234, 2001.
38. Kim HK, Thornton AF, Greenberg HS, et al: Results of re-irradiation of primary intracranial neoplasms with three dimensional conformal therapy. Am J Clin Oncol 20:358–363, 1997.
39. Kelly PJ, Rappaport ZH, Bhagwati SN, et al: Reoperation for recurrent malignant gliomas: What are your indications? Surg Neurol 47:39–42, 1997.
40. Hudes RS, Corn BW, Werner-Wasik M, et al: A phase I dose escalation study of hypofractionated stereotactic radiotherapy as salvage therapy for persistent or recurrent malignant gliomas. Int J Radiat Oncol Biol Phys 43:293–298, 1999.
41. Huncharek M, Muscat J: Treatment of recurrent high grade astrocytoma: Results of a systematic review of 1,415 patients. Anticancer Res 18:1303–1311, 1998.
42. Shepherd SF, Laing RW, Cosgrove VP: Hypofractionated stereotactic radiotherapy in the management of recurrent glioma. Int J Radiat Oncol Biol Phys 37:393–398, 1997.
43. Halligan JB, Stelzer KJ, Rostomily RC, et al: Operation and permanent low activity ^{125}I brachytherapy for recurrent high grade astrocytomas. Int J Radiat Oncol Biol Phys 35:541–547, 1996.
44. Tatter SB, Shaw EG, Rosenblum ML, et al: An inflatable balloon catheter and liquid ^{125}I radiation source (GliaSite Radiation Therapy System) for treatment of recurrent malignant glioma: Multicenter safety and feasibility trial. J Neurosurg 99:297–303, 2003.

45. Shrieve DC, Alexander E, Wen PC, et al: Comparison of stereotactic radiosurgery and brachytherapy in the treatment of recurrent glioblastoma multiforme. Neurosurgery 36:275–284, 1995.

46. Cho KH, Hall WA, Berbi BJ, et al: Single dose versus fractionated stereotactic radiotherapy for recurrent high grade gliomas. Int J Radiat Oncol Biol Phys 45:1133–1141, 1999.

47. Kim JH, Lew YS, Kolozsvary A, et al: Arsenic trioxide enhances radiation response of 9L glioma in the rat brain. Radiat Res 160:662–666, 2003.

48. Hara A, Nishimura Y, Sakai N, et al: Effectiveness of intraoperative radiation therapy for recurrent supratentorial low grade glioma. J Neurooncol 25:239–243, 1995.

49. Paganelli G, Bartolomei M, Ferrari M, et al: Pre-targeted locoregional radioimmunotherapy with ^{90}Y-biotin in glioma patients: Phase I study and preliminary therapeutic results. Cancer Biother Radiopharm 16:227–235, 2001.

50. Reardon DA, Akabani G, Coleman RE, et al: Phase II trial of murine^{131} I-labeled antitenascin monoclonal antibody 81C6 administered into surgically created resection cavities of patients with newly diagnosed malignant gliomas. J Clin Oncol 20:1389–1397, 2002.

51. Jaeckle KA, Hess KR, Yung WK, et al: North American Brain Tumor Consortium: Phase II evaluation of temozolomide and 13-*cis*-retinoic acid for the treatment of recurrent and progressive malignant glioma: A North American Brain Tumor Consortium study. Oncology 21:2305–2311, 2003.

52. Jenkins RB, Curran W, Scott CB, Cairncross G: Pilot evaluation of 1p and 19q deletions in anaplastic oligodendrogliomas collected by a national cooperative cancer treatment group. Am J Clin Oncol 24:506–508, 2001.

53. Soffietti R, Ruda R, Bradac GB, et al: PCV chemotherapy for recurrent oligodendrogliomas and oligoastrocytomas. Neurosurgery 43:1066–1073, 1998.

54. Fine HA, Dear KBG, Loeffler JS, et al: Meta-analysis of radiation therapy with and without adjuvant chemotherapy for malignant gliomas in adults. Cancer 71:2585–2597, 1993.

55. Levin VA, Silver P, Hannigan J, et al: Superiority of post radiotherapy adjuvant chemotherapy with CCNU, procarbazine, and vincristine (PCV) over BCNU for anaplastic gliomas: NCOG 6G61 final report. Int J Radiat Oncol Biol Phys 18:321–324, 1990.

56. Hassenbusch SJ, Nardone EM, Levin VA, et al: Stereotactic injection of DTI-015 into recurrent malignant gliomas: Phase I/II trial. Neoplasia 5:9–16, 2003.

57. Yung WKA, Mechtler L, Gleason MJ: Intravenous carboplatin for recurrent malignant glioma: A phase II study. J Clin Oncol 9:860–864, 1991.

58. Prados MD, Russo C: Chemotherapy of brain tumors. Semin Surg Oncol 14:88–95, 1998.

59. Hayes RL, Koslow M, Hiesiger EM, et al: Improved long term survival after intracavitary interleukin-2 and lymphokine-activated killer cells for adults with recurrent malignant glioma. Cancer 76:840–852, 1995.

60. Shand N, Weber F, Mariani L, et al: A phase 1–2 clinical trial of gene therapy for recurrent glioblastoma multiforme by tumor transduction with herpes simplex thymidine kinase gene followed by ganciclovir. Hum Gene Ther 10:2325–2335, 1999.

61. Shah AC, Benos D, Gillespie GY, Markert JM: Oncolytic viruses: Clinical applications as vectors for the treatment of malignant gliomas. J Neurooncology 65:203–226, 2003.

62. Harsh GR, Deisboeck TS, Louis DL, et al: Thymidine kinase activation of ganciclovir in recurrent malignant gliomas: A gene marking and neuropathological study. J Neurosurg 92:804–811, 2000.

63. Olivi A, Grossman SA, Tatter S, et al: Dose escalation of carmustine in surgically implanted polymers in patients with recurrent malignant glioma: A New Approaches to Brain Tumor Therapy CNS Consortium trial. J Clin Oncol 21:1845–1849, 2003.

64. Wood GW, Holladay FP, Turner T, et al: A pilot study of autologous cancer cell vaccination and cellular immunotherapy using anti-CD3 stimulated lymphocytes in patients with recurrent grade III/IV astrocytoma. J Neurooncol 48:113–120, 2000.

65. Brem H, Piantadosi S, Berger PC, et al: Placebo controlled trial of safety and efficacy of intraoperative controlled delivery by biodegradable polymers of chemotherapy for recurrent gliomas. Lancet 345:1008–1012, 1995.

66. Subach BR, Witham TF, Kondziolka D, et al: Morbidity and survival after BCNU wafer implantation for recurrent glioblastoma: A retrospective case matched cohort series. Neurosurgery 45:17–22, 1999.

67. Boiardi A, Eoli M, Pozzi A, et al: Locally delivered chemotherapy and repeated surgery can improve survival in glioblastoma patients. Ital J Neurol Sci 20:43–48, 1999.

68. Ammirati M, Vick N, Liao Y, et al: Effect of the extent of surgical resection on survival and quality of life in patients with supratentorial glioblastomas and anaplastic astrocytomas. Neurosurgery 21:201–206, 1987.

69. Wallner KE, Galicich JH, Malkin MG: Inability of computed tomography appearance of recurrent malignant astrocytoma to predict survival following reoperation. J Clin Oncol 7:1492–1496, 1989.

70. Sipos L, Afra D: Reoperations of supratentorial anaplastic astrocytomas. Acta Neurochir (Wien) 39:99–104, 1997.

71. Ammirati M, Galicich JH, Arbit B: Reoperation in the treatment of recurrent intracranial malignant gliomas. Neurosurgery 21:607–614, 1987.

72. Berger MS, Tucker A, Spence A, Winn HR: Reoperation for glioma. Clin Neurosurg 39:172–186, 1992.

73. Harsh GR, Levin VA, Gutin PH, et al: Reoperation for recurrent glioblastoma and anaplastic astrocytoma. Neurosurgery 21:615–621, 1987.

74. Karnofsky D, Burchenal JH, Armistead GC Jr, et al: Triethylene melamine in the treatment of neoplastic disease. Arch Intern Med 87:477–516, 1951.

75. Guyotat J, Signorelli F, Frappaz D, et al: Is reoperation for recurrence of glioblastoma justified? Oncol Rep 7:899–904, 2000.

76. Daneyemez M, Gezen F, Canakci Z, et al: Radical surgery and reoperation in supratentorial glial tumors. Minim Invasive Neurosurg 41:209–213, 1998.

77. Patel S, Breneman JC, Warnick RE, et al: Permanent iodine-125 interstitial implants for the treatment of recurrent glioblastoma multiforme. Neurosurgery 46:1123–1128, 2000.

78. Chandler KL, Prados MD, Malec M, Wilson CB: Long-term survival in patients with glioblastoma multiforme. Neurosurgery 32:716–720, 1993.

79. Rostomily RC, Spence AM, Duong D: Multimodality management of recurrent adult malignant gliomas: Results of a phase II multiagent chemotherapy study and analysis of cytoreductive surgery. Neurosurgery 35:378–388, 1994.

80. Stromblad LG, Anderson H, Malmstrom P: Reoperation for malignant astrocytomas: Personal experience and a review of the literature. Br J Neurosurg 7:623–633, 1993.

81. Latif AZ, Signorini D, Gregor A, et al: Application of the MRC brain tumour prognostic index to patients with malignant glioma not managed in randomized control trial. J Neurol Neurosurg Psychiatry 64:747–750, 1998.

82. Brandes AA, Vastola F, Monfardini S: Reoperation in recurrent gliomas: Literature review of prognostic factors and outcome. Am J Clin Oncol 22:387–390, 1999.

83. Bohinski RJ, Kokkino AK, Warnick RE, et al: Glioma resection in a shared-resource magnetic resonance operating room after optimal image-guided frameless stereotactic resection. Neurosurgery 48:731–742, 2001.

84. Clarke CA, Barick TR, Murphy MM, Bell BA: White matter fiber tracking in patients with space-occupying lesions of the brain: A new technique for neurosurgical planning? Neuroimage 20:1601–1608, 2003.

85. Hernes TA, Ommedal S, Lie T, et al: Stereoscopic navigation-controlled display of preoperative MRI and intraoperative 3D ultrasound in planning and guidance of neurosurgery: New technology for minimally invasive image-guided surgery approaches. Minim Invasive Neurosurg 46:129–137, 2003.

86. Roux FE, Boulanouar K, Lotterie JA, et al: Language functional magnetic resonance imaging in preoperative assessment of language areas: Correlation with direct cortical stimulation. Neurosurgery 52:1335–1345, 2003.

87. Quinones-Hinojosa A, Ojemann SG, Sanai N, et al: Preoperative correlation of intraoperative cortical mapping with magnetic resonance imaging landmarks to predict localization of the Broca area. J Neurosurgery 99:311–318, 2003.

88. LeRoux PD, Berger MS, Ojemann GA, et al: Correlation of intraoperative ultrasound tumor volumes and margins with preoperative computerized tomography scans. J Neurosurg 71:691–698, 1989.

89. Young B, Oldfield EH, Markesbery WR, et al: Reoperation for glioblastoma. J Neurosurg 55:917–921, 1981.

51 Surgical Management of Convexity, Parasagittal, and Falx Meningiomas

BERND M. HOFMANN and RUDOLF FAHLBUSCH

INTRODUCTION AND HISTORICAL SURVEY

Cushing and Eisenhardt[1] defined a class of benign neoplasms that arise from meninges of the brain and the spinal cord and account for approximately 15% of the tumors of the central nervous system. Cushing[2] also was the first to publicize a case of a parasagittal meningioma, which was excised in 1910. About 90% of intracranial meningiomas are located supratentorially, less than 10% within the posterior fossa, and less than 2% within the ventricular system. One third of the supratentorial meningiomas originate along the superior sagittal sinus or the falx, one third over the convexity, and one third from the basal region. Calcification of these tumors and involvement of the surrounding bone can occur. This chapter covers only meningiomas around the convexity and falx or the superior sagittal sinus.

Peak incidence of this subset of meningiomas is between 50 and 70 years of age. Women are affected two to three times more often than men, whereas malignant meningiomas are slightly more frequent in men. According to newer figures,[3] the annual incidence is about 6/100,000 population.

To define origin more clearly, meningiomas arise from arachnoid cap cells, but their causation is not known so far. Patients who have undergone radiotherapy show an increased incidence of meningiomas (even multiple ones), and these patients also show an increased rate of recurrence and of malignant and atypical tumor types. Genetic studies of such cases revealed a loss of DNA from chromosome 22. This chromosome normally carries a tumor suppressor gene, and this mutation is also found in patients with neurofibromatosis type 2 (NF2). This explains why patients suffering from NF2 show an increased incidence of meningiomas. According to the literature,[4] multiple meningiomas are found in as many as 8% of all patients suffering from a meningioma and most of these are associated with NF2. Among the latter, concurrent appearance of neurinomas is typical.

DEFINITION AND CLASSIFICATION

Anatomic distinction among (1) convexity, (2) parasagittal, and (3) falx meningiomas is more difficult than clinical distinction, especially in meningiomas of parasagittal and falcine origin.

Historically, convexity meningiomas have been classified into seven subgroups according to the overlying brain area: precoronar, coronar, postcoronar, pararolandic, parietal, temporal, and occipital. About 70% of these tumors are located anterior to the rolandic fissure. Pure temporal and occipital localization are more rare. These subdivisions arose because the coronar suture was used to define the precentral area, with the involvement of eloquent areas assessed by anatomic landmarks. A location anterior to the coronar suture clearly indicates a position anterior to the motor strip, while the term postcoronal localizes the tumor as adjacent to or within the central area. Today, magnetic resonance imaging (MRI) and functional mapping (see later) allows a more precise localization, including recognition of a tumor close to speech areas in the frontal lobe (Broca's area) and parietal lobe (Wernicke's area). New technologies are currently allowing a redefinition of the classification of convexity meningiomas.

Parasagittal meningiomas occur seven times more frequently than falx meningiomas, according to a series of Cushing. Hyperostosis often occurs with parasagittal meningiomas but not with falcine ones.[1] The two types of meningiomas can be distinguished according to their involvement with and relationship to the superior sagittal sinus; however, the specific localization along this sinus (i.e., anterior, medial, or posterior third) plays the most important role in both. The superior sagittal sinus extends from the crista galli to the confluens sinuum in the sagittal plane and is contained within the dura at the junction with the falx cerebri. It is attached to the cranial vault and lies within a shallow groove of the inner table of the bone, while its three walls form a triangle based in the cranial vault. The sinus communicates with venous lacunae, mostly found in the parietal region, and arachnoid granules project into them. The sinus is anatomically divided into three parts. The anterior part includes the area from the crista galli to the coronal suture, the medial part extends up to the lambdoid suture, and the posterior part terminates with the confluens sinuum.

Parasagittal meningiomas are defined as filling the angle between falx and the meninges of the convexity, so that there is no layer of mesial or superficial cortex separating the tumor from the sinus. These brain structures are displaced outward. Falcine meningiomas arise from the falx and are completely concealed by overlying cerebral cortex. There might be involvement of only the wall itself or the lumen of the superior sagittal sinus as well. Convexity meningiomas are defined as arising from the dura of the cranial vault; they involve no dural sinuses and have no relationship to the falx or the skull base. Usually there is a rim of brain between the superior sagittal sinus and the tumor (Fig. 51-1).

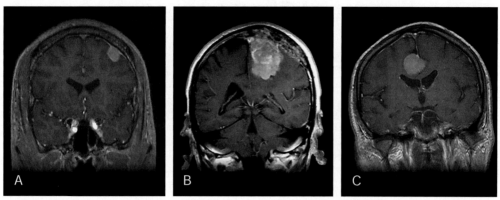

FIGURE 51-1 Vicinity to superior sagittal sinus as criteria of localization of (*A*) convexity, (*B*) parasagittal, and (*C*) falcine meningioma.

A review of the literature[5] revealed that about 35% of parasagittal meningiomas are located in the anterior, about 55% in the medial, and about 10% in the posterior part, whereas 43% of falcine meningiomas are found in the anterior and 57% in the medial part. Localization plays a major role in surgical treatment and is characteristic for an individual patient's symptoms.

SYMPTOMS

Patients suffering from meningiomas that are growing may show general symptoms of raised intracranial pressure such as headache, seizures, and organic psychosyndrome. Neurologic deficits are in accord with the eloquent areas involved. Tumors of the convexity around the precentral cortex may cause contralateral palsy and motor seizures, while tumors of the postcentral area may result in sensory deficits and Jacksonian seizures, eventually preceded by motor or sensory aura and followed by a residual postictal paresis (Todd's paralysis). If certain areas of the temporal (Wernicke's area) or frontal lobe (Broca's area) of the dominant hemisphere are affected, speech disturbances may follow; seizures are caused by tumors overlying the temporal lobe (especially temporomesial), and a homonymous hemianopsia is found with tumors overlying the occipital lobe. Brain shift may result in larger temporal meningiomas compressing the contralateral peduncle to the edge of the tentorium, with resulting ipsilateral spastic weakness of the leg and visual field defects.

A recent report found that 40.7% of patients suffering from convexity meningiomas had seizures.[6]

Parasagittal and falcine meningiomas of the middle third of the superior sagittal sinus are initially accompanied by motor or sensory seizures that may spread, with eventual subsequent loss of sensory and residual Todd's paresis. Seizures were found in 27.5% of all patients suffering from meningioma in this localization.[6] If controlled by anticonvulsants without further diagnosis, a paresis of the contralateral leg may follow. In large tumors, signs of raised intracranial pressure and hemiparesis are observed.

Patients with meningiomas involving the posterior third of the superior sagittal sinus complain mostly of headache followed by hemianopsia or visual field deficits, depending on the location and size of tumor. The latter symptom very often goes unnoticed by the patient. Some patients suffer from visual hallucinations as well.

Parasagittal and falcine meningiomas within the anterior third of the sinus can grow very large and cause personality changes.

Progress in imaging techniques and the increased application of neuroradiologic imaging for screening purposes have led to an increase in the diagnosis of incidental meningiomas. These special cases require careful consideration about the indications for and timing of surgery. Elderly patients presenting with meningiomas deserve similar consideration with regard to subtotal removal or such treatment options as radiotherapy or medical treatment. These situations are discussed later in this chapter.

PREOPERATIVE DIAGNOSTICS AND SPECIAL CONSIDERATIONS

Plain skull x-ray films demonstrating hyperostosis and involvement of the skull have been replaced by computed tomography (CT) and MRI scans.

Computed tomography has the advantage of demonstrating bony alternations (hyperostosis, invasion) and normally leads to the diagnosis of meningioma. These tumors are hypodense in plain films and show intense and rapid enhancement. Calcification is found in 25% of all meningiomas and ranges from diffuse appearance to dense sclerosis.[7] MRI dominates the diagnostic procedures. With gadolinium enhancement, it provides an excellent imaging of these tumors. Meningiomas are isointense or hypointense to brain in T1-weighted images and show rapid, mostly homogeneous enhancement with gadolinium. In some cases, a "dura tail" enhancement of surrounding meninges is visible on MRI. A rim of subarachnoid space can be seen in nonenhanced slices. Peritumoral edema is common but not necessarily found in all cases. Furthermore, dislocation of sulci and gyri, especially in eloquent areas and, confirmed with MR angiography or phlebography, venous drainage, sinus patency, and displacement of major arteries can be visualized. When performing functional imaging, these scans can be used for intraoperative, frameless (functional) neuronavigation. MRI-related advanced technologies are discussed in the following paragraphs.

Meningiomas are usually found to be solid tumors, but cystic ones exist in 6.3% of the cases and can be confused with metastasis.[8]

Digital subtraction angiography (DSA) is indicated to demonstrate the degree of vascularization, to demonstrate by phlebogram the free passage of the superior sagittal sinus in all of its three segments (anterior, medial, posterior), and to localize the main draining bridging vessels toward the sinus, with regard to a potential goal of embolization. Angiography is performed by selective catheterization of the internal and external carotid arteries. Blood supply of the tumor is chiefly drawn from the dural-based arterioles arising from the external carotid artery (mainly the medial meningeal artery). In some tumors, supplementary blood supply is drawn from pial vessels ("pial parasitization"), necessitating internal carotid angiography as well. Selective catheterization is helpful in distinguishing falcine from parasagittal meningiomas as well as in determining the side of their dural attachment. In falcine meningiomas the blood supply is not likely to derive from the external carotid artery. Contrast enhancement within the neoplasm usually appears early and remains long into the venous phase. Information obtained from angiography includes the following: Where does the primary blood supply originate and how are these vessels located relative to the operative approach? Is the tumor extremely vascularized, and is embolization of one or more major feeders possible without risking such neurologic deficits as loss of vision if, for example, the central retinal artery is inadvertently embolized? Is any necrosis of the skin to be expected? Is the superior sagittal sinus occluded by tumor mass, and what is the relationship to major draining veins? Are there any signs of collateralization that suggest an (at least partially) occluded sinus? Some problems must be borne in mind.

For example, the sagittal sinus will be receiving a large amount of unopacified blood from the contralateral side and therefore may not be visible on angiography.

Signs of a occluded sinus, as outlined by Marc and Schlechter,[9] are: (1) nonvisualization of a segment of the superior sagittal sinus; (2) failure of the cortical veins to reach the sinus in this area; (3) delayed venous drainage in the area of obstruction; (4) reversal of normal venous flow with large collaterals connecting anterior-superior with superior sagittal sinus distal to the obstruction or with the transverse sinus or middle cerebral vein. It is important to know whether the sinus is patent, because (inadvertent) acute occlusion of the superior sagittal sinus can lead to life-threatening complications such as venous infarction, hemiparesis, or death.

In any case, angiograms should be examined carefully by the surgeon and the decision about embolization made in advance in consultation with an interventional neuroradiologist.

Embolization should take place 24 hours (to 3 days) before operation. Although controversial, the benefits of embolization are believed to be reduction of blood loss and a shortening of the surgical procedure. In the latest study,[10] performed in two university hospitals, intraoperative blood loss was reduced only if the entire tumor could be embolized. There was no significant difference in duration of surgical procedure and extent of resection. Embolization shows some benefit in basal meningiomas but not in superficial ones. In any case, care must be taken not to cause neurologic deficits by obliterating important vessels. In addition, there is a risk of brain swelling and bleeding within the tumor bed following endovascular procedure, necessitating acute surgery. Figure 51-2A and B (preoperative MRI and angiography)

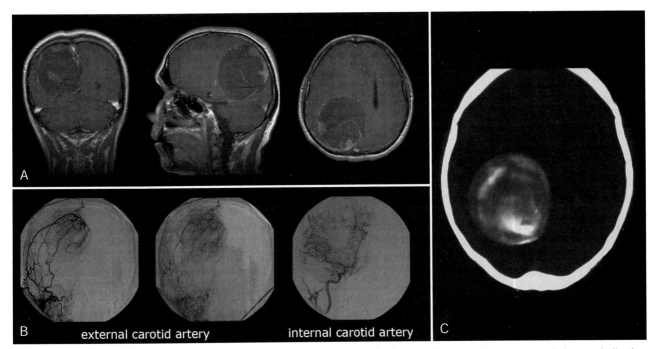

FIGURE 51-2 A 54-year-old female with a right parieto-occipital meningioma with tumor hemorrhage during embolization, raised intracranial pressure, and requiring immediate excision of the tumor. *A,* Contrast-enhanced MRI preoperatively (bleeding after embolization already present). *B,* External and internal right carotid angiography showing tumor vascularization. *C,* CT scan immediately after embolization showing extravasation.

represents a case of a 54-year-old female suffering from psychosyndrome and loss of memory caused by a large right parieto-occipital meningioma. Preoperative embolization led to acute bleeding (see Fig. 51-2C; CT scans following bleeding), with loss of consciousness requiring emergent tumor extirpation.

Preoperative information revealing cleavage between the arachnoid membrane and the tumor capsule can be drawn from T2-weighted MRI and angiography and may lead to special considerations concerning effort of tumor resection.[11,12] It is well known that a well-defined boundary between tumor capsule and arachnoid membrane leads to a simple resection of the tumor accompanied by a low risk of vulneration of the brain. It is essential to perform an extrapial tumor resection to avoid devascularization of the underlying cortex, which may result in small cortical hemorrhages and loss of function. No cleavage plane is found in tumors drawing vascularization from pial vessels (and consecutively from the internal carotid artery), which is shown in angiography and expressed in perifocal edema on MRI. In tumor vascularization arising from the external carotid artery, a cleavage plane is usually found during resection. When a tumor shows a diameter less than 3 cm, extrapial resection is possible in general; in contrast, it has been found that a tumor larger than 3 cm in diameter is associated with a higher risk of pial vascularization and therefore the need to perform subpial resection. An irregular border of the tumor usually suggests pial vascularization. Unfortunately, there is no statistically significant visibility of tumor-brain interface on T2-weighted images on MRI and thus no opportunity to determine a safe surgical plane for resection. Generally speaking, in one third of patients no extrapial plane can be found; therefore, 30% of these patients had an unfavorable neurologic outcome as subpial resection had to be carried out. If it is possible to carry out extrapial resection, unfavorable outcome (Karnofsky score <80) occurs in only 25% of patients. This issue must be addressed during the planning of surgical treatment, especially if eloquent areas are involved. It may be wise to leave some tumor remnants around eloquent areas to avoid neurologic deterioration.

ADVANCED TECHNOLOGIES

Anatomic navigation requires segmentation of the tumor and of important structures in the vicinity of the tumor such as arteries (a. pericallosa) or veins. This is used to allow the surgeon to keep trephination small and well directed. The trajectory guides us in virtual and physical space to the tumor and avoids damage of normal brain. In eloquent areas, functional brain mapping for localization of the precentral and postcentral gyrus, sensory and motor speech areas and pyramidal tract can be extremely helpful. Functional brain mapping can be performed by functional MRI (fMRI; 1.5 T high field) or by magnetic encephalography (MEG). Using MEG, magnetic changes in brain tissue can be visualized while a patient is performing several tasks activating motor, sensory, or speech areas. The combination of anatomic and functional data, called functional neuronavigation, provides a very useful tool in preoperative surgical planning. According to data obtained by functional neuronavigation, in selected cases tumor remnants were left within the central region to avoid higher morbidity.

In special cases, intraoperative MRI can be useful to determine the extent of resection. Tumor remnants remaining within the superior sagittal sinus, for example, can be visualized and additional treatment strategies chosen. In some cases the extent of resection can be easily enlarged without vulneration of important structures and causing bleeding from any important vessel, especially the tumor-involved sinus. Furthermore, updating of functional neuronavigation data with respect to intraoperative brain shift is possible.

If functional neuronavigation is not available, localization of the central area, respectively the central sulcus, is possible by using somatosensory evoked potentials (SEPs). In this procedure, the contralateral median nerve is electrically stimulated and typical "phase reversal" is observed in a consecutive of four or more cortical leads using a strip of platelet electrodes placed above the suspected central sulcus. As a result of the improving accuracy of functional imaging and neuronavigation, the use of this method is fading; yet it is still sometimes used to confirm information gained from these newer technologies.[13] The use of functional neuronavigation is demonstrated in the Illustrative Reports.

INDICATIONS FOR SURGERY AND AIMS OF THE OPERATION

General Indications

The diagnosis of a meningioma does not inevitably lead to surgical removal, especially not when the finding is incidental or the patient is older.

Surgery for meningioma is indicated when there are seizures or neurologic deficits due to size and extent of tumor and/or increase in intracranial pressure. Space-occupying lesions include not only solid tumor but also edema. Perifocal edema is mainly present in a special subgroup (secretory meningiomas), even if they are small, but it is seen in other tumors as well. This edema also has epileptogenic potential.

Tumors that are mainly growing osteophytically and that are extending and also perforating the skin are comparatively rare in occurrence but do indicate surgery from a cosmetic viewpoint as well as to prevent infections.

Incidental Findings

Incidental meningiomas are found in 2.3% of the population during autopsy series. The frequent use of CT and MRI as screening methods has resulted in an increase in the identification of incidental meningiomas. It is commonly thought that these tumors do not grow throughout life and that they generally show a very low rate of growth. Absolute growing rates are between 0.03 and 2.62 cm^3/year, while relative growing rates are between 0.48% and 72.2%. Many efforts have been made to determine both the kinetics of and influences on tumor growth. It is significantly shown that tumors found in elderly patients show a slower growth pattern than those found in younger people. Indications for a slower growth pattern include spots of calcification and isointense or hypointense signals in T2-weighted MRI. Furthermore, there is a mild positive correlation between tumor volume and absolute growth. According to these findings, MRI should be performed every 3 to 6 months in younger and every 6 to 12 months in older patients. Larger intervals are used by the authors. Surgical resection should be performed in respect to tumor growth but obligatorily if the tumor growth rate is greater than 1 cm³/year.[14,15]

In multiple meningiomas, which occur in about 8% of patients, only the tumors causing clinical symptoms or tumors that show a tendency to grow should be surgically treated.

Elderly Patients

Even if age per se is not a contraindication to surgery, one should consider not only the higher risk of anesthesia but also the higher mortality and morbidity associated with advanced age. The most important variable influencing the decision in elderly patients seems to be neurologic status and general health condition.[16] If one or both are low and there is either no tumor growth or only mild signs of it, then observation is justified. In cases of any sign of growth, conservative treatment such as radiation therapy (underlying certain restrictions) or medical treatment (hydroxyurea, see later) to prevent progression is indicated.

Within a newer study of patients older than 70 years,[17] 18 patients suffering from a parasagittal and 16 suffering from a convexity meningioma, as well as patients with other tumor localizations were examined. Neurologic deficit improved in 57.6%, was unchanged in 16.6%, and deteriorated in 18.2%, while 7.6% died within 30 days after surgery. Postoperative complications in 66 patients consisted of hematoma (10 patients), pneumonia (6), seizures (5), ischemia (5), coagulation disorders (4), and gastrointestinal bleeding (3). The smaller the tumor size (<3 cm) the more rapidly surgery was performed (<4 hours); furthermore, a lesser degree of perifocal edema was invariably associated with a better neurologic outcome. Outcome in patients suffering from recurrent tumor was worse. Surgical resection was suggested in patients expressing criteria following American Society of Anesthesiologists (ASA) physical status grade I or II and a Karnofsky index of 70 or more. Because of the patients' age and thus the lower risk of significant tumor regrowth, total resection was not the ultimate goal. Furthermore, adjuvant treatment such as that discussed earlier seemed to be adequate to achieve tumor control.

Indication Depending on Localization

Indications for surgery on convexity meningiomas are neurologic deficits or epilepsy. In case of incidental findings, operation should be performed if tumor growth is proved; this might be indicated by surrounding edema, especially if signs of increased intracranial pressure are present, such as headache, nausea, or papilledema. Furthermore, surgery should be performed in asymptomatic tumors that are adjacent to eloquent areas and are removed easily in an early stage but are expected to become more difficult to remove after growing further.

Convexity meningiomas show the highest potential to be cured, especially if they are well encapsulated. Total excision is possible in most cases because of the easy accessibility and the absence of complex surrounding structures, except for eloquent regions of the underlying brain, which can be spared for the most part.

In parasagittal and falx meningiomas the indication for surgery is more difficult to determine. The decision depends chiefly on the timing and radicality of resection, since these tumors have a lower rate of cure and a higher rate of recurrence. They are more difficult to resect, not only because they are surrounded by such complex structures as sinuses, eloquent areas, arteries (pericallosal artery), and major draining veins, but because they are comparatively inaccessible if overlain by brain, especially in the case of falcine meningiomas. The aims of and indications for surgery must, therefore, be considered in more detail.

The primary goal of the operation is total tumor removal; in cases where this is not possible, as much tumor as possible should be removed, because whatever tumor tissue is left behind gives rise to regrowth. Attachments to bone and dura should be removed as well. The walls of the sinus are kept intact without compromising circulation within it. An occluded sinus can be removed (which is necessary to reduce rate of recurrence), but anastomotic veins must be preserved. Even if patent, the anterior third of the superior sagittal sinus can be ligated by the surgeon and removed. If the tumor invades the sinus but does not obliterate it, it is wise to leave tumor remnants attached at the sinus and await further growth. If the sinus becomes occluded with time, it can be easily removed during reoperation.

Better imaging techniques allow earlier detection of meningiomas and a better chance for cure. The smaller the tumor, the more easily it can be removed, even if accessibility is difficult. It is reasonable to observe asymptomatic meningiomas for a period of 3 to 12 months. If the Karnofsky index or neurologic status shows deterioration, then surgery should be performed. In case of any neurologic deficit attributed to the tumor, one should perform surgery without observation.

PREOPERATIVE MANAGEMENT

Preoperative management includes treatment of brain edema by steroids (1 week pretreatment with 8 mg dexamethasone three times daily and the same dose before surgery), detection of tumor vascularization by angiography, anticonvulsant medication, and optimizing treatment for concomitant disease such as diabetes or hypertension. Furthermore, assessment of cardiac and pulmonary function, including preoperative pulmonary coaching is necessary, especially in elderly patients.

When tumors are large or highly vascularized, preparation for autologous transfusion should be considered if the patient decides on elective surgery.

Embolization is carried out in highly vascularized tumors 1 to 3 days before operation. This may result in malignant brain swelling or bleeding within the tumor, which requires immediate tumor resection to avoid further morbidity or mortality.

Anesthesiologic treatment immediately before surgery consists of placing an indwelling urinary catheter and applying calf compression to prevent thromboembolism. A single injection of preoperative antibiotic is administered. Only in exceptional cases are diuretic agents (20 mg furosemide [Lasix]) and mannitol are given preoperatively or intraoperatively to control cerebral edema.

OPERATIVE TECHNIQUES

Even in these times of neuronavigation, it remains common sense to use bony landmarks such as coronal and sagittal

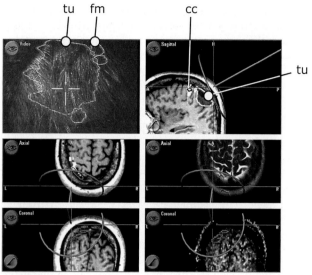

FIGURE 51-3 Functional neuronavigation for localizing the tumor and planning the skin incision. cc, central cortex; fm, functional markers; tu, tumor.

sutures, orbital rim, outer ear, and meatus in tumor localization, and experienced neurosurgeons do still use these landmarks. On the historical way to modern neuronavigation, external marking of the tumor margins was found to be helpful.

Functional neuronavigation, however, represents the best and most powerful method, helpful in localizing the tumor and planning skin incision as well as bone flap (Fig. 51-3). Apart from solid mass, extension of the tumor within the dura must be taken into consideration. Intradurally, in case the tumor overlies eloquent areas of the brain or, in larger tumors, if important vessels are hidden by the tumor, it permits the surgeon to localize and spare these structures (Fig. 51-4). While creating the surgical opening, the feasibility of reinsertion of the bone flap and of dural closure must already be under consideration.

POSITIONING

Some general considerations with reference to positioning the patient must be observed. The patient must be positioned in such a way that the tumor is located at the top of the surgical field. Performing procedures within a steep-face orientation are to be avoided whenever possible. Some authors prefer positioning the patient so as to allow the tumor to shift away from midline under the influence of gravity. This results in a movement of the tumor mass toward the surgeon. Other authors, in contrast, prefer a position of the head that minimizes brain retraction under the influence of gravity. The latter positioning causes the brain to "fall away" from the tumor and depict the borderline between both. Tearing of adjoining vessels by excessive tension of the tumor is considered a diasadvantage of this method and must be avoided. The operation on large meningiomas, especially those of parasagittal and falcine origin, could require several hours, and it is thus important to provide for the comfort of both patient and surgeon.

According to the localization of the tumor, a supine, park bench or prone position is chosen while the head should be elevated over the heart. The head is secured in a three-pin fixation and attached to the table. Adequate fixation should be checked to avoid inadvertent movement during surgery. Fixation provides movement of table, head, and body of the patient as a single unit; rapid repositioning of the patient to prevent bleeding from the sinus or occurrence of an air embolism is made possible by adjustment of the operating table.

With convexity meningiomas, the patient's head is tilted such that the tumor is positioned at the top of the surgical field. With falcine and parasagittal tumors, the sagittal plane of the head is positioned parallel to the wall and perpendicular to the ceiling. If the tumor is at the frontal third of the sagittal sinus, the patient is positioned prone with a flat head; with tumors involving the middle third of the sinus, the head is slightly flexed, allowing the surgeon to look at the vertex (Fig. 51-5). Tumors behind the lambdoid suture are approached via a three-quarters sitting or prone position. Excessive neck flexion, which can lead to diminished venous

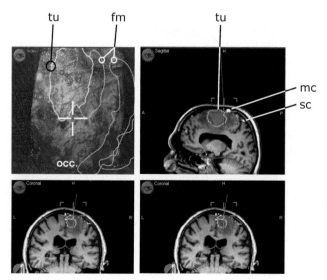

FIGURE 51-4 Functional neuronavigation during surgery in eloquent areas. fm, functional markers; mc, motor cortex; sc, sensory cortex; tu, tumor.

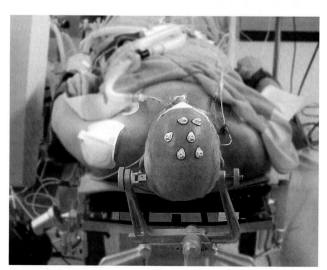

FIGURE 51-5 Positioning of the patient with a tumor at the anterior third of the falx.

return within jugular veins, is avoided while the patient is positioned and fixation is carried out. The latter should be performed in consideration of an ergonomic posture and the handed side of the surgeon. A surface on which the surgeon can rest his or her arms, or an armrest fixed at the operating chair can be helpful.

After positioning has been accomplished, pressure points such as the brachial plexus, peripheral nerves, and eyes are padded and adequately positioned. Shaving is carried out in accordance with prevailing preferences and the patient's agreement. Some surgeons do not perform any shaving, but in the authors' opinion partial shaving and, with large tumors, total shaving should be carried out. Scrub solution must not run into eyes or onto the cautery plate (which could cause burns); the operative field is scrubbed and draped with adhesive plastic film and draping. Midline (with parasagittal and falcine meningiomas), line of incision, and other key landmarks are marked sterile before draping.

SKIN FLAP

While designing the skin incision, several issues must be kept in mind: (1) adequate exposure of the tumor, (2) sufficient vascular supply of the scalp, and (3) possible modifications of the incision in case of inaccurate localization of the tumor or insufficient access to critical structures and in case of tumor recurrence beyond the present tumor margins (Fig. 51-6). Planning of the incision should be given serious consideration, even if this is the first operation, since if repeat surgery for recurrence becomes necessary, pure vascularization can result in problems and require long-term reconstructive surgery. A (vascularized) pericranial or temporalis flap should be provided for dural closure, and a satisfactory cosmetic result should also be a concern. Linear or S-shaped incisions centered on the lesion provide adequate exposure; not only is blood supply considered, but they are also easily modified during initial or recurrent surgery. Flaps, which have to be based on their vascular pedicle, should not exceed a length-to-width ratio of 3:2 and should be widest at their base. Later incisions are more difficult to modify and should only slightly exceed the size of the bone flap. On the whole, flaps should be made too big rather than too small, so that any modifications due to incorrect

planning can be avoided. With frontal or frontotemporal tumors, scalp flaps risk crossing the forehead and leaving cosmetic deformities; therefore a bicoronal incision is preferable. The temporal branch of the facial nerve is spared if the incision ends at the top of the zygomatic arch and is barely in front of the ear as well as if its course within the temporal fat pad is reflected in combination with the temporalis muscle or at least if the fat pad above the muscle is left at the skin. A flap that must cross the sinus, in contrast, is used in falcine and parasagittal tumors. Skin is incised sharply down to the pericranium, which is left intact. Large arterioles and veins are cauterized, and clips including skin and galea aponeurotica are also placed to avoid oozing hemorrhage. The scalp is now stripped off the pericranium and reflected by using fish hooks or one or two sutures clamped to the draping. The pericranium is incised (some authors use monopolar cautery) and based at its vascular supply, elevated, soaked in saline, and reflected to the skin flap. It is placed under tension to avoid shrinking, using dural stitches. Later it can be used for dural closure as pediculated or free flap. Tumor feeders arising from the scalp, commonly seen in highly vascularized convexity meningiomas, are cauterized and cut as soon as they are noticed.

BONE FLAP

It is best in meningioma surgery to create a free bone flap for at least two reasons: (1) pediculated flaps receive excessive blood supply by branches of the external carotid artery, which might be enlarged by taking part in the tumor supply; (2) these flaps are bulky and difficult to handle.

Bone flaps should be made generous, especially if there is tumor located in eloquent areas, both to avoid inadvertent vulneration of brain and to respect localization of larger bridging veins, which have to be spared as well. This is an important issue if these veins overlie and block access to the tumor. Changes within the bony structure (e.g., perforation by tumor invasion or by appositional ossification) can provide initial evidence with respect to tumor localization in convexity meningiomas. In falcine or parasagittal meningiomas, the bone flap must cross the superior sagittal sinus to the contralateral side to provide access to the full area of the sinus and, especially in meningiomas growing through the falx, to the contralateral part of the tumor. By cutting the bone in line with the sinus, the latter is easily opened accidentally, and in this case hemostasis is difficult to achieve. Burr holes are placed circumferentially outside the tumor margins (Fig. 51-7), or, if the tumor is small, a single burr hole is placed. For the average-sized parasagittal tumor, one burr hole on the contralateral side opposite the sinus is sufficient. Bone edges are waxed and a blunt, bent dissector is used to detach dura from bone either in the direction of the next burr hole, or in the case of a single burr hole, in the direction toward the following bone cut. Stripping of the dura in the direction of the tumor may cause bleeding and should be avoided.

The burr holes are now connected by using a craniotome or Gigli's wire saw. Use of a Gigli's saw avoids dural tears and gives the advantage of producing a beveled edge, which protects the bone flap from depression and is especially used in frontal craniotomies. The air-driven osteotome, in contrast, avoids bleeding from the bone edge by occluding diploic

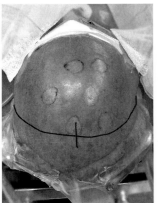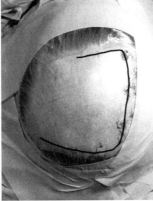

FIGURE 51-6 Skin incision in falcine meningioma. *Left:* Bicoronal flap due to baldness. *Right:* Temporal-based skin flap crossing midline.

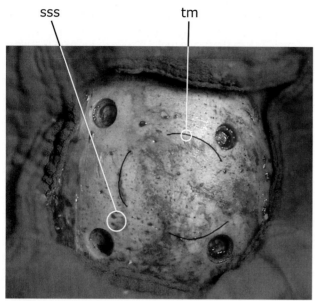

FIGURE 51-7 Bone flap in right frontal falcine meningioma. sss, superior sagittal sinus underneath sagittal suture; tm, tumor margin.

channels with fine bone dust. Care should be taken to use the full extent of the exposure by connecting the outer margins of the burr holes. The final cut should be made at the side closest to the venous sinus, so as to be able to turn out the flap quickly and control possible bleeding rapidly.

Using an elevator, the bone flap is gently elevated, if possible under vision, while the dura overlying the tumor is detached from the bone with a blunt dissector. During this step, care must be taken not to tear the dura, which is sometimes difficult if the tumor is adherent to the inner table. In case this occurs above the sagittal sinus, tumor-invaded bone should be separated from the bone flap by using a rongeur or an air-driven diamond drill, leaving bone adjacent to the sinus. Bleeding diploic channels are packed with wax, whereas hemorrhages from arachnoid granulations or the sagittal sinus are compressed with absorbable gelatin sponge or oxidized cellulose temporarily covered by cotton pads, applying gentle pressure with suction. After obliterating the space between dura and bone at the edges of the flap using oxidized cellulose, the dura is either tacked to the bone, using small burr holes, or to the adjacent subcutaneous tissue. Meticulous hemostasis is performed, the wound is irrigated with saline, and moist skin towels are applied to the margin of the skin wound before the dura is opened.

Handling of the bone flap is of secondary importance and can be performed after removal of the tumor. If invasive tumor or a thickening of the bone is found, hyperostosis is drilled away and, in case there is infiltration of the entire bone flap, it is left out and replaced by cranioplasty. Alternatively, an outer table craniotomy is performed to remove bone in hyperossified meningioma.

For cases in which the tumor has broken through bone, another bone incision is performed circumferentially in the immediate vicinity of the breakthrough and a doughnut-shaped bone flap removed. Residual bone is resected along with adjacent dura and possibly tumor parts.

DURAL OPENING

For cases in which the tumor is highly vascularized and is fed from dural vessels, the first priority is given to rapid suturing and/or coagulation of these feeders. Second, the surgeon must avoid a tense dura or brain swelling; after incision of the dura, the latter will lead to cortex herniation and, if not treated immediately, subsequent brain infarction. Head elevation, hyperventilation, continuous administration of steroids, and mannitol are applied in this case. Only with uncontrolled high intracranial pressure, ventriculostomy and cerebrospinal fluid diversion is an option.

The dura should be opened 0.5 cm away from the tumor margin, which can be defined by ultrasonography or neuronavigation. The dura is elevated a short distance outside the tumor margin with a sharp hook or a dura stitch, and the incision is carried out using a knife. The dural incision is carried on circumferentially to the tumor using blunt-tipped scissors; in parasagittal or falcine meningiomas it is hinged to the sagittal sinus (Fig. 51-8). During opening, one must avoid damage to draining veins that run around the tumor, especially in eloquent areas (Fig. 51-9). After resection of the tumor, the dura should be excised at least 5 to 10 mm away from the tumor margin, because tumor remnants have been shown to be present in normal similarly appearing dura[18] in up to 40% of all tumors. Moreover, a dura tail may be the result of either hypervascularization or tumor invasion. Therefore, dura removal must be performed either in accordance with angiographic and radiographic contrast enhancement, or in that extent, tumorous tissue is found within dura. This might become difficult in individual cases, and if there is any doubt about total resection, several histologic samples should be taken. Furthermore, dura opening must be performed at a size that allows the removal of en plaque tumors or tumor cells spread within the arachnoid.[19,20] It is obvious that cauterization of the dural edges is the second-best choice to avoid recurrences.

After the initial opening, some surgeons also find it helpful to put stitches through the edges of resected dura,

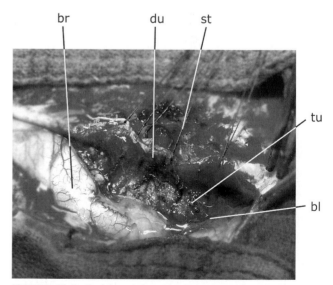

FIGURE 51-8 Incision of dura (du) and mobilization of tumor (tu). br, brain; st, dura stitch; bl, borderline of the tumor.

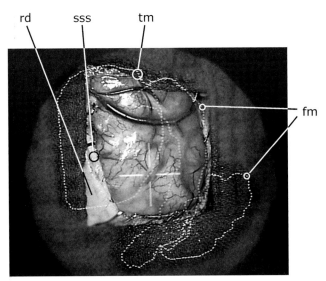

FIGURE 51-9 Intraoperative situs after dura opening. fm, functional markers; rd, reflected dura; sss, superior sagittal sinus; tm, tumor margin.

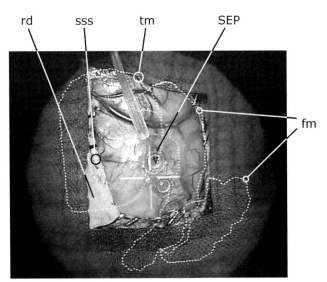

FIGURE 51-10 Insertion of an SEP electrode to localize the central sulcus: fm, functional markers; rd, reflected dura; SEP, electrode for cortical somatosensory evoked potentials mapping; sss, superior sagittal sinus; tm, tumor margin.

so that dura and tumor can be handled by gentle traction and manipulation. This will avoid the need for retraction applied directly to tumor or brain (Fig. 51-8).

TUMOR EXCISION

General considerations are addressed before tumor excision. First of all one must decide whether resection en bloc seems possible or if blood supply has to be diminished and intracapsular debulking has to be performed. This depends on size and localization of the tumor. Both procedures are carried out using microsurgical techniques without the use of brain retractors and cotton pads. With falcine tumors, one first separates the tumor from its origin or reduces the tumor mass. After that, one has to decide where to begin preparation to spare eloquent areas; the usual recommendation is that this preparation starts far beyond the eloquent areas. Localization of these areas is provided by SEPs or by neuronavigation (Figs. 51-10 and 51-11). With precentral meningiomas, resection is started frontal to the tumor. Postcentral tumors are separated from eloquent areas first, while with parasagittal meningiomas resection starts at the convexity and is finished at the falx or superior sagittal sinus. After gentle pulling at the dura, a border between arachnoidea and tumor becomes visible. A cleavable tumor-arachnoid plane is found in one half to two thirds of all patients—more often in those who show no pial vessel parasitization.[11] If a tumor capsule exists, preparation is carried out easily, whereas in case of tumor growth along vessels without a clear capsule present, preparation might become very difficult. Blunt dissection using cautery forceps and microscissors is performed while this cleavable plane is followed extrapially. Furthermore, these instruments are also used to depict, coagulate, and cut fine arachnoidal adhesive bands and small tumor vessels arising from pia mater (Fig. 51-12). In recurrent meningiomas, which frequently show atypical features, more aggressive surgical resection may be required, possibly the same as that used with malignant meningiomas. The latter tumors show frank invasion

of the brain, and the extent of surgery will determine the patient's outcome, not the least with respect to recurrence. Insertion of retractors must be avoided and is only exceptionally and temporarily done.

Magnification provided by microscope is common to the experience of every surgeon and can be used from the very beginning of preparing the tumor borderline or later, when separation of supplying vessels in the deep areas, especially in eloquent areas, is necessary. Overestimation with the microscope can be very time consuming and sometimes confusing, while underestimation can lead to sacrifice of important vessels.

Branches of the middle cerebral artery may be adherent to the tumor capsule overlying the sylvian fissure. These vessels

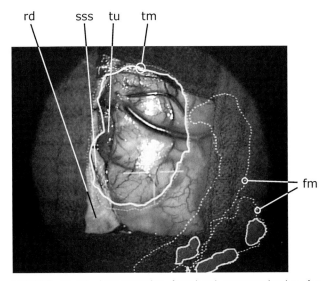

FIGURE 51-11 Intraoperative functional neuronavigation for tumor localization and functional cortex mapping (microscopic view). fm, functional markers; rd, reflected dura; sss, superior sagittal sinus; tm, tumor margin (whole extent of tumor partially covered by brain); tu, tumor.

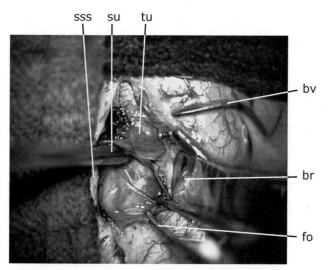

FIGURE 51-12 Preparation of tumor within arachnoidal plane. br, brain retractor; bv, bridging vein; fo, bipolar cautery forceps; sss, superior sagittal sinus; su, suction; tu, tumor.

must be dissected meticulously, and preparation of the capsule should start in uninvolved areas. Large draining veins in eloquent areas such as the rolandic vein must be preserved as well.

Recommendations made in the past to resect brain in the case of larger tumors and overlying brain tissue seems now to be avoidable.

Except for the smallest tumors, after starting to develop the space between the tumor capsule and the arachnoidal plane, it is helpful to exenterate the core of the tumor piecemeal (intracapsular debulking), using diathermy cutting loops (Fig. 51-13) in firmer tumor or an ultrasonic aspirator. Care must be taken not to sacrifice the tumor capsule and adjacent brain. The thinned capsule now can be retracted to this created space. It is wise to alternate between excavating the tumor and developing the border between arachnoidea and tumor capsule to avoid direct damage of the brain or underlying

arteries by debulking or detracting, especially in large tumors. In soft, avascular, and necrotic tissue it might be possible to debulk tumor by suction and curettage.

In highly vascularized and angioblastic tumors, bleeding can cause major difficulties that might be reduced by preoperative embolization. Furthermore, in meningiomas fibrin products are broken down more rapidly because of high fibrinolytic activity.[21] In case of intracapsular bleeding, pressure is applied transitorily by cotton balls; if that measure does not control the bleeding, then thrombin-soaked, absorbable gelatin sponge, oxidized cellulose, or microfibrillar collagen hemostats are applied with gentle pressure. Experienced surgeons will tolerate milder bleeding in favor of a rapid tumor enucleation.

In infiltrating tumors of the falx that are compromising the medial side at both hemispheres, the falx is resected along the anterior and posterior margin of the tumor and the meningioma is resected from the contralateral brain as just described (Figs. 51-14 and 51-15). Nutrient vessels coming off the pericallosal arteries and the inferior sagittal sinus are coagulated and divided, but care is taken not to injure the major vessels.

In some cases, total tumor removal might not be possible. The main reasons are sinus infiltration and the impossibility of extrapial resection of the tumor overlying eloquent areas. One possible strategy is to control any tumor remnant, especially if there is no rapid growth. Figure 51-16 shows an MRI scan of a 73-year-old male who was operated on for a meningioma WHO I° (World Health Organization classification; see section on Histologic Results) 7 years ago. Because of invasive tumor growth into the right central region, a small tumor remnant was left in situ to avoid paresis. During follow-up, there is no neurologic deficit and no tumor progression. This case demonstrates that it is not always necessary to achieve complete tumor removal in all circumstances by running the risk of evoking neurologic deficits. In older patients, observation of tumor growth and in younger patients, adjuvant treatment such as radiotherapy, radiosurgery, or medical treatment are the treatments of choice.

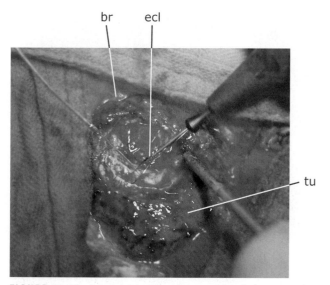

FIGURE 51-13 Internal debulking of tumor using diathermy cutting loop. br, brain; ecl, electrocautery loop; tu, tumor.

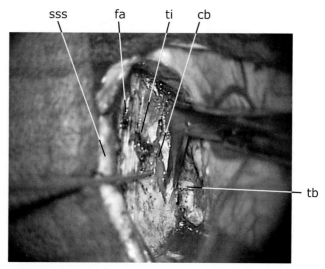

FIGURE 51-14 Resection of tumor insertion at falx. fa, falx; cb, contralateral brain; sss, superior sagittal sinus; tb, tumor bed after resection of tumor; ti, tumor insertion.

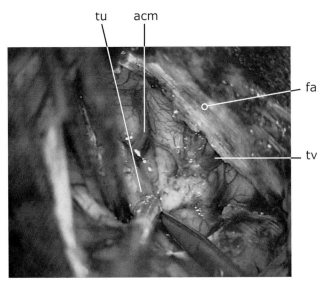

FIGURE 51-15 Microscopic view after resecting the tumor from its falcine origin. acm, callosomarginal artery; fa, falx; tu, retracted tumor; tv, tumor supplying vein.

The extent of tumor removal is graded according to Simpson[22] and is characteristic for regrowth and recurrence rates:

Grade 1. Complete removal with excision of the dural attachment.

Grade 2. Complete removal with endothermic coagulation of the dural attachment.

Grade 3. Complete resection without resection or coagulation of dural attachments or extradural extensions.

Grade 4. Partial removal, leaving tumor in situ.

Grade 5. Simple decompression or biopsy.

After tumor resection, care is taken to achieve hemostasis. Some authors tend to cover tumor bed with oxidized cellulose.

CLOSURE

For cases in which no infiltration exists, the dura is closed either directly or by using the harvested pericranial flap or temporal fascia to avoid cerebrospinal fluid leakage, brain herniation, cortical scarring, or wound infection. In our opinion, an artificial or heterologous dura graft is the second-best choice (Fig. 51-17). Before final closure, the subdural space is filled with saline. The bone flap is reinserted, using nonreabsorbable sutures (Vicryl) rather than stainless-steel miniplates. If the bone flap has to be removed

FIGURE 51-16 Residual tumor within central region, showing no progression during observation. (*upper row*) MRI 3 years after operation. (*lower row*) MRI 7 years after operation.

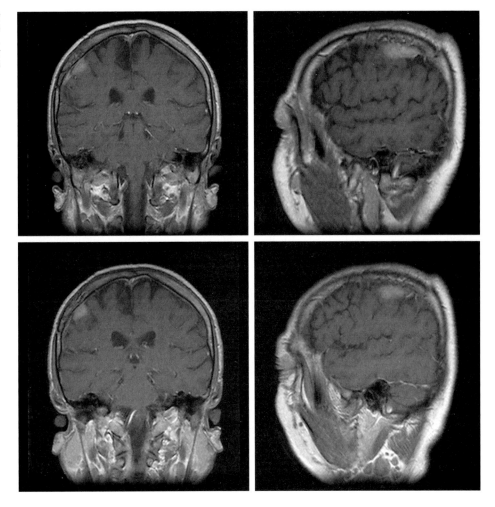

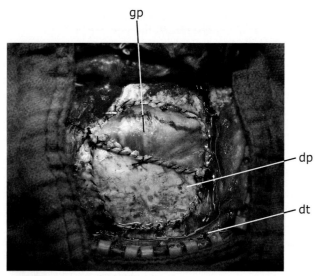

FIGURE 51-17 Dural closure. dp, dural patch; dt, dural tacks; gp, galea patch.

because of invasiveness, methacrylic cranioplasty is performed in small openings, taking care of correct placement. One or more central dura tacks are carried out, and the subcutaneous and cutaneous layers are closed after insertion of a subgaleal drain, which will remain for 1 or 3 days, depending on the size and materials of the cranioplasty. With large resections, a delayed osteoplasty is performed after 8 to 10 days; in case of large defects of the dura it is carried out after 6 to 8 weeks. This leads to better healing.

INTERVENTIONS AT THE SUPERIOR SAGITTAL SINUS

Surgery at the superior sagittal sinus presents a challenge because of the dire consequences of an acute closure within the middle and posterior third, becoming necessary during an acute bleeding episode. Spastic diplegia or death may result if this happens.

The anterior third of the sinus, ranging from the crista galli to the coronar suture, can be ligated and divided. There is little controversy about whether an occluded sinus should be excised or should be left in situ after removal of the tumor. In case of the latter, important collateral venous channels passing through the falx to the inferior sinus would have been spared.

This is in contrast to tumors involving the middle and posterior part of the sinus. It is easy to solve the problem if the meningioma is attached to one wall of the sinus without significant infiltration to dura; the tumor is peeled off the wall and the dura is coagulated at the point of attachment.

According to Hakuba,[23] parasagittal meningiomas are divided into eight subgroups. Types I and II can be resected and the patency of the sinus remains, whereas in types III to VIII multiple walls are involved and resection is only possible by grafting the walls. Otherwise, bits of tumor must be left in situ. Operative technique is described by this author as follows. In case the tumor is only attached to the wall of the sinus (type I), the tumor is peeled off and the site of the attachment is simply coagulated. If the tumor involves one corner of the sinus (type II), the sinus is opened and the tumor removed while an incision is made 2 mm away from each edge of the meningioma. Thereafter, compression of the wall of the sinus by a forceps or a clamp is performed and the sinus closed by continuous nylon sutures. If tumor involves one or two walls widely (types III and IV), after debulking of the tumor mass the sinus is opened and tumor within the sinus is removed. Leaving a rim of 2 mm, the involved wall is removed and replaced by a vein graft. In case of excessive bleeding, the sinus is compressed manually or, in cases where the posterior third of the sinus is involved, a temporary silicone tube shunting is performed. A semisitting position to decrease pressure within the sinus seems to be helpful. If the sinus is stenotic because of tumor (types V and VI), Hakuba suggests resecting the intrasinus portion and the involved wall of the sinus and then performing reconstruction, using an external jugular vein graft. Large draining veins and their connection to the sinus are reconstructed as well.[24,25] Brain protection using barbiturates is essential in this case, but it remains an open question whether these reconstructions can work very well, at least in the long run. If the sinus is completely obliterated by tumor mass (types VII and VIII) and collateralization is sufficient, the tumor and the infiltrated wall are resected without any problems. The stump of the sinus is occluded beyond the tumor margin by using temporary clamps; then double ligature using nonabsorbable stitches or a reconstruction using an external jugular vein graft is performed. In performing vein bypass grafts, there is a rate of late thrombosis reaching almost 50%.[23,26] Some authors[27] use a laser to remove meningioma remnants from the wall of the sinus until it is bleeding and repair the wall.

According to newer literature, Sindou[28] operated on 80 patients suffering from tumors invading the superior sagittal sinus; the recurrence rate was 2.5%, having an overview of 1 to 17 years (mean, 8 years). His surgical treatment followed the guidelines already described. Among the 80 patients, 70 (87.5%) had good outcome, while 3 (3.6%) who exhibited infiltrating types V to VI died from venous infarction and brain edema but did not undergo sinus reconstruction. Seven patients showed aggravated neurologic deficit following closure of the rolandic vein. Patients were operated on in a semisitting position, and a large opening was made to allow a good overview; the sinus was opened, even in cases where there was no hint of tumor invasion, just to be certain that there was no intrinsic growth. Postoperative heparin was administered to allow endothelialization of the sinus for at least 21 days; blood pressure, blood volume, and blood viscosity were monitored. In case of brain swelling, the operation was stopped and continued only after the edema had resolved. Notably, all Goretex and one third of autologous bypasses thrombosed, but this was, except for one case, slowly so collateral pathways developed and no severe neurologic deficit resulted.

More conservative treatment is suggested by other authors.[29] A patent but tumor-infiltrated sinus is enclosed in a sleeve fashioned from convexity and falcine dura. Further tumor growth cannot spread beyond and cause obliteration of the sinus. If case collateralization takes place, the sinus can be removed during subsequent surgery.

From the authors' point of view, if multiple sinus walls are involved by tumor but the sinus is patent, and resection and repair are precluded, residual tumor is left behind. This permits retarded occlusion of the sinus and the development of collaterals. The patient is followed up within short intervals, and if reoperation becomes necessary, then the sinus is resected while care is taken to prevent damage to collateral vessels. With the advent of new techniques in radiosurgery, it is possible to leave residual tumor within the infiltrated sinus. Depending on the localization of tumor and the age of the patient, first tumor growth is observed and in case of tumor progression or younger aged patient, radiosurgery using gamma knife or linear accelerator (LINAC) is performed. These treatments lead to an adequate tumor control as well.[30–33]

POSTOPERATIVE CARE AND COMPLICATIONS

Except with larger meningiomas, the anesthesiologist strives for a smooth extubation by avoiding increases in blood and intracranial pressures. With larger tumors, especially when brain swelling has occurred, ventilation might become necessary for several days. In these cases, postoperative CT scan should be performed. In our opinion, CT scans are not necessary in uneventful cases. During the patient's stay in the intensive care unit, neurologic status (level of consciousness, focal neurologic deficits, and seizure activity), vital signs, pulmonary function, electrolytes, and fluid intake are monitored. The patient's head is elevated 20 to 30 degrees, and corticosteroid therapy at full dose (supported by H_2-receptor antagonists) is continued for up to 2 weeks to cover the period of maximal brain swelling and then tapered. Facultative mannitol or furosemide might be necessary as well. To avoid thromboembolism, coagulation is inhibited by administering heparin from day 4 after surgery. If epilepsy is preexisting, anticonvulsant drugs are continued. The main concern is to avoid and rule out elevated intracranial pressure caused by thrombosis, hematoma, or brain edema. Any new or deteriorated hemiplegia, seizure, or any change in consciousness lead to an immediate CT evaluation and adequate treatment of mass effect (e.g., caused by rebleeding) consisting of reoperation or treatment of brain swelling consisting of medical therapy.

Complications involving hemorrhage and blood loss constitute the most important single cause of death following meningioma surgery. Attention must be directed toward bleeding from the scalp, from highly vascularized bone, from tumor, from dura mater, and, finally, from the superior sagittal sinus and its bridging veins. Meticulous coagulation and in some cases embolization of tumor feeders can diminish the risk. In case of hyperostosis, the bone flap should be elevated carefully to avoid dural tear and sacrificing of bridging veins consecutively. Removal of the tumor from the sinus can also lead to severe bleeding and cause difficulties in closure. As mentioned before, resection or closing of the medial and posterior third of the sinus sagittalis (if it is patent) or of bridging veins can lead to severe neurologic deficits such as hemiplegia or death following hemorrhagic infarction. In large falcine meningiomas there is a relationship to greater inner veins and the corpus callosum; sacrificing these can also lead to major complications such as death or disturbances in the connection between right and left

hemispheres. Compromising the arachnoidea can lead to seizures; of course, any direct injury of the brain that can lead to contralateral deficits (i.e., hemiparesis, changes in sensibility, motor or sensory aphasia, visual disturbances, deterioration of memory function) should be avoided, such as accidental closure of a major bridging vein.

If the bone flap becomes infected, it must be removed and antibiotics given for at least 14 days. A cranioplasty must subsequently be performed, but this should not be done before 3 months after extraction.

Operative mortality for parasagittal meningiomas ranges from 3.7% to 12.6% and for falcine meningiomas from 2.3% to 13.4% in various studies. Giombini and co-workers[34] observed in his study a mortality rate of 3.7% in patients with parasagittal and of 13.4% in patients with falcine meningiomas. The main causes were brain swelling and pulmonary complications, followed by hematoma, cardiac failure, and infection. Nonlethal complications such as flap infection, cerebrospinal fluid leakage, thrombophlebitis of the inferior limbs, bronchopneumonia, cerebral swelling, intracranial hematoma, hydrocephalus, and renal failure were observed less frequently. In 29% to 43% of all cases, deep vein thrombosis was reported to develop.[35] An overview of complication rates is given in Table 51-1. In elderly patients, mortality and morbidity is somewhat higher (30-day mortality 16%; complication rate 39%), but no detailed information about falcine, parasagittal, or convexity meningiomas is provided.[36] In these patients postoperative confusion is common, but any severe adverse event must be ruled out. Fatal pulmonary embolism occurs in about 1.2% of all cases following meningioma surgery.[37] One case of postoperative mutism following resection of a parasagittal meningioma caused by injury of the supplementary motor cortex is reported in the literature.[38]

HISTOLOGIC RESULTS

Meningiomas can be divided into three types: benign (WHO I°), constituting about 91% of cases; atypical (WHO II°) 7%; and malignant (WHO III°) 2%.

Generally speaking, meningiomas are marked by characteristic whorl formations around a central hyaline material. This eventually calcifies and forms psammoma bodies. Bundles of elongated fibroblasts with narrow nuclei that interlace the whorls and psammoma bodies are found.

TABLE 51-1 ▪ Overview of Postoperative Complications

Complication	Parasagittal Meningioma	Falcine Meningioma
Postoperative bleeding	0.9% (severe)	0.3% (minor)
Brain swelling	2.6% (lethal)	1.3% (nonlethal)
Pulmonary complications	2.0% (lethal)	1.6% (nonlethal)
Cardiac failure	0.9% (lethal)	0.0% (nonlethal)
Infection	0.3% (lethal)	2.2% (nonlethal)
CSF leakage	0.0% (lethal)	0.0% (nonlethal)
Thrombophlebitis	0.0% (lethal)	1.9% (nonlethal)
Hydrocephalus	0.3% (lethal)	0.3% (nonlethal)
Renal failure	0.0% (lethal)	0.3% (nonlethal)
Mortality	3.7%	13.4%

CSF, cerebrospinal fluid.
Data from reference 34.

Among benign meningiomas, there is a wide range of appearances. Most common are meningothelial, fibrous, and transitional meningiomas. Furthermore, there are psammomatous, angiomatous, microcystic, secretory, clear cell, chordoid, lymphoplasmacyte-rich, and metaplastic types known. Meningothelial types show cell lobules surrounded by thin collagenous septa. Furthermore, they show generally oval nuclei, some of which show central clearing, and thin chromatin is found in nuclei. In fibrous meningiomas, tumor cells form wide fascicles and are predominantly spindle-shaped. Whorls and psammoma bodies are uncommon in either type. Transitional types express mixed features of meningothelial and fibrous meningiomas.

Atypical meningiomas show several of the following features, according to the WHO classification: frequent mitoses, increased cellularity, small cells with high nucleus-to-cytoplasm ratios and/or prominent nucleoli, uninterrupted patternless or sheetlike growth, and foci of necrosis. Malignant meningiomas, moreover, show a high mitotic index and conspicuous necrosis.[40]

With respect to the molecular biology of meningiomas, convexity meningiomas seem to be associated with abnormalities in chromosome 22q. Furthermore, this is a typical finding especially in the transitional and fibrous subtypes, which are consequently more often found in convexity than meningothelial subtypes; the latter are more often located at the skull base and show no changes in chromosome 22.[41] Deletion of the short arm of chromosome 1 and therefore loss of expression of alkaline phosphatase is an important prognostic factor in tumor recurrence.[42,43] Tumors showing this deletion tend to recur in 60% of the cases.[44] Ki-67 labeling can be used to determine malignancy. In grade I meningiomas the mean Ki-67 index is 0.7%, in grade II it is 2.1%, and in grade III it is 11%. According to the literature, the higher the tumor grade is, the higher the recurrence rate as well.[45]

PROGNOSIS AND FURTHER TREATMENT

Prognosis depends on the extent of resection as well as histologic and cytogenetic characteristics of the tumor.

In convexity meningiomas, the prognosis is very good. Easy access to the tumor provides a good opportunity for total resection. It seems clear that the risk of recurrence is related directly to the extent of resection. Complete resection, even if there is en plaque growth, excludes recurrences in almost all cases.

With respect to parasagittal and falx meningiomas, there are a few series that provide evidence about prognosis. The 5-year survival rate in one study was 82.5%, although survival during the first year depends on the postoperative course and complications. The survival rate depends also on the preoperative clinical condition. The better this is, the better the survival rate will be. After the first year, the prognosis is related to the extent of tumor removal, clinical condition, hyperostosis, and histologic type. In the same study the 15-year survival rate was 62.6%. The recurrence rate for parasagittal meningiomas is twice as high as that for convexity tumors. This may depend on the potential for parasagittal tumors to invade the superior sagittal sinus. As expected, subtotal tumor removal or coagulation instead

of excision of dural insertion leads to a higher recurrence rate.[37] Tumor remnants (e.g., left within the wall of the sinus) tend to regrow. Regrowth is also possible if microscopic residuals remain in situ or, as described in one study, within the arachnoid membrane.[46] These remnants seem to secrete vascular endothelial growth factor, which induces neovascularization and tumor regrowth.[47] In this case, a higher grade of tumor is not as closely associated with incidence of recurrence as is tumor remnant. For that reason, reoperation in recurrent cases should be performed whenever possible, especially if the sinus becomes totally occluded and can be resected or if total resection can be achieved. It is self-evident that in reoperation the morbidity rate is higher. Unfortunately, there are no actual figures available about recurrence rate; the latest ones date from the 1980s. For example, Mirimanoff and co-workers[48] found a recurrence rate in parasagittal and falx meningioma of 18% at 5 years and 24% at 10 years; Jaaskelainen[49] described a recurrence rate in parasagittal meningiomas of 21% after 20 years; and Melamed and co-workers[50] found recurrences in 20.5% of parasagittal and 5.9% in falx meningiomas.

Because the recurrence rate is invariably higher with atypical or malignant meningiomas, thorough follow-up is essential. The earlier a recurrence is detected, the smaller is the tumor size and the better the chance that subsequent treatment will succeed. This is the case even with benign tumors when reoperation is the treatment of choice. In case of recurrence, higher grade meningiomas show increased glucose utilization and are noted on positron emission tomography scans. In this case, reoperation followed by radiotherapy is performed. When tumor diameter is less than 2.5 cm, stereotactic radiosurgery can be performed, using gamma knife (^{60}Co γ-ray source) or LINAC systems; among the latter, software and planning systems such as Novalis' shaped beam radiosurgery appear also in our hands to be very modern and precise. Single-dose irradiation concepts are under investigation. A review of early results up to 1 year after gamma knife radiosurgery showed tumor growth in 1, control of tumor size in 32, and decrease of size in 7 patients. In parasagittal meningiomas the complication rate was 8.7% in seizures, paresis, and headache, respectively.[51] According to another author, the complication rate was 25.0%.[52] Permanent brachytherapy following surgery in recurrent grade II or III meningiomas is considered as ultima ratio and shows no significant benefit compared to other treatment.[53]

In slow-growing or recurrent tumors that are not accessible to surgery either because of the age and general condition of the patient or because of localization, chemotherapy using hydroxyurea (Litalir) produces promising results in control of tumor growth in a selected subgroup of patients (20% to 30%).[54]

To give a prediction on epilepsy is more difficult. Patients suffering from convexity or parasagittal meningiomas are affected more often than patients suffering from tumors at other localizations within the cranium. Whether seizure disorders were preexisting or only subsequent to surgery, they are difficult to treat because of their involvement with highly functional areas and their relationship to major draining veins. In preexisting seizures, time since onset and frequency of seizures may predict outcome. The etiology of new seizures may be recurrence or intraoperative complications such as excessive retraction of brain tissue,

FIGURE 51-18 MRI in left convexity meningioma. Views shown are (A) coronal, (B) sagittal, and (C) axial.

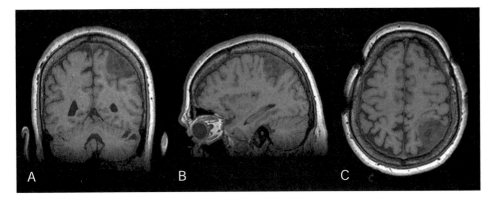

sacrificing of larger draining bridging veins, or subpial dissection. In these cases, anticonvulsive treatment must be continued and its discontinuation should not be attempted before 1 year following surgery.

According to the latest series[34] examining patients operated on for parasagittal and falx meningiomas, 47% of the patients were fit for work and 6% were completely disabled. According to a series[55] from 2001 examining patients who underwent meningioma surgery of unspecified localization, about 60% suffered from mild to moderate impairment of quality of life and about 20% showed moderate to severe impairment. It can be argued that currently better surgical technique may lead to better prognosis, but this has not yet been proven.

Gamma knife radiosurgery is supported as optional therapy for meningioma surgery. Because of the higher risk of peritumorous changes and the risk of malignant transformation, only older patients for whom anesthesia presents a high risk should be treated in this way,[52] especially because convexity or even parasagittal and falcine meningiomas can be treated surgically with a low risk of mortality or morbidity.

Illustrative Cases

CONVEXITY MENINGIOMA

A 58-year-old female was suffering from paresthesia within the left hand. An evaluation of the cervical spine detected no pathology, so an MRI scan of the brain was performed. A left parieto-occipital, partly cystic meningioma was found. Episodes of focal seizures remained unclear. Neurologic examination revealed no further deficit.

An MRI study detected a left parieto-occipital, partly cystic meningioma measuring 3.3 × 3.1 × 2.5 cm and surrounded by perifocal edema (Fig. 51-18). Tumor vascularization was found from the medial meningeal artery (Fig. 51-19). fMRI revealed a distance to the central sulcus of 2.5 cm and to the postcentral gyrus of 1.5 cm. The speech area was farther away. With DSA, vascularization was found to originate not only from the medial meningeal artery but also from a few small cerebral arteries.

Functional neuronavigation (Fig. 51-20) was used for surgical planning and performing a small parietal bone flap. After opening of the dura, a thickened arachnoid layer was found and dissected. Small tumor feeders arising from the cortex were coagulated, but no clear capsule was found in later stages of the operation. A bridging vein at the occipital tumor pole and a large parietal draining vein were preserved. Finally, after the meningioma could be removed totally (Fig. 51-21), the dura was excised at 1.5 cm distance from the tumor and the margins were coagulated. Intraoperative MRI confirmed total removal of the tumor. A patch consisting of galea and periost was used for dural closure. The postoperative course was uneventful, and a histologic workup showed an angiomatous meningioma classified as WHO I°.

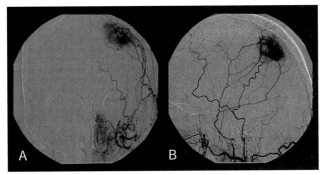

FIGURE 51-19 DSA in left convexity meningioma. Views shown are (A) coronal and (B) sagittal. Tumor vascularization arises from medial meningeal artery.

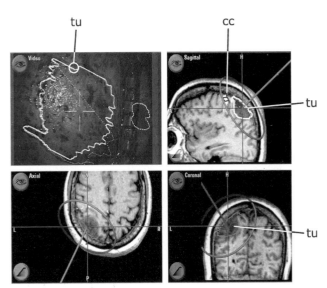

FIGURE 51-20 Microscopic view using functional neuronavigation in surgical planning and performing trephination. cc, central cortex; tu, tumor.

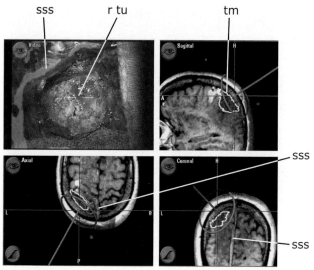

FIGURE 51-21 Operative result. Resected tumor has been placed back into the tumor bed. r tu, resected tumor; sss, superior sagittal sinus (displayed by neuronavigation); tm, tumor margin.

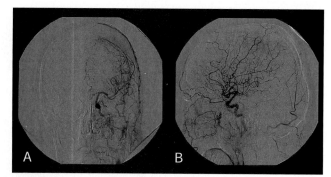

FIGURE 51-23 DSA in left parasagittal meningioma. Views shown are (A) coronar and (B) sagittal. Note: vascularization from branches of internal and external carotid artery and tumor-infiltrated scalp.

PARASAGITTAL MENINGIOMA

A 76-year-old male in good general condition was complaining of a weakness of the right leg lasting for 8 months. MRI revealed a parasagittal meningioma. On the day of admission, a paresis of the right leg was found and a local elevation of the skull above the tuber parietale was observed. There was no loss of consciousness and no further neurologic deficit (in particular, no sensible deficit or seizures). MRI detected a 5 × 4 × 4 cm left parasagittal meningioma compressing central gyri. Both dura and bone were infiltrated (Fig. 51-22). Vascularization was from the internal and external carotid arteries. The superior sagittal sinus was patent (Fig. 51-23).

After performing an osteoclastic flap, the infiltrated dura was pediculated to the superior sagittal sinus. Cortical veins in front and behind the tumor were preserved and an internal debulking was performed using electrocautery loops. Arachnoid membranes were found in the frontal and parietal parts of the tumor; there was no distinct border to the depressed central gyri visible. The brain was edematous at this side. Adhesions to the

superior sagittal sinus were scraped off by using a sharp dissector and coagulated, but the sinus itself was not invaded. Pathologic vascularization relating to the falx was coagulated as well. The dura was resected and a fascia lata patch from the right leg was used for dural closure. Total Simpson Grade II° resection was achieved. Histologic examination revealed a transitional meningioma of WHO I° classification. The postoperative course remained uneventful; the patient recovered quickly and a slight but much improved paresis was found on the day of discharge. A methacrylate flap was performed 6 months later.

FALCINE MENINGIOMA

Sudden loss of consciousness led to the diagnosis of a falcine meningioma in a 62-year-old man. One week before admission to hospital, his condition deteriorated. The patient was complaining of headache, dizziness, and loss of coordination, especially within the left hand. There was a weakness in the left arm and a tendency to fall to the left side. Neurologic examination revealed a slight paresis of the left leg, a dysmetria and a dysdiadochokinesia at the left hand, and a moderate psychosyndrome. With an MRI scan a right falcine meningioma was found at the precentral area (Fig. 51-24). The size of the tumor was 4 × 2.5 × 2.5 cm, and it was located 1.5 cm in front of the precentral gyrus, as was

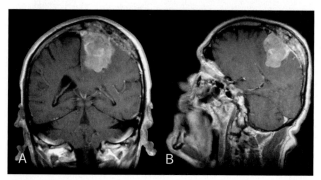

FIGURE 51-22 MRI in left parasagittal meningioma. Views shown are (A) coronar and (B) sagittal.

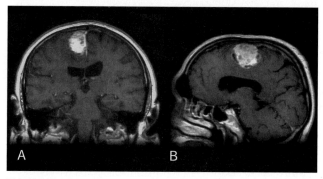

FIGURE 51-24 MRI in right falcine meningioma. Views shown are (A) coronar and (B) sagittal.

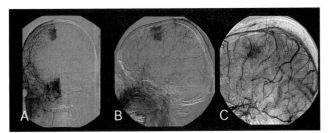

FIGURE 51-25 DSA in right falcine meningioma. Views shown are (*A*) coronar and (*B*) sagittal, arterial phase; (*C*) sagittal, venous phase. Note that superior sagittal sinus is patent.

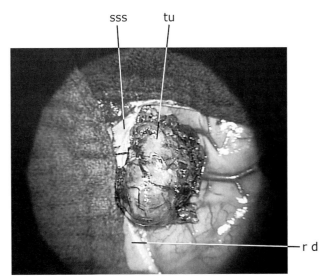

FIGURE 51-27 Resected tumor placed back into tumor bed. r d, retracted dura; sss, superior sagittal sinus; tu, tumor.

shown by functional neuronavigation. Diffusion weighted imaging showed a distance to the pyramidal tract of about 1.5 cm as well. Perifocal edema was found to involve the precentral cortex. There was no contact between the tumor and the pericallosal artery, but the corpus callosum was slightly shifted by perifocal edema. Angiography revealed little vascularization arising from the medial meningeal artery; the tumor was draining to the superior sagittal sinus, which was patent (Fig. 51-25).

A small craniotomy was performed using a bifrontal incision because of baldness (see Fig. 51-6, *left*). The tumor was discovered after a small rim of cortex was retracted and a bridging vein in front of the tumor was sacrificed (Fig. 51-26). Brain had to be retracted slightly to develop tumor margins (see Fig. 51-12). An arachnoid layer was followed for tumor resection; during this procedure small feeding vessels were coagulated and dissected. The corpus callosum was almost reached by tumor mass. The pericallosal artery was covered by an arachnoid membrane as well and could be preserved easily.

After resecting the tumor from its origin at the falx cerebri, it was removed in total (Fig. 51-27). The tumor origin at the falx was resected as well (see Fig. 51-14), so total tumor removal (Simpson Grade I) was achieved (Fig. 51-28). The postoperative course was uneventful, and histologic evaluation revealed an atypical meningioma (WHO II°).

Acknowledgments

We are indebted to PD Dr. C. Nimsky and PD Dr. O Ganslandt for providing screenshots taken during neuronavigational operations and Mr. F. Bittner for editing of pictorial material. Neuronavigation was performed by using VectorVision.

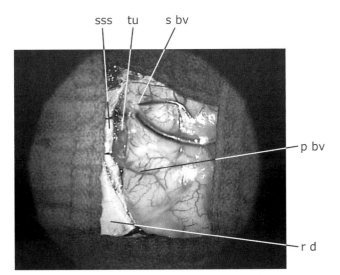

FIGURE 51-26 Anterior bridging vein has to be sacrificed to achieve complete tumor removal. p bv, posterior bridging vein, r d, retracted dura; s bv, sacrificed bridging vein; sss, superior sagittal sinus; tu, tumor.

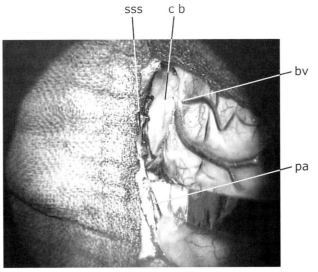

FIGURE 51-28 Microscopic view after tumor removal and resection of its falcine origin. bv, bridging vein; cb, contralateral brain; pa, pericallosal artery; sss, superior sagittal sinus.

REFERENCES

1. Cushing H, Eisenhardt L: Meningiomas: Their Classification, Regional Behavior, Life History and Surgical End Results. Springfield, IL: Charles C Thomas, 1938.
2. Cushing H: Meningiomas: Macewen memorial lecture, 1927. Glasgow: Jackson Wylie & Company, 1927.
3. Lantos PL, VandenBerg SR: Tumours of the nervous system. In Graham DI, Lantos PL (eds): Greenfield's Neuropathology 9, 6th ed. London: Arnold, 1996, pp 583–879.
4. Al-Mefty O: Meningiomas. New York: Raven Press, 1991.
5. Wilkins R: Parasagittal meningiomas. In Al-Mefty O (ed): Meningiomas. New York: Raven Press, 1991, pp 329–344.
6. Lieu AS, Howng SL: Intracranial meningiomas and epilepsy: Incidence, prognosis and influencing factors. Epilepsy Res 38:45–52, 2000.
7. Osborne A: Meningiomas and Other Nonglial Neoplasms: Diagnostic Neuroradiology. St. Louis: CV Mosby, 1996, pp 579–625.
8. Weber J, Gassel AM, Hoch A, et al: Intraoperative management of cystic meningiomas. Neurosurg Rev 26:62–66, 2003.
9. Marc JA, Schlechter MM: Cortical venous rerouting in parasagittal meningiomas. Radiology 112:85–92, 1974.
10. Bendszus M, Rao G, Burger R, et al: Is there a benefit of preoperative meningioma embolisation? Neurosurgery 47:1306–1312, 2000.
11. Sindou M, Alaywan M: Most intracranial meningiomas are not cleavable tumors: Anatomic-surgical evidence and angiographic predictability. Neurosurgery 42:476–480, 1998.
12. Alvernia J, Sindou M: Preoperative neuroimaging findings as a predictor of the surgical plane of cleavage: Prospective study of 100 consecutive cases of intracranial meningioma. J Neurosurg 100:422–430, 2004.
13. Romstock J, Fahlbusch R, Ganslandt O, et al: Localisation of the sensimotor cortex during surgery for brain tumors: Feasibility and waveform patterns of somatosensory evoked potentials. J Neurol Neurosurg Psychiatry 72:221–229, 2002.
14. Nakamura M, Roser F, Michel J, et al: The natural history of incidental meningiomas. Neurosurgery 53:62–71, 2003.
15. Yoneoka Y, Fujii Y, Tanaka R: Growth of incidental meningiomas. Acta Neurochir (Wien) 142:507–511, 2000.
16. Lieu AS, Howng SL: Surgical treatment of intracranial meningiomas in geriatric patients. Kaohsiung J Med Sci 14:498–503, 1998.
17. Buhl R, Ahmad H, Behnke A, et al: Results in the operative treatment of elderly patients with intracranial meningioma. Neurosurg Rev 23:25–29, 2000.
18. Nakau H, Miyazawa T, Tamai S, et al: Pathological significance of meningeal enhancement (flare sign) on meningiomas in MRI. Surg Neurol 48:584–591, 1997.
19. vonDeimling A, Kraus J, Stangl A, et al: Evidence for subarachnoid spread in the development of multiple meningiomas. Brain Pathol 5:11–14, 1995.
20. Stangl A, Wellenreuther R, Lenartz D, et al: Clonality of multiple meningiomas. J Neurosurg 86:853–858, 1997.
21. Tovi D, Pandolfi M, Astedt B: Local hemostasis in brain tumours. Experientia 31:977–978, 1975.
22. Simpson D: The recurrence of intracranial meningiomas after surgical treatment. J Neurol Neurosurg Psychiatry 20:22–39, 1957.
23. Hakuba A: Reconstruction of dural sinus involved in meningiomas. In Al-Mefty O (ed): Meningiomas. New York: Raven Press, 1991, pp 371–382.
24. Menovsky T, DeVries J: Cortical vein end-to-end anastomosis after removal of a parasagittal meningioma. Microsurgery 22:27–29, 2002.
25. Murata J, Sawamura Y, Saito H, et al: Resection of a recurrent parasagittal meningioma with cortical vein anastomosis: A technical note. Surg Neurol 48:592–597, 1997.
26. Al-Mefty O, Yamamoto Y: Neurovascular reconstruction during and after skull base surgery. Contemp Neurosurg 15:1–9, 1993.
27. Ransohoff J: Removal of convexity, parasagittal and falcine meningiomas. Neurosurg Clin N Am 5:293–297, 1994.
28. Sindou M: Meningiomas invading the sagittal or transverse sinuses, resection with venous reconstruction. J Clin Neurosci 8(Suppl 1): 8–11, 2001.
29. Hartmann K, Klug W: Recurrence and possible surgical procedures in meningiomas of the middle and posterior parts of the superior sagittal sinus. Acta Neurochir (Wien) 31:283, 1975.
30. Harris A, Lee J, Omalu B, et al: The effect of radiosurgery during management of aggressive meningiomas. Surg Neurol 60:298–305, 2003.
31. Pollock B, Stafford S, Utter A, et al: Stereotactic radiosurgery provides equivalent tumor control to Simpson grade 1 resection for patients with small- to medium-size meningiomas. Int J Radiat Oncol Biol Phys 55:1000–1005, 2003.
32. Stafford S, Pollock B, Foote RL, et al: Meningioma radiosurgery: Tumor control, outcomes and complications among 190 consecutive patients. Neurosurgery 49:1029–1037, 2001.
33. Ojeman S, Sneed P, Larson D, et al: Radiosurgery for malignant meningioma: Results in 22 patients. J Neurosurg 93(Suppl 3):62–67, 2000.
34. Giombini S, Solero CL, Lasio G, et al: Immediate and late outcome of operations for parasagittal and falx meningiomas. Surg Neurol 21:427–435, 1984.
35. Powers SK, Edwards MSB: Prevention and treatment of thromboembolic complications in a neurosurgical patient. In Wilkins RH, Rengachary SS (eds): Neurosurgery. New York: McGraw-Hill, 1985, pp 406–410.
36. Black P, Kathiresan S, Chung W: Meningioma surgery in the elderly: A case-control study assessing morbidity and mortality. Acta Neurochir (Wien) 140:1013–1017, 1998.
37. Kallio M, Sankila R, Hakulinen T, et al: Factors affecting operative and excess long-term mortality in 935 patients with intracranial meningioma. Neurosurgery 31:427–435, 1992.
38. Crutchfield JS, Sawayaa R, Meyers CA, et al: Postoperative mutism in neurosurgery. Report of two cases. J Neurosurg 81:115–121, 1994.
39. Louis DN, Budka H, von Deimling A: Meningiomas. In Kleihues P, Cavenee WK (eds): Pathology and genetics: Tumours of the nervous system. Lyons: International Agency for Research on Cancer, 1997, pp 134–141.
40. Kleihues P, Cavenee WK: Pathology and genetics of tumours of the nervous system. Oxford: Oxford University Press, 2000.
41. Kros J, de Greve K, van Tilborg A, et al: NF2 status of meningiomas is associated with tumour localization and histology. J Pathol 194:367–372, 2001.
42. Ketter R, Henn W, Niedermayer I, et al: Predictive value of progression-associated chromosomal aberrations for the prognosis of meningiomas: A retrospective study of 198 cases. J Neurosurg 95:601–607, 2001.
43. Muller P, Henn W, Niedermayer I, et al: Deletion of chromosome 1p and loss of expression of alkaline phosphatase indicate progression of meningiomas. Clin Cancer Res 5:3569–3577, 1999.
44. Steudel W, Feld R, Henn W, et al: Correlation between cytogenetic and clinical findings in 215 human meningiomas. Acta Neurochir Suppl (Wien) 65:73–76, 1996.
45. Kolles H, Niedermayer I, Schmitt C, et al: Triple approach for diagnosis and grading of meningiomas: Histology, morphometry of Ki-67/Feulge stainings, and cytogenetics. Acta Neurochir (Wien) 137:174–181, 1995.
46. Kamitani H, Mauzawa H, Kanazawa I, et al: Recurrence of convexity meningiomas: Tumor cells in the arachnoid membrane. Surg Neurol 56:228–235, 2001.
47. Yamasaki F, Yoshioka H, Hama S, et al: Recurrence of meningiomas. Cancer 89:1102–1110, 2000.
48. Mirimanoff RO, Dosretz DE, Linggood RM, et al: Meningioma: Analysis of recurrence and progression following neurosurgical resection. J Neurosurg 62:18–24, 1985.
49. Jaaskelainen J: Seemingly complete removal of histologically benign intracranial meningioma: Late recurrence rate and factors predicting recurrence in 657 patients: A multivariate analysis. Surg Neurol 26:461–469, 1986.
50. Melamed S, Sahar A, Beller AJ: The recurrence of intracranial meningiomas. Neurochirurgie 22:47–51, 1979.
51. Singh V, Kansal S, Vaishya S, et al: Early complications following gamma knife radiosurgery for intracranial meningiomas. J Neurosurg 93(Suppl 3):57–61, 2000.
52. Chang JH, Chang JW, Choi JY, et al: Complications after gamma knife radiosurgery for benign meningiomas. J Neurol Neurosurg Psychiatry 74:226–230, 2003.
53. Ware M, Larson D, Sneed P, et al: Surgical resection and permanent brachytherapy for recurrent atypical and malignant meningioma. Neurosurgery 54:55–64, 2004.
54. Schrell UM, Rittig MG, Anders M, et al: Hydroxyurea for treatment of unresectable and recurrent meningiomas. II: Decrease in the size of meningiomas in patients treated with hydroxyurea. J Neurosurg 86:840–844, 1997.
55. Mohsenipour I, Deusch E, Gabl M, et al: Quality of life in patients after meningioma resection. Acta Neurochir (Wien) 143:547–553, 2001.

52 Neuroendoscopic Approach to Intraventricular Tumors

MICHAEL R. GAAB, HENRY W. S. SCHROEDER, and JOACHIM M. K. OERTEL

With the development of endoscopic systems properly adapted to neurosurgical demands, endoscopic techniques have been used increasingly in the treatment of various neurosurgical conditions since the late 1980s. Initially, noncommunicating hydrocephalus was the main indication for an intracranial neuroendoscopic procedure. However, with increasing experience and technical advances in endoscopic instrumentation, cystic as well as solid lesions have been treated endoscopically.[1-23]

Intraventricular tumors are ideal lesions for the application of an endoscope. Located in a cerebrospinal fluid (CSF)–filled preformed cavity, which allows a clear view, they can be very well visualized. Intraventricular tumors often cause CSF pathway obstruction and ventricular enlargement, which gives sufficient space for maneuvering with endoscopes and instruments. However, ventricular dilatation is not a prerequisite for an endoscopic approach. With the aid of computerized neuronavigation, endoscopes can be inserted even into very small ventricles with high accuracy.[24,25] Thanks to further improvements in endoscopic hemostasis, including the development of bipolar diathermy probes and suitable laser devices,[26] selected highly vascularized tumors can also be completely resected.

Treatment of tumors arising in the ventricular system, however, remains a difficult neurosurgical challenge. These tumors must be approached over a considerable distance through normal brain tissue. In general, intraventricular lesions are treated by microsurgical resection.[27] Advantages of the endoscopic approach are that dissection and brain retraction can be reduced to a minimum. Craniotomies can be avoided because endoscopes are inserted through simple burr holes. Working through an operative sheath protects the surrounding structures such as fornix, hypothalamus, and vessels. To a certain extent, the procedure is comparable to Kelly's microsurgical stereotactic tube approach,[28,29] but the endoscope sheath is much smaller (6.5 vs. 20 mm) and therefore less invasive. Along with tumor resection, CSF pathways can be simultaneously restored using the same endoscopic approach by performing ventriculostomies, septostomies, or stent implantations.[2,16,19]

ENDOSCOPIC EQUIPMENT

For the endoscopic treatment of intraventricular tumors, a sophisticated and complex neuroendoscopic system is necessary. It should include various rigid and flexible endoscopes, effective instruments, bright cold light sources, a high-resolution digital video camera system, and an irrigation device. Combination with a guidance system is desirable. We use the universal GAAB neuroendoscopic system developed by the senior author and manufactured by Karl Storz GmbH & Co. (Tuttlingen, Germany).

Endoscopes

The endoscopes are inserted through an operating sheath (outer diameter 6.5 mm; GAAB I system) that is initially introduced with the aid of a trocar (Fig. 52-1). This allows for intraoperative change of endoscopes without the need to reinsert the endoscopes through brain tissue, thus eliminating unnecessary damage to the surrounding brain. We prefer to use rigid rod-lens endoscopes (Hopkins II; 4 mm outer diameter) because of their brilliant optical quality, extreme wide-angle view, and ease of orientation and guidance. These endoscopes give an excellent overview of the intraventricular anatomy. Accurate assessment of tumor vascularization and the relation of the lesion to major vessels or other important structures are easily obtained. Even in the case of minor bleeding, which might blur the view, the surgeon can stay oriented, which is extremely difficult with the poor optics of a fiberscope. There are rigid endoscopes with four different angles of view available (0, 30, 45, 70, and 120 degrees; Fig. 52-2). The 0- and 30-degree endoscopes are used for inspection and manipulation, and the 45-, 70-, and 120-degree endoscopes for inspection only ("looking around a corner"). The main difference compared with other neuroendoscopic systems is the operating endoscope (wide-angle, straightforward endoscope

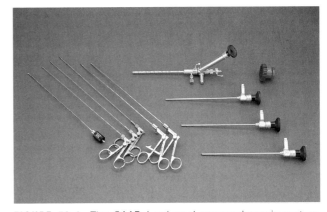

FIGURE 52-1 The GAAB I universal neuroendoscopic system. (Copyright © Karl Storz-Endoskope, Germany.)

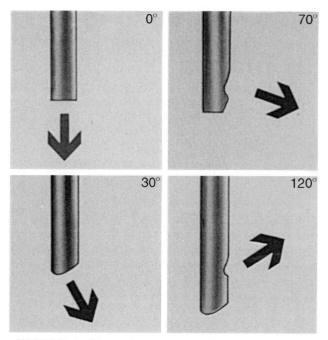

FIGURE 52-2 Diagnostic scopes with different angles of view.

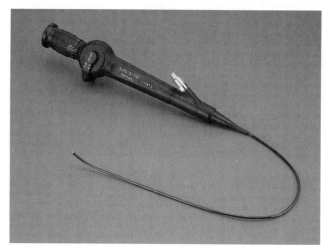

FIGURE 52-3 Steerable neurofiberscope. (Copyright © Karl Storz-Endoskope, Germany.)

with angled eyepiece), which has no separate working channel but allows use of the whole inner diameter (approximately 6 mm) of the endoscopic sheath. This enables effective tissue removal. For removal of larger pieces of tumor, the forceps are withdrawn simultaneously with the endoscope after grasping tumor tissue. If manipulations "around a corner" are needed, we use steerable fiberscopes of two different diameters (2.5 and 3.5 mm; Fig. 52-3). An instrument channel of 1.2 mm is integrated. The high mobility of the tips (170 and 180 degrees upward, and 120 and 100 degrees downward movement) and wide angle of view (65 and 110 degrees) facilitates easy navigation through the ventricular spaces. These endoscopes are especially useful for inspecting the fourth ventricle through the aqueduct. In addition, a miniature endoscope (4-mm operating sheath outer diameter) for pediatric purposes has been developed (Fig. 52-4). This endoscope (GAAB II system) is based on semirigid minifiber optics (10,000 fibers/mm^2) and incorporates an instrument channel as well as two separate channels for irrigation inflow and outflow. Using rigid 1.3-mm instruments, third ventriculostomies, aqueductoplasties, cystostomies, and tumor biopsies can be performed.

Instruments

Various mechanical instruments of different sizes (1.7 and 2.7 mm outer diameter), including scissors, hooks, puncture needles, and biopsy and grasping forceps, are used for dissection and tissue removal (Fig. 52-5). The operating endoscope with the angled eyepiece as well as the miniature endoscope allow manipulations with rigid instruments in a straight line. This makes good tactile feedback from the tissue and easy guidance of the tools possible. For hemostasis and dissection, bipolar as well as monopolar diathermy probes and a laser guide that enables bending of the laser fiber tip are available (Fig. 52-6). However, we almost exclusively use the bipolar diathermy in our neuroendoscopic procedures. Balloon catheters of 3- or 4-French size are applied for enlarging ventriculostomies or other fenestrations.

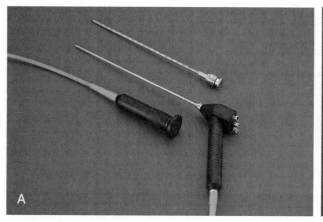

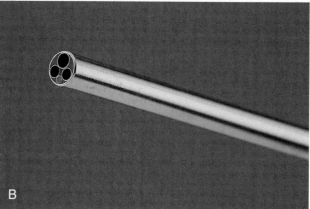

FIGURE 52-4 *A,* GAAB II miniature semirigid fiberscope. *B,* Tip of endoscope (0.8-mm optics, one working channel, two irrigation channels: inflow and outflow). (Copyright © Karl Storz-Endoskope, Germany.)

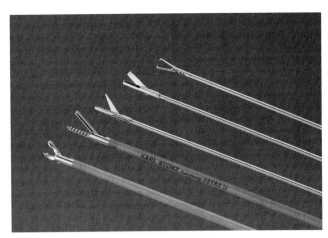

FIGURE 52-5 Endoscopic scissors and biopsy and grasping forceps. (Copyright © Karl Storz-Endoskope, Germany.)

Irrigation

In intraventricular endoscopy, the Clear Vision Device (Karl Storz GmbH & Co., Tuttlingen, Germany) is used. The flow of irrigation fluid is controlled with a foot switch. We use lactated Ringer's solution at 36°C to 37°C because postoperative increases in body temperature, often seen after abundant irrigation with saline, are rarely encountered. It is of utmost importance to make sure that the outflow channel is open to prevent dangerous increases in intracranial pressure.

Light Sources, Cameras, and Video System

Xenon light sources provide the best illumination because the color temperature of xenon light resembles that of sunlight (6000 K). The light is transmitted by glass fiber or fluid (better light transmission but more susceptible to kinking) cables from the light source to the endoscope. Although this system is called cold light fountain, the endoscope tip may become extremely hot.

Digital one-chip (horizontal resolution >450 lines) or three-chip (horizontal resolution >750 lines, separate processing of the three primary colors) mini-video cameras are attached by a sterile optical bridge to the endoscope. Camera and bridge are draped with a sterile covering. This allows sterile intraoperative exchange of endoscopes using the same camera. Several functions of the digital video cameras, such as adjusting contrast, white balance, and selection of different filters (e.g., anti-Moire filter for fiberscopes to minimize the pixel appearance of the image), can be controlled directly by the surgeon pressing buttons on the camera. Of course, high-resolution video monitor screens are necessary to display the endoscopic picture obtained by the video cameras without loss of image quality. We use a Sony Trinitron monitor (horizontal resolution 800 lines, nonflickering, 100 Hz). Each endoscopic procedure is digitally recorded (AIDA system, Karl Storz GmbH & Co., Tuttlingen, Germany). The saved pictures and sequences can be modified on a computer and incorporated into slides or illustrations. A video printer completes the documentation equipment.

For certain endoscopic procedures, the simultaneous use of two endoscopes is desirable. The images from both endoscopes can be displayed on one video monitor with the aid of a digital picture-in-picture device (Twinvideo), allowing the surgeon to obtain the input of both endoscopes by looking at one screen.

For convenience and ease of use, all the aforementioned video equipment can be placed on a mobile cart. Figure 52-7 shows an example of a videocart containing two monitors, one light source, an endoscopic camera, and the AIDA system for digital recording and printing.

INDICATIONS FOR ENDOSCOPIC SURGERY

All intraventricular lesions that do not exceed a certain size limit are candidates for an endoscopic approach. However, it is difficult to determine the exact size limit of a tumor for an effective endoscopic resection. Endoscopic piecemeal

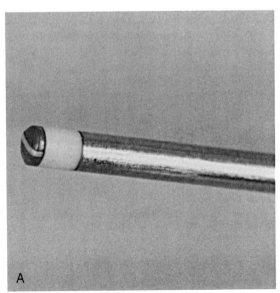

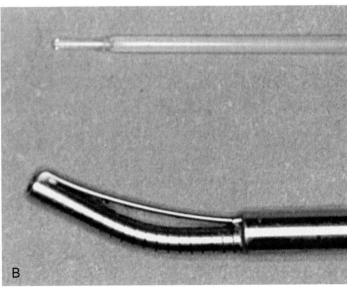

FIGURE 52-6 *A,* Tip of a bipolar diathermy probe. *B,* Tip of a movable laser guide and a laser fiber tip.

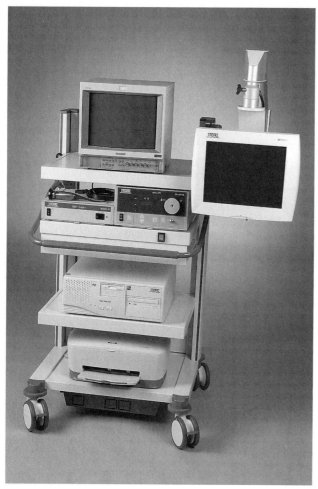

FIGURE 52-7 Endoscopic equipment on a mobile videocart including the AIDA digital recording system. (Copyright © Karl Storz-Endoskope, Germany.)

removal may become time consuming and ineffective if the tumor is too large. The benefits of a minimally invasive approach are then outweighed by the length of the operation. A solid tumor should not exceed 2 to 3 cm in diameter; cystic lesions can be effectively treated even if they are much larger. Tumor consistency and vasculature are additional considerations. Extirpation of soft lesions is easier and more rapid than removal of firm ones. The ideal indication for an endoscopic treatment is a small and avascular tumor located in the lateral or third ventricle, especially if the lesion causes CSF pathway obstruction resulting in enlargement of the ventricles. Ventricular dilatation gives sufficient space for manipulation of the endoscopes and instruments. However, using a computerized navigation system or ultrasound guidance, even very narrow ventricles can be approached accurately with an endoscope. With the aid of bipolar diathermy or (in selected cases) the neodymium:yttrium aluminum garnet (Nd:YAG) laser, even highly vascularized tumors such as cavernomas and hemangiomas can be removed. Large tumors with accompanying hydrocephalus, in which an endoscopic resection is not feasible, are indications for ventriculostomy or aqueductal stenting to restore CSF circulation. Tumor tissue sampling can be carried out on any tumor visible at the

ventricular surface. The use of a second working portal permitting the insertion of larger instruments and thus accelerating tumor removal has been advocated.[5,30] We do not routinely recommend two portals because it makes the approach more invasive and manipulations more difficult. If endoscopic tumor removal turns out to be ineffective, we do not hesitate to change in midprocedure to an open microsurgical operation. With a small keyhole approach and endoscope-assisted microsurgical techniques, an effective and minimally invasive tumor removal without extensive brain dissection, as proposed by Perneczky and colleagues,[31,32] is feasible. To date, in our series and using our system with one large working space, a second port has never been necessary.

General Operative Technique

Once general anesthesia has been induced, the patient is commonly placed supine with the head in three-pin fixation and slight anteflexion. If infrared-based computer neuronavigation is to be used, a camera bar and dynamic reference frame are mounted. After patient registration and verification of accuracy (landmark test), the operating field is prepared and draped, allowing immediate changing to microsurgical intervention in case of ineffective tumor removal or complications. The operating microscope and microsurgical instruments are prepared for use. Just before starting the operation, the patient receives a bolus of 40 mg of dexamethasone intravenously if no contraindications exist. Four milligrams of dexamethasone are given every 6 hours for 2 days after surgery. Antibiotics are not administered routinely.

The entry point usually is selected according to information obtained by preoperative assessment of computed tomography (CT) scan or magnetic resonance imaging (MRI).[2] For lesions occupying the posterior part of the third ventricle or in ventricles that are very narrow, computerized neuronavigation has replaced the previously used frame-based stereotaxy to determine the ideal access route to the target.[24] In cooperation with Carl Zeiss and Karl Storz companies, we developed a universal guiding system for endoscopic purposes (Fig. 52-8 A, B). At present, all current neuronavigation systems (infrared, active, and passive) can be adapted as well to the trocar for initial puncture as well as to the operating sheath or any scope for intraventricular guidance (Fig. 52-8C). With the aid of neuronavigation, the endoscopic sheath can be inserted precisely into the ventricles even if they are very small. Furthermore, this technique allows accurate planning of the approach—for example, in a straight line through the foramen of Monro to the aqueduct without injuring the fornix. Frameless computer navigation allows freehand movement of the endoscope with real-time control of the endoscope tip's position and of the approach trajectory. The degree of accuracy is between 2 and 3 mm, which is sufficient for endoscopic purposes. After reaching the target point with neuronavigational guidance, minor position corrections can be made under endoscopic view.

If the ventricles or foramens of Monro are asymmetric in size, the approach should be made through the larger ventricle or foramen. If feasible, the entry point should be located opposite the dominant hemisphere. Once a 3-cm straight scalp incision has been made, a 10-mm burr hole

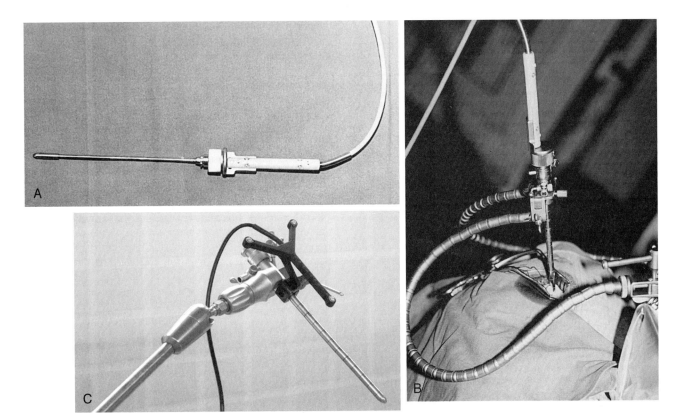

FIGURE 52-8 *A,* A trocar with an LED bar for computerized neuronavigation. *B,* An operating sheath inserted with the aid of navigational guidance. *C,* Light-emitting diode (Radionics) is attached to the trocar for intraoperative guidance.

is placed. After opening the dura, the operating sheath containing the trocar is introduced freehand with or without navigational guidance into the lateral ventricle and fixed with the endoscope holder (Karl Storz GmbH & Co., Tuttlingen, Germany) or simply with two Leyla retractor arms (Fig. 52-9). The trocar is then removed and the rigid diagnostic endoscope inserted after white-balancing the camera. After inspection of the ventricle and identification of the main landmarks (i.e., choroid plexus, fornix, and veins), the tumor with its feeding arteries is visualized. Once the tumor has been explored, the diagnostic endoscope is replaced by the operating endoscope (Fig. 52-10). Capsule vessels are coagulated with the aid of a bipolar diathermy probe. Tumor specimens are taken for histologic investigation. Depending on the size of the lesion, tumor resection usually begins with intracapsular debulking or

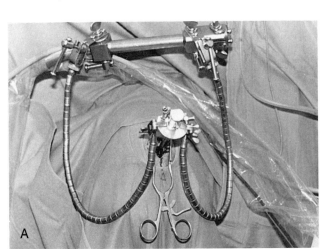

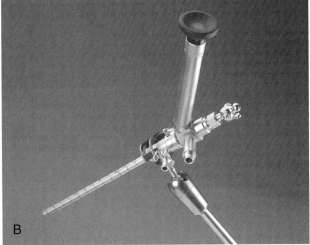

FIGURE 52-9 *A,* An endoscopic sheath fixed with standard microsurgical self-retaining retractors. *B,* The commercially available endoscope holder by the Karl Storz Company. (*B,* Copyright © Karl Storz-Endoskope, Germany.)

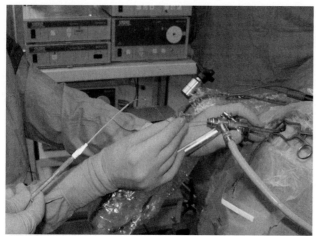

FIGURE 52-10 An operating endoscope guided with the left hand and a balloon catheter guided with the right hand.

dissection in the plane between tumor and brain tissue. Feeding arteries should be identified early and cauterized before bleeding blurs the view. In special cases with highly vascularized lesions, the Nd:YAG laser might be useful.[33] Then, a chisel laser fiber is used in noncontact mode for tumor debulking and vessel coagulation. Tumor dissection is then performed with the chisel fiber or a conical fiber in contact mode for cutting. Laser-assisted resection requires vigorous irrigation to avoid thermal injury to the adjacent brain tissue.[34] After dissection of the tumor from the surrounding brain, the lesion is removed in piecemeal fashion with the aid of various grasping and biopsy forceps. The large operating sheath of our instrument allows removal of solid tumor pieces 6 mm in diameter, and even larger pieces of soft tumors. Details about the entry points for the different tumor locations are given later and in Table 52-1.

All endoscopic tumor operations are performed under continuous irrigation because each tumor resection causes some bleeding. A separate irrigation tube is used to focus the irrigation on the source of bleeding. For forced irrigating, a 20-mL syringe is helpful. Small hemorrhages usually cease spontaneously after a few minutes of irrigation. Rarely, irrigation for 20 minutes is necessary to stop a larger venous

TABLE 52-1 ■ Endoscopic Approaches for Different Tumor Locations

Tumor Location	Entry Point
Lateral ventricle—frontal horn	2–3 cm parasagittal, coronal to 2 cm precoronal
Lateral ventricle—Sella media	2–3 cm parasagittal, coronal to 2 cm precoronal
Lateral ventricle—trigone	2–3 cm parasagittal, 4–6 cm precoronal
Foramen of Monro	3–5 cm parasagittal, 2–4 cm precoronal
Third ventricle—anterior part	1–2 cm parasagittal, coronal
Third ventricle—posterior part	1–2 cm parasagittal, 4–6 cm precoronal
Fourth ventricle—floor of third ventricle (combined approach)	1–2 cm parasagittal, 2–3 cm precoronal

hemorrhage and to clear the view. It is ill-advised to remove the endoscope in case of bleeding; rather, stay in place, rinse, and wait. Larger vessels that are at risk of injury during tumor dissection should be cauterized with the bipolar diathermy probe before bleeding occurs. In rare cases of severe hemorrhage, aspiration of CSF is needed to obtain a dry field. With this "dry-field" technique, bleeding vessels are more easily identified and hemostasis is quickly achieved. To avoid a dangerous increase in intracranial pressure, care must be taken to maintain sufficient outflow of irrigation fluid.

After tumor removal, the resection site is inspected with the diagnostic endoscope to check that there is no active bleeding. The ventricles are vigorously irrigated to remove any clots. The operating sheath is then withdrawn simultaneously with the endoscope to look for potential bleeding at the foramen of Monro or in the cortical puncture channel. In general, no external ventricular drainage is placed. We pack the burr hole with a gelatin sponge and tightly suture the galea to prevent subgaleal CSF accumulation and fistula formation. The skin is closed with running atraumatic sutures. CSF accumulation despite these measures indicates increased intracranial pressure chiefly due to obstructed CSF flow. The patient usually is observed overnight in the intensive care unit.

Tumors of the Lateral Ventricle

Tumors of the lateral ventricle are mostly benign or low-grade lesions such as gliomas, meningiomas, plexus papillomas, and hemangiomas.[35] Lesions located in the frontal horn may obstruct the foramen of Monro, resulting in unilateral hydrocephalus. The choroidal arteries usually supply the lesions.[36]

The patient is positioned supine with the head tilted slightly forward. For lesions of the frontal horn and ventricular body, a standard precoronal (3-cm paramedian) burr hole is placed. Tumors of the trigone are approached through a burr hole located more anteriorly to reach the target in a straight line through the ventricular body. A posterior approach is advisable only if marked ventricular dilatation provides enough space for manipulation with endoscope and instruments. The CSF-filled working space in front of the tumor is usually very limited, making the inspection of the lesion, orientation, and dissection more difficult or even impossible. To date, our experience with tumors arising in the temporo-occipital region of the lateral ventricle is limited to two cases. In one case, the histologic diagnosis of a multifocal intraventricular glioblastoma without CSF outflow obstruction could not be obtained by repeated spinal taps. An endoscopic biopsy was taken via a transcortical very anterior approach. The second case consisted of an choroid plexus cyst and is illustrated in Figure 52-11.

In general, we prefer a transcortical insertion of the endoscope into the lateral ventricle. In a few patients, the endoscope was introduced using a transcallosal approach; this resulted in permanent memory loss in one patient, probably related to fornical damage. We abandoned this approach for inserting the endoscope because it requires a small craniotomy and microsurgical dissection for exposing the corpus callosum (instead of a simple burr hole) and makes initial orientation more difficult. The transcortical

FIGURE 52-11 Thalamic diffuse astrocytoma. *A*, Preoperative coronar T1-weighted enhanced MRI scan showing diffuse right thalamic anaplastic astrocytoma with subsequent blockage of the foramen of Monro. *B*, Endoscopic view at the ventricular wall covered by a tumor layer. *C*, Bipolar coagulation before tumor biopsy. *D*, Mild hemorrhage after biopsy from the lesion.

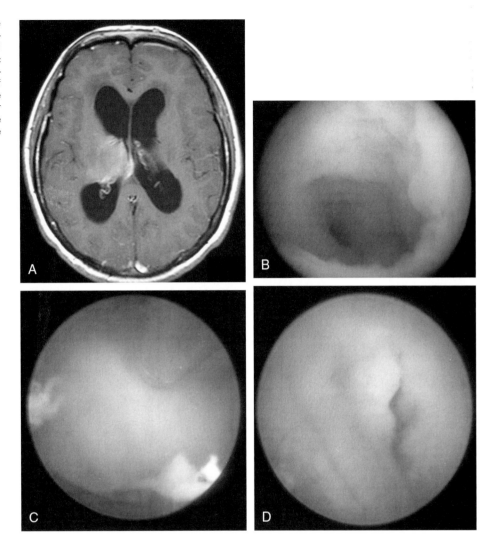

burr hole approach has proven to be fast, easy, and safe because of well-known landmarks. A higher seizure rate has been reported after the transcortical approach,[37,38] although we have seen no increased seizure rate after the transcortical insertion of an endoscope in more than 600 cases.

Once the endoscopic sheath has been inserted into the lateral ventricle, the tumor is visualized. The relation of the tumor to the choroid plexus should be ascertained before starting tumor dissection. Because tearing of the choroid plexus may lead to bleeding at a distance from the operating field,[39] the choroid attachment of the lesion should be coagulated first with the aid of the bipolar probe or the Nd:YAG laser (see Fig. 52-11). Care must be taken to avoid injury to the thalamus, caudate nucleus, and fornices. Patency of the foramen of Monro usually is achieved after tumor resection. If the foramen is still occluded, CSF circulation can be restored by performing a septostomy through the septum pellucidum. The septostomy can be made with the aid of laser, diathermy, scissors, and balloon catheters. The size of this fenestration should be approximately 10 mm². When the ventricles are very small or ventricular collapse occurs after ventricular puncture, there might be not enough working space for instrument manipulations. The endoscopic procedure must then be abandoned and the tumor removed microsurgically.

Tumors of the Third Ventricle

Tumors located in the third ventricle are among the most difficult lesions to expose and remove. A variety of approaches have been advocated in the literature, including the transsphenoidal, anterior and posterior transventricular, anterior and posterior transcallosal, subfrontal, frontotemporal, occipital transtentorial, and infratentorial supracerebellar approaches.[40–45] Division of the anterior column of the fornix,[40] division of the thalamostriate vein,[46] interfornical midline division of the ventricular roof,[44,47] and a subchoroid approach[48,49] have been recommended for entering the third ventricle. The choice of approach depends on the surgeon and the tumor location. When working in the third ventricle, brain retraction should be minimized to avoid injury to important structures such as thalamus, fornix, veins, and hypothalamus. With endoscopic techniques, there is little need for retraction.[50]

Frameless computerized neuronavigation aids in determining the exact entry point and the approach trajectory along which the endoscope is passed in a straight line through the foramen of Monro to the target without injuring the surrounding brain tissue. Neuronavigation has proven especially helpful for lesions in the posterior third ventricle.

Tumors originating in the third ventricle include astrocytomas (Fig. 52-12), ependymomas, epidermoids, colloid cysts (Fig. 52-13), craniopharyngiomas, pituitary adenomas, medulloblastomas, and gliosis (Fig. 52-14). In the pineal region, germinomas, nongerminomatous germ cell tumors, pinealocytomas, pinealoblastomas, and pineal cysts occur.[42]

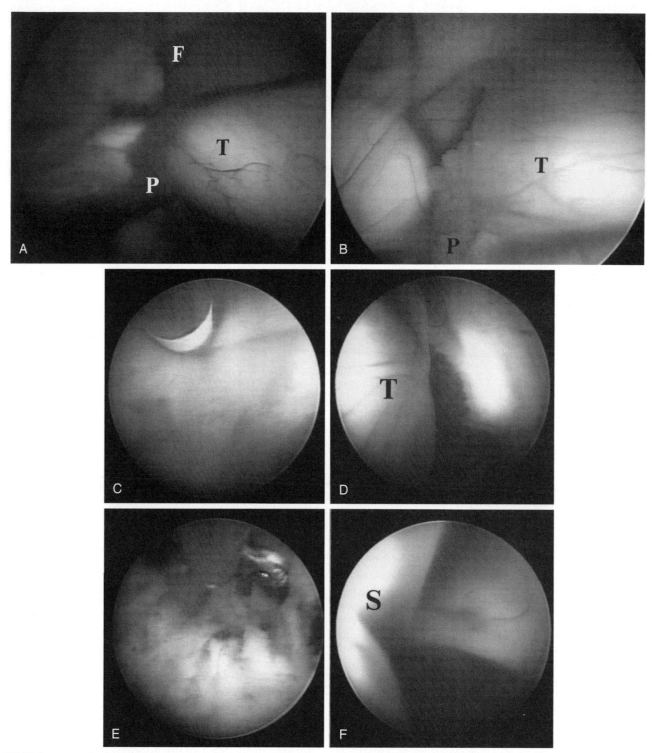

FIGURE 52-12 Benign astrocytoma within the foramen of Monro. *A,* View into the left lateral ventricle showing a tumor (T) medial from the choroid plexus (P) with an obstructed foramen of Monro (F). *B,* Closer view with an occluded foramen of Monro with a tumor (T) and choroid plexus (P). *C,* Septostomy in the septum pellucidum with a bipolar probe. *D,* View through the septostomy showing a tumor (T) bulging into the right lateral ventricle. *E,* Tumor resection using biopsy forceps. *F,* A stent (S) is inserted into the foramen of Monro.

(Continued)

FIGURE 52-12 Cont'd *G,* Axial T1-weighted enhanced MRI scan showing a tumor with bilateral obstruction of the foramen of Monro and hydrocephalus. *H,* Axial T1-weighted enhanced MRI scan obtained 10 months after surgery showing partial tumor resection (the fornices are spared!) and relief of hydrocephalus.

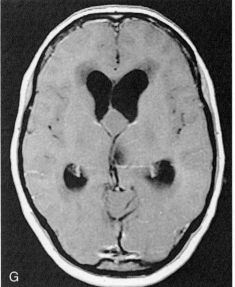
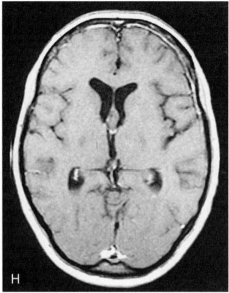

The patient is placed in the supine position with the head slightly flexed. Tumors of the third ventricle are approached by a transcortical, transventricular, transforaminal route, regardless of anterior or posterior location. This is the standard approach in ventriculoscopy with clear landmarks. If the tumor is located in the anterior part of the ventricle, the entry point is at the coronal suture.[19,51] If the tumor arises in the posterior part, the burr hole is made more anteriorly to pass the foramen of Monro in a straight line.[19,52,53] For endoscopic procedures, we do not use the infratentorial supracerebellar approach,[43] which we prefer for microsurgical operations in the pineal region. Because a simple burr hole is not sufficient to identify the transverse sinus, a small craniotomy must be made. Thick arachnoid membranes often cover the pineal region and hinder accurate orientation. These membranes are more easily and safely divided microsurgically than endoscopically. Finally, the superior cerebellar bridging veins and deep incisural veins are at risk when introducing an endoscope.[54] These veins must be cauterized and divided. Hence, a strictly endoscopic infratentorial supracerebellar approach is inconvenient and poses a considerable risk. A better alternative is an endoscope-assisted microsurgical approach, as recommended by Perneczky.[55]

Tumors of the third ventricle are removed according to the guidelines earlier described. When advancing the operating sheath through the foramen of Monro, care should be taken to avoid the fornix and the adjacent veins. Tilting the endoscopic sheath in the foramen of Monro can be done only with great caution, especially when the foramen is small. Cystic lesions are first punctured and the contents aspirated. Cyst collapse facilitates dissection from the adjacent brain. Capsule vessels are coagulated. Residual parts of the capsule firmly attached to the roof of the ventricle should be coagulated rather than vigorously removed, because pulling may cause severe venous bleeding. After tumor removal, patency of CSF pathways should be verified. First, the entry of the aqueduct must be inspected to

ensure there is no blockade by tumor debris. If the tumor resection is incomplete and residual tumor tissue may progress and occlude the CSF pathways in the future, a stent should be inserted. In tumors of the posterior part of the third ventricle, such as in the pineal region, a short stent between the fourth and third ventricles is sufficient to maintain CSF circulation. However, if the tumor occupies the entire third ventricle and blocks the foramen of Monro as well as the aqueduct, the stent should extend from the lateral to the fourth ventricle. Unilateral obstruction of the foramen of Monro can be managed by fenestration in the septum pellucidum (septostomy). Sometimes both stenting and septostomy are required to preserve CSF circulation.

Frame-based stereotactic MRI- or CT-guided tumor biopsy is a well-established and safe option to obtain tumor tissue specimens. However, stereotactic puncture of tumors near the foramen of Monro has the potential for fornical and venous injury.[56] Stereotactic biopsy of pineal lesions places the great vein and the internal veins at risk. Endoscopic biopsy offers some advantages over stereotactic biopsy. First, the lesions can be inspected. Changes in coordinates (e.g., after cyst aspiration) can be recognized early. Second, the procedure can be performed under direct vision and therefore be better controlled. Bleeding can be seen and hemostasis quickly achieved. For pineal lesions in particular, we prefer the endoscopic approach for obtaining a biopsy. Despite reports on large series of stereotactic biopsies of pineal lesions[57,58] describing this technique as safe and reliable, we are concerned about the "blind" sampling of tissue in this area. We favor neuroendoscopic exploration and biopsy under direct view. Through the same burr hole, occluded CSF pathways can easily be restored by stenting of the aqueduct or third ventriculostomy. Thus endoscopy offers simultaneous histologic verification and permanent restoration of blocked CSF pathways. After reaching an accurate histologic diagnosis, further treatment, such as microsurgical operation, irradiation, chemotherapy, or radiosurgery, is initiated.

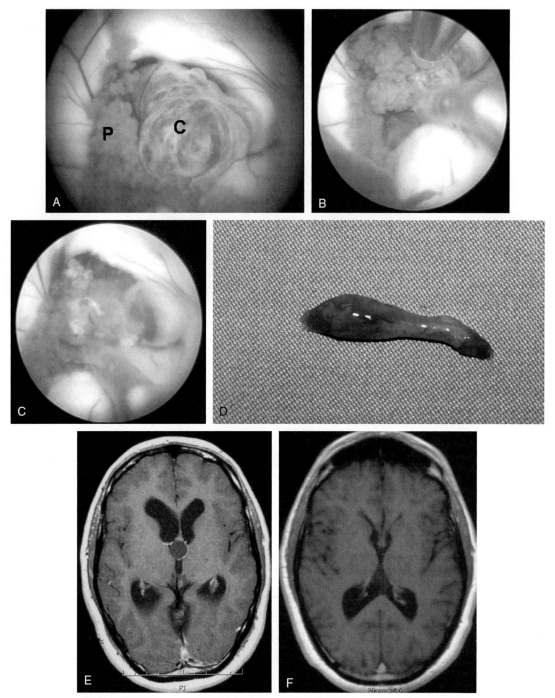

FIGURE 52-13 A colloid cyst in the ventricle. *A,* A colloid cyst (C) bulging into the lateral ventricle through the foramen of Monro (P: choroid plexus). *B,* Coagulation of the capsule vessels and the choroids plexus with a bipolar probe. *C,* After opening the cyst, the yellow colloid contents drain into the lateral ventricle. *D,* Colloid cyst after extraction. *E,* Axial T1-weighted enhanced MRI scan showing the colloid cyst obstructing the foramen of Monro and ventricular dilatation. *F,* Postoperative axial T1-weighted enhanced MRI scan showing complete colloid cyst removal and a decrease in ventricular size.

Tumors of the Fourth Ventricle

In our experience, tumors of the fourth ventricle are rarely suitable for an endoscopic resection because the ventricular space is very limited. However, because these lesions often become initially symptomatic with signs of increased intracranial pressure caused by obstructive hydrocephalus, a third ventriculostomy is indicated. In selected cases, biopsies are taken through the enlarged aqueduct. For cases in which a combined procedure of approaching the lesion and

taking a biopsy and performing a third ventriculostomy to restore CSF circulation is indicated, we place the burr hole 1 to 2 cm parasagittal and 2 to 3 cm precoronal. After insertion of the operating sheath through the foramen of Monro, we switch to the flexible endoscope and inspect the lesion through the enlarged aqueduct. A biopsy is taken and a standard third ventriculostomy follows. However, in any case, the indication for this combined approach is narrow. The periaqueductal brain in particular is easily subjected to injury. At present, our experience with

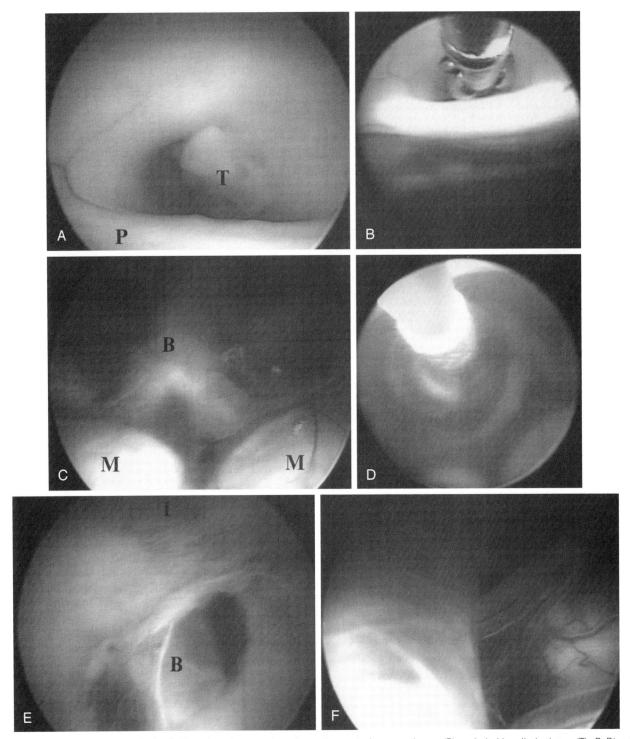

FIGURE 52-14 Aqueductal gliosis. *A*, Entry into the aqueduct above the posterior commissure (P) occluded by gliotic tissue (T). *B*, Biopsy with forceps. *C*, Translucent floor of the third ventricle with mammillary bodies (M) and a clearly visible basilar artery (B). *D*, Ventriculostomy with a Fogarty balloon catheter. *E*, Ventriculostomy behind the infundibular recess (I); basilar artery (B). *F*, View through a ventriculostomy into the interpeduncular cistern showing the basilar artery with pontine branches. (*Continued*)

this combined procedure is limited to two cases (both astrocytomas). In those, both procedures were performed without complications.

Results

One hundred and three patients harboring an intraventricular lesion underwent endoscopic treatment at our department between February 1993 and December 2003 (February 1993 until January 2003 at the University of Greifswald; February 2003 until December 2005 at the Hannover Nordstadt Hospital). Histologic examination revealed 21 colloid cysts, 23 astrocytomas and glioblastomas, 8 craniopharyngiomas, 5 subependymomas, 4 ependymomas, 4 intraventricular arachnoid cyst, 8 pineal cyst, 3 metastases, 3 glioses, 3 plexus papilloma, 2 germinomas, 2 medulloblastoma, 2 lymphoma, 2 cavernoma, 1 arteriovenous hemangioma, 1 pineocytoma/pineoblastoma (intermediate type), 1 pineoblastoma,

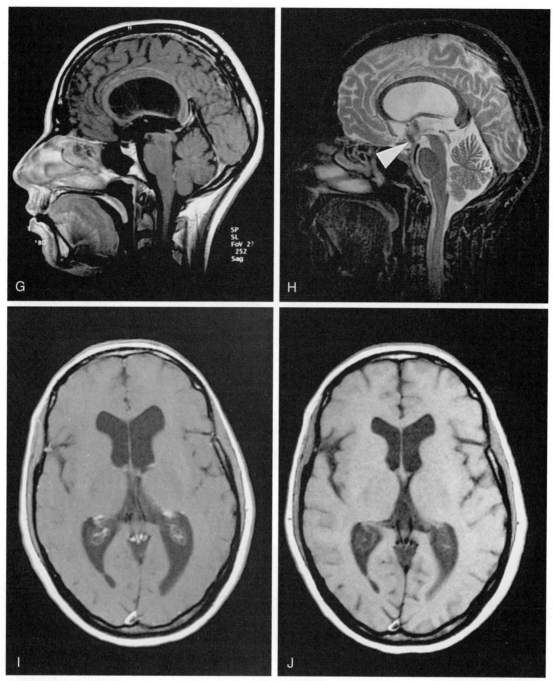

FIGURE 52-14   Cont'd *G*, Sagittal T1-weighted enhanced MRI scan revealing a nonenhancing lesion within the aqueduct. *H*, Sagittal T2-weighted MRI scan obtained 6 months postoperatively revealing a patent third ventriculostomy with a flow void sign (*arrow*). *I*, Axial T1-weighted enhanced MRI scan showing ventricular enlargement. *J*, An axial T1-weighted enhanced MRI scan obtained 6 months postoperatively showing a decrease in size of the ventricle.

1 pituitary adenoma, 1 neuroblastoma, 1 melanoma, 1 choroid plexus cyst, 1 epidermoid, 1 ganglioglioma, and 1 sarcoma. In two specimens, chronic ventriculitis was detected. In one, no pathological diagnosis could be made. The follow-up period ranges from 1 month up to 9 years.

None of the endoscopic procedures had to be stopped because of significant bleeding or poor orientation. Two minor and one major venous hemorrhage occurred in procedures for colloid cysts but could be controlled endoscopically. In another colloid cyst case, the endoscopic procedure was

abandoned because of recurrent bleeding and the lesion microsurgically removed. Because of very firm tissue consistency, the endoscopic resection of two subependymomas larger than 2 cm in diameter was ineffective; the endoscopic procedure was also discontinued and the tumors microsurgically removed. These two operations lasted 135 and 210 minutes, respectively. The mean surgical time for the strictly endoscopic procedures was 91 minutes, ranging from 30 to 270 minutes. One very small colloid cyst could not be detected endoscopically. Because the foramen of Monro was not narrowed, no further measures were undertaken. All other cystic lesions were completely evacuated and the membranes widely resected. In two colloid cysts, capsule remnants firmly attached to the roof of the third ventricle were not removed. However, MRI has not shown colloid cyst recurrence in any of the patients (follow-up periods of 3 to 105 months). Astrocytomas were partially resected. Patients with malignant tumors were referred for stereotactic precision irradiation or radiosurgery, and benign tumors were controlled with repeated MRI.

Total endoscopic removal of solid lesions was performed on the two cavernomas, the three plexus papillomas, the two medulloblastomas, the arteriovenous hemangioma, and one subependymoma. Follow-up MRIs have demonstrated no tumor recurrences. One craniopharyngioma, initially histologically classified as an epidermoid, recurred after 12 months. However, small ventricles indicated a patent septostomy and stent. Thirty four third ventriculostomies and eight septostomies were performed. Ten stents were inserted. In 28 patients, a tumor biopsy was taken. The hydrocephalus-related symptoms of increased intracranial pressure were relieved in all patients.

Complications

There was no mortality related to the endoscopic procedure in this series.[59,60] Twelve patients died from progression of the tumor within the follow-up period. Two patients died after microsurgical extirpation of the tumor (giant pituitary adenoma and craniopharyngioma) because of diencephalic dysfunction. Significant bleeding blurred the view in six cases. In five, these hemorrhages were controlled endoscopically using the dry-field technique. In one case, the endoscopic procedure was abandoned and continued microsurgically. The postoperative course was uneventful in these six cases. Memory loss attributed to fornical damage was observed in two cases, and in one it remained permanent. Meningitis occurred in one patient and was treated with antibiotics. Because an external ventricular drainage was inserted 2 days before the endoscopic procedure, the meningitis was probably related to the external ventricular drainage rather than to the endoscopy. In one patient, a transient mutism occurred. We observed one transient trochlear palsy after biopsy of an aqueductal tumor, and one patient experienced transient confusion after biopsy of a suprasellar germinoma.

CONCLUSIONS

In our experience, the endoscopic management of intraventricular tumors has proven to be effective and safe. The symptoms of obstructive hydrocephalus were relieved in all patients. All third ventriculostomies have remained patent. All stents have remained patent, and no dislocation has been observed. Shunting was completely avoided. The endoscopic procedure had to be abandoned and continued microsurgically in only three patients, and a histologic tumor diagnosis was obtained in all but three contrast-enhancing lesions.

With the application of neuroendoscopic techniques, the invasiveness of microsurgical procedures can be further reduced with similar or even better results. In selected cases, cystic and solid intraventricular tumors can be removed completely using endoscopic techniques. Craniotomies are not required and brain retraction is minimized. Another advantage of the endoscopic approach is the rapid and straightforward access to the lesion. The combination of endoscopes with frameless computerized neuronavigation has improved the accuracy of the approach. The endoscopic procedures have usually been shorter than the analogous microsurgical procedure. The surgeon should be aware of potential complications, however, and all preparations should be made for immediate microsurgical intervention in case of complications or ineffectiveness of the endoscopic approach. In our experience, intraventricular hemorrhage rapidly blurring the view is the major risk in endoscopic brain surgery. This risk might be reduced with the introduction of new techniques preserving even the smallest blood vessels in the near future.[61,62] However, in case of recurrent bleeding, we recommend there be no hesitation to switch to an open microsurgical approach.

In our opinion, endoscopic techniques should be applied in the treatment of selected intraventricular lesions. In the future, endoscopic techniques will probably also be used for the treatment of paraventricular and intraparenchymal lesions. The combination of real-time computer-aided neuronavigation and intraoperative ultrasound (image fusion) will increase the accuracy of the approach and help control the extent of tumor removal.

REFERENCES

1. Caemaert J, Abdullah J, Calliauw L, et al: Endoscopic treatment of suprasellar arachnoid cysts. Acta Neurochir (Wien) 119:68–73, 1992.
2. Gaab MR, Schroeder HWS: Neuroendoscopic approach to intraventricular lesions. J Neurosurg 88:496–505, 1998.
3. Schroeder HWS, Gaab MR, Niendorf W-R: Neuroendoscopic approach to arachnoid cysts. J Neurosurg 85:293–298, 1996.
4. Bauer BL, Hellwig D: Minimally invasive endoscopic neurosurgery: A survey. Acta Neurochir Suppl (Wien) 61:1–12, 1994.
5. Cohen AR: Endoscopic ventricular surgery. Pediatr Neurosurg 19:127–134, 1993.
6. Auer LM, Holzer P, Ascher PW, et al: Endoscopic neurosurgery. Acta Neurochir (Wien) 90:1–14, 1988.
7. Eiras Ajuria J, Alberdi Vinas J: Traitement endoscopique des lesions intracranienne: A propos de 8 cas. Neurochirurgie 37:278–283, 1991.
8. Hor F, Desgeorges M, Rosseau GL: Tumour resection by stereotactic laser endoscopy. Acta Neurochir Suppl (Wien) 54:77–82, 1992.
9. Merienne L, Leriche B, Roux FX, et al: Utilisation du laser Nd-YAG en endoscopie intracranienne: Experience preliminaire en stereotaxie. Neurochirurgie 38:245–247, 1992.
10. Decq P, Yepes C, Anno Y, et al: L'Endoscopie neurochirurgicale: Indications diagnostiques et thérapeutiques. Neurochirurgie 40:313–321, 1994.
11. Fukushima T, Ishijima B, Hirakawa K, et al: Ventriculofiberscope: A new technique for endoscopic diagnosis and operation. J Neurosurg 38:251–256, 1973.
12. Fukushima T: Endoscopic biopsy of intraventricular tumors with the use of a ventriculofiberscope. Neurosurgery 2:110–113, 1978.
13. Griffith HB: Endoneurosurgery: Endoscopic intracranial surgery. Adv Tech Stand Neurosurg 14:2–24, 1986.
14. Grunert P, Perneczky A, Resch K: Endoscopic procedures through the foramen interventriculare of Monro under stereotactical conditions. Minim Invasive Neurosurg 37:2–8, 1994.
15. Abdullah J, Caemaert J: Endoscopic management of craniopharyngiomas: A review of 3 cases. Minim Invasive Neurosurg 38:79–84, 1995.
16. Oka K, Yamamoto M, Nagasaka S, et al: Endoneurosurgical treatment for hydrocephalus caused by intraventricular tumors. Childs Nerv Syst 10:162–166, 1994.
17. Jho H-D, Carrau RL: Endoscopic endonasal transsphenoidal surgery: Experience with 50 patients. J Neurosurg 87:44–51, 1997.

18. Caemaert J, Abdullah J: Endoscopic management of colloid cysts. Tech Neurosurg 1:185–200, 1996.

19. Schroeder HWS, Gaab MR: Intracranial endoscopy. Neurosurg Focus 6 (issue 4): Article 1, April 1999.

20. Abdou MS, Cohen AR: Endoscopic treatment of colloid cysts of the third ventricle. J Neurosurg 89:1062–1068, 1998.

21. Rodziewicz GS, Smith MV, Hodge CJ, Jr: Endoscopic colloid cyst surgery. Neurosurgery 46:655–662, 2000.

22. Teo C: Complete endoscopic removal of colloid cysts: Issues of safety and efficacy. Neurosurg Focus 6 (issue 4): Article 9, April 1999.

23. Decq P, Le Guerinel C, Brugieres P, et al: Endoscopic management of colloid cysts. Neurosurgery 42:1288–1296, 1998.

24. Schroeder HWS, Wagner W, Tschiltschke W, et al: Frameless neuronavigation in intracranial endoscopic neurosurgery. J Neurosurg 94:72–79, 2001.

25. Alberti O, Riegel T, Hellwig D, et al: Frameless navigation and endoscopy. J Neurosurg 95:541–543, 2001.

26. Hellwig D, Haag R, Bartel V, et al: Application of new electrosurgical devices and probes in endoscopic neurosurgery. Neurol Res 21:67–72, 1999.

27. Collmann H, Kazner E, Sprung C: Supratentorial intraventricular tumors in childhood. Acta Neurochir Suppl (Wien) 35:75–79, 1985.

28. Kelly PJ, Kall BA, Goerss S, et al: Computer-assisted stereotaxic laser resection of intra-axial brain neoplasms. J Neurosurg 64:427–439, 1986.

29. Kelly PJ: Volumetric stereotactic surgical resection of intra-axial brain mass lesions. Mayo Clin Proc 63:1186–1198, 1988.

30. Jallo GI, Morota N, Abbott R: Introduction of a second working portal for neuroendoscopy: A technical note. Pediatr Neurosurg 24:56–60, 1996.

31. Perneczky A, Fries G: Endoscope-assisted brain surgery. Part I: Evolution, basic concept, and current technique. Neurosurgery 42:219–225, 1998.

32. Fries G, Perneczky A: Endoscope-assisted brain surgery. Part 2: Analysis of 380 procedures. Neurosurgery 42:226–232, 1998.

33. Schroeder HWS, Gaab MR, Niendorf W-R, et al: Neuroendoscopy in the treatment of brain tumors [Abstract]. Zentralbl Neurochir 57 (Suppl):50, 1996.

34. Goebel KR: Fundamentals of laser science. Acta Neurochir Suppl (Wien) 61:20–33, 1994.

35. Lapras C, Deruty R, Bret P: Tumors of the lateral ventricles. Adv Tech Stand Neurosurg 11:103–167, 1984.

36. Kempe LG, Blaylock R: Lateral-trigonal intraventricular tumors: A new operative approach. Acta Neurochir (Wien) 35:233–242, 1976.

37. McKissock W: The surgical treatment of colloid cyst of the third ventricle. Brain 74:1–9, 1951.

38. Little JR, MacCarty CS: Colloid cysts of the third ventricle. J Neurosurg 39:230–235, 1974.

39. Piepmeier JM, Westerveld M, Spencer DD, et al: Surgical management of intraventricular tumors of the lateral ventricles. In Schmidek HH, Sweet WH (eds): Operative Neurosurgical Techniques, 3rd ed. Philadelphia: WB Saunders, 1995, pp 725–738.

40. Rhoton AL, Jr, Yamamoto I, Peace DA: Microsurgery of the third ventricle. Part 2: Operative approaches. Neurosurgery 8:357–373, 1981.

41. Carmel PW: Tumours of the third ventricle. Acta Neurochir (Wien) 75:136–146, 1985.

42. Sawaya R, Hawley DK, Tobler WD, et al: Pineal and third ventricle tumors. In Youmans JR (ed): Neurological Surgery, 3rd ed. Philadelphia: WB Saunders, 1990, pp 3171–3203.

43. Stein BM: The infratentorial supracerebellar approach to pineal lesions. J Neurosurg 35:197–202, 1971.

44. Apuzzo MLJ, Chikovani OK, Gott PS, et al: Transcallosal, interfornicial approaches for lesions affecting the third ventricle: Surgical considerations and consequences. Neurosurgery 10:547–554, 1982.

45. Camins MB, Schlesinger EB: Treatment of tumours of the posterior part of the third ventricle and the pineal region: A long-term follow-up. Acta Neurochir (Wien) 40:131–143, 1978.

46. Hirsch JF, Zouaoui A, Renier D, et al: A new surgical approach to the third ventricle with interruption of the striothalamic vein. Acta Neurochir (Wien) 47:135–147, 1979.

47. Busch E: A new approach for the removal of tumours of the third ventricle. Acta Psychiatr Scand 19:57–60, 1944.

48. Viale GL, Turtas S: The subchoroid approach to the third ventricle. Surg Neurol 14:71–76, 1980.

49. Cossu M, Lubinu F, Orunesu G, et al: Subchoroidal approach to the third ventricle: Microsurgical anatomy. Surg Neurol 21:325–331, 1984.

50. Otsuki T, Jokura H, Yoshimoto T: Stereotactic guiding tube for open-system endoscopy: A new approach for the stereotactic endoscopic resection of intra-axial brain tumors. Neurosurgery 27:326–330, 1990.

51. Schroeder HWS, Gaab MR: Endoscopic resection of colloid cysts. Neurosurgery 51:1441–1445, 2002.

52. Schroeder HWS, Gaab MR: Endoscopic aqueductoplasty: Technique and results. Neurosurgery 45:508–518, 1999.

53. Schroeder HWS, Oertel J, Gaab MR: Endoscopic aqueductoplasty in the treatment of aqueductal stenoses. Childs Nerv Syst 20:821–827, 2004.

54. Cohen AR: Comment on Ruge JR, Johnson RF, Bauer J: Burr hole neuroendoscopic fenestration of quadrigeminal arachnoid cyst: Technical case report. Neurosurgery 38:837, 1996.

55. Perneczky A: Comment on Ruge JR, Johnson RF, Bauer J: Burr hole neuroendoscopic fenestration of quadrigeminal cistern arachnoid cyst: Technical case report. Neurosurgery 38:837, 1996.

56. Lewis AI, Crone KR, Taha J, et al: Surgical resection of third ventricle colloid cysts: Preliminary results comparing transcallosal microsurgery with endoscopy. J Neurosurg 81:174–178, 1994.

57. Regis J, Bouillot P, Rouby-Volot F, et al: Pineal region tumors and the role of stereotactic biopsy: Review of the mortality, morbidity, and diagnostic rates in 370 cases. Neurosurgery 39:907–914, 1996.

58. Kreth FW, Schatz CR, Pagenstecher A, et al: Stereotactic management of lesions of the pineal region. Neurosurgery 39:280–291, 1996.

59. Schroeder HWS, Niendorf WR, Gaab MR: Complications of endoscopic third ventriculostomy. J Neurosurg 96:1032–1040, 2002.

60. Schroeder HWS, Oertel J, Gaab MR: Incidence of complications in neuroendoscopic surgery. Childs Nerv Syst 20:878–883, 2004.

61. Oertel J, Gaab MR, Pillich D-T, et al: Comparison of waterjet dissection and ultrasonic aspiration: An in vivo study in the rabbit brain. J Neurosurg 100:498–504, 2004.

62. Oertel J, Gaab MR, Knapp A, et al: Water jet dissection in neurosurgery: Experimental results in the porcine cadaveric brain. Neurosurgery 52:153–159, 2003.

53 Approaches to Lateral and Third Ventricular Tumors

S. BULENT OMAY, JOACHIM BAEHRING, and
JOSEPH PIEPMEIER

SUMMARY

Tumors of the lateral and third ventricles grow slowly and are often benign; thus by the time that the patient presents to the surgeon, they may have reached a significant size. Clinical findings vary according to the specific location and the biologic behavior of the tumor and range from nonspecific headaches to peculiar syndromes such as drop attacks. Infiltrative gliomas (astrocytoma, oligodendroglioma, mixed glial tumors) are the most common neoplasm affecting lateral and third ventricles.

There are multiple surgical approaches to these tumors, but all attempt to use the pathways around the brain that least disturb and minimally displace normal anatomy. Before embarking on an approach, the surgeon should be familiar with both the ventricular anatomy and the types and behavior of lesions of the lateral and third ventricles. The lateral and third ventricles can be accessed by transcallosal, transcortical, and, in some cases, supracerebellar, subfrontal, pterional, and transtentorial approaches. Endoscopic approaches are available and very promising in some cases.

Approaches to the lateral and third ventricles are difficult and potentially dangerous procedures and have a significant morbidity and mortality. Because of the numerous types of approaches and the varied pathology involved, it is difficult to make generalizations regarding morbidity. The complications are very specific to the type of tumor and its location.

Most commonly encountered postoperative complications are cognitive deficits, hydrocephalus, and seizures.

CLINICAL PRESENTATION

The lateral ventricles are surrounded by the large commissural (corpus callosum) and projection fiber systems of the frontal lobe (corticospinal tract), parietal lobe (thalamocortical projections of the sensory system), and the temporal and the occipital lobes (optic radiation). The boundaries of the third ventricle are formed by the functionally diverse anatomic structures of the diencephalon. There is a wide range of clinical syndromes caused by lateral and third ventricular neoplasms that is dependent on tumor location, size, and amount of perifocal edema; the clinical course is determined by the tumor type.

Some rules are useful to the clinician. A brain tumor should be considered in patients with a new headache or change in quality of a chronic headache, focal neurologic symptoms, or cognitive loss. The clinical presentation is nonspecific and can be acute (strokelike due to intratumoral hemorrhage, pressure valve effect of a colloid cyst) or subacute (slowly progressive headache that is typically worst on awakening, personality changes, memory loss). Seizures are much less common than in hemispheric tumors and indicate tumor growth beyond the confines of the ventricles.

Depending on tumor location, patients with tumors restricted to the ventricular lumen, sooner or later are bound to develop symptoms of cerebrospinal fluid (CSF) flow obstruction. Cognitive decline or personality changes are accompanied by progressive headache. Patients may not come to medical attention until nausea, vomiting, hiccoughing, yawning, and increasing somnolence occur. In infants, before closure of the calvarial sutures, hydrocephalus is accompanied by enlargement of head circumference. Communicating hydrocephalus in patients with intraventricular tumors is the result of spinal fluid overproduction (choroid plexus papilloma) or decreased reabsorption.

A peculiar syndrome of intermittent spinal fluid obstruction is seen in patients with colloid cyst of the interventricular foramen. Sudden onset of severe headache with nausea, vomiting, somnolence, incontinence, imbalance, or drop attacks (sudden loss of tone without loss of consciousness), sometimes elicited by a Valsalva maneuver and relieved by particular head positions is characteristic.

Asymmetrical hydrocephalus is observed in patients with tumors of the body and temporal and occipital horns of the lateral ventricle. Focal neurologic symptoms arise when the tumor involves adjacent structures. A subcortical hemiparesis with equal involvement of arm and leg results from infiltration of the centrum semiovale. Tumors surrounding the atrium, the occipital horn, or the temporal horn give rise to visual field defects that are the more congruent and dense the closer that they are to the primary visual cortex. Infiltration of the corpus callosum is the basis for disconnection syndromes such as alexia without agraphia or transcortical dysphasias.

Even more variable are syndromes caused by tumors of or surrounding the third ventricle. Thalamic deficits are rarely complete, and even diffuse infiltration can remain asymptomatic in slow-growing tumors. Unilateral tumors cause contralateral hypesthesia and hemiataxia. Hemiparesis results from infiltration of the posterior limb of the internal capsule. Thalamic pain syndromes are characterized by hyperpathia and allodynia. Language disturbances are complex and involve receptive and expressive functions. Bilateral involvement of nuclei of the reticular activating system causes somnolence in the absence of spinal fluid obstruction. Psychomotor slowing and profound memory impairment have been described, usually with bilateral lesions. Destruction of subthalamic and basal ganglionic structures elicits extrapyramidal syndromes. Infiltration of the hypothalamus disrupts the hypothalamopituitary hormonal axis and results in numerous vegetative signs or symptoms such as hyperthermia and hypothermia due to dysfunction of central temperature regulatory mechanisms and electrolyte imbalances (central diabetes insipidus, syndrome of inappropriate secretion of antidiuretic hormone). Hyperphagia has been linked to destruction of a satiety center located in the ventromedial nucleus of the hypothalamus. Emaciation due to destruction of a hypothalamic appetite center has not been clearly established in adults. In children, a syndrome denoted as the diencephalic syndrome (progressive emaciation despite normal food intake) occurs with hypothalamic tumors. Other manifestations of hypothalamic neoplasms are hypersexuality or loss of sexual interest, pubertas praecox in children, disturbances of affect control (pathologic laughing or crying), amnestic syndromes, somnolence, or disturbance of sleep-wake cycles. Gliomas of the optic chiasm result in blurred vision, various visual field defects, and proptosis. Infrachiasmatic mass lesions present with headaches projecting to the center of the forehead. Pressure on the optic chiasm from below is the basis for a bitemporal hemianopsia, the classic visual field defect from a pituitary adenoma. Partial field defects affecting the upper quadrants of the temporal visual fields may be an early sign. In addition to nonspecific, pressure-related effects, symptoms caused by pituitary tumors reflect their hormone-producing status. Hemorrhage into a pituitary tumor, pituitary apoplexy, may constitute a neurosurgical emergency and presents with severe headache, panhypopituitarism, and visual field defect. Pituitary carcinomas and meningiomas of the lesser wing of the sphenoid bone infiltrate the cavernous sinus and result in ocular dysmotility due to compression of cranial nerves III, IV, and VI and facial paresthesias. Cerebrovascular complications are rare and more commonly reflect the effects of surgical intervention or radiation.

Tectal syndromes are observed with pineal region tumors. Parinaud's syndrome with conjugate upgaze inhibition, light-near dissociation of pupillary contraction, pathologic lid retraction (Collier's sign), and retraction nystagmus is rarely complete, but partial variants are common. Parenchymal invasion of the mesencephalon is the basis for nuclear third nerve palsies. As there is a higher incidence of intraventricular tumors in patients with phakomatoses, other physical findings may facilitate the diagnosis of ventricular neoplasms. Subependymal giant cell astrocytoma, a manifestation of tuberous sclerosis, and optic glioma in neurofibromatosis are associated with characteristic skin findings.

DIAGNOSIS AND CONSIDERATIONS FOR MANAGEMENT

Epidemiology

Tumors involving the ventricular system arise within the ventricle or protrude into it from surrounding structures. The majority of lateral ventricular tumors are low-grade, slow-growing tumors. There is an age- and location-dependent presentation of most tumor types. In adults,

low-grade neuroepithelial neoplasms (infiltrative gliomas, ependymal tumors) predominate (50%). One third of growths arise from the choroid plexus (meningioma, papilloma). Neuronal (neurocytomas), germ cell tumors (GCTs), and dysembryoplastic mass lesions (epidermoid) account for another 10% of lateral ventricular tumors. The remainder is composed of metastases, cysts originating from the ventricular wall or the septum pellucidum, and rare lesions such as lymphoma, schwannoma,[1] sarcoma,[2] intraventricular cavernoma,[3] hemangioendothelioma, hemangioblastoma,[4] and mixed glial-neuronal tumors.[5,6] Half of lateral ventricular neoplasms arise in the trigone, and 35% affect the body of the lateral ventricle. Ten percent are confined to the frontal horns and the remaining 5% to the temporal horn. Tumors restricted to the ventricular lumen are more common in children, and a larger proportion are malignant (more than one third). The most common histopathologic subtype is subependymal giant cell astrocytoma followed by tumors of the choroid plexus, ependymoma, and astrocytic tumors (commonly pilocytic astrocytoma).[7] Like lateral ventricular tumors, most of those occurring in the third ventricle are low grade. The most common purely intraventricular third ventricular mass lesion is the colloid cyst of the interventricular foramen.

Specific Tumor Types

Infiltrative gliomas (astrocytoma, oligodendroglioma, mixed glial tumors) are the most common neoplasms affecting lateral and third ventricles (Fig. 53-1). They arise from the surrounding subependymal white matter, the optic pathway, or glial elements of the basal ganglia and expand into the ventricle. Less common is their origin in intraventricular structures.[8] Magnetic resonance imaging identifies gliomas as hyperintense (compared with white matter) on T2-weighted sequences and hypointense on unenhanced T1-weighted images. Contrast enhancement is an ominous sign indicating an area of malignant degeneration. Vasogenic edema surrounding the tumor contributes to the mass effect on the ventricular system in high-grade tumors. High-grade tumors are also characterized by areas of necrosis

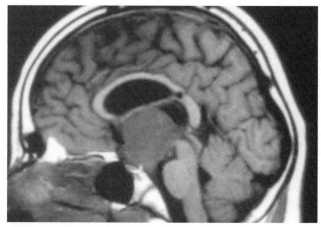

FIGURE 53-1 Midline sagittal magnetic resonance imaging of a glioma arising from and filling the third ventricle.

that are T1 hypointense and do not enhance. Although anterior third ventricular and lateral ventricular astrocytomas are usually only amenable to biopsy, a more aggressive surgical approach is generally employed for the posteriorly located neoplasms.

Gliomas of the optic pathway present during the first decade of life and are generally low grade. The pilocytic subtype predominates. In one third of cases, they are associated with neurofibromatosis 1.[9] Resection can be performed, resulting in potential cure with good quality of life in tumors of the optic nerve. Hypothalamic infiltration renders the tumor unresectable. Adjuvant radiation prolongs progression-free survival but is associated with endocrine dysfunction and memory loss. Chemotherapy has been used to defer irradiation.[10]

Subependymal giant cell astrocytoma is almost invariably located near the foramen of Monro.[11] A benign tumor, it occurs in 6% of patients with tuberous sclerosis. On magnetic resonance imaging, the mass appears as a T2-hyperintense, calcified subependymal lesion enhancing with gadolinium. Surgical removal is curative and indicated when CSF flow is obstructed.

The anterior third ventricle is a common location of supratentorial juvenile pilocytic astrocytoma. It generally arises from the anterior floor of the third ventricle or optic pathways.[12] On imaging studies, nodules of contrast enhancement can be distinguished from cystic areas. The tumor is benign, but due to its location, the risk of tumor- or treatment-related morbidity is considerable.

The histogenetic origin of chordoid glioma remains unknown. This rare tumor grows in the third ventricle of adults. Women are more commonly affected. The excellent prognosis reflects the extent of surgical resection. The tumor tends to adhere to neighboring structures, increasing the risk of surgical morbidity and incomplete removal.[13,14]

Ependymomas occur along the neuraxis, usually within or in proximity to the ventricles or subarachnoid space. Intracranial ependymoma is more common in children (infratentorial more frequent than supratentorial) and spinal ependymoma in adults. Infratentorial growth typically occurs within the fourth ventricle. Supratentorial ependymomas are more commonly located outside the ventricular system. Of the few intraventricular tumors, the majority is found within the trigone of the lateral ventricle. Third ventricular ependymomas are rare.[11] Only a small fraction of ependymomas is high grade. Calcification and intratumoral cysts give rise to a heterogeneous appearance and enhancement pattern on magnetic resonance imaging. Complete surgical removal is indicated and may cure the patient with a low-grade ependymoma. Radiation therapy is beneficial to patients with residual symptomatic tumor after operation, at recurrence, or with aggressive histology.[15] Leptomeningeal tumor dissemination requires craniospinal irradiation. Chemotherapy is provided when all other approaches have failed.[16]

Subependymomas are benign tumors in proximity to the ventricular system.[11] The fourth ventricle is the most common location followed by the septum pellucidum and the lateral ventricles (Fig. 53-2). The tumor is well demarcated and may contain areas of calcification and cysts. Not uncommonly, its detection is incidental, and surgical

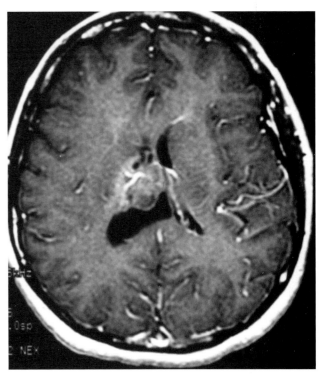

FIGURE 53-2 Axial enhanced magnetic resonance imaging of a subependymoma arising in the right lateral ventricle causing obstruction.

resection, though curative, is rarely needed unless it exhibits significant growth or obstruction to CSF flow.

Choroid plexus papilloma is one of the most common lateral ventricular tumors in children, although its overall incidence, especially in adults, is low.[17] The majority of tumors are located in the atrium and the velum medullare superius of the fourth ventricle (Fig. 53-3). Third ventricular masses, attached to its roof, are rare. On imaging studies, the tumor is characterized by its papillary growth pattern and homogeneous contrast enhancement. Cure is achieved through complete resection. Choroid plexus carcinoma is much less common than its benign counterpart. Adjuvant radiation to the tumor bed or, when leptomeningeal seeding occurs, the craniospinal axis, and chemotherapy are required.

Neurocytomas are rare tumors of neuronal origin that are typically found at the inferior septum pellucidum near the foramen of Monro between the second and fourth decades of life. Fifteen percent of tumors involve both the lateral and third ventricles.[11] On imaging studies, the tumor has a lobulated appearance and may contain cysts and calcification. Contrast enhancement is variable and heterogeneous (Fig. 53-4). The tumor is broadly adherent to the interventricular septum or the ventricular wall. In less than 50% of patients, surgical cure is accomplished. However, long-term tumor control can be achieved with partial resection. Rare are cases with anaplastic features for which conventional or stereotactic radiation and chemotherapy are available.[18–20]

Meningioma is the most common atrial mass and presents during the fourth to fifth decades of life.[5,11] Less common is

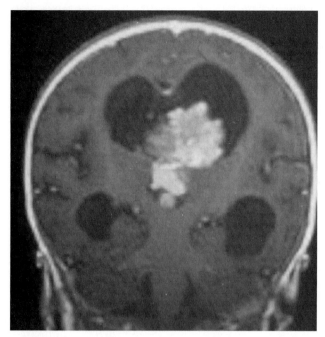

FIGURE 53-3 Coronal enhanced magnetic resonance imaging of a choroid plexus papilloma arising from the left lateral ventricle and extending into the third ventricle.

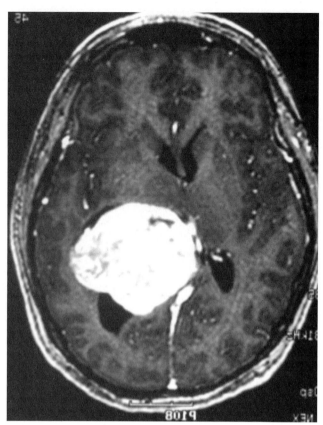

FIGURE 53-5 Axial enhanced magnetic resonance imaging of a meningioma arising in the trigone of the right lateral ventricle and causing obstruction.

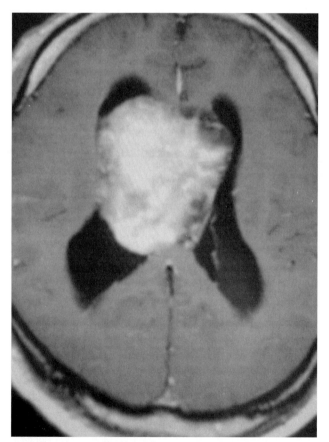

FIGURE 53-4 Axial enhanced magnetic resonance imaging of a central neurocytoma filling the right lateral ventricle and distending into the left with ipsilateral obstruction.

third ventricular location. A computed tomography (CT) scan shows an isodense, well-circumscribed tumor, which may be calcified and enhances brightly (Fig. 53-5). These tumors are treated surgically, and complete resection is the goal.[21]

Germ cell tumors (GCTs) of the central nervous system are rare tumors of childhood and adolescence predominantly affecting males. Manifestation after the second decade is exceptional. The most common GCT occurring in the central nervous system is germinoma, which shares a common histology with testicular seminoma and ovarian dysgerminoma (Fig. 53-6). Less common are nongerminomatous GCTs (teratoma, embryonal carcinoma, yolk sac tumor [endodermal sinus tumor], choriocarcinoma, and mixed GCTs). The entire group has a proclivity for midline structures, the sellar and suprasellar region, walls of the third ventricle, and the pineal gland, and subependymal and leptomeningeal spread. Lateral ventricular GCTs are rare.[22] Surgical access is difficult and often limits intervention to biopsy. Treatment planning depends on careful analysis of resected tissue and evaluation of serologic and CSF levels of β-human chorionic gonadotropin, α-fetoprotein, and placental alkaline phosphatase. On magnetic resonance imaging, GCTs appear as avidly enhancing masses. Teratomas, composed of tissue derived from all three germinal layers, display heterogeneous signal characteristics. Traditionally, treatment of GCTs has included surgical resection or biopsy followed by radiation therapy. Neuro-oncologists make

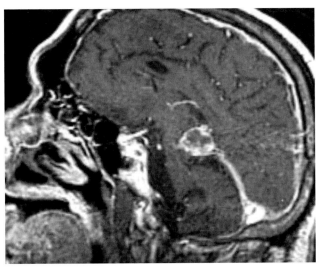

FIGURE 53-6 Midline enhanced sagittal magnetic resonance imaging of a germ cell tumor of the posterior third ventricle.

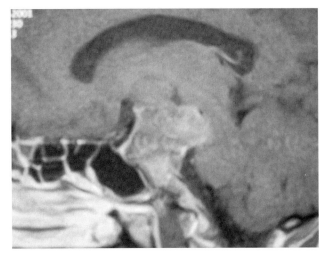

FIGURE 53-7 Midline enhanced sagittal magnetic resonance imaging of a craniopharyngioma filling the anterior third ventricle.

increasing use of platinum-based chemotherapy, allowing for limitation of surgical intervention and reduction of radiation dose and field. Whereas the prognosis for germinomas and mature teratomas is excellent, only 10% to 15% of patients with embryonal carcinoma, yolk sac tumor, or choriocarcinoma survive 3 years after diagnosis.[23–25]

Pineocytoma, pineal parenchymal tumors of intermediate differentiation, and pineoblastoma are rare tumors of the pineal gland.[26,27] The more malignant tumors are seen in younger patients; more than 90% of the pineoblastoma patients are younger than age 23, whereas after the age of 40 years, one third of the masses are tumors of low or intermediate grade.[28] On CT scan, pineocytomas are well circumscribed and display homogeneous enhancement and occasional calcifications. Pineoblastomas have a similar appearance but invade adjacent structures. There is uncertainty regarding the role of surgery. CT- or magnetic resonance imaging–based stereotactic biopsies are performed in many centers. Tertiary neurosurgical hospitals advocate complete tumor resection. Radiation therapy to the pineal region and the craniospinal axis is provided to patients with high-grade neoplasms, residual tumor after surgery, and subarachnoid dissemination. As for other neuroblastic neoplasms, platinum- and nitrogen mustard–based chemotherapy is used in the setting of malignant pineal parenchymal tumor that is disseminated at onset or at recurrence. Its neoadjuvant use may decrease morbidity of surgery or irradiation in selected cases.

Craniopharyngiomas are tumors derived from Rathke's pouch epithelium and constitute 3% to 5% of all intracranial neoplasms (Fig. 53-7). Whereas expansion into the anterior third ventricle and hypothalamus is common, pure intraventricular growth occurs in less than 10% of cases. Two types are distinguished. Adamantinomatous craniopharyngioma is seen in the pediatric population and displays a more aggressive behavior. The papillary type is more common in adults.[29] A CT scan shows an often cystic (in 90%), multilobulated calcified mass. Enhancement is present in the solid portions and cyst wall. Magnetic resonance imaging appearance is variable and depends on cyst content.[30]

Complete resection is curative, although the infiltrative nature of these tumors at their diencephalic interface makes that goal difficult to attain.[31–33]

Primary lymphoma of the central nervous system constitutes 2% of primary brain tumors. The disease has a propensity to infiltrate subependymal structures (Fig. 53-8). The hypothalamus, pineal gland, and choroid plexus are involved frequently. The vast majority of infiltrates enhance on imaging studies. Due to their cell density, they appear hyperdense to white matter on CT and show restricted proton diffusion on MRI. Diagnosis usually

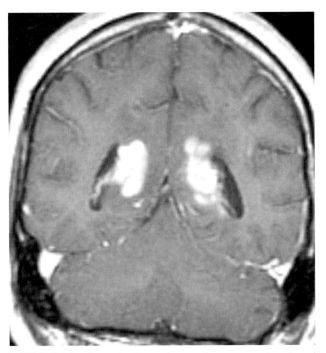

FIGURE 53-8 Coronal enhanced magnetic resonance imaging of primary central nervous system lymphoma in the subependymal layer of both lateral ventricles.

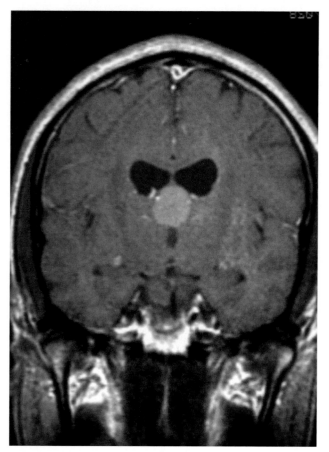

FIGURE 53-9 Coronal enhanced magnetic resonance imaging of a colloid cyst of the third ventricle.

requires stereotactic tissue acquisition; when lesions are inaccessible, diagnosis can be established through cytopathologic evaluation or immunoglobulin gene rearrangement analysis of spinal fluid in a small subset of patients. Methotrexate-based chemotherapy is the treatment of choice. There is no indication for surgical removal. Radiation is increasingly reserved for chemoresistant disease to avoid its neurotoxic effects.[34]

Metastases to the ventricular system are infrequent, accounting for less than 5% of secondary brain tumors. They only pose a diagnostic challenge when they occur in isolation, and an underlying malignancy is not known. They have been reported in the choroid plexus of the lateral, third, and fourth ventricles; the pituitary gland; and the anterior part of the third ventricle as well as the pineal gland.[35] Choroid plexus metastases predominantly arise from renal and lung carcinoma in adults, whereas in children, Wilms' tumor and retinoblastoma predominate.[11] On a CT scan, they are generally hyperdense with marked enhancement. Surgery is rarely indicated unless there is diagnostic uncertainty.

Histiocytosis with central nervous system manifestations affect children more commonly, and this entity also has a predilection for the floor of the third ventricle. There is a male preponderance, and clinically patients present with pituitary dysfunction and bony skeletal lesions. Surgery, when performed, is for biopsy because these lesions are radiosensitive.

There are several nonneoplastic entities that can present in the third and lateral ventricles, and these need to be considered as part of the differential diagnosis.

The most common third ventricular mass lesion in adults is the colloid cyst (Fig. 53-9). This likely congenital, slowly expanding lesion can present at any age but typically manifests itself in midadulthood. It is located in the anterior roof of the third ventricle at the level of the foramen of Monro.[36] Cyst content determines appearance on imaging studies. On CT scan, a round, homogeneous hyperdense mass is seen at the level of the foramen of Monro. On T2-weighted magnetic resonance images, the cyst can be either hypo- or hyperintense.[37,38] Indication for surgery is determined by the presence of symptoms, cyst size, and patient's age. As sudden deaths have been reported in patients with a colloid cyst, resection is recommended in young patients with lesions exceeding 1.5 cm in diameter even if they are asymptomatic.[39]

Epidermoids and dermoids are uncommon dysembryoplastic third ventricular mass lesions that grow by displacing surrounding tissue rather than invading it (Figs 53-10 and 53-11). On a CT scan, these tumors are hypodense and do not enhance. The dermoids contain fat (hyperintense on T1) and can be calcified, whereas the epidermoids do not. Epidermoids are hyperintense on diffusion-weighted images (Fig. 53-12). Surgical resection is curative. Spontaneous or intraoperative leakage of cyst material into the CSF gives rise to an aseptic meningitis.

SURGICAL ANATOMY

The lateral and third ventricles are divided into specific areas that help define both the pathology and the surgical approaches. Specific types of tumors tend to occur regularly

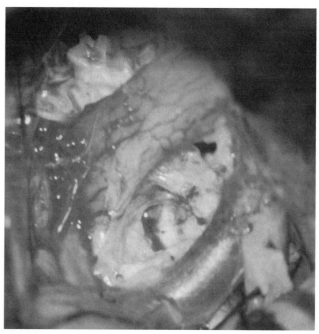

FIGURE 53-10 Intraoperative view of an epidermoid distending the right optic nerve, carotid artery, and anterior third ventricle.

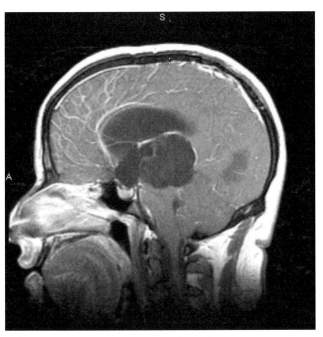

FIGURE 53-11 Midline sagittal enhanced magnetic resonance imaging of a epidermoid arising in the posterior third ventricle.

in specific anatomic areas of the third and lateral ventricles that assist the differential diagnosis.

Lateral Ventricular Anatomy

The lateral ventricles are C-shaped, CSF-filled cavities that can be divided into five areas: (1) the frontal horns, (2) the bodies, (3) the atria, (4) the occipital horns, and (5) the temporal horns. The frontal horns are triangular extensions of the lateral ventricles anterior to the foramen of Monro and are bounded laterally by the head of the caudate, anteriorly and superiorly by the corpus callosum, and medially by the septum pellucidum. Posteromedially, the foramen of Monro marks the posterior extent of the frontal horns, and the boundary consists of the forniceal columns that run just anterior to the foramen of Monro as they bend inferiorly to start their descent toward the mammillary bodies. The floor consists of the rostrum of the corpus callosum as it curves underneath the frontal horn (Fig. 53-13). The frontal horn contains no choroid plexus but has on its wall surface two important veins that help with the surgical orientation. On its infero-medial border, the anteroseptal vein leads into the medial foramen of Monro, where it enters the velum interpositum in the roof of the third ventricle to join the internal cerebral vein (ICV). Laterally, the anterior caudate vein runs medioinferiorly to join the thalamostriate vein near the foramen of Monro.

The body of the lateral ventricles begins at the posterior edge of the foramen of Monro and extends posteriorly to

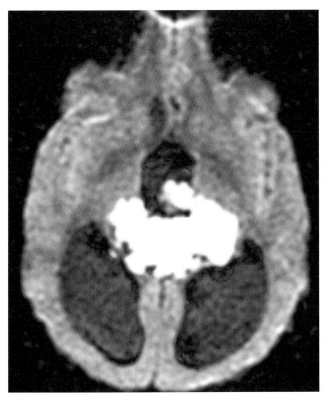

FIGURE 53-12 Axial diffusion weighted image of an epidermoid in the posterior third ventricle.

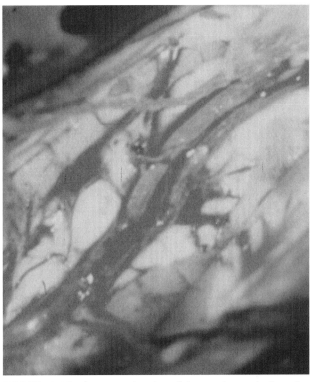

FIGURE 53-13 Intraoperative view of the anterior cerebral arteries over a distended corpus callosum.

the anterior border of the splenium of the corpus callosum, an area where the septum pellucidum tapers off. The body of the ventricle is covered superiorly by the corpus callosum and laterally by the body of the caudate. There are two sets of veins that travel on the lateral wall of the body: the more anterior thalamocaudate (the size of which is inversely proportional to the thalamostriate vein) and the posterior caudate vein, which drains into the thalamostriate. Inferiorly, the junction of the lateral wall and floor of the body of the ventricle is demarcated by the striothalamic sulcus, which separates the caudate from the thalamus (Fig. 53-14). In this sulcus, one finds the thalamostriate vein coursing anteriorly to the foramen of Monro. The vein generally curves around the foramen of Monro to drain into the ICVs. The curve of this vein can often be seen on cerebral angiography and is called the venous angle. One should note that occasionally this vein drains more posteriorly through the choroidal fissure directly into the ICV without going through the foramen of Monro. Medial to this vein, the thalamus protrudes to make up the ventricular floor. Medial to the thalamus, separating the thalamus from the body of the fornix, is the choroidal fissure. This fissure is obscured by the choroid plexus, in which the superior

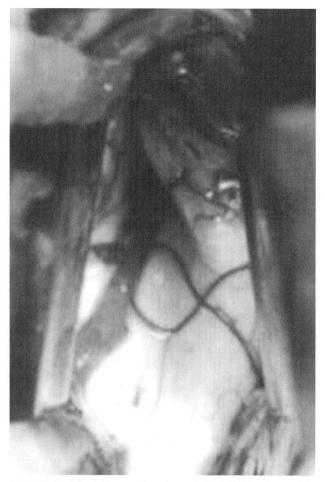

FIGURE 53-14 Intraoperative view of the left lateral ventricle showing the choroid plexus, thalamostriate vein, and septum pellucidum.

choroidal vein, which starts posteriorly in the atrium and may anastomose with the inferior choroidal vein, flows toward the foramen of Monro. The medial posterior choroidal artery, which enters the ventricular system just lateral to the pineal and travels anteriorly in the roof of the third ventricle in the velum interpositum, can be seen in the lateral ventricle as it ascends through the foramen of Monro and bends posteriorly to run in the direction of the choroid plexus. Coming from the atrial side of the ventricle, the lateral posterior choroidal artery courses anteriorly toward the foramen of Monro and may anastomose with the medial posterior choroidal artery. Medially, the two leaves of the septum pellucidum separate the two ventricles. On their surface, one can see the posterior septal veins, which run inferiorly, pierce the choroid fissure, and drain into the ICVs.

The trigone or atrium of the lateral ventricles is a confluence of the body and temporal and occipital horns. The atrium begins as a continuation of the body at the posterior edge of the thalamus and ends further posteriorly as the bulb of the corpus callosum blends into the occipital lobe. The splenium (superiorly) and the tapetum of the corpus callosum (more posteriorly) make up the roof of the atrium. Because the roof bends into the lateral wall posteriorly, the tapetum covers this lateral wall segment. More anteriorly, the caudate tail covers the lateral wall as it curves downward, on its way toward the temporal lobe. On the surface of the lateral wall, just below the ependyma, the lateral atrial veins can be seen running inferiorly and medially toward the choroid fissure. This vein starts posteriorly in the occipital horn and empties, once through the choroidal fissure, in the basal vein, ICV, or great vein of Galen. The anterior boundary of the atrium starts just medial to the caudate tail with the pulvinar eminence. Medial to the pulvinar, covered by choroid, is the crus of the fornix. At the atrial level of the choroid plexus, two choroidal arteries can often be seen, one curving with the choroid medially and the anterior choroidal artery, which can course into the body of the ventricle. More laterally, the lateral posterior choroidal artery, which may have several branches, runs to supply the atrium and body of the choroid. The choroid plexus itself forms a triangular enlargement at the trigone called the glomus of the choroid plexus. The medial wall of the atrium has two prominences. The upper prominence consists of the forceps major fibers and is called the bulb of the corpus callosum. The lower prominence is called the calcar avis and is simply the ventricular protrusion of the calcarine sulcus. The floor similarly consists of the upward protrusion of the collateral sulcus forming the collateral trigone. On the surface of the medial wall, the medial atrial vein can be seen coursing toward the choroid fissure to pierce it and drain into the great vein of Galen, basal vein, or ICV.

The occipital horn is a posterior extension of the atrium and can vary in size. Medially, the wall consists of the same structures that make up the atrial medial wall, namely, the forceps major superior and, inferiorly, the calcar avis. Likewise, the collateral trigone forms the floor of the occipital horn. The roof and lateral wall blend into one and are both covered by the tapetum. There is no choroid in the occipital horn. The veins of the occipital horn are the posterior extension of the lateral and medial atrial veins.

The temporal horn is an extension of the lateral ventricles into the medial temporal lobe. The floor displays two prominences: (1) laterally the collateral eminence formed by the underlying deep collateral sulcus and (2) medial to that, the hippocampus, which protrudes prominently into the floor. Seen running longitudinally over the hippocampal surface is a set of veins called the transverse hippocampal veins. These veins penetrate through the space between the fimbria and hippocampus into the ambient cistern, where they drain into the anterior and posterior hippocampal veins. The latter drain into the basal vein. The lateral wall, which angles into the roof of the temporal horn, is lined by the tapetum. In the medial part of the roof, the tail of the caudate projects anteriorly toward the amygdaloid nucleus. In this area, on the ventricular surface, the inferior ventricular vein runs in an anteromedial direction to exit through the choroid fissure at the level of the so-called inferior choroidal point and drain into the basal vein near the lateral geniculate body. Medial to the caudate tail, forming the medial wall of the temporal horn, is the thalamus and, inferior to it, the fimbria of the fornix. The choroid fissure separates the thalamus from the fornix. The choroid plexus is attached as it continues anteriorly to end just posterior to the amygdaloid nucleus at the inferior choroidal point. The anterior choroidal artery enters the choroidal fissure at approximately this point and courses posteriorly in the plexus. More posteriorly, the lateral posterior choroidal artery enters the fissure and is seen more laterally in the choroid plexus. Starting at about the level of the atrium and draining anteriorly toward the "inferior choroidal point," the inferior choroidal vein is seen on the surface of the choroidal fissure. It drains into the basal vein. The temporal horn ends blindly anteriorly in the amygdaloid nucleus, on the surface of which can be seen the amygdalar vein, which drains into the inferior ventricular vein.[40–44]

Third Ventricular Anatomy

The third ventricle communicates with the lateral ventricles via the foramen of Monro and drains posteriorly into Sylvius' aqueduct. Approximately one third of the third ventricle is located anterior to the foramen of Monro and extends inferiorly to the optic chiasm. The anterior wall consists mainly of the lamina terminalis, which is a thin sheet of pia and gray matter that runs between the optic chiasm inferiorly to the rostrum of the corpus callosum superiorly. The columns of the fornix are found at the superior lateral margins, and the anterior commissure crosses the anterior wall at its upper end. The lateral wall of the third ventricle is formed inferiorly by the hypothalamus and superiorly and posteriorly by the thalamus. At the upper and posterior end of the third ventricle, a thalamic projection, the massa intermedia often connects (in 75% of cases) with its counterpart on the other side. The floor of the third ventricle starts anteriorly and inferiorly at the optic chiasm; progressing posteriorly, the floor dips into the infundibular recess. The floor slants superiorly and posteriorly over the tuber cinereum and then the two mammillary bodies and posterior perforated substance, which is located anterior to the cerebral peduncles. Posterior to the level of the peduncles is the aqueduct, which is surrounded by the tegmentum of the midbrain. The roof of the third ventricle starts anteriorly at the foramen of Monro and ends posteriorly in the suprapineal recess. The roof is separated from the lateral

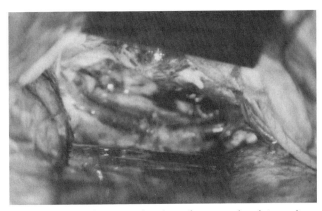

FIGURE 53-15 Intraoperative view of a transvelum interpositum approach to the third ventricle.

wall by the choroidal fissure, which runs in the cleft between the upper part of the thalamus and the fornix. Over the anterior part of the roof, the fornices run in parallel and are often attached into the body of the fornix, whereas over the posterior roof, the fornices separate into the forniceal crura, and the roof is draped by interforniceal-connecting white matter called the hippocampal commissure. However, the fornices and hippocampal commissure in the roof of the third ventricle are covered by a loose trabecular pial tissue that forms a double layer called the tela choroidea (Fig. 53-15). Between these two layers of tela choroidea is a space, the velum interpositum, through which the ICVs and the medial posterior choroidal arteries course. The ICVs start at the posterior edge of the foramen of Monro and run posteriorly to exit the velum interpositum just above the pineal body. The third ventricular choroid plexus is attached to the roof by the tela choroidea, which communicates through the choroidal fissure with the lateral ventricular tela choroidea. The posterior wall of the third ventricle begins at Sylvius' aqueduct anteriorly and inferiorly. Proceeding in a posterior and superior direction, the posterior wall of the third ventricle contains the posterior commissure, the pineal body, the habenular commissure, and the suprapineal recess above.[45–47]

SURGICAL OPTIONS FOR THE LATERAL VENTRICLES

There are numerous surgical approaches to the ventricular system. The optimal choice of the best route is largely dictated by the location and extent of the tumor, the presence of hydrocephalus, preoperative neurologic deficits, and the anticipated operative goals. The shortest possible route to the tumor may not be the best approach. Thus any preexisting ventriculomegaly may serve to provide access to the lesion through a cortical or callosal incision. Particular attention should be directed toward the vasculature, including the cortical draining veins, and, whenever possible, their drainage patterns should be preserved. Adequate identification of the variation in cortical venous drainage patterns as well as the deep veins of the galenic system often can be obtained with magnetic resonance arteriography and magnetic resonance venography. Finally, the surgeon's experience

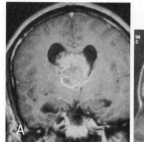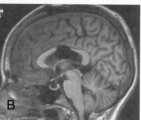

FIGURE 53-16 Coronal enhanced magnetic resonance imaging (MRI) of a midbody central neurocytoma (*A*). *B*, Postoperative MRI after transcallosal resection of the neurocytoma shows the location and extent of the callosal sectioning.

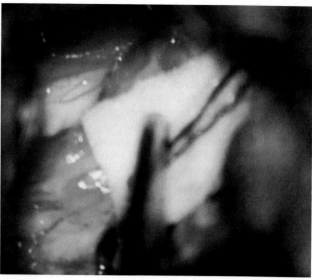

FIGURE 53-17 Intraoperative view of an intraventricular tumor (under the instrument) and the interface with the ependymal surface.

and comfort level with specific operative approaches must be included in the design of a surgical approach.

Transcallosal Approaches to the Lateral Ventricle

The transcallosal approach is commonly used to access the lateral and third ventricles. This route is useful for lesions arising within the body of the lateral ventricle as well as for access to the third ventricle (Fig. 53-16). The preoperative cerebral angiogram or a magnetic resonance venogram is important in the preoperative planning. Cortical veins draining into the sagittal sinus can be a significant obstacle to interhemispheric access. Furthermore, the ventricular venous and arterial structures can be distorted by the tumor and should be noted preoperatively. The patient is placed in a supine position, with the head slightly flexed. Alternatively, the patient's head is fixed in a lateral position with the affected hemisphere toward the floor to use gravity to assist with retraction. A bicoronal incision is made just posterior to the coronal suture. The craniotomy is often centered on the coronal suture. Midline exposure should extend up to the superior sagittal sinus. The dura is opened and reflected medially up to the sagittal sinus. Often, cortical draining veins enter the dura before reaching the midline. These veins may be preserved by opening the dura on both sides around the veins and leaving the venous access to the sagittal sinus intact. If exuberant arachnoid granulations are encountered, they can be divided with sharp dissection and bipolar cautery. Once the midline is reached, the falx is followed to its depth. At this point, the operating microscope is used. At the inferior edge of the falx, small cingulate gyrus veins may be encountered as they drain into the inferior sagittal sinus. These veins may be sacrificed. The arachnoid below the falx may be adherent, and this arachnoid must be divided carefully not to injure the cingulate gyrus on either side. After placing protective patties over the brain surface, the frontal lobe is retracted laterally. Once the corpus callosum is reached, the two pericallosal arteries are visualized (see Fig. 53-13). Ventricular access between the two arteries helps to prevent vascular injury. The callosotomy can be started just posterior to the genu and developed 3 cm posteriorly to gain access to the lateral ventricle. Occasionally, the opposite lateral ventricle is entered, and orientation is

achieved by locating septal vein and the thalamostriate vein running to the foramen of Monro. The interface between the tumor and the ependymal surface should be identified and preserved as this prevents losing the plane of dissection (Fig. 53-17). Since many lateral ventricular tumors can reach a very large size, resection proceeds by first doing internal debulking, then isolating the tumor capsule away from surrounding ventricular structures.[40,48–51]

The posterior transcallosal approach gains access to the roof and medial part of the atrium of the lateral ventricles. This is achieved, however, at the expense of splitting the splenium of the corpus callosum and is contraindicated for patients with a preoperative right homonymous hemianopia. Because the lateral ventricle extends laterally in this region, the lateral part of the atrium is not well visualized by this route. Preoperatively, as in the anterior approaches, a magnetic resonance arteriogram or cerebral angiogram helps to guide the placement of the craniotomy by visualizing the dominant cortical draining vessels. The patient is positioned in the three-quarter prone position, with the parietal area of the operated side in the dependent position. The anterior extent of the craniotomy is at the posterior edge of the post-central gyrus, and, depending on the venous anatomy, the posterior edge is approximately 4 cm posterior to that. The craniotomy exposes the superior sagittal sinus and extends laterally 3 to 4 cm. The dura is reflected medially, and care is taken to maintain the large draining veins. The parietal lobe is gently retracted (approximately 2 cm) away from the falx. Once arachnoid adhesions are opened, the distal pericallosal arteries and the splenium are identified. Below the splenium, the ICVs join Galen's vein, and these can be seen once the splenium is cut. The splenium is incised with a bipolar cautery, and this incision must be made lateral to the midline because the atrium of the lateral ventricle deviates laterally. Access into the atrium is now achieved; however, tumors not found in the medial part of the atrium will be hard to resect by this route, and the surgeon should consider the posterior transcortical route for lateral atrial tumors.[40,52,53]

One of the contraindications to transcallosal surgery is crossed dominance, a condition in which the hemisphere controlling the dominant hand is opposite the hemisphere mediating language and speech.[5,39,54] Crossed dominance can occur when there is evidence of extracallosal dysfunction, particularly after cerebral injury (surgery, trauma, infection) during childhood resulting in relocation of function. These patients may be at risk of writing and speech deficits after callosal sectioning. Another contraindication can arise if the splenium of the corpus callosum is sectioned in the presence of a homonymous hemianopia in the dominant hemisphere, causing alexia.

Transcortical Approaches

The anterior transcortical approach (middle frontal gyrus) is used commonly for lesions found specifically in the anterior part of the lateral and third ventricular system, especially when associated with hydrocephalus. In addition, this approach is preferred over the transcallosal route for large, dominant, draining cortical veins. The craniotomy is similar to the one used for the transcallosal approach and uses a bicoronal incision, a preferably right-sided craniotomy, lateral to the midline, measuring 4 to 6 cm in length. The superior and middle frontal gyri need to be exposed, but usually the middle frontal gyrus is accessed. Intraoperative ultrasound can provide guidance for direct ventricular access. Once confirmed, a 2- to 3-cm gyral incision is made and developed down into the ventricle. The operative microscope is used after the ventricular chamber is opened. Dissection proceeds by developing the tumor interface with the ependymal surface (see Fig. 53-17). Access into the third ventricle, if necessary, can be achieved by further developing this approach and

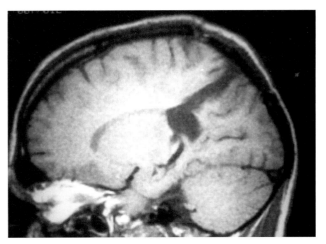

FIGURE 53-19 Postoperative magnetic resonance imaging of the transcortical approach to the tumor in Figure 53-18.

combining it with transforaminal or subchoroidal dissection into the third ventricle (described later).[40,55-57]

The posterior transcortical approach (superior parietal lobule) is the preferred route to the atrium of the lateral ventricle and allows access to both medial and lateral segments of the atrium (Figs 53-18 through 53-20). The patient is positioned in the three-quarter prone position with the parietal area of interest at the highest point in the field. The craniotomy extends, as in the posterior transcallosal approach, from the posterior margin of the postcentral gyrus, posteriorly approximately 4 cm. A preoperative magnetic resonance arteriogram or angiogram is helpful when determining the position of major draining veins. The craniotomy does not have to cross midline. Once the cortex is

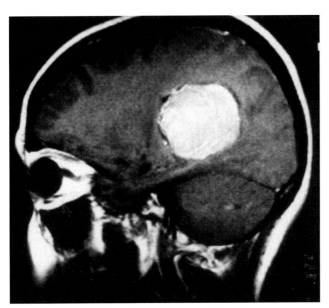

FIGURE 53-18 Sagittal enhanced magnetic resonance imaging of a meningioma of the trigone.

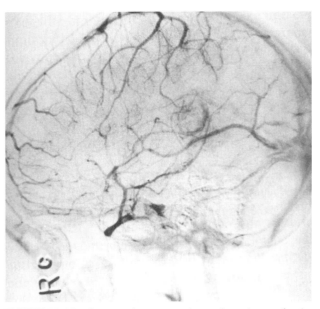

FIGURE 53-20 Preoperative venous phase of arteriogram for the tumor in Figure 53-18.

exposed, the cortical incision is made along the superior parietal gyrus. If the ventricular system is enlarged, before the cortical incision, it is useful to access the ventricle with a ventriculostomy. The atrium is more lateral at this location, and the direction of the dissection should reflect that. Once inside the atrium, should the tumor allow, the surgeon can visualize the thalamus anteriorly, the choroid plexus more medially, and the crus of the fornix. It should be remembered that the optic radiations course laterally to the atrium, and one should avoid dissecting into that area. The tumor should be debulked piecemeal before separating it from surrounding structures. Care should be taken to avoid blood pooling in the ventricles, which can lead to postoperative obstructive hydrocephalus. The vascular pedicle of the tumor should be identified and coagulated at the earliest possible time to avoid excessive bleeding.[40,58]

Inferior Temporal Approach

This approach is used to gain access to temporal horn lesions. The patient is placed supine, with the head tilted away by 45 degrees and extended. A reverse question mark incision is made starting at the level of the zygoma just anterior to the ear, then curving posteriorly over the ear and anteriorly toward the forehead. The temporalis muscle is mobilized anteriorly, and the craniotomy is extended inferiorly to the level of the zygoma. The dura is opened with its base anteriorly. Access to the ventricle is achieved either by first performing an anterolateral temporal lobectomy to include no more than the anterior 5 cm of the temporal lobe from the tip or by making a cortical incision in the middle or inferior temporal gyrus. The more inferior temporal approaches are often used for lesions residing in the temporal horn or lateral atrium of the dominant hemisphere. Debulking of the tumor is followed by dissection away from surrounding tissues.[40]

The transtemporal approach to the atrium or lateral horn is a transcortical route for lesions that are located laterally in the atrium or within the temporal horn (Fig. 53-21). The patient is positioned either supine with the head tilted at least 60 degrees away from the craniotomy side or in the lateral position. The reverse question mark incision runs approximately 5 cm posteriorly over the ear and behind it. The temporal craniotomy is performed across the base, just above the plane with the transverse sinus posteriorly. Extreme care should be taken not to injure the dura at this level because the vein of Labbe travels underneath to drain at the junction of the transverse and sigmoid sinus. Once the dura is exposed, on the nondominant side, an incision into the posterior middle or inferior temporal gyrus will gain access to the atrium. The incision should be along the axis of the gyrus. Once the ventricle is accessed, the tumor is removed piecemeal, then separated away from surrounding tissues. On the dominant side, the approach can be varied to avoid impairment in language abilities. The inferior temporal bone and mastoid air cells can be drilled or rongeured to gain access to the subtemporal area. The cortical incision is then made in the occipitotemporal gyrus. Although this avoids more of the optic radiations and is further removed from the speech cortex, this route requires more temporal lobe retraction. Care should be taken to avoid stretching or kinking the vein of Labbe. Furthermore, on closure of the subtemporal craniotomy, the mastoid air cells must be waxed,

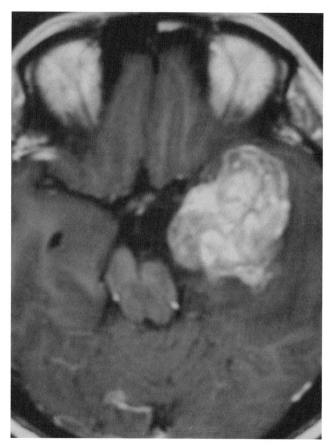

FIGURE 53-21 Axial enhanced magnetic resonance imaging of a choroid plexus papilloma of the temporal horn.

and closure must be watertight to avoid postoperative CSF leakage.

APPROACHES TO THE THIRD VENTRICLE

Transcallosal Approaches: Transforaminal, Transchoroidal, Subchoroidal, and Interforniceal

The transcallosal approaches to the third ventricle are a continuation of the approaches described earlier for access into the lateral ventricles. The anterior transcallosal approach is the most commonly used for access to the third ventricle and affords an excellent, low morbidity pathway to the level of the lateral ventricle. This strategy provides several paths of dissection to open into the third ventricular chamber. The structures that are most at risk of injury with third ventricular tumors are the fornices and the vessels within the velum interpositum (the ICVs and the medial posterior choroidal arteries). These approaches are adequate for lesions extending to or posterior to the foramen of Monro. Lesions that are anterior to the foramen of Monro and inferior in the third ventricle may not be as readily accessible by this route.

Access to the anterior part of the third ventricle via the transcallosal route can be accomplished through an enlarged the foramen of Monro. This transforaminal approach is particularly useful for tumors that dilate the foramen of Monro. Colloid cysts can be removed in this fashion with minimal manipulation of the foramen and the encircling fornix. The use of angled view ventriculoscopes has allowed visualization of third ventricular structures. However, access to the third ventricle is limited by the size of the foramen of Monro, and when this limitation prohibits further removal of the tumor, one of four approaches to the third ventricle can be developed from this vantage point. The first method is enlargement of the foramen of Monro by unilateral transection of the fornix. This allows anterior access into the third ventricle. This approach, however, has been associated with potential significant morbidity in memory impairment. Thus it is not a recommended route.[59–63]

A second approach is the interforniceal route to the third ventricle, which gains access by splitting the fornices in the sagittal plane, along the direction of their fibers. In this approach, the septum pellucidum is opened wide and used as a guide to the midline. The great advantage of this approach is that posterior dissection can be carried out to expose the entire third ventricle. The ICVs have no reported branches between them and must be separated. The disadvantage of this method is the potential bilateral damage to the fornices, which are closely adherent over the body of the fornix.[55,64,65] Consequently, the interforniceal approach is best used for patients who have a cavum septum pellucidum.

The transchoroidal and subchoroidal routes are two related approaches that seek to gain access to the midline and posterior third ventricle without disturbing the forniceal body or columns (see Fig. 53-21). In the subchoroidal approach, the lateral ventricular choroid is separated from the thalamus. The tenia choroidea is cut, and the choroid plexus is reflected medially. The thalamostriate vein at the foramen of Monro is the anterior extent of the dissection, whereas posteriorly the exposure can be developed as far as the atrium. Once the tenia choroidea is cut, the velum interpositum and the ICVs are visualized. The velum is cut lateral to the ICVs, and both veins are displaced medially. The limitation in exposure with this maneuver can be the ipsilateral thalamic veins, which, if sacrificed, may lead to hemorrhagic thalamic infarcts. The advantage of this approach is the relative distance away from the body of the fornix and less manipulation of the ICVs.

In the transchoroidal route, the choroidal dissection is performed medial to the lateral ventricular choroid, through the tenia fornicis, separating the choroid from the body of the fornix. The choroid plexus is reflected laterally. This minimizes contact with the posterior choroidal artery and the superficial thalamic veins. Once the choroid is reflected laterally, the velum interpositum, the ICVs, and the medial posterior cerebral arteries are visualized. At this point, the ICVs are separated, and a plane is developed between them. There are no reported bridging veins between these vessels; nevertheless, because they run closely together, they require manipulation and intermittent compression to gain access to the third ventricle. The last layer in this approach to be split is the third ventricular choroid plexus, which must also be separated in the midline. Finally, one should keep in mind that the anatomy is often

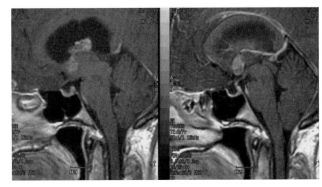

FIGURE 53-22 Sagittal enhanced magnetic resonance imaging images of a meningioma arising in the lateral ventricle and extending into the third ventricle through the foramen of Monro.

distorted; in this case, the preoperative radiographic studies are particularly useful.[42,45,66,67]

Subfrontal Approach

This approach is useful for midline suprasellar and anterior third ventricular lesions (Figs. 53-22 and 53-23). The exposure can be unilateral or bilateral, with olfaction being at risk. The patient is positioned supine, and a bicoronal incision in used. The unilateral craniotomy starts laterally at the pterion, runs just above the orbital ridge, and goes past the midline. For bilateral subfrontal approaches, the craniotomy extends from pterion to pterion. The flap is developed 4 to 5 cm above the orbital ridge. The brain is relaxed with mannitol and CSF drainage, while the frontal lobe is retracted gently. To reduce retraction and increase the upward angle of vision, the orbital ridges can be removed. For unilateral approaches, the ipsilateral olfactory nerve is often sacrificed. Care should be taken to coagulate small draining veins because they may rupture during retraction. Past the planum sphenoidale, the optic nerves, the chiasm, and both internal carotids are visualized. The tumor is generally evident

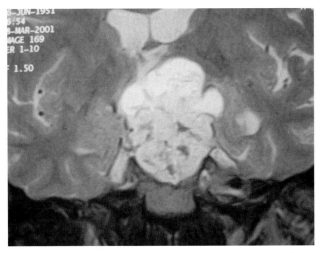

FIGURE 53-23 Coronal T2-weighted magnetic resonance imaging of a chordoma filling the anterior third ventricle.

at this stage. The A1 branches must be identified bilaterally to the level of the anterior communicating artery. If the tumor has a cystic component, such as in a craniopharyngioma, it is useful to decompress the cyst at this point. Care should be taken not to allow cystic contents to escape into the ventricle or subarachnoid space because it can cause aseptic meningitis. If the tumor does not contain a cystic component, then internal decompression is highly beneficial in reducing tension on surrounding structures during dissection of the capsule. The resection can be performed through the prechiasmatic space, the opticocarotid triangle, or the retrocarotid space. The latter two routes are the reasons for a wide craniotomy extending to the pterion. In patients with a prefixed chiasm, resection is particularly difficult to accomplish, and opening of the lamina terminalis must be performed. The lamina is opened above the chiasm and below the anterior cerebral vessels. In suprasellar tumors that extend upward into the anterior third ventricle, the anterior floor of the third ventricle is pushed upward. Thus, on opening the lamina, the tumor is covered by a thin third ventricular floor, which every effort should be made to save. Occasionally, the tumor can be accessed and delivered through either the prechiasmatic space or the opticocarotid triangle.[68–71]

Interhemispheric Approach

This approach is closely related to the subfrontal approach and allows access to suprasellar and anterior third ventricular lesions. The head position and incision are similar to those used in the subfrontal approach. A bifrontal craniotomy is performed, with the inferior margin as close to the anterior fossa floor base as possible. The dural incision cuts across midline; thus the anterior inferior segment of the superior sagittal sinus is sacrificed, as is the falx at this level. The olfactory nerves can be saved in most cases by dissecting the tracts away from the retracting frontal lobes. This approach affords good visualization of both optic nerves and carotid arteries and optimizes the access to the prechiasmatic space. However, this approach does put the frontal venous drainage system at risk.[72–74]

Pterional Approach

This approach is a common one to suprasellar tumors that extend into the anterior third ventricle. The weakness of this approach is the poor visualization of the ipsilateral third ventricular extension and contralateral opticocarotid and retrocarotid space. The positioning is supine, with the head tilted approximately 45 degrees to the left and in approximately 20 degrees of extension. The incision follows a hairline curve from the zygoma anterior to the ear to the frontal region. It is important to stay flush with the pterional base; alternatively, an orbital osteotomy maximizes the upward angle. The Sylvian fissure may need to be opened. Once CSF is released and brain relaxation is achieved, gentle retraction is applied to the frontal lobe. The tumor is accessed through the retrocarotid space, the opticocarotid triangle, and the prechiasmatic space. In addition, the lamina terminalis can be accessed and opened.[75]

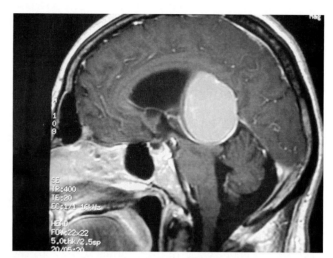

FIGURE 53-24 Sagittal enhanced magnetic resonance imaging of a meningioma compressing the posterior third ventricle with obstructive hydrocephalus.

SPECIFIC APPROACHES TO THE POSTERIOR THIRD VENTRICLE

Lesions in and around the posterior third ventricle, especially those of the pineal region, are accessed via several approaches that aim to maintain the integrity of the ICVs and Galen's vein and avoid injury to the midbrain (Fig. 53-24). Most of these patients present with hydrocephalus, which must be relieved at the time of surgery, either with shunting or ventriculostomy. Spinal drainage in cases of obstructive hydrocephalus is not indicated because compartmentalization of CSF may lead to herniation.

Infratentorial Supracerebellar Approach

This approach is well suited for midline tumors in the pineal region and avoids retraction or manipulation of the supratentorial brain. The approach is not adequately suited if the tumor infiltrates laterally or superiorly above the tentorium. The patient can be placed in the sitting position, the three-quarter prone position, or the prone position. The sitting position is optimal for brain relaxation; the cerebellum falls away, while venous drainage is optimized. If this position is chosen, armrests are crucial for the surgeon to avoid rapid fatigue. Furthermore, the patient is susceptible to air embolism in this position; thus a central line, carbon dioxide monitor, and compression stockings are advised. The incision is midline, and the wide suboccipital craniotomy is performed bilaterally to the level of the mastoids, thus exposing the transverse sinus and torculum. Inferiorly, the craniotomy is developed to a distance of approximately 1 cm from the foramen magnum. The dura is opened with its base superiorly. Retraction may be applied superiorly to the underside of the tentorium in the midline, while gentle inferior retraction can be placed on the vermis. Care should be taken to coagulate and divide cerebellar bridging veins because they drain superiorly into the tentorium. The arachnoid is thick and should be divided before the parapineal vessels and the tumor are visualized. The precentral cerebellar vein connects the vermis to Galen's vein. This vein can be sacrificed to gain access to the pineal. Resection of the tumor proceeds inferior to Galen's vein, the ICVs, and Rosenthal's basal vein. The quadrigeminal plate should be well visualized inferiorly. After resection, a postoperative shunt or ventriculostomy must be left to avoid immediate postoperative obstructive hydrocephalus.[76,77]

Occipital Transtentorial Approach

This approach is used for pineal and posterior third ventricular lesions with either supratentorial or infratentorial components because it allows a wide exposure. The patient can be placed in either the sitting or semiprone position, with the right side lower. However, whereas the sitting position helps in the infratentorial approach by allowing the cerebellum to fall away, the three-quarter prone position helps the occipital lobe to fall away, thus reducing need for retraction. The trapdoor incision is made with its base inferiorly and across the midline. The occipital craniotomy must extend across the midline and below the transverse sinus; it measures approximately 5 cm above the transverse sinus and lateral to the midline. The dura is opened with its base on the sinuses. Minimal retraction on the occipital lobe is necessary with adequate CSF drainage and brain relaxation. When retracting, the inferior tentorial surface should be retracted rather than the falx to avoid injuring the calcarine fissure. There are no significant draining veins from the medial occipital lobe into the tentorium, although there is a dominant cortical vein draining into the transverse sinus, the inferior cerebral vein, which should be lateral to the working area. The transection of the tentorium proceeds in a posterior to anterior direction by first making an incision proximally and then proceeding in a line approximately 1 cm off midline toward the tentorial edge. The tentorium is well vascularized, and hemostasis may require a bipolar cautery and clips. The thick arachnoid should be separated at the edge of the tentorium to avoid undue bleeding of small vessels. Once the tentorium is cut, it is gently retracted laterally with a suture. The deep veins around the pineal are surrounded in a thick arachnoid, which once cut reveal the anatomy. If necessary, the precentral cerebellar vein should be sacrificed to increase the working space. Tumor resection can proceed between the ICVs and Rosenthal's basal vein. A variation on this approach, the retrocallosal approach, can be developed if further exposure is necessary. The falx can be cut approximately 1 cm in anterior to the insertion of the vein of Galen into the sinus, after coagulating or clipping the inferior sagittal sinus. Retraction on the falx allows further exposure. The splenium does not have to be cut but can be gently retracted upward to allow extra exposure. Once the tumor is resected or debulked, the tentorium is simply returned to its position but does not need to be sutured.[78,79]

Posterior Transcallosal and Interhemispheric Approaches

This approach is suited for lesions in the mid to posterior third ventricle. The patient is placed in the lateral decubitus position; the side of approach (usually the right) is allowed to fall away. The craniotomy is centered more superiorly toward the area of the lambdoid suture, and the superior sagittal sinus is exposed. Generally, in the posterior third of the superior sagittal sinus, there are few noteworthy draining veins; however, an angiogram might be helpful in this position. The craniotomy is approximately 8 cm in the sagittal plane and extends laterally approximately 4 to 5 cm in a triangular fashion. The dura is opened with its base midline, and the hemisphere is separated from the falx. Lesions compressing the posterior third ventricle can be reached by this approach (see Fig. 53-20). The exposure of the corpus callosum must be made between the two pericallosal arteries from the splenium anteriorly for a distance of approximately 6 cm. A 3-cm corpus callosotomy is performed in the midline, leaving 2 to 3 cm of splenium intact posteriorly. The fornices should be just lateral to the midline, and care should be taken not to injure them. After the corpus callosum is cut, the tela choroidea is encountered, and the ICVs should be visible. A wide plane between the two can be developed to allow lateral displacement of the two vessels. Internal tumor debulking is performed before separating the tumor capsule away from the ventricular walls.[41,80–82]

ENDOSCOPIC APPROACH TO THE VENTRICLES

Minimally invasive neurosurgery is becoming the choice of approach in particular kinds of central nervous system lesions. The improvement of endoscopic techniques and instruments and good long-term results in endoscopically treated patients have established endoscopic approaches as an alternative to microsurgical techniques in selected cases.[83] The ventricular system seems to be a very suitable ground for neuroendoscopy being a fluid-filled space Useful applications of neuroendoscopy in the ventricular system are tumor biopsy under direct visualization and restoration of CSF flow by endoneurosurgically opening natural pathways.[84] The intraventricular lesions treated most commonly using an endoscopic approach are colloid cysts of the third ventricle. The details of the neuroendoscopy technique is beyond the scope of this chapter, but essentially the technique, although variations are possible, is as follows: Through a right or left frontal burr hole, a working sleeve is inserted. Placement can be controlled stereotactically or with ultrasound guidance. A video unit connected to a rigid endoscope with a 30-degree angled optical system is used. Microscopic instruments and bipolar coagulation inserted through the sleeve can be controlled in the visual field of the scope. This provides enough space and flexibility to separate tumor tissue or membranes and remove intraventricular tumors through the tube.[85] The advantages of using neuroendoscopy in selected cases, especially third ventricular tumors, are much greater when compared with transcallosal and transcortical craniotomy, stereotactic aspiration of the cyst contents, and indirect palliation of the associated hydrocephalus, with CSF diversion. Although microsurgery for most patients can completely extirpate their tumors, complications have been more frequently reported than with less invasive approaches. These complications include the risks that go along with frontal lobe retraction or incision and potential injury to deep venous and neural structures, such as the ICVs and fornices. Stereotactic puncture is minimally invasive, but colloid cyst contents may be too solid, thus making aspiration almost impossible. Furthermore, the lesion can be engulfed by neural or vascular structures, such as the choroid plexus, or covered by the large veins at the venous angle, which cannot be appreciated during stereotactic surgery. Frequently, the cyst or the adjacent tissue must be dissected or coagulated to adequately expose the tumor so safe resection is possible. Clearly, blind puncture of the colloid cyst would put these structures at risk. Ventricular shunting seems to be the least desirable therapeutic option because multiple catheters may be required if the lateral ventricles are not in communication and shunting does not necessarily relieve symptoms resulting from the tumor. The aggressive endoscopic approach using modern instrumentation, including bipolar cauterization, allows complete or nearly complete removal of the cyst wall and should result in a low recurrence rate, mostly without the consequences described.[86]

The choice of the procedure must be tailored to the tumor location within the third ventricle, the degree of ventriculomegaly, and the need to perform a septostomy.[84] Endoscopic colloid cyst resections can be challenging or impossible in some situations. First, the presence of small ventricles is a notably difficult situation technically. Second, recurrent colloid cysts would likely be a technical challenge because of the inevitable cicatrix formation within the ventricles. The risk of neurovascular injury and poor visualization endoscopically might make this approach difficult. Finally, small third ventricular lesions located within the roof posterior to the foramen of Monro would be difficult to remove with the rigid endoscope and would be associated with an increased risk of injury to the fornix. Consequently, these lesions might be better treated using a flexible endoscope.[86]

Bleeding is a major problem in endoscopic surgery. With well-adapted tools, this problem can be controlled without wide exposure, but one should be prepared to perform a craniotomy if necessary.[85]

Endoscopy can be used in selected cases in ventricular surgery, but even in appropriate cases, the risks of incomplete tumor removal, bleeding, and small operative corridor must be weighed against the 3-dimensional visualization of the operative microscope, wider operative field, greater chance of total resection, and better hemostasis.

COMPLICATIONS

Approaches to the lateral and third ventricles are difficult and potentially dangerous procedures and have a significant morbidity and mortality. Because of the numerous types of approaches and the varied pathology involved, it is difficult to make generalizations regarding morbidity. The complications are very specific to the type of tumor and its location.

Mortality

Surgery of the lateral and third ventricle has carried an extremely high mortality rate in the past (as high as 75%). With advances in microsurgery and improved understanding of anatomic pathways, the 30-day postoperative mortality at present is 5% to 12%. Among the immediate causes of the mortality were cerebral hemorrhage, infarction, brain swelling, and pulmonary embolus.

Cognitive Deficits

Many patients undergoing lateral and third ventricular surgery exhibit immediate postoperative impairment of cognitive functions. Some of these symptoms are related to the corpus callosum disconnection and include disturbed consciousness, a transient state of mutism, memory impairment and apathy, contralateral leg weakness, incontinence, and disinhibition. These symptoms can be seen in as many as 75% of patients but tend to resolve spontaneously within 3 weeks. Permanent changes in cognition are reported in 5% to 10%. Neuropsychological testing is useful in these cases. Persistent focal neurologic deficits such as impairment of motor function or a visual field cut are reported in 8% to 30% of cases.

Seizures

Postoperative seizures are more common in patients who undergo transcortical procedures, and past reports have indicated that approximately one third of patients have seizures in the postoperative period. In patients undergoing transcallosal procedures, the incidence is unknown, although it is presumed to be lower. Although most approaches avoid transversing cortical tissue, retraction injuries to the brain may account for postoperative seizures.

Hydrocephalus

Most of the lateral and third ventricular tumors present with hydrocephalus. Yet often, despite good resection of the tumor, hydrocephalus persists in as many as 33% of patients. These patients require shunting. Furthermore, these shunts often (>20% cases) malfunction, likely because of the higher protein content in the CSF of these postoperative patients, and there is an increased risk of shunt infection. Overshunting can add to the problem of postoperative subdural hematoma collections, which are found in approximately 40% of patients. Only one fourth of these require surgery for drainage of the subdural collection; nevertheless, this implies that approximately 10% of patients who under-go ventricular surgery will require drainage of a subdural collection later on. The more pronounced the preoperative ventriculomegaly, the higher is the risk of this complication.[83,87–91]

Multiple factors influence the successful outcome of surgery of the lateral and third ventricles. The approaches described have been developed to allow access to the ventricular system while minimizing manipulation of the surrounding brain. Among the numerous factors that are involved in choosing a particular surgical approach to these tumors are the location in the ventricles, the size, vascularity, feeding the blood supply, the presumptive pathology, and the surgeon's comfort level with a particular approach. Although treatment of these lesions can be complex and often difficult, a good surgical outcome, which

TABLE 53-1 ▪ Complication after Surgery for Third Ventricular Tumors

	Approach	
Complication	**Transcortical**	**Transcallosal**
Seizures	9%	0%
Hemiparesis	4%	2.5%
Memory loss	4%	33%
Infection	4%	12%
Death	17%	5.8%

maximizes the patient's quality of life, can now be anticipated in most cases.

Comparison of Transcortical and Transcallosal Approaches

An extensive review of complications related to surgery for third ventricular tumors was published in 1993.[52] The incidence of complications for reports published after 1980 is shown in Table 53-1.

The variability in the incidence of complications noted in Table 53-1 is not sufficiently reliable for recommending one operative approach over another. Because the frequency of unintended injury is in part related to surgical experience, the surgeon should chose the operative approach that is more familiar.

Partial sectioning of the corpus callosum rarely results in persistent neurologic problems; however, patients occasionally experience a disconnection syndrome with larger callosal incisions.[54] Contralateral hemiparesis, mutism, and hemineglect are common transient disconnection symptoms that routinely recover within days to weeks. Patients with a history of cortical injury and potential cortical reorganization may be at increased risk after callosal sectioning. Sectioning the splenium in a patient with a dominant hemisphere homonymous hemianopia can result in alexia and visual anomia. Patients with ipsilateral hand motor and speech dominance can result in agraphia and dysphasia. When dominant memory function resides in the hemisphere contralateral to speech, severe memory impairments can occur. These unique circumstances are uncommon but may be present, particularly in patients who have deficits from previous surgery or a history of a significant head injury, particularly during childhood.

REFERENCES

1. Erdogan E, Onguru O, Bulakbasi N, et al: Schwannoma of the lateral ventricle: Eight-year follow-up and literature review. Minim Invasive Neurosurg 40:50–53, 2003.
2. Baehring JM, Alemohammed S, Croul SE: Malignant fibrous histiocytoma presenting as an intraventricular mass five years after incidental detection of a mass lesion. J Neurooncol 52:157–160, 2001.
3. Reyns N, Assaker R, Louis E, Lejeune JP: Intraventricular cavernomas: Three cases and review of the literature. Neurosurgery 44:648–654, 1999.
4. Isaka T, Horibe K, Nakatani S, et al: Hemangioblastoma of the third ventricle. Neurosurg Rev 22:140–144, 1999.
5. Piepmeier JM: Tumors and approaches to the lateral ventricles. Introduction and overview. J Neurooncol 30:267–274, 1996.
6. Yin Foo LG, Scott G, Blumbergs PC, et al: Ganglioglioma of the lateral ventricle presenting with blepharospasm—Case report and review of the literature. J Clin Neurosci 8:279–282, 2001.
7. Zuccaro G, Sosa F, Cuccia V, et al: Lateral ventricle tumors in children: A series of 54 cases. Childs Nerv Syst 15:774–785, 1999.
8. Markwalder TM, Huber P, Markwalder RV, Seiler RW: Primary intraventricular oligodendrogliomas. Surg Neurol 11:25–28, 1979.
9. Khafaga Y, Hassounah M, Kandil A, et al: Optic gliomas: A retrospective analysis of 50 cases. Int J Radiat Oncol Biol Phys 56:807–812, 2003.
10. Tow SL, Chandela S, Miller NR, Avellino AM: Long-term outcome in children with gliomas of the anterior visual pathway. Pediatr Neurol 28:262–270, 2003.
11. Koeller KK, Sandberg GD: From the archives of the AFIP. Cerebral intraventricular neoplasms: Radiologic-pathologic correlation. Radiographics 22:1473–1505, 2002.
12. Forsyth PA, Shaw EG, Scheithauer BW, et al: Supratentorial pilocytic astrocytomas: A clinicopathologic, prognostic, and flow cytometric study of 51 patients. Cancer 72:1335–1342, 1993.
13. Raizer JJ, Shetty T, Gutin PH, et al: Chordoid glioma: Report of a case with unusual histologic features, ultrastructural study and review of the literature. J Neurooncol 63:39–47, 2003.
14. Brat DJ, Scheithauer BW, Staugaitis SM, et al: Third ventricular chordoid glioma: A distinct clinicopathologic entity. J Neuropathol Exp Neurol 57:283–290, 1998.
15. Schild SE, Nisi K, Scheithauer BW, et al: The results of radiotherapy for ependymomas: The Mayo Clinic experience. Int J Radiat Oncol Biol Phys 42:953–958, 1998.
16. Chamberlain MC: Ependymomas. Curr Neurol Neurosci Rep 3:193–199, 2003.
17. Rickert CH, Paulus W: Tumors of the choroid plexus. Microsc Res Tech 52:104–111, 2001.
18. Schild SE, Scheithauer BW, Haddock MG, et al: Central neurocytomas. Cancer 79:790–795, 1997.
19. Brandes AA, Amist inverted question marka P, Gardiman M, et al: Chemotherapy in patients with recurrent and progressive central neurocytoma. Cancer 88:169–174, 2000.
20. Yasargil MG, von Ammon K, von Deimling A, et al: Central neurocytoma: Histopathological variants and therapeutic approaches. J Neurosurg 76:32–37, 1992.
21. Fornari M, Savoiardo M, Morello G, Solero CL: Meningiomas of the lateral ventricles: Neuroradiological and surgical considerations in 18 cases. J Neurosurg 54:64–74, 1981.
22. Goetz CM, Schmid I, Pietsch T, et al: Mixed malignant germ cell tumour of the lateral ventricle in an 8-month-old girl: Case report and review of the literature. Childs Nerv Syst 18:644–647, 2002.
23. Matsutani M, Sano K, Takakura K, et al: Combined treatment with chemotherapy and radiation therapy for intracranial germ cell tumors. Childs Nerv Syst 14:59–62, 1998.
24. Sawamura Y, Shirato H, Ikeda J, et al: Induction chemotherapy followed by reduced-volume radiation therapy for newly diagnosed central nervous system germinoma. J Neurosurg 88:66–72, 1998.
25. Schild SE, Haddock MG, Scheithauer BW, et al: Nongerminomatous germ cell tumors of the brain. Int J Radiat Oncol Biol Phys 36:557–563, 1996.
26. Baumgartner JE, Edwards MS: Pineal tumors. Neurosurg Clin N Am 3:853–862, 1992.
27. Kleihues P, Louis DN, Scheithauer BW, et al: The WHO classification of tumors of the nervous system. J Neuropathol Exp Neurol 61:215–225, 2002.
28. Chang SM, Lillis-Hearne PK, Larson DA, et al: Pineoblastoma in adults. Neurosurgery 37:383–390, 1995.
29. Crotty TB, Scheithauer BW, Young WF Jr, et al: Papillary craniopharyngioma: A clinicopathological study of 48 cases. J Neurosurg 83:206–214, 1995.
30. Ahmadi J, Destian S, Apuzzo ML, et al: Cystic fluid in craniopharyngiomas: MR imaging and quantitative analysis. Radiology 182:783–785, 1992.
31. Behari S, Banerji D, Mishra A, et al: Intrinsic third ventricular craniopharyngiomas: Report on six cases and a review of the literature. Surg Neurol 60:245–252, 2003.

32. Van Effenterre R, Boch AL: Craniopharyngioma in adults and children: A study of 122 surgical cases. J Neurosurg 97:3–11, 2002.

33. Yasargil MG, Curcic M, Kis M, et al: Total removal of craniopharyngiomas. Approaches and long-term results in 144 patients. J Neurosurg 73:3–11, 1990.

34. Baehring JM, Hochberg FH: Central nervous system lymphoma in AIDS and non-AIDS patients. In Black P, Loeffler J (eds): Cancer of the Nervous System. Philadelphia: Lippincott Williams & Wilkins, 2004, pp 589–603.

35. Kakita A, Kobayashi K, Aoki N, et al: Lung carcinoma metastasis presenting as a pineal region tumor. Neuropathology 23:57–60, 2003.

36. Lach B, Scheithauer BW, Gregor A, Wick MR: Colloid cyst of the third ventricle: A comparative immunohistochemical study of neuraxis cysts and choroid plexus epithelium. J Neurosurg 78:101–111, 1993.

37. Wilms G, Marchal G, Van Hecke P, et al: Colloid cysts of the third ventricle: MR findings. J Comput Assist Tomogr 14:527–531, 1990.

38. Armao D, Castillo M, Chen H, Kwock L: Colloid cyst of the third ventricle: Imaging-pathologic correlation. AJNR Am J Neuroradiol 21:1470–1477, 2000.

39. Desai KI, Nadkarni TD, Muzumdar DP, Goel AH: Surgical management of colloid cyst of the third ventricle—A study of 105 cases. Surg Neurol 57:295–302, 2002.

40. Timurkaynak E, Rhoton AL Jr, Barry M: Microsurgical anatomy and operative approaches to the lateral ventricles. Neurosurgery 19:685–723, 1986.

41. Ono M, Rhoton AL Jr, Peace D, et al: Microsurgical anatomy of the deep venous system of the brain. Neurosurgery 15:621–657, 1984.

42. Nagata S, Rhoton AL Jr, Barry M: Microsurgical anatomy of the choroidal fissure. Surg Neurol 30:3–59, 1988.

43. Fuji K, Lenkey C, Rhoton AL Jr: Microsurgical anatomy of the choroidal arteries: Lateral and third ventricle. J Neurosurg 52:165–188, 1980.

44. Yamamoto I, Rhoton AL Jr, Peace D: Microsurgery of the third ventricle: Microsurgical anatomy. Neurosurgery 8:334–356, 1981.

45. Wen WT, Rhoton AL Jr, de Oliveira E: Transchoroidal approach to the third ventricle: An anatomic study of the choroidal fissure and its clinical application. Neurosurgery 42:1205–1219, 1998.

46. Rhoton AL Jr: Microsurgical anatomy of the third ventricular region. In Apuzzo MLJ (ed.): Surgery of the Third Ventricle, 2nd ed. Baltimore: Williams & Wilkins, 1998, pp 89–158.

47. Piepmeier JM, Sass KJ: Surgical management of lateral ventricular tumors. In Paoletti P, Takakura K, Walker M, et al (eds): Neuro-oncology. Kluver: Dordrecht, 1991, pp 333–335.

48. Sugita K, Kobayashi S, Yokoo A: Preservation of large bridging veins during brain retraction. J Neurosurg 57:856–860, 1982.

49. Shucart WA, Stein BM: Transcallosal approach to the anterior ventricular system. Neurosurgery 3:339–343, 1978.

50. Geffen G, Walsh A, Simspson D, Jeeves M: Comparison of the effects of transcortical removal of intraventricular tumors. Brain 103:773–788, 1980.

51. Sass K, Novelly R, Spencer D, Spencer S: Mnestic and attention impairments following corpus callosotomy section for epilepsy. J Epilepsy 1:61–66, 1988.

52. Piepmeier J, Spencer D, Sass K, George T: Lateral ventricular masses. In Apuzzo MLJ (ed.): Brain Surgery: Complications Avoidance and Management. New York: Churchill Livingstone, 1993, pp 581–600.

53. Dandy WE: Operative experience in cases of pineal tumor. Arch Surg 33:19–46, 1936.

54. Piepmeier JM: Tumors and approaches to the lateral ventricles. J Neurooncol 30:267–274, 1996.

55. Little JR, MacCarty CS: Colloid cysts of the third ventricle. J Neurosurg 40:230–235, 1974.

56. Viale GL, Turtas S: The subchoroidal approach to the third ventricle. Surg Neurol 14:71–76, 1980.

57. Shucart W: The anterior transcallosal and transcortical approaches. In Apuzzo MLJ (ed.): Surgery of the Third Ventricle, 2nd ed. Baltimore: Williams & Wilkins, 1998, pp 369–389.

58. Rhoton AL Jr, Yamamoto I, Pease DA: Microsurgery of the third ventricle. Part 2: Operative approaches. Neurosurgery 8:357–373, 1981.

59. Ehni G, Ehni BL: Considerations in transforaminal entry. In Apuzzo MLJ (ed.): Surgery of the Third Ventricle, 2nd ed. Baltimore: Williams & Wilkins, 1998, pp 391–419.

60. Garcia-Bengochea F, Friedman WA: Persistent memory loss following section of the anterior fornix in humans: A historical review. Surg Neurol 27:361–364, 1987.

61. Sweet WH, Talland GA, Ervin FR: Loss of recent memory following section of fornix. Trans Am Neurol Assoc 84:76–82, 1959.

62. Tucker DM, Roeltgen DP, Tully R, et al: Memory dysfunction following unilateral transection of the fornix: A hippocampal disconnection syndrome. Cortex 23:465–472, 1988.

63. Ture U, Yasargil MG, Al-Mefty O: The transcallosal-transforaminal approach to the third ventricle with regard to the venous variations in this region. J Neurosurg (Wien) 87:706–715, 1997.

64. Wang AM, Power TC, Rumbaugh CL: Lateral ventricular meningioma. Comput Radiol 9:355–358, 1985.

65. Nitta M, Symon L: Colloid cyst of the third ventricle: A review of 36 cases. Acta Neurochir (Wien) 76:99–104, 1985.

66. Lavyne MH, Patterson RH Jr: Sub-choroidal trans-velum interpositum approach to mid third ventricular tumors. Neurosurgery 12:86–94, 1983.

67. Petrucci RJ, Bucheit WA, Woodruff GC, et al: Transcallosal parafornical approach for third ventricle tumors: Neurophysiological consequences. Neurosurgery 20:457–464, 1987.

68. Patterson RH Jr: The subfrontal transsphenoidal and trans-lamina terminalis approaches. In Apuzzo MLJ (ed.): Surgery of the Third Ventricle, 2nd ed. Baltimore: Williams & Wilkins, 1998, pp 471–487.

69. Choux M, Lena G, Genitori L: Craniopharyngioma in children. Neurochirurgie 37:1–174, 1991.

70. Tomita T, McLone D: Radical resection of childhood meningiomas. Pediatr Neurosurg 19:6–14, 1993.

71. King TT: Removal of intraventricular craniopharyngiomas through the lamina terminalis. Acta Neurochir (Wien) 45:277–286, 1979.

72. Susuki J, Katakura R, Mori T: Interhemispheric approach through the lamina terminalis to tumors of the anterior part of the third ventricle. Surg Neurol 22:157–163, 1984.

73. Kasama A, Kano T: A pitfall in the interhemispheric translamina terminalis approach for the removal of craniopharyngioma: Significance of preserving draining veins. Surg Neurol 32:116–120, 1989.

74. Yasui N, Nathal E, Fujiwara H, et al: The basal interhemispheric approach for acute anterior communicating aneurysms. Acta Neurochir (Wien) 118:91–97, 1992.

75. Yasargil MG, Curcic M, Kis M, et al: Total removal of craniopharyngiomas: Approaches and long term results in 144 patients. J Neurosurg 73:3–11, 1990.

76. Stein BM: The infratentorial supracerebellar approach to pineal lesions. J Neurosurg 35:197–202, 1971.

77. Bruce JN, Stein BM: Surgical management of pineal region tumors. Acta Neurochir (Wien) 134:130–135, 1995.

78. Reid WS, Clark WK: Comparison of the infratentorial and transtentorial approaches to the pineal region. Neurosurgery 3:1–8, 1978.

79. Clark WK, Batjer HH: The occipital transtentorial approach. In Apuzzo MLJ (ed.): Surgery of the Third Ventricle, 2nd ed. Baltimore: Williams & Wilkins, 1998, pp 721–741.

80. Dandy WE: An operation for removing pineal tumors. Surg Gynecol Obstet 33:113–119, 1921.

81. Ono M, Rhoton AL Jr, Barry M: Microsurgical anatomy of the region of the tentorial incisura. J Neurosurg 60:365–399, 1984.

82. Westerveld M, Sass K, Spencer S, Spencer D: Neuropsychological function following corpus callosotomy for epilepsy. In Devinsky T (ed.): Epilepsy and Behavior. New York: Alan Liss, 1991, pp 203–212.

83. Hellwig D, Bauer BL, Schulte M, et al: Neuroendoscopic treatment for colloid cysts of the third ventricle: The experience of a decade. Neurosurgery 52:525–533, 2003.

84. Souweidane MM, Sandberg DI, Bilsky MH, Gutin PH: Endoscopic biopsy for tumors of the third ventricle. Pediatr Neurosurg. 33:32–37, 2000.

85. Oppel F, Hoff HJ, Pannek HW: Endoscopy of the ventricular system: Indications, operative procedure and technical aspects. In Hellwig D, Bauer BL (eds): Minimally Invasive Techniques for Neurosurgery. Berlin: Springer, 1998, pp 97–100.

86. King WA, Ullman JS, Frazee JG, et al: Endoscopic resection of colloid cysts: Surgical considerations using the rigid endoscope. Neurosurgery 44:1103–1109, 1999.

87. Bruce DA: Complications of third ventricular surgery. Pediatr Neurosurg 17:325–330, 1991.

88. Alesh F, Kitz K, Koos WT, et al: Diagnostic potential of stereotactic biopsy of midline lesions. Acta Neurochir (Wien) Suppl 53:33–36, 1991.

89. Stein BM, Bruce JN: Surgical management of pineal region tumors. Clin Neurosurg 39:509–532, 1992.

90. Camacho A, Abernathey CD, Kelly PJ, Laws ER Jr: Colloid cysts: Experience with the management of 84 cases since the introduction of computer tomography. Neurosurgery 24:693–700, 1989.

91. Bellotti C, Pappada G, Sani R, et al: The transcallosal approach for lesions affecting the lateral and third ventricles: Surgical considerations and results in a series of 42 cases. Acta Neurochir (Wien) 111:103–113, 1991.

54 Transcallosal Approach to Tumors of the Third Ventricle

ROBERTO M. VILLANI and GIUSTINO TOMEI

Tumors of the third ventricle include a wide variety of pathologic entities that can arise either within the ventricular cavity or from the neural structures that form the ventricle. According to anatomic site, tumors of the third ventricle are classified as primarily intraventricular (e.g., colloid cyst, ependymoma, craniopharyngioma) when their attachment to the ventricular wall is minimal and well circumscribed and secondarily intraventricular when they arise from the wall of the ventricle and secondarily occupy the cavity (e.g., glioma, craniopharyngioma, lymphoma).[1]

Tumors that originate within the neural elements of the different structures of the third ventricle (e.g., glial tumors affecting the thalamus and the hypothalamus; tumors growing from the intraventricular ependyma; germinomas; medulloblastomas) are classified as intra-axial. Extra-axial ventricular lesions are histologically benign tumors with a limited area of implantation to the ventricular wall. They include lesions of developmental, neoplastic, vascular, and infectious origin (e.g., colloid cyst, dermoids and epidermoids, arteriovenous malformations, cysticercosis, lymphocytic hypophysitis).[1]

Although these tumors are relatively rare,[2-5] it is important to diagnose them before surgery and to distinguish, on the basis of neuroradiologic investigation, intra-axial from extra-axial neoplasms. Tumors arising from the base and invading and compressing from outside the third ventricular chamber (meningiomas, craniopharyngiomas, epidermoids, gliomas) (Fig. 54-1) should not be considered as tumors properly of the third ventricle.

The surgical approach to the region of the third ventricle should be tailored first according to the location of the tumor and second to the surgeon's experience and preference. In our experience, tumors arising from the anterior base and secondarily invading the third ventricle are better approached through pterional, subfrontal, or translamina terminalis routes.[6] When the tumor cannot be entirely removed via this approach, the anterior subfrontal approach can be combined with a superior approach (i.e., transcallosal or transcortical).[7,8] Tumors of the pineal region, compressing the posterior part of the third ventricle, are better exposed through an infratentorial supracerebellar or suboccipital transtentorial entry.[9,10] This approach has been recently described as being a suitable entry corridor for reaching a colloid cyst of the third ventricle.[11]

Lesions located in the anterior or middle third ventricular chamber as well as those tumors that occupy the entire cavity of the third ventricle are approached via an anterior transcallosal route.[1,7,12-26]

As for all central nervous system tumors, the first aim of surgery for masses in the third ventricle remains the improvement of neurologic signs and symptoms through as complete an excision as possible of the tumor. Second, because of the large variety of neoplasms encountered in this area, a precise histologic diagnosis for optimal completion of therapy is required. The third goal is the reopening of cerebrospinal fluid (CSF) pathways, because in more than 50% of cases the tumor occludes the foramen of Monro and can produce an acute or chronic hydrocephalus.[6]

Because the cavity of the third ventricle can be reached only by incision of neural structures, the complications of surgery of these tumors are the result of manipulation and alteration of a number of neural structures that form the third ventricular chamber and the brain areas surrounding it.[14,15,27-30]

The appropriate corridor to reach tumors of the third ventricle should be chosen on the basis of precise neuroradiologic assessment: particular attention must be paid to the location of the mass and its relationship with the ventricular cavity, particularly with the fornix, the foramen of Monro,

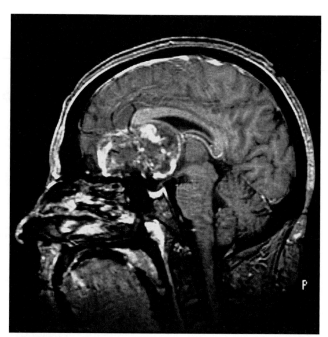

FIGURE 54-1 Sagittal T1-weighted magnetic resonance image of a large tumor arising from the anterior skull base and secondarily invading the third ventricle.

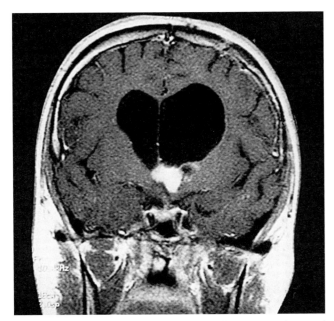

FIGURE 54-2 Coronal T1-weighted magnetic resonance image of a pilocytic astrocytoma of the third ventricle involving the foramen of Monro.

and the infundibulum. The size of the lateral and third ventricles, the thickness of the corpus callosum, and the anatomic characteristics of the septum have to be clearly borne in mind. Other important findings to be considered are the size of the mass and its relationship with the foramen of Monro (Figs. 54-1 to 54-4), the site of implant, the presence or absence of a CSF layer surrounding the mass, and the relationship of the mass with the vascular structures, particularly, the internal cerebral vein.

The anterior approach to the third ventricle can be performed using either the transcortical or transcallosal route.[1,2,7,8,12,13,15–18,30–34] The transfrontal transcortical approach to the lateral and then the third ventricle requires an incision of the brain parenchyma. This procedure, along

with many other disadvantages,[13] is followed by postoperative epilepsy in more than 20% of cases.[2]

The anterior transcallosal approach to the third ventricle does not seem to be responsible for significant postoperative deficits per se[2,12,13,16,30]: this approach has been the method of choice for treating tumors of the third ventricle in our institution since the late 1980s. Since 1999, with the introduction of endoscopic procedures, colloid cysts of the third ventricle have been approached and removed endoscopically.[35–38]

The transcallosal approach is the most straightforward, shortest corridor to the third ventricle. The corpus callosum can be reached by simple retraction of the right hemisphere through a corridor between the bridging veins; cortical incision is not required. Incision of the anterior portion of the corpus callosum for a limited length (2 cm) allows entry into either or both lateral ventricles, providing exposure of the two foramina of Monro.[24] The surgeon is then presented with different entry options for direct access to deep-seated lesions in the third ventricle, providing greater flexibility in the anteroposterior exposure of the ventricular cavity. Last, the transcallosal approach can be used even in the presence of a normal, not enlarged, lateral ventricle.

Because surgery of the diencephalic region still represents a major technical challenge in the surgical treatment of tumors of this area, the surgeon, in evaluating the operative approach to tumors of the third ventricle, should take into consideration the appropriateness of the tumor exposure through the chosen entry route, the risks associated with that particular corridor, and the transient or permanent postoperative deficits likely to follow. The region of the third ventricle remains difficult to explore, and the operative field is often extremely limited. The most challenging problems are bleeding in the tumor bed and the dissection and separation of the external layer of the neoplasm from the surrounding neural structures. Surgery of the third ventricle requires a detailed knowledge of the anatomic landmarks and the intrinsic characteristics of the different tumors that involve this structure.[19,21,32,39,40]

FIGURE 54-3 Coronal T1- and T2-weighted magnetic resonance images of a tumor involving the entire cavity of the third ventricle.

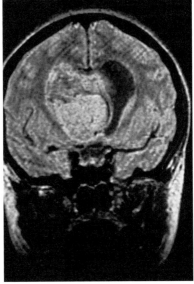
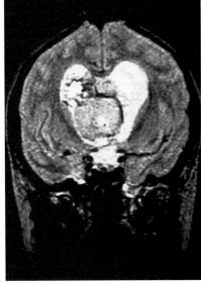

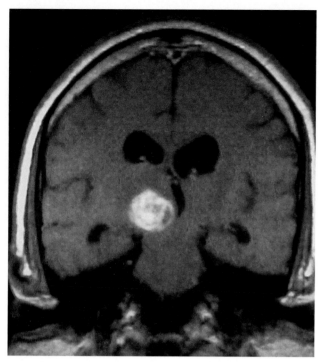

FIGURE 54-4 Coronal T1-weighted magnetic resonance image of a thalamic tumor elevating and obliterating the unilateral foramen of Monro.

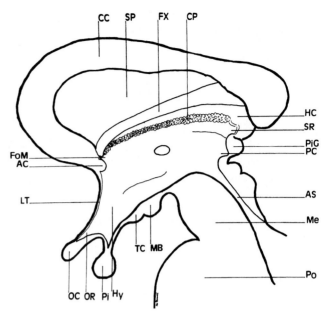

FIGURE 54-5 Schematic drawing of the midsagittal section of the third ventricle. CC, corpus callosum; SP, septum pellucidum; FX, fornix; CP, choroid plexus; HC, hippocampal commissure; SR, suprapineal recess; PiG, pineal gland; PC, posterior commissure; AS, aqueduct of Sylvius; Me, mesencephalon; Po, pons; MB, mamillary body; TC, tuber cinereus; Hy, hypothalamus; Pi, pituitary gland; OR, optic recess; OC, optic chiasm; LT, lamina terminalis; AC, anterior commissure; FoM, foramen of Monro.

Results using the transcallosal approach to these tumors are satisfying; most of them can be completely removed, and long-term follow-up reveals good outcomes.[2]

SURGICAL ANATOMY

The third ventricle is a narrow midline cavity of the brain located between the two thalami and under the body of the lateral ventricles[18,19,32,39-41] (Fig. 54-5). The cavity of the third ventricle communicates anterosuperiorly with the lateral ventricles through each foramen of Monro and posteriorly with the fourth ventricle through the aqueduct of Sylvius.

The third ventricular cavity can be approached and its inner structure exposed using different surgical options. The upper part of the third ventricle comprises the fornix. The septum pellucidum connects the inner surface of the corpus callosum to the upper surface of the body of the fornix. The septum is tallest anteriorly and shortest posteriorly, disappearing near the junction of the body and the posterior columns of the fornix. At the posterior end of the septum pellucidum, the crura and the hippocampal commissure fuse with the lower surface of the corpus callosum.

The fornix consists of a body, two anterior limbs (the columns), and two posterior columns. The two anterior columns, viewed superiorly, form the foramina of Monro that open between the fornix and the thalamus into the lateral ventricles on each side and extend inferiorly into the third ventricle.

At the level of the opening of each foramen of Monro, the two anterior columns split away and terminate in the mamillary bodies. The anterior commissure fills the gap between the two anterior columns, below the foramina of Monro. The anterior commissure is connected to the optic chiasm by the lamina terminalis. The anterior wall of the third ventricle runs from the foramina of Monro to the optic chiasm.

The posterior limbs (crura) of the fornix are interconnected by the hippocampal commissure, which is fused with the lower surface of the corpus callosum. Beneath the fornix is the tela choroidea, which is formed by two thin leptomeningeal membranes (the superior and inferior membranes) that contain a space called the velum interpositum, in which the vascular layer of the third ventricle runs.[18,39,40] Beneath the velum interpositum is the choroid plexus of the third ventricle. The tela choroidea, through the choroidal fissure, forms a continuum with the choroid plexus of the lateral ventricle. The choroidal fissure is an incisura between the lateral edge of the fornix and the superomedial surface of the thalamus, and the choroid plexus of the lateral ventricle is attached to it. The attachment of the choroid plexus of the lateral ventricle to the fornix and to the thalamus is made by ependyma that, from the wall of the lateral ventricle, also covers the choroid plexus. The medial portion of the ependymal layer that attaches the plexus of the lateral ventricle to the fornix is called the taenia fornicis, and the lateral portion that attaches to the thalamus is called the taenia choroidea.[40]

The posterior aspect of the third ventricular cavity is covered by the tela choroidea beneath the hippocampal commissure. Viewed from the inner cavity of the ventricle, starting from above to below, the following structures are evident: the suprapineal recess extending from the posterior layer of the tela choroidea to the pineal gland; the pineal gland, which protrudes into the cavity; the pineal recess extending posteriorly toward the quadrigeminal cistern; and the two commissures of the posterior part of the third ventricle (the abenula and the posterior commissure), which cross the midline and the orifice of the aqueduct of Sylvius.

The oval medial surface of the thalamus (superiorly) and the hypothalamus (inferiorly), delineated from each other by the hypothalamic sulcus, form the lateral wall of the ventricle. The superomedial border of the thalamus is marked by the eminence of the striae medullaris thalami, close to the attachment of the tela choroidea. On the oval surface of the thalamus, almost in its midposition, the massa intermedia often interconnects the two opposite thalami.

The floor of the third ventricle is formed by the hypothalamus anteriorly and by the mesencephalon posteriorly. The anteroinferior margin of the cavity of the third ventricle is formed by a prominence due to the optic chiasm. Behind this prominence, the infundibular recess extends into the infundibulum, and more posteriorly, the inner surface of the floor of the third ventricle is indented by the prominences of the mamillary bodies. The portion of the floor between the mamillary bodies and the aqueduct of Sylvius corresponds to the posterior perforated substance and the medial part of the cerebral peduncle.

Different vascular structures run within and around the third ventricle.[18,39–41] Between the two sheets of the tela choroidea (the superior and inferior membranes) lies the vascular layer of the roof of the third ventricle, in which the medial posterior choroidal arteries and the internal cerebral veins are located. The space in which the vascular layer of the third ventricle is located is known as the velum interpositum.

The medial posterior choroidal artery arises proximally from the posterior cerebral artery, which, in its course toward the quadrigeminal cistern and at the level of the pineal gland, gives rise to the medial branch for supply of the choroid plexus of the third ventricle.

The internal cerebral vein originates at the level of the foramen of Monro from the confluence of multiple veins. The internal cerebral veins course from anterior to posterior in the midline between the two layers of the tela choroidea. At the level of the superolateral surface of the pineal gland, the two internal cerebral veins diverge from the midline and, more posteriorly, converge to form the vein of Galen.

On each side, the internal cerebral vein receives subependymal tributary veins that run in the wall of the lateral ventricle and collect blood from periventricular white and gray matter and converge into the internal cerebral vein at the level of the foramen of Monro. Three main groups of tributary veins are recognized: the medial group, the lateral group, and the direct lateral and medial veins. The septal vein is the principal medial vein; it crosses the septum pellucidum and the fornix. The lateral group includes the caudate veins, which cross the caudate nucleus and the thalamus from posterolateral to anteromedial, and the thalamostriate vein, which collects blood from the caudate veins. The thalamostriate vein courses from the posterolateral to the anteromedial aspect of the ependymal layer of the frontal horn between the caudate nucleus and the thalamus. At the level of the foramen of Monro, it curves medially and joins the internal cerebral vein.

The direct lateral vein runs across the caudate nucleus and the thalamus more posteriorly than the thalamostriate vein; the direct medial vein crosses the posterior part of the septum pellucidum, passes the fornix, and enters posteriorly to the internal cerebral vein.

Below the floor of the third ventricle, the tip of the basilar artery and the posterior part of the circle of Willis are located. Branches of the posterior communicating and posterior cerebral arteries (thalamogeniculate and thalamoperforating arteries) reach the thalamus, the hypothalamus, and the internal capsule. The internal capsule and the posteroinferior aspect of the thalamus also receive branches from the anterior choroidal artery.

The anterior and anterior communicating arteries are intimately related to the lamina terminalis of the anterior wall of the third ventricle; they give rise to perforating branches for the hypothalamus, fornix, septum pellucidum, and striatum.

The anterior cerebral artery, along its course around the corpus callosum, sends tributaries to the corpus callosum, septum pellucidum, and fornix.

FUNCTIONAL ANATOMY

Compromised memory function is one of the more frequent postoperative deficits reported in surgery of the third ventricle. Although clinicopathologic studies have never clearly defined the precise anatomic substrates of memory, many structures around and within the third ventricle have been reported to be involved in memory disturbances.

Corpus Callosum

The corpus callosum is a midline structure that interconnects the two hemispheres. Although the limbic system is responsible for temporary storage of short-term memory (see later), the rostral tract of the corpus callosum is implicated in memory retrieval, which depends on interhemispheric interaction and association.

It is well documented in the literature that section of the entire corpus callosum is followed by the disconnection syndrome (i.e., akinetic mutism, motor apraxia, tactile agnosia, auditory suppression, hemialexia, and hemianopia).[31,42–45] The section of the corpus callosum that spares the splenium does not produce disconnection syndrome: mutism is rare and transient and so are the language, auditory, and somesthesic effects. Section of the splenium of the corpus callosum commonly causes left hemialexia with and without agraphia. Section of the anterior two thirds of the corpus callosum does not produce the disconnection syndrome; memory deficits are of a lesser degree compared with those in patients undergoing complete commissurotomy.

Limited section (2.5 cm) of the anterior portion of the corpus callosum does not produce measurable memory deficits.[1,2,30]

Hippocampus, Fornix, Septum, Thalamus, and Gyrus Cinguli: The Limbic System

Alteration of the limbic system is almost always reported in many pathologic conditions (e.g., trauma, tumor, infarction, encephalitis, Alzheimer's disease, and Korsakoff's syndrome) that produce memory deficits.[45] Manipulation or significant lesions of the dorsal, lateral, and ventral aspects of the third ventricle can disrupt the major connections between the components of the limbic system, which, besides being manipulated during surgery, can be invaded by or can be the site of origin of tumors of the third ventricle.

The limbic system is composed of complex neural pathways that interconnect the various components to each other and includes the hippocampus, fornix, septum, thalamus, hypothalamus, and cingulate gyrus.[45-48]

The limbic system is the main system for the temporary storage of short-term memory traces, from which long-term memory is eventually consolidated at the cortical level. Moreover, the limbic system is responsible for spatial orientation of recent memory and, because it projects to endocrine and autonomic centers, also affects vegetative functions.

Lesions of the different neural components of the limbic system, as well as disconnection of each center from the others, have been reported to be responsible for memory deficits, spatial disorientation, inability to interact with the environment, and alteration of behavior. Involvement of the hippocampal formation, mainly when bilateral, is followed by severe impairment of learning ability and loss of recent memory.

Although the role of the fornix and the consequences of its dissection in determining memory disturbances are still under debate, there is both clinical and experimental evidence that sectioning of the anterior columns of the fornix produces memory disturbances.[2,12,47-49]

Experimental lesions of the septum have led to a reduced ability to interact and pay attention to the environment, and produce hyperemotional responses. The medial and lateral nuclei of the septum are located in its anterior portion, in front of the anterior commissure. Fenestration of the septum to access the contralateral ventricle therefore must be performed in its highest portion, posterior to the foramen of Monro.

The thalamus and the dorsomedial thalamic nuclei seem to be more important in the process of recent memory storage than the hippocampus. Thalamic lesions result in severe memory disturbances and reduced initiative.

Other structures crucial to recent memory are the anterior commissure, the superior thalamic peduncle, and the thalamostriate pathway.

Hypothalamus

The hypothalamus forms the floor of the third ventricle below the foramina of Monro and extends from the preoptic area to the mamillary bodies.[50] It contains a complex group of nuclei that play an important role in the regulation of anterior and posterior pituitary functions.

The tuberoinfundibular neurons are contained in the tuber cinereum, which, along with the median eminence of the infundibulum, gives rise to the pituitary stalk. The projection of these areas to the brain stem and forebrain is the anatomic basis for coordination of autonomic and behavioral responses to pituitary secretion.

The hypothalamic-hypophysial system plays a leading role in the regulation of homeostasis, endocrinologic patterns, and behavioral state. Alteration of this system results in dysregulation of water balance and body temperature;

alterations in level of alertness and consciousness and the sleep-wake cycle; modification of pituitary functions (i.e., panhypopituitarism or hypopituitarism, hypogonadism, obesity, hypothyroidism, compromised adrenal function, hypotension), and changes in behavioral state.

OPERATIVE APPROACH

Preparation

Appropriate diagnosis and treatment of air embolism should be planned and a central venous catheter along with Doppler ultrasound and end-tidal PCO_2 monitoring must be placed. If tumor characteristics permit, a spinal needle for CSF drainage may be placed and mannitol used to relax the brain and obtain a wider exposure, necessitating less reflection of the brain.

The patient is positioned in the supine position with the back raised and the head flexed (35 degrees) and fixed by a pin-type headholder (Fig. 54-6). Care must be taken to prevent any change in head position during surgery. The position of the head has to be secured and the angle of the head has to be memorized by the surgeon to allow correct entry into the desired ventricle, neither too rostral nor too caudal to the foramen of Monro.

Tumors of the third ventricle are removed using standard microsurgical techniques.

Bone Flap

The corpus callosum is approached surgically through a frontal bone flap on the right side. The skin incision can be either linear or S-shaped or shaped like a question mark, with a tract parallel to the midline from anterior to posterior and then curving caudally toward the zygoma (Fig. 54-7).

The free bone flap can be either quadrangular (four holes) or triangular (three holes; our preferred method), with each margin not greater than 5 cm in length. The medial margin of the bone flap can be placed either 1 cm

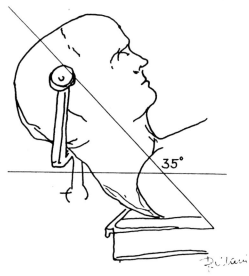

FIGURE 54-6 Positioning of the patient: the head is fixed and flexed 35 degrees from the longitudinal axis.

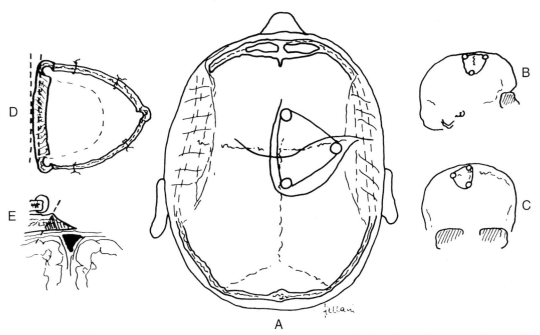

FIGURE 54-7 *A,* Different options of skin incision in relationship with the burr holes of the bone flap and the coronal suture. *B* and *C,* Lateral and anteroposterior views of the triangular bone flap for the access to the anterior portion of the corpus callosum. *D,* Line of incision for the dura opening. *E,* Coronal view of the medial margin of the bone flap cut obliquely. The inner table and the spongiosa (*hatched tract*) is removed over the midline, allowing a good visualization of the superior sagittal sinus. Leaving the outer table intact, the bone flap can be well repositioned.

left of the midline or exactly along the midline, overlapping and exposing the sagittal sinus. The medial margin of the bone flap is cut in an oblique way. The inner table and the spongiosa covering the midline is then removed, providing good visualization of the superior sagittal sinus. With the outer table left intact, a good repositioning of the bone flap can be obtained (see Fig. 54-7).

The two burr holes along the midline are placed so that the medial anteroposterior margin of the bone flap will be anterior to the coronal suture for two thirds of its length and posterior for one third. Placing the posterior burr hole more than 2 cm posterior to the coronal suture can lead to positioning of the retractor just at the level of the supplementary motor area, thus increasing the chance of postoperative hemiparesis.

A U-shaped incision of the dura is made with its base along the sagittal sinus (see Fig. 54-7). The dural incision should reach the edges of the sagittal sinus and the flaps reflected and secured on the opposite side, thus permitting good visualization of the medial part of the frontal lobe and the falx. Dural flaps should not be so tight as to close the superior sagittal sinus.

Approaching the Corpus Callosum

The medial aspect of the right frontal lobe should be retracted after the medial margin of the hemisphere is freed from Pacchioni granulations and cortical veins entering the sagittal sinus. These veins should be dissected and displaced from the sinus, without sacrificing them if possible, making an entry corridor through the bridging veins. Preoperative angiography can give useful information regarding the number and dimension of the cortical veins,

and their relationship with the superior sagittal sinus. The bone flap can then be tailored according to the distribution of the veins, coagulation of which should be avoided because it can result in cerebral infarction, sometimes favored by the cerebral edema that follows positioning of the retractor over the hemisphere. Edema and infarction can be responsible for postoperative hemiparesis.

Displacement of the medial aspect of the hemisphere should not exceed 3 cm in length (the width of the retractor). If the tension on the brain is considered excessive, CSF drainage through the spinal needle or infusion of mannitol usually results in improved brain relaxation and eases the positioning of the retractors.

Entering the interhemispheric space, care must be taken in maintaining cortical pial layer integrity and identifying the cingulate gyri. The two cingulate gyri are often attached to each other and can be misidentified and confused with the corpus callosum. Entering the gyrus cinguli, besides making the approach to the corpus callosum more difficult, would result in direct injury to this structure. The cingulate gyrus is more vascularized than the callosum and contains gray matter. When the two cingulate gyri are displaced, one medially and one laterally, the main trunks of anterior cerebral arteries are visualized. Pericallosal arteries are easily displaced either to the left or to the right, or one to the right and one to the left. Dissection from the cingulate gyri sometimes requires the sacrifice of small tributaries from the pericallosal arteries.

At this point, the cortex must be protected with cottonoids, and a self-retaining retractor with a 2-cm blade can be positioned. A second retractor over the falx can also be set out, so that the falx is pushed toward the left and the view is enlarged (Fig. 54-8). The superficial layer of the

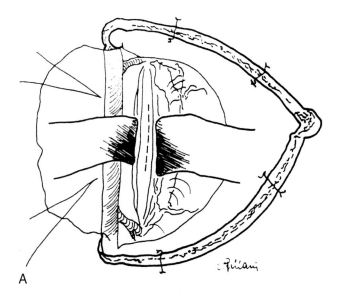

A

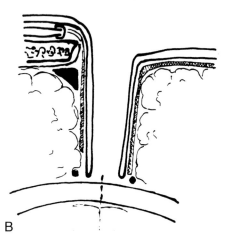

B

FIGURE 54-8 Positioning of the retractors (over the hemisphere and the falx) to expose the corpus callosum after pericallosal and callosomarginal arteries have been divaricated. *A,* Superior view. *B,* Coronal view.

corpus callosum appears whiter than the surrounding cortical structure, bright, and almost avascular, apart from some small running veins.[39,51]

After accurate cauterization of the pial layer of the corpus callosum, a vertical incision 2 cm long is made. The landmarks for a correct incision of the corpus callosum are the coronal suture for exact orientation of the angulation of the foramen of Monro, and the caudal border of the falx for the midline, thus avoiding incorrect entry into the left or right lateral ventricle. The incision of the corpus callosum can be placed over the midline or just to its left or right, according to what entry route into the third ventricle is desired, or which lateral ventricle the surgeon wants to reach.

The corpus callosum is penetrated by blunt dissection and suctioning. Its thickness can be calculated from sagittal magnetic resonance images (MRIs); it varies greatly according to the degree of ventricular dilatation. The ependymal layer of the lateral ventricle is then easily recognized because

the color and consistency of the tissue change. Opening the ependyma is followed by CSF leakage and visualization of the lateral ventricular cavity.

Entering the Lateral Ventricle

At this point, it may be difficult for the surgeon to recognize whether the entry has been made into the left or right lateral ventricle. Precise landmarks are the choroid plexus, which runs from the lateral to the medial aspect of the lateral ventricle and terminates at the level of the foramen of Monro, and the thalamostriate and septal veins. However, in some circumstances, because of decompression of the entered ventricle, the septum pellucidum can be bent inward and obscure the view of the medial structures of the ventricle. The septum can be moved medially or can be widely fenestrated in its posterior part, allowing a complete exposure of both lateral ventricles.

When the desired lateral ventricle is exposed, the retractors are deeply advanced and the lateral and medial borders of the corpus callosum retracted.

Corridors to the Third Ventricle

Two main corridors provide access to the third ventricular cavity: the transforaminal and the interforniceal entry[1,2,12,13,15,19-20,25,30,31,49] (Fig. 54-9). The choice of appropriate entry largely depends on the position, size, and anatomic characteristics of the tumor (e.g., vascularization, consistency, adherence to surrounding structures) and its relationship to the foramen of Monro. The entry should be carefully evaluated and planned by the surgeon in light of detailed MRI in different planes.[21]

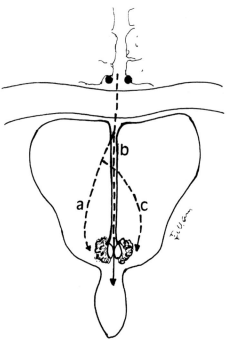

FIGURE 54-9 Diagram showing the two main options to enter the third ventricle cavity through the transcallosal approach: transforaminal (a) and interforniceal (b). Opening the septum allows the visualization of the contralateral foramen of Monro (c).

Transforaminal Entry

Lesions in the third ventricle can alter the foramen of Monro: it can be enlarged because of coexistent hydrocephalus, or it can be slitlike. Moreover, some tumors arising from the thalamus can elevate the floor of the lateral ventricle and obliterate the foramen (see Fig. 54-4).

Only tumors visible by direct microsurgical inspection of the foramen and that enlarge the foramen or come out from it (see Fig. 54-2) can be treated via a transforaminal entry (Fig. 54-10): we do not recommend the section of one or both fornices to enlarge the exposure anteriorly, or removal of tissue from the posteroinferior aspect of the foramen to gain a better posterior view, because severe postoperative deficits can arise.[44] To gain a better view of the posterior aspects of the foramen of Monro, we prefer alternative routes (see later). However, as reported by Ture and colleagues,[32] the foramen of Monro can be posteriorly enlarged without tissue damage if the location of the junction between the anterior septal and internal cerebral veins is posterior.

The foramen provides access to the tumor, and space is gained by sharp dissection, gentle retraction, and intracapsular suction of the mass, getting the surface free from the surrounding cerebral structures by a progressive shrinking of the capsule itself. Any traction to the mass must be avoided because it can facilitate bleeding, mainly from the posterior portion of the tumor mass.

Anterosuperior detachment of the tumor could lead to some damage to the fornix from the manipulation of this structure; on the other hand, injury to the tela choroidea and internal cerebral veins remains the main risk during both the posterior enlargement of the foramen of Monro and the detachment of the posterior part of the tumor.

Difficulty in separating the tumor capsule from the choroid plexus, tela choroidea, and internal cerebral veins

can lead to bleeding from the roof of the third ventricle, and sometimes the bleeding cannot be appreciated until the entire ventricle is filled with blood. Hemorrhage from a blind surface of the ventricle can be managed only with great difficulty; repeated rinsing and positioning of a piece of sponge and gently pushing, using a curved dissector as counterforce, can be very helpful.

After completion of tumor removal, care must be taken to determine the presence of tumor remnants or clots that can produce acute obstruction of the foramina of Monro or aqueduct of Sylvius. We recommend an accurate rinse and direct visualization of the third ventricular cavity using a mirror or an endoscope.

Interforniceal Entry

The interforniceal approach must be planned before surgery using accurate neuroradiologic assessment. MRI in different planes and cerebral angiography or MR angiography can afford important information about vascular anatomy and, particularly, the anatomy of the corpus callosum, septum pellucidum, and fornices and their relationship with the mass in the ventricular cavity. Interforniceal entry is the corridor of choice for tumors located in the mid third portion of the third ventricular chamber, or for tumors that occupy the entire cavity of the third ventricle (see Fig. 54-3).

After dissection of the corpus callosum, the surgeon has two options: identification and separation of the leaves of the septum before entering the lateral ventricle, or entering the lateral ventricle and sectioning the septum pellucidum.

After completion of the corpus callosum dissection and appreciation of the ependymal layer and underlying lateral ventricle, the line of attachment of the septum can sometimes be recognized.[12,13,25] The two leaves of the septum can then be split away (this maneuver can be easily performed

FIGURE 54-10 *A,* View into the anterior aspect of the right lateral ventricle. Visualization of the septum pellucidum, fornix, foramen of Monro, thalamostriate vein, and choroid plexus of the lateral ventricle. *B,* High magnification of the operative field: foramen of Monro (∗), septal (a) and thalamostriate (b) veins, and the choroid plexus of the lateral ventricle. *C,* Scheme of the subchoroidal approach.

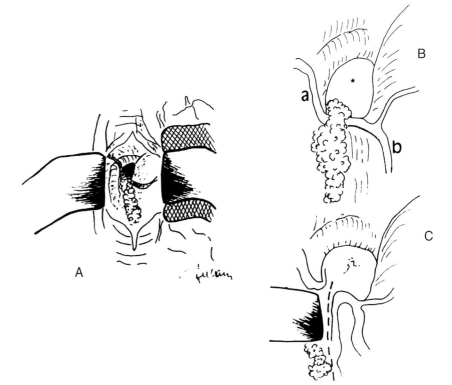

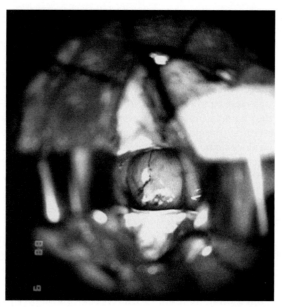

FIGURE 54-11 Operative field of the transcallosal interforniceal approach: the tumor mass becomes apparent as soon as the fornices are divaricated.

if a cavum vergae is present), after which the median raphe of the fornices can be reached. However, in the presence of large masses that completely fill the cavity of the third ventricle, the roof of the third ventricle can be raised up by the tumor. In this case, the septum is no longer evident and the fornices are in direct contact with the corpus callosum, and sometimes spread apart; thus once the dissection of the corpus callosum is completed, the surgeon can continue the dissection over the midline, obtaining entry to the third ventricle between the two fornices (see Fig. 54-3).

When the leaves of the septum are not identifiable from the ependymal layer of the lateral ventricle before entering it, the surgeon can enter the lateral ventricle and then, after identification of the different structures, can fenestrate the septum just posterior to the foramen of Monro and the septal vein, thus opening the contralateral ventricle.[12,13,22] Because the septum is attached to the dorsomedial aspect of the fornices, it serves as a landmark for the midline, allowing a precise midline entry between the two fornices. These have to be bluntly and gently dissected for approximately 2 cm of posterior extension, starting just posterior to the foramen of Monro.

The anterior and posterior boundaries of the interforniceal incision are represented by the anterior commissure and hippocampal commissure, respectively, which must be preserved because any lesion of these structures can lead to permanent memory deficits.

Once the interforniceal space is opened, the cavity of the third ventricle is apparent and the tumor is recognized. Entering the roof of the third ventricle through the interforniceal corridor, the surgeon must bear clearly in mind the anatomy of different vascular and nervous structures: tumors located in the middle portion of the third ventricle can displace the vascular layer, mainly the internal cerebral veins and medial posterior choroidal arteries, and modify their normal anatomy. Should these vessels be immediately

recognized once dissection of the fornices is completed, the veins and arteries can be gently dissected and lateralized from the tela choroidea.

Standard microsurgical techniques are required to remove the tumor; when visible and distinguishable from surrounding normal tissue, the superficial layer of the mass can be coagulated and then incised, and the inner content progressively aspirated with an ultrasound aspirator. Difficulties in the total removal of intraventricular masses arise with tumors whose boundaries are not clearly separate and distinct from normal tissue. Particular attention must be focused on the lateral and anteroposterior boundaries of the tumor during its separation from the vascular structures of the roof (internal cerebral veins and posterior choroidal arteries), the lateral walls of the third ventricle (thalamus), and the anteroinferior portion of the floor of the third ventricle (hypothalamus). Removal of the more posterior portion of the tumor, sometimes not visible through the direct transcallosal interforniceal route, can be achieved by modifying the microscope's angulation or altering the patient's head positioning.

As soon as the inferior part of the tumor is completely removed, basal structures may be visualized progressively: from the posterior to anterior aspects, the surgeon can appreciate the prepontine cistern, basilar circulation vessels (basilar tip, posterior cerebral, and anterosuperior cerebellar arteries), clivus, posterior clinoids, anterior circulation vessels (anterior cerebral and communicating arteries), and dorsum sellae.

Alternative and Combined Routes

When the surgeon is planning alternative routes to the third ventricle other than the aforementioned entries, detailed preoperative neuroradiologic evaluation of the anatomic relationships of the tumor is required. Tumors that are entirely confined in the third ventricle, located in its posteroinferior third, and do not alter either the foramen of Monro or the fornix and septum pellucidum, can be approached through a subchoroidal or transchoroidal route.[20,25,40,52–54] In addition, if a transforaminal or interforniceal entry has been chosen and these corridors do not enable complete removal of the tumor, these alternative entry routes can be combined with that initially chosen.

The subchoroidal and transchoroidal approaches use the corridor between the inferolateral aspects of the fornices and the medial aspects of the thalamus. This thin space is filled by the choroid plexus, the velum interpositum, and the venous and arterial system of the diencephalon. There are two main options in relation to the thalamostriate vein: the anterior (subchoroidal) and the posterior (transchoroidal) approaches.

Subchoroidal Transvelum Interpositum Approach

As soon as the right lateral ventricle is entered and all the structures well recognized, the choroid plexus of the lateral ventricle is anteriorly moved and elevated so that the dorsomedial aspect of the thalamus is exposed.[53]

To gain and enlarge the view, the plexus can be coagulated and shrunk and the leptomeninges of the velum interpositum gently cut (see Fig. 54-10). This procedure allows the surgeon to visualize the confluence of the septal and thalamostriate veins into the internal cerebral vein and the group of subependymal thalamic veins (mainly the anterior and posterior groups) that run on the anterior and superior aspects of the thalamus and drain to the thalamostriate and internal cerebral veins, respectively. The thalamostriate vein (sometimes with the septal vein) can be coagulated and cut: advancing the retractors along the medial wall of the thalamus and the inferior border of the fornix, a good access to the cavity of the third ventricle is gained. In this access, a corridor is created beneath the choroidal plexus of the lateral ventricle and the internal cerebral vein and above the superomedial aspect of the thalamus.

Transchoroidal Approach

Transchoroidal approaches enter the third ventricle through the velum interpositum behind the thalamostriate vein, and do not require its cutting.[52,54] The corridor may be created either by dividing the attachment of the choroid plexus of the lateral ventricle from the fornix in its superior portion at the level of the choroidal fissure, or by separating the inferior aspect of the choroid plexus from the internal cerebral vein, the leptomeninges of the tela choroidea, and the superomedial aspect of the thalamus. Both these corridors enter the cavity of the third ventricle posterior to the thalamostriate vein and the foramen of Monro.

In the transchoroidal superior approach, the taenia fornicis can be easily identified because it is formed by the ependymal layer that covers the lateral ventricle and the plexus and is located between the inferolateral portion of the fornix and the superomedial aspect of the plexus of the lateral ventricle.[40] Once the taenia fornicis is opened, the superior membrane of the tela choroidea becomes apparent. The tela has to be opened so that the internal cerebral vein and the medial posterior choroidal artery can be exposed, separated, and gently moved laterally. Beneath these vessels are the inferior membrane of the tela choroidea and the plexus of the third ventricle: their dissection should start medial to the internal cerebral vein, from the posterior aspect of the third ventricle cavity toward the foramen of Monro. When dissection of the different layers of the tela choroidea is completed, the entire cavity of the third ventricle can be visualized. However, the presence of a mass in the third ventricle can grossly alter the anatomy of the various layers of the third ventricular roof: it may not be possible to distinguish the two membranes from each other, and the vein and the artery can be displaced upward, inward, or laterally.

In the transchoroidal inferior approach, the taenia choroidea is opened. In this approach, manipulation of the upper thalamic surface and the veins than run in its superficial layer could increase the risk for their damage.[40]

The major risks in both transchoroidal entries are possible damage to the internal cerebral and thalamic veins as well as to the fornix, which sometimes must be elevated, and to the thalamus, which has to be displaced laterally to allow the entry to the third ventricular cavity.

Based on our experience, the different options for transvelum interpositum access should be tailored during surgery. Sectioning the thalamostriate vein and the septal vein could lead to infarction of the thalamic and septal structures.

This complication can increase the risk for postoperative hemiparesis and severe memory disturbances. Thus thalamostriate and septal veins should be spared as often as possible and the approach to the posterior portion of the third ventricle should be gained first through a posterior enlargement of the foramen of Monro, with an anterior opening of the velum interpositum in there is a posterior location and junction between the anterior septal and internal cerebral veins,[40] or through a superior transchoroidal approach that initially spares the thalamostriate vein.

Closure

When the tumor has been removed as completely as possible and meticulous hemostasis of the operative field obtained, an intraventricular catheter is placed into the cavity of the third ventricle, which is then filled with saline. The retractors are gently removed under direct vision and the borders of the line of incision of the corpus callosum along with the medial aspect of the hemisphere are carefully inspected for bleeding. The closure of the dura, resecuring of the bone flap, positioning of drainage, and closure of the galea and skin are performed using standard surgical procedures.

The intraventricular catheter can then be connected to an external transducer for continuous intracranial pressure monitoring.

COMPLICATIONS

Most of the complications of third ventricular surgery are related to the location of the lesion rather than to the approach.[2,20,24,25,29]

Intraventricular and other intracranial hemorrhages (epidural and intracerebral) are rarely observed but require immediate reoperation to detect the source of bleeding. Massive intraventricular hemorrhage from the ependyma layer, choroid plexuses, and tumor remnants can be prevented by meticulous coagulation of any source of bleeding, continuous irrigation of the ventricular cavity, and adequate cauterization of tumor remnants when complete excision of the tumor is thought to be contraindicated. Indirect (using a mirror or an endoscopic device) or direct microscopic visualization of the ventricular cavity is highly recommended at the end of the operation. This allows the surgeon to visualize the possible presence of a blind site of bleeding, or occlusion of the aqueduct of Sylvius or the foramen of Monro. We routinely perform an immediate postoperative computed tomography (CT) scan to evaluate the presence of intracranial hemorrhages. Positioning of an intraventricular catheter, besides continuously measuring the intracranial pressure over the postoperative course, allows immediate drainage when a sudden increase of intracranial pressure is detected.

Postoperative pneumocephalus is often observed after third ventricular surgery and does not represent a major complication. Persistent CSF subdural collection is often observed in the transcortical transventricular approach to the third ventricle, but is rare in the transcallosal approach, and has never been observed in our series.

Bacterial meningitis and ventriculitis are rare: the use of prophylactic antibiotics is questionable in preventing infectious complications. Serial CSF cell count and culture and identification of the infectious agent seem the best procedures for choosing a correct antibiotic regimen. Broad-spectrum antibiotic therapy should be started if there is an increase in CSF cells and proteins. Although the diagnosis is sometimes difficult, aseptic meningitis must be presumed when CSF cultures are persistently negative and CSF cell count and chemistry do not suggest infection. Aseptic meningitis can be observed after the removal of a colloid cyst or in the case of partial removal of an intra-axial tumor, and requires corticosteroid treatment.

Despite total removal of tumor masses in the third ventricle, the reopening of the foramina of Monro, and the avoidance of intraventricular bleeding, reestablishment of CSF pathways is not always obtained. Ventricular dilatation is present in more than 50% of patients with third ventricular tumors, and one third of these require a permanent CSF shunt.[2,7,20]

Early postoperative seizures are rarely observed after the transcallosal approach and are controlled with anticonvulsant therapy. Late epilepsy, observed in more than 20% of patients who undergo surgery through a transcortical transventricular route, has never been observed in our series of patients who underwent surgery via a transcallosal approach.[2]

Large or confined areas of brain edema or infarction, due to either direct venous drainage compromise or arterial occlusion or indirect occlusion by the retractor, are the main factors responsible for postoperative hemiparesis.[13,15,30,31] Hemiparesis is usually transient,[2,13] unless large portions of the hemispheres are involved.[33] Although vascular manipulation is a significant factor in this complication, postoperative hemiparesis may also be directly related to the tumor masses themselves, which may have required prolonged manipulation of the walls of the third ventricle to be removed.[14,15] Accordingly, surgery of large intra-axial tumors that invade and distend the walls of the ventricle as well as extra-axial neoplasms that are strictly adherent to the ventricular walls could result in secondary injury to the thalamus, internal capsule, and deep diencephalic structures.

In our experience, diencephalohypothalamic involvement remains a major complication of third ventricular surgery because it produces severe metabolic derangement, gastrointestinal bleeding, diabetes insipidus, alterations of alertness and consciousness, and an akinetic mutism-like status.

Akinetic mutism is reported with variable incidence in the literature[2,13,17,23,27–31,33,34,42–44] and is the result of involvement of the inferior frontal lobes and cingulate gyri outside the third ventricular region.[2,30,31,34,35]

Memory disturbances have been reported frequently in patients submitted to transcallosal or transcortical approaches to third ventricular tumors; they usually involve short-term memory and in general are transient.[2,12–15,30,45–49,55–58] Incision of the anterior part of the corpus callosum for the limited length necessary to provide access to the third ventricle (Fig. 54-12) does not seem, in itself, to produce permanent and measurable memory deficits.[2,13,30,31,53] Psychological and memory disturbances are often observed as presenting symptoms in patients with third ventricular tumors, and in many instances they disappear after surgery.[2]

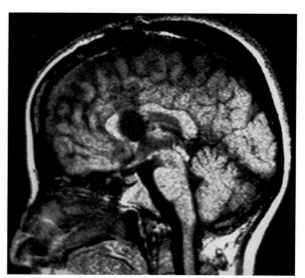

FIGURE 54-12 Postoperative sagittal T1-weighted magnetic resonance image of a third ventricle tumor completely removed. The incision of the corpus callosum is evident.

Permanent memory losses are mainly related to the maneuvers necessary for removal of the tumor, rather than to the approach itself.[14,15] In our experience, permanent memory loss was observed in a patient with postoperative alteration of the septal and forniceal areas.[2,46–49,54–55]

A disconnection syndrome or impairment of the frontal functions (i.e., attention, intelligence, and verbal fluency) usually is not observed at long-term neuropsychological evaluation of patients submitted to the transcallosal approach.[2,19]

PERSONAL SERIES

Between 1984 and 2003, 231 patients with tumors located in and around the third ventricle were observed at our institution: 112 were operated on through different surgical approaches (transcortical transventricular, 23; transcallosal transventricular, 47; translamina terminalis, 4; pterional, 21; suboccipital transtentorial, 5; suboccipital supracerebellar, 4; endoscopic procedures, 8). Of 47 patients who underwent surgery through a transcallosal route, 17 were male and 30 were female. Age ranged from 4 to 70 years.

Headache was the most common initial complaint, usually referred to the frontal or retro-orbital area (38 cases; 81%); in four patients headache was paroxysmal or intermittent and positional (8.5%). Obesity, impotence, dysmenorrhea, diabetes insipidus, and sleep-wake cycle alterations were evident in 11 patients (23%). Five patients (10.5%) had temporary loss of vision or diplopia. An epileptic seizure was the first symptom in one patient (2%).

Signs of increased intracranial pressure (papilledema with and without decreased visual acuity) were evident in 25 patients (53%). Hypothalamohypophysial dysfunction (partial or panhypopituitarism) was demonstrated in 23% of cases (11 patients). Gait disturbances and pyramidal tract signs were evident in seven patients (15%). Decreased visual acuity or visual field defects were seen in seven patients (15%). An organic mental syndrome (confusion, memory loss, and urinary incontinence) was reported in

10 cases (21%); in addition, 1 patient was lethargic and 1 was comatose.

Lesions distending the foramen of Monro were approached by a transforaminal entry (26 cases; 55%; see Fig. 54-2). Sixteen patients harboring large masses distending and occupying the entire cavity of the third ventricle were approached by an interforniceal route (34%; see Fig. 54-3). An interseptal or transseptal route provided complete exposure of the ventricular cavity, and the midline basal structures were largely exposed. Tumor masses located posterior to the foramen of Monro that were not visualized through a transforaminal route were approached by a transchoroidal or subchoroidal entry (five cases; 10.5%; see Fig. 54-4).

Four patients (8.5%) underwent a second operation: two were 10 and 6 years of age and had incomplete removal of tumor (one pilocytic and one low-grade glioma) demonstrated on postoperative MRI. They underwent a second procedure 3 and 5 months, respectively, after the first procedure, and the tumors were completely removed.

The remaining two patients were reoperated on 17 months and 5 years, respectively, after the first procedure for a regrowth of the tumor (one astrocytoma and one oligodendroglioma).

Complete resection of the mass, documented on postoperative CT or MRI, was achieved in all 18 patients with extra-axial tumors. In patients with intra-axial tumors (29 cases), total removal was achieved in 61% (29 patients) with the first procedure and in 66% after the second approach.

Histologic assessment of the third ventricular tumors of our series revealed that 61.7% of the tumors (29 patients) were intra-axial and 38.3% were extra-axial (18 cases) (Table 54-1). Among the former, low-grade gliomas (fibrillary and protoplasmatic variants of astrocytoma and giant cell astrocytoma) and pilocytic astrocytomas were more frequently observed. Rare tumors included ependymoma, ependymoblastoma, neurocytoma, and glioblastoma. Colloid cysts (10 cases) were the most common variant among the extra-axial tumors, whereas craniopharyngiomas (4 cases) were less frequently observed. Rare tumors included

metastasis, ectopic pituitary adenoma, epidermoid and lymphocytic hypophysitis.

As a result of the first surgical procedure, two patients died (4.2%). In one case, the patient with a lymphocytic hypophysitis, the postoperative course was characterized by an akinetic mutism-like status and a diencephalic syndrome (diabetes insipidus, electrolyte imbalance, hyperthermia), and the patient died 72 days after surgery. The second patient, with an ependymoma, died of postoperative hematoma 3 days after surgery.

Major postoperative complications were hemiparesis (five patients; 10.6%) and diabetes insipidus (seven patients; 15%). Hemiparesis was moderate and had resolved in four patients by the 6-month follow-up. Persistent diabetes insipidus was present in one patient. Four of the seven patients with preoperative psychic disturbances experienced a normalization of mental performance. Epileptic seizures never appeared in the postoperative course of these patients. Patients who underwent a second procedure had no mortality or significant morbidity.

In spite of an anatomically opened foramen of Monro after the surgical procedure, 13 of 23 patients with preoperative hydrocephalus had persistent ventricular enlargement; in 11 patients, a permanent CSF shunt was implanted.

CONCLUSIONS

Reaching the third ventricular cavity obliges the surgeon to choose a route that invariably requires an incision of the brain parenchyma. Therefore, the method of choice is that which causes the least amount of clinically relevant brain damage. In the transcallosal approach, microsurgical techniques limit the damage because a 2-cm opening of the corpus callosum allows visualization and treatment of intraventricular lesions with sufficient safety.

Anatomically, the transcallosal approach has various advantages. The vascularization of the corpus callosum is modest and thus an incision does not cause great vessel sacrifice. Moreover, both ventricles can be reached through the same incision, and the dimension of the ventricles does not represent a contraindication to this approach. Last, dissection of the corpus callosum carries little or no incidence of postoperative epilepsy. Clinical and neuropsychological evaluations have documented that section of the corpus callosum limited to its anterior third does not, in itself, cause significant deficits in personality or behavior.

Evaluation of damage by partial dissection of the corpus callosum should be compared with those observed after the transcortical-transventricular approach to third ventricular tumors. However, none of the series reported in the literature allow for this because there is always a lesion involving the third ventricle, the removal of which necessarily implicates those structures of the third ventricle that are decisively involved in mnestic and neuropsychic functions.

However, with our data and clinical experience, we believe that the transcallosal approach is the route of first choice to approach tumors of the third ventricle because of its limited mortality and late postoperative morbidity. Although this decision also implies some technical and surgical considerations, the restricted access and the spatial limitations of the transcallosal route, along with the necessary attention to the manipulation of several structures

---

TABLE 54-1 ▪ Histology of Third Ventricular Tumors: 47 Cases Approached through the Transcallosal Route

Intra-axial (*n* = 29)	
Pilocytic astrocytoma	5
Low-grade glioma*	12
Giant cell astrocytoma	2
Subependymoma	5
Ependymoma	2
Neurocytoma	1
Glioblastoma	2
Extra-axial (*n* = 18)	
Colloid cyst	10
Craniopharyngioma	4
Pituitary adenoma†	1
Lymphocytic hypophysitis	1
Epidermoid	1
Metastasis	1

*Fibrillary and protoplasmatic variants.
†Ectopic.

(i.e., the bridging veins, the cortex of the medial aspect of the right hemisphere, the superior sagittal sinus, the pericallosal arteries, and the veins of the corpus callosum), have never prevented the treatment of these neoplasms.

Cases of subtotal or partial removal of tumor are always caused by the difficulty or impossibility of recognizing clear anatomic landmarks, and are never due to the limited corridor of access. Even lesions with heavy bleeding have not caused insurmountable problems of hemostasis, first because spontaneous hemorrhage usually ceases after tumor removal is completed, and second because the operative field is sufficiently exposed to allow direct hemostasis with traditional methods.

Surgical indications for the transcallosal route are confined to tumors that occupy the anterior and middle portion of the third ventricle, as well as those that completely fill the cavity of the third ventricle. The transcallosal route can be combined with subfrontal or interhemispheric approaches when the latter do not enable the surgeon completely to remove tumors arising from the base and secondarily invading the third ventricle.

Tumors of the posterior part of the third ventricle that primarily or secondarily invade the ventricle are better approached through transtentorial suboccipital or infratentorial supracerebellar routes, the discussion of which is beyond the scope of this chapter.

REFERENCES

1. Apuzzo MLJ, Zee CS, Breeze RE, Day JD: Anterior and mid-third ventricular lesions: A surgical overview. In Apuzzo MLJ (ed): Surgery of the Third Ventricle, 2nd ed. Baltimore: Williams & Wilkins, 1998, pp 635–680.
2. Villani R, Papagno C, Tomei G, et al: Transcallosal approach to tumors of the third ventricle: Surgical results and neuropsychological evaluation. J Neurosurg Sci 41:41–50, 1997.
3. Kim DG, Chi JG, Park SH, et al: Intraventricular neurocytoma: Clinicopathological analysis of seven cases. J Neurosurg 76, 1992.
4. Lee TT, Manzano GR: Third ventricular glioblastoma multiforme: Case report. Neurosurg Rev 20:291–294, 1997.
5. Schwartz TH, Kim S, Glick RS, et al: Supratentorial ependymomas in adult patients. Neurosurgery 44:721–731, 1999.
6. Maira G, Anile C, Colosimo C, et al: Craniopharyngiomas of the third ventricle: Trans lamina terminalis approach. Neurosurgery 47:857–863, 2000.
7. Desai KI, Nadkarni TD, Mumumdar DP, et al: Surgical management of colloid cyst of the third ventricle—A study of 105 cases. Surg Neurol 57:295–302, 2002.
8. Solaroglu I, Besckonakli E, Kaptanoglu E, et al: Transcortical-transventricular approach in colloid cysts of the third ventricle: Surgical experience in 26 cases. Neurosurg Rev 27:89–92, 2004.
9. Sano K: Pineal masses: General considerations. In Apuzzo MLJ (ed): Brain Surgery: Complication Avoidance and Management, vol 1. Edinburgh: Churchill Livingstone, 1993, pp 463–473.
10. Takakura K, Matsumani M: Pineal region masses: Selection of an operative approach. In Apuzzo MLJ (ed): Brain Surgery: Complication Avoidance and Management, vol 1. Edinburgh: Churchill Livingstone, 1993, pp 473–485.
11. Konovalov AN, Pitskhelauri DI: Infratentorial supracerebellar approach to the colloid cyst of third ventricle. Neurosurgery 49:1116–1123, 2001.
12. Apuzzo MLJ, Chikovani O, Gott P, et al: Transcallosal interforniceal approaches for lesions affecting the third ventricle: Surgical considerations and consequences. Neurosurgery 10:547–554, 1982.
13. Apuzzo LJ, Amar AP: Transcallosal interforniceal approach. In Apuzzo MLJ (ed): Surgery of the Third Ventricle, 2nd ed. Baltimore: Williams & Wilkins, 1998, pp 421–452.
14. Woiciechowsky C, Vogel S, Lehmann R, et al: Transcallosal removal of lesions affecting the third ventricle: An anatomic and clinical study. Neurosurgery 36:117–123, 1995.
15. Woiciechowsky C, Vogel S, Meyer BU, et al: Neuropsychological and neurophysiological consequences of partial callosotomy. J Neurosurg Sci 41:75–80, 1997.
16. Hutter BO, Spetzger U, Bertalanffy H, et al: Cognition and quality of life in patients after transcallosal microsurgery for midline tumors. J Neurosurg Sci 41:123–129, 1997.
17. Bellotti C, Pappada G, Sani R, et al: The lesions affecting the lateral and third ventricle: Surgical considerations and results in a series of 42 cases. Acta Neurochir (Wien) 111:103–107, 1984.
18. Rhoton AL, Yamamoto I, Peace DA: Microsurgery of the third ventricle. Part 2: Operative approaches. Neurosurgery 8:357–373, 1981.
19. Winkler PA, Weis S, Buttner A, et al: The transcallosal interforniceal approach to the third ventricle: Anatomical and microsurgical aspects. Neurosurgery 40:973–981, 1997.
20. Behari S, Banerji D, Mishra A, et al: Intrinsic third ventricular craniopharyngioma: Report of six cases and a review of the literature. Surg Neurol 60:245–252, 2003.
21. Winkler PA, Weis S, Wenger E, et al: Transcallosal approach to the third ventricle: Normative morphometric data based on magnetic resonance imaging scans with special reference to the fornix and forniceal insertion. Neurosurgery 45:309–317, 1999.
22. Lawton MT, Golfinos JG, Spetzler RF: The contralateral transcallosal approach: Experience with 32 cases. Neurosurgery 39:729–735, 1996.
23. Benes V: Advantages and disadvantages of the transcallosal approach to third ventricle. Childs Nerv Syst 6:437–439, 1990.
24. Konovalov AN, Gorelyshev SK: Surgical treatment of anterior third ventricle tumours. Acta Neurochir 118:33–39, 1992.
25. Paleologos TS, Wadley JP, Kitchen ND, et al: Interactive image-guided transcallosal microsurgery for anterior third ventricle cysts. Minim Invasive Neurosurg 44:157–162, 2001.
26. Jeffre RL, Besser M: Colloid cyst of the third ventricle: A clinical review of 39 cases. J Clin Neurosci 8:328–331, 2001.
27. Winkler PA, Ilmberger J, Krishnan KG, et al: Transcallosal interforniceal-transforaminal approach for removing lesions occupying the third ventricular space: Clinical and neuropsychological results. Neurosurgery 46:879–890, 2000.
28. Friedman MA, Meyers CA, Sawaya R: Neuropsychological effects of third ventricle tumors surgery. Neurosurgery 52:791–798, 2003.
29. Asgari S, Engelhorn T, Brondies A, et al: Transcortical or transcallosal approach to ventricle-associate tumours: A clinical study on the prognostic role of surgical approach. Neurosurg Rev 26:192–197, 2003.
30. Nakasu Y, Isozumi T, Nioka H, et al: Mechanism of mutism following the transcallosal approach to third ventricle. Acta Neurochir 110:146–153, 1991.
31. Ehni G, Ehni B: Considerations in transforaminal entry. In Apuzzo MLJ (ed): Surgery of the Third Ventricle, 2nd ed. Baltimore: Williams & Wilkins, 1998, pp 391–419.
32. Ture U, Yasargil MG, Al-Mephty O: The transcallosal-transforaminal approach to the third ventricle with regard to the venous variations in this region. J Neurosurg 87:706–715, 1997.
33. Shucart W: The anterior transcallosal and transcortical approach. In Apuzzo MLJ (ed): Surgery of the Third Ventricle, 2nd ed. Baltimore: Williams & Wilkins, 1998, pp 369–389.
34. Nakasu Y, Isozumi T, Nioka H, et al: Mechanism of mutism following the transcallosal approach to the ventricles. Acta Neurochir (Wien) 110:146–153, 1991.
35. Abdou MS, Cohen AR: Endoscopic treatment of colloid cysts of the ventricle: Technical note and review of the literature. J Neurosurg 89:1062–1068, 1998.
36. Sgaramella E, Sotgiu S, Crotti FM: Neuroendoscopy: One year of experience—personal results, observations and limits. Minim Invasive Neurosurg 46:215–219, 2003.
37. Schroeder HW, Gaab MR: Endoscopic resection of colloid cysts. Neurosurgery 51:1441–1444, 2002.
38. Hellwig D, Bauer BL, Schulte M, et al: Neuroendoscopic treatment for colloid cyst of third ventricle: The experience of a decade. Neurosurgery 52:525–533, 2003.
39. Rhoton AL Jr: The lateral and third ventricle. Neurosurgery 51(Suppl):207–271, 2002.
40. When HT, Rhoton AL Jr, de Olivera E: Transchoroidal approach to the third ventricle: An anatomic study of the choroidal fissure and its clinical application. Neurosurgery 42:1205–1219, 1998.
41. Yamamoto I, Rhoton AL, Peace DA: Microsurgery of the third ventricle. Part 1: Microsurgical anatomy. Neurosurgery 8:334–356, 1981.

42. Bogen JE: Physiological consequences of complete or partial commissural section. In Apuzzo MLJ (ed): Surgery of the Third Ventricle, 2nd ed. Baltimore: Williams & Wilkins, 1998, pp 167–186.

43. Habib M: Syndromes de deconnexion calleuse et organization fonctionelle du corps calleux chez l'adulte. Neurochirurgie 44(Suppl 1): 102–109, 1998.

44. Sauerwein HC, Lassonde M: Neuropsychological alterations after split-brain surgery. J Neurosurg Sci 41:59–66, 1997.

45. Damasio AR, Van Hoesen GW, Tranel D: Pathological correlates of amnesia and the anatomical basis of memory. In Apuzzo MLJ (ed): Surgery of the Third Ventricle, 2nd ed. Baltimore: Williams & Wilkins, 1998, pp 187–204.

46. Garretson HD: Memory in man: A neurosurgeon's perspective. In Apuzzo MLJ (ed): Surgery of the Third Ventricle, 2nd ed. Baltimore: Williams & Wilkins, 1998, pp 211–214.

47. Gaffan D: Recognition impaired and association intact in the memory of monkeys after transection of the fornix. J Comp Physiol Psychol 86:1100–1109, 1974.

48. Gaffan D, Gaffan EA: Amnesia in man following transection of the fornix: A review. Brain 114:2611–2618, 1991.

49. McMackin D, Cockburn J, Ansow P, et al: Correlation of fornix damage with memory impairment in six cases of colloid cyst removal. Acta Neurochir (Wien) 135:12–18, 1995.

50. Page RB: Functional anatomy of the human hypothalamus. In Apuzzo MLJ (ed): Surgery of the Third Ventricle, 2nd ed. Baltimore: Williams & Wilkins, 1998, pp 233–251.

51. Kakou M, Velut S, Destrieux C: Vascularisation arterielle et veineuse du corp calleux. Neurochirurgie 44(Suppl 1):31–37, 1998.

52. Nagata S, Rhoton AL, Barry M: Microsurgical anatomy of the choroidal fissure. Surg Neurol 30:3–59, 1988.

53. Lavyne MH, Patterson RH: The subchoroidal trans-velum interpositum approach. In Apuzzo MLJ (ed): Surgery of the Third Ventricle, 2nd ed. Baltimore: Williams & Wilkins, 1998, pp 453–469.

54. Viale GL, Turtas S: The subchoroidal approach to the third ventricle. Surg Neurol 14:71–76, 1980.

55. Von Cramon DY, Markowitsch HJ, Schuri U: The possible contribution of the septal region to memory. Neuropsychologia 31:1158–1180, 1993.

56. Diamond SJ, Scammel RH, Brouwers EYM, et al: Functions of the centre section (trunk) of the corpus callosum in man. Brain 100:543–562, 1977.

57. Gordon HW: Neuropsychological sequelae of partial commissurotomy. In Boller F, Grafman J (eds): Handbook of Neuropsychology. New York: Elsevier, 1990, pp 85–87.

58. Petrucci RJ, Buchleit WA, Woodruff GC, et al: Transcallosal parafornicial approach for third ventricle tumors: Neuropsychological consequences. Neurosurgery 20:457–464, 1987.

55 Pineal Region Masses: Clinical Features and Management

JEFFREY N. BRUCE

HISTORY

Walter Dandy[1] was the first to undertake a scholarly analysis of surgery in the pineal region. His supratentorial parafalcine approach to the pineal region was the culmination of extensive preclinical animal studies. The exact head position that he used is unclear from his writings, but it appears that some operations were done in a semisitting position, whereas others were done with the hemisphere on the side of the approach uppermost, retracted against gravity. Once the pineal region was reached, he sectioned the corpus callosum and dissected the deep venous system, which unfortunately often resulted in venous damage and central brain edema. Without an operating microscope, steroids, and sophisticated anesthesia, the surgical mortality rate was prohibitively high. Other, just as illustrious, neurosurgeons of that era dismissed the feasibility of operative intervention for pineal tumors because of the technical difficulties encountered and the probability that most of these tumors could not be totally removed because of their malignant and invasive characteristics.

It is remarkable that before Dandy's numerous efforts, Krause[2] in 1926 operated on three patients with lesions in the area of the pineal gland that were probably astrocytomas (perhaps one was a teratoma). There was no operative mortality, and the operative approach was through the posterior fossa over the cerebellum. Considering the limited instrumentation, lack of a microscope or good lighting, and suboptimal anesthesia, these were operative triumphs.

Since that time, a number of different approaches have been advocated including those around the occipital lobe and over the tentorium as described by Poppen.[3] The approach through a dilated lateral ventricle proposed by Van Wagenen[4] was difficult and never gained wide acceptance. The continued difficulty in achieving successful surgical results led to a more conservative approach for pineal region tumors consisting of a shunt for hydrocephalus and radiotherapy for presumed malignancy.[5] Unfortunately, this resulted in numerous publications containing anecdotal information, and an excellent opportunity was lost to study the natural history of the wide variety of tumor types in the pineal region.

In the 1970s, the increasing use of the operating microscope rekindled interest in direct surgical approaches to the pineal region, particularly among Japanese and American neurosurgeons.[6–9] This led to considerable debate over the best surgical route to the pineal region.[7] More important than the route, however, was the fact that debates stimulated interest in operating on these tumors to identify their nature and remove them whenever possible.[10,11] The most recent development in pineal surgery has been the use of stereotactic biopsy as another option for obtaining tissue for histologic diagnosis.[12,13]

The more aggressive approach to pineal region tumors resulted in greater awareness of the histologic diversity of these tumors that exist along an extensive continuum from benign to highly malignant.[14,15] Some of these tumors are mixed in nature, simultaneously containing benign as well as malignant elements or even glial and pineal cell constituents.[14,15] It is now generally accepted that, despite advances in radiographic imaging and increased experience with tumor markers, preoperative diagnostic tests are insufficient and accurate determination of histologic typing requires operative intervention.[16–19]

CLINICAL FEATURES

Epidemiology

Pineal region tumors are rare, accounting for less than 1% of human central nervous system tumors, with somewhat higher percentages in the Japanese population.[15,20,21] Germ cell tumors occur more frequently in the pediatric population, whereas pineal cell tumors are most prevalent in young adults.[22,23] Germ cell tumors have a strong predilection for men over women, although other pineal region tumor types are distributed with equal gender representation.[22–24]

Heritable examples of pineal region tumors are exceptional occurrences, although the childhood syndrome of trilateral retinoblastoma has a familial association.[25,26] This genetically inherited syndrome is characterized by simultaneous pineoblastoma and bilateral retinoblastoma and has been associated with gene deletions and common embryologic origins among the tumors.[24,27]

Pathology

The various cell types that comprise the mature pineal gland account for the diversity of histologic tumor subtypes that can occur in the pineal region. Lobules of pinealocytes surrounded by astrocytes form the pineal parenchyma with ependymal cells of the third ventricle lining the anterior border of the gland. Pineal tumors are grouped into four main categories: (1) germ cell tumors, (2) pineal cell tumors, (3) glial cell tumors, and (4) miscellaneous tumors (covering a wide range of histology) (Table 55-1). Each category contains tumors existing along a continuum from benign to malignant and can include mixed tumors of more than one cell type.[10,28,29] The term *pinealoma* was originally

TABLE 55-1 ▪ **Summary of Pathologic Findings in 191 Patients Undergoing Surgery for Pineal Region Tumors at the New York Neurological Institute (1981–2001)**

Tumor Pathologic Type	No.
Germ Cell	**62 (32%)**
Germinoma	30
Teratoma	9
Lipoma	2
Epidermoid	1
Mixed malignant germ cell	16
Immature teratoma	2
Embryonal cell carcinoma	2
Pineal Cell	**48 (25%)**
Pineocytoma	27
Pineoblastoma	11
Mixed pineal cell	10
Glial Cell	**52 (27%)**
Astrocytoma	27
Anaplastic astrocytoma	3
Glioblastoma	4
Ependynoma	14
Oligodendroglioma	2
Choroid plexus neoplasms	2
Miscellaneous	**29 (15%)**
Pineal cyst	9
Meningioma	10
Other malignant	5
Other benign	4
Total	**191**

used by Krabbe and is a misnomer because it originally pertained to germ cell tumors.[30] Eventually this term was applied more generically to refer to any tumors of the pineal region. The term is now obsolete, in favor of *pineal region tumors* when a general reference is desired or an individual tumor's histology in that region when specificity is preferred (e.g., astrocytoma of the pineal region).[15]

Presentation

Tumors in the pineal region, regardless of their histology, may become symptomatic by three possible mechanisms: (1) increased intracranial pressure from hydrocephalus, (2) direct cerebellar or brain stem compression, or (3) endocrine dysfunction.[14,31,32] Headache, the most common presenting symptom, occurs after obstruction of the third ventricle outflow at Sylvius' aqueduct. More advanced hydrocephalus can result in nausea, vomiting, papilledema, obtundation, and other cognitive deficits.

Direct brain stem compression may lead to disturbances of extraocular movements, classically known as Parinaud's syndrome.[33,34] Parinaud's features include paralysis of upgaze or convergence, retractory nystagmus, and light-near pupillary dissociation. Compression or infiltration of the dorsal midbrain and periaqueductal area can cause paralysis of downgaze, ptosis, and lid retraction. Double vision from fourth nerve palsy is rare but may occur. Extraocular movement dysfunction may also be caused by hydrocephalus, in which case improvement would be expected after ventricular shunting. Involvement of the superior cerebellar

peduncles can lead to ataxia and dysmetria. Hearing disturbances can occasionally occur, probably from compression of the inferior colliculi.[35,36]

Endocrine dysfunction is rare and may be caused by direct tumor involvement in the hypothalamus or from secondary effects of hydrocephalus.[37] Diabetes insipidus and other neuroendocrine disturbances are often indicative of hypothalamic infiltration by tumor, even when not radiographically visualized.[23,38] Precocious puberty has been historically associated with pineal region tumors; however, true documented cases are rare.[30,37,39,40] This syndrome is limited to boys with ectopic β-human chorionic gonadotropin (β-hCG) secretion from choriocarcinomas or germinomas with syncytiotrophoblastic cells.[23,37] The β-hCG secondarily stimulates androgen secretion by the Leydig cells of the testes resulting in the premature sexual maturation characteristics of what is more appropriately termed *pseudopuberty*.

Pineal apoplexy is a rare but often dramatic presentation after spontaneous hemorrhage into a vascular pineal tumor.[41–44] Highly vascular tumors such as pineal cell tumors and choriocarcinomas are most commonly associated with this phenomenon, which can occur postoperatively with devastating consequences in an incompletely resected tumor.[45]

Laboratory Diagnosis

α-Fetoprotein and β-hCG are markers of germ cell malignancy and should be measured in serum and cerebrospinal fluid, if possible, as part of the preoperative workup in patients with pineal region tumors.[15,31,32,46] Elevation of germ cell markers is pathognomonic for the presence of a malignant germ cell tumor, and under these circumstances, histologic verification is unnecessary as surgery does not improve the outcome with radiation and chemotherapy.[31] In patients with marker-positive germ cell tumors, measurement of marker levels can also be useful to monitor therapeutic response and as a sensitive early sign of tumor recurrence. It is important to note that the absence of germ cell markers should be interpreted cautiously because malignant germ cell tumors such as germinomas and embryonal cell carcinomas cannot be ruled out.[15,31]

α-Fetoprotein, normally associated with fetal yolk sac elements, is markedly elevated with endodermal sinus tumors, whereas smaller elevations occur with embryonal cell carcinomas and immature teratomas.[23,32,46–52] β-hCG, normally secreted by placental trophoblastic tissue, is markedly elevated with choriocarcinomas, with smaller elevations associated with embryonal cell carcinomas and those occasional germinomas containing syncytiotrophoblastic giant cells.[15,23,32,46,48,50,53–56] Most germinomas are nonsecretory and carry a better prognosis than β-hCG-positive germinomas.[57,58]

Other tumor markers including placental alkaline phosphatase, c-*kit* proto-oncogene, carcinoembryonic antigen, lactate dehydrogenase, and B5 monoclonal antibody have been investigated with pineal tumors but have not been as clinically relevant as α-fetoprotein and β-hCG.[32,48,59–62] Markers of pineal cell tumors such as S antigen and melatonin have been more useful for immunohistochemical applications in tissue diagnosis.[63–69]

Imaging

The standard diagnostic workup includes magnetic resonance imaging (MRI), with and without contrast, which has proven to be the most accurate diagnostic examination and provides information on tumor type and the anatomic relationships of the tumor with its surroundings (Fig. 55-1). Some tumors can be suspected from the appearance of the scans, particularly teratomas, which contain multiple germ layers (Fig. 55-2). Angiography is only performed if the MRI suggests a vascular lesion such as an aneurysm of Galen's vein or arteriovenous malformation. Despite this broad diagnostic armamentarium, the exact histologic nature of the tumor cannot be reliably determined without surgery.[14,16–18,31,70]

The radiographic workup provides relevant information about the following:

1. Size of tumor: lateral and superior extent
2. Vascularity of the lesion and the nature of its contents (whether homogeneous or heterogeneous)
3. Irregularities of margination and the probability of invasion
4. Anatomic relationships of the tumor and the surrounding structures, including involvement of the third ventricle and position within the third ventricle, extension into or above the corpus callosum, superolateral extension into the region of the ventricular trigone, involvement or compression of the quadrigeminal region and aqueduct, relationship to the anterior cerebellar vermis, and location of the deep venous system

The increasing use of MRI has revealed a large number of patients with lesions of the pineal gland that are mostly cystic but contain a small amount of solid tissue (Fig. 55-3). In most cases, the aqueduct has not been compromised and

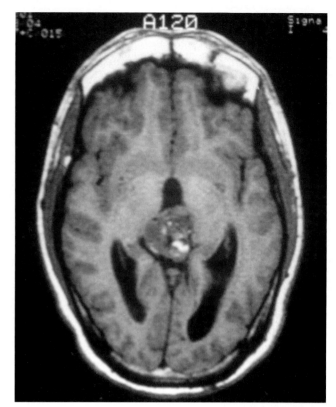

FIGURE 55-2 Magnetic resonance imaging with contrast (axial view) demonstrates the typical variegated pattern of a mixed germ cell tumor of the pineal region. The heterogeneity of lesions such as this in the pineal region can lead to misdiagnosis from sampling error.

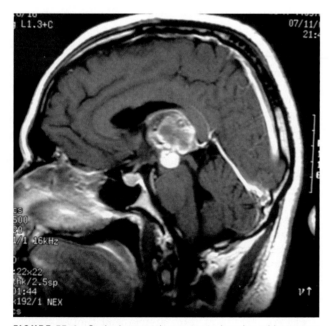

FIGURE 55-1 Sagittal magnetic resonance imaging with contrast shows a large pineal region tumor. The anatomic relationships of the tumor are well identified including the third ventricle, aqueduct, and quadrigeminal plate.

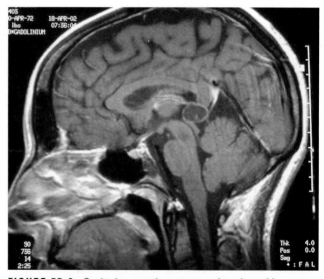

FIGURE 55-3 Sagittal magnetic resonance imaging with contrast shows an incidental pineal cyst discovered during the workup for unrelated headaches. The aqueduct is not compromised, and there is no hydrocephalus. Pineal cysts are anatomic variants and do not require treatment except in rare instances when they become symptomatic.

the patients are not symptomatic from their lesion. Initially, they were considered to be low-grade cystic astrocytomas but, after surgical removal, were found to be composed of normal astrocytes and normal pineal cells.[71] Histologically, these are pineal cysts and are normal anatomic variations of the pineal gland. As experience with pineal cysts has increased, it is clear that they should be managed conservatively with serial MRI scans and without surgery. Surgery is reserved for lesions that are symptomatic, progressing in size, or causing aqueductal obstruction.

SURGICAL CONSIDERATIONS

Surgical Anatomy

Most tumors arise from and are attached to the undersurface of the velum interpositum, which includes the choroid plexus, deep venous system, and choroidal arteries (see Fig. 55-6). Depending on the degree of invasion of these important midline structures, the attachment may be minimal or comprehensive. Tumors rarely extend above the velum interpositum for any significant distance. Therefore, the blood supply comes from within the velum interpositum, mainly through the posterior medial and lateral choroidal arteries with anastomoses to the pericallosal arteries and quadrigeminal arteries.[72,73]

Some tumors extend to the Monro's foramen, but most are centered at the pineal gland, extending to the midportion of the third ventricle and posteriorly to compress the anterior portion of the cerebellum. In rare instances, the internal cerebral veins are ventral to the tumor, which can be recognized through the MRI (Fig. 55-4). Mostly, however, Galen's vein, internal cerebral veins, Rosenthal's vein, and precentral cerebellar vein surround or cap the periphery of these tumors. The quadrigeminal plate may give rise to an exophytic astrocytoma or be infiltrated by the more malignant tumors of the pineal region, encompassing the aqueduct in the course of tumor growth. Most tumors are not highly vascular, with the exception of pineoblastomas,

hemangioblastomas, and hemangiopericytomas (angioplastic meningiomas). The most important aspects of the anatomy, which can be gleaned by radiographic imaging, are the relationship of the tumor to the third ventricle and quadrigeminal cistern, and the lateral and superior extent of the tumor. These features determine the route of the operation and the degree of difficulty likely to be encountered during surgery.[73]

Management of Hydrocephalus

Most patients present with obstructive hydrocephalus, a problem that may be managed in several ways. When a complete tumor removal is anticipated and a permanent shunt may not be necessary, the hydrocephalus can be managed with a ventricular drain placed at the time of tumor surgery. The ventricular drain can be removed or converted to a permanent shunt on postoperative day 2 or 3, depending on which circumstances prevail. Occasionally, no drain is necessary and the hydrocephalus resolves after complete tumor removal.[31,74] The drain can be removed or converted to a shunt in the postoperative period as the circumstances dictate. Patients with more advanced symptomatology should be managed with a computed tomography–guided stereotactic endoscopic third ventriculostomy to allow a gradual reduction in intracranial pressure and resolution of symptoms.[75] This method is preferable to ventriculoperitoneal shunting as it eliminates potential complications such as infection, overshunting, and peritoneal seeding of malignant cells.

Operative Approaches: Biopsy versus Open Resection

The wide diversity of pathology that can occur in the pineal region makes histologic diagnosis a necessity to optimize patient management decisions.[8,13,14,19,74,76–88] Tissue histology has important implications for decisions concerning adjuvant therapy, metastatic workup, prognosis, and long-term follow-up. Cerebrospinal fluid cytology and radiographic examination are not sufficiently consistent to supplant the need for tissue diagnosis.[16,70,89–92] The exception to mandatory histologic diagnosis is patients with elevated germ cell markers who can be treated with chemotherapy and radiation without a biopsy.[31,93] Some of these patients require a delayed surgical resection to remove residual radiographic abnormalities that may represent residual tumor.[94]

Specimens for tissue diagnosis can be obtained by either a stereotactic biopsy or an open operation.[14,31] Passionate advocates for either approach can be found; however, it is important to recognize the relative advantages and disadvantages of each and use them in a complementary fashion for appropriate patients rather than having an inflexible dedication to one. Procedural decisions will be influenced by the radiographic and clinical features of the tumor and the surgeon's experience.

Experienced neurosurgeons using current microsurgical techniques can expect favorable results with open surgery.[19] Open procedures have the advantage of obtaining larger amounts of tissue to provide more extensive tissue sampling. This is particularly important for pineal region tumors where heterogeneity and mixed cell populations are common.

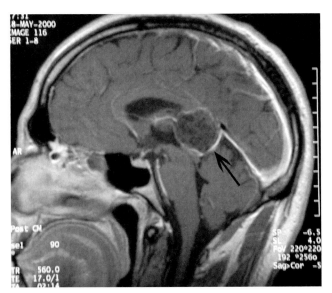

FIGURE 55-4 Sagittal magnetic resonance imaging view shows a pineal tumor situated dorsal to the internal cerebral veins (*arrow*).

This diversity is problematic for even experienced neuropathologists who can best resolve the subtleties of histologic diagnosis when free from the constraints of limited tissue sampling.[14,51,74,95,96] Additionally, open procedures provide a clinical advantage by facilitating tumor removal. This is particularly important for the one third of patients with benign pineal tumors, in whom resection is usually complete but can also be useful for patients with malignant tumors in whom debulking may provide a more favorable response to adjuvant therapy and a better long-term prognosis.[28,87,97–101] Additional advantages of aggressive tumor debulking include the potential to relieve hydrocephalus without additional procedures and the ability to control the risks of postoperative hemorrhage into an incompletely resected tumor bed. A disadvantage of open procedures is the relatively higher surgical morbidity compared with that of stereotactic biopsy, at least in the short term. This short-term disadvantage, however, may be a reasonable concession for the long-term advantage of better tumor control.

Any discussion about the relative risks and benefits of open procedures must recognize that the highly favorable outcome for patient with pineal tumor assumes an advanced level of experience, judgment, and expertise. These sophisticated surgical procedures are not recommended for novice surgeons as they can expect significantly less favorable outcomes. Stereotactic procedures, in contrast, can be appealing because of their ease of performance; however, the pineal region is among the most hazardous areas in the brain to safely biopsy, and careful forethought must be given to planning the target and trajectory to minimize hemorrhagic risks.[12,13,86,102–104] The potential for hemorrhage is increased because of several mechanisms including bleeding from any of several pial surfaces that must be traversed, bleeding in highly vascular tumors, damage to the deep venous system, and bleeding into the ventricle where the tissue turgor is insufficient to tamponade minor bleeding.[12,74,95,105,106] Despite this increased risk, several series have validated the effectiveness of stereotactic biopsy for these tumors.[13,103]

Stereotactic biopsy is ideally suited for patients with multiple lesions or clinical conditions that contraindicate open surgery and general anesthesia.[31] Biopsy may also be preferable for tumors that are clearly invading the brain stem. However, the degree of invasion is not always easily discernible and tumors may have a surgically dissectable capsule that is not predicted on preoperative imaging studies.

Stereotactic Biopsy

Stereotactic biopsies of pineal tumors are more complicated and have a reduced margin of error compared with tumors in other locations.[105,107] Nevertheless, several series by experienced neurosurgeons have validated stereotactic biopsy as a suitable alternative to open procedures.[13,103,108] Advances in radiographic imaging and software planning provide several alternatives for safely planning biopsy trajectories. Computed tomography–guided procedures are acceptable because of their high degree of accuracy and common availability. Although nearly any stereotactic frame system is sufficient, target-centered stereotactic frame

systems such as the CRW (Cosman-Roberts-Wells) have the versatility to facilitate even complex biopsies. Local anesthesia with mild sedation is safe and usually sufficient to perform biopsies.

The most common surgical trajectory to the pineal region is via an anterolaterosuperior approach anterior to the coronal suture and lateral to the mid-pupillary line.[109] This trajectory passes through the frontal lobe and the internal capsule. The ependyma of the lateral ventricle and the internal cerebral vein should be avoided. An alternative approach is a posterolaterosuperior approach through the parieto-occipital junction, which is best suited for large tumors that have a lateral extension.

Whenever possible, multiple serial biopsy specimens should be obtained. Obviously, the risks of bleeding for each additional specimen must be considered, taking into account the size of the mass. A frozen section intraoperatively may be useful in verifying pathologic tissue, however, the high diversity of tissue types reduces the accuracy of a frozen tissue diagnosis.

Endoscopy

Advances in endoscopic technique have led to investigations of biopsies via this method.[110–115] Endoscopy is sometimes performed in conjunction with an endoscopic third ventriculostomy to relieve hydrocephalus. Performing a ventriculostomy and biopsy simultaneously requires the use of a flexible endoscope because of the limited trajectory to the tumor through Monro's foramen. A rigid endoscope can be used but would necessitate a second burr hole and trajectory with a more inferior entry point on the forehead. The risks of an endoscopic biopsy are considerable due to the limited tissue sampling and difficulty achieving hemostasis within the ventricle. Even minor bleeding can obscure the operative field, making it difficult to identify the target. In general, given these limitations, a stereotactic biopsy is preferable to endoscopic biopsy in situations in which diagnostic tissue is desired.

SURGICAL APPROACHES
Operative Considerations

Common approaches to the pineal region include infratentorial supracerebellar, occipital transtentorial, and transcallosal interhemispheric.[31,116,117] These approaches are described in the next two chapters. The best approach to use depends on the anatomic location or spread of the tumor along with a degree of familiarity and confidence that the surgeon has with a given approach.

Generally, the infratentorial supracerebellar approach is preferred for several reasons (Fig. 55-5A):

1. The approach is to the center of the tumor, which begins at the midline and grows eccentrically.
2. The approach is ventral to the velum interpositum and the deep venous system to which the tumor is often adherent. This minimizes the risk of damage to the vascular drainage of this critical region.
3. The exposure in the sitting position is comparable with that of other routes.
4. No normal tissue is violated on route to the tumor.

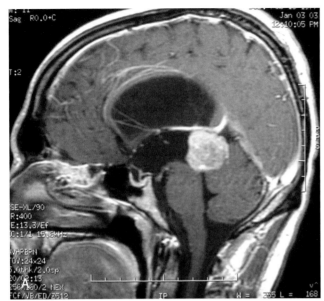

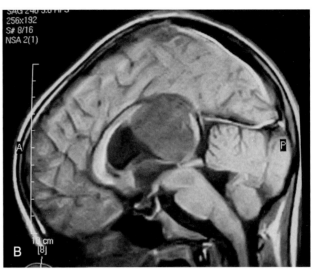

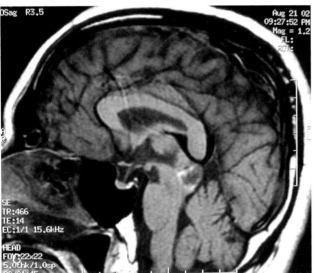

FIGURE 55-5 Midsagittal gadolinium enhanced magnetic resonance images illustrate the preferred surgical approaches. *A,* Meningioma of the velum interpositum with dorsal displacement of internal cerebral veins is best approached via the infratentorial-supracerebellar corridor. *B,* Pilocytic astrocytoma arising from the corpus callosum with ventral displacement of the internal cerebral veins is best approach via the posterior-interhemispheric corridor. *C,* Tectal glioma is best approached via the occipital transtentorial corridor to facilitate access to the inferior portion of the tumor.

Either the transcallosal interhemispheric or occipital transtentorial approaches are used under the following circumstances (see Fig. 55-5):

1. Tumors that extend superiorly, involving or destroying the posterior aspect of the corpus callosum and deflecting the deep venous system in a dorsolateral direction
2. Tumors that extend laterally to the region of the trigone
3. In rare cases in which the tumor displaces the deep venous system in a ventral direction (often seen with meningiomas)

Under these circumstances, the transcallosal interhemispheric approach can provide extensive exposure, although the subtentorial portion of the tumor on the contralateral side of the approach is not easily visualized. This approach requires retraction of the parietal lobe and the disruption of bridging veins between parietal lobe and the sagittal sinus, creating the potential for venous infarct and retraction injury. Additionally, the veins of the deep venous

system usually overlie the tumor, forcing the surgeon to work around them to avoid injury. Like the transcallosal approach, the occipital transtentorial approach has the disadvantage of encountering the deep venous system overlying the tumor. Once the tentorium is divided, however, this approach permits a wide view of the pineal region with particularly good visualization of the quadrigeminal plate. A major drawback is the high frequency of visual field deficits associated with this approach.[118]

Various positions have been described for these approaches. The sitting position is used most often for the infratentorial supracerebellar and occipital transtentorial approaches. This position enables gravity to work in the surgeon's favor by helping tumor dissection from the roof of the third ventricle and minimizing blood pooling in the operative field. It does carry the risk of air embolus or ventricular and cortical collapse with subsequent subdural hematoma or air.[45,119] However, with proper precautions, these complications are infrequent. The occipital transtentorial approach often uses the three-quarter prone and lateral decubitus position, which, although avoiding many of the complications of the sitting position, does not allow gravity to work in the surgeon's favor.[31,116,117] The Concorde position was developed to combine aspects of both the prone and semisitting positions but still has the disadvantage of blood pooling in the operative field.[120]

COMPLICATIONS OF SURGERY

Serious complications of pineal tumor surgery, regardless of the route used, are related to the nature of the tumor and its potential for intra- or postoperative hemorrhage.[45,119] Hemorrhage has played a major role in most of the surgery-related deaths and can occur with a delay of as long as several postoperative days. This phenomenon is most prevalent with malignant pineal cell tumors (pineoblastomas), which tend to be soft and highly vascular. Hemorrhage can occur before surgery as a so-called pineal apoplexy or can be associated with stereotactic biopsy.[42,43]

Complications of the sitting position, particularly with the posterior fossa approach, include air embolism, hypotension, and cortical collapse when hydrocephalus of significant degree is relieved by tumor removal.[45,119] The incidence of cortical collapse can be reduced by preoperative shunting or third ventriculostomy to allow the ventricular system a chance to accommodate over several days before the major operation. This phenomenon can occur in varying degrees and, although striking on the postoperative computed tomography scan, gradually improves without major neurologic complications for the patient. Subdural shunting is rarely required to relieve chronic hygromas resulting from this complication.

The complications of the interhemispheric approach are related to retraction of the parietal lobe with transient sensory or stereognostic deficits on the opposite side.[119] These have not been serious or permanent. Unlike the occipital transtentorial approach, the interhemispheric approach has not been associated with visual field defects.

Regardless of the operative approach used, various pupil abnormalities, difficulty focusing or accommodating, interocular palsies, and limitation of upward gaze can be expected whenever the tumor is dissected from the quadrigeminal region. These deficits improve gradually but may last for many months or as long as a year before normal function returns. Manipulation of the brain adjacent to the third ventricle can lead to impaired consciousness. The fourth cranial nerve is generally caudal to the tumor and is rarely identified or injured. Ataxia has been minimal and usually transient. The incidence and severity of deficits are increased with prior radiation therapy, presence of symptoms preoperatively, and a high degree of malignant and invasive characteristics.[45,101] Shunt malfunction or blockage of a ventriculostomy can occur in as many as 20% of patients after surgery.

SURGICAL RESULTS

Among large series of pineal region tumors in the microscopic era, operative mortality ranges from 0 to 8% and permanent morbidity from 0 to 25%.[19,50,74,83,85,86,97,99,121–123] Pineal region tumors are among the most difficult surgical challenges, and outcome will vary significantly with the expertise and experience of the individual surgeon.

For benign tumors, surgical resection is the treatment of choice with complete surgical removal likely to result in excellent long-term survival and likely cure.[19,97,124–126] With malignant tumors, the impact of surgery is less delineated, although the degree of resection can correlate with improved prognosis.[19,28,97,99,100,123]

ADJUVANT THERAPY

Postoperative Staging

All patients with malignant pineal cell tumors, germ cell tumors, and ependymomas should have a postoperative staging to look for spinal metastasis. In the past, these patients were screened with a myelogram and computed tomography scan; however, spinal MRI with contrast is now the procedure of choice.[28,127] Cerebrospinal fluid cytology is performed but is rarely helpful for guiding management decisions.

Prophylactic spinal radiation is controversial in patients with pineal region tumors. Previously, complete cranial-spinal irradiation was recommended for all malignant pineal tumors; however, the current trend is to avoid spinal radiation unless there is documented evidence of spinal seeding.[14,23,74,91,127–133] Overall, the incidence of spinal seeding is relatively small, and it is not clear that spinal radiation prevents failure in the spine when no tumor is present on postoperative staging. In patients with radiographic documentation of spinal seeding, a dose of 3500 cGy is recommended to the spine.

Radiation Therapy

Patients with malignant germ cell or pineal cell tumors require radiation therapy. The recommended radiation dose is 5500 cGy given in 180-cGy daily fractions with 4000 cGy to the ventricular system and an additional 1500 cGy to the tumor bed.[15,32,134] Recent studies suggest that using a more limited field of radiation that avoids the adverse side effects of ventricular exposure may be sufficiently efficacious; however, these studies lack long-term follow-up.[131]

Radiation therapy may be withheld for the rare, histologically benign pineocytoma or ependymoma that has been completely resected.[28,97,126] This distinction is based on the intraoperative observation of a well-circumscribed tumor that is well differentiated histologically. Surgical resection alone provides excellent long-term control in this group; however, careful follow-up is necessary so that radiation or radiosurgery can be offered at the first sign of recurrence.

Germinomas are the most radiosensitive malignant tumors in the central nervous system, with current expectations of 90% long-term control after a full course of radiation therapy.[133,135] Older published series, with more long-term follow-up, report 5-year survival rates of more than 75% and 10-year survival rates of 69% when radiation doses of 5000 cGy have been used.[74,134,136] With less than 5000 cGy, a higher incidence of local failure can be expected.[90,134] Germinomas associated with elevated β-hCG levels may have a less favorable prognosis.[57,58]

The extended long-term survival in these patients makes them vulnerable to delayed side effects of radiation.

Cognitive deficits, hypothalamic and endocrine dysfunction, cerebral necrosis, and de novo tumor formation are some of the reported delayed complications of cranial radiation therapy.[74,140–144] Pediatric patients are particularly vulnerable to adverse radiation effects.[145–149] In an effort to reduce the dose of radiation and minimize these effects, treatment strategies combining reduced radiation with chemotherapy are being investigated.[137–139]

Chemotherapy

Patients with nongerminomatous malignant germ cell tumors have benefited most from advances in chemotherapy (Fig. 55-6). Current chemotherapy regimens have resulted in reasonable expectations for long-term survival. Additionally, patients with germinomas containing syncytiotrophoblastic giant cells have a less favorable prognosis and may benefit from more aggressive treatment with chemotherapy in addition to radiotherapy.[57,58]

Most of the germ cell chemotherapy regimens have been extrapolated from experience treating germ cell tumors of extracranial origin in which success has been remarkable.[150–154] Unfortunately, these successes have not been as favorable for intracranial tumors.[23,53,57,74,84,155–159] Most successful chemotherapy regimens are derived from the protocols for testicular cancer using the Einhorn regimen of cisplatin, vinblastine, and bleomycin, although other combinations involving cyclophosphamide or etoposide have been investigated.[32,155,160] Recent studies, using VP-16 (etoposide) in place of vinblastine and bleomycin to avoid the pulmonary toxicity have shown improved response rate with less morbidity.[57,83,157,158] Currently a regimen of cisplatin or carboplatin with etoposide is among the most widely used.

The role of radiation therapy combined with chemotherapy in these tumors is unclear.[161] Although radiation therapy is generally given before chemotherapy, the optimal timing has not been defined. Whether radiation therapy improves survival over chemotherapy alone is not clear; however, several reports show increased survival in aggressively treated patients using a combination of chemotherapy, radiation, and surgery.[23,49,159,162–165] An aggressive approach seems reasonable given the poor prognosis of these tumors and strategies for second-look surgeries to remove tumors that remain after adjuvant therapy may improve long-term survival.[94,166] For pure germinomas, the exquisite radiosensitivity of these tumors has made chemotherapy less compelling except for patients with recurring or metastatic disease. This success has spurred interest in the use of chemotherapy as a means of reducing the overall dose of radiation.[138,139,167] Although this is a sound philosophy, the long-term results have not withstood the same test of time established for radiation therapy alone.

Chemotherapy for pineal cell tumors has mostly been relegated to recurrent or disseminated pineal cell tumors.[22,32,84,168] There have been some responses in treatment combinations consisting of various combinations of vincristine, lomustine, cisplatin, etoposide, cyclophosphamide, actinomycin D, and methotrexate. Success with these various regimens has been limited, and therefore no clear-cut recommendations have been given.[169] Recent

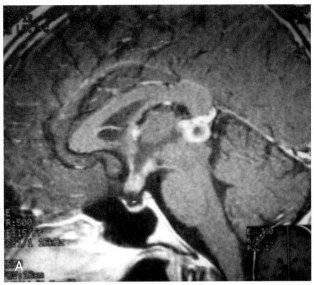

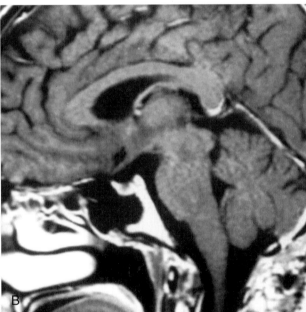

FIGURE 55-6 Malignant germ cell tumors respond well to chemotherapy. *A,* Sagittal magnetic resonance imaging of malignant germ cell tumor involving the pineal region and floor of the third ventricle before chemotherapy. *B,* Same tumor after one course of chemotherapy with no radiographically visible residual.

reports suggest that combined radiation and chemotherapy may be beneficial for pediatric patients with malignant pineal cell tumors.[168]

Radiosurgery

One of the more recent developments in pineal region treatment has been the application of radiosurgical techniques.[13,77,170,171] Several studies have clearly documented the relative safety of this method, although long-term follow-up results are currently lacking. Radiosurgery is generally limited to tumors less than 3 cm in diameter.

Distinct differences in radiobiologic effects between radiosurgery and conventional fractionated radiation must be considered when choosing optimal therapeutic strategies. Germinomas, for example, have excellent long-term response to fractionated radiation, and it is unlikely that radiosurgery will improve on these results. Additionally, because radiosurgery provides no therapeutic coverage to the ventricular system, tumors such as pineal cell and germ cell tumors are particularly vulnerable to ventricular recurrence. Radiosurgery may have its greatest benefit in providing a local boost to the tumor bed so that the radiation exposure to the ventricles and surrounding brain can be reduced.[77] It may also be useful for tumors that recur locally.

CONCLUSIONS

Advances in the treatment of pineal region tumors have led to significant improvements in survival as well as quality of life. The wide diversity of histologic subtypes in the pineal region necessitates a tissue diagnosis to optimally guide management decisions (the only exception being patients with elevated germ cell markers). A variety of operative approaches including stereotactic procedures can facilitate this with a reasonable risk. Surgical removal of benign or encapsulated tumors results in excellent long-term outcome. Most patients with malignant tumors will benefit from surgical removal as well, although successful surgical outcomes are dependent on advanced surgical expertise and experience. Adjuvant therapy with radiation and/or chemotherapy can be highly beneficial for most malignant pineal region tumors, with malignant germ cell tumors among the most responsive. Radiosurgery is a more recent addition to the armamentarium and may be most helpful for recurrent tumors.

REFERENCES

1. Dandy WE: Operative experience in cases of pineal tumor. Arch Surg 33:19–46, 1936.
2. Krause F: Operative Frielegung der Vierhugel, nebst Beobachtungen uber Hirndruck und Dekompression. Zentrabl Chir 53:2812–2819, 1926.
3. Poppen JL: The right occipital approach to a pinealoma. J Neurosurg 25:706–710, 1966.
4. Van Wagenen WP: A surgical approach for the removal of certain pineal tumors. Surg Gynecol Obstet 53:216–220, 1931.
5. Abay EO II, Laws ER Jr, Grado GL, et al: Pineal tumors in children and adolescents: Treatment by CSF shunting and radiotherapy. J Neurosurg 55:889–895, 1981.
6. Page LK: The infratentorial-supracerebellar exposure of tumors in the pineal area. Neurosurgery 1:36–40, 1977.
7. Reid WS, Clark WK: Comparison of the infratentorial and transtentorial approaches to the pineal region. Neurosurgery 3:1–8, 1978.
8. Stein BM: The infratentorial supracerebellar approach to pineal lesions. J Neurosurg 35:197–202, 1971.
9. Lazar ML, Clark K: Direct surgical management of masses in the region of the vein of Galen. Surg Neurol 2:17–21, 1974.
10. Sano K: Pineal region tumors: Problems in pathology and treatment. Clin Neurosurg 30:59–89, 1984.
11. Stein BM, Fetell MR: Therapeutic modalities for pineal region tumors. Clin Neurosurg 32:445–455, 1985.
12. Pecker J, Scarabin J-M, Vallee B, Brucher J-M: Treatment in tumours of the pineal region: Value of stereotaxic biopsy. Surg Neurol 12:341–348, 1979.
13. Dempsey PK, Kondziolka D, Lunsford LD: Stereotactic diagnosis and treatment of pineal region tumours and vascular malformations. Acta Neurochir (Wien) 116:14–22, 1992.
14. Bruce JN: Management of pineal region tumors. Neurosurg Q 3:103–119, 1993.
15. Bruce JN, Connolly ES, Stein BM: Pineal and germ cell tumors. In Laws ER (ed): Brain Tumors, 2nd ed. London: Churchill Livingstone, 2001, pp 771–800.
16. Ganti SR, Hilal SK, Silver AJ, et al: CT of pineal region tumors. AJNR Am J Neuroradiol 7:97–104, 1986.
17. Müller-Forell W, Schroth G, Egan PJ: MR imaging in tumors of the pineal region. Neuroradiology 30:224–231, 1988.
18. Tien RD, Barkovich AJ, Edwards MSB: MR imaging of pineal tumors. AJNR Am J Neuroradiol 11:557–565, 1990.
19. Bruce JN, Ogden AT: Surgical strategies for treating patients with pineal region tumors. J Neurooncol 69:221–236, 2004.
20. Koide O, Watanabe Y, Sato K: A pathological survey of intracranial germinoma and pinealoma in Japan. Cancer 45:2119–2130, 1980.
21. Zimmerman RA, Bilaniuk LT: Age-related incidence of pineal calcification detected by computed tomography. Neuroradiology 142:659–662, 1982.
22. Schild SE, Scheithauer BW, Schomberg PJ, et al: Pineal parenchymal tumors: Clinical, pathologic, and therapeutic aspects. Cancer 72:870–880, 1993.
23. Jennings MT, Gelman R, Hochberg F: Intracranial germ-cell tumors: Natural history and pathogenesis. J Neurosurg 63:155–167, 1985.
24. Russell DS, Rubinstein LJ: Tumours of specialized tissues of central neuroepithelial origin. In Rubinstein LJ (ed): Pathology of Tumours of the Nervous System. Baltimore: Williams & Wilkins, 1989, pp 351–420.
25. Russell DS, Rubinstein LJ: Tumours and tumour-like lesions of maldevelopmental origin. In Rubinstein LJ (ed): Pathology of Tumours of the Nervous System. Baltimore: Williams & Wilkins, 1989, pp 664–765.
26. Bader JL, Meadows AT, Zimmerman LE, et al: Bilateral retinoblastoma with ectopic intracranial retinoblastoma: Trilateral retinoblastoma. Cancer Genet Cytogenet 5:201–213, 1982.
27. Murphree A, Benedict W: Retinoblastoma: Clues to human oncogenesis. Science 223:1028–1033, 1984.
28. Stein BM, Bruce JN: Surgical management of pineal region tumors. Clin Neurosurg 39:509–532, 1992.
29. Horowitz MB, Hall WA: Central nervous system germinomas. Arch Neurol 48:652–657, 1991.
30. Krabbe KH: The pineal gland, especially in relation to the problem on its supposed significance in sexual development. Endocrinology 7:379–414, 1923.
31. Bruce J: Pineal tumors. In Winn H (ed): Youman's Neurological Surgery, vol 1. Philadelphia: WB Saunders, 2004, pp 1011–1029.
32. Sawaya R, Hawley DK, Tobler WD, et al: Pineal and third ventricular tumors. In Youmans J (ed): Neurological Surgery. Philadelphia: WB Saunders, 1990, pp 3171–3203.
33. Parinaud H: Paralysis of the movement of convergence of the eyes. Brain 9:330–341, 1886.
34. Posner M, Horrax G: Eye signs in pineal tumors. J Neurosurg 3:15–24, 1946.
35. Missori P, Delfini R, Cantore G: Tinnitus and hearing loss in pineal region tumours. Acta Neurochir 135:154–158, 1995.
36. DeMonte F, Zelby A, Al-Mefty O: Hearing impairment resulting from a pineal region meningioma. Neurosurgery 32:665–668, 1993.
37. Fetell MR, Stein BM: Neuroendocrine aspects of pineal tumors. In Abrams GM (ed): Neurologic Clinics: Neuroendocrinology and Brain Peptides, vol 4. Philadelphia: WB Saunders, 1986, pp 877–905.
38. Grote E, Lorenz R, Vuia O: Clinical and endocrinological findings in ectopic pinealoma and spongioblastoma of the hypothalamus. Acta Neurochir 53:87–98, 1980.
39. Zondek H, Kaatz A, Unger H: Precocious puberty and chorioepithelioma of the pineal gland with report of a case. J Endocrinol 10:12–16, 1953.
40. Borit A: History of tumors of the pineal region. Am J Surg Pathol 5:613–620, 1981.
41. Herrick MK, Rubinstein LJ: The cytological differentiating potential of pineal parenchymal neoplasms (true pinealomas): A clinicopathological study of 28 tumours. Brain 102:289–320, 1979.
42. Higashi K, Katayama S, Orita T: Pineal apoplexy. J Neurol Neurosurg Psychiatry 42:1050–1053, 1979.
43. Burres KP, Hamilton RD: Pineal apoplexy. Neurosurgery 4:264–268, 1979.
44. Steinbok P, Dolmen C, Kaan K: Pineocytomas presenting as subarachnoid hemorrhage: Report of 2 cases. J Neurosurg 47:776–780, 1977.

45. Bruce J, Stein B: Supracerebellar approaches in the pineal region. In Apuzzo M (ed): Brain Surgery: Complication Avoidance and Management. New York: Churchill Livingstone, 1993, pp 511–536.

46. Allen JC, Nisselbaum J, Epstein F, et al: Alphafetoprotein and human chorionic gonadotropin determination in cerebrospinal fluid: An aid to the diagnosis and management of intracranial germ-cell tumors. J Neurosurg 51:368–374, 1979.

47. Allen JC, Bosl G, Walker R: Chemotherapy trials in recurrent primary intracranial germ cell tumors. J Neurooncol 3:147–152, 1985.

48. Arita N, Ushio Y, Hayakawa T, et al: Serum levels of alpha-fetoprotein, human chorionic gonadotropin and carcinoembryonic antigen in patients with primary intracranial germ cell tumors. Oncodev Biol Med (Amsterdam) 1:235–240, 1980.

49. Bamberg M, Metz K, Alberti W, et al: Endodermal sinus tumor of the pineal region: Metastasis through a ventriculoperitoneal shunt. Cancer 54:903–906, 1984.

50. Jooma R, Kendall BE: Diagnosis and management of pineal tumors. J Neurosurg 58:654–665, 1983.

51. Ho DM, Liu H-C: Primary intracranial germ cell tumor: Pathologic study of 51 patients. Cancer 70:1577–1584, 1992.

52. Wilson ER, Takei Y, Bikoff WT, et al: Abdominal metastases of primary intracranial yolk sac tumors through ventriculoperitoneal shunts: Report of three cases. Neurosurgery 5:356–364, 1979.

53. Haase J, Norgaard-Pedersen B: Alpha-fetoprotein (AFP) and human chorionic gonadotropin (HCG) as biochemical markers of intracranial germ cell tumors. Acta Neurochir (Wien) 53:269–274, 1979.

54. Neuwelt EA, Glasberg M, Frenkel E, Clark WK: Malignant pineal region tumors. J Neurosurg 51:597–607, 1979.

55. Page R, Doshi B, Sharr M: Primary intracranial choriocarcinoma. J Neurol Neurosurg Psychiatry 49:93–95, 1986.

56. Bloom H: Primary intracranial germ cell tumours. Clin Oncol 2:233–257, 1983.

57. Yoshida J, Sugita K, Kobayashi T, et al: Prognosis of intracranial germ cell tumours: Effectiveness of chemotherapy with cisplatin and etoposide (CDDP and VP-16). Acta Neurochir (Wien) 120:111–117, 1993.

58. Uematsu Y, Tsuura Y, Miyamoto K, et al: The recurrence of primary intracranial germinomas: Special reference to germinoma with STGC (syncytiotrophoblastic giant cell). J Neurooncol 13:247–256, 1992.

59. Shinoda J, Yamada H, Sakai N, et al: Placental alkaline phosphatase as a tumor marker for primary intracranial germinoma. J Neurosurg 68:710–720, 1988.

60. Suzuki Y, Tanaka R: Carcinoembryonic antigen in patients with intracranial tumors. J Neurosurg 53:355–360, 1980.

61. Metcalfe S, Sikora K: A new marker for testicular cancer. Br J Cancer 52:127–129, 1985.

62. Miyanohara O, Takeshima H, Kaji M, et al: Diagnostic significance of soluble c-kit in the cerebrospinal fluid of patients with germ cell tumors. J Neurosurg 97:177–183, 2002.

63. Korf HW, Klein DC, Zigler JS, et al: S-antigen-like immunoreactivity in a human pineocytoma. Acta Neuropathol (Berl) 69:165–167, 1986.

64. Korf HW, Bruce JA, Vistica B, et al: Immunoreactive S-antigen in cerebrospinal fluid: A marker of pineal parenchymal tumors? J Neurosurg 70:682–687, 1989.

65. Vorkapic P, Waldhauser F, Bruckner R, et al: Serum melatonin levels: A new neurodiagnostic tool in pineal region tumors? Neurosurgery 21:817–824, 1987.

66. Wurtman RJ, Kammer H: Melatonin synthesis by an ectopic pinealoma. N Engl J Med 274:1233–1237, 1966.

67. Miles A, Tidmarsh S, Philbrick D, Shaw D: Diagnostic potential of melatonin analysis in pineal tumors. N Engl J Med 313:329–330, 1985.

68. Arendt J: Melatonin as a tumour marker in a patient with pineal tumour. BMJ 26:635–636, 1978.

69. Barber S, Smith J, Hughes R: Melatonin as a tumour marker in a patient with pineal tumour. Lancet ii:328, 1978.

70. Zimmerman R: Pineal region masses: Radiology. In Rengachary S (ed): Neurosurgery, vol 1. New York: McGraw-Hill, 1985, pp 680–686.

71. Fetell MR, Bruce JN, Burke AM, et al: Non-neoplastic pineal cysts. Neurology 41:1034–1040, 1991.

72. Quest DO, Kleriga E: Microsurgical anatomy of the pineal region. Neurosurgery 6:385–390, 1980.

73. Yamamoto S, Kageyama N: Microsurgical anatomy of the pineal region. J Neurosurg 53:205–221, 1980.

74. Edwards MSB, Hudgins RJ, Wilson CB, et al: Pineal region tumors in children. J Neurosurg 66:689–697, 1988.

75. Goodman R: Magnetic resonance imaging-directed stereotactic endoscopic third ventriculostomy. Neurosurgery 32:1043–1047, 1993.

76. Fauchon F, Jouvet A, Paquis P, et al: Parenchymal pineal tumors: A clinicopathological study of 76 cases. Int J Radiat Oncol Biol Phys 46:959–968, 2000.

77. Casentini L, Colombo F, Pozza F, Benditt A: Combined radiosurgery and external radiotherapy of intracranial germinomas. Surg Neurol 34:79–86, 1990.

78. Chapman PH, Languid RM: The management of pineal area tumors: A recent reappraisal. Cancer 46:1253–1257, 1980.

79. Fuller B, Kapp D, Cox R: Radiation therapy of pineal region tumors: 25 new cases and a review of 208 previously reported cases. Int J Radiat Oncol Biol Phys 28:229–245, 1993.

80. Graafian SL, Paulos FP, Rudolph AR, et al: Mixed germ-cell tumor of the pineal region. J Neurosurg 66:300–304, 1987.

81. Hoffman H, Yoshida M, Becker L, et al: Pineal region tumors in childhood: Experience at the Hospital for Sick Children. In Humphreys R (ed): Concepts in Pediatric Neurosurgery 4. Basel: S. Charger, 1983, pp 360–386.

82. Hoffman HJ, Yoshida M, Becker LE, et al: Experience with pineal region tumors in childhood. Neurol Res 6:107–112, 1984.

83. Neuwelt EA: An update on the surgical treatment of malignant pineal region tumors. Clin Neurosurg 32:397–428, 1985.

84. Packer RJ, Sutton LN, Rodenstock JG, et al: Pineal region tumors of childhood. Pediatrics 74:97–101, 1984.

85. Rout D, Sharman A, Radhakrishnan VV, Rao VRK: Exploration of the pineal region: Observations and results. Surg Neurol 21:135–140, 1984.

86. Pluchino F, Broggi G, Fornari M, et al: Surgical approach to pineal tumors. Acta Neurochir (Wien) 96:26–31, 1989.

87. Shokry A, Janzer RC, Von Hochstetter AR, et al: Primary intracranial germ-cell tumors: A clinicopathological study of 14 cases. J Neurosurg 62:826–830, 1985.

88. Suzuki J, Iwabuchi T: Surgical removal of pineal tumors (pinealomas and teratomas): Experience in a series of 19 cases. J Neurosurg 23:565–571, 1965.

89. D'Andrea DA, Packer RJ, Rorke LB, et al: Pineocytomas of childhood: A reappraisal of natural history and response to therapy. Cancer 59:1353–1357, 1987.

90. Kersh CR, Constable WC, Eisert DR, et al: Primary central nervous system germ cell tumors: Effect of histologic confirmation on radiotherapy. Cancer 61:2148–2152, 1988.

91. Wood JH, Zimmerman RA, Bruce DA, et al: Assessment and management of pineal-region and related tumors. Surg Neurol 16:192–210, 1981.

92. Bruce JN, Stein BM: Management of pineal region tumors. In Barrow DL (ed): The Practice of Neurosurgery. Baltimore: Williams & Wilkins, 1996, pp 875–887.

93. Choi JU, Kim DS, Chung SS, Kim TS: Treatment of germ cell tumors in the pineal region. Childs Nerv Syst 14:1–8, 1998.

94. Weiner HL, Lichtenbaum RA, Wisoff JH, et al: Delayed surgical resection for central nervous system germ cell tumors. Neurosurgery 50:727–734, 2002.

95. Chandrasoma PT, Smith MM, Apuzzo MLJ: Stereotactic biopsy in the diagnosis of brain masses: Comparison of results of biopsy and resected surgical specimen. Neurosurgery 24:160–165, 1989.

96. Kraichoke S, Cosgrove M, Chadrasoma PT: Granulomatous inflammation in pineal germinoma. Am J Surg Pathol 12:655–660, 1988.

97. Bruce JN, Stein BM: Surgical management pineal region tumors. Acta Neurochir (Wien) 134:130–135, 1995.

98. Schild SE, Scheithauer BW, Haddock MG, et al: Histologically confirmed pineal tumors and other germ cell tumors of the brain. Cancer 78:564–571, 1996.

99. Sano K: Pineal region and posterior third ventricular tumors: A surgical overview. In Apuzzo M (ed): Surgery of the Third Ventricle. Baltimore: Williams & Wilkins, 1987, pp 663–683.

100. Sawamura Y, de Tribolet N, Ishii N, Abe H: Management of primary intracranial germinomas: Diagnostic surgery or radical resection? J Neurosurg 87:62–66, 1997.

101. Lapras C, Patet JD: Controversies, techniques and strategies for pineal tumor surgery. In Apuzzo MLJ (ed): Surgery of the Third Ventricle. Baltimore: Williams & Wilkins, 1987, pp 649–662.

102. Conway LW: Stereotaxic diagnosis and treatment of intracranial tumors including an initial experience with cryosurgery for pinealomas. J Neurosurg 38:453–460, 1973.

103. Kreth F, Schatz C, Pagenstecher A, et al: Stereotactic management of lesions of the pineal region. Neurosurgery 39:280–291, 1996.

104. Moser R, Backlund E: Stereotactic techniques in the diagnosis and treatment of pineal region tumors. In Neuwelt E (ed): Diagnosis and Management of Pineal Region Tumors. Baltimore: Williams & Wilkins, 1984, pp 236–253.

105. Field M, Witham TF, Flickinger JC, et al: Comprehensive assessment of hemorrhage risks and outcomes after stereotactic brain biopsy. J Neurosurg 94:45–51, 2001.

106. Peragut JC, Dupard T, Graziani N, Sedan R: De la prévention des risques de la biopsie stéréotaxique de certaines tumeurs de la région pinéale: A propos de 3 observations. Neurochirurgie 33:23–27, 1987.

107. Favre J, Taha JM, Burchiel KJ: An analysis of the respective risks of hematoma formation in 361 consecutive morphological and functional stereotactic procedures. Neurosurgery 50:48–57, 2002.

108. Regis J, Bouillot P, Rouby-Volot F, et al: Pineal region tumors and the role of stereotactic biopsy: Review of the mortality, morbidity, and diagnostic rates in 370 cases. Neurosurgery 39:907–914, 1996.

109. Maciunas R: Stereotactic biopsy of pineal region lesions. In Black P (ed): Operative Neurosurgery, vol 1. London: Churchill Livingstone, 2000, pp 841–848.

110. Oi S, Shibata M, Tominaga J, et al: Efficacy of neuroendoscopic procedures in minimally invasive preferential management of pineal region tumors: A prospective study. J Neurosurg 93:45–53, 2000.

111. Oka K, Kin Y, Go Y, et al: Neuroendoscopic approach to tectal tumors: A consecutive series. J Neurosurg 91:964–970, 1999.

112. Ferrer E, Santamarta D, Garcia-Fructuoso G, et al: Neuroendoscopic management of pineal region tumours. Acta Neurochir 139:2–20, 1997.

113. Gaab MR, Schroeder HW: Neuroendoscopic approach to intraventricular lesions. J Neurosurg 88:496–505, 1998.

114. Pople IK, Athanasiou TC, Sandeman DR, Coakham HB: The role of endoscopic biopsy and third ventriculostomy in the management of pineal region tumours. Br J Neurosurg 15:305–311, 2001.

115. Gangemi M, Maiuri F, Colella G, Buonamassa S: Endoscopic surgery for pineal region tumors. Minim Invasive Neurosurg 44:70–73, 2001.

116. Bruce J: Posterior third ventricular tumors. In Black P (ed): Operative Neurosurgery, vol 1. London: Churchill Livingstone, 2000, pp 769–775.

117. Bruce J, Stein B: Supracerebellar infratentorial approach. In Black P (ed): Operative Neurosurgery, vol 1. London: Churchill Livingstone, 2000, pp 815–824.

118. Nazzaro JM, Shults WT, Neuwelt EA: Neuro-ophthalmological function of patients with pineal region tumors approached transtentorially in the semisitting position. J Neurosurg 76:746–751, 1992.

119. Bruce JN, Stein BM: Complications of surgery for pineal region tumors. In McCormick PC (ed): Postoperative Complications in Intracranial Neurosurgery. New York: Thieme, 1993, pp 74–86.

120. Kobayashi S, Sugita K, Tanaka Y, Kyoshima K: Infratentorial approach to the pineal region in the prone position: Concorde position. J Neurosurg 58:141–143, 1983.

121. Herrmann H-D, Winkler D, Westphal M: Treatment of tumours of the pineal region and posterior part of the third ventricle. Acta Neurochir (Wien) 116:137–146, 1992.

122. Pendl G: Case material. In Pendl G (ed): Pineal and Midbrain Lesions. Wien: Springer-Verlag, 1985, pp 128–207.

123. Lapras C, Patet JD, Mottolese C, Lapras C Jr: Direct surgery of pineal tumors: Occipital-transtentorial approach. Prog Exp Tumor Res 30:268–280, 1987.

124. Konovalov AN, Pitskhelauri DI: Principles of treatment of the pineal region tumors. Surg Neurol 59:250–268, 2003.

125. Rubinstein LJ: Cytogenesis and differentiation of pineal neoplasms. Hum Pathol 12:441–448, 1981.

126. Vaquero J, Ramiro J, Martinez R, et al: Clinicopathological experience with pineocytomas: Report of five surgically treated cases. Neurosurgery 27:612–619, 1990.

127. Rippe JD, Boyko OB, Friedman HS, et al: Gd-DTPA-enhanced MR imaging of leptomeningeal spread of primary intracranial CNS tumor in children. AJNR Am J Neuroradiol 11:329–332, 1990.

128. Amendola B, McClatchey K, Amendola M: Pineal region tumors: analysis of treatment results. Int J Radiat Oncol Biol Phys 10:991–997, 1984.

129. Bruce JN, Fetell MR, Stein BM: Incidence of spinal metastases in patients with malignant pineal region tumors: Avoidance of prophylactic spinal irradiation. J Neurosurg 72:354A, 1990.

130. Disclafani A, Hudgins RJ, Edwards SB, et al: Pineocytomas. Cancer 63:302–304, 1989.

131. Dattoli MJ, Newall J: Radiation therapy for intracranial germinoma: The case for limited volume treatment. Int J Radiat Oncol Biol Phys 19:429–433, 1990.

132. Rao Y, Medini E, Haselow R, et al: Pineal and ectopic pineal tumors: The role of radiation therapy. Cancer 48:708–713, 1981.

133. Wolden SL, Wara WM, Larson DA, et al: Radiation therapy for primary intracranial germ-cell tumors. Int J Radiat Oncol Biol Phys 32:943–949, 1995.

134. Sung DI, Harisiadis L, Chang CH: Midline pineal tumors and suprasellar germinomas: Highly curable by irradiation. Radiology 128:745–751, 1978.

135. Matsutani M, Sano K, Takakura K, et al: Primary intracranial germ cell tumors: A clinical analysis of 153 histologically verified cases. J Neurosurg 86:446–455, 1997.

136. Sano K, Matsutani M: Pinealoma (germinoma) treated by direct surgery and postoperative irradiation. Child Brain 8:81–97, 1981.

137. Aoyama H, Shirato H, Ikeda J, et al: Induction chemotherapy followed by low-dose involved-field radiotherapy for intracranial germ cell tumors. J Clin Oncol 20:857–865, 2002.

138. Sawamura Y, Shirato H, Ikeda J, et al: Induction chemotherapy followed by reduced-volume radiation therapy for newly diagnosed central nervous system germinoma. J Neurosurg 88:66–72, 1998.

139. Allen JC, Kim JH, Packer RJ: Neoadjuvant chemotherapy for newly diagnosed germ-cell tumors of the central nervous system. J Neurosurg 67:65–70, 1987.

140. Duffner P, Cohen M, Thomas P, Lansky S: The long-term effects of cranial irradiation on the central nervous system. Cancer 56:1841–1846, 1985.

141. Hodges LC, Smith LJ, Garrett A, Tate S: Prevalence of glioblastoma multiforme in subjects prior to therapeutic radiation. J Neurosci Nurs 24:79–83, 1992.

142. Nighoghossian N, Confavreaux C, Sassolas G, et al: Insuffisance hypothalamique apres irradiation demence tardive, subaigue et curable. Rev Neurol (Paris) 144:215–218, 1988.

143. Noell K, Herskovic A: Principles of radiotherapy of CNS tumors. In Rengachary S (ed): Neurosurgery, vol 1. New York: McGraw-Hill, 1985, pp 1084–1095.

144. Sakai N, Yamada H, Andoh T, et al: Primary intracranial germ-cell tumors: A retrospective analysis with special reference to long-term results of treatments and the behavior of rare types of tumors. Acta Oncol 27:43–50, 1988.

145. Sands SA, Kellie SJ, Davidow AL, et al: Long-term quality of life and neuropsychologic functioning for patients with CNS germ-cell tumors: From the First International CNS Germ-Cell Tumor Study. Neurooncology 3:174–183, 2001.

146. Rowland JH, Glidewell OJ, Sibley RF, et al: Effects of different forms of central nervous system prophylaxis on neuropsychologic function in childhood leukemia. J Clin Oncol 2:1327–1335, 1984.

147. Jenkin D, Berry M, Chan H, et al: Pineal region germinomas in childhood treatment considerations. Int J Radiat Oncol Biol Phys 18:541–545, 1990.

148. Bendersky M, Lewis M, Mandelbaum DE, Stanger C: Serial neuropsychological follow-up of a child following craniospinal irradiation. Dev Med Child Neurol 30:808–820, 1988.

149. Donahue B: Short- and long-term complications of radiation therapy for pediatric brain tumors. Pediatr Neurosurg 18:207–217, 1992.

150. Einhorn L: Testicular cancer as a model for curable neoplasm. Cancer Res 41:3275–3280, 1981.

151. Hainsworth J, Greco F: Testicular germ cell neoplasms. Am J Med 75:817–832, 1983.

152. Logothetis CJ, Samuels ML, Selig DE, et al: Chemotherapy of extragonadal germ cell tumors. J Clin Oncol 3:316–325, 1985.

153. McLeod DG, Taylor HG, Skoog SJ, et al: Extragonadal germ cell tumors: Clinicopathologic findings and treatment experience in 12 patients. Cancer 61:1187–1191, 1988.

154. Pinkerton CR, Pritchard J, Spitz L: High complete response rate in children with advanced germ cell tumors using cisplatin-containing combination chemotherapy. J Clin Oncol 4:194–199, 1986.

155. Parsa AT, Pincus DW, Feldstein N, et al: Pineal region tumors. In Packer R (ed): Tumors of the Pediatric Central Nervous System. New York: Thieme, 2001, pp 308–325.

156. Prioleau G, Wilson C: Endodermal sinus tumor of the pineal region. Cancer 38:2489–2493, 1976.

157. Patel SR, Buckner JC, Smithson WA, et al: Cisplatin-based chemotherapy in primary central nervous system germ cell tumors. J Neurooncol 12:47–52, 1992.
158. Kobayashi T, Yoshida J, Ishiyama J, et al: Combination chemotherapy with cisplatin and etoposide for malignant intracranial germ-cell tumors: An experimental and clinical study. J Neurosurg 70:676–681, 1989.
159. Takakura K: Intracranial germ cell tumors. Clin Neurosurg 32:429–444, 1985.
160. Einhorn LH, Donohue J: Cis-diaminedichloroplatinum, vinblastine, and bleomycin combination therapy in disseminated testicular cancer. Ann Intern Med 87:293–298, 1977.
161. Merchant TE, Davis BJ, Sheldon JM, Leibel SA: Radiation therapy for relapsed CNS germinoma after primary chemotherapy. J Clin Oncol 16:204–209, 1998.
162. Chan H, Humphreys R, Hendrick E, et al: Primary intracranial choriocarcinoma: A report of two cases and a review of the literature. Neurosurgery 15:540–545, 1984.
163. Herrmann H-D, Westphal M, Winkler K, et al: Treatment of non-germinomatous germ-cell tumors of the pineal region. Neurosurgery 34:524–529, 1994.
164. Hoffman HJ, Otsubo H, Bruce E, et al: Intracranial germ-cell tumors in children. J Neurosurg 74:545–551, 1991.
165. Robertson PL, DaRosso RC, Allen JC: Improved prognosis of intracranial non-germinoma germ cell tumors with multimodality therapy. J Neurooncol 32:71–80, 1997.
166. Friedman JA, Lynch JJ, Buckner JC, et al: Management of malignant pineal germ cell tumors with residual mature teratoma. Neurosurgery 48:518–523, 2001.
167. Allen J, DaRosso R, Donahue B, Nirenberg A: A phase II trial of preirradiation carboplatin in newly diagnosed germinoma of the central nervous system. Cancer 25:26–32, 1994.
168. Jakacki RI, Zeltzer PM, Boyett JM, et al: Survival and prognostic factors following radiation and/or chemotherapy for primitive neuroectodermal tumors of the pineal region in infants and children: A report of the Childrens Cancer Group. J Clin Oncol 13:1377–1383, 1995.
169. Chang SM, Lillis-Hearne PK, Larson DA, et al: Pineoblastoma in adults. Neurosurgery 37:383–391, 1995.
170. Hasegawa T, McInerney J, Kondziolka D, et al: Long-term results after stereotactic radiosurgery for patients with cavernous malformations. Neurosurgery 50:1190–1198, 2002.
171. Backlund E-O, Rahn T, Sarby B: Treatment of pinealomas by stereotaxic radiation surgery. Acta Radiol Ther Physiol Biol 13:368–376, 1974.

Alternate Surgical Approaches to Pineal Region Neoplasms

KEIJI SANO

Because the pineal body is located in the center of the cranial cavity, René Descartes (1596–1650), the greatest philosopher of 17th-century France, thought that the pineal body might be the seat of the soul. This concept is, of course, wrong. The pineal body, however, is certainly the seat of various kinds of neoplasms. Because of the central location of the pineal body, the distance between it and the surface of any portion of the scalp is almost the same, regardless of the surgical approach taken to the pineal region (Fig. 56-1). Therefore, the surgical approach to this region should be chosen according to the size and extension of the neoplasm so that removal of the neoplasm will be most extensive or complete and damage to the normal brain will be minimal. Neoplasms in the pineal region occupy 3.5% of all intracranial primary neoplasms in Japan (996 of 28,424 cases).[1] These neoplasms are mostly composed of the so-called germinomas or tumors of the two-cell pattern type, which form 2.3% of all primary intracranial neoplasms, according to the most recent Japanese statistics.[1] In the same statistics, pineocytomas make up 0.1%; pineoblastomas, 0.2%; teratomas, including malignant teratomas, 0.8%; and choriocarcinomas, 0.1% of all intracranial primary neoplasms. Therefore, in the pineal region, germ cell tumors and tumors of pineal parenchymal origin are predominantly found.

This chapter discusses the surgery and management of a germinoma, a germinoma with syncytiotrophoblastic giant cells, an embryonal carcinoma, an endodermal sinus tumor (yolk sac tumor), a choriocarcinoma, a mature teratoma, an immature teratoma, a teratoma with malignant transformation, the so-called mixed germ cell tumor, and a pineocytoma with lymphocytic infiltration. I believe that only a germinoma derives from primordial germ cells and, hence, is a true germ cell tumor.[2–4] Among neoplasms of the two-cell pattern type in the pineal region, a germinoma (a true germ cell tumor) and a pineocytoma with lymphocytic infiltration may be based on the difference of the tumor cell–stroma relationship and placental alkaline phosphatase stain (positive in a germinoma and negative in a pineocytoma with lymphocytic infiltration).[2,5] Both types of neoplasm are radiosensitive, however, and their biologic behaviors are similar.

THERAPEUTIC PRINCIPLES

Diagnosis of a medium-sized or large tumor arising in the pineal region and the posterior third ventricle is not difficult because of the presence of increased intracranial pressure, paralysis of conjugate upward gaze (Parinaud's sign), and pseudo-Argyll-Robertson pupil (reacting to accommodation but not to light). In the later stages, ataxia, choreic movements, or spastic weakness of the limbs may appear. Cerebral angiography is useful in the detection of the extent and vascularization of the tumor. Calcification on plain craniograms may sometimes be pathognomonic, especially in patients younger than 10 years of age. The most powerful noninvasive diagnostic tools, however, are computed tomography and magnetic resonance imaging.

Levels of α-fetoprotein (AFP), human chorionic gonadotropin (hCG), and carcinoembryonic antigen should be determined in the serum or the cerebrospinal fluid in all cases. The first two tumor markers (AFP and hCG) are especially informative about the nature of tumors in this region.

If hCG is present, the tumor must be a choriocarcinoma, a mixed germ cell tumor with choriocarcinomatous elements, or a germinoma with syncytiotrophoblastic giant cells. The last tumor type is not as malignant as choriocarcinoma and mixed tumors with choriocarcinomatous elements, which are very malignant. The levels of serum hCG in choriocarcinoma cases are more than 2000 mIU/mL, whereas those in cases of a germinoma with syncytiotrophoblastic giant cells are less than 1000 mIU/mL.[6] If AFP is present, the tumor must be an endodermal sinus tumor (yolk sac tumor) or a mixed germ cell tumor with endodermal sinus tumor elements. Prognosis of choriocarcinoma or endodermal sinus tumor, especially the former, is poor, even after surgical removal of the tumor and postoperative radiotherapy of the whole neuraxis.[2,3,6] Chemotherapeutic agents, such as cisplatin, vinblastine, bleomycin, etoposide, ifosfamide, and their combinations, are reported to be useful.[6]

If AFP and hCG are not present, the tumor may be a germinoma, an embryonal carcinoma, a mature teratoma, an immature teratoma, a teratoma with malignant transformation, a mixed germ cell tumor with a combination of these tumor elements, or a pineal parenchymal tumor (pineocytoma, pineoblastoma, or pineocytoma with lymphocytic infiltration[2]). AFP and hCG are not present in a pure embryonal carcinoma, which is rare. This tumor, however, is more frequently found as a mixed tumor with an endodermal sinus tumor or a choriocarcinoma. In these cases, AFP or hCG is present.

If 20 Gy of local radiation effectively abolishes the tumor, as confirmed by computed tomography or magnetic resonance imaging, the tumor may be a germinoma or a two-cell pattern type of tumor of pineal parenchymal origin, which I call pineocytoma with lymphocytic infiltration or which used to be called a pinealoma, in honor of Krabbe.[7] In this case, radiation should be continued to 50 Gy. However, if the tumor diameter is more than 2 cm (or sometimes more than 1.5 cm), direct surgery and removal of the tumor

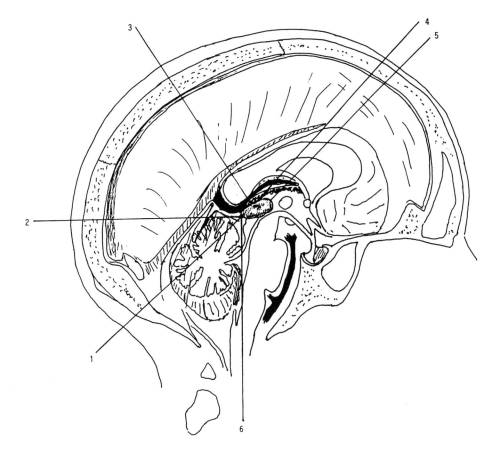

FIGURE 56-1 Various approaches to tumors in the pineal region and the posterior third ventricle: (1) infratentorial supracerebellar, (2) occipital transtentorial, (3) posterior transcallosal or posterior transventricular, (4) anterior transcallosal transventricular transvelum interpositum, (5) transcallosal interforniceal, (6) lateral paramedian infratentorial.

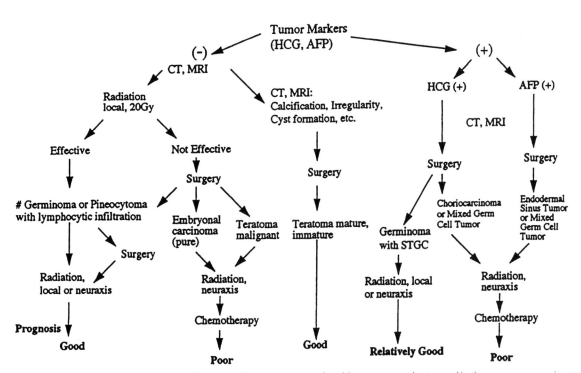

FIGURE 56-2 Flowchart of treatments of pineal tumors. Pineocytomas or pineoblastomas may be treated in the same way as pineocytomas with lymphocytic infiltration.

followed by radiation or chemotherapy are recommended. (For a germinoma and a pineocytoma with lymphocytic infiltration, local radiation is usually sufficient treatment.) A mature teratoma and an immature teratoma can be cured only by removal of the tumor, and the prognosis is good after this treatment. An embryonal carcinoma and a teratoma with malignant transformation usually have a poor prognosis, even after surgical removal and postoperative radiotherapy of the whole neuraxis.[6] The chemotherapeutic agents mentioned earlier are also recommended in these patients. A flowchart of therapies for various tumors is presented in Figure 56-2.

Stereotactic or endoscopic biopsy of tumors of this region has recently been gaining in popularity. However, I am not particularly enthusiastic about this procedure because different parts of the same tumor of this region may show different histology; hence, biopsy of a small piece of the tumor may mislead the clinician as to the true nature of the tumor. Therefore, I prefer exploration and removal or debulking (unless removal is possible) of the tumor. Cytologic examination of the cerebrospinal fluid is important for diagnosis. If malignant neoplastic cells are identified cytologically, the patient may develop disseminated metastases in the cerebrospinal fluid space. For diagnostic purposes, I recommend millipore filter-cell culture[8] of the cerebrospinal fluid. This method is more sensitive than conventional cytologic studies. Therefore, a positive culture result does not necessarily mean that the probability of disseminated metastases is very high. During follow-up, repeated examinations of the tumor markers are useful to detect recurrence of the tumor that is producing these markers at the earliest possible stage.

ANATOMIC CONSIDERATIONS

The artery supplying the pineal body is the medial posterior choroidal artery (ramus choroideus posterior medialis). This artery arises from the posterior cerebral artery lateral to its junction with the posterior communicating artery (pars postcommunicalis); runs in the ambient cistern, parallel to the posterior cerebral artery; supplies the pineal body and superior and inferior colliculi; and then runs forward in the tela choroidea of the third ventricle. It then turns backward at the foramen of Monro, runs in the choroid plexus of the lateral ventricle, and anastomoses with the lateral posterior choroidal arteries, sending branches to the anterior thalamic nucleus, the medial geniculate body, and the pulvinar. This artery is usually single (69%) but is sometimes double (23.9%), triple (6.2%), or quadruple (0.9%).[9]

There are usually two lateral posterior choroidal arteries (rami choroidei posteriores laterales) (but there are one to four). They arise from the posterior cerebral artery (pars postcommunicalis), run in the ambient cistern, go through the choroidal fissure, run into the choroid plexus of the lateral ventricle, and anastomose with the medial posterior choroidal artery and the anterior choroidal artery, sending branches to the lateral geniculate body and parts of the thalamus. The arteria laminae tecti (arteria quadrigemina)[9] arises from the posterior cerebral artery medial to its junction with the posterior communicating artery (pars precommunicalis), runs in the ambient cistern, and supplies the superior colliculus. A branch of the superior cerebellar artery supplies the inferior colliculus. From the peripheral trunk of the posterior cerebral

TABLE 56-1 ▪ **Arteries Supplying the Pineal and Neighboring Regions**

From the posterior cerebral artery (arteria cerebri posterior)
  From the pars precommunicalis
    Arteria laminae tecti (arteria quadrigemina)
      Colliculus superior
  From the pars postcommunicalis
    Medial posterior choroidal artery (ramus choroideus posterior medialis)
      Pineal body
      Corpora quadrigemina
      Tela choroidea ventriculi tertii
      Thalamus
    Lateral posterior choroidal arteries (rami choroidei posteriores laterales)
      Choroid plexus of the lateral ventricle
      Lateral geniculate body
      Thalamus
  From the peripheral trunk
    Arteria occipitalis medialis
      Calcarine artery (ramus calcarinus)
        Sulcus calcarinus
      Parieto-occipital artery (ramus parieto-occipitalis)
        Sulcus parieto-occipitalis and its area
    Posterior pericallosal artery
From the superior cerebellar artery (arteria cerebelli superior)
    Colliculus inferior

artery, the arteria occipitalis medialis arises and sends the calcarine artery (ramus calcarinus) to the calcarine sulcus, and the parieto-occipital artery (ramus parieto-occipitalis) to the parieto-occipital sulcus and its area. These arteries are listed in Table 56-1 and are diagrammed in Figure 56-3. The arteries supplying various portions of the brain stem and the thalamus should always be preserved at surgery.

The draining veins from the pineal body and the habenular trigone were named the superior and inferior pineal veins by Tamaki and colleagues[10] and flow into the vein of Galen or the internal cerebral veins. The veins from the superior and inferior colliculi, the superior and inferior quadrigeminal veins (per Tamaki and colleagues[10]), or the tectal veins (per Matsushima and colleagues[11]) flow into the vein of Galen or the superior vermian vein. The basal veins of Rosenthal flow directly into the vein of Galen (28%[9]), into the internal cerebral veins (34%), into the confluence of the bilateral internal cerebral veins (28%), or directly into the straight sinus (approximately 9%). Many veins draining the frontal base, the lateral ventricle, and the hippocampus flow into the basal veins.

The anterior septal vein, the anterior caudate vein, the choroidal vein of the choroid plexus, and the thalamostriate (terminal) vein flow into the internal cerebral vein at the posterior rim of the foramen of Monro. In addition, the internal cerebral vein receives the posterior septal vein, the medial atrial vein (trigonal vein), and the direct lateral veins. The internal cerebral veins flow into the vein of Galen, which is 0.5 to 1.5 cm long and flows into the straight sinus (sinus rectus). The precentral cerebellar vein (one present in 46%, two in 54%) and the superior vermian veins (one present in 70%, two in 30%) flow into the vein of Galen or directly into the straight sinus. These veins are listed in Table 56-2 and are diagrammed in Figure 56-4. The veins draining portions of the brain stem and thalamus should always be preserved at surgery.

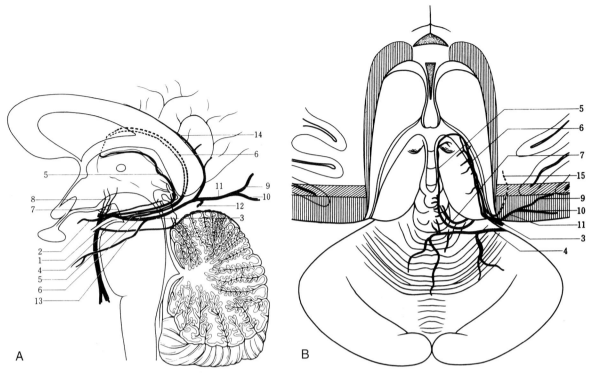

A   B

FIGURE 56-3   Lateral view (*A*) and view from above (*B*). Arteries supplying the pineal region and its neighborhood: 1, a. basilaris (basilar artery); 2, a. communicans posterior (posterior communicating artery); 3, a. cerebri posterior (posterior cerebral artery); 4, a. cerebelli superior (superior cerebellar artery; 5, ramus choroideus posterior medialis (medial posterior choroidal artery); 6, rami choroidei posteriores laterales (lateral posterior choroidal arteries); 7, a. laminae tecti, sive A. quadrigemina (quadrigeminal artery); 8, thalamoperforating arteries; 9, ramus parieto-occipitalis (parieto-occipital artery); 10, ramus calcarinus (calcarine artery); 11, a. occipital medialis; 12, a. temporalis posterior (posterior temporal artery); 13, a. temporalis anterior (anterior temporal artery); 14, a. pericallosa posterior (posterior pericallosal artery); 15, a. choroidea anterior. (From Sano K: Surgery of pineal tumors-anatomical consideration of various approaches. Neurol Surg (Tokyo) 12:1119–1129, 1984.)

TABLE 56-2 ▪ Veins Draining the Pineal and Neighboring Regions

Great cerebral vein of Galen (vena cerebri magna)
  Pineal veins (superior and inferior)
    Pineal body
    Trigonum habenulae
  Quadrigeminal veins (superior and inferior) (tectal veins)
    Corpora quadrigemina
  Superior vermian vein
    Superior vermis
  Precentral cerebellar vein
    Cerebellum
    Superior cerebellar peduncle
  Posterior pericallosal vein
  Internal occipital vein
  Internal cerebral veins (venae cerebri internae)
    Septal veins (anterior and posterior)
      Septum pellucidum
    Anterior caudate vein
      Caput nuclei caudati
    Thalamostriate vein (vena thalamostriata, terminal vein)
    Choroidal vein (vena choroidea)
      Choroid plexus of the lateral ventricle
    Medial atrial vein (trigonal vein)
      Trigonum of the lateral ventricle
    Direct lateral veins
  Basal veins of Rosenthal (venae basales)
    Vena cerebri media profunda
    Venae centrales (striatae) inferiores
    Vena cerebri anterior
    Vena apicis cornus temporalis (hippocampal vein)
    Vena atrii lateralis (lateral atrial vein)
    Vena cornus temporalis (atriotemporal vein)

OPERATIVE APPROACHES TO THE PINEAL REGION

Historical Perspectives

Horsley was probably the first to try to remove a pineal tumor. He used the infratentorial supracerebellar approach, but with poor results. He therefore recommended supratentorial approaches. In 1913, Fedor Krause successfully removed a huge tumor in the region of the quadrigeminal plate from a 10-year-old boy by the infratentorial supracerebellar approach, which he reported on with Oppenheim, who diagnosed the case.[12] The tumor was reported to be a fibrosarcoma or an encapsulated mixed cell sarcoma but seems, however, to have been a teratoma or a meningioma, according to modern pathologic designation. The boy was reported to have been well at least until World War I. In 1926, Krause[13] added two more patients, who were operated on by the same approach; in these two, however, he could not remove the tumors. In 1956, Zapletal[14] reported using practically the same approach. He reported on four cases: a malignant astrocytoma in the quadrigeminal region, a medulloblastoma of the upper vermis, an epidermoid, and a pineal tumor. The last one was successfully removed. In 1971, using microsurgical techniques, Stein[15] revived and elaborated this infratentorial supracerebellar approach, which has been widely used since then.

The parietal transcallosal approach was performed by Dandy[16] in 1921, then by Kunicki[17] and others. In 1931, Van Wagenen[18] proposed the posterior transventricular approach. This approach, however, has been used only rarely.

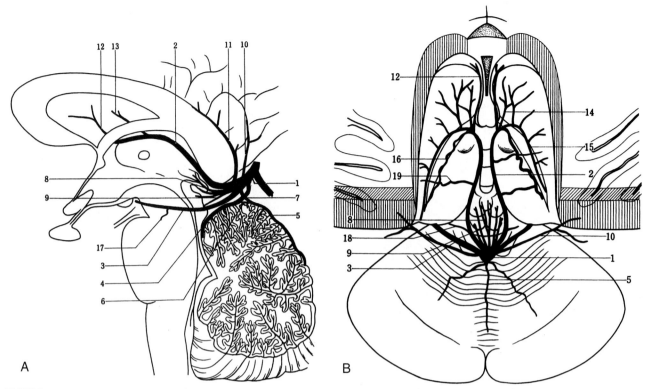

FIGURE 56-4   Lateral view (*A*) and view from above (*B*). Veins draining from the pineal region and its neighborhood: 1, v. cerebri magna (great cerebral vein of Galen); 2, v. cerebri interna (internal cerebral vein); 3, v. basalis (basal vein of Rosenthal); 4, precentral cerebellar vein; 5, supraculminate vein; 6, pre- and intraculminate veins; 7, superior vermian vein; 8, superior and inferior pineal veins (Tamaki and colleagues); 9, superior and inferior quadrigeminal (tectal) veins; 10, internal occipital vein; 11, posterior pericallosal vein; 12, anterior septal vein; 13, posterior septal vein; 14, anterior caudate vein; 15, v. thalamostriata (thalamostriate vein, terminal vein); 16, choroidal vein (v. choroidea); 17, lateral mesencephalic vein; 18, medial atrial vein (trigonal vein); 19, direct lateral vein. (From Sano K: Surgery of pineal tumors-anatomical consideration of various approaches. Neurol Surg 12:1119–1129, 1984.)

The occipital or parieto-occipital approach along the falx with or without splitting the tentorium and with or without splitting the splenium of the corpus callosum has been done by Heppner,[19] Poppen and Marino,[20] Glasauer,[21] Jamieson,[22] Lazar and Clark,[23] and many others. Special credit should be given to Jamieson, who established the occipital transtentorial approach. For huge tumors in the pineal region or the posterior third ventricle, Sano[5,24–27] proposed the anterior transcallosal transventricular transvelum interpositum approach. Most recently in 1990, Van den Bergh[28] proposed the lateral paramedian infratentorial approach, which is a modification of the infratentorial supracerebellar approach. The unilateral cerebellopontine angle is explored, and from there, the tentorial notch is reached over the unilateral cerebellar hemisphere so that the tumor can be dissected between the internal cerebral vein and the basal vein of Rosenthal. Other approaches, such as the subchoroidal approach[29,30] and the transcallosal interforniceal approach,[31] are primarily used for lesions in the middle or anterior third ventricle. These may, however, be used for tumors in the pineal posterior third ventricular region.

Among various operative approaches to neoplasms in this region, I prefer the occipital transtentorial approach proposed by Poppen and Marino,[20] Jamieson,[22] and others; the infratentorial supracerebellar approach proposed by Krause and Oppenheim,[12,13] Zapletal,[14] and Stein[15]; or the lateral paramedian infratentorial approach proposed by

Van den Bergh,[28] if the neoplasm is medium sized or small. If, however, the neoplasm is large enough to reach anterior to the adhesio interthalamica, the anterior transcallosal transventricular transvelum interpositum approach, originally described as the frontal transcallosal approach by Sano,[5,24–27] is recommended.

The infratentorial supracerebellar approach is described in another chapter. The parietal transcallosal approach[16] inevitably requires splitting of the splenium to cause disconnection syndrome. In the subchoroidal approach, the thalamostriate vein must be sacrificed; this process may damage the thalamus. The transcallosal interforniceal approach provides a narrow operative field, and, in addition, there is a danger of a lesion of both fornices. Therefore, in this chapter, only the occipital transtentorial, the lateral paramedian infratentorial, and the anterior transcallosal transventricular transvelum interpositum approaches are described.

Occipital Transtentorial Approach

For the occipital transtentorial approach to a pineal neoplasm, I prefer to use the incision (usually on the nondominant side, i.e., on the right side) illustrated in Figures 56-5 and 56-6. The midline portion of the incision can be elongated to the suboccipital region if opening the posterior fossa for supracerebellar approach is necessary to add. Recently, Ziyal and colleagues[32] reported a combined

FIGURE 56-5 Occipital transtentorial approach (S) and parietal transcallosal approach (D). (From Sano K: Pineal region tumors: Problems in pathology and treatment. Clin Neurosurg 30:59–91, 1983.)

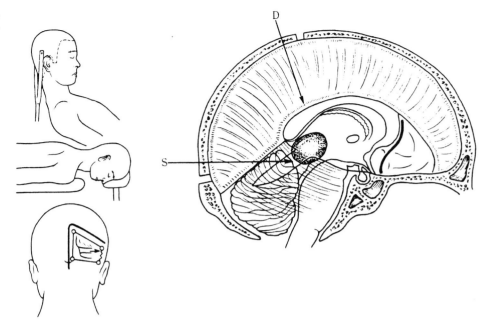

supra/infratentorial transsinus approach. However, sectioning the transverse sinus is not necessary in my opinion.

Craniotomy is close to the superior sagittal and the transverse sinuses. If necessary, the bone edge over the sinus is rongeured off. The patient is either in the prone position (the operating table should be slightly tilted to the side of craniotomy, i.e., the right side, so that the right occipital lobe sinks laterally and falls off the falx) or in the lounging position, as seen in Figure 56-5. The occipital horn is punctured through the dura mater, and a silicone rubber tube is inserted into the posterior portion of the lateral ventricle and secured to the dura (Fig. 56-7). The tube drains cerebrospinal fluid during the operation and makes lateral retraction of the occipital lobe unnecessary or easier. The dura is opened by an H-shaped incision close to the superior sagittal sinus.

The operating microscope is used from this stage. The tentorium is split close to the straight sinus, and the superior surface of the cerebellum is exposed. The arachnoid over the

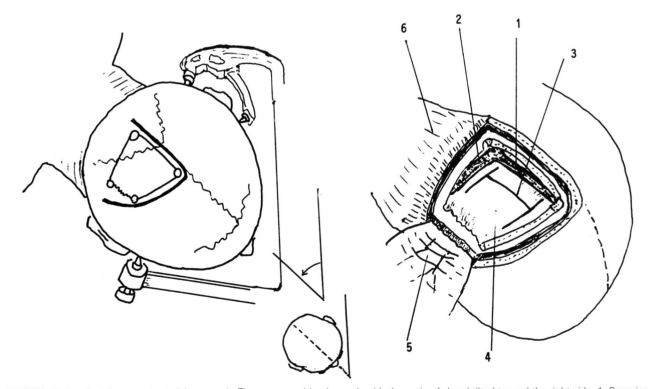

FIGURE 56-6 Occipital transtentorial approach. The prone position is used, with the patient's head tilted toward the right side. 1, Superior sagittal sinus; 2, transverse sinus; 3, dural incision; 4, dura; 5, bone flap; 6, skin flap.

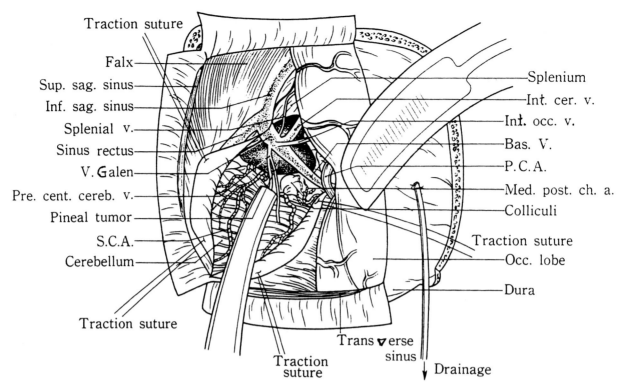

FIGURE 56-7   Occipital transtentorial approach (detailed view). Tumor (*dotted black*) is visible in front of the vein of Galen and the vein of Rosenthal. Sup. sag. sinus, superior sagittal sinus; Inf. sag. sinus, inferior sagittal sinus; Splenial v., splenial vein or posterior pericallosal vein; V. Galen, vein of Galen; Pre. Cent. Cereb. v., precentral cerebellar vein; S.C.A., superior cerebellar artery; Int. occ. v., internal occipital vein; Int. cer. v., internal cerebral vein; Bas. v., basal vein of Rosenthal; P.C.A., posterior cerebral artery; Med. post. ch. a., medial posterior choroidal artery; Occ. lobe, occipital lobe. (From Sano K: Surgery of pineal tumors-anatomical consideration of various approaches. Neurol Surg 12:1119–1129, 1984.)

deep veins, which is tough and opaque, is sharply dissected. A pineal tumor is often visible rostral to the vermis, underneath the vein of Galen (see Fig. 56-7). If the tumor is located further rostrally, the splenium of the corpus callosum is split by suction to expose the tela choroidea of the third ventricle. If the tumor is large, it is often already breaking through the tela choroidea; if not, the tela is incised along the midline or close to the nondominant occipital lobe after cauterization with a bipolar coagulator.

This approach enables the operator to use the low (parieto) occipital approach (as proposed by Poppen and Marino[20] and Jamieson[22]) and, if necessary, the high parieto-occipital approach (as proposed by Dandy[16] and others) or the additional infratentorial supracerebellar approach.

If the tumor is a pineocytoma with lymphocytic infiltration or a germinoma (a germinoma is usually slightly tougher in consistency than the former), the tumor is removed piecemeal with or without the use of an ultrasonic aspirator. If the tumor is a teratoma, removal en bloc is sometimes feasible. After tumor removal, the other end of the silicone rubber tube (which has been inserted into the lateral ventricle) is brought into the lateral cistern or the pontine cistern to ensure an unobstructed cerebrospinal fluid pathway. This step is performed because the rostral portion of the aqueduct is often compressed by the tumor, and even after removal of the tumor, the effect of the compression may remain for a period of time. Care should always be taken not to disseminate tumor debris in the subarachnoid space or the ventricular system in any approach used.

This approach provides an excellent view both above and below the tentorial notch. However, reaching the part of a large tumor extending to the opposite side may be difficult. Rarely, a danger of damaging the occipital lobe exists, as does a danger of damaging the splenium of the corpus callosum, resulting in disconnection syndrome. The approach is indicated in surgery of tumors that straddle the tentorial notch or are located above the notch. The advantages and disadvantages of this approach are listed in Table 56-3.

Lateral Paramedian Infratentorial Approach

The infratentorial supracerebellar approach is difficult when the tentorium is very steep, and if the patient is in the sitting position, an air embolism may occur despite various

---

TABLE 56-3 ▪ Occipital Transtentorial Approach

Advantage	Provides an excellent view both above and below the tentorial notch
Disadvantages	May damage the occipital lobe
	May damage the splenium of the corpus callosum
	May be difficult to reach parts of lesions extending to the opposite side
Indication	Tumors that straddle the tentorial notch or those located above the notch

FIGURE 56-8 Position of the patient for lateral paramedian infratentorial approach. 1, Skin incision.

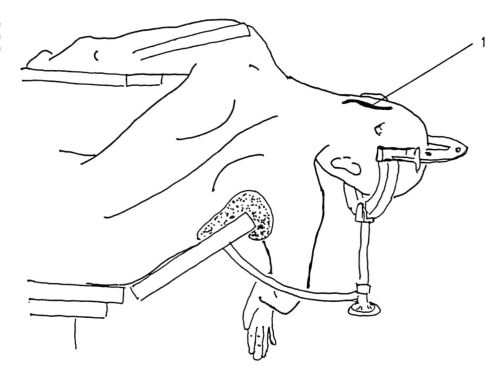

precautionary measures, such as Doppler probe, central venous catheter, and modest pressure ventrilation.

In 1990, Van den Bergh[28] proposed a new infratentorial approach. The patient is positioned on the side, usually the right side; if, however, the tumor extends to the right side, then positioning is on the left side. The upper part of the trunk is raised approximately 30 degrees by upward inclination of the operating table. The head is flexed with the neck stretched and then rotated 45 degrees in a face-down fashion (Fig. 56-8). Care should be taken that the jugular veins remain unobstructed during flexion and rotation.

A flat, S-shaped incision is made just behind the mastoid process. The muscles are stripped away to expose the occipital bone. An oval craniectomy is made close to the sigmoid sinus laterally, to the transverse sinus superiorly, and caudally close to the foramen magnum (Fig. 56-9). The dura is opened in a cruciate fashion.

The superior surface of the cerebellar hemisphere is eased gently down. Bridging veins between it and the tentorium or the transverse sinus are electrocoagulated and severed. The petrosal vein and the precentral cerebellar vein are preserved. Thus, the tentorial incisura is easily reached. The arachnoid of the ambient cistern and the upper edge of the cerebellum are sharply dissected, permitting the cerebellum to descend further without retraction. The pineal tumor usually appears between the internal cerebral veins and the

FIGURE 56-9 Lateral paramedian infratentorial approach. Site of craniectomy. (From Van den Bergh R: Lateral-paramedian infratentorial approach in lateral decubitus for pineal tumours. Clin Neurol Neurosurg 92:311–316, 1990.)

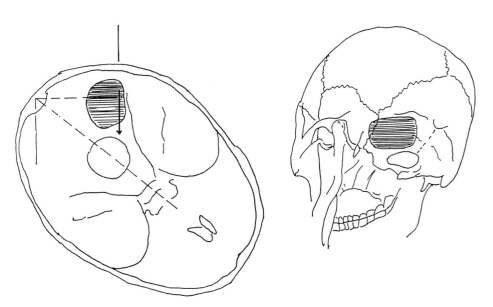

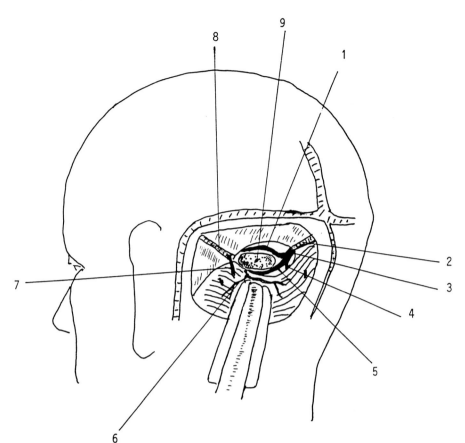

FIGURE 56-10 Lateral paramedian infratentorial approach. 1, Internal cerebral vein; 2, straight sinus; 3, vein of Galen; 4, precentral cerebellar vein; 5, basal vein of Rosenthal; 6, superior cerebellar artery; 7, petrosal vein; 8, superior petrosal sinus; 9, tumor. (From Van den Bergh R: Lateral-paramedian infratentorial approach in lateral decubitus for pineal tumours. Clin Neurol Neurosurg 92:311–316, 1990.)

basal veins of Rosenthal (Fig. 56-10). The superior cerebellar artery appears at the rostral edge of the cerebellar hemisphere and gives branches to the cerebellar hemisphere and the vermis. This artery should be preserved. Elevating the straight sinus and the transverse sinus is unnecessary. The lateral paramedian infratentorial approach may replace the infratentorial supracerebellar approach if it is performed by an experienced surgeon. The advantages and disadvantages of this approach are described in Table 56-4.

Anterior Transcallosal Transventricular Trans-velum Interpositum Approach

The patient is positioned supine, with the head elevated 20 degrees in pin fixation. A coronal or horseshoe-shaped skin incision is made on the right (nondominant) side, in the frontal region. A quadrangular bone flap extending to the midline and anterior to the coronal suture is elevated (Fig. 56-11A and B). The dura is hinged toward the midline.

TABLE 56-4 ▪ Lateral Paramedian Infratentorial Approach

Advantage	Minimal damage to neural tissues
Disadvantages	Narrow space
	Difficult to reach portions of tumor extending to the inferoposterior part of the third ventricle
Indications	Small tumors in the pineal region and the quadrigeminal area
	Biopsy

The right frontal lobe is retracted away from the falx to expose the corpus callosum and the anterior cerebral arteries. The anterior part of the corpus callosum is split between these arteries, 3 to 4 cm in length, and the surgeon proceeds posteriorly to open the pars centralis of the right lateral ventricle (Fig. 56-12A and B). The velum interpositum (tela choroidea of the choroidal fissure) is cut just lateral to the tenia fornicis and medial to the choroid plexus of the lateral ventricle (Fig. 56-13A and B), as seen under the microscope. The velum tissue between the internal cerebral vein and the choroid plexus of the lateral ventricle is very thin and easily cut (Fig. 56-14). The bilateral fornices and the internal cerebral veins are retracted to the medial side to explore the tumor between these structures and the right thalamus (Fig. 56-15). Section of the choroid plexus or the thalamostriate vein is not necessary. Thus, the tumor and the surrounding structures are viewed from above and from the front. Microsurgical manipulation of the tumor is easy because of the ample space provided. This approach provides an excellent view of tumors in the third ventricle and allows the surgeon to manage parts of tumors extending to the lateral ventricle. However, damage to the anterior portion of the corpus callosum occurs and may also occur to the fornix on the right side by retraction. This approach is indicated in cases of huge tumors in the pineal region or the posterior third ventricle that extend anterior to the adhesio interthalamica. The advantages and disadvantages of this approach are listed in Table 56-5. After this approach and its anatomic consideration were described,[24–27] Wen and colleagues[33] reported and proposed a very similar transchoroidal approach.

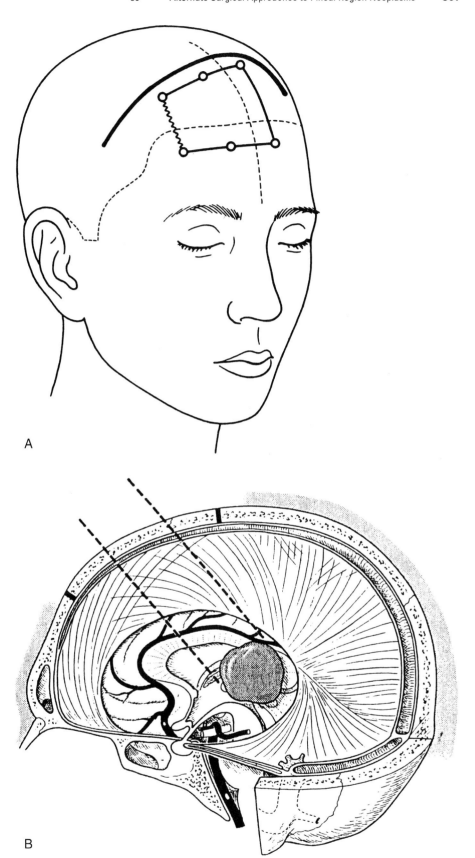

FIGURE 56-11 Anterior transcallosal transventricular trans-velum interpositum approach. Skin incision and craniotomy (*A*) and approach to a tumor (*B*). (From Sano K: Surgery of pineal tumors—anatomical consideration of various approaches. Neurol Surg 12: 1119–1129, 1984.)

A

B

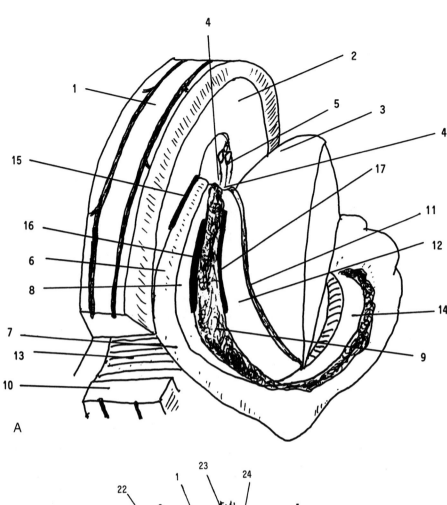

A

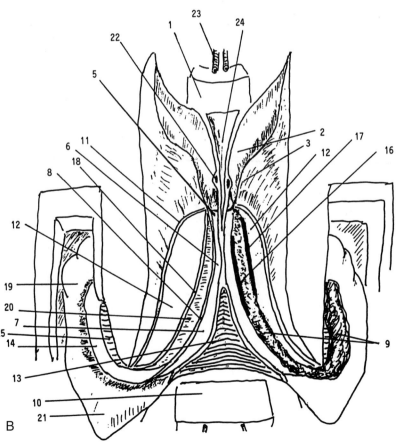

B

FIGURE 56-12 Anatomy of the lateral ventricle. Right lateral ventricle opened (*A*) and corpus callosum stripped off (*B*). 1, Corpus callosum; 2, septum pellucidum; 3, head of the caudate nucleus; 4, foramen of Monro; 5, columna fornicis; 6, corpus fornicis; 7, crus fornicis; 8, tenia fornicis; 9, choroid plexus of the lateral ventricle; 10, splenium of the corpus callosum; 11, vena thalamostriata; 12, lamina affixa; 13, commissura fornicis (hippocampal commissure); 14, fimbria hippocampi; 15, development of the interforniceal plane; 16, trans-velum interpositum approach; 17, development of the subchoroidal plane; 18, tenia choroidea; 19, hippocampus; 20, surface of the thalamus with the tela choroidea stripped off; 21, calcar avis; 22, anterior septal vein; 23, anterior cerebral artery; 24, cavum septi pellucidi; 25, gyrus dentatus. (Modified from Apuzzo MLJ, Chkovani OK, Gott PS, et al: Transcallosal interforniceal approaches for lesions affecting the third ventricle: Surgical considerations and consequences. Neurosurgery 10: 547–554, 1982.)

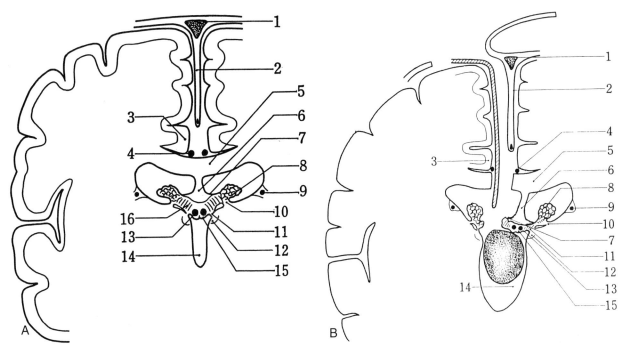

FIGURE 56-13 Anatomy of the velum interpositum (*A*) and trans-velum interpositum approach and a tumor in the third ventricle (*B*). 1, Sinus sagittalis superior; 2, falx; 3, gyrus cinguli; 4, arteria cerebri anterior; 5, corpus callosum; 6, fornix; 7, tenia fornicis; 8, plexus choroideus ventriculi lateralis; 9, vena thalamostriata, stria terminalis, and lamina affixa; 10, tenia choroidea; 11, tenia thalami; 12, stria medullaris thalami; 13, vena cerebri interna; 14, ventriculus tertius; 15, plexus choroideus ventriculi tertii; 16, tela choroidea ventriculi tertii (8 + 16 + 15: velum interpositum). (From Sano K: Surgery of pineal tumors-anatomical consideration of various approaches. Neurol Surg 12:1119–1129, 1984.)

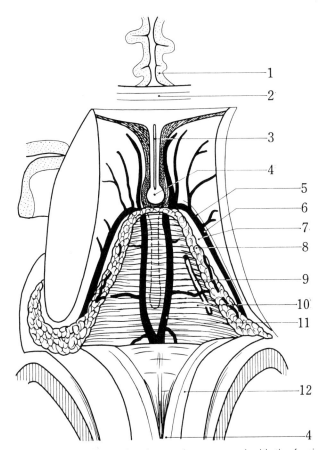

FIGURE 56-14 The velum interpositum exposed with the fornix stripped away. Incision of the velum interpositum just lateral to the tenia fornicis on the right side. 1, Gyrus cinguli; 2, corpus callosum; 3, septum pellucidum; 4, fornix; 5, stria terminalis; 6, vena thalamostriata; 7, lamina affixa; 8, plexus choroideus ventriculi lateralis; 9, section of the velum interpositum; 10, velum interpositum; 11, vena cerebri interna; 12, tenia fornicis. (From Sano K: Surgery of pineal tumors-anatomical consideration of various approaches. Neurol Surg 12:1119–1129, 1984.)

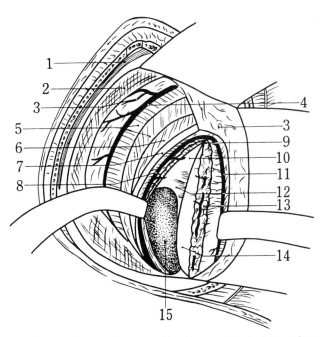

FIGURE 56-15 Anterior transcallosal transventricular trans-velum interpositum approach. Actual operative view. 1, Sinus sagittalis superior; 2, falx; 3, gyrus cinguli; 4, arteria cerebri anterior sinistra; 5, corpus callosum; 6, septum pellucidum; 7, fornix; 8, vena cerebri interna dextra; 9, foramen of Monro; 10, ventriculus tertius; 11, vena thalamostriata dextra and lamina affixa; 12, adhesio interthalamica; 13, plexus choroideus ventriculi lateralis dexter; 14, thalamus dexter; 15, tumor. (From Sano K: Surgery of pineal tumors-anatomical consideration of various approaches. Neurol Surg 12:1119–1129, 1984.)

TABLE 56-5 ▪ Anterior Transcallosal Transventricular Trans-velum Interpositum Approach	
Advantages	Provides an excellent view of lesions in the (posterior) third ventricle
	Allows surgeon to manage parts of lesions extending to the lateral ventricle
Disadvantages	Causes damage to the anterior portion of the corpus callosum
	May cause damage to the fornix
Indications	Huge tumors in the pineal region or in the posterior third ventricle
	Tumors extending anterior to the level of the adhesio interthalamica

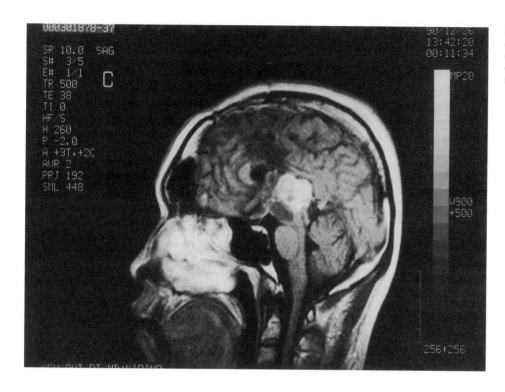

FIGURE 56-16 Gadolinium-diethylenetriaminepentaacetic acid enhancement of a recurrent endodermal sinus tumor in a 21-year-old man.

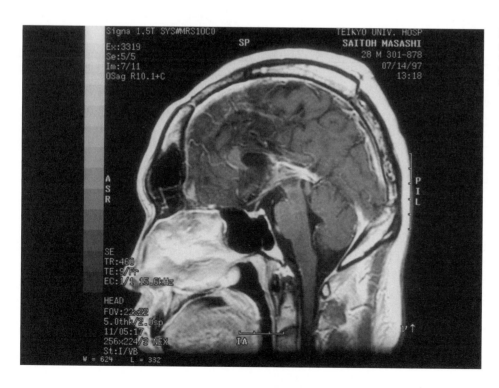

FIGURE 56-17 The same patient as in Figure 56-16 six years after total removal of the tumor. The veins are enhanced by gadolinium-diethylenetriaminepentaacetic acid.

In all patients, steroids are administered before, during, and after the operation. Postoperative irradiation is indicated in cases of a germinoma or a pineocytoma with lymphocytic infiltration and usually consists of ^{60}Co or LINAC (linear accelerator), the total dose being 50 to 60 Gy (daily dose, 1 to 2 Gy). The field of irradiation is 6 × 6 cm to 8 × 8 cm, centering on the pineal region. In malignant neoplasms, whole-brain irradiation and spinal cord irradiation are added, but even in these cases, the total dose does not exceed 50 to 60 Gy. Chemotherapy may also be used before or after radiation therapy.[6] Figure 56-16 is a gadolinium-diethylenetriaminepentaacetic acid–enhanced magnetic resonance imaging scan of a 21-year-old man with a recurrent endodermal sinus tumor with teratomatous tissue. His tumor was macroscopically totally removed 5 years before this scan by the anterior transcallosal transventricular trans-velum interpositum approach. He was treated by radiotherapy and chemotherapy consisting of cisplatin, vinblastine, and bleomycin. The radiotherapy and chemotherapy did not reduce the bulk of the tumor. The tumor was totally removed 7 months later by the occipital transtentorial approach. Figure 56-17 is a magnetic resonance imaging scan taken 6 years after the second operation. No tumor recurrence is observed, although the veins are enhanced by gadolinium-diethylenetriaminepentaacetic acid. Malignant tumors such as teratomas with malignant transformation, endodermal sinus tumors, and choriocarcinomas often recur despite surgery, radiotherapy, and chemotherapy and may require second surgery.

REFERENCES

1. Committee of Brain Tumor registry of Japan: Brain tumor registry of Japan. Neurol Med Chir (Tokyo) 32:395–438, 1992.
2. Sano K, Matsutani M, Seto T: So-called intracranial germ cell tumours: Personal experiences and a theory of their pathogenesis. Neurol Res 11:118–126, 1989.
3. Sano K: So-called intracranial germ cell tumors: Are they really of germ cell origin? Br J Neurosurg 9:391–401, 1995.
4. Sano K: Pathogenesis of intracranial germ cell tumors reconsidered. J Neurosurg 90:258–264, 1999.
5. Sano K: Pineal region tumors: Problems in pathology and treatment. Clin Neurosurg 30:59–91, 1983.
6. Matsutani M, Sano K, Takakura K, et al: Primary intracranial germ cell tumors: A clinical analysis of 153 histologically verified cases. J Neurosurg 86:446–455, 1997.
7. Krabbe KH: The pineal gland, especially in relation to the problem of its supposed significance in sexual development. Endocrinology 7:379–414, 1923.
8. Sano K, Nagai M, Tsuchida T, Hoshino T: New diagnostic method of brain tumors by cell culture of the cerebrospinal fluid-millipore filter-cell culture method. Neurol Med Chir (Tokyo) 8:17–27, 1966.
9. Lang J: Praktische Anatomie. Kopf Teil B Gehirn- und Augenschadel. Berlin/Heidelberg/New York: Springer-Verlag, 1979.
10. Tamaki N, Fujiwara K, Matsumoto S, Takeda H: Veins draining the pineal body: An anatomical and neuroradiological study of "pineal veins." J Neurosurg 39:448–454, 1973.
11. Matsushima T, Rhoton AL, Jr, de Oliveira E, Peace D: Microsurgical anatomy of the veins of the posterior fossa. J Neurosurg 59:63–105, 1983.
12. Oppenheim H, Krause F: Operative Erfolge bei Geschwülsten der Sehhügel- und Vierhügelgegend. Berl Klin Wochenschr 50:2316–2322, 1913.
13. Krause F: Operative Freilegung der Vierhügel nebst Beobachtungen über Hirndruck und Dekompression. Zentralbl Chir 53:2812–2819, 1926.
14. Zapletal B: Ein neuer operativer Zugang zum Gebiet der Incisura Tentorii. Zentralbl Neurochir 16:64–69, 1956.
15. Stein BM: The infratentorial supracerebellar approach to pineal lesions. J Neurosurg 35:197–202, 1971.
16. Dandy W: An operation for the removal of pineal tumors. Surg Gynecol Obstet 33:113–119, 1921.
17. Kunicki A: Operative experience in 8 cases of pineal tumor. J Neurosurg 17:815–823, 1960.
18. Van Wagenen WP: A surgical approach for the removal of certain pineal tumors: Report of a case. Surg Gynecol Obstet 53:216–220, 1931.
19. Heppner F: Zur Operationstechnik bei Pinealomen. Zentralbl Neurochir 19:219–224, 1959.
20. Poppen JL, Marino R, Jr: Pinealomas and tumors of the posterior portion of the third ventricle. J Neurosurg 28:357–364, 1968.
21. Glasauer FE: An operative approach to pineal tumors. Acta Neurochir (Wien) 22:177–180, 1970.
22. Jamieson KG: Excision of pineal tumors. J Neurosurg 35:550–553, 1971.
23. Lazar ML, Clark K: Direct surgical management of masses in the region of the vein of Galen. Surg Neurol 2:17–21, 1974.
24. Sano K: Surgery of pineal tumors—anatomical consideration of various approaches. Neurol Surg (Tokyo) 12:1119–1129, 1984.
25. Sano K: Treatment of tumors in the pineal and posterior third ventricular region. In Samii M (ed): Surgery in and around the Brain Stem and the Third Ventricle. Berlin/Heidelberg: Springer-Verlag, 1986, pp 309–317.
26. Sano K: Pineal region and posterior third ventricular tumors: A surgical overview. In Apuzzo MLJ (ed): Surgery of the Third Ventricle, 2nd ed. Baltimore: Williams & Wilkins, 1998, pp 801–819.
27. Sano K: Alternate surgical approaches to pineal region neoplasms. In Schmidek HH, Sweet WH (eds): Operative Neurosurgical Techniques, 3rd ed. Philadelphia, WB Saunders, 1995, pp 743–754.
28. Van den Bergh R: Lateral-paramedian infratentorial approach in lateral decubitus for pineal tumours. Clin Neurol Neurosurg 92:311–316, 1990.
29. Layne MH, Patterson RH: Subchoroidal trans-velum interpositum approach to mid-third ventricular tumors. Neurosurgery 12:86–94, 1983.
30. Viale GL, Turtas S: The subchoroidal approach to the third ventricle. Surg Neurol 14:71–76, 1980.
31. Apuzzo MLJ, Chikovani OK, Gott PS, et al: Transcallosal interforniceal approaches for lesions affecting the third ventricle: Surgical considerations and consequences. Neurosurgery 10:547–554, 1982.
32. Ziyal IM, Sekhar LN, Salas E, et al: Combined supra/infratentorial transsinus approach to large pineal region tumors. J Neurosurg 88:1050–1057, 1998.
33. Wen HT, Rhoton AL, Jr, de Oliveira E: Transchoroidal approach to the third ventricle: An anatomic study of the choroidal fissure and its clinical application. Neurosurgery 42:1205–1219, 1998.

57

Supracerebellar Approach for Pineal Region Neoplasms

JEFFREY N. BRUCE

Pineal region tumors encompass a diverse group of tumors that can arise from pineal parenchymal cells, supporting cells of the pineal gland, or glial cells from the midbrain and medial walls of the thalamus.[1,2] These tumors occupy a central position that is equidistant from various cranial points traditionally used as routes of exposure. The deep central location places these tumors in intimate contact with important components of the deep venous system that lie dorsally, including the Galen's vein, the precentral cerebellar vein, and the internal cerebral veins.[3] In some instances, there may be a dense attachment to these structures and the tela choroidea. The tumor is often fed by small-caliber branches of the posterior choroidal arteries and branches of the quadrigeminal arteries. These vessels generally do not supply any areas of the brain outside the tumor.

Although pineal region tumors affect a relatively small number of patients, a comparatively large volume of literature has been generated about these neoplasms because of their variable histology and the difficult surgical challenge that they present. This difficulty is underscored by Cushing's[4] statement, "Personally, I have never succeeded in exposing a pineal tumor sufficiently well to justify an attempt to remove it." Several other surgeons have emphasized the high mortality rate after pineal tumor surgery.[5–7] Later, the advent of the operating microscope, a better understanding of pineal region anatomy, and improvement of sophisticated surgical techniques led to a rediscovery of microsurgical approaches to these lesions.[8–11] With experience, the mortality and morbidity rates from the various surgical approaches dropped steadily and led to the current management philosophy for pineal tumors, which relies on an aggressive surgical approach for the removal of benign tumors and decompression and accurate histologic diagnosis of malignant tumors.[2,12,13]

CLASSIC SURGICAL TECHNIQUES

Over the years, various supratentorial and infratentorial approaches have been developed by several prominent neurosurgeons including Dandy's[14] interhemispheric approach, Van Wagenen's[15] transventricular approach, and Poppen's[16] occipital transtentorial approach. The supracerebellar infratentorial approach was first described in 1926, when Krause reported three cases, each a different variety of tumor in the pineal or quadrigeminal region, which he approached through the posterior fossa, over the cerebellar hemispheres, and under the tentorium.[17]

As Krause recognized, because most of these tumors are centrally located, the posterior fossa approach with the patient in the sitting position provides a natural advantage

by providing a midline central exposure.[2] Furthermore, because most tumors lie primarily beneath the deep venous system, this exposure reduces the risk of venous injury. Overall, it provides exposure commensurate with supratentorial approaches and avoids injury to the parietal or occipital lobes and subsequent deficits in sensation or peripheral vision. However, when the tumor extends dorsally above the incisura or extends laterally to the trigone of the lateral ventricle, the posterior fossa approach is not recommended (Fig. 57-1). The tentorium may be cut, but it is still difficult to reach the periphery of the tumor. Overall, this approach provides excellent access and is associated with excellent surgical results.[2,13,18]

Although the supracerebellar approach is versatile enough to be useful for most pineal tumors, its successful application requires a sophisticated level of microsurgical expertise and operative judgment generally associated with experienced neurosurgeons.

PREOPERATIVE EVALUATION

Most of the relevant clinical features of pineal regions tumors are covered in Chapter 56. In general, high-resolution magnetic resonance imaging with gadolinium is mandatory in the evaluation of all pineal region tumors. Despite advances in radiographic imaging, histologic subtypes

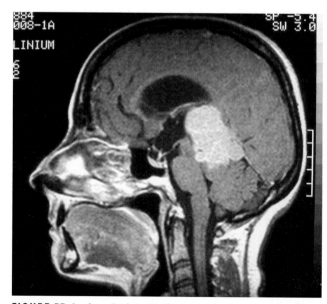

FIGURE 57-1 A sagittal magnetic resonance imaging scan shows a large pineal region tumor extending well above the level of the incisura. A supratentorial approach is recommended for this tumor.

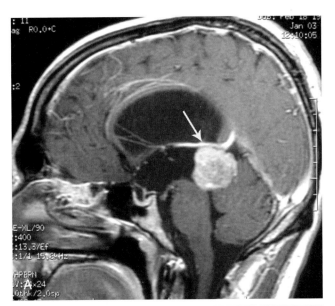

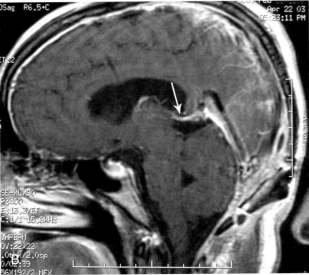

FIGURE 57-2 *A,* A sagittal magnetic resonance imaging scan shows a large pineal tumor ventral to the deep venous system (*arrow*) and causing compression of the aqueduct with resultant hydrocephalus. *B,* Postoperative magnetic resonance imaging after tumor removal that left the deep venous system intact (*arrow*).

cannot be predicted consistently based on radiographic characteristics.[19–21] Magnetic resonance imaging can precisely define the size of the tumor, its vascularity, and its relationship to surrounding structures. Planning the operative approach depends on knowing the tumor's position within the third ventricle, its lateral and supratentorial extension, the degree of brain stem involvement, and the position relative to the deep venous system (Fig. 57-2). Tumor invasiveness can sometimes be inferred by the degree of margination and irregularity on magnetic resonance imaging; however, the true degree of encapsulation can only be determined at surgery. Computed tomography scans can provide details of calcification, blood-brain barrier breakdown, and degree of vascularity, as well as the presence of hydrocephalus. Magnetic resonance imaging, however, nearly always allows better visualization of the tumor than computed tomography. Angiography is unnecessary unless a vascular anomaly is suspected.

Markers for malignant germ cell elements such as α-fetoprotein and human chorionic gonadotropin should be measured in the cerebrospinal fluid and blood as part of the routine preoperative workup.[2,22,23] In addition to aiding in arriving at the correct diagnosis, the presence of these markers can be helpful in monitoring the patient's response to therapy and to detect early tumor recurrence. By definition, patients with elevated germ cell markers have malignant germ cell tumors and do not require a histologic diagnosis before commencing with chemotherapy or radiation therapy.[2]

SURGICAL CONSIDERATIONS

Surgical intervention to obtain diagnostic tumor tissue is mandatory because of the wide variety of tumor subtypes that occur in the pineal region, each having implications for prognosis and selection of clinical management options.[2,23] Selection of a surgical approach for an individual patient depends on clinical features and radiographic findings. For most pineal tumors, the infratentorial supracerebellar approach performed in the sitting position is the method of choice (Fig. 57-3). It offers the advantage of approaching the tumor from a midline trajectory while avoiding the inconvenience of working around the deep venous vessels that generally lie dorsal to the mass. With this approach, gravity is helpful in assisting with the tumor dissection. When the tumor is eccentric or grows laterally to the region of the trigone or superiorly to the corpus callosum, the posterior parietal-interhemispheric approach is recommended. Using this approach, a portion of the posterior corpus callosum is sectioned to reach the tumor. With the supratentorial approach, however, tumor extension to the contralateral side or into the posterior fossa can be difficult to visualize. The tentorium on the ipsilateral side can be sectioned to increase exposure of the posterior fossa component.

Stereotactic biopsy can be useful in addition to diagnostic biopsy in patients with disseminated tumor or those in whom extensive medical problems pose excessive surgical risks.[2,12,24] Some tumors that appear to invade the brain stem or thalamus likewise may benefit from stereotactic biopsy. Overall, however, the routine use of stereotactic biopsy is prohibited by problems of sampling error and the difficulties of making an accurate diagnosis through the study of small specimens.[25,26] Furthermore, it ignores the advantages that open operation can provide in resecting benign tumors and debulking

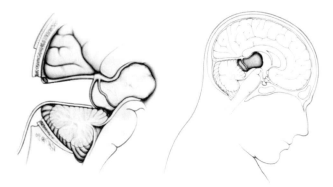

FIGURE 57-3 Drawing of the sagittal view shows the position of the pineal tumor with gravity facilitating retraction of the cerebellum to access the infratentorial supracerebellar corridor.

malignant tumors. Small tumors in particular are prone to risks of hemorrhage from damage to the deep venous system, whereas extremely vascular tumors, such as pineal cell tumors, are vulnerable to hemorrhage as well.

OPERATIVE TECHNIQUE: SUPRACEREBELLAR APPROACH

Most patients with pineal tumors have increased intracranial pressure and hydrocephalus resulting from obstruction or compromise of the aqueduct. Hydrocephalus must be relieved before attempting any direct approach to the tumor. Stereotaxic-guided third ventriculostomy is preferred over shunting procedures because it avoids the need for hardware, reduces the risk of ventricular collapse, and minimizes tumor seeding.[27] Treating hydrocephalus a week or two before surgical tumor removal allows the ventricular system sufficient time to gradually decompress. In situations of mild hydrocephalus in which the tumor is likely to be resected, a ventricular drain can be placed at the time of craniotomy and then converted to a shunt on the second or third postoperative day if the hydrocephalus persists.

There are several positions that can be used for the infratentorial supracerebellar approach. Unless the patient is younger than 2 years of age and has a severe degree of hydrocephalus, the sitting position is preferred.[2,28] The three-quarter prone and lateral decubitus position and the Concorde position are possible alternatives; however, they do not allow gravity to work in the surgeon's favor.[29,30]

The sitting position is accomplished by raising the back of the table to its maximal position. The patient's head, neck, and shoulders are brought forward by a pin-vise head fixation device such as the Mayfield headholder. The head must be strongly flexed so that optimal exposure of the tentorial notch can be achieved with the greatest comfort to the surgeon. The patient is tilted somewhat forward after being positioned on the operating table so that the surgeon actually works over the back of the patient's shoulders to the posterior fossa (Fig. 57-4). A Doppler probe, central venous catheter, end-tidal PCO_2 evaluation, and modest positive pressure ventilation are used to recognize and avoid air embolism, which can occur during the bony opening or when large venous sinuses are exposed.

A self-retaining retractor, such as Greenberg's Universal Retractor, is fixed via a bar to the operating table on the left side. The bars are then arranged in a rectangular configuration framing the operative field, facilitating placement of a retractor in the inferior position to depress the cerebellum. A cottonoid tray is fixed to the self-retaining retractor system and held by one of the retractor's arms.

A long midline incision is used, extending approximately from the spinous process of the third vertebral body up into the occipital region, so that the pericranium and muscle attachments can be elevated on each side without disrupting their continuity. Freeing up the muscle layer facilitates closure later. A wide craniotomy is performed to include the lateral sinuses and torcula but without extending to the foramen magnum. Generally, using a high-speed air drill to perform a suboccipital craniotomy is preferred so that the bone flap may be replaced at the end of the procedure. A craniotome is used to turn the flap after first exposing each of the dural sinuses to avoid tears. Brain relaxation and cerebellar

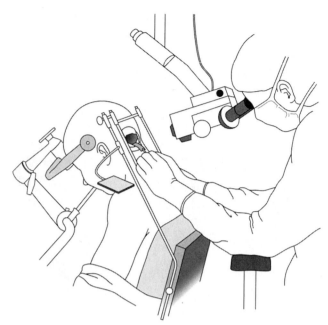

FIGURE 57-4 Diagram of the patient position and operative setup for the supracerebellar approach.

retraction can be facilitated by mannitol, ventricular drainage, or removal of cerebrospinal from the cisterna magna. It is preferable to open the dura on either side of the midline so that the cerebellar falx and accompanying cerebellar sinus can be ligated and divided. The dural opening should extend bilaterally up to the lateral sinus (Fig. 57-5).

Once the dura is opened, all bridging veins over the dorsal surface of the cerebellum, including the hemispheres and vermis, can be sacrificed to free the cerebellum from the tentorium. The weight of cottonoids and a copper retractor, along with gravitational forces that are exerted in the sitting position, allow sufficient depression of the cerebellum to establish an unobstructed corridor to the pineal region under the tentorium (see Fig. 57-3).

At this point, the operating microscope should be brought to the operating table. A microscope capable of varying the objective length from 275 to 400 mm is desirable because the operating distance for the surgeon changes throughout the operation, going from the dorsal surface of the cerebellum to the center of the third ventricle. The use of a freestanding armrest is also helpful in minimizing fatigue.

The arachnoid in the quadrigeminal region and around the incisura is usually thickened and opaque in the presence of tumors and must be opened by microdissection techniques to expose the surface of the tumor. The precentral cerebellar vein, which can be seen extending from the edge of the vermis to Galen's vein, should be cauterized and divided. Galen's great vein and the internal cerebral veins are well above the tumor and are not encountered in these initial maneuvers. Laterally, the medial aspect of the temporal lobe and Rosenthal's veins can be seen as they course upward toward the confluence of veins in these regions. The thickened arachnoid should be opened widely to appreciate the underlying anatomy. Using sharp dissection, the arachnoidal opening must be kept close to the anterior surface of the vermis and cerebellar hemisphere to avoid injuring the deep venous system, keeping in mind that the initial trajectory is

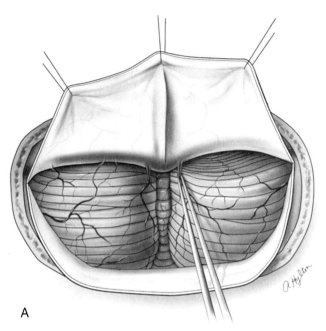

A

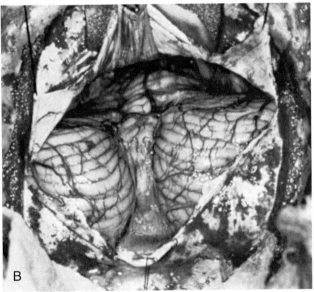

B

FIGURE 57-5 *A*, Drawing shows the dural opening and sacrifice of bridging veins. *B*, Full dural opening and the cerebellum, which is sagging because of gravity after the bridging veins have been divided.

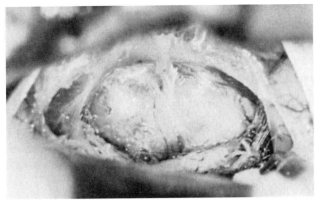

FIGURE 57-6 Operative view shows exposure of the posterior surface of a tumor in the pineal region.

the tumor. With tumors of firm consistency, a Cavitron with a long, curved tip can be helpful for debulking. The instrument is large and can be difficult to maneuver into the operative field, especially if an objective lens of less than 275 mm is used in the microscope.

In general terms, the trajectory of the operation is toward the velum interpositum (Fig. 57-7). This must be considered when attempting to remove segments of the tumor in the inferior portion of the third ventricle or directly over the quadrigeminal plate in relation to the anterior lobe of the cerebellum. The most difficult dissection involves the inferior portion of the tumor, where it is adherent to the collicular region of the dorsal midbrain. Small dental mirrors and angled instruments may be required to remove this portion of the tumor. Similarly, these techniques may be helpful for supratentorial tumor extensions. Further exposure can be gained by incising the tentorium if necessary.

Even with unresectable tumors, considerable benefit can be gained from internal decompression of the tumor or from sufficient tumor resection to expose the posterior third ventricle. Tumors that are benign or encapsulated can usually be removed completely. For most malignant tumors, an

toward Galen's vein. The anterior portion of the cerebellum is retracted by the inferior self-retaining retractor to expose the posterior surface of the tumor (Fig. 57-6). The tumor may be invested and supplied by branches of the choroidal arteries. The tumor capsule is then cauterized and opened by sharp dissection. Depending on its consistency, the tumor is removed with tumor forceps, small curets, suction, or cautery. A portion of the tumor should be sent for frozen tissue diagnosis early in the dissection. Although it may be helpful for intraoperative management, the frequent inaccuracy of frozen section diagnosis for these tumors should be kept in mind when making intraoperative decisions.

Because many of these tumors extend well into the third ventricle, even to the region of Monro's foramen, long instruments are required to reach the anterior margins of

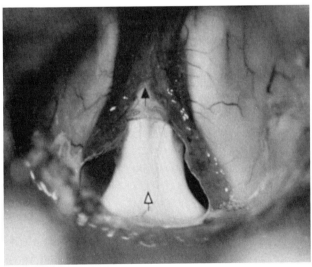

FIGURE 57-7 View of the interior of the third ventricle shows the columns of the fornix (*open arrow*) and the tela choroidea (*closed arrow*) after removal of a large pineal region tumor.

aggressive resection is desirable to improve the efficacy of adjuvant therapy, and complete resection is sometimes possible. One exception may be for germinomas in which the exquisite radiosensitivity leaves surgical resection with little impact on long-term outcome.[31] With tumors that are incompletely resected, particularly vascular ones such as pineal cell tumors, meticulous hemostasis is crucial. Surgicel is the preferred hemostatic agent, and it should be placed carefully so that it does not float and obstruct the aqueduct when the third ventricle fills with cerebrospinal fluid.

At the conclusion of the operation, after decompression of the tumor and the ventricular system, the dura can be closed to support the cerebellum. When a craniotomy has been performed, the bone flap is secured back in place with wires or miniplates. A greater degree of dural and bony closure seems to lower the incidence of postoperative aseptic meningitis.

OPERATIVE COMPLICATIONS

Impairment of extraocular movements, particularly limitation of upward gaze and convergence, can be expected whenever the tumor is dissected from the quadrigeminal region.[13,32] Other deficits, including pupillary abnormalities and difficulty focusing or accommodating may also occur. These deficits are generally transient, but in some instances, they may last for several months. The incidence of ataxia has been minimal and usually transient. Manipulation of the brain in the adjacent third ventricle or in the periaqueductal region of an infiltrating tumor can cause altered consciousness, which in severe instances can take the form of akinetic mutism. The incidence and severity of postoperative deficits are increased when significant symptoms are present after surgery, if previous radiation therapy has been given, and with tumors having highly malignant and invasive characteristics.

The most serious complication of pineal tumor surgery is postoperative hemorrhage, which can occur with a delay of as long as several postoperative days.[32] It is seen most often with subtotally resected pineal cell tumors, which tend to be soft and highly vascular. Hemorrhage has also been associated with stereotactic biopsy and has been known to occur before surgery as so-called pineal apoplexy.[33,34]

Other complications related to the supracerebellar infratentorial approach in the sitting position include collapse of the ventricular system and entry of air into the ventricular system and subdural space.[32] These conditions generally improve with time and rarely is anything done to correct them. The incidence of air embolism causing complications is very low. Shunt malfunction can occur in as many as 20% of patients after surgery. This problem can be minimized by leaving a catheter from the third ventricle into the cisterna magna at the time of surgery.

RESULTS

Ninety-three operations for pineal region tumors have been performed at the New York Neurological Institute between 1990 and 2001 (Table 57-1). Surgery resulted in an excellent outcome more than 90% of the time, and a histologic diagnosis was made in all patients. For nearly all the benign tumors, surgery alone was curative. Among all tumors, benign

and malignant, a radical or gross total resection was possible 72% of the time (Table 57-2).

The only surgery-related death occurred as a result of a pulmonary embolism 3 weeks after surgery in a woman with a subtotally resected ependymoma whose clinical course was complicated by a postoperative hemorrhage. Permanent major morbidity occurred in 2% of patients and was most commonly associated with malignant tumors, previous radiation therapy, and the presence of significant preoperative neurologic impairment. Most patients had temporary disturbances in extraocular movements that gradually improved over time.

Overall, long-term results have been uniformly excellent for all tumors that were benign, which comprised one third of all pineal tumors. Because of the encapsulated nature of benign tumors, nearly all were completely removable with microsurgical techniques. No recurrences have been seen in patients with benign tumors that have been completely resected at the initial operation. Complete resection should be the operative goal in these patients.

For patients with malignant tumors, the long-term prognosis depends mostly on the histologic diagnosis. The role of aggressive surgical resection for malignant pineal region tumors has not been validated to a statistically significant standard. Our anecdotal experience has been that patients with malignant tumors that can be radically resected have a better long-term prognosis, improved response to adjuvant therapy, and reduced postoperative complications.

SUMMARY

Optimal management decisions in patients with pineal region tumors are incumbent on making an accurate histologic diagnosis. Therefore, surgical exploration is mandated

TABLE 57-1 ▪ **Outcome after Surgery for Pineal Region Tumors at the New York Neurological Institute (1990–2001)**

Histology	Minor/No Morbidity	Major Morbidity		
		Transient	Permanent	Death
Benign	32	0	0	0
Malignant	47	11	2	1
Total	79 (85%)	11 (12%)	2 (2%)	1 (1%)

TABLE 57-2 ▪ **Surgical Results for Pineal Region Tumors at the New York Neurological Institute (1990–2001)**

Histology	Biopsy	Subtotal Resection	Radical Subtotal Resection	Gross Total Resection
Benign	0	0	1	31
Malignant	3	23	8	27
Total	3 (3%)	23 (25%)	9 (10%)	58 (62)

in all patients. The benefits of surgery extend beyond diagnostic purposes because one third of pineal tumors are benign and treatable with surgery alone. Malignant tumors may benefit from surgical debulking to reduce tumor burden before adjuvant therapy, and gross total resection is often possible.

The supracerebellar infratentorial approach offers several advantages over supratentorial techniques. By providing a midline trajectory beneath the deep venous system and taking advantage of the effects of gravity in the sitting position, the supracerebellar approach reduces the risk of complications and facilitates tumor removal. Improvements in microsurgical technique and neuroanesthesia have resulted in excellent surgical outcomes after pineal surgery.

REFERENCES

1. Bruce JN, Connolly ES, Stein BM: Pineal and germ cell tumors. In Laws ER (ed): Brain Tumors, 2nd ed. London: Churchill Livingstone, 2001, pp 771–800.
2. Bruce J: Pineal tumors. In Winn H (ed): Youman's Neurological Surgery, vol 1, 5th ed. Philadelphia: WB Saunders, 2004, pp 1011–1129.
3. Quest DO, Kleriga E: Microsurgical anatomy of the pineal region. Neurosurgery 6:385–390, 1980.
4. Cushing H: Intracranial Tumors: Notes upon a Series of Two Thousand Verified Cases with Surgical Mortality Pertaining Thereto. Springfield, IL: Charles C Thomas, 1932.
5. Camins MB, Schlesinger EB: Treatment of tumours of the posterior part of the third ventricle and the pineal region: A long term follow-up. Acta Neurochir (Wien) 40:131–143, 1978.
6. Cummins F, Taveras J, Schlesinger E: Treatment of gliomas of the third ventricle and pinealomas: With special reference to the value of radiotherapy. Neurology 10:1031–1036, 1960.
7. Horrax G, Daniels J: The conservative treatment of pineal tumors. Surg Clin North Am 22:649–659, 1942.
8. Suzuki J, Iwabuchi T: Surgical removal of pineal tumors (pinealomas and teratomas): Experience in a series of 19 cases. J Neurosurg 23:565–571, 1965.
9. Sano K: Pineal region tumors: problems in pathology and treatment. Clin Neurosurg 30:59–89, 1984.
10. Reid WS, Clark WK: Comparison of the infratentorial and transtentorial approaches to the pineal region. Neurosurgery 3:1–8, 1978.
11. Page LK: The infratentorial-supracerebellar exposure of tumors in the pineal area. Neurosurgery 1:36–40, 1977.
12. Bruce JN, Ogden AT: Surgical strategies for treating patients with pineal region tumors. J Neurooncol 69:221–236, 2004.
13. Bruce JN, Stein BM: Surgical management pineal region tumors. Acta Neurochir (Wien) 134:130–135, 1995.
14. Dandy WE: Operative experience in cases of pineal tumor. Arch Surg 33:19–46, 1936.
15. Van Wagenen WP: A surgical approach for the removal of certain pineal tumors. Surg Gynecol Obstet 53:216–220, 1931.
16. Poppen JL: The right occipital approach to a pinealoma. J Neurosurg 25:706–710, 1966.
17. Krause F: Operative Frielegung der Vierhugel, nebst Beobachtungen uber Hirndruck und Dekompression. Zentrabl Chir 53:2812–2819, 1926.
18. Stein BM, Bruce JN: Surgical management of pineal region tumors. Clin Neurosurg 39:509–532, 1992.
19. Tien RD, Barkovich AJ, Edwards MSB: M.R. imaging of pineal tumors. AJNR Am J Neuroradiol 11:557–565, 1990.
20. Müller-Forell W, Schroth G, Egan PJ: MR imaging in tumors of the pineal region. Neuroradiology 30:224–231, 1988.
21. Ganti SR, Hilal SK, Silver AJ, et al: CT of pineal region tumors. AJNR Am J Neuroradiol 7:97–104, 1986.
22. Bjornsson J, Scheithauer B, Okazaki H, Leech R: Intracranial germ cell tumors: Pathobiological and immunohistochemical aspects of 70 cases. J Neuropathol Exp Neurol 44:32–46, 1985.
23. Bruce JN: Management of pineal region tumors. Neurosurg Q 3:103–119, 1993.
24. Kreth F, Schatz C, Pagenstecher A, et al: Stereotactic management of lesions of the pineal region. Neurosurgery 39:280–291, 1996.
25. Kraichoke S, Cosgrove M, Chadrasoma PT: Granulomatous inflammation in pineal germinoma. Am J Surg Pathol 12:655–660, 1988.
26. Edwards MSB, Hudgins RJ, Wilson CB, et al. Pineal region tumors in children. J Neurosurg 66:689–697, 1988.
27. Goodman R: Magnetic resonance imaging-directed stereotactic endoscopic third ventriculostomy. Neurosurgery 32:1043–1047, 1993.
28. Bruce JN, Stein BM: Infratentorial approach to pineal tumors. In Wilson CB (ed): Neurosurgical Procedures: Personal Approaches to Classic Operations. Baltimore: Williams & Wilkins, 1992, pp 63–76.
29. Ausman JI, Malik GM, Dujovny M, Mann R: Three-quarter prone approach to the pineal-tentorial region. Surg Neurol 29:298–306, 1988.
30. Kobayashi S, Sugita K, Tanaka Y, Kyoshima K: Infratentorial approach to the pineal region in the prone position: Concorde position. J Neurosurg 58:141–143, 1983.
31. Sawamura Y, de Tribolet N, Ishii N, Abe H: Management of primary intracranial germinomas: Diagnostic surgery or radical resection? J Neurosurg 87:262–266, 1997.
32. Bruce J, Stein B: Supracerebellar approaches in the pineal region. In Apuzzo M (ed): Brain Surgery: Complication Avoidance and Management. New York: Churchill Livingstone, 1993, pp 511–536.
33. Burres KP, Hamilton RD: Pineal apoplexy. Neurosurgery 4:264–268, 1979.
34. Peragut JC, Dupard T, Graziani N, Sedan R: De la prévention des risques de la biopsie stéréotaxique de certaines tumeurs de la région pinéale: a propos de 3 observations. Neurochirurgie 33:23–27, 1987.

Section X

Brain Stem Tumors

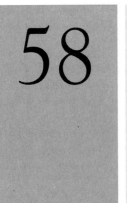

58 Surgical Management of Brain Stem, Thalamic, and Hypothalamic Tumors

ALEXANDER N. KONOVALOV, SERGEY K. GORELYSHEV, and ELENA A. KHUHLAEVA

Surgery of primary axial tumors of the brain stem, thalamic, and hypothalamic regions presents serious problems. Until recently most of these tumors have been considered unremovable and even untreatable. Lesions of the midline are more common in children than in adults and represent approximately 57% of pediatric brain tumors.[1] Despite localization in deep-seated, vitally important structures of the brain, some of these tumors are reachable and, because of their benign nature and well-defined borders, can be removed. Magnetic resonance imaging (MRI) and computed tomography (CT) make possible the visualization of these tumors, and microsurgical techniques permit their successful excision.

The Moscow Burdenko Neurosurgical Institute is a major referral center where patients with severe brain lesions including diencephalic and brain stem tumors (BSTs) often come as a "court of last resort."

In this chapter, we discuss two groups of midline primary brain tumors: tumors of the hypothalamus and of the brain stem.

In this analysis, we include only those patients who were operated on by the first author (A.N.K.) because this permits a better understanding of the possibilities and limitations of surgery (Table 58-1).

CHIASMAL/HYPOTHALAMIC GLIOMAS

There is no clear definition in the literature of hypothalamic gliomas and terms such as optic pathway gliomas, optico/hypothalamic gliomas. We prefer to use the term chiasmal/hypothalamic gliomas (CHGs) to describe tumors originating from chiasm and floor of the third ventricle.

At the Burdenko Institute of Neurosurgery, the first operations aimed at the surgical removal of CHGs started in 1982, and by the end of 2002, their number reached 216 cases. During this same period, the total number of patients with CHGs investigated and observed was 319 cases (Table 58-2).

Our surgical experience devoted to the gliomas of chiasm and floor of third ventricle covers three periods: 1982 to 1986, 1987 to 1992, and 1993 to 2002.

During the first period (1982 to 1986), the indications for radical surgery were rather narrow and included patients predominantly with giant gliomas (37 operations). The mortality rate during this period was approximately 19%.

In the second period (1987 to 1992), the indications for surgery became wider and included all cases with nodular tumors (88 operations). Postoperative mortality decreased to 6% (Fig. 58-1).

Since 1993, the mortality rate has been 0%, and we consider surgery to be a method of choice in the treatment of nodular gliomas of chiasma and floor of the third ventricle despite their size and topographic variation (94 operations), whereas diffuse tumors still remain inoperable.

One hundred three patients were not operated on. In 60 patients surgery was not performed due to the limited indications during the first period. This group mainly included patients with gliomas of chiasm infiltrating adjacent brain structures (groups II, III, and IV). Shunting procedures were performed in 42 patients, irradiation in 6 patients, and 12 patients were observed without treatment.

The age of the operated patients varied from 2.5 to 50 years old with a significant predominance of children (86%; 188 children, 28 adults). The overall sex distribution is nearly equal (112 males, 104 females).

TABLE 58-1 ▪ Diencephalic and Brain Stem Tumors (N = 614)

Localization	No. of Operations
Hypothalamic gliomas	216
Gliomas of the thalamus	92
Brain stem tumors	306
Total	614

TABLE 58-2 ▪ Total Number of Patients with CHG Treated from 1982 to 2002

Nodular gliomas, tumor removal	216	
Nodular gliomas, palliative procedures*	60	Shunting: 42
		Irradiation: 6
		Observation: 12
Diffuse gliomas with neurofibromatosis, no surgery	43	
Total	319	

*These modalities of treatment were used in the period 1982 to 1986.

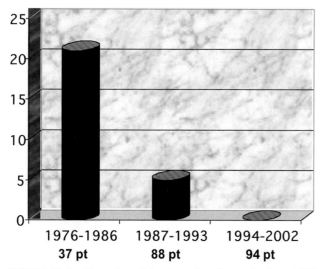

FIGURE 58-1 Illustration of the dynamics of mortality from 1976 to 2002. During the past 10 years, there has been no mortality.

Topography

CHGs include nodular-type and diffuse-type tumors involving the chiasm and floor of the third ventricle. We outline two main groups of tumors.

The nodular type is classified into five groups according to the predominant direction of growth and possible place of origin along visual pathways (Fig. 58-2 and Table 58-3).

The first group consists of tumors with predominant anterior expansion (Fig. 58-3), probably arising at the anterior corner of the chiasm. Some of these tumors reach giant size and form masses that displace the frontal lobes and may grow into the middle fossa. These tumors are often solid or partially cystic. In addition to real tumor cysts, large, well-delineated arachnoid cysts are seen in some cases that develop as a result of tumor infiltration of arachnoid and disturbances in cerebrospinal fluid circulation in the sylvian fissure and basal cisterns.

The second group consists of tumors that grow anteriorly, infiltrating part of the chiasm as well as penetrating the third

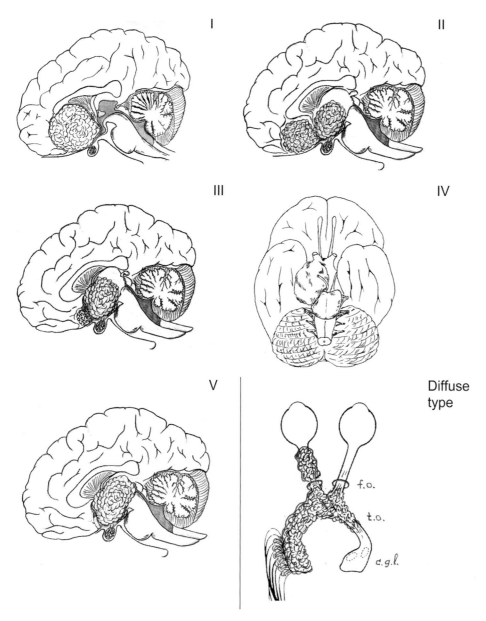

FIGURE 58-2 Topography of hypothalamic tumors. *I,* Tumors with predominant anterior growth; *II,* tumors that grow anteriorly and penetrate the third ventricle; *III,* tumors with the main part occupying the third ventricle but infiltrating the chiasma as well; *IV,* tumors of the optic tract; *V,* gliomas of the floor of the third ventricle. Diffuse tumors infiltrate optic pathways, including the visual nerves, both parts of the chiasma, and the optic tracts.

Diffuse type

TABLE 58-3 ▪ Distribution of Patients with Different Types of CHG

Tumor Type	Percent of Patients
Tumors of the chiasma	
Group I	22
Group II	18
Group III	22
Tumors of the optic tract: group IV	19
Tumors of the floor of the third ventricle: group V	18

ventricle (Figs. 58-4 and 58-5). The anterior cerebral (A_1) and anterior communicating arteries partially separate these two tumor components.

The third group (retrochiasmal type) consists of tumors that predominantly spread into the third ventricle. These tumors may have their origin at the posterior part of chiasma near the optic tract (Figs. 58-6 and 58-7).

The fourth group consists of tumors that originate and grow along the optic tract and may destroy half of the chiasm and penetrate the subcortical nuclei and thalamus (Figs. 58-8 and 58-9).

The separate group of tumors originates in the floor of the third ventricle (the fifth group) and may infiltrate all the walls of the third ventricle including its roof. The chiasm is stretched on the anterior pole of the tumor (Figs. 58-10 to 58-12).

This classification has practical importance because the surgical approach depends on the precise localization of the tumor. However, many other classifications have been developed by pathologists and neurosurgeons.

The classification that to some extent resembles ours was described by Bregeat[2] in 1978.

Diffuse tumors infiltrate optic pathways including the visual nerves, both parts of the chiasma, and the optic tracts. In most patients, they are associated with clinical signs of neurofibromatosis 1 (NF-1) (except children younger than 2 to 3 years old in whom the signs of NF-1 have not yet developed). Diffuse infiltration of both parts of the visual pathways differentiates them from the nodular type of CHGs (Fig. 58-13).

Pathology

In accordance with the recent World Health Organization classification of brain tumors, hypothalamic tumors in most of our cases are pilocytic astrocytomas grade I (64% of patients). In some cases, the patterns of malignancy were revealed in pilocytic astrocytomas (grade II): frequent mitosis, pronounced endothelial proliferation, and necrotic foci (28%). These tumors often infiltrate adjacent arachnoid and grow around the carotid artery and its branches, which become embedded in the tumor tissue.

Anaplastic astrocytomas are rare (8%) and more often localized in the third ventricle (group V).

Recently, a new group of tumors, previously classified as pilocytic astrocytomas, with unique histologic features and aggressive behavior has been identified (pilomyxoid astrocytomas). These tumors have unusual histomorphology and a mixture of ependymal and piloid-like astrocytic features and a myxoid stroma similar to that of myxopapillary ependymomas.[3–7] Choroid glioma is another recently described histopathologic entity that has been added to the World Health Organization glioma classification scheme

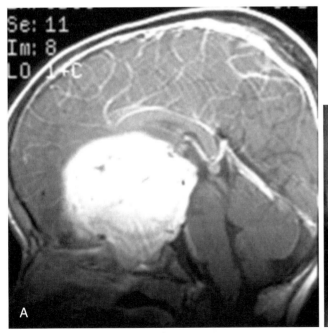
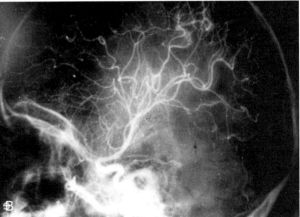

FIGURE 58-3 A giant tumor of group I. *A,* Sagittal T1-weighted magnetic resonance imaging after gadolinium injection shows marked enhancement of the tumor, which displaces the third ventricle backward. *B,* Carotid angiography shows the prominent caudal displacement of anterior cerebral artery by the tumor nodule.

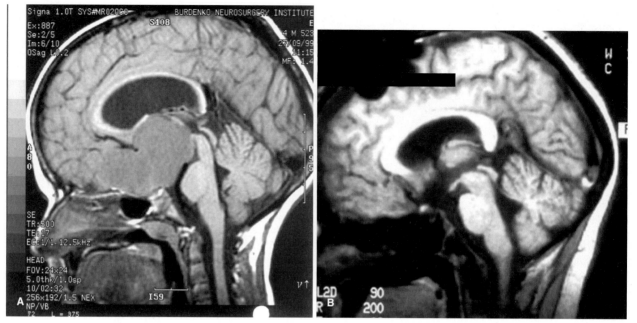

FIGURE 58-4   A tumor that partially destroys the chiasm and grows anteriorly and penetrates the third ventricle (group II). The anterior cerebral (A_1) and anterior communicating artery separate chiasmal and retrochiasmal parts of the tumor. *A,* Magnetic resonance imaging (MRI) before surgery. *B,* Sagittal T1-weighted MRI shows the total removal of the tumor.

and must be included in the differential diagnosis of a suprasellar mass.[8–11] However, we have not yet identified similar tumors in our patients.

Gliomas of the chiasma are often surrounded by large cysts (30% of all cases), formed by thickened arachnoid, that usually contain normal or slightly xanthochromic cerebrospinal fluid (Fig. 58-14A).

Calcifications and small cysts in the tumor tissue are not infrequent in CHGs (10% to 20%), which may confuse the differentiation from craniopharyngiomas (see Fig. 58-14B).

Clinical Picture

Nodular Gliomas

The first clinical manifestation of these tumors is usually revealed 2 years before presentation. It is very difficult to notice the deterioration of vision in young children, although hypothalamic and endocrine disorders are not common in children younger than 7 years old.

Visual deterioration is seen in nearly in all patients, and in most cases, visual disturbances are asymmetrical. Symmetrical bilateral visual disturbances were more common either in patients with gliomas of the ventricle floor or in the last stages of visual impairment.

Bitemporal hemianopsia is characteristic of patients with gliomas of the ventricle floor and homonymous hemianopsia in patients with gliomas of the optic tract. Defects in the temporal half of the visual field of the "better" eye combined with practical blindness in the other eye is typical for chiasmal gliomas (the first three groups).

The signs of increased intracranial pressure are present in half of patients, predominantly in those with the tumors occupying the third ventricle, where they are usually the first signs of a disease.

Hemiparesis is typical only for the gliomas of the optic tract and is related to compression of the subcortical nuclei and internal capsule by the tumor.

Although visual impairment and hydrocephalus are widely described in literature, only limited data are available on endocrine disturbances in these lesions.[12–14] Endocrine disturbances in patients with CHGs are very mild (in comparison with other tumors in this region). Thus growth disorders are rather rare, except in children with precocious puberty; growth hormone deficiency is uncommon.

Sexual development is also nearly normal, but a specific syndrome, precocious puberty, is seen in 8% of children. This condition is due to the high level of sex hormones (testosterone, estradiol, luteinizing hormone, follicle-stimulating hormone), but the cause of its hypersecretion in nonactive tumors remains unclear and may be related to the high level of transforming growth factor α in astrocytes of hypothalamus.[11a,11b]

In contrast, obesity is significantly more common in these patients but is seen predominantly in adults. Diencephalic cachexia is noted exceptionally in infants (12%).

Signs of hypothireosis and hypocortisolism are rare (6% to 8% of patients); diabetes insipidus is not common (8%) in comparison with craniopharyngiomas.

In contrast to other suprasellar tumors, endocrine deficiencies are surprisingly rare in opticohypothalamic gliomas despite their large size.[12] This may be used as a criterion in the differential diagnosis of these lesions, in addition to the radiographic findings.[15]

The clinical picture varies according the type of tumor (Table 58-4). The first symptoms in gliomas of the chiasma and optic tract (groups I to IV) are visual disturbances. At the time of the patient's admission, the disturbances are always pronounced, asymmetrical, and associated with primary optic atrophy.

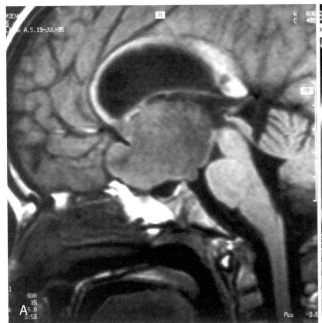

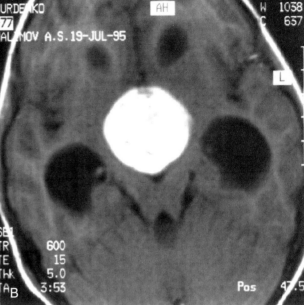

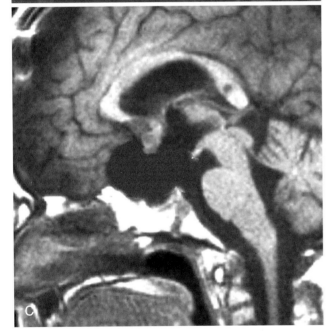

FIGURE 58-5 A case of a tumor that destroyed the chiasm and penetrated the third ventricle up to foramen of Monro (group II). *A*, T1-weighted magnetic resonance imaging (MRI) before surgery. *B, C*, Sagittal T1-weighted MRI shows the total removal of the tumor.

The manifestation of the disease in patients with gliomas of optic tract and the floor of the third ventricle (group V) begins with intracranial hypertension and is characterized by mild, symmetrical visual disturbances with papilledema and hydrocephalus.

Diffuse Tumors

Diffuse tumors have the following characteristics:

1. Infiltrative pattern of growth along visual pathways
2. Bilateral expansion of the chiasma and optic nerves and tracts
3. Association with NF type I
4. Variable, even decelerating tumor growth rate and stabilization in half of patients
5. High incidence of precocious puberty (25%)

6. Manifestation in young age (younger than 2 to 3 years old)
7. Abnormal sex distribution (male:female = 1:2)
8. Association with other congenital malformations (30%)

Computed Tomography and Magnetic Resonance Imaging Diagnostic Methods

CT and MRI are very effective diagnostic methods for detecting hypothalamic tumors. MRI allows the surgeon to clarify the relationship of the tumor to the skull base and vital brain structures (e.g., the brain stem and the third ventricle structures). MRI, used in combination with CT, allows the topographic type of tumor to be defined and enables

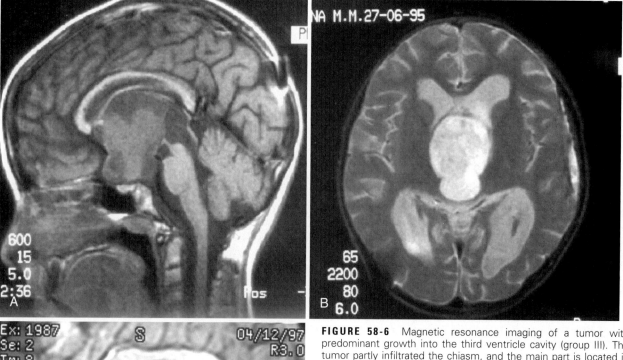

FIGURE 58-6 Magnetic resonance imaging of a tumor with predominant growth into the third ventricle cavity (group III). The tumor partly infiltrated the chiasm, and the main part is located in the cavity of the third ventricle. *A*, Before surgery (T1). *B*, Before surgery (T2). *C*, After surgery, small remnants of a tumor are seen near the chiasm.

the surgeon to choose the appropriate surgical approach. Hypothalamic gliomas usually look like highly intense masses on T2-weighted MRI scans (see Figs. 58-6B and 58-8A), whereas T1-weighted images show isointense lesions (see Figs. 58-4A, 58-5A, and 58-12A). Large tumors may be heterogenic on T1-weighted imaging (see Figs. 58-6A and 58-7A).

T1-weighted MRI after gadolinium injection usually shows marked enhancement of the tumor (see Figs. 58-3A, 58-45B, and 58-11A). A tumor cyst is characterized by low signals on T1-weighted scans (see Figs. 58-8B and 58-14A).

In most cases, CT allows discrimination between gliomas and other suprasellar tumors. Gliomas are usually homogeneous, hyperdense, and, occasionally, isodense or hypodense tumors.

Nevertheless, some gliomas show the signs characteristic of craniopharyngiomas: large cysts and calcifications (see Fig. 58-14A). Cysts may be intratumoral (20% of patients) or paratumoral (30% of patients) (see Figs. 58-8B, 58-12C, and 58-14A).

Surgical Removal of Chiasmal/Hypothalamic Gliomas

Experience in the surgical removal of these tumors is limited. Several neurosurgeons advocate the radical (subtotal) removal as the first attempt to treat these tumors[16–37] (Table 58-5).

Hoffman and colleagues[30–32] "advocate an aggressive surgical approach to these tumors for diagnostic and therapeutic purposes." They believe that patients with progressive

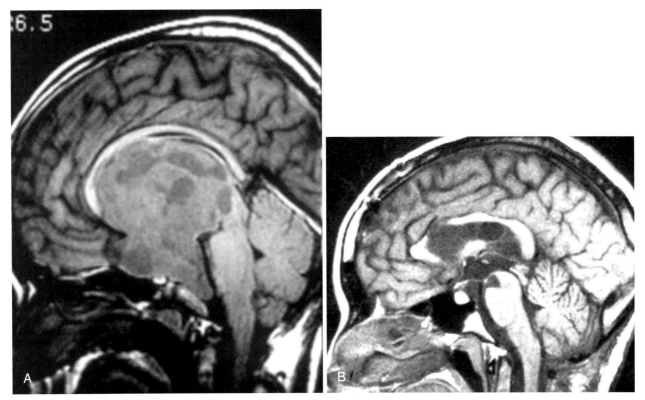

FIGURE 58-7   The tumor infiltrates the chiasm; the main part is in the cavity of the third ventricle (group III). The brain stem is vastly displaced backward. *A,* Before surgery. *B,* After the removal of the tumor via the transcallosal approach (no remnants of a tumor are seen).

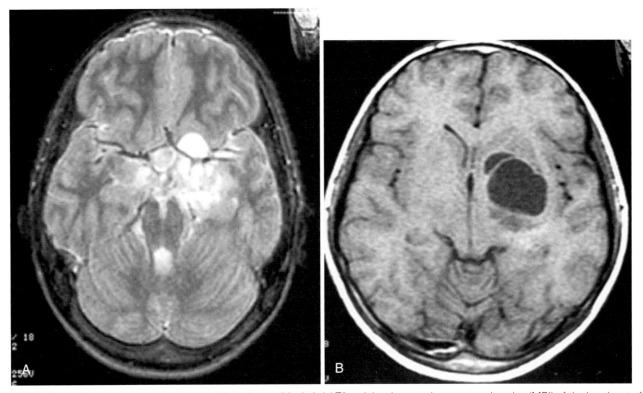

FIGURE 58-8   Glioma of the optic tract and chiasm (group IV). *A,* Axial T2-weighted magnetic resonance imaging (MRI) of the basal part of the tumor destroying the left part of the chiasm and left optic tract. *B,* Axial T1-weighted MRI of a tumor cyst that compresses the thalamus (lateral type of growth).

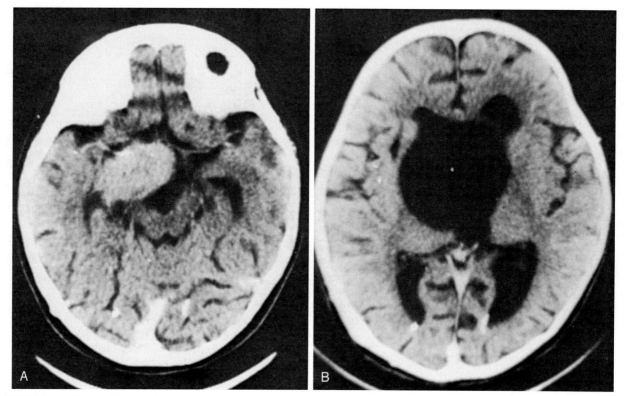

FIGURE 58-9 Glioma of the optic tract and chiasm (group IV). The tumor destroyed half of the chiasm, grew along the right optic tract, and formed a giant cyst that compressed the third ventricle (medial type).

visual and neurologic deterioration and a rapidly expanding suprasellar mass lesion should be treated surgically.

According to Medlock and Scott,[27] the indications for surgery are to debulk symptomatic tumors (>50 mm) that are exophytic or cystic and to relieve obstruction at the foramen of Monro.

Radical (70% to 95%) resection without operative mortality was achieved by Wisoff[33] (11 of 16 patients) and by Valdueza and colleagues[34] (12 of 20 patients).

Lapras[38] analyzed this problem at the European Congress in Moscow in 1991 and concluded that radical surgery is preferable to palliative methods and irradiation.

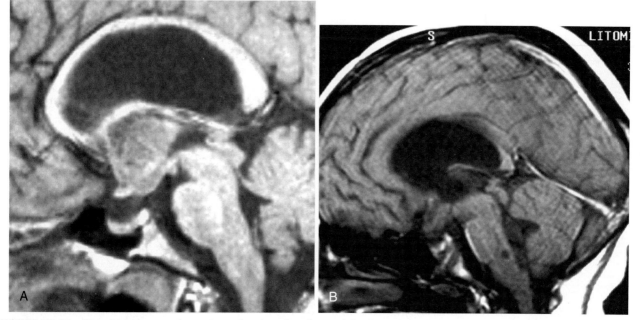

FIGURE 58-10 T1-weighted magnetic resonance imaging of a glioma of the floor of the third ventricle (group V). The tumor is entirely situated in the cavity of the third ventricle. During surgery, the chiasm without signs of infiltration was seen stretched on the anterior pole of the tumor. A, Before surgery. B, After removal of the tumor (tiny remnants of a tumor are seen).

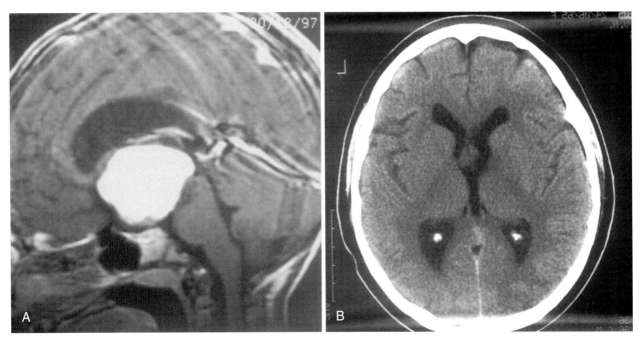

FIGURE 58-11   *A,* Magnetic resonance imaging with contrast (Magnevist) of a glioma of the floor of the third ventricle (group V) before surgery. The tumor is situated in the cavity of the third ventricle. *B,* After the tumor has been removed.

Albright and Sclabassi[23] also support the surgical treatment of these lesions and uses the ultrasound Cavitron and visual evoked potentials for safer removal of chiasmatic gliomas in children.

Helcl[39] considers that up-to-date criteria for surgical treatment of chiasmal gliomas in children are exploration of the chiasmal region and biopsy with radical surgery only in extrinsic gliomas of the chiasmal region and a conservative surgical approach to intrinsic chiasmal gliomas.

Peculiarities of tumor removal and surgical approaches differ due to the exact topography of CHGs.

Chiasmal Gliomas with Anterior Growth: Group I (See Fig. 58-3)

A subfrontal unilateral approach is usually adequate for radical removal of chiasmal gliomas. After debulking the main part of the tumor with an ultrasonic aspirator, additional space appears, and almost all parts of the tumor become accessible.

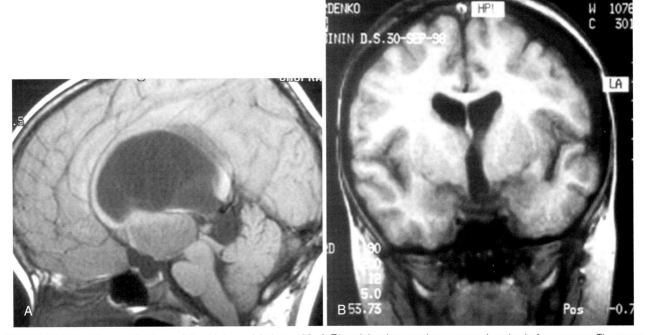

FIGURE 58-12   Glioma of the floor of the third ventricle (group V). *A,* T1-weighted magnetic resonance imaging before surgery. The tumor entirely occupies the cavity of the third ventricle. *B,* Total removal of the tumor. (See comments in case report.)

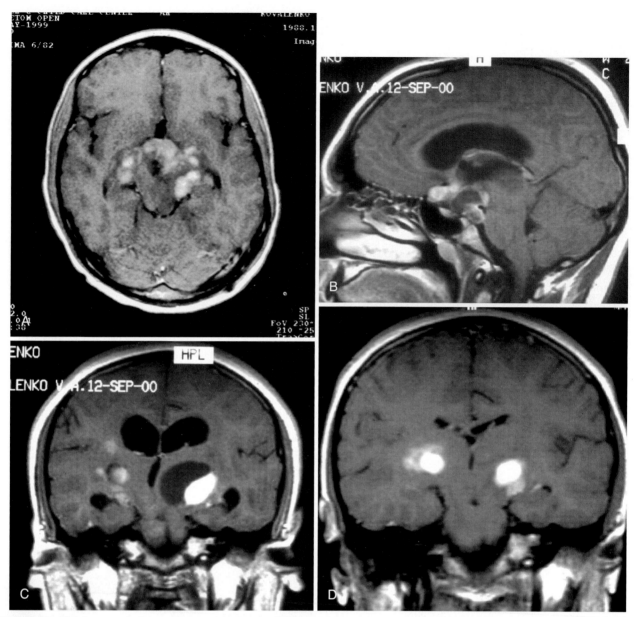

FIGURE 58-13   An example (magnetic resonance imaging [MRI] with Magnevist) of a diffuse tumor that grew bilaterally along the visual pathways. *A,* Axial MRI shows infiltration of the chiasma and both optic tracts. *B,* Diffuse infiltration of the chiasma. *C, D,* Frontal MRI reveals infiltration of both tracts, with a small cyst adjacent to the left one. Note the infiltration without enlargement of the right tract seen only after enhancement.

The tumor often grows asymmetrically: one optic nerve and half of the chiasm are predominantly infiltrated by the tumor, whereas the other optic nerve and contralateral part of a chiasm is simply displaced. If there is no or very poor vision on the side of the predominant tumor growth, this optic nerve may be cut at the level of its entrance to the optic channel, which facilitates further tumor removal and helps to expose the ophthalmic artery, from which the main tumor feeders arise. Coagulation of these arteries diminishes blood loss during tumor ablation.

It is usually possible to differentiate, under the microscope, the normal tissue of the optic pathways and to separate it from the tumor. Care is necessary to reveal and preserve the

pituitary stalk, which is usually displaced downward and backward by the tumor.

Tumors that Grow Anteriorly and to the Third Ventricle: Group II (See Figs. 58-4 and 58-5)

This type of tumor usually needs either a subfrontal or a combined approach to remove it.

In cases of a relatively small retrochiasmal part (see Fig. 58-4), the subfrontal approach alone may permit successful tumor ablation. The removal of the anterior part of the tumor is performed as previously described. The most difficult stage of the surgery is usually the removal of a part of the tumor that is hidden behind the carotid bifurcation and the

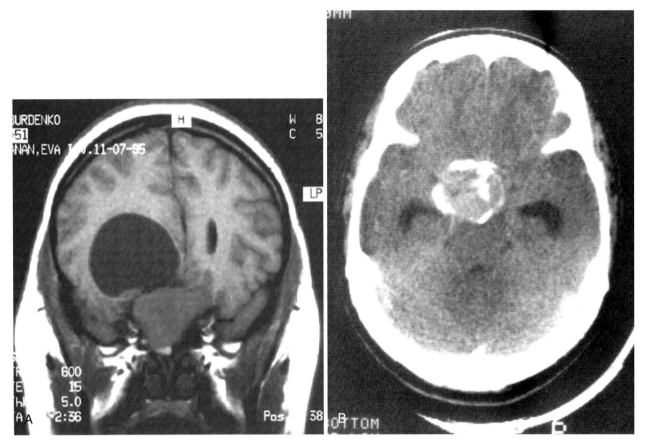

FIGURE 58-14   Chiasmal/hypothalamic glioma surrounded by large cysts (*A*) and calcifications in the tumor tissue (*B*) should be differentiated from craniopharyngiomas.

anterior cerebral arteries. It is necessary to manipulate in the narrow space between perforating arteries. The posterior part of the tumor is usually softer and can easily be removed by aspiration. If the tumor infiltrates the adjacent membranes and the surrounding main arteries are embedded in the tumor tissue, surgery becomes more difficult and requires hours of meticulous dissection.

Tumors that infiltrate both the chiasm and occupy the third ventricle up to the foramen of Monro (see Fig. 58-5) should usually be removed by a combined approach (either a

TABLE 58-4 ▪ Clinical Signs of Different Types of CHG (before Surgery)

Clinical Signs	Group				
	I	*II*	*III*	*IV*	*V*
No. of patients	34	28	33	29	27
Histology					
Grade 1	75%	64%	60%	65%	55%
Grade 2			25%–30%		
Grade 3	0	7%	9%	8%	15%
Visual deterioration (acuity of vision)	100%	100%	100%	38%	52%
Asymmetrical visual deterioration	91%	82%	72%	76%	27%
Intraorbital extension of a tumor	18%	10%	0	0	0
Hemianopsia		Irregular		Homonymous	Bitemporal
Intracranial hypertension	43%	55%	64%	48%	72%
Precocious puberty	0	8%	4%	4%	4%
Weight		Nearly normal (0.62–1.1 SDS BMI)			Adult/child obesity
Diabetes insipidus	2.8%	7.1%	7.6%	6.8%	8.1%
Growth		Nearly normal (−0.3 to +2.0 SDS)			
Hemiparesis	0	0	0	24%	0

BMI, body mass index; SDS, standard deviation score.

TABLE 58-5 ▪ Results of Surigcal Treatment of CHG

Author	Year of Publication	No. of Operations	Visual Deterioration	Mortality
Fowler, Matson	1957	7	0	29%
Tym	1961	5	0	0
Chutorian	1963	8	0	13%
Glaser	1974	13	23%	0
Iraci	1981	15	0	0
Kanamori	1985	9	0	33%
Fletcher	1986	13	8%	0
Wong	1987	19	6%	5%
Rodriguez	1990	28	0	11%
Wisoff	1990	18	0	0
Hoffman	1993	33	?	0
Valdueza	1994	20	20%	0
Janss	1995	26	0	4%
Yasargil	1996	61	?	0
Medlock	1997	20	5%	0
Konovalov	2003	216	23%	8% (0%)*

*Past 10 years.

transcallosal and subfrontal one or a transcallosal and pterional approach).

Tumors with Predominant Growth into the Third Ventricle: Groups III and V (See Figs. 58-6 and 58-7 and 58-10 to 58-12)

The transcallosal approach is the best way to reach tumors with predominant growth into the third ventricle.[21,40,41] The corpus callosum is divided between the anterior cerebral arteries with an incision 1 to 1.5 cm long. The tumor can then be reached and removed through one or both of the foramina of Monro (in the latter case, the septum pellucidum must be opened). The upper surface of a tumor can also be exposed by division of the columns of the fornix.

Ultrasonic aspiration is helpful when removing the main bulk of a tumor. Tumors usually infiltrate the anterior wall and the floor of the third ventricle; in some cases, they also infiltrate the lateral walls and occlude the foramen of Monro. Even in these cases, subtotal tumor removal is usually possible, leaving only a thin layer of tumor that infiltrates the adjacent brain tissue. After the tumor has been removed through the hole in the floor of the third ventricle, the basilar artery and its branches (which lie behind the arachnoid membrane) can usually be seen.

Some of these tumors are richly supplied by vessels coming from the anterior wall and the ventricle floor, which are coagulated during tumor removal.

Gliomas of the Optic Tract: Group IV (See Figs. 58-8 and 58-9)

Tumors of the optic tract have an asymmetrical localization, and the main part of the tumor is hidden behind the carotid artery and its bifurcation. A pterional transsylvian approach is preferable for their removal. Although the operating field

is narrow and the posterior communicating and anterior choroidal arteries hinder a wide exposure of the lateral surface of the tumor, it can be radically removed up to the border of normal-looking brain structures.

These tumors may also infiltrate the thalamus and displace the third ventricle. In these cases, a transcallosal or a combined approach (transcallosal and pterional) may be used. The presence of cysts simplifies the removal of the tumor.

Selection of the appropriate approach depends on the size and precise location of the tumor. In some cases, a very unusual approach was chosen: the tumor was removed via the posterior fossa above the cerebellum and with the dissection of the tentorium to reach the basal medial surface of the temporal lobe.

Diffuse Tumors

Diffuse CHGs were seen in 43 patients with NF-1. Half of them remained stable, in contrast to none in the group without NF. We are sure that NF CHG is a separate entity from non-NF optic pathway gliomas, with different imaging features and prognosis, thereby warranting a specific diagnostic, clinical, and therapeutic approach.[42]

Radical surgery is impossible in most cases due to their type of growth (see Fig. 58-13). Shunting procedures can be performed if necessary and a biopsy is performed in unclear cases, whereas the role of radiotherapy and chemotherapy in this type of chiasmal/hypothalamic tumor is being investigated.

Recently, many authors have come to the conclusion that patients with anterior visual pathway gliomas associated with NF-1 should not be treated unless there is clear clinical or neuroimaging evidence of progression, which takes place only in 10% to 50% of cases).[43-56] Close observation is usually the most appropriate management, whereas 90% to 100% of children with CHGs without NF-1 will require some form of therapy.[57]

Spontaneous regression of chiasmal gliomas associated or not with NF has been occasionally described.[58-66] The largest series is described by Parsa and colleagues,[67] who analyzed 13 cases documented by serial neuroimaging in which tumor reduction and improvement of vision were seen in the majority of cases. In two of our patients with NF-1, spontaneous tumor progression was followed by spontaneous regression in several years. This bimodal dynamics of tumor growth is rare but highlights the variable natural history of low-grade gliomas in children with NF-1 and the difficulty in elaborating the appropriate treatment.[62,64-66]

As estimated from the respective apoptosis data, tumor regression may occur when the rate of cell loss is greater than that of tumor growth[68] or with a decrease in mucin content in the tumor.

RESULTS

We consider total removal in cases in which no remnants of a tumor were noted at the end of surgery as well as on postoperative CT/MRI. Nevertheless, we realize that a zone of infiltration of visual pathways surely remains in all cases. This was achieved in 20% of cases.

Subtotal removal is when small remnants of a tumor capsule are left near the chiasm, floor of the third ventricle, carotid arteries, or pituitary stalk. On postoperative CT/MRI, the size of these tumor remnants does not exceed 15% of initial tumor volume, a situation noted in 25% of our cases.

Partial removal is when most of the tumor (more than 50% of volume) was, however, removed (55% of patients).

During the past 10 years, there was no mortality, both in children and in adults for all types of tumors (0%). The main cause of death previously was hemorrhage into the remaining tumor and disturbance of the cerebral circulation with ischemia in different vascular territories. The improvement in our results is due to better diagnostics in the regions, which leads to a better patient state and smaller tumor size, greater surgical experience, and less radical surgery. The latter factor has allowed us to achieve better functional results, including vision, whereas the progression-free survival rate has remained nearly unchanged.

In the postoperative period, morbidity is due to endocrinologic dysfunction, water-electrolyte disturbances, and subdural fluid collections.

Removal of hypothalamic tumors often results in changes in water-electrolyte regulation, with diabetes insipidus in 12% of cases. In contrast to patients with craniopharyngiomas (in whom diabetes insipidus is one of the most common surgical complications), in those with hypothalamic gliomas, the syndrome of inappropriate vasopressin secretion is frequently observed.

Removal of hypothalamic gliomas often results in brain collapse, subdural cerebrospinal fluid, and blood collection, which require additional surgical intervention in 5% of cases (external drainage or shunting procedures). Their occurrence is not due to the surgical approach, and risk factors likely to contribute to this complication are preoperative ventriculomegaly (frontal horn index >0.40) and tumor size (>5 cm in diameter).

Because these tumors can destroy the chiasm, we feared that surgery would produce additional serious visual impairment. Our results show that these concerns were overestimated: visual function in the early postoperative period improved in 14% of patients, remained unchanged in 63%, and deteriorated in 23% of patients (half of whom were almost blind before surgery).

Surgery on diencephalic gliomas may provide astonishing results. We have operated on some patients who were in a desperate state: they were cachectic and had a severe hypothalamic insufficiency. Nevertheless, some of these patients (mainly young children) not only survived the surgery but also showed quick and marked improvement, as seen in the following case report.

CASE REPORT

A 3-year-old boy was admitted to the Institute in October 1999 with diencephalic cachexia with normal psychological development (Fig. 58-15A). On admission, the child weighed 9.5 kg (−4.1 standard deviation score [SDS] body mass index [BMI]) and showed signs of increased intracranial pressure. Visual function was preserved. MRI revealed a tumor entirely occupying the cavity of the third ventricle (see Fig. 58-12A). The tumor was completely removed by the transcallosal approach (see Fig. 58-12B), with the corpus callosum divided between the anterior cerebral arteries with an incision 1.5 cm long. The tumor was removed through the right foramen of Monro with ultrasonic aspiration. The tumor infiltrated the anterior wall and the floor of the third ventricle. After the tumor was removed, the basilar artery and its branches were seen through the hole in the floor of the third ventricle, which was covered by arachnoid membrane. Mild water-electrolyte disturbances occurred in the postoperative period.

At the time of discharge from the Burdenko Neurosurgical Institute, the boy was active, with no signs of neurologic morbidity; diabetes insipidus regressed. The weight of the child during 3 weeks increased to 11 kg.

A year after surgery (at 4 years old), the development of the boy is normal, weight gain is approximately 8 kg (17.5 kg, normal for this age: SDS BMI = +0.7) (Fig. 58-15B). MRI revealed no signs of recurrence.

Two years later (at the age of 5), the weight reached 25.5 kg, which exceeds normal values (+3.0 SDS BMI). In the 3 years after surgery, the BMI began to normalize and the boy's weight reached 23 kg (0.7 SDS BMI), with no signs of recurrence; visual acuity is 0.8 to 0.9 in both eyes (Fig. 58-15C)

Adjuvant Treatment Modalities

Gamma radiotherapy with rotation was performed in 47 patients after surgery. They received 45 to 52 Gy to the tumor volume. There were recurrences in three patients.

Some of the authors believe that radiotherapy is an effective adjuvant treatment modality. It was shown that irradiation in the dose more then 45 Gr is effective in stabilization or improvement of vision and prevention of tumor progression.[16,34–37,69–83]

A preliminary report devoted to gamma knife treatment of diencephalic gliomas has been published.[84]

Radiotherapy is not recommended in young children because of its severe adverse effects on cognitive and neuroendocrine function, and therefore chemotherapy becomes a component of the management of diencephalic gliomas,[57,80,85–100] although its effectiveness is lower than that of radiotherapy. Chemotherapy is used (1) as initial treatment in children younger than 4 years, (2) as a palliative method that can postpone the need for radiotherapy, and (3) in patients with recurrent CHGs. Usually carboplatin or a combination of carboplatin and vincristine is recommended.[99] Osztie and colleagues[101] suggest a new approach using combined intra-arterial and intravenous carboplatin-based chemotherapy for patients in whom surgery or conventional chemotherapy has failed. Fouladi and colleagues[80] reviewed 73 children and recommend observation in asymptomatic patients with platinum-based chemotherapy in younger patients, and irradiation in older symptomatic patients.

Long-Term Results

In the follow-up period, visual functions improved in 28% of patients and remained unchanged in 50%. Thus the

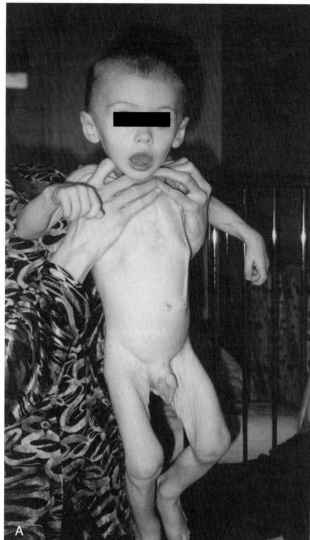

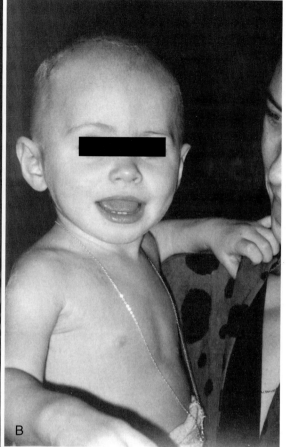

Age(years)	0	1	2	3	4	5	6
Weight (Kg)	2,8	7,1	8,3	9,5	17,5	25,5	23
SDS		-3,2	-3,0	-4,1	+0,7	+3,0	+1,0

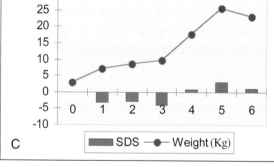

FIGURE 58-15 Case report. A 3-year-old boy with a glioma of the floor of the third ventricle with diencephalic cachexia (*A*). The same patient a year after surgery (*B*) (photo by N. Mazerkina, M.D.). Dynamics of weight and body mass index after surgery (*C*).

number of patients whose vision improved doubled in several years. Deterioration was seen in 22% of patients (deterioration of vision in the follow-up period is due to recurrence). The prognosis for vision is much worse in patients with predominantly chiasma-located tumors.

Signs of endocrine dysfunction in the follow-up period are not common.[44,102] In our series, growth retardation and diabetes insipidus (12%) were rare, but most patients develop severe obesity and some develop precocious puberty (18%). Weight gain is observed in all patients (100%) during the first 1.5 years and may reach +5 to 9 SDS BMI, but then it shows a tendency to normalize.

Follow-up evaluation (mean, 7 years; range, 1 to 16 years) showed that the tumor recurs in 25% of case and a second operation was performed in 13 cases. The surgery for recurrences appeared to be rather safe with low morbidity, mortality, and risk of visual deterioration and recurrence. Aspiration and shunting procedures for cystic tumors are ineffective.

The progression-free survival and observed survival probabilities were calculated using the Kaplan-Meier method, and differences between curves were evaluated by the Mantel-Cox and log rank tests. The obtained significant variables in the univariate analysis were analyzed using the Cox proportional hazards model.

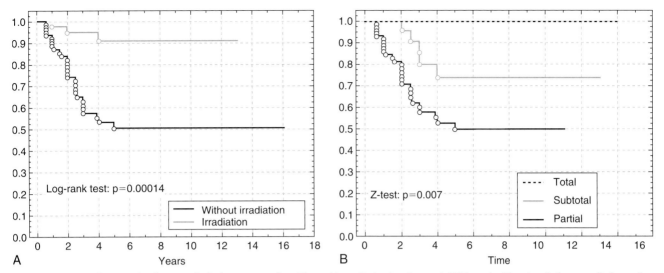

FIGURE 58-16 Progression-free survival after surgery for chiasmal/hypothalamic glioma. *A,* With and without radiotherapy. *B,* According to the radicality of surgery.

Overall and progression-free survival probabilities for the entire group are 93% and 77%, respectively, at 5 years and 89% and 75%, respectively, at 10 years.

Differences in progression-free survival probabilities between the group with surgical treatment (50%) and combined therapy (90%) at 5 and 10 years are statistically significant (log rank test: $p = 0.00014$) (Fig. 58-16A).

A progression-free survival advantage was found in favor of patients with partial removal of tumors treated with radiotherapy compared with no radiotherapy, with 5-year and 10-year progression-free survival rates of 86% versus 27% (log rank test: $p = 0.0002$).

Radicality of surgery dramatically influences the long-term outcome with 5- and 10-year progression-free survival probabilities for the radical, subtotal, and partial surgery of 51%, 74%, and 100%, respectively (Z test: $p = 0.007$) (see Fig. 58-16B).

Differences in overall and progression-free survival probabilities between grade I and II astrocytomas are not statistically significant both after surgical and combined treatment. All patients with anaplastic astrocytomas were irradiated and all of them are alive.

In the Cox multivariate analysis, use of radiation therapy, the radicality of tumor removal, and the presence of degenerative signs in tumor tissue (calcifications and cysts) significantly influence progression-free survival.

Indications for Surgery

We consider the surgery to be a method of choice in the treatment of nodular CHGs irrespective of size. Adjuvant radiotherapy is indicated in cases with signs of tumor malignancy, after partial removal even of benign tumors, and in cases of tumor recurrence.

Radical surgery is impossible in most diffuse tumors. Shunting procedures can be performed if necessary and a biopsy specimen is obtained in unclear cases, whereas the

role of radiotherapy and chemotherapy in this type of chiasmal/hypothalamic tumors is being investigated.

THALAMIC TUMORS

The indications for surgery on thalamic tumors are controversial. Steiger and colleagues[103] have concluded that radical resection of thalamic tumors is feasible with microsurgical techniques despite neighboring critical structures. The thalamus has a unique configuration within the basal ganglia. It has three free surfaces, and only the ventrolateral border is in contact with vital functional structures: the subthalamic nuclei and the internal capsule. In adults, these tumors are mostly malignant, diffuse-growing grade III and IV gliomas; therefore, the possibility of radical tumor removal is limited. However, in children, focal benign tumors (grades I and II) occur quite often, and these tumors may be removed totally with a more favorable outcome. Some authors show favorable results after microsurgical thalamic tumor resection.[103–109] For example, Kelly,[110] using stereotactic resection, has achieved good results in 32 cases of such circumscribed thalamic tumors.

In the case of a thalamic tumor of an infiltrative type without clear tumor-brain interface, surgery is limited to partial tumor ablation.

In our practice, we differentiate several topographic variants of thalamic tumors: (1) anterior tumors localized at the level of the foramen of Monro, (2) posterior tumors occupying the posterior part of the thalamus and the pulvinar, (3) lateral tumors, and (4) total tumors, when a large tumor occupies the whole thalamus and spreads into adjacent structures. Another group of tumors consists of those that occupy both the thalamus and the midbrain. Tumor distribution according to these variants and histology are summarized in Tables 58-6 and 58-7.

The clinical manifestation of these tumors is related to the tumor location. Tumors of the anterior part of the thalamus occlude the ipsilateral foramen of Monro (rarely on both sides), producing asymmetrical lateral ventricle distention.

TABLE 58-6 ▪ Topographic Variants of Thalamic Tumors (92 Cases)

Variant	No.	Percent
Anterior	16	19
Lateral	26	28
Total	24	25
Posterior	13	14
Thalamus and midbrain	13	14

Posterior thalamic lesions primarily compress the aqueduct, which results in the symmetrical dilatation of the lateral ventricles.

Clinical symptoms other than those of intracranial hypertension depend mainly on compression or invasion of the surrounding structures (e.g., internal capsule, quadrigeminal plate, peduncles).

Surgery

An attempt at radical tumor resection should be made in all focal, slowly progressive tumors that are mainly benign tumors. We also operate on malignant lesions that have no diffuse spread to adjacent structures. In most cases, the results of CT and MRI investigations help us to distinguish a tumor that is benign and focal from one that is diffuse and malignant. If clinical and neuroimaging data are not diagnostic, stereotactic biopsy is indicated to clarify the situation.

There are several approaches to thalamic tumor resection: transcallosal, transcortical, via a transsylvian fissure, posterior interhemispheric, and a combination of these. The choice of appropriate approach depends on the topographic variant of tumor growth. In anterior thalamic tumors, we prefer to explore using the transcallosal approach. It is necessary to maintain the microscope direction in the foramen of Monro projection. Orientation in the lateral ventricle may be difficult: the main landmarks, the foramen of Monro and the choroidal plexus, may be hidden by the bulging tumor. In that case, the positions of the thalamostriate, septal, and nucleus caudatus veins help to determine the position of the foramen of Monro. A small incision in the thalamic superior surface (usually in front of the thalamostriate vein) is necessary to explore the tumor. We use retractors with 5-mm retractor blades to displace the cortical margins. Tumor ablation is performed mainly with ultrasound aspiration and bipolar coagulation of the tumor tissue.

TABLE 58-7 ▪ Histology of Thalamic Tumors (92 Cases)

Histology	No.	Percent
Pilocytic astrocytoma	10	12
Fibrillary astrocytoma	42	45
Anaplastic astrocytoma	26	28
Glioblastoma	6	6
Ganglioastrocytoma	2	3
Others	6	6

The radicality of tumor resection depends on the existence of a distinct brain tumor interface. Even in a left-sided tumor, we prefer right-sided transcallosal access. The opposite-side approach in some cases is more convenient because the trajectory of the surgical approach is straighter with less brain retraction.

In the case of posterior thalamic and pulvinar tumors, we prefer a posterior occipital approach, which requires sectioning the tentorium when the tumor penetrates the peduncle.

Large tumors that occupy the whole thalamus need transcortical exploration (frontotemporal or parietal) for their resection. Ventriculomegaly has made such an approach feasible.

Pterional basal access provides limited exposure to the tumor through small spaces between branches of the carotid artery and optic tract. That is why it is necessary to combine this approach with the upper transcallosal approach. Some of the tumors may be also reached by splitting the sylvian fissure. Some examples of thalamic tumor removal via different routes are illustrated in Figures 58-17 and 58-18.

Ventricular Shunting

When tumors interfere with cerebrospinal fluid circulation and produce ventricular dilatation, a shunt may be necessary. When dealing with focal resectable tumors, we prefer to start with direct tumor removal. In the case of a malignant tumor or a patient in critical condition due to intracranial hypertension, it is necessary to start with a shunting procedure. Surgical results are summarized in Table 58-8.

Three patients died after surgery. One patient died as result of exacerbation of intracranial inflammation (the patient had a shunt placed previously in another hospital, and the surgery had been complicated by meningitis). In two other cases, death was caused by hemorrhage into the tumor remnants.

Clinical conditions improved in 48% of patients immediately after surgery, and further improvement was observed in another 20% of operated patients. In the pediatric group, results were much better, mainly because focal thalamic tumors are common in the pediatric population.

BRAIN STEM TUMORS

Brain stem tumors account for approximately 15% to 20% of all pediatric brain tumors. In the past, BSTs were considered to be a single pathologic entity, and patients were usually treated with radiotherapy without confirmation of tumor histology. In cases of intracranial hypertension, shunting procedures were performed and surgery was rare and limited to tumor biopsy or evacuation of a cystic lesion. One of the first descriptions of brain stem tumor removal was that of Pool,[111] who resected a tumor of the aqueduct in 1968. The advent of CT and MRI demonstrated that BSTs are not a homogeneous entity and that some distinct tumor types are identifiable according to growth pattern, microscopic pathology, and location. At the same time, improvement in neurosurgical techniques and perioperative care made surgery for brain stem lesions a reality. In 1986, Stroink and colleagues[112] presented the results of surgical treatment of BSTs in 35 patients who underwent a suboccipital craniectomy

FIGURE 58-17 Magnetic resonance imaging (MRI) demonstrates a cystic thalamic-midbrain tumor (*A*). Postoperative MRI after subtotal removal of pilocytic astrocytoma via transcallosal approach (*B*).

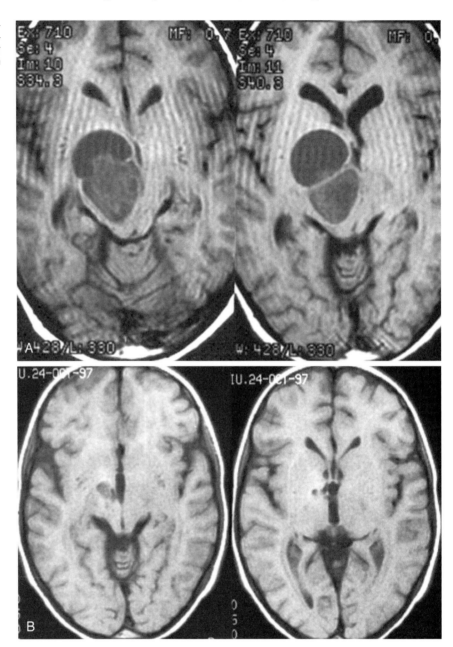

for histologic evaluation, decompression, subtotal resection of the tumor, and/or cyst aspiration. They differentiated several groups of these tumors based on the location of the tumor, whether the tumor was intrinsic or extrinsic to the brain stem, and its contrast-enhancing CT features. Surgery was considered in cases of contrast-enhancing tumors growing exophytically into the fourth ventricle and in focally intrinsic tumors with bright contrast enhancement.

In 1986, Epstein and McCleary[113] summarized their experience of radical excision of intrinsic nonexophytic brain stem gliomas in 34 children. They classified these tumors into focal, diffuse, and cervicomedullary subgroups and recommended primary radical excision for cervicomedullary neoplasms, which were often benign, and for focal BSTs. Such treatment could result in improvement in a patient's condition. Radiation therapy, chemotherapy,

or both were considered appropriate treatment for diffuse tumors located above the medulla.

Later, several series of patients with successfully removed BSTs were reported.[114–122]

One of the most detailed descriptions of the surgical technique for BST removal (especially for cervicomedullary tumors) was given by Jallo and colleagues.[123] Almost all cervicomedullary tumors are considered to be well-delineated benign lesions that should be operated on. In 2000, Bricolo[124] presented the results of surgical treatment of 125 patients with intrinsic BSTs, 75% of which were focal. He concluded that aggressive direct surgery can obtain complete removal of many focal brain stem gliomas with good clinical results.

Different classifications of BSTs were proposed. These classifications aimed to identify different types of tumors and outline those that could benefit from surgery.

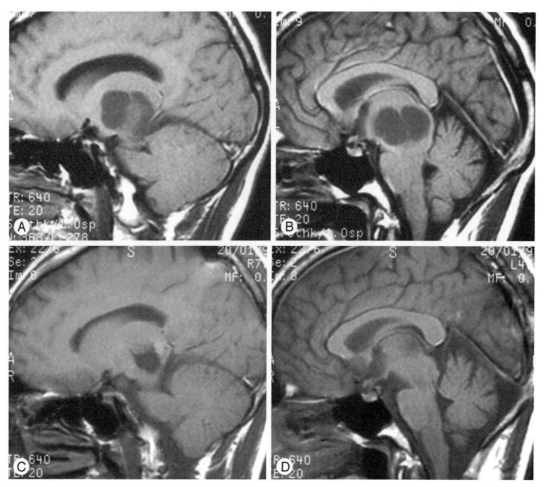

FIGURE 58-18 *A, B,* Preoperative magnetic resonance imaging (MRI) shows a posterior tumor of the thalamus. *C, D,* Postoperative MRI after radical resection using the interhemispheric occipital approach.

According to MRI data, BSTs are divided into four groups: (1) focal, (2) cervicomedullary, (3) dorsally exophytic, and (4) diffuse.

Despite intensive investigations and numerous publications devoted to indications for surgery of BSTs, this subject remains controversial.

In 1984, we started to operate on patients with primary BSTs to establish the indications and contraindications for surgery. Since then, approximately 1200 patients (total number) with BSTs have been examined in the outpatient department of the Moscow Burdenko Neurosurgical Institute. In all these cases, the diagnosis was verified with CT, MRI, or both. In 306 patients, we attempted radical tumor removal. Only these cases are discussed in this chapter.

One of the main goals of our investigations was to discover the types of tumor growth.

TABLE 58-8 ▪ Results of Thalamic Tumor Surgery

	Percent of Cases (92 Cases = 100%)	Benign Tumors (60 Cases = 100%)	Malignant Tumors (32 Cases = 100%)
Total resection	49	70	8
Subtotal resection	31	23	46
Partial resection or biopsy	20	7	46
Postoperative			
Improvement	48	51	37
No change	16	17	17
Impairment	32	28	42
Death	3.4	1	2
Follow-up			
Dead	50	26	24
Alive	42	34	8
Median survival (yr)	5.1	5.8	2.3

Pathologic examination was performed in 93 cases by A. G. Korshunov. These included patients who died (predominantly before 1984) without surgery, after exploration of the posterior fossa, or after an attempt at partial removal of the BST. According to pathologic data, we identified three main types of tumor growth.

Diffuse-growing tumors (78%) are not demarcated from surrounding brain stem structures (Fig. 58-19A). Neurons and axons of the brain stem tissue persist between tumor cells in different parts of the tumor. These tumors are astrocytic gliomas, most of which are high-grade gliomas.

Some infiltrative-growing tumors (11% of all investigated tumors) look macroscopically like well-circumscribed tumors; however, in reality, the tumor cells infiltrate brain stem structures. The neural tissue in this zone is totally destroyed by the tumor. Pathologically, these tumors are primitive neuroepithelial tumors and glioblastomas. They are called pseudofocal tumors.

Expansive-growing tumors (22%), in which the border of the tumor is well defined (see Fig. 58-19B), and brain stem structures are demarcated from the tumor by a compact layer of tumor astrocytes axons (tumor capsula). Pathologic examination reveals pilocytic astrocytomas (grade I); 40% of these tumors contain vascular hamartomas and are called angioastrocytomas.

From the surgical point of view, it is important to outline extrinsic and intrinsic tumors. Extrinsic tumors protrude in the fourth ventricle or one of subarachnoid cisterns. Intrinsic tumors are located completely inside the brain stem and do not penetrate its surface.

Diagnosis

MRI has become the primary diagnostic modality and is the diagnostic gold standard in assessing patients with BSTs.[125-127]

MRI and CT permit detection of the tumor's edges and suggest the type of tumor growth (tumor growth pattern) and histology. Based on MRI, CT morphologic criteria, and clinical signs, the following groups of BSTs may be defined.

Classification of BSTs According to Type of Tumor Growth and Possibility of Surgical Removal

DIFFUSE TUMORS

MRI shows the enlargement and deformation of the brain stem without delineation of the tumor edges. Most diffuse tumors involve a large area of the brain stem: the pons and the midbrain or medulla oblongata. The basilar artery may be included in tumor tissue. Diffuse tumors have a low or isointense signal on T1-weighted MRI and an increased signal on T2-weighted MRI (Fig. 58-20A–C). Hyperintensity on T1-weighted MRI is due to hemorrhage; 60% of them show an absence or a low degree of contrast enhancement. Contrast enhancement in diffuse tumors is considered to be a sign of malignant degeneration (see Fig. 58-20D).

However, in the initial stage, diffuse-growing tumors can imitate the focal tumor (Fig. 58-21).

FOCAL TUMORS

T1-weighted MRI shows a well-demarcated lesion of isodense or slightly low signal intensity. T2-weighted MRI

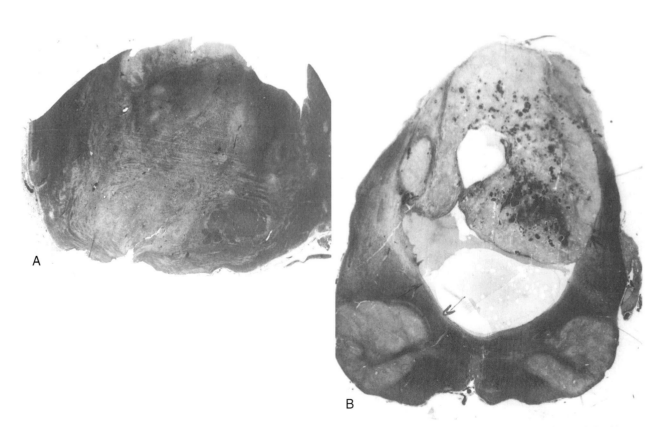

FIGURE 58-19 Types of tumor growth. *A,* A diffuse-growing tumor in the pons. *B,* An expansive-growing tumor in the medulla oblongata.

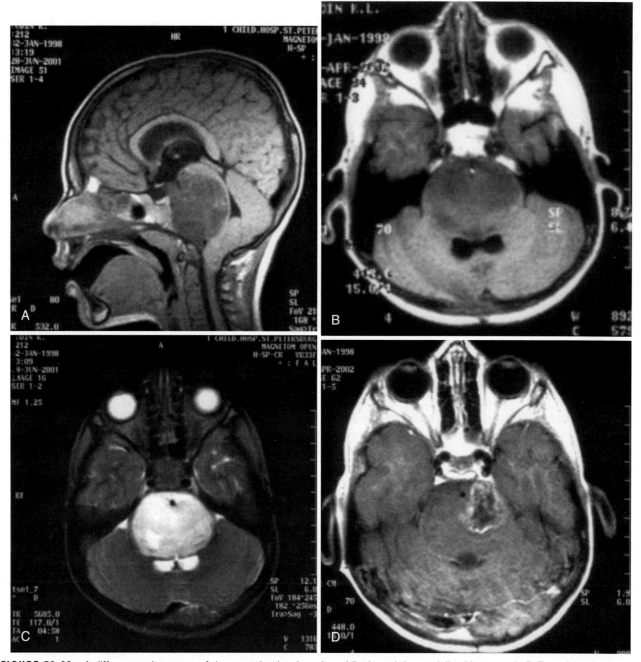

FIGURE 58-20   A diffuse-growing tumor of the pons that involves the midbrain and the medulla oblongata. *A, B,* T1-weighted magnetic resonance imaging (MRI) shows the expanded hypointense brain stem. *C,* Axial T2-weighted MRI shows a hypointense pons. The basilar artery is included in the tumor tissue. *D,* Slight contrast enhancement (necrosis) in the basal part of the pons.

demonstrates the mass of increased signal. Edema is not typical. Benign focal tumors show different variants of evident contrast enhancement, which correlates with piloid astrocytoma histology (Figs. 58-22 to 58-24) but may be also nonenhanced lesions.

Some malignant tumors (glioblastomas, primitive neuroepithelial tumors) infiltrate the brain stem structures but may look like a focal one (pseudofocal tumor). MRI and CT show focal enhancement after contrast injection, with normal signal characteristics from the peritumoral area, imitating the focal lesion (Fig. 58-25). MRI also identifies whether a

tumor is extrinsic or intrinsic to the brain stem and shows the presence of a cyst.

EXOPHYTICALLY GROWING BRAIN STEM TUMORS

In the literature, two main groups of these tumors are outlined: (1) dorsally exophytic tumors growing into the fourth ventricle and (2) cervicomedullary tumors with exophytic growth into the cisterna magna and the fourth ventricle. According to Epstein, these tumors are usually benign well-delineated lesions that may be successfully removed.[113] Our experience shows that these tumors can be focal and well

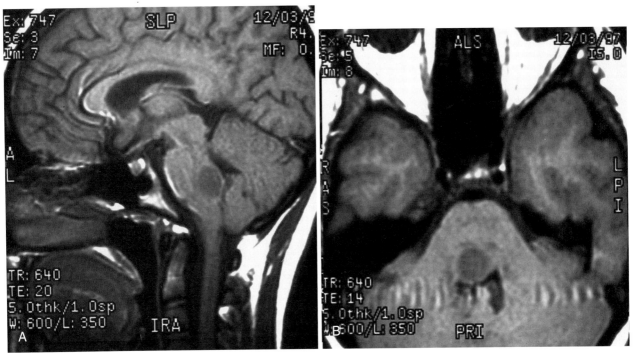

FIGURE 58-21 Small diffuse tumor of the pons. Pathologic examination of the tumor tissue revealed the persistence of brain stem tissue among the tumor cells (fibrillary astrocytoma and confirmed diffuse type of tumor growth. Sagittal (*A*) and axial (*B*) T1-weighted magnetic resonance imaging shows a small hypointense lesion in the pons tegmentum, imitating a focal tumor. The duration of illness is 4 months. The presenting symptom is sixth nerve deficit.

circumscribed as well as diffuse-growing lesions bulging not only into the fourth ventricle (Fig. 58-26) but also into the cerebellopontine angle and prepontine and other cisterns.

Intrinsic BSTs do not penetrate the brain stem surface.

Other lesions of the brain stem that should be differentiated from brain stem gliomas are ependymomas, hematomas, hemangioblastomas, metastatic tumors, epidermoid cysts, and granulomas. In cases in which the nature of the brain stem lesion is in doubt, stereotactic biopsy is indicated.

Clinical Manifestation

The clinical manifestation of brain stem gliomas depends on such factors as the tumor location, type of growth, and degree of malignancy. Diffuse malignant tumors are characterized by a short duration of the disease (median, 6 months), rapid deterioration of the patient's clinical state, and severe signs of brain stem damage, which include cranial nerve palsy and signs of long tract damage. Signs of intracranial hypertension usually occur in the later stages of the disease.

For focal tumors, slow progression of neurologic signs (median, 2.4 years), corresponding with tumor location, is more typical. In some cases of benign tumors, local signs of brain stem damage are very mild.

Midbrain tumors present with oculomotor deficit, ataxia, hemiparesis, and hydrocephalus. Hydrocephalus can be the only sign in cases of tectal and tegmental tumors.

For dorsally exophytic tumors, failure to thrive due to vomiting and signs of high intracranial pressure are typical.

Cervicomedullary tumors present with torticollis, long tract signs, and lower cranial nerve deficits.

We found that different variants of hyperkinesis are typical of midbrain tumors. The main neurologic signs revealed at the time of admission in our series of patients are presented in Table 58-9.

Indications for Surgery

We consider that surgery is indicated in all cases of focal (suggestive of benign) tumors, tumors with evident exophytic component, and pseudofocal and cystic tumors. Other than those, we had to operate on some patients who had malignant diffuse intrinsic tumors. If the tumor growth pattern remains unclear after MRI, clinical evaluation surgery or stereotactic biopsy may be recommended.

Surgery

In the period from 1984 to January 2003, 306 patients were selected for surgery with the aim of radical tumor removal. These patients consisted of 115 adults and 191 children, who presented with a history of illness duration of between 1 month and 25 years. The longest duration of the disease occurred in cases of benign focal tumors, such as angioastrocytomas. At the time of admission, most patients were severely disabled with a Karnofsky score of less than 50.

TUMOR LOCATION ALONG THE BRAIN STEM

For selection of the most appropriate approach to the tumor, we identified several groups of BSTs according to their predominant location identified by CT and MRI.

1. Caudal BSTs: spinomedullary (24 patients), medullary (34 patients), medullary-pontine (46 patients), and pontine (70 patients).

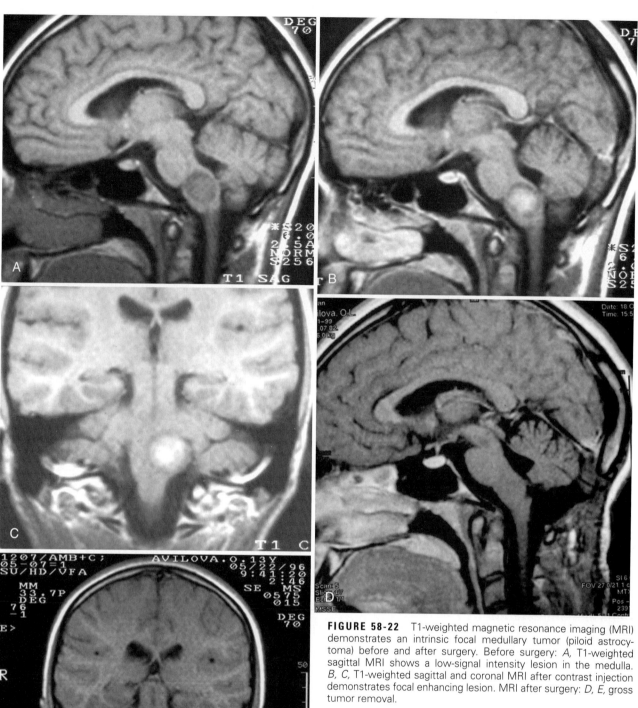

FIGURE 58-22   T1-weighted magnetic resonance imaging (MRI) demonstrates an intrinsic focal medullary tumor (piloid astrocytoma) before and after surgery. Before surgery: *A,* T1-weighted sagittal MRI shows a low-signal intensity lesion in the medulla. *B, C,* T1-weighted sagittal and coronal MRI after contrast injection demonstrates focal enhancing lesion. MRI after surgery: *D, E,* gross tumor removal.

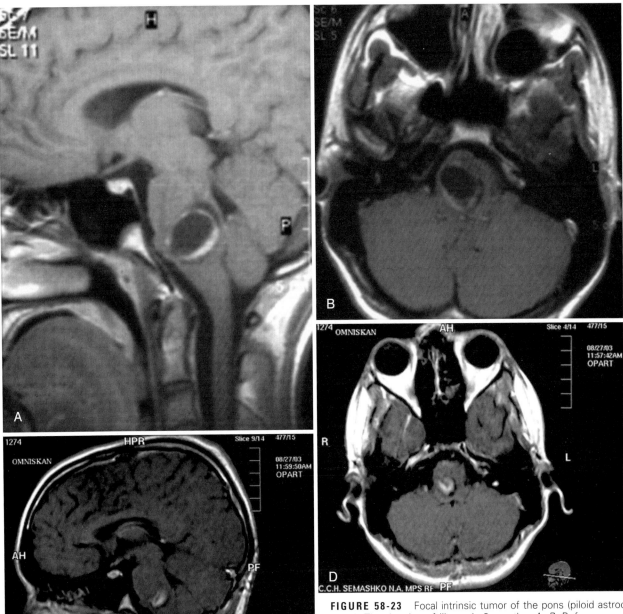

FIGURE 58-23 Focal intrinsic tumor of the pons (piloid astrocytoma). The duration of illness is 3 months. *A, B,* Before surgery: sagittal and axial T1-weighted magnetic resonance imaging (MRI) after contrast enhancement shows a ring-enhancing lesion and nonenhancing core. *C, D,* One month after surgery: sagittal and axial T1-weighted MRI shows subtotal tumor removal.

(Continued)

2. Rostral BSTs: pontine-midbrain (54 patients), midbrain tegmentum or peduncle (40 patients), and tectal plate and aqueductal tumors (38 patients). In 25 cases, midbrain tumors spread to the posterior thalamus.

We identified tumors according to the intrinsic or extrinsic type. In 49% of patients, the tumor was intrinsic to the brain stem. The exophytic part of the tumor localized in the fourth ventricle in 32% of patients, in the cerebellopontine angle in 9%, and the cisterna ambiens in 10% of patients.

The exact extension of the tumor was determined predominantly by MRI and to a lesser extent by enhanced CT and verified during surgery. MRI is mandatory in cases of cervicomedullary tumors and intrinsic tectal plate tumors that are poorly diagnosed by CT.

Surgical Technique

Patient's Position

In most cases, we prefer to operate on patients with BSTs in the sitting position with all necessary precautions against

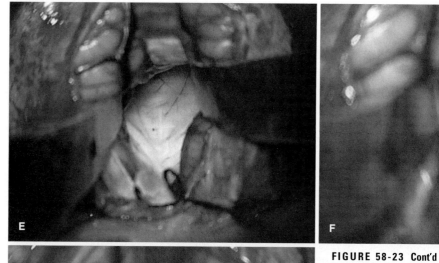

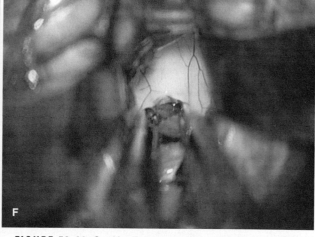

FIGURE 58-23 Cont'd *E,* Intraoperative view of the patient. The floor of the fourth ventricle is deformed. *F,* After identification of facial colliculus by direct electrical stimulation, the incision of the brain was performed. *G,* Subtotal tumor removal.

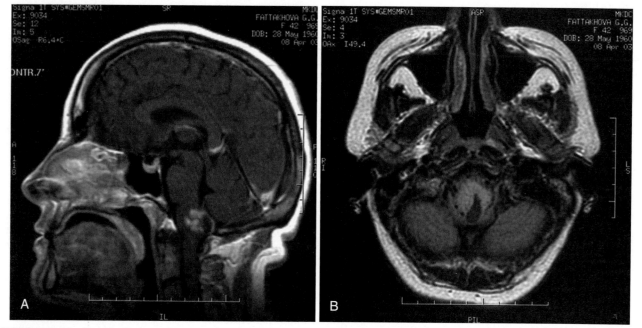

FIGURE 58-24 Focal intrinsic cystic tumor of the medulla (piloid astrocytoma). The duration of illness is 20 years. *A, B,* Before surgery: sagittal and axial T1-weighted magnetic resonance imaging (MRI) after contrast enhancement shows a heterogeneous enhancing lesion with a cyst.

(Continued)

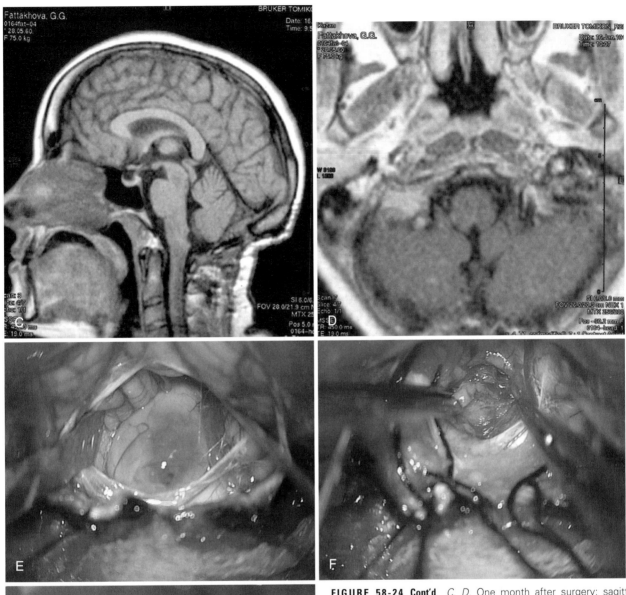

FIGURE 58-24 Cont'd *C, D,* One month after surgery: sagittal and axial T1-weighted MRI shows gross total tumor removal. Intraoperative view: *E,* cyst in the dorsal part of the tumor; *F,* after evacuation of the cyst tumor removal is performed; *G,* cavity after tumor removal.

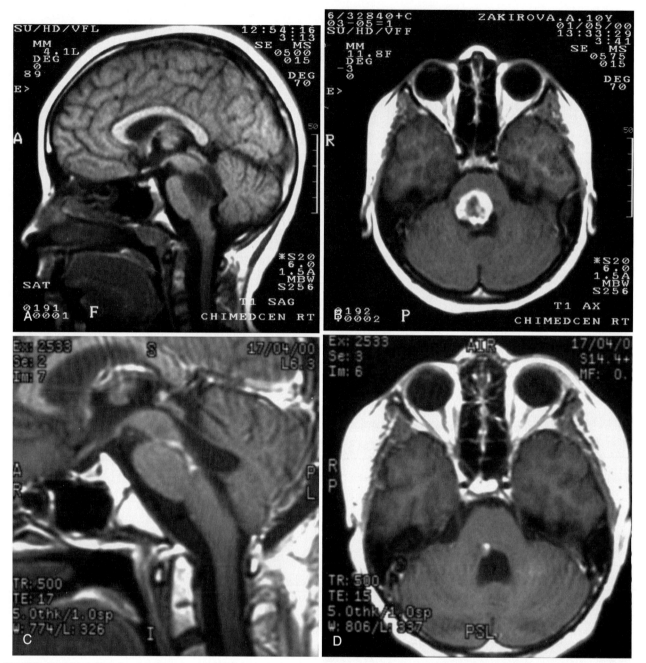

FIGURE 58-25 Infiltrative-growing tumor (glioblastoma) with focal contrast enhancement (pseudofocal tumor). *A,* Sagittal T1-weighted magnetic resonance imaging (MRI) shows a hypointense lesion in the pons tegmentum. *B,* Axial T1-weighted MRI after contrast enhancement reveals a nonhomogeneous enhancing ring with a hypointense core. *C, D,* T1-weighted MRI shows gross tumor removal. The duration of illness is 3 months.

air embolism. This position is most convenient when the tumor is located in the upper pons and midbrain. The prone position is preferable for small children and patients with extensive hydrocephalus.

Brain Stem Monitoring

During BST surgery,[128,129] we monitor somatosensory and the auditory evoked potentials and use direct stimulation of the motor nuclei of cranial nerves III, VI, VII, IX, X, and XII. Registration of somatosensory and auditory evoked potentials is not very reliable. More information comes from mapping

from the floor of the fourth ventricle with direct stimulation of cranial nerve motor nuclei.

Tumor removal often causes bradycardia and an increase or decrease in blood pressure, usually during manipulation in the vicinity of the nuclei of cranial nerves V and IX. These reactions disappear when manipulation in that region ceases.

Approaches

Surgical approaches depend on the location and size of the tumor. Tumors located in the tectal plate are exposed with either the supracerebellar subtentorial or occipital

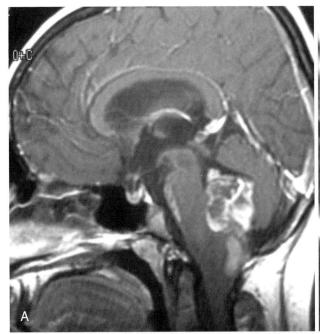

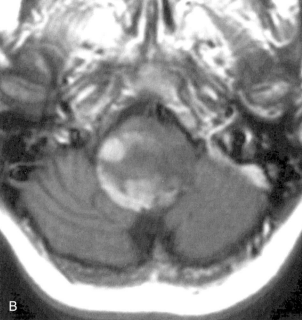

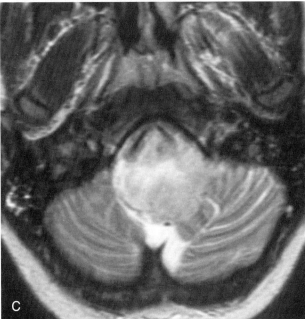

FIGURE 58-26 Diffuse tumor with exophytic component. The tumor arises from the pons and medulla oblongata, occupies the fourth ventricle (ganglioastrocytoma). *A,* Sagittal T1-weighted magnetic resonance imaging (MRI) after contrast injection shows nonhomogeneous enhancement of the exophytic part of the tumor in the fourth ventricle. *B,* Axial T1-weighted MRI after contrast injection demonstrates the enlargement of the medulla infiltrated by the tumor and nonhomogeneous enhancement of the lesion. *C,* Axial T2-weighted MRI shows a nonhomogeneous hypointense lesion in the enlarged medulla.

TABLE 58-9 ▪ **Brain Stem Tumors: Neurologic Signs in 306 Patients at the Time of Admission**

Caudal Brain Stem		*Rostral Brain Stem*	
Neurologic Signs	**%**	**Neurologic Signs**	**%**
Hemiparesis	22	Hemiparesis	30
Monoparesis	2	Ataxia	17
Ataxia	33	Unilateral hyperkinesis	15
9th, 10th nerve deficit	38	Oculomotor disorders	43
8th nerve deficit	14	Parinaud's syndrome	33
6th nerve deficit	23	Behavioral problems	18
Lateral gaze palsy	13	High ICP	27
High ICP	25		

ICP, intracranial pressure.

supratentorial approach with section of the tentorium laterally and along the rectus sinus.

Gliomas that predominantly occupy the midbrain tegmentum, brain peduncle, or both can be approached either by the occipital transtentorial, lateral subtentorial, or subtemporal approach (Fig. 58-27).

If the tumor grows into the fourth ventricle or is identified as an aqueductal tumor, the medial posterior fossa access is preferable. Some tumors that grow in the region of the aqueduct are easily reached through the fourth ventricle (Fig. 58-28).

In some cases, a combination of different approaches permits the surgeon to accomplish radical tumor ablation. For example, the supracerebellar approach can be combined

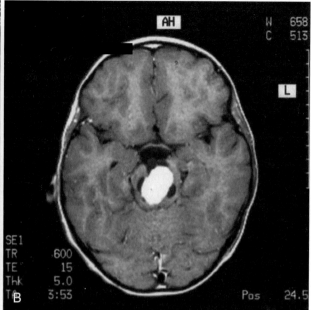

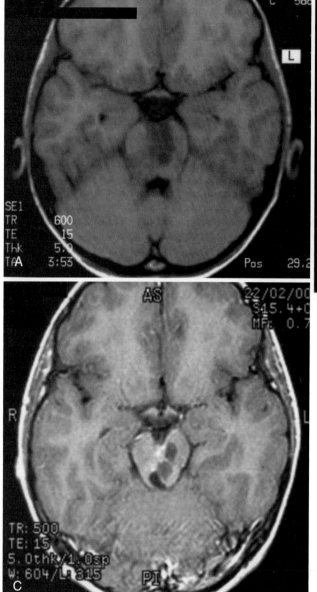

FIGURE 58-27   Focal low-grade astrocytoma of the left part of the midbrain tegmentum approached via the occipital transtentorial route before and after surgery. *A, B,* Before surgery, T1-weighted axial magnetic resonance imaging (MRI) shows a hypointense mass in the left part of the midbrain. *B,* T1-weighted axial MRI shows focal contrast enhancement of midbrain lesion. *C,* T1-weighted axial MRI scan after surgery demonstrates total removal of the tumor.

with the approach through the fourth ventricle, the occipital transtentorial approach can be combined with the supracerebellar, and so forth. In cases in which the tumor penetrates into the thalamus, the transcallosal approach may be used.

The most difficult task is to access tumors that are located predominantly in the anterior part of the pons and the peduncle. In such cases, the pterional route, using a subtemporal approach with tentorial section, or the presigmoid route may be selected.

Caudal BSTs (involving the pons, medulla oblongata, and upper segments of the spinal cord) can be explored and removed using the osteoplastic posterior fossa approach.

In cases of spinomedullary tumors that occupy the cervical part of the spinal cord, we prefer a laminotomy with repositioning of the vertebral arches after tumor removal.

When approaching dorsally exophytic tumors that occupy the fourth ventricle, it is not necessary to cut the vermis. For adequate exploration of the fourth ventricle, it is necessary only to coagulate and divide the plexus in the region of the foramen of Magendie.

Technique of Tumor Removal

Ultrasound aspiration is the most efficient method for glial BST removal, especially if the tumor is solid. Soft tumors may be evacuated using bipolar coagulation and simultaneous aspiration of coagulated tissue. Coagulation changes the color and density of the tumor (it becomes more solid and pale), and for determination of the border between the tumor and brain stem structures, thorough aspiration of coagulated tissue is necessary. When dealing with brain stem lesions, we prefer not to use the retractor to open the

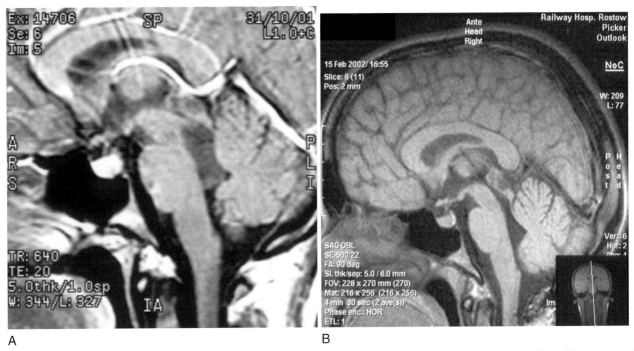

FIGURE 58-28   The nonenhancing tumor of the aqueduct removed through the fourth ventricle. *A,* Before surgery: T1-weighted magnetic resonance imaging (MRI) after contrast enhancement shows a nonenhancing tumor of the aqueduct arising from the tectal plate. *B,* MRI 3 weeks after the subtotal removal of the tumor. The tectal plate is infiltrated by the tumor.

brain stem wound. If the tumor has an exophytic component, the surgery starts with its removal. Radicality of tumor ablation in such cases depends on the possibility of distinguishing the interface between the tumor and the surrounding brain. Infiltration of the brain stem in this group of tumors is variable. Tumors arising from the subependymal portion of the pons or medulla with no or minimal brain stem invasion (focal tumors) and protruding in the fourth ventricle constitute a subgroup of dorsally exophytic tumors that are always benign and can be operated on successfully.[130–132] Most of the tumor is located in the fourth ventricle and is easily removed with the Cavitron (Fig. 58-29) It is necessary to differentiate these tumors from diffuse tumors with an exophytic component that can be debulked only occasionally (see Fig. 58-26). Therefore, if the definite tumor–brain stem interface is absent, complete resection of the tumor is not feasible.

If the tumor contains a cyst or cysts, evacuation of the cystic fluid greatly facilitates removal of the tumor because the surgeon gains additional space for manipulation (see Fig. 58-24). When the cavity after evacuation of a cyst or removal of a tumor is large, we use a spatula with narrow blades (3 to 5 mm width) just to support the cavity walls. Routinely, we use blades of a bipolar coagulating forceps as a retractor.

In approximately half of our cases, the tumor was intrinsic to the brain stem, and it was necessary to make an incision in the surface of the brain stem. The length of this incision may vary, but it is usually relatively small (<1 cm). That is enough to reach and remove even large tumors (see Figs. 58-22 and 58-23). These incisions are placed nearest to the surface of the tumor. It is important to approach the tumor at a distance from the nuclei of cranial nerves VII, IX, and X. This location can be determined with the help of fourth ventricle floor mapping. The brain stem can be violated

with low risk by entering through some safe areas including the supracollicular, infracollicular, and lateral mesencephalic sulcus; the median sulcus above the facial colliculus; the suprafacial, infrafacial, and area acustica; the posterior median fissure below the obex; the posterior intermediate sulcus; and the posterior lateral sulcus.[124]

When the tumor penetrates the subarachnoid space, it may come into contact with important arteries. In some cases, these vessels are included in the tumor tissue. The surgeon must be cautious when removing a tumor that penetrates the ventral part of the brain stem and contacts vertebral or basilar arteries and their branches.

Some tumors are well supplied with blood, and these vessels must be coagulated while the tumor is being removed. In some cases, such coagulation may result in ischemic damage of the surrounding brain tissue.

Critical in the removal of brain stem gliomas is differentiation between tumor and brain tissue. If tumor infiltrates the brain stem, its removal may result in increased neurologic morbidity, with disturbances of vital neurologic functions. In such cases, radical tumor removal is impossible.

We do not want to describe in detail the risks of surgery in all groups of patients with BSTs but do comment on our experience with cervicomedullary tumor surgery (24 patients). Jallo and colleagues[132] described these tumors. These tumors are almost invariably low-grade tumors amenable to radical surgery. The rostral axial extension of the tumor is restricted by long tracts and the obex without infiltration of the medulla and the pons (Fig. 58-30A). We also have favorable results in some patients in this group (Fig. 58-31). In most spinomedullary tumors, there were neurologic or MRI signs of medulla oblongata involvement (see Fig. 58-30B) that made the radical surgery risky and

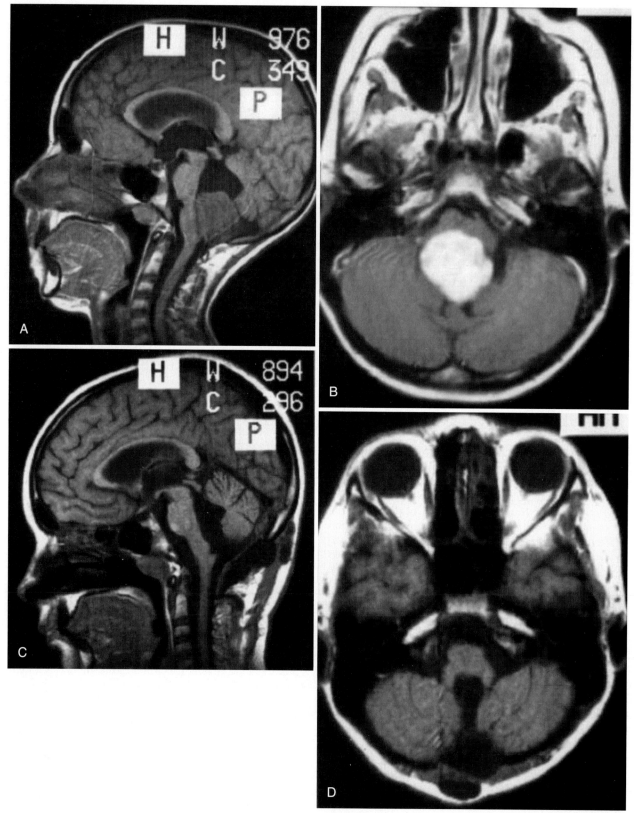

FIGURE 58-29   Dorsally exophytic pilocytic astrocytoma of the medulla oblongata in a 12-year-old girl with vomiting, nausea, and weight loss. The duration of the disease is not less than 10 years. Magnetic resonance imaging (MRI) before (*A, B*) and after (*C, D*) surgery. *A*, Sagittal T1-weighted MRI shows a hypointense mass arising from the dorsal surface of the medulla oblongata. *B*, Axial T1-weighted MRI after gadolinium injection shows marked enhancement of the tumor. *C, D*, Sagittal and axial T1-weighted MRI shows the total removal of the tumor.

(Continued)

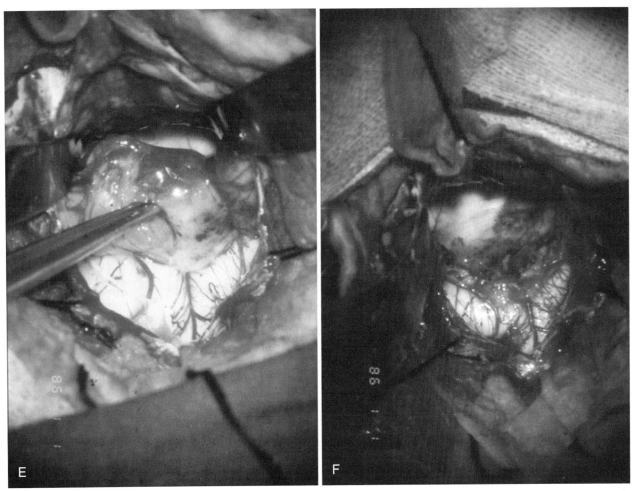

FIGURE 58-29 Cont'd *E, F,* Intraoperative view of the patient. Compact exophytic tumor was resected en bloc. Total tumor removal.

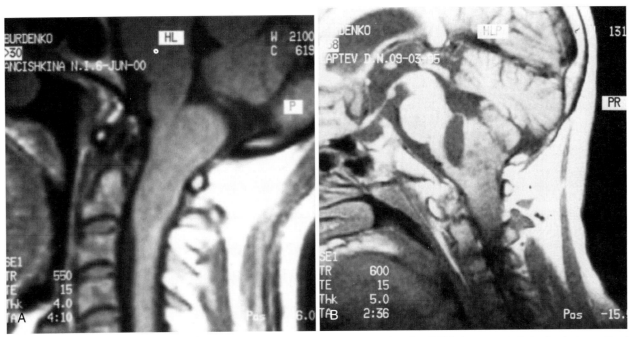

FIGURE 58-30 Variants of spinomedullary tumor growth. *A,* Magnetic resonance imaging (MRI) shows posteriorly directed growth of a solid spinomedullary tumor (piloid astrocytoma). Rostral tumor growth is limited by long pathways. *B,* Predominantly solid diffuse spinomedullary tumor (grade III) arising from the medulla oblongata and cervical part of the spinal cord. MRI demonstrates the growth from cervical cord to the upper part of the medulla.

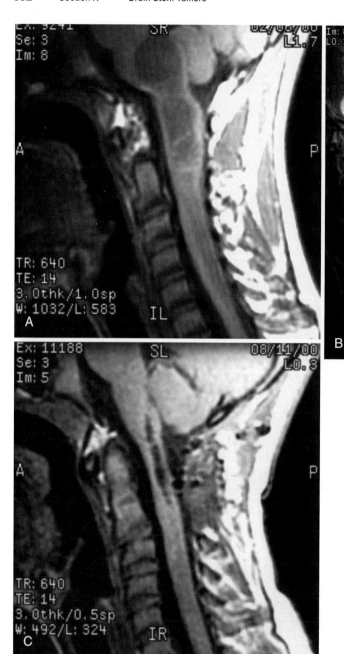

postoperative mortality dangerously high (16%). Squires and colleagues[133] also described a case of a diffuse infiltrating astrocytoma in the cervicomedullary region. It seems that careful analysis of the clinical manifestation and MRI data is of special importance for better operative planning and optimal management of this group of BSTs.

RESULTS AND CONCLUSIONS

The results of BST removal are presented in Tables 58-10 to 58-12. Some comments are in order.

1. The more unfavorable results are observed in patients with spinomedullary tumors and gliomas of medulla oblongata and lower pons (see Table 58-10). Postoperative mortality is the highest in this group.

TABLE 58-10 ■ Caudal Brian Stem Tumors: Neurologic Status 1.5 Months* after Surgery Related to Tumor Location

	Sp. Med	Med	Med P	Pons
Improved	10 (42%)	17 (50%)	18 (39%)	36 (51%)
Unchanged	5 (21%)	7 (21%)	11 (24%)	16 (23%)
Deteriorated + improved†	5 (21%)	1 (3%)	5 (11%)	9 (13%)
Deteriorated	0 (0%)	5 (15%)	3 (6%)	7 (10%)
Death	4 (16%)	4 (11%)	9 (20%)	2 (3%)
Total = 174	24	34	46	70

*Mean time of discharge after surgery.
†Some neurologic symptoms increased, some decreased.
Sp. Med, spinomedullary; M, medullary; P Mid, pontine midbrain.

TABLE 58-11 ▪ Rostral Brain Stem Tumors: Neurologic Status 1.5 Months* after Surgery Related to Tumor Location

	P Mid	Mid	Tect
Improved	29 (54%)	24 (61%)	21 (55%)
Unchanged	11 (20%)	3 (6%)	8 (21%)
Deteriorated + improved†	5 (9%)	6 (15%)	6 (16%)
Deteriorated	6 (11%)	5 (13%)	2 (5%)
Death	3 (6%)	2 (5%)	1 (3%)
Total = 132	54	40	38

*Mean time of discharge after surgery.
†Some neurologic symptoms increased, some decreased.
 P Mid, pontine midbrain; Mid, tegmentum, crus cerebri;
Tect, aqueductal and tectal.

Preoperative and postoperative disturbances of vital functions such as breathing and swallowing often necessitate long-term artificial ventilation, which cannot be effective enough to save a patient's life. Much better results may be achieved in patients with rostral BSTs (see Table 58-11).

2. Sixteen percent of patients in our series had malignant pseudofocal tumors. Removal of malignant tumors produces worse results in comparison with removal of benign tumors: there was improvement after surgery in only 40% of patients with malignant tumors. The recurrence-free period in patients with gliomas (grade IV) and primitive neuroepithelial tumors did not exceed 12 months.

3. Results are the best after the removal of focal (benign) tumors (84% of patients). Improvement after surgery in patients with benign tumors was more than 60% and depended on the location of the lesion.

4. Surgery in adults is more dangerous than in children (see Table 58-12).

The widespread classification of BSTs according to which they are divided into four groups (focal, diffuse, cervicomedullary, and dorsally exophytic) needs to be some commented on. The term focal tumor in this classification means that the brain stem lesion is well delineated on MRI

TABLE 58-12 ▪ Brain Stem Tumors: Neurologic Status 1.5 Months* after Surgery Related to the Tumor Location and Age

	Caudal BSTs		Rostral BSTs	
	Children	Adults	Children	Adults
Improved	57 (51%)	24 (38%)	52 (64%)	22 (42%)
Unchanged	19 (17%)	20 (32%)	11 (14%)	11 (21%)
Deteriorated + improved†	13 (12%)	7 (11%)	7 (9%)	10 (19%)
Deteriorated	12 (11%)	3 (5%)	8 (10%)	5 (10%)
Death	10 (9%)	9 (14%)	2 (3%)	4 (8%)
Total = 306	111	63	80	52

*Mean time of discharge after surgery.
†Some neurologic symptoms increased, some decreased.
 BSTs, brain stem tumors.

and CT. But CT and MRI together with clinical evaluation only allow the type of tumor growth (tumor growth pattern) to be supposed, and it is verified only during surgery and pathologic examination of the tumor tissue.

Location of the tumor per se is not the indication for surgery. Spinomedullary and dorsally exophytic tumors are no more than one of the variants of tumor topography. A tumor of any topographic variant can be focal or diffuse. Spinomedullary tumors should be also classified as focal and diffuse.

We conclude that surgical removal of primary BSTs is indicated in cases of focal benign and some diffuse tumors with an exophytic component. Surgery may result in marked long-lasting improvement. Nevertheless, the results of BST surgery are far from satisfactory and new attempts to improve them are necessary.

REFERENCES

1. Koos WT, Horaczek A: Statistics of intracranial midline tumors in children. Acta Neurochir Suppl (Wien) 35:1–5, 1985.
2. Bregeat P: Quelques reflexions sur les gliomes hypothalamique. Adv Ophtal 36:130–137, 1978.
3. Tihan T, Fisher PG, Kepner JL, et al: Pediatric astrocytomas with monomorphous pilomyxoid features and a less favorable outcome. J Neuropathol Exp Neurol 58:1061–1068, 1999.
4. Fuller CE, Frankel B, Smith M, et al: Suprasellar monomorphous pilomyxoid neoplasm: An ultrastructural analysis. Clin Neuropathol 20:256–262, 2001.
5. Arslanoglu A, Cirak B, Horska A, et al: MR imaging characteristics of pilomyxoid astrocytomas. AJNR Am J Neuroradiol 24:1906–1908, 2003.
6. Lieberman KA, Wasenko JJ, Schelper R, et al: Tanycytomas: A newly characterized hypothalamic-suprasellar and ventricular tumor. AJNR Am J Neuroradiol 24:1999–2004, 2003.
7. Komotar RJ, Burger PC, Carson BS, et al: Pilocytic and pilomyxoid hypothalamic/chiasmatic astrocytomas. Neurosurgery 54:72–79, 2004.
8. Pomper MG, Passe TJ, Burger PC, et al: Chordoid glioma: A neoplasm unique to the hypothalamus and anterior third ventricle. AJNR Am J Neuroradiol 22:464–469, 2001.
9. Castellano-Sanchez AA, Schemankewitz E, Mazewski C, Brat DJ: Pediatric chordoid glioma with chondroid metaplasia. Pediatr Dev Pathol 4:564–567, 2001.
10. Pasquier B, Peoc'h M, Morrison AL, et al: Chordoid glioma of the third ventricle: A report of two new cases, with further evidence supporting an ependymal differentiation, and review of the literature. Am J Surg Pathol 26:1330–1342, 2002.
11. Taraszewska A, Bogucki J, Andrychowski J, et al: Clinicopathological and ultrastructural study in two cases of chordoid glioma. Folia Neuropathol 41:175–282, 2003.
11a. Ojeda SR, Prevot V, Heger S, et al: Glia-to-neuron signaling and the neuroendocrine control of female puberty. Ann Med 35:244–255, 2003.
11b. Junier MP, Hill DF, Costa ME, et al: Hypothalamic lesions that induce female precocious puberty activate glial expression of the epidermal growth factor receptor gene: Differential regulation of alternatively spliced transcripts. J Neurosci 13:703–713, 1993.
12. Martinez R, Honegger J, Fahlbusch R, Buchfelder M: Endocrine findings in patients with optico-hypothalamic gliomas. Exp Clin Endocrinol Diabetes 111:162–167, 2003.
13. Kanumakala S, Warne GL, Zacharin MR: Evolving hypopituitarism following cranial irradiation. J Paediatr Child Health 39:232–235, 2003.
14. Rivarola, Belgorosky A, Mendilaharzu H, Vidal G: Precocious puberty in children with tumours of the suprasellar and pineal areas: Organic central precocious puberty. Acta Paediatr 90:751–756, 2001.
15. Bisson E, Khoshyomn S, Braff S, Maugans T: Hypothalamic-opticochiasmatic gliomas mimicking craniopharyngiomas. Pediatr Neurosurg 39:159–165, 2003.
16. Symon L, Pell MF, Habib AH: Radical excision of craniopharyngioma by the temporal route: A review of 50 patients. Br J Neurosurg 5:539–549, 1991.

17. Gillett GR, Symon L: Hypothalamic glioma. Surg Neurol 28:291–300, 1987.

18. Apuzzo ML, Levy ML, Tung H: Surgical strategies and technical methodologies in optimal management of craniopharyngioma and masses affecting the third ventricular chamber. Acta Neurochir Suppl (Wien) 53:77–88, 1991.

19. Koos WT, Perraczky A, Horaczek A: Problems of surgical technique for the treatment of supratentorial midline tumors in children. Acta Neurochir Suppl (Wien) 35:31–41, 1985.

20. Gower DJ, Pollay M, Shuman RM, Brumback RA: Cystic optic glioma. Neurosurgery 26:133–136, 1990.

21. Carmel PW: Tumors of the III ventricle. Acta Neurochir (Wien) 75:136–146, 1985.

22. Stein BM: Third ventricle tumors. Clin Neurosurg 17:315–331, 1985.

23. Albright AL, Sclabassi RJ: Cavitron ultrasonic surgical aspiration and visual evoked potential monitoring for chiasmal gliomas in children. J Neurosurg 63:138–140, 1985.

24. Schuster H, Koos WT, Zaunbauer F: Results of microsurgical treatment of gliomas of the optic system and hypothalamus in children. Mod Probl Paediatr 18:211–215, 1977.

25. Maspes P, Geuna E: Resultats du traitement chirurgical de 182 cas de tumeurs du III ventricule. Neurochirurgie 12:633–636, 1966.

26. Pecker J, Faivre J, Guy G: Indications chirurgicales dans les tumeur du plancher du III ventricule. Neurochirurgie 12:653–660, 1966.

27. Medlock MD, Scott RM: Optic chiasm astrocytomas of childhood. Pediatr Neurosurg 27:129–136, 1997.

28. Konovalov AN, Gorelyshev SK, Serova NK: Surgery of giant gliomas of chiasm and III ventricle. Acta Neurochir (Wien) 130:71–79, 1994.

29. Konovalov AN, Gorelyshev SK: Surgical treatment of anterior third ventricle tumours. Acta Neurochir (Wien) 118:33–39, 1992.

30. Alshail E, Rutka GT, Becker LE, Hoffman HJ: Optic chiasmatic-hypothalamic glioma. Brain Pathol 7:799–806, 1997.

31. Rutka JT, Hoffman HJ, Drake JM, Humphreys RP: Suprasellar and sellar tumors in children and adolescence. Neurosurg Clin N Am 3:803–820, 1992.

32. Hoffman HJ, Humphreys RP, Drake JM, et al: Optic pathway/hypothalamic gliomas: A dilemma in management. Pediatr Neurosurg 19:186–195, 1993.

33. Wisoff JH: Management of optic pathway tumors of childhood. Neurosurg Clin N Am 3:791–802, 1992.

34. Valdueza JM, Lohmann F, Dammann O, et al: Analysis of 20 primarily surgically treated chiasmatic/hypothalamic pilocytic astrocytomas. Acta Neurochir (Wien) 126:44–50, 1994.

35. Erkal HS, Serin M, Cakmak A: Management of optic pathway and chiasmatic-hypothalamic gliomas in children with radiation therapy. Radiother Oncol 45:11–15, 1997.

36. Nishio S, Takeshita I, Fujiwara S, et al: Optico-hypothalamic glioma: An analysis of 16 cases. Childs Nerv Syst 9:334–338, 1993.

37. Rodriguez LA, Edwards MS, Levin VA: Management of hypothalamic gliomas in children: An analysis of 33 cases. Neurosurgery 26:242–246, 1990.

38. Lapras C: Paper presented at the 9th European Congress of Neurosurgery, 1991, Moscow.

39. Helcl F: Surgical treatment of chiasmal gliomas in children. Bratisl Lek Listy 98:166–169, 1997.

40. Long DM, Chou SN, Shelley N: Transcallosal removal of the craniopharyngiomas within the III ventricle. J Neurosurg 39:563–567, 1973.

41. Stein BM: Transcallosal approach to third ventricle tumors. In Schmidek HH, Sweet WH (eds): Operative Neurosurgical Techniques. New York: Grune & Stratton, 1982.

42. Czyzyk E, Jozwiak S, Roszkowski M, Schwartz RA: Optic pathway gliomas in children with and without neurofibromatosis 1. J Child Neurol 18:471–478, 2003.

43. Balcer LJ, Liu GT, Heller G, et al: Visual loss in children with neurofibromatosis type 1 and optic pathway gliomas: Relation to tumor location by magnetic resonance imaging. Am J Ophthalmol 131:442–445, 2001.

44. Collet-Solberg PF, Sernyak H, Satin-Smith M, et al: Endocrine outcome in long-term survivors of low-grade hypothalamic/chiasmatic glioma. Clin Endocrinol (Oxf) 47:79–85, 1997.

45. Cummings P, Baumann-Schroder U, Hazim W, et al: Long-term outcome of gliomas of the visual pathway in type 1 neurofibromatosis. Klin Monatsbl Augenheilkd 215:349–354, 1999.

46. Deliganis AV, Geyer JR, Berger MS: Prognostic significance of type 1 neurofibromatosis (von Recklinghausen disease) in childhood optic glioma. Neurosurgery 38:1114–1119, 1996.

47. Grill J, Couanet D, Cappelli C, et al: Radiation-induced cerebral vasculopathy in children with neurofibromatosis and optic pathway glioma. Ann Neurol 45:393–396, 1999.

48. Kuenzle C, Weissert M, Roulet E, et al: Follow-up of optic pathway gliomas in children with neurofibromatosis type 1. Neuropediatrics 25:295–300, 1994.

49. Listernick R, Charrow J, Greenwald M, Mets M: Natural history of optic pathway tumors in children with neurofibromatosis type 1: A longitudinal study. J Pediatr 125:63–66, 1994.

50. Listernick R, Charrow J, Greenwald MJ, Esterly NB: Optic gliomas in children with neurofibromatosis type 1. J Pediatr 114:788–792, 1989.

51. Listernick R, Charrow J, Gutmann DH: Intracranial gliomas in neurofibromatosis type 1. Am J Med Genet 26;89:38–44, 1999.

52. Listernick R, Darling C, Greenwald M, et al: Optic pathway tumors in children: The effect of neurofibromatosis type 1 on clinical manifestations and natural history. J Pediatr 127:718–722, 1995.

53. Listernick R, Louis DN, Packer RJ, Gutmann DH: Optic pathway gliomas in children with neurofibromatosis 1: Consensus statement from the NF1 Optic Pathway Glioma Task Force. Ann Neurol 41:143–149, 1997.

54. Tow SL, Chandela S, Miller NR, Avellino AM: Long-term outcome in children with gliomas of the anterior visual pathway. Neuro-Ophthalmology Unit, Wilmer Eye Institute, the Johns Hopkins Hospital, Baltimore.

55. Steinbok P: Optic pathway tumors in children. J Chin Med Assoc 66:4–12, 2003.

56. Kornreich L, Blaser S, Schwarz M, et al: Optic pathway glioma: Correlation of imaging findings with the presence of neurofibromatosis. AJNR Am J Neuroradiol 1963–1969, 2001.

57. Allen JC: Initial management of children with hypothalamic and thalamic tumors and the modifying role of neurofibromatosis-1. Pediatr Neurosurg 32:154–162, 2000.

58. Colosimo C, Cerase A, Maira G: Regression after biopsy of a pilocytic opticochiasmatic astrocytoma in a young adult without neurofibromatosis. Neuroradiology 42:352–356, 2000.

59. Gottschalk S, Tavakolian R, Buske A, et al: Spontaneous remission of chiasmatic/hypothalamic masses in neurofibromatosis type 1: Report of two cases. Neuroradiology 41:199–201, 1999.

60. Perilongo G, Carollo C, Salviati L, et al: Diencephalic syndrome and disseminated juvenile pilocytic astrocytomas of the hypothalamic-optic chiasm region. Cancer 80:142–146, 1997.

61. Rubtsova IV, Parsa CF, Hoit WF: Spontaneous regression of familial glioma of the optic nerve in a boy with suspected neurofibromatosis 1 (Recklinghausen's disease). Vestn Oftalmol 114:48–51, 1998.

62. Schmandt SM, Packer RJ, Vezina LG, Jane J: Spontaneous regression of low-grade astrocytomas in childhood. Pediatr Neurosurg 32:132–136, 2000.

63. Takeuchi H, Kabuto M, Sato K, Kubota T: Chiasmal gliomas with spontaneous regression: proliferation and apoptosis. Childs Nerv Syst 13:229–233, 1997.

64. Schmandt SM, Packer RJ, Vezina LG, Jane J: Spontaneous regression of low-grade astrocytomas in childhood. Pediatr Neurosurg 32:132–136, 2000.

65. Zizka J, Elias P, Jakubec J: Spontaneous regression of low-grade astrocytomas: An underrecognized condition? Eur Radiol 11:2638–2640, 2001.

66. Perilongo G, Moras P, Carollo C, et al: Spontaneous partial regression of low-grade glioma in children with neurofibromatosis-1: A real possibility. J Child Neurol 14:352–356, 1999.

67. Parsa CF, Hoyt CS, Lesser RL, et al: Spontaneous regression of optic gliomas: Thirteen cases documented by serial neuroimaging. Arch Ophthalmol 119:516–529, 2001.

68. Takenchi H, Kabuto M, Sato K, Kubota T: Chiasmal gliomas with spontaneous regression: Proliferation and apoptosis. Childs Nerv Syst 13:229–233, 1997.

69. Mohadjer M, Etou A, Milios E, et al: Chiasmatic optic glioma. Neurochirurgia (Stuttg) 34:90–93, 1991.

70. Bataini JP, Delanian S, Ponvert D: Chiasmal gliomas: Results of irradiation management in 57 patients and review of literature. Int J Radiat Oncol Biol Phys 21:615–623, 1991.

71. Capo H, Kupersmith MJ: Efficacy and complications of radiotherapy of anterior visual pathway tumors. Neurol Clin 9:179–203, 1991.

72. Gould RJ, Hilal SK, Chutorian AM: Efficacy of radiotherapy in optic gliomas. Pediatr Neurol 3:29–32, 1987.

73. Cohen ME, Duffner PK: Optic pathway tumors. Neurol Clin 9:467–477, 1991.

74. McLaurin RL, Breneman J, Aron B: Hypothalamic gliomas: Review of 18 cases. Concepts Pediatr Neurosurg 7:19–29, 1987.

75. Wechsler-Jentzsch K, Witt JH, Fitz CR, et al: Unresectable gliomas in children: Tumor-volume response to radiation therapy. Radiology 169:237–242, 1988.

76. Friedman HS, Oakes WJ: Recurrent brain tumors in children. Pediatr Neurosci 13:233–241, 1987.

77. Scott E, Mickle JP: Pediatric diencephalic gliomas—a review of 18 cases. Pediatr Neurosci 13:225–232, 1987.

78. Turpin G, Heshmati HM, Scherrer H, et al: Tumeurs hypothalamiques primitives (en dehors des craniopharyngiomes): Étude endocrinienne et évolutive post-radiotherapie. A propos de 17 observations. Ann Med Interne (Paris) 137:395–400, 1986.

79. Packer RJ, Ater J, Allen J, et al: Carboplatin and vincristine chemotherapy for children with newly diagnosed progressive low-grade gliomas. J Neurosurg 86:747–754, 1997.

80. Fouladi M, Wallace D, Langston JW, et al: Survival and functional outcome of children with hypothalamic/chiasmatic tumors. Cancer 97:1084–2092, 2003.

81. Grabenbauer GG, Schuchardt U, Buchfelder M, et al: Radiation therapy of optico-hypothalamic gliomas (OHG)—radiographic response, vision and late toxicity. Radiother Oncol 54:239–245, 2000.

82. Erkal HS, Serin M, Cakmak A: Management of optic pathway and chiasmatic-hypothalamic gliomas in children with radiation therapy. Radiother Oncol 45:11–155, 1997.

83. Khafaga Y, Hassounah M, Kandil A, et al: Optic gliomas: A retrospective analysis of 50 cases. Int J Radiat Oncol Biol Phys 56:807–812, 2003.

84. Ganz JC, Smievoll AI, Thorsen F: Radiosurgical treatment of gliomas of the diencephalon. Acta Neurochir Suppl (Wien) 62:62–66, 1994.

85. Bernstein M, Laperriere NJ: A critical appraisal of the role of brachytherapy for pediatric brain tumors. Pediatr Neurosurg 16:213–218, 1991.

86. Mohadjer M, Etou A, Milios E, et al: Chiasmatic optic glioma. Neurochirurgia (Stuttg) 34:90–93, 1991.

87. Kretschmar CS, Linggood RM: Chemotherapeutic treatment of extensive optic pathway tumors in infants. J Neurooncol 10:263–270, 1991.

88. Petronio J, Edwards MS, Prados M, et al: Management of chiasmal and hypothalamic gliomas of infancy and childhood with chemotherapy. J Neurosurg 74:701–708, 1991.

89. Packer RJ, Sutton LN, Bilaniuk LT, et al: Treatment of chiasmatic/hypothalamic gliomas of childhood with chemotherapy. Ann Neurol 23:79–85, 1988.

90. Shuper A, Horev G, Kornreich L: Visual pathway glioma: An erratic tumour with therapeutic dilemmas. Arch Dis Child 76:259–263, 1997.

91. Garvey M, Packer R: An integrated approach to the treatment of chiasmatic-hypothalamic gliomas. J Neurooncol 28:167–183, 1996.

92. Sutton LN, Molloy PT, Sernyak H: Long-term outcome of hypothalamic/chiasmatic astrocytomas in children treated with conservative surgery. J Neurosurg 83:583–589, 1995.

93. Chamberlain MC: Recurrent chiasmatic-hypothalamic glioma treated with oral etoposide. Arch Neurol 52:509–513, 1995.

94. Janss AJ, Grundy R, Cnaan A, et al: Optic pathway and hypothalamic/chiasmatic gliomas in children younger than age 5 years with 6 years follow-up. Cancer 75:1051–1059, 1995.

95. Nishio S, Morioka T, Takeshita I, et al: Chemotherapy for progressive pilocytic astrocytomas in the chiasmo-hypothalamic regions. Clin Neurol Neurosurg 97:300–306, 1995.

96. Mahoney DH, Jr, Cohen ME, Friedman HS, et al: Carboplatin is effective therapy for young children with progressive optic pathway tumors: A Pediatric Oncology Group phase II study. Neuro-oncology 2:213–220, 2000.

97. Silva MM, Goldman S, Keating G, et al: Optic pathway hypothalamic gliomas in children under three years of age: The role of chemotherapy. Pediatr Neurosurg 33:151–158, 2000.

98. Steinbok P, Hentschel S, Almqvist P, et al: Management of optic chiasmatic/hypothalamic astrocytomas in children. Can J Neurol Sci 29:132–138, 2002.

99. Kageji T, Nagahiro S, Horiguchi H, et al: Successful high-dose chemotherapy for widespread neuroaxis dissemination of an optico-hypothalamic juvenile pilocytic astrocytoma in an infant: A case report. J Neurooncol 62:281–287, 2003.

100. Rilliet B, Vernet O: Gliomas in children: A review. Childs Nerv Syst 16:735–741, 2000.

101. Osztie E, Varallyay P, Doolittle ND, et al: Combined intraarterial carboplatin, intraarterial etoposide phosphate, and IV Cytoxan chemotherapy for progressive optic-hypothalamic gliomas in young children. AJNR Am J Neuroradiol 22:818–823, 2001.

102. Brauner R, Malandry F, Rappaport R, et al: Growth and endocrine disorders in optic glioma. Eur J Pediatr 149:825–828, 1990.

103. Steiger HJ, Gots C, Schmid-Elsaesser R, Stumme W: Thalamic astrocytomas: Surgical anatomy and results of a pilot series using maximum microsurgical removal. Acta Neurochir (Wien) 142:1327–1337, 2000.

104. Nishio S, Morioca T, Suzuki S, et al: Thalamic gliomas: A clinicopathologic analysis of 20 cases with reference to patient age. Acta Neurochir (Wien) 139:336–342, 1997.

105. Albright AL, Sclabassi RJ: Use of the Cavitron ultrasonic surgical aspirator and evoked potentials for the treatment of thalamic and brain stem tumors in children. Neurosurgery 17:564–568, 1985.

106. Drake JM, Joy M, Goldenberg A, Kreindler D: Computer- and robot-assisted resection of thalamic astrocytomas in children. Neurosurgery 29:27–33, 1991.

107. Hoffman HJ, Soloniuk DS, Humphreys RP, et al: Management and outcome of low-grade astrocytomas of the midline in children: A retrospective review. Neurosurgery 33:964–971, 1993.

108. Villarejo F, Amaya C, Perez Diaz-C, et al: Radical surgery of thalamic tumors in children. Childs Nerv Syst 10:111–114, 1994.

109. Souweidane MM, Hoffman HJ: Current treatment of thalamic gliomas in children. J Neurooncol 28:157–166, 1996.

110. Kelly PJ: Stereotactic biopsy and resection of thalamic astrocytomas. Neurosurgery 25:185–195, 1989.

111. Pool JL: Gliomas in the region of the brain stem. J Neurosurg 29:164–167, 1968.

112. Stroink AR, Hoffman HJ, Hendric EB, et al: Diagnosis and management of pediatric brain stem gliomas. J Neurosurg 65:745–750, 1986.

113. Epstein F, McCleary EL: Intrinsic brain stem tumors in childhood: Surgical indications. J Neurosurg 64:11–15, 1986.

114. Konovalov AN, Atieh J: The surgical treatment of primary brain stem tumors. In Schmidek HH, Sweet WH (eds): Operative Neurosurgical Techniques, 2nd ed. New York: Grune & Stratton, 1988, pp 709–737.

115. Heffez DS, Zinreich SJ, Long DM: Surgical resection of intrinsic brain stem lesions: An overview. Neurosurgery 27:789–798, 1990.

116. Pendl G, Vorcapic P: Microsurgery of intrinsic midbrain lesions. Acta Neurochir Suppl (Wien) 53:137–143, 1991.

117. Bricollo A, Turrazzi S, Cristofori I, et al: Direct surgery for brain stem tumours. Acta Neurochir Suppl (Wien) 53:148–158, 1991.

118. Vandertop WP, Hoffman HJ, Drake JM, et al: Focal midbrain tumors in children. Neurosurgery 31:186–194, 1992.

119. Behnke J, Christen HJ, Bruck W, et al: Intra-axial endophytic tumors in the pons and/or medulla oblongata. II: Intraoperative findings, postoperative results, and 2-year follow-up in 25 children. Childs Nerv Syst 13:122–134, 1997.

120. Abbott R, Shiminski-Maher T, Epstein FJ: Intrinsic tumors of the medulla: Predicting outcome after surgery. Pediatr Neurosurg 25:41–44, 1996.

121. Xu QW, Bao WM, Mao RI, et al: Surgical treatment of solid brain stem tumors in adults: A report of 22 cases. Surg Neurol 48:30–36, 1997.

122. Farmer JP, Montes JL, Freeman CR, et al: Brain stem gliomas: A 10-year institutional review. Pediatr Neurosurg 34:206–214, 2001.

123. Jallo GI, Freed D, Roonpraunt C, Epstein FJ: Current management of brainstem gliomas. Ann Neurosurg 3:1–17, 2003.

124. Bricolo A: Surgical management of intrinsic brain stem gliomas. In Spetzler F (ed): Operative Techniques in Neurosurgery. Brain Stem Surgery, vol 3, 2000, pp 137–154.

125. Zimmerman RA: Neuroimaging of primary brain stem gliomas: Diagnosis and course. Pediatr Neurosurg 25:45–53, 1996.

126. Fischbein NJ, Prados MD, Wara W: Radiologic classification of brain stem tumors: Correlation of magnetic resonance imaging appearance with clinical outcome. Pediatr Neurosurg 24:9–23, 1996.

127. Beltramello A, Lombardo MC, Massoto B, Bricolo A: Imaging of brain stem tumors: In Spetzler F (ed): Operative Techniques in Neurosurgery. Brain Stem Surgery, vol 3, 2000, pp 87–105.

128. Morota N, Deletis V, Epstein F, et al: Brain stem mapping: Neurophysiological localization of motor nuclei on the floor of the fourth ventricle. Neurosurgery 37:922–930, 1995.

129. Strauss C, Romstock J, Nimsky C: Intraoperative identification of motor areas of the rhomboid fossa using direct stimulation. J Neurosurg 79:393–399, 1993.

130. Hoffman HJ: Dorsally exophytic brain stem tumors and midbrain tumors. Pediatr Neurosurg 24:256–262, 1996.

131. Pollack IF, Hoffman HJ, Hemphreys RP, et al: The long-term outcome after surgical treatment of dorsally exophytic brain stem gliomas. J Neurosurg 78:859–863, 1993.

132. Jallo GI, Kothbauer KF, Epstein FJ: Surgical management of cervicomedullary and dorsally exophytic brain stem tumors. In Spetzler F (ed): Operative Techniques in Neurosurgery. Brain Stem Surgery, vol 3, Philadelphia: WB Saunders 2000, pp 131–136.

133. Squires LA, Constantini S, Epstein F: Diffuse infiltrating astrocytoma of the cervicomedullary region: Clinicopathological entity. Pediatr Neurosurg 27:153–159, 1997.

Section XI

Posterior Fossa Tumors

59

Surgical Management of Cerebellar Hemorrhage and Cerebellar Infarction

ANTONINO RACO

Indication for surgery in patients with cerebellar hemorrhage and infarction remains a controversial topic. Although the treatment of cerebellar hemorrhage has quite a long history in neurosurgical practice, infarction of the cerebellum only recently has been recognized as a surgical emergency. Several algorithms of treatment have been proposed in the past 15 years for patients harboring cerebellar spontaneous hematomas. Those are mainly based on the size of hematoma, the state of consciousness of the patient, and the obliteration of the cisterns of the posterior fossa. Indication for surgery for cerebellar infarction is dependent, again, on the alertness of the patient and the effacement of the quadrigeminal cistern. A more gradual surgical approach is favored in those patients, and possibly half of the cases may be solved just by positioning an external ventricular drainage.

INTRODUCTION

The management of patients with cerebellar infarction or cerebellar hemorrhage remains controversial.[1-18] Before the introduction of computed tomography (CT), the differential diagnosis between the two entities, on clinical grounds alone, was prohibitively difficult.[19,20] Because the coexistence or preponderance of signs and symptoms of brain stem compression further complicate the clinical presentation, diagnosis was frequently possible only at postmortem examination.

The treatment of vascular cerebellar syndromes, particularly hemorrhage, is not a new topic.[21-23] Yet only recently, thanks to the advent of CT and subsequently magnetic resonance imaging (MRI), have neurosurgeons recognized that not only cerebellar hemorrhage but also cerebellar infarction is sometimes a surgical emergency.[24,25]

SURGICAL ANATOMY

The brain stem and the cerebellum are supplied by three pairs of arteries: (1) the posterior inferior cerebellar artery (PICA), (2) the anterior inferior cerebellar artery (AICA), and (3) the superior cerebellar artery (SCA). The three vessels in their arcuate course give branches that supply the brain stem. These arteries anastomose not only with the contralateral arteries, by means of their distal branches, but also with the ipsilateral contiguous arteries. Their terminal branches run along the folia and penetrate into the cerebellar fissures, spreading out into specific areas.[26]

Posterior Inferior Cerebellar Artery

The PICA normally originates from the vertebral artery (82%) 1 to 3 cm caudally from the point where the two vertebral arteries unite in the basilar trunk. In a few cases, it may originate from the basilar artery (10%), from a trunk in common with the AICA (6%), or from the AICA itself (2%).[27]

From its origin, the PICA runs transversally and backward around the bulbus; it then turns upward, continuing along the sulcus, which separates the dorsal part of the bulbus from the cerebellar tonsil. Between the cranial part of the tonsil and the inferior medullary veil, it takes a brusque turn backward and downward, thus forming the tonsillar, choroidal, and bulbar branches.[27] In this way, it reaches the inferior surface of the cerebellum between the vermis and the tonsils, where it divides into two branches, a medial branch and a lateral branch. The medial branch, which is generally smaller, supplies a triangular area with a dorsal base and a ventral apex facing toward the fourth ventricle. This area includes the inferior vermis, nodulus, uvula, pyramis, tuber, and sometimes clivus and the internal part of the inferior semilunar lobe, gracile lobule, and the tonsil.[28]

When the medial branch of the PICA also supplies all or part of the lateral medullary territory,[29] its occlusion leads to Wallenberg's syndrome, although this is an uncommon occurrence (13%).[30] In some cases, anatomic variations may be observed in the territory of distribution: the medial ramus may be the only branch to supply the dorsolateral bulbar region and sometimes the retro-olivar area.[31,32]

The lateral branch of the PICA is larger than the medial branch and supplies the inferior surface of the cerebellar hemisphere and tonsil.[27] Because this branch never supplies the bulbus, its occlusion may go unnoticed.[28]

The hemispheric branches of the PICA always form anastomoses with the hemispheric branches of the AICA and the SCA.

Anterior Inferior Cerebellar Artery

The AICA normally originates from the inferior third of the basilar artery (75% of cases) and sometimes from the middle third. However, it may originate from the vertebral artery or the basilar artery by means of a trunk in common with the PICA.[33] Sometimes, it is double (26%).[33] According to Lazorthes,[34] it is absent in 4% of the population.

From its origin, it runs along the caudal part of the pons, supplying it with branches, and then crosses the abducens nerve; it then reaches the cerebellopontine angle, where it meets the acoustic-facial bundle. At the point where it crosses the acoustic-facial bundle (after giving rise to the labyrinthine artery), it divides into two branches. One branch runs laterally low down toward the anterior inferior portion of the cerebellar hemisphere. The other branch runs laterally and horizontally, forming a loop around the acoustic-facial bundle, to reach the flocculus, the middle cerebellar peduncle, and the middle part of the cerebellar hemisphere, thus forming vessels that supply these structures and the adjacent portion of the pons.

The AICA, therefore, feeds two distinct brain stem territories: (1) the proximal trunk supplies the lateral part of the pons and (2) the lateral branches supply both the middle cerebellar peduncle and the tegmental part of the inferior two thirds of the pons.[33]

The cerebellar structures supplied include the flocculus. This is the only area of the brain stem to be supplied exclusively by the AICA, except in 3% to 5% of cases.[33] In 40% of the population, the AICA terminates in this zone; in the remainder, following the sulcus separating the semilunar lobe and the anterior lobe, it gives rise to terminal branches that supply the nearby lobes: anterior, simplex, superior, and inferior semilunaris; gracilis; and biventer.[34,35]

The AICA may substitute a hypoplastic PICA, supplying its entire distribution territory.[25,28] The terminal branches of the AICA also anastomose with branches of the SCA and PICA.

Superior Cerebellar Artery

Of the three arteries supplying the cerebellum, the SCA is the most constant in caliber and in distribution territory. In most cases, it is single (86%) and less frequently double (14%).[27] It originates from the basilar artery shortly before its bifurcation or, in a few cases (4%),[27] from the posterior cerebral artery.

From its origin, it proceeds dorsally into the perimesencephalic cistern, running along the anterior edge of the pontomesencephalic sulcus, or within it, surrounding the cerebral peduncle. At this point, it gives rise to most of the collateral branches. Its initial segment is separated from the posterior cerebral artery by the common oculomotor nerve. It then divides into two principal branches, a medial branch and a lateral branch, which run parallel to the trochlear nerve.[26]

The medial branch, which runs between the inferior colliculus and the medial portion of the rostral edge of the cerebellum, divides into the vermian and paravermian arteries and occasionally into the intermediate arteries. The vermian arteries supply the ipsilateral rostral half of the vermis. The paravermian branches supply the medial part of the tentorial surface of the cerebellar hemisphere.

The lateral trunk runs around the lateral portion of the rostral edge of the cerebellum. It gives rise to between one and four lateral hemispheric branches and supplies the lateral portion of the tentorial surface of the cerebellum. In general, the SCA supplies most of the tentorial surface of the cerebellum, including the superior vermis, the dentate nucleus, and the superior cerebellar peduncle.[27]

The SCA connects with the AICA and PICA through anastomotic branches. Those between the PICA are particularly long. The anastomoses formed by these posterior cranial fossa vessels explain why clinically evident cerebellar infarction is comparatively less common than hemorrhage.

HISTORICAL BACKGROUND

Spontaneous cerebellar hemorrhage has only recently been identified as a distinct nosologic entity.[22,36] Morgagni and Lieutard were probably the first to recognize a spontaneous cerebellar hemorrhage, which was reported by Sédillot[37] in 1813. The first detailed descriptions of the disease date back to the 18th century. One paper, published in the *Lancet* in 1861, was written by Brown-Sequard[38]; another study was done by Hillairet.[39]

In 1906, Ballance[40] was the first person to describe the successful removal of a cerebellar hemorrhage. More recently, Mitchell and Angrist[36] reviewed a Queen Square series of 115 cases of intracerebral hemorrhage and reported on 15 patients with cerebellar hematoma.

The modern era of treatment for spontaneous cerebellar hemorrhage began with report of McKissock and colleagues[22] in 1960, which was an update of the Queen Square experience based on 34 patients, followed by the report of Fisher and colleagues[20] in 1965. However, at that time, the choice of treatment still depended on clinical criteria that were much less reliable than the imaging methods available today. The advent of CT brought about a great improvement in the surgical results and overall management of these patients. As stated by Little and colleagues[41] in 1978, "the findings of CT investigations proved very helpful in defining appropriate therapy." They allowed the operating surgeon to distinguish patients with pure cerebellar hematomas amenable to surgical treatment from those with primitive brain stem hemorrhage and secondary ventricular involvement. Despite their poor quality compared with modern imaging, the first-generation CT images always permitted a differential diagnosis by exclusion with cerebellar infarction. In this context, the article written by Norris and colleagues[19] in 1969 is interesting for its historical value. One of the paper's subheadings, "Problems in Differential Diagnosis," gives an idea of the difficulties that our neurosurgical colleagues encountered approximately 30 years ago.

Other recent contributions, no longer regarding the diagnosis but the treatment of cerebellar hemorrhage, came from Weisberg[42] in 1986 and Taneda and colleagues[24] in 1987. Weisberg[42] was the first to apply the concept of the tight posterior fossa (TPF) to clinical practice. After reviewing the case records of 20 consecutive patients with CT evidence of cerebellar hemorrhage, he selected 14 patients who had CT features of TPF, which was defined as effacement of the basal cisterns in the posterior fossa and ventricular enlargement consistent with obstructive hydrocephalus. All patients who harbored a TPF had rapid neurologic deterioration, whereas none of the six patients who did not have a TPF deteriorated; all recovered without surgery. One year later, in a large series of 75 patients with cerebellar hemorrhage diagnosed by CT scanning, Taneda and colleagues[24] assessed the relationship between the outcome and the CT appearance of the quadrigeminal cistern. They concluded that "the CT grade of quadrigeminal cistern obliteration is an accurate indicator of outcome and is highly useful in selecting appropriate treatment for patients with cerebellar hemorrhage."

Previously, in 1984, Laun and colleagues[18] had already reviewed their personal experience with seven patients with infarction of the PICA and showed how obliteration of the cisterns of the quadrigeminal plate and Galen's vein was the determining factor when assessing the indications for suboccipital decompressive craniotomy.

During the past decade or so, many investigators have proposed guidelines for the surgical treatment of cerebellar hemorrhage, among them Auer and colleagues,[9] Kobayashi and colleagues,[11] Luparello and Canavero,[12] Salvati and colleagues,[1] and Kirollos and colleagues.[7] Yet none have managed to set the gold standard, namely, to select with absolute certainty the criteria valid for opting between surgical or conservative treatment in these patients.

Compared with hemorrhage in this site, cerebellar infarction attracted neurosurgical interest much more recently. The first to acknowledge cerebellar infarction as a neurosurgical emergency were probably Fairburn and Oliver[43] and Lindgren[44] in 1956. Among the several papers dealing with this subject since then, those published in 1975 by Duncan and colleagues[45] and Sypert and Alvord[46] deserve mention. In a clinicopathologic (two cases) and clinicosurgical description (one case), the former describes the most common type of cerebellar infarction, that of the PICA. Duncan and colleagues[45] emphasized the difficulties in the clinical diagnosis between pure cerebellar infarction and symptoms attributable to concomitant involvement of the brain stem. Interestingly, the clinical diagnosis made in two of the three cases was a benign labyrinthine disorder. The paper by Sypert and Alvord[46] considering 28 patients with acute, massive cerebellar infarction provided a detailed clinicopathologic correlation, which is up to date even today. Evidence of the difficult clinical diagnosis is that the studies published before the advent of CT scan came mainly from large autopsy series.[46] Indeed, Sypert and Alvord emphasized the similarities between the clinical pictures of cerebellar infarction and acute cerebellar hemorrhage, subdural or epidural hematoma, rapidly growing cerebellar tumor, and abscess in the posterior cranial fossa.

During the same period, a French journal published a detailed review of the literature based on 79 cases, including 11 personal ones; the salient feature was the low number of cases operated on (only 17).[8] The papers published in the ensuing years show how the introduction of CT scanning and MRI into clinical practice allowed an early differential diagnosis and hence suitable treatment. It thus represented a turning point in the management of patients with cerebellar infarction. These diagnostic methods have also led to classification of cerebellar infarctions based on anatomic-radiographic criteria and correlations.

In 1995, Mathew and colleagues[13] reported a surgical series of patients with cerebellar infarction predominantly treated conservatively or by external ventricular drainage. Chen and colleagues[17] surgically treated 11 patients with massive cerebellar infarction, by suboccipital decompressive craniectomy and ventricular drainage. In recent years, the papers by Amarenco and colleagues[33,47-50] on cerebellar infarction deserve credit for their new perspective and their contribution to knowledge about the angioarchitecture of

the posterior cranial fossa, as well as for their extremely interesting anatomic clinical correlations, supported by MRI findings. These studies have shed light on the physiopathologic mechanisms underlying territorial and nonterritorial infarction (i.e., a cerebellar infarct <2 cm).[51]

In cerebellar hemorrhage, debate concerns mainly the identification and correlation of the criteria indicating surgical or conservative treatment: the neurologic status of the patient, the size of the hematoma, and the presence of a TPF. Conversely, fewer reports address the surgical management of cerebellar infarction, and this remains controversial. Whereas some investigators believe that most cases respond satisfactorily to external ventricular drainage,[10,13] others advocate treating cerebellar infarcts as space-occupying lesions.[17]

PATHOLOGY

Patients with cerebellar hemorrhage are generally hypertense; some have Charcot-Bouchard microaneurysms of the posterior circulation.[52] Cole and Yates[53] demonstrated these lesions on the larger cerebellar cortical vessels that run along the folia and penetrate deeply within the cerebellar fissures. Most lesions were multiple aneurysms located at the point where the perforating arteries branch in the region of the dentate nucleus.

Using a technique for serial sectioning of the surgical specimen, Wakai and Nagai,[54] in 14 patients with lobar intracerebral hemorrhage or cerebellar hemorrhage without vascular abnormalities on angiograms, detected definite microaneurysms in five patients and probable ones in two others. Histopathologic studies may disclose small angiomas known as cryptic vascular malformations, which are no longer identifiable after massive hemorrhage.[55]

The cerebellar hemorrhage typical of a microaneurysm is generally located deep in the region of the dentate nucleus. The vessels most frequently involved are the SCA and the AICA. Most patients are elderly and frequently present with concomitant systemic diseases, such as diabetes, liver disease, and hematologic disorders.

Conversely, patients with cerebellar infarction mainly have embolic disease. The finding of atrial flutter and cardiac ischemia in these patients evinces the cardiac origin of this disease. In their study of 88 cases, Amarenco and colleagues[48] found that 43% of infarcts were cardioembolic and 35% were atherosclerotic.

Symptomatic cerebellar infarction mainly affects the vertebral artery, usually unilaterally but in rare cases bilaterally, at the origin of the PICA. The PICA is, therefore, the most frequently affected vessel.

Reports have evaluated the concept of territorial infarcts involving the full territory of a cerebellar artery or its branches, as opposed to border zone or nonterritorial infarcts.[51] Territorial infarction has a thromboembolic mechanism, frequently due to cardioembolism. Nonterritorial infarcts may be caused by small emboli, usually in a clinical setting of hypercoagulation; sometimes the mechanism is hemodynamic. Amarenco and Caplan affirmed that most SCA infarcts are embolic.[56] AICA infarcts arise equally from embolic and atherosclerotic occlusions, whereas PICA infarcts are predominantly atherosclerotic.

Nonterritorial infarcts rarely present a surgical indication. Of all territorial infarcts, those of the PICA most frequently require surgical treatment not only because they are the most common but also for anatomic reasons.

As Sypert and Alvord[46] emphasized in their detailed anatomicopathologic study, more than 40% of patients with cerebellar infarction have hypertension. In their series of 88 cases, Amarenco and colleagues[48] noted that as many as 64% were hypertense.

PREOPERATIVE AND POSTOPERATIVE DIAGNOSTIC PROTOCOL

On admission to our hospital, patients with cerebellar hemorrhage are evaluated neurologically by means of standard neurologic tests as well as by other grading systems such as the Glasgow Coma Scale (GCS).[57] A scrupulous general clinical examination, together with a complete battery of laboratory tests, completes the initial evaluation.

The preoperative diagnostic imaging workup includes a CT study of the brain as well as an MRI, if necessary and feasible. In doubtful cases, magnetic resonance angiography completes the diagnostic protocol. CT or MRI allows assessment of a series of variables that we believe to be important for prognostic evaluation and therapeutic purposes. These are essentially as follows:

Location of the hemorrhage (vermian, hemispheric, or both)
Size of the hemorrhage (the two major diameters in millimeters)
Presence of blood in the ventricles (particularly the fourth ventricle)
Invasion of blood into the brain stem
Presence of hydrocephalus
Signs of brain stem impairment
Presence and extent of perilesional edema
Evidence of TPF, according to the criteria established by Weisberg[42]

Weisberg defined the anatomic and radiographic features of TPF as obliteration of the basal cisterns in the posterior cranial fossa; enlargement of the third ventricle and lateral ventricles, including the temporal horns; and effacement of the fourth ventricle (inconstant).

In addition to the imaging criteria, we also assess the presence of preexisting or concomitant medical problems, including diabetes, arterial hypertension, hematologic disorders, and liver disease. We base our clinical assessment not only on the evolution of disease but also on a serial study using the same criteria used for the initial evaluation (general clinical and neurologic evaluation, GCS score, and laboratory tests).

In the Department of Neurology and Neurosurgery, we also see patients with suspected cerebellar infarction. However, unlike patients with hemorrhage who undergo priority transferral to the neurosurgical department, those with suspected infarcts are admitted to a neurologic ward or neurologic stroke unit, depending on their initial status. After admission, detailed background information is obtained on preexisting or concomitant medical conditions and family history. We then evaluate on CT and MRI the following parameters that are essential for prognosis and therapy:

Location of the infarct
Size of the infarct
Involvement of one or more arterial districts
Secondary hemorrhagic infarction of the ischemic area

Presence of hydrocephalus
Presence and amount of perilesional edema
Signs of brain stem compression

During the ensuing days, the initial assessment is repeated (preferably using the GCS).[57]

PERSONAL EXPERIENCE

During the past 10 years in our department, we have treated 70 patients with cerebellar hemorrhage (39 men and 31 women, with a mean age of 64 years) and 52 patients with cerebellar infarction (26 men and 26 women, with a mean age of 58 years). Patients with cerebellar hemorrhage showed a slight male preponderance, whereas the median age was almost the same in both groups (Table 59-1).

Our patients with cerebellar hemorrhage typically presented with a clinical picture of rapid onset. Their symptoms began on average 13 hours before admission. On admission, most patients showed rapidly deteriorating neurologic status: 60% of the patients were in coma, and 22% had unmistakable signs of intracranial hypertension. In patients with cerebellar infarction, the initial symptoms had a less sudden onset. Between the onset of the clinical picture and the patient's admission to the hospital, an average of 19 hours had elapsed. Our patients with cerebellar infarction typically presented clinically with symptoms of dizziness, nausea, vomiting, and sometimes headache, whereas those with cerebellar hemorrhage first had a headache, which was described as a piercing and continuous pain centered in the neck and typically radiating toward the posterior cervical region (Table 59-2). Cerebellar symptoms were predictably common in both diseases.

TABLE 59-1 ▪ Clinical Characteristics of the 122 Patients with Cerebellar Hemorrhage and Infarction in Our Series

Cerebellar Hemorrhage (70 Cases)	Cerebellar Infarction (52 Cases)
Male, 39 (56%)	Male, 26 (50%)
Female, 31 (44%)	Female, 26 (50%)
Median age, 64 yr	Median age, 58 yr
Median presentation, 13 hr	Median presentation, 19 hr

TABLE 59-2 ▪ Presenting Symptoms and Glasgow Coma Scale Score in 122 Patients

Cerebellar Hemorrhage (70 Patients)		Symptoms	Cerebellar Infarction (52 Patients)	
56 (80%)		Headache	21 (40%)	
44 (65%)		Nausea, vomiting	24 (46%)	
15 (21%)		Vertigo	22 (44%)	
GCS, 3–6	6 (8%)		GCS, 3–6	4 (8%)
GCS, 7–11	30 (43%)		GCS, 7–11	11 (21%)
GCS, 12–13	16 (23%)		GCS, 12–13	27 (52%)
GCS, 14–15	18 (26%)		GCS, 14–15	10 (19%)

CGS, Glasgow Coma Scale

TABLE 59-3 ▪ Risk Factors for Cerebellar Hemorrhage and Infarction in Our Series

Cerebellar Hemorrhage (70 Patients)		Cerebellar Infarction (52 Patients)	
Hypertension	42 (60%)	Hypertension	21 (40%)
Diabetes	13 (19%)	Recent cardiac infarction	9 (17%)
Hematologic disease	12 (17%)	Hematologic disease	3 (6%)
Liver disease	7 (10%)	Atrial flutter	4 (8%)
		Endocarditis with vegetations	2 (4%)
		Patent foramen ovale	2 (4%)

Most of our patients with cerebellar hematomas were hypertensive; some had diabetes, hematologic disorders, or liver disease. Conversely, patients with cerebellar infarction sometimes had potentially embolic disease, such as recent cardiac infarctions or atrial flutter, endocarditis with vegetations, or a patent foramen ovale. Again, some of these patients (40%) were hypertensive (Table 59-3). Spontaneous cerebellar hemorrhages occurred more frequently at a vermian site than at a hemispheric site. Later blood invasion into the fourth ventricle or into the lateral ventricles was common. Approximately half of these patients had coexisting hypertensive hydrocephalus. In 38% of cases, these abnormalities led to the diagnosis of a TPF (Table 59-4).

The criteria for establishing the surgical indications for cerebellar hemorrhage in our department are extremely strict. For this reason, in this series, patients with hemispheric hematomas that exceeded a maximal diameter of 40 mm and a minimal diameter of 30 mm or vermian hematomas more than 35 mm and less than 25 mm and with a GCS score of less than 13 underwent surgery. The identification of a TPF reduced by 10 mm the diameters indicating surgery. The remaining patients received conservative treatment with 18% mannitol solution and corticosteroids. Surgery consisted of removal of the hematoma. A lobectomy was undertaken only for hematomas that occupied more than 80% of the total lobar volume. Patients who had been in deep coma for several hours before admission to the

TABLE 59-4 ▪ Associated Hydrocephalus, Site of the Hematoma and Artery Involved in the Infarction in 122 Patients

Cerebellar Hemorrhage (70 Patients)		Cerebellar Infarction (52 Patients)	
Hydrocephalus	29 (41%)	Hydrocephalus	11 (22%)
Hemorrhage, vermian	24 (34%)	Infarction AICA*	5 (10%)
		Infarction SCA*	2 (4%)
Hemorrhage, hemispheric	39 (56%)	Infarction PICA*	29 (56%)
Hemorrhage, both	7 (10%)	Infarction Massive*	12 (23%)
Tight posterior fossa	19 (38%)		

*Three cases (7%). The artery responsible for the infarction could not be detected with certainty.
PICA, posterior inferior cerebellar artery; AICA, anterior inferior cerebellar artery; SCA, superior cerebellar artery.

TABLE 59-5 ▪ Management of the 122 Patients with Cerebellar Hemorrhage and Infarction

Cerebellar Hemorrhage (70 Patients)	Cerebellar Infarction (52 Patients)
20 Treated conservatively	30 Treated conservatively
7 TLD	2 TLD
43 Treated surgically	20 Treated surgically
30 SC + EVD	6 SC + EVD
13 SC	5 SC
	9 EVD

Nine patients with cerebellar hemorrhage and one patient with cerebellar infarct had a definitive ventriculoperitoneal shunt placement.
TLD, treatment-limiting decision; EVD, external ventricular drainage; SC, suboccipital craniectomy.

hospital did not undergo surgery. Of the 30 patients treated by craniectomy and placement of external drainage, nine patients subsequently needed placement of a permanent ventriculoperitoneal shunt (Table 59-5). Most of the patients needed postoperative mechanical ventilation, which was continued on average for 48 hours. Preoperative and postoperative antibiotic prophylaxis practically eliminated the risks of local surgical sepsis but had no effect on the risk of bronchopulmonary infection, which is a frequent postoperative complication in our series. Hypertensive hydrocephalus, which is always treated promptly, did not influence the prognosis. Vermian hematomas had no less favorable an outcome than did hemispheric hematomas, possibly because we used distinct criteria for establishing the surgical indications for the two sites. Age did not unfavorably affect the course of the illness. Conversely, the presence of two or more general risk factors significantly influenced both mortality and the subsequent quality of life, despite preoperative attempts to restore normal function (e.g., by infusion of plasma and platelet supplements in patients with blood or coagulation disorders) before undertaking surgical treatment.

More than half of our patients with cerebellar hemorrhage had a good postoperative functional recovery. The overall mortality rate was 27% (Table 59-6).

The surgical indications for cerebellar infarction, unlike those for hemorrhage, depend almost entirely on the patient's clinical conditions. In this series, we resorted to surgery much less frequently in patients with cerebellar infarction than in patients with hematoma. Most patients

TABLE 59-6 ▪ Management and Mortality in the 122 Patients with Cerebellar Hemorrhage and Infarction

Cerebellar Hemorrhage (70 Patients)		Cerebellar Infarction (52 Patients)	
Overall mortality	19 (27%)	Overall mortality	8 (16%)
Operated cases	11 (16%)	Operated cases	3 (6%)
Treated conservatively	2 (3%)	Treated conservatively	2 (4%)
Not treated (coma depassé)	6 (9%)	Not treated (coma depassé)	2 (4%)

received conservative treatment with dexamethasone and mannitol. Patients whose clinical condition required surgery underwent placement of temporary ventricular drainage.

Eleven of 52 patients in this series underwent suboccipital craniectomy and removal of necrotic tissue; in six of them, an external ventricular drainage was previously placed. Another nine patients were treated only by external ventricular drainage (see Table 59-5) One patient needed placement of a permanent ventriculoperitoneal shunt.

Two thirds of our patients with cerebellar infarction had a good postoperative recovery. The overall mortality rate was 16% (see Table 59-6).

Case Reports

CASE REPORT 1

This 71-year-old man, with a history of untreated hypertension, presented with the sudden onset of a piercing occipital headache. This man, who was initially admitted to another hospital, had a brain CT scan that detected a 40 × 30-mm hematoma in the right cerebellar hemisphere with effacement of cisterns, slight ventricular dilatation, and secondary intraventricular hemorrhage (Fig. 59-1A to C). While undergoing the scan, the patient

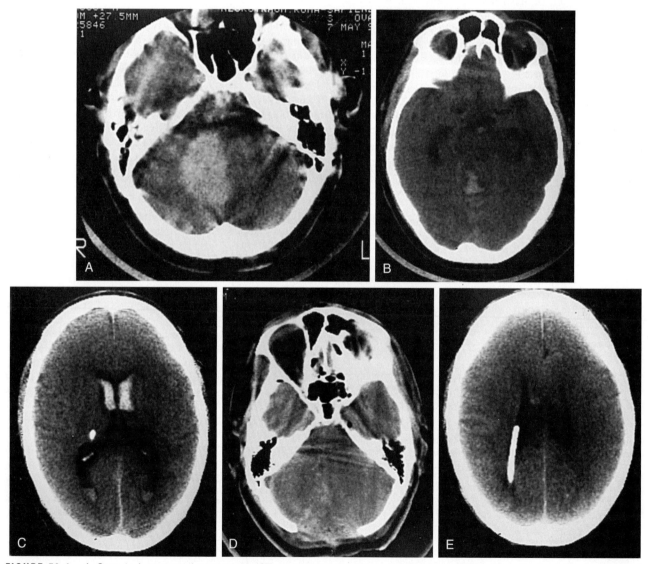

FIGURE 59-1   *A*, Case 1: A computed tomography (CT) scan shows a large acute right hemispheric cerebellar hematoma. *B*, Case 1: A CT scan shows effacement of the perimesencephalic cistern and initial dilatation of the temporal horns of the lateral ventricle. *C*, Case 1: A CT scan demonstrates a supratentorial intraventricular hemorrhage in the same patient. *D*, Case 1: A postoperative CT scan shows evacuation of the hematoma. *E*, Case 1: A postoperative CT scan shows ventricular drainage, which is inserted through the right occipital horn and left in place, partially resolving obstructive hydrocephalus.

presented progressive impairment of consciousness, and he was therefore transferred on an emergency basis to our department for treatment. Because the patient was stuporous on admission and unable to obey commands, cerebellar function could not be tested: Babinski's sign was detectable bilaterally and breathing was arrhythmic.

The size of the hematoma, the effacement of cisterns in the posterior fossa, and the evolving clinical picture called for an immediate emergency surgical procedure. The patient underwent a right suboccipital craniectomy, the hematoma was removed, and a drainage system was inserted through the occipital horn in the right lateral ventricle and left in situ. After surgery, the patient's clinical status immediately improved. The patient was discharged 9 days later; he was mildly ataxic and had right cerebellar incoordination (see Fig. 59-1D, E).

CASE REPORT 2

This 29-year-old woman with a history of diabetes presented to our emergency department after falling off her bicycle because of the onset of dizziness, severe nausea, and vomiting. On admission to the hospital, a neurologic examination showed severe impairment of consciousness, bilateral cerebellar incoordination, and cerebellar dysarthria.

The CT scan showed a large cerebellar hematoma that measured 5.5 × 3.8 cm with extensive intraventricular spread of blood above and below the tentorium. It also showed marked ventricular dilatation with a blood clot within the lateral ventricles and the third ventricle (Fig. 59-2A and B). In the meantime, the patient's overall neurologic status deteriorated and decerebrate posture developed.

The patient underwent an emergency removal of the hematoma and insertion of a ventricular drainage system through the right frontal horn (see Fig. 59-2C and D). Mechanical ventilation was maintained for 48 hours. Approximately 72 hours after surgery, the patient's neurologic conditions improved, and a permanent ventriculoperitoneal shunt was placed. Nine days later, the patient was able to walk again. Two years later, she lives a normal life without neurologic sequelae.

CASE REPORT 3

A young boy, aged 9, was admitted to our pediatric department for investigation of a progressive syndrome characterized by vertigo, nausea, and vomiting. The boy had an acute headache. His body temperature was slightly increased (37.6°C). He had previously been diagnosed as having polymyositis. The other interesting finding was a family history of cerebral stroke. Three years earlier, the patient's father had suffered an MRI-documented left middle cerebral artery stroke, which left him with right hemiparesis. The patient's chest radiographs, electrocardiogram, and blood tests were unremarkable. The neurologic examination revealed mild ataxia and cerebellar incoordination.

An MRI scan done on the third day showed a cerebellar infarction in the right PICA territory, whereas magnetic resonance angiography showed the absence of PICA filling on the right side (Fig. 59-3A to C).

Conservative therapy was begun with 60 mL of 18% mannitol solution every 6 hours and 1.5 mg dexamethasone every 8 hours plus gastric protection with cimetidine. Bed rest was continued for another week, and the patient's symptoms slowly subsided. Residual symptoms consisted of mild ataxia and right dysmetria.

CASE REPORT 4

A 64-year-old woman with diabetes experienced the sudden onset of nausea and vomiting followed by vertigo. She was admitted to the emergency department of our hospital, where neurologic examination revealed gait ataxia and right-sided pyramidal tract signs. She complained of a persistent occipital headache. An electrocardiogram showed an atrial flutter, whereas the echocardiogram disclosed nothing remarkable. The result of the CT scan was negative. Nevertheless, therapy was begun with 4 mg dexamethasone every 8 hours. Within 2 days, the symptoms had abated except for the headache. Another CT scan (Fig. 59-4A) detected a hypodense lesion in the medial left cerebellar hemisphere that was compatible with occlusion of the left PICA. For the next 3 days, 100 mL of 18% mannitol solution every 6 hours was added to the patient's therapy. An MRI scan (see Fig. 59-4B) confirmed the CT findings. The patient did not undergo magnetic resonance angiography. She had a complete functional recovery and was discharged 5 days later.

DISCUSSION

For its definition as a distinct nosologic entity, cerebellar hemorrhage had to await the coming of the CT era. The diagnostic and semeiotic means available before the advent of CT scanning made cerebellar hemorrhage extremely difficult to recognize. Hence, the surgical indications, relying as they did on indirect signs of the lesion alone, were also extremely imprecise. This shortcoming explains the considerable discrepancy between the various mortality rates reported in the literature throughout the years, from 73.5% reported by McKissock and colleagues[22] in 1960 to 20% reported by Luparello and Canavero[12] in 1995.

Spontaneous cerebellar hemorrhages occur predominantly in the older age groups, from the sixth to the eighth decades,[9,11,13,15,24] both in our experience and in published series. However, this preference for elderly patients does not necessarily correspond with a less favorable prognosis, either in terms of mortality or quality of life nor does the patient's clinical status on admission influence operative mortality as long as surgery is done immediately.

In our experience, the location of the hematoma in the vermis rather than the cerebellar hemispheres did not seem to influence the prognosis compared with other recent reports,[11,12] nor did hypertensive hydrocephalus seem to affect the prognosis unfavorably as long as the condition was diagnosed and treated without delay. The presence of

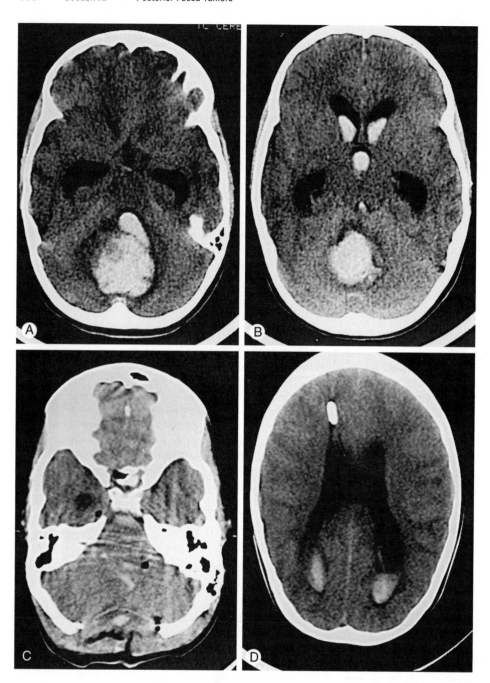

FIGURE 59-2 *A,* Case 2: A computed tomography (CT) scan shows a large acute vermian hematoma with marked dilatation of the temporal horn of the lateral ventricles. *B,* Case 2: A CT scan shows the disappearance of the perimesencephalic cistern and an intraventricular blood clot. *C,* Case 2: A CT scan shows the evacuation of the hematoma. *D,* Case 2: The CT scan demonstrates a ventricular catheter inserted through the right frontal horn.

general risk factors (e.g., diabetes, arterial hypertension, hematologic disorders, and liver disease), if considered singly, had no significant influence on survival. However, a combination of two or more risk factors statistically worsened the prognosis, as did the invasion of blood into the brain stem.

Neuroradiographic diagnosis plays an essential role in the staging of patients with hemorrhage.[9,10,11,14,24,41] For early recognition of the disease, because MRI yields no better results than CT scanning, its higher costs hardly justify its use as an emergency procedure. Blood invasion into the brain stem, the presence of hypertensive hydrocephalus, blood in the ventricular system, and the size of the hematoma can be easily evaluated on unenhanced CT scans. For characterizing the bleeding in doubtful cases, MRI gives more detailed information on small vessel malformations and is ideal for studying the brain stem. Magnetic resonance angiography also allows noninvasive evaluation of eventual vascular abnormalities in this region.

As opposed to expansive lesions in the posterior cranial fossa, the role of perilesional edema is unimportant. It also has little practical value because it is overshadowed by the role played by the compressive and destructive phenomena triggered by the hematoma.

Much controversy surrounds the indications for surgical treatment, especially the choice of criteria for the surgical

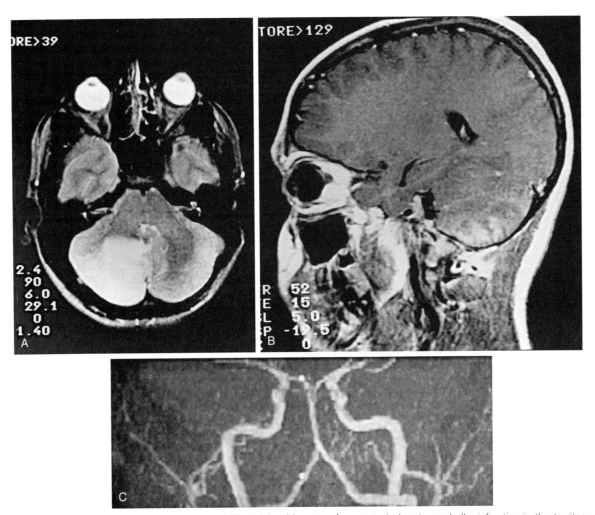

FIGURE 59-3   *A,* Case 3: Magnetic resonance axial T2-weighted images of an acute ischemic cerebellar infarction in the territory of the right posteroinferior cerebellar artery (PICA). *B,* Case 3: Sagittal T1-weighted images with gadolinium enhancement in the same patient. *C,* Case 3: Angiomagnetic resonance imaging in a coronal section shows the absence of filling of the right PICA.

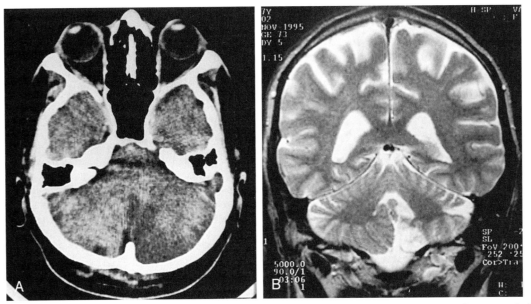

FIGURE 59-4   *A,* Case 4: A computed tomography (CT) scan performed 48 hours after the onset of symptoms of acute cerebellar infarction in the left posteroinferior cerebellar artery (PICA) territory. *B,* Case 4: Coronal T2-weighted magnetic resonance images of the same patient show occlusion of the left medial branch of the PICA.

indications.[1,4,7,9–13,20,24,41,42] Obviously, the more prognostic factors assessed, the more reliable they are for predicting the outcome. Conversely, unduly strict adherence to these criteria may cause the surgeon's personal judgment acquired by experience to go unheeded.

Our experience suggests that a vermian hematoma larger than 35 × 25 mm or a hemispheric hematoma larger than 40 × 30 mm represents an indication for surgery because hematomas of this size invariably lead to altered consciousness. The rationale for the distinction in size between vermian and hemispheric hematomas is that vermian hematomas lie closer to the brain stem and cerebrospinal fluid (CSF) pathways. Whether patients who belong in one of the two aforementioned categories but have a GCS score of 13 or more should undergo surgery remains debatable, as reported also by Kobayashi and colleagues.[11] Although we have not personally dealt with a similar clinicoradiographic presentation, we would implement a "watchful, armed wait-and-see" strategy. This type of management seems to be justified by the scarce clinical and neuroimaging progression observed in almost all our patients who were not operated on and whose initial clinical conditions were satisfactory.

Although we have no experience with CT-guided stereotactic fibrinolysis techniques for removal of the hematoma, published data imply that this procedure is effective for hematomas that are considered borderline, namely, those on the borderline between conservative and surgical treatment.[14]

Third ventriculocisternostomy according to Roux and colleagues[58] is a maneuver that may be used even in an emergency in those patients with cerebellar hematomas who do not need evacuation of the clot.

In our series, there were no cases of "spontaneous" cerebellar hemorrhage after supratentorial craniotomy, which was first described by Koenig and colleagues[59] and then by Van Loon and colleagues[15] in two of 49 cases of their series. In the series described by Toczek and colleagues,[60] this event accounted for almost 5% of complications after temporal lobectomy.

On the same subject, Honegger and colleagues[61] recently reported an incidence of cerebellar hemorrhage of 0.6% in all patients undergoing supratentorial surgery; this figure reached 12.9% in those patients who underwent temporal lobe resection. Friedman and colleagues,[62] in their retrospective study on 42 patients with remote cerebellar hemorrhage, focused on the risk factors (i.e., preoperative aspirin use and moderately elevated intraoperative systolic blood pressure) for developing remote cerebellar hemorrhage. The authors emphasized as well the benign course of the lesion, which in most cases was an incidental finding on postoperative CT.

Remote cerebellar hemorrhage has also been reported after spinal surgery.[63] Dural opening with loss of CSF is the mechanism invoked in the pathogenesis of this condition, whereas patient positioning during surgery does not seem to play a causative role.

One concept that requires careful evaluation is the presence of a TPF.[42] Obliteration of the cisterns does not only depend on the size of the hematoma. Hematomas of similar size may exert widely differing amounts of compression on the cisterns. The amount of compression probably depends also on various factors, including the patient's age, the amount of cerebellar atrophy, and the anatomy of the posterior cranial fossa. Therefore, identification of a TPF justifies

changing the aforementioned surgical criteria, reducing by 10 mm the diameters indicating surgical treatment.

Kirollos and colleagues[7] recently reported a prospective treatment protocol based on the appearance on CT of the fourth ventricle, adjacent to the hematoma. The appearance of the fourth ventricle was divided in three grades (normal, compressed, or completely effaced). Although the completely effaced fourth ventricle was considered a mandatory indication for surgery, neither the level of consciousness of the patient nor the size of the hematoma was initially considered when choosing the appropriate treatment.

The duration of hospitalization of these patients depends on how delicate and functionally important the surrounding brain is. The role of mechanical ventilation, when necessary, is predictably important for improving the prognosis for these patients. Conversely, prophylactic postoperative mechanical ventilation seems to be unnecessary if blood gas analysis values and assessment of autonomous ventilation immediately after the operation come within even the lowest values of the normal range.

Our strategy in managing comatose patients with cerebellar hemorrhage differs from that of others.[16] Patients who are admitted in deep coma or with flaccid paralysis or loss of brain stem reflexes that lasts for more than 2 hours do not undergo surgery.

Of the simple, standardized methods for assessing the outcome of patients with cerebellar hemorrhage on admission, the one most commonly used is the GCS.[57] Even though the use of such a scale renders clinical evaluation less precise and less descriptive, it helps greatly with comparison of results. Despite these advantages, use of the GCS for the preoperative evaluation of patients with cerebellar hemorrhage is open to criticism. The GCS was conceived for patients with head injuries, many of whom present with neurologic deterioration "due to a supratentorial pathology and consequent transtentorial herniation."[57] This scale focuses on the level of consciousness and motor responsiveness of the patient. Heros emphasized how "unresponsiveness and posturing" have different prognostic implications when the cause is a posterior fossa mass rather than herniation from a supratentorial mass.[64]

Particularly gratifying, considering their poor conditions on admittance, was the return of our patients to social activities. Most of the elderly patients almost reverted to their prepathologic level of activity.

Acknowledgment of direct surgical treatment of cerebellar infarct as a lifesaving maneuver is even more recent than treatment of cerebellar hemorrhage. In most cases, conservative treatment was preferred, particularly in the past, and the first surgically treated cases date back only as far as the mid-1950s.[43,44] The true incidence of infarction of a cerebellar hemisphere is unknown and difficult to assess.[47] Contrary to previous beliefs, cerebellar infarction seems to be much more frequent than cerebellar hemorrhage, at least in CT studies[10] and postmortem series.[46] In the report of Amarenco and colleagues[48] of 190 cases of cerebellar stroke, 85% were infarcts and 15% were hemorrhages. One explanation is the high incidence of asymptomatic (nonterritorial) cerebellar infarcts in diagnostic and postmortem series. Alternatively, some symptomatic cerebellar infarcts may be misdiagnosed.

In surgical series, similar numbers of patients with hemorrhage and with infarction undergo operation. Of 60 cases reported by Turgut and colleagues,[65] 39 were spontaneous cerebellar hemorrhages and 21 were infarcts; of the 89 cases reported by Mathew and colleagues,[13] 50 were infarcts and 39 were cerebellar hemorrhages. This finding implies that, despite autopsy observations and a wealth of CT and MRI studies, cerebellar infarcts still receive less attention than they deserve. In cases of infarction, MRI shows an area of increased signal on T2-weighted images, whereas CT scans depict an area of hypodensity that is not usually detected in the first hours. Because of the limited CT scan resolution owing to the bony artifacts in the posterior cranial fossa, many cerebellar infarcts are overlooked initially.

Cerebellar infarcts may be due not only to atherosclerosis or acute vertebral artery occlusion of cardioembolic origin but also to various pathogenic causes, including cervical manipulation,[66] trauma,[67] use of drugs such as cocaine,[68] and intra-extracranial dissection of vertebral arteries.[69] They may also represent the presenting symptom of polycythemia[70] or the result of the prolonged, although reversible, vasospasm that is sometimes associated with some migraine syndromes or linked to congenital odontoid aplasia.[71]

Our series highlighted several differences between patients with cerebellar hemorrhage and infarction. First, patients with cerebellar infarction had a slightly lower average age than did patients with spontaneous cerebellar hemorrhage. In addition, patients with hemorrhage had a worse neurologic status evaluated according to the GCS.[47] Signs of brain stem compression also appear later in infarction than in hemorrhage. Cerebellar dysfunction is more frequent because the neurosurgeon has longer to evaluate the course of the illness in patients with infarction who tend to go into coma later and less frequently than patients with hemorrhage.

In the past few years, many published papers have addressed the clinical topographic correlations supplied by CT and above all by MRI.[47,72] For this reason, we now know exactly which clinical pictures correspond with occlusion of the various arteries that supply the cerebellum.[73] In SCA infarcts, the clinical presentation is characterized by gait and limb ataxia, which are often accompanied by nystagmus.[70] In patients whose infarcts involve the lateral branch of the SCA, dysmetria, dysarthria, and axial lateropulsion predominate.[50] Vertigo and headache are much less common.

AICA infarcts are characterized by a pure vestibular syndrome or otherwise by dysmetria, Horner's syndrome, vestibular signs, contralateral pain and temperature sensory loss in the limbs, and facial sensory impairment.[33]

Last, patients with PICA infarcts present with vertigo, headache, and gait imbalance. Nystagmus is a predominant sign and is sometimes associated with Wallenberg's syndrome with ipsilateral limb ataxia.[73] A comparison of the results of our series with other published data shows that cerebellar infarction requires open surgery less frequently than does hemorrhage because in some cases medical treatment[23] or external ventricular drainage will suffice.[10] In cerebellar hemorrhage, hydrocephalus is generally due to secondary blood extravasation into the fourth ventricle, whereas in cerebellar infarction, it arises from necrotic tissue obstructing the CSF pathways. This could explain why in our series cerebellar hemorrhages more often required a permanent ventriculoperitoneal shunt. Only 1 of 15 patients with cerebellar infarcts treated by an external shunt required

a permanent ventriculoperitoneal shunt. Because none of them had intraventricular blood, once medical treatment or external drainage had resolved the acute edematous phase, CSF circulation returned to normal. Conversely, nine of our patients with cerebellar hemorrhage needed a permanent ventriculoperitoneal shunt.

The choice of the most appropriate surgical treatment in patients with cerebellar infarction is still controversial. Many neurosurgeons have emphasized the success of surgical resection of the necrotic tissue in the infarcted territory.[19,43–45] Others have reported good results with ventricular drainage and conservative management.[10]

Other noteworthy publications on the surgical management of cerebellar infarction include two studies[74,75] by the same authors. The first,[74] a pilot study conducted retrospectively, compares the results in a group of patients in deep coma (stuporous or with posturing or cardiovascular instability and pinpoint pupils) with cerebellar infarcts treated by ventriculostomy. The results were significantly worse than those observed in a clinically matched group of patients who were treated prospectively with decompressive craniotomy. The second,[75] conducted as a prospective observational multicenter trial, supports the notion that the level of consciousness is the most powerful predictor of outcome, superior to any other clinical sign and treatment assignment. These investigators, nevertheless, favor a gradual therapeutic approach that consists of medical therapy for awake patients, ventriculostomy for patients with hydrocephalus, and decompressive craniotomy for patients with signs and symptoms of brain stem compression.[74]

A paper recently published on stroke tried to define the neuroimaging criteria predictive of deterioration in patients with cerebellar infarction and mass effect.[3] According to the authors, although hydrocephalus, brain stem deformity, and basal cistern compression may herald deterioration, vertical displacement of the tonsils or aqueduct demonstrated on MRI examination did not predict deterioration.

We also opted for "specific" and "gradual" therapy. It depended specifically on clinical evaluation of the patients' neurologic conditions to detect signs of endocranial hypertension or brain stem compression. Therapy also included CT scanning or MRI to detect hydrocephalus or brain stem compression. Patients who, despite conservative therapy, fail to show neurologic improvement or display radiographic signs of brain stem compression should undergo decompressive craniectomy and removal of the necrotic tissue.

In "awake" patients without symptoms of endocranial hypertension or signs of compression of the brain stem and ventricles, therapy to reduce edema is indicated, accompanied by frequent clinical and radiographic monitoring.[9,18,74] We disagree with those who warn that in cerebellar infarction positioning an external ventricular drainage system carries a real risk of upward transtentorial herniation. This undesirable complication can be virtually avoided by regulating CSF flow while simultaneously monitoring the patient's neurologic condition.

External drainage may also be criticized because it fails to decompress the brain stem. However, the good results obtained in our series (as in others) demonstrate that, in most cases, deterioration of the patient's neurologic status and level of consciousness coincided with the increase of intracranial pressure caused by obstructive hydrocephalus.[10]

In cerebellar hemorrhage, conversely, the risks of an upward transtentorial herniation invariably contraindicate external ventricular drainage without a preceding decompressive craniectomy. In the series described by Van Loon and colleagues,[15] two of 26 patients treated by immediate ventricular drainage had upward herniation, and one of these patients died. In the series of McKissock and colleagues,[22] all nine patients who were treated by ventricular drainage alone died; in some of these patients, sudden deterioration occurred after ventricular tapping. Transtentorial upward herniation, therefore, remains a possible event in patients with cerebellar hemorrhage treated solely by ventricular drainage.

A recently published paper on neuropsychological disturbances in patients with cerebellar infarcts deserves attention.[76] Fifteen patients with isolated cerebellar infarcts were submitted to a neuropsychological test battery, and the results were compared with those of a control group. Patients with cerebellar infarcts exhibited significantly lower neuropsychological performance compared with the control group. At 1-year follow-up, performance tended to improve. The cerebellum may play a role in addition to that of control of the motor function, which is not fully clarified.

Surgical Technique

The surgical treatment of cerebellar hemorrhage and infarction is generally a straightforward, standardized technique. In our department, we do not routinely use anesthetic gases. Anesthesia is induced with the aid of barbiturates such as sodium thiopental or propofol and maintained with the use of an analgesic (fentanyl) and a neuroleptic. Muscle relaxation is obtained and maintained with pancuronium bromide and vecuronium.

After being intubated by the oral or nasotracheal route, the patient is placed supine on the operating table. We prefer nasotracheal intubation whenever we consider that the patient's condition could benefit from postoperative mechanical ventilation.

Monitoring involves a series of variables, including cardiac activity, blood gases, arterial pressure, urinary output, and rectal temperature.

The head is completely shaved and immobilized using the three-point headrest. For a predominantly vermian hematoma that only partially involves the cerebellar hemisphere, a median incision is made 2 cm above the inion as far as the spinous process of the fourth cervical vertebra. A Y-shaped incision is made in the deep fascia; the V-shaped portion of the incision of the fascia is lifted up and retracted posteriorly with silk sutures, and, using the electric scalpel, the median raphe is identified and cut to expose the spinous process of C2. The muscles with insertion on the occipital squama are partly incised, again with a Y-shaped incision, and superiorly retracted with the fascia. They are then partly detached laterally and maintained in situ with a self-retaining retractor. Once the occipital squama has been exposed, several burr holes are made, and a bone forceps is used to complete the craniectomy. Our experience suggests a wide craniectomy.

A Y-shaped incision of the dura mater is made, retracting the V-shaped flap superiorly and posteriorly with 3-0 silk sutures; the fixed flaps are retracted and suspended with 3-0 silk sutures. If the hematoma principally involves the cerebellar hemisphere, we prefer a paramedian incision; subsequently, the technique is similar to that used for exposing a neurinoma of the eighth cranial nerve. Although the craniectomy need not be extended as far as the transverse sinus and sigmoid sinus,[71] it should be wide enough to allow treatment of an unsuspected pathologic condition, such as a hemorrhagic tumor or a vascular malformation.

Once the cerebellar surface has been exposed, a cortical incision is made that provides the most direct access yet the least injury to the cerebellar parenchyma and vessels. The hematoma is evacuated using a suction and irrigation technique. When most of the hematoma has been removed, the surgical microscope is brought into the operating field and the remaining clots are removed using forceps; thus, possible sources of bleeding are identified and coagulated. In our experience, bleeding rarely arises from a single source such as a single artery; it originates most often from the cavity walls and can be controlled using a hemostatic gelatin sponge or fibrillar collagen that is left in situ.

Hemostasis should be meticulous. To identify any persistent bleeding site, we usually increase the patient's blood pressure approximately 20 mm Hg over the monitored preoperative pressure. As a further check for eventual residual bleeding, the cavity is irrigated several times with a saline solution before closure. The dura mater is then closed with a continuous suture. Several dural suspension stitches are placed along the border of the craniectomy, and the watertightness of the dura mater is checked. The trapezius muscle, the muscles attached to the occipital protuberance, and the paraspinous muscles are sutured in two layers, and the skin is sutured using resorbable 3-0 silk thread.

The surgical techniques for cerebellar hemorrhage and cerebellar infarction use similar opening and closure stages. The cerebellar tissue at the site of the infarct is removed using low-suction aspiration and bipolar coagulation. The site of infarction is easy to recognize owing to its soft, fluffy consistency.

The amount of bleeding is usually moderate, and the infarcted or shifted cerebellar tonsil or tonsils are generally removed to favor proper restoration of CSF circulation. In patients with cerebellar infarcts and those with hemorrhage who have preoperative ventricular dilatation, an external ventricular shunt is usually placed using the standard technique and left in situ for 48 to 72 hours.

Postoperative Care

Our patients go to the intensive care unit for the first 24 hours after surgery. Patients who are in satisfactory preoperative neurologic condition are extubated immediately after surgery, and their arterial pressure, pulse, electrocardiogram, water and electrolyte balance, and blood gases are closely monitored. The most important single aim is to avoid peaks of arterial hypertension. Patients in critical neurologic condition remain under mechanical ventilation and receive full doses of corticosteroids and mannitol; they undergo a CT scan within the first 24 hours. As soon as their neurologic condition has improved, patients are transferred to the neurosurgical ward until they are discharged from the hospital. During this time, they undergo serial CT scans.

CONCLUSIONS

Vascular cerebellar syndromes occur predominantly in the elderly. The most frequent cause of cerebellar hemorrhage is arterial hypertension; the most frequent cause of infarction is cardioembolic disease. In our experience, hemorrhages require surgical treatment more frequently than do infarcts, mainly on an emergency basis. Cerebellar infarcts are diagnosed more frequently today than in the past. Most of them involve the territory of the PICA. The majority responds well to conservative management or external ventricular drainage for 48 to 72 hours. Comparatively few need a decompressive suboccipital craniectomy. The choice of surgical option is based on neurologic evaluation of consciousness.

The essential criteria for the surgical assessment of intracerebellar hemorrhages are the diameter of the hematoma (40 × 30 mm in hemispheric lesions and 35 × 25 mm in vermian lesions), the presence of a TPF (reducing the aforementioned diameters by 5 mm) and a GCS score of less than 13.

Blood invasion of the brain stem and the presence of two or more general risk factors considerably worsen survival. The presence of hypertensive hydrocephalus, if diagnosed and treated promptly, does not adversely influence the prognosis. Patients who are in a deep coma should be treated conservatively. Despite an often dramatic clinical onset, not all patients have an unfavorable course. Even patients with low preoperative GCS scores sometimes make a surprisingly good functional recovery.

REFERENCES

1. Salvati M, Cervoni L, Raco A, et al: Spontaneous cerebellar hemorrhage: Clinical remarks on 50 cases. Surg Neurol 55:156–161, 2001.
2. Raco A, Caroli M, Isidori A, et al: Management of acute cerebellar infarction: One institution's experience. Neurosurgery 53:1061–1066, 2003.
3. Koh MG, Fhan TG, Atkinson JL, et al: Neuroimaging in deteriorating patients with cerebellar infarcts and mass effect. Stroke 31:262–267, 2000.
4. Pollack L, Rabey JM, Gur R, et al: Indication to surgical management of cerebellar hemorrhage. Clin Neurol Neurosurg 100:99–103, 1998.
5. Cohen Z, Ram Z, Knoller N, et al: Management and outcome of non traumatic cerebellar hemorrhage. Cerebrovasc Dis 14:207–213, 2002.
6. Wijdicks E, St. Louis E, Atkinson J, et al: Clinician biases toward surgery in cerebellar hematomas: An analysis of decision making in 94 patients. Cerebrovasc Dis 10:93–96, 2000.
7. Kirollos R, Tyagi A, Ross S, et al: Management of spontaneous cerebellar hematomas: A prospective treatment protocol. Neurosurg 49:1378–1387, 2001.
8. George B, Cophignon J, George C, et al: Surgical aspects of cerebellar infarction: Based upon a series of 79 cases. Neurochirurgie 24:83–88, 1978.
9. Auer LM, Auer T, Sayama I: Indications for surgical treatment of cerebellar hemorrhage and infarction. Acta Neurochir (Wien) 79:74–79, 1986.
10. Shenkin HA, Zavala M: Cerebellar strokes mortality, surgical indications and result of ventricular drainage. Lancet 2:429–432, 1982.
11. Kobayashi S, Sato A, Kageyama Y, et al: A treatment of hypertensive cerebellar hemorrhage: Surgical or conservative management. Neurosurgery 34:246–251, 1994.
12. Luparello V, Canavero S: Treatment of hypertensive cerebellar hemorrhage-surgical or conservative management? Neurosurgery 37:552–553, 1995.
13. Mathew P, Teasdale G, Bannan A, et al: Neurosurgical management of cerebellar hematoma and infarct. J Neurol Neurosurg Psychiatr 59:287–292, 1995.
14. Neubauer U, Schwenk B: Therapy and prognosis in spontaneous cerebellar hematomas. Adv Neurosurg 21:57–60, 1993.
15. Van Loon J, Van Calenbergh F, Goffin J, et al: Controversies in the management of spontaneous cerebellar hemorrhage: A consecutive series of 49 cases and review of the literature. Acta Neurochir (Wien) 122:187–193, 1993.
16. Waidhauser E, Hamburger C, Marguth F: Neurosurgical management of cerebellar hemorrhage. Neurosurg Rev 13:211–217, 1990.
17. Chen HJ, Lee TC, Wei CP: Treatment of cerebellar infarction by decompressive suboccipital craniectomy. Stroke 23:7, 1992.
18. Laun A, Busse O, Calatayud V, et al: Cerebellar infarcts in the area of the supply of the pica and their surgical treatment. Acta Neurochir (Wien) 71:295–306, 1984.
19. Norris JW, Eisen AA, Branch CL: Problems in cerebellar hemorrhage and infarction. Neurology 19:1043–1050, 1969.
20. Fisher CM, Picard EH, Polak A, et al: Acute hypertensive cerebellar hemorrhage. J Nerv Ment Dis 140:38–57, 1965.
21. Abud-Ortega AF, Rajput A, Rozdilsky B: Observations in five cases of spontaneous cerebellar hemorrhage. CMAJ 106:40, 1972.
22. McKissock W, Richardson A, Walsh L: Spontaneous cerebellar hemorrhage: A study of 34 cases treated surgically. Brain 38:1–9, 1960.
23. Lehrich JR, Winkler GF, Ojemann RG: Cerebellar infarction and brain stem compression: Diagnosis and surgical treatment. Arch Neurol 22:490–498, 1970.
24. Taneda M, Hayakawa T, Mogami H: Primary cerebellar hemorrhage: Quadrigeminal cistern obliteration on CT scans as a predictor of outcome. J Neurosurg 67:545–552, 1987.
25. Scotti G, Spinnler H, Sterzi R, et al: Cerebellar softening. Ann Neurol 8:2, 1980.
26. Sobotta J, Becher H: Atlas der anatomie des Menschen. Munich: Urban & Schwarzenberg, 1988.
27. Marinkovic S, Kovacevic M, Gibo H, et al: The anatomical basis for the cerebellar infarcts. Surg Neurol 44:450–461, 1995.
28. Amarenco P, Roullet E, Hommel M, et al: Infarction in the territory of the medial branch of the posterior inferior cerebellar artery. J Neurol Neurosurg Psychiatry 53:730–735, 1990.
29. Fisher CM, Karnes WE, Kubik CS: Lateral medullary infarction: The pattern of vascular occlusion. J Neuropathol Exp Neurol 29:323–379, 1961.
30. Amarenco P, Hauw JJ, Henin D, et al: Les infarctus du territoire de l'artere cerebelleuse postero-inferieure: Etude clinico-pathologique de 28 cas. Rev Neurol (Paris) 145:277–286, 1989.
31. Duvernoy HM: Human Brain Stem Vessels. Berlin: Springer-Verlag, 1978.
32. Goodhart SP, Davison C: Syndrome of the posterior-inferior cerebellar arteries and of anterior-inferior cerebellar arteries and their branches. Arch Neurol Psychiatry 35:501–524, 1936.
33. Amarenco P, Hauw JJ: Cerebellar infarction in the territory of the anterior and inferior cerebellar artery. Brain 113:139–155, 1990.
34. Lazorthes G: Vascularisation et Circulation Cérébrales. Paris: Masson, 1961.
35. Takahashi M: The anterior inferior cerebellar artery. In Newton TH, Potts DG: Radiology of the Skull and Brain, vol 2, book 2. St. Louis: CV Mosby, 1974, pp 1796–1808.
36. Mitchell N, Angrist A: Spontaneous cerebellar hemorrhage: Report of fifteen cases. Am J Pathol 18:935–946, 1942.
37. Sédillot J: Epanchement de sang dans le lobe droit du cervelet suivi de la mort. J Gen Med Chir Pharm 47:375–379, 1813.
38. Brown-Sequard CE: Diagnosis of hemorrhage in the cerebellum. Lancet 2:391, 1861.
39. Hillairet JB: De L'haemorrhagie cerebelleuse. Arch Gen Med 1:149–169, 324–340, 411–432, 549–568, 1858.
40. Ballance H: A case of a traumatic hemorrhage into the left lateral lobe of the cerebellum, treated by operation with recovery. Surg Gynecol Obstet 3:223–225, 1906.
41. Little JR, Tubman DE, Ethier R: Cerebellar hemorrhage in adults. J Neurosurg 48:574–578, 1978.
42. Weisberg LA: Acute cerebellar hemorrhage and CT evidence of tight posterior fossa. Neurology 36:858–860, 1986.
43. Fairburn B, Oliver LC: Cerebellar softening: A surgical emergency. BMJ 1:1335–1336, 1956.
44. Lindgren SO: Infarctions simulating brain tumors in the posterior fossa. J Neurosurg 13:575–581, 1956.
45. Duncan GW, Parker SW, Fisher CM: Acute cerebellar infarction in the pica territory. Arch Neurol 32:364–368, 1975.
46. Sypert GW, Alvord EC Jr: Cerebellar infarction: A clinico-pathological study. Arch Neurol 32:357–363, 1975.

47. Amarenco P: The spectrum of cerebellar infarctions. Neurology 41:973–979, 1991.
48. Amarenco P, Hauw JJ, Gautier JC: Arterial pathology in cerebellar infarction. Stroke 21:1299–1305, 1990.
49. Amarenco P, Hauw JJ: Cerebellar infarction in the territory of the superior cerebellar artery: A clinicopathologic study of 33 cases. Neurology 40:1383–1390, 1990.
50. Amarenco P, Roullet E, Goujon C, et al: Infarction in the anterior rostral cerebellum (the territory of the lateral branch of the superior cerebellar artery). Neurology 41:253–258, 1991.
51. Amarenco P, Levy C, Cohen A, et al: Causes and mechanism of territorial and nonterritorial cerebellar infarcts in 115 consecutive patients. Stroke 25:105–112, 1994.
52. Russel RWR: Observation on intracranial aneurysm. Brain 86:425–442, 1963.
53. Cole FM, Yates IO: The occurrence and significance of intracerebral micro-aneurysms. J Pathol Bact 93:393–411, 1967.
54. Wakai S, Nagai M: Histological verification of microaneurysms as a cause of cerebral hemorrhage in surgical specimen. J Neurol Neurosurg Psychiatry 52:595–599, 1989.
55. McCormick WF, Nafzinger JD: Cryptic vascular malformations of the central nervous system. J Neurosurg 5:892–894, 1966.
56. Amarenco P, Caplan LR: Vertebrobasilar occlusive disease: Review of selected aspects, III: Mechanisms of cerebellar infarctions. Cerebrovasc Dis 3:66–73, 1993.
57. Teasdale G, Jennet B: Assessment and prognosis of coma after head injury. Acta Neurochir (Wien) 34:45–55, 1976.
58. Roux FE, Boetto S, Tremoulet M: Third ventriculocisternostomy in cerebellar haematomas. Acta Neurochir (Wien) 144:337–342, 2002.
59. Koenig A, Laas R, Hermann HD: Cerebellar hemorrhage as a complication after supratentorial craniotomy. Acta Neurochir (Wien) 88:104–108, 1997.
60. Toczek MT, Morrell J, Silverberg GA, et al: Cerebellar hemorrhage complicating temporal lobectomy: Report of four cases. J Neurosurg 85:718–722, 1996.
61. Honegger J, Zentner J, Spreer J, et al: Cerebellar hemorrhage arising postoperatively as a complication of supratentorial surgery: A retrospective study. J Neurosurg 96:248–254, 2002.
62. Friedman JA, Piepgras DJ, Duke DA, et al: Remote cerebellar hemorrhage after supratentorial surgery. Neurosurgery 49:1327–1340, 2001.
63. Friedman JA, Ecker RD, Piepgras DJ, et al: Cerebellar hemorrhage after spinal surgery: Report of two cases and literature review. Neurosurgery 50:1361–1364, 2002.
64. Heros RC: Surgical treatment of cerebellar infarction [Editorial]. Stroke 23:937–938,1992.
65. Turgut M, Ozcan OE, Ertuck O, et al: Spontaneous cerebellar strokes: Clinical observations in 60 patients. Angiology 47:841–848, 1996.
66. Jeret JS, Bluth M: Stroke following chiropractic manipulation. Report of 3 cases and review of the literature. Cerebrovasc Dis 13:210–213, 2002.
67. Tyagi AK, Kirollos RW, Marks PV: Posttraumatic cerebellar infarction. Br J Neurosurg 9:683–686, 1995.
68. Aggarwal S, Byrne BD: Massive ischemic cerebellar infarction due to cocaine use. Neuroradiology 33:449–450, 1992.
69. Caplan LR, Baquis MD, Pessin MS, et al: Dissection of the intracranial vertebral artery. Neurology 38:868–877, 1988.
70. Hilzenrat N, Zilberman D, Sikuler E: Isolated cerebellar infarction as a presenting symptom of polycythemia vera. Acta Haematol 88:204–206, 1992.
71. Philips PC, Lorentsen KJ, Shropshire LC, et al: Congenital odontoid aplasia and posterior circulation stroke in childhood. Ann Neurol 23:410–413, 1988.
72. Chaves CJ, Caplan LR, Chung CS, et al: Cerebellar infarcts in the New England Medical Center Posterior Circulation Stroke Registry. Neurology 44:1385–1390, 1994.
73. Kase CS, Norrvig B, Levine S, et al: Cerebellar infarction: Clinical and anatomic observations in 66 cases. Stroke 24:76–83, 1993.
74. Rieke K, Krieger D, Adams HP, et al: Therapeutic strategies in space-occupying cerebellar infarction based on clinical, neuroradiological and neurophysiological data. Cerebrovasc Dis 3:45–55, 1993.
75. Jauss M, Krieger D, Horning C, et al: Surgical and medical management of patients with massive cerebellar infarctions: Results of the German-Austrian cerebellar infarction studies. J Neurol 246:257–264, 1999.
76. Neau J-PH, Arroyo-Anllo E, Bonnaud V, et al: Neuropsychological disturbances in cerebellar infarcts. Acta Neurol Scand 102:363–370, 2000.

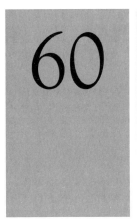

60 Surgical Management of Cerebellar Astrocytomas in Adults

KHALID M. ABBED and E. ANTONIO CHIOCCA

EPIDEMIOLOGY

Cerebellar astrocytomas constitute only 3.5% of all primary brain tumors and only 8% of all gliomas, but they represent nearly 35% to 40% of all posterior fossa tumors and 30% of gliomas occurring during childhood.[1–3] They are rare in the first year of life, and there are few published reports of cerebellar astrocytomas in middle-aged and elderly adults.[4–8] When cerebellar astrocytomas occur in adults, they are more often associated with anaplastic changes and have a less favorable prognosis compared with children. There is no sex predominance nor is there any obvious racial predilection.[5] The differential diagnosis of posterior fossa tumors in adults includes metastases, vestibular schwannoma, meningioma, hemangioblastoma, epidermoid, brain stem glioma, ependymoma, chordoma, paraganglioma, sarcoma, and choroids plexus papilloma.

HISTOPATHOLOGIC CHARACTERISTICS

Over the years, a number of grading and classification systems for diffusely infiltrating (fibrillary) astrocytomas have been proposed. The classic Kernohan system is a four-point scale with grade 1 representing the most benign tumors and grade 4 representing the most malignant ones (glioblastoma multiforme); it is based on the degree of presence of several histologic features such as nuclear pleomorphism, anaplasia, and number of mitoses. The World Health Organization (WHO) classification is a three-tiered modified system whose classification criteria is based on cellularity, nuclear and cellular pleomorphism, endothelial proliferation, mitotic figures, and necrosis (Table 60-1).

The low-grade astrocytomas (Kernohan grades 1 and 2, WHO grade II) make up 10% to 15% of astrocytomas and occur primarily in the cerebral hemispheres of children and young adults between 20 and 40 years of age. Median survival is usually between 7 and 10 years, and the most common cause of death is degeneration into a higher-grade neoplasm.

The anaplastic astrocytomas (Kernohan grade 3, WHO grade III) constitute one third of astrocytomas and occur typically in the cerebral white matter of patients in their 40s to 60s. Anaplastic astrocytomas have a poor prognosis, with an average 2-year survival.

Glioblastoma multiforme (GBM) (Kernohan grade 4, WHO grade VI) is the most common primary brain tumor, encompassing 50% of all astrocytomas. Like the anaplastic astrocytomas, they most commonly occur in the cerebral white matter of older patients. GBMs spread rapidly and have the worst prognosis of the primary brain tumors, with a median survival of 8 months.

Cerebellar astrocytomas are most often histologically pilocytic astrocytomas (WHO grade I), which are a morphologically distinct astrocytoma subtype that differs significantly from the diffusely infiltrating (fibrillary) astrocytomas with regards to age of presentation, common locations of occurrence, and prognosis.

Pilocytic astrocytomas constitute 5% to 10% of all gliomas and are the second most common pediatric brain tumor. They occur most often during the first and second decades of life, with a second incidence peak in young adulthood. These astrocytomas most commonly occur around the third and fourth ventricles and in the optic chiasm and hypothalamus. One third of pilocytic astrocytomas occur in the cerebellar vermis or hemispheres, and they only occasionally occur in the cerebral hemispheres. These tumors have a good prognosis with an 85% to 100% 5-year survival rate.

CLINICAL PRESENTATION

The clinical presentation and symptoms caused by cerebellar astrocytomas in adults can be secondary to obstructive hydrocephalus and/or cerebellar dysfunction. The patient's complaints are often nonspecific in nature and, because of the slow, indolent growth pattern of these tumors, the symptoms tend to occur in a gradual fashion.

There is usually some degree of ventriculomegaly, but because of the slow pattern of growth, it is usually well compensated for by the patient. The most common initial

TABLE 60-1 ▪ The Approximate Equivalents of the Traditional Four-tiered Kernohan Classification System of Astrocytomas and the Three-tiered Modification of the WHO Sytem

Kernohan Grade	WHO Designation
	Pilocytic astrocytoma and subependymal giant cell (grade I)
1 and 2	Low-grade/Benign astrocytoma (grade II)
3	Anaplastic astrocytoma (grade III)
4	Glioblastoma multiforme (grade IV)

symptom is headache,[9] which is often associated with nausea, vomiting, and lethargy. Herniation of the cerebellar tonsils and subsequent pressure on the brain stem and lower cranial nerves may cause neck pain and stiffness. The sign of a head tilt is rare in adults, compared with children. Papilledema and compression of the sixth cranial nerve may lead to complaints of blurry or double vision. In children, signs such as opisthotonic posture bradycardia, depressed respiratory rate, hypertension, and depressed consciousness indicate increased intracranial pressure and impending deterioration. In adults, alteration in mental status will precede brain stem compression signs, indicating impending neurologic catastrophe.

Cerebellar dysfunction is common in patients with cerebellar astrocytomas. The resulting signs and symptoms are dependent on the location of the tumor. Midline cerebellar masses typically produce truncal ataxia and a subsequent broad-based unsteady gait. Hemispheric lesions, on the other hand, tend to cause limb ataxias, presenting as dysmetria, dysdiadochokinesia, nystagmus, hypotonia, and hyporeflexia ipsilateral to the tumor.

PREOPERATIVE IMAGING STUDIES

The studies of choice for the diagnosis and management of cerebellar tumors are computed tomography (CT) and magnetic resonance imaging (MRI). MRI has a number of advantages over CT, including better sensitivity for detecting posterior fossa lesions (because of the lack of bone artifact), better definition of the displacement of normal structures, multiplanar reconstruction, and a lack of radiation exposure to the patient. CT, however, is usually much easier and quicker to obtain than is MRI, especially for critically ill patients.

The radiographic appearance of cerebellar astrocytomas is variable (Fig. 60-1A and Fig. 60-2A). On nonenhanced CT scans, these tumors are typically round or oval, well-circumscribed, hypo- or isodense masses with smooth margins and often no associated vasogenic edema. Calcifications are rare because only about 10% of all pilocytic astrocytomas have calcifications.[10] Contrast enhancement is usually strong but variable, because some lesions are solid and enhance homogenously whereas others are grossly cystic with a small enhancing mural nodule located in the cyst wall. The wall of most cystic astrocytomas is composed of nonneoplastic, partially gliotic compressed white matter, and thus it typically does not enhance. Occasionally, however, the cyst wall may enhance; this is indicative of tumor infiltration of the wall.

On MRI, most cerebellar astrocytomas are hypo- or isointense on T1-weighted images and hyperintense on T2-weighted images. Solid tumors and the mural nodules of the cystic tumors enhance strongly but often nonhomogeneously.[10] The enhancement patterns are typically similar on CT and MRI.

Angiography is usually used when a cerebellar hemangioblastoma is suspected or when there is evidence of a vascular malformation. In the case of cerebellar astrocytomas, angiograms demonstrate an avascular mass effect with stretching and draping of otherwise normal vessels. If a mural nodule is present, it may show significant neovascularity.

Magnetic resonance angiography (MRA) is also a useful tool in the diagnosis and analysis of brain tumors, because it can help define the relationship between the tumor and adjacent vasculature noninvasively. The administration of gadolinium allows further analysis of tumors and offers additional information about the cerebral hemodynamics with relatively little cost and risk.

Magnetic resonance spectroscopy (MRS) allows for direct, noninvasive investigation of tumor metabolism and provides insight into the composition and distribution of cellular metabolites. It has shown great potential in the diagnosis of tumor grades and in differentiating tumor recurrence from radiation changes.

PREOPERATIVE MANAGEMENT

Upon the diagnosis of a cerebellar astrocytoma, it must be determined whether the patient would benefit from preoperative corticosteroids and from preoperative diversion of cerebrospinal fluid. In the majority of patients, corticosteroid therapy (with dexamethasone or an equivalent) controls the symptoms of increased intracranial pressure (e.g., headache, nausea, and vomiting) in less than 24 hours and remains efficacious for several days, often alleviating the need for shunting. Complications of preoperative steroid use are rare.

However, emergency diversion of cerebrospinal fluid may be necessary if the patient presents with severe, symptomatic hydrocephalus. In this case, an external ventricular drain (EVD) is placed emergently.

An EVD has several advantages over preoperative ventriculoperitoneal shunting (VPS), including the ability to gradually decompress the ventricular system by varying the outflow pressures and thereby decreasing the risk of upward transtentorial herniation of the cerebellum. Perhaps most importantly, it has been shown that only 30% to 40% of cerebellar astrocytoma patients who have gross total resection without residual blockage of the aqueduct or fourth ventricle will require permanent postoperative shunting.[11]

SURGICAL PROCEDURE

The patient may be positioned in the prone position, the lateral decubitus position, or the sitting position. Each of these positions has certain advantages and disadvantages (Table 60-2). The decision as to which position to use is often based largely on the prior experience of the neurosurgeon. The head of the patient should be approximately 10 to 15 cm above the heart. Preoperative steroids (usually 10 mg of dexamethasone), mannitol (usually 50 mg at the beginning of the case and 50 mg prior to opening of the dura), lasix (usually 20 mg), and antibiotics (cefazolin, 1 g) are administered prior to skin incision.

If needed (because of concerns for ventriculomegaly complicating the surgical exposure or because of symptomatic hydrocephalus), an EVD may be placed on the operating table after induction and positioned via an occipital burr hole. The burr hole is placed 3 to 4 cm from the midline and 6 to 7 cm above the inion. The catheter is then inserted with a trajectory parallel to the skull base by aiming for the middle of the forehead. In adults, an insertion length of about 10 to 12 cm will put the tip just anterior to Monro's foramen. During insertion, the stylet should be used initially as the catheter penetrates the occipital parenchyma. After the initial 6 cm, the stylet is removed and the catheter is inserted the remaining length. As a precaution, sometimes a burr hole can be drilled without placement of an EVD. The EVD can then be placed for intraoperative or postoperative emergencies related to acute hydrocephalus.

If there is no concern about ventriculomegaly on preoperative imaging, or if the patient is relatively asymptomatic, a prophylactic EVD is not necessary. If cerebellar herniation becomes an intraoperative issue, another maneuver is to raise the head of the patient, although this may increase the

risk of air embolism. In cases where such a maneuver fails, rapid removal of cerebellar hemispheric tissue may forestall impending herniation.

If frameless stereotactic navigation is employed, coordinates can be acquired before draping and prepping the patient. One advantage of frameless stereotaxy is that it may guide the surgeon's ability to minimize the size of the skin incision and bony removal, particularly for small lesions.

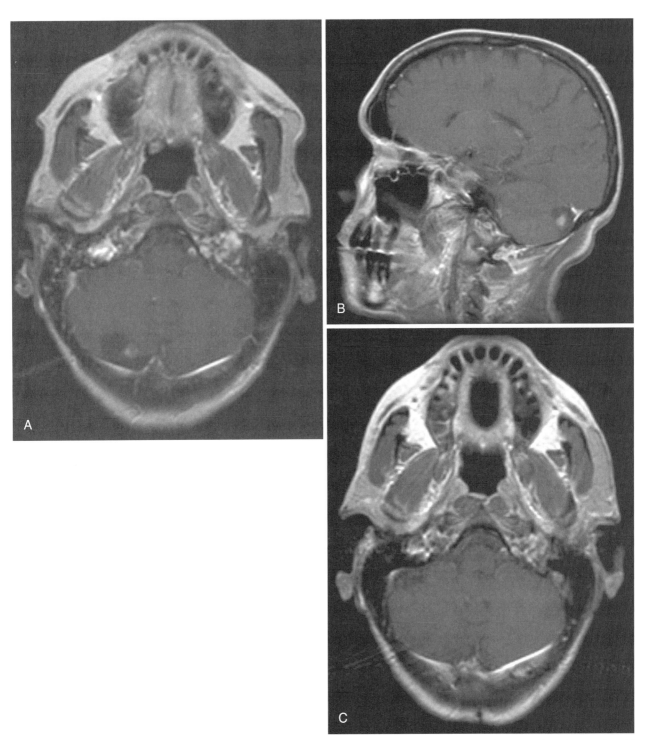

FIGURE 60-1 *A,* Axial T1 postgadolinium MRI showing 2.6-cm cystic right posterior cerebellar lesion with 7-mm enhancing mural nodule. *B,* Sagittal T1 postgadolinium MRI showing cystic right posterior cerebellar lesion with 7-mm enhancing mural nodule. *C,* A 17 months postoperative axial T1 postgadolinium MRI showing no recurrence of tumor.

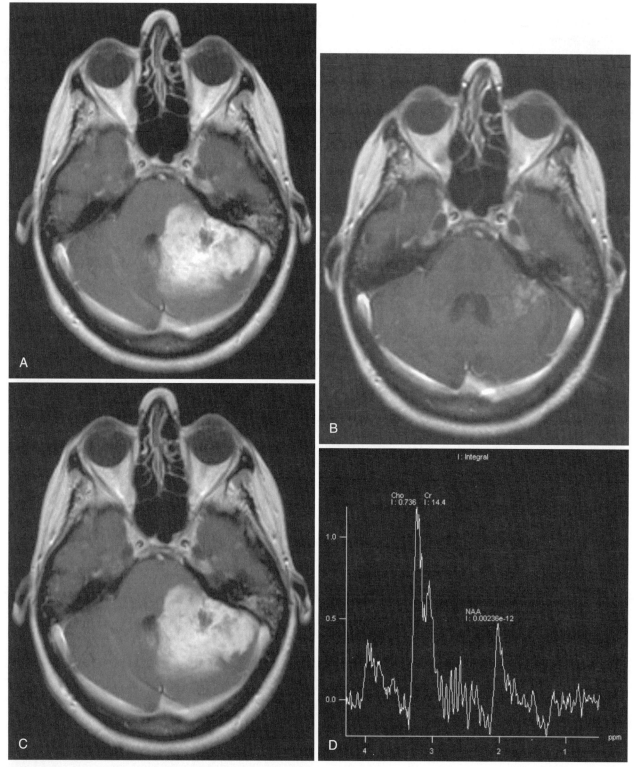

FIGURE 60-2 *A,* Axial T1 postgadolinium MRI showing enhancement in the left cerebellar hemisphere, middle cerebellar peduncle, and vermis with a focal cystic region in the hemisphere. *B,* Axial T1 postgadolinium MRI after two cycles of Temodar chemotherapy showing less prominent enhancement. *C,* Axial T1 postgadolinium MRI 6 months after initiation of Temodar chemotherapy showing a marked increase in the size of the enhancing mass centered in the left cerebellum. *D,* MR spectroscopy of enhanced left cerebellar lesion showing increased choline-to-creatine ratio and depressed NAA peak consistent with recurrent tumor.

(Continued)

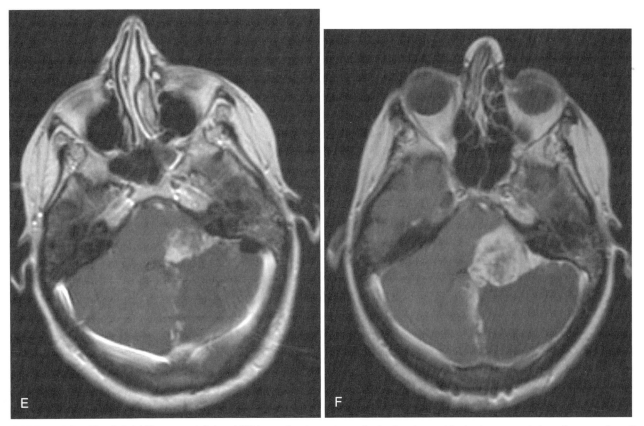

FIGURE 60-2 Cont'd *E*, Axial T1 postgadolinium MRI immediately postoperatively showing residual enhancement along the resection site greatest in the left pons and left middle cerebellar peduncle. *F*, Axial T1 postgadolinium MRI 1 month postoperatively showing significant interval increase in enhancement involving the anterior and medial aspects of the left cerebellar resection cavity extending into the pons.

A midline skin incision extending from the external occipital protuberance to the midcervical region is first made with a No. 10 skin blade and then continued deeply through the avascular median raphe with the cautery. The occipital bone is exposed by stripping the periosteum deep to the occipital muscles away with a periosteal elevator. Any venous bleeding should be controlled promptly. The posterior fossa is then opened by either craniotomy or craniectomy. For relatively large lesions, the bony removal should be wide, with its superior margin overlying the inferior torcula to provide adequate exposure of the superior

cerebellum; it should then be extended caudally into the foramen magnum on both sides. Dural attachments to the foramen magnum may require sharp dissection to detach them from the overlying bone.

The posterior arch of C1 should be exposed for large lesions, but may not need to be resected because depressed cerebellar tonsils, if present, often retract upward after the tumor mass is removed. If, however, the cerebellar tonsils remain impacted, it may be necessary to resect the arch of C1 to adequately decompress the medulla and upper cervical spinal cord.

The dura is opened in a Y-shaped configuration crossing the occipital and circular sinuses, which may be occluded with Weck clips. The dura is then reflected laterally. If the cerebellum is bulging from the durotomy, cerebrospinal fluid should be drained. This can be done by unclamping the EVD (if one has been placed), by opening the cisterna magna, or by raising the head of the patient.

A linear corticectomy is made overlying the tumor, and the astrocytoma is resected by microdissection, suction, and bipolar cautery. Gross total resection of all contrast-enhancing tissue should be the goal. With the classic cystic cerebellar astrocytoma, this is usually easily accomplished because the tumor-brain interface is usually well demarcated. The classic nonenhancing cyst wall has been confirmed by pathologic inspection to be nonneoplastic; thus it need not be resected to effect cure. However, enhancing cyst walls have been shown to contain tumor cells, and these must be removed for resection to be considered complete.[12]

TABLE 60-2 ▪ Advantages and Disadvantages of Patient Positions

Patient Position	Advantage	Disadvantage
Prone	Reduced risk of air embolism	Increased pressure on facial structures
Lateral decubitus	Decreased risk of air embolism; good airway access	May be interference from weight of upper cerebellar hemisphere, surgeon
Sitting	Allows good blood and CSF drainage from surgical field; affords best access to superior cerebellar vermis	Highest risk of air embolism; surgical discomfort with arm, hands elevated

In the case of solid tumors, dissection around the tumor's perimeter is performed. An ultrasonic aspirator may also be used to debulk the tumor from within. If the tumor infiltrates the brain stem via the cerebellar peduncles, complete tumor resection is virtually impossible. These tumors should not be followed into the brain stem because the risk of causing further neurologic deficit is too great.

After tumor removal, the dura should be closed in a watertight fashion. A dural substitute or pericranial graft may be required, because the dura often shrinks during the surgery.

Intraoperative MRI (iMRI) and MRI-guided frameless stereotaxy are recent additions to the neurosurgeon's armamentarium to assist in maximizing resections safely. iMRI enables the neurosurgeon to evaluate the extent of a resection at the time of surgery, thus allowing for further tumor removal during the same surgical procedure in the case of tumor residual. In a recent review, Schulder and Carmel[13] reported that in 112 patients with intracranial tumors, intraoperative imaging resulted in additional tumor removal in 40 (36%) of the patients; in another 35 (31%), imaging confirmed that the goals of the surgery had been accomplished, thus avoiding potentially harmful dissection. The MRI-guided frameless stereotaxy allows the neurosurgeon to navigate the surgical field more accurately. The combination of iMRI and MRI-guided frameless stereotaxy allows for more accurate neuronavigation. For example, the effects of brain shift can be compensated for by an update of the navigation system with intraoperative MRI data.

There are several types of iMRI machines. A widely used type is the Polestar magnet (Medtronic). One disadvantage of this system is that its geometry renders its use for infratentorial tumors relatively difficult, although newer models may provide a solution to this problem.

POSTOPERATIVE MANAGEMENT

Steroids are not continued or are tapered off over 1 to 3 days, if the patient was not on steroids preoperatively. Steroids are tapered more gradually if the patient was being treated with steroids preoperatively for a relatively long time (weeks). Postoperative antibiotics covering skin flora are continued for 24 hours or, if an EVD is in place, until the EVD is removed.

Patients with an EVD should be gradually weaned by raising the drip chamber over several days followed by a clamping trial for 24 hours. If the patient tolerates the clamping trial, the EVD is removed. If the patient is unable to be weaned from the EVD, as indicated by signs and symptoms of intracranial hypertension and persistent ventriculomegaly on serial imaging, a permanent shunt should be placed.

One of the most important factors in the outcome of patients with cerebellar astrocytomas is the extent of tumor removal.[14] This fact, combined with the fact that neurosurgeons often overestimate the amount of tumor removed during surgery,[15] makes it extremely important to schedule early (within 2 to 3 days) postoperative imaging (preferable with a pre- and postcontrast MRI, or else a CT) to determine the degree of tumor resection.

Cerebellar mutism is an unusual complication of posterior fossa surgery that consists of transient loss of speech usually beginning 1 to 3 days postoperatively without any other language disorder or cranial nerve dysfunction. The mutism may last for months but is always transient. It is usually seen in children but has been described in adults.[16] The majority of the reported cases of mutism have been of midline cerebellar tumors. The cause may be related to dissection or to retraction in the region of the dentate nucleus.

Case Reports

CASE REPORT 1
PILOCYTIC ASTROCYTOMA

A 71-year-old female with a past medical history of ovarian cancer status post TAH BSO in 1985 was seen by an orthopedic surgeon for complaints of pain in the back of the head and neck radiating to the shoulders and bilateral, right greater than left; and complaints of numbness in the second through fifth digits. The patient also noted a 4- or 5-year history of worsening balance with occasional falls and "tripping for no apparent reason."

The patient's examination was notable for slower fine finger movements with the left hand and difficulty with dysdiadochokinesis bilaterally. Finger-nose-finger testing was without significant dysmetria. Heel-to-shin testing was slightly ataxic on the left, and foot tapping was also slower on the left. She had decreased vibratory sense distally in the feet and in the ankles. Pinprick had no clear gradient, and her gait was normal, including tandem and walking on her heels and toes.

A cervical MRI was performed and showed multilevel degenerative disc disease with narrowing of bilateral neural foramina and moderate central canal stenosis (most prominently at C4–C5) and an incidental cystic cerebellar mass. A dedicated brain MRI was then performed and showed a 2.6-cm cystic right (despite her examination, which suggested more left cerebellar dysfunction) posterior cerebellar mass with a 7-mm enhancing nodule (see Figs. 60-1A and B).

The patient underwent a suboccipital craniotomy for resection of the tumor, and the pathology was consistent with grade I pilocytic astrocytoma. A postoperative MRI showed complete resection, and serial follow-up MRI scans have shown no sign of recurrence (see Fig. 60-1C).

CASE REPORT 2
ANAPLASTIC ASTROCYTOMA

A 45-year-old female with a history of presumptive low-grade pontine astrocytoma (no biopsy had been performed), who received involved field radiation therapy and PCV chemotherapy 11 years ago, had been functioning normally in all respects and had no evidence of tumor recurrence or radiation injury on serial imaging.

However, over the ensuing 6 months, she developed left arm and leg instability, tilting to the left side, and a mild left facial paresis. An MRI at this time revealed an enhancing lesion in the left cerebellar hemisphere, middle cerebellar peduncle, and vermis with a focal cystic region in the hemisphere (see Fig. 60-2A). A positron-emission tomography scan showed decreased activity within the left cerebellar hemisphere.

The patient was started on Temodar chemotherapy, and an MRI performed 2 months later showed that the previously noted enhancing abnormality was much less prominent (see Fig. 60-2B). The patient also improved clinically.

This improvement, both radiologic and clinical, was short-lived, however, because monthly MRI scans and physical examinations revealed progressive worsening of the lesion. Finally, 6 months after the initiation of the Temodar chemotherapy, the patient developed profound left arm and leg dysmetria, gait imbalance with multiple falls, and hiccups. Her MRI at this time showed a marked increase in the size of the enhancing mass centered in the left cerebellum (see Fig. 60-2C), and the MR spectroscopy demonstrated an elevated choline-to-creatine ratio and a depressed N-acetylaspartate (NAA) peak (see Fig 60-2D).

The patient was taken to the operating room and underwent a suboccipital craniotomy for tumor resection. During the removal of tumor from the middle cerebellar peduncle, the patient had brief episodes of asystole. The decision to halt further resection was thus made. Pathology revealed a grade III astrocytoma. The postoperative MRI showed residual enhancement along the resection site, greatest in the left pons and left middle cerebellar peduncle as expected (see Fig. 60-2E).

One month postoperatively, her MRI showed significant interval increase in enhancement involving the anterior and medial aspects of the left cerebellar resection cavity extending into the pons (see Fig. 60-2F). Two months postoperatively, the patient expired.

OUTCOME

The most important predictive parameters in determining patient outcome and survival length in patients with cerebellar astrocytomas is the degree of tumor resection and the tumor histology.[2,14,17-19]

Complete excision of pilocytic astrocytomas is generally considered curative, and the degree of tumor removal has been shown to affect prognosis.[15,18] The postoperative recurrence rate is low; however, because of the slow growth rate of these tumors and the rare possibility of malignant transformation,[20] patients should be followed over many years (see Fig. 60-2).

In general, the prognosis for patients with pilocytic astrocytomas is excellent, with an overall 10-year survival rate of 83% and an overall 20-year survival rate of 70%.[21] In contrast, patients with the diffuse (fibrillary) type of astrocytoma have 10-year and 20-year survival rates of 7%.[2]

Some pathologic characteristics of prognostic significance have been identified. The tumor characteristics associated with a favorable prognosis include microcysts, leptomeningeal deposits, oligodendroglial fibers, and Rosenthal fibers. Astrocytomas with these findings have been categorized as Winston type A, and patients with these lesions have a 10-year survival rate of 94%.[22] In contrast, patients whose tumors have perivascular pseudorosettes, mitoses, necrosis, hypercellularity, or calcifications without type A findings (Winston type B) have a 10-year survival rate of 29%.[22] Recently, classification systems for tumors based on their global gene expression profiles and/or cytogenetic anomalies have shown correlations with responses

to therapy and outcome.[23,24] This suggests that future treatments could be guided by the tumor's genetic characteristics.

ADJUVANT THERAPIES

The role for adjuvant radiation therapy remains unclear. Postoperative radiation therapy is not generally recommended for patients with low-grade cerebellar astrocytoma after complete resection[2,9,25]; it is, however, recommended for high-grade, poorly differentiated tumors. Unfortunately, patients with anaplastic forms of cerebellar astrocytoma have a poor outcome regardless of treatment.

Because of the small number of cases and the slow progression rate of the tumor, a definitive answer on the role of radiation therapy in subtotally resected low-grade astrocytomas will be difficult to establish. Garcia and colleagues[18] found that although radiation tended to lower the recurrence rate of these tumors, it did not significantly improve survival. Conversely, Conway and colleagues[26] and Akyol and colleagues[27] both concluded that postoperative irradiation after an incomplete resection improved prognosis.

Because the role for postoperative radiation therapy in incompletely resected low-grade tumors is uncertain and unproved, one strategy is careful observation and reoperation (when possible) with radiation therapy reserved for recurrences. Although there is no strong evidence to support the use of chemotherapy in cerebellar astrocytomas, this modality may be reserved for recurrences after radiation and/or additional surgery.

TUMOR RECURRENCE

A common clinical problem that occurs with glioma patients who have undergone surgical and radiation therapy is differentiating the cause of clinical or radiographic evidence of progression, which can be caused by tumor recurrence, radiation necrosis, a combination of both, or a radiation-induced tumor. All of these entities appear as contrast-enhancing, space-occupying mass lesions surrounded by edema, and as a result, CT and MRI cannot differentiate these entities reliably.

Several noninvasive methods exist to aid in differentiating tumor recurrence from radiation necrosis; these include positron emission tomography (PET), single photon emission computed tomography (SPECT), and MRS (see Fig. 60-2D). PET allows the differentiation of radiation necrosis (which is hypometabolic) from high-grade recurrent tumors with necrosis (which is hypermetabolic) with sensitivities from 80% to 90% and specificities from 50% to 90%.[28] However, the sensitivities are much lower with low- or intermediate-grade gliomas because of low uptake of fluoro-2-deoxy-D-glucose.

Thallium-201 SPECT scans measure metabolically active tissues by cell-specific tracer uptake in malignant cells. Because ^{201}Tl accumulates in viable tumor cells but not in normal brain tissue or other nonneoplastic tissue such as radiation necrosis, it is a useful method to differentiate between tumor recurrence and radiation necrosis.[29]

Unlike PET and SPECT, MR spectroscopy does not use high-energy radiation or require radiolabeled tracers: it provides metabolic information about brain tumors by analyzing spectral patterns of several metabolites. The concentration of NAA appears to be related to neuron and axon density, choline (Cho)-containing compounds seem to correlate with alteration in phospholipid membrane turnover, lipid and lactate (Lip-Lac) may be found in areas of abnormal or anaerobic metabolism or necrosis, and creatine (Cr) may be seen in regions rich in energy metabolism. The ratios of these metabolites, based on their spectral patterns, have been shown to be reliable indicators of whether tissues are composed of pure tumor or pure necrosis, but they are less reliable when tissues are composed of varying degrees of mixed tumor and necrosis.[30,31]

The gold standard for differentiating tumor recurrence from radiation necrosis in patients with irradiated gliomas remains tissue biopsy. Because gliomas are histologically heterogeneous, a main concern regarding stereotactic biopsy has been how accurately the biopsy specimens reflect the histologic characteristics of the tumor as a whole. Forsyth and colleagues reported that stereotactic biopsy, even when performed by different neurosurgeons at several institutions, had accuracy rates ranging from 76% to 100%, with a median of 95%.[32] In their study, stereotactic biopsy results were predictive of survival outcomes (i.e., patients with recurrent tumor had the shortest survival times, all patients with pure radiation necrosis survived, and patients with a mixture of tumor and radiation necrosis had an intermediate survival time), providing indirect evidence for the accuracy of the diagnosis.[32]

REFERENCES

1. Obrador S, Blazquez MG: Benign cystic tumours of the cerebellum. Acta Neurochir (Wien) 32:55–68, 1975.
2. Hayostek CJ, Shaw EG, Scheithauer B, et al: Astrocytomas of the cerebellum: A comparative study of pilocytic and diffuse astrocytomas. Cancer 72:856–869, 1993.
3. Pagni CA, Giordana MT, Canavero S: Benign recurrence of a pilocytic cerebellar astrocytoma 36 years after radical removal: Case report. Neurosurgery 28:606–609, 1991.
4. Cushing H: Experiences with the cerebellar astrocytomas: A critical review of 76 cases. Surg Gynecol Obstet 52:129–204, 1931.
5. Kehler U, Arnold H, Muller H: Long-term follow-up of infratentorial pilocytic astrocytomas. Neurosurg Rev 13:315–320, 1990.
6. Ilgren EB, Stiller CA: Cerebellar astrocytomas: Clinical characteristics and prognostic indices. J Neurooncol 4:293–308, 1987.
7. Hassounah M, Siqueira EB, Haider A, Gray A: Cerebellar astrocytoma: Report of 13 cases aged over 20 years and review of the literature. Br J Neurosurg 10:365–371, 1996.
8. Morreale VM, Ebersold MJ, Quast LM, Parisi JE: Cerebellar astrocytoma: Experience with 54 cases surgically treated at the Mayo Clinic, Rochester, Minnesota, from 1978 to 1990. J Neurosurg 87:257–261, 1997.
9. Abdollahzadeh M, Hoffman HJ, Blazer SI, et al: Benign cerebellar astrocytoma in childhood: Experience at the hospital for sick children, 1980–1992. Child's Nerv Syst 10:380–383, 1994.
10. Lee Y-Y, Van Tassel P, Bruner JM, et al: Juvenile pilocytic astrocytomas: CT and MR characteristics. AJNR Am J Neuroradiol 10:363–370, 1989.
11. Culley DJ, Berger MS: Requirements of ventriculoperitoneal shunts following posterior fossa tumor surgery: A retrospective analysis. Neurosurgery 34:402–407, 1994.
12. Suzuki M, Takashima T, Kadoya M, et al: Contrast enhancement of cystic portions in brain tumors on delayed image of gadolinium-DTPA-enhanced MR imaging. Radiat Med 9:14, 1991.
13. Schulder M, Carmel PW: Intraoperative magnetic resonance imaging: Impact on brain tumor surgery. Cancer Control 10(2):115–124, 2003.
14. Gjerris F, Klinken L: Long-term prognosis in children with benign cerebellar astrocytoma. J Neurosurg 49:179–184, 1978.
15. Schneider JH Jr, Raffel C, McComb JG: Benign cerebellar astrocytomas of childhood. Neurosurgery 30:58–62, 1992.
16. Salvati M, Missori P, Lunardi P, et al: Transient cerebellar mutism after posterior cranial fossa surgery in an adult: Case report and review of literature. Clin Neurol Neurosurg 93:313–316, 1991.
17. Ampil FL: Prognostic factors in childhood intracranial neoplasms. Radiat Med 5:202–206, 1987.
18. Garcia DM, Marks JE, Latifi HR, et al: Childhood cerebellar astrocytomas: Is there a role for postoperative irradiation? Int J Radiat Oncol Biol Phys 18:815–818, 1990.
19. Ilgren EB, Stiller CA: Cerebellar astrocytomas. Part II. Pathologic features indicative of malignancy. Clin Neuropathol 6:201–214, 1987.
20. Casadei GP, Arrigoni GL, D'Angelo V, et al: Late malignant recurrence of childhood cerebellar astrocytoma. Clin Neuropathol 9:295–298, 1990.
21. Wallner KE, Gonzales MF, Edwards MS, et al: Treatment results of juvenile pilocytic astrocytoma. J Neurosurg 69:171–176, 1988.
22. Winston K, Giles FH, Leviton A, et al: Cerebellar gliomas in children. J Natl Cancer Inst 58:833–838, 1977.
23. Mason W, Louis DN, Cairncross JG: Chemosensitive gliomas in adults: Which ones and why? J Clin Oncol 15:3423–3426, 1997.
24. Pomeroy SL, Tamayo P, Gaasenbeek M, et al: Prediction of central nervous system embryonal tumor outcome based on gene expression. Nature 415:436–442, 2002.
25. Undjian S, Marinov M, Georgiev K: Long-term follow-up after surgical treatment of cerebellar astrocytomas in 100 children. Child's Nerv Syst 5:99–101, 1989.
26. Conway PD, Oechler HW, Kun LE, et al: Importance of histologic condition and treatment of pediatric cerebellar astrocytoma. Cancer 67:2772–2775, 1991.
27. Akyol FH, Atahan IL, Zorlu F, et al: Results of post-operative or exclusive radiotherapy in grade I and grade II cerebellar astrocytoma patients. Radiother Oncol 23:245–248, 1992.
28. Schlemmer HP, Bachert P, Henze M, et al: Differentiation of radiation necrosis from tumor progression using proton magnetic resonance spectroscopy. Neuroradiology 44(3):216–222, 2002.
29. Vos MJ, Hoekstra OS, Barkhof F, et al: Thallium-201 single-photon emission computed tomography as an early predictor of outcome in recurrent glioma. J Clin Oncol 21(19):3559–3565, 2003.
30. Rock JP, Hearshen D, Scarpace L, et al: Correlations between magnetic resonance spectroscopy and image-guided histopathology, with special attention to radiation necrosis. Neurosurg 51:912–920, 2002.
31. Rabinov JD, Lee PL, Barker FG, et al: In vivo 3-T MR spectroscopy in the distinction of recurrent glioma versus radiation effects: Initial experience. Radiology 225:871–879, 2002.
32. Forsyth PA, Kelly PJ, Cascino TL, et al: Radiation necrosis or glioma: Is computer-assisted stereotactic biopsy useful? J Neurosurg 82:436–444, 1995.

61

Surgical Management of Tumors of the Fourth Ventricle

JONATHAN P. MILLER and ALAN R. COHEN

INTRODUCTION

Tumors of the fourth ventricle offer a unique challenge to the neurosurgeon because they lie deep in the brain in close proximity to a number of vital structures. Although recent diagnostic and therapeutic advances have dramatically improved outcome for patients affected with these tumors, there are still many difficulties for which new solutions are always being offered. The purpose of this chapter is to provide a systematic and comprehensive review of tumors that occur in the region of the fourth ventricle. The first section reviews the relevant anatomy. The second section describes the surgical approach to fourth ventricular tumors and common complications associated with surgical resection. The third section describes in detail the epidemiology, clinical presentation, radiology, pathology, surgical techniques, and prognosis for specific fourth ventricular tumors.

ANATOMY

The fourth ventricle is a broad, tent-shaped cerebrospinal fluid (CSF) cavity located behind the brain stem and in front of the cerebellum in the center of the posterior fossa (Fig. 61-1). CSF enters through the cerebral aqueduct, which opens into the fourth ventricle at its rostral end. The ventricle widens caudally until its maximal width at the level of the lateral recesses, from which CSF exits through the two foramina of Luschka into the cerebellopontine cisterns on either side. The ventricle narrows again to its caudal terminus at the obliterated central canal of the spinal cord, called the obex from the Latin for "barrier." The foramen of Magendie is just posterior to the obex and allows CSF to exit into the cerebellomedullary cistern, which is continuous with the cisterna magna. There are no arteries or veins within the cavity of the fourth ventricle. All the vessels associated with this region are in the fissures located just outside the fourth ventricular roof.

The glistening white floor of the fourth ventricle is the posterior surface of the brain stem (Fig. 61-2). The border between the pons and medulla is approximately at the level of the foramina of Luschka. The superior (pontine) part of the floor begins at the aqueduct and expands to the lower margin of the cerebellar peduncles. The inferior (medullary) part of the floor begins just below the lateral recesses at the attachment of the tela choroidea to the taenia choroidea and extends to the obex, limited laterally be the taeniae, which mark the inferolateral margins of the floor. Between these is the intermediate part, which extends into the lateral recesses on either side. There is a longitudinal

midline sulcus in the fourth ventricular floor called the median sulcus. On either side of the median sulcus is the sulcus limitans, which also runs longitudinally parallel to the median sulcus. The sulcus limitans is an important landmark for functional anatomy of nuclei beneath the ventricular floor, as motor nuclei are medial and sensory nuclei lateral to the sulcus limitans. Medial to the sulcus limitans on either side of the median sulcus is the median eminence, a collection of four paired elevations in the fourth ventricular floor that are collectively referred to as the calamus scriptorius

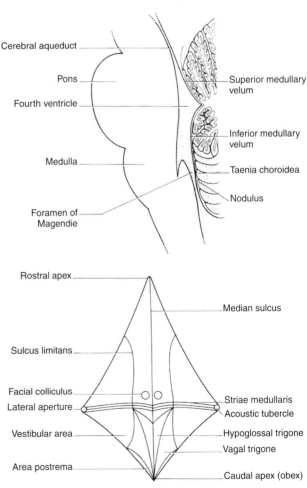

FIGURE 61-1 Fourth ventricle viewed from the side (*top*) and from behind (*bottom*). Landmarks such as the vertical median sulcus and oblique calamus scriptorius give the caudal floor the appearance of a fountain pen. (From Cohen AR: Surgical Disorders of the Fourth Ventricle. Cambridge, MA: Blackwell Science, 1996.)

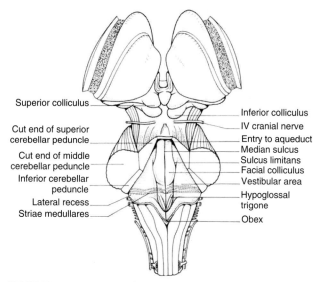

Superior colliculus

Cut end of superior cerebellar peduncle

Cut end of middle cerebellar peduncle

Inferior cerebellar peduncle

Lateral recess

Striae medullares

Inferior colliculus

IV cranial nerve

Entry to aqueduct

Median sulcus

Sulcus limitans

Facial colliculus

Vestibular area

Hypoglossal trigone

Obex

FIGURE 61-2 Fourth ventricle after removal of the cerebellum. (From Cohen AR: Surgical Disorders of the Fourth Ventricle. Cambridge, MA: Blackwell Science, 1996.)

because they resemble the head of a fountain pen (see Fig. 61-1). Rostral to caudal, the median eminence consists of the facial colliculus, which overlies the facial nucleus; the hypoglossal triangle, which overlies the hypoglossal nucleus; the vagal triangle, which overlies the dorsal nucleus of the vagus; and the area postrema, a tongue-shaped structure that is part of the brain stem emetic center. Lateral to the sulcus limitans is the vestibular area, so named because is overlies the vestibular nuclei. This area is widest in the neighborhood of the lateral recess, where the striae medullaris cross transversely the inferior cerebellar peduncles to disappear into the median sulcus. The auditory tubercle in the lateral part of the vestibular area overlies the dorsal cochlear nucleus and cochlear nerve.

The roof of the fourth ventricle is tent shaped, rising to an apex called the fastigium that divides the superior roof from the inferior roof. The median part of the superior roof, called the superior medullary velum, consists of a thin lamina of white matter between the cerebellar peduncles. Just behind its outer surface is the lingula, the uppermost division of the vermis. The lateral walls of the superior roof are formed by the superior and inferior cerebellar peduncles, which lie between the fourth ventricle and the middle cerebellar peduncle. The rostral midline of the inferior roof is formed by the nodule, which lies directly in front of the uvula, the lower part of the vermis that hangs down between the tonsils (mimicking the appearance of the pharynx). Lateral to the nodule is the inferior medullary velum, a thin sheet of neural tissue that stretches over the fourth ventricle to connect the nodule to the flocculi on either side just superior to the outer extremity of the lateral recess. The inferior medullary velum is thus part of the primitive flocculonodular lobe of the cerebellum. The caudal inferior roof consists of the tela choroidea, two thin arachnoid-like membranes sandwiching a vascular layer of choroidal vessels to which the choroid plexus is attached. The junction between the tela choroidea and the nodule/inferior medullary velum (telovelar junction) is at the level of the lateral recess.

The tela choroidea is attached to the ventricular floor at narrow white ridges called taeniae choroidea, which meet at the obex and extend upward to turn laterally over the inferior cerebellar peduncles into each lateral recess, forming its lower border. As a result, the choroid plexus (extending from the ventricular surface of the tela) forms an upside-down L shape on either side of midline. There are a medial segment of choroid plexus that extends longitudinally from the foramen of Magendie up to the nodule and a lateral segment that extends transversely from the rostral ends of the medial segments out to the foramen of Luschka. The three fourth ventricular outlet foramina (Magendie and Luschka) are located in the tela choroidea itself, and frequently choroid plexus protrudes from these foramina.

External to the fourth ventricle are three deep V-shaped fissures between the cerebellum and brain stem that enclose subarachnoid cisterns and through which course the principal arteries and veins of the posterior fossa. These three fissures are intimately related to the structures of the posterior fossa. Located between the midbrain and cerebellum, the cerebellomesencephalic fissure (also called the precentral cerebellar fissure) is the most rostral of the three and is intimately associated with the superior part of the fourth ventricular roof. This fissure is shaped like a V in the axial plain with the point facing posteriorly. The brain stem and fourth ventricle line the inner surface along with the lingula of the vermis, dorsal superior cerebellar peduncles, and rostral middle cerebellar peduncles. The outer surface of the V consists of the cerebellum, specifically the culmen and wings of the central lobule. The trochlear nerves run through the cerebellomesencephalic fissure, as do the superior cerebellar arteries. The superior cerebellar arteries leave the brain stem between cranial nerves IV and V to enter the fissure, and then after several sharp hairpin turns give rise to the precerebellar arteries that pass along the superior cerebellar peduncle to reach the superior fourth ventricle and dentate nucleus. Upon leaving the fissure, the arteries supply end branches to the tentorial surface of the cerebellum. Venous drainage from the superior fourth ventricle occurs primarily through Galen's vein. The vein of the cerebellomesencephalic fissure (also called the precentral cerebellar vein) is formed by the union of the paired veins of the superior cerebellar peduncle and ascends through the quadrigeminal cistern to drain into Galen's vein either directly or through the superior vermian vein.

The cerebellopontine fissures are intimately related to the lateral recesses of the fourth ventricle. They are produced by the folding of the cerebellum laterally around the sides of the pons and middle cerebellar peduncles. Each cerebellopontine fissure is shaped like a V in the coronal plain with the point facing laterally. The outer surface of the V is made up of the petrosal surfaces of the cerebellum, and the inner surface is made up of the middle cerebellar peduncles. The lateral recess and foramen of Luschka open into the medial part of the inferior limb of the V near the flocculus. Several cranial nerves run through the cerebellopontine fissure, including the trigeminal (through the superior limb) and the facial, glossopharyngeal, and vagus (through the inferior limb). The anterior inferior cerebellar arteries (AICA) also run through these fissures. Each AICA courses posteriorly around the pons then sends branches to nerves of the acoustic meatus and choroid plexus protruding from the foramen of Luschka before passing around the flocculus on the middle cerebellar peduncle to supply the petrosal surface of the cerebellum. Venous blood from the cerebellopontine fissure and lateral recess primarily drains into the superior petrosal sinus. The vein of the cerebellopontine fissure is formed by the convergence of several veins on the apex of the fissure, including the vein of the middle cerebellar peduncle into which the vein of the inferior cerebellar peduncle drains. This vein courses near the superior limb of the fissure to drain into the superior petrosal sinus rostral to the facial and glossopharyngeal nerves.

The cerebellomedullary fissure is directly behind the inferior roof of the fourth ventricle. It is the most caudal of the three fissures and extends between the cerebellum and medulla. Like the cerebellomesencephalic fissure, it is shaped like a V in the axial plain with the point facing posteriorly. The ventral wall consists of the inferior roof of the fourth ventricle (inferior medullary velum and tela choroidea) and the posterior medulla. The dorsal wall consists of the uvula in the midline and the tonsils (paired ovoid structures attached to the cerebellar hemispheres along their superolateral borders) and biventral lobules laterally. The fissure communicates with the cisterna magna around the superior poles of the tonsils through the telovelotonsillar cleft (tonsils to tela/velum) and supratonsillar cleft (superior extension of this cleft over the superior pole of tonsil). The posterior inferior cerebellar arteries (PICAs) course around the medulla to reach the cerebellar tonsil and lower half of the floor of the fourth ventricle. They then loop superiorly at the caudal pole of the tonsil (caudal loop) to ascend in the fissure as far as the upper pole of the tonsil, and then loop again inferiorly over the inferior medullary velum (cranial loop). Branches of the artery radiate outward from the borders of the tonsils to supply the suboccipital surface of the cerebellum. Most of the venous blood from this region drains anteriorly into the superior petrosal sinus through the vein of the cerebellopontine fissure, although some drains posteriorly into the tentorial sinuses converging on the torcular Herophili. The vein of the cerebellomedullary fissure originates on the lateral edge of the nodule and uvula and courses laterally near the telovelar junction to reach the cerebellopontine angle.

SURGICAL TECHNIQUE

Surgical Approach

The safest and most direct approach to the fourth ventricle is the midline suboccipital approach. The operative corridor to the fourth ventricle using this approach is somewhat superiorly directed. Preoperatively, all imaging and laboratory results should be reviewed carefully. Antibiotics should be given with incision. Preoperative treatment with steroids can decrease vasogenic edema, alleviate headache and neck pain, decrease the incidence and severity of aseptic meningitis and the posterior fossa syndrome, and decrease nausea and vomiting allowing for better hydration and nutrition before surgery. It is helpful to have an automatic retractor system available.

Intraoperative monitoring may be helpful if there is danger of violating the brain stem or cranial nerves. The most sensitive measure of alteration of brain stem function is the pulse and blood pressure because cardiovascular reflexes are mediated by structures near the fourth ventricle such as the nucleus tractus solitarius and dorsal motor nucleus of the vagus. Any alterations in vital signs while working near the floor of the fourth ventricle should be considered a serious warning sign to stop manipulation. The best option for direct monitoring of brain stem function is brain stem auditory evoked potentials, in which an auditory click is measured at earlobe and vertex electrodes. This produces five waves that correspond, respectively, to the proximal cochlear nerve, distal cochlear nerve, cochlear nucleus, superior olive, and lateral lemniscus/inferior colliculus. Evidence of pontomesencephalic transmission of the impulse implies that the brain stem has not been compromised. However, this pathway is fairly lateral and may be preserved in spite of serious damage to the central core of the brain stem. Another monitoring technique, somatosensory evoked potentials, follows sensory signals through the medial lemniscus, but this is also some distance from the floor of the fourth ventricle, and somatosensory evoked potentials are even less sensitive than brain stem auditory evoked potentials. Finally, electromyography with direct stimulation of the facial nerve or lateral rectus can be used to verify integrity of the cranial motor nerves if tumor abuts or envelops them.

There are three possibilities for positioning: prone, lateral oblique, and sitting. The prone position is optimal for very young children, but there is some controversy over which is the best position for older children and adults. Each of the positions requires the head to be pinned using a Mayfield or Sugita headholder as long as the patient is more than 2 years old. The pins are coated with an antibiotic ointment and placed 2 cm above the ear in the unshaven scalp. It is important to avoid the squamous temporal bone and shunt tubing if present. Use of pins in infants can lead to skull penetration producing depressed fracture, dural laceration, hematoma, or postoperative abscess. Therefore, rather than using pins, very young children should be placed face down with the head on a padded horseshoe, ensuring there is no pressure on the eyes. All three positions require some amount of neck flexion, so caution should be used if there is known preexisting neck pathology, especially a craniocervical anomaly, spinal instability, significant cervical spondylosis, or herniation of the cerebellar tonsils on preoperative imaging.

The most commonly used position for the midline suboccipital approach (especially in very young patients) is the prone position, in which the patient is rolled after induction of anesthesia so that the face is toward the floor (Fig. 61-3). There are many advantages to this position: the anatomy is clearly visualized, it is easy for two operators to work together because one operator can stand on each side, and the multiple complications of the sitting position do not occur. The most significant disadvantage of the prone position is venous congestion that can lead to more significant blood loss, pooling of blood in the operative field, and soft-tissue swelling of the face. This congestion is much worse if the head is rotated and flexed and is improved somewhat by elevating the head above the level of the heart. Also, nasotracheal rather than orotracheal intubation can minimize compression of the base of tongue and impairment of venous drainage of the tongue and pharynx. The weight is distributed to minimize

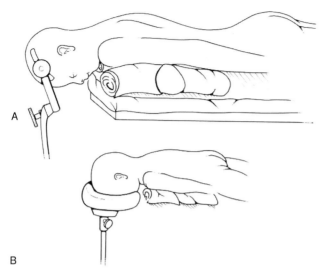

FIGURE 61-3 Prone position. The neck is in moderate flexion with the head higher than the heart. The surgeon and assistant stand on either side of the patient's neck. *A*, Skeletal fixation with a pin headholder. *B*, Padded horse shoe headrest for young patients. (From Cohen AR: Surgical Disorders of the Fourth Ventricle. Cambridge, MA: Blackwell Science, 1996.)

pressure points that can lead to skin breakdown and neuropathy, especially at the ulnar nerve at the elbow, common peroneal nerve across fibular head, and lateral femoral cutaneous nerve at the iliac crest. Two longitudinal padded roles are placed under the patient, and the knees and ankles are padded. The neck is placed in the military tuck position with moderate flexion of the upper cervical spine (to open up the space between the foramen magnum and the arch of C1) and less flexion of the lower cervical spine (to bring the occiput parallel with the patient's back). The chin and chest are at least two fingers apart. Finally, the table is positioned so that the neck is parallel to floor and the head is above the heart. The shoulders can be gently retracted toward the feet with some tape, and a strap under the buttocks is helpful to prevent sliding. The surgeon and assistant then operate from either side using the microscope, and the scrub nurse's Mayfield table can be placed over the patient's back.

The lateral oblique or lateral decubitus position is similar to the prone position except that the patient is lying on his or her side. This allows superior visualization of pathology high in the fourth ventricle, in the lateral recesses, and in the cerebellopontine angle. The posterior fossa contents do not sink inward as they do in the prone position, and the operative distance is more comfortable for the surgeon. The principal disadvantage of the lateral oblique position is that the anatomy is not centered so the surgeon must visualize all structures rotated. Also, it is constantly necessary to support the upper cerebellar hemisphere to maintain exposure, although the lower hemisphere naturally falls away. The patient is placed on his or her side with the dependent arm ventral on the table. A soft roll or intravenous bag wrapped in foam is placed in the axilla of the dependent arm to prevent brachial plexus injury or vascular compression, and the dependent leg is padded with special attention paid to the fibular head of the upper leg to avoid peroneal palsy.

The third option for positioning is the sitting position, in which the patient is positioned sitting upright so that the operative corridor is parallel to the floor (Fig. 61-4). The sitting position offers a very clear operative field because blood and cerebrospinal fluid drain out of the operative site. However, there are many risks to the sitting position.[1] The most significant dangers are cardiovascular instability and hypotension, air embolism, and subdural hematoma. All patients should have an agitated saline echocardiogram to exclude right-to-left shunt through a patent foramen ovale that could complicate air embolism, and the presence of such a shunt is an absolute contraindication for the sitting position. Precordial Doppler ultrasound monitor and end-tidal CO_2 should be monitored throughout the case. The risk of subdural hematoma is greatly increased by presence of a shunt, and if possible the shunt should be occluded before attempting an operation in the sitting position. Other risks of the sitting position include tension pneumocephalus, cervical myelopathy, thermal loss (especially in children), surgeon fatigue, and sudden loss of CSF from enlarged lateral and third ventricles after removal of a fourth ventricle mass lesion. When applying the headholder, the pin sites must be covered with Vaseline gauze to minimize entry of air[2] and the head taped to the headholder for extra support in case the pins become dislodged. The patient is elevated slowly into the sitting position so that the foramen magnum is at the surgeon's eye level with both of the patient's legs flexed at the knees to prevent postoperative sciatica. The instrument table is placed over the patient's head. Infants too young for pins may be taped to a padded headrest to support the forehead and chin, but it is probably safer to use the prone position. Throughout the operation, the patient should be carefully monitored for signs of hypotension or air embolism. If air embolism occurs, the wound should be packed with a saline-soaked sponge, and anesthesia should

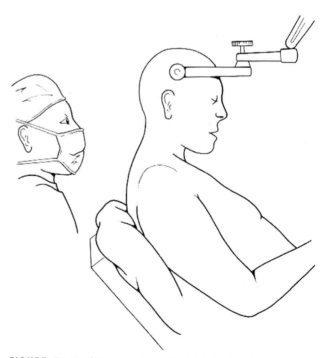

FIGURE 61-4 Sitting position. Skeletal fixation is maintained using a pin headholder with the neck moderately flexed. (From Cohen AR: Surgical Disorders of the Fourth Ventricle. Cambridge, MA: Blackwell Science, 1996.)

aspirate the atrial catheter to attempt to remove the embolus from the left atrium. If the embolus is severe, the patient should be placed in left decubitus position; otherwise, as soon as the patient is stable, the wound may be slowly exposed while covering the potential source of air with Gelfoam and Surgicel. If careful preparation is undertaken and complications dealt with promptly, the sitting position can be relatively safe.[3,4]

After positioning, the back of the head is shaved to expose the suboccipital region and the scalp is degreased with acetone and alcohol and then cleansed with a povidone-iodine solution. A linear midline incision is outlined 1 to 2 cm above the external occipital protuberance down to the level of C4. The operative field is walled off with towels, draped with iodoform adhesive, and infiltrated with 0.25% lidocaine with 1/400,000 epinephrine (or 0.1% lidocaine with 1/1,000,000 epinephrine in infants younger than 1 year old). If there is concern that it will be necessary to rapidly decompress the lateral ventricles intraoperatively or postoperatively, a burr hole may be drilled in the right posterior parietal region.

The incision is made with a no. 10 blade applying firm digital compression, and bleeding points are coagulated (Fig. 61-5). The incision should be midline, but if the tumor is lateral, a hockey stick incision can be used to allow for a wider craniectomy. The skin is undermined superficial to the fascia on both sides of the superior half of the incision in preparation to create a fascial flap for closure (Fig. 61-6). The skin is then elevated with toothed forceps or a skin hook and a plane of dissection developed with knife or monopolar coagulation, sparing the occipital artery and nerve whenever possible. Even a slight deviation off midline will produce brisk bleeding from the muscles once deeper tissues are exposed. When anatomic landmarks are identified to confirm that the operative course is truly midline, cerebellar or Weitlaner retractors are placed to

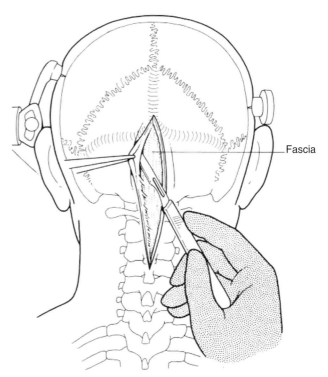

FIGURE 61-6 Fascial exposure. Skin flaps are mobilized by undermining the subcutaneous plane to prepare a fascial flap for closure. (From Cohen AR: Surgical Disorders of the Fourth Ventricle. Cambridge, MA: Blackwell Science, 1996.)

maintain exposure. As deeper layers are exposed, curved retractors may be used.

Next, the fascia is incised using a Y-shaped incision, keeping the lateral ends of the Y below the ligamentous insertion (Fig. 61-7). Although a linear midline fascial incision without the upper limbs of the Y allows use of the avascular plane between the splenius capitis and semispinalis capitis muscles, it is often difficult to reapproximate such an incision tightly at the superior nuchal line. Muscle flaps are then developed with monopolar cautery and periosteal elevators, stripping the muscle from the bone as far as the mastoid emissary vein. This exposure is maintained with two curved cerebellar retractors and the rostral flap is placed under tension using a 3-0 silk suture to reflect it rostrally (Fig. 61-8). The muscle insertions are stripped off the spinous process and laminae of C2. Finally, the junction between the pericranium and dura at the foramen magnum is sharply dissected and then the posterior fossa dura is separated from the inner table of the occipital bone using a curet.

The suboccipital craniotomy is begun with burr holes on either side of midline just below the transverse sinuses, approximately 3 cm from midline (Fig. 61-9). A third burr hole can be placed below the torcular in older patients. In children, the dura is not firmly adherent to the skull, so it is safe to drill close to or even on top of the sinuses, but more caution must be used with adults. The dura near the burr hole is then stripped using a Penfield dissector, and the bone is removed using a high-speed drill. The superior and lateral limits of the craniotomy are the transverse and sigmoid sinuses (Fig. 61-10). Inferiorly, the craniotomy should always include the posterior edge of the foramen magnum

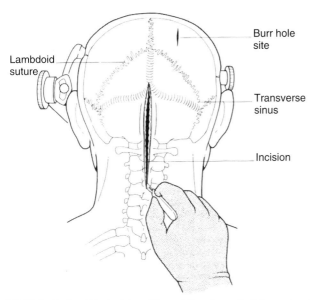

FIGURE 61-5 Skin incision. The midline linear incision extends from just above the inion to the midcervical region. (From Cohen AR: Surgical Disorders of the Fourth Ventricle. Cambridge, MA: Blackwell Science, 1996.)

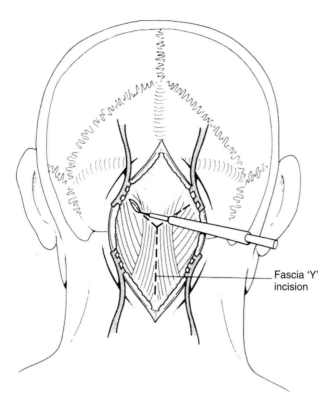

FIGURE 61-7 Fascial incision. The fascia and muscle are incised in the shape of a Y. The inferior limb of the Y passes through the avascular ligamentum nuchae. (From Cohen AR: Surgical Disorders of the Fourth Ventricle. Cambridge, MA: Blackwell Science, 1996.)

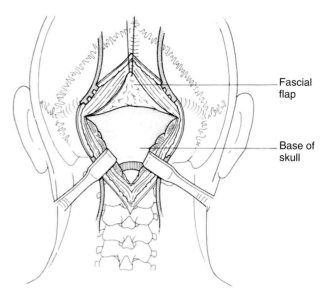

FIGURE 61-8 Bone exposure. The occipital bone at the base of the skull is exposed widely using monopolar cautery and periosteal elevators. (From Cohen AR: Surgical Disorders of the Fourth Ventricle. Cambridge, MA: Blackwell Science, 1996.)

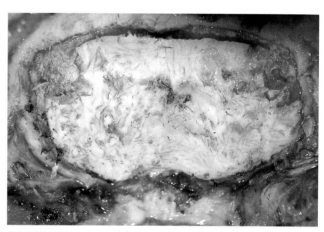

FIGURE 61-9 Suboccipital craniotomy. Burr holes are placed, and a high-speed drill is used to connect them. The bone flap is elevated after the dura is carefully stripped. (From Cohen AR: Surgical Disorders of the Fourth Ventricle. Cambridge, MA: Blackwell Science, 1996.)

to prevent laceration of the brain against the closed bony rim when cerebellar elements are retracted downward and minimize damage from herniation if hematoma or swelling should occur postoperatively. The midline bone is removed last because it is often very vascular and contains a keel that can be quite deep. This keel must be stripped of dura with a Penfield dissector, using extreme caution near the occipital sinus in the midline and the annular sinus near the foramen magnum. All exposed bone edges should be waxed, especially in the sitting position. Because of the irregular contour of

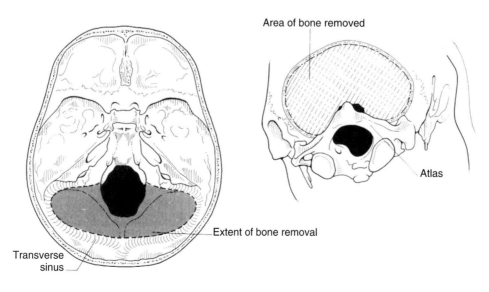

FIGURE 61-10 Suboccipital craniotomy. The craniotomy may be extended superiorly to the transverse sinus, laterally to the sigmoid sinuses, and inferiorly to the foramen magnum. (From Cohen AR: Surgical Disorders of the Fourth Ventricle. Cambridge, MA: Blackwell Science, 1996.)

the inner bone surface in adult patients, it is sometimes necessary to perform a craniectomy rather than a craniotomy, removing the bone in a piecemeal fashion.

To expose the posterior arch of C1, the soft tissues overlying it are reflected laterally using a small periosteal elevator, stripping the inferior arch first because the vertebral artery is on its superior aspect. It is sometimes easier to do this after C2 has been exposed. The periosteum can sometimes be swept off the arch of C1 using an index finger covered with gauze. Monopolar cautery should be used with caution when dissecting the soft tissue over C1 (especially at the superolateral surface) to prevent injury to vertebral artery. It is important to remember that C1 can be bifid and is often cartilaginous in infants and young children. C1 laminectomy is helpful for lesions that herniate beneath the foramen magnum. To remove the lamina, small angled curets can be used to strip the deep surface of the bone, and then the bone itself is removed with an angled Kerrison punch or Leksell rongeur (Fig. 61-11). Because extending a laminectomy below C2 in young children increases the risk of swan neck deformity,[5] it is prudent to remove the smallest amount of bone possible. For most tumors, it is usually only necessary to remove as far as one level above the most caudal aspect of the tumor.

Before the dural incision, the wound should be irrigated and retractor systems and microscope prepared (Fig. 61-12). If the dura is tense, the intracranial pressure can be reduced with external ventricular drainage (if available), hyperventilation, or mannitol, although mannitol should be used with caution in the sitting position as it has been implicated in the development of subdural hematomas. All techniques for dural incision require crossing the occipital and annular sinuses, which may be very large in infants younger than age 2 and can persist until 25 years of age. A Y-shaped incision allows wide visualization and can be extended if necessary (Fig. 61-13). One superior limb should be incised first with a no. 15 blade. The incision should start just inferior to the transverse sinus and travel obliquely to the midline, stopping short of the occipital sinus. The other superior limb is incised next, and then they are connected over the midline. If there is significant bleeding from the midline occipital sinus, it should be controlled with obliquely placed hemostatic clips or suture ligatures (Fig. 61-14). Either way, both the superficial and deep layer of the dura must be incised or the sinus will be tented open. The vertical limb of the Y is opened last using scissors so that the dura can be tented if bleeding is seen. The vertical incision extends to the foramen magnum so that it will extend below the falx cerebelli, which is occasionally present in childhood. If bleeding is very troublesome, the dura can be opened para-midline. The dura is then covered with a moist collagen sponge or wet Gelfoam sandwich to prevent desiccation and anchored to the fascia with 4-0 Neurolon suture. This allows wide exposure of the cerebellar vermis and hemispheres (Figs. 61-15 and 61-16). The arachnoid is opened next over the cisterna magna to allow drainage of CSF (Fig. 61-17). If the tumor is in the cerebellar hemisphere, another dural incision can be extended laterally to more fully expose the involved cerebellum.

Techniques for intradural exposure and resection of the tumor will vary depending on the location and size of the tumor and is discussed in more detail for each individual tumor. Gentle separation of the cerebellar tonsils will

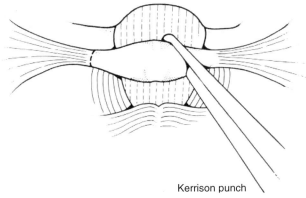

Kerrison punch

FIGURE 61-11 Removal of atlas (C1). This step may facilitate removal of some fourth ventricular tumors. To prevent injury to an aberrant vertebral artery, it is best to avoid use of monopolar cautery near the arches of C1 and C2. (From Cohen AR: Surgical Disorders of the Fourth Ventricle. Cambridge, MA: Blackwell Science, 1996.)

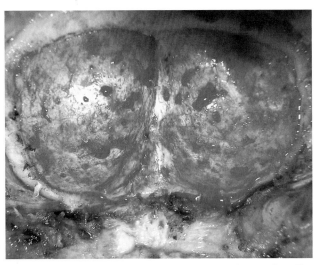

FIGURE 61-12 Dural exposure after removal of bone flap. The arch of C1 has been preserved in this patient.

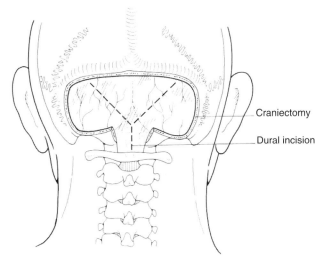

Craniectomy

Dural incision

FIGURE 61-13 Dural incision. The vertical limb of the Y-shaped incision, which overlies the occipital sinus, is opened last. (From Cohen AR: Surgical Disorders of the Fourth Ventricle. Cambridge, MA: Blackwell Science, 1996.)

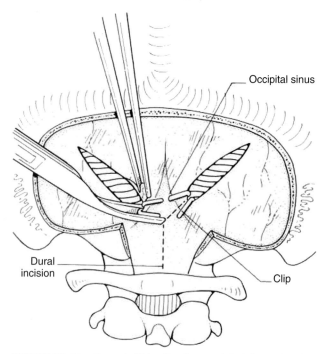

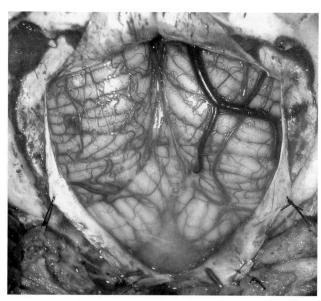

FIGURE 61-14 Control of bleeding from occipital sinus with clips. (From Cohen AR: Surgical Disorders of the Fourth Ventricle. Cambridge, MA: Blackwell Science, 1996.)

FIGURE 61-16 Exposure of cerebellar hemispheres and vermis. The tumor (in this case, a medulloblastoma) can be seen between the hemispheric tonsils in the lower midline of the exposure.

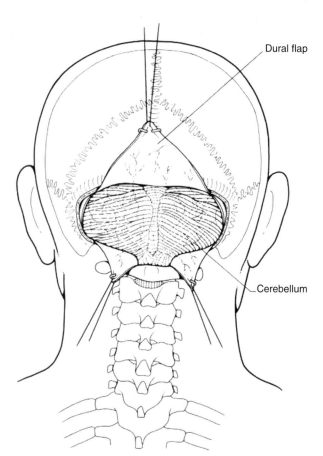

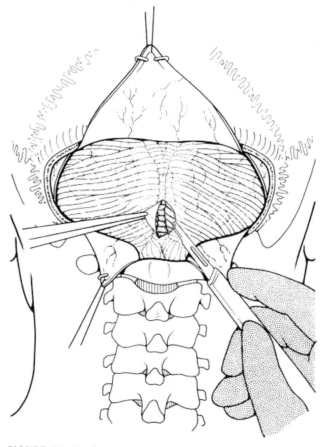

FIGURE 61-15 Exposure of cerebellar hemispheres and vermis. (From Cohen AR: Surgical Disorders of the Fourth Ventricle. Cambridge, MA: Blackwell Science, 1996.)

FIGURE 61-17 Opening the cisterna magna. This allows drainage of cerebrospinal fluid and relaxes the posterior fossa. (From Cohen AR: Surgical Disorders of the Fourth Ventricle. Cambridge, MA: Blackwell Science, 1996.)

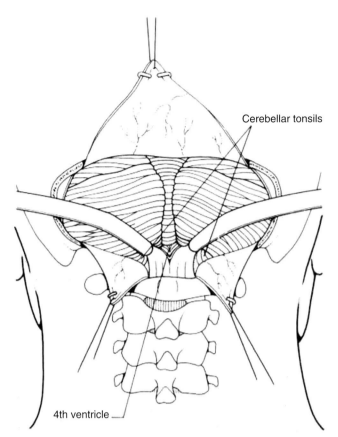

FIGURE 61-18 Cerebellar tonsils

4th ventricle

FIGURE 61-18 Exposure of the fourth ventricle. Retraction of the cerebellar tonsils widens the vallecula, which allows visualization of the caudal fourth ventricle. Automatic retractors may be used to facilitate exposure. (From Cohen AR: Surgical Disorders of the Fourth Ventricle. Cambridge, MA: Blackwell Science, 1996.)

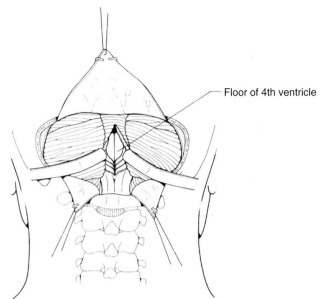

Floor of 4th ventricle

FIGURE 61-19 Splitting the vermis. Incision of the cerebellar vermis allows exposure of lesions situated more rostrally. Alternatively, some fourth ventricular tumors can be approached without splitting the vermis by opening the cerebromedullary fissure on each side. (From Cohen AR: Surgical Disorders of the Fourth Ventricle. Cambridge, MA: Blackwell Science, 1996.)

expose the cerebellomedullary fissure through the opened vallecula, giving an unimpeded view of the inferior roof of the fourth ventricle (Fig. 61-18). Narrow malleable automatic retractors can be used to maintain separation of the tonsils; the retractor system should be kept close to the patient so as not to interfere with the subsequent operation. The operating microscope is brought into the field, and the anatomy is identified. In particular, the location of the caudal loops of the PICAs should be carefully noted because they are often tethered to the tonsils and the walls of the cerebellomedullary fissure by small perforating branches. The foramen of Magendie and the small tuft of choroid plexus protruding from it will be clearly seen, as well as any tumor that protrudes from the foramen. The thin layers forming the lower part of the roof can be opened to expose the cavity of the fourth ventricle. Often this will provide sufficient exposure, but if not, it is sometimes helpful to retract the inferior vermis rostrally or incise the caudal vermis, avoiding the gutter between the vermis and the hemisphere to prevent injury to the inferior vermian veins there (Fig. 61-19). Lateral lesions may require removal of one tonsil by dividing the pedicle attaching the superolateral margin of the tonsil to the biventral lobule. To reach the lateral roof or lateral recess, part of the cerebellar hemisphere can be resected without significant morbidity as long as the dentate nuclei are not violated. If the tumor is not adherent to the floor of

the fourth ventricle, cottonoid patties should be placed beneath the tumor to protect the delicate brain stem structures just beneath the floor. These cottonoids should be placed under direct vision and never used as a tool to dissect the tumor from the floor of the fourth ventricle. After the tumor has been removed, the glistening white floor of the fourth ventricle should be clearly visible. The retractors are then removed, and the cerebellar hemispheres are allowed to fall back into place. If there is extension of the tumor through one of the foramina of Luschka into the cerebellopontine cistern, the ipsilateral tonsil and cerebellar hemisphere can be retracted medially to expose it. Sometimes it is necessary to do a secondary retromastoid approach to completely resect the tumor.

The dura is closed using a running 4-0 Neurolon or polypropylene after approximating the dural edges with interrupted sutures (Fig. 61-20). A Valsalva maneuver will identify potentially dangerous venous bleeding. The dural closure should be watertight if possible, starting peripherally then working centrally to gradually overcome the tension. If the dura is not watertight, there is increased risk of pseudomeningocele due to a ball-valve effect or hydrocephalus from arachnoid adhesions produced by blood from the muscles. Sometimes the dura will be dried and shrunken by the end of the operation, especially if measures have been taken to obliterate the occipital sinus. In this case, the remaining defect can be covered with a pericranial or fascial graft (Fig. 61-21). Freeze-dried bovine pericardium or human allograft dura can also be used, but use of autogenous material is less likely to produce postoperative aseptic meningitis.[6] If clips were used on the midline occipital sinus, they can be removed as the dura is sutured. The suture line may be covered with thrombin-soaked Gelfoam. If a craniotomy was performed, the bone flap can be secured

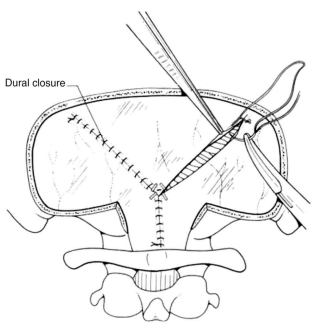

FIGURE 61-20   Dural closure. After the pathology is removed and hemostasis is obtained, the Y incision is closed with a running suture, starting peripherally. The lower midline limb is closed last. (From Cohen AR: Surgical Disorders of the Fourth Ventricle. Cambridge, MA: Blackwell Science, 1996.)

with wires, plates and screws, or sutures. Alternatively, the defect can be covered with a titanium screen held in place by gently compressing the screen and allowing it to insert itself between the dura and inner margins of the bony defect. The fascia is closed with interrupted absorbable sutures to approximate the muscle and fascia (Fig. 61-22). If the fascia is dried and difficult to approximate, the skeletal fixation apparatus can be loosened and the neck extended to facilitate closure. An adequate amount of tissue must be

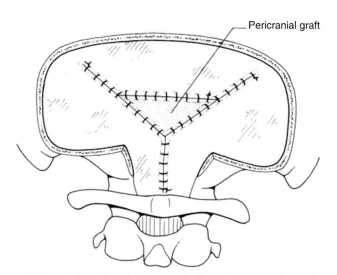

FIGURE 61-21   Use of a dural graft. If the dura cannot be easily brought together, a graft of pericranium or fascia can be used to complete the closure. (From Cohen AR: Surgical Disorders of the Fourth Ventricle. Cambridge, MA: Blackwell Science, 1996.)

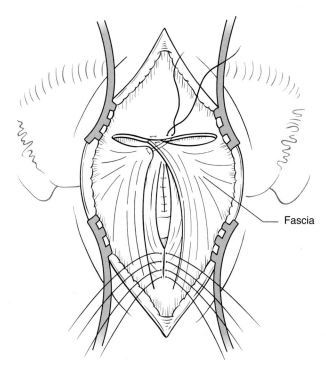

FIGURE 61-22   Fascial closure. The muscle and fascia are closed in layers using interrupted absorbable sutures. (From Cohen AR: Surgical Disorders of the Fourth Ventricle. Cambridge, MA: Blackwell Science, 1996.)

left at the superior fascial flap to prevent buttonholes at superior nuchal line. The scalp is then closed in layers, ending with a subcutaneous reapproximation using interrupted absorbable sutures with inverted knots. If in the sitting position, all layers should start from the caudal end of the wound so that the tails do not hang in the way. The wound is then closed with sutures or staples (Fig. 61-23). The wound is covered with a sterile dressing, and the patient is extubated in a supine position.

Complications

Hydrocephalus is common with fourth ventricular tumors and is one of the most significant causes of morbidity and mortality associated with these tumors.[7,8] In the past, many patients with tumors and hydrocephalus underwent temporizing preoperative shunting to treat hydrocephalus and prevent pseudomeningocele, CSF leak, and meningitis from fistulas. However, more recently, it has been observed that shunting is associated with many complications, and the increased incidence of subdural hematoma, infection, and brain stem compression from upward herniation may outweigh its benefits.[9-12] Also, the advent of advanced radiographic imaging has allowed diagnosis of fourth ventricular tumors much earlier than before, when patients were frequently moribund with dehydration and malnutrition from vomiting and hydrocephalus needed to be urgently treated. Today, only approximately 10% to 20% of patients with cerebellar and posterior fossa tumors require permanent shunting[7,8,13] and most of these have slow-growing tumors

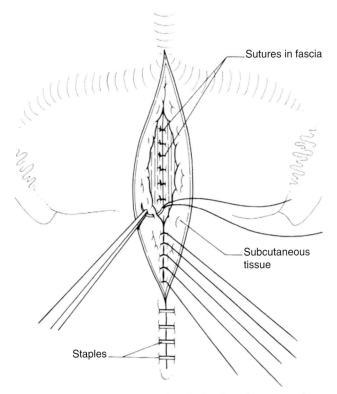

Sutures in fascia

Subcutaneous
tissue

Staples

FIGURE 61-23 Skin closure. After closing the subcutaneous layer with interrupted inverted absorbable sutures, the skin is closed with staples or monofilament nylon suture material. (From Cohen AR: Surgical Disorders of the Fourth Ventricle. Cambridge, MA: Blackwell Science, 1996.)

such as astrocytomas because more acute tumors distend the ventricles for a short period of time and do not allow outlet adhesions to form. Risk factors for shunt dependence include younger age, larger preoperative ventricle size, and more extensive tumors. In many cases, preoperative high-dose steroids will produce satisfactory improvement in hydrocephalus. Otherwise, an appropriate alternative to shunting is perioperative external ventricular drainage,[14] especially if a patient is lethargic or obtunded. This allows for precise pressure monitoring and control of drainage rate to prevent upward herniation and, if continued postoperatively, clearance of debris, proteinaceous blood, and air from the operation. Although external ventricular drainage does reduce the need for permanent shunts, the infection rate may be as high as 10%, so it should be used judiciously. If a shunt is required for a malignant tumor, there may be an increased risk of extraneural metastasis through the shunt tubing (especially to the peritoneum),[15] although some studies have suggested that such metastases may occur as often in patients without shunts.[16]

Pneumocephalus in the ventricles and subdural space is common after fourth ventricular surgery, especially when patients are operated in the sitting position[17] although it also occurs after prone operations. It is much more common when patients have preoperative hydrocephalus and frequently results from overzealous drainage of CSF through an external ventricular drain intraoperatively. Because nitrous oxide can diffuse into air-filled spaces, it is possible

that nitrous oxide contributes to tension pneumocephalus, although this is controversial. If tension pneumocephalus is recognized intraoperatively, the patient should be placed in the Trendelenburg position and the operative bed irrigated to replace air with the irrigating fluid. Symptomatic postoperative tension pneumocephalus can be treated with a small frontal burr hole to relieve the pressure caused by the trapped air. Intraventricular air may cause ventriculoperitoneal shunt malfunction due to airlock.

Postoperative pseudomeningoceles affect 10% to 15% of all children with posterior fossa tumors. Normally, these are small collections of fluid that respond well to serial lumbar punctures. Occasionally, they can put the closure under tension and eventually produce a leak, which carries a risk of meningitis. Pseudomeningocele may be a manifestation of hydrocephalus and in some cases may require a CSF diversion shunt to control.

Aseptic meningitis, also called posterior fossa fever, is a rare occurrence after posterior fossa surgery, especially for epidermoids or dermoids that rupture intraoperatively leaking cholesterol cyst fluid, although it also occurs after resection of astrocytoma or medulloblastoma. It may be a presenting symptom preoperatively but much more common as a postoperative complication.[18,19] Patients usually present approximately 1 week after surgery with fever, headache, irritability, and CSF pleocytosis. It can be difficult in some cases to differentiate aseptic meningitis from true bacterial meningitis, which should always be carefully excluded before treating for aseptic meningitis. The condition resolves with steroid or antiinflammatory treatment and serial lumbar punctures to remove CSF.

Transient or permanent cranial nerve palsies sometimes occur after surgery of the fourth ventricle. These deficits are usually immediately evident in the recovery room. The most common deficit is palsy of cranial nerves VI and VII caused by disruption of the fourth ventricular floor along the facial colliculus where the intrapontine course of the facial nerve loops around the abducens nucleus. If this area is dissected or excavated, the deficit will often be permanent, but even gentle diathermy with low-current bipolar can produce a partial paralysis with total or nearly total recovery. In most cases, patients with temporary facial weakness should be treated to prevent corneal desiccation with artificial tears, temporary tarsorrhaphy, or gold weight implantation in the upper eyelid. Permanent weakness has been treated with facial-hypoglossal anastomosis, which can partially restore upper eyelid function. Abducens palsy is best treated with an eye patch to prevent diplopia (or amblyopia if the patient is younger than 5 years of age); if the condition persists beyond a few months, eye muscle surgery may be appropriate. Cranial nerve XII palsy can occur from injury to the hypoglossal trigone. Although less common than facial palsy, this is a very serious complication because it is usually bilateral because the nuclei are close together by the median raphe. Patients present with dysarthria, swallowing apraxia, and continuous drooling. When combined with cranial nerve VII or IX/X deficits, even aggressive treatment with tracheostomy and feeding tubes may not prevent serious complications due to aspiration.

Skewed ocular deviation is a rare condition that is sometimes seen after fourth ventricular surgery during which the aqueductal opening is manipulated. This usually occurs with damage to the region of the cerebral aqueduct. It is thought to occur because vertical yoking of eye movements involves pathways that pass through the periaqueductal gray matter in the mesencephalic tegmentum. This condition usually resolves within weeks after surgery and can be avoided by gentleness when working around the aqueduct.

The posterior fossa syndrome, also called posterior fossa mutism or pseudobulbar palsy, is characterized by the delayed onset of mutism, emotional lability, and supranuclear lesions that occurs within a few days after midline posterior fossa operations.[20] The syndrome has been seen in as many as 15% of intraventricular approaches to lesions near the brain stem but has also been described with supracerebellar infratentorial approach to the pineal region and retromastoid lateral cerebellar approach to the side or front of the brain stem. Patients present with global confusion, disorientation, combativeness, paranoia, or visual hallucinations. They are generally alert and will follow simple commands but will sometimes refuse to speak or present scanning speech. Orofacial apraxia, drooling, dysphagia, pharyngeal dysfunction, and flat affect are common, but there is no actual weakness, hence the term pseudobulbar palsy. Because of the delay in onset, it has been suggested that edema from operative manipulation may play a role, for example, through transmission of retractor pressure from the medial cerebellum through fiber pathways along the middle and superior cerebellar peduncles into the upper pons and midbrain. There are no consistent neuropathologic findings, and most patients have some improvement over several weeks to months.[20-22]

Generalized and focal seizures have been described after posterior fossa surgery. The incidence is higher in faster growing tumors and in the presence of ventricular drainage or shunting. Late-onset seizures may be related to remote hemorrhage, meningitis, or hydrocephalus.

Ipsilateral limb ataxia, dysmetria, dysdiadokinesis, and hypotonia usually result from damage to the cerebellar hemisphere, especially the dentate nucleus, which is located along the superolateral margin of the roof of the fourth ventricle adjacent to the upper pole of the tonsil. Most injuries to the dentate nucleus occur during dissection of a hemispheric tumor. Retraction during dissection of the superior vermis can injure the superior cerebellar peduncle, producing similar symptoms. Unless the dentate is completely ablated, most patients recover well within a few months with only minor residual intention tremor that does not interfere with motor development.

Because the superior and inferior cerebellar peduncles make up the lateral walls of the superior roof of the fourth ventricle, they are susceptible to damage during intraventricular procedures. The superior cerebellar peduncle contains pathways connecting the dentate nucleus to the red nucleus and thalamus, so damage to the superior cerebellar peduncle produces a clinical syndrome similar to damage of the dentate nucleus with ipsilateral ataxia and intention tremor. Injury to the inferior cerebellar peduncle produces a syndrome similar to ablation of the flocculonodular lobe with equilibrium disturbances, truncal ataxia, staggering gait, and oscillation of head and trunk on assuming an erect position without ataxia of voluntary movement of the extremities. Injury to the middle cerebellar peduncle (which causes ataxia and dysmetria) is rare during intraventricular

procedures but can occur during an approach to the cerebellopontine cistern.

Postoperative dysarthria can result when resections extend into the paravermian part of the cerebellar hemisphere. This occurs more frequently from left hemisphere injury than from vermal or right hemisphere injury.

Acute urinary retention is an uncommon complication of dissection of the fourth ventricular floor near the striae medullaris, presumably due to injury to the pontine micturition center in the pontine tegmentum, the structure that integrates the cortex with sacral and pelvic sensory pathways that apprise bladder filling status.[23] Patients with this condition demonstrate an inability to initiate voiding despite a full bladder with high intravesicular pressure. Because the pontine micturition center is deep in the pons near the reticular activating system, this symptom is usually associated with a disturbance in sensorium but can occur in conscious patients. It is usually reversible but does not respond to detrusor augmenting agents or α-adrenergic blockers. Patients are best managed by intermittent catheterization.

Patients treated with radiation sometimes have significant learning disabilities[24] and should undergo follow-up neuropsychiatric evaluation. Radiation treatment has also been associated with endocrine dysfunction, growth dysfunction, hypothyroidism, delayed or precocious puberty, and secondary malignancy.[25] Patients who have extensive laminectomies are predisposed to development of swan neck deformity, and should be kept in a soft cervical collar for 6 to 8 weeks until the paraspinal muscles reattach and be monitored with cervical spine radiographs every few months for a few years to check for spinal deformities.

Injury to major vessels is rare with fourth ventricular surgery. The most likely artery to be injured is the PICA. Most patients with PICA injury present with postoperative flocculonodular dysfunction with nausea, vomiting, nystagmus, vertigo, and inability to stand or walk without appendicular dysmetria. Venous injury is extremely rare even if veins are sacrificed due to diffuse anastomosis in this region. Veins near the tonsils, vermis, and inferior roof can be safely sacrificed. Medial retraction of the cerebellar hemisphere to expose the lateral recess and cerebellopontine cistern can stretch bridging veins to the sigmoid sinus, but it is seldom necessary to sacrifice them. Most venous infarctions of the posterior fossa have followed sacrifice of the petrosal veins or veins of the cerebellomesencephalic fissure (including the precentral cerebellar vein).

SPECIFIC TUMORS

Medulloblastoma

The term medulloblastoma was initially introduced by Bailey and Cushing[26] who noted the highly cellular architecture of small round basophilic cells that showed various degrees of differentiation along neuronal and glial lines. They assumed that the cell of origin (the medulloblast) was a primitive cell capable of both neural and glial differentiation. More recently, it has been theorized that these are related to tumors with similar histology in other locations, such as in the pineal gland (pineoblastoma), ependyma (ependymoblastoma), retina (retinoblastoma), and elsewhere (neuroblastoma). The term primitive neuroectodermal tumor was used to describe these tumors. A medulloblastoma would therefore be described as a primitive neuroectodermal tumor of the fourth ventricle.

Medulloblastoma is the most common malignant primary brain tumor in children, accounting for 20% to 25% of all childhood primary brain tumors and 40% of all childhood posterior fossa tumors.[27,28] Peak incidence is 3 to 5 years of age; half of all medulloblastoma patients are younger than 10 years of age at diagnosis, and three-quarters are younger than age 15. Medulloblastoma is uncommon in infancy, and less than 5% of patients present younger than 1 year of age. There is a second peak between 20 and 40 years, so that medulloblastoma accounts for 5% of all adult posterior fossa tumors and 1% of all adult brain tumors. Adult medulloblastomas are more likely to be hemispheric than midline, likely due to the lateral migration of cells of the granular layer of cerebellum from the inferior medullary velum. Adult medulloblastomas are also more likely to be cystic or necrotic, have poorly defined margins, and have less contrast enhancement.[29] They may even involve the cerebellar surface and resemble meningiomas. There is a slight male preponderance in most clinical series, and for reasons that are unclear, medulloblastomas have a significantly higher incidence in North America than elsewhere in the world.[30] Medulloblastomas frequently metastasize in the subarachnoid space, and some dissemination is evident in 20% to 30% of all patients and 50% of young patients at diagnosis.[31,32] Familial medulloblastoma has been reported.[33]

Medulloblastomas grow quickly, so onset of symptoms is usually fairly acute; most patients are symptomatic less than 2 months before the tumor is diagnosed, and very few report symptoms for longer than 6 months. Most patients initially experience symptoms of increased intracranial pressure from CSF obstruction. Symptoms typically begin with intermittent headache (often worst in the morning) followed by vomiting and eventually gait problems.[34] Gait difficulties include wide-based gait and inability to tandem walk; these findings are often subtle and not appreciated by the child or the parents but frequently alert the physician to the presence of a neurologic lesion. Clinical signs include ataxia for midline tumors or dysmetria/dysdiadokinesia for lateral tumors. Most patients have papilledema by the time that they present for evaluation. Less common signs include diplopia from abducens palsy, facial paresis or lower cranial nerve palsy from tumor invasion, head tilt from tumor extension into the upper spinal canal, or impaction of the cerebellar tonsils at the foramen magnum against the first two cervical nerve roots. Because medulloblastomas can metastasize along the subarachnoid space, some patients present with cranial or spinal nerve root symptoms from distant metastases or even seizures from cortical metastases. Patients who present with signs of metastatic disease have a limited life expectancy.

Medulloblastomas usually appear as midline solid tumors on neuroimaging, although cystic change is sometimes observed. Eighty-five percent are midline vermian lesions, usually arising from the vermis or inferior medullary velum and growing into the fourth ventricle, sometimes appearing to be entirely intraventricular.[32] Adult lesions are much more likely to be in a lateral location. Computed tomography (CT) demonstrates a homogeneous hyperdense lesion that enhances intensely and diffusely after contrast administration

with occasional heterogeneously enhancing regions due to necrosis, although rarely medulloblastomas do not enhance at all on CT.[35] Calcification will be apparent in 10% of medulloblastomas,[36] but the presence of calcium or cystic change is more typical of ependymomas. On magnetic resonance imaging (MRI), the lesion is hypointense to isointense to brain on T1 and hyperintense or hypointense on T2 with heterogeneous signal due to microcysts, necrotic cavities, tumor vessels, or calcification (Fig. 61-24). The tumor displays irregular enhancement with MRI contrast material,[36,37] and enhanced MRI will disclose small cortical or basal metastases in 5% to 10% of cases. Sagittal MRI can help delineate the relationship of the tumor to the vermis, midbrain tectum, Galen's vein, and cervicomedullary junction. Additionally, sagittal MRI can differentiate true intraventricular tumors from extraventricular vermian tumors: intraventricular tumors will widen the aqueduct and displace the quadrigeminal plate posterosuperiorly, whereas dorsal lesions will kink the quadrigeminal plate giving it a C-shaped appearance.[38] Uncommonly, the tumor will be seen to extend out of foramen of Luschka, but this is far more typical of ependymomas. In young children, medulloblastomas are often radiographically indistinguishable from ependymomas by radiographic appearance alone. Because of the frequency of craniospinal metastases, all patients should undergo contrast MRI of the entire craniospinal axis.

Grossly, medulloblastomas are discrete, soft tumors, although adult lesions tend to be firmer and more adherent to leptomeninges. Medulloblastomas can be divided into two broad histologic patterns: classic and desmoplastic. Classic medulloblastomas, which make up three fourths of the total, are seen to have dense, diffusely monotonous sheets of cells with intensely basophilic nuclei and scant cytoplasm (small round blue cells). There is regional variability in the size and shape of cells, number of mitoses, and appearance of nuclei, and necrosis is common. Desmoplastic medulloblastomas have a higher proportion of fibrous stroma associated with perivascular collagen skeleton of tumor. Sometimes there are uniform compact lines of cells around islands of relative hypocellularity; when this is seen, the compact rims stain heavily with reticulin and the hypocellular areas stain for glial fibrillary acidic protein (GFAP). Occasionally, individual cells resembling oligodendrocytes are seen, having perinuclear halos and staining with tubulin and synaptophysin. The desmoplastic variant is more common in older patients. In young patients, location is not associated with histology, but older patients are more likely to have desmoplastic histology in more lateral tumors.[39] In both histologic patterns, there are occasionally neuroblastic areas with histology similar to neuroblastomas with Homer-Wright rosettes (rings of nuclei surrounding a central zone of fibrillary processes) and perivascular pseudorosettes that resemble those in ependymomas except that they do not stain for GFAP. Mature ganglion cells are sometimes seen, although it is controversial whether these represent further neuronal differentiation or engulfing of deep cerebellar nuclei by the tumor. Also seen are islands of glial development characterized by clusters of GFAP-staining cells, with pink cytoplasm commonly seen as circular whirls of cells with bipolar processes. These may represent entrapped or reactive astrocytes.

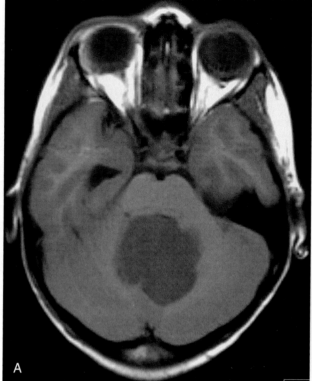

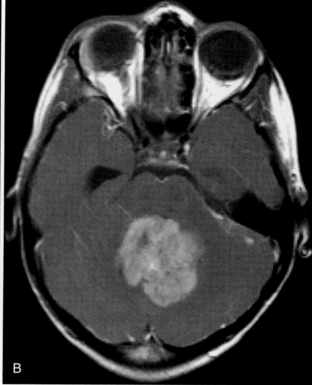

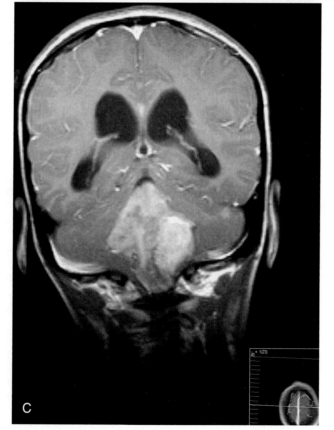

FIGURE 61-24 *A,* Medulloblastoma, T1 without contrast. The midline hypointense lesion usually arises from the inferior medullary velum. *B,* Medulloblastoma, T1 with contrast. The lesion enhances brightly and heterogeneously. *C,* Medulloblastoma, T1 with contrast, coronal section. The tumor is seen to fill the fourth ventricle and displace the cerebellar hemispheres laterally.

To resect a medulloblastoma, the posterior fossa is exposed as described previously. Because most medulloblastomas arise from the vermis or inferior medullary velum, the tumor will often be immediately visible, either protruding through the foramen of Magendie or immediately deep to the vermis. If the tumor protrudes through the foramen, it often will fill the cisterna magna and even extend into the upper cervical canal. If the tumor is deep to the vermis, the tonsils will usually be displaced backward, and it may be necessary to retract the cerebellar tonsils or biventricular lobules using self-retaining retractors to visualize the inferior vermis. By exposing the cerebellomedullary fissure on each side, it is sometimes possible to resect the tumor without dividing the cerebellar vermis, although sometimes midline incision of the vermis is necessary to obtain adequate exposure. Gentle retraction of the cerebellar hemispheres will expose the intraventricular tumor, which generally appears purple-gray, friable, and quite vascular.

Even with a vermian incision, it is seldom possible to expose the entire tumor. Therefore, the next step is to debulk the central portion of the tumor using blunt or sharp dissectors with microscissors and microsuction aspiration. Desmoplastic tumors cannot be aspirated with microsuction, so ultrasonic aspiration can be used for these tumors, but this must be used with caution around the brain stem because of increased destruction of tissue. Bleeding is controlled with bipolar cautery. To expedite removal of the tumor and minimize blood loss, the tumor can be divided into four quadrants; as soon as bleeding becomes troublesome from one quadrant, a micropatty is placed there and attention turned to a different quadrant, and so on. By the time the dissection returns to the first quadrant, the bleeding will have slowed enough to allow continued resection. After the tumor has been debulked, the shell of tumor is carefully stripped off the brain stem from inferior to superior using a small brain retractor and separated from the brain stem using cottonoid patties. Cottonoid patties should be placed along the fourth ventricular floor as early as possible to protect the brain stem, and it is important to constantly ensure that the trajectory is correct to prevent diving into the brain stem at an angle. When the brain stem is protected with a cottonoid patty, the inferior half of the tumor can then be safely removed. The tumor is rarely adherent or invasive to the brain stem, but when it is, gross total resection should not be attempted due to the risk of permanent cranial nerve defects. Rather, any focal areas of adhesion are separated using bipolar cautery and covered with a cottonoid. Later, when the tumor is entirely removed, the residual tumor tissue can be carefully aspirated parallel to the plane of the fourth ventricular floor until only a thin lining remains, and this lining can be coagulated with bipolar cautery to reduce the viability of remaining cells.

The next step is to resect the lateral and anterior portions of the tumor. The lateral and superior attachments of the tumor usually blend with the paravermian brain so there is seldom a plane between tumor and normal brain. As a result, most residual tumor fragments are left in this area. Because there are minimal postoperative neurologic deficits that result from removing a thin rim of cerebellum, the dissection should be carried out on the brain side of the brain-tumor interface so that all the tumor is resected and hemostasis is easier to obtain. At the end of the dissection,

there will be a bed of clean white brain. The lateral dissection is extended onto the ependymal surface, where the tumor attaches to the cerebellum, and this margin is defined upward and forward until the dilated caudal aqueduct is reached, producing a conical dissection field. Finally, the anterosuperior tumor pole is removed, leaving the tip of the tumor covering the opening of the caudal aqueduct until the end of the operation so that no blood from the dissection will enter the lateral or third ventricle.

If only a small amount of tumor extends laterally through the foramen of Luschka, it can usually be aspirated under direct vision from the ventricular side because the tumor is not adherent to the ependyma. A large extraventricular segment that extends to the pons or mesencephalic peduncle may rarely require a secondary retromastoid approach after main tumor debulking with extension of the craniectomy and dural opening to lateral venous sinuses. The cerebellar hemisphere is retracted medially and dissection extended along the plane of the petrous bone to expose the lateral part of the tumor. It is important to identify the lower cranial nerves because they are sometimes encapsulated by the tumor.

Because medulloblastoma often spreads through the subarachnoid space and the tumors are highly radiosensitive, radiotherapy to the entire neuraxis is considered standard, even when there are no obvious lesions on postoperative imaging.[31] Best survival rates are obtained with 3600 to 4000 cGy to whole craniospinal axis supplemented to 5400 to 5600 cGy to the primary site and 1800 to 3000 cGy extra to any area of lump disease. Young children have a high incidence of postradiation neurocognitive deficits so radiation should be delayed or eliminated in very young patients; various studies have suggested lower dose[40] or chemotherapy until the brain is mature enough to handle radiation.[28] Trials using various chemotherapy regimens have demonstrated improved survival with chemotherapy, especially for locally extensive or widely disseminated tumors.[28,41,42]

Prognosis for patients with medulloblastoma is related to size, invasiveness, and dissemination of tumor at diagnosis; age of the patient; and postoperative residual tumor. Large tumors have been shown to have a lower 5-year disease-free survival.[42] Brain stem invasion also carries a poorer prognosis and is problematic for preoperative staging because it cannot be predicted based on MRI.[42,43] Presence of dissemination through the neuraxis is the single most significant predictor of outcome for all histologic types of medulloblastoma. Even microscopic dissemination (determined by lumbar puncture performed at least 10 days postoperatively) carries a significantly lower 5-year survival.[28] Extraneural metastases to bone and even lymph nodes have been reported, but the incidence is too low to warrant screening all medulloblastoma patients.[44] Young patients are much more likely to have dissemination, but patients younger than 4 years of age have a worse prognosis, out of proportion to the increased dissemination rates.[41] Finally, completeness of resection is thought to affect the subsequent behavior of the tumor,[43,45] and presence of more than 1 mm³ of residual tumor has been associated with worse survival. Histology has not been shown to affect prognosis except for rare tumor subtypes at the extreme ends of the histologic spectrum; specifically, medulloblastomas with extensive nodularity and large cells/anaplastic medulloblastomas are associated with better and worse clinical outcomes, respectively. However, histologic features have not been shown to correlate with clinical outcome for the vast majority of medulloblastomas that lie between these extremes.[46]

Overall, with surgery and radiation, 5-year disease-free survival rates approach 80%.[28] Medulloblastomas have classically been said to follow Collin's law, which says that a cure has been obtained if there is no tumor recurrence over period equal to the age at diagnosis plus 9 months. However, one third of survivors at 5 years have recurrence, and one third of the recurrences are outside the period predicted by Collin's law. Most recurrence occurs in the cerebellum or along CSF pathways. Surveillance imaging has been shown to improve survival.[32,47]

Atypical Teratoid/Rhabdoid Tumor

Atypical teratoid/rhabdoid tumors share many clinical and pathologic features with medulloblastomas but appear to be unique entity with a more aggressive course and worse prognosis.[48] They may occur anywhere in the neuraxis but are most commonly found in the cerebellum, and clinical presentation is similar to that of medulloblastomas. Most patients are younger than 2 years of age at diagnosis. One third of patients have subarachnoid dissemination on presentation. Histologically, they are composed at least partly of rhabdoid cells but also have areas typical for medulloblastoma and malignant mesenchymal or epithelial tissue. They stain for epithelial membrane antigen, vimentin, and smooth muscle actin. They are associated with abnormalities of chromosome 22, whereas medulloblastomas typically have an i(17q) abnormality.[48] Prognosis is dismal, and most patients die within 1 year of diagnosis regardless of treatment.[49]

Astrocytoma

In the pediatric population, astrocytomas account for approximately one fourth of all brain tumors and one third of posterior fossa tumors. These tumors occur most often during the first 20 years of life, with peak incidence at 5 to 8 years of age, and very few patients are younger than 1 year or older than 40. Males and females are affected equally.[50,51] Unlike astrocytomas of the cerebrum, they are chronic and slowly progressive tumors that usually present subacutely and can be resected with minimal morbidity with a very high rate of cure.

Because they are slow-growing tumors, onset of symptoms is usually far more insidious than medulloblastomas and ependymomas. In 1931, Cushing[52] remarked with amazement that "tumors of such high magnitude in such a critical situation and so certain to produce early hydrocephalus can be tolerated for so many years with so comparatively insignificant symptoms." Most patients have had symptoms for many months by the time the tumor is diagnosed, and some undergo extensive gastrointestinal or neuropsychological investigation before the tumor is diagnosed. Although outside the lumen of the fourth ventricle, astrocytomas frequently disrupt the flow of CSF, so the most common presenting symptoms are those of increased intracranial pressure such as headache, vomiting, abducens palsy, and papilledema. Other common symptoms include altered gait, clumsiness, and head tilt. Common signs include papilledema, ataxia that is often unilateral, appendicular dysmetria, nystagmus,

and macrocephaly that occasionally dates back several years even to infancy. Severe neck pain, opisthotonus, bradycardia, hypertension, and altered neurologic function are less common but require immediate attention, and rarely patients will present with signs of acute hydrocephalus such as stupor or coma, projectile vomiting, and oculomotor and facial palsies. Blindness was once a very common presenting symptom (present on presentation in 23 of the 76 patients reviewed by Cushing) but is rarely seen today.[50]

On imaging, astrocytomas are solid, cystic, or mixed lesions that arise from the medial hemisphere or vermis[53,54]; one third are entirely in one cerebellar hemisphere (Fig. 61-25). When in the midline, they can be difficult to differentiate from medulloblastomas and ependymomas. MRI will usually disclose a round to oval mass with well-defined margins and of mixed intensity, hypointense to surrounding brain on T1 and hyperintense on T2. On CT, the tumor is hypodense or isodense to surrounding brain. Unlike low-grade supratentorial astrocytomas, the tumor enhances brightly with CT and MRI contrast material. If the tumor is cystic, there may be an enhancing mural nodule and the cyst fluid will be slightly denser than CSF on T2-weighted images. The cyst wall is sometimes denser than surrounding brain but does not contain tumor unless it enhances (Figs. 61-26 and 61-27). Calcification and peritumoral edema are infrequently observed.[54] Skull radiographs are generally not helpful, although they may show signs of chronically increased intracranial pressure such as thinning or asymmetrical bulging of occipital squama, chronic splitting of cranial sutures, or demineralization of sella turcica.

Grossly, astrocytomas are firm with discrete borders. Approximately half will have some degree of cystic degeneration (compared with 80% of supratentorial astrocytomas). There is usually one cyst with a prominent mural nodule, although honeycombing of small cysts is also seen. The cyst wall is most commonly smooth and glistening, although sometimes there will be a coating of tumor or raised tumor nodules on the inner surface of the cyst (seen more often when there is enhancement of the cyst wall on neuroimaging). Histologically, areas of loose glial tissue resembling cerebral protoplasmic astrocytes with round or oval nuclei are intermixed with compact areas of fusiform, fibrillated cells that often have elongated eosinophilic bodies called Rosenthal fibers. When the cells conform to white matter tracts, they have an elongated hairlike structure and are described as pilocytic (hair cell). The cells stain weakly for GFAP and have bundles of intermediate filaments in perikaryon and cell processes, both of which confirm their identity as astrocytes.

Some posterior fossa astrocytomas have histology and clinical behavior that deviate from those of the typical pilocytic astrocytoma described previously. These tumors resemble low-grade astrocytomas of the cerebral hemispheres.[55–57] They have diffusely homogeneous histology, lack microcysts and Rosenthal fibers, and are characterized by pseudorosettes, high cell density, necrosis, mitoses, and calcification. The incidence of these tumors is much lower than pilocytic astrocytomas, and they are more common in older patients, especially those who have previously received radiation.[55,58] They have a much higher rate of malignant degeneration,[51] and high-grade anaplastic astrocytomas and even glioblastomas have been reported in the posterior fossa.[59–61]

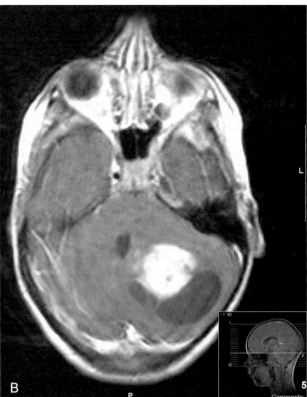

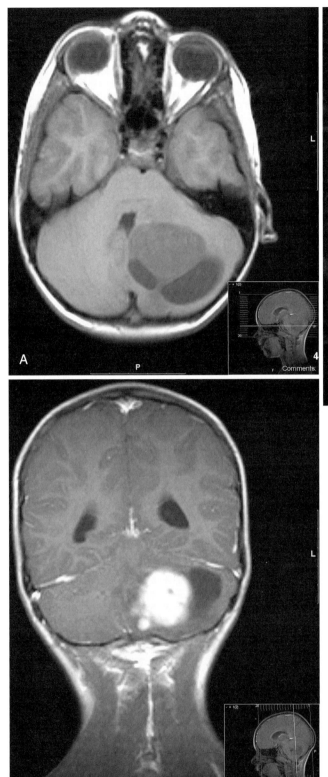

FIGURE 61-25 *A*, Astrocytoma, T1 without contrast. The hemispheric lesion is slightly hypodense to brain and has a cystic component. *B*, Astrocytoma, T1 with contrast. The solid portion of the tumor enhances irregularly. *C*, Astrocytoma, T1 with contrast, coronal section. These tumors are much more likely to involve the cerebellar hemisphere.

Even when histologically low grade, they may infiltrate into cerebellar nuclei or peduncles and often lack clear tumor margins making gross tumor resection difficult. Survival rates with these tumors are lower than the typical astrocytomas,[59] and there are reports of diffuse leptomeningeal spread[55] and

even spread to the muscles of the neck requiring several local surgical procedures to control.[62]

After exposing the posterior fossa, the tumor is usually immediately apparent as enlargement of the vermis or unilateral hemisphere with distended folia. The cerebellar

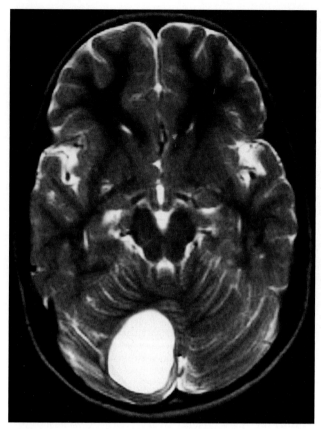

FIGURE 61-26 Astrocytoma, T2. The cyst associated with this tumor is often much larger than the mural nodule.

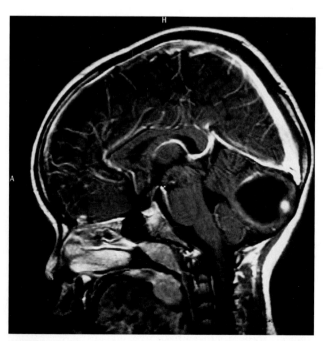

FIGURE 61-27 Astrocytoma, T1 with contrast, sagittal section. Note the small enhancing mural nodule posteriorly. If the cyst wall does not enhance, removal of the nodule is usually all that is necessary.

tonsils may be pushed down on the side of the tumor. Intraoperative ultrasonography can be used transdurally to be certain bony exposure is adequate or after dura has been opened to demonstrate the closest location of tumor to cerebellar surface to minimize the amount of cerebellar tissue that must be removed to provide adequate exposure of the tumor. After incising the vermis or hemisphere, the tumor is removed with the ultrasonic aspirator until normal cerebellar tissue is seen. Very large tumors will cause the compressed cerebellum to relax inward after debulking so self-retaining retractors are helpful to keep the tumor bed open. If there is a cystic component to the tumor, the cyst is entered and cyst fluid quickly suctioned, supporting the hemisphere with self-retaining retractors to prevent collapse away from the tentorium with rupture of bridging veins. The mural nodule is then identified and removed using the ultrasonic aspirator. If the tumor is mixed or enhancement of the cyst wall is seen, the entire cyst wall should be removed and normal cerebellar tissue exposed; otherwise, simple removal of the mural nodule is curative. To prevent contamination of the CSF with blood and cyst fluid (which can produce chemical meningitis that increases the likelihood of postoperative communicating hydrocephalus), the cisterna magna and fourth ventricle should not be opened unless it is necessary to do so to achieve gross total resection. All walls of the tumor bed are then carefully inspected to ensure that there is no residual tumor. Finally, before closing, it is important to ensure that bridging tentorial veins are not stretched. These veins can be safely sacrificed but tearing one later can lead to a life-threatening hematoma. All patients should get a postoperative contrast-enhanced scan within the first 24 hours to evaluate the extent of resection, provide a baseline if hydrocephalus should develop, and evaluate for cerebellar/brain stem retraction edema or clinically silent hematomas. If more than 1 cm^3 has been left behind, early reexploration to remove the residual tumor is indicated.

True pilocytic astrocytomas are almost always resectable by modern techniques and have excellent prognosis with no adjuvant therapy if gross total resection is possible.[53,56] Postoperative MRI is particularly poor at differentiating residual astrocytoma from postsurgical changes, so early postoperative imaging to obtain a baseline is probably not helpful.[63] If there is a small amount of residual tumor, serial imaging can be used to follow its growth. Although there are several well-documented cases of low-grade astrocytoma undergoing malignant degeneration several years after surgical resection, this is probably quite rare and each of the documented cases had received radiation therapy. Radiation therapy has not been shown to be successful in the management of these tumors[64] and is associated with significant side effects, although focused radiation may be helpful for surgically inaccessible or rapidly growing lesions.[65] Combined chemotherapy and radiotherapy for high-grade cortical astrocytomas has been shown to decrease rates of metastasis for children with high-grade astrocytomas. As with pilocytic astrocytomas, patients with more complete resections of infiltrative tumors fare better.

Recurrence of posterior fossa astrocytomas is related to the extent of resection, location, invasiveness, and histology of the original tumor.[51,67] Age of the patient does not appear to have any effect on outcome. Recurrence is most common at the primary site, and if any tumor is left behind, symptoms almost invariably recur. Cystic tumors can usually be totally extirpated, but solid tumors tend to regrow after prolonged remission, even if grossly resected. Solid midline tumors are most likely to recur because they more often extend toward the cerebellar peduncles, aqueduct, or brain stem, which may prevent total excision. Invasion of the subarachnoid space often occurs, but this does not indicate a poor prognosis as with most other tumors. Astrocytomas do not follow Collin's law for tumor recurrence and can have recurrences long after complete resection.[68] Overall 10-year survival for astrocytomas is close to 100% with complete resection, and 20-year survival is more than 70%.[56,67]

Ependymoma

Ependymoma is the third most common infratentorial tumor of childhood, representing 10% to 20% of all posterior fossa brain tumors, although in children younger than 3 years of age, they represent 30% of all posterior fossa tumors. They occur very rarely in adults.[69] Because ependymomas arise from the cells lining the ventricles, they can appear in any of the ventricles or ependymal streaks (obliterated portions of ventricles). Sixty-five percent of these tumors are infratentorial, and the most common location is in the middle to lower fourth ventricle or at the junction of the lateral inferior medullary velum and foramen of Luschka. Males are affected approximately twice as often as females, and 60% of all patients are younger than 5 years old at diagnosis.[70] Recently, it was suggested that ependymomas may have a viral etiology because DNA sequences identical to segments of the SV40 virus have been identified in childhood ependymomas,[71,72] and ependymomas can be induced in rodents by intracerebral inoculation of SV40.[73] For unclear reasons, they are much more common in India than elsewhere in the world.[30]

Ependymomas are relatively fast-growing tumors and present more acutely than astrocytomas but not as acutely as medulloblastomas. Median duration of symptoms is 2 to 3 months. The most common presenting symptoms are nausea and vomiting from increased intracranial pressure, ataxia, and nystagmus. Some patients have repeated vomiting in the absence of hydrocephalus due to direct stimulation of the brain stem emetic center. At presentation, one third to one half of ependymomas will have grown through the foramen of Luschka or central canal with direct extension into the upper cervical spine, and this can produce nuchal rigidity, torticollis, posterior neck pain, or head tilt. Infiltration of brain stem or direct tumor involvement within lateral brain stem recesses can produce cranial nerve deficits, and this is associated with a particularly poor outcome.[70,74] Finally, ependymomas do metastasize (although not as often as medulloblastomas), and patients rarely present with signs of metastatic spinal cord or nerve root compression.[74,75]

Ependymomas usually appear isodense to brain on both MRI and CT, although they may be hypodense on CT, hypointense on T1-, and hyperintense on T2-weighted MRI.[76] They are almost always seen on the floor of the fourth ventricle with the body of the ventricle expanded around the tumor and are often quite large by the time they are discovered (Fig. 61-28). They frequently extend through the foramen of Luschka into the cerebropontine angle or through the foramen of Magendie, occasionally compressing the upper

cervical cord. This extraforaminal extension is an important diagnostic feature because other tumors in the differential diagnosis (medulloblastoma, astrocytoma, and choroid plexus papilloma) almost never do this (Fig. 61-28B). Calcifications are seen in one fourth of ependymomas on CT, although a greater percentage of tumors have microcalcification[77]; these calcifications are usually soft and do not pose a problem during tumor removal, so preoperative CT is not necessary. MRI appearance is usually heterogeneous from calcification, cysts, blood products, necrotic foci, and tumor vascularity. Enhancement on both CT and MRI is more heterogeneous than most other tumors in this area, and peritumoral edema is often seen on T2-weighted images.[76]

Grossly, the tumor is gray, well circumscribed, and homogeneous or less often lobulated and is seen to arise directly from the floor of the fourth ventricle. Microscopically, ependymomas are quite heterogeneous and can have highly variable histology within a single tumor. The two most common ependymoma histologic patterns are cellular and epithelial. Cellular (or glial) ependymomas consist of sheets of glia-appearing cells interrupted by perivascular pseudorosettes, in which fusiform cells with tapered fibrillary processes that stain for GFAP surround blood vessels. The pseudorosettes produce perivascular eosinophilic zones free of nuclei, giving the tumor a "leopard skin" appearance under low magnification. Epithelial ependymomas have cells with discernible boundaries that are arranged in canals and form true rosettes, reflecting the cell's origin as ventricular lining. As with normal ependyma, these cells have basal bodies that anchor cilia and intracytoplasmic spherical or rod-shaped structures called blepharoplasts. Other rare histologic variants include papillary in which tumor cells are seen to cover glial tissue, tanycytic with elongated cells that resemble astrocytes, and clear cell in which cells have perinuclear halos like oligodendrocytes. Regardless of histologic pattern, ependymomas frequently have small cystic areas, regions of necrosis, evidence of acute or chronic hemorrhage, and calcification. More than half of infratentorial ependymomas have evidence of microcalcification, which is important to differentiate the tumor from medulloblastoma,[77] and the chromatin is much denser than is seen with astrocytomas. Occasionally, focal areas of anaplastic degeneration are seen with increased mitoses, cellular anaplasia, vascular proliferation, necrosis, and fewer perivascular pseudorosettes, although this happens much more often with supratentorial ependymomas. Unlike astrocytomas and medulloblastomas, in which histologic grade and proliferative potential correlate with prognosis, it is controversial whether histologic grade affects prognosis; this is likely to be because of the diversity of pathology seen. A high mitotic index and the presence of focal areas of dense cellularity are associated with poor prognosis, but calcium and ependymal rosettes have no impact.

The so-called ependymoblastoma, which has been reclassified as an entirely separate embryonal primitive neuroectodermal tumor, usually occurs supratentorially in young children and consists of sheets of poorly differentiated cells with frequent mitoses and distinctive rosettes of pseudostratified cells surrounding a lumen and surrounded by terminal bars. Median survival for ependymoblastoma is a few months, and patients frequently have diffuse spread through the subarachnoid space by presentation.[79]

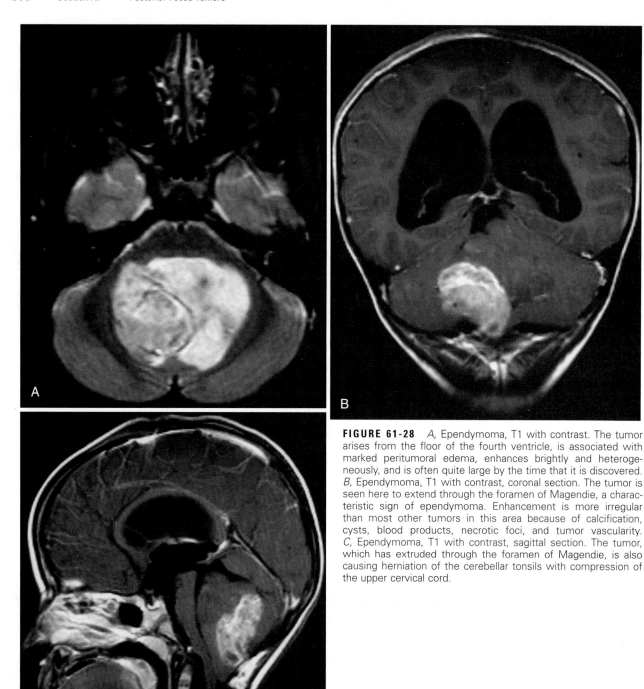

FIGURE 61-28 *A*, Ependymoma, T1 with contrast. The tumor arises from the floor of the fourth ventricle, is associated with marked peritumoral edema, enhances brightly and heterogeneously, and is often quite large by the time that it is discovered. *B*, Ependymoma, T1 with contrast, coronal section. The tumor is seen here to extend through the foramen of Magendie, a characteristic sign of ependymoma. Enhancement is more irregular than most other tumors in this area because of calcification, cysts, blood products, necrotic foci, and tumor vascularity. *C*, Ependymoma, T1 with contrast, sagittal section. The tumor, which has extruded through the foramen of Magendie, is also causing herniation of the cerebellar tonsils with compression of the upper cervical cord.

Because ependymomas usually arise from the floor of the fourth ventricle and are frequently adherent to the lower cranial nerves, it is often quite difficult to achieve gross total resection, and in the past, surgery was limited to removing enough of the tumor to allow free flow of CSF. More recently, the benefits of total resection have been shown to outweigh the risks, as there is a significant difference in survival depending on extent of resection.[70,74] The posterior fossa is exposed by standard techniques. If there is extension of the tumor through the foramen of Magendie, it will be apparent in the cisterna magna immediately after the dura is opened. Any tumor tissue extending into the cervical canal is gently aspirated from the surface of the cord with suction or ultrasonic aspiration. This is usually easy to do because the tumor does not invade the pia. The cerebellar hemispheres are then retracted laterally and resection continued along the floor of the fourth ventricle until the point of origin is determined (usually caudal to the stria medullaris). Ependymomas rarely submerge deep into the brain stem, so a 1-mm-thick carpet of tumor should be left at its point of attachment and resection continued parallel to the floor of the fourth ventricle using the ultrasonic aspirator. It is vitally important to identify the glistening white fourth ventricular floor before attempting to remove the tumor from its point of attachment. If the tumor extends through the foramen of Luschka, the area of origin will usually be found at the junction of the lateral medullary velum and the medial foramen of Luschka. In this case, the tumor should be resected from within the fourth ventricle as far laterally as possible and then the retractors removed from the fourth ventricle and placed underneath the cerebellar tonsil to expose the cerebellomedullary cistern where the rest of the tumor may be visualized and resected. Ependymomas are quite soft and can usually be safely aspirated off the lower cranial nerves, but it is important not to violate the PICA and its lateral medullary branches, although the lateral medullary veins can be safely sacrificed if inadvertently entered. Any changes in cardiac rate or rhythm (more common when dissecting on the left side) can be abolished by soaking a micropatty in 1% lidocaine and placing it on the cranial nerve near the root entry zone for a few minutes. Removing tumors from deep within the cerebellopontine angle may require partial resection of the lateral cerebellar hemisphere to facilitate exposure. Occasionally, the tumor arises from the roof rather than the floor of the fourth ventricle and will invade the roof and inferior vermis without attachment to the floor of the fourth ventricle. This often allows for complete tumor removal, but excessive resection of the inferior vermis or nodulus increases the risk of damage to the superior cerebellar peduncle, producing postoperative ataxia or the posterior fossa syndrome. Recurrent ependymomas are usually invasive or adherent, so it is challenging to distinguish invasive disease from normal anatomy. As a result, resection of recurrent disease is almost always incomplete.[74]

Because recurrence is most common at the primary site, radiotherapy with 4500 to 5600 cGy to the primary site has shown to significantly improve overall rate and duration of disease-free survival in patients with incompletely resected ependymoma in several retrospective studies.[80,81] Most authors therefore recommend local radiotherapy even if gross total resection is confirmed by postoperative MRI and staging is negative for leptomeningeal spread,[80] although one recent study recommends withholding further treatment unless there is evidence of tumor recurrence.[74] If there are no radiographically evident metastases, craniospinal irradiation probably does not improve outcome because only 3% of patients with low-grade tumors later show clinical evidence of metastatic disease (although one third have dissemination at autopsy). Also, most spinal seeding occurs only after recurrence at the primary site, and craniospinal irradiation has not been shown to prevent spinal metastases.[82] However, anaplastic ependymomas are much more likely to be disseminated and should be treated with craniospinal irradiation,[74] although it may not help.[83] If disseminated disease is confirmed, most authors recommend 3600 cGy to the entire axis with an additional boost of 1980 cGy to the local site and areas of macroscopic dissemination.[80]

There are not many data concerning chemotherapy for ependymomas. Although chemotherapy does transiently reduce tumor bulk and stabilize tumor growth in patients with recurrent disease, no chemotherapeutic regimen has been shown to be effective after radiation at the time of initial diagnosis.[81,84]

Prognosis for patients with ependymoma is poor compared with that of medulloblastomas and astrocytomas, although survival studies are difficult to interpret because most include anaplastic histology and supratentorial tumors. Most studies show that long-term survival is strongly correlated with amount of residual tumor as judged by postoperative MRI. For example, 5-year disease-free survival approaches 70% to 90% if there is no evidence of residual tumor compared with 0% to 30% if residual tumor is untreated.[70,80,85] Other studies show no effect.[81] Because ependymomas tend to insinuate into crevices within and about the fourth ventricle, the surgeon's assessment overestimates completeness of resection as much as one third of the time, and so MRI should be used to determine completeness of resection. Therefore, any presence of residual enhancing tissue on imaging studies after completion of radiation should be explored and resected if possible. Overall, 5-year survival is variously quoted at 15% to 50% for children and 50T to 75% for adults with fourth ventricle ependymomas.[70,85] Histology and age of the patient do not significantly affect survival,[70,74] although anaplastic ependymomas have a worse outcome[68] and female patients do better.[80] Midline tumors have a better 5-year survival than lateral ependymomas, out of proportion to their ease of resection.[86] Disseminated ependymomas, approximately 5% of low-grade and 15% of anaplastic tumors,[82] have a particularly poor prognosis, with 5-year survival rates near 12%.

Brain Stem Glioma

Brain stem gliomas are much more common in children than adults and make up approximately 10% to 20% of intracranial pediatric tumors and 15% to 30% of all posterior fossa tumors.[87,88] They are a heterogeneous group of tumors with many distinct clinical and pathologic varieties. The duration of symptoms before presentation varies widely but is generally 3 to 5 months with insidious onset. Unlike the tumors described previously, increased intracranial pressure is infrequent except as very late manifestation. Most patients present with a triad of a cerebellar deficit, pyramidal tract deficit, and involvement of cranial nerve nuclei; more than half have clinically detectable facial weakness, pharyngeal weakness, trigeminal deficit, or paresis of conjugate gaze by admission. The vast majority of brain stem gliomas are astrocytomas, with gangliogliomas and oligodendrogliomas making up the remainder. Histologically, they resemble fibrillary or pilocytic astrocytomas of cerebellar hemispheres, although they can show anaplastic components and cytoarchitecture of glioblastoma multiforme. Brain stem tumors can be classified into three general categories based on location: tumors of the midbrain (including tectal gliomas and focal midbrain tumors, not discussed here), dorsally exophytic brain stem tumors, and cervicomedullary tumors.

Pontine tumors have the highest prevalence in the first decade but can present in adults as old as 40. They tend to be infiltrative with indistinct borders and are always malignant regardless of histology at diagnosis[89] and spread early through the leptomeningeal space[90] and even extraneurally.[91] Pontine tumors usually present with cranial nerve palsies followed by pyramidal tract signs, ataxia, and hydrocephalus in the most advanced stages. Imaging demonstrates diffuse pontine enlargement with hypodense signal to the brain on CT, hypointense on T1-weighted MRI and hyperintense on T2-weighted MRI. Calcification and hemorrhagic foci are unusual. They are often seen to extend into the midbrain, medulla, or cerebellum and can encircle the basilar artery.[92] They rarely enhance on CT (occasionally there are areas of focal enhancement) but do enhance with MRI (Fig. 61-29). These tumors are surgically inaccessible, and surgical intervention does not alter survival.[93,94] Radiation therapy is standard treatment, and many patients initially exhibit a striking response in terms of alleviation of symptoms and even radiographic resolution of tumor. However, within 6 to 12 months of starting radiation, there is nearly always recurrence with diffuse leptomeningeal spread. Chemotherapy has not been shown to improve survival time. Most patients are dead within 2 years of diagnosis, and the overall 5-year survival rates are less than 10%.[94]

A subset (approximately 20%) of patients with pontine gliomas will have dorsal exophytic growth in which the tumor has eroded the ependyma to produce a wide-based, lobulated intraventricular mass that does not involve the cerebellum.[95,96] These patients have more chronic and insidious symptoms such as failure to thrive, headaches, and loss of balance, but hydrocephalus is often an earlier finding. They have a lower rate of malignancy than diffuse pontine tumors and a much better prognosis. These tumors may be amenable to surgical resection using microsurgical techniques to achieve maximal subtotal removal.

Focal pontine astrocytomas have been described that are confined to half or part of half of the pons, sometimes extending into the fourth ventricle. These are more common in type 1 neurofibromatosis and have a variable natural history.[97–99] They are amenable to surgical debulking and may not require immediate intervention after surgery; some patients do well with an aggressive surgical approach.

Cervicomedullary tumors generally present in young children, with average age at onset of 6 to 7 years. They almost never extend above the pontomedullary junction because their superior growth is limited by crossing fibers in the lower medulla and pontomedullary junction.[100] They generally grow outward and extend into the fourth ventricle as a cystic or solid exophytic growth and can eventually produce hydrocephalus from compression of the fourth ventricle or its outlet foramina. The symptoms are insidious and often present for months or years. Most patients initially experience dysfunction of the lower cranial nerves manifested by difficulty swallowing, nasal speech, or recurrent aspiration. Sometimes they have torticollis or neck pain, and half will have some spinal cord dysfunction, usually insidious motor findings or paresthesias. MRI demonstrates the lesions quite well, but CT is of little use because of the artifact created by the bones of the posterior fossa. These tumors are surgically accessible.[101]

Because most surgically accessible brain stem gliomas extend to posterior aspect of brain stem or bulge into the fourth ventricle or cervicomedullary cistern, the standard fourth ventricle approach is useful to address them. For cervicomedullary tumors, intraoperative ultrasound should be used to identify the rostral and caudal poles of neoplasm before opening the dura, and the initial myelotomy should initially be made in the middle of the tumor.[102] In all cases, the tumor should be carefully removed from the inside out using ultrasonic aspiration, laser, microsuction, or irrigating bipolar forceps. It is possible to work to the brain interface when resecting pontine or cervical lesions, but when resecting medullary tumors, it is prudent to stop after only one half to three fourths of the tumor is removed so that there is no chance that normal medullary structures will be violated. In particular, the cranial nerve nuclei should be carefully avoided. Monitoring (especially somatosensory evoked potentials) is helpful to ensure that important structures are not inadvertently damaged. It is important to avoid excessive manipulation and to consider every deviation in pulse or blood pressure to be a warning sign. Postoperatively, the most common threat to good recovery is respiratory difficulties, especially for medullary lesions. Therefore, patients should be monitored carefully and extubated only after fully awake. Postoperative radiation therapy may be helpful. If the tumor is focal and benign and gross total resection is obtained, many patients can have extended disease-free survival.

Choroid Plexus Papilloma

Choroid plexus papillomas are rare tumors, accounting for 2% to 3% of pediatric intracranial tumors and 0.5% of adult tumors.[103,104] Unlike most fourth ventricular brain tumors that are more common in the pediatric population, fourth ventricular papillomas are more common in adults and most

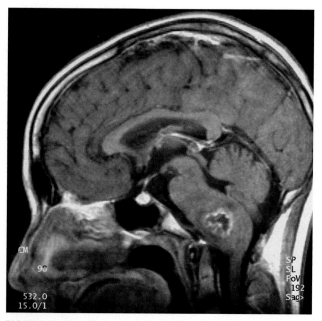

FIGURE 61-29 Brain stem glioma, T1 with contrast, sagittal section. The tumor is seen to enlarge the pons, which is a characteristic sign of brain stem glioma. Unless the tumor extends to the posterior aspect of the brain stem or bulges into the fourth ventricle or cervicomedullary cistern, it is not resectable.

pediatric choroid plexus papillomas are in the lateral ventricles. The third ventricle is an uncommon location at any age. Males slightly outnumber females in most clinical series. When in the fourth ventricle, they usually occur in the cavity, although rarely they are found in the lateral recess[105] or in the cerebellopontine angle arising from the small tuft of choroid plexus that extends through the foramen of Luschka.[106,107] Carcinomas of the choroid plexus account for approximately 20% of choroid plexus tumors and are usually found in the lateral ventricles,[103,108,109] but they occasionally involve the fourth ventricle. These malignant tumors almost invariably occur in young children, often during the first few days of life, and carry a grave prognosis with wide dissemination at or shortly after presentation.

Most choroid plexus papillomas present with symptoms of increased intracranial pressure such as headache, gait disturbances, and abducens palsy. Excessive formation of CSF is responsible for much of the hydrocephalus, although obstruction to CSF flow by the tumor or at the level of the arachnoid granulations due to hemorrhage is probably a more common cause. Because of CSF overproduction, affected infants often have papilledema despite an open fontanelle and macrocephaly disproportional to the size of the tumor. When in the cerebellopontine angle, dysfunction of lower cranial nerves and cerebellar ataxia are the main clinical findings.[106,107] In adults, these tumors usually do not produce excessive CSF and are sometimes discovered incidentally at autopsy.

On imaging, choroid plexus papillomas are usually seen as intraventricular masses. On CT, they are hyperdense and enhance brightly and homogeneously with contrast.[110] Calcifications are common in childhood papillomas but are rare during infancy.[111] MRI demonstrates hypointensity on T1 and heterogeneous hyperintensity on T2. The tumor can be highly vascular, and angiography is useful for preoperative planning when faced with an extremely brightly enhancing tumor or one that demonstrates high vascularity on MRI to identify feeding vessels and develop a plan for early devascularization of the tumor. There is often hypertrophy of the feeding artery, which is usually the PICA, although anterior inferior cerebellar artery supplies some tumors arising from choroid plexus far in the lateral recess. An important diagnostic clue is engulfing of the choroid glomus by tumor, which usually suggests choroid plexus papilloma.[112] Choroid plexus carcinomas are less homogeneous on neuroimaging due to necrosis, intratumoral hemorrhage, and cysts.[113]

Grossly, the papilloma is well defined, lobulated, mulberry-like, and reddish purple, with a firm and vascular basal portion. Microscopically, these tumors strongly resemble normal choroid with a single layer of cuboidal epithelium that occasionally appears somewhat crowded and taller seated on a simple fibrovascular stroma with little or no abnormal mitotic activity. Calcification is common in these tumors and is extensive in 10%. Some atypical histologic features such as enlargement, irregularity, hyperchromasia, mitoses, and loss of papillary growth pattern are present in half of these tumors but have no prognostic significance. In infants, there is occasionally evidence of ependymal differentiation with piling of ependymal cells or presence of cilia and blepharoplast. In these patients, it can be difficult to differentiate the tumor from papillary ependymomas. Rarely, the tumors have a cystic portion within the tumor or

in the brain parenchyma filled with CSF, presumably secreted by the papilloma. The so-called oncocytic variant of papilloma resembles oncocytomas in other organs, with cytoplasm packed with mitochondria. Carcinoma of the choroid plexus is recognizable by heterogeneity, necrosis, invasiveness, cellular pleomorphism, and mitotic figures. The tumor has a tendency to form multilayered epithelium and invades the parenchyma.[111] This malignant tumor may be confused with metastatic adenocarcinoma, especially when it occurs in adults, and sometimes the only indication that it is a choroid tumor at all is the presence of cilia, microvilli, and zonula adherens on electron microscopy.

Complete surgical resection of fourth ventricular choroid plexus papillomas is frequently possible because the tumor typically does not invade the parenchyma or floor of the fourth ventricle. Because they are very vascular tumors, it is important to prepare for significant blood loss. The fourth ventricle is exposed by standard techniques. Because of their extreme vascularity, it is important to identify feeding vessels during the resection. If the tumor is small, it may be possible to identify its point of attachment to normal choroid plexus and devascularize the tumor by coagulating and sectioning the tonsillar and vermian choroidal branches of the PICA. Larger tumors may have feeding arteries embedded in the core of the tumor and occasionally envelope the PICA, so the intraventricular papillary portion (which is less vascular than the core) is first shrunk with bipolar cautery or ultrasonic aspirator, and then the feeding branches are identified and coagulated. Forceful retraction of the tumor should be avoided because there is sometimes a major draining vein on the dome of the papilloma and inferior vermian veins may be arterialized due to intratumoral shunting; these can produce significant hemorrhage if violated. It may be necessary to section the inferior vermis to reach the rostral end of the tumor. If there is extension through the foramen of Luschka into the cerebellopontine angle, the intraventricular part is resected first, and then the rest of the tumor is exposed by elevating the ipsilateral tonsil and hemisphere. There may be displacement of cranial nerves and brain stem, but the papilloma can usually be easily be separated from these structures.[106]

At one time, radiation therapy was commonly used for unresectable or recurrent papillomas, but it is controversial whether it is effective.[114-116] Because there are risks associated with radiation (especially in children), adjuvant radiotherapy is not warranted for these tumors, although some authors assert that radiotherapy may be effective in treating invasive benign tumors that could not be resected.[104] Choroid plexus carcinomas, on the other hand, should receive radiation to the entire craniospinal axis because these tumors often disseminate along CSF pathways; most long-term survivors of choroid plexus carcinoma were treated with radiation.[109,115] Chemotherapy may be appropriate for young patients in whom radiation is too risky.

Benign papillomas have a good prognosis. Total resection is usually curative without recurrence, and symptoms generally do not recur even after subtotal resection. Overall, the 5-year survival rates for papillomas are nearly 100%.[103,104,114-116] Choroid plexus carcinomas have a much poorer prognosis because gross total resection is usually impossible due to frequent infiltration of the brain stem and cerebellar peduncles and extreme vascularity. The tumor often disseminates through CSF pathways, and it usually occurs in very young children, which limits use of adjuvant radiotherapy. Although there are reports of gross total resection of choroid plexus carcinomas without recurrence,[103,109] they tend to recur even after total resection. Most authors agree that the degree of resection is the most important variable, followed by histology (cellular atypia, microscopic invasion, or mitosis).[116] Five-year survival rates vary significantly among reports but are generally less than 50%, with carcinomas of the fourth ventricular choroid plexus having a worse prognosis than those in the lateral ventricles.[109,114]

Hemangioblastoma

Hemangioblastomas are benign, slow-growing vascular tumors that are found exclusively in the neuraxis.[117] The most common location is the cerebellum, followed by the brain stem (usually on the floor of the fourth ventricle near the cervicomedullary junction) and spinal cord. They rarely occur supratentorially, but when they do and are dural based, it is difficult to distinguish them from angioblastic meningiomas. They account for 1% to 2% of all intracranial neoplasms and 7% to 12% of adult post fossa tumors. Isolated sporadic hemangioblastomas are more common in adults 30 to 40 years of age. Males slightly outnumber females.

Ten to 20% of hemangioblastomas occur as part of the von Hippel-Lindau syndrome. This syndrome was initially described in 1904 when von Hippel identified two patients with vascular retinal tumors. In 1926, Lindau noted an association with retinal tumors, cerebellar tumors, and visceral cysts.[118] It is now known that von Hippel-Lindau syndrome is an autosomal dominant condition with varying degrees of penetrance, similar to neurofibromatosis and other neurocutaneous syndromes.[119,120] In addition to multiple hemangioblastomas (which occur in 40% of patients with von Hippel-Lindau), there are multiple angiomatoses of the retina; visceral cysts; and tumors, especially of kidney and pancreas; pheochromocytoma; and papillary cystadenoma of epididymis or mesosalpinx (called tubular adenomata by Lindau). Recently, the gene for von Hippel-Lindau has been mapped to a small region of chromosome 3p25–p26,[121] and a protein called pVHL identified that is a moderator of mRNA elongation and may be responsible for the syndrome. Whether associated with von Hippel-Lindau or not, hemangioblastomas are always benign tumors, and although there is occasional local subarachnoid seeding after surgery, distant metastases have never been reported.

As with most other tumors of the posterior fossa, the most common presenting symptoms are increased intracranial pressure and ataxia. Because the most common location is in the fourth ventricle at the level of the obex, some patients present with intractable nausea and vomiting from direct irritation of the area postrema in the fourth ventricular floor. The mass effect is usually due to cystic enlargement rather than the solid tumor itself.[122] In 10% of patients with hemangioblastoma, there will be a secondary polycythemia due to erythropoietin secreted by stromal tumor cells.[123,124] This is more common with solid tumors, but cyst fluid from hemangioblastomas often contains erythropoietin. Resection of the tumor usually improves this polycythemia. Any patient known to have retinal angioma and polycythemia

should be scanned to rule out hemangioblastoma. If there is evidence of von Hippel-Lindau, it is necessary to image the entire neuraxis to search for multiple lesions. First-degree relatives should also be screened because as many as 20% will have the disease.

On CT and MRI, most fourth ventricular hemangioblastomas appear cystic with a mural nodule that is located next to the pial surface of the brain (usually inferior or lateral), but they can be solid or mixed (supratentorial and spinal lesions tend to be solid). The nodule (which contains the tumor) invariably enhances, but the cyst wall does not. CT demonstrates an isodense tumor with hypodense cystic fluid. On MRI, the solid portion of the tumor is hypointense to brain tissue on T1 and slightly hyperintense on T2, and the cyst fluid is isointense or hyperintense to CSF on T1 and hyperintense on T2 to CSF (Fig. 61-30). Most hemangioblastomas produce peritumoral edema visible on T2-weighted MRI, and there are often flow voids that indicate enlarged draining veins (Fig. 61-31). There may be hemorrhage with a hemorrhagic fluid level within the tumor cyst or blood products such as hemosiderin within the solid tumor.[126] Tumors can be multiple with additional lesions in the brain stem and spinal cord; when in the spinal cord, they strongly resemble a syrinx except that they enhance dramatically with contrast. Leptomeningeal hemangioblastosis has been reported.[127] Because the tumors are extremely vascular, conventional or magnetic resonance angiography is essential in preoperative planning for successful removal of hemangioblastomas to identify the location of feeding vessels and develop a plan for early devascularization to avoid serious hemorrhage.

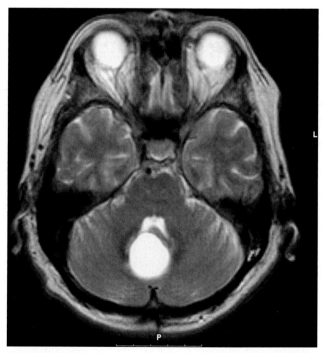

FIGURE 61-30 Cystic hemangioblastoma, T2. When in the posterior fossa, hemangioblastomas are usually cystic. This lesion had an enhancing subpial mural nodule that represented the tumor itself.

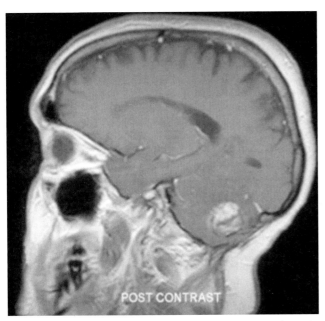

FIGURE 61-31 Solid hemangioblastoma, T1 with contrast, sagittal section. The tumor enhances brightly. Flow voids are seen that represent tumor vascularity.

For very large or vascular tumors, preoperative embolization of major feeding vessels may reduce intraoperative hemorrhage. Revascularization of the tumor occurs rapidly, so the embolization should be carried out no more than 1 to 2 days before the operation. Patients with multiple small hemangioblastomas may be treated with embolization alone.

Grossly, hemangioblastomas are smooth, orange tumors from high lipid content, and the cut surface is beefy red from rich vascularity with multiple cysts. When cystic, there is always a mural nodule. The cyst fluid is golden yellow to brown and highly proteinaceous and clots readily after aspiration. The inner surface of the cyst wall is smooth and made up of glial cells and compressed cerebellar tissue; the tumor itself never lines the cyst wall. Microscopically, the tumor consists of endothelial cells, pericytes, and stromal cells, but it is not known which of these cells participate in the neoplastic process or whether these cells interconvert. The most characteristic feature is the presence of numerous capillary channels that form an anastomosing plexiform pattern lined by a single layer of plump endothelial cells. This capillary network compartmentalizes larger, pale stromal cells with lipid vacuoles in the cytoplasm. Lindau thought that these were endothelial cells that had ingested lipids that resulted from generation of myelin, but immunologic studies have shown that they do not originate from endovascular cells; because they sometimes stain with GFAP and S100, it is possible that they are glial in origin. The nuclei are round, elongated, and sometimes multiple; this does not affect prognosis. There is no tumor capsule, but the margin is well defined, and even if invasion occurs, complete resection is usually possible. There is often surrounding reactive astrocytosis. On frozen section, hemangioblastomas can be confused with cerebellar astrocytomas or metastatic renal cell cancer (which coexists in 25% of patients with von Hippel-Lindau). Mast cells are common

in hemangioblastomas and uncommon in other tumors, and negative staining for glycogen and epithelial membrane antigen should be able to differentiate hemangioblastoma from metastatic renal cancer.

Because hemangioblastomas are always benign and total removal is curative, surgical removal is the treatment of choice for fourth ventricle hemangioblastomas.[117] Perioperative steroids are helpful because of the extensive swelling, and the sitting position may make hemorrhage easier to deal with intraoperatively. The fourth ventricle is exposed by standard techniques, then different techniques are used to remove the tumor itself depending on whether it is cystic or solid. If the tumor is cystic, the cyst should be entered and the fluid drained. The mural nodule is then identified and dissected away from the cyst cavity using bipolar coagulating forceps. Occasionally, the preoperative angiogram will identify a large feeding artery on the external surface of the cyst that must be divided before resecting the tumor; otherwise, the cyst wall should be left intact because it is not made up of tumor tissue but compressed gliotic cerebellum. If the tumor is solid, it is essential to avoid violating the tumor itself because this will lead to brisk hemorrhage. The dissection should be carried out between the external surface of the tumor and adjacent compressed gliotic cerebellum. Even after the major arterial supply has been controlled, there will frequently be many small perforating arteries or arterioles feeding the tumor that require coagulation. As soon as the dissection planes meet behind the tumor, it can be rolled out of the cerebellar bed and bleeding controlled. If the tumor tissue is violated before separation from the adjacent cerebellum, the tumor should be rapidly dissected from the cerebellar bed and hemorrhage controlled afterward; attempting hemostasis within the center of the tumor is futile and only leads to continued hemorrhage and delayed swelling.

All patients should get a postoperative enhanced MRI to determine whether complete resection has been achieved. If no residual tumor remains, most patients have no recurrence, except in the case of von Hippel-Lindau. Partial resection usually leads to recurrence. Adjuvant radiotherapy is generally ineffective; although gamma knife treatment can sometimes cause the solid portion of the tumor to stop growing or even to shrink, the cystic component does not respond and usually requires surgical treatment.[128]

Epithelial Cysts: Epidermoids and Dermoids

Epidermoid and dermoid cysts occur intracranially as result of nests of epithelial cells remaining intracranially during embryogenesis, probably due to failure of separation between neural and cutaneous ectoderm at the time of closure of the neural groove.[129] Epidermoids, also called pearly tumors or cholesteatomas, include only ectodermal elements. They are usually lateral in location; 50% are parapontine, and they frequently affect the cerebellopontine angle, suprasellar cistern, and cranial base.[130,131] By contrast, dermoid cysts include elements of all three germ layers and include skin appendages. They tend to be located along the central neuraxis anywhere from the pituitary to distal spinal cord, although the most common location is in the posterior fossa, especially the fourth ventricle. Dermoids are sometimes associated with a dermal sinus tract that extends from the skin toward the tumor with an associated suboccipital skull defect,[132] and there will usually be a cutaneous marker such as hair, telangiectasia, pigmentation, or increased subcutaneous tissue. Together, epidermoids and dermoids account for 1% of intracranial masses, and epidermoids are somewhat more common in most clinical series. Males and females are affected equally.

Although congenital in origin, epidermoids and dermoids can become symptomatic at any age, although dermoids tend to manifest earlier, usually in childhood. Both tumors grow very slowly and by linear rather than exponential growth because they enlarge by deposition of stratified squamous epithelium and its products (such as keratin and cholesterol) into the center rather than mitotic proliferation as with true neoplasms. Dermoids grow somewhat faster because, in addition to growth by desquamation, they also fill with secretions of sebaceous glands, sweat glands, and hair follicles. Symptoms are related to site of the cyst and are not specific. Most become symptomatic due to mass effect, although epidermoids occasionally burrow into the brain stem. Epidermoids occasionally rupture, causing sterile meningitis. Dermoids associated with a dermal sinus most often present with localized swelling, redness, tenderness, and purulent drainage from inflammation or infection of the dermal sinus. This often occurs several times before a neurosurgical consult is obtained. Some patients present with meningitis or cerebellar abscess because the sinus tract can act as a portal for bacterial entry into the subarachnoid space,[133,134] and subsequent scarring can lead to hydrocephalus.

On CT, an epidermoid cyst appears as a nonenhancing hypodense mass with frondlike margins that interdigitate into normal brain structures. Dermoids have a similar appearance but are somewhat higher density and may also contain calcification or fat, and sometimes the cyst wall enhances with contrast. Both epidermoids and dermoids have well-defined margins and contain a central low-density area similar to CSF but with frequently nonhomogeneous contents ("dirty CSF"). On MRI, epidermoids appear homogeneous, hypointense to brain on T1-weighted images, and hyperintense to CSF on T2-weighted images. Dermoids appear more heterogeneous because of a greater variety of constituents (keratin debris has high attenuation and dermal elements have low attenuation), so their appearance varies considerably on different T2-weighted images, but they are sometimes hyperintense to brain on T1 due to the presence of fatty tissue. Sometimes it is possible to see a dermal sinus tract. Both cyst types conform to adjacent anatomy but may produce some mass effect; they almost never produce edema.[135] Hydrocephalus can occur but is rarer than with other fourth ventricular tumors. Because the imaging appearance is so variable (especially for dermoids), the differential diagnosis can be extensive and includes abscess, cystic astrocytoma, hemangioblastoma, and even medulloblastoma or cystic ependymoma.

Grossly, epidermoids are pearly white from desquamated keratin, while dermoids are buttery yellow from pilosebaceous contents and sometimes contain hair. Because the connection between the dermal and neural ectoderm is small and there is minimal disturbance of mesoderm, adjacent structures are usually not affected by the malformation. Epidermoids (but not dermoids) are sometimes seen to invaginate into adjacent brain, and the capsule of either can become adherent to surrounding neural structures, especially after infection or inflammation from fatty acids of degenerating material within the capsule. Microscopically, epidermoids are seen to be composed of stratified squamous epithelium, and dermoids also have skin appendages such as hair follicles, sebaceous glands, and sweat glands. Dermoids sometimes have areas of cystic degeneration. Malignant degeneration (squamous cell cancer) can occur and is more common in epidermoids. Cysts of the fourth ventricle are almost invariably dermoids; if no skin appendages are seen on pathologic analysis, it is possible that the specimen does not include the whole tumor or dermal elements have been destroyed by inflammation.

Morbidity and the degree of invasiveness of the tumor dictate decisions regarding surgical treatment. If surgically excised, these cysts must be totally removed because subtotal resection usually leads to recurrence. The capsule may separate easily or be densely adherent (especially if infected due to dermal sinus tract); either way, every effort should be made to keep the capsule intact to prevent spillage of cyst contents or purulent material into subarachnoid space, which can lead to severe chemical meningitis. If the cyst does rupture intraoperatively, the area should be copiously irrigated with corticosteroid irrigant and the patient should receive intravenous steroids postoperatively. Cysts that are densely adherent to the floor of the fourth ventricle or cervicomedullary junction can be gently coagulated with the bipolar forceps to minimize the risk of recurrence. If a dermal sinus tract is present, it must be explored, even if imaging does not indicate any abnormality, although the absence of bony defect on exploration excludes the possibility of intracranial extension. An elliptical incision is made around the opening of the dermal sinus tract and the bone is removed inferiorly because the tract always extends inferiorly below the torcular. The tract is then removed in toto. The sinus tract is often intimately related to torcula so it is important to be prepared for major venous bleeding. Postoperatively, all patients should undergo an MRI scan with contrast to obtain a baseline; if residual cyst is seen, immediate re-exploration is warranted. Overall, the long-term prognosis for patients with fourth ventricular dermoid or epidermoid cysts is quite good.[136]

In addition to epidermoids and dermoids, neuroepithelial and endodermal cysts can occur in the region of the fourth ventricle. Neuroepithelial cysts result from embryologic folding of primitive ventricular lining into or out of ventricles. These include ependymal cysts and colloid cysts that usually involve the anterior third ventricle but can rarely occur in the fourth ventricle.[137–139] They secrete solid or viscous exudate that results in gradual enlargement. Endodermal cysts are slow-growing, endothelial-lined cysts that are most often located in the spinal canal but can occur in the fourth ventricle. They are likely due to an error in embryogenesis, probably early in gastrulation because their location tends to follow the location of the primitive notochord.[140,141] Each of these is very slow growing but can become symptomatic from mass effect due to local compression or obstruction of the ventricular system; many remain asymptomatic and are discovered only incidentally or at autopsy. Treatment options for symptomatic cysts include excision, fenestration, and shunting.

Meningioma

Meningiomas can rarely produce a fourth ventricular mass. Overall, meningiomas are quite common and account for more than 15% of all primary intracranial tumors, but intraventricular meningiomas account for only 0.5% to 2% of all meningiomas, and most intraventricular meningiomas are in the trigone of the lateral ventricle. Fourth ventricular meningiomas without dural attachment are quite rare.[142–145] The first reported case of a fourth ventricular meningioma that was removed by Ernest Sachs in 1936 in a patient with diminished hearing, leading Cushing to suggest coexistent neurofibromatosis.[146] Since then, there have been only a few dozen additional cases reported. Meningiomas are believed to arise from arachnoid cap cells, which are specialized cells found on the outer aspect of the arachnoid layer, particularly at arachnoid granulations, because the distribution of the location of meningiomas parallels the frequency of arachnoid cap cells in normal meninges.[147] It is possible that these cells are dragged into ventricles by vessels piercing the ependymal layer during choroid plexus development. Most fourth ventricular meningiomas arise from the choroid plexus or inferior tela choroidea, although they can extend into the posterior fossa from the posterior petrous ridge, clivus, tentorium, foramen magnum, or cerebellar hemisphere convexity. The blood supply is usually from the PICA.

Meningiomas primary affect adults, and peak occurrence is during the fifth decade. Females are affected more often than males. Typically, fourth ventricular meningiomas are asymptomatic until large enough to obstruct CSF flow. The vast majority are larger than 3 cm by the time of presentation. The most common symptoms are headache, vomiting, nystagmus, cerebellar dysfunction such as ataxia and dysmetria, cranial nerve palsies, and behavioral change.[144]

Because they are so rare, there are few descriptions of radiographic appearance of fourth ventricular meningiomas. In general, meningiomas are isodense on CT and T1-weighted MRI and bright on T2-weighted MRI; they enhance brightly with contrast. There is usually no peritumoral edema. There is often calcification, and sometimes flow voids representing large blood vessels surround the tumor. Angiography can be used to identify tumor-feeding vessels.

Grossly, meningiomas are firm, well-circumscribed, globular or lobulated yellow to pink-gray tumors. They are usually homogeneous in consistency and can be cystic or gritty from calcification. Microscopically, meningiomas are divided into four categories: meningothelial, fibroblastic, transitional (between meningothelial and fibroblastic), and angioblastic. Meningothelial meningiomas have uniform sheets of cells with indistinct borders, occasional orientation into whorls, foamy yellow areas (called xanthomatous), and basophilic calcifications called psammoma ("sand") bodies. Fibroblastic meningiomas have spindle cells with elongated interwoven bundles of cell bodies with collagen and reticulin fibers. Angioblastic meningiomas have pathology very similar to that of hemangiopericytomas and hemangioblastomas, and some believe that they are not meningiomas at all. Among fourth ventricular meningiomas, pathologic analysis has been roughly equally divided between meningothelial, fibroblastic, and transitional.[143]

A few have been largely psammomatous, one osteoblastic,[148] one associated with Sturge-Weber syndrome,[149] and one with an associated inflammatory reaction.[150]

Because they are well circumscribed with distinct borders, fourth ventricular meningiomas can usually be completely resected. After exposing the fourth ventricle, the blood supply is identified (usually from the choroid plexus in lateral recess) and coagulated. The tumor is then resected in piecemeal fashion, progressively folding the capsule inward and using cottonoid patties to define the border between the brain and tumor and protect the fourth ventricle. If the meningioma is very large, it may be necessary to debulk internally using suction or ultrasonic aspiration before identifying the attachment site to the choroid plexus. Alternatively, if very small, it is sometimes possible to remove the tumor en bloc. Most patients do quite well after complete resection with few recurrences.

Subependymoma

Fourth ventricular subependymomas are rare neoplasms that account for less than 1% of all tumors in adults.[151,152] Peak incidence is 40 to 60 years of age, and males are affected more often than females. They are usually found on the caudal fourth ventricular floor or roof of the fourth ventricle but have also been described in the lateral recess of the fourth ventricle, the lateral ventricles, and rarely the third ventricle. They are frequently asymptomatic and usually found incidentally at autopsy but can grow large enough to produce hydrocephalus or mass effect causing visual abnormalities, ataxia, or cranial nerve palsies.[153] They have been associated with the Chiari II malformation.[154]

On CT, subependymomas are asymmetrical, lobulated, often calcified intraventricular masses that enhance moderately with contrast. MRI reveals a mass that is hypointense on T1 and hyperintense on T2, with little or no surrounding edema. Compared with lateral and third ventricular subependymomas, fourth ventricular subependymomas are more likely to have calcification and enhance (heterogeneously) with contrast.[155] Grossly they can be firm or friable but are usually gray and soft with occasional cystic change and hemorrhage.[151] Small subependymomas often have a small area of attachment to the ventricular wall with sharp demarcation from the underlying brain, but larger tumors will often have several secondary sites of attachment.[151] Microscopically, subependymomas have a lobulated appearance with clusters of astrocytic nuclei in a dense fibrillary background of neuroglial fibers.[156] There are no cytologic features of malignancy such as mitoses, but the tumor can infiltrate the brain.

It is controversial whether these tumors arise from subependymal glia, astrocytes of the subependymal plate, ependyma, a mixture of astrocytes and ependymal cells, or simply a nonneoplastic reaction to another process such as meningitis. Initially, it was believed that the subependymomas originated from subependymal glia because microscopically the cells resemble fibrillary subependymal astrocytes. However, mixed ependymoma/subependymoma tumors have been described in which areas typical for subependymoma are adjacent to areas typical for ependymoma.[152] Also, electron microscopic analysis of subependymoma reveals blepharoplasts, intermediate junctions, and microvilli that suggest ependyma, along with intermediate filaments that suggest astrocytoma.[157]

If the patient is asymptomatic and there is no sign of brain stem compression, it is appropriate to follow with serial MRI scans to monitor growth of the tumor. Subependymomas occasionally become symptomatic and warrant surgical treatment. After internal debulking with ultrasonic aspiration or laser, the tumor is gradually folded in on itself and dissected from the surrounding brain. There is usually a well-defined plane between the tumor and normal brain, but occasionally the tumor will be infiltrative and adherent, presumably due to an ependymal component of the tumor. In these cases, it is extremely important not to pull on the capsule attached to the fourth ventricle because respiratory failure from brain stem manipulation is the most common perioperative cause of death in patients with subependymoma.[152] If the patient is elderly and presents with obstructive hydrocephalus without brain stem compression from a mass with a radiographic appearance consistent with subependymoma, insertion of a ventriculoperitoneal shunt and observation with MRI may be a good alternative to removing the tumor surgically.

Most patients who survive surgery to completely resect a pure subependymoma do well with no recurrence,[151] although the natural history of incomplete resection is not known.[153] The presence of an ependymal component carries a worse prognosis and should be treated as a true ependymoma.

Lhermitte-Duclos Disease

Lhermitte-Duclos disease is characterized by a cerebellar mass of abnormal ganglion cells producing circumscribed regions of enlarged cerebellar folia.[36,158] It is unclear whether it represents a congenital cerebellar malformation, hamartoma, phakomatosis, arrest of cell migration, graded hypertrophy of granular cell neurons, or true neoplasm. Immunohistochemical analysis confirms that the cells are derived from granule cells with a minor population of Purkinje cells, and they have no significant proliferative activity, which suggests that the disease is a nonneoplastic malformation predominantly derived from granule cells.[159] Because little is known about its pathogenesis, many names have been used to describe this lesion,[158] including dysplastic gangliocytoma, hamartoma, hamartoblastoma, neurocytic blastoma, diffuse ganglioneuroma, myelinated neurocytoma, granulomolecular cerebellar hypertrophy, gangliocytoma myelinicum diffusum, and purkinjioma.

Most patients with Lhermitte-Duclos disease also have megencephaly. Other associated malformations include hydromyelia, cortical heterotopia, leontiasis ossea, neurofibromatosis, microgyria, hemihypertrophy, numerous hemangiomata, and polydactyly.[160] It is known to be familial in some cases,[161] and there is an association between Lhermitte-Duclos disease and Cowden disease,[162–165] an autosomal dominant condition characterized by multiple cutaneous trichilemmomas, oral papillomatosis, and increased incidence of breast, colon, and adnexa malignancies. The association suggests that both conditions may represent a single disorder of cellular development, perhaps a phakomatosis involving all three germ layers with a tendency for malignant degeneration of lesions.[163]

Peak incidence is between 20 and 40 years of age,[158] but patients can present with this disease at any age, even at birth.[166] There is no sex predominance. In most cases, the lesion grows slowly and produces few symptoms until the abnormal bulk of the cerebellum becomes large enough to obstruct CSF flow and produce brain stem compression. Most patients have a history of several months of progressive headache, vomiting, gait disturbance, and cranial nerve dysfunction. The lesion almost always becomes progressively larger and is rarely an incidental finding at autopsy.

Imaging demonstrates unilateral cerebellar enlargement with a gyriform pattern within the lesion corresponding with the enlarged folia (Fig. 61-32). Most patients have hydrocephalus from fourth ventricular compression at the time of presentation. On CT, the mass is hypodense with ill-defined borders and no enhancement. There is sometimes thinning of occipital squama and focal areas of calcification.[167,168,170] On MRI, the lesion is well defined, hypointense on T1, and hyperintense on T2. The lesion usually does not enhance on CT or MRI,[168,171] but there is occasionally peripheral enhancement due to proliferation of veins near the edge of the tumor in the molecular layer and leptomeninges.[172,173] Except for the lack of enhancement, the mass can closely resemble a low-grade astrocytoma.[170,174] The preserved folial pattern and lack of enhancement produces a striated "tiger-striped cerebellum" pattern that is characteristic of this tumor.[175,176]

Grossly, Lhermitte-Duclos disease appears as broad, pale cerebellar folia confined to one hemisphere or a portion of one hemisphere.[36,177] Microscopically, there is a thick outer layer of well-developed myelinated nerve fibers, encompassing an inner layer of abnormal densely packed neurons that superficially resemble Purkinje cells. There is no layering of Purkinje cells and granular neurons, the folia central white

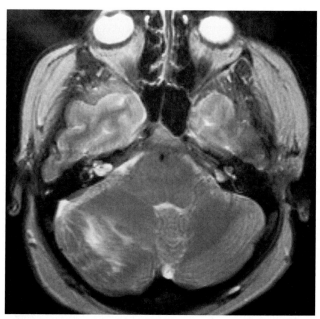

FIGURE 61-32 Lhermitte-Duclos disease, T2. Note the enlarged cerebellar folia on the right and mass effect on the fourth ventricle. This patient also had hydrocephalus.

matter is often absent, and the transition between normal and abnormal areas is gradual.

Because the lesion almost always continues to enlarge progressively, patients who become symptomatic from Lhermitte-Duclos disease invariably require surgery. On exposure of the cerebellum, the large, pale, broadened gyri should be immediately apparent. The affected tissue is usually hypovascular and easily removed with ultrasonic aspiration.[177] Because there is no clear plane between the involved and normal cerebellum, the preoperative MRI should be used to determine the extent of resection. Recurrence years after initial resection has been reported,[159,178–180] so complete resection should be attempted and patients should get periodic follow-up MRI scans. Otherwise, no adjuvant treatment is necessary.

Metastasis

Brain metastases occur in approximately one fourth of all patients with metastatic cancer, so metastases outnumber all other brain tumors in adults. This is true in the posterior fossa as well, in which 15% of metastases are located (equal to the proportional weight of brain tissue in the posterior fossa).[181,182] In adults, the most common metastases to brain tissue are lung (30%), breast (20%), melanoma (10%), kidney (10%), and gastrointestinal tract (5%). Some cancers, like melanoma, metastasize to the brain very commonly, so melanoma brain metastases are often found even though it is a relatively rare tumor. Others, like gastrointestinal tumors, rarely metastasize to the brain but are so common that they are frequently found in the brain. Any tumor that metastasizes to the brain can be found in the posterior fossa, but gastrointestinal, bladder, and uterine tumors do so slightly more often than the others do, and lymphoma sometimes presents as a subependymal mass that extends into the ventricle. When they occur in the posterior fossa, metastatic tumors often become symptomatic from fourth ventricular compression, and most patients present with signs of increased intracranial pressure and hydrocephalus. In children, the most common metastatic tumors are neuroblastoma, rhabdomyosarcoma, Wilms' tumor, and acute lymphoblastic leukemia (chloromas).

The radiographic appearance of metastatic tumors is highly variable. CT may show hyperdensity (from dense cellularity of most metastatic tumors) or hypodensity, and MRI may be hyperintense, hypointense, or isointense on both T1 and T2 weighting. Metastases usually occur at the gray-white junction and are often multiple, although renal and gastrointestinal metastases tend to be solitary. Because they have no blood-brain barrier, virtually all metastatic tumors enhance on CT and MRI, either diffusely or at the tumor margins (ring enhancing); there are sometimes nonenhancing central areas consistent with necrosis.[183,184] Hemorrhage is more characteristic of some tumors, especially melanoma, choriocarcinoma, renal cell cancer, and lung cancer. Adjacent tissue usually has significant vasogenic edema that follows white matter tracts that is often so extensive that the tumor will be obscured on CT or T2-weighted MRI. The histology of metastases is similar to that of the tumor of origin. They differ from primary brain tumors in that they contain more collagen and have more distinct borders with adjacent normal brain.

Brain metastases are usually tertiary metastases from previously metastatic locations in the lung, liver, or lymph nodes; therefore, presence of metastasis in the brain suggests advanced cancer, and the prognosis is very poor. Survival rates vary with different tumors, but few patients survive more than 1 year. Surgery for metastatic disease can prolong patients' survival and quality of life, especially if the metastasis is solitary, which is true in approximately 50% of cases.[181] Radiation is often used as primary or adjunctive therapy.

Other Tumors of the Fourth Ventricle

Teratomas rarely occur in the fourth ventricle or cerebellar vermis, either alone or in combination with the more common pineal location.[185–188] Clival chordomas, arising from the remnants of the primitive notochord, can spread along the floor of the posterior fossa to compress the brain stem and cranial nerves and require adjuvant radiotherapy because complete surgical excision is rarely possible. Nerve root fibromas of the lower cranial nerves often affect the cerebellopontine angle, especially in neurofibromatosis type 2, which includes bilateral vestibular schwannomas and silent fibromas of the vagus and trigeminal nerves. Gangliogliomas have been described in the cerebellum and brain stem.[189,190] Finally, single cases of fourth ventricular myxofibroxanthoma[191] and hemangioma calcificans[192] have been reported.

CONCLUSION

Tumors that arise in the fourth ventricle present the neurosurgeon with a unique challenge because there are many vital neural structures in close proximity to the lesions. Most posterior fossa tumors occur in children, and medulloblastoma, astrocytoma, and ependymoma are the most common. In adults, the most common lesions are metastasis and hemangioblastoma. Improvements in surgical technique and instrumentation have resulted in better outcomes for patients with these tumors.

REFERENCES

1. Porter JM, Pidgeon C, Cunningham AJ: The sitting position in neurosurgery: A critical appraisal. Br J Anaesth 82:117–128, 1999.
2. Pang D: Air embolism associated with wounds from a pin-type headholder: Case report. J Neurosurg 57:710–713, 1982.
3. Harrison EA, Mackersie A, McEwan A, et al: The sitting position for neurosurgery in children: A review of 16 years' experience. Br J Anaesth 88:12–17, 2002.
4. Orliaguet GA, Hanafi M, Meyer PG, et al: Is the sitting or the prone position best for surgery for posterior fossa tumours in children? Paediatr Anaesth 11:541–547, 2001.
5. Steinbok P, Boyd M, Cochrane D: Cervical spine deformity following craniotomy and upper cervical laminectomy for posterior fossa tumors in children. Childs Nerv Syst 5:25–28, 1989.
6. Culley DJ, Berger MS, Shaw D, et al: An analysis of factors determining the need for ventriculoperitoneal shunts following posterior fossa tumor surgery in children. Neurosurgery 34:402–448, 1994.
7. Gnanalingham KK, Lafuente J, Thompson D, et al: The natural history of ventriculomegaly and tonsillar herniation in children with posterior fossa tumours—an MRI study. Pediatr Neurosurg 39:246–253, 2003.
8. Raimondi AJ, Tomita T: Hydrocephalus and infratentorial tumors. Incidence, clinical picture, and treatment. J Neurosurg 55:174–182, 1981.
9. Epstein F, Murali R: Pediatric posterior fossa tumors: Hazards of the "preoperative" shunt. Neurosurgery 3:348–350, 1978.

10. Waga S, Shimizu T, Shimosaka S, et al: Intratumoral hemorrhage after a ventriculoperitoneal shunting procedure. Neurosurgery 9:249–252, 1981.

11. Vaquero J, Cabezudo JM, De Sola RG, et al: Intratumoral hemorrhage in posterior fossa tumors after ventricular drainage: Report of two cases. J Neurosurg 54:406–408, 1981.

12. McLaurin RL: Disadvantages of the preoperative shunt in posterior fossa tumors. Clin Neurosurg 30:286–294, 1983.

13. Dias MS, Albright AL: Management of hydrocephalus complicating childhood posterior fossa tumors. Pediatr Neurosci 15:283–290, 1989.

14. Rappaport ZH, Shalit MN: Perioperative external ventricular drainage in obstructive hydrocephalus secondary to infratentorial brain tumours. Acta Neurochir (Wien) 85:118–121, 1989.

15. Magtibay PM, Friedman JA, Rao RD, et al: Unusual presentation of adult metastatic peritoneal medulloblastoma associated with a ventriculoperitoneal shunt: A case study and review of the literature. Neuro-oncol 5:217–220, 2003.

16. Berger MS, Baumeister B, Geyer JR, et al: The risks of metastases from shunting in children with primary central nervous system tumors. J Neurosurg 74:872–877, 1991.

17. Suri A, Mahapatra AK, Singh VP: Posterior fossa tension pneumocephalus. Childs Nerv Syst 16:196–199, 2000.

18. Carmel PW, Frazer R, Stein B: Aseptic meningitis following posterior fossa surgery in children. J Neurosurg 41:44–48, 1974.

19. De Chadarevian JP, Becker WJ: Mollaret's recurrent aseptic meningitis: relationship to epidermoid cysts. J Neuropathol Exp Neurol 39:661–669, 1980.

20. Wisoff JH, Epstein FJ: Pseudobulbar palsy after posterior fossa operation in children. Neurosurgery 15:707–709, 1984.

21. Pollack IF, Polinko P, Albright AL, et al: Mutism and pseudobulbar symptoms after resection of posterior fossa tumors in children: Incidence and pathophysiology. Neurosurgery 37:885–893, 1995.

22. Pollack IF: Posterior fossa syndrome. Int Rev Neurobiol 41:411–432, 1997.

23. McGuire EJ: The innervation and function of the lower urinary tract. J Neurosurg 65:278–285, 1986.

24. Packer RJ, Sutton LN, Atkins TE, et al: A prospective study of cognitive function in children receiving whole-brain radiotherapy and chemotherapy: 2 year results. J Neurosurg 70:707–713, 1989.

25. Duffner PK, Cohen ME, Thomas PRM, et al: The long-term effects of cranial irradiation in the central nervous system. Cancer 56:1841–1847, 1985.

26. Bailey P, Cushing H: Medulloblastoma cerebelli: A common type of midcerebellar glioma of childhood. Arch Neurol Psychiatry 14:192–224, 1931.

27. Farwell JR, Dohrmann GJ, Flannery JT: Medulloblastoma in childhood: An epidemiological study. J Neurosurg 61:657–664, 1984.

28. Packer RJ, Cogen P, Vezina G, Rorke LB: Medulloblastoma: Clinical and biologic aspects. Neuro-oncol 1:232–250, 1999.

29. Malheiros SM, Carrete H Jr, Stavale JN: MRI of medulloblastoma in adults. Neuroradiology 45:463–467, 2003.

30. Breslow N, Langholz B: Childhood cancer incidence: Geographical and temporal variations. Int J Cancer 32:702–716, 1983.

31. Scheurlen W, Kuhl J: Current diagnostic and therapeutic management of CNS metastasis in childhood primitive neuroectodermal tumors and ependymomas. J Neurooncol 38:181–185, 1998.

32. Koeller KK, Rushing EJ: From the archives of the AFIP: Medulloblastoma: A comprehensive review with radiologic-pathologic correlation. Radiographics 23:1613–1637, 2003.

33. von Koch CS, Gulati M, Aldape K: Familial medulloblastoma: Case report of one family and review of the literature. Neurosurgery 51:227–233, 2002.

34. Park TS, Hoffman HJ, Hendrick EB, et al: Medulloblastoma: Clinical presentation and management—experience at the Hospital for Sick Children, Toronto 1950–1980. J Neurosurg 58:543–552, 1983.

35. Segall HD, Zee CS, Naidich TP, et al: Computed tomography in neoplasms of the posterior fossa in children. Radiol Clin North Am 20:237–253, 1982.

36. Koeller KK, Henry JM: From the archives of the AFIP: Superficial gliomas: Radiologic-pathologic correlation. Armed Forces Institute of Pathology. Radiographics 21:1533–1556, 2001.

37. Meyers SP, Kemp SS, Tarr RW: MR imaging features of medulloblastoma. AJR Am J Roentgenol 158:859–865, 1992.

38. Nemoto Y, Inoue Y, Fukuda T, et al: Displacement of the quadrigeminal plate in tumors of the fourth ventricle. J Comput Assist Tomogr 13:769–772, 1989.

39. Arseni C, Ciurea AV: Statistical survey of 276 cases of medulloblastoma (1935–1978). Acta Neurochir (Wien) 57:159–162, 1981.

40. Packer RJ, Sutton LN, D'Angio G, et al: Management of children with primitive neuroectodermal tumors of the posterior fossa/medulloblastoma. Pediatr Neurosci 12:272–282, 1985-86.

41. Evans A, Jenkin D, Sposto R, et al: The treatment of medulloblastoma. J Neurosurg 72:572–582, 1990.

42. Packer RJ, Sutton LN, Goldwein JW, et al: Improved survival with the use of adjuvant chemotherapy in the treatment of medulloblastoma. J Neurosurg 74:433–440, 1991.

43. Chan AW, Tarbell NJ, Black PM, et al: Adult medulloblastoma: Prognostic factors and patterns of relapse. Neurosurgery 47:623–631, 2000.

44. Lefkowitz I, Packer R, Ryan S, et al: Late recurrence of primitive neuroectodermal tumor/medulloblastoma. Cancer 62:826–830, 1988.

45. Packer RJ, Rood BR, MacDonald TJ, et al: Medulloblastoma: Present concepts of stratification into risk groups. Pediatr Neurosurg 39:60–67, 2003.

46. Perry A: Medulloblastomas with favorable versus unfavorable histology: How many small blue cell tumor types are there in the brain? Adv Anat Pathol 9:345–350, 2002.

47. Saunders DE, Hayward RD, Phipps KP, et al: Surveillance neuroimaging of intracranial medulloblastoma in children: How effective, how often, and for how long? J Neurosurg 99:280–286, 2003.

48. Rorke LB, Packer RJ, Biegel JA, et al: Central nervous system atypical teratoid/rhabdoid tumors of infancy and childhood: Definition of an entity. J Neurosurg 85:56–65, 1996.

49. Bambakidis NC, Robinson S, Cohen M, et al: Atypical teratoid/rhabdoid tumors of the central nervous system: Clinical, radiographic and pathologic features. Pediatr Neurosurg 37:64–70, 2002.

50. Campbell JW, Pollack IF: Cerebellar astrocytomas in children. J Neurooncol 28:223–231, 1996.

51. Schneider JH Jr, Raffel C, McComb JG, et al: Benign cerebellar astrocytomas of childhood. Neurosurgery 30:58–63, 1992.

52. Cushing H: Experiences with the cerebellar astrocytomas: A critical review of 76 cases. Surg Gynecol Obstet 52:129–204, 1931.

53. Morreale VM, Ebersold MJ, Quast LM, et al: Cerebellar astrocytoma: Experience with 54 cases surgically treated at the Mayo Clinic, Rochester, Minnesota, from 1978 to 1990. J Neurosurg 87:257–261, 1997.

54. Lee YY, Van Tassel P, Bruner JM, et al: Juvenile pilocytic astrocytomas: CT and MR characteristics. AJNR Am J Neuroradiol 10:363–370, 1989.

55. Endo H, Kumabe T, Jokura H, et al: Leptomeningeal dissemination of cerebellar malignant astrocytomas. J Neurooncol 63:191–199, 2003.

56. Fernandez C, Figarella-Branger D, Girard N, et al: Pilocytic astrocytomas in children: Prognostic factors—a retrospective study of 80 cases. Neurosurgery 53:544–553, 2003.

57. Gilles FH, Winston K, Fulchiero A, et al: Histological features and observational variation in cerebellar gliomas in children. J Natl Cancer Inst 58:175–181, 1977.

58. Griffin TW, Beaufait D, Blasko JC: Cystic cerebellar astrocytomas in childhood. Cancer 44:276–280, 1979.

59. Gupta V, Goyal A, Sinha S, et al: Glioblastoma of the cerebellum: A report of 3 cases. J Neurosurg Sci 47:157–165, 2003.

60. Kuroiwa T, Numaguchi Y, Rothman MI, et al: Posterior fossa glioblastoma multiforme: MR findings. AJNR Am J Neuroradiol 16:583–589, 1995.

61. Obana W, Cogen P, Davis R, et al: Metastatic juvenile pilocytic astrocytoma. J Neurosurg 75:972–975, 1991.

62. Kepes JJ, Lewis RC, Vergara GG: Cerebellar astrocytoma invading the musculature and soft tissues of the neck. J Neurosurg 52:414–418, 1980.

63. Rollins NK, Nisen P, Shapiro KN: The use of early postoperative MR in detecting residual juvenile cerebellar pilocytic astrocytoma. AJNR Am J Neuroradiol 19:151–156, 1998.

64. Burkhard C, Di Patre PL, Schuler D, et al: A population-based study of the incidence and survival rates in patients with pilocytic astrocytoma. J Neurosurg 98:1170–1174, 2003.

65. Tarbell NJ, Loeffler JS: Recent trends in the radiotherapy of pediatric gliomas. J Neurooncol 28:233–244, 1996.

66. Bertolone SJ, Yates AJ, Boyett JM: Children's Cancer Group. Combined modality therapy for poorly differentiated gliomas of the posterior fossa in children: A Children's Cancer Group report. J Neurooncol 63:49–54, 2003.

67. Desai KI, Nadkarni TD, Muzumdar DP, et al: Prognostic factors for cerebellar astrocytomas in children: A study of 102 cases. Pediatr Neurosurg 35:311–317, 2001.

68. Austin E, Alvord E: Recurrences of cerebellar astrocytomas: a violation of Collin's law. J Neurosurg 68:41–47, 1988.

69. Guyotat J, Signorelli F, Desme S, et al: Intracranial ependymomas in adult patients: Analyses of prognostic factors. J Neurooncol 60:255–268, 2002.

70. van Veelen-Vincent ML, Pierre-Kahn A, Kalifa C, et al: Ependymoma in childhood: Prognostic factors, extent of surgery, and adjuvant therapy. J Neurosurg 97:827–835, 2002.

71. Croul S, Otte J, Khalili K: Brain tumors and polyomaviruses. J Neurovirol 9:173–182, 2003.

72. Bergsagel D, Finegold M, Batel J, et al: DNA sequences similar to those of simian virus 40 in ependymoma and choroid plexus tumors of childhood. N Engl J Med 326:989, 1992.

73. Kirschstein R, Gerger P: Ependymomas produced after intracerebral inoculation of SV40 into newborn hamsters. Nature 195:299, 1962.

74. Nazar GB, Hoffman HJ, Becker JE, et al: Infratentorial ependymomas in childhood: Prognostic factors and treatment. J Neurosurg 72:408–417, 1990.

75. Nakasu S, Ohashi M, Suzuki F, et al: Late dissemination of fourth ventricle ependymoma: A case report. J Neurooncol 55:117–120, 2001.

76. Lefton DR, Pinto RS, Martin SW: MRI features of intracranial and spinal ependymomas. Pediatr Neurosurg 28:97–105, 1998.

77. Swartz JD, Zimmerman RA, Bilaniuk LT: Computed tomography of intracranial ependymomas. Radiology 143:97–101, 1982.

78. Chiu J, Woo S, Ater J, et al: Intracranial ependymoma in children: Analysis of prognostic factors. J Neurooncol 13:283, 1992.

79. Ross G, Rubinstein L: Lack of histopathological correlation of malignant ependymomas with postoperative survival. J Neurosurg 70:31–36, 1989.

80. Oya N, Shibamoto Y, Nagata Y, et al: Postoperative radiotherapy for intracranial ependymoma: Analysis of prognostic factors and patterns of failure. J Neurooncol 56:87–94, 2002.

81. Goldwein JW, Glauser TA, Packer RJ, et al: Recurrent intracranial ependymomas in children—survival, patterns of failure, and prognostic factors. Cancer 66:557, 1990.

82. Vanuytsel L, Brada M: The role of prophylactic spinal irradiation in localized intracranial ependymoma. Int J Radiat Oncol Biol Phys 21:825–830, 1991.

83. Goldwein JW, Corn BW, Rinlay JL, et al: Is craniospinal irradiation required to cure children with malignant (anaplastic) intracranial ependymomas? Cancer 67:2766–2771, 1991.

84. Paulino AC: Radiotherapeutic management of intracranial ependymoma. Pediatr Hematol Oncol 19:295–308, 2002.

85. Smyth MD, Horn BN, Russo C, et al: Intracranial ependymomas of childhood: Current management strategies. Pediatr Neurosurg 33:138–150, 2000.

86. Kiyonobu I, Matsushima T, Inoue TYN, et al: Correlation of microanatomical localization with postoperative survival in posterior fossa ependymomas. Neurosurgery 32:38–44, 1993.

87. Berger M, Edwards M, Lamasters D, et al: Pediatric brain stem tumors: Radiographic, pathological, and clinical correlations. Neurosurgery 12:298–302, 1983.

88. Littman P, Jarret P, Bilanuk L, et al: Pediatric brainstem gliomas. Cancer 45:2787–2792, 1980.

89. Mantravadi R, Phatak R, Bellur S, et al: Brainstem gliomas: an autopsy study of 25 cases. Cancer 49:1294–1296, 1982.

90. Packer RJ, Alien JC, Deck M, et al: Brainstem glioma: Clinical manifestation of meningeal gliomatosis. Ann Neurol 14:177–182, 1983.

91. Yanagawa Y, Miyazawa T, Ishihara S, et al: Pontine glioma with osteoblastic skeletal metastases in a child. Surg Neurol 46:481–484, 1996.

92. Packer RJ, Zimmerman RA, Luerssen TG, et al: Brainstem gliomas of childhood: Magnetic resonance imaging. Neurology 35:397–401, 1985.

93. Epstein F, McCleary EL: Intrinsic brain-stem tumors of childhood: Surgical indications. J Neurosurg 64:11–15, 1986.

94. Farmer JP, Montes JL, Freeman CR, et al: Brainstem gliomas: A 10-year institutional review. Pediatr Neurosurg 34:206–214, 2001.

95. Pollack IF, Hoffman HJ, Humphreys RP, et al: The long-term outcome after surgical treatment of dorsally exophytic brain-stem gliomas. J Neurosurg 78:859–863, 1993.

96. Stroink AR, Hoffman HJ, Hendrick EB, et al: Transependymal benign dorsally exophytic brain stem gliomas in childhood: Diagnosis and treatment recommendations. Neurosurgery 20:439–444, 1987.

97. Bilaniuk LT, Molloy PT, Zimmerman RA, et al: Neurofibromatosis type 1: Brain stem tumours. Neuroradiology 39:642–653, 1997.

98. Milstein JM, Geyer JR, Berger MS, et al: Favorable prognosis for brain-stem gliomas in neurofibromatosis. J Neurooncol 7:367–371, 1989.

99. Vandertop WP, Hoffman HJ, Drake JM, et al: Focal midbrain tumors in children. Neurosurgery 31:186–194, 1992.

100. Epstein FJ, Farmer JP: Brain stem glioma growth patterns. J Neurosurg 78:408–412, 1993.

101. Young Poussaint T, Yousuf N, Barnes PD, et al: Cervicomedullary astrocytomas of childhood: Clinical and imaging follow-up. Pediatr Radiol 29:662–668, 1999.

102. Epstein F, Wisoff J: Intra-axial tumors of the cervicomedullary junction. J Neurosurg 67:483–487, 1987.

103. Ellenbogen RG, Winston KR, Kupsky WJ: Tumors of the choroid plexus in children. Neurosurgery 25:327–335, 1989.

104. Tomita T, McLone D, Flannery A: Choroid plexus papillomas of neonates, infants, and children. Pediatr Neurosci 14:23–30, 1988.

105. Ken JG, Sobel DF, Copeland B, et al: Choroid plexus papillomas of the foramen of Luschka: MR appearance. AJNR Am J Neuroradiol 12:1201–1203, 1991.

106. Picard C, Copty M, Lavoie G, et al: A primary choroid plexus papilloma of the cerebellopontine angle. Surg Neurol 12:123–127, 1979.

107. Talacchi A, De Micheli E, Lombardo C, et al: Choroid plexus papilloma of the cerebellopontine angle: A twelve patient series. Surg Neurol 51:621–629, 1999.

108. Shinoda J, Kawaguchi M, Matsuhisa T, et al: Choroid plexus carcinoma in infants: Report of two cases and review of the literature. Acta Neurochir (Wien) 140:557–563, 1998.

109. Packer R, Perilongo G, Johnson D, et al: Choroid plexus carcinoma in childhood. Cancer 69:580–585, 1992.

110. Shin JH, Lee HK, Jeong AK, et al: Choroid plexus papilloma in the posterior cranial fossa: MR, CT, and angiographic findings. Clin Imaging 25:154–162, 2001.

111. Ho DM, Wong TT, Liu HC, et al: Choroid plexus tumors in childhood: Histopathologic study and clinicopathologic correlation. Childs Nerv Syst 7:437–441, 1991.

112. Coates TL, Hinshaw DB, Peckman N, et al: Pediatric choroid plexus neoplasms: MR, CT, and pathologic correlation. Radiology 173:81–88, 1989.

113. Vasquez E, Ball WS Jr, Prenger EC, et al: Magnetic resonance imaging of fourth ventricular choroid plexus neoplasms in childhood. Pediatr Neurosurg 17:48–52, 1991–1992.

114. McEvoy AW, Harding BN, Phipps KP, et al: Management of choroid plexus tumours in children: 20 years experience at a single neurosurgical centre. Pediatr Neurosurg 32:192–199, 2000.

115. Wolff JE, Sajedi M, Brant R, et al: Choroid plexus tumours. Br J Cancer 87:1086–1091, 2002.

116. McGirr SJ, Ebersold MJ, Scheithauer BW, et al: Choroid plexus papillomas: Long-term follow-up results in a surgically treated series. J Neurosurg 69:843–849, 1988.

117. Weil RJ, Lonser RR, DeVroom HL, et al: Surgical management of brainstem hemangioblastomas in patients with von Hippel-Lindau disease. J Neurosurg 98:95–105, 2003.

118. Lindau A: Studien uber Kleinhirncysten. Bau, Pathogenese und Beziehungen zur Angiomatosis Retinae. Acta Pathol Microbiol Scand Suppl 1:1–128, 1926.

119. Friedrich CA: Von Hippel-Lindau syndrome: A pleomorphic condition. Cancer 86(11 Suppl):2478–2482, 1999.

120. Neumann HPH, Eggert HR, Weigel K, et al: Hemangioblastomas of the central nervous system: A 10-year study with special reference to von Hippel-Lindau syndrome. J Neurosurg 70:24–30, 1989.

121. Seizinger BR, Smith DI, Filling-Katz MR, et al: Genetic flanking markers refine diagnostic criteria and provide insights into the genetics of von Hippel Lindau disease. Proc Natl Acad Sci USA 88:2864–2868, 1991.

122. Wanebo JE, Lonser RR, Glenn GM, et al: The natural history of hemangioblastomas of the central nervous system in patients with von Hippel-Lindau disease. J Neurosurg 98:82–94, 2003.

123. Waldmann TA, Levin EH, Baldwin M, et al: The association of polycythemia with a cerebellar hemangioblastoma: The production of an erythropoiesis stimulating factor by the tumor. Am J Med 31:318–324, 1961.

124. Tachibana O, Yamashima T, Yamashita J, et al: Immunohistochemical study of erythropoietin in cerebellar hemangioblastomas associated with secondary polycythemia. Neurosurgery 28:24–26, 1991.

125. Elster AD, Arthur DW: Intracranial hemangioblastomas: CT and MR findings. J Comput Asst Tomogr 12:736–739, 1988.

126. Lee SR, Sauches J, Mark AS, et al: Posterior fossa hemangioblastomas: MR imaging. Radiology 171:463–468, 1989.

127. Reyns N, Assaker R, Louis E, et al: Leptomeningeal hemangioblastomatosis in a case of von Hippel-Lindau disease: Case report. Neurosurgery 52:1212–1215, 2003.

128. Niemela M, Lim YJ, Soderman M, et al: Gamma knife radiosurgery in 11 hemangioblastomas. J Neurosurg 85:591–596, 1996.

129. Guidetti B, Gagliardi FM: Epidermoid and dermoid cysts: Clinical evaluation and late surgical results. J Neurosurg 47:12–18, 1977.

130. Berger MS, Wilson CB: Epidermoid cyst of the posterior fossa. J Neurosurg 62:214–219, 1985.

131. Rosario M, Becker DH, Conley FK: Epidermoid tumors involving the fourth ventricle. Neurosurgery 9:9–13, 1981.

132. Goffin J, Plets C, Van Calenbergh F, et al: Posterior fossa dermoid cyst associated with dermal fistula: Report of 2 cases and review of the literature. Childs Nerv Syst 9:179–181, 1993.

133. Logue V, Till K: Posterior fossa dermoid cysts with special reference to intracranial infection. J Neurol Neurosurg Psychiatry 15:1–12, 1952.

134. Akhaddar A, Jiddane M, Chakir N, et al: Cerebellar abscesses secondary to occipital dermoid cyst with dermal sinus: Case report. Surg Neurol 58:266–270, 2002.

135. Barloon TJ, Jacoby CG, Schultz DH: MR of fourth ventricular epidermoid tumors. Am J Neuroradiol 9:794–796, 1988.

136. Tancredi A, Fiume D, Gazzeri G: Epidermoid cysts of the fourth ventricle: Very long follow up in 9 cases and review of the literature. Acta Neurochir (Wien) 145:905–911, 2003.

137. Muller A, Buttner A, Weis S: Rare occurrence of intracerebral colloid cyst: Case report. J Neurosurg 91:128–131, 1999.

138. Jan M, BaZozo V, Velut S: Colloid cyst of the fourth ventricle: Diagnostic problems and pathogenic considerations. Neurosurgery 24:939–942, 1989.

139. Parkinson D, Childe AE: Colloid cyst of the fourth ventricle: Report of a case of two colloid cysts of the fourth ventricle. J Neurosurg 9:404–409, 1952.

140. Bejjani GK, Wright DC, Schessel D, et al: Endodermal cysts of the posterior fossa: Report of three cases and review of the literature. J Neurosurg 89:326–235, 1998.

141. Harris C, Dias M, Brockmeyer D, et al: Neurenteric cysts of the posterior fossa: Recognition, management, and embryogenesis. Neurosurgery 29:893–898, 1991.

142. Akimoto J, Sato Y, Tsutsumi M, et al: Fourth ventricular meningioma in an adult—case report. Neurol Med Chir (Tokyo) 41:402–405, 2001.

143. Ceylan K, Ilbay K, Kuzeyli M, et al: Intraventricular meningioma of the fourth ventricle. Clin Neurol Neurosurg 94:181–184, 1992.

144. Chaskis C, Buisseret T, Michotte A, et al: Meningioma of the fourth ventricle presenting with intermittent behaviour disorders: A case report and review of the literature. J Clin Neurosci 8(Suppl 1):59–62, 2001.

145. Iseda T, Goya T, Nakano S, et al: Magnetic resonance imaging and angiographic appearance of meningioma of the fourth ventricle—two case reports. Neurol Med Chir (Tokyo) 37:36–40, 1997.

146. Cushing H, Eisenhardt L: Meningiomas: Their Classification, Regional Behavior, Life History, and Surgical End Results. Springfield, IL: Charles C Thomas, 1938, pp 139–140.

147. Black P: Meningiomas. Neurosurgery 32:643–657, 1993.

148. Johnson MD, Tulipan N, Whetsell WO: Osteoblastic meningioma of the fourth ventricle. Neurosurgery 24:587–590, 1989.

149. Gokalp HZ, Ozkal E, Erdogan A, et al: A giant meningioma of the fourth ventricle associated with Sturge-Weber disease. Acta Neurochir (Wien)57:115–120, 1981.

150. Ferrara M, Bizzozero L, D'Aliberti G, et al: Inflammatory meningioma of the fourth ventricle: Case report. J Neurosurg Sci 38:59–62, 1994.

151. Scheithauer BW: Symptomatic subependymoma: Report of 21 cases with review of the literature. J Neurosurg 49:689–696, 1978.

152. Jooma R, Torrens MJ, Bradshaw J, et al: Subependymoma of the fourth ventricle: Surgical treatment in 12 cases. J Neurosurg 62:508–512, 1985.

153. Lombardi D, Scheithauer BW, Meyer FB, et al: Symptomatic subependymoma: A clinicopathological and flow cytometric study. J Neurosurg 75:583–588, 1991.

154. Piatt JH Jr, D'Agostino A: The Chiari II malformation: Lesions discovered within the fourth ventricle. Pediatr Neurosurg 30:79–85, 1999.

155. Chiechi MV, Smirniotopoulos JG, Jones RV: Intracranial subependymomas: CT and MR imaging features in 24 cases. AJR Am J Roentgenol 165:1245–1250, 1995.

156. Gandolfi A, Brizzi RE, Tedeschi F, et al: Symptomatic subependymoma of the fourth ventricle: Case report. J Neurosurg 55:841–844, 1981.

157. Moss TH: Observations on the nature of subependymoma: an electron microscopic study. Neuropathol Appl Neurobiol 10:63–75, 1984.

158. Nowak DA, Trost HA: Lhermitte-Duclos disease (dysplastic cerebellar gangliocytoma): A malformation, hamartoma or neoplasm? Acta Neurol Scand 105:137–145, 2002.

159. Hair LS, Symmans F, Powers JM, et al: Immunohistochemistry and proliferative activity in Lhermitte-Duclos disease. Acta Neuropathol 84:570–573, 1992.

160. Reznick M, Schoenen J: Lhermitte-Duclos disease. Acta Neuropathol 59:88–94, 1983.

161. Ambler M, Pogacar S, Sidman R: Lhermitte-Duclos disease (granule cell hypertrophy of the cerebellum): Pathological analysis of the first familial case. J Neuropathol Exp Neurol 28:622–647, 1969.

162. Vinchon M, Blond S, Lejeune JP, et al: Association of Lhermitte-Duclos and Cowden disease: Report of a new case and review of the literature. J Neurol Neurosurg Psychiatry 57:699–704, 1994.

163. Padberg GW, Schot JDL, Vielvoye GJ, et al: Lhermitte-Duclos disease and Cowden disease: A single phakomatosis. Ann Neurol 29:517–523, 1991.

164. Albrecht S, Haber RM, Goodman JC, et al: Cowden syndrome and Lhermitte-Duclos disease. Cancer 70:869–876, 1991.

165. King MA, Coyne TJ, Spearritt DJ, et al: Lhermitte-Duclos disease and Cowden disease: A third case. Ann Neurol 32:112–113, 1992.

166. Roessmann U, Wongmongkolrit T: Dysplastic gangliocytoma of the cerebellum in a newborn. J Neurosurg 60:845–847, 1984.

167. Vieco PT, del Carpio-O'Donovan R, Melanson D, et al: Dysplastic gangliocytoma (Lhermitte-Duclos disease): CT and MR imaging. Pediatr Radiol 22:366–369, 1992.

168. Ashley DG, Zee CS, Chandrasoma PT, et al: Case report. Lhermitte-Duclos disease: CT and MR findings. J Comput Assist Tomogr 14:984–987, 1990.

169. Smith RR, Grossman RI, Goldberg HI, et al: MR imaging of Lhermitte-Duclos disease: A case report. AJNR Am J Neuroradiol 10:187–189, 1989.

170. Choudhury AR: Short report. Preoperative magnetic resonance imaging in Lhermitte-Duclos disease. Br J Neurosurg 4:225–230, 1990.

171. Spaargaren L, Cras P, Bomhof MA, et al: Contrast enhancement in Lhermitte-Duclos disease of the cerebellum: Correlation of imaging with neuropathology in two cases. Neuroradiology 45:381–385, 2003.

172. Awwad EE, Levy E, Martin DS, et al: Atypical MR appearance of Lhermitte-Duclos disease with contrast enhancement. AJNR Am J Neuroradiol 16:1719–1720, 1995.

173. Carter JE, Merren MD, Swann KW, et al: Preoperative diagnosis of Lhermitte-Duclos disease by magnetic resonance imaging: Case report. J Neurosurg 70:135–137, 1989.

174. Meltzer CC, Smirniotopoulos JG, Jones RV, et al: The striated cerebellum: An MR imaging sign in Lhermitte-Duclos disease (dysplastic gangliocytoma). Radiology 194:699–703, 1995.

175. Wolansky LJ, Malantic GP, Heary R, et al: Preoperative MRI diagnosis of Lhermitte-Duclos disease: Case report with associated enlarged vessel and syrinx. Surg Neurol 45:470–475, 1996.

176. Faillot T, Sichez JP, Brault JL, et al: Lhermitte-Duclos disease (dysplastic gangliocytoma of the cerebellum): Report of a case and review of the literature. Acta Neurochir (Wien)105:44–49, 1990.

177. Stapleton SR, Wilkins PR, Bell BA, et al: Short report. Recurrent dysplastic cerebellar gangliocytoma (Lhermitte-Duclos disease) presenting with subarachnoid haemorrhage. Br J Neurosurg 6:153–156, 1992.

178. Hashimoto H, Iida J, Masui K, et al: Recurrent Lhermitte-Duclos disease—case report. Neurol Med Chir (Tokyo) 37:692–696, 1997.

179. Williams DW 3rd, Elster AD, Ginsberg LE, et al: Recurrent Lhermitte-Duclos disease: Report of two cases and association with Cowden's disease. AJNR Am J Neuroradiol 13:287–290, 1992.

180. Patchell R, Tibbs P, Walsh J, et al: A randomized trial of surgery in the treatment of single metastases to the brain. N Engl J Med 322:494–500, 1990.

181. Soffietti R, Ruda R, Mutani R: Management of brain metastases. J Neurol 249:1357–1369, 2002.

182. Potts DG, Abbott GF, von Sneidem JV: National Cancer Institute Study: Evaluation of computed tomography in the diagnosis of intracranial neoplasms: III. Metastatic tumors. Radiology 136:657–664, 1980.

183. Bisese JH: MRI of cranial metastases. Semin Ultrasound CT MRI 13:473–483, 1992.

184. Iwasaki I, Horie H, Yu TJ, et al: Intracranial teratoma with a prominent rhabdomyogenic element and germinoma in the fourth ventricle. Neurol Med Chir (Tokyo) 24:51–55, 1984.

185. Desai K, Nadkarni T, Muzumdar D, et al: Midline posterior fossa teratoma—case report. Neurol Med Chir (Tokyo) 41:94–96, 2000.

186. Drapkin AJ, Rose WS, Pellmar MB: Mature teratoma in the fourth ventricle of an adult: Case report and review of the literature. Neurosurgery 21:404–410, 1987.

187. Aoyama I, Makita Y, Nabeshima S, et al: Intracranial double teratomas. Surg Neurol 17:383–387, 1982.

188. Harada K, Okamoto H, Fujioka Y, et al: Teratoma in the fourth ventricle of an elderly adult: Case report. Neurol Med Chir (Tokyo) 24:499–503, 1984.

189. Lagares A, Gomez PA, Lobato RD, et al: Ganglioglioma of the brainstem: Report of three cases and review of the literature. Surg Neurol 56:315–322, 2001.

190. Bills DC, Hanieh A: Hemifacial spasm in an infant due to fourth ventricular ganglioglioma: Case report. J Neurosurg 75:134–137, 1991.

191. Chen MN, Nakazawa S, Shimura T, et al: Myxofibroxanthoma of the fourth ventricle: Case report. Neurol Med Chir (Tokyo) 25:564–567, 1985.

192. Kobayashi H, Kawano H, Ito H, et al: Hemangioma calcificans in the fourth ventricle. Neurosurgery 14:737–739, 1984.

62 Radiosurgery of Vestibular Schwannomas

JOHN C. FLICKINGER, DOUGLAS KONDZIOLKA,
and L. DADE LUNSFORD

INTRODUCTION

Radiosurgery is an attractive, low-morbidity alternative to microsurgical resection of vestibular schwannoma (acoustic neuroma), with similar long-term tumor control rates.[1–10] For many years, these tumors were widely believed to be insensitive to radiation, leaving surgery as the only effective management strategy. By 1987, when Wallner reported a small series supporting conventional postoperative fractionated radiotherapy for vestibular schwannomas, radiosurgery programs were already under way at Harvard and the University of Pittsburgh, based on early reports of success with arteriovenous malformation (AVM) and vestibular schwannoma radiosurgery in Sweden.[5,6,11] Over the next 10 to 15 years, the results of radiosurgery reproduced in multiple centers around the world changed the belief that vestibular schwannomas were radioresistant and moved radiosurgery into a major role in the primary management of these tumors.

Benign tumors like vestibular schwannomas can sometimes be observed sometimes for years without any tumor growth. The slow growth rate of benign tumors also means that recurrences can occur 10 years or more after initial radiotherapy.[12] Large series with lengthy follow-up are required to define tumor control rates and to distinguish between radiation effect and natural history. Outcome studies of radiosurgery with longer term follow-up continue to appear; however, these studies still need to be extended and enlarged, particularly using current techniques with lower marginal tumor doses.[3,5,6]

EVOLUTION OF TREATMENT TECHNIQUES

Radiosurgical treatment techniques have evolved considerably over the years. These changes include improvements in stereotactic imaging, in treatment planning, and refinements in dose prescription. The early work at Karolinska started with hand dose calculations. Tumor imaging, beginning with pneumoencephalography and angiography, and even with the early generation computed tomography (CT) that followed, was inadequate for fully defining tumors (by today's standards). The intracanalicular portion of the tumor was usually not covered in the treatment plan.

By 1987, the early computer-generated treatment plans would take more than an hour if more than one isocenter was required. Because of difficulties in treatment planning, all institutions limited the number of isocenters treated, to the extent possible. Treatment volumes were less conformal than today, when multiple isocenters are used freely. Gamma knife vestibular schwannoma treatment plans usually consisted of one isocenter for the smaller intracanalicular tumor portion in the porus acousticus (usually treated with 4-mm diameter collimators) and, if possible, one isocenter for the extracanalicular (intracranial) portion (Fig. 62-1). More than one isocenter was used for the extracanalicular portion only when the 18-mm diameter collimator couldn't cover the diameter of that portion, or if the tumor was highly irregular in shape. Early LINAC treatment plans usually consisted of one isocenter centered in the extracanalicular portion of the tumor.

By 1992, high-resolution stereotactic imaging had been used for stereotactic targeting by gamma knife centers for 1 year, and image fusion techniques were being developed for use with stereotactic CT scans (which also had improved resolution by then). Treatment-planning programs were faster and fully integrated with imaging; therefore elaborate, highly conformal, multi-isocenter treatment plans could be developed in minutes. Gamma knife centers began using 6 to 13 isocenters in more than half the cases to achieve a high degree of conformality. The use of multiple isocenters to achieve conformality is a form of intensity-modulated radiotherapy. Figure 62-1 shows a typical gamma knife plan for vestibular schwannoma radiosurgery based on stereotactic MR imaging. By 1992, LINAC centers were adopting multiple isocenter techniques, switching to multiple static conformal fields to improve conformality, or switching to fractionated techniques with more gentle radiation doses.[2,3] Later years saw the introduction of inverse treatment planning, which can make treatment planning with multiple isocenters easier.

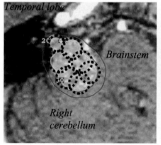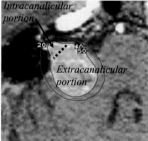

FIGURE 62-1 A typical multiple isocenter radiosurgery plan for a vestibular schwannoma with stereotactic MR imaging. Each individual isocenter is pictured on the left with the composite distribution shown on the right. The 20%, 40%, and 50% isodose volumes are displayed.

Prescription doses for radiosurgery have moved downward over the years. Much of the early experience with Karolinska used minimum tumor doses of 20 Gy. Initially, minimum tumor doses of 16 to 20 Gy, according to tumor volume, were prescribed at Pittsburgh. Prescription doses were lowered slowly over the years because of the fear of compromising long-term tumor control for lower morbidity; so far, that has not occurred. The prescription doses (marginal doses) most commonly used today are in the range of 12 to 13 Gy, with no compromise in tumor control seen in retrospective analysis.[2,5,6] How far radiosurgery doses for vestibular schwannoma may safely be lowered is unclear. Fractionated stereotactic radiotherapy has been used with apparent success with doses as low as 20 Gy in five fractions.[13-23] The single-fraction equivalent for a dose of 20 Gy in five fractions, predicted by the linear quadratic formula with alpha/beta ratios of 0, 2.5, or 5, would be 8.9, 9.2, or 11.1 Gy, respectively. In a University of Florida series,[4] Foote observed a trend ($p = 0.207$) for poorer tumor control with radiosurgery doses of less than 10 Gy; this argues against using doses this low.

EARLY RADIOSURGERY EXPERIENCE

The early radiosurgical experience in treating vestibular schwannomas is well documented in Kondziolka's analysis of the University of Pittsburgh experience from 1987 to 1992.[8] The authors recently reanalyzed this experience with further follow-up.

From 1987 to 1992, 157 patients underwent gamma knife radiosurgery for unilateral vestibular schwannoma at the University of Pittsburgh. During the initial years, only patients who were poor surgical candidates or who refused recommended surgical resection were accepted for treatment. After the first 2 years, when preliminary results confirmed the safety and efficacy seen in Sweden, more patients who were reasonable surgical candidates were accepted for treatment. The median age for this series was 60 years (range, 28 to 83 years). The number of prior surgical resections was zero in 117 patients, 1 in 26 patients, 2 in 12 patients, and 3 or 4 resections in 2 patients. Of the last operations performed before radiosurgery, 7 tumors recurred after "total" resections, 29 were irradiated after subtotal resection, and in 4 cases records were unclear whether the procedure was a complete or partial resection. The most common presenting symptom was hearing loss (60 patients), followed by tinnitus (35 patients). Facial weakness was present in 33 patients prior to radiosurgery, and decreased facial sensation was also seen in 33 patients.

The median treatment volume was 2.7 cm³ with a range of 0.08 to 18.0 cm³. The median marginal dose prescribed was 16 Gy (range, 12 to 20 Gy) with a median maximum dose of 32 Gy (range, 20.6 to 50.0 Gy). The median prescription isodose volume was 50%, with a range of 40% to 70%. The 50% isodose volume was delivered to 126 patients, 40% to 45% was delivered to 6 patients, and 55% to 70% was delivered to 24 patients.

Follow-up physical examinations with CT or MR images were requested every 6 months for the first 2 years, and then yearly afterwards. Tumor sizes were carefully measured on follow-up films with calipers. Tumor enlargement or regression was defined as a 2-mm change in tumor diameter from treatment baseline. For patients with preserved hearing, audiograms were requested at similar intervals for the first 3 years, but follow-up audiograms were performed more selectively after 3 years.

The median follow-up was 9.1 years; it was 10.2 years for patients alive at the time of last follow-up (excluding intercurrent deaths). Three patients had a surgical procedure after radiosurgery (these were at 19, 33, and 40 months). The first patient had a prior subtotal resection of a vestibular schwannoma that may have been related to a prior mantle radiotherapy field extending up to the mastoids. In the second patient, follow-up imaging documented growth of the extracanalicular portion of the tumor. The third patient had a cystic recurrence initially drained and then partially resected. An additional patient had surgery for an adjacent arachnoid cyst even though the tumor had not enlarged. Serial imaging studies after radiosurgery (n = 157) showed a decrease in tumor size in 114 patients (73%), no change in 40 patients (25.5%), and an increase in 3 patients (1.9%) who had later resection. Counting the arachnoid cyst progression as a failure of radiosurgical management, the long-term actuarial tumor control rate was 97.0 ± 1.3% (Fig. 62-2).

Facial weakness developed after radiosurgery in 26 of 157 patients (16.6%), (none worse than House-Brackman Grade 3 at last follow-up). In 5 patients, facial weakness improved after radiosurgery. Reduced facial sensation developed in 25 of 157 patients (15.9%) after radiosurgery, whereas facial sensation improved in 6 patients. The Gardner-Robertson hearing grade remained unchanged in 43 of 85 patients (51%) with testable hearing preradiosurgery. Serviceable hearing (Grade 1 or 2) remained in 15 of 32 patients (47%) with Gardner-Robertson Grade 1 or 2 hearing prior to radiosurgery.

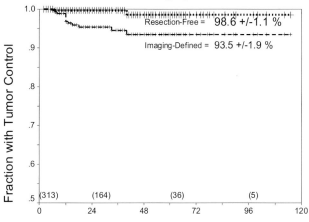

FIGURE 62-2 Actuarial tumor control in 313 unilateral vestibular schwannoma patients undergoing radiosurgery at the University of Pittsburgh with marginal tumor doses of 12 to 13 Gy. Imaging-defined control refers to imaging-defined tumor control, which strictly counts any temporary or sustained increase in tumor diameter of 1 mm or more as failure, even if the tumor later shrinks. The numbers in parentheses refer to the number of patients with follow-up greater than the corresponding time.

Ten patients with vestibular schwannomas later developed other intracranial tumors, including 2 with pituitary tumors or meningiomas, 2 with brain metastasis, and 1 with another schwannoma. All of these were in remote brain locations. No patient developed a radiation-induced malignant or benign tumor.

This series clearly documents the long-term safety and efficacy of radiosurgery for vestibular schwannomas. Despite the higher rates of cranial nerve injury seen after radiosurgery in this early series compared with those seen with present techniques, these results represent a substantial improvement over surgical management with equal or better long-term tumor control.

RECENT REPRESENTATIVE RADIOSURGERY SERIES

Results for modern radiosurgery techniques are found in recently published series from Marseille, Pittsburgh, and Osaka.[3,9,10] Regis recently published a carefully documented comparison of 110 surgery and 97 radiosurgery (12 or 14 Gy) vestibular schwannoma patients with close follow-up (4-year minimum)[9] (Fig. 62-3). Facial nerve preservation was 100% in the radiosurgery group, compared with 63% in the microsurgery group. Functional hearing preservation was 70% in the radiosurgery group. A larger study from their group on 211 patients undergoing radiosurgery for unilateral vestibular schwannoma found a hearing preservation rate of 73%. They found that hearing preservation was related to preoperative Gardner Robertson stage 1 (versus 2), planning with multiple isocenters, and marginal tumor doses of less than 13 Gy. A stage 1 intracanalicular tumor with Gardner and Robertson Class 1 hearing, treated with a marginal dose of less than 13 Gy had a greater than 95% chance of functional conservation at 2 years.

The authors recently reviewed 313 patients with previously untreated unilateral vestibular schwannomas who underwent gamma knife radiosurgery at the University of Pittsburgh between February 1991 and February 2001 with marginal tumor doses of 12 to 13 Gy (median, 13 Gy).[3] Maximum doses were 20 to 26 Gy (median, 26 Gy). Treatment volumes were 0.04 to 21.4 cm^3 (median = 1.1 cm^3). Median follow-up was 24 months (maximum, 115 months; 36 patients had 60 months of follow-up). The actuarial 6-year resection-free clinical tumor control rate (defined as no requirement for surgical intervention) was 98.6% ± 1.1%. Two patients required surgical resection; one had a complete resection for continued solid tumor growth, and the other required partial resection for an enlarging adjacent subarachnoid cyst (despite control of the irradiated tumor). The 6-year actuarial rates for preserved facial nerve strength, normal trigeminal nerve function, unchanged hearing-level, and useful hearing were 100%, 95.6% ± 1.8%, 70.3% ± 5.8%, and 78.6% ± 5.1%, respectively. Among the eight patients developing new trigeminal neuropathy (5 to 48 months postradiosurgery), six developed numbness (6-year actuarial rate, 2.5% ± 1.5%) and the other two developed new typical trigeminal neuralgia (6-year actuarial rate, 1.9% ± 1.5%). The risk of developing any trigeminal neuropathy correlated with increasing tumor volume ($p = 0.038$).

Iwai and colleagues analyzed the outcome of low-dose gamma knife radiosurgery (8 to 12 Gy; median, 12 Gy) in 51 consecutive vestibular schwannoma patients treated from 1992 to 1996, with median follow-up of 60 months (range, 19 to 96 months).[10] Resection-free tumor control was 96%. Freedom from any new facial weakness or new numbness was 100% and 100%, respectively, although 4% of patients with preexisting facial neuropathy experienced worsening of facial numbness postradiosurgery. Preservation of Class 1 or 2 (serviceable) hearing was achieved in 56% of patients.

FRACTIONATED STEREOTACTIC RADIOTHERAPY

Williams recently published the Johns Hopkins experience with fractionated stereotactic radiotherapy in 125 vestibular schwannoma patients with more than 1-year follow-up (out of 249 patients treated between 1996 and 2001).[23] For tumors less than 3.0 cm in diameter, 25 Gy was given in 5 consecutive 5-Gy fractions (111 patients); tumors of 3.0 cm in diameter received 30 Gy in 10 fractions (14 patients). With a median follow-up of 21 months (range, 12 to 68 months), tumor control and facial nerve preservation were both 100%. Two patients developed transient decreases in facial sensation. Hearing preservation was seen in approximately 70% of patients.

Sakamoto reported the experience of Hokkaido University in Sapporo, Japan, with stereotactic fractionated radiotherapy in 65 vestibular schwannoma patients who received 44 to 50 Gy in 22 to 25 fractions with a mean follow-up of 37 months (range, 6 to 97 months).[20] The 5-year actuarial tumor control rate, calculated from the 44 patients with more than 2-year follow-up, was 92%. Transient facial nerve palsy and transient trigeminal nerve palsy developed in 4.6% and 9.2% of those 44 patients, respectively. Transient trigeminal nerve palsy developed significantly more often in cystic versus solid tumors (25% versus 2%).

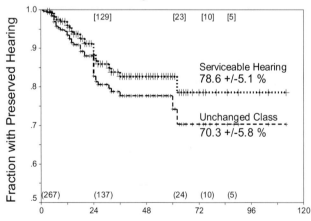

Actuarial Hearing Preservation

Serviceable Hearing
78.6 +/-5.1 %

Unchanged Class
70.3 +/-5.8 %

FIGURE 62-3 Actuarial hearing preservation in 267 unilateral vestibular schwannoma patients with preoperative hearing out of 313 patients undergoing radiosurgery at the University of Pittsburgh with marginal tumor doses of 12 to 13 Gy. Unchanged Class refers to preservation of the same Gardner Robertson hearing class (I to IV). The numbers in parentheses refer to the number of patients with follow-up greater than the corresponding time.

TABLE 62-1 ▪ Tumor Control and Cranial Nerve Preservation Rates for a Number of Representative Series for Radiosurgery and Stereotactic Fractionated Radiotherapy and of Vestibular Schwannoma

Institution	No. of Patients	Median FU MO (range)	Median Marginal Tumor Dose in Gy (range)/ No. Fractions	Tumor Control	Complications in Cranial Nerves V, VII, and VIII (Temporary/Permanent Rates)
SRS					
Pittsburgh[3]	313	24 (1–115)	13 (12–13) Gy/1 fr	98.6%	V 4%, VII 0%, VIII 30%
Osaka[10]	51	60 (8–96)	12 (8–12) Gy/1 fr	92%	V 2%, VII 0%, VIII 44%
Marseille[9]	97	? (36–108?)	12–14 Gy/1 fr	97%	V 4%, VII 0% VIII 30%
Jefferson[13]	69	27 ± 15 (SE)	12 (*range?*)	98%	V 5%, VII 2% VIII 67%
Amsterdam[18]	49	33 (12–107)	10 or 12.5 Gy/1 fr	100%	V 8%, VII 7% VIII 25%
SRT					
Jefferson[13]	56	27 ± 22 (SE)	50 Gy/25 fr	92%*	V 7%, VII 2%, VIII 30%*
Amsterdam[18]	80	33 (12–107)	20 Gy/4–5 fr	94%	V 2%, VII 3%, VIII 39%
Stanford[18]	33	24 (6–48)	21 Gy/3 fr	97%	V 16%, VII 3%, VIII 23%
Staten Island[16,19]	38	24 (24–32)	20 Gy/4–5 fr	100%	V 0%, VII 3%, VIII 23%
Sapporo[20,21]	65	37 (6–97)	36–50 Gy/20–23 fr	92%	V 0/12%, VII 0/5%, VIII 53%?
Johns Hopkins[11]	125	21 (12–68)	25 Gy/5 fr, 30 Gy/10 fr	100%	V 0/2%, VII 0%, VIII 30%
Heidelberg[15]	42	42 (17–131)	57.6 ± 2.5 Gy at 1.8–2 Gy/fr	97.7%	V 4%, VII 0%, VIII 15%
Loma Linda[14]	29	34 (7–98)	54,60 CGE,30–33 fr	100%	V 0%, VII 0%, VIII 69%

*Actuarial at 4 years.
  CGE, Cobalt-Gy-equivalent for protons.

Other fractionated stereotactic radiotherapy series are listed in Table 62-1.

Single Institution Comparisons of SRS and SRT

Single institution comparisons of stereotactic radiosurgery (SRS) and stereotactic fractionated radiotherapy (SRT) were recently published by Jefferson University in Philadelphia and VU University Medical Center in the Netherlands.[14,17] The Jefferson experience compared 69 patients who had radiosurgery with 56 patients who had fractionated radiotherapy (50 Gy/25 fractions).[14] The first 25 acoustic tumor patients were treated at Jefferson with a linear accelerator: 14 without hearing underwent radiosurgery, and 11 with hearing received fractionated radiotherapy with 9 4-Gy fractions. The authors state that the patients receiving nine fractions of 4 Gy will be the subjects of a separate report, but it is unclear whether the LINAC radiosurgery patients were included in the total of 69 radiosurgery patients. They state that the radiosurgery patients were treated with a gamma unit "almost invariably" with a marginal dose of 12 Gy to the 50% isodose volume. Some of the radiosurgery patients received higher prescription doses than 12 Gy, but there are no details provided in the paper. The team found that the rates of facial and trigeminal neuropathy were similar in both the radiosurgery and fractionated radiotherapy groups (see Table 62-1), but the rate of hearing loss was significantly higher in the radiosurgery group. Because there were a limited number of patients with serviceable hearing in each group (12 radiosurgery and 21 radiotherapy patients), and because follow-up was limited, it is by no means clear that long-term hearing preservation will be significantly different between the groups. Hearing loss in the radiosurgery arm was dramatically worse than in other series with similar doses (see Table 62-1).

Meijer and colleagues in Amsterdam recently reported another single-institution comparison of radiosurgery and fractionated SRT for vestibular schwannoma.[14,17] Some 49 edentulous patients (mean age, 63 years), unable to reliably use a bite block in a relocatable/noninvasive stereotactic frame, were selected for linear accelerator radiosurgery to either 10- or 12.5-Gy marginal dose, prescribed to the 80% isodose. Some 80 patients with intact dentition (mean age, 43 years) underwent stereotactic fractionated radiotherapy to 20 Gy in four or five fractions prescribed to the 80% isodose volume. They found a higher 5-year rate of trigeminal neuropathy with radiosurgery versus radiotherapy (8% versus 2%, p = 0.048). Five-year actuarial tumor control was similar (100% radiosurgery versus 94% SRT), as was facial neuropathy (7% radiosurgery versus 3% SRT) and hearing loss (25% radiosurgery versus 39% SRT). The higher-than-expected rates of facial and trigeminal neuropathy for the 13-0 to 12.5 Gy radiosurgery group, compared with published low-dose radiosurgery results with the gamma knife, may reflect less than fully conformal treatment plans.

RARE SEQUELAE AFTER RADIOSURGERY AND RADIOTHERAPY

The most common delayed effects of radiosurgery (i.e., facial weakness, numbness, and hearing loss) develop almost exclusively within 2 to 3 years after radiosurgery. Radiation-induced tumors, on the other hand, can arise 5 to 30 years after radiotherapy. The actuarial incidence of radiation-induced tumors after fractionated conventional radiotherapy for pituitary adenomas is 1% to 2% in series with 20- to 30-year follow-up.[12] Similar doses of 40- to 60-Gy have been used in these series (usually 45- to 50-Gy in 25 to 28 fractions), with treatment volumes averaging 5 cm in diameter, and a target in the skull base not very far from that for vestibular schwannomas. The most common radiation induced tumors in these series are meningiomas and primary gliomas (e.g., glioblastoma and anaplastic astrocytoma). There are case reports of secondary tumors arising after radiosurgery, but the true incidence is not known.[24] There are no good data on the effect of fractionation on second tumor formation. Because tumor induction appears to involve multiple mutations, it is reasonable to guess that it increases the risk of second tumor formation. With the smaller tumor volumes treated in radiosurgery and in the use of single fraction radiation, it is reasonable to estimate the risk of second tumor formation after radiosurgery to be in the range of 1 in 500 (0.2%) with 30-year follow-up. With the effect of fractionation and slightly larger treatment volumes used with fractionated stereotactic radiosurgery (compared with radiosurgery), the authors would estimate the second tumor risk at somewhere between 0.2% to 2.0%.

Primary vestibular schwannoma radiosurgery is performed without first verifying tissue diagnosis. Rarely, a clinically diagnosed "vestibular schwannoma" has progressed after radiosurgery and then was found to be a malignant tumor after salvage surgical resection. The likelihood of this occurring seems to be in the range of 1 in 500 to 1 in 1000. This raises the question of whether the tumor initially was benign and underwent malignant transformation, or whether the tumor was malignant to start with and simply wasn't controlled by radiosurgery.

Routine pregnancy tests should be performed prior to radiosurgery on any female patients capable of childbearing. This is because even a low dose of scatter radiation to the pelvis is capable of increasing the risks of birth defects if the patient is pregnant.

SALVAGE PROCEDURES AFTER FAILED RADIOSURGERY

It appears to be more difficult to preserve facial nerve function in patients who need salvage surgery after failing radiosurgery than with initial surgical resection. This may be mostly because facial nerve preservation is harder for recurrent tumors that have first failed surgery and then fail salvage radiosurgery (because of the combined effects of prior surgery and radiation). Arguing that initial surgical resection is a better strategy than initial radiosurgery because of problems preserving facial nerves with reoperation is misleading, because recurrence rates after radiosurgery are low (compared with surgery) and facial nerve injury rates are much lower (zero) than initial surgery. Even if all salvage resections after radiosurgery resulted in facial paralysis (which they do not), far fewer patients would end up with facial weakness in the long run by starting out with radiosurgery.

Now that radiosurgery is being performed with lower radiation doses, it is reasonable to ask whether repeat radiation treatment with either radiosurgery or stereotactic fractionated treatment should be performed. There is no reported experience with repeat radiosurgery for vestibular schwannomas. Favorable tumor control has been reported with re-treating other benign tumor like meningiomas and pituitary adenomas with repeat radiosurgery, as well as with repeat fractionated radiotherapy.[25,26] The chief drawback with repeating radiation is the lack of tissue confirmation in patients originally managed with radiosurgery. A limited partial resection or biopsy followed by repeat radiation is another management strategy.

CONCLUSIONS

Stereotactic radiosurgery has proven itself to be an alternative to surgical resection of vestibular schwannomas. Because of the low morbidity and high long-term tumor control rates with radiation treatment compared with surgery, radiation is now seen by most patients and radiation oncologists as the preferred initial management for vestibular schwannomas. Early results with stereotactic fractionated radiotherapy indicate outcomes similar to those of radiosurgery using modern techniques and marginal doses of 13 Gy.

REFERENCES

1. Andrews DW, Suarez O, Goldman HW, et al: Stereotactic radiosurgery and fractionated stereotactic radiotherapy for the treatment of acoustic schwannomas: Comparative observations of 125 patients treated at one institution. Int J Radiat Oncol Biol Phys 50(5):1265–1278, 2001.
2. Flickinger JC, Kondziolka D, Niranjan A, Lunsford LD: Results of acoustic neuroma radiosurgery: An analysis of 5 years' experience using current methods: J Neurosurg 94(1):1–6, 2001.
3. Flickinger JC, Kondziolka D, Niranjan A, et al: Acoustic neuroma radiosurgery with marginal tumor doses of 12 to 13 Gy. Int J Radiat Oncol Biol Phys 57(2 Suppl):S325, 2003.
4. Foote KD, Friedman WA, Buatti JM, et al: Analysis of risk factors associated with radiosurgery for vestibular schwannoma. J Neurosurg 95(3):440–449, 2001.
5. Kondziolka D, Lunsford LD, McLaughlin MR, Flickinger JC: Long-term outcomes after radiosurgery for acoustic neuromas. N Engl J Med 339:1426–1433, 1998.
6. Noren G, Greitz D, Hirsch A, Lax I: Gamma knife surgery in acoustic tumors. Acta Neurochirurgica 58(Suppl):104–107, 1993.
7. Pollock BE, Lunsford LD, Kondziolka D, et al: Outcome analysis of acoustic neuroma management: A comparison of microsurgery and stereotactic radiosurgery. Neurosurgery 36(1):215–225, 1995.
8. Foote KD, Friedman WA, Buatti JM, et al: Analysis of risk factors associated with radiosurgery for vestibular schwannoma. J Neurosurg 95(3):440–449, 2001.
9. Regis J, Pellet W, Delsanti C, et al: Functional outcome after gamma knife surgery or microsurgery for vestibular schwannomas. J Neurosurg 97(5):1091–1100, 2002.
10. Iwai Y, Yamanaka K, Shiotani M, Uyama T: Radiosurgery for acoustic neuromas: Results of low-dose treatment. Neurosurgery 53(2):282–287, 2003.
11. Wallner KE, Sheline GE, Pitts LH, et al: Efficacy of irradiation for incompletely excised acoustic neurilemomas. J Neurosurgery 67(6):858–863, 1987.
12. Breen P, Flickinger JC, Kondziolka D, Martinez AJ: Radiotherapy for nonfunctional pituitary adenoma: Analysis of long-term tumor control. J Neurosurg 89(6):933–988, 1998.
13. Andrews DW, Suarez O, Goldman HW, et al: Stereotactic radiosurgery and fractionated stereotactic radiotherapy for the treatment of acoustic schwannomas: Comparative observations of 125 patients treated at one institution. Int J Radiat Oncol Biol Phys 50(5):1265–1278, 2001.
14. Bush DA, McAllister CJ, Loredo LN, et al: Fractionated proton beam radiotherapy for acoustic neuroma. Neurosurgery 50(2):270–273, 2002.
15. Fuss M, Debus J, Lohr F, et al: Conventionally fractionated stereotactic radiotherapy (FSRT) for acoustic neuromas. Int J Radiat Oncol Biol Phys 48(5):1381–1387, 2000.
16. Lederman G, Lowry J, Wertheim S, et al: Acoustic neuroma: Potential benefits of fractionated stereotactic radiosurgery. Stereo Funct Neurosurg 69(1–4 Pt 2):175–182, 1997.
17. Meijer OW, Vandertop WP, Baayen JC, Slotman BJ: Single-fraction vs. fractionated linac-based stereotactic radiosurgery for vestibular schwannoma: A single-institution study. Int J Radiat Oncol Biol Phys 56(5):1390–1396, 2003.
18. Poen JC, Golby AJ, Forster KM, et al: Fractionated stereotactic radiosurgery and preservation of hearing in patients with vestibular schwannoma: A preliminary report. Neurosurgery 45(6):1299–1305, 1999.

19. Rashid H, Lowry J, Wertheim S, et al: Improved results for acoustic neuroma (AN) treated with fractionated stereotactic radiosurgery (FSR). Int J Radiat Oncol Biol Phys 42:211, 1998.

20. Sakamoto T, Shirato H, Takeichi N, et al: Annual rate of hearing loss falls after fractionated stereotactic irradiation for vestibular schwannoma. Radiother Oncol 60(1):45–48, 2001.

21. Shirato H, Sakamoto T, Sawamura Y, et al: Comparison between observation policy and fractionated stereotactic radiotherapy (SRT) as an initial management for vestibular schwannoma. Int J Radiat Oncol Biol Phys 44:545–550, 1999.

22. Varlotto JM, Shrieve DC, Alexander E 3rd, et al: Fractionated stereotactic radiotherapy for the treatment of acoustic neuromas: Preliminary results. Int J Radiat Oncol Biol Phy 36(1):141–145, 1996.

23. Williams JA: Fractionated stereotactic radiotherapy for acoustic neuromas. Int J Radiat Oncol Biol Phys 54(2):500–504, 2002.

24. Hanabusa K, Morikawa A, Murata T, Taki W: Acoustic neuroma with malignant transformation: Case report. J Neurosurg 95(3):518–521, 2001.

25. Flickinger JC, Deutsch M, Lunsford LD: Repeat megavoltage irradiation of pituitary and suprasellar tumors. Int J Radiat Oncol Biol Phys 17:171–175, 1989.

26. Bhatnagar A, Heron DE, Kondziolka D, et al: Analysis of repeat stereotactic radiosurgery for progressive primary and metastatic CNS tumors. Int J Radiation Oncology Biol Phys 53(3):527–532, 2002.

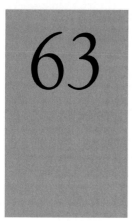

63 Suboccipital Transmeatal Approach to Vestibular Schwannoma

ROBERT G. OJEMANN and ROBERT L. MARTUZA

OVERALL MANAGEMENT PLAN

Three management options are considered when a patient with a vestibular schwannoma is evaluated: (1) surgery, (2) radiosurgery or fractionated radiation therapy, and (3) observation. To decide on the best management plan for each patient, the physician must obtain the patient's history; this is necessary to form a clear idea of the patient's course and of how the symptoms are affecting the patient's life, to make an objective assessment of any neurologic deficit, for careful review of the radiographic studies to ensure they are adequate, and to help determine whether any additional studies are needed. The management options are then evaluated. The physician must have up-to-date knowledge about these alternatives. What will be the impact of the proposed treatment on the patient's daily life? Will the treatment improve or arrest the progression of symptoms? Can further growth or recurrence of the tumor be prevented? What are the risks of the treatment? Do the short-term and long-term benefits justify these risks? The physician and patient should discuss the patient's hopes and expectations about the treatment. The informational brochures from the Acoustic Neuroma Association have been a great help to many patients and their families as they consider these questions.

In some patients, little doubt exists as to the treatment course. In other patients, the decision may be difficult because the symptoms are minimal or nonprogressive, the growth rate is unpredictable, no treatment plan is free of risk, and the long-term results of the radiosurgery and radiation therapy options continue to be evaluated. Vestibular schwannomas usually enlarge slowly. It has been well documented that some tumors stop growing, a few grow rapidly, and spontaneous regression rarely occurs.[1-3]

The indications for considering surgery are as follows:

1. Recent or worsening symptoms, except in some elderly patients with a tumor having 2 cm or less intracranial extension
2. Enlargement of the tumor in a patient who is being observed, except in some elderly patients with a tumor having 2 cm or less intracranial extension
3. Enlargement of a tumor after radiosurgery once the initial swelling reaction has subsided
4. The patient's decision after discussion of the treatment options

The indications for considering stereotactic radiosurgery or fractionated stereotactic radiotherapy are as follows:

1. An elderly patient with an enlarging tumor or recent symptoms and 2 cm or less intracranial extension
2. Hearing loss or enlarging tumor in the only hearing ear
3. Residual tumor or regrowth after subtotal removal
4. Major medical illness that significantly increases the risk of operation
5. The patient's decision after discussion of the treatment options

The indications for considering observation with careful audiologic and radiologic monitoring are as follows:

1. A long history of unilateral auditory symptoms referable to the tumor
2. An elderly patient with mild symptoms
3. An incidental finding of the tumor on a scan performed for some other reason
4. The patient's decision after discussion of the treatment options

SURGICAL MANAGEMENT

Overview

The microsurgical removal of a vestibular schwannoma can be performed by a suboccipital, translabyrinthine, or middle fossa approach. Good results after the removal of vestibular schwannomas have been reported with all three approaches by experienced groups of surgeons.[4] A thorough understanding of the anatomy of the cerebellopontine angle and petrous bone and of the relationship of anatomic structures to the tumor is essential.[4-7] The authors prefer the suboccipital approach for most patients because of the wide visualization it allows, the ability to save hearing, and the good results that we[4,8-19] and others[6,20-31] have reported. The middle fossa approach is used for intracanalicular tumors that extend to the lateral end of the internal auditory canal when an attempt is being made to save hearing. The translabyrinthine approach is used for small tumors when there is no useful hearing. In a few patients, the authors have used a combined suboccipital-translabyrinthine-transtemporal approach for large tumors growing far anteriorly. A similar approach has been described by Haddad and Al-Mefty,[32] in which a petrosal exposure can be combined

920

with a translabyrinthine and transcochlear approach. Gormley and colleagues[26] also use a transpetrosal-retrosigmoid approach in some patients with large tumors. Evaluation of a large number of hospitals and operations showed that the short-term results of surgical excision of vestibular schwannomas were superior with higher-volume hospitals and surgeons.[33]

Other modifications of the suboccipital approach have been described. Shelton and associates[34] combine a suboccipital approach with a mastoidectomy in some patients when they are attempting to save hearing. Poe and co-workers[35] have used a translabyrinthine drill-out from the suboccipital approach to combine the advantages of both exposures. Darrouzet and colleagues[25] describe a widened retrolabyrinthine approach exposing the temporal dura, sigmoid sinus, and retrosigmoid dura with removal of a portion of the mastoid bone. With some large tumors, Comey and associates[36] have suggested that a staged operation may be of benefit.

The authors' operative approach and techniques for the suboccipital transmeatal approach have been described and illustrated in detail in previous publications.[4,16–19,37,38] The operation is performed in collaboration with an otologic surgeon, who exposes the internal auditory canal and dissects the tumor in that area. The suboccipital approach has also been described by several other groups.[5,7,21,22,39–41]

Preoperative Evaluation

In most patients, the diagnosis of vestibular schwannomas is established with magnetic resonance imaging (MRI) after gadolinium enhancement. Usually, MRI is the only imaging study needed. It has been suggested that computed tomography (CT) images with bone windows may be valuable in planning a hearing-saving operation, but this remains to be proven.[42,43] Pure-tone audiometry and speech discrimination testing are usually performed as part of the patient's initial evaluation.[44] The information from these tests is used to help determine the probability of saving useful hearing and to evaluate hearing in the opposite ear.

Management of Preoperative Hydrocephalus

Occasionally, patients with vestibular schwannomas have enlarged ventricles and no symptoms of hydrocephalus. No special treatment is needed for these patients.

High-pressure hydrocephalus is now uncommon in the patient with a vestibular schwannoma, but if it is present, the symptoms usually improve with steroid therapy. A ventricular drain may be needed at operation and for a few days postoperatively. Rarely does a patient need a ventriculoperitoneal shunt. Removal of the tumor often improves cerebrospinal fluid (CSF) flow to adequately treat the hydrocephalus.

Occasionally, an elderly patient is seen with a large tumor and large ventricles and with symptoms suggesting normal-pressure hydrocephalus. If the only other symptom is hearing loss, a ventriculoperitoneal shunt may be the only treatment needed. If symptoms of increasing cranial nerve or brain stem compression are also present, treatment consists of placement of a ventriculoperitoneal shunt and subtotal removal of the tumor, usually in the same operation. These patients generally have a good long-term result.

Monitoring

Continuous electrophysiologic monitoring of facial nerve function during the operation has become an established procedure.[4,17,38,45,46] The benefits of this monitoring have been documented.[47] Several different anesthetic techniques have been used to allow this monitoring. In one, a continuous drip of a muscle relaxant is carefully administered so that facial nerve function can be assessed. The dosage is monitored by following the twitches elicited with ulnar nerve stimulation. Another technique is to use continuous administration of a low dose of propofol. Facial nerve function is monitored by continuous recording of electromyographic activity with two recording electrodes, one in the orbicularis oculi and the other in the orbicularis oris muscles (Fig. 63-1). The muscle contractions, which can occur from stimulation of the facial nerve during coagulation when the electrodes are inactive, are recorded from a motion sensor placed on the cheek. Monopolar stimulation is used to locate the seventh nerve. Fifth nerve function is monitored with an electrode placed in the masseter muscle.

Monitoring of auditory function can be done using electrocochleography, brain stem auditory evoked potential recording, direct cochlear nerve recording, or a combination of these techniques. The authors have used a system developed by Levine.[48–50] A transtympanic electrode is placed for electrocochleography, scalp electrodes are inserted for brain stem auditory evoked potential monitoring, and a microphone system is placed in the external ear canal to provide the sound stimulus (see Fig. 63-1). More recently, we have utilized a wick electrode placed onto the tympanic membrane. In most cases, this obviates the need for a transtympanic electrode.

Perioperative Medical Therapy

Steroids are usually started before the induction of anesthesia. A high steroid dose is continued every 6 hours during the operation, then gradually tapered over 4 to 7 days depending on the size of the tumor and neurologic and facial nerve function. The blood glucose level is monitored. An antibiotic is given intravenously starting just before surgery and is continued for 24 hours after surgery. To prevent deep venous thrombosis, alternating compression thigh-high air boots are placed.

After anesthesia is induced, an indwelling Foley catheter is inserted, and 10 to 20 mg of furosemide is administered intravenously. During preparation and exposure of the dura, a 20% solution of mannitol is given intravenously in a dose of 0.5 to 1.0 g/kg over 20 to 30 minutes.

Patient Position

The semisitting, prone, supine-oblique, lateral or park bench, and lateral-oblique positions have been used for suboccipital removal of vestibular schwannomas.[4] The authors' experience with the semisitting position has been described previously.[11–12] No major permanent morbidity is related to this position, but occasional problems with air embolus and hypotension are encountered. Because of the risk of hypotension in older patients, a supine-oblique position was used. In addition to preventing hypotension and air embolism,

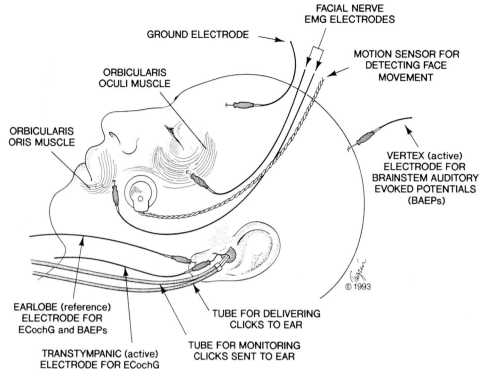

FIGURE 63-1 Monitoring of facial and cochlear nerve function during operation. (Copyright 1993, Edith Tagrin.)

other advantages of this position are excellent visualization of the cerebellopontine angle, ease of tumor removal, and comfort of the surgeon. This position is now used for removal of all but a few cerebellopontine angle tumors. If severe cervical spondylosis or limitation of neck motion exist from a previous injury, a lateral position is used. The intermittent pulsation of CSF into the operative area is not a problem

and, in fact, keeps the neural and vascular structures from drying.

The operating table is reversed so that the surgeon can sit behind the patient's head with his or her feet under the table. The patient lies supine with the shoulder that is ipsilateral to the tumor slightly elevated (Fig. 63-2). The head is turned parallel to the floor, elevated, and held with a

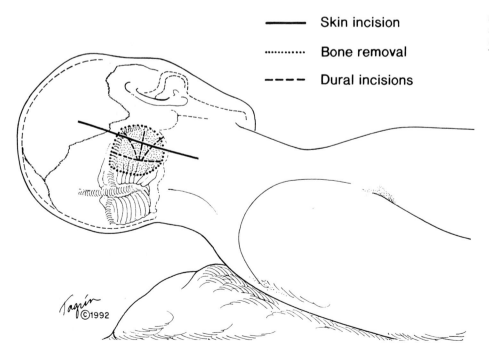

——— Skin incision

·········· Bone removal

- - - - Dural incisions

FIGURE 63-2 Position, skin incision, craniotomy opening, and dural incisions. (Copyright 1992, Edith Tagrin.)

three-point skeletal-fixation headrest. During the operation, the surgeon's line of sight to the brain stem or internal auditory canal may be altered by rotating the table from side to side. It is important that the patient is strapped securely in the bed and that the elbow and knee areas are padded to prevent neural compression from rotation. An armrest is placed for the surgeon's arm nearest the vertex. The other arm rests on the patient.

Incision and Exposure

A vertical linear incision is centered 1 cm medial to the mastoid process (see Fig. 63-2). Other types of incisions that have been reported include an inverted J-shaped or L-shaped incision, an S-shaped incision, and various semi-curved incisions.[4] A graft of pericranial tissue about 4 cm in diameter is taken from the occipital region. This graft is used in closing the cerebellar convexity dura at the end of the operation. The suboccipital muscles and fascia are incised in line with the incision and are carefully separated from their attachments to the bone by use of subperiosteal dissection and electrocautery. Special care is taken to occlude the arterial vessels as they are encountered in the muscle. An emissary vein is usually exposed in the region of the medial mastoid area.

The bone over the lateral two thirds of the cerebellar hemisphere is exposed. Visualizing the midline bone or rim of the foramen magnum is usually not necessary. A burr hole is placed immediately inferomedial to the asterion, the dura is carefully separated from the overlying bone, and a free bone flap is cut (see Fig. 63-2). Care is taken not to take this initial opening too far laterally so as to avoid venous bleeding from the emissary veins or sigmoid sinus. The initial opening often exposes the edge of the transverse sinus. Further bone is removed as needed to expose the edge of the transverse sinus, the proximal sigmoid sinus, and the edge of the petrous bone laterally. This exposure allows the edge of the sinus to be retracted when the sutures are placed to hold the dural flaps, and it gives a direct line of sight down the posterior surface of the petrous bone. The mastoid air cells are usually entered and are occluded with bone wax.

The dura is opened vertically a few millimeters from the medial edge of the craniotomy. Stellate dural incisions provide superior, lateral, and inferior flaps of dura, which are held back with sutures (Fig. 63-3; see also Fig. 63-2).

The cerebellum is gently elevated, the arachnoid opened, and CSF allowed to drain (see Fig. 63-3). This process usually relieves any bulging of the cerebellum and allows exposure of the cerebellopontine angle with minimal retraction. For medium and large tumors, the tip of a small catheter is placed in the cistern and sutured to the inferior medial corner of the dural opening to drain CSF continuously during the operation. The cerebellum is covered with a rubber sheet and Tefla, upon which are placed self-retaining Greenberg retractors. The operating microscope is positioned.

Removal of Small Tumors and Hearing Preservation

Under the microscope, arachnoid over the tumor is opened and, if needed, the petrosal vein is coagulated and divided.

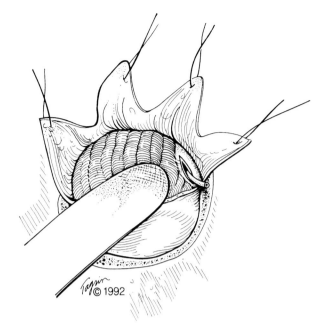

FIGURE 63-3 Retraction of the dural flaps, elevation of the cerebellum, opening of the arachnoid, drainage of cerebrospinal fluid, and insertion of a catheter in the cistern. (Copyright 1992, Edith Tagrin.)

The retractors are repositioned. It is best to leave the protective arachnoid over the lower cranial nerves, but at times it may be necessary to open the arachnoid to facilitate the exposure. With small tumors, the eighth nerve complex is seen coming into the inferomedial side of the tumor. Although the facial nerve is usually on the anterior surface of the tumor, the capsule is stimulated to determine if there is an unusual course for the facial nerve. If there is a significant intracranial extension of the tumor, an internal decompression is done using sharp dissection or an ultrasonic aspirator.

The next step is exposure of the tumor in the internal auditory canal. Gelatin sponge (Gelfoam) is placed in the subarachnoid spaces to prevent dissemination of bone dust. Dura is removed over the region of the internal auditory canal, and bone is carefully removed by use of an air drill with constant suction-irrigation for cooling. The surgeon needs to remember that occasionally a high jugular bulb is exposed during the bone removal. Care is taken not to enter the labyrinth because this usually causes loss of hearing. If a semicircular canal is entered, it should be immediately closed with wax because hearing may still be preserved.[51] Once the internal auditory canal is exposed, the dura is opened over the tumor. An internal decompression of the tumor is done using sharp dissection so that the capsule can be mobilized with minimal pressure.

Dissection depends on an assessment of the relationship of the tumor to the vestibular and cochlear nerves. In most patients, the vestibular nerve fibers entering the medial edge of the tumor are divided, the cochlear and facial nerves are identified, and the dissection proceeds from medial to lateral. In a few patients, defining the cochlear nerve medially may be difficult. The tumor is then carefully rotated near the lateral end of the canal while the surgeon looks for the seventh nerve anteriorly and superiorly and

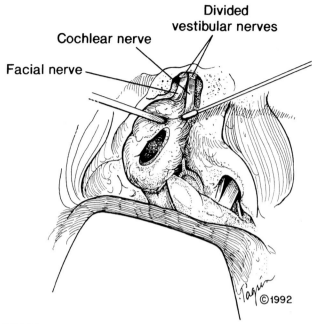

Facial nerve

Cochlear nerve

Divided vestibular nerves

©1992

FIGURE 63-4 Exposure of a tumor and the seventh and eighth cranial nerves in the internal auditory canal. (Copyright 1992, Edith Tagrin.)

the cochlear nerve anteriorly and inferiorly (Fig. 63-4). Stretching or putting tension on the cochlear nerve must be avoided to prevent avulsion of the fibers. The position of the seventh nerve is confirmed with stimulation.

Dissection along the facial and cochlear nerves is performed with fine straight or curved microdissectors or canal knives and sharp dissection with microscissors. The tumor capsule is elevated laterally and superiorly. Dissection is alternated from different directions, depending on what direction provides the best exposure, the easiest plane of dissection, and the least traction on the nerves. When the cochlear and facial nerves have been clearly defined, the vestibular nerves coming into the tumor are divided on the lateral aspect of the tumor. In some patients, the lateral end of the tumor may not be exposed because of the limitation in bone removal. In these patients, the tumor is transected near the end of the canal, and the lateral extent of the tumor is removed with a small ring curet. To overcome the problem of inadequate visualization of the lateral end of the internal auditory canal, endoscopy may be used to ensure that all tumor has been removed and to visualize air cells that need to be occluded.[52-55] The authors have used this procedure and agree that excellent visualization can be achieved.

To maximize the possibility of preserving hearing, the arachnoid over the cochlear nerve should be preserved whenever possible. During the dissection, intermittent bleeding may occur along the nerves. A fine suction and irrigation keeps the field clean and does not damage the nerves. Most of the bleeding stops spontaneously or with temporary placement of Surgicel or Gelfoam. When hearing is to be saved, the surgeon should attempt to preserve any significant arterial vessel entering the internal auditory meatus. If the evoked responses or electrocochleogram diminish, temporary application of a papaverine-soaked

paddy and changing dissection to a different location are warranted.

Removal of Medium-Sized and Large Tumors

Arachnoid between the posterior capsule of the tumor and cerebellum and over the lower cranial nerves is opened. On rare occasion, a separate cystic collection of CSF containing xanthochromic fluid and surrounded by thickened arachnoid may occasionally be loculated in relation to the tumor capsule. The petrosal vein or one of its branches, which usually comes off the cerebellum or middle cerebellar peduncle to the petrosal sinus just above the tumor, is coagulated and divided as needed. To complete the initial exposure of most of the posterior capsule, self-retaining retractors are repositioned. On occasion, an operculum of cerebellum may extend over the tumor, making it necessary to shrink or resect this cerebellar tissue with bipolar coagulation.

The posterior capsule is stimulated to locate the facial nerve. The facial nerve is usually on the anterior surface of the tumor, and no response occurs to this first stimulation. In some patients, the nerve is displaced superiorly, particularly in its lateral course. In this situation, a response may be seen on the initial stimulation over the superior capsule. Anteromedial displacement of the facial nerve along the brain stem and over the anterosuperior aspect of the tumor may also occur, and the facial nerve may be displaced against the fifth nerve. Rarely, the nerve is inferior or across the posterior surface. The facial nerve was displaced posteriorly in only 1 patient in a series of 461 patients.[17]

The ninth, tenth, and eleventh cranial nerves are identified, and arachnoid is carefully dissected to aid exposure of the inferomedial capsule. With larger tumors, the ninth and tenth nerves are carefully reflected off the tumor capsule. A small rubber dam is placed over these nerves for protection during the rest of the operation.

The next step is internal decompression of the tumor, which is performed intermittently as needed. This process allows all the pressure to be placed on the tumor capsule while separating it from the cranial nerves and brain stem. Ultrasonic aspiration, bipolar coagulation, and sharp dissection are used for internal decompression. In some patients, one or more cysts may be encountered within the tumor.

Dissection begins inferiorly and medially. In medium-sized tumors, the eighth nerve complex can usually be defined with moderate dissection (Fig. 63-5). These nerves are rarely seen initially in larger tumors. After carefully reflecting the capsule laterally and superiorly into the area of decompression, the surgeon looks for the eighth nerve complex along the inferomedial capsule. Being a right-handed surgeon, this author uses a fine suction in the left hand to retract the tumor and to keep the area of dissection clean. Care is taken to locate the facial nerve, which can be just under the eighth nerve complex or may be several millimeters away. It can usually be recognized by its white or gray color, which is different from the adjacent brain stem. In many patients, the facial nerve is seen by elevating the eighth nerve complex, but when the seventh nerve is pushed against the brain stem and displaced anteriorly and medially, it is found by looking above the eighth nerve. If the seventh nerve has not been localized, intermittent

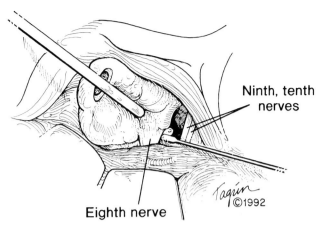

FIGURE 63-5 Visualization of the eighth cranial nerve on the inferior medial capsule after internal decompression of the tumor. (Copyright 1992, Edith Tagrin.)

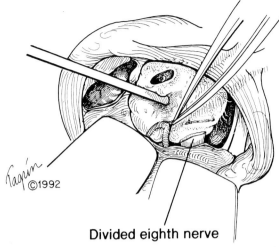

FIGURE 63-7 Division of the eighth cranial nerve and coagulation of a small arterial branch entering the tumor with preservation of the anterior inferior cerebellar artery branch. (Copyright 1992, Edith Tagrin.)

stimulation is used. The vestibular and cochlear nerve fibers entering the tumor are divided using bipolar coagulation and sharp dissection. The surgeon must look carefully for a branch of the anterior-inferior cerebellar artery, which may loop just behind these nerves.

If the facial nerve is not seen anterior to the divided eighth nerve complex, it is usually located by reflecting the inferior and medial tumor capsule further laterally and superiorly (Fig. 63-6). Spontaneous electromyographic activity may indicate when the surgeon is near that nerve. Usually the facial nerve forms a solid band on the tumor capsule, but more laterally it may be spread out over a wide area and, occasionally, it is surrounded by the tumor.

As the dissection of the capsule progresses, not only is further internal decompression performed as indicated, but also sections of the tumor capsule are removed to allow room to reflect the capsule laterally. Arterial vessels adjacent to the tumor are preserved by division of only the branches entering the tumor (Fig. 63-7). Alternating dissection of the

inferomedial capsule, with dissection superiorly and medially to define the fifth nerve and brain stem attachments, may be advantageous (Fig. 63-8). Vascular attachments are often in the region of the fifth nerve root entry zone. Small rubber dams may be placed on the brain stem for protection as the dissection progresses.

Dissection extends along the seventh nerve toward the internal auditory meatus (Fig. 63-9). When the point is reached where the bone over the internal auditory canal is impeding further dissection or the dissection is difficult, attention is directed to the tumor in the internal auditory canal. The exposure is the same as that described for small tumors except that the bone is removed to expose the lateral end of the canal entering the labyrinth, if necessary.

After separation of the tumor from the facial nerve in the internal auditory canal, the attachments along the edge of the internal auditory meatus are divided. The facial nerve

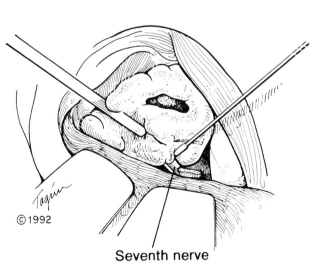

FIGURE 63-6 Identification of the seventh cranial nerve anterior to the divided eighth cranial nerve. (Copyright 1992, Edith Tagrin.)

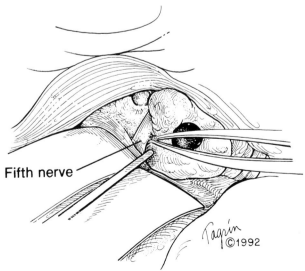

FIGURE 63-8 Exposure of the proximal segment of the fifth nerve. (Copyright 1992, Edith Tagrin.)

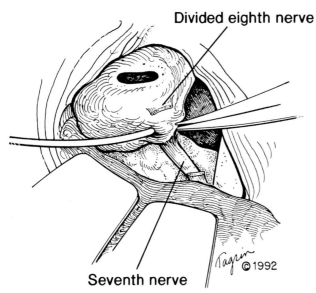

Divided eighth nerve

Seventh nerve

Tagrin © 1992

FIGURE 63-9 Dissection along the seventh cranial nerve. (Copyright 1992, Edith Tagrin.)

starts to turn anteriorly or anterosuperiorly as the posterior fossa is entered. The surgeon can then decide how best to proceed. The dissection may be continued medially along the brain stem and cerebellar peduncle, and the arachnoid and vascular attachments are divided as they are encountered, gradually freeing the facial nerve. Occasionally a large branch of the anterior-inferior cerebellar artery is embedded in the tumor capsule, but it can usually be dissected free by division of the small branches directly supplying the tumor. In large tumors, the trochlear nerve and superior cerebellar artery may be adherent superiorly, the sixth nerve adherent anteriorly, and the ninth and tenth nerves adherent inferiorly. The objective is to reduce the bulk and attachments of the tumor so that the surgeon is dealing only with dissection from the facial nerve and brain stem. The facial nerve is usually most adherent to the tumor capsule in the posterior fossa near the internal auditory meatus, where the nerve may be splayed over the anterior-superior capsule, or it may occasionally be surrounded by tumor. Dissection in this area is often complicated by vascular and fibrous attachments. The surgeon must adapt to the characteristics of the tumor, and working alternately from various angles may be necessary.

If the tumor is large, the capsule may be so intimately adherent to the brain stem and cranial nerves that a plane cannot be developed. In such cases, a thin layer of tumor capsule is left (radical subtotal removal).[17]

Closure

Once the tumor is removed, hemostasis is checked. The area of bone removal over the internal auditory meatus is carefully waxed to occlude air cells. An adipose tissue graft taken via a superficial incision on the lower abdomen is carefully placed in the area where bone has been removed. Surgicel is used to hold this graft in place and may also be used to cover the area of resected or retracted cerebellum.

The dura is closed in a watertight fashion, using the graft of pericranial tissue taken at the beginning of the operation. One or two tenting sutures are placed to tack this up to the bone or cranioplasty. The dura is covered with absorbable gelatin sponge (Gelfoam). The bone flap is replaced and held with titanium miniplates and screws (which do not interfere with future imaging) and a dural tenting suture. A cranioplasty is done to occlude all of the bone defects; this may consist of acrylic or of titanium mesh plus autologous bone (chips and dust from the opening). The wound is thoroughly irrigated with an antibiotic solution before closure. Careful attention should be given to muscle reapproximation.

MANAGEMENT OF POSTOPERATIVE COMPLICATIONS

Hematoma and Cerebellar Infarction

During the initial exposure, particular attention is paid to occlusion of the arterial vessels in the muscles as they are encountered. During closure, the muscles are again carefully checked for bleeding. Postoperatively, blood pressure is controlled, beginning in the operating room with an intravenous antihypertensive medication, and is monitored continuously for as long as necessary.

If the cerebellum is unusually full at the end of the operation, and good CSF drainage has occurred, cerebellar infarction or hematoma should be ruled out. In this situation, the lateral 1 to 2 cm of cerebellum may need to be resected. If there is doubt about the situation, the incision should be closed, and the patient should be kept intubated and taken immediately for a CT scan.

If the patient does not recover promptly from anesthesia, or if an unexpected significant neurologic deficit or a delayed neurologic deterioration occurs, a CT scan is performed immediately to look for cerebellar hematoma or infarction. Prompt removal of a significant hematoma or area of infarction can lead to a dramatic recovery.

Cerebrospinal Fluid Leak

If a CSF leak develops, a lumbar drain is placed for 72 hours, and this often resolves the problem. When the leak persists, a transmastoid repair using an adipose tissue graft is performed.

Hydrocephalus

In the postoperative period, the patient may develop neurologic symptoms that suggest hydrocephalus, or a tense subgaleal fluid collection may be present. Ventricular size is observed by CT scan. Persistent hydrocephalus is a rare complication. Most patients recover spontaneously, a few require a temporary lumbar drain, and only occasionally do patients require a ventriculoperitoneal shunt.

Meningitis

When postoperative fever with headache or stiffness in the neck occurs, the possibility of either bacterial or aseptic meningitis must be considered. CT with contrast enhancement is performed to look for local infection. A lumbar puncture is performed, and broad-spectrum antibiotics are started. Subsequent treatment is guided by the results of the

CSF examination and cultures. If the findings suggest an aseptic meningitis, steroids are administered.

Wound Infection

When the infection is superficial and the organism is sensitive to antibiotics, removing the bone flap may not be necessary. If the infection is extensive, débridement of the wound and removal of the bone flap need to be done.

Neurologic Disability

If any significant postoperative disability occurs, the patient is seen by physical and occupational therapists. Some patients note mild unsteadiness that clears over several days to several weeks. More severe impairment in walking and difficulties with coordination and dysarthria take longer to reverse, and permanent disability may result. If transient difficulty in focusing the eyes or diplopia occurs, it usually clears over days to a few weeks. Dizziness and vertigo are common complaints in the initial postoperative period, but these symptoms usually resolve quite rapidly.

Increased loss of facial sensation is usually not a problem except in the few patients who also have a facial paralysis (see following section on facial nerve function). Recovery from the facial numbness is variable.

Difficulty swallowing because of impaired function in the ninth and tenth nerves should be carefully evaluated with a modified barium swallow and followed by a specialist in swallowing disorders. Often the patient can be given instructions that facilitate his or her swallowing and prevent aspiration. If there is severe impairment in swallowing, a gastrostomy may need to be performed.

Medical Complications

To prevent deep venous thrombosis, the authors use alternating-compression, thigh-high air boots, which are continued until the patient is ambulatory. Electrocardiographic changes and any cardiopulmonary symptoms are immediately evaluated by a cardiologist.

Headache

Persistent headache remains a significant problem in a small percentage of patients. MRI rarely shows a structural abnormality such as hydrocephalus. Harner and co-workers[56] found the incidence of significant headache was 23% at 3 months and 9% at 2 years after operation. Possible causes of headache that have been suggested include aggravation of preexisting vascular headache, degenerative disease in the cervical spine, occipital nerve neuroma, myofascial scar, scar between the neck muscle and dura, and subarachnoid bone dust. A reduced incidence of headache with the use of methyl methacrylate cranioplasty has been reported.[56] Catalano and associates[57] found that preventing the free circulation of bone dust by keeping the arachnoid relatively intact and using pieces of Gelfoam to block off the subarachnoid space during intradural drilling caused the most dramatic reduction in headache. Their patients also had a cranioplasty. Headache usually improves with time and responds to a program of physical therapy and medication.

RESULTS FOR UNILATERAL VESTIBULAR SCHWANNOMA SURGICAL REMOVAL

Overall Function

Good results using the suboccipital (posterior fossa) approach for removal of unilateral vestibular schwannomas have been reported by the authors' group[4,8–19] as well as others.[6,20–31] A series of 461 patients with unilateral vestibular schwannomas, operated by a suboccipital approach in conjunction with an otologist, has been reviewed.[17] The size of the tumor has been recorded as intracanalicular or by size of the extension into the posterior fossa. The functional results of the operation are reported as good, fair, or poor. The term *good* is used for patients who were free of major neurologic deficit and who returned to their preillness level of activity. Seventh and eighth nerve function was not considered. *Fair* described patients who were functionally independent but who were unable to return to their previous full activity because of a neurologic deficit, or who had a significant preoperative neurologic deficit that, although improved, continued to cause disability. Many of these patients returned to work and are leading normal lives. The term *poor* described patients who were dependent because of a major new or preoperative neurologic disability. Overall, 99% were independent in their activities. All patients with intracanalicular tumors or tumors extending 1 cm into the posterior fossa had a good result, as did 96% in the 1- to 1.9-cm group and 93% in the 2- to 2.9-cm group. Even patients with large tumors had an 80% chance of having a good outcome. The most common reasons for the fair results were impaired balance, gait, or coordination. Dysarthria or diplopia occurred in a few patients. In 6 of the 43 fair patients, a significant preoperative deficit improved but still limited the patient's activity. In a small percentage of patients, a significant headache problem lasted longer than expected and prevented full recovery, placing them in the fair result category.

In this series, there were two poor results (0.5%) and two deaths occurred (operative mortality, 0.5%). The operative mortality in most large series is close to 1%, and a high percentage of the patients return to normal activities.

Extent of Tumor Removal and Recurrence

The goal of the operation is total removal of the tumor. This goal must be tempered, however, by surgical judgment, which considers the need to preserve and improve function as well as the long-term results. The authors' experience indicates that a place exists for subtotal and radical subtotal removal of vestibular schwannomas because the recurrence rate has been low, and in larger tumors, the incidence of postoperative neurologic problems has been low, especially in elderly patients.

The term *radical subtotal removal* describes a procedure in which a small fragment of tumor is left, usually because it is densely adherent to the facial nerve or brain stem.[17] The term *subtotal removal* describes extensive removal of tumor in which a portion of the rim of the capsule is left attached to the brain stem and cranial nerves.

The reasons for performing a radical subtotal or subtotal removal include adherence of the tumor to the facial nerve or brain stem, age (70 years or greater), treatment of a tumor affecting an only-hearing ear, and the patient's request. After carefully considering all the treatment options, some patients now request a less-than-total removal to reduce the risk to the facial nerve and the risk of neurologic disability.

The recurrence rates after radical subtotal and subtotal removal have been carefully evaluated. A series of 76 patients who underwent radical subtotal removal of a vestibular schwannoma (average size, 3.1 cm) because of dense adherence to the facial nerve or brain stem had a mean radiologic follow-up of 7.4 years.[58] In 76% (57 of 75) there was no radiographic evidence of growth. The mean time from initial surgery to regrowth was 3.1 years, and delayed radiosurgery was effective in arresting growth of the tumor.

Wazen and co-workers[59] found that in 9 of 13 patients (aged 66 to 81 years) who had subtotal removal, no growth occurred in the residual tumors in follow-up periods ranging from 6 months to 15 years. Klemink and associates[60] reported on 20 patients who had incomplete removal of the tumor to reduce operative risks. Two groups were defined: (1) a subtotal group (resection of less than 95% of the tumor), and (2) a near-total group (resection of 95% or more of the tumor). The subtotal group included mostly elderly patents (mean age, 68.5 years) with large tumors, and the near-total group consisted of young patients (mean age, 45.8 years). The mean length of follow-up was 5 years, and only one patient showed regrowth during this period. Lownie and Drake[61] reported that 9 of 11 patients followed for 10 to 22 years after radical intracapsular removal had no recurrence. The two recurrences were at 2 and 3 years postoperatively. The low incidence of recurrence, and the ability to treat recurrence effectively when it does occur, suggests that a radical subtotal or subtotal removal should be considered in some patients with large tumors, particularly in the elderly.

Recurrence can also occur after apparent total removal of the tumor. The reported recurrence rate is under 1%.[17,28]

Facial Nerve Function

With the development of microsurgical techniques and intraoperative monitoring of facial nerve function, preservation of facial nerve function has been possible in a high percentage of patients. Sampath and associates[46] have summarized the results of several large series. The House-Brackmann facial nerve grading system is used to record facial nerve function (Table 63-1).[62] In one series, evaluation of facial nerve function approximately 1 year after operation or the last time the patient was seen before 1 year postoperatively revealed good function (grade I or II) as follows: intracanalicular, 26 patients (96%); up to 0.9 cm intracranial extension, 37 patients (100%); 1.0 to 1.9 cm intracranial extension, 122 patients (96%); 2 to 2.9 cm intracranial extension, 96 patients (77%); 3 to 3.9 cm intracranial extension, 102 patients (60%); and greater than 4 cm intracranial extension, 71 patients (58%).[17]

The facial nerve is so involved with tumor in some patients that it cannot be saved. A decision has to be made about whether to leave a small piece of tumor capsule with the nerve (radical subtotal removal), to divide the nerve

TABLE 63-1 ▪ House-Brackmann Facial Nerve Grading System*

Grade	Description
I	Normal
II	Mild; slight weakness only on close inspection
III	Moderate; obvious but not disfiguring difference
IV	Moderately severe; obvious weakness
V	Severe; barely perceptible motion
VI	Complete paralysis

*Data from House JW, Brackmann DE: Facial nerve grading system. Otolaryngol Head Neck Surg 93:146–147, 1985.

and approximate the ends, or to perform a nerve graft with the sural nerve. Recovery after graft or anastomosis usually returned the face to at best a grade III, which is defined as a moderate weakness with an obvious but not disfiguring difference in the two sides of the face. Samii and Matthies[38] have reported on a large series of facial nerve reconstructions. The authors have left tumor in patients who, in the preoperative discussion, requested this to reduce the risk of facial paralysis, although they knew that they might need further treatment in the future. The results of long-term follow-up on these patients are encouraging (see previous section and reference 58).

Delayed onset of facial weakness can occur from a few hours to 2 weeks after removal of a vestibular schwannoma.[17,63–65] Most patients make an excellent recovery, often within a few weeks, and usually there is a full recovery by 6 months.

When the patient awakens from anesthesia with a facial paralysis, or develops a delayed complete facial paralysis, the cornea must be protected. Initially the eyelids may almost close, but as muscle tone is lost in the lower eyelid, the opening becomes wider. Beginning immediately after surgery, the eyelids are approximated with tape. Artificial tears are used regularly during the day, and an ophthalmic ointment is used at night. The use of a tarsorrhaphy, a gold weight in the upper eyelid, or both is essential to the maintenance of a healthy cornea and prevention of visual loss and incapacitating pain. Which oculoplastic procedure is best suited for a particular patient depends on the patient's age, skin laxity, and presence or absence of corneal anesthesia. These procedures have the advantage of being reversible. When loss of corneal sensation occurs, the cornea is at great risk, and a medial and lateral tarsorrhaphy may be necessary for protection. When facial paralysis does not recover, improved function may result from use of a modification of the classic hypoglossal-facial anastomosis, with partial division of the hypoglossal nerve and anastomosis of half of the nerve to the lower branch of the facial nerve. This procedure can be combined with one of the eye procedures and a temporalis transposition flap.[66]

Cochlear Nerve Function

Preservation of useful hearing depends on the size of the tumor, the level of preoperative hearing, and the involvement of the internal auditory artery branches with the tumor. The question of what constitutes useful serviceable hearing has been discussed by several authors. The most common criteria are a speech reception threshold of less than 50 dB with a speech discrimination score of 50% or more.[67]

Publications from the authors' group have reported on the preservation of hearing.[4,8,9,14,15,17,68] Several publications from other centers have discussed hearing preservation with the suboccipital transmeatal approach.[22–24,27,29,69–77]

In patients with intracanalicular tumors, the rate of saving useful hearing in a series of reasonable size has ranged from 33% to greater than 90%.[17,27,29,74] As the tumor grows into the posterior fossa and enlarges, this rate drops. Patients with tumors that have an extension into the posterior fossa of 2 cm or more have a low probability of hearing preservation even if preoperative hearing is excellent.

In an attempt to help preserve hearing during removal of a vestibular schwannoma, monitoring of auditory evoked responses has been studied using a system developed by Levine.[14,17,48–50] Electrocochleography monitors the status of the cochlea and the auditory nerve peripheral to the tumor, and brain stem auditory evoked potential recording measures the neural activity central to the tumor. The goal of monitoring is to give an indication of early hearing compromise that is reversible and that allows the surgeon to alter the dissection.[4,15,17,78] This reversible hearing compromise has likely been the case in some patients in whom a change in the evoked response occurred that recovered when the dissection was stopped or altered. In some patients, no change occurs in the evoked responses. Monitoring has not made a difference in the outcome when abrupt loss of function has occurred without warning, presumably as a result of interruption of vascular supply.

Slavit and colleagues[76] compared two matched series of patients with and without auditory monitoring and concluded that there is a benefit from intraoperative monitoring. In an attempt to improve the use of monitoring in preserving cochlear nerve function, several techniques have been tried. Direct recording from the eighth nerve has been used, but this technique can be used only in patients with small tumors, and movement of the electrode remains a problem.[78] Matthies and Samii[79] using auditory brain stem response (ABR) waves I, III, and V, reported that "useful recognition of significant waveform changes is possible and enables changes of microsurgical maneuvers to favor (ABR) recovery." Compton and colleagues,[70] Rowed and Nedzelski,[27] and Koos and associates[29] found monitoring to be of little help, however, and Post and co-workers[80] were not sure if there was help from the monitoring.

The long-term results of hearing preservation have been evaluated.[68,73] McKenna and co-workers,[68] reporting on our series of 18 patients with follow-up periods ranging from 3.4 to 10.4 years (mean, 5.4 years), found 4 patients (22%) with a significant decline in hearing. Changes did not correlate with tumor size, preoperative hearing, intraoperative changes in hearing, interval between initial symptoms and surgery, sex, or age. Chee and colleagues[31] found that over a mean follow-up period of 113 months, 40% (12 of 30 patients) had a significant deterioration in hearing.

Concern about recurrence after removal of an acoustic neuroma with preservation of the cochlear nerve has been discussed in the literature. Thedinger and colleagues[81] emphasize that inadequate exposure of the lateral end of the internal auditory canal may be associated with leaving a remnant of tumor. Samii and Matthies[74] reported a recurrence rate of 1.4% in 260 patients who had removal of vestibular schwannomas with hearing preservation. Post and associates[80] had a 4% recurrence rate in 56 patients. The authors' results show a 2% incidence of recurrence in this group of patients. A few patients have an area of gadolinium enhancement in the internal auditory canal on postoperative MRI. Whether this manifestation represents residual tumor or postoperative scar is unknown, but follow-up scans have usually remained unchanged, and the report of Weisman and colleagues[82] suggests that this finding is usually not caused by tumor.

Tinnitus may persist after removal of an acoustic neuroma. There does not seem to be any difference in the incidence of tinnitus between patients who had the cochlear nerve preserved to save hearing and those in whom the cochlear nerve was divided for tumor removal.[83]

REFERENCES

1. Bederson JB, von Ammon K, Wichmann WW, et al: Conservative treatment of patients with acoustic neuroma. Neurosurgery 28:646–651, 1991.
2. Nedzelski JM, Canter RJ, Kassel EE, et al: Is no treatment good treatment in the management of acoustic neuromas in the elderly? Laryngoscope 96:825–829, 1986.
3. Valvassori GE, Shannon M: Natural history of acoustic neuroma. Skull Base Surg 1:165–167, 1991.
4. Ojemann RG, Martuza RL: Acoustic neuroma. In Youmans JR (ed): Neurological Surgery, 3rd ed. Philadelphia: WB Saunders, 1990, pp 3316–3350.
5. Camins MB, Oppenhiem JS: Anatomy and surgical techniques in the suboccipital transmeatal approach to acoustic neuromas. Clin Neurosurg 38:567–588, 1992.
6. Rhoton AL Jr: Microsurgical anatomy of the brain stem surface facing an acoustic neuroma. Surg Neurol 25:326–339, 1986.
7. Rhoton AL Jr: Microsurgical anatomy of the cerebellopontine angle. In Wilkins RH, Rengachary SS (eds): Neurosurgery. New York: McGraw-Hill, 1996, pp 1063–1084.
8. Nadol JB Jr, Levine RA, Ojemann RG, et al: Preservation of hearing in surgical removal of acoustic neuromas of the internal auditory canal and cerebellar pontine angle. Laryngoscope 97:1287–1294, 1987.
9. Nadol JB Jr, Chiong CM, Ojemann RG, et al: Preservation of hearing and facial nerve function in resection of acoustic neuroma. Laryngoscope 102:1153–1158, 1992.
10. Ojemann RG, Montgomery WW, Weiss AD: Evaluation and surgical treatment of acoustic neuroma. N Engl J Med 287:895–899, 1972.
11. Ojemann RG: Microsurgical suboccipital approach to cerebellopontine angle tumors. Clin Neurosurg 25:461–479, 1978.
12. Ojemann RG, Crowell RM: Acoustic neuromas treated by microsurgical suboccipital operations. Prog Neurol Surg 9:334–373, 1978.
13. Ojemann RG: Comments on Fischer G, Costantini JL, Mercier P: Improvement of hearing after microsurgical removal of acoustic neuroma. Neurosurgery 7:158–159, 1980.
14. Ojemann RG, Levine RA, Montgomery WM: Use of intraoperative auditory evoked potentials to preserve hearing in unilateral acoustic neuroma removal. J Neurosurg 61:938–948, 1984.
15. Ojemann RG: Strategies to preserve hearing during resection of acoustic neuroma. In Wilkins RH, Rengachary SS (eds): Neurosurgery Update I. New York: McGraw-Hill, 1990, pp 424–427.
16. Ojemann RG: Suboccipital approach to acoustic neuromas. In Wilson CB (ed): Neurosurgical Procedures: Personal Approaches to Classic Techniques. Baltimore: Williams & Wilkins, 1992, pp 78–87.
17. Ojemann RG: Management of acoustic neuroma (vestibular schwannoma). Clin Neurosurg 40:498–535, 1993.
18. Ojemann RG: Acoustic neurinoma (vestibular schwannoma)-the suboccipital approach. In Kaye AH, Laws ER Jr (eds): Brain Tumors. Edinburgh: Churchill Livingstone, 1995, pp 623–641.
19. Ojemann RG: Acoustic neuroma (vestibular schwannomas). In Youmans JR (ed): Neurological Surgery, 4th ed. Philadelphia: WB Saunders, 1996, pp 2841–2867.

20. Symon L, Bordi LT, Comptor JJ, et al: Acoustic neurinoma: A review of 392 cases. Br J Neurosurg 3:343–347, 1989.

21. Baldwin DL, King TT, Morrison AW: Hearing conservation in acoustic neuroma surgery via the posterior fossa. Laryngol Otol 104:463–467, 1990.

22. Ebersold MJ, Harner SG, Beatty CW, et al: Current results of retrosigmoid approach to acoustic neurinoma. J Neurosurg 76:901–909, 1992.

23. Klemink JL, LaRouare MJ, Kileny PR, et al: Hearing preservation following suboccipital removal of acoustic neuromas. Laryngoscope 100:597–601, 1990.

24. Fisher G, Fisher C, Remond J: Hearing preservation in acoustic neuroma surgery. J Neurosurg 76:910–917, 1992.

25. Darrouzet V, Guerin J, Aouad N, et al: The widened retrolabyrinthine approach: A new concept in acoustic neuroma surgery. J Neurosurg 86:812–821, 1997.

26. Gormley WB, Sekkhar LN, Wright DC, et al: Acoustic neuromas: Results of current surgical management. Neurosurgery 41:50–60, 1997.

27. Rowed DW, Nedzelski JM: Hearing preservation in removal of intracanicular acoustic neuroma via the retrosigmoid approach. J Neurosurg 86:456–461, 1997.

28. Samii M, Matthies C: Management of 1000 vestibular schwannomas (acoustic neuromas): Surgical management and results with an emphasis on complications and how to avoid them. Neurosurgery 40:11–23, 1997.

29. Koos WT, Day JD, Matula C, et al: Neurotopographic considerations in microsurgical treatment of small acoustic neuromas. J Neurosurg 88:506–512, 1998.

30. Tonn JC, Schlake HP, Goldbrunner R, et al. Acoustic neuroma surgery as an interdisciplinary approach: A neurosurgical series of 508 patients. J Neurol Neurosurg Psychiatry 69:147–148, 2000.

31. Chee GH, Nedzelski JM, Rowed D: Acoustic neuroma surgery: the results of long-term hearing preservation. Oto Neuratol 24:672–676, 2003.

32. Haddad GF, Al-Mefty O: The road less traveled: Transtemporal access to the CPA. Clin Neurosur 41:150–167, 1994.

33. Barker FG II, Carter BS, Ojemann RG, et al: Surgical excision of acoustic neuroma: Patient outcome and provider caseload. Laryngoscope 43:1332–1343, 2003.

34. Shelton C, Alavi S, Li JC, et al: Modified retrosigmoid approach: Use for selected acoustic tumor removal. Am J Otol 16:672–678, 1994.

35. Poe DS, Tarlov EC, Gadre AK: Translabyrinthine drillout from suboccipital approach to acoustic neuroma. Am J Otol 14:215–219, 1993.

36. Comey CH, Janetta PJ, Sheptak PE, et al: Staged removal of acoustic tumors: Technique and lessons learned from a series of 83 patients. Neurosurgery 37:915–921, 1995.

37. Ojemann RG: Retrosigmoid approach to acoustic neuroma (vestibular schwannoma) Neurosurg 48:553–558, 2001.

38. Samii M, Matthies C: Management of 1000 vestibular schwannomas (acoustic neuromas): The facial nerve-preservation and restitution of function. Neurosurgery 40:684–695, 1997.

39. Eisenberg MB, Catalano PJ, Post KD: Management of acoustic schwannomas. In Tindall GT, Cooper PR, Barrow DL (eds): The Practice of Neurosurgery. Baltimore: Williams & Wilkins, 1996, pp 995–1004.

40. Buchheit WA, Getch CC: Tumors of the cerebellopontine angle: Clinical features and surgical management via retrosigmoid approach. In Wilkins RH, Rengachary SS (eds): Neurosurgery. New York: McGraw-Hill, 1996, pp 1085–1094.

41. Malis LI: Nuances in acoustic neuroma surgery. Neurosurg 49:337–341, 2001.

42. Matthies C, Samii M, Krebs S: Management of vestibular schwannomas (acoustic neuromas): Radiological features in 202 cases—their value for diagnosis and their predictive importance. Neurosurgery 40:469–482, 1997.

43. Yokoyama T, Venura K, Ryu H, et al: Surgical approach to the internal auditory meatus in acoustic neuroma surgery: Significance of preoperative high resolution computed tomography. Neurosurgery 39:965–970, 1996.

44. Martuza RL, Parker SW, Nadol JB Jr, et al: Diagnosis of cerebellopontine angle tumors. Clin Neurosurg 32:177–213, 1985.

45. Eldridge R, Parry D: Summary: Vestibular Schwannoma (Acoustic Neuroma) Consensus Development Conference. Neurosurgery 30:962–964, 1992.

46. Sampath P, Holliday MJ, Brem H, et al: Facial nerve injury in acoustic neuroma (vestibular schwannoma) surgery: Etiology and prevention. J Neurosurg 87:60–66, 1997.

47. Jellinek DA, Tan LC, Symon L: The import of continuous electrophysiological monitoring on preservation of the facial nerve during acoustic neuroma surgery. Br J Neurosurg 5:19–24, 1991.

48. Levine RA, Ojemann RG, Montgomery WM: Monitoring auditory evoked potentials during acoustic neuroma surgery: Insights into the mechanism of the hearing loss. Ann Otol Rhinol Laryngol 93:116–123, 1984.

49. Levine RA: Surgical monitoring applications of the brainstem auditory evoked response and electrocochleography. In Owen J, Donohoe C (eds): Clinical Atlas of Auditory Evoked Potentials. New York: Grune & Stratton, 1988, pp 103–106.

50. Levine RA: Monitoring auditory evoked potentials during cerebellopontine angle tumor surgery: Relative value of electrocochleography, brain-stem auditory evoked potentials, and cerebellopontine angle recordings. In Schramm J, Moelle AN (eds): Intraoperative Neurophysiologic Monitoring. Berlin: Springer-Verlag, 1991, pp 193–204.

51. Tatagiba M, Samii M, Matthies C, et al: The significance for postoperative hearing of preserving the labyrinth in acoustic neurinoma surgery. J Neurosurg 77:677–684, 1992.

52. McKennan KX: Endoscopy of the internal auditory canal during hearing conservation in acoustic neuroma surgery. Am J Otol 14:259, 1993.

53. Tatagita M, Matthies C, Samii M: Microendoscopy of the internal auditory canal in vestibular schwannoma surgery. Neurosurgery 38:737–740, 1996.

54. Valtonen JH, Poe DS, Heilman CD, et al: Endoscopically assisted prevention of cerebrospinal fluid leak in suboccipital acoustic neuroma surgery. Am J Otol 18:381–383, 1997.

55. Goksu N, Bayazit Y, Kemaloglu Y: Endoscopy of the posterior fossa and dissection of acoustic neuroma. J Neurosurg 91:776–780, 1999.

56. Harner SG, Beatty CW, Ebersold MJ: Impact of cranioplasty on headache after acoustic neuroma removal. Neurosurgery 36:1097–1100, 1995.

57. Catalano PJ, Jacobowitz O, Post KD: Prevention of headache after retrosigmoid removal of acoustic tumors. Am J Otol 17:904–908, 1996.

58. Kalkanis SN, Ojemann RG, McKenna MJ, et al: Subtotal resection for acoustic neuromas: Long-term results. Neurosurgery 51:552, 2002.

59. Wazen J, Silverstein H, Norroll H, et al: Preoperative and postoperative growth rate in acoustic neuromas documented with CT scanning. Otolaryngol Head Neck Surg 93:151–155, 1985.

60. Klemink JL, Langman AW, Niparko JK, et al: Operative management of acoustic neuromas: The priority of neurologic function over complete resection. Otolaryngol Head Neck Surg 104:96–99, 1991.

61. Lownie SP, Drake CG: Radical intracapsular removal of acoustic neuroma: Long-term follow-up review of 11 patients. J Neurosurg 74:422–425, 1991.

62. House JW, Brackmann DE: Facial nerve grading system. Otolaryngol Head Neck Surg 93:184–193, 1985.

63. Lalwani AK, Butt FY, Jackler RK, et al: Delayed onset of facial nerve dysfunction following acoustic neuroma surgery. Am J Otol 16:758–764, 1995.

64. Megerian CA, McKenna MJ, Ojemann RG: Delayed facial paralysis after acoustic neuroma surgery: Factors influencing recovery. Am J Otol 17:630–633, 1996.

65. Grant GA, Rostomily RR, Kim DK, et al: Delayed facial palsy after resection of vestibular schwannoma. J Neurosurg 97:93–96, 2002.

66. Cheney ML, McKenna MJ, Megerian CA: Early temporalis muscle transposition for the management of facial paralysis. Laryngoscope 105:993–1000, 1995.

67. Silverstein H, McDaniel A, Norrell H, Haber Kamp T: Hearing preservation after acoustic neuroma surgery with intraoperative direct eighth cranial nerve monitoring: A classification of results. Otolaryngol Head Neck Surg 95:285–291, 1986.

68. McKenna MJ, Halpin C, Ojemann RG, et al: Long-term hearing results in patients after surgical removal of acoustic tumors with hearing preservation. Am J Otol 13:134–136, 1992.

69. Cohen NL: Retrosigmoid approach for acoustic tumor removal. Otolaryngol Clin North Am 25:295–310, 1992.

70. Compton JS, Bordi LT, Chesseman AD, et al: The small acoustic neuroma: A chance to preserve hearing. Acta Neurochir (Wien) 98:115–117, 1989.

71. Glasscock ME III, Hays JW, Monor LB, et al: Preservation of hearing in surgery for acoustic neuromas. J Neurosurg 78:872–870, 1993.

72. Pensak ML, Tew JM Jr, Keith RW, et al: Management of the acoustic neuroma in an only hearing ear. Skull Base Surg 1:93–96, 1991.

73. Rosenberg RA, Cohen NL, Ransohoff J: Long term hearing preservation after acoustic neuroma surgery. Otolaryngol Head Neck Surg 97:270–274, 1987.

74. Samii M, Matthies C: Management of 1000 vestibular schwannomas (acoustic neuromas): Hearing function in 1000 tumor resections. Neurosurgery 40:248–262, 1997.

75. Shelton C, Hitselberger WE, House WF, et al: Hearing preservation after acoustic tumor removal: Long term results. Laryngoscope 100:115–119, 1990.

76. Slavit DH, Hamer SC, Harper CM Jr, et al: Auditory monitoring during acoustic neuroma removal. Arch Otolaryngol Head Neck Surg 117:1153–1157, 1991.

77. Umezu H, Aiba T, Tsuchida S, et al: Early and late postoperative hearing preservation in patients with acoustic neuromas. Neurosurgery 39:267–272, 1996.

78. Matthies C, Samii M: Direct brainstem recording of auditory evoked potentials during vestibular schwannomas resection: Nuclear BAEO recording. J Neurosurg 86:1057–1062, 1997.

79. Matthies C, Samii M: Management of vestibular schwannomas (acoustic neuromas): The value of neurophysiology for intraoperative monitoring of auditory function in 200 cases. Neurosurgery 40:459–468, 1997.

80. Post KD, Eisenberg MB, Catalano PS: Hearing preservation in vestibular schwannoma surgery: What factors influence outcome? J Neurosurg 83:191–196, 1994.

81. Thedinger BS, Whittaker CK, Luetje CM: Recurrent acoustic tumor after a suboccipital removal. Neurosurgery 29:681–687, 1991.

82. Weisman JL, Hirsch BE, Fukai MB, et al: The evolving MR appearance of structure in the internal auditory canal after removal of acoustic neuroma. AJNR Am J Neuroradiol 18:313–323, 1997.

83. Goel A, Sekhar LN, Langheinrich W, et al: Late course of preserved hearing and tinnitus after acoustic neurilemoma surgery. J Neurosurg 77:685–689, 1992.

64 Translabyrinthine Approach to Vestibular Schwannomas

LARS POULSGAARD

Vestibular schwannomas can be surgically accessed via a subtemporal, a translabyrinthine, or a suboccipital and retrosigmoid approach.[1,2] The number of centers that has mastered all approaches has increased. The translabyrinthine approach was reintroduced approximately 35 years ago[3] and is successfully used by several otologic specialist centers.[4–6] After developments in skull base surgery, neurosurgeons have become aware of the advantages of the translabyrinthine approach for vestibular schwannomas and for other skull base lesions.

ADVANTAGES OF THE TRANSLABYRINTHINE APPROACH

The most obvious advantages of the translabyrinthine route are the direct approach that it offers to the cerebellopontine angle and the fact that the cerebellum requires a minimum of retraction. The tumor is lifted away from the brain stem, avoiding pressure on the brain stem and cerebellum.

It has been stated that the usefulness of the translabyrinthine approach is limited to small tumors. In fact, no tumor is too large to be approached by the translabyrinthine route.[7–9] In large and giant tumors, it is a significant advantage to be able to go directly to the center of the tumor; after debulking the center of the tumor, the neoplasm collapses and is displaced toward the opening by the surrounding brain structure.

The procedure offers excellent exposure of the lateral end of the internal auditory meatus and allows identification of the facial nerve as it enters the fallopian canal. This identification ensures complete tumor removal from that area and the best chance to preserve the facial nerve.

We find it convenient that two surgeons may help each other in the removal of the tumor. As pointed out later, this approach offers two surgeons comfortable placement during a lengthy procedure.

DISADVANTAGES OF THE TRANSLABYRINTHINE APPROACH

The procedure destroys the labyrinth and, as a consequence, hearing. This approach is not used if preservation of hearing is attempted. Only a limited number of patients with vestibular schwannomas have hearing worth preserving, however. If the tumor exceeds 2 cm in size, the chances of preserving hearing are known to be poor.[10]

If the patient has had active otitis media in the past, the approach involves crossing a potentially infected field, and alternative exposure should be considered. In the case of a mastoid cavity, a total obliteration with blind sac closure of the external auditory canal should be performed and healed before the translabyrinthine approach can be done. Finally, the procedure is generally more time consuming than the suboccipital or middle fossa approach, a fact that must be considered if a limited duration of the operation is desirable.

SURGICAL ANATOMY

The bone opening for the translabyrinthine approach is done in the mastoid part of the temporal bone (Fig. 64-1). The mastoid is filled with air cells, and the air cells are connected to the middle ear through the tympanic antrum. In the translabyrinthine approach, the bone is removed between the sigmoid sinus and the external ear canal. The sigmoid sinus is located in the sigmoid sulcus in the temporal bone. From the posterior aspect of the sigmoid sinus, emissary veins run through the mastoid foramen to subgaleal veins.[11–13]

Removing the air cells creates a space that is bounded posteriorly by the wall of the sigmoid sulcus, superiorly by the tegmen tympani, and anteriorly by the prominence of the lateral semicircular canal. Above the prominence of the lateral semicircular canal, the antrum communicates with the tympanic cavity. The facial canal runs close to the mastoid

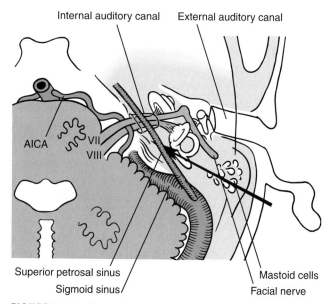

FIGURE 64-1 Illustration of the approach to the cerebellopontine angle through the mastoid and labyrinth. The *arrow* indicates the surgical view after an extended mastoidectomy.

wall of the tympanic cavity. The genu of the facial canal is just inferior to the lateral semicircular canal, and it continues inferiorly to emerge below the skull base at the stylomastoid foramen (Fig. 64-2). The sigmoid sulcus meets the roof of the cavity at a sharp sinodural angle from which the superior petrosal sulcus runs anteriorly. When removing the bone in the sinodural angle, the superior petrosal sinus is exposed in a dural duplex.

The lateral semicircular canal is an important landmark for the location of the entire labyrinth. After removing all three semicircular canals, the vestibule is open. The vestibule is the bone cavity that harbors the soft-tissue part of the labyrinth utricle and saccule. Through the aperture of the vestibular aqueduct runs the endolymphatic duct that connects the utricle to the endolymphatic sac. The internal auditory canal contains four separate nerves: two vestibular nerves, the facial nerve, and the cochlear nerve. Located laterally are the superior and inferior vestibular nerves separated at the fundus by a bony crest, the transverse crest. Anterior to the superior vestibular nerve, the facial nerve enters the fallopian canal. Laterally, the facial nerve is separated from the superior vestibular nerve by a small vertical bony septum, the vertical crest, or Bill's bar (Fig. 64-3).

Most vestibular schwannomas arise from one of the vestibular nerves in the internal auditory canal. The facial nerve is often displaced in the internal auditory canal, and its location may vary. The nerve can always be identified laterally in the internal auditory canal.

After maximal translabyrinthine bone removal and opening of the dura, the cerebellopontine angle with its nerves and vessels is seen. Superiorly, the exit of the fifth cranial

nerve is seen on the pontine surface near the cerebellum. The exits of cranial nerves VI, VII, and VIII are located on a vertical line on the medulla oblongata near the crossing to the pons. The exit of the eighth nerve is just anterior and superior to the flocculus. The entry zone for the abducens nerve is anteriorly on the medulla oblongata. It runs in a superior direction anteriorly on the pons to enter the Dorello canal.

The blood vessels in the cerebellopontine angle display greater variability than do the nerves. The posterior-inferior cerebellar artery emerges from the vertebral artery. Loop formations of this artery are often seen to extend cranially to the level of the ninth and eighth nerves, and in these cases, it may be seen using the translabyrinthine approach. The anterior-inferior cerebellar artery extends from the basilar artery, and in most cases, it forms a loop that protrudes against or into the internal auditory canal. From the loop of the anterior-inferior cerebellar artery, the labyrinthine and the subarcuate arteries extend.

PREPARATION FOR SURGERY

A cephalosporin is given intravenously just before surgery and repeated every 3 hours. The patient is placed in a supine position on the operating table. The patient's head is turned toward the opposite side and maintained in position with a Sugita head frame. Excessive rotation of the head should be avoided because it may cause venous obstruction in the neck. Decreased mobility of the neck in elderly patients may make sufficient rotation of the head difficult to achieve. This problem may be solved by lifting the ipsilateral shoulder with a pillow and by rotating the whole table.

Continuous electrophysiologic monitoring of facial nerve function is performed during the operation.[14–16] This monitoring has become an established procedure and is mandatory in our operations. To accomplish this, electrodes are placed in the frontal and oral orbicular muscles.

We use a floor-standing operating microscope with the two surgeons sitting opposite each other on each side of the patient's head. This setup enables both surgeons to be in a comfortable sitting position with a direct view in the microscope. The lead surgeon sits on the same side as the tumor. In left-sided tumors, the drill is placed between the two surgeons, and in right-sided tumors, the drill is placed between the

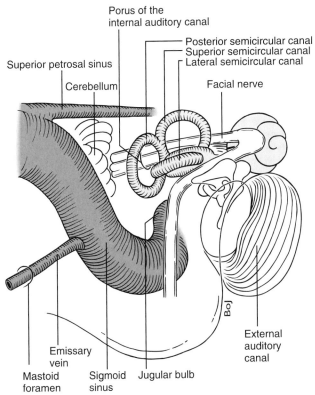

FIGURE 64-2 The relationship between the labyrinth, the internal acoustic canal, the facial nerve, and the sigmoid sinus.

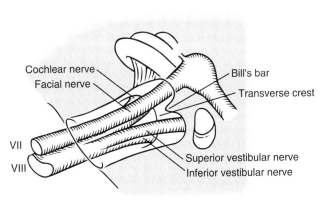

FIGURE 64-3 The contents of the internal acoustic canal, which shows the relation of the facial nerve to Bill's bar.

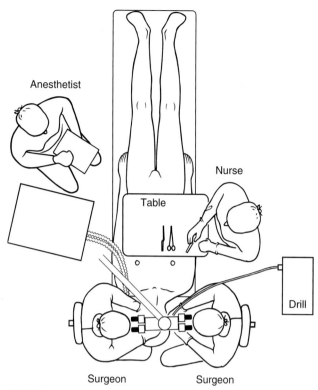

FIGURE 64-4 Room arrangement for the translabyrinthine approach. Note the position of the two surgeons. Both have comfortable access to the microscope.

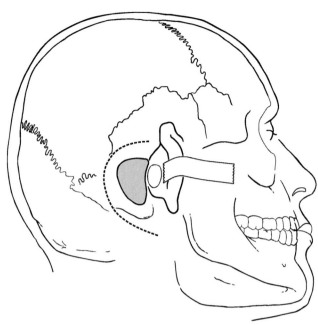

FIGURE 64-5 Skin incision behind the right ear. The area planned for a mastoidectomy is indicated.

scrub nurse and the surgeon on the right side (Fig. 64-4). The anesthesiologist is placed at the lower left side of the table at the level of the hip of the patient.

The surgical view of the cerebellopontine angle occurs along the posterior fossa dura. Posteriorly, it is limited by the sigmoid sinus and anteriorly by the horizontal part of the facial nerve. The operating microscope can be moved in all directions, and the table can be tilted in all directions, which ensures visualization of all surgical planes.

SURGICAL PROCEDURE

Although some surgeons advocate routine cannulation of the lateral ventricle to relieve hydrocephalus or prevent surgically induced hydrocephalus, we do not find this necessary because even in large tumors, it is easy to access the cistern magna beneath the tumor, open the arachnoid, and allow cerebrospinal fluid (CSF) to drain. The incision is made using the cutting cautery to decrease the amount of bleeding from the skin. The incision starts at the upper edge of the helix, superior to the linea temporalis; it continues 4 to 5 cm posteriorly and turns inferiorly and ends near the tip of the mastoid process (Fig. 64-5).

The incision is made first only through the skin. Second, a curved incision is made in the muscle fascia and pericranium. This incision is made similar to the skin incision, but with a smaller radius than the skin incision. This procedure enables a watertight closure of the muscle fascia and pericranium layer. The skin and muscle/pericranium layer are elevated and turned anteriorly over the auricle, where it is covered with a piece of moist gauze and fixed with hooks attached to the

Sugita head frame. Because of the size of the skin incision, it is not necessary to retract the skin at the superior, posterior, or inferior margin.

Mastoidectomy

An extended mastoidectomy is performed with removal of bone over the sigmoid sinus and the middle cranial fossa (see Fig. 64-5). In cases with an anteriorly placed sigmoid sinus or in cases with large tumors, we also remove bone over the posterior cranial fossa behind the sigmoid sinus.[17,18] The extended bone removal ensures good visualization of the entire surgical field. The power drill, driven by either an electric motor or an air turbine, is an essential tool in the translabyrinthine procedure. The cortical bone covering the mastoid region is removed by a large cutting drill. In cases with pronounced pneumatization, a large hole can be made quickly and safely. The anterior margin for cortical bone removal is just behind the external ear canal. The opening is gradually widened backward to the sigmoid sinus and upward to the dura in the middle cranial fossa. Removal of bone over the sigmoid sinus must be done carefully. If the cutting drill tears the sigmoid sinus, profuse bleeding ensues, requiring packing with Surgicel. Large emissary veins often drain into the posterior aspect of the sigmoid sinus. They can be identified through the bone as it is removed. The emissary veins must be controlled with bipolar coagulation and are filled with bone wax. With a drill, the sigmoid sinus is skeletonized.

There are several methods to skeletonize the sigmoid sinus, including the eggshell method, creation of Bill's island of bone, and total bone removal. The aim of the eggshell method is to make the sigmoid sinus wall compressible without removing all bone. By continuous drilling with a large diamond drill and successive pressing of the bone with a dissector, the bony sinus wall becomes compressible because of the many microfractures in the eggshell bone. The preserved periosteum covering the sinus helps to avoid lesions in the sinus.

The method recommended by House and Hitselberger[19] is to leave a small island of bone (Bill's island) over the sigmoid sinus to protect the surface from the trauma of retraction. With a diamond drill, the bone around the outlined island is removed, leaving a part of the sinus wall with an oval piece of bone. The sinus wall and the bony island can then be depressed, and the sinus wall that corresponds to the bony island is protected. We find this method less appropriate because of the risk of lesions in the sinus wall that may be produced by the sharp edge of the bony island.

We prefer total bone removal. This method is initiated by carefully drilling away all the bone covering a small part of the sinus. Through this hole, the adjacent sinus wall can be depressed with a Freer raspatory, and the edge of the bone can safely be removed with Kerrison bone punches without damage of the sinus wall. This method ensures an easily compressible sinus wall.

With blunt dissection, the adjacent dura in the middle and posterior cranial fossa is loosened, and the remaining bone may be removed by either bone punches or a drill.

Labyrinthectomy

As soon as the mastoid cortical bone has been removed and the sigmoid sinus and the middle fossa dura have been outlined, the operating microscope is used. The facial nerve is an important landmark, and its position must be established early in the surgical dissection. After skeletonizing the middle fossa dura, the antrum is opened, and the compact bone of the labyrinth is visualized. We do not routinely remove the incus.

It is essential to open the antrum and to identify the lateral semicircular canal (Fig. 64-6). This canal is a main landmark, and once the position of this canal and antrum is known, the 3-dimensional anatomy of the facial nerve is known. After identification of the facial nerve, the labyrinthectomy is performed. The bone in the sinodural angle is removed followed by opening along the superior petrosal sinus until the labyrinthine bone is encountered. The lateral semicircular canal is drilled away until the ampulla is reached anteriorly. Then the posterior and superior canals are identified and removed to their entrance in the vestibule. After opening of the vestibule, the facial nerve is skeletonized from the genu inferiorly to near the stylomastoid foramen. It is not necessary to remove all the bone around the nerve. We always make a small window in the fallopian canal near the second genu to ensure the position of the nerve and to ensure correct function of the facial nerve monitoring device. To avoid injury to the facial nerve, a thin, eggshell bone is left on the nerve. Only posteriorly, where access is needed to approach the cerebellopontine angle, is the nerve exposed.

After removal of all semicircular canals, the labyrinthectomy is completed, and the vestibule is opened. The endolymphatic duct must be excised from the endolymphatic sac on the posterior fossa dura. The vestibule is removed, and the cribriform area in the saccule marks the most lateral extent of the internal auditory meatus. In the center of the labyrinth, the subarcuate artery is located, and it is usually bleeding when it is opened by the drill.

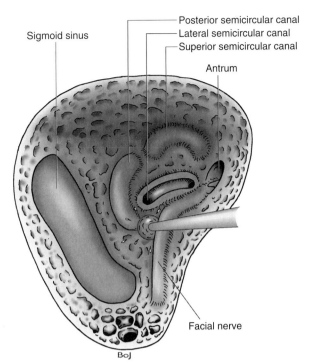

FIGURE 64-6 The facial nerve and the sigmoid sinus have been skeletonized. The lateral semicircular canal is opened.

Internal Auditory Canal Dissection

The dura of the internal auditory canal is identified posteriorly, where it continues as dura of the posterior cranial fossa. The dura at the opening of the canal can be loosened from the bone with slightly bent sharp dissectors. The bone around the canal is gently removed with a diamond drill. A more than 180-degree arc of bone around the canal is removed. At this point, it is important to remove as much bone as possible on both sides below and above the meatus because this helps in accessing the superior and inferior borders of the tumor. Care is taken not to open the dura covering the nerves and tumor in the canal. If the dura is accidentally damaged, the facial nerve should be identified by stimulation.

All bone between the internal meatus and the jugular bulb is removed. The location of the jugular bulb is extremely variable. When it is positioned low, all bone removal necessary for tumor removal can be performed without seeing the jugular bulb. In other cases, it is positioned high and occurs as a bluish spot in the bone after removing the ampulla of the posterior semicircular canal. The surgeon should always be aware of the blue color of the jugular bulb when drilling medial to the facial nerve and inferior to the posterior semicircular canal. All bone covering the jugular bulb must be removed in cases with a high-positioned jugular bulb, in which the bulb is an obstacle to proper bone removal from the inferior aspect of the internal acoustic meatus.

The technique of bone removal from the jugular bulb is the same as described for the sigmoid sinus. With the eggshell method, the bone can be thinned so much that the jugular bulb can be compressed and allow further removal of bone from the inferior part of the porus. Bone is removed until the cochlear aqueduct is identified. The cochlear aqueduct enters the posterior fossa directly inferior to the midportion of the internal auditory canal above the jugular bulb. It is an important landmark because it identifies the location of cranial nerves IX, X, and XI in the neural compartment of the jugular foramen. Bone dissection should be confined to the area superior to the cochlear aqueduct to avoid injury to these nerves. After removal of bone on the inferior part of the internal auditory canal, the dissection is carried out on the superior and anterior parts.

The facial nerve often underlies the dura along the anterior-superior aspect of the internal auditory canal, and extreme care must be taken not to allow the burr to slip into the canal. The facial nerve is especially vulnerable at this point. The lateral end of the internal auditory canal is divided by the transverse crest in an inferior and a superior compartment (Fig. 64-7). The bone around the inferior compartment can be drilled away to the most lateral extent of the canal without risk of facial nerve injury. In the superior compartment, bone removal allows identification of a bar of bone (Bill's bar), which separates the superior vestibular nerve from the facial nerve. The bone is removed at the porus and the medial part of the internal auditory canal first, and the more difficult lateral part is left until last when most of the bone removal has been completed.

All bone between the middle fossa dura and the internal auditory canal must be removed. With the visualization of the most lateral end of the internal auditory canal, the bone

work is completed. Until this point, all the dissection has been extradural and the morbidity of the approach consequently low.

Dural Opening

The dural incision is started superiorly in the sinodural angle near the sigmoid sinus continuing down to the porus (see Fig. 64-7). Care is taken to avoid vessels on the surface of the tumor. Posteriorly, the petrosal vein lies just beneath the dura. This vein originates in the cerebellum and drains into the superior petrosal sinus near the level of the internal auditory canal. If the dura is pulled laterally with a small hook, the space between the cerebellum and the dura is enlarged, and injury to the vessels may be avoided. At the porus, a small incision is made on both sides of the porus. Around the porus, the dura often forms a distinct constriction ring that usually adheres to the surface of the tumor, and there are small vessels going from the dura to the tumor. The dural ring must be divided, and a further incision is made over the dura in the meatus. In the meatus, the dura is often extremely thin, and sometimes it is opened while removing the bone around the meatus. The small vessels in the thickened dura at the porus can be coagulated with bipolar coagulation. Cottonoids are advanced into the plane between the tumor and cerebellum. It is important to develop this plane accurately because doing so separates the major vessels of the cerebellopontine angle from the tumor. To widen the opening, retractors, attached to the Sugita head frame, are placed on the dura of the middle fossa and on a cottonoid on the cerebellum and the sigmoid sinus.

Tumor Removal

After opening the dura, the posterior part of the tumor is exposed. Rarely, the facial nerve may lie on the posterior surface of the tumor, and this surface must be carefully inspected for nerve bundles. In large tumors, it is essential to begin tumor removal with intracapsular debulking to reduce tumor size and subsequently develop the extracapsular dissection planes. In small tumors, the surgeon can readily identify the inferior and superior extracapsular dissection planes of the tumor. An ultrasonic aspirator is useful for debulking and removing intracapsular tumor.

Identification of the Facial Nerve in the Fundus of the Internal Auditory Canal

In approximately 15% of vestibular schwannomas, the fundus of the internal auditory canal is empty, and all four nerves are visible and easy recognizable. In these cases, bone work in the internal auditory canal does not need to be as extensive as described. The identification of the vertical crest (Bill's bar) is not necessary. Exact determination of the facial nerve is done with stimulation.

In the remaining cases, the fundus of the internal auditory canal is filled up with tumor, and identification of the facial nerve is more difficult. During bone removal, the medial part of the fallopian canal is opened, which uncovers a labyrinthine segment of the facial nerve. Bill's bar separates the facial nerve anteriorly from the superior vestibular nerve. A fine hook is inserted lateral to Bill's bar and gently placed beneath the superior vestibular nerve and Bill's bar.

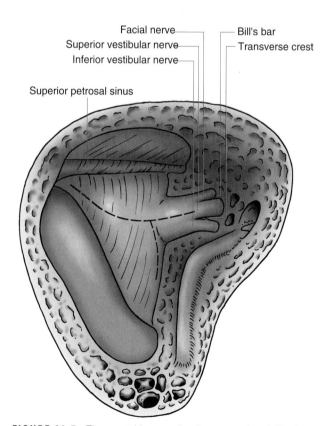

Facial nerve
Superior vestibular nerve
Inferior vestibular nerve
Bill's bar
Transverse crest
Superior petrosal sinus

FIGURE 64-7   The mastoidectomy has been completed. The internal auditory canal is opened and allows the facial nerve to be identified. The *broken lines* indicate the dural incisions.

The superior vestibular nerve can then be pulled out from its canal. Likewise, the two nerves inferior to the transverse crest (the inferior vestibular nerve and the cochlear nerve) are pulled out from their canals along with the tumor (Fig. 64-8). Positive identification of the facial nerve at the lateral end of the internal auditory canal is one of the principal advantages of the translabyrinthine approach.

Freeing the Tumor from the Facial Nerve in the Internal Auditory Canal

The arachnoid sheath completely surrounds the tumor, nerves, and vessels in the meatus, and the arachnoid strands that attach the facial nerve to the tumor must be divided. The meatal part of the tumor is gently retracted backward. Small hooks or fine microscissors are used to free the facial nerve from the arachnoid fibers that bind the nerve to the tumor. Because cutting of the arachnoid occurs along the facial nerve, it is important to have identified the inferior and the superior edges of the nerve accurately. Usually, it is relatively easy to develop the dissection plane between the facial nerve and the tumor in the internal auditory canal, but difficulties often arise at the porus. Around the entire circumference of the porus, dural adhesions to the tumor make dissection of the facial nerve from the tumor difficult. The exact position of the facial nerve in the porus must be established before the adhesions between dura and the tumor are removed. Inferiorly, freeing of the tumor from the porus is simpler because damage to the cochlear nerve is insignificant. Superiorly, the facial

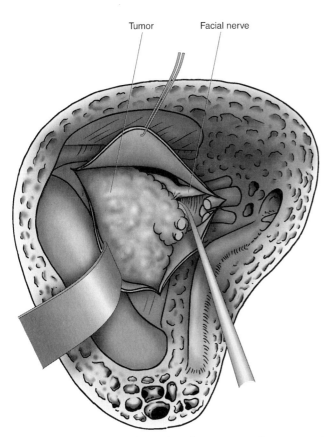

FIGURE 64-8 After dural opening, the tumor can be separated from the facial nerve in the internal auditory canal. The vestibular nerves and the cochlear nerve are divided laterally in the internal auditory canal.

nerve may be at risk. At times, it is difficult to isolate the facial nerve at the porus. In these cases, it is wise to carry out a partial tumor removal, then identify the facial nerve medially, and follow the nerve laterally until the porus is reached. During this work, the surgeon must be careful not to push the tumor forward or medially because stretching the facial nerve, especially at the porus level, can damage the nerve. Early mobilization of the tumor from the internal auditory canal has the advantage that the landmarks are well defined and are not obscured with blood, as tends to happen later in the surgical dissection.

Reducing Tumor Size

In large tumors, there is inadequate space in the cerebellopontine angle to mobilize the tumor in the superior, inferior, and lateral directions, which is necessary to identify and free the facial nerve. In these cases, the posterior surface of the tumor capsule is incised in a superior-inferior direction, and an intracapsular removal is gently performed with the ultrasonic aspirator.

Isolation of the Tumor

With tumors of all sizes, it is important to work in the proper cleavage plane between the tumor and the arachnoid. Tumor growth pushes the arachnoid membrane of the pontocerebellar cistern and causes it to double in the distal part of the internal auditory canal and in the cerebellopontine angle. In large tumors, there is duplication of the cerebellar cistern and the cerebellomedullary cistern, causing formation of the third and fourth arachnoid layers. Through these layers, cranial nerves IX, X, and XI run at the inferior aspect of the tumor. The petrosal veins run through the layers of cisterna cerebelli at the superior-posterior aspect of the tumor.

Tumor Removal

The principle for removal of large tumors is intracapsular gutting to reduce tumor bulk followed by mobilization and removal of the adjacent capsule segment. The point of attack must be changed progressively, and as the limits of mobilization are reached at one point, the surgeon moves to another. Once the interior part of the tumor has been extensively removed, the capsule is displaced into the tumor space. Opening of the arachnoid layers and dissecting within these layers facilitates the isolation of the tumor. Semisharp dissectors and sometimes small cottonoids are used in the proper dissection plane to separate the tumor from the surrounding structures. The dissection is made from four directions: inferior, superior, medial, and lateral.

Inferior Dissection

Dissection at the inferior aspect of the tumor usually leads into the large cerebellomedullary cistern, which allows CSF to escape. This step improves the operative condition, and if any difficulties are encountered because of lack of room in the posterior fossa, draining the cerebellomedullary cistern as soon as possible is valuable.

On the inferior aspect of the tumor, it is possible to localize cranial nerves IX and X, which are best identified near the jugular foramen medial to the jugular bulb. These nerves must be freed from the tumor and isolated. Sometimes they are not well seen because they tend to lie around the corner of the opening. During manipulation of cranial nerves IX and X, changes in the pulse rate may occur. Stopping the manipulation restores the pulse rate.

The posterior-inferior cerebellar artery is at the inferior aspect of the tumor and must be carefully separated from the tumor capsule and preserved. The labyrinthine artery supplies branches to the facial nerve and should be preserved. Dissection inferior to the tumor continues until the brain stem is reached and is completed with removal of that portion of the capsule.

Superior Dissection

The facial nerve is normally located anteriorly to the tumor, but it is not unusual to find the facial nerve over the top of the tumor. If the precise location of the facial nerve is unknown, when starting the dissection at the superior aspect of the tumor, it is imperative to inspect the tumor surface carefully and to use the nerve stimulator to identify the nerve and avoid injury.

The petrosal vein and cranial nerve V are located in the superior aspect of the tumor. These structures must be identified and carefully separated from the tumor. The trigeminal nerve is a broad white structure running in the inferior-posterior direction. Near the brain, the nerve lies in close contact with the tumor capsule but is usually easy to separate from the tumor. Handling the nerve must be avoided if recovery of sensory loss in the face is to be achieved. The petrosal vein and vein branches are stretched over the tumor and enter the superior petrosal sinus. To stay in the proper cleavage, it is better to separate the vein from the tumor rather than coagulate the vessels. The coagulation seals the layers together and makes later separation difficult. The superior dissection is continued until the pons is reached and the attachment of the trigeminal nerve to the brain stem is visualized.

Medial Dissection

The medial dissection is the most difficult part of the tumor removal because of the risk of damaging the facial nerve or the pons. After the posterior part of the tumor is debulked, a small portion of tumor capsule is left attached to the cerebellum and the pons. The tumor capsule is lifted, and the proper cleavage plane is identified. In large tumors, the posterior pole may protrude far under the cerebellum and deep into the brain stem. This protrusion requires maximal rotation of the operating table toward the surgeon to visualize the dissection plane. The vessels are dissected away, and the branches that extend into the capsule are coagulated and divided. The capsule and tumor remnant are pushed anteriorly, and arachnoid and veins are dissected from the capsule. When the brain stem has been reached from all directions and the has gradually been removed, the remaining small portion of tumor covers a part of the brain stem, facial nerve, and cochlear nerve.

Anterior Dissection and Final Tumor Removal

In small tumors, the main approach is from the anterior aspect. In these cases, the facial nerve can easily be located at the brain stem, and the precise position of the nerve is easy to

ascertain early. Separating the tumor from the facial nerve is done from the porus and against the brain stem.

In large tumors, the dissection of the facial nerve is done in an anterior-posterior direction. The small portion of tumor that covers the facial nerve from the brain stem to the porus is the most difficult to remove (Fig. 64-9). The anterior part of the tumor capsule usually contains a number of small vessels from arteries and vein, and dissection can easily provoke bleeding. Veins are often present around the facial nerve's entry zone from the brain stem. Coagulation of the bleeding vessels is dangerous and must be precise to avoid facial nerve injury.

For several reasons, the dissection on the anterior aspect of the tumor is troublesome and time consuming:

1. The facial nerve is often stretched and spread out over the largest prominence of the tumor, which sometimes makes the nerve nearly invisible.
2. The facial nerve is not protected by an epineurium and is vulnerable to injury.
3. At the porus, the facial nerve is often embedded in the tumor capsule, causing problems when loosening the tumor.

Care must be taken not to leave fragments of tumor on the nerve because the dissection continues inside the tumor and obscures the location of the nerve, which may be lost.

Once the facial nerve has been separated from the tumor, the last bit of tumor is removed from the brain stem. The adhesions between the tumor and the brain stem are not

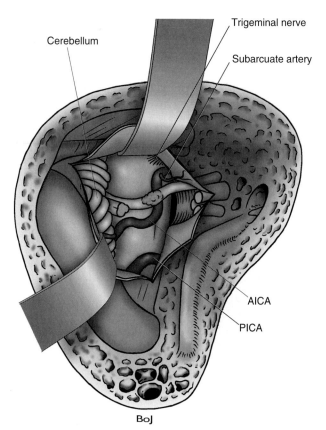

Cerebellum

Trigeminal nerve

Subarcuate artery

AICA

PICA

BoJ

FIGURE 64-9 The tumor has been removed. A small tumor remnant is left on the facial nerve.

usually dense, but if they are, clearing the brain stem of tumor demands particularly careful dissection. Once the tumor has been removed, the field is inspected, and the facial nerve is examined with the stimulator. If a signal can be obtained by stimulating the nerve at the brain stem, it is likely that the patient will have normal facial nerve function. The wound is then irrigated with saline, and all bleeding points are controlled. Absolute hemostasis is required and may take some time.

Facial Nerve Repair

If the nerve has been divided during operation, one may get an acceptable level of function by anastomosing the nerve ends, provided that the central stump can be found and isolated. If the nerve ends can reach each other, they are anastomosed end to end and fixed with a suture and Tisseel.[20–22] If a gap exists, a great auricular nerve or sural nerve graft is used to bridge the gap between the nerve ends.

Closure

An essential part of the wound closure involves preventing rhinorrhea. CSF may escape through the middle ear and the eustachian tube. The middle ear is packed with a small piece of muscle. The dural opening and the mastoid cavity are filled up with large pieces of adipose tissue taken from the abdomen. Fibrin glue is injected around the adipose tissue. The muscle fascia/pericranium flap is closed watertight with absorbable sutures. The postauricular skin incision is closed in two layers with absorbable subcutaneous suture and nylon suture in the skin. We do not use a subgaleal drain but make a solid compression of the wound by gauze supported by a solid elastic bandage.

POSTOPERATIVE MANAGEMENT AND COMPLICATIONS

Surgery on large tumors in posterior fossa is not without risks.[23–25] Large tumors sometimes adhere strongly to the surface of the cerebellum and the brain stem. Dissection of the tumor from the surroundings may elicit cerebellar edema and infarction. Veins can often be coagulated, but sometimes packing is necessary, especially of the bulb of the sigmoid sinus and the petrosal vein. Hematomas or reactive edema of the cerebellum may necessitate immediate response. Close observation of the patient is necessary in the initial postoperative phase by trained nurses in the intensive care unit. Acute hydrocephalus resulting from obstruction of CSF drainage from the ventricles may occur because of edema or hematoma at the level of the fourth ventricle.

Hematoma

Postoperative hematoma after a translabyrinthine approach is a rarity but a serious complication. This complication is the cause of most of the mortality seen after translabyrinthine removal of vestibular schwannomas. Even when excellent hemostasis appears to have been achieved, however, postoperative hemorrhage may still occur[26] and seems most likely among elderly patients and patients with large tumors.

The hematoma is most likely to occur shortly after the operation but may be seen days after surgery.

The clinical course is often insidious. If the patient does not regain consciousness after surgery or if the patient after a period with normal sensorium develops decreasing consciousness, a hematoma must be suspected. If the symptoms develop quickly, it may be necessary to open the wound immediately. If the symptoms develop more slowly, computed tomography can confirm the diagnosis. We always perform a control computed tomography scan the day after surgery to avoid clinical deterioration or death because of slowly progressive hematomas.

Cerebellar Edema

Rarely, cerebellar edema may develop during surgery, unprovoked and early in the procedure. This complication may hinder further attempts at tumor removal. In such cases, it is necessary to keep the patient on moderate hyperventilation and only slowly take the patient off the respirator. Also, patients who do not wake up or who deteriorate after surgery in whom computed tomography excludes significant hematoma may benefit from moderate hyperventilation.

Acute Hydrocephalus

Acute dilatation of the cerebral ventricles may be observed either immediately postoperatively or in the following days. Failure to wake up or decreasing consciousness should arouse suspicion, and a computed tomography scan should be obtained. If the complication is diagnosed soon after surgery, ventricular drainage is undertaken. If the complication arises slowly and later after surgery, a permanent CSF shunt may be considered.

Facial Paralysis

Facial paralysis is often difficult to detect immediately postoperatively, when full wakefulness and cooperation are absent and, for unknown reasons, eye closure may be present. If the face is paralyzed, eye care is of great importance. In the first days after surgery, the eye is covered with a protective shield and viscous eyedrops are used. Shortly thereafter, a tarsorrhaphy is performed. The patient is warned to protect the eye and to wear protective spectacles. An ophthalmologist should be consulted.

Even though the nerve seems anatomically intact at the end of the operation, some patients exhibit postoperative facial paralysis. These patients still have a good chance for some function of the facial nerve. At least 6 months of observation should be allowed before any further treatment is considered. If permanent facial paralysis exists, a faciohypoglossal anastomosis is carried out after a delay of approximately 1 year.[27]

Cerebrospinal Fluid Leakage

CSF leakage is a common complication after vestibular schwannoma surgery,[28] and it is seen in 5% to 15% of the cases. The leakage may occur either through the skin at the wound site or via the nose. Rhinorrhea is much more common than leakage through the wound. The diagnosis of postoperative CSF rhinorrhea is often obvious within a few days of surgery, but its recognition may be delayed. Some patients report only a sensation of postnasal dripping or a salty taste in the mouth. In these cases, the diagnosis may be subtle. The patient should be tested in a head-down position for watery escape from the nose before discharge.

When rhinorrhea is diagnosed, a lumbar drain is inserted for 3 to 5 days; however, the success with CSF drainage is not as high as in the wound leakage, probably because the defect is located in the bone, which is not as easily overgrown as is a defect in soft tissue. If the lumbar drainage fails to close the defect, reoperation and resealing the communication to the middle ear with muscle graft or bone wax in the communicating air cells is necessary.

CSF escape through the postauricular wound may be prevented by meticulous closure of the wound followed by a tight head bandage. If wound leakage occurs, spinal drainage is often sufficient to solve the problem, and reoperation is rarely necessary.

Meningitis

Because the translabyrinthine approach is time consuming and involves opening of an air-filled cavity, meningitis is among the more common complications, occurring in 5% to 10% of cases. The peak incidence is seen from the third to the fifth postoperative day. Delayed meningitis is often caused by an undiagnosed otorhinorrhea. Early recognition of meningitis with demonstration of high polymorphonuclear cell count in the CSF usually ensures rapid resolution.

A high or persistent fever combined with severe headache or signs of altered mental status is likely to be caused by meningitis. Because postoperative fever and headache are common after the translabyrinthine procedure, the clinician should have a low threshold for performing a lumbar puncture when suspicion of meningitis arises.

A large proportion of postoperative meningitis after vestibular schwannoma surgery is aseptic in nature.[29] It is not always clear from the CSF findings whether an infection is present. If there is any doubt, the patient should be treated with intravenous antibiotics.

CONCLUSIONS

The results from translabyrinthine and retrosigmoid approaches are comparable, with less than 2% mortality, 97% total removal, anatomic preservation of facial nerve in 90% to 95%, and a functioning facial nerve in more than 70% 1 year after surgery.[4,30–32] Except for hearing preservation, the published results do not favor one method over the other, and preference of one method should be based mostly on personal experience.

No comparison exists regarding the clinical outcome of the two approaches in vestibular schwannomas larger than 3.5 cm. In such cases, hearing preservation is seldom an issue. The standard retrosigmoid approach, as used in most neurosurgical departments for other pathologies in the cerebellopontine angle, does not, in our opinion, offer the same control of the tumor surfaces, especially the relation to the brain stem, as that achieved by a large, translabyrinthine exposure.

SUMMARY

Three different surgical approaches can be used for vestibular schwannoma surgery: subtemporal, suboccipital, and translabyrinthine.

In patients with nonserviceable hearing, the translabyrinthine approach offers the most direct route to the cerebellopontine angle and can be used for removal of tumors regardless of the size.

The patient is placed in a supine position with the head turned toward the opposite side. Intraoperative facial nerve monitoring is mandatory. A curved skin incision is made behind the ear, and the skin and muscle/pericranium layer are retracted anteriorly.

An extended mastoidectomy is performed. The facial nerve is identified close to the lateral semicircular canal. The nerve is exposed by making a small window in the fallopian canal. After complete removal of the labyrinth, a more than 180-degree arc of bone around the internal auditory canal is removed. Dura is open from the internal auditory canal to the sinodural angle near the sigmoid sinus.

After opening the dura, the posterior part of the tumor is exposed. Small tumors can be removed en bloc after careful dissection of the facial nerve away from the tumor. In large tumors, it is essential to begin removal with intracapsular debulking to reduce the tumor size and subsequently develop the extracapsular dissection planes. Around the entire circumference of the porus, dural adhesions to the tumor make dissection of the facial nerve difficult.

When tumor removal has been accomplished, absolute hemostasis must be obtained.

To prevent rhinorrhea, the middle ear is packed with a small piece of muscle, and the dural opening and the mastoid cavity are filled up with large pieces of adipose tissue taken from the abdomen. Fibrin glue is injected around the adipose tissue. The muscle fascia/pericranium flap is closed watertight, and the skin incision is closed in two layers.

Complications after using the translabyrinthine approach may be serious or even fatal. Close observation of the patient is necessary in the initial postoperative phase by trained nurses in the intensive care unit. Hematomas or reactive edema of the cerebellum may necessitate immediate response.

Acknowledgment

The author is indebted to Bo Jespersen, M.D., who provided all illustrations for this chapter.

REFERENCES

1. Helms J: Indications for the suboccipital, translabyrinthine, and transtemporal approaches in acoustic neuroma surgery. In Tos M, Thomsen J (eds): Proceedings of the First International Conference on Acoustic Neuroma. Amsterdam: Kugler, 1992, pp 501–502.
2. Jackler RK, Pitts LH: Selection of surgical approach to acoustic neuroma. Otolaryngol Clin North Am 25:361–387, 1992.
3. House WF (ed): Monograph. Transtemporal microsurgical removal of acoustic neuromas. Arch Otolaryngol Head Neck Surg 80:597–756, 1964.
4. Sterkers JM, Corlieu C, Sterkers O: Acoustic neuroma surgery (1300 cases), the translabyrinthine method. In Tos M, Thomsen J (eds): Acoustic Neuroma. Amsterdam: Kugler, 1992, pp 377–378.
5. Tos M, Thomsen J, Harmsen A: Results of translabyrinthine removal of 300 acoustic neuromas related to tumour size. Acta Otolaryngol Suppl (Stockh) 452:38–51, 1988.

6. King TT, Morrison AW: Translabyrinthine and transtentorial removal of acoustic tumours: Results of 150 cases. J Neurosurg 52:210–216, 1980.

7. Mamikoglu B, Wiet RJ, Esquivel CR: Translabyrinthine approach for the management of large and giant vestibular schwannomas. Otol Neurotol 23: 224–227, 2002.

8. Briggs RJS, Fabinyi G, Kaye AH: Current management of acoustic neuromas: Review of surgical approaches and outcomes. J Clin Neurosci 7: 521–526, 2000.

9. Briggs RJ, Luxford WM, Atkins JS Jr, Hitselberger WE: Translabyrinthine removal of large acoustic neuromas. Neurosurgery 34:785–790, 1994.

10. Yates PD, Jackler RK, Satar B, et al: Is it worthwhile to attempt hearing preservation in larger acoustic neuromas? Otol Neurotol 24:460–464, 2003.

11. Rhoton AL Jr: Microsurgical anatomy of the brainstem surface facing an acoustic neuroma. Surg Neurol 25:326–339, 1986.

12. Rhoton AL Jr, Tedeschi H: Microsurgical anatomy of acoustic neuroma. Otolaryngol Clin North Am 25:257–294, 1992.

13. Anson BJ, Donaldson JA: Surgical Anatomy of the Temporal Bone and Ear, 2nd ed. Philadelphia: WB Saunders, 1973.

14. Hammerschlag PE, Cohen NL: Intraoperative monitoring of the facial nerve in acoustic cerebellopontine angle surgery. Otolaryngol Head Neck Surg 103:681–684, 1990.

15. Syms CA 3rd, House JR 3rd, Luxford WM, Brackmann DE: Preoperative electroneuronography and facial nerve outcome in acoustic neuroma surgery. Am J Otol 18:401–403, 1997.

16. Harner SG, Daube JR, Beatty CW, Ebersold MJ: Intraoperative monitoring of the facial nerve. Laryngoscope 98:209–212, 1988.

17. Day JD, Chen DA, Arriaga M: Translabyrinthine approach for acoustic neuroma. Neurosurgery 54:391–395, 2004.

18. Tos M, Thomsen J (eds): Translabyrinthine Acoustic Neuroma Surgery: A Surgical Manual. Stuttgart: Georg Thieme, 1991.

19. House WF, Hitselberger WE: Translabyrinthine approach. In House WF, Leutje CM (eds): Acoustic Tumors. Baltimore: University Park Press, 1979, pp 43–87.

20. Barrs DM, Brackmann DE, Hitzelberger WE: Facial nerve anastomosis in the cerebellopontine angle: A review of 24 cases. Am J Otol 5:269–272, 1984.

21. Fisch U, Dobie RA, Gmur A, Felix H: Intracranial facial nerve anastomosis. Am J Otol 8:23–29, 1987.

22. Luetje CM, Whittaker CK: The benefits of VII-XII neuroanastomosis in acoustic tumor surgery. Laryngoscope 101:1273–1275, 1991.

23. Benecke JE: Complications of acoustic tumor surgery and their management. Semin Hear 10:341–345, 1989.

24. Sterkers JM: Life-threatening complications and severe neurologic sequelae in surgery of acoustic neurinoma. Ann Otolaryngol Chir Cervicofac 106:245–250, 1989.

25. Slattery WH III, Francis S, House KC: Perioperative morbidity of acoustic neuroma surgery. Otol Neurotol 22:895–902, 2001.

26. House WF, Hitselberger WE: Fatalities in acoustic tumor surgery. In House WF, Leutje CM (eds): Acoustic Tumors. Baltimore: University Park Press, 1979, pp 235–264.

27. Ebersold MJ, Quast LM: Long-term results of spinal accessory nerve-facial nerve anastomosis. J Neurosurg 77:51–54, 1992.

28. 28. Selesnick SH, Liu JC, Jen A, Newman J: The incidence of cerebrospinal fluid leak after vestibular schwannoma surgery. Otol Neurotol 25:387–393, 2004.

29. Ross D, Rosegay H, Pons V: Differentiation of aseptic and bacterial meningitis in postoperative neurosurgical patients. J Neurosurg 69:669–674, 1988.

30. Ebersold MJ, Harner SG, Beatty CW, et al: Current results of the retrosigmoid approach to acoustic neurinoma. J Neurosurg 76:901–909, 1992.

31. Mass SC, Wiet RJ, Dinces E: Complications of the translabyrinthine approach for the removal of acoustic neuromas. Arch Otolaryngol Head Neck Surg 125:801–804, 1999.

32. Thomsen J, Tos M, Bàrgesen SE, Màller H: Surgical results after removal of 504 acoustic neuromas. In Tos M, Thomsen J (eds): Proceedings of the First International Conference on Acoustic Neuroma. Amsterdam: Kugler, 1992, pp 331–335.

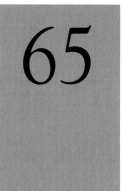

65 Vestibular Nerve Section in the Management of Intractable Vertigo

SETH I. ROSENBERG and HERBERT SILVERSTEIN

When medical management of a patient with Ménière's disease fails to control episodic vertigo, and hearing is better than 80 dB pure tone average and 20% speech discrimination, posterior fossa vestibular neurectomy has been utilized by the authors since 1978.[1] Complications have been minor, and facial paralysis, meningitis, or death has not occurred in series by the authors.[1-7] In numerous studies, it has been demonstrated that vertiginous attacks have been cured or improved in greater than 90% of the authors' patients, with preservation of hearing in most cases.[1-7] A review of the literature suggests that increasing emphasis is being placed on hearing preservation in surgery for vertigo, and that more neuro-otologic surgeons are using the vestibular nerve section through the posterior fossa as their procedure of choice to cure vertigo caused by inner ear disease.[8] A survey of the American Otologic Society and the American Neurotologic Society in 1990 indicated that almost 3000 vestibular nerve sections had been performed in the United States, and 95% of these were done through the posterior fossa by retrolabyrinthine, retrosigmoid, or combined approaches.[5] In this series, representing the experience of 59 surgeons, the cure rate for vertigo exceeded 90%, as did the reported patient satisfaction rate.[5]

The modern trend toward interdisciplinary surgical approaches often combines the talents of both neurosurgeon and neuro-otologist during cranial nerve operations. The neurosurgeon's role in vestibular neurectomy may range from primary surgeon to operative assistant, but in any event, the neurosurgeon must have a clear understanding of the disease process involving the vestibular system and of the treatment options and surgical technique. The surgical anatomy and techniques involved in vestibular nerve section are also applicable to most posterior skull base operations.

HISTORICAL PERSPECTIVE

In 1904, Frazier[9] was the first to perform an eighth cranial nerve section through the posterior fossa to relieve the symptoms of aural vertigo in a patient with Ménière's disease. After 1924, when Dandy[10,11] began his surgical series, the eighth nerve section received more widespread attention. Anatomic dissections of the eighth nerve by McKenzie[12,13] in 1930 permitted him to be the first to section the vestibular nerve selectively, preserving the cochlear nerve in 117 patients. In 1932, Dandy began to perform the selective vestibular nerve section for a variety of balance disorders. His personal series of 624 procedures is still the largest in the world literature.[14] These procedures were performed without the benefit of microsurgical techniques and instrumentation. One half of Dandy's patients underwent a total eighth nerve section, and approximately 10% experienced a permanent facial paralysis. Although the procedure boasted excellent control of vertigo, it was not widely accepted because of the magnitude of these complications.

After Dandy's death in 1946, the vestibular nerve section fell into disuse until 1961, when House described a neurosurgical extradural approach to the internal auditory canal through the middle fossa.[15] Via this approach, the superior vestibular nerve could be exposed and sectioned. Because of the poor control of vertigo with this procedure, Fisch[16,17] and Glasscock[18,19] modified it to include sectioning of the inferior vestibular nerve and excision of Scarpa's ganglion. This modification yielded excellent control of vertigo, with preservation of hearing in many cases. Although the middle fossa vestibular nerve section was performed often by Fisch[16,17] and Garcia-Ibanez and Garcia-Ibanez,[20] it never achieved widespread popularity in either Europe or the United States. For many otologists, the middle fossa vestibular nerve section was formidable, and anatomic landmarks were difficult to determine reliably. The exposure was difficult and fraught with complications, including injury to the facial nerve, the cochlea, or the labyrinth. Generally, patients older than 60 years were not candidates because of the difficulty in elevating the thin dura from the skull and the risk of postoperative hematoma.

In 1972, Hitselberger and Pulec[21] described the retrolabyrinthine approach for section of the trigeminal nerve in the posterior fossa. The procedure was further modified by Brackmann and Hitselberger[22] in 1978 to allow for various posterior fossa operations. In 1978, during the removal of a glossopharyngeal neurilemmoma through the posterior fossa, the senior author (H.S.) noted the close proximity of the eighth nerve complex to the dural opening.[1] More importantly, he noted a well-delineated cleavage plane between the vestibular and cochlear constituents of the nerve. Gross anatomic and microscopic laboratory studies have confirmed that the vestibular nerve section can be performed routinely through the posterior fossa. The retrolabyrinthine exposure offered excellent exposure to the cerebellopontine angle with minimal cerebellar retraction, permitting vestibular nerve section within the posterior fossa. Since its introduction, posterior fossa vestibular nerve section (including the retrolabyrinthine approach and its subsequent modifications, the retrosigmoid-internal auditory canal approach and the combined retrolabyrinthine-retrosigmoid approach) has become the most popular means of selective vestibular nerve section.[5] Today, this exposure is widely used for vestibular nerve section and for the removal of acoustic neuromas in which hearing preservation is the goal. Many skilled otologists and neurosurgeons continue to perform retrolabyrinthine or middle fossa vestibular nerve sections with results quite similar to those achieved by the combined approach.[5] As endoscopic techniques and equipment improve, the possibility of endoscopic posterior fossa vestibular nerve section is a possibility. In contrast to the anecdotal results reported in earlier days of vestibular nerve sections, results today are objectively documented and established so that careful postoperative evaluation and comparisons are possible.[24,25]

DIFFERENTIAL DIAGNOSIS OF VESTIBULAR DISORDERS

Rarely is the neurosurgeon the initial consultant for the patient experiencing dizziness, but it is important for the neurosurgeon to be able to establish a correct diagnosis and have an understanding of vestibular disorders. The cause of the vertigo must be determined before any treatment is undertaken. The differentiation between peripheral and central vertigo is the first step in arriving at a diagnosis. Peripheral vertigo arises from the inner ear or vestibular nerve, whereas the origin of central vertigo is the brain stem or cerebellum. History and physical examination, combined with audio vestibular testing and diagnostic imaging, result in an accurate diagnosis.

Peripheral vertigo is characterized by an intense subjective sensation of spinning, accompanied by nystagmus. The vertigo is often induced by positional changes (benign paroxysmal positional vertigo), and the vertigo and nystagmus rarely persist for 30 seconds, even when position is maintained. If the provocative moves are repeated, the signs and symptoms progressively lessen with each trial (fatigability). In contrast, central positional vertigo may occur with head movements in the recumbent patient, but the patient does not have the intense vertigo experienced with peripheral disorders. The vertigo persists as long as the position is maintained and lacks latency of onset and fatigability. Peripheral vertigo can be relieved by vestibular nerve section, whereas central vertigo cannot.

Ménière's disease classically affects middle-aged adults, producing a triad of symptoms. Early symptoms include fluctuating unilateral hearing loss and tinnitus; later in the course of the disease, vertiginous attacks appear. The vertiginous attacks last from minutes to hours, disabling the victim, who prefers to lie immobilized in a dark, quiet place. Often the individual vertiginous attack is preceded by a sensation of increasing pressure or fullness in the involved ear. Vertigo attacks may undergo remissions and exacerbations and finally disappear as the disease burns out, whereas hearing and vestibular functions progressively deteriorate. Occasionally, vestibular symptoms may predominate from the start, with minimal hearing loss, a condition that leads

to a diagnosis of vestibular Ménière's disease. Rarely, drop attacks, with or without vertigo, may occur as a manifestation of Ménière's disease.[18] Patients experiencing such attacks describe the sensation as a feeling of being pushed or shoved to the ground without loss of consciousness.

Otologic testing in patients with Ménière's disease reveals a hearing loss in the low frequencies with a recovery at 2000 Hz early in the course of disease. Electronystagmography demonstrates a reduced caloric response in the affected ear, but imaging studies reveal no abnormalities. Profound hearing loss in all frequencies may occur, producing loss of serviceable hearing in the involved ear. In 15% to 40% of patients, the disease may involve both ears.

Most investigators agree that Ménière's disease results from endolymphatic hydrops or distention of the endolymphatic spaces, ultimately resulting in fibrosis of the labyrinth. The vertiginous episodes occur with the rupture of the endolymphatic membranes, allowing potassium-rich endolymph to mix with the potassium-poor perilymph. The potassium influx produces depolarization of the vestibular nerve endings, producing vertigo and nystagmus. As repair proceeds, symptoms resolve, and hearing may improve to near normal, although each attack results in progressive degenerative changes in the cochlear and vestibular nerve endings.

The clinician must differentiate between Ménière's disease and other episodic peripheral vertigo disorders; the results of vestibular nerve section for Ménière's disease exceed the relief afforded for other conditions. Other important causes of acute vertiginous disorders include vestibular neuronitis and chronic labyrinthitis. Vestibular neuronitis occurs as a single or recurrent vertiginous episode without hearing loss. The cause appears to be an inflammatory process, possibly viral, involving the vestibular ganglia. Chronic labyrinthitis follows middle ear inflammatory disease or trauma to the labyrinth. Chronic labyrinthitis may result in recurrent episodes of vertigo but may also be associated with chronic disequilibrium.

Benign paroxysmal positional vertigo (cupulolithiasis) must not be confused with Ménière's disease or other chronic vestibular disorders. In patients with benign positional vertigo, rapid changes in position result in brief vertiginous episodes. In the provocative test for this disorder, the patient quickly assumes the lateral supine position (Hallpike's maneuver). Symptoms occur only when the ear containing the diseased labyrinth is on the down side. Vertigo occurs and rotatory nystagmus appears. The nystagmus is fatigable on repeated provocative testing, and the disease is commonly self-limited. Disabling or persistent symptoms may require section of the nerve to the ampulla of the posterior semicircular canal.

The role of vascular cross-compression involving the vestibular nerve deserves mention. Dandy,[11] in discussing Ménière's disease in 1937, stated: "In about 20 percent of the cases, a large artery (one of the branches of the superior-inferior cerebellar artery) lies against the nerve and, I think, is the cause of deafness and dizziness in this disease." Jannetta and associates[26] championed the cross-compression theory as the cause of vertigo that does not fit any other diagnostic profile. Typical symptoms consist of a constant positional vertigo or a disequilibrium so severe that patients are disabled or constantly nauseated. Patients characteristically have motion intolerance, particularly when riding in an automobile or while pushing a shopping cart and gazing along the shelves. No demonstrable loss of auditory or vestibular function occurs. In the opinion of Jannetta and associates,[26] vascular compression of the vestibular nerve at the brain stem is responsible for this disorder. Vessels further distal along the course of the vestibular nerve are common and are not a source of the problem.

Disorders of the central nervous system, including multiple sclerosis or brain stem tumor, may produce acute central vertigo. Additional symptoms, signs, and imaging study results differentiate these disorders. Vertebral artery insufficiency rarely produces vertiginous attacks in the absence of other neurologic signs or symptoms. Acute occlusion of the labyrinthine artery may produce sudden hearing loss and vertigo, but the vertigo is self-limited once central accommodation occurs. Hearing loss is usually permanent.

TREATMENT OF PERIPHERAL VESTIBULAR DISORDERS

Nonsurgical treatment forms the cornerstone of therapy for Ménière's disease and other peripheral labyrinthine disorders. Neurologists, internists, and otolaryngologists depend on vestibular depressant drugs, salt restriction, and diuretics to control symptoms. Time alone may produce a complete remission of symptoms. Recently, chemical perfusion of the inner ear with gentamicin as an in-office procedure has been used as a second line of therapy for Ménière's disease.[27] The unpredictability and the profound discomfort as well as the interruption of lifestyle that accompanies the episodic vertigo attacks compel the patient to seek surgical treatment. When the vertiginous attacks begin to interfere with everyday function, surgery is considered.

Indications and Contraindications

Dandy reportedly performed a vestibular neurectomy on patients with a variety of dizzy disorders, some within 1 week of the onset of the vertigo.[14] Indications for surgery today are continued intractable vertigo attacks that have not responded to multiple trials of medical treatment. Approximately 20% of patients with Ménière's disease become surgical candidates. The selection of the initial procedure largely depends on the neuro-otologist's evaluation of the patient's hearing. With good hearing (i.e., 80 dB or greater pure tone average or less than 20% discrimination), preservation of auditory function is an additional goal of surgery; selective vestibular nerve section is the procedure of choice. Because preservation of any hearing in the involved ear is important, even in patients with poor hearing, vestibular nerve section is usually the initial procedure chosen. Occasionally, in a patient with poor hearing, some surgeons choose labyrinthectomy or eighth nerve section as the initial procedure.

Although the most common inner ear disorder treated by vestibular nerve section is classic Ménière's disease, the procedure is also useful in selected cases of recurrent vestibular neuronitis, traumatic labyrinthitis, and vestibular Ménière's disease. In deciding when to operate, the patient's perception of his or her disability is an important consideration. Some patients may have infrequent severe episodes

of vertigo that do not affect their lifestyles sufficiently to warrant a major surgical procedure. Others, even those who have only a few attacks per year, may be so severely affected that they live in constant apprehension of the next attack. For some patients, attacks of vertigo may pose an occupational hazard that may jeopardize themselves, their co-workers, or the public. Often, a patient decides to have surgery when he or she no longer has an aura preceding the onset of the vertigo.

Before surgery can be considered, objective evidence of unilateral inner ear disease should be documented with audiometry, electronystagmography, or electrocochleography. Early in the course of classic Ménière's disease, there is an ipsilateral low-frequency sensorineural hearing loss with good discrimination. As the disease progresses, the audiogram may flatten out or become downsloping, and the discrimination may deteriorate. During quiescence, electronystagmography may show normal or reduced caloric function in the involved ear. In the rare case in which an acute attack may be observed, spontaneous nystagmus toward the affected side and ipsilateral vestibular hyperfunction may be observed during the irritative phase. This activity is followed by a longer paralytic phase, characterized by spontaneous nystagmus away from the affected side and reduced vestibular response to caloric testing. Electrocochleography classically shows an elevated ratio of the summation potential-to-compound action potential, thought to be indicative of endolymphatic hydrops with distention of the basilar membrane.

The surgical candidate should be in good health, and between vertigo attacks the patient should have balance adequate to perform a tandem gait reasonably well. Elderly patients with good balance function are surgical candidates; however, they usually require more postoperative time and vestibular rehabilitation to regain good equilibrium than do younger patients. Vestibular nerve section has been performed on patients in their late 70s with excellent results and no additional morbidity.

Contraindications to vestibular nerve section include physiologic old age, poor general health, ataxia, unsteadiness, multisensory deficit syndrome, and other evidence of central nervous system involvement. Patients with ataxia or disequilibrium of central nervous system origin or a multisensory syndrome accommodate poorly after vestibular nerve section. Patients with these conditions may benefit from vestibular rehabilitation therapy. Those with severe disability are referred for a specialized rehabilitation program, but most respond well to home exercise regimens and are encouraged to maintain the most active lifestyle possible. Poor hearing in the ear opposite to the one producing vertigo is a strong contraindication to vestibular neurectomy; the chance of hearing loss as a result of surgery must be considered. Bilateral Ménière's disease is another contraindication to vestibular neurectomy. Previous transmastoid surgery of the endolymphatic sac is not a contraindication to surgery.

The surgical candidate must be well educated in postoperative expectations. Several preoperative sessions with a surgeon are necessary to answer all the patient's questions. The patient must understand that the major purpose of the surgery is to relieve vertiginous attacks; tinnitus will likely be unaffected, and hearing loss may continue to progress, following the natural course of Ménière's disease. The greatest fear most patients profess is facial paralysis; this consequence must be discussed frankly and openly. Unless the possibility of cere-brospinal fluid (CSF) rhinorrhea and its treatment has been introduced before surgery, the uninformed patient assumes this to be a catastrophic complication if it occurs. The acute vertigo and the more subacute disequilibrium experienced after vestibular nerve section, both of which subside spon-taneously, must be carefully explained. The nurses caring for the patient after surgery must also be well versed in the postoperative course. Anxiety from an inexperienced nurse can rapidly be transferred to the patient.

Surgical Anatomy

Multiple superbly illustrated microdissections of the cranial nerves in humans were published in 1865 by Bischoff.[28] Figure 65-1 reproduces some of these illustrations of the sev-enth and eighth cranial nerves and the nervus intermedius.

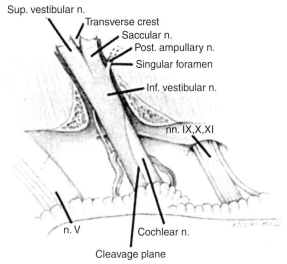

FIGURE 65-2 Within the right internal auditory canal, the superior vestibular nerve obscures the facial nerve, whereas the inferior vestibular nerve hides the cochlear nerve. The distance from the singular foramen to the transverse crest is 2 ± 0.7 mm; the trans-verse crest would not be exposed during surgery.

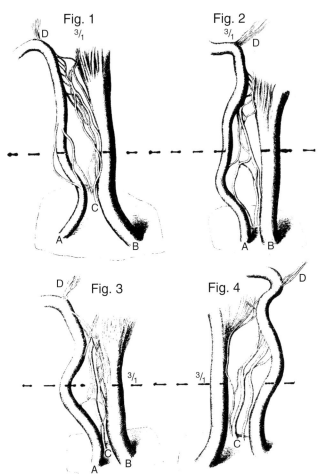

FIGURE 65-1 Dissection of nerves VII, VIII, and intermedius beginning at their emergence from the brain stem at A, B, and C, respectively, extending to their terminations within the petrous bone for nerves VIII and intermedius and to the knee of nerve VII at the point where it branches off the greater superficial petrosal nerve. Branches of the intermedius nerve unite about as often with nerve VIII as with nerve VII. Rarely, this union occurs in the cere-bellopontine cistern. The *dashed line* through each drawing marks the approximate level of the opening into the internal auditory canal. (Courtesy of Bischoff EPE: Mikrospichen Analyse der Anastomosen der Kopfnerven. München: J.J. Leniner 1865, Tab. XLIII, p 52.)

McKenzie's[13] dissections led to the first practical localiza-tion of the vestibular portion of the eighth nerve in the cerebellopontine angle. Using McKenzie's[12] 1936 illustra-tions as an anatomic guide, a surgeon today could success-fully perform a differential section of the vestibular nerve in the cerebellopontine angle. It is best to understand the changing anatomic relationships between the cochlear, vestibular, and facial nerves and the nervus intermedius throughout their course from the brain stem to their bony exits in the depths of the internal auditory canal. Throughout most of their course, minor individual anatomic variations occur; however, all nerves are constant in their position at the distal end of the internal auditory canal. Near the terminal end of the canal, which during surgery can be seen only by drilling away the bone that forms the posterior wall of the internal auditory canal, the superior and inferior vestibular nerves lie caudal (posterior), closest to the surgeon, obscuring the facial and cochlear nerves from view (Fig. 65-2). Terminally, the vestibular nerves are separated by the transverse (falciform) crest. Anterior to and in front of the superior vestibular nerve lies the facial nerve. Below the facial nerve, the cochlear nerve lies in front of the inferior vestibular nerve. As the facial nerve enters its bony canal, it is separated from the superior vestibular nerve by the vertical crest, or Bill's bar (named in honor of William House).

The inferior vestibular nerve is formed by the fusion of the saccular and posterior ampullary nerves in the depths of the internal auditory canal. The saccule (innervated by the saccular nerve) has no apparent significant physiologic function in humans, which has important implications when section of the inferior vestibular nerve is considered. After innervating the saccule, the saccular nerve enters the terminal end of the internal auditory canal through its fenestrated posterior-inferior quadrant. Within 1 to 2 mm proximal to the terminal bony fenestrations, the saccular nerve is joined by the posterior ampullary nerve, which enters

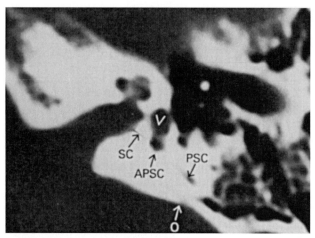

FIGURE 65-3 A computer-generated axial tomogram of the temporal bone demonstrates the singular canal (SC), the posterior semicircular posterior canal (PSC) and its ampulla (APSC), the vestibule (V), and the operculum (O) covering the endolymphatic duct.

the posterior wall of the internal auditory canal through a small bony opening, the singular foramen (Fig. 65-3). The posterior ampullary nerve (singular nerve) innervates only the ampulla of the posterior semicircular canal. Almost immediately after the inferior vestibular nerve is formed, it begins to fuse with the cochlear nerve just medial to the falciform crest. Because of this early fusion, attempts to

section the entire inferior vestibular nerve, even within the depths of the internal auditory canal, carry a significant risk of injury to the cochlear nerve. By the midportion of the internal auditory canal, the inferior vestibular nerve–cochlear nerve complex and superior vestibular nerve commonly fuse into a single bundle, the eighth nerve.

As the nerves course through the internal auditory canal and the cerebellopontine cistern, rotation occurs. By the midportion of the internal auditory canal, the cochlear nerve has rotated more caudally (posteriorly) and dorsally to emerge from the porus acusticus closest to the surgeon, and the combined vestibular portions of the nerve have rotated rostrally away from the surgeon. Rotation continues so that when the nerves reach the midportion of the cerebellopontine cistern, the cochlear nerve has rotated a full 90 degrees and is within full view of the surgeon (Fig. 65-4). As the eighth nerve emerges into the cerebellopontine cistern, a fine cleavage plane usually exists between the cochlear and vestibular nerves. Subtle color difference also assists the surgeon in identifying the separate components of the eighth nerve. The vestibular portion of the nerve, rostral and closest to the trigeminal nerve, appears grayer than the inferior white cochlear component that is closest to the ninth nerve. Maintaining its rostral position, the vestibular portion of the nerve enters the brain stem rostral to the auditory portion through the middle cerebellar peduncle, and the auditory portion of the nerve enters the brain stem caudal and slightly more dorsally, where the restiform body disappears under the middle peduncle.

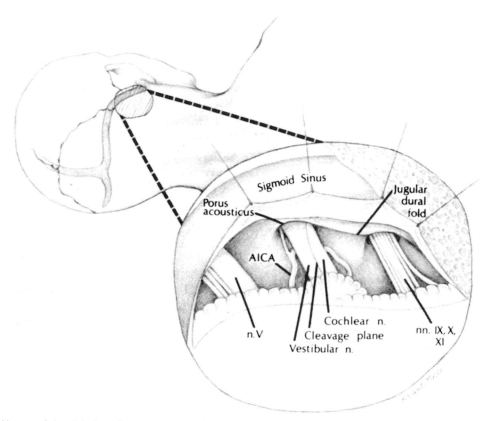

FIGURE 65-4 Nerves of the right lateral posterior cranial fossa demonstrating the cochleovestibular cleavage plane. The facial nerve is hidden beneath the eighth nerve.

The facial nerve also participates in the rotation from the brain stem to its bony canal. The facial nerve emerges from the brain stem ventral and usually caudal to the eighth nerve; it is usually obscured from the surgeon's view by the eighth nerve throughout its course from the brain stem to the porus acusticus. Within the internal auditory canal, the seventh nerve rotates from caudal to rostral and from ventral to dorsal in its relationship to the cochlear portion of the eighth nerve before entering the bony facial canal. The nervus intermedius commonly originates as several twigs from the brain stem between the seventh and eighth nerves. Within the cerebellopontine cistern, the nervus intermedius fibers are intimately associated with the eighth nerve, usually attached to the ventral cleavage plane between the auditory and vestibular divisions of the nerve. In the midportion of the internal auditory canal, the nervus intermedius departs from the eighth nerve, joining the seventh nerve as it enters the facial canal.

A clear understanding of the rotation and changing relationship between the vestibular and cochlear portions of the eighth nerve is essential for surgeons performing surgery in the cerebellopontine angle. Before McKenzie's work, the changing position of the eighth nerve components was described but lacked practical value.[29] After the vestibular nerve section lost its popularity in the 1940s, the anatomy became less important, and more recent anatomic descriptions were misleading because they failed to note the rotation of the seventh and eighth nerves.[30] The resurrection of vestibular neurectomy and the possibility of hearing preservation during the removal of an acoustic neurinoma refocused attention on the importance of the eighth nerve rotation.[31,32]

Rasmussen[33] was among the first to describe the histologic morphology of the eighth cranial nerve. He demonstrated the occasional complete separation between the cochlear and vestibular portions in the eighth nerve, and the total intermingling of fibers within a single trunk in other specimens. The histologic difference between the two components of the nerve accounts for the surgical color difference. The cochlear fibers are uniform in size and more compact, appearing white under surgical magnification, whereas the loose fibers of the vestibular nerve produce a grayer color. Current histologic descriptions of the cleavage plane between the cochlear and vestibular nerves vary. Silverstein and colleagues[31] described an identifiable cleavage plane in 75% of specimens, realizing that in some cases vestibular fibers might still be contained within the cochlear portion of the nerve. Natout and co-workers[34] described an overlapping zone between the two divisions, in which the vestibular fibers were interspersed between the adjacent cochlear fibers. Schefter and Harner[35] studied the eighth nerve in 10 cadavers; they found no separation between the cochlear and vestibular fibers within the cerebellopontine angle in 5 specimens, and in the remaining cases, the eighth nerve was divided into many fascicles. No cochleovestibular cleavage plane was found in their study. Surgical outcome studies tend to favor at least some separation in most patients.

Operating Room Setup

Before surgery, a thin-section computed tomography (CT) scan of the temporal bones is performed in addition to auditory and vestibular testing. This scan provides useful anatomic information about the labyrinths, venous sinuses, singular canals, and internal auditory canals.

Retrolabyrinthine and combined retrolabyrinthine-retrosigmoid operations for relief of peripheral vertigo are generally performed by teams of neurosurgeons and neuro-otologists. The positions of the patient, the surgeon, and the anesthesiologist during the surgery are identical to those used for the retrolabyrinthine and the combined retrolabyrinthine-retrosigmoid operations. The patient rests supine on an electrically controlled operating table, with the head turned and comfortably flexed away from the side of the surgery. Occasionally, pin-fixation head immobilization must be used, particularly in patients with thick, short necks. The patient need not be positioned in the "park-bench" position or prone, provided that an electric operating table is available to enable rotation. The surgeon sits directly behind the patient's head, with the anesthesiologist further down on the same side of the operating table. The surgical nurse is positioned directly opposite the surgeon, and the surgical microscope base is positioned at the head of the operating table. Electronic equipment is stacked at the foot of the operating table.

Intraoperative facial nerve monitoring is performed using the Silverstein Facial Nerve Monitor/Stimulator Model S8 (WR Medical Electronics, Stillwater, MN) and the Brackmann EMG Monitor (WR Medical Electronics, Stillwater, MN). The Silverstein monitor relies on an ultrasensitive piezoelectric strain gauge placed in the ipsilateral oral commissure that responds to facial movement. The electromyographic monitor senses facial myoelectric activity through bipolar electrodes placed in the facial musculature; the electrodes are typically placed in the ipsilateral orbicularis oris and orbicularis oculi muscles. The operation of these monitors has been described elsewhere. Intraoperative facial nerve stimulation is performed with the Silverstein Stimulator Probe (WR Medical Electronics, Stillwater, MN) and the Silverstein micro insulated neuro-otologic instruments (Storz Instruments, St. Louis, MO) using constant-current square wave pulse stimulation. Brain stem auditory evoked responses and direct eighth nerve potentials can be recorded during the operation. Cochlear nerve recordings are not considered to be an essential element in vestibular nerve section, but the use of this technique in these cases gives the surgeon a comfortable familiarity that is essential for acoustic neuroma surgery in which hearing preservation is the goal.

All patients receive perioperative intravenous antibiotics, starting immediately before incision and continuing for 24 hours. Intracranial pressure is lowered by the administration of mannitol (1.5 g/kg), and hypocarbia is produced by controlled hyperventilation. The mannitol is administered when the drilling begins. A urinary catheter is placed, and the urine output is monitored.

Surgical Procedure

Adipose tissue is harvested from the left lower quadrant, and a suction drain is used to prevent hematoma formation. This tissue is used to obliterate the postauricular surgical defect in the retrolabyrinthine and combined retrolabyrinthine-retrosigmoid vestibular nerve section procedures.

The retrolabyrinthine and the combined retro-labyrinthine-retrosigmoid operations begin with elevation of an anteriorly based, 4 × 5-cm U-shaped postauricular skin muscle flap. The flap, including the mastoid-occipital peri-osteum, is elevated in one layer. Anteriorly the spine of Henle should be visible. The mastoid emissary vein is commonly divided in the exposure, and bone wax is usually necessary to control the bleeding from the mastoid. Bleeding from the occipital artery should be controlled by suture ligation to avoid further intraoperative bleeding and postoperative hematoma formation.

Retrolabyrinthine Vestibular Nerve Section

A complete mastoidectomy is performed, and the lateral venous sinus is skeletonized. The dura in front of and 1 cm behind the lateral venous sinus is exposed (Fig. 65-5). Bleeding from the lateral venous sinus is controlled by placing compressed Avitene and Gelfoam sponge over the bleeding site and holding it in place with a neurosurgical cottonoid sponge. Bleeding from a large emissary vein is controlled with bipolar cautery or an Avitene-Gelfoam pack. The endolymphatic sac is completely exposed, and the posterior semicircular canal is identified. The vertical segment of the facial nerve is delineated, and the retrofac-ial cells are opened. The dura over the posterior fossa is exposed from the middle fossa to the jugular bulb, and from the lateral venous sinus to the posterior semicircular canal. The sigmoid sinus is compressed and retracted with the Silverstein lateral venous sinus retractor (Storz Instruments, St. Louis, MO), and the dura is incised around the endolymphatic sac anterior to the sigmoid sinus, forming a C-shaped flap based on the labyrinth. The use of mannitol helps reduce the size of the cerebellum, allowing a wider exposure of the cerebellopontine angle.

A Penrose drain is placed over the cerebellum, which is then gently retracted with a Penfield elevator until the arachnoid is opened with an arachnoid knife (Storz Instruments, St. Louis, MO) to allow CSF to escape. As the cerebellopontine cistern is drained, the cerebellum falls away from the temporal bone to allow good exposure of the cere-bellopontine angle and cranial nerves V, VII, VIII, IX, X, and XI without cerebellar retraction. Care must be taken not to traumatize the petrosal veins located above the fifth nerve and near the tentorium. Because of brain shrinkage from mannitol, these veins are stretched and can rupture easily. Bleeding is controlled with Avitene or bipolar cautery.

In 75% of cases, a good cochleovestibular cleavage plane exists between the cochlear and vestibular fibers of the eighth nerve in the cerebellopontine angle; the cochlear fibers constitute the caudal portion of the nerve, and the vestibular fibers constitute the cephalad portion. The ori-entation is important; the fifth cranial nerve is identified cephalad, and the ninth, tenth, and eleventh nerves are identified caudally. The facial nerve should be identified. Occasionally the facial nerve is adherent to the vestibular nerve and must be separated from the vestibular nerve with a round knife. After the cleavage plane is identified under high magnification, an incision is made in the cleavage plane, the cochlear and vestibular fibers are separated, and the vestibular nerve is transected. The vestibular and cochlear nerves are separated longitudinally with an elec-trified sickle knife and nerve separator (Storz Instruments, St. Louis, MO), and the vestibular nerve is transected with microscissors and sickle knife. Transecting 75% of the vestibular nerve with microscissors and completing the transection with the sickle knife helps avoid injury to the facial nerve and the internal auditory artery. The cephalad half of the eighth nerve is transected when a cleavage plane

FIGURE 65-5 Removal of the right retro-labyrinthine bone exposes the sigmoid sinus and presigmoid sinus dura of the posterior fossa.

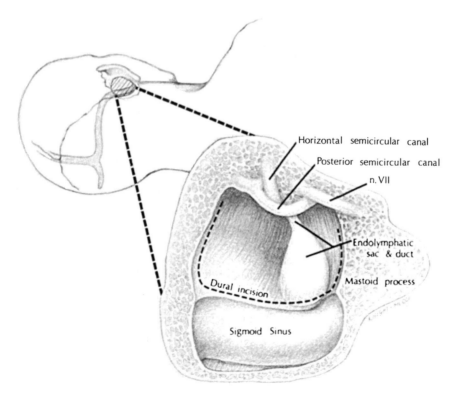

Horizontal semicircular canal
Posterior semicircular canal
n. VII
Endolymphatic sac & duct
Mastoid process
Dural incision
Sigmoid Sinus

cannot be readily identified. When this technique is used, most vestibular fibers are transected, and most cochlear fibers are spared. The dural incision is completely closed with 4-0 silk sutures. Temporalis fascia is placed over the dural incision using fibrin glue, and the mastoid cavity is obliterated with abdominal adipose tissue and fibrin glue. The skin is closed with skin staples.

Retrosigmoid-Internal Auditory Canal Vestibular Nerve Section

Either a U-shaped postauricular incision or a traditional neurosurgical straight suboccipital incision may be used. A round posterior fossa craniotomy 3 cm in diameter is made posterior to the lateral sinus. After the dura is opened with a posteriorly based U-shaped incision, the cerebellum is gently retracted with a self-retaining retractor blade to give exposure to the seventh and eighth cranial nerves and the internal auditory canal. The dura is closed in a watertight fashion, and the skin incision is closed. No fat graft is placed.

Combined Retrolabyrinthine-Retrosigmoid Vestibular Nerve Section

A limited mastoidectomy is performed to expose 3 cm of the lateral venous sinus from the transverse sinus inferiorly. The lateral venous sinus is skeletonized, and the posterior fossa dura is exposed for 1.5 cm posterior to the lateral sinus (see Fig. 65-4). A dural incision is made 3 mm behind and parallel to the lateral sinus for 3 cm, and the lateral sinus is retracted anteriorly by means of stay sutures placed in the dural margin. A Penrose drain is placed against the cerebellum, and the cerebellum is gently retracted with a Penfield elevator. The landmark to the arachnoid over the cerebellopontine cistern is a white fold of dura, the jugular dural fold, attached to the temporal bone just lateral to the jugular foramen above the exit of the ninth nerve. The jugular dural fold is identified anterior to the endolymphatic sac on the inner surface of the temporal bone. The eighth nerve is found approximately 1 cm anterior to the cephalad extent of the jugular dural fold. The arachnoid layer is gently dissected, and the cerebellopontine cistern is entered. After the CSF is released from the cerebellopontine angle, the cerebellum falls away from the temporal bone, allowing good exposure of the cerebellopontine angle without cerebellar retraction.

The eighth nerve is examined, and the cleavage plane is sought between the cochlear and vestibular fibers. If the cochleovestibular cleavage plane is identified, the vestibular nerve section is performed as in the retrolabyrinthine approach. Sometimes the flocculus of the cerebellum is adherent to and hides much of the eighth nerve in the cerebellopontine angle. The flocculus must be dissected away from the eighth nerve with a round knife. If no cleavage plane is identified, an anteriorly based, U-shaped dural flap is elevated from the posterior surface of the temporal bone between the operculum and the porus acusticus. With diamond burrs, the posterior wall of the internal auditory canal is removed to the singular canal, exposing the branches of the vestibular nerve. Usually, 7 to 8 mm of bone is removed. This length is determined from the preoperative CT scan. The superior vestibular nerve and the posterior ampullary nerve are divided. The inferior vestibular nerve fibers that

innervate the saccule are spared because of their close association with cochlear fibers. Because the saccule has no known vestibular function in humans, sparing these fibers does not result in postoperative vertigo attacks. The dura is closed in a watertight fashion, any exposed mastoid air cells are filled with bone wax, and the defect is filled with abdominal adipose tissue. The skin is closed with skin staples.

Postoperative Care

Immediately after surgery, patients experience acute vertigo, nausea, and vomiting similar to a Ménière's attack. As vestibular compensation occurs in the central nervous system, however, vertigo resolves rapidly over 3 to 4 days; the common complaint of disequilibrium improves more slowly. Patients with near-normal preoperative vestibular function experience the greatest immediate postoperative vertigo and nausea after labyrinthine denervation. Early ambulation appears to hasten vestibular compensation, although immediately after surgery, patients usually have a wide-based gait and tend to fall to the operated side. One year after surgery, some patients may experience mild transient unsteadiness after abrupt head movement. Third-degree horizontal nystagmus beating away from the operated ear is seen early and diminishes quickly. It is not unusual, however, for a patient to have first-degree nystagmus for several days. Diplopia occurs in a small number of patients: it is difficult to document and clears rapidly, apparently caused by ocular dysmetria or a skew deviation.

Complications

Early postoperative bleeding in the posterior fossa requires prompt assessment by a neurosurgeon. The wound may have to be opened immediately. Meningismus with mild temperature elevation occurring soon after surgery usually represents chemical meningitis caused by small amounts of blood in the CSF.

Spiking fever with nuchal rigidity and headache requires lumbar puncture for a CSF culture and sensitivity testing. The patient should then be treated empirically for meningitis, and the antibiotic coverage should be narrowed later on the basis of culture results. As yet, the authors have not encountered this complication.

Wound infection secondary to serum collected beneath the postauricular skin flap is treated with incision, drainage, culture, and appropriate antibiotics. This complication has been reduced by keeping the skin muscle flap in one layer during its elevation. Perioperative antibiotic administration has reduced wound infections to less than 1% of cases.

Postoperative CSF leak occurs in less than 5% of all patients.[3,4] It was the most common early complication of retrolabyrinthine vestibular nerve section, occurring in approximately 10% of patients, and was seen occurring through the wound or as persistent rhinorrhea. When a leak is detected, lumbar drainage is immediately instituted and maintained for 3 to 5 days, avoiding re-exploration of the wound in most cases. Because the dura cannot be closed in a watertight fashion in the retrolabyrinthine approach, no way has been found to eliminate CSF leaks; however, the use of cryoprecipitate autologous fibrin glue appears to have reduced their incidence. The retrosigmoid-internal auditory canal and combined retrolabyrinthine-retrosigmoid approaches allow a watertight dural closure, and CSF leakage is rarely encountered.

Facial paralysis and transient facial weakness have been reported and are rare. The authors have not experienced either complication in their series.

RESULTS

The retrolabyrinthine vestibular nerve section was developed in 1978 to replace the middle fossa vestibular nerve section. Results of this procedure have been good. In a review of 67 patients, 88% were completely cured of their vertigo, and 7% were substantially improved. Hearing has been maintained within 20 dB of the preoperative level in 70%. Some patients experienced mild conductive loss in the low frequencies, which is presumed to be caused by bone dust or fat herniating into the attic and impeding ossicular motion. CSF leak occurred in 10% of patients and responded to lumbar drainage. Wound infection occurred in 3%. There were no cases of meningitis, facial paralysis, or death.

In 1985, the retrosigmoid-internal auditory canal vestibular nerve section was developed in an effort to improve results.[4] Because the cleavage plane between the cochlear and vestibular fibers is more completely developed within the internal auditory canal, a more complete and selective vestibular nerve section can be performed there. This approach resulted in a 92% cure rate for vertigo in 14 patients, with hearing results similar to those with the retrolabyrinthine approach. Fifty percent of patients, however, experienced prolonged severe headaches that were difficult to control with non-narcotic analgesics. Two years after surgery, 25% of patients still experienced headaches requiring medication. The authors have speculated that removal of the dura from the bone at the porus, and bone dust produced by drilling the internal auditory canal may have resulted in a prolonged arachnoiditis. Owing to the unacceptably high incidence of severe postoperative headaches, the authors abandoned the retrosigmoid-internal auditory canal approach in 1987. Only 15 procedures were performed.

The combined retrolabyrinthine-retrosigmoid vestibular neurectomy was developed in 1987.[3] This procedure incorporates the advantages of both of its predecessors. Depending on the presence of a good cochleovestibular cleavage plane in the cerebellopontine angle, the vestibular nerve section may be performed there, or the internal auditory canal may be opened and the superior vestibular and posterior ampullary nerves sectioned. Less bone removal is required, and surgical time is shortened. Also, a watertight dural closure may be accomplished. In the authors' series, vertigo has been cured in 90% of patients, and hearing has been preserved to within 20 dB of preoperative levels in 84%. When the internal auditory canal was not opened, only 1% of patients developed headaches. Since October 1988, the internal auditory canal has not been drilled. Three of five patients requiring internal auditory canal exposure developed moderate headaches. There have been no cases of CSF leak, meningitis, facial paralysis, or death.

After vestibular nerve section in patients with vertigo attacks from labyrinthitis or vestibular neuronitis, the surgical results are slightly less impressive than in patients with Ménière's disease. Nguyen and colleagues[36] and Kemink[37] reported only a 70% improvement or complete resolution of symptoms in the non-Ménière's group of patients with chronic vertigo. There is a lack of correlation between surgical outcome and the surgeon's assessment of either the completeness of the vestibular neurectomy or the clarity of the cleavage plane.

Beyond relief of vertigo, some patients report relief of chronic unsteadiness, aural pressure, and tinnitus. The possibility of relief of any one of these symptoms, no matter how troublesome, in the absence of vertigo attacks, does not justify the performance of vestibular neurectomy.

Failure of surgery to relieve vertigo attacks requires reevaluation of vestibular function. Approximately 3% of patients require additional surgery. If a patient continues to have vertigo attacks arising from the side of the original surgery, a decision must be made regarding further surgery. Labyrinthectomy, transcanal eighth nerve section, or middle fossa or posterior fossa total eighth nerve section should be performed. All of these procedures result in hearing ablation, but the results of vertigo relief are quite good.

OUTCOMES STUDY

An important outcome measurement in any treatment modality is whether or not the patient feels better and considers himself or herself cured. In an effort to ascertain whether the patient's perception of the surgical outcome agrees with the surgeon's criteria of success, a comprehensive outcomes questionnaire was developed.[38,39] The questionnaire, which addresses patient lifestyle and incidence of vertigo, balance function, hearing, tinnitus, aural fullness, and incidence of failures or complications, was sent to all patients who underwent posterior fossa vestibular neurectomy. Of the patients that responded, 88% believed that the vertigo caused by their Ménière's disease was cured after surgery, and 78% believed that their hearing was maintained. After surgery, 95% believed that their balance function "rarely" or "never" prevented them from doing their normal daily activities. Overall, patient perception of outcome after posterior fossa vestibular neurectomy was similar to the surgeon's and to what has been previously reported.

CONCLUSIONS

In the nearly 90 years since Frazier first performed an eighth cranial nerve section through the posterior fossa for the treatment of Ménière's disease, the surgical management of Ménière's disease has come full circle. With refinements in surgical technique and advancements in instrumentation, optics, illumination, and neuromonitoring, a procedure that was once resoundingly condemned by the otologic community is now regarded as the procedure of choice in patients with serviceable hearing. The vestibular nerve section has experienced a renaissance. The posterior fossa vestibular nerve section has undergone an evolution, and the combined retrolabyrinthine-retrosigmoid vestibular nerve section represents the highest form. It is a significant improvement over its predecessors, and is the authors' procedure of choice in properly selected patients.

REFERENCES

1. Silverstein H, Norrell H: Retrolabyrinthine surgery: A direct approach to the cerebellopontine angle. Otolaryngol Head Neck Surg 88:462–469, 1980.

2. Silverstein H, Norrell H, Smouha E: Retrosigmoid-internal auditory canal approach vs. retrolabyrinthine approach for vestibular neurectomy. Otolaryngol Head Neck Surg 97:300–307, 1987.

3. Silverstein H, Norrell H, Smouha E, et al: Combined retrolabyrinthine-retrosigmoid approach for vestibular neurectomy. Am J Otol 10:166–169, 1989.

4. Silverstein H, Norrell H, Rosenberg S: The resurrection of vestibular neurectomy: A 10–year experience with 115 cases. J Neurosurg 72:533–539, 1990.

5. Silverstein H, Wanamaker H, Flanzer J, Rosenberg S: Vestibular neurectomy in the USA 1990. Am J Otol 13:23–30, 1992.

6. Rosenberg S, Silverstein H, Norrell H, et al: Hearing results after posterior fossa vestibular neurectomy. Otolaryngol Head Neck Surg 114:32–37, 1996.

7. Silverstein H, Arruda J, Rosenberg S: Vestibular neurectomy. In Harris JP (ed): Ménière's Disease. Amsterdam: Kugler, 1998, pp 263–273.

8. Roland PS, Meyerhoff WL: Should the membranous labyrinth be destroyed because of vertigo? Otolaryngol Head Neck Surg 95: 550–553, 1986.

9. Frazier CH: Intracranial division of the auditory nerve for persistent aural vertigo. Surg Gynecol Obstet 15:52–59, 1912.

10. Dandy WE: Ménière's disease: Its diagnosis and method of treatment. Arch Surg 16:1127–1152, 1928.

11. Dandy WE: Treatment of Ménière's disease by section of only the vestibular portion of the acoustic nerve. Bull Johns Hopkins Hosp 53:52–55, 1933.

12. McKenzie KG: Intracranial division of the vestibular portion of the auditory nerve for Ménière's disease. Can Med Assoc J 34:369–391, 1936.

13. McKenzie KG: Ménière's syndrome: A follow-up study. Clin Neurosurg 2:44–49, 1955.

14. Green RE: Surgical treatment of vertigo, with follow-up on Walter Dandy's cases. Clin Neurosurg 6:141–152, 1958.

15. House WE: Surgical exposure of the internal auditory canal and its contents through the middle cranial fossa. Laryngoscope 71:1363–1385, 1961.

16. Fisch U: Vestibular and cochlear neurectomy. Trans Am Acad Ophthalmol Otolaryngol 78:252–254, 1977.

17. Fisch U: Vestibular nerve section for Ménière's disease. Am J Otol 5:543–545, 1984.

18. Glasscock ME: Vestibular nerve section. Arch Otolaryngol 97:112–114, 1973.

19. Glasscock ME, Kveton JF, Christiansen SG: Middle fossa neurectomy: An update. Otolaryngol Head Neck Surg 92:216–220, 1984.

20. Garcia-Ibanez E, Garcia-Ibanez IL: Middle fossa vestibular neurectomy: A report of 373 cases. Otolaryngol Head Neck Surg 88:486–490, 1988.

21. Hitselberger WE, Pulec JL: Trigeminal nerve (anterior root) retrolabyrinthine selective section. Arch Otolaryngol 96:412–415, 1972.

22. Brackmann DE, Hitselberger WE: Retrolabyrinthine approach: Technique and newer applications. Laryngoscope 88:286–297, 1978.

23. Rosenberg SI, Silverstein H, Willcox TO, Gordon MA: Endoscopy in otology and neurotology. Am J Otol 15:168–172, 1994.

24. Pearson BW, Brackmann DE: Committee on hearing and equilibrium guidelines for reporting treatment results in Ménière's disease. Otolaryngol Head Neck Surg 93:579–581, 1985.

25. Monsell EM, Balkany TA, Gates GA, et al: Committee on hearing and equilibrium guidelines for the diagnosis and evaluation of therapy in Ménière's disease. Otolaryngol Head Neck Surg 113:181–185, 1995.

26. Jannetta PJ, Moller MB, Moller AR: Disabling positional vertigo. N Engl J Med 310:1700–1705, 1984.

27. Jackson LE, Silverstein H: Chemical perfusion of the inner ear. Otolaryngol Clin North Am 35:639–653, 2002.

28. Bischoff EPE: Mikrospichen Analyse der Anastomosen der Kopfnerven. Munchen: JJ Leniner, 1865.

29. Courville CB: Applied anatomy of the VIIIth nerve and its environs, the cerebellopontine angle.

30. Rhoton A: Neurosurgery of the internal auditory meatus. Surg Neurol 2:311–318, 1974.

31. Silverstein H, Norrell H, Haberkamp T, McDaniel AB: The unrecognized rotation of the vestibular and cochlear nerves from the labyrinth to the brain stem: Its implications to surgery of the eighth cranial nerve. Otolaryngol Head Neck Surg 95:543–549, 1986.

32. Malkasian DR, Rand RW: Microsurgical neuroanatomy. In Rand RW (ed): Microneurosurgery, 2nd ed. St. Louis, CV Mosby, 1978, pp 37–70.

33. Rasmussen AT: Studies of the VIIIth cranial nerve of man. Laryngoscope 50:67–83, 1949.

34. Natout MAY, Terr LI, Linthicum FH Jr, House WF: Topography of the vestibulocochlear nerve fibers in the posterior cranial fossa. Laryngoscope 97:954–958, 1987.

35. Schefter RP, Harner SG: Histologic study of the vestibulocochlear nerve. Ann Otolaryngol 95:146–150, 1986.

36. Nguyen CD, Brackmann DE, Crane RT, et al: Retrolabyrinthine vestibular nerve section: Evaluation of technical modification in 143 cases. Am J Otol 13:328–332, 1992.

37. Kemink IL: Retrolabyrinthine vestibular nerve section: A preliminary report. Am J Otol 5:549–551, 1984.

38. Rosenberg SI, Silverstein H, Hester TO, Deems D: Outcomes research after posterior fossa vestibular neurectomy-a 20 year experience. Proceedings of the 4th International Symposium on Ménière's Disease: 803–811, April, 1999.

39. Jackson LE, Silverstein H: Vestibular nerve section. Otolaryngol Clin North Am 35:655–673, 2002.

66 Surgical Management of Lesions of the Clivus

GIULIO MAIRA and ROBERTO PALLINI

INTRODUCTION

The clivus is a region of the skull characterized anatomically by its central and deep location at the skull base and surgically by the difficulty in reaching this structure.

Tumors that arise purely from the clivus are rare, but the region can be involved with numerous processes extending from the structures near the clivus, mainly from the petrousclival line. Tumors may be limited to a part of the clivus or they may involve the entire clivus. Tumors may also extend superiorly to the suprasellar region; inferiorly to the foramen magnum and cervical spine; and laterally to the cavernous sinus, subtemporal region, or pontocerebellar angle.

Different pathologic lesions can develop in this region.[1] Lesions can be benign (e.g., meningiomas, epidermoid cyst, cholesterol granuloma, or glomus jugulare tumors with major petroclival involvement); of a low-grade malignancy (e.g., chordomas and chondrosarcomas); or of a high-grade malignancy (e.g., squamous cell cancer, adenocarcinoma, basal cell carcinoma, osteogenic sarcoma, or metastases). Some of these tumors have an intradural location, whereas others are extradural.

The lesions that most often involve this region are meningiomas (commonly intradural), followed (much less commonly) by chordomas, which are often extradural. The former grow from the dura that covers the clivus or the passage from the clivus and the petrous bone (petroclivus fold),[2] whereas the latter originate directly from embryonic residues enclosed in the bone of the clivus.[3-6]

Tumors in the region of the clivus may involve the lowest seven cranial nerves. Cranial nerve VI can be within the tumor itself, where it runs through Dorello's canal in the lateral region of the clivus. The brain stem can be displaced dorsally or laterally. The basilar artery is usually displaced contralaterally; however, occasionally it is shifted dorsally or is encased by the tumor.

Major advances in imaging modalities over the last two decades have permitted a more precise delineation of the anatomic extension of these tumors. In most cases, the nature of the lesion can be suspected in advance.

Tumors in the region of the clivus are difficult to treat using conventional neurosurgical approaches. Until a few decades ago, owing to the relative inaccessibility of the clivus and its close proximity to the brain stem and surrounding neurovascular structures, the results of surgical treatment were so dismal that these tumors were often considered to be incurable.[1]

Advances in microsurgery of the skull base have resulted in the development and refinement of approaches to petroclival and clival lesions,[7-57] better methods for tumor removal, and innovative techniques[44,45,58-62] to minimize injury to neural and vascular structures during tumor removal. These factors enable the surgeon to treat these tumors more effectively, aiming at a radical excision with an acceptable morbidity and mortality.

In some cases, the combined effort of the neurosurgeon with other disciplines interested in skull base surgery (e.g., otolaryngology or maxillofacial surgery) constitutes real progress in the realization of special approaches that aim at improving the exposure of the tumor and reducing trauma to the brain during surgery.

In general, surgical approaches to the clival region have followed two main strategies. The first strategy utilizes conventional approaches, which are technically simple and are characterized by a low approach-related morbidity. The disadvantages of these approaches include the limited surgical field, long working distance, and the need for brain retraction, which all make tumor dissection difficult. The second strategy implies the use of complex approaches that require specific anatomic knowledge on cadaveric dissections; are time consuming because of the extensive bone removal; and are themselves related with some morbidity in terms of hearing loss, facial nerve dysfunction, and postoperative cerebrospinal fluid (CSF) leak. These approaches do facilitate tumor dissection owing to the wide surgical field and short working distance.

In recent years, a third option has been developed in which simple conventional approaches, such as the retrosigmoid or subtemporal routes, are combined with conservative petrosectomies to create key openings to the tumor area while preserving hearing and providing adequate exposure to the petroclival and prepontine regions. Such approaches appear suited for treating petroclival meningiomas. In clival chordomas, however, the extensive bony involvement by the tumor forces the surgeon to choose between a partial removal through a simple anterior approach (e.g., the transsphenoidal approach or Le Fort I maxillotomy) and an attempt for total tumor resection using more complex anterior or anterolateral approaches. Nevertheless, surgeons who have extensive experience with the transsphenoidal route for pituitary tumors have shown that gross total removal of clival chordomas can be achieved in up to 70% of cases with low morbidity and excellent long-term survival.

SURGICAL ANATOMY

The clivus is located at the midline, which is the deeper part of the skull base. The clivus constitutes the inclined anteroinferior surface of the posterior cranial fossa and

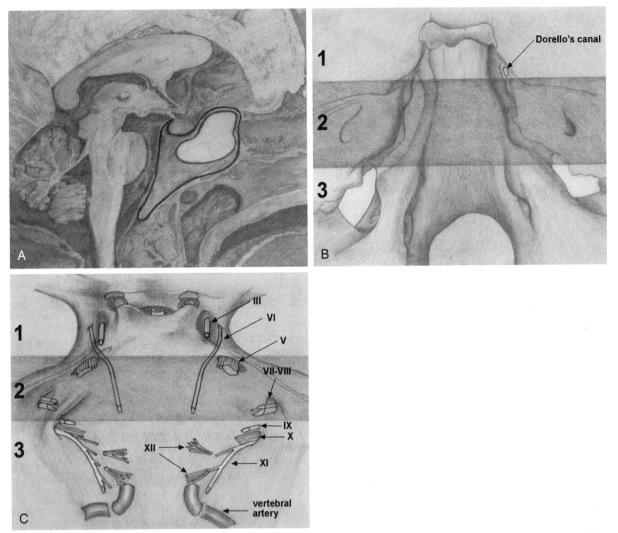

FIGURE 66-1 *A,* Anatomy of the clivus and adjacent structures. *B,* Anatomic division of the clivus in upper (1), middle (2), and lower (3) regions. *C,* The clivus and cranial nerves III, V to XII.

extends from the dorsum sellae to the foramen magnum (Fig. 66-1A). It is formed by a sphenoidal part (corresponding to the superior third) that extends from the dorsum sellae to the spheno-occipital synchondrosis, and by an occipital part (corresponding to the inferior two thirds) that reaches the anterior intraoccipital synchondroses.[3,63]

Surgical access to the clivus is complicated by the presence of osseous barriers corresponding to the sphenoid and facial bones (anteriorly and inferiorly) and to the petrous bones (laterally). Posteriorly and laterally, there are critical structures, including the basilar artery, brain stem, cavernous sinus, petrous carotid arteries, temporal lobes, and cranial nerves.

Owing to the complexity of the clivus and its surrounding structures, the knowledge of their anatomy is essential to plan a correct surgical approach for patients who have a tumor in this region.

The clivus is usually divided into the upper, middle, and lower clivus[25] (see Fig. 66-1B and C); or into superior and inferior halves of the clivus.[64]

The upper clivus is the part above the crossing of the trigeminal and the abducens nerves from the posterior to

the middle cranial fossa; this part includes the dorsum sellae and the posterior clinoid processes. This area is bounded anteriorly by the sella turcica and sphenoid sinus; posteriorly by the basilar artery and the midbrain; and laterally by the cavernous sinus, the temporal lobes, and (from superior to inferior) cranial nerves III through VI.

The middle clivus is the part between the exits of the trigeminal and the glossopharyngeal nerves; it is bounded anteriorly by the upper nasopharynx and retropharyngeal tissues, posteriorly by the basilar artery and the pons, and laterally by the petrous apices and by cranial nerves VII and VIII.

The lower clivus is the part from the glossopharyngeal nerve to the foramen magnum. This part is bounded anteriorly by the lower nasopharynx and retropharyngeal tissues; posteriorly by the vertebral artery and the medulla; and laterally by the sigmoid sinus, jugular bulb, and cranial nerves IX to XII.

The superior and inferior halves of the clivus extend, respectively, above the internal auditory canal and below it.

The topographic anatomy of the clivus makes several surgical approaches feasible.[1,11,34,35,37,41,65,66] The choice of an approach to remove a tumor from this region must take into account the nature of the lesion (i.e., whether the lesion is intradural or extradural, its position in respect to the clivus, and its lateral extension).

The surgical approaches to the clivus are divided into three general groups: (1) anterior, (2) anterolateral, and (3) posterolateral.

Anterior approaches are mainly used for extradural lesions that primarily involve the clivus and extend extracranially (e.g., chordoma and chondrosarcoma). For these tumors, the anterior approaches are usually extradural and include transnasal-transsphenoidal, transethmoidal, transoral-transpalatal, transmaxillary, and transcervical. A subfrontal transbasal extraintradural anterior approach can also be indicated for huge tumors with maximal involvement of the clival area and surrounding structures (e.g., chordoma, pituitary tumors, and craniopharyngiomas).

Anterolateral approaches are mainly utilized for intradural tumors that involve the upper and middle clivus and that extend into the surrounding regions. The fronto-temporal transsylvian approach exposes lesions of the upper clivus with extension in the suprasellar region. The subtemporal transtentorial approach exposes lesions of the upper and midclival region, with extension in the middle fossa and tentorial edge (a zygomatic osteotomy and anterior petrosectomy increase the exposure inferiorly and toward the clivus).

Posterolateral approaches are mainly utilized for tumors involving the medial and lower part of the clivus with extension to the petrous bone, cerebellopontine angle, foramen magnum, or upper cervical region. These approaches include the combined subtemporal suboccipital presigmoid with posterior petrosectomy (retrolabyrinthine, translabyrinthine, transcochlear, and total petrosectomy); the retrosigmoid; and the extreme lateral transjugular transcondylar approach.

EXTRADURAL LESIONS: CHORDOMAS

Chordomas are the most common extradural tumors of the clivus; they arise from remnants of the embryonic notochord and are located in all places where the notochord existed (i.e., the entire clivus, sella turcica, foramen magnum, C1, and nasopharynx).[3,5] From there, they may spread to the upper cervical region, petrous bone, posterior fossa, cavernous sinus, middle fossa, nasopharynx, and sphenoid sinus.[3,5]

Chordomas grow slowly but may present the characteristics of a malignant tumor in being locally aggressive with a tendency for regrowth.[67] About 20% of chordomas recur as early as 1 year after surgery in spite of extensive surgical resection.[48,68] Ten percent of chordomas show histologic signs of malignancy.[5] Although it is considered difficult to identify histologic features indicative of aggressiveness,[69,70] recent studies indicate that some molecular features of these tumors are associated with an aggressive biological behavior.[47,48,68,71,72] Metastases are relatively rare.[68,70]

Chordomas infiltrate the bone and spread into the epidural space, seeding the dura with microscopic deposits well beyond the limits of the tumor bulk.[5,73] For this reason, they may invade the dura and become adherent to the arachnoid and pia mater. The tumor is often gelatinous and soft, with a jelly-like consistency, but it may also appear as a very firm cartilaginous mass.

Chordomas are usually classified according to the portion of clivus involved by the tumor and by the extension to surrounding structures (e.g., upper clivus, middle clivus, lower clivus, and craniocervical junction tumors, with or without invasion of sphenoid, cavernous sinus, and petrous bone).[1,3]

Computed tomography (CT) scan and magnetic resonance imaging (MRI) are the most important radiologic tools for diagnosis. The CT scan reveals the destruction of bone, whereas the MRI shows the extension of the tumor, which appears isodense with the brain and with a variable contrast enhancement after gadolinium.[4]

The most commonly involved cranial nerve is the sixth, and diplopia is the most common presenting symptom, particularly in the midclivus chordomas. Other symptoms include headache, pituitary dysfunction, visual field defects, cerebellar syndrome, torticollis, and brain stem syndrome.[74]

Surgical Treatment

Its deep position (at the central base of the skull) and its tendency to infiltrate the bone make total removal of the clivus chordoma difficult. However, in recent years, owing to the development of innovative and complex approaches to the clival area[29,30,34,35,37,41,42,75–79] and to the extensive application of standard procedures to this area,[12,13,16,36,38,74,80–85] many possibilities are at the disposal of the surgeon attempting radical removal of these tumors.

Because chordomas are basically extradural and midline tumors, they displace the neuraxis dorsally or dorsolaterally. Anterior midline extradural approaches are generally preferred (Fig. 66-2).[20,46,52,73,80,86–90] These approaches allow a

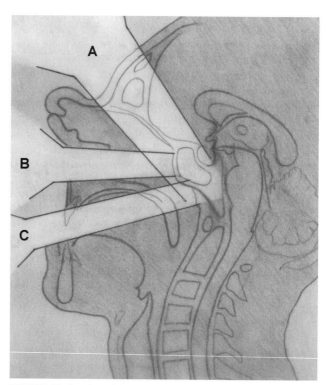

FIGURE 66-2   Anterior approaches to the clivus: subfrontal transbasal approach (*A*); transsphenoidal approach (*B*); and transoral approach (*C*).

midline exposure of the clivus and a short working distance, avoiding any retraction of the brain.

The choice of surgical approach depends on the location and extension of the tumor. Even when only anterior extracranial approaches are considered, many options exist. These include the transbasal,[13] extended subfrontal,[89] transseptal transsphenoidal,[16,74,81,82] transsphenoethmoidal,[80] transmaxillary transnasal,[91] transfacial,[92] facial translocation,[93] transmaxillary,[94,95] midfacial degloving,[88] transoral,[12] mandible-splitting transoral,[82] transcervical transclival,[96] and anterior cervical[97] approaches; Le Fort I osteotomy[98]; unilateral Le Fort I osteotomy[99]; total rhinotomy; and pedicled rhinotomy.[100]

All these approaches are devoted to removing all clival lesions localized on the midline without important lateral extent. In the case of massive lateral extension, so that a midline approach is insufficient for the removal of all the tumor, more complex lateral approaches can be utilized as a primary or secondary procedure.[1,5] These include, for lesions of the upper clivus, the subtemporal, transcavernous, and transpetrous apex approach; for lesions of the midclivus,

a subtemporal and infratemporal approach; and for lesions of the lower clivus with lateral extension to the occipital condyle, jugular foramen, and cervical area, the extreme lateral transcondylar approach.[26,43,101]

According to the level of the clival lesion, the approaches that the authors often utilize include the following:

1. For chordomas located in the upper and middle clivus, the transsphenoidal approach is favored.
2. For lesions of the lower clivus that involve the foramen magnum, C1, and C2, the transoral approach is preferred, with or without splitting the palate.
3. For tumors in the lower clivus, foramen magnum, and first cervical spinal bodies, with important lateral extension, the Le Fort I osteotomy can be used with a midline incision of the hard and soft palate and lateral swinging of the two flaps of the hard palate.
4. For huge tumors involving all the clival area, the sphenoid, and the sellar region and extending anteriorly to the optic nerves, the transbasal or extended subfrontal route is utilized.

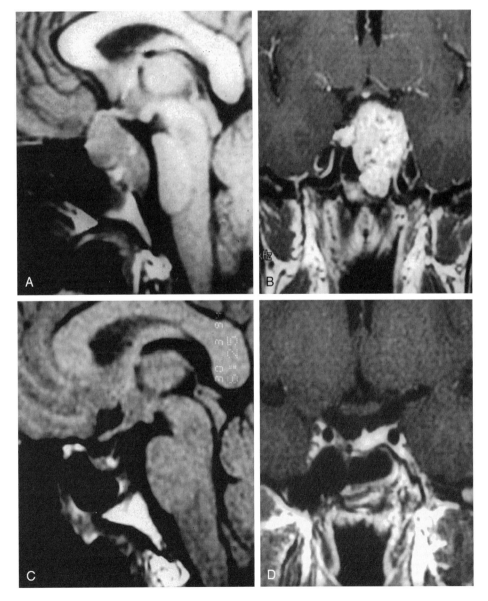

FIGURE 66-3 The transsphenoidal approach. An upper and middle clivus chordoma with retroclival diffusion and pontine compression. Contrast-enhanced magnetic resonance imaging is used. *A,* Preoperative sagittal image. *B,* Preoperative coronal image. *C,* Postoperative sagittal image. *D,* Postoperative coronal image.

5. For lesions that involve the lower clivus and the upper cervical region, and that extend laterally into the occipital condyle and the jugular bulb on one side, the extreme lateral, transcondyle approach is particularly well suited.

Other anterior approaches can be utilized, including the following:

1. The transsphenoethmoidal approach[80] provides access to the entire sphenoid sinus, prepontine space, and superior clivus; a limited medial maxillectomy improves access to the inferior clivus.
2. The transfacial approach[92] is indicated for extradural tumors confined on the midline and extending from the level of the sellar floor to the foramen magnum. This approach offers direct access to the clivus along its rostrocaudal extent up to the anterior arch of C1; with depression of the palate, the odontoid can also be visualized. The main advantage is to add, by this single facial route, the possibilities of the transsphenoidal and transoral routes, avoiding any injury to the hard and soft palate. The disadvantages are a facial scar and osteotomy of the facial skeleton.

Transsphenoidal Approach

The transsphenoidal approach provides excellent exposure to chordomas of the sphenoid sinus, sella turcica, and upper and middle clivus (see Fig. 66-2), minimizing the morbidity of more complex surgical approaches[13,16,74,84] with a route that, when necessary, can easily be repeated. The technique utilized for the sublabial, transseptal transsphenoidal procedure has already been described.[102] Extensive experience obtained with pituitary tumors[103,104] and with craniopharyngiomas[105] has made this route safe and effective, even for other pathologies (Figs. 66-3 to 66-6). Some papers have been published about the results obtained regarding chordomas.[74,82,83] These reports clearly indicate that gross

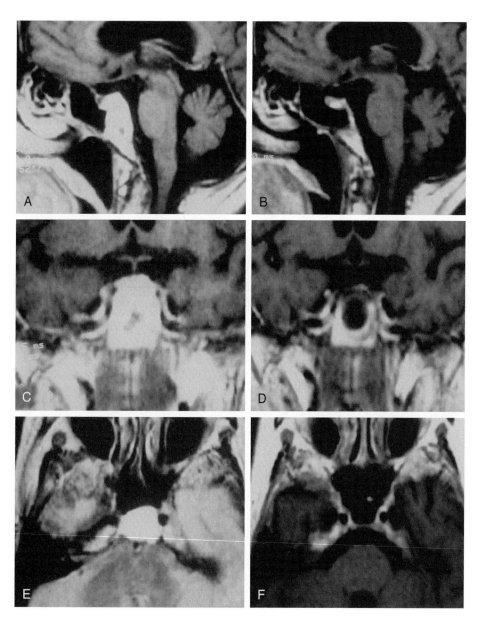

FIGURE 66-4 The transsphenoidal approach. An upper and middle clivus chordoma with a retroclival intradural diffusion (E). Contrast-enhanced magnetic resonance imaging is used. A, Preoperative sagittal image. B, Postoperative sagittal image. C, Preoperative coronal image. D, Postoperative coronal image. E, Preoperative axial image. F, Postoperative axial image.

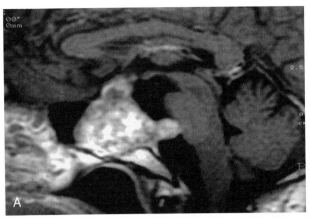

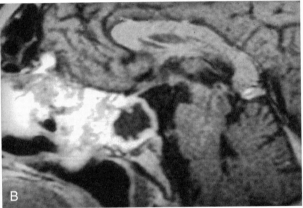

FIGURE 66-5 The transsphenoidal approach. An upper and middle clivus chordoma with an intradural retroclival nodule compressing the brain stem. Contrast-enhanced magnetic resonance imaging is used. *A,* Preoperative sagittal image. *B,* Early postoperative sagittal image (1 month after surgery).

total removal of the tumor can be achieved in up to 70% of cases, with excellent long-term survival and no evidence of disease in all patients at a mean of 38.6 months after surgery.[74]

The main disadvantages of this approach are represented by the limited lateral exposure and the deep and narrow field. Nevertheless, the correct use of long and angled curets can allow a skillful surgeon to remove even large tumors (greater than 4 cm) that are not strictly confined to the midline.[68] Application of endoscopy to the transsphenoidal route may increase the approach and allow even very extended tumors to be removed.[45]

When the tumor is found to be located extraintradurally, an opening of the dura mater can be realized to remove the intradural tumor. Afterward, an accurate reconstruction must be realized. The authors usually use a dural patch and glue or fat tissue graft and human fibrin.

Transoral Approach

The transoral route is indicated for extradural lesions of the inferior clivus confined to the midline, protruding into the posterior pharyngeal region, and extended to C1 to C2 (see Fig. 66-2). The approach provides a good exposure with limited surgical trauma.[65,106] This route has been used for many years for epidural tumors of the cervical spine.[107]

Many reports have described the utilization of this surgical route to treat clivus chordomas.[108–110]

A modified transoral version has been described for these lesions.[95,98] It combines the Le Fort I osteotomy with a midline incision of the hard and soft palate and allows lateral swinging of the two flaps of the hard palate based on their own palatine artery and nerves. The advantage is extensive exposure of the region, inferiorly and laterally (Fig. 66-7); the wound must be closed carefully in order to preserve occlusion and functioning of the palate. A unilateral Le Fort I osteotomy can be realized for laterally growing tumors.[99] Neuronavigation in transoral approach has been found to be a useful tool for planning and checking the limits of resection and for reducing morbidity in chordoma surgery.[44]

Subfrontal Transbasal Approach or Extended Frontal Approach

This route can be utilized for chordomas with both intradural and extradural extension and with extensive involvement of the clivus and surrounding structures.[5] The approach is a modification of the "transbasal approach" of Derome.[13,111,112] After a bifrontal craniotomy (including the orbital roof and nasal bones), the anterior skull base is exposed extradurally on both sides (Fig. 66-8; see also Fig. 66-2). The planum sphenoidale and part of the anterior wall of the sella are removed. The clivus is reached anterior to the sella and exposed up to the rim of the foramen magnum (see Fig. 66-2). If the lesion presents an intradural expansion, the frontal dura is opened. It also allows for the removal of tumors that extend near to the clivus (i.e., the frontal suprasellar region, orbits, paranasal sinuses, and temporal fossa). This approach has been also used for different tumors such as craniopharyngiomas (Fig. 66-9), meningiomas, or pituitary tumors.

Extreme Lateral Transcondylar Approach

The approach is useful for the management of both intradural and extradural lesions that involve the lower clival and foramen magnum regions (Fig. 66-10), with extension into the occipital condyles and the jugular bulb on one side and the upper cervical spine.[15,26,113,114] The technical steps of the approach are well described by many authors.[8,26,43,66,101,112] The main advantage of this route is the direct view that it offers to the ventral aspect of the foramen magnum without requiring brain stem retraction.

The patient is placed in a full lateral decubitus position, with the head in the neutral position. After skin incision and muscle dissection, the lateral mass of C1 is exposed and the vertebral artery is unroofed in the foramen transversarium of C1. Then a C1 laminotomy and suboccipital craniotomy are performed. The occipital condyle and the lateral mass of C1 are partly removed. The vertebral artery is transposed during the dural opening.

Postoperative Adjunctive Radiotherapy

Although the definitive modality for treating clival chordomas is surgical resection, an adjunctive treatment can be considered in selected cases. A correlation between radiation dose and length of the disease-free interval has been

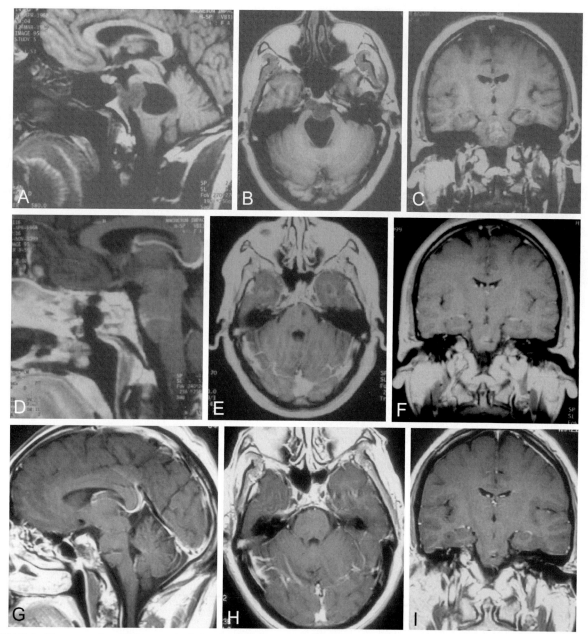

FIGURE 66-6 The transsphenoidal approach. A chordoma of the middle clivus with intradural retroclival extension causing an unusual intra-axial CSF cystic dilation. Contrast enhanced T1-weighted magnetic resonance images. *A,* Preoperative sagittal image. *B,* Preoperative axial image. *C,* Preoperative coronal image. *D,* Postoperative sagittal image (6 months after surgery). *E,* Postoperative axial image (6 months after surgery). *F,* Postoperative coronal image (6 months after surgery). *G,* Postoperative sagittal image (5 years after surgery). *H,* Postoperative axial image (5 years after surgery). *I,* Postoperative coronal image (5 years after surgery).

indicated,[115] but the prevailing opinion is somewhat skeptical as to the actual efficacy of postoperative radiotherapy in the management of chordomas.[116–118] Conventional external beam radiotherapy, after partial or subtotal removal, does not seem to affect the regrowth of the tumor.[119] Nevertheless, a better prognosis for small remnants is achieved with proton beam therapy.[120] Although used in small series, stereotactic radiosurgery, carbon ion radiotherapy, and radiofrequency ablation appear promising options for adjunctive treatment of chordoma tumors.[121–123]

INTRADURAL LESIONS: MENINGIOMAS

Meningiomas of the clivus and apical petrous bone are the most common intradural neoplasms of this region. Their natural history is characterized by a slow but progressive growth that eventually enables these tumors to achieve an enormous size before manifesting neurologic symptoms related to distortion of the brain stem or cranial nerves III to XII. The growth pattern of these tumors may be unpredictable, and factors that influence their growth remain unknown.[124]

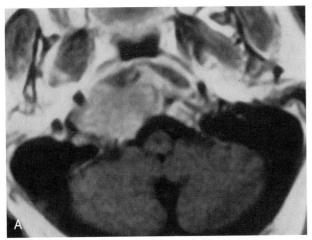

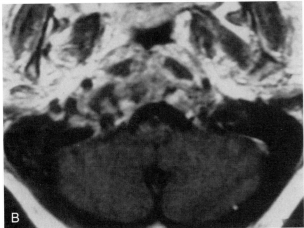

FIGURE 66-7 A modified transoral approach. Le Fort I osteotomy with a midline incision of the hard and soft palate. The middle and lower clivus chordoma are shown with left lateral expansion. Contrast-enhanced magnetic resonance imaging is used. *A*, Preoperative axial image. *B*, Postoperative axial image.

According to Yasargil and associates,[2] these meningiomas may be attached "at any of the lateral sites along the petroclival borderline, where the sphenoidal, petrous and clival bones meet." These authors suggested that such basal tumors could be divided into clival, petroclival, and sphenopetroclival, according to their points of insertion and extent.

Clival meningiomas originate from the clival dura. They are rare and commonly encase the basilar artery and its branches. Petroclival meningiomas are tumors that originate in the upper two thirds of the clivus at the petroclival junction, medial to the entry of the trigeminal root in Meckel's cave.[2,125,126] These meningiomas often displace the basilar artery and the brain stem on the opposite side; however, in up to 25%, there is encasement of the artery.[127] Sphenopetroclival meningiomas are the most extensive of these lesions, involving the clivus and the petrous apex. These meningiomas invade the posterior cavernous sinus and the sphenoid sinus, and grow into the middle and posterior fossae.[126]

Classification of meningiomas of this area can also be based on the anatomic location of the tumor with reference to the clivus (i.e., upper, middle, or lower) and to the

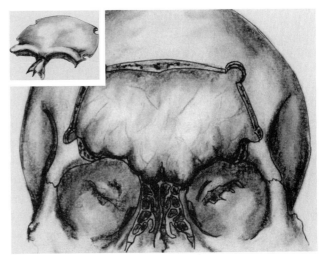

FIGURE 66-8 A subfrontal transbasal approach using a bifrontal craniotomy, including the orbital roof and nasal bones.

size and volume of the tumor (i.e., medium, up to 2.5 cm in average diameter; large, 2.5 to 4.5 cm; and giant, more than 4.5 cm).[128]

Structures that are in close proximity to the clivus may often be involved because of the growth of the tumor. Meningiomas of the upper clivus may involve the cavernous sinus, sella turcica, Meckel's cave, and tentorial notch; meningiomas of the middle clivus may involve the cerebellopontine angle; meningiomas of the lower clivus may involve the jugular bulb, hypoglossal foramina, and upper cervical region.

The location and volume of the tumor, its consistency and vascularity, the presence or absence of a subarachnoid plane between the meningioma and the brain stem, arterial and nervous displacement or encasement, and correct choice of the surgical approach are the factors that, ultimately, decide the extent of the surgical resection and the quality of the results.

Surgical Treatment

For safe excision of these deep tumors, an adequate exposure (with a low or basal approach to limit or avoid brain retraction) is necessary. The combined supratentorial and infratentorial approach, which Malis called the petrosal approach,[9,20,129] was the first progress in the surgical exposure of the petroclival region. Thereafter, several surgical approaches were proposed to reach tumors in this region.[66,12,130–132] In these approaches, the petrous part of the temporal bone is often removed to reduce retraction of the temporal lobe and cerebellum and to provide better exposure of the clivus and ventral surface of the brain stem.

Surgical removal of the petrous bone was first used by King in 1970.[133] Limited anterior resection (anterior transpetrosal approach), with preservation of hearing, was reported by Kawase and associates in 1985.[134] Since then, the transpetrosal approach has received many modifications and has become a relevant part of the surgical approaches to the clivus and brain stem.* As suggested by Miller and associates,[139]

---

*References 14,18,22,23,29–32,34,35,37,38,40–42,78,135–138.

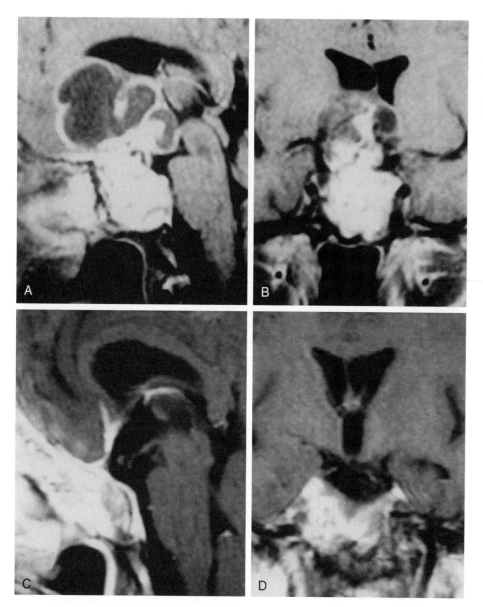

FIGURE 66-9 A subfrontal transbasal approach. An intraextradural craniopharyngioma with sellar, suprasellar, and retroclival extension is shown. Contrast-enhanced magnetic resonance imaging is used. *A,* Preoperative sagittal image. *B,* Preoperative coronal image. *C,* Postoperative sagittal image. *D,* Postoperative coronal image.

transpetrosal approaches can be divided basically into two types: (1) anterior petrosectomy, for lesions of the petrous apex and superior half of the clivus, and (2) posterior petrosectomy, for lesions of the petroclival area and cerebellopontine angle.

Meningiomas of the petroclival region are reached through several routes that pass through the middle or posterior fossa (Fig. 66-11 and Table 66-1):

1. Anterolateral route: frontotemporal transsylvian approach (usually combined with an orbitozygomatic osteotomy) for tumors of the upper clivus and tentorial notch
2. Lateral route: anterior subtemporal approach with zygomatic osteotomy and anterior petrosectomy, for tumors of the petrous apex and upper half of the clivus
3. Posterolateral route:
    - Posterior subtemporal suboccipital presigmoid approach with posterior petrosectomy for centrolateral

midclival and petrous apex lesions. (In case of extensive meningiomas, this route can be combined with the anterior subtemporal approach.)
- Retrosigmoid approach for lateral, small, and medium-sized tumors of the midclivus (which are eventually combined with the previous approach)
- Extreme lateral transcondylar approach for tumors of the lower clivus, foramen magnum, and cervical spine

Frontotemporal Transsylvian Approach

This approach provides good exposure for removal of small tumors in the upper clivus and tentorial notch. If necessary, exposure of the floor of the middle fossa can be also obtained by performing a zygomatic or orbitozygomatic osteotomy with inferior displacement of the temporalis muscle.[17,140,141]

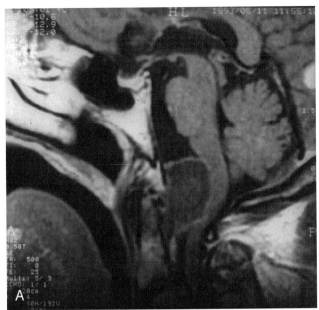

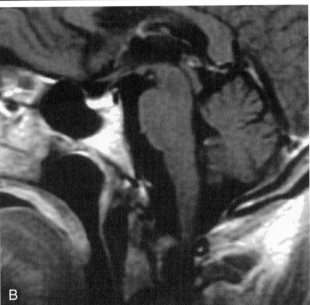

FIGURE 66-10 An extreme lateral transcondylar approach. Lower clivus and upper cervical chordoma. Contrast-enhanced magnetic resonance imaging is used. *A,* Preoperative sagittal image. *B,* Postoperative sagittal image.

Anterior Subtemporal Approach with Anterior Petrosectomy

This approach is indicated for lesions of the tip of the petrous bone or for those involving the middle upper clival area that do not extend behind the internal auditory canal.[19] This approach is also indicated when the greater part of the tumor is in the middle fossa, involving the cavernous sinus.[25,41,128]

An anterior temporal craniotomy is performed, followed by an orbitozygomatic osteotomy to extend the exposure of the conventional craniotomy anteriorly or inferiorly. The superior orbital fissure and the foramen ovale are exposed. To increase exposure at the petrous apex and midclivus, a part of the petrous bone is removed. Kawase and co-workers[19] described a

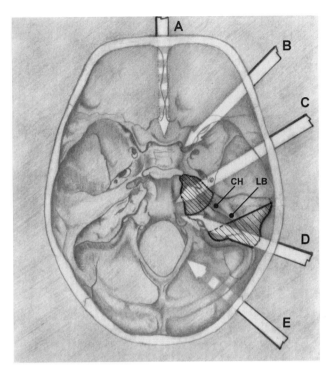

FIGURE 66-11 Approaches to the clivus: Anterior approaches (*A*); frontotemporal approach (*B*); anterior subtemporal approach with an anterior petrosectomy (*C*); presigmoid retrolabyrinthine approach with a posterior petrosectomy (*D*); extreme lateral transcondylar approach (*E*). (CH, cochlea; LB, labyrinth.)

triangle in the petrous bone (lateral to the trigeminal nerve and medial to the internal auditory meatus) that can be drilled, thus providing a route toward the lesions located in the region of the midclivus (see Fig. 66-11). Anteroinferiorly to this area is the horizontal segment of the petrous carotid artery. The petrous apex can be drilled at the Glasscock triangle (demarcated laterally by a line from the foramen spinosum toward the arcuate eminence ending at the facial hiatus; medially by the greater petrosal nerve; and, at the base, by the third trigeminal nerve division).[139] The exposure can be further increased by anterior displacement of the carotid artery or by drilling the region

TABLE 66-1 ▪ Choice of Surgical Approach in Relation to the Location of the Tumor

Location of Lesion	Surgical Approach
Upper clivus	1. Frontotemporal approach with orbitozygomatic osteotomy
	2. Subtemporal approach with a zygomatic osteotomy and an anterior petrosectomy
Upper and middle third of the clivus	1. Subtemporal craniotomy with an anterior petrosectomy
	2. Subtemporal-suboccipital craniotomy with a posterior petrosectomy
Lower third of the clivus	Extreme lateral transcondylar approach
Middle and lower third of the clivus	Combined posterior petrosectomy with an extreme lateral approach
Entire clivus through the level of the foramen magnum	Far lateral/combined supratentorial and infratentorial approach (including posterior petrosectomy or total petrosectomy)

of the cochlea and thus sacrificing hearing. During this procedure, care should be taken not to damage the abducens nerve that runs through Dorello's canal just medial to this area.

The approach to the clivus can be obtained by the simple fenestration of the petrous bone and attached tentorium[19] or with an intradural transtentorial approach.[64,137] In the latter case, an intradural and extradural subtemporal approach is combined with division of the tentorium and with intradural removal of the petrous bone from its apex to the cochlea.

Taniguchi and Perneczky[138] suggested the application of the keyhole concept during surgery of petroclival lesions; this involves the reduction of the conventional approach to its essential parts. The concept to restrict petrous bone removal to obtain the necessary exposure in individual cases has also been applied by several neurosurgeons.[29,34,42,56,62]

Subtemporo-Suboccipital Presigmoid Approach with a Posterior Petrosectomy

In 1992, Spetzler and associates[27] summarized neurosurgical approaches that required a posterior petrosectomy into three groups:

- Group 1: approach that preserves hearing
- Group 2: approaches involving sacrifice of hearing
- Group 3: approaches involving mobilization of the facial nerve

Approach That Preserves Hearing

The presigmoid, retrolabyrinthine, transmastoid approach is most suitable for tumors of the clivus with extension in the middle and posterior fossa. This approach provides excellent exposure of the region ventral to the midbrain and pons. Described by Hakuba and associates[142] in 1977 and refined by Al-Mefty and associates,[7,30] this approach requires a low posterior temporal craniotomy and a lateral retrosigmoid craniotomy.[135] A mastoidectomy is performed to expose the sigmoid sinus, the dura mater of the posterior cranial fossa situated anteriorly to the sinus, and the labyrinth. The sinus must be unroofed along its entire course to provide adequate length for mobilization, and the labyrinthine complex must be skeletonized completely from mastoid cells in order to gain as much space as possible (Fig. 66-12). A labyrinthectomy minimally improves access to the posterior fossa; its use should be avoided unless hearing has been irreversibly lost. Some authors have suggested the use of a partial labyrinthectomy to widen the exposure from the presigmoid route without affecting hearing.[34,143]

The dura mater of the posterior cranial fossa is incised anteriorly to the sigmoid sinus, and this incision is joined to that of the dura mater of the middle cranial fossa, thus preserving the sigmoid sinus as described by Al-Mefty.[135] The superior petrosal sinus is then resected, and the tentorium is incised (see Fig. 66-12). The fourth nerve is identified by moving the edge of the tentorium. A crucial

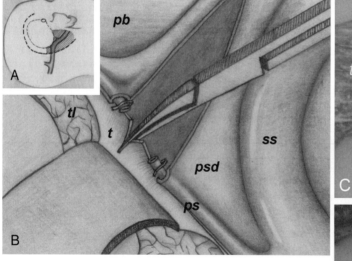
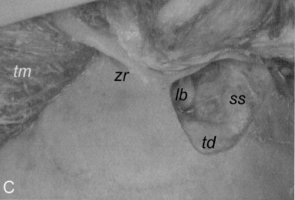
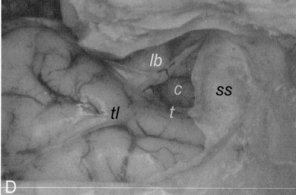

FIGURE 66-12 Presigmoid retrolabyrinthine approach. *A,* Temporal craniotomy, retrolabyrinthine craniectomy and petrosectomy. *B,* Incision of tentorium after opening of the presigmoid and temporal dura. *C,* Cadaveric specimen, right side. Temporalis muscle reflected, extralabyrinthine petrosectomy with exposure of presigmoid dura. *D,* Cadaveric specimen, right side. Temporal and presigmoid dura opened, superior petrosal sinus ligated and cut, tentorium incised. (c, cerebellum; lb, labyrinthine block; pb, petrous bone; ps, petrous sinus; psd, presigmoid dura; ss, sigmoid sinus; t, tentorium; td, temporal dura; tl, temporal lobe; tm, temporalis muscle; zr, zygomatic root.)

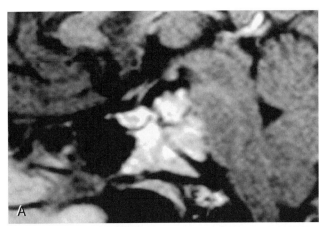

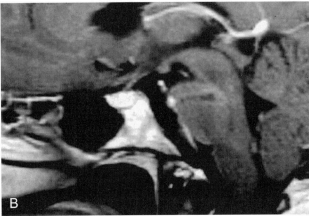

FIGURE 66-13 A presigmoid retrolabyrinthine approach. Central meningioma of the upper and middle clivus. Contrast-enhanced magnetic resonance imaging is used. *A,* Preoperative sagittal image. *B,* Postoperative sagittal image.

step in the petrosal approach is the identification and preservation of the venous drainage of the posterior temporal lobe (i.e., the vein of Labbè and other basal veins). The transverse sinus may be divided to obtain improved exposure of structures below the auditory canal; this can be performed for patients who have good patency of the contralateral venous sinuses.

The advantages of this approach include minimal cerebellar and temporal lobe retraction and shortening of the operative distance to the tumor by 3 cm when compared with the retrosigmoid approach. The surgeon has surgical access more anterior and closer to the clivus, the latter factor being very important for the removal of lesions with a central location anterior to the brain stem (Figs. 66-13 and 66-14). Disadvantages are temporal lobe retraction and the possibility of injury to the vein of Labbè. Furthermore, paralysis of the lower cranial nerves constitutes one of the major sources of morbidity. Exposure of the lower clivus is limited by the jugular bulb, especially when it is high.

Access to the foramen magnum and inferior clivus can be improved by adding a retrosigmoid dural opening with anterolateral retraction of the sinus. If the lesion extends forward, one has to consider combining this approach with an anterior subtemporal zygomatic approach. Variants include the partial labyrinthectomy petrous apicectomy approach,[41,56] extended lateral subtemporal approach,[38] and anterior subtemporal medial transpetrosal approach.[42]

Approaches Involving Sacrifice of Hearing

The presigmoid translabyrinthine approach is an anterior extension of the presigmoid retrolabyrinthine approach. The approach involves the removal of the semicircular canals, thus enhancing the exposure. The transcochlear approach involves the anterior extension of the translabyrinthine approach.[32,144]

A combination of the transcochlear approach with more extensive bone removal and anterior mobilization of the petrous internal carotid artery is called a total petrosectomy approach.[66]

Approaches Involving Mobilization of the Facial Nerve

Various elaborate transpetrous approaches have been described, some of which involve mobilization of the facial nerve. A total petrosectomy approach has been described by Sekhar and associates.[128,137] The approach requires unroofing of the entire facial nerve and its posterior mobilization and anterior displacement of the petrous carotid artery.

Retrosigmoid Approach

A retrosigmoid approach is generally indicated for lateral, small, and medium-sized tumors of the midclivus. The approach is easy but it requires the surgeon to work between the cranial nerves and blood vessels in the cerebellopontine angle and does not provide adequate exposure of more medial or contralateral extensions of the lesion.[145] Samii, who advocates the simple retrosigmoid route even for large petroclival meningiomas,[36] has recently described an elegant variant, the retrosigmoid intradural suprameatal approach, in which the suprameatus petrous bone is drilled, thus providing access to Meckel's cave and the middle fossa.[37] Samii's school is going to develop surgical "corridors" along the dural structures of the sphenopetroclival area in order to reach the lateral sellar compartment via the posterior fossa.[55]

Extreme Lateral Transcondylar Approach

This approach has already been described among the approaches for extradural lesions.

Far Lateral/Combined Approach

This approach combines the far lateral approach with subtemporal and transpetrosal exposures to gain an extensive view of the entire petroclival region in the event of tumors involving the entire clivus and also extending to the craniocervical region.[146,147] The model incorporates a subtemporal craniotomy and posterior petrous bone resection into the far lateral approach to obtain an unobstructed view of the entire clivus and ventral brain stem.

Surgical Adjuvants

1. Vascular embolization: Preoperative embolization of the external carotid artery feeders can be helpful in reducing intraoperative bleeding.
2. Intraoperative lumbar drainage of CSF: Drainage of CSF is an important adjuvant to help relaxation of the brain.

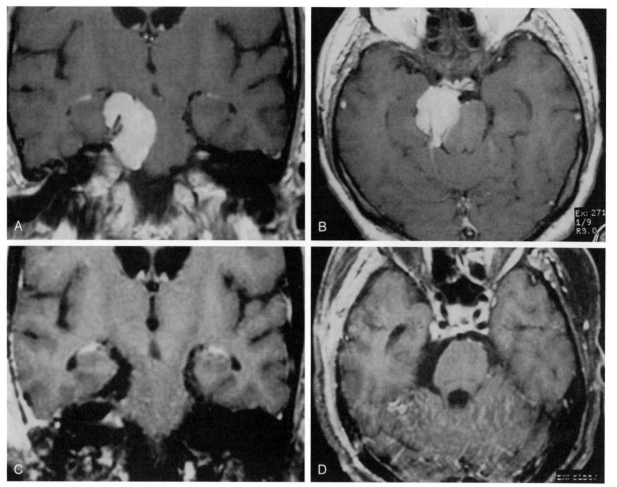

FIGURE 66-14 A presigmoid retrolabyrinthine approach. Petroclival meningiomas. Contrast-enhanced magnetic resonance imaging is used. *A,* Preoperative coronal image. *B,* Preoperative axial image. *C,* Postoperative coronal image. *D,* Postoperative axial image.

3. Intraoperative monitoring of the brain and cranial nerve functions: This includes somatosensory evoked potential, auditory brain stem evoked potential, and monitoring of cranial nerves III, IV, VI, VII, X, XI, and XII.

4. Frameless stereotactic navigation: This improves the exposure and reduces the risks.

5. Contact neodymium:yttrium-aluminum-garnet laser: This increases the achievement of total removal, which can be realized faster and with less bleeding.[58]

6. Arterial bypass: When the tumor encases the petrous or cavernous carotid artery, if the patient fails the balloon occlusion test and vascular ligation is necessary, a vascular reconstruction is mandatory using a saphenous vein graft bypass or using an extracranial-intracranial arterial bypass.[148]

7. Adequate reconstruction of the skull base to prevent CSF leakage: This is done by placing a pericranial flap or autologous fat and biologic glue.

8. Radiosurgery can be helpful for treating small remnants in critical areas.

9. Postoperative hydroxyurea therapy has been shown to stabilize and even to reduce the size of residual petroclival meningiomas.[149,150]

REFERENCES

1. Sekhar LN, Goel A, Sen CN: Extradural clival tumors. In Apuzzo MLJ (ed): Brain Surgery: Complication Avoidance and Management. New York: Churchill Livingstone, 1993, pp 2221–2244.
2. Yasargil MG, Mortara RW, Curcic M: Meningiomas of the posterior cranial fossa. In Krayenbuhl H (ed): Advances and Technical Standards in Neurosurgery, vol 7. New York: Springer-Verlag, 1980, pp 4–115.
3. Lang J: Anatomy of clivus. In Samii M, Draf W (eds): Surgery of the Skull Base. Berlin: Springer-Verlag, 1989, pp 90–101.
4. Meyers SP, Hirsch WL, Curtin HD, et al: Chondrosarcomas of the skull base: MR imaging features. Radiology 184:103–108, 1992.
5. Gay E, Sekhar LN, Wright DC: Chordomas and chondrosarcomas of the cranial base. In Kaye AH, Laws ER Jr (eds): Brain Tumors. Edinburgh: Churchill Livingstone, 1995, pp 777–794.
6. Goel A: Chordomas and chondrosarcomas: Relationship to the internal carotid artery. Acta Neurochir (Wien) 133:30–35, 1995.
7. Al-Mefty O, Fox JL, Smith RR: Petrosal approach for petroclival meningiomas. Neurosurgery 22:510–517, 1988.
8. Bertalanffy H, Seeger W: The dorsolateral, suboccipital, transcondylar approach to the lower clivus and anterior portion of the craniocervical junction. Neurosurgery 129:815–821, 1991.
9. Bonnal J, Louis R, Combalbert A: L'abord temporal transtentoriel de l'angle ponto-cerebelleux et du clivus. Neurochirurgie 10:3–12, 1964.
10. Bricolo A, Turazzi S, Cristofori L, et al: Microsurgical removal of petroclival meningiomas: A report of 33 patients. Neurosurgery 31:813–828, 1992.
11. Cantore GP, Ciappetta P, Delfini R: Choice of neurosurgical approach in the treatment of cranial base lesions. Neurosurg Rev 17:109–125, 1994.

12. Crockard HA, Sen CN: The transoral approach for the management of intradural lesions at the craniovertebral junction: Review of 7 cases. Neurosurgery 28:88–98, 1991.
13. Derome PJ, Guiot G: Surgical approaches to the sphenoidal and clival area. In Krayenbuhl H (ed): Advances and Technical Standards in Neurosurgery, vol 6. New York: Springer-Verlag, 1979, pp 101–136.
14. Fisch U, Kumar A: Infratemporal surgery of the skull base. In Rand RW (ed): Microneurosurgery, 3rd ed. St. Louis: CV Mosby, 1985, pp 421–454.
15. George B, Dematons C, Copignon J: Lateral approach to the anterior portion of the foramen magnum: Application to surgical removal of 14 benign tumors: Technical note. Surg Neurol 29:484–490, 1988.
16. Hardy J: L'abord transsphenoidal des tumeurs du clivus. Neurochirurgie 23:287–297, 1977.
17. Hakuba A, Liu S, Nishimura S: The orbitozygomatic infratemporal approach: A new surgical technique. Surg Neurol 26:271–276, 1986.
18. Hakuba A, Nishimura S, Jang BJ: A combined retroauricular and preauricular transpetrosal-transtentorial approach to clivus meningiomas. Surg Neurol 30:108–116, 1988.
19. Kawase T, Shiobara R, Toya S: Anterior transpetrosal-transtentorial approach for sphenopetroclival meningiomas: Surgical method and results in 10 patients. Neurosurgery 28:869–876, 1991.
20. Malis LI: Surgical resection of tumors of the skull base. In Wilkins RH, Rengashary SS (eds): Neurosurgery, vol 1. New York: McGraw-Hill, 1985, pp 1011–1021.
21. Malis L: The petrosal approach. Clin Neurosurg 37:528–540, 1990.
22. Samii M, Ammirati M: The combined supratentorial presigmoid sinus avenue to the petroclival region: Surgical technique and clinical applications. Acta Neurochir (Wien) 95:6–12, 1988.
23. Samii M, Ammirati M, Maharan A, et al: Surgery of petroclival meningiomas: Report of 24 cases. Neurosurgery 24:12–17, 1989.
24. Sekhar LN, Jannetta PJ, Burkhart LE, et al: Meningiomas involving the clivus: A six year experience with 41 patients. Neurosurgery 27:764–781, 1990.
25. Sekhar LN, Sen CN, Snyderman CH, et al: Anterior, anterolateral and lateral approaches to extradural petroclival tumors. In Sekhar LN, Janecka IP (eds): Surgery of Cranial Base Tumors. New York: Raven Press, 1993, pp 157–223.
26. Sen CN, Sekhar LN: An extreme lateral approach to intradural lesions of the cervical spine and foramen magnum. Neurosurgery 27:197–204, 1990.
27. Spetzler RF, Daspit CP, Pappas CTE: The combined supra and infratentorial approach for lesions of the petrous and clival regions: Experience with 46 cases. J Neurosurg 76:588–599, 1992.
28. Symon L: Surgical approaches to the tentorial hiatus. Advances and Technical Standards in Neurosurgery 9:69–112, 1982.
29. Seifert V, Raabe A, Zimmermann M: Conservative (labyrinth-preserving) transpetrosal approach to the clivus and petroclival region—indications, complications, results and lessons learned. Acta Neurochir (Wien) 145:631–642, 2003.
30. Cho CW, Al-Mefty O: Combined petrosal approach to petroclival meningiomas. Neurosurgery 51:708–716, 2002.
31. Kirazli T, Oner K, Ovul L, et al: Petrosal presigmoid approach to the petro-clival and anterior cerebellopontine region (extended retro-labyrinthine, transtentorial approach). Rev Laryngol Otol Rhinol (Bord) 122(3):187–190, 2001.
32. Angeli SI, De la Cruz A, Hitselberger W: The transcochlear approach revisited. Otol Neurotol 22:690–695, 2001.
33. Roberti F, Sekhar LN, Kalavakonda C, et al: Posterior fossa meningiomas: Surgical experience in 161 cases. Surg Neurol 56:8–20, 2001.
34. Horgan MA, Delashaw JB, Schwartz MS, et al: Transcrusal approach to the petroclival region with hearing preservation: Technical note and illustrative cases. J Neurosurg 94:660–666, 2001.
35. Abdel Aziz KM, Sanan A, van Loveren HR, et al: Petroclival meningiomas: Predictive parameters for transpetrosal approaches. Neurosurgery 47:139–150, 2000.
36. Samii M, Tatagiba M, Carvalho GA: Resection of large petroclival meningiomas by the simple retrosigmoid route. J Clin Neurosci 6:27–30, 1999.
37. Samii M, Tatagiba M, Carvalho GA: Retrosigmoid intradural suprameatal approach to Meckel's cave and the middle fossa: surgical technique and outcome. J Neurosurg 92:235–241, 2000.
38. Goel A: Extended lateral subtemporal approach for petroclival meningiomas: Report of experience with 24 cases. Br J Neurosurg 13:270–275, 1999.
39. Lang DA, Neil-Dwyer G, Garfield J: Outcome after complex neurosurgery: The caregiver's burden is forgotten. J Neurosurg 91:359–363, 1999.
40. Spallone A, Makhmudov UB, Mukhamedjanov DJ, et al: Petroclival meningioma: An attempt to define the role of skull base approaches in their surgical management. Surg Neurol 51:412–419, 1999.
41. Sekhar LN, Schessel DA, Bucur SD, et al: Partial labyrinthectomy petrous apicectomy approach to neoplastic and vascular lesions of the petroclival area. Neurosurgery 44:537–550, 1999.
42. MacDonald JD, Antonelli P, Day AL: The anterior subtemporal, medial transpetrosal approach to the upper basilar artery and pontomesencephalic junction. Neurosurgery 43:84–89, 1998.
43. Babu RP, Sekhar LN, Wright DC: Extreme lateral transcondylar approach: Technical improvements and lessons learned. J Neurosurg 81:49–59, 1994.
44. Vougioukas VI, Hubbe U, Schipper J, et al: Navigated transoral approach to the cranial base and the craniocervical junction: Technical note. Neurosurgery 52:247–250, 2003.
45. de Divitiis E, Cappabianca P, Cavallo LM: Endoscopic transsphenoidal approach: Adaptability of the procedure to different sellar lesions. Neurosurgery 51:699–705, 2002.
46. Crockard HA, Cheeseman A, Steel T, et al: A multidisciplinary team approach to skull base chondrosarcomas. J Neurosurg 95:184–189, 2001.
47. Crockard HA, Steel T, Plowman N, et al: A multidisciplinary team approach to skull base chordomas. J Neurosurg 95:175–183, 2001.
48. Colli B, Al-Mefty O: Chordomas of the craniocervical junction: Follow-up review and prognostic factors. J Neurosurg 95:933–943, 2001.
49. Mortini P, Mandelli C, Franzin A, et al: Surgical excision of clival tumors via the enlarged transcochlear approach: Indications and results. J Neurosurg Sci 45:127–139, 2001.
50. Colreavy MP, Baker T, Campbell M, et al: The safety and effectiveness of the Le Fort I approach to removing central skull base lesions. Ear Nose Throat J 80:315–320, 2001.
51. Bejjani GK, Sekhar LN, Riedel CJ: Occipitocervical fusion following the extreme lateral transcondylar approach. Surg Neurol 54:109–115, 2000.
52. Diaz-Gonzalez FJ, Padron A, Foncea AM, et al: A new transfacial approach for lesions of the clivus and parapharyngeal space: The partial segmented Le Fort I osteotomy. Plast Reconstr Surg 103:955–959, 1999.
53. Nakase H, Ohnishi H, Matsuyama T, et al: Two-stage skull base surgery for tumours extending to the sub- and epidural spaces. Acta Neurochir (Wien) 140:891–898, 1998.
54. Carpentier A, Polivka M, Blanquet A, et al: Suboccipital and cervical chordomas: The value of aggressive treatment at first presentation of the disease. J Neurosurg 97:1070–1077, 2002.
55. Iaconetta G, Fusco M, Samii M: The sphenopetroclival venous gulf: A microanatomical study. J Neurosurg 99:366–375, 2003.
56. Chanda A, Nanda A: Partial labyrinthectomy petrous apicectomy approach to the petroclival region: An anatomic and technical study. Neurosurgery 51:147–159, 2002.
57. Ozveren MF, Uchida K, Aiso S, et al: Meningovenous structures of the petroclival region: Clinical importance for surgery and intravascular surgery. Neurosurgery 50:829–836, 2002.
58. Maira G, Anile C, Vignati A, et al: Advances in treatment of supratentorial meningiomas of the skull base by microsurgical and laser techniques. In Samii M (ed): Skull Base Surgery. Basel: Karger, 1994, pp 190–193.
59. Hirohata M, Abe T, Morimitsu H, et al: Preoperative selective internal carotid artery dural branch embolisation for petroclival meningiomas. Neuroradiology 45:656–660, 2003.
60. Schul C, Wassmann H, Skopp GB, et al: Surgical management of intraosseous skull base tumors with aid of Operating Arm System. Comput Aided Surg 3:312–319, 1998.
61. Villavicencio AT, Gray L, Leveque JC, et al: Utility of three-dimensional computed tomographic angiography for assessment of relationships between the vertebrobasilar system and the cranial base. Neurosurgery 48:318–326, 2001.
62. Kocaogullar Y, Avci E, Fossett D, et al: The extradural subtemporal keyhole approach to the sphenocavernous region: Anatomic considerations. Minim Invasive Neurosurg 46:100–105, 2003.
63. Lang J: Skull Base and Related Structures: Atlas of Clinical Anatomy. New York: Schattauer, 1995, pp 85–86.

64. Harsh GR, Sekhar LN: The subtemporal, transcavernous, anterior transpetrosal approach to the upper brain stem and clivus. J Neurosurg 77:709–717, 1992.

65. Day JD, Koos WT, Matula C, et al: Color Atlas of Microneurosurgical Approaches, vol 1. New York: Thieme, 1997, pp 160–171.

66. Sekhar LN, Goel A: Intradural clival lesion. In Apuzzo MLJ (ed): Brain Surgery: Complication Avoidance and Management. New York: Churchill Livingstone, 1993, pp 2245–2264.

67. Saeger W, Ludecke DK, Muller S, et al: Chordome des clivus: Histologie, Ultrastruktur und Klinik. Tumor Diagnostik Therapie 4:74–79, 1983.

68. Pallini R, Maira G, Pierconti F, et al: Chordoma of the skull base: Predictors of tumor recurrence. J Neurosurg 98:812–822, 2003.

69. Goel A, Kobayashi S: Chordomas: A clinical review. In Kobayashi S, Goel A, Hongo K (eds): Neurosurgery of Complex Tumors and Vascular Lesions. New York: Churchill Livingstone, 1997, pp 293–306.

70. Chambers PW, Schwinn CP: A clinicopathologic study of metastasis. Am J Clin Pathol 72:765–776, 1979.

71. Deniz ML, Kilic T, Almaata I, et al: Expression of growth factors and structural proteins in chordomas: Basic fibroblast growth factor, transforming growth factor alpha, and fibronectin are correlated with recurrence. Neurosurgery 51:753–760, 2002.

72. Rosenberg AE, Nielsen GP, Keel SB, et al: Chondrosarcoma of the base of the skull: A clinicopathologic study of 200 cases with emphasis on its distinction from chordoma. Am J Surg Pathol 23:1370–1378, 1999.

73. Crumley RL, Gutin PH: Surgical access for clivus chordoma: The University of California, San Francisco, experience. Arch Otolaryngol Head Neck Surg 115:295–300, 1989.

74. Maira G, Pallini R, Anile C, et al: Surgical treatment of clival chordomas: The transsphenoidal approach revisited. J Neurosurg 85:784–792, 1996.

75. Al-Mefty O, Fox JL, Rifai A, et al: A combined infratemporal and posterior fossa approach for the removal of giant glomus tumors and chondrosarcomas. Surg Neurol 28:423–431, 1987.

76. Canalis RF, Black K, Martin N, et al: Extended retrolabyrinthine transtentorial approach to petroclival lesions. Laryngoscope 101:6–13, 1991.

77. Gay E, Sekhar LN, Rubinstein E, et al: Chordomas and chondrosarcomas of the cranial base: Results and follow-up of 60 patients. Neurosurgery 36:887–897, 1995.

78. Goel A: Extended middle fossa approach for petroclival lesions. Acta Neurochir (Wien) 135:78–83, 1995.

79. Sen CN, Sekhar LN, Schramm VL, et al: Chordoma and chondrosarcoma of the cranial base: An 8-year experience. Neurosurgery 25:931–941, 1989.

80. Lalwani AK, Kaplan MJ, Gutin PH: The transsphenoethmoid approach to the sphenoid sinus and clivus. Neurosurgery 31:1008–1014, 1992.

81. Laws ER Jr: Transsphenoidal surgery for tumors of the clivus. Otolaryngol Head Neck Surg 92:100–101, 1984.

82. Laws ER Jr: Clivus chordomas. In Sekhar LN, Janecka IP (eds): Surgery of Cranial Base Tumors. New York: Raven Press, 1993, pp 679–685.

83. Raffel C, Wright DC, Gutin PH, et al: Cranial chordomas: Clinical presentation and results of operative and radiation therapy in twenty-six patients. Neurosurgery 17:703–710, 1985.

84. Rougerie J, Guiot G, Bouche J, et al: Les voies d'abord du chordome du clivus. Neurochirurgie 13:559–570, 1967.

85. Jung HW, Yoo H, Paek SH, et al: Long-term outcome and growth rate of subtotally resected petroclival meningiomas: Experience with 38 cases. Neurosurgery 46:567–574, 2000.

86. Harris JP, Godin MS, Krekorian TD, et al: The transoropalatal approach to the atlantoaxial-clival region: Considerations for the head and neck surgeon. Laryngoscope 99:467–474, 1989.

87. Menezes AH, VanGilder JC: Transoral-transpharyngeal approach to the anterior craniocervical junction: Ten-year experience with 72 patients. J Neurosurg 69:895–903, 1988.

88. Price JC: The midfacial degloving approach to the central skull base. Ear Nose Throat J 65:174–180, 1986.

89. Sekhar LN, Nanda A, Sen CN, et al: The extended frontal approach to tumors of the anterior, middle, and posterior skull base. J Neurosurg 76:198–206, 1992.

90. Williams WG, Lo LJ, Chen YR: The Le Fort I-palatal split approach for skull base tumors: Efficacy, complications, and outcome. Plast Reconstr Surg 102:2310–2319, 1998.

91. Rabadan A, Conesa H: Transmaxillary-transnasal approach to the anterior clivus: A microsurgical anatomical model. Neurosurgery 30:473–481, 1992.

92. Swearingen B, Joseph M, Cheney M, et al: A modified transfacial approach to the clivus. Neurosurgery 36:101–105, 1995.

93. Janecka IP, Sen CN, Sekhar LN, et al: Facial translocation: A new approach to the cranial base. Otolaryngol Head Neck Surg 103:413–419, 1990.

94. James D, Crockard HA: Surgical access to the base of the skull and upper cervical spine by exterior maxillotomy. Neurosurgery 29:411–416, 1991.

95. Anand VK, Harkey HL, Al-Mefty O: Open-door maxillotomy approach for lesions of the clivus. Skull Base Surg 1:217–225, 1991.

96. Stevenson GC, Stoney RJ, Perkins RK, et al: A transcervical transclival approach to the ventral surface of the brain stem for removal of a clivus chordoma. J Neurosurg 24:544–551, 1996.

97. George B, Lot G, Velut S, et al: Pathologie tumoral du foramen magnum. Neurochirurgie 39(Suppl 1):1–89, 1993.

98. Sasaki CT, Lowlicht RA, Astrachan DI, et al: Le Fort I osteotomy approach for skull base tumors. Laryngoscope 100:1073–1076, 1990.

99. Bowles AP, Al-Mefty O: The transmaxillary approach to clival chordomas. In Al-Mefty O, Origitano TC, Harkey HL (eds): Controversies in Neurosurgery. New York: Thieme, 1996, pp 115–121.

100. Joseph M: Pedicled rhinotomy for exposure of the clivus. In Schmidek HH, Sweet WH (eds): Operative Neurosurgical Techniques. Philadelphia: WB Saunders, 1995, pp 469–475.

101. Al-Mefty O, Borba LA, Aoki N, et al: The transcondylar approach to extradural nonneoplastic lesions of the craniovertebral junction. J Neurosurg 84:1–6, 1996.

102. Hardy J: Transsphenoidal microsurgery of the normal and pathological pituitary. Clin Neurosurg 16:185–217, 1969.

103. Hardy J: Transsphenoidal microsurgery of prolactinomas: Report on 355 cases. In Tolis G, Stefanis C, Mountokalakis T, et al (eds): Prolactin and Prolactinomas. New York: Raven Press, 1983, pp 431–440.

104. Maira G, Anile C, De Marinis L, et al: Prolactin-secreting adenomas: Surgical results and long-term follow-up. Neurosurgery 24:736–743, 1989.

105. Maira G, Anile C, Rossi GF, et al: Surgical treatment of craniopharyngiomas: An evaluation of the transsphenoidal and pterional approaches. Neurosurgery 36:715–724, 1995.

106. Miller E, Crockard HA: Transoral transclival removal of anteriorly placed meningiomas at the foramen magnum. Neurosurgery 20:966–968, 1987.

107. Mullan S, Naunton R, Hekmat-panach J, et al: The use of an anterior approach to ventrally placed tumours in the foramen magnum and vertebral column. J Neurosurg 24:536–543, 1966.

108. Delgado TE, Garrido E, Harwick R: Labiomandibular, transoral approach to chordomas in the clivus and upper spine. Neurosurgery 8:675–679, 1981.

109. Gutkelch AN, Williams RG: Anterior approach to recurrent chordomas of the clivus. Neurosurgery 36:670–672, 1972.

110. Krayenbuhl H, Yasargil MG: Chondromas. Progr Neurol Surg 6:435–463, 1975.

111. Derome P, Visot A, Monteil JP, et al: Management of cranial chordomas. In Sekhar LN, Schramm VL (eds): Tumors of the Cranial Base. Mount Kisco: Futura, 1987, pp 607–622.

112. Pallini R, Patel S, Salvinelli F, et al: Petroclival tumors. Anterolateral Approaches. In Salvinelli F, De La Cruz A (eds): Otoneurosurgery and Lateral Skull Base Surgery. Philadelphia: Saunders, 1996, pp 457–472.

113. Perneczky A: The posterolateral approach to the foramen magnum. In Samii (ed): Surgery In and Around the Brain Stem and Third Ventricle. New York: Springer-Verlag, 1986, pp 460–466.

114. Spetzler RF, Graham TW: The far lateral approach to the inferior clivus and upper cervical region: Technical note. BNI Q 6:35–38, 1990.

115. Heffelfinger MJ, Dahlin DC, MacCarty CS, et al: Chordomas and cartilaginous tumors at the skull base. Cancer 32:410–420, 1973.

116. Kondziolka D, Lunsford LD, Flickinger JC: The role of radiosurgery in the management of chordoma and chondrosarcoma of the cranial base. Neurosurgery 29:38–46, 1991.

117. Samii M: Comments. In Gay E, Sekhar LN, Rubinstein E, et al: Chordomas and chondrosarcomas of the cranial base: Results and follow-up of 60 cases. Neurosurgery 36:896–897, 1995.

118. Suit HD, Goitein M, Munzenrider J, et al: Definitive radiation therapy for chordoma and chondrosarcoma of base of skull and cervical spine. J Neurosurg 56:377–385, 1982.
119. Keisch ME, Garcia DM, Shibuya RB: Retrospective long-term follow-up analysis in 21 patients with chordoma of various sites treated at a single institution. J Neurosurg 75:374–377, 1991.
120. Austin-Seymour M, Muzenrider J, Goitein M, et al: Fractionated proton radiation therapy of chordoma and low-grade chondrosarcoma of the base of the skull. J Neurosurg 70:13–17, 1989.
121. Crockard A, Macaulay E, Plowman PN: Stereotactic radiosurgery. VI: Posterior displacement of the brainstem facilitates safer high dose radiosurgery for clival chordoma. Br J Neurosurg 13:65–70, 1999.
122. Schulz-Ertner D, Haberer T, Jakel O, et al: Radiotherapy for chordomas and low-grade chondrosarcomas of the skull base with carbon ions. Int J Radiat Oncol Biol Phys 53:36–42, 2002.
123. Neeman Z, Patti JW, Wood BJ: Percutaneous radiofrequency ablation of chordoma. Am J Roentgenol 179:1330–1332, 2002.
124. Van Havenbergh T, Carvalho G, Tatagiba M, et al: Natural history of petroclival meningiomas. Neurosurgery 52:55–62, 2003.
125. Goel A, Nitta J, Kobayashi S: Surgical approaches to clival lesions. In Kobayashi S, Goel A, Hongo K (eds): Neurosurgery of Complex Tumors and Vascular Lesions. New York: Churchill Livingstone, 1997, pp 181–210.
126. Al-Mefty O: Operative Atlas of Meningiomas. Philadelphia: Lippincott Raven, 1998.
127. Long DM: Surgical approaches to tumors of skull base: An overview. In Wilkins RH, Rengachary SS (eds): Neurosurgery Update. I: Diagnosis, Operative Technique and Neuro-oncology. New York: McGraw-Hill, 1990, pp 266–276.
128. Sekhar LN, Javed T, Jannetta PJ: Petroclival meningiomas. In Sekhar LN, Janecka IP (eds): Surgery of Cranial Base Tumors. New York: Raven Press, 1993, pp 605–659.
129. Luyendijk W: Operative approaches to the posterior fossa. In Krayenbuhl H (ed): Advances and Technical Standards in Neurosurgery, vol 3. New York: Springer-Verlag, 1976, pp 81–101.
130. Mayberg MR, Symon L: Meningiomas of the clivus and apical petrous bone: Report of 35 cases. J Neurosurg 65:160–167, 1986.
131. Samii M, Draf W: Surgery of the skull base. Berlin: Springer-Verlag, 1989, pp 209–348.
132. Cantore GP, Delfini R, Ciappetta P: Surgical treatment of petroclival meningiomas: Experience with 16 cases. Surg Neurol 42: 105–111, 1994.
133. King TT: Combined translabyrinthine-transtentorial approach to acoustic nerve tumors. Proc R Soc Med 63:780–782, 1970.
134. Kawase T, Toya S, Shiobara R, et al: Transpetrosal approach for aneurysms of the lower basilar artery. J Neurosurg 63:857–861, 1985.
135. Al-Mefty O: Surgery of the Cranial Base. Boston: Kluwer, 1988, pp 239–258.
136. Sen CN, Sekhar LN: The subtemporal and preauricular infratemporal approach to intradural structures ventral to the brain stem. J Neurosurg 73:345–354, 1990.
137. Sekhar LN, Pomeranz S, Janecka IP, et al: Temporal bone neoplasms: A report on 20 surgically treated cases. J Neurosurg 76:578–587, 1992.
138. Taniguchi M, Perneczky A: Subtemporal keyhole approach to the suprasellar and petroclival region: Microanatomic considerations and clinical applications. Neurosurgery 41:592–601, 1997.
139. Miller CG, van Loveren HR, Keller JT, et al: Transpetrosal approach: Surgical anatomy and technique. Neurosurgery 33:461–469, 1993.
140. Pellerin P, Lesoin F, Dhellemmes P, et al: Usefulness of the orbitofrontomalar approach associated with bone reconstruction for frontotemporosphenoid meningiomas. Neurosurgery 15:715–718, 1984.
141. Zabramski JM, Kiris T, Sankhla SK, et al: Orbitozygomatic craniotomy: Technical note. J Neurosurg 89:336–341, 1998.
142. Hakuba A, Nishimura A, Tanaka K, et al: Clivus meningiomas: Six cases of total removal. Neurol Med Chir (Tokyo) 17:63–77, 1977.
143. Hirsch BE, Cass SP, Sekhar LN, et al: Translabyrinthine approach to skull base tumors with hearing preservation. Am J Otol 14:533–543, 1993.
144. House WF, Hitselberger WE: The transcochlear approach to the skull base. Arch Otolaryngol 102:334, 1976.
145. Lang J Jr, Samii M: Retrosigmoidal approach to the posterior cranial fossa: An anatomical study. Acta Neurochir (Wien) 111:147–153, 1991.
146. Baldwin HZ, Miller CG, van Loveren HR, et al: The far lateral-combined supra- and infratentorial approach: A human cadaveric prosection model for routes of access to the petroclival region and ventral brain stem. J Neurosurg 81:60–68, 1994.
147. Baldwin HZ, Spetzler RF, Wascher TM, et al: The far lateral-combined supra- and infratentorial approach: Clinical experience. Acta Neurochir (Wien) 134:155–158, 1995.
148. Linskey ME, Sekhar LN, Sen C: Cerebral revascularization in cranial base surgery. In Sekhar LN, Janecka IP (eds): Surgery of Cranial Base Tumors. New York: Raven Press, 1993, pp 45–68.
149. Schrell UM, Rittig MG, Anders M, et al: Hydroxyurea for treatment of unresectable and recurrent meningiomas. II: Decrease in the size of meningiomas in patients treated with hydroxyurea. J Neurosurg 86:840–844, 1997.
150. Mason WP, Gentili F, Macdonald DR, et al: Stabilization of disease progression by hydroxyurea in patients with recurrent or unresectable meningioma. J Neurosurg 97:341–346, 2002.

67

Surgical Treatment of Neurofibromatosis

JAMES H. TONSGARD, PRISCILLA SHORT, BAKHTIAR YAMINI, and DAVID M. FRIM

Neurofibromatosis types 1 and 2 (NF1 and NF2) are genetic diseases that commonly affect the brain, peripheral nerves, spinal roots, spinal cord, and dura. While the type of neurologic complications in NF1 and NF2 are also found in patients without NF, management frequently is different. It is important for the neurosurgeon to be aware of not only the range of neurologic complications that occur in NF but also their clinical course in NF patients. This chapter covers the neurologic complications, the indications for surgery, and the surgical approach to the tumor types found in NF1 and NF2. The details of the techniques of tumor removal are similar to those used for removal of the same tumors in patients without NF. Because NF1 and NF2 have very different complications, the two diseases are presented separately.

NEUROFIBROMATOSIS TYPE 1

Neurofibromatosis type 1 is an autosomal dominant genetic disorder caused by a mutation or deletion of the neurofibromin gene on the long arm of chromosome 17.[1] The diagnosis of NF1 requires the presence of two or more major criteria: six or more café-au-lait spots, two cutaneous neurofibromas, one plexiform neurofibroma, certain bony abnormalities, an optic glioma, iris Lisch nodules, or a first-degree relative with NF1.[2] While there are no silent carriers of NF, clinical manifestations are variable even within the same family.[3] Because NF1 may affect virtually any organ system and some complications such as plexiform neurofibromas commonly involve adjacent organs, a multidisciplinary team is essential for management. Such a team should include a pediatrician, neurologist, geneticist, neurosurgeon, orthopedist, plastic surgeon, and oncologist. NF1 is a progressive disorder. Some complications worsen with age. Moreover, complications of NF1 are usually age specific. Plexiform neurofibromas are felt to be congenital, although they may not require surgical intervention until later in life. Optic gliomas usually present between 18 months and 7 years of age.[4] Cutaneous neurofibromas commonly occur in teenagers or young adults, and malignant peripheral nerve sheath tumors are a complication of young adults.[5]

Neurologic Complications of NF1 and Indications for Neurosurgical Intervention

The neurologic complications of NF1 include headaches, learning disabilities, seizures, peripheral nerve tumors, spinal nerve root tumors, dural ectasias, deafness, optic gliomas, areas of high-intensity signal on magnetic resonance imaging (MRI), tumors of the brain parenchyma, and aqueductal stenosis.[6] Migraine headaches are a common feature.[7] Learning disabilities and hyperactivity occur in at least one half of patients.[8] Deafness occurs in 10% of NF1 patients and is not caused by tumors.[9] Brain tumors and optic gliomas occur in a small percentage of patients. The incidence is increased compared with the normal population.[10] All patients with NF1 develop peripheral nerve tumors.

Peripheral Nerve Tumors

Five types of peripheral nerve tumors occur in NF1: schwannomas, discrete neurofibromas (sometimes called cutaneous or dermal neurofibromas), diffuse neurofibromas, plexiform neurofibromas, and malignant peripheral nerve sheath tumors. Schwannomas are infrequently found in patients with NF1. This tumor is more typical of NF2 and is discussed in the section on NF2. Diffuse neurofibromas most commonly present as boggy caplike lesions of the scalp that involve the subcutaneous tissue, stopping at the fascia.[11] Diffuse neurofibromas of the scalp do not progress beyond the hairline and are best left alone.

Discrete neurofibromas and plexiform neurofibromas involve a proliferation of fibroblasts, Schwann cells, perineural cells, mast cells, extracellular matrix, axons, and blood vessels.[12] These two tumors differ histologically primarily in the extent of extracellular matrix. Plexiform neurofibromas have more extracellular matrix. Both tumors cause expansion of the nerve. Nerve fibers run through the tumor. Plexiform neurofibromas may involve small peripheral nerves, large peripheral nerves, nerve trunks, plexus, or spinal roots. Either motor or sensory nerves or both are affected. Plexiform neurofibromas may be associated with markedly dilated veins. Plexiform neurofibromas involve the skin with or without involvement of underlying muscle, or they may be confined to deeper tissues. Plexiform tumors are felt to be congenital or to appear within the first year of life. Growth is highly variable. Some tumors remain static, others relentlessly increase, while others undergo spurts of growth and periods of quiescence. Plexiform neurofibromas may appear discrete and isolated, diffuse and infiltrative, or nodular with multiple grapelike clusters.[13] Plexiform neurofibromas commonly infiltrate adjacent muscle and will sometimes infiltrate adjacent organs such as bladder or esophagus. Plexiform neurofibromas occur in at least 50% of all patients.[14] Large areas of hyperpigmentation with fine hair may overlie plexiform neurofibromas.

Discrete or cutaneous neurofibromas occur in all patients with NF1. These tumors usually appear in teenagers or adults.[15] Early appearance of large numbers of neurofibromas is associated with complete deletion of the NF1 gene.[16] Isolated neurofibromas may involve both motor and sensory nerves in the epidermis and/or dermis.

Malignant peripheral nerve sheath tumors (MPNSTs) occur in 4% of all patients with NF1. These tumors arise within plexiform neurofibromas usually between the ages of 15 and 40.[5] Earlier onset is uncommon but occurs. MPNSTs may be multifocal in some patients. MPNSTs are highly malignant with rapid hematogenous dissemination. Outcome for patients with MPNSTs is poor. The best outcome is associated with radical resection.[17]

Indications for Removal of Peripheral Nerve Tumors

Neurofibromas, either discrete or plexiform, should be removed or resected only if they are symptomatic. Discrete neurofibromas may be associated with some discomfort and/or itching as they grow. Rarely, isolated neurofibromas will cause compression of a motor nerve with distal weakness. Discrete neurofibromas should be removed if they produce significant discomfort or are located in exposed areas that are stigmatizing. Discrete neurofibromas may recur near the site of removal, but usually not for several years if removal is complete. Resection of plexiform neurofibromas is more difficult. Plexiform neurofibromas frequently have diffuse projections that make complete removal impossible. Moreover, plexiform neurofibromas sometimes involve large nerves or nerve roots, so that complete resection results in disability. Nevertheless, resection of plexiform neurofibromas should be considered if they cause cosmetic disfigurement, pain, or compromise of function. No successful chemotherapy has been identified for plexiform neurofibromas. Growth of plexiform neurofibromas is sometimes stimulated by radiation therapy. Histologic identification is not an indication for surgery unless the tumor is suspected to be malignant.

Malignant peripheral nerve sheath tumors are commonly associated with pain. There are no reliable radiologic characteristics to distinguish MPNSTs from plexiform neurofibromas.[12] While MPNSTs commonly enhance with contrast and lack a homogeneous appearance, the same is true of some benign plexiform tumors. A helpful distinguishing feature is that MPNSTs commonly take up gallium in radioisotope scans.[18,19] Because MPNSTs arise within plexiform neurofibromas, in which only a small portion of the tumor is malignant, biopsies can be negative. Computed tomography (CT)-directed needle biopsy is preferred when MPNST is suspected. MPNSTs do not respond well to chemotherapy or radiation therapy.[20]

Spinal Nerve Root Tumors and Dural Ectasias

Tumors of spinal roots are plexiform neurofibromas. One nerve root or multiple roots may be affected. Nerve root involvement is associated with enlargement of the neural foramen on MRI or scalloping of vertebral bodies on radiography. Virtually any nerve root may be affected, but high cervical and lower lumbar spine are the most common sites. Nerve root tumors may extend through the neural foramen and expand and compress the cord, or they may remain static. Surgery is indicated if there is pain or compression of the spinal cord.

Dural ectasias are a weakening or expansion of the dural covering of a spinal root that is independent of a nerve root tumor. Dural ectasias commonly erode the vertebral body and may produce large dilated pockets anterior to the vertebral body (so-called anterior meningoceles). This is associated with pain, scoliosis, and sometimes vertebral instability.[21] Dural ectasias increase in size or remain static. Surgery is indicated if there is intractable pain or vertebral instability.

Brain Tumors, Magnetic Resonance Imaging Abnormalities, and Hydrocephalus

High-intensity signals are present on T2 images in the MRI of the brain in roughly 50% of all patients with NF1. Common locations are the basal ganglia, cerebellum, midbrain, and pons. The lesions do not enhance and are less easily visible on T1 images. They are not visible on CT scans. These areas of increased signal are sometimes referred to as unidentified bright objects, heterotopias, or hamartomas. The latter terms are misleading, since the etiology of the lesions is unclear.[22] They may be more common in children with learning disabilities but also occur in children without any cognitive difficulties. Areas of hyperintensity are dependent on age. They are less common after age 20.[23] In younger patients the hyperintense signals may increase or decrease over time. They are not tumors and do not require radiologic follow-up or biopsy.

Optic glioma occurs in 15% of patients with NF1.[24] Optic gliomas are pilocytic astrocytomas (WHO grade I).[25] They commonly affect the chiasm as well as one of the optic nerves. Bilateral involvement is common. The tumors may extend into the hypothalamus or along the optic radiations.[4] Because they can extend beyond the optic nerve, they are usually referred to as optic pathway tumors. Impairment of vision occurs in only 20% to 30% of patients.[26] If treatment is required, chemotherapy is preferred.[27] The tumors do not require biopsy. The age of onset is between 16 months and 7 years of age. Screening for optic gliomas is done with regular eye exams rather than imaging. Optic gliomas are almost never symptomatic after age 7.[4]

Tumors of the brain parenchyma (not including optic pathway tumors) occur in 2% of patients with NF1.[28] Cerebellum and brain stem are the most common locations.[29] Brain stem tumors involve the midbrain, pons, or medulla. They commonly have an exophytic component. Some enhancement with contrast may be seen. The natural history of brain stem tumors is usually benign.[30] Almost all are grade I astrocytomas. They may be associated with recurrent coughing, intermittent difficulty swallowing, or choking, but they are not associated with any weakness or cranial nerve palsies. Rarely, they produce obstructive hydrocephalus. Once a brain stem tumor has been identified, it is prudent to obtain imaging at intervals for a few years to prove that the lesion is stable.[31] Brain tumors in other locations can vary from grade I to grade IV astrocytomas. In general, brain tumors in NF1 are more indolent than in normal individuals. Some tumors even regress over time. Highly malignant gliomas also occur in NF1. Tumors should not be biopsied unless they are clearly symptomatic or show progression over time.

Aqueductal stenosis is a rare complication of NF1. Symptoms include headache, vomiting, progressive gait disturbance, incontinence, and cognitive difficulties.[32] The onset may be insidious and recognition delayed. Surgical intervention usually results in significant improvement even when the symptoms appear to be long-standing.

Surgical Approach to the Lesions of Neurofibromatosis Type 1

Peripheral Nerve Lesions

Tumors of small peripheral nerves are usually discrete neurofibromas. The surgical approach is a direct linear incision along the length of the nerve. Care must be taken to dissect down to the expanded nerve sheath, incise it, and deliver the lesion through the incision. Electrical nerve stimulation is useful to ensure that motor function is identified and preserved. In the absence of any motor function, nerve sectioning above and below the lesion with complete removal is appropriate. The cut nerve endings should be sewn into a nearby muscle to reduce the likelihood of painful postresection neuroma. When motor function is identified in the nerve entering the neurofibroma, we advocate intracapsular removal, incising the tumor sheath to deliver the intracapsular portion and remove it in its entirety, leaving the residual nerve in continuity. Often the bulk of the functional nerve is expanded and external to the tumor capsule. Function can be preserved by leaving the capsule in continuity with the nerve. After resection, the wound is closed in layers.

Large Nerves and Plexus

Neurofibromas of large peripheral nerves, such as the sciatic, common peroneal, or the divisions of the brachial and lumbosacral plexus, are more complicated to approach than tumors of small cutaneous nerves. Tumors of large nerves are invariably plexiform tumors. The anatomic structures entering and leaving the area of the tumor must be carefully identified and dissected before tumor resection is attempted. The approach to the brachial plexus and lumbosacral plexus is similar to that of any lesion in those areas. However, plexiform neurofibromas often adhere to and follow the nerve trunks as an axis of growth. The tumors often envelope the entire plexus and adjacent tissue. Maximal debulking should be attempted while preserving function. The dissection must proceed along the anatomic plane of the nerve, and electrical stimulation and monitoring of all of the involved nerves in the plexus is mandatory. Some success has been reported with a more radical approach to plexiform neurofibromas of the plexus with postresection nerve grafting. We do not advocate that approach because of the potential for disability, long recovery period, and likelihood of recurrence.

Spinal Nerve Root Tumors

Spinal nerve root tumors are plexiform neurofibromas that grow from the nerve root into the intraspinal space either intradurally or epidurally and exit through the neural foramen, producing a dumbbell appearance. The tumors may occur at any level of the spine. Because some patients have enlargement of multiple nerve roots, care must be taken to identify tumors that are symptomatic. Only those lesions that are symptomatic or threaten to become symptomatic should be approached. Spinal cord compression or canal compromise is the most reliable indication for surgery.

In the cervical spine, spinal root tumors are usually approached posteriorly to relieve spinal cord compression. A laminectomy is performed through a midline incision. In young adults and children, an osteoplastic laminoplasty provides stability to the spine. Additionally, the presence of bony lamina provides a landmark for dissection if patients require reoperation for recurrent tumor.

Intradural tumors without any extradural component are approached similarly to any nerve sheath tumor in the intradural space. They are usually dorsal or dorsolateral to the spinal cord but occasionally occur more ventrally. A midline or paramedian durotomy is performed once adequate exposure has been achieved by bony decompression. The nerve root involved is identified and stimulated. If it is a sensory root, which is usually the case, the root is sectioned proximal to the tumor. The tumor bulk is removed as the tumor is followed into the neural foramen. When there is minimal extension of the tumor beyond the neural foramen, the bulk of the tumor is removed from the intraspinal space. Residual tumor in the foramen is left to ensure adequate cerebrospinal fluid (CSF) closure. The dura is closed either primarily or with an expansile duraplasty patch graft and the lamina replaced where appropriate. This approach presumes that tumor regrowth, though likely, will be slow and easily monitored. We do not resect small residual epidural tumor. Radical excision does not enhance symptomatic relief. Epidural tumor is highly vascular, and radical resection may cause significant bleeding. Radical resection entails removal of lateral or ventral dura resulting in CSF leakage. Moreover, recurrence from small amounts of residual tumor is rare.

When the plexiform neurofibroma is primarily extradural, the approach is posterior with wide unilateral or bilateral bony decompression. The tumor is dissected in the epidural space. The epidural venous structures above and below are cauterized and divided. The tumor capsule is entered sharply and removed intracapsularly. We recommend the intracapsular approach to epidural tumors to preserve nerve root function. Removal of the tumor with its capsule and dural sheath will interrupt both sensory and motor nerve function. In the thoracic region radical removal can performed, but radical removal in the cervical and lumbar region would cause significant morbidity.

Spinal Nerve Root Tumors with Large Extra-axial Components

Spinal nerve root tumors with significant extra-axial extension are particularly challenging. In the cervical spine, extension of the tumor may compress the trachea or invade the esophagus. In the lumbosacral region, extra-axial tumor commonly compresses the rectum or invades the bladder.[14] An interdisciplinary surgical team is essential for resection of these tumors. The intraspinal portion of the procedure is performed in identical fashion to purely spinal tumors whether they be intradural or epidural. However, patient position and the incisions are dictated by the extra-axial portion of the tumor.

In the cervical spine where all the nerve roots carry significant function, the tumor is removed intracapsularly. Upon decompression of the intraspinal space, the posterior incision is closed and a separate incision is made for resection of the extra-axial extension into the neck. The diffuse nature of plexiform neurofibromas frequently results in poorly defined margins of adjacent organs. Care must be taken to avoid entry into the trachea, esophagus, and great vessels. The goal of tumor resection in the neck is usually decompression of the airway. Plexiform neurofibromas almost never compromise the great vessels. Preservation of function of adjacent structures limits the extent of removal of the tumor.

In the thoracic region, when the extra-axial extent of the tumor is large, tumor removal is accomplished in the lateral position using either one or two adjacent incisions— one for thoracotomy and a second (or an extension of the first) for laminectomy. The patient is positioned for a thoracotomy, and the approach to the intrapleural space is performed by a thoracic surgeon. The neural foramina are identified in the pleural space. The extra-axial portion of the tumor is removed, along with its pleural investment with dissection along major vascular structures. The enlarged spinal foramina can be approached from the front by the neurosurgeon. When the foramina are wide and the intraspinal tumor is small, the resection can be completed from the anterolateral approach by foraminotomy and partial vertebrectomy. When the intraspinal extent is large or difficult to reach through the neural foramina from the front, we enlarge the incision or make a separate midline posterior incision. The lateral position for laminectomy (or osteoplastic laminoplasty) permits a standard approach to the epidural or intradural components of the tumor. In general, plexiform neurofibromas in the thoracic space requiring a transthoracic approach can be resected in their entirety, if there is no intradural extension, by sectioning the nerve root as it exits the dural sac. Intraspinal tumor can be delivered through the widened foramen along with a portion of the extraspinal intraforaminal tumor, achieving a near-complete resection. This is one of the few situations in which removal of the involved neural structure causes minimal residual functional loss.

Tumors in the lumbosacral region with large extra-axial extensions are best approached in the lateral position through a large flank incision. The tumor is dissected through the retroperitoneum and the lumbosacral plexus identified. The extra-axial portion of the tumor is followed to the neural foramen and removed. If the tumor cannot be adequately removed from the lateral approach, the intraspinal portion of the tumor is approached posteriorly. This can be accomplished during the same procedure through a laminectomy by lengthening the flank incision or by creating a separate midline lumbar incision. Occasionally the flank incision is closed and the patient is repositioned for a posterior approach. If the retroperitoneal surgery is extensive, the spinal portion of the tumor can be removed at a later date in the prone position. Since the lumbar and sacral nerves are functionally important, tumors of these nerves must be approached intracapsularly. Resection should be limited to decompression and debulking. Recurrence is unusual.

Lesions of the Cranial Vault and Brain

Patients with NF1 may have a variety of parenchymal abnormalities on MRI. Of the parenchymal brain lesions in NF1, only symptomatic tumors with radiologic characteristics of malignancy or progression require surgical intervention. Treatment of these lesions entails biopsy and aggressive resection, where possible, followed by adjunctive chemotherapy and radiotherapy. The treatment protocols are identical to high-grade astrocytomas in normal individuals. Treatment of the optic pathway tumors is not surgical. Diagnostic biopsy is not required. When optic pathway tumors progress, chemotherapy may be indicated.[27]

The aqueductal stenosis that is associated with NF1 is treated as any congenital aqueductal stenosis lesion. Endoscopic third ventriculocisternostomy is the approach of choice. If that procedure is not available or a large optic glioma limits access to the floor of the third ventricle, standard lateral ventricular shunting adequately treats this problem.

NEUROFIBROMATOSIS TYPE 2

Neurofibromatosis type 2 is an autosomal dominantly inherited disease due to a mutation or deletion in the long arm of chromosome 22 of the merlin gene.[33] The diagnosis depends on the presence of bilateral eighth-nerve tumors or the presence of a unilateral eighth-nerve tumor before 30 years of age in an individual with a first-degree relative with NF2 or two of the following: neurofibroma, meningioma, glioma, schwannoma, or juvenile posterior cataract.[9] NF2 is characterized by the presence of multiple central nervous system (CNS) tumors. The clinical hallmark is bilateral vestibular nerve schwannomas. Patients may have multiple supratentorial meningiomas and schwannomas of the cranial nerves in addition to vestibular tumors. Meningiomas occur along the spine, and schwannomas may develop along spinal nerve roots.[34] Roughly a third of NF2 patients have intramedullary tumors of the spinal cord or brain stem that are either ependymomas or astrocytomas.[35] Juvenile posterior subcapsular cataracts and retinal hamartomas occur in 80% of patients.[36] Skin tumors occur in patients with NF2 but are not particularly prominent.

The clinical presentation of NF2 is usually unilateral deafness. Facial weakness, visual impairment, dizziness, or painful peripheral nerve lesions may also be presenting complaints.[37] Spinal cord compression or seizures are late symptoms. There appear to be at least two clinical phenotypes in NF2. Patients with the Gardner phenotype have few intracranial tumors, little or no spinal involvement, and no retinal hamartomas. The onset of symptoms is after 20 years of age and the life span is longer than 40 years. The Wishart phenotype is more severe, with multiple intracranial and intraspinal tumors and retinal hamartomas. Onset is before 20 years of age and life span is less than 40 years. There is no statistically significant evidence for an intermediate (Lee/Abbott) phenotype.[37] Although there is considerable variability in clinical manifestations in patients with NF2, there is at least some consistency of phenotype within family members.[9]

Neurofibromatosis type 2 is completely distinct from NF1, although rare patients may have features of both diseases. Patients with a unilateral vestibular schwannoma and multiple ipsilateral brain tumors may have somatic mosaic inactivation of the NF2 gene.[38] Two additional disorders must be distinguished from NF2: schwannomatosis is characterized by multiple schwannomas of the peripheral, spinal, or cranial nerves without evidence of a vestibular schwannoma.[39] This can be either a sporadic or autosomal dominant disorder. Meningiomatosis is an autosomal dominant disorder characterized by multiple meningiomas along the spinal cord as well as supratentorially.[40]

Tumors Associated with Neurofibromatosis Type 2

Schwannomas

Schwannomas are typically nodular masses surrounded by a fibrous capsule consisting of epineurium and some nerve fibers. The tumors consist predominantly of Schwann cells with alternating patterns of cellularity.[41] Glandular or cystic areas sometimes occur. Schwannomas are virtually never malignant. Unlike neurofibromas, in which axons run through the tumor, schwannomas are usually extrinsic to the nerve and separate from the majority of the axons. However, when schwannomas involve small nerves, the tumor frequently engulfs the nerve, making separation from the nerve difficult. Schwannomas of the vestibular nerves are histologically identical to schwannomas of other nerves. Frequently, vestibular schwannomas are multinodular.[42] Although these tumors were originally called acoustic neuromas, they arise from the vestibular nerve. They usually impair hearing, but vestibular symptoms may also be prominent at the time of presentation. Schwannomas of the other cranial nerves are found in at least 25% of patients, particularly the third and fifth cranial nerves.[9] Schwannomas of the spinal nerves are present in the majority of patients.[37]

Meningiomas

Meningiomas arise from arachnoid cells of the leptomeninges. Meningiomas in patients with NF2 are predominantly fibrous, but meningothelial tumors also occur.[43] Orbital meningiomas may occur in childhood and must be distinguished from optic gliomas. Meningiomas of the cerebellar pontine angle are occasionally confused with vestibular schwannomas. Meningiomas of the skull base produce brain stem compression and are an important cause of mortality in NF2. Meningioma en plaque occurs in some patients with NF2 late in their disease.

Astrocytomas, Ependymomas, and Hamartomas

Astrocytomas and ependymomas occur in as many as a third of NF2 patients.[32] The most common site is the brain stem or cervical cord.[44] These tumors are typically indolent in NF2. Evidence of rapid growth or symptoms related to the tumors is an indication for surgery, but radiation and chemotherapy are usually not indicated. Hamartomas of the brain are frequently found in patients with NF2. They are a mixture of Schwann cells, glia, and meningeal cells.[45]

Indications for Neurosurgery

Neurofibromatosis type 2 is not a surgically curable disease. Lesions recur and progress. The entire CNS can be involved. The tumors of NF2 do not respond to chemotherapy. Radiation therapy can be considered for lesions that are not surgically accessible. Lesions are usually addressed surgically when they are symptomatic. There are special considerations involved in the surgery of the vestibular schwannomas that are discussed later. In patients with the more benign phenotype with few and slow-growing tumors, surgical intervention is reserved for prevention of impending symptoms or for

symptomatic tumors. In its most aggressive form, however, the disease can progress rapidly and cause severe disability that leads to death. In that situation, surgical intervention is palliative to improve quality of life.

A variety of surgical approaches with different goals and complications are available for vestibular schwannomas. It is important to discuss goals for surgery and define the degree of aggressiveness of the surgical approach with the patient before surgery. Aggressive removal of vestibular schwannomas may cause facial nerve injury. Facial nerve injury may be extremely distressing to patients and predisposes to ocular injury. These complications should be discussed with patients. Surgical removal of intramedullary spinal cord tumors is indicated when there are signs of spinal cord compression. Because multiple tumors may develop over time along the length of the spinal cord, the number of surgical interventions is limited. Schwannomas of the spinal nerves rarely cause problems. Surgery on these tumors should be avoided.

Surgical Approach to the Lesions of Neurofibromatosis Type 2

Vestibular Schwannoma (Acoustic Neuroma)

The technical approach to a vestibular schwannoma in an NF2 patient is identical to sporadic tumors. However, surgical decisions in NF2 patients are affected by the presence of bilateral disease and the knowledge that the disease is not surgically curable. Surgical approaches include radical resection, partial removal, and decompression. Suboccipital retrosigmoid, translabyrinthine, or middle cranial fossa approaches can all be appropriately used for tumor removal. The arguments for these various approaches are outlined elsewhere in this text. The translabyrinthine approach permits greater exposure of the tumor but results in deafness. The middle cranial fossa approach is used primarily for decompression. We prefer the suboccipital retrosigmoid approach with the goal of hearing sparing.[46] This operation entails drilling open the posterior aspect of the internal auditory meatus, followed by subtotal resection of the tumor, preserving facial nerve function at all costs. Electrophysiologic monitoring of the eighth cranial nerve helps to preserve hearing.

We advocate early surgery on one side if one of the vestibular tumors is less than 1.5 cm in diameter. When the tumor is small, early surgery reduces the size of the tumor and preserves hearing and facial nerve function. If the tumors are greater than 1.5 cm, we prefer to wait until there is significant motor dysfunction due to brain stem compression. When motor dysfunction is present in patients with large bilateral tumors, we recommend subtotal resection of one of the tumors. If brain stem compression is predominantly unilateral, subtotal resection of the larger tumor relieves brain stem compression and preserves facial nerve function and hearing. However, when patients have very large bilateral tumors and bilateral brain stem compression, the appropriate operation may be a radical subtotal resection on one side, sacrificing hearing and preserving facial nerve function. In the latter situation, aggressive tumor removal may compromise facial nerve function.

In patients with large vestibular tumors, the presence of additional CNS tumors may affect the surgical approach to a vestibular tumor. If there are multiple large CNS tumors and the vestibular schwannoma is causing brain stem compression, subtotal resection of the vestibular tumor for brain stem decompression alone may be more appropriate than radical resection. Since vestibular schwannomas may remain stable for prolonged periods, simple decompressive subtotal resection can provide symptomatic relief for several years.

In children and young adults, the vestibular tumors may be small. If one of the tumors is less than 1.5 cm in size, we recommend operating on the smaller tumor. Resection is performed with the goal of preserving hearing on that side. Successful resection of the smaller tumor with preservation of hearing on that side, permits radical resection of the contralateral tumor at a later time when hearing loss on that side will not affect quality of life.

Other Intracranial Tumors

The technical surgical approach to the removal of brain tumors in patients with NF2 is identical to the same tumor in normal individuals. However, the potential for multiple recurrent CNS tumors and multiple surgeries must be considered before deciding on surgery. Tumors are only removed when they are symptomatic. Meningiomas in NF2 are removed for cortical compression causing neurologic deficit or for seizure generation. En plaque meningiomas, even when very large and diffusely compressive, should be watched in patients with NF2, especially if there is a large additional tumor burden.

Spinal Cord Lesions

The surgical approach to intramedullary spinal tumors of NF2 is identical to intramedullary spinal tumor in normal individuals. The levels of interest are exposed by generous bony removal, the dura is opened and retracted, a midline myelotomy is performed, and pial retraction stitches are placed after the tumor has been reached by gentle dissection under the microscope. Ependymomas in NF2 are usually well circumscribed. They can be debulked and dissected from normal spinal cord tissue with care. Although the spinal cord may appear thinned and compressed, recovery from a first surgery is generally good.

Hydrocephalus

Hydrocephalus can occur either from tumor obstruction of CSF pathways or from tumor protein production within the CSF, causing reduced CSF absorption. Hydrocephalus is treated with tumor removal or ventriculoperitoneal shunting. Frequently, hydrocephalus is observed postoperatively after removal of an intraventricular or subarachnoid tumor (e.g., vestibular schwannoma). Despite treatment with anti-inflammatory glucocorticoids, the malabsorption of CSF, presumed to be from inflammatory insult at the villus absorptive surface, rarely resolves. Knowledge of the type of hydrocephalus, obstructive versus absorptive, as well as consideration of the presumed elevated CSF protein in the presence of multiple CNS tumors, may affect choice of shunting valve system.

CONCLUSIONS

The neurofibromatoses are not surgically curable diseases. Unfortunately, the limited usefulness of adjuvant therapy leaves surgery as the primary treatment to alleviate symptoms.

While surgery provides symptomatic relief, it may not alter the course of disease. Surgery should be limited to the removal of tumors that are symptomatic or that threaten to cause symptoms. The technical surgical approach to the tumors of NF1 and NF2 is generally similar to the approach of the same tumor in patients without NF. However, the decision of when to operate and to what level of aggressiveness is often affected by the disease and is of critical importance in NF. Even though the relentless progression of disease may at times be discouraging, the ability of neurosurgery to alleviate symptoms and improve longevity and quality of life is significant.

REFERENCES

1. Cawthon RM, Weiss R, Xu G, et al: A major segment of the neurofibromatosis type 1 gene: cDNA sequence, genomic structure, and point mutations. Cell 62:193–201, 1990.
2. Neurofibromatosis Conference Statement: National Institutes of Health Consensus Development Conference. Arch Neurol 45:575–578, 1988.
3. Carey JC, Laud, Hall BD: Penetrance and variability of neurofibromatosis: A genetic study of 60 families. Birth Defects 15:271–281, 1979.
4. Listernick R, Charrow J, Greenwald MJ, et al: Natural history of optic pathway tumors in children with neurofibromatosis type 1: A longitudinal study. J Pediatr 125:63–66, 1994.
5. Ducatman BS, Scheithauer BW, Piepgras DG, et al: Malignant peripheral nerve sheath tumors: A clinicopathologic study of 120 cases. Cancer 57:2006–2021, 1986.
6. Gutmann DH: Abnormalities of the nervous system. In Friedman JM, Gutmann DH, MacCollin M, et al (eds): Neurofibromatosis: Phenotype, Natural History, and Pathogenesis. Baltimore: Johns Hopkins University Press, 1999, pp 190–202.
7. North K: Neurofibromatosis type 1: Review of the first 200 patients in an Australian clinic. J Child Neurol 8:395–402, 1993.
8. North K, Joy P, Yuille D, et al: Cognitive function and academic performance in children with Neurofibromatosis type 1. Dev Med Child Neurol 37:427–436, 1995.
9. Mulvihill JJ, Parry DM, Sherman JL: NIH Conference. Neurofibromatosis 1 (Recklinghausen disease) and neurofibromatosis 2 (bilateral acoustic neurofibromatosis): An update. Ann Intern Med 113:39–52, 1990.
10. Cohen BH, Rothner AD: Incidence, types, and management of cancer in patients with neurofibromatosis. Oncology 3:23–38, 1989.
11. Weiss SW, Goldblum JR (eds): In Enzinger and Weiss's Soft Tissue Tumors, 4th edition. St. Louis: Mosby, 2001, pp 1132–1137.
12. Fisher ER, Vuzevski VD: Cytogenesis of schwannoma (neurilemmoma), neurofibroma, dermatofibroma, and dermatofibrosarcoma as revealed by electron microscopy. Am J Clin Pathol 49:141–154, 1968.
13. Friedrich RE, Korf B, Funsturer C, et al: Growth type of plexiform neurofibromas in NF1 determined on magnetic resonance images. Anticancer Res 23:949–952, 2003.
14. Tonsgard JH, Kwak SM, Short MP, et al: CT imaging in adults with neurofibromatosis-1: Frequent asymptomatic plexiform lesions. Neurology 50:1755–1760, 1998.
15. Huson SM, Harper PS, Compston DAS: Von Recklingausen neurofibromatosis: A clinical and population study in southeast Wales. Brain 111:1355–1381, 1988.
16. Tonsgard JH, Yelavarthi KK, Cushner S, et al: Do NF1 gene deletions result in a characteristic phenotype? Am J Med Genet 73:80–86, 1997.
17. Sordillo PP, Helson L, Hajdu SI: Malignant schwannoma: Clinical characteristics, survival, and response to therapy. Cancer 47:2503–2509, 1981.
18. Hammond JA, Dreidger AA: Detection of malignant change in neurofibromatosis (von Recklinghausen's disease) by gallium-67 scanning. Can Med Assoc J 119:352–353, 1978.
19. Kloos RT, Rufini V, Gross MD, et al: Bone scans in neurofibromatosis: Neurifibroma, plexiform neuroma, and neurofibrosarcoma. J Nucl Med 37:1778–1783, 1996.
20. Edmonson JH, Ryan LM, Blum RH, et al: Randomized comparison of doxorubicin alone versus ifosfamide plus doxorubicin or mitomycin, doxorubicin, and cisplatin against advanced soft tissue sarcomas. J Clin Oncol 11:1269–1275, 1993.
21. Erkulvrawatr S, El Gammai T, Hawkins J, et al: Intrathroacic meningoceles and neurofibromatosis. Arch Neurol 36:557–559, 1979.

22. Duffner PK, Cohen ME, Seidel FG, et al: The significance of MRI abnormalities in children with neurofibromatosis. Neurology 39:373–378, 1989.

23. Aoki S, Barkovich AJ, Nishimura K, et al: Neurofibromatosis types 1 and 2: Cranial MR findings. Radiology 172:527–534, 1989.

24. Listernick R, Charrow J, Greenwald MJ, et al: Optic gliomas in children with neurofibromatosis type 1. J Pediatr 114:788–792, 1989.

25. Kleihues P, Soylemezoglu F, Schauble B, et al: Histopathology, classification, and grading of gliomas. Glia 15:211–221, 1995.

26. Lewis RA, Gerson LP, Axelson KA, et al: Von Recklinghausen neurofibromatosis: Incidence of optic gliomata. Ophthalmology 91:929–935, 1984.

27. Packer RJ, Ater J, Allen J, et al: Carboplatin and vincristine chemotherapy for children with newly diagnosed progressive low-grade gliomas. J Neurosurg 86:747–754, 1997.

28. Sorensen SA, Mulvihill JJ, Nielsen A: Long-term follow-up of von Recklinghausen neurofibromatosis: Survival and malignant neoplasms. N Engl J Med 314:1010–1015, 1986.

29. Ilgren EB, Kinnier-Wilson LM, Stiller CA: Gliomas in neurofibromatosis: A series of 89 cases with evidence for enhanced malignancy in associated cerebellar astrocytomas. Pathol Ann 20:331–358, 1985.

30. Bilaniuk LT, Malloy PT, Zimmerman RA, et al: Neurofibromatosis type 1: Brainstem tumors. Neuroradiology 39:642–653, 1997.

31. Pollack IF, Shultz B, Mulvihill JJ: The management of brainstem gliomas in patients with neurofibromatosis 1. Neurology 46:1652–1660, 1996.

32. Horwich A, Riccardi VM, Fracke U: Aqueductal stenosis leading to hydrocephalus—an unusual manifestation of neurofibromatosis. Am J Med Genet 14:577–581, 1983.

33. Trofatter JA, MacCollin MM, Rutter JL, et al: A novel moesin-, ezrin-, radixin-like gene is a candidate for the neurofibromatosis 2 tumor suppressor. Cell 75:826, 1993.

34. Evans DGR, Huson SM, Donnai D, et al: A clinical study of type 2 neurofibromatosis. Quart J Med 84:603–618, 1992.

35. Mautner VF, Tatagiba M, Lindenau M, et al: Spinal tumors in patients with neurofibromatosis type 2: MR imaging study of frequency, multiplicity, and variety. Am J Roentgenol 165:951–955, 1995.

36. Bouzas EA, Parry DM, Eldridge R, et al: Visual impairment in patients with neurofibromatosis 2. Neurology 43:622–623, 1993.

37. Parry DM, Eldridge R, Kaiser-Kupfer MI, et al: Neurofibromatosis 2 (NF2): Clinical characteristics of 63 affected individuals and clinical evidence of heterogeneity. Am J Med Genet 52:450–461, 1994.

38. Evans DGR, Wallace A, Wu C, et al: Somatic mosaicism: A common cause of classic disease in tumor-prone syndromes? Lessons from type 2 neurofibromatosis. Am J Hum Genet 63:727–736, 1998.

39. MacCollin M, Woodfin W, Kronn D, et al: Schwannomatosis: A clinical and pathologic study. Neurology 46:1072–1079, 1996.

40. Pulst SM, Rouleau G, Marineau C, et al: Familial meningioma is not allelic to neurofibromatosis 2. Neurology 43:2096–2098, 1993.

41. Sobel RA: Vestibular (acoustic) schwannomas: Histologic features in neurofibromatosis 2 and in unilateral cases. J Neuropathol Exp Neurol 52:106–113, 1993.

42. Hamada Y, Iwaki T, Fukui M: A comparative study of embedded nerve tissue in six NF2-associated schwannomas and 17 nonassociated NF2 schwannomas. Surg Neurol 48:395–400, 1997.

43. Louis DN, Ramesh V, Gusella J: Neuropathology and molecular genetics of neurofibromatosis 2 and related tumors. Brain Pathol 5:163–172, 1995.

44. McCormick P, Torres R, Post K, et al: Intramedullary ependymoma of the spinal cord. J Neurosurg 72:523–532, 1990.

45. Rubinstein L: The malformative central nervous system lesions in the central and peripheral forms of neurofibromatosis: A neuropathological study of 22 cases. Ann N Y Acad Sci 486:14–29, 1986.

46. McKenna M, Halpin C, Ojemann R, et al: Long-term hearing results in patients after surgical removal of acoustic tumors with hearing preservation. Am J Otolaryngol 13:134–136, 1992.

68 Posterior Fossa Meningiomas

JACK P. ROCK, SAMUEL RYU, and TOOMAS ANTON

INTRODUCTION

Posterior fossa meningiomas are uncommon lesions that are most often slow-growing neoplasms manifesting in clinically indolent fashion. Based on clinical and radiographic information, the differential diagnosis is relatively straightforward; however, the range of management options can be considerable, including observation, surgery, and radiation in various forms and combinations. Although chemotherapeutic agents have been and continue to be investigated, this form of therapy is generally considered only for intractable, atypical, and malignant tumors and is not part of the general armamentarium in the majority of patients. Although the surgical management of meningiomas located in the posterior fossa is challenging, patient-based outcomes studies suggest that long-term results can be encouraging.[1]

Posterior fossa meningiomas can be found anywhere in the posterior fossa, and individualized management recommendations depend primarily on size, growth rate, clinical presentation, and location (i.e., surgical accessibility). Tumors are primarily classified by their anatomic origin along the suboccipital surface of the cerebellum, the lateral (i.e., lateral to the internal auditory meatus) petrous bone, the petroclival junction, clivus, foramen magnum, pineal region, tentorium, jugular foramen, or fourth ventricle (Table 68-1). Surgical accessibility varies based on location, with the most straightforward originating on the suboccipital surface of the cerebellum and lateral petrous bone; the more difficult originating on the tentorial surface, in the fourth ventricle, and cerebellopontine angle (CPA); and the most difficult originating at the petroclival junction. Each location is associated with different clinical implications regarding presentation and treatment strategy. Contemporary radiation therapy and radiosurgical decisions also depend on tumor location and the proximity of the tumor to critical neural elements. This chapter reviews the topic of posterior fossa meningioma from diagnosis though management and follow-up, in terms of both general and specific approaches relative to the various anatomic sites.

GENERAL CLINICAL PRESENTATION AND DIAGNOSIS

The clinical presentation of posterior fossa meningiomas varies according to the location and size of the tumor, but because meningiomas are, for the most part, slow-growing tumors, size plays less of a role in presentation and more of a role in choice of treatment strategy. Anatomically speaking, the presenting clinical symptoms most often are related to involvement of cranial nerves and to a lesser degree the cerebellum, brain stem (i.e., long tracts), and fourth ventricle (i.e., hydrocephalus). Headaches are a common but nonspecific symptom. More specific clinical features based on location will be discussed in the individual sections (see Table 68-1).

The diagnosis of meningioma is generally made radiographically, and most tumors share certain imaging characteristics. Plain radiographs, although no longer commonly utilized, often demonstrate bony hyperostosis; bony erosion; calcification; and, occasionally, evidence of enlarged vascular channels. Computerized transaxial tomography (CT) most often shows a hyperdense tumor signal (75% of cases) that intensely and homogeneously enhances after contrast administration. Cystic regions within the tumor can be seen but are uncommon, and peritumoral low-density suggestive of edema is noted in up to 60% of tumors. Calcification can also be noted on CT, but hemorrhage is distinctly uncommon. Magnetic resonance imaging (MRI) will most often reveal an isointense lesion on T1-weighted imaging, which is heterogeneous on T2-weighted imaging. These tumors almost always intensely enhance after gadolinium administration. The dural tail sign is one of the most revealing characteristics of meningioma even though it is not pathognomonic (Fig. 68-1). A high-intensity signal noted on T2-weighted imaging is typical of peritumoral edema. Cerebral angiography commonly (but not invariably) reveals an intense vascular supply, primarily from the dural arteries; a prolonged stain in the late venous phase of the angiogram is also common. Given the efficacy of magnetic resonance angiography (MRA) and venography (MRV) for diagnosis and surgical planning, formal cerebral angiography is used less often today, but it is still required for preoperative embolization.

Although the differential diagnosis of posterior fossa tumors is extensive, the common radiographic features of meningioma will usually serve to establish the diagnosis between the more common lesions. The most common tumors encountered along the dural margins of the posterior fossa include schwannomas, epidermoids, and metastases. Ependymomas and choroid plexus papillomas, in the fourth ventricle; and primary pineal tumors and germ cell tumors, in the pineal region, must also be considered.

Preoperative Evaluation

Most posterior fossa meningiomas are radiologically evaluated in a similar fashion, although smaller tumors may not require extensive testing. The standard diagnostic workup includes

TABLE 68-1 ▪ Posterior Fossa Meningiomas

Location	Incidence	Symptoms	Common Surgical Approaches
Occipital	10%	Headaches, cerebellar syndrome, increased ICP, hemianopsia, visual hallucinations	Suboccipital craniotomy +/− occipital craniotomy
Lateral petrous	8–10%	V, VII, VIII cranial neuropathies, brain stem and cerebellar compression syndrome	Retrosigmoid craniotomy
Cerebellopontine angle	10–15%	V, VII, VIII cranial neuropathies, brain stem and cerebellar compression syndromes	Retrosigmoid craniotomy Translabyrinthine craniotomy
Petroclival	10–38%	III, IV, V, VI, VII, VIII, IX, X, XI cranial neuropathies, brain stem and cerebellar compression syndromes, spasticity, headache	Petrosal craniotomy variants +/− anterior petrosectomy
Jugular foramen	Rare	IX, X, XI cranial neuropathies, brain stem compression syndrome	Retrosigmoid craniotomy Transjugular variants
Foramen magnum	4–20%	Increased ICP, IX, X, XI, XII cranial neuropathies, brain stem and spinal cord compression syndromes	Suboccipital craniotomy +/− C1 laminectomy, transoral Far lateral approach
Pineal	6–8%	Increased ICP, visual symptoms, cerebellar dysfunction	Infratentorial-supracerebellar craniotomy Occipital transtentorial craniotomy Supra/infratentorial transsinus approach
Fourth ventricle	Rare	Headache, increased ICP	Midline suboccipital craniotomy
Tentorial	30%	III, V, VI, VII, VIII cranial neuropathies, headache, increased ICP, brain stem and cerebellar compression syndromes, psychomotor epilepsy	Subtemporal craniotomy, petrosal craniotomy variants, retrosigmoid craniotomy

MRI, with and without contrast administration; MRA; MRV; and, for lesions involving the petrous bone, thin-cut temporal bone CT scan may be useful. Tumor extensions are best appreciated on contrast-enhanced MRI, and MRA will generally demonstrate the degree of tumor vascularity. When optimally performed, MRV will demonstrate (although in not as detailed a fashion as angiography) the venous anatomy, including the dominance of the transverse and

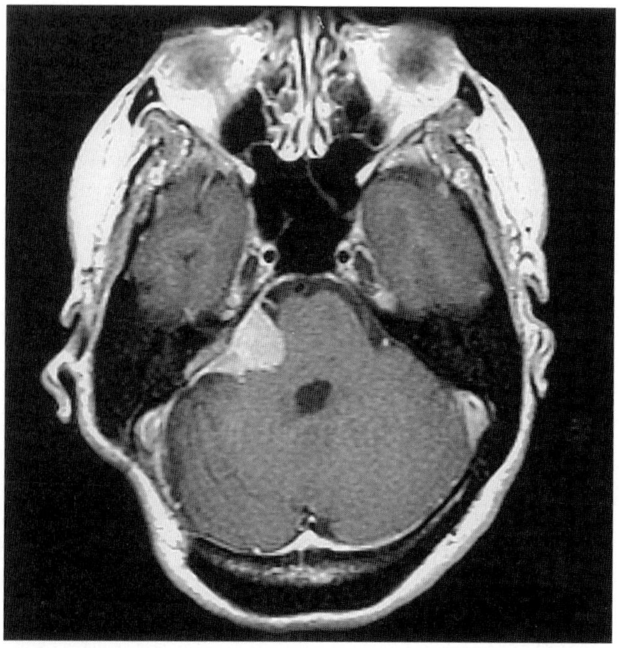

FIGURE 68-1   The thin layer of enhancement extending posterior to this cerebellopontine angle tumor is referred to as the dural tail, and although commonly noted with meningiomas, may also be seen with other tumor types.

sigmoid sinuses, the size of the jugular bulb, the superior and inferior petrosal sinuses, and the temporal lobe drainage pattern. Temporal bone CT will indicate the extent of hyperostosis or erosion, and will also demonstrate the relationship between the size of the jugular bulb and the surrounding bony anatomy.

Cerebral Angiography and Embolization

The need for preoperative cerebral angiography as a diagnostic and surgical planning tool has largely been supplanted by MRA and MRV. In most cases, the vascular supply to the tumor comes from arteries related to meningeal tumor origins. In the posterior fossa, arterial branches from the petrous and cavernous segments of the carotid, as well as branches from the vertebrobasilar and external carotid systems, constitute the main supply.

Given the limited space in the posterior fossa, the surgical removal of a highly vascular lesion can be fraught with difficulty (e.g., increased blood loss leading to morbidity), and although ideally the surgeon will select an approach that allows eradication of the tumor's vascular supply early in the operation, this is not always possible or sufficient. In these instances, preoperative arterial embolization can be very helpful, especially for selected tumors in the posterior fossa[2] (Fig. 68-2). The primary reservations regarding embolization generally include the fact that the arterial supply from the external carotid can be controlled during the approach, the risk of stroke, retroperitoneal hematoma, and secondary tumor necrosis and swelling (possibly leading to clinical deterioration). In addition, because the vascular supply is commonly made up of internal and external vessels, external carotid embolization may shift vascular supply to more difficult to control internal carotid branches. Nevertheless, the experiences of the authors and others suggest that embolization can be very helpful.[3,4] Most authors conclude

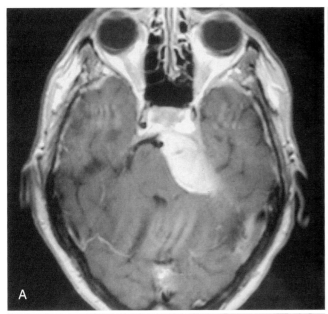

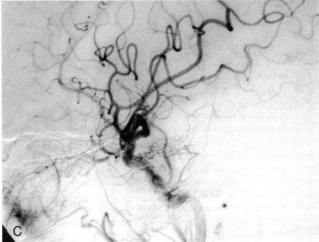

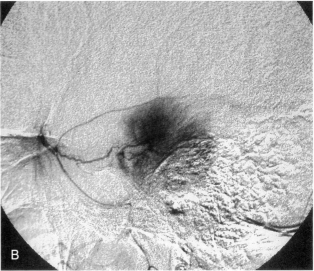

FIGURE 68-2 *A*, Petroclival meningioma. *B*, Preoperative angiogram with prominent vascular supply through the tentorial arteries. *C*, Angiogram postembolization. The patient was operated on 72 hours after embolization, and the tumor was significantly necrotic and removable by standard suction.

that to be most helpful, embolization must achieve complete or near-complete eradication of the vascular supply to the tumor: partial interruption of the blood supply may still leave the surgeon with a significant intraoperative bleeding challenge.

An additional issue relates to the timing of the surgical procedure relative to embolization. After an investigation of 50 patients, Chun and colleagues observed that more favorable results of embolization were noted with delays of longer than 24 hours, although the optimal delay was not specified.[5] It has become the practice with all posterior fossa tumors at Henry Ford Hospital to delay the surgical procedure 48 to 72 hours from the time of embolization; and because of the potential risk (albeit rare) of clinical deterioration from tumor swelling, the patient is admitted to the hospital until surgery.

General Treatment Considerations

The general management considerations surrounding meningiomas located in the posterior fossa run parallel to those for treating these lesions located in other regions of the brain. Because meningiomas are for the most part slow-growing neoplasms, urgent and emergent management decisions are seldom required. Recent reports on residual disease after surgical resection of petroclival tumors indicate that the average growth rate is 0.37 cm/year; this is associated with a median time to progression of 36 months, a median progression-free survival of 66 months, and a 5-year progression-free survival rate of 60%.[6] Older age, menopause, and previous radiation therapy can be associated with slower growth. Despite this indolent nature the neoplasms seem to grow relentlessly, often by en-plaque growth along tissue planes, the dura, and through basal cranial foramina, thereby making accurate growth assessment by CT or MRI a challenge. For practical purposes, four management options are available: (1) observation alone, (2) surgical resection, (3) radiation therapy or radiosurgery, and (4) some combination of surgery and radiation.

Observation

Observation is usually selected when the patient is neurologically intact, the lesion is small, and especially if the patient is elderly or has significant comorbidities. Observation remains reasonable even when the diagnosis is histologically unproven, because these lesions usually can be correctly diagnosed with MRI. Given the known natural history, when a lesion grows more than a couple of millimeters in a 6-month period, either the accuracy of the diagnosis will be questionable or the tumor growth more aggressive; in either case, surgical treatment would be the most judicious recommendation. Another consideration leading to a decision to observe rather than treat in an asymptomatic patient would be the surgeon's experience and the consequent risks of resection in addition to the risks of possible postoperative radiation therapy for lesions nestled tightly amid important neurologic structures in the posterior fossa. Whatever the reasons for choosing observation as a management strategy, when this form of management is selected, relatively frequent MRI imaging (i.e., 6- to 12-month intervals) is recommended because, although the lesions are generally slow growing, occasionally rapid growth can occur.

Intervention as Opposed to Observation

Although it is difficult to set absolute standards for intervention, examples include the young patient without, or especially, with neurologic symptoms and signs; a large tumor (generally greater than 3 cm); the asymptomatic patient's preference for removal; and documented neurologic and/or radiographic progression. The recommendation to intervene then leads to selection of a treatment alternative that seems most reasonable from both the physician's and the patient's points of view.

SURGERY

Realistically, most surgeons focus primarily on the removal of the significant bulk (i.e., Simpson grade 3) of the tumor and "decompression" of neurologic structures including the brain stem and cranial nerves.[7] Although it is known that recurrence will often follow when the tumor is not totally removed, the morbidity associated with attempts at total resection is clearly higher. However, in the modern era, and in the hands of experienced surgeons, the extent of resection has dramatically improved and has been associated with a marked decrease in morbidity.[8] In large part, this decrease in morbidity relates to the use of skull base surgical approaches that rely on bone removal as opposed to brain retraction to create tumor exposure.

There are general concepts that are important for the successful removal of most meningiomas; these include adequate bony exposure, early eradication of vascular supply, debulking of tumor mass, and maintenance of the arachnoid plane. A sufficient bony exposure greatly facilitates surgical manipulation and allows the surgeon an opportunity to move from one section of the tumor to another. Although it is preferable to internally debulk most tumors so that the tumor capsule can be more easily separated from adjacent normal structures, for many vascular lesions, an approach that provides access to and early elimination of the vascular supply is desirable (Fig. 68-3). Once the vascular supply is eliminated, a far less challenging resection may be possible.

Although not essential, image guidance can facilitate tumor resections, especially those along the petrous bone and in the petroclival region. For the experienced surgeon, the surgical anatomy is so familiar that simply by maintaining the arachnoid planes one can appreciate the boundaries of

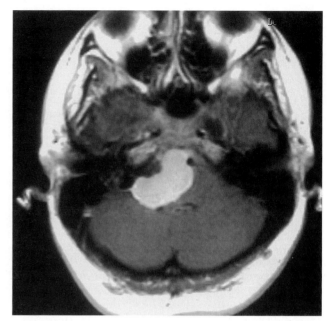

FIGURE 68-3 Petroclival tumor extending into the cerebellopontine angle. Although the lesion can be reached through a retrosigmoid exposure, the petrosal approach allowed ready access to and eradication of the feeding arteries. Note on the axial image that the basilar artery is displaced but not narrowed. The tumor readily separated from the artery in this case, and perforating vessels were preserved.

the lesion; however, for those with less experience, image guidance can help with orientation, save considerable time by providing a map around petrous bone and clival structures, and indicate the extent of the residual lesion as the resection proceeds.

Caused partially by the location of the cells of origin of meningiomas, these tumors are commonly situated next to cerebral venous structures, the preservation of which is often critical. Generally, acute occlusion of major draining veins or sinuses as a result of surgical approach and/or dissection is likely to lead to cerebral edema and significant neurologic deficit, and should be avoided. Despite this, instances of resection of the tumor-infiltrated walls of a patent sagittal sinus with successful repair, complete tumor resection, and maintenance of sinus patency have been reported.[9] In addition, division of the sigmoid and transverse sinuses during petrosal and pineal approaches, respectively, have been reported.[10,11] In principle, however, it is safest to avoid division of major veins and sinuses. It is quite reasonable to consider radical subtotal resections, leaving patent venous structures intact and following the patient to monitor growth of the residual tumor with consideration of radiation in a delayed fashion.

RADIATION

Conventional Radiation Therapy. Meningiomas are best managed with total excision, if that is achievable with acceptable morbidity. However, about one third of meningiomas are not fully resectable because of tumor location, size, and proximity to adjacent tissue and vascular structures. The posterior fossa is also a common site of residual postoperative disease.[12] Because subtotal resection is associated with a higher chance of clinically significant recurrence than is total resection, postoperative radiotherapy has been common practice and is associated with improved local tumor control and low morbidity.[13,14] The goals of radiotherapy are to prevent tumor progression, prolong the interval to recurrence, and improve survival whether administered as adjuvant or primary therapy.

As primary therapy, radiation therapy has been shown to be efficacious for tumor control and long-term relapse-free survival.[15–18] The standard recommendation for external beam radiotherapy is a dose of 5400 to 6000 cGy in fractionated doses of 180 to 200 cGy to the entire tumor plus a 2 cm margin. Histologically benign meningiomas have most often been treated with a lower dose of about 5400 cGy, and malignant meningiomas have been treated with 6000 cGy. To these dosing standards, the recent addition of intensity modulated radiation therapy (IMRT) has significantly improved the delivery process. IMRT allows for the administration of multiple and highly conformal radiation beams to be delivered to the tumor volume while significantly decreasing the dose to immediately adjacent tissue (e.g., the optic tracts, acoustic and facial nerves, and brain stem). Three-dimensional radiography coupled with CT- or MRI-assisted computerized treatment planning and precise tumor localization and patient immobilization techniques have all served to improve progression-free survival as compared with the techniques used previously.[19]

In the past, radiotherapy has been used primarily as an adjuvant for treatment of meningioma after subtotal resection, for infiltrating tumor into the adjacent brain parenchyma, and after multiple recurrences. Although postoperative radiotherapy has never been evaluated in a randomized trial, there have been large retrospective analyses, and the results of these strongly support its role following subtotal resection.[14,15] Recurrence rates of 60% after subtotal resection (vs. 32% after subtotal resection plus radiotherapy at mean follow-up of 78 months), and 5-year freedom-from-recurrence of 59% after subtotal resection alone (vs. 77% after postoperative radiation therapy) have been noted.[13] These studies also found that median time-to-recurrence was doubled by radiotherapy (i.e., 66 months vs. 125 months) and this analysis was notable in that many of the irradiated patients had more adverse factors such as surgically unfavorable sites (e.g., posterior fossa) than did patients treated with surgery alone.

In another report, findings for skull base meningiomas (including those in the posterior fossa) did not differ significantly in terms of progression-free survival from similar findings for other, more favorable sites.[12] An interesting observation suggests that progression-free survival rate at 5 years for those patients treated before 1980 was 77%, versus 98% for those treated after 1980 when CT and MRI became available for tumor localization and treatment planning.[19] The Royal Marsden Hospital experience also supported the role for postoperative radiotherapy, particularly following subtotal resection.[18] All patients were treated to a total dose of 5000 to 5500 cGy over 6 to 6.5 weeks. Interestingly, there was no significant difference in disease-free survival of minimum postoperative residual versus bulky residual; with actuarial disease-free survivals at 5, 10, and 15 years, patients with minimum residual tumor had survival rates of 78%, 67%, and 56%, respectively, whereas patients with bulky residual tumor had survival rates of 81%, 68%, and 61%, respectively. As salvage therapy for patients with recurrent or progressive disease, radiotherapy may be used either alone or as an adjuvant to surgical resection. In these cases, local control with the radiotherapy appears equal to or superior to that seen with reresection alone.[14,20,21] With a total dose of 4500 to 5500 cGy using older megavoltage radiation, the crude salvage rate was 50% as compared with 37% for reoperation alone.[20] More recent reports showed 10-year tumor control rates in the range of 80% with adjuvant radiotherapy following reoperation, as opposed to 10% to 30% for surgery alone.[21] Although the local control rate following salvage radiotherapy compares favorably with rates seen with immediate postoperative radiotherapy, these data should not be interpreted as a sole justification for withholding radiation in the early postoperative period. Given the natural history of many meningiomas, progression, although common, is often extremely slow, and the decision as to when to radiate (i.e., immediate postoperative period vs. time of recurrence) is a matter for the treating physician and patient. In the authors' practice, radiation is generally postponed to the time of demonstrable radiographic or clinical progression.

Stereotactic Radiation Therapy and Radiosurgery. Despite the favorable results obtained with conventional fractionated radiotherapy for subtotally resected, unresectable, and "inoperable" meningiomas, the use of radiosurgery evolved as both adjuvant and primary therapy; however, controversy exists. The arguments against the routine use of radiosurgery are largely based on the lack of long-term radiosurgical data and on the fear of potential delayed radiation injury to the brain tissue. However, considering the encapsulation of most benign meningiomas, the relatively low risk of infiltration into the adjacent brain tissue, the steep dose gradient characteristics, and the low reported morbidity (albeit after relatively short-term follow-up), the use of radiosurgery has become firmly established and is readily applied to meningiomas in the posterior fossa. Another significant concern has been the likelihood that secondary tumors will develop in the wake of radiosurgery, although very few reports have appeared in the literature to date.[22] Fractionated radiosurgery has also become readily available (Fig. 68-4), largely as a result of noninvasive patient immobilization methods including "head mask" frame (i.e., noninvasive) and frameless image-guidance systems.

A recent report evaluating fractionated stereotactic radiotherapy showed survival rates of 97% for 5 years and 96% for 10 years after treatment, with local failure seen in only 3 out of 189 patients with World Health Organization (WHO) grade I meningiomas (22.5% located in the posterior fossa).[23] These researchers noted tumor shrinkage (i.e., more than 50% reduction) in 14% of patients, and resolution of preexisting cranial nerve symptoms in 28% of patients. Clinically significant treatment-related toxicity was seen in 1.6% of the patients.[23] Outcomes data for radiosurgery are available for intracranial meningiomas, generally, as well as for those located in the posterior fossa. Engenhart reported an experience of radiosurgery in 17 patients with histologically proven benign meningiomas. Using a linear accelerator radiosurgery system, a maximum single dose of 10 to 50 Gy was used, with mean dose of 29 Gy prescribed to the 80% isodose line matching the tumor volume.[24] The dose was chosen based on tumor volume, location, and the radiosensitivity of the

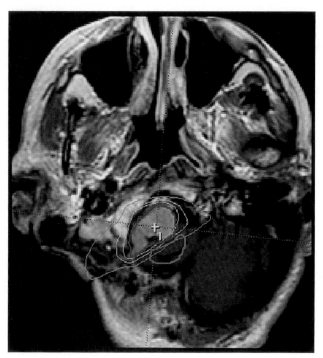

FIGURE 68-4 Fractionated radiosurgical treatment plan for a foramen magnum meningioma.

adjacent brain tissue. Freedom from tumor progression was noted in 80% of patients, and late complications included transient neurologic deficits with perifocal brain edema and one case of visual loss.

Also relating to intracranial meningiomas in general, Kondziolka reported 2-year radiosurgical tumor control rates of 96% in 50 patients.[25,26] The radiosurgery dose was 10 to 25 Gy (mean, 17 Gy) to the tumor margin using a gamma knife unit; the doses were chosen based on tumor volume, location, previous radiotherapy dose, and adjacent critical normal tissue (e.g., optic chiasm). Tumors greater than 35 mm in diameter and located within 5 mm from the optic chiasm were excluded for radiosurgery. Three patients experienced delayed neurologic complications, thought to be consistent with radiation injury, at 3 to 12 months following radiosurgery.[25–27] In another report from the Mayo clinic on radiosurgical results for meningioma (in which 77% of 206 tumors were located at the cranial base), median tumor margin dose was 16 Gy and survival rates at 5 and 7 years were 94% and 92%, respectively.[28] The overall tumor control rate was 89% at 5 years, with 56% of tumors decreasing in size. Taken together, the available data relating intracranial meningiomas (with the endpoint as freedom from progression after radiosurgery) indicate that tumor control appears to be in the range of 90% with tumor shrinkage noted in approximately one third of radiosurgical patients.

Meningiomas in the posterior fossa often will require radiation as either adjuvant or primary therapy. The radiosurgical experiences for acoustic and other schwannomas, as well as those for various benign and malignant tumors, have provided an important database regarding the responses of the cranial nerves and brain stem. For practical purposes, most cranial nerves are tolerant to radiosurgical doses up to

16 Gy, whereas the optic nerves, chiasm, and tracts seem more sensitive, and lower doses up to 10 Gy seem reasonable.[29] Of note, the radiosurgical response may vary depending on the length of nerve irradiated; the microenvironment of the nerve (e.g., ischemia); the degree of compression by the tumor; prior surgery and radiotherapy effects; retreatment and treatment intervals; and additional host factors[30,31] (Fig. 68-5). Motor morbidity rates appear to be less than 5%. However, the assessment of sensory nerve function poses more difficult problems, depending on the tumor type and location. For example, whereas the radiosurgical impact on cochlear nerve function may be less significant when dealing with meningiomas, radiosurgical dosing for acoustic neuroma has undergone a gradual decrease, possibly as a result of the intimate relation of tumor to nerve. One recent report on 55 patients with skull base meningiomas (3 petrous apex, 4 tentorium, 2 clivus, 5 CPA, and 3 jugular foramen) with average follow-up of 48.4 months, noted tumor stabilization in 69%, shrinkage in 29%, and enlargement in 2%.[32] Mean tumor volume was 7.33 cm³, and doses ranged from 12 to 25 Gy. All complications were transient, including seven trigeminal pareses and three patients with diplopia. Radiosurgical data on 62 patients with petroclival meningiomas treated with tumor margin doses of 11 to 20 Gy documented tumor shrinkage in 23%, stabilization in 68%, and growth in 8%.[33] Median follow-up was 37 months.

For tumor residuals intimately attached to the dural sinuses, similar principles apply. Based on the current literature, it is reasonable to use radiosurgery for tumor located adjacent or inside a dural sinus. There does not appear to be increased risk of weakening of the walls of the sinus, venous infarction, or other vascular-related complications, and it seems unlikely that radiosurgery will lead to progressive sinus occlusion. Larger experience and longer-term follow-up will be needed to answer these questions.

Combined Surgery and Radiation

Ultimately, it seems logical to consider a combination of surgical resection and postoperative radiation treatment for the management of many of these patients. In this way, the surgeon can remove the bulk of the tumor and the residual tumor can be treated with radiation or simply observed until progression is documented. A word of caution: although subtotal resection followed by radiation may be in the patient's best interest from a neurologic point of view, the larger the surgical remnant, especially those in close proximity to critical structures (e.g., optic nerves or brain stem), the more challenging and potentially risky the radiation treatment prescription and risk.

Perioperative Issues

There are several issues that, although not exclusively related to meningiomas, are commonly encountered in dealing with meningioma.

Preoperative Edema and Postoperative Swelling

Many patients present with meningiomas that have significant associated peritumoral edema. The edema appears as a low-intensity signal on T1-weighted MRI and as a high-intensity signal on T2-weighted MRI images. Unlike that seen with gliomas, with meningioma this signal does not

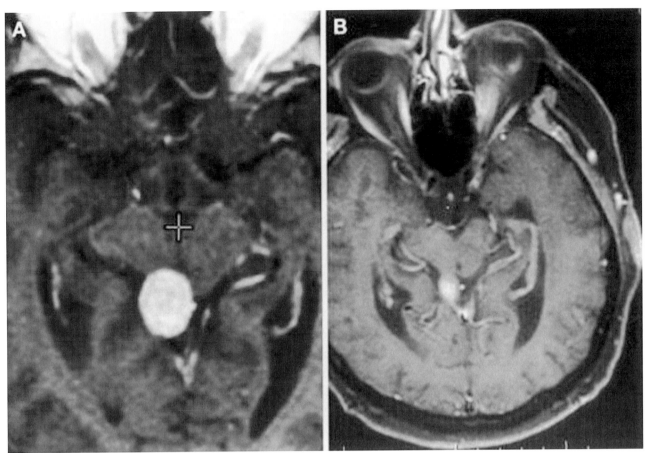

FIGURE 68-5 *A*, Axial contrast-enhanced magnetic resonance images showing tentorial meningioma at the time of radiosurgery in 1992. *B*, Tumor regression 10 years later. (From Kondziolka D, Nathoo N, Flickinger JC, et al: Long-term results after radiosurgery for benign intracranial tumors. Neurosurgery 53[4]:815–822, 2003.)

represent tumor infiltration but rather increased water concentration. Increased water content may lead to significant mass effect and must be considered in preparation for tumor removal. Edema can complicate the initial and postoperative stages of the operation. In the former, edematous brain will force its way out as the dura is opened; this can lead to unnecessary frustration and cortical resection in the early stages of the operation. In the postoperative stage, inadequate attention to peritumoral edema can lead to greatly increased pressure in the posterior fossa, herniation, and death. Significant preoperative edema is best managed by the administration of steroids; this should begin several days prior to the operation. When steroids (typically, decadron 4 mg every 8 hours) are begun several days prior to the operation, the likelihood of difficulty in the initial phases of the operation is low even though the peritumoral T2 signal remains unchanged.

The postoperative problems secondary to edema are best dealt with during the operation by ensuring sufficient bony exposure, thereby limiting the extent of cerebellar retraction, which can aggravate the edema. A difficult tumor dissection may distract the surgeon, and when tumor removal requires greater and greater retraction, it is often best to resect the portion of the commonly contused cerebellum underlying the retractor rather than leave it in. This area can further swell and create significant, if not

fatal, postoperative problems. Steroids are continued into the postoperative period and osmotic diuretics (i.e., mannitol) may also be useful. Standard skull base approaches specifically for petroclival tumors now substitute bony removal for cerebellar retraction as the primary means to achieve the necessary exposure for safe tumor resection.

Large Tumor without Preoperative Edema and Postoperative Swelling

An uncommon but important observation relates to large tumors without surrounding edema on preoperative MRI. Very often after uneventful tumor resection (i.e., slack brain after total resection and no apparent venous injury), the patient will do well for the first day and then become progressively more sleepy, after which CT will demonstrate extensive brain edema that has filled the resection cavity. The reason for this observation is not entirely clear, but aggressive management of elevated intracranial pressure with osmotic diuretics and possibly reintubation is required; reoperation for dural grafting and brain resection may be necessary.

Tumor En-plaque Extension beyond Typical Craniotomy

Meningiomas grow along the meninges, and a bony resection that closely conforms to the overtly contrast-enhancing mass of the tumor may often be insufficient.

Because the tumor extends along the meninges, it is best to make a larger bony opening and therefore have the opportunity to remove the lateral en-plaque extensions of the tumor if necessary. Image guidance can be helpful in these situations.

Hyperostosis

Although still somewhat controversial, the hypertrophic bony changes often noted adjacent to meningiomas are known in many instances to be secondary to tumor invasion. Previous theories have suggested that these bony changes were related to vascular disturbances, "irritation" of the bone, osteoblastic stimulation by tumor, and direct tumor-derived bone formation.[34] The authors' own experience, as well as the plentiful evidence in the literature, demonstrate that in many, if not in all cases, these changes are secondary to tumor invasion. The practical issue then relates to the potential for tumor recurrence, and it is well-known that the best chance of cure follows radical tumor resection including the involved dura and bone (i.e., Simpson grade 1).

Venous Obstruction and Infarction

More obvious with supratentorial tumors, venous infarction can also complicate surgery in the posterior fossa. Adequate exposure and internal debulking (when possible) of the tumor are the best means of avoiding this complication. After debulking, the tumor falls away or can be more easily separated from the adjacent vein. The effects of disrupting the venous sinuses (deep and superficial draining veins) are not completely predictable. The veins near the roof of the fourth ventricle (i.e., around the cerebellar vermis and tonsils, petrosal veins, and the veins of cerebellomedullary fissure) can usually be sacrificed without major consequences. However, sacrificing the vein of Galen, torcula, dominant lateral, or sigmoid sinuses is considered high risk.[10,11] Resection of a meningioma involving unilateral transverse sinus is feasible when the contralateral traverse sinus is open and close to the size of involved sinus. If a significant size discrepancy exists, prior to division of the involved transverse sinus, temporary sinus occlusion and pressure measurement should be considered.[11] When present, significant changes in manometric pressures during temporary occlusion and acute but temporary brain swelling indicate high risk.

When a dural sinus is partially occluded, the surgeon will usually decide to radically remove the tumor mass but leave the patent sinus intact. Eventually, with continued tumor growth, the sinus will occlude, and if adjuvant therapy is either not recommended or is ineffective, total resection can be considered at that time.

Tumor-Brain Interface

In most situations, the tumor does not adhere significantly to the brain surface. Although limited adhesions do exist, these are easily divided, and the tumor separates by simply advancing a cotton patty along the tumor-brain interface. The surgeon must pay attention so that small veins and arteries along this plane are not unnecessarily disrupted. On the other hand, invasive tumors (i.e., generally atypical and malignant subtypes) do invade the pial and brain surface, and great care must be exercised during dissection (especially along the brain stem) to remain on the tumor's immediate surface.

Hydrocephalus

Hydrocephalus is one of the common presenting symptoms of posterior fossa meningiomas, particularly those located in the fourth ventricle. Although not all cases of hydrocephalus associated with posterior fossa meningiomas are obstructive, careful consideration must be given prior to lumbar puncture, which can have serious ramifications. When surgical resection is delayed, it may be appropriate to relieve the hydrocephalus either by temporary ventriculostomy, ventriculoperitoneal shunt, or third ventriculostomy. On many occasions, removal of the tumor with temporary postoperative ventricular drainage will serve to adequately manage hydrocephalus. At the authors' center, external ventriculostomy is the preferred method for managing hydrocephalus because intracranial pressure can be better monitored after resection of the tumor and, ultimately, if there is no longer need for a shunt, it can be removed easily.

Specific Locations in the Posterior Fossa

Occipital and Lateral Petrous Surface of the Posterior Fossa

Tumors located along the midline and lateral aspect of the occipital surface and lateral petrous bone (i.e., lateral to the internal auditory meatus) are, surgically speaking, the least problematic (Fig. 68-6). Meningiomas in this region often present with symptoms of cerebellar dysfunction and headache, but they may also present as an incidental finding during workup for unrelated central nervous system symptoms. Occasionally these tumors present with signs of elevated intracranial pressure. A suboccipital craniectomy/craniotomy is generally sufficient, and standard surgical techniques are employed to remove the tumor. The main surgical challenge is not to inadvertently open a patent dural sinus, although

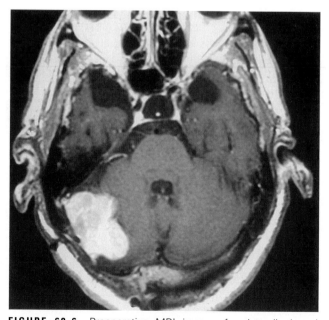

FIGURE 68-6 Preoperative MRI image of a laterally based meningioma that originated from the suboccipital surface and was easily removed through a retrosigmoid incision and laterally oriented craniotomy without morbidity. Although the tumor separated from the transverse sinus, infiltration was apparent; radiation was not administered, and frequent follow-up is required.

a simple suture or graft will generally suffice as closure. The surgeon must realize that collateral venous drainage around an occluded sinus may be critical and should be protected. For those lesions located on the petrous bone lateral to the CPA, careful attention to the nerves coursing into the internal auditory meatus is required, and electrophysiologic monitoring of both the facial and acoustic nerves is recommended. Although these lateral petrous tumors may be seen on MRI to be adjacent but lateral to the facial and acoustic nerve complex, the ability to stimulate the facial nerve, especially as it is located behind the tumor (i.e., in the surgeon's view), can be very reassuring. It is important after the resection is complete to assess whether the adjacent cerebellum has been too heavily retracted or contused. In either case, resection of the injured brain may be prudent to avoid the postoperative risks associated with swelling.

Tentorial Surface

The clinical presentation of patients with tentorial meningioma is generally nonspecific. When the tumor originates in the anterior region of the tentorium, compression of the trigeminal and abducens nerves may lead to tic doloreaux and occulomotor paresis, but trochlear nerve signs are uncommon. Tumors originating from the posterior region of the tentorium rarely present with other than headache and, perhaps, mild cerebellar signs. Occasionally, as a result of occlusion of the dural sinuses, a meningioma may present with signs of elevated intracranial pressure and visual loss (Fig. 68-7).

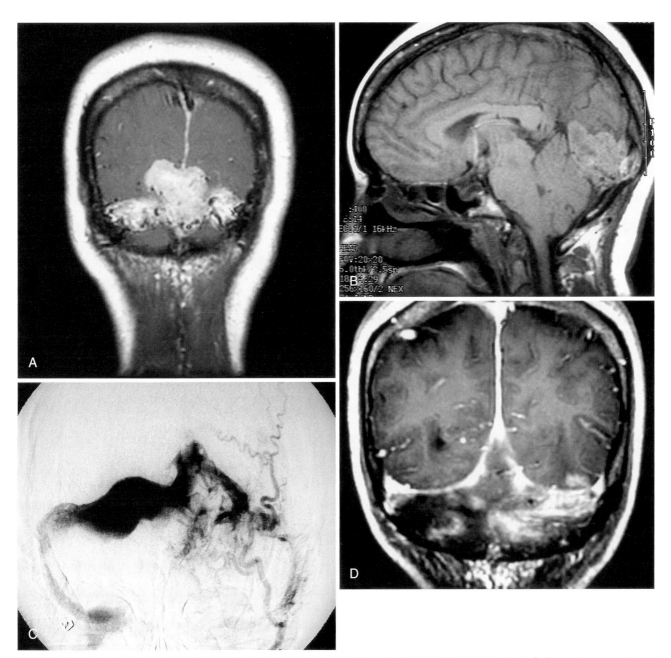

FIGURE 68-7 *A,* Coronal enhanced image of tentorial meningioma. *B,* Sagittal image of the same lesion. *C,* Pretreatment angiogram depicting the intense tumor stain and extensive collateral drainage. *D,* Coronal image 9 months postradiation treatment with 60 Gy.

An additional but rare clinical presentation involves that of trigeminal neuralgia and hemifacial spasm secondary to a tumor that arises on the posterior portion of the tentorium but not involving the CPA.[35] In this case the presumed cause of the neurologic symptoms and signs was rotation of the brain stem secondary to the large size of the tumor such that the cranial nerves were brought in contact with an ectatic vertebral artery. All symptoms and signs resolved after tumor removal.

Tumors originating from the posterior portion of the tentorium and extending into the posterior fossa are easily resected via standard suboccipital or retrosigmoid approaches. The tumor rarely invades the underlying cerebellum, and standard surgical techniques, as just noted for tumors located on the suboccipital and lateral petrosal surfaces, are sufficient. For those lesions extending toward the CPA, care must be taken to determine the location of the seventh and eighth cranial nerves, but generally this is not a significant obstacle to total resection, and every effort to preserve and even improve hearing should be made because this is a much more realistic goal with meningiomas (as opposed to

acoustic schwannomas). Small lesions arising more anteriorly along the tentorium are usually adequately managed with a standard subtemporal approach, but for larger tumors, some variation on the transpetrosal approaches described in the following may be necessary.

Although not a unique feature of tentorial meningiomas, an interesting surgical challenge concerns the handling of the dural venous sinuses. Generally, resection of these sinuses is not recommended if there is any indication of patency on angiography, MRV, or by direct intraoperative observation. However, when the sinus is completely occluded, it can be resected, but attention to the collateral venous drainage is critical because disruption of significant collateral drainage can be fatal.[36] Collignon recently reported a case of occlusion of the torcula and bilateral transverse sinuses with hemangiopericytoma (Fig. 68-8).[37] The patient presented with visual blurring and bilateral papilledema, which was managed by bilateral occipital and suboccipital craniotomy. The tumor was noted to be filling the sinuses without extension beyond the walls of the sinuses. Total resection was achieved, and control of venous bleeding was

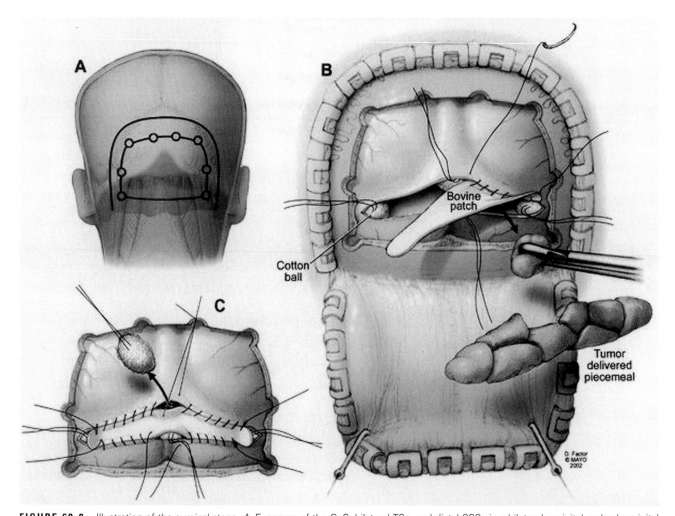

FIGURE 68-8   Illustration of the surgical steps. *A,* Exposure of the CoS, bilateral TSs, and distal SSS via a bilateral occipital and suboccipital craniotomy. *B,* The TSs are opened and the tumor is removed in a piecemeal fashion. Cotton balls control sinus bleeding while the venous sinuses are repaired with the aid of a bovine patch. *C,* Completion of the sinus repair after sequential removal of the cotton balls. (From Collignon FP, Cohen-Gadol AA, Piepgras DG: Hemangiopericytoma of the confluence of sinuses and the transverse sinuses. J Neurosurg 99:1085–1088, 2003.)

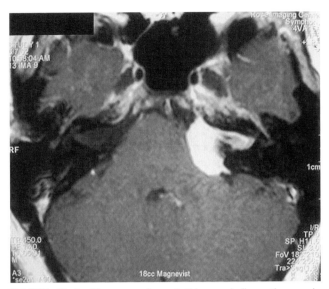

FIGURE 68-9 The extension of this cerebellopontine angle meningioma into the internal auditory canal is a relatively uncommon feature. Note also the normal diameter of the canal, an uncommon feature for acoustic schwannoma.

accomplished with cotton balls, after which the sinus was repaired with bovine pericardial graft. Radiation therapy was used adjunctively, and 4 months after surgery the sinus remained patent, the patient was well, and papilledema had resolved. Although this unique case and others demonstrates the feasibility of sinus resection, it should not be undertaken lightly.

Cerebellopontine Angle

The CPA is the most common location for posterior fossa meningiomas, which are thought to originate from arachnoid cap cells in this region. The primary differential diagnostic consideration is acoustic neuroma, which arises from schwann cells on the vestibular division of the statoacoustic nerve. Patients generally present in their fourth and fifth decades of life.[38] The clinical presentation, as for meningiomas as a whole, depends on the site of origin and direction of growth. Tumors growing superior to the internal auditory meatus commonly present with trigeminal symptoms (notably numbness and/or neuralgia), whereas those growing alongside the meatus may present with auditory and facial nerve dysfunction, the latter being distinctly uncommon with vestibular schwannoma. Those tumors growing inferior to the meatus may present with dysfunction of the lower cranial nerves (i.e., IX through XII). Symptoms and signs secondary to brain stem and cerebellar compression, owing to the slow growth of the typical meningioma, are a late occurrence and often are not apparent even with very large tumors. CPA meningiomas cannot be distinguished from other tumor types based on clinical presentation alone, even though hearing loss and vestibular dysfunction are far less common with meningioma than with acoustic schwannoma.

MRI is the study of choice, although various auditory tests (e.g., pure-tone audiometry, speech discrimination, acoustic reflex, and brain stem auditory evoked responses) are commonly performed in neuro-otology practice, where many patients presenting with hearing loss are first evaluated.

MRI findings (i.e., extra-axial CPA mass) can include an enlarged CPA cistern, gray-white distortion of the adjacent cerebellum, and an indication of contrast enhancement extending along the skull base beyond the main tumor mass (i.e., dural tail) (Fig. 68-9). Calcification and cystic change are more common and less common, respectively, with meningiomas, whereas expansion of the porus acousticus is uncommon for the meningiomas. Although a typical acoustic schwannoma has the appearance of an ice cream cone, with sharply demarcated and rounded borders along the CPA portion with tumor extension filling the fundus of the internal auditory canal (IAC), meningiomas most often fill the CPA cistern with lateral extensions, irregular borders, and distinctly less notable growth into the IAC.

Because the epicenter of the tumor is the IAC, a standard lateral suboccipital approach will generally provide sufficient exposure for complete tumor removal.[39] The patient is placed in a "park-bench" position with the head slightly flexed and tilted toward the floor, after which the nose is rotated toward the floor. Mannitol and spinal drainage may facilitate the exposure and help to maintain this exposure, especially with larger tumors and longer dissections. The facial and acoustic nerves are routinely monitored. Given the fact that the cranial nerves do not generally adhere to the tumor capsule, hearing preservation and even improvement should be reasonable expectations.

The craniotomy is centered about 1 cm behind the mastoid process, and exposure of the sigmoid sinus will allow decreased retraction and about 0.5 to 1 cm of additional exposure anterior to the cerebellum. After durotomy and throughout subsequent dissection, attention must always be directed to brain stem auditory responses that will act as a guide to the impact of cerebellar retraction on hearing function, which may easily be lost by direct medial retraction. The microscopic tumor dissection begins by assessment of cranial nerve and brain stem/cerebellar relationships. Once the cranial nerves have been identified, small cotton patties can be introduced into the tumor/cranial nerve/brain stem/cerebellar planes. The vascular supply to these tumors generally originates from vessels traversing the petrous bone and tentorium, and commonly will be difficult to interrupt early in the dissection because the trajectories of the facial and acoustic nerves must be clearly defined before coagulating across the base of the tumor. With smaller tumors, interruption of the vascular supply will greatly facilitate the subsequent dissection. With large tumors, internal debulking may be required to create "space" around tumor boundaries. As a rule, safe removal of posterior fossa tumors requires extensive internal debulking. After the majority of the tumor has been removed from the CPA, and the facial, acoustic, and trigeminal nerves are isolated, the portion located in the fundus of the IAC can be removed. The limits to bony removal along the IAC (i.e., generally less than 10 mm but may be precisely determined on preoperative temporal bone CT) are set by the location of the common crus of the posterior and superior semicircular canals. Disruption of this structure will lead to deafness. At this point, the surgical resection is usually terminated (Simpson grade II). When possible, the surrounding dura that is invaded by tumor should be removed, but the resection will generally not be absolutely complete, and careful MRI follow-up over the next 5 to 10 years is required.

Other surgical approaches can be considered, but these have their own limitations. The translabyrinthine approach may be suitable when hearing is absent and may allow for early devascularization, but the bony drilling is time consuming. The standard petrosal approach will generally be too extensive for most lesions limited to the CPA, and the subtemporal approach is too limited for most of these tumors.

Petroclival

Anatomically, the petroclival region extends along the midline from the level of the posterior clinoid process to the jugular foramen and laterally to the CPA, incorporating cranial nerves III through XI and the brain stem. In a recent publication, Cho described hearing loss, facial and trigeminal pareses, gait disturbance, dysarthria, spasticity, and headache as the predominant clinical findings in patients with petroclival meningiomas prior to surgery.[40]

Surgically speaking, meningiomas centered in the petroclival region are among the most challenging lesions to manage. Although there are many feasible surgical approaches to this region (e.g., transbasal, transoral, frontotemporal, subtemporal-transtentorial, combined subtemporal-suboccipital, transpetrous variations, and transsphenoidal), all except the transpetrous approaches have limitations in accessing only a limited portion of the tumor. For lesions straddling a significant portion of the petroclival region, the most useful approach involves an exposure around and/or through the petrous bone.

Pioneered by Malis, transpetrous approaches provide exposure above and behind the petrous bone into the middle and posterior fossa, respectively.[41] Subsequent modifications of this approach provided additional exposure by incorporating various extents of petrous bone resection (i.e., retrolabyrinthine) which, in keeping with standard skull base techniques, markedly decreases the need for temporal lobe, cerebellar, and brain stem retraction, thereby minimizing morbidity and allowing for total to near-total tumor resection.[42] This approach follows a route anterior to the sigmoid sinus and shortens the distance from the operator to the tumor. The approach also increases the risk to hearing loss by inadvertent drilling into the posterior semicircular canal; however, even this approach cannot easily visualize the most anteromedial portion of tumors extending along the midline clivus.

The anterior transpetrous approach is well-suited for smaller lesions centered medial and superior to the internal auditory meatus (IAM) and is based on the original description of the extended middle fossa approach.[40,43,44] In 1991, Spetzler reported the results of various extents of petrous bone resection (i.e., retrolabyrinthine, translabyrinthine, and transcochlear) for 46 lesions including 18 petroclival meningiomas.[10] A recent report describes the addition of an anterior transpetrous bony removal (i.e., anteromedial to the cochlea, posteromedial to the petrous carotid, and inferior and medial to the gasserian ganglion) to a standard petrosal approach.[40] The authors report that in five of seven tumors, total resection was accomplished with neither mortality nor a decrease in performance status, and only one patient lost hearing.

In the combined approach, the patient is placed in a supine position with a bolster under the shoulder and the head is turned about 30 to 45 degrees to the contralateral side.[40] The supra- and infratentorial craniotomy utilizes four burr holes placed above and below the transverse-sigmoid junction plus one hole immediately above the zygoma, another at the superior temporal line, and one hole in the posterior fossa. The plate can frequently be removed as one piece. Next, a mastoidectomy with retrolabyrinthine bony removal is performed. The middle fossa dura is elevated, and the middle meningeal artery and greater superficial petrosal nerve are divided. The horizontal portion of the carotid is then exposed, and after identification and elevation of the third division of the trigeminal nerve, the anteromedial petrous apex (i.e., anteromedial to the cochlea) is removed, exposing the upper clivus. The dura is then opened above and below the superior petrosal sinus (SPS). The SPS is divided after the surgeon has carefully examined the MRV to ensure that no significant temporal bridging vein will be interrupted.[45] This maneuver exposes the middle and inferior clival regions. The tumor can now be appreciated, and piecemeal removal follows with initial attention to the vascular supply. By working back and forth between the inferior and superior extremes of this exposure, the surgeon often can radically remove the tumor and safely work around vascular and nervous elements. The initial phases of the dissection may be facilitated by image guidance, especially regarding the anterior transpetrous resection. The approach provides excellent exposure for lesions centered on the midline and extending in an ipsilateral direction, as well as for extensions across the midline. The most anteromedial portions of the tumor may occasionally be better visualized through the retrosigmoid portion of the exposure toward the end of the dissection (see Fig. 68-3). If hearing is to be preserved, this combined approach will generally be required (especially for larger tumors); however, when hearing is not an issue, the translabyrinthine and transcochlear bony variations add considerably to the exposure.

Jugular Foramen

The jugular foramen region is a relatively uncommon origin for meningiomas.

Symptoms and signs reflect the local anatomy with involvement of cranial nerves IX to XI (occasionally V and VIII), and larger tumors may be associated with brain stem compression.[46] Because of the nature of the preoperative neurologic deficits, otolaryngology evaluation should be performed to establish a preoperative baseline, but postoperative testing will also be required and is more critical.

Monitoring of cranial nerves VII, VIII, IX, XI, and XII should be performed because these nerves may be hidden (especially IX and XI) by the tumor capsule. Al-Mefty describes a suprajugular, retrojugular, and transjugular approach for tumors in this region, with the patency and dominance of the jugular bulb dictating the choice.[47] The infralabyrinthine suprajugular approach requires a mastoidectomy followed by skeletonization of the superior petrosal and sigmoid sinuses and jugular bulb, after which the tumor is dissected from the cranial nerves (Fig. 68-10). In the retrojugular approach, a lateral suboccipital craniotomy and mastoidectomy with skeletonization of the sigmoid sinus and jugular bulb are followed by removal of a portion of the occipital condyle and jugular tubercle. A durotomy posterior to the sigmoid sinus provides the exposure for tumor removal. In the transjugular variation, a mastoidectomy that exposes the sigmoid sinus, jugular bulb, and

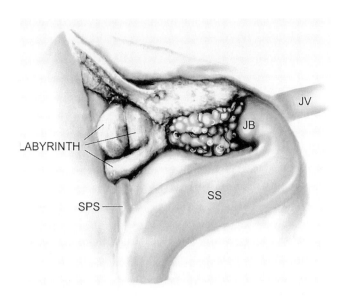

FIGURE 68-10 Drawing of the suprajugular approach. Note the infralabyrinthine position of the tumor; the SS; the JB, which is patent; the JV; the superior petrosal sinus (SPS); and the labyrinth (right side is shown). (From Arnautovic KI, Al-Mefty O: Primary meningiomas of the jugular fossa. J Neurosurg 97:12–20, 2002.)

jugular vein and suboccipital craniotomy is performed. The posterior belly of the digastric muscle and the stylohyoid muscle are divided, after which the styloid process is removed. The sigmoid sinus and jugular vein are ligated above and below the tumor, respectively, and the tumor is dissected from the cranial nerves and carotid artery (Fig. 68-11). In this series of eight patients (nine surgeries), worsened or new deficits in three patients were reported, and some degree of recovery or stabilization was noted in all eight patients.[46]

Foramen Magnum

Meningiomas at the foramen magnum arise from the dura of the craniocervical junction; they account for 4.2% to 20% of posterior fossa meningiomas, depending on the referral status of the reporting institution[47] (Fig. 68-12).

These tumors tend to go undiagnosed or misdiagnosed for long periods because of the variety of presenting symptoms. Tumors can present with cerebellar signs, evidence of increased intracranial pressure, lower cranial nerve deficits, and brain stem or spinal cord signs mimicking cervical myelopathy with radicular signs and dysesthesias. In addition, symptoms of suboccipital pain may be seen.

As with all meningiomas, MRI is the study of choice and is complemented by MRA and MRV, although thin-section CT will better define bony involvement. Selective angiography can be used to determine the blood supply and the utility of preoperative embolization. The vascular supply to these tumors is predominantly from the ascending pharyngeal artery and the middle meningeal artery, whereas the dura posterior to foramen magnum is supplied by the occipital artery and the posterior meningeal branch of the vertebral artery. Those tumors located ventral to the dentate ligaments should be differentiated from those arising dorsally because of significant differences in clinical presentation, in the degree of operative difficulty, and in the likelihood of postoperative morbidity. The primary difference lies in the fact that truly ventral tumors originate anterior to the lower cranial (i.e., IX–XII), upper cervical nerves, posterior inferior cerebellar artery, and brain stem, all of which make surgical removal far more challenging.

Surgical approaches have included the standard posterior midline suboccipital approach with C1 laminectomy, the transoral approach, and the transcondylar approach.[48–50] For true ventral lesions, the posterior midline approach is insufficient for anything better than a Simpson grade IV removal, and it can be associated with significant morbidity because the spinal cord and lower brain stem will be interposed between the surgeon and the pathology. However, for lesions arising more laterally and dorsal to the dentate ligaments and displacing the spinal cord and brain stem medially, standard midline approaches may well be sufficient, although removal of the most medial extents of the tumor can be difficult in the final phases of the operation when the brain stem and spinal cord expand into the operative field. Theoretically reasonable from an anatomic viewpoint, the transoral approach provides very limited

FIGURE 68-11 Drawing of the transjugular approach. Note the tumor occluding the JB, which is open; the SS and JV, both of which are ligated; the SPS; the internal carotid artery (ICA); the lower cranial nerves (ninth through eleventh nerves) extracranially; and the labyrinth (right side is shown) (From Arnautovic KI, Al-Mefty O: Primary meningiomas of the jugular fossa. J Neurosurg 97:12–20, 2002.)

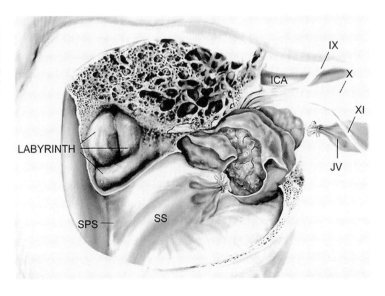

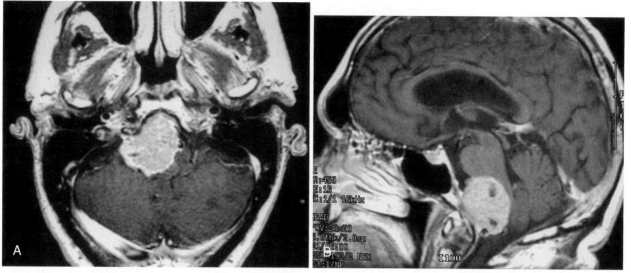

FIGURE 68-12 Enhanced T1-weighted MRI images of a foramen magnum meningioma. Although the tumor has created space along the lateral aspect of the brain stem, a more lateral approach will provide ample exposure for removal of the midline portion of the tumor toward the end of the procedure.

exposure, carries the serious risk of postoperative CSF leak through the oropharyngeal mucosa, and is best left to surgeons experienced with transoral techniques.[49] The transcondylar approach has been detailed by Sen and others[50–52] and is most suitable for practically all meningiomas in this location.

Preoperative considerations include the precise origin of the tumor, the relationship of the vertebral artery to the tumor, the relative sizes (i.e., contribution to stability) of the occipital-C1 joint, the vascular anatomy, the patency of the vertebral arteries (i.e., noted with MRA and MRV), and the status of lower cranial nerve function (especially swallowing). Patients are placed in a "park-bench" position and are monitored for somatosensory and possibly auditory brain stem function along with cranial nerves X through XII. The transcondylar approach for ventrally situated tumors will generally require transposition of the vertebral artery, which must be carefully rotated such that thrombosis will not occur during the commonly lengthy procedure. To create the greatest extent of exposure, especially for tumors with extension across the midline, one half to two thirds of the condyle may be removed. Only rarely will this require surgical stabilization. The final element in the initial exposure involves the extent of venous engorgement in the so-called suboccipital cavernous sinus, as detailed by Caruso, which can complicate the dissection.[53] From this point careful attention to the cranial nerves traversing the tumor capsule is required while the tumor is debulked and dissected. In a review of 18 patients with ventral foramen magnum tumors followed for a mean of 40 months after first-time surgery, Al-Mefty described 75% gross total (Simpson I–II), 12.5% with near-total (Simpson III), and 12.5% with subtotal excision (Simpson IV).[47] Ninth and tenth cranial nerve deficits were the most common consequence, and there was no 30-day operative mortality.

Pineal

Meningiomas in the pineal region are a rare entity constituting approximately 6% to 8% of neoplasms.[54] Most meningiomas arise from the tentorial edge or from the junction of tentorium and falx, although some instances of lesions with no dural attachment have been reported, in which case the tumor is believed to arise from the tela-choroidea in the roof of the third ventricle.[55,56] Presenting symptoms are quite variable reflecting, in part, the local anatomy. Common presenting symptoms are related to increased intracranial pressure (i.e., secondary to either tumor size or to deep venous occlusion) and/or the visual system.[57] As with many meningiomas in various locations, headache is a common but nonspecific finding. Involvement of the tectal region may manifest as various degrees of upgaze paresis, pupillary and convergence abnormalities culminating occasionally in a complete Parinaud syndrome. Additionally, symptoms and signs of cerebellar dysfunction may also occur but are uncommon. When the tumor compresses the cerebral aqueduct, hydrocephalus may develop.

The imaging study of choice is contrast-enhanced MRI with MRA and MRV, although with larger tumors cerebral angiography may be more useful for arterial and venous delineation (i.e., internal cerebral veins, basal vein of Rosenthal, vein of Galen, sinuses, and superficial venous system). Preoperative embolization, although rare, may also be considered (Fig. 68-13). Feeding vessels are commonly the medial and lateral posterior choroidal arteries as well as the tentorial arteries. Given the usual operative choices (i.e., infratentorial-supracerebellar and occipital transtentorial approaches), a clear understanding of the arterial and venous anatomy may be important because early arterial occlusion during the surgical procedure is not always possible.

In the past, surgical treatment of pineal region meningiomas has been associated with significant morbidity and mortality; however, as with meningiomas in all other locations, recent subspecialization and improvements in surgical techniques have markedly reduced these morbidities.[58] The main surgical approaches currently used are infratentorial-supracerebellar and occipital-transtentorial, with a supra/infratentorial-transsinus approach recently reported.[11] When significant obstructive hydrocephalus is detected preoperatively, insertion of a ventriculoperitoneal shunt

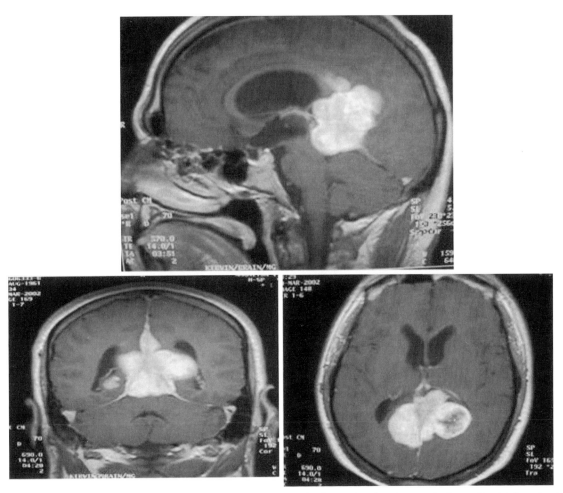

FIGURE 68-13 Sagittal, axial, and coronal T1-weighted MRI images of a large pineal region meningioma. Dural tails extend in three directions on the coronal image. This tumor was resected (i.e., Simpson grade III) via an occipital-transtentorial approach.

may be considered; however, endoscopically guided third ventriculostomy is becoming the procedure of choice.

With the occipital-transtentorial approach, it is preferable to approach the tumor from the nondominant side, but tumor shape and vascular anatomy primarily determine this orientation. The patient may be sitting or semisitting, but the authors prefer a three-quarter prone position with the operated side down.[59] The occipital lobe is gently retracted laterally, with attention paid to the bridging veins because their injury can lead to hemianopsia. After a paramedian tentorial incision, the tumor should come into view. The advantages of this approach are surgeon comfort (i.e., for those unfamiliar with the sitting position); disadvantages include limited space, potential for retraction injury to occipital lobe, off-midline anatomic orientation, and venous anatomy oriented between the surgeon and the tumor.

The advantages of the infratentorial-supracerebellar approach are the midline orientation, excellent tumor visibility below the venous system, and minimal cerebellar retraction. The main disadvantages of this approach, done with the patient in the sitting position, are limited exposure of tumors extending above the deep venous complex; and fatigue in the surgeon's arm and hand, although with appropriate flexion of the patient's head and back, this can

be minimized.[60] As for any operation with the patient in a sitting position, air embolism is a possibility.[57]

For large tumors in the pineal region, a combined supra/infratentorial-transsinus approach has been described.[11] A craniotomy in three pieces is made over the torcula and transverse sinuses, with subsequent section of transverse sinus and tentorium. This approach provides a wide surgical corridor and large exposure with access to the tumor extending into the third ventricle, minimal retraction of cerebellum and occipital lobes, and a comfortable position for the surgeon.[11]

Fourth Ventricular

Meningiomas located in the fourth ventricle are rare and usually present with signs of obstructive hydrocephalus; rarely they present with cranial neuropathies secondary to compression of cranial nerves and nuclei in the floor of the ventricle (Fig. 68-14). The surgical approach generally requires a midline suboccipital craniotomy with vermian split and early devascularization of the tumor. Care to limit iatrogenic compression of the structures in the floor and not to intrude through the floor of the ventricle is paramount. With larger tumors it is generally recommended to monitor somatosensory and brain stem auditory evoked responses along with lower cranial nerves (i.e., VI to XII).

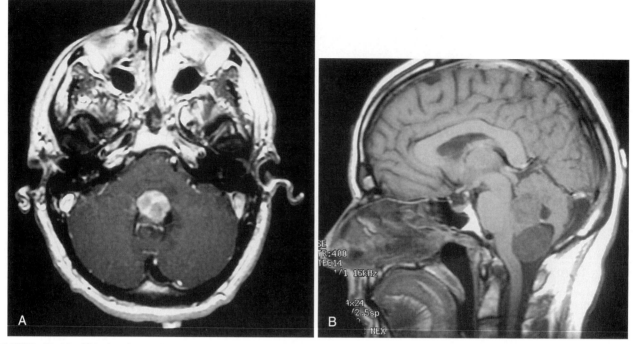

FIGURE 68-14 This fourth ventricular meningioma was totally resected by splitting the cerebellar vermis. *A*, Axial enhanced image; *B*, sagittal nonenhanced image.

CONCLUSIONS

Management strategies for patients with meningiomas in the posterior fossa have undergone considerable evolution during the past 25 years. For meningiomas (in general, as well as for those located in the posterior fossa), complete surgical resection remains the treatment of choice. For those tumors located at the petroclival junction, the jugular foramen, the CPA, or the pineal region, resection is best accomplished in centers with subspecialized and frequent experience. However, given the indolent natural history of these tumors, the diagnostic accuracy of radiography when combined with clinical data, the surgical challenges associated with posterior fossa tumors, and the modern refinements in radiation delivery methods along with the extensive literature documenting tumor control and limited morbidity, it has now become reasonable to consider radical subtotal resection combined with some form of adjuvant radiation therapy for many tumors and, for smaller tumors, radiosurgery alone as a primary therapy.

REFERENCES

1. Akagami R, Napolitano M, Sekhar LN: Patient-evaluated outcome after surgery for basal meningiomas. Neurosurgery 50:941–949, 2002.
2. Bendszus M, Rao G, Burger R, et al: Is there a benefit to preoperative meningioma embolization. Neurosurgery 47:1306–1312, 2000.
3. Dean B, Flom RA, Wallace RC, et al: Efficacy of endovascular treatment of meningiomas: Evaluation of matched samples. AJNR Am J Neuroradiol 15:1675–1680, 1993.
4. Macpherson P: The value of pre-operative embolization of meningioma estimated subjectively and objectively. Neuroradiology 33:334–337, 1991.
5. Chun JY, McDermott MW, Lamborn KR, Wilson CB, Higashida R, Berger MS: Delayed surgical resection reduces intraoperative blood loss for embolized meningiomas. Neurosurgery 50:1231–1237, 2002.
6. Jung H, Yoo H, Paek SH, Choi KS: Long-term outcome and growth rate of subtotally resected petroclival meningiomas: Experience with 38 cases. Neurosurgery 46:567–575, 2000.
7. Simpson D: The recurrence of intracranial meningioma after surgical treatment. J Neurol Neurosurg Psychiatry 20:22, 1957.
8. Kinjo T, Al-Mefty O, Imad K: Grade zero removal of supratentorial convexity meningiomas: Clinical study. Neurosurgery 33:394–399, 1993.
9. Bonnal J, Brotchi J: Reconstruction of the superior sagittal sinus in parasagittal meningiomas. In Schmidek HH (ed): Meningiomas and their Surgical Management. Philadelphia: WB Saunders, 1991, pp 221–229.
10. Spetzler RF, Daspit P, Pappas CT: The combined supra- and infratentorial approach for lesions of the petrous and clival regions: Experience with 46 cases. J Neurosurg 76:588–599, 1992.
11. Ziyal IM, Sekhar LN, Salas E, Olan WJ: Combined supra/infratentorial-transinus approach to large pineal region tumors. J Neurosurg 88:1050–1057, 1998.
12. Mirimanoff RA, Dorseretz DE, Linggood RM, et al: Meningioma: Analysis of recurrence and progression following neurosurgical resection. J Neurosurg 62:18–24, 1985.
13. Barbaro NM, Gutin PH, Wilson CB, et al: Radiation therapy in the treatment of partially resected meningiomas. Neurosurgery 20:525–528, 1987.
14. Taylor BW, Marcus RB, Friedman WA, et al: The meningioma controversy: Postoperative radiation therapy. Int J Radiat Oncol Biol Phys 15:299–304, 1988.
15. Forbes AR, Goldberg ID: Radiation therapy in the treatment of meningioma: The Joint Center for Radiation Therapy experience. J Clin Oncol 2:1139–1143, 1984.
16. Carella RJ, Ransohoff J, Newall J: Role of radiation therapy in the management of meningioma. Neurosurgery 10:332–339, 1982.
17. Condra K, Buatti J, Mendenhall WM, et al: Benign meningiomas: Primary treatment selection affects survival. Int J Radiat Oncol Biol Phys 39:427–436, 1997.
18. Glaholm J, Bloom HJG, Crow JH: The role of radiotherapy in the management of intracranial meningiomas: The Royal Marsden Hospital experience with 186 patients. Int J Radiat Oncol Biol Phys 18:755, 1990.
19. Goldsmith BJ, Wara WM, Wilson CB, et al: Postoperative irradiation for subtotally resected meningioma. J Neurosurg 80:195–201, 1994.
20. Wara WM, Sheline GE, Newman H, et al: Radiation therapy of meningiomas. Am J Roentgenol Rad Ther Nucl Med 123:453, 1975.
21. Mirabell R, Linggood RM, de la Monte S, et al: The role of radiotherapy in the treatment of subtotally resected meningiomas. J Neurooncol 13:157, 1992.

22. Loeffler JS, Niemierko A, Chapman PH: Second tumors after radiosurgery: Tip of the iceberg or a bump on the road? Neurosurgery 52:1436–1442, 2003.
23. Debus J, Wuendrich M, Pirzkall A, et al: High efficacy of fractionated stereotactic radiotherapy of large base of skull meningiomas: Long-term results. J Clin Oncol 19:3547–3553, 2001.
24. Engenhart R, Kimming BN, Hover KH, et al: Stereotactic single high dose radiation therapy of benign intracranial meningiomas. Int J Radiat Oncol Biol Phys 19:1021–1026, 1991.
25. Kondziolka D, Lunsford LD: Radiosurgery of meningioma. Neurosurg Clin N Am 3:219–230, 1992.
26. Kondziolka D, Lundsford LD, Flickinger JC: Stereotactic radiosurgery of meningiomas. In Lundsford LD, Kondziolka D, Flickinger JD (eds): Gamma Knife Brain Surgery, vol 14. Basel: Karger, 1998, pp 104–113.
27. Flickinger JC, Lundsfors LD, Kondziolka D: Dose prescription and dose-volume effects in radiosurgery. Neurosurg Clin N Am 3:51–59, 1992.
28. Stafford SL, Pollock BE, Foote RL, et al: Meningioma radiosurgery: Tumor control, outcomes, and complications among 190 consecutive patients. Neurosurg 49:1029–1038, 2001.
29. Tishler RB, Loeffler JS, Lundsford LD, et al: Tolerance of cranial nerves of the cavernous sinus to radiosurgery. Int J Radiat Oncol Biol Phys 27:215–221, 1993.
30. Ryu S, Gorty S, Kazee AM, et al: "Full dose" re-irradiation of human cervical spinal cord. Am J Clin Oncol 23:29–31, 2000.
31. Kondziolka D, Nathoo N, Flickinger JC, et al: Long-term results after radiosurgery for benign intracranial tumors. Neurosurgery 53:815–822, 2003.
32. Chang SD, Adler JR: Treatment of cranial base meningiomas with linear accelerator radiosurgery: A clinical study. Neurosurgery 41:1019–1027, 1997.
33. Subach BR, Lunsford LD, Kondziolka D, et al: Management of petroclival meningiomas by stereotactic radiosurgery. Neurosurgery 42:437–445, 1998.
34. Pieper DR, Al-Mefty O, Hanada Y, Buechner D: Hyperostosis associated with meningioma of the cranial base: Secondary changes or tumor invasion. Neurosurgery 44:742–747, 1999.
35. Ogasawara H, Oki S, Kohno H, et al: Tentorial meningioma and painful tic convulsive. J Neurosurg 82:895–897, 1995.
36. Sindou M: Meningiomas invading the sagittal and transverse sinuses, resection and venous reconstruction. J Clin Neurosci 8(Suppl 1):8–11, 2001.
37. Collignon FP, Cohen-Gadol AA, Piepgras DG: Hemangiopericytoma of the confluence of the sinuses and the transverse sinus. J Neurosurg 99:1085–1088, 2003.
38. Sekhar LN, Janetta PJ: Cerebellopontine angle meningiomas. J Neurosurg 60:500, 1984.
39. Rock JP, Monsell EM, Schmidek HH: Meningiomas of the cerebellopontine angle. In Schmidek HH (ed): Meningiomas and their Surgical Management. Philadelphia: WB Saunders, Harcourt Brace Jovanovich, Inc., 1991, pp 417–425.
40. Cho CW, Al-Mefty O: Combined petrosal approach to petroclival meningiomas. Neurosurgery 51:708–716, 2002.
41. Malis LI: Surgical resection of tumors of the skull base. In Wilkin RH, Rengachary SS (eds): Neurosurgery, vol 1. New York: McGraw-Hill, 1985, pp 1011–1021.
42. Al-Mefty O, Fox JL, Smith RR: Petrosal approach for petroclival meningiomas. Neurosurgery 22:510–517, 1988.
43. House WF, Hitselberger WE, Horn KL: The middle fossa transpetrous approach to the anterior-superior cerebellopontine angle. Am J Otol 7:1–4, 1986.
44. Kawase T, Shiobara R, Toya S: Anterior transpetrosal- transtentorial approach for sphenoclival meningiomas: Surgical methods and results in 10 patients. Neurosurgery 28:869–976, 1991.
45. Sakata K, Al-Mefty O, Yamamoto I: Venous consideration in the petrosal approach: Microsurgical anatomy of the temporal bridging vein. Neurosurgery 47:153–161, 2000.
46. Arnautovic KI, Al-Mefty O: Primary meningiomas of the jugular fossa. J Neurosurg 97:12–20, 2002.
47. Arnautovic KI, Al-Mefty O, Husain M: Ventral foramen magnum meningiomas. J Neurosurg (Spine 1) 92:71–80, 2000.
48. Yasargil MG, Mortara RW, Curcic M: Meningiomas of basal posterior cranial fossa. Adv Tech Stand Neurosurg 7:1–15, 1980.
49. Miller E, Crockard HA: Transoral transclival removal of anteriorly-placed meningiomas at the foramen magnum. Neurosurgery 20:966–968, 1987.
50. Sen CN, Sekhar LN: An extreme lateral approach to intradural lesions of the cervical spine and foramen magnum. Neurosurgery 27:197–204, 1990.
51. Babu RP, Sekhar LN, Wright DC: Extreme lateral transcondylar approach: Technical improvements and lessons learned. J Neurosurg 81:49–59, 1994.
52. George B, Lot G: Anterolateral and posteriolateral approaches to the foramen magnum: Technical description and experience from 97 cases. Skull Base Surg 5:9–19, 1995.
53. Caruso RD, Rosenblaum AE, Chang JK, et al: Craniocervical junction venous anatomy on enhanced MRI images: The suboccipital cavernous sinus. AJNR Am J Neuroradiol 20:1127–1131, 1999.
54. Asari S, Maeshiro T, Tomita S: Meningiomas arising from the falcotentorial junction: Clinical features, neuroimaging studies, and surgical treatment. J Neurosurg 82:726–738, 1995.
55. Madari AA, Crochard HA, Stevens JM: Pineal region meningioma without dural attachment. Br J Neurosurg 10:305–307, 1996.
56. Roda JM, Perez-Higueras A, Oliver B: Pineal region meningiomas without dural attachment. Surg Neurol 17:147–151, 1982.
57. Konovalov AN, Spallone A, Pitzkhelauri DI: Meningioma of the pineal region: A surgical series of 10 cases. J Neurosurg 85:586–590, 1996.
58. Bruce JN, Stein BM: Surgical management of pineal region tumors. Acta Neurochir (Wien) 134:130–135, 1995.
59. Ausman JI, Malik GM, Dujovny M: Three-quarter prone approach to the pineal-tentorial region. Surg Neurol 29:298–306, 1988.
60. Bloomfield SM, Sonntag VKH, Spetzler RF: Pineal region lesions. BNI Q1:10–23, 1985.

Petroclival Meningiomas

ALBINO BRICOLO and SERGIO TURAZZI

Among the meningeal tumors of the basal posterior cranial fossa, petroclival meningiomas offer the greatest technical challenge to the neurosurgeon. Because of their rarity, their critical location in the center of the posterior skull base, and their proximity to the brain stem, cranial nerves III to XII, and arteries of the posterior circulation, the petroclival remains the most formidable of all meningiomas.[1-17]

Petroclival meningiomas arise in the area of the spheno-occipital synchondrosis, and in addition to the clivus and petrous apex, these tumors may involve the medial tentorium, Meckel's cave, the middle cranial fossa, the parasellar area, the petrosal and cavernous sinuses, and the transmission foramens of cranial nerves III to XII. Such tumors, often wedged in the brain stem, may encase cranial nerves and basilar and carotid arteries and their roots, perforate the dura, and invade the underlying bone.

Much was written in the 1990s about these tumors, particularly by skull base surgeons who have developed numerous complex approaches such that there is no aspect of the cranial base and underlying brain that cannot be exposed if required by the circumstance.[18] Unfortunately, these advances in "access surgery" have not obtained the results anticipated by initial enthusiasts, and thus the intimidating reputation of these lesions has been reduced but not eliminated.

Advances in neuroimaging, microsurgery, and approaches to the skull base have provided better preoperative definition of these tumors while making their removal easier and less conducive to iatrogenic damage. Developments and improvements of microsurgical techniques, tools, and associated skull base approaches have also permitted total resection of these tumors with modest rates of morbidity and, specifically, mortality, because until the time of Olivercrona mortality was at an unacceptable level on the basis of the general acceptance

that tumors of the clivus were inoperable. Surgical morbidity remains consistent in all contemporary published series, although in clinical reality, at least in our experience, quite a few patients operated on for this lesion are not satisfied with the outcome and the surgeon's performance.

These slow-growing tumors tend to produce worrisome symptoms only after reaching considerable size and extension. Two aspects of petroclival meningiomas continue to plague the neurosurgeon: (1) the tumor is histologically benign and causes relatively mild neurologic impairment with which the patient can learn to live; and (2) major surgery is required for removal, with some risk that the patient will be neurologically worse after surgery (Fig. 69-1).

In this chapter, the surgical management of petroclival meningiomas is discussed with reference to our experience. Current and relevant literature is also reviewed.

PATHOLOGIC ANATOMY AND CLASSIFICATION

Petroclival meningiomas are considered rare tumors, accounting for approximately 3% to 10% of all posterior fossa meningiomas. However, the actual incidence of these lesions is difficult to establish because they are difficult tumors and are typically treated only by a few leading neurosurgical centers specializing in skull base surgery. In addition, incidence data are unreliable because of the lack of precise definition. Thus it is opportune first to discuss the criteria used to define petroclival meningiomas among the broad group of posterior skull base meningiomas, emphasizing that until a general consensus is established regarding this crucial problem, published series will continue to remain poorly comparable.

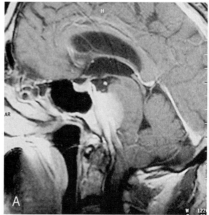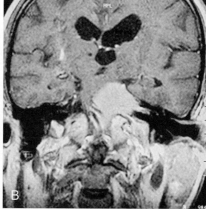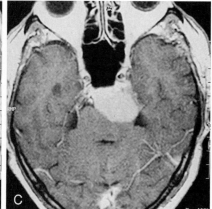

FIGURE 69-1 Sagittal (*A*), coronal (*B*), and axial (*C*) postcontrast T1-weighted MRI scan demonstrating a medium-sized petroclival meningioma with extensive adhesion to the clivus and involving the basilar artery. The patient complained only of transient diplopia and facial numbness. This case is typical not only for the characteristics of the tumor but also for the management decision. The encasement of the abducens, the trigeminal nerve, and the basilar artery are most likely; thus surgery should be carefully evaluated.

Since the historical contribution of Cushing and Eisenhardt in 1938 (see reference 19), meningiomas have been classically grouped according to the dural site at origin, and with this broad grouping, some petroclival meningiomas were perhaps included in their "gasseropetrosal" group. With regard to posterior fossa meningiomas, the landmark classification adopted for many years was proposed in 1953 by Castellano and Ruggiero[20] based on Olivercrona's material. This classification, which was rigorously based on the site of dural attachment, also benefited from the often readily available postmortem material. In this classification, posterior fossa meningiomas were categorized as: (1) cerebellar convexity, (2) tentorium, (3) posterior surface of the petrosal bone, (4) clival, and (5) foramen magnum.

The advent of modern diagnostic imaging techniques and the introduction of surgical microscopes allowed surgeons to operate on numerous meningiomas as well as to identify other criteria for subgrouping. As a consequence, in 1980, Yasargil and colleagues[17] proposed a new classification of posterior base meningiomas based on their extensive surgical experience: (1) clival, (2) petroclival, (3) sphenopetroclival, (4) foramen magnum, and (5) cerebellopontine angle (CPA). This new classification was fundamental because Yasargil and colleagues were the first to deny the existence of a pure midline clivus meningioma, and they introduced the term petroclival, adding that "our impression is that these tumors arise along the petro-clival line . . . (lateral clivus)." These authors, capturing the difficulties inherent in precisely grouping meningiomas of the basal posterior fossa, pointed out that the separation of basal meningiomas into precise topographic areas is artificial because there are always transitional cases.

Today, however, there is still a problem with the so-called petroclivals, a term that became relatively popular in the 1990s. The boundaries of this group of tumors lack precise definition, and as a result many authors prefer to describe such tumors as "meningiomas involving the clivus." Couldwell and associates[6] define petroclivals as those meningiomas with basal attachment at or medial to the skull base foramens of cranial nerves V through IX, X, and XI. Al-Mefty and Smith[3] emphasized that only those

meningiomas arising medial to the trigeminal nerve should be included in the petroclival group to differentiate them from those arising more laterally; the latter may be included in the broad family of CPA meningiomas, which are easily removed.

Identification of the origin of the dural attachment is not always possible on magnetic resonance imaging (MRI) or even during surgery, although it has been demonstrated that the difficulty of surgical removal increases with a progressively deeper and more centrally situated tumor origin. Reasons for this include: (1) the more medial the tumor, the greater the conflict with the brain stem; (2) more cranial nerves are involved; and (3) there is a closer relationship with the basilar artery and its branches. These factors also determine the degree of surgical difficulty and the approach; therefore, issues of naming and classification cannot be regarded as merely a semantic dispute.

Our working hypothesis is that meningiomas at the posterior cranial base must be grouped not only according to the dural attachment, but with respect to the manner in which the cranial nerves are displaced by the tumor. Because the cranial nerves have a constant entry and exit zone at the brain stem and the basal foramens, they are the most reliable "witnesses" of the growth pattern of the meningioma.

We have reconstructed the pathologic microsurgical anatomy of the last 150 posterior basal meningiomas on which we operated by reviewing neuroimaging and intraoperative data. In the small area comprising the clivus and the petrous pyramid, crowded by cranial nerves and arteries, five homogeneous subgroups of meningiomas, differing in topography as well as in displacement or encasement of neurovascular structures, can be identified: (1) petroclival, (2) anterior petrous, (3) posterior petrous, (4) jugular foramen, and (5) foramen magnum meningiomas (Fig. 69-2). The cranial nerves and arteries have a relatively constant relationship to each of these subgroups of meningiomas, as shown in Tables 69-1 and 69-2.

When the tumor is exposed through the classic suboccipital retrosigmoid approach with the patient in a semisitting position, the relationship of the tumor to the cranial nerves gives an immediate understanding of the site of dural origin, and consequently the related difficulties in its removal

FIGURE 69-2 The site of the dural origin of the five groups of posterior skull base meningiomas: petroclival (1), anterior petrous (2), posterior petrous (3), jugular foramen (4), and foramen magnum (5).

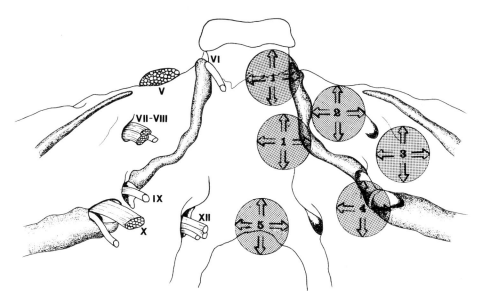

TABLE 69-1 ▪ **Position of the Cranial Nerves in Posterior Skull Base Meningiomas**

	Cranial Nerves						
Meningioma	**III**	**IV**	**V**	**VI**	**VII, VIII**	**IX, X, XI**	**XII**
Petroclival	Superior Medial	Superior Lateral	Posterior Superior	Medial Anterior	Posterior	Inferior Posterior	Inferior
Anterior petrous	Medial Superior	Superior Medial	Anterior Medial	Medial Anterior	Posterior Inferior	Inferior	—
Posterior petrous	—	—	Anterior	Anterior	Anterior	Anterior Inferior	—
Jugular foramen	—	—	—	Medial	Superior	Posterior Lateral	Inferior
Foramen magnum	—	—	—	Posterior	Superior Posterior	Posterior Superior	Posterior

(Fig. 69-3). The position of cranial nerves VII and VIII is a fundamental landmark for dividing these meningiomas into two main groups: those originating anterior to the acoustic meatus, which displace the cranial nerves VII and VIII complex posteriorly; and those growing from the dura posterior to the meatus, which displace cranial nerves VII and VIII anteriorly.

Both the petroclival and the anterior petrous displace cranial nerves VII and VIII posteriorly, and the lower cranial nerves posteriorly and inferiorly. What differentiates the two groups is the position of the trigeminal nerve: in petroclival meningiomas, its position is posterior-superior, whereas in the anterior petrous group, it is anterior-superior. In addition, simple visual examination of cranial nerve V, if the nerve is visible over the posterior surface of the tumor, ensures that its dural origin is in the clival area. Thus it is more than reasonable that the term petroclival meningioma be limited to this particular type of tumor, although some anterior petrous meningiomas may be included in this group because of their extensive dural insertion around the petroclival line and the trigeminal encasement (Figs. 69-4 and 69-5).

In contrast to acoustic neuromas, which displace adjacent nerves and vessels, posterior skull base meningiomas often engulf or encase arteries and cranial nerves encountered during their growth. This propensity to envelope functionally important neurovascular structures is the major cause of the significant morbidity commonly reported after surgical excision. Therefore, based on the surgical and

pathologic anatomy, it is reasonable to classify these tumors into five groups, which are homogeneous in more ways than one: (1) by their dural origin, (2) by their spatial relationship to adjacent nerves and arteries, and (3) by the frequency with which they encase specific cranial nerves and arteries (Tables 69-3 and 69-4).

We reclassified our previous 150 cases of posterior cranial base meningiomas according to the aforementioned criteria, and the resulting distribution is given in Table 69-5.

CLINICAL PRESENTATION

Patients with petroclival meningiomas are first seen by neurosurgeons in a variety of clinical conditions, ranging from isolated trigeminal neuralgia or numbness to multiple cranial nerve deficits associated with ataxia and somatomotor and sensory deficits. The clinical syndrome is of insidious onset, often mimicking other pathologic processes; in elderly patients, the presenting symptoms are often attributed to vertebrobasilar insufficiency.

Headache, gait ataxia, facial dysesthesia, vertigo, and reduced hearing are the more frequent presenting symptoms, with the trigeminal nerve as the single structure most often involved from onset. Later symptoms (those appearing more recently and leading to diagnostic suspicion), in addition to gait ataxia, include double vision, swallowing difficulty, and somatomotor deficits of various types. Papilledema and changes in mental status are rare.

TABLE 69-2 ▪ **Position of the Arteries in Posterior Skull Base Meningiomas**

Meningiomas	**Posterior Cerebral Artery**	**Superior Cerebellar Artery**	**Basilar Artery**	**AICA**	**PICA**	**Vertebral Artery**
Petroclival	Superior Medial	Superior Medial	Posterior Medial	Posterior Medial	Posterior Inferior	Posterior Inferior
Anterior petrous	Superior Medial	Medial	Medial	Anterior Medial	Inferior Medial	Medial
Posterior petrous	—	—	Anterior Medial	Anterior	Anterior	Anterior Medial
Jugular foramen	—	—	Medial	Superior	Inferior	Medial Inferior
Foramen magnum	—	—	—	Superior	Posterior	Posterior Lateral

AICA, anterior inferior cerebellar artery; PICA, posterior inferior cerebellar artery.

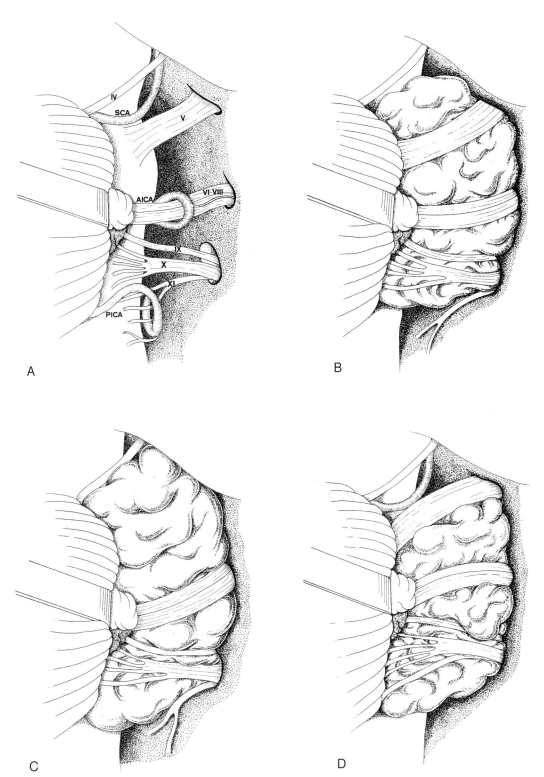

A

B

C

D

FIGURE 69-3 Schematic illustration of the cerebellopontine angle (A). The cerebellum has been retracted to show (from top to bottom): the trochlear nerve (IV), the superior cerebellar artery (SCA), the trigeminal (V), facial and vestibulocochlear (VII–VIII) with the anterior inferior cerebellar artery (AICA), the glossopharyngeal (IX), vagus (X), and spinal accessory (XI) nerves with the posterior inferior cerebellar artery (PICA). Petroclival meningiomas (B) displace posteriorly the trigeminal, and cranial nerves VII and VIII and IX and X, whereas in anteropetrous meningiomas (C) the trigeminal nerve is displaced anteriorly and thus remains hidden by the tumor. The distinction between the two types of tumors is not always clear, because the trigeminal nerve may assume an intermediate position (D) or may be encased by the tumor.

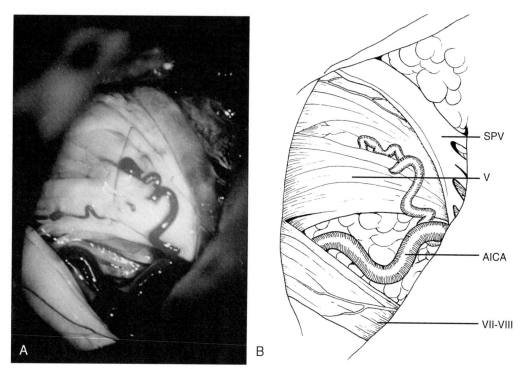

FIGURE 69-4   *A* and *B,* Intraoperative microphotographs and diagrammatic sketches of a typical petroclival meningioma exposed using a left suboccipital lateral retrosigmoid approach with the patient in a semisitting position. The tumor originating from the clival area remains anterior to the trigeminal (V) and faciovestibulocochlear nerves (VII–VIII), which are shown to be stretched over the tumor. AICA, anterior inferior cerebellar artery.

In our first series of 33 petroclival meningiomas published in 1992 (see reference 4), the onset of symptoms usually occurred later on in the disease, varying from 7 months to 17 years (on average, 35 months for combined symptoms). The two most frequent early complaints were trigeminal neuralgia (43 months) and impaired hearing (35 months), whereas the two more common complaints nearer diagnosis were diplopia (4 months) and facial weakness (3 months). At the time of objective examination shortly before surgery, the clinical picture was usually dominated by deficits of the

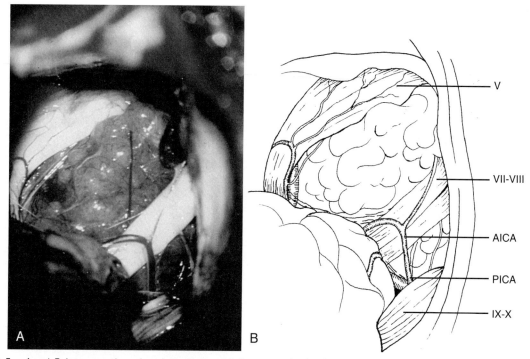

FIGURE 69-5   *A* and *B,* Intraoperative microphotographs and diagrammatic sketches of a meningioma exposed using a right retrosigmoid approach. In this case, the trigeminal nerve (V) is displaced upward, thus the mass may still be considered as a petroclival meningioma. AICA, anterior inferior cerebellar artery; PICA, posterior inferior cerebellar artery.

TABLE 69-3 ▪ **Frequency of Cranial Nerve Encasement in Posterior Skull Base Meningiomas**

Meningioma	Cranial Nerves						
	III	IV	V	VI	VII, VIII	IX, X, XI	XII
Petroclival	+	+	+ +	+ + +	+ +	+	—
Anterior petrous	—	+	+ + +	+ +	+ +	—	—
Posterior petrous	—	—	—	—	+	—	—
Jugular foramen	—	—	—	—	+	+ + +	+
Foramen magnum	—	—	—	—	—	+ +	+ +

intermediate cranial nerves, which were present in varying degrees in nearly all patients, with concomitant cerebellar signs in 60% of patients. Cranial nerve V was affected both earlier and more often (67% of patients), followed by cranial nerves IX, X, and XI (45%). The typical sign of a petroclival meningioma is a relatively fair preservation of hearing, in contrast to severe trigeminal involvement and impairment of the cranial nerves below VIII, with accompanying cerebellar signs. The preoperative performance status, as expressed by the Karnofsky scale, was higher than 70 in 23 patients (70%) and lower than 70 in 10 (30%).

IMAGING EVALUATION

Computed tomography (CT), angiography, and MRI each play an important role in the preoperative evaluation of petroclival meningiomas, and none of these diagnostic methods has been able adequately to replace the other (Fig. 69-6). The general imaging characteristics of petroclival meningiomas do not differ from those of other meningiomas. Regarding skull base meningiomas and those of the clivus, it is particularly useful to apply or assemble all the information derived from the three investigative methods.

The most important information the surgeon needs to know before surgery includes the site and extension of dural attachment; tumor size, consistency, and vascularity; bone involvement; tumor–brain stem interface; the position and eventual encasement of the arteries; and extension of the tumor outside the proper petroclival area, particularly any involvement of the cavernous sinus. MRI, the latest entrant in the arsenal of diagnostic tools, is the single examination that answers many of these questions (Figs. 69-7 to 69-10).

The inability to define an arachnoid cleavage plane between extra-axial tumors and the brain stem is one of the most troubling situations confronting the surgeon, and is one of the primary reasons for abandoning a radical procedure, as well as being the major cause of postoperative

complications.[13–15,17,21–23] Sekhar and colleagues[15] pointed out that some of these meningiomas have poor planes of dissection because of microvascular invasion of the brain stem pial layer. They concluded that this situation, which prohibits complete removal, can be predicted by the presence of brain stem edema on preoperative MRI, demonstrated by high signal intensity on T2-weighted images, together with the lack of evidence of an arachnoid plane.

Sekhar and colleagues[15] also found a good correlation between radiologic and operative findings when signs of vascular encasement and tumoral blood supply from the basilar artery were seen in angiographic studies.

When MRI is not available, CT can be most useful; using high-resolution CT scanning, preoperative differentiation of petroclival meningiomas from other pathologic processes of the region is possible. CT scanning also permits the construction and display of 3-dimensional images, which may allow better judgment of the relationship of the meningioma with the tentorium and other structures (Fig. 69-11).

Cerebral angiography is considered by many[24] to be mandatory for the preoperative workup of tumors of this type, whereas some surgeons consider it necessary only for those cases with expected encasement of the basilar artery and its branches or direct vascularization of the tumor from the basilar artery.[4,6,15]

Angiography gives indirect evidence of the tumor mass in terms of dislocation of the basilar artery and its branches (posterior cerebral and superior, anterior, and posterior inferior cerebellar arteries); in addition, it reveals any "choking" of the basilar and carotid arteries by the tumor and provides some information about tumoral blood supply, although the extent of tumor vascularization is not always easy to determine. The tumors are supplied in various degrees by the meningohypophysial trunk of the internal carotid artery (ICA), the posterior branch of the middle meningeal artery, the meningeal branch of the vertebral artery, the clivus artery originating from the carotid siphon, the petrosal

TABLE 69-4 ▪ **Frequency of Arteries Encasement in Posterior Skull Base Meningiomas**

Meaningiomas	Posterior Cerebral Artery	Superior Cerebellar Artery	Basilar Artery	AICA	PICA	Vertebral Artery
Petroclival	+	+ + +	+ + +	+ + +	+	+
Anterior petrous	+	+ +	+ +	+ +	—	—
Posterior petrous	—	—	—	—	—	—
Jugular foramen	—	—	—	+	+ + +	+
Foramen magnum	—	—	—	—	+ + +	+ +

AICA, anterior inferior cerebellar artery; PICA, posterior inferior cerebellar artery.

TABLE 69-5 ▪ Grouping the Posterior Skull Base Meningiomas*

Group	N (%)
Petroclival	84 (56%)
Anterior petrous	16 (11%)
Posterior petrous	27 (18%)
Jugular foramen	5 (3%)
Foramen magnum	18 (12%)

*In the authors' series of the last 150 posterior skull base meningiomas treated.

branches of the meningeal arteries, and the ascending pharyngeal branches of the external carotid artery. In 30% of patients in our first series,[4] definite tumor staining was visible in the capillary and venous phases of angiography (Figs. 69-12 and 69-13).

PATIENT SELECTION AND MANAGEMENT

Treatment strategies for difficult tumors such as the petroclival meningioma are complex issues, because the patient may have a large tumor and minimal symptoms, the natural history is far from homogeneous, and total removal is difficult to achieve. Although the remarkable evolution of surgical techniques and facilities has led most authors to consider the results of this surgery acceptable, some express a more critical attitude.[6,15,23,25–27] Although data on the natural history of unoperated patients are unavailable, follow-up in postoperative patients confirms progressive growth of the tumor at variable rates[11,20]; it is well known, however, that some tumors can remain dormant for many years (Fig. 69-14).

As stated by Sekhar and colleagues,[14] "when and whether to operate a newly discovered tumor in patients with minimal symptoms can be a difficult decision." Important preoperative factors affecting patient outcomes include tumor size, degree of neurologic involvement, and patient age. Because tumor size is the most important factor affecting postoperative outcome in nonelderly, symptomatic patients with small or medium-sized tumors, surgery should be recommended even when symptoms are minimal. In this group of patients, total excision can be achieved with minimal morbidity and a low risk of moderate neurologic dysfunction. However, the surgeon should be cautious in considering the small tumor as "easy and without risk of morbidity," because these small tumors have not created a sufficient space to reach and remove them.

Patients with large, recurrent, or previously irradiated tumors have higher operative risks and the likelihood of worsened postoperative neurologic status, along with a reduced chance of obtaining total or satisfactory tumor removal.

Another issue in preoperative patient evaluation is the selection of approach based on tumor extension and site, and any neurologic dysfunction such as deafness.[16] Although objective criteria should be weighed and kept in mind, the operative choice is determined based on the surgeon's personal experience and preference.

The main issue in this difficult procedure is to determine at what point and at what price radical removal can be achieved. This problem, perhaps more of a management issue than of a technical nature, is also decided according to the surgeon's experience and personal philosophy.[28] Brain stem invasion by the tumor with an obscured arachnoid layer, vascular encasement (primarily the basilar artery and perforators), and cavernous sinus invasion are obstacles to radical removal that require intraoperative judgment and technique. When the tumor cannot be easily dissected, a subtotal removal is recommended, with the residual monitored or treated by radiosurgery. Theoretical considerations and preoperative planning must be confronted by intraoperative practicability.

SURGICAL MANAGEMENT

The removal of petroclival meningiomas continues to be regarded as a formidable challenge, because the morbidity rates of published series remain high and mortality rates, though lower in the 1990s, are not zero. Furthermore, despite

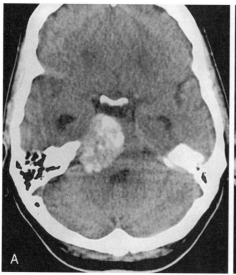 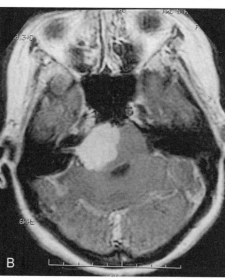

FIGURE 69-6 A plain CT scan (*A*) may show an extensive and dense calcification in a petroclival meningioma, which is not demonstrated by MRI (*B*).

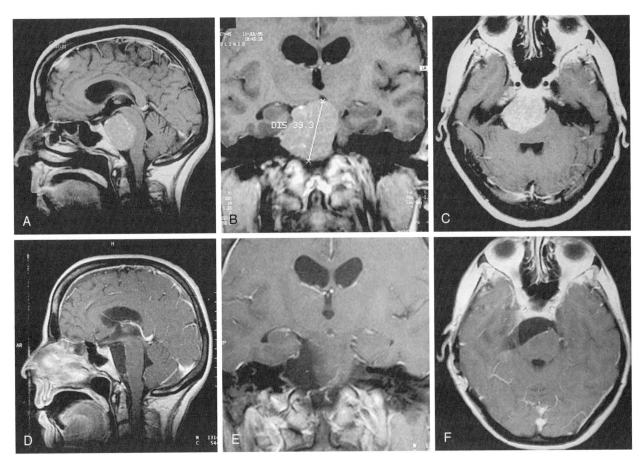

FIGURE 69-7   Preoperative sagittal (*A*), coronal (*B*), and axial (*C*) postcontrast T1-weighted MRI scan of a petroclival meningioma radically removed (*D–F*) through a lateral suboccipital retrosigmoid approach. The tumor–brain stem interface at surgery was well delineated by a good arachnoid plane. The patient, who was neurologically intact before surgery, remained asymptomatic after surgery.

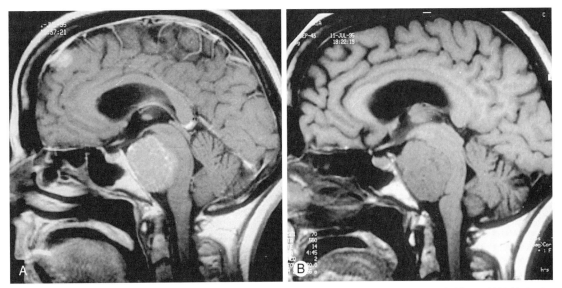

FIGURE 69-8   Sagittal contrast-enhanced (*A*) and plain (*B*) T1-weighted MRI scans of the same patient as in Figure 69-7. Notice how contrast administration may sometimes hide the natural tumor–brain stem interface. The possibility that contrast-enhanced images can be misleading, suggesting brain stem edema or invasion, must be taken into consideration.

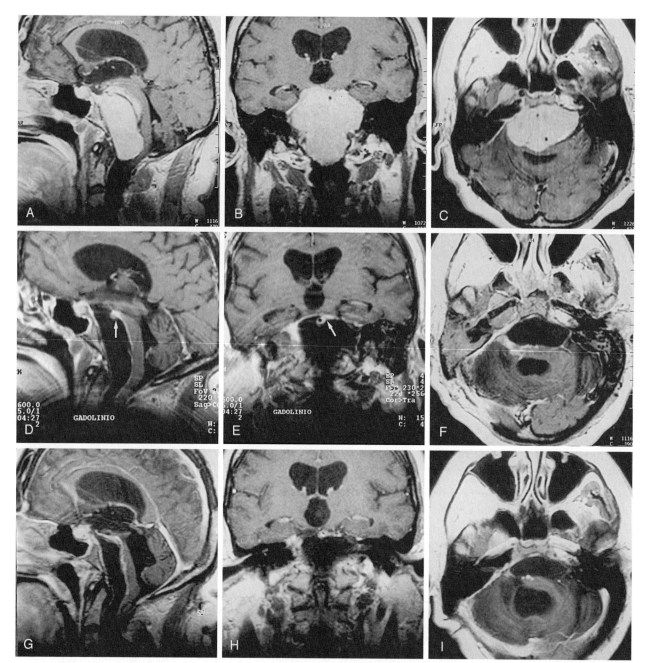

FIGURE 69-9 Preoperative sagittal (*A*), coronal (*B*), and axial (*C*) postcontrast T1-weighted MRI scan of a giant panclival meningioma removed through a right suboccipital retrosigmoid dorsolateral approach. The signal voids represent the vertebral basilar artery and its branches encased by the tumor; thus careful microdissection is required to avoid vessel injury. In this patient, the right vertebral artery, which was completely engulfed by the tumor, was dissected and freed while the top of the basilar artery and both anterior inferior cerebellar arteries (AICAs) were encased in a solid, calcified piece of tumor that was left in place. Comparable 4-week postoperative MRI scans (*E–G*) demonstrate removal of the tumor with a small remnant (*arrows*). The patient, who was severely disabled before surgery, recovered well after a difficult perioperative course. Today, 4 years after surgery, the patient is almost self-sufficient and able to care for a large family. Notice the signs of brain stem atrophy on an MRI scan performed at a 4-year follow-up (*H–I*), which contrast with the capability to perform daily functions.

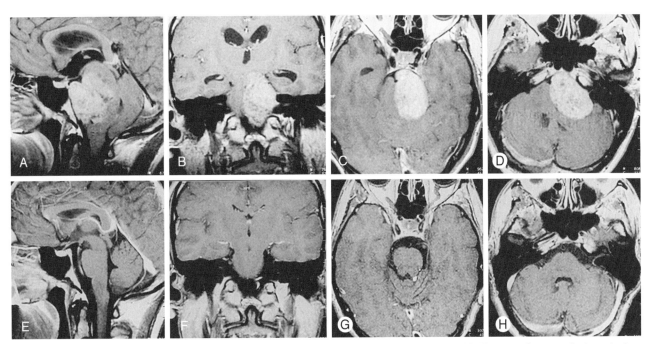

FIGURE 69-10 Preoperative sagittal (*A*), coronal (*B*), and axial (*C* and *D*) postcontrast T1-weighted MRI scans of a petroclival meningioma that was totally (*E–H*) and easily removed through a lateral suboccipital retrosigmoid approach. The tumor's soft consistency and its weak adherence to the brain stem, cranial nerves, and arteries were favorable for radical removal with no morbidity.

demanding and time-consuming surgery, radical removal of these lesions is reported only in approximately 60% of cases, and occasional recurrence of disease indicates that radicality was only apparent; knowledge of the natural history of basal meningiomas and longer follow-up periods are therefore required.

In an attempt to attain the primary goal of surgery, which is radical removal with low morbidity and mortality, new,

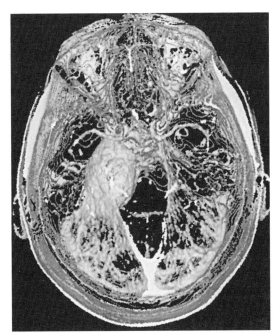

FIGURE 69-11 A 3-dimensional contrast-enhanced CT reconstructed scan demonstrating the relationship of a petroclival meningioma with the tentorium, the clivus, and the basilar artery.

complex approaches and surgical techniques have been developed without regard to specialty-imposed surgical boundaries (mixing the competence of neurosurgeons and ear, nose, and throat surgeons). General surgical aggressiveness, which characterizes skull base surgery, enhanced by interdisciplinary work and innovation, have produced a myriad of new approaches and variations; however, such methods have only slightly reduced the intrinsic difficulty of removing a tumor that infiltrates the cranial nerves, encases the arteries and veins, and has a poor arachnoid plane with the brain stem.

Controversy has developed over the use of new, complex skull base approaches as opposed to more rational and modern adaptations of older and simpler neurosurgical approaches discredited because they belong to the premicrosurgical era. Only recently has a more analytic and critical evaluation of the most advantageous approaches emerged. The numerous published approaches for posterior skull base meningiomas can be categorized into three groups: middle fossa, lateral suboccipital, and combined supratentorial-infratentorial.

Middle Fossa Approach

This approach is suitable for tumors involving the cavernous sinus, the upper clival area, and some of the middle clival area (sphenopetroclival meningiomas). The extradural approach to cavernous sinus lesions, proposed by Dolenc,[29,30] was later extended by the same author for middle and upper clivus meningiomas by drilling the petrous apex and dividing the tentorium. The anterior middle fossa approach was described in 1991 by Kawase and associates[31] as the "anterior transpetrosal transtentorial approach" for sphenopetroclival meningiomas.

The area of pyramid resection in Kawase's procedure is bounded by the trigeminal nerve inferiorly and anteriorly,

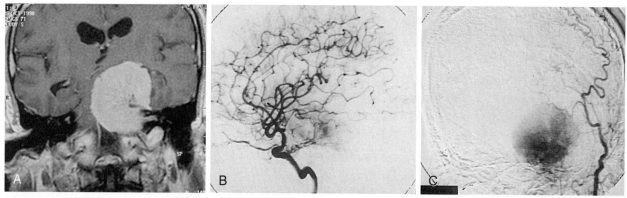

FIGURE 69-12   Coronal (*A*) T1-weighted post-gadolinium MRI scan showing a huge petroclival meningioma. Left internal carotid angiography (*B*) illustrates the early-filling vessels (tentorial marginal arteries of Bernasconi and Cassinari), and left external carotid angiography (*C*) shows the abundant amount of blood brought to the tumor by the ascending pharyngeal artery, which may be embolized.

the eminentia arcuata posteriorly, the major petrosal groove laterally, and the carotid and internal auditory canal inferiorly. However, because this approach still resulted in a fairly restricted access to the clival area, in 1994 Kawase and associates[32] proposed its extension with a petrosectomy.

Sekhar and colleagues[14] termed this approach the frontotemporal transcavernous and sometimes combined it with orbitozygomatic osteotomy to minimize brain retraction. When the tumor has been removed from the cavernous sinus, the clival area is reached by removing the dorsum sellae, the posterior clinoid process, and the petrous apex, the lowest limit of exposure being the horizontal segment of the ICA. The tumor is removed by working between the supraclinoidal ICA and cranial nerve V. The advantage of this approach is

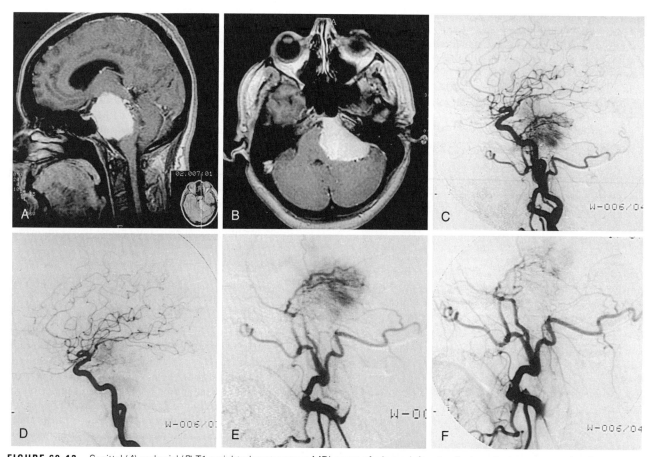

FIGURE 69-13   Sagittal (*A*) and axial (*B*) T1-weighted postcontrast MRI scans of a large, left petroclival meningioma suggesting the presence of rich vasculature at the tumor–brain stem interface with possible violation of the arachnoid and pial sheaths. Left common (*C*) and internal (*D*) carotid angiography illustrates the early-filling vessels in a corkscrew configuration. Left external carotid angiography before (*E*) and after (*F*) embolization.

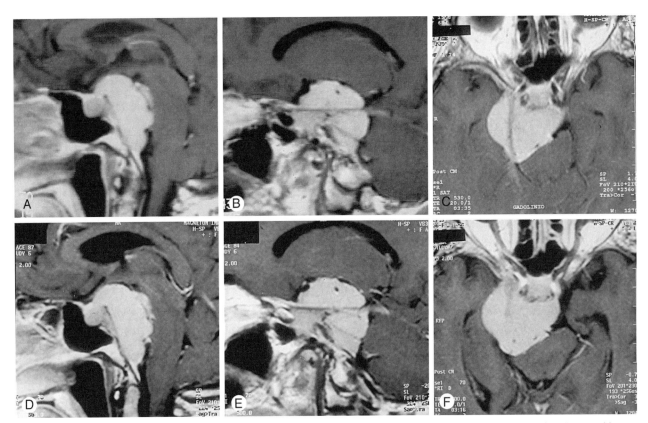

FIGURE 69-14 Sagittal (*A*), parasagittal (*B*), and axial (*C*) T1-weighted postcontrast MRI scan performed in March 1992 in a 67-year-old woman who was neurologically intact and who complained only of a transient headache. The patient refused surgery and preferred to return periodically for follow-up. This large petroclival cavernous meningioma remained asymptomatic and practically unchanged in volume, as demonstrated in the last MRI scan (*D–F*), which was performed in October 1998. The patient is still neurologically intact and leads a normal active life.

that it allows the surgeon to work in the upper clival area without retraction of the posterior temporal lobe, and the tumor can be devascularized early.

The middle fossa approach can also be extended posteriorly to the subtemporal and the preauricular infratemporal approach, which requires resection of the mandibular condyle and exposure of the petrous ICA.[14,33,34]

Suboccipital Retrosigmoid Approach

The lateral suboccipital approach has been a common method of access to tumors of the CPA since Dandy[35] proposed it in 1925. Today, using this access, we are able to remove pathologic processes radically and atraumatically in the deeper petroclival region, and it remains a preferred choice in our practice because it offers the simplest access to the CPA and lateral clivus.[36] The main disadvantage of this route is the difficulty of removing dural and extradural structures invaded by the tumor when approached from such a confined surgical field surrounded by cranial nerves and the already distorted brain stem.[17,31]

As a rule, we place the patient in a semisitting position with the head flexed and rotated toward the side of the lesion (Fig. 69-15A). Particular care must be taken to extend bone drilling upward and laterally to unroof the lateral and sigmoid sinuses all the way to the jugular bulb (see Fig. 69-15B). With that done, the incised dura is drawn upward and sideways with retraction sutures arranged to pull the sinuses out of the surgeon's hands (see Fig. 69-15C). This creates a very

lateral access to the CPA parallel to the posterior aspect of the fossa petrosa and to the insertion angle of the tentorium of the petrosal ridge, making it possible to initiate tumor exeresis by devascularization through coagulation of the dural attachment, first on the posterior surface of the petrous bone, then on the clivus. We then proceed to debulk the tumor with the ultrasonic aspirator throughout the fissure of the tentorium and cranial nerves V, VII and VIII, and IX and X (see Fig. 69-15D). The tumor is thus detached in succession from the cranial nerves and the brain stem; last, its insertion or site of attachment is demolished on the petrous apex, tentorium, and upper clivus.

The greatest possible care is taken to identify and preserve the arachnoid layers next to the cranial nerves, the brain stem, and the arteries (Fig. 69-16). At this stage of the procedure, coagulation is mostly abandoned and replaced by continuous irrigation with saline solution. When the CPA is completely freed of the tumor, an open space remains between the brain stem and the free margin of the tentorium through which the supratentorial space can be accessed. By this exposure, the surgeon can reach and remove even the more rostral projection of the tumor into the middle cranial fossa and parasellar area by dissecting it away from cranial nerves IV and III and from the arteries of the circle of Willis.

Supratentorial subtemporal and parasellar tumor expansion does not in itself disqualify or contradict this simple, well-tested approach that has rewarded surgeons with excellent results. Access to this area is prepared by the tumor itself, located as it is in the tentorial hiatus, which can be enlarged

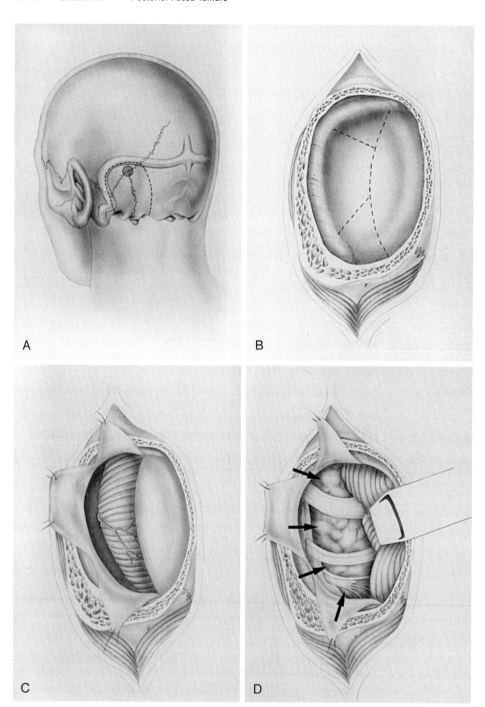

A

B

C

D

FIGURE 69-15 The simplest surgical approach to the petroclival area is the lateral suboccipital retrosigmoid route, preferably with the patient in a semisitting position. A retromastoid craniotomy (A) extended to unroof the lateral and sigmoid sinuses is performed (B), and a three-flap duratomy is retracted outside the surgical corridor (C) to improve the exposure and reduce the need for cerebellar retraction (D). The tumor is devascularized at its dural attachment and removed working through different routes (arrows) between the tentorium, cranial nerve V, cranial nerves VII and VIII, and cranial nerves IX and X.

by resecting the tentorial flap. Thus the upper pole of the tumor, if not attached to the parasellar dura, can be dislocated downward and removed by separating it from the arachnoid of the interpeduncular, carotid, and chiasmatic cisterns, even though in some cases the excessive slope of the tentorium could direct the surgeon away from the floor of the middle cranial fossa, leaving the tumor lodgment out of view.

The working field is divided into narrow routes or corridors by cranial nerves crossing the CPA to their emerging foramens. The larger portion of the tumor is removed by dissecting between the inferior aspect of the tentorium and the vestibulocochlear nerves and trigeminal nerve. The middle clivus can be approached between cranial nerves VII and VIII

and the caudal cranial nerves, and the lower clivus is reached by dissection below the caudal nerves.

The tumor enlarges the narrow space between the brain stem and the posterior surface of the pyramid laterally and the tentorium superiorly, making it possible to gain access to the clival area without intolerable retraction of the cerebellum and the already distorted brain stem. The elevation of the tentorium produced by the tumor creates a sizable space used for access to the tentorial incisure. The gap of the lateral suboccipital approach can be further enlarged upward by incising the tentorium laterally along the tentorial edge and downward, combining a transcondylar-C1 laminectomy approach.[14,37–39] In tumors that involve the lower clivus and

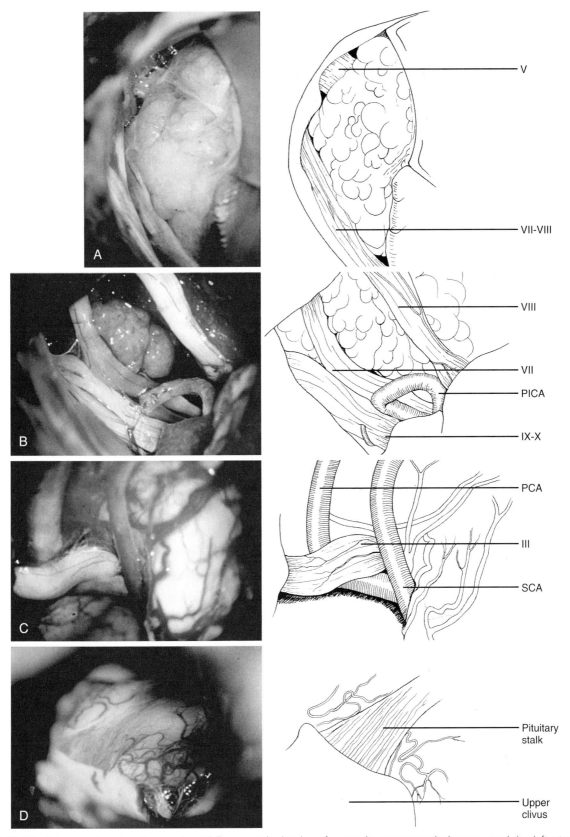

FIGURE 69-16 Intraoperative microphotographs and diagrammatic sketches of an anterior petrous meningioma exposed via a left retrosigmoid approach. *A*, The trigeminal nerve (V) is displaced anteriorly, and cranial nerves VII and VIII posteriorly and inferiorly. *B*, The faciovestibulocochlear (VII–VIII), glossopharyngeal (IX), and vagus nerves (X) and the posterior inferior cerebellar artery are dissected over the caudal extension of the tumor. *C*, After the tumor has been removed, the oculomotor nerve is seen emerging from the mesencephalon between the posterior cerebral artery (PCA) and the superior cerebellar artery (SCA). *D*, The pituitary stalk entering the sella is viewed from above.

foramen magnum, after retrosigmoid craniectomy, the medial two thirds of the mastoid process and the posterior half of the occipital condyle are removed. The sigmoid sinus is then completely exposed and the C1 lamina is removed to the foramen transversarium. This approach provides sufficient lateral exposure of the tumor lying anterior to the brain stem without retraction of neural structures, and fusion procedures are not required because stability is not affected (Fig. 69-17).

Combined Supratentorial and Infratentorial Approach

Meningiomas arising from the petroclival area occasionally extend above the tentorium to the cavernous sinus, and at the same time below to the foramen magnum. These tumors cannot be resected totally using a subtemporal or infratentorial approach alone; a combined supratentorial and infratentorial operation, as pioneered by Malis,[9] should be adopted.

Lateral approaches based on varying degrees of petrous bone resection combined with lateral suboccipital and subtemporal craniotomies have been termed the posterior subtemporal and the pure sigmoid transpetrosal approaches,[12,14] the petrosal approach,[1,40] the combined retroauricular and preauricular transpetrosal-transtentorial approach,[7] the combined supratentorial and infratentorial approach,[16] and the combined supraparapetrosal and infraparapetrosal approach.[41]

Bone removal ranges from the simpler retrolabyrinthine, presigmoid drilling to a total petrosectomy with transposition of the facial nerve. Simple bone-destructive approaches, sometimes in two-stage operations, can be tailored to the extension of the tumor and the presumed goal of surgery.

In the simpler and more rapid form described by Samii and colleagues,[12] a posterior subtemporal craniotomy is extended by lateral suboccipital craniotomy of the posterior cranial fossa; this provides the advantages of both approaches, and additional space at the petrous bone can be obtained through an extralabyrinthine presigmoidal mastoidectomy (Fig. 69-18).

The skin incision is basically an extended retromastoid incision that curves upward and forward into the temporal area. The temporal part of the craniotomy is performed first and must be extended to the floor of the middle fossa and below the transverse sinus, which has been carefully unroofed by its groove. Next, a suboccipital craniotomy is done with a large cutting drill.

The last bony structures over the sigmoid sinus are removed with a cutting burr, exposing the presigmoid dura and the sinodural angle. Drilling is continued along the pyramid toward its apex. The dura is then opened in such a way that the temporal lobe with the superior anastomotic

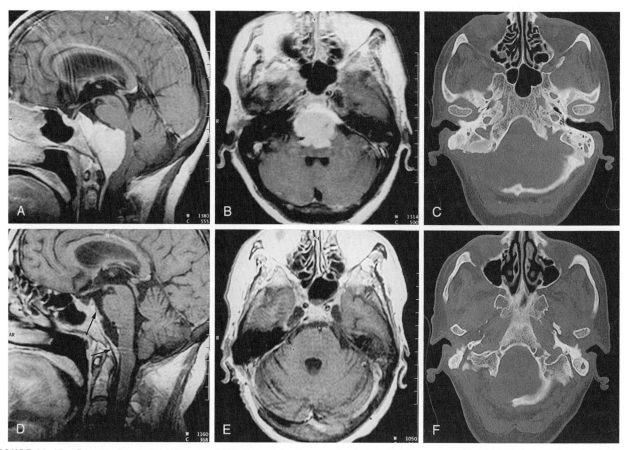

FIGURE 69-17 Preoperative sagittal (*A*) and axial (*B*) T1-weighted contrast-enhanced MRI scans of a large middle-lower clival meningioma approached and removed via a right retrosigmoid dorsolateral approach. Comparable 2-month postoperative images (*D* and *E*) demonstrate the gross total removal. *Arrows* indicate a possible tumoral residual infiltration. The postoperative CT scans (*C* and *F*) show the extent of bone removal.

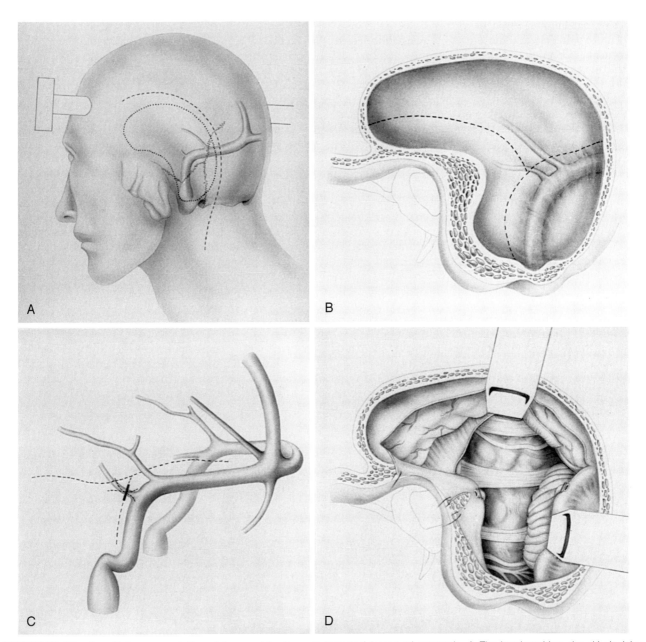

FIGURE 69-18 An artist's representation of the combined suprainfratentorial petrosal approach. *A,* The head position, the skin incision (*dashed lines*), and the extent of the craniotomy (*dotted line*) are shown. *B,* A temporal suboccipital bone flap is elevated exposing the transverse and sigmoid sinuses, and a mastoidectomy is performed exposing the sigmoid sinus until the jugular bulb and the dura anterior to the sigmoid sinus. The petrous pyramid is drilled to expose the sinus dural angle and the superior petrosal sinus, barely stripping the labyrinth and staying out of the fallopian canal to avoid deafness and injury to the facial nerve. If the hearing is absent, a total labyrinthectomy is performed, which allows an increase of the anterolateral exposure of the tumor. *C,* The dura is opened along the floor of the temporal fossa using great care to preserve and protect the superior anastomotic vein and then along the anterior border of the sigmoid sinus. *D,* The superior petrous sinus is divided, and the tentorium is completely transected. One retractor is placed under the posterior flap of the tentorium to maintain suspended the temporal lobe, and the second is placed anteriorly to the sigmoid sinus to assist the spontaneous falling back of the cerebellum. Cranial nerves III to IX and X are exposed over the lateral aspect of the tumor.

vein (vein of Labbé) can be elevated and the sigmoid sinus and cerebellum displaced posteriorly.

Next, the superior petrosal sinus is interrupted and the tentorium is incised along the petrous ridge close to its line of attachment. In this area, the large temporolateral superior anastomotic vein flows into the sinus system, and the surgeon must take great care not to injure it and to preserve its discharge into the sinus. The dural incision is then prolonged downward along the anterior margin of the sigmoid sinus,

crossing the superior petrosal sinus, which can be divided without any associated risk. The posterior portion of the temporal lobe is then gently lifted with a self-retractor, taking particular care to maintain discharge of the superior anastomotic vein into the sinus. The tentorium is then transected from lateral to medial in a line parallel to the petrous ridge as much as necessary to open the tentorial notch. Care should be taken to identify and preserve the trochlear nerve, which penetrates into the free edge of the tentorium.

The tentorial division produces a good exposure of the upper clivus as well as of the anterior and lateral aspect of the brain stem, the basilar artery and its highest branches, and cranial nerves III, IV, and V. At this point, a second retractor is placed anterior to the sigmoid sinus to keep both the posterior edge of the transected tentorium and the cerebellum posterior and medial. Cerebellar retraction can be very slight because after transecting the tentorium, the cerebellum spontaneously withdraws from the posterior surface of the pyramid. Through this opening, the surgeon gains a good view of cranial nerves V to IX and of the medium and lower clivus. Neurosurgeons are particularly indebted to Al-Mefty and colleagues[1] and Samii and co-workers[12] for conceiving, carrying out, and clearly describing this elegant, tissue-preserving, and ample avenue to the skull base using a unilateral temporal suboccipital craniectomy and drilling of the petrosal bone to gain access to the tumor through the presigmoid (retrolabyrinthine) and subtemporal transtentorial approach (Fig. 69-19). This approach allows the surgeon to work approximately 2 cm closer to the tumor than would be possible through the retrosigmoid approach, and to remain in front of the brain stem (Fig. 69-20). Division of the tentorium reduces the need for retraction of the cerebellum and temporal lobe, preserves drainage of the superior anastomotic vein, and creates an excellent exposure, opening a vista

from the lowest cranial nerves to the sella. The combined posterior-subtemporal-suboccipital-presigmoid-transpetrous (retrolabyrinthine) approach without sinus division has proved to be the most efficient and least dangerous way to reach and possibly remove clival tumors that involve a large portion of the skull base from the lower clivus to the parasellar area (Fig. 69-21).

This access can be further enlarged by ligation and division of the transverse sinus laterally to the entrance of the superior anastomotic vein.[7,10–12,14,17] This is the simplest approach for centrolateral clival meningiomas. The advantage of this approach is that the surgeon can start working on the tumor in a reasonably short time, and mild cerebellar and tentorial retraction is well tolerated.

The translabyrinthine and total petrosectomy approach provides a wide exposure of the petroclival area but results in loss of hearing and varying degrees of facial palsy, and requires highly skilled bone work and reconstructive technique on the surgeon's part.

RESULTS

A review of the major operative series in the microsurgical era indicates that the percentage of patients with petroclival meningiomas obtaining complete removal varies from

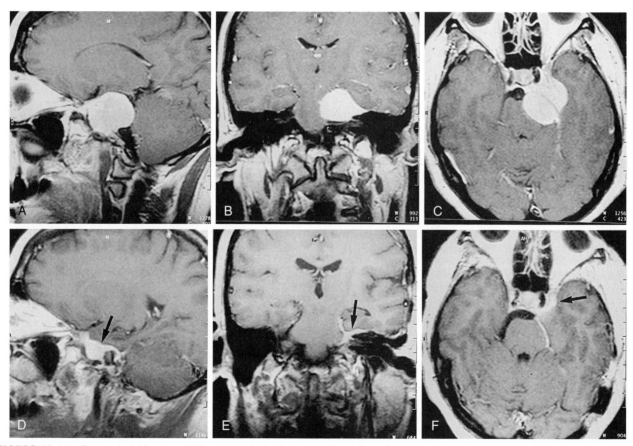

FIGURE 69-19 Parasagittal (*A*), coronal (*B*), and axial (*C*) postcontrast T1-weighted MRI scans demonstrate a medium-sized petroclival-cavernous meningioma. The tumor was approached and removed (*D–F*) through a combined temporal-suboccipital presigmoid petrosal route leaving a remnant in the cavernous sinus (*arrows*). The patient had an uneventful postoperative course with the exception of transient trigeminal herpes. The residual tumor was treated by gamma knife radiosurgery without waiting for signs of regrowth.

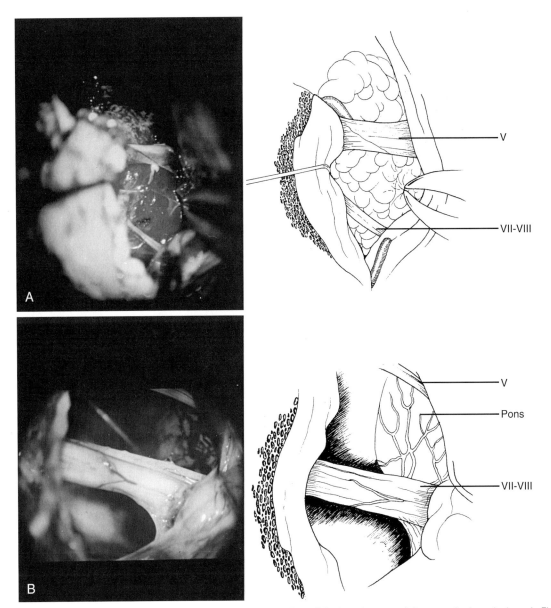

FIGURE 69-20 Intraoperative microphotographs and diagrammatic sketches of the lateral aspect of the petroclival meningioma in Figure 69-19 exposed using the combined subtemporal-presigmoid petrosal approach. *A*, The trigeminal nerve (V) is displaced posteriorly and laterally, and the faciovestibulocochlear complex (VII–VIII), partially engulfed by the tumor, posteriorly and inferiorly. *B*, After tumor removal, the faciovestibulocochlear appears reanimated.

25% to 100% (Table 69-6). Based on these data, it can be estimated that so-called gross-total excision is obtained in approximately 60% of all reported cases.

Reported mortality rates in the series range from 17% to 0%. This low rate of mortality demonstrates the progress achieved in the surgical technique of tumor removal. Illustrating this progress, a review by Hakuba and colleagues[8] of 31 reported patients operated on before 1977 showed a mortality rate as high as 68%.

Operative morbidity tends to be high, exceeding 50% in most contemporary series. The actual morbidity rate is difficult to evaluate, because most authors report transient and permanent complications in a different manner. However, it may be estimated that permanent morbidity of various degrees is present in roughly half of the cases operated on, and the incidence of severe disability is not negligible (15% to 20% of cases).

Major complications of surgery for petroclival meningiomas include (in order of frequency) cranial nerve dysfunction, long-tract deficits, cerebrospinal fluid leakage, stupor and coma, and sinus thrombosis.[2–4,14,15,42] In almost all cases, the patient is in worse clinical and neurologic condition after surgery than before, and needs constant, meticulous assistance. What contributes more than anything else to postoperative neurologic deterioration is the onset of new cranial nerve deficits or the aggravation of preexisting deficits. Only 8 (24%) of 33 patients in our first series emerged from surgery without any change in cranial nerve function; all others showed the onset of at least one new cranial nerve deficit, and 12 showed definite aggravation of preexisting deficits. Fortunately, many patients with either kind of deterioration showed some evidence of improvement within the first month after surgery, such that morbidity of this type was materially reduced at 4 weeks. The most dangerous type of

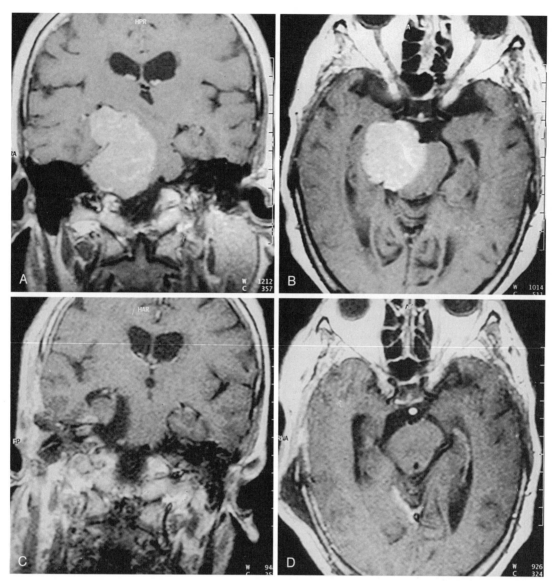

FIGURE 69-21   Preoperative coronal (*A*) and axial (*B*) postcontrast T1-weighted MRI scans of a large petroclival meningioma that was totally removed by a combined temporal-suboccipital presigmoid petrosal approach. Early postoperative comparable imaging (*C* and *D*) verify radicality.

impairment is palsy of cranial nerves IX and X, causing severe dysphagia and requiring utmost care to prevent aspiration pneumonia. A lesser but still significant contribution to overall neurologic deterioration is caused by the onset or aggravation of somatomotor deficits. In our series, hemiparesis developed in four patients, abating in two within a few weeks. Altered states of consciousness, deregulation of brain stem functions, and functional impairment of the lowest cranial nerves were causes of respiratory problems, requiring mechanical ventilation beyond the second postoperative day in six patients and necessitating tracheostomy in two.

Cerebrospinal fluid leakage facilitated by the opening of the mastoid air cells is usually successfully treated by lumbar drainage for 1 week or more. Thrombosis of the transverse or sigmoid sinus is a life-threatening complication that must be immediately recognized and treated with intravenous heparin.[13]

RECURRENCES

Unfortunately, surgical results of petroclival meningiomas are negatively affected by tumor remants. Tumor recurrence means that some remaining tumor tissue was capable of regrowing into a tumor mass. In approximately 30% of patients in reported series with subtotal tumor removal, recurrence was due either to incomplete excision or to regrowth after seemingly total removal. The broad dural base of most petroclival meningiomas and their tendency to grow en plaque with extensive bone and dural infiltration account for the high recurrence rate.

Although the goal of surgery should be complete removal of the lesion, these tumors also may be well controlled for a long period after a large and efficacious subtotal removal. In the series reported by Sekhar and associates,[15] only one of the five patients (20%) with residual tumor required

TABLE 69-6 ▪ **Reported Series of Petroclival Meningiomas**

Authors	Year	No. of Patients	Total Removal (%)	Operative Morbidity* (%)	Mortality† (%)
Hakuba et al[7]	1977	6	100	—	17
Yasargil et al[17]	1980	20	35	50	15
Mayberg and Symon[11]	1986	35	26	54	9
Al-Mefty et al[1]	1988	13	85	31	0
Nishimura et al[47]	1989	24	—	91	8
Samii et al[12]	1989	24	71	46	0
Sekhar et al[14]	1990	41	78	22	2
Al–Mefty and Smith[3]	1991	18	83	—	0
Bricolo et al[4]	1992	33	79	76	9
Samii and Tatagiba[13]	1992	36	75	42	—
Spetzler et al[16]	1992	46	91	56	0
Sekhar et al[15]	1994	75	60	60	0
Cantore et al[48]	1994	16	80	38	0
Couldwell et al[6]	1996	109	69	51	4
Thomas and King[49]	1996	16	44	—	0
Zentner et al[23]	1997	19	68	58	5
Bricolo and Turazzi[45]	1999	110	66	47	4

*Operative morbidity is reported differently according to author. This table attempts to report the average occurrence of early postoperative dyfunction. A percentage of these are transient.

†A number of patients who died after surgery because of postoperative complications may not have been included.

reoperation. In the series of Mayberg and Symon,[11] 4 of 26 patients (15%) with subtotal removal had clinical progression and eventually died. In 1994, Kawase and associates[32] reported a rapid regrowth in 3 (7%) of 42 patients between 1 and 4 years after surgery, and stable residual tumor in 7 patients (17%).

Treatment of residual tumor depends on many variables: a small tumor remnant left unresected because of neural or vascular structural encasement may be observed or treated by radiosurgery; the same can be done in elderly patients when a small amount of tumor remains after surgery. For larger tumor remnants, Sekhar and colleagues[14] propose an early second operation before development of scar tissue. This aggressive surgical treatment seems justified because of unsatisfactory results and side effects of radiation therapy, which, however, still maintains a role in the treatment of large and fast-growing recurrences.

Prevention of recurrences may interfere with surgical wound closure. Ear, nose, and throat surgeons[43] who have resolved the problem of repairing large dural defects in the skull base by placing large pieces of autologous fat, claim the necessity of "as large as possible" dural removal to obtain true radicality and proper treatment of skull base meningiomas.

FINAL REMARKS AND CONCLUSION

Evaluation of our experience in the surgical management of more than 100 petroclival meningiomas and review of major contemporary series demonstrate that it is not easy nor the rule to attain good clinical results after removal of such tumors. Surgical technical advancements associated with improved neuroanesthesia, postoperative intensive care, and rehabilitation make it possible to obtain much better results than in the past, and today surgical mortality rates approach 0%. However, morbidity, primarily from cranial nerve neuropathies, remains significant and unacceptable for more than a few patients.

The primary factors limiting total removal (Table 69-7) and reduction of operative morbidity are basically the same ones faced by many skull base surgeons who tend to use more extensive approaches.[44] It is our belief that the real limitation in obtaining radical and safe removal is not inadequate exposure but rather the anatomicopathologic characteristics of the tumor.

Meningiomas of the clivus and petrous apex continue to pose a surgical challenge, and the optimal surgical management remains controversial. In a retrospective study, we reviewed all our experience in this field (Table 69-8).[45] In approximately 19 years (1981 to July 1999), 110 meningiomas of the petroclival region were treated. Separating the data into two groups by decades, the following changes in the latter decade can be noted: (1) a slight increase in the use of a complex approach, (2) a reduction of the rate of total resection, and (3) a significant reduction in operative morbidity. From these changes one can deduce that the "learning curve" has taught neurosurgeons to be less aggressive in tumor removal in an effort to avoid injury to the involved neurovascular structures. This attitude, also shared by others,[46] guarantees better clinical outcome based on the current technical capability.

A number of issues related to surgical management of petroclival meningiomas are still unresolved. We believe that

TABLE 69-7 ▪ **Combined Factors Opposing Total Removal in 37 of the Last 110 Petroclival and Anterior Petrous Meningiomas in the Authors' Series**

Factors	N
Tumor extension	16
Arterial encasement	18
Cranial nerve	24
Absent arachnoid plane	12
Dural invasion	8
Intraoperative failure	2

TABLE 69-8 ▪ Authors' Series of 110 Consecutive Petroclival Meningiomas

Period	No. of Patients	Restrosigmoid Approach	Skull Base Approach	Total Removal	Operative Morbidity	Mortality
1981–1990	33	23 (70%)	10 (30%)	26 (79%)	25 (72%)	3 (9%)
1991–1999	77	49 (64%)	28 (36%)	47 (61%)	29 (37%)	2 (3%)
Total	110	72 (65%)	38 (35%)	73 (66%)	54 (47%)	5 (4%)

preservation of function should take priority, and this remains the most important factor governing the procedure. Radical tumor removal at all costs, at the risk of adding permanent dysfunction to a preexisting picture of brain stem distress, does not seem to be the appropriate strategy. If safe radical excision of a tumor is not feasible because of its invasive nature, little room is left for complete removal, and severe brain stem indentation and arterial and cranial nerve encasement represent unresolved technical difficulties.

Although total eradication certainly remains the prime objective of surgery, the surgeon must also consider that a number of subtotally removed petroclival meningiomas remain stationary, often for long periods, and radiosurgery can control eventual regrowth.

Acknowledgments

The authors thank Ms. Marina Longani for the illustrations, Ms. Cristina Bertolin for her preparation of the photographic material, and Ms. Victoria Praino for editing.

REFERENCES

1. Al-Mefty O, Fox JL, Smith RR: Petrosal approach for petroclival meningiomas. Neurosurgery 22:510–517, 1988.
2. Al-Mefty O, Ayoubi S, Smith RR: The petrosal approach: Indications, technique, and results. Acta Neurochir Suppl (Wien) 53:166–170, 1991.
3. Al-Mefty O, Smith RR: Clival and petroclival meningiomas. In Al-Mefty O (ed): Meningiomas. New York: Raven Press, 1991, pp 517–537.
4. Bricolo A, Turazzi S, Cristofori L, et al: Microsurgical removal of petroclival meningiomas: A report of 33 patients. Neurosurgery 31:813–828, 1992.
5. Bricolo A: Radical surgical removal of clival meningiomas. In Al-Mefty O (ed): Controversies in Neurosurgery. New York: Thieme, 1996, pp 110–114.
6. Couldwell WT, Fukushima T, Giannotta S, et al: Petroclival meningiomas: Surgical experience in 109 cases. J Neurosurg 84:20–28, 1996.
7. Hakuba A, Nishimura S, Tanaka K, et al: Clivus meningioma: Six cases of total removal. Neurol Med Chir (Tokyo) 17:63–77, 1977.
8. Hakuba A, Nishimura S, Jang BJ: A combined retroauricular and preauricular transpetrosal-transtentorial approach to clivus meningiomas. Surg Neurol 30:108–116, 1988.
9. Malis LI: The petrosal approach. Clin Neurosurg 37:528–540, 1991.
10. Malis LI: Suboccipital subtemporal approach to petroclival tumors. In Wilson CB (ed): Neurosurgical Procedures: Personal Approaches to Classic Operations. Baltimore: Williams & Wilkins, 1992, pp 41–51.
11. Mayberg M, Symon L: Meningiomas of the clivus and apical petrous bone: Report of 35 cases. J Neurosurg 65:160–167, 1986.
12. Samii M, Ammirati M, Mahran A, et al: Surgery of petroclival meningiomas: Report of 24 cases. Neurosurgery 24:12–17, 1989.
13. Samii M, Tatagiba M: Experience with 36 surgical cases of petroclival meningiomas. Acta Neurochir (Wien) 118:27–32, 1992.
14. Sekhar LN, Jannetta PJ, Burkhart LE, et al: Meningiomas involving the clivus: A six-year experience with 41 patients. Neurosurgery 27:764–781, 1990.
15. Sekhar L, Swamy NKS, Jaiswal V, et al: Surgical excision of meningiomas involving the clivus: Preoperative and intraoperative features as predictors of postoperative functional deterioration. J Neurosurg 81:860–868, 1994.
16. Spetzler RF, Daspit CP, Pappas CTE: The combined supra- and infratentorial approach for lesions of the petrous and clival regions: Experience with 46 cases. J Neurosurg 76:588–599, 1992.
17. Yasargil MG, Mortara RW, Curcic M: Meningiomas of basal posterior cranial fossa. Adv Tech Stand Neurosurg 7:3–115, 1980.
18. Uttley D: Skull base surgery. Br J Neurosurg 9:437–439, 1995.
19. Cushing HW, Eisenhardt L: Meningiomas: Their Classification, Regional Behavior, Life History and Surgical End Results. Springfield, IL: Charles C Thomas, 1938, pp 3–387.
20. Castellano F, Ruggiero G: Meningiomas of the posterior fossa. Acta Radiol (Suppl) 104:3–157, 1953.
21. Spetzler RF, Daspit CP, Pappas CTE: Combined approach for lesions involving the clivus and cerebellopontine angle: Experience with 23 cases. Presented at the International Symposium on Processes of the Cranial Midline, Vienna, May 21–25, 1990.
22. Couldwell WT, Weiss MH: Surgical approaches to petroclival meningiomas. I: Upper and midclival approaches. Contemp Neurosurg 16:1–6, 1994.
23. Zentner J, Meyer B, Vieweg U, et al: Petroclival meningiomas: Is radical resection always the best option? J Neurol Neurosurg Psychiatry 62:341–345, 1997.
24. McDermott MW, Wilson CB: Meningiomas. In Youmans J (ed): Neurological Surgery. Philadelphia: WB Saunders, 1997, pp 2782–2825.
25. Ojemann RG: Skull base surgery: A perspective. J Neurosurg 76:569–570, 1992.
26. Pomeranz S, Umansky F, Elidan J, et al: Giant cranial base tumors. Acta Neurochir (Wien) 129:121–126, 1994.
27. Holmes B, Sekhar L, Sofaer S, et al: Outcome analysis in cranial base surgery: Preliminary results. Acta Neurochir (Wien) 134:136–138, 1995.
28. Samii M, Tatagiba M: Petroclival approach. In Donald PJ (ed): Surgery of the Skull Base. Philadelphia: Lippincott-Raven, 1998, pp 423–442.
29. Dolenc VV: Direct microsurgical repair of intracavernous vascular lesions. J Neurosurg 58:826–831, 1983.
30. Dolenc VN: Anatomy and Surgery of the Cavernous Sinus. New York: Springer-Verlag, 1989.
31. Kawase T, Shiobara R, Toya S: Anterior transpetrosal-transtentorial approach for sphenopetroclival meningiomas: Surgical method and results in 10 meningiomas. Neurosurgery 28:869–875, 1991.
32. Kawase T, Shiobara R, Ohira T: Middle fossa transpetrosal-transtentorial approaches for petroclival meningiomas: Selective pyramid resection and radicality. Acta Neurochir (Wien) 129:113–120, 1994.
33. Al-Mefty O, Anand VK: Zygomatic approach to skull-base lesions. J Neurosurg 73:668–673, 1990.
34. Sen CN, Sekhar LN: The subtemporal and preauricular infratemporal approach to intradural structures ventral to the brain stem. J Neurosurg 73:345–354, 1990.
35. Dandy W: An operation for the total removal of cerebellopontine (acoustic) tumors. Surg Gynecol Obstet 41:129–148, 1925.
36. Bricolo A, Turazzi A, Talacchi A, et al: Simple neurosurgical approaches to the clivus. In Samii M (ed): Skull Base Surgery. First International Skull Base Congress, Hannover, 1992. Basel: Karger, 1994, pp 1055–1064.
37. Bertalanffy H, Gilsbach J, Seeger W, et al: Surgical anatomy and clinical application of the transcondylar approach to the lower clivus. In Samii M (ed): Skull Base Surgery. First International Skull Base Congress, Hannover, 1992. Basel: Karger, 1994, pp 1045–1048.
38. Sen CN, Sekhar LN: An extreme lateral approach to intradural lesions of the cervical spine and foramen magnum. Neurosurgery 27:197–204, 1990.
39. Al-Mefty O, Borba LAB, Aoki N, et al: The transcondylar approach to extradural nonneoplastic lesions of the craniovertebral junction. J Neurosurg 84:1–6, 1996.
40. King AK, Black KL, Martin NA, et al: The petrosal approach with hearing preservation. J Neurosurg 79:508–514, 1993.

41. Fukushima T: Combined supra- and infra-parapetrosal approach for petroclival lesions. In Sekhar LN, Janecka IP (eds): Surgery of Cranial Base Tumors. New York: Raven Press, 1992, pp 661–670.

42. Bricolo A, Turazzi S, Cristofori L, et al: Surgical treatment of meningiomas in the petroclival area: Experience in 28 cases [Abstract]. Presented at the First Asian-Oceanic International Congress on Skull Base Surgery, Tokyo, June 18–20, 1991.

43. Sanna M, Mazzoni A, Saleh EA, et al: Lateral approaches to the median skull base through the petrous bone: The system of the modified transcochlear approach. J Laryngol Otol 108:1036–1044, 1994.

44. Lang DA, Neil-Dwyer G, Garfield J: Outcome after complex neurosurgery: The caregiver's burden is forgotten. J Neurosurg 91:359–363, 1999.

45. Bricolo A, Turazzi S: Surgical management of petroclival meningiomas: Experience on 110 cases [Abstract]. Presented at XLVIII Congress of the Italian Neurosurgical Society, Catanzaro, September 12–15, 1999.

46. David CA, Spetzler RF: Petroclival meningiomas. BNI Q 15:5–14, 1999.

47. Nishimura S, Hakuba A, Jang B, et al: Clivus and apicopetroclivus meningiomas: Report of 24 cases. Neurol Med Chir 29:1004–1011, 1989.

48. Cantore G, Delfini R, Ciappetta P: Surgical treatment of petroclival meningiomas: Experience with 16 cases. Surg Neurol 42:105–111, 1994.

49. Thomas NWM, King TT: Meningiomas of the cerebellopontine angle: A report of 41 cases. Br J Neurosurg 10:59–68, 1996.

70 Surgical Management of Glomus Jugulare Tumors

CARL B. HEILMAN, JON H. ROBERTSON,
GALE GARDNER, and NIKOLAS BLEVINS

The optimal management of a glomus jugulare tumor remains a challenge. This chapter presents a comprehensive review of this formidable lesion while emphasizing the relevant surgical anatomy and the importance of developing an individualized treatment plan for a particular lesion.

Glomus jugulare tumors are believed to arise from glomus bodies in the region of the jugular bulb. The first description of glomus tissue is credited to Valentin, who in 1840 noted a small cellular formation near the origin of the tympanic nerve that he thought was a ganglion.[1] In 1878, Krause[2] further described glomus tissue as being microscopic, indistinguishable from the carotid body, and occurring along the tympanic branch of the glossopharyngeal nerve in the inferior tympanic canaliculus. Valentin's and Krause's work received little attention. It was not until 1941 that glomus tissue was rediscovered by Guild.[3] Guild coined the term glomus jugularis, or jugular body, to describe the paraganglionic tissue that is composed largely of capillary or precapillary vessels interspersed with numerous epithelioid cells and that is found along the jugular bulb in human temporal bone sections. The relationship between the "glomus jugularis" described by Guild and the "carotid body–like" tumor in the temporal bone was first recognized by Rosenwasser[4] in 1945. In 1953, after serially sectioning 88 human temporal bones, Guild[5] noted that approximately 50% of jugular bodies were situated in the adventitia of the jugular bulb dome. The remainder occurred with equal frequency along the course of the tympanic branch of the glossopharyngeal nerve (Jacobson's nerve) or the auricular branch of the vagus nerve (Arnold's nerve). This explained the observation that "glomus tumors" occur in the middle ear (glomus tympanicum tumors) as well as in the region of the jugular bulb (glomus jugulare tumors).

Rockley and Hawke[6] in 1990 published a systematic study of the exact anatomic distribution of glomus bodies in the temporal bone (Fig. 70-1). They noted that glomus bodies, which measured up to 1 mm in diameter, were found only along the course of parasympathetic nerves of the ear (Arnold's or Jacobson's nerve) or their identifiable branches. Histologically, the glomus bodies appeared as nests of epithelioid cells surrounded by a connective tissue capsule. On the surface of the capsule were tortuous arterioles, whereas thin-walled venous sinusoids coursed through the substance of the glomus body. Rockley and Hawke[6] concluded that dividing glomus tumors into two groups (glomus tympanicum and glomus jugulare tumors) was an artificial distinction based on observed clinical presentation rather than on actual anatomic distribution of glomus bodies. Tumors arising distally on Jacobson's nerve or on the promontory would manifest clinically as glomus tympanicum tumors. Tumors arising more proximally on Jacobson's nerve in the inferior tympanic canaliculus or adjacent to the jugular bulb would expand into the jugular bulb and manifest as glomus jugulare tumors. The discovery by Rockley and Hawke[6] of glomus bodies located along the course of Arnold's nerve adjacent to the facial nerve could account for the occasional clinical presentation of a glomus tumor in the descending facial canal.

The exact physiologic function of the glomus body remains unknown. Its histologic similarity to carotid and aortic bodies has suggested a chemoreceptor role responding to hypoxia, hypercarbia, or acidosis. Other possibilities are a role in regulating microcirculatory blood flow or the homeostasis of gas composition and pressure in the middle ear. On the basis of their anatomic study, Rockley and Hawke[6] suggested that temporal glomus bodies regulate the

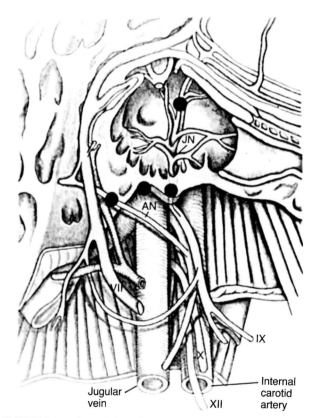

FIGURE 70-1 Lateral view of the temporal bone through the region of the jugular bulb demonstrating the anatomic location of the glomus bodies (*black dots*). AN, Arnold's nerve; JN, Jacobsen's nerve.

blood flow to the promontory with a secondary effect on gas pressure in the middle ear.

EPIDEMIOLOGY

Although glomus jugulare tumors are second to vestibular schwannomas as the most common tumor involving the temporal bone, they are still uncommonly seen in neurosurgical practice. The age of presentation ranges from the second to the ninth decade, although most tumors manifest in middle age, with the disease affecting women more often than men.[7-9] In one study of 231 cases, glomus jugulare tumors were six times more common in women than in men.[7]

Most glomus jugulare tumors are benign, slow-growing neoplasms that are highly vascular and locally invasive. Symptoms may exist from months to decades before the diagnosis.[7,8,10,11] In 1992, van der Mey and colleagues[11] reported a series of 52 patients with glomus jugulotympanicum tumors, of whom 20 underwent subtotal tumor removal and 13 patients were followed without treatment. All of these patients, except three who were lost to follow-up, were alive and without serious complaints with an average follow-up of 13.5 years (range, 1–32 years). Clinically, their disease was not progressive, with the exception of one case that required additional surgery 5 years after incomplete surgical removal. Occasionally, however, the tumor is aggressive and grows rapidly; in rare cases (1% to 3%), it can metastasize to regional lymph nodes or distant sites.[7,12-19]

Glomus jugulare tumors can be bilateral or associated with other chemodectomas[20-22] (Fig. 70-2). In most series, familial glomus jugulare tumors compose a minority; however, in a report by van der Mey and colleagues[11] from the Netherlands, familial cases of all glomus tumors (including carotid body tumors) made up approximately 50% of the entire series.

Catecholamine biosynthesis and secretion has been reported in approximately 4% of patients with glomus jugulare tumors.[23-29] Excess catecholamines may be responsible for hypertension preoperatively or for wide fluctuations in blood pressure during surgical manipulation. Preoperative 24-hour urinary studies to screen for vanillylmandelic acid, metanephrine, free catecholamine, and 5-hydroxyindole acetic acid (5-HIAA) may help predict which patients will have blood pressure fluctuations during tumor removal.

PRESENTATION

The locally invasive and highly vascular nature of glomus jugulare tumors accounts for their clinical presentation. They usually present with progressive unilateral hearing loss from invasion of the mesotympanum and pulsatile tinnitus secondary to the tumor's rich vascularity. Other symptoms depend on the direction of tumor growth. Invasion of the cochlea or labyrinth produces sensorineural hearing loss or vertigo, respectively. Lower cranial nerve dysfunction, manifested as hoarseness or dysphagia, occurs more commonly with larger tumors but is generally well tolerated because of its gradual onset and simultaneous compensation. In a series of 102 patients reported by Makek and associates,[30] cranial nerve VII was affected at presentation in 33% of patients. This cranial nerve was the most often affected on presentation in their series, followed by cranial nerves X, IX, XII, and XI. In a series of 59 patients reported by Jackson and associates[31] in 1990, however, preoperative facial weakness was present in only 8%. Notably, the lack of preoperative nerve dysfunction does not preclude finding neural invasion at the time of surgery.[30] A complete jugular foramen syndrome is unusual unless advanced disease is present. Large glomus jugulare tumors may grow anteriorly and encase the carotid artery, producing Horner's syndrome, or extend

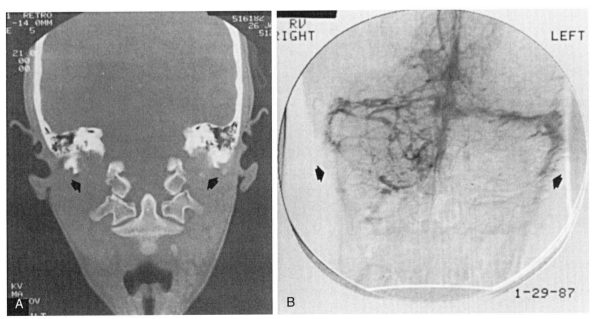

FIGURE 70-2 *A*, Coronal computed tomography scan of the skull base demonstrating bilateral glomus jugulare tumors. Note the irregular bone edges of the jugular foramina, which is typical for this locally invasive tumor (*arrows*). *B*, An anteroposterior venogram of the head in the same patient, demonstrating bilateral jugular bulb occlusion (*arrows*).

medially and superiorly up into the cavernous sinus. Intracranial extension, either through the jugular foramen or via expansion in the epidural space along the posterior aspect of the petrous bone, may cause fifth and sixth cranial nerve dysfunction, brain stem compression, and hydrocephalus. Extracranial extension into and along the jugular vein may produce a mass visible in the oropharynx or palpable in the neck. Rarely, patients can present with palpitations and flushing from secretion of catecholamines.[32]

SURGICAL ANATOMY

The jugular foramen in the posterolateral skull base is bounded anterolaterally by the petrous portion of the temporal bone and posteromedially by the occipital bone. The two jugular foramina are asymmetric, with the right side being larger in more than two thirds of cases.[33,34] This is believed to be secondary to the asymmetry in the size of the transverse and sigmoid sinuses. The foramen is subdivided into two compartments by a fibrous or, less frequently, bony septum that connects the jugular spine of the petrous bone with the jugular process of the occipital bone. In a systematic study of 129 dry skulls, Di Chiro and colleagues[33] noted a bony septum unilaterally in 13.2% and bilaterally in 4.7%. The posterolateral compartment, called the pars venosa, is larger and contains the jugular bulb, cranial nerves X and XI, and the posterior meningeal artery. The smaller anteromedial compartment, called the pars nervosa, contains cranial nerve IX and the venous channels of the inferior petrosal sinus (Fig. 70-3).[35] The exact anatomic location of cranial nerves IX, X, and XI as they traverse the jugular foramen is variable, but in essentially every case, they are medial to the jugular bulb. The ninth cranial nerve travels alone, medial and slightly superior to cranial nerves X and XI, which are intimately associated with each other. In rare cases (6%), the glossopharyngeal nerve leaves the skull through a separate bony canal rather than through the pars nervosa.[34]

The venous anatomy of the jugular foramen is formed by the continuation of the horizontal limb of the sigmoid sinus into the jugular bulb. The jugular bulb then rises above the horizontal segment of the sigmoid sinus. Surrounding the dome of the jugular bulb in the temporal bone are numerous anatomic structures, including the posterior semicircular canal, the middle ear, the medial aspect of the external auditory canal, and cranial nerve VII. In 1975, Graham[36] reported that in some cases, the jugular bulb rose 0.75 inch above the horizontal limb of the sigmoid sinus, whereas in other cases it rose not more than 0.25 inch. The jugular bulb lies inferior to the middle ear and, when small, is separated from the middle ear by bone. The bone separating a large jugular bulb from the middle ear may be thin or dehiscent, with the venous wall of the bulb occasionally reaching the round window.[36] The facial nerve descends in the fallopian canal on the lateral aspect of the jugular bulb, often as close as 1 mm.

An understanding of the anatomy of the inferior petrosal sinus is critical during removal of glomus jugulare tumors. The inferior petrosal sinus is usually the largest vessel to empty into the jugular bulb, with the exception of the sigmoid sinus. The inferior petrosal sinus opens into the anterior medial aspect of the jugular bulb usually by several channels coursing through the fibrous septum separating the pars nervosa and pars venosa. Occasionally, the vein of the cochlear aqueduct or a branch from the occipital sinus empties into the jugular bulb as well.[36] These multiple channels are a source of bleeding that must be controlled during the final stages of tumor excision without causing injury to the underlying cranial nerves.

As the contents of the jugular foramen leave the skull base, they are surrounded by vital structures, including the internal carotid artery (ICA), the facial nerve, and the hypoglossal nerve. Several relatively constant anatomic relationships are essential to successful dissection in this region. The stylomastoid foramen containing the facial nerve is located just lateral and posterior to the base of the styloid process. The glossopharyngeal nerve exits the medial and superior aspect of the jugular foramen and then passes lateral to the ICA. The spinal accessory nerve leaves the jugular foramen medial to the jugular vein. This nerve usually passes anterior to the jugular vein extracranially before passing under the sternocleidomastoid muscle. The hypoglossal nerve leaves the hypoglossal canal and passes around behind the vagus nerve before coursing anteriorly over the ICA toward the tongue. In summary, the nerves exiting the jugular foramen all travel medial to the jugular bulb, and all cranial nerves seen with this dissection (VII, IX, X, XI, and XII) pass lateral to the ICA.

MANAGEMENT OF GLOMUS JUGULARE TUMORS

Patients presenting with a mass consistent with a glomus jugulare tumor should be evaluated by audiometry to determine the function of the middle and inner ear. In older patients with a large tumor, in whom blood pressure fluctuations would increase the risk of surgery, a 24-hour urinary catecholamine screen should be performed to rule out a catecholamine-secreting tumor. If elevated levels of catecholamines are detected, preoperative treatment with an alpha blocker and beta-blockade therapy during surgery are recommended. Magnetic resonance imaging (MRI), with and without gadolinium enhancement, provides excellent definition of the tumor and its relationship to both neural and vascular structures, particularly if there is intracranial extension. However, enhancement in the jugular foramen on MRI scans can occur with relatively static blood flow through a large jugular bulb in the absence of a tumor.[37] This enhancement can be erroneously interpreted as a glomus jugulare tumor if MRI alone is used for diagnosis. Thin-section computed tomography (CT) is the preferred method for determining the extent of bony involvement.

Cerebral arteriography is useful for evaluating the tumor's blood supply, involvement of the ICA, and demonstration of the venous anatomy. It is important to know whether the sigmoid sinus and jugular bulb are occluded by the tumor, whether the opposite sigmoid sinus is patent, and whether there is communication across the torcula. Arteriography can also demonstrate an associated glomus vagale or carotid body tumor that is not seen on the CT or MRI scan. If sacrifice of the ICA is a possibility, arteriography combined with balloon test occlusion with cerebral blood flow studies can further evaluate collateral blood flow. In addition, the vascularity of the tumor and the potential for embolization can be assessed.

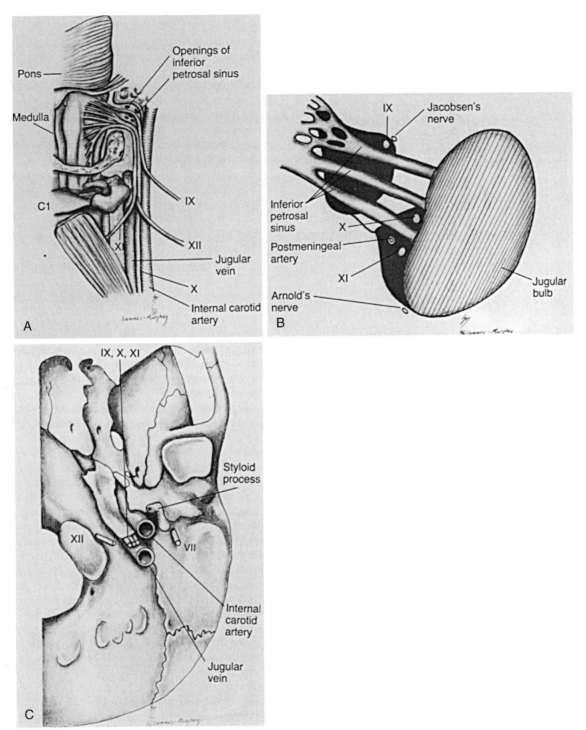

FIGURE 70-3 *A,* Lateral view of the jugular foramen with the jugular vein and bulb removed. *B,* Cross section of the jugular foramen. *C,* Basal view of the skull base focusing on the region of the jugular foramen. (Copyright © Semmes-Murphey Clinic.)

Embolization

The use of preoperative embolization has been a major advance in the successful surgical management of glomus jugulare tumors.[38–40] Embolization has been shown to reduce operative blood loss, decrease the need for blood transfusion, and shorten operating time.[41–44] Preoperative embolization may increase the likelihood of complete tumor excision. In addition, embolization possibly decreases the incidence of postoperative cranial nerve palsy by improving visibility of the lower cranial nerves and by decreasing the need for bipolar coagulation in the region of the jugular foramen during tumor removal.

The main blood supply of glomus jugulare tumors is from the inferior tympanic branch of the ascending pharyngeal artery and the stylomastoid artery. The stylomastoid artery arises from the occipital artery in 60% of patients and from the posterior auricular artery in 40% (see references 44 and 45). Occlusion of tumor vessels through these arteries is often the main goal of embolization. Large tumors may parasitize branches from either the ICA or the vertebral artery. Embolization of these vessels is advisable only in rare circumstances because of their small size and the risk of intracranial embolization. We have found that venous embolization of the inferior petrosal sinus and sigmoid sinus just upstream from the tumor can be performed in selective cases and may decrease venous bleeding during surgery.

Surgery

The surgical management of glomus jugulare tumors has evolved gradually over the past 4 decades. Surgeons have been challenged by the tumor's rich vascularity, the complex regional anatomy, and the potential for injury to the carotid artery or lower cranial nerves. In the 1950s, radiation therapy alone or in combination with limited surgery became the preferred treatment because of the morbidity and mortality associated with radical surgery. Advances in neuroimaging in the 1960s led to better understanding of the tumor's size and anatomic location, which led to a renewed interest in surgical resection.

In 1964, Shapiro and Neues[46] established the general strategy for resecting a glomus jugulare tumor by combining a mastoidectomy with lateral skull base exposure through the neck. By rerouting the facial nerve, they were able to remove a tumor with minimal blood loss and no significant neurologic deficit. In the 1970s, the operating microscope, neuroanesthesia, and a better understanding of the surgical anatomy contributed to improved surgical results. Further refinements in technique led to the development of combined lateral skull base approaches[47,48] and the infratemporal fossa approach,[49] both of which emphasized exposure and control of the ICA. These approaches, with minor improvements, are the mainstays of surgical treatment today.

Although some authors continue to recommend radiation therapy as the initial treatment for all glomus jugulare tumors, we believe that in the young and middle-aged patients, the current definitive therapy is surgical. In elderly patients or those with major medical problems, we recommend radiosurgery or a "wait and see" policy.

In general, patients who present with complete ninth and tenth nerve palsy have compensated for this deficit because of its gradual onset. In our experience, these patients tolerate surgery extremely well. The patient with a large tumor and normal lower cranial nerve function, however, is more likely to have postoperative difficulty with swallowing and aspiration because of the acute onset of vagus nerve dysfunction.

Surgical Approaches

The choice of surgical approach is based on the anatomic extent of the tumor and, to some extent, the patient's preoperative hearing function. A glomus tympanicum or glomus hypotympanicum tumor can be approached through the ear canal or mastoid, respectively. Glomus jugulare tumors require more extensive exposure and cannot be adequately approached through the mastoid alone.

LATERAL SKULL BASE APPROACH

The lateral skull base approach is used for medium glomus jugulare tumors that extend up to the petrous portion of the ICA. After the induction of general anesthesia, with the patient supine, the head is turned away from the operative side. A retroauricular C-shaped incision is made that extends into the neck along the anterior border of the sternocleidomastoid muscle (Fig. 70-4). The greater auricular nerve is identified, divided, and tagged for reanastomosis or potential later use as a nerve graft. The ear canal is transected at the bony-cartilaginous junction. The ear canal skin is dissected off the ear canal cartilage and pulled out through the ear canal. It is then closed from the outside in an everted fashion with a running absorbable suture. A portion of the canal cartilage is removed from the membranous ear canal. Mastoid periosteum is then rotated over the opening of the ear canal and sutured down to complete a two-layer closure. An incision is then made in the periosteum of the skull, parallel and just inferior to the lower border of the temporalis muscle. A periosteal flap is then elevated inferiorly and kept in continuity with the sternocleidomastoid muscle as it is dissected off its attachment to the mastoid bone. This mastoid periosteal flap will be sutured to the inferior border of the temporalis muscle at the time of closure.

Attention is then turned to the neck. The ICA and adjacent cranial nerves are exposed medial to the sternocleidomastoid muscle. The facial vein must often be divided. The carotid bifurcation, external carotid artery, ICA, jugular vein, hypoglossal nerve, ansa hypoglossi, spinal accessory nerve, and vagus nerve are identified. The posterior belly of the digastric muscle is released from the digastric groove of the mastoid bone. If possible, the posterior belly of the digastric muscle and adjacent soft tissue are left attached to the soft tissue surrounding the facial nerve as it exits the stylomastoid foramen. This helps to preserve the facial nerve's blood supply and decreases the incidence of postoperative facial nerve paralysis. However, with large tumors, this muscle and attached soft tissue obstructs exposure and can be removed if necessary. The occipital artery is divided. The ICA and the jugular vein are dissected free of soft tissue and isolated. The distal styloid process and attached tendons are removed with a rongeur, and care is taken to protect the underlying ICA and ninth cranial nerve. The base of the styloid process is left in place at this point as a landmark. The glossopharyngeal nerve is identified. The transverse process of C1 lateral to the foramen transversaria can be removed to improve exposure if necessary. The soft tissue between the base of the skull and the transverse process of C1 is removed carefully to protect the underlying vertebral artery. The base of the styloid process is removed, along with the soft tissue at the lateral edge of the jugular foramen.

A simple mastoidectomy is then performed with a high-speed drill and suction irrigation. Care is taken to avoid entering the semicircular canals or the cochlea unless sensorineural function has previously been destroyed by the tumor. The bone of the posterior aspect of the external auditory canal is removed. The tympanic membrane, malleus, and incus are removed after disarticulation of the incostapedial joint. The mastoid and tympanic segments of the facial nerve are skeletonized. If possible, the facial nerve is left in a thin fallopian bridge.[50] Alternatively, the facial nerve can be drilled free of its bony canal from the geniculate ganglion

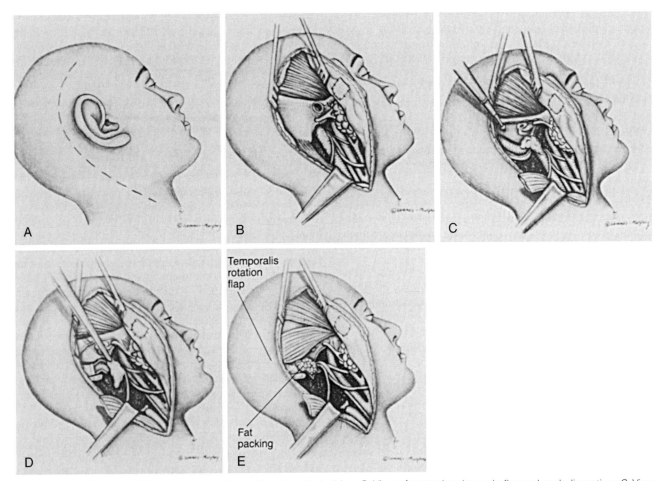

FIGURE 70-4 Lateral skull base approach. *A*, Location of a skin incision. *B*, View after turning the scalp flap and neck dissection. *C*, View after the temporal bone dissection. *D*, Ligation of the sigmoid sinus and jugular vein with removal of the tumor. *E*, Reconstruction of the wound with fat packing and rotation of the temporalis muscle. (Copyright, © Semmes-Murphey Clinic.)

to the stylomastoid foramen and transposed anterior and superior to the middle ear. This maneuver provides an unobstructed view of the tumor but essentially guarantees at least a temporary postoperative facial nerve paralysis. If the facial nerve was weak before surgery and is infiltrated by tumor, the involved portion of the nerve can be resected and grafted. If the facial nerve is transposed, it is placed proximally into a bony groove drilled into the epitympanum and distally into a groove in the substance of the parotid gland, as described by Fisch.[49]

The sigmoid sinus is then skeletonized, and the dura anterior and posterior to it is exposed. The bone of the lateral skull base between the digastric groove and the jugular foramen is removed.

The bony wall of the tympanum and hypotympanum is drilled away, exposing the petrous segment of the ICA. The eustachian tube is sealed with bone wax, fascia, and fibrin glue. The ICA is exposed from the neck to the horizontal segment in the petrous bone. The tumor is coagulated and mobilized inferiorly away from the carotid artery down toward the hypotympanum. Care is taken to avoid traumatizing the stapes.

The sigmoid sinus is then occluded in its descending portion above the tumor mass. This can be performed by packing Surgicel between the bone and the sigmoid sinus

until the sigmoid sinus is occluded. Alternatively, the sigmoid sinus can be ligated with a 2-0 silk suture. Suture ligation, however, often violates the arachnoid and might increase the likelihood of cerebrospinal fluid (CSF) leak. The jugular vein is then ligated in the neck beyond the tumor extension. The lateral wall of the sigmoid sinus is then incised, and the inside of the sigmoid is packed with Surgicel down toward the jugular bulb. The lateral wall of the sigmoid is removed from the point of sinus occlusion down to the tumor. Typically, there is a preserved plane of dissection between the tumor and the medial wall of the jugular bulb. Bleeding from the inferior petrosal sinus or occipital sinus is controlled by packing with Surgicel. Care should be taken to avoid bipolar coagulation and excessive pressure on the Surgicel, because this force will be transmitted to the underlying cranial nerves. The tumor is then removed by working circumferentially in the plane between the tumor and the lower cranial nerves. The tumor cavity is inspected, and any remaining tumor remnants are removed. The dura of the posterior cranial fossa must be removed if it is in contact with tumor. The dural defect is closed with a graft of pericranium or temporalis fascia.

All remaining remnants of mastoid mucosa are drilled away, and the mastoid cavity is packed with fat and covered by downward rotation of the posterior temporalis muscle and upward mobilization of the previously prepared sternocleidomastoid-periosteal flap. The skin edges are closed in layers, and a Hemovac drain is placed if the dura was not violated. A spinal drain is placed at the end of the procedure if a dural graft was required.

MODIFIED LATERAL SKULL BASE APPROACH

In selected patients with relatively small tumors and good preoperative hearing, an attempt at preservation of middle ear function is reasonable.[51] The skin incision and cervical dissection proceeds as described for the lateral skull base approach. A mastoidectomy is performed, but in this case the posterior bony canal wall, tympanic membrane, and ossicles are preserved (Fig. 70-5). The tympanic segment of the facial nerve is left in place, and only the mastoid segment is mobilized. Alternatively, the facial nerve can be preserved in a thin canal of bone known as the fallopian bridge technique as described by Pensak and Jackler.[50] The facial nerve is not transposed but may be moved 1 cm forward and back during tumor removal. The tumor is mobilized out of the middle ear mainly through the facial recess. Tumor removal then proceeds as described for the lateral skull base approach.

INFRATEMPORAL FOSSA APPROACH

The development of the infratemporal fossa approach by Fisch has been a significant advance in the resection of large tumors.[38,49] This approach is similar to the lateral skull base approach, but the exposure is carried farther in front of the ear canal into the infratemporal fossa. With this exposure, the bone over the glenoid fossa is removed, and the ICA is exposed from its extracranial portion up to the cavernous sinus (Fig. 70-6). The base of the skull can be removed anteriorly up to the foramen ovale or, with sectioning of this nerve, up to the foramen rotundum.

INTRACRANIAL EXTENSION

Intracranial extension can be removed via a retrosigmoid, presigmoid retrolabyrinthine, translabyrinthine, or

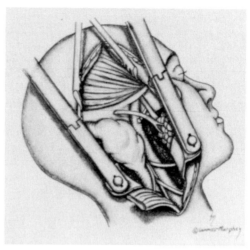

FIGURE 70-6 Infratemporal fossa approach with removal of the glenoid fossa, the floor of the middle cranial fossa, and complete release of the internal carotid artery from the petrous bone. The eustachian tube and the third division of the trigeminal nerve are visible. (Copyright © Semmes-Murphey Clinic.)

transcochlear approach, depending on the size and location of the tumor.

Radiation

The role of radiation therapy in the management of glomus jugulare tumors remains controversial. No prospective controlled trial comparing radiation therapy with surgery has been performed as yet. Long-term tumor control has been reported by many authors,[8,9,52–55] although recurrence after radiation therapy is not rare.[56–59] We use radiation therapy as the primary treatment modality in elderly patients with symptomatic tumors and in middle-aged patients with medical problems that substantially increase the risk of surgery. We have also made use of postoperative radiation therapy for the rare case of subtotal tumor removal.

The argument against radiation therapy is primarily that the patient is not cured of the disease, and if the tumor recurs years or decades later, the morbidity of surgery in an irradiated field is thought to be increased. Radiation-induced osteonecrosis of the temporal bone has been reported rarely after conventional radiation[60] but probably will not be seen with radiosurgery. The development of new radiation-induced neoplasms is often mentioned as a risk of radiation but is probably rare. Glomus jugulare tumors rarely decrease in size following radiation therapy, and lack of growth is considered to indicate successful treatment.[8,9,55]

In 1997, Foote and colleagues reported on the use of stereotactic radiosurgery for nine patients with glomus tumors with an average of 20 months of follow-up.[61] In eight of the nine patients, the tumor remained stable in size. In one of the nine patients, the tumor decreased in size. However, none of the tumors enlarged with follow-up ranging from 7 to 65 months. In addition, seven of the nine patients reported a subjective decrease in symptoms, and there was no acute or chronic toxicity. In 1998, Liscak and associates reported on the use of Leksell gamma knife radiosurgery for 14 patients with glomus jugulare and tympanicum tumors.[62] Eleven patients were available for follow-up ranging between

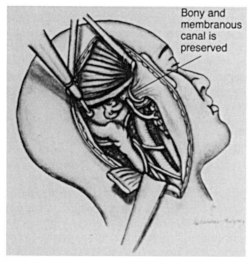

FIGURE 70-5 Surgical exposure with maintenance of the external auditory canal—the so-called canal wall-up approach. The facial nerve is only partially mobilized in its mastoid segment. (Copyright © Semmes-Murphey Clinic.)

Bony and membranous canal is preserved

6 and 42 months, with an average of 20.5 months. Of the 11 patients, 4 showed a decrease in tumor volume, but 7 patients showed no change. A decrease in symptoms was reported by 5 of the 11 patients. However, three patients had a further impairment in hearing, and two patients required a second radiosurgery treatment for infrabasal spread of tumor that was not delineated on the preoperative CT scan. Radiosurgery planning with MRI might eliminate this problem. The effectiveness of radiosurgery for the symptom of pulsatile tinnitus is not well known. In the series of Liscak and colleagues,[62] angiography was performed on follow-up in three patients. One patient showed no pathologic vascularity at 1 year after radiosurgery. The other two patients had either a partial decrease or no effect on pathologic tumor vascularity at 12 months and 22 months, respectively. Tumor embolization followed by radiosurgery may prove to be effective for controlling pulsatile tinnitus.

Histologic studies of previously irradiated glomus tumors have concluded that the tumor cells appear unaffected by the irradiation. The primary effect of radiation is thought to be vascular injury.[63,64] In addition, catecholamine secretion has not been shown to be affected by radiation therapy.[29] The primary argument against surgery is the risk of lower cranial nerve palsy with dysphagia and subsequent aspiration. In general, radiation therapy has not been shown to induce lower cranial nerve injury.

COMPLICATIONS OF SURGERY

Complications after surgery for glomus jugulare tumors are mainly a function of the tumor's size, vascularity, and anatomic location, combined with the patient's preoperative condition, the surgeon's skill, and the choice of surgical approach. Complications can be minimized by proper patient selection, excellent surgical technique, and knowledge of regional anatomy. Preoperative embolization can decrease intraoperative blood loss. This both aids in visualization of vital neurovascular structures and decreases the need for electrocautery around the lower cranial nerves as they pass through the jugular foramen. The major complications following surgery for glomus jugulare tumors are as follows:

Cranial nerve injury
Wound healing or CSF leak
Bleeding or vascular injury
Infection or meningitis

Other complications are catecholamine secretion, eustachian tube dysfunction, trismus, deep vein thrombosis with or without pulmonary embolism, and associated medical problems.

Cranial Nerve Injury

Cranial nerve preservation after surgery is directly related to surgical technique, unless the tumor has invaded a specific cranial nerve. One would expect that a benign tumor would merely compress cranial nerves, but in a retrospective review of 83 patients with glomus temporale tumors, Makek and colleagues[30] detected neural infiltration in 30 of the tumors reviewed. They concluded that as tumor size increased, cranial nerve invasion increased as well. In addition, normal nerve function before surgery did not rule out the possibility of finding neural invasion at surgery.

The cranial nerves most commonly affected by the growth of glomus jugulare tumors are the facial nerve and the lower cranial nerves (IX, X, XI, and XII). If the facial nerve is normal preoperatively, good function can be expected if tumor removal can be accomplished without transposition of the facial nerve. In moderate to large tumors, however, transposition of the facial nerve often results in a temporary paralysis, probably as a result of interruption of the nerve's blood supply in the tympanic and mastoid segments. In 1994, Green and associates reported good recovery of facial nerve function (House grades I or II out of VI) in 95% of patients in a series of 52 patients with previously untreated patients with glomus jugulare tumors.[65]

If neural invasion of the facial nerve is evident, resection of the involved segment is necessary, with reconstruction by end-to-end anastomosis of the remaining facial nerve or use of an interposition nerve graft. If the proximal stump of the facial nerve is lost at surgery, which might occur with a large intracranial extension, then an early hypoglossal to facial anastomosis should be considered if the hypoglossal nerve has functional integrity.

Postoperative facial nerve palsy should be managed aggressively with eye lubricants, an eye patch, and consideration of gold weight insertion in the upper lid or lateral canthoplasty. In most cases, satisfactory recovery of the facial nerve occurs if continuity of the facial nerve was maintained at surgery.

Lower cranial nerve palsies are potentially the most serious complication after surgery for glomus jugulare tumors. A complete injury to the vagus nerve near the skull base is probably the least well tolerated. In a review of the subject, Tucker[66] pointed out that an acute vagal palsy at the skull base results in dysfunction of the entire upper aerodigestive tract, including airway control, swallowing, and phonation. Paralysis of the palate combined with some loss of pharyngeal sensation causes incoordination of swallowing, because the pharyngeal muscles fail to contract properly in combination with relaxation of the cricopharyngeus muscles. This may result in repeated aspiration with subsequent pneumonia and can be fatal if not promptly recognized and treated effectively. The aggregate loss of function of several lower cranial nerves may compound the risk of aspiration and, even if incomplete, may result in considerable short-term morbidity.

Injury to the lower cranial nerves can be minimized by not using cautery around the nerves as they pass medial to the tumor in the jugular foramen. In addition, Surgicel packing of the orifices of the inferior petrosal sinus must be performed carefully to avoid injury to the underlying cranial nerves. We think that preoperative embolization decreases intraoperative blood loss, improves visualization, and minimizes the need for electrocautery around the lower cranial nerves.

A patient with an acute postoperative vagal palsy should be evaluated by swallowing studies. If aspiration is present, early placement of a percutaneous endoscopic gastrostomy (PEG) tube should be considered. The patient should have hand-held suctioning devices available to assist in the control of saliva. Swelling of the vocal cords in the immediate postoperative period due to the endotracheal tube may sometimes mask an underlying vocal cord paralysis. As the swelling of the vocal cord resolves, the patient develops problems with hoarse voice and aspiration. Tracheostomy may be required in some patients, but because it further impairs swallowing function by limiting the upward movement of the larynx, we often try to avoid it. If the vagus nerve was preserved at surgery and recovery is expected in time, Gelfoam can be injected into the vocal cord to temporarily improve the patient's voice and cough. If unilateral vagus nerve function is permanently lost, a more permanent medialization of the vocal cord can be accomplished by either injecting Teflon or performing a laryngoplasty.[67]

Most patients compensate for unilateral lower cranial nerve injury in 1 to 4 months. Persistent nasal regurgitation of food may be corrected with a palatoplasty, in which the paralyzed segment of the soft palate is unilaterally sutured to the posterior pharyngeal wall. Persistent dysphagia with recurrent aspiration despite vocal cord augmentation may on rare occasions require a cricopharyngeal myotomy.

Refinements in surgical technique and the successful management of lower cranial nerve palsies have decreased the morbidity associated with the surgical treatment of glomus jugulare tumors. In 1991, Jackson and colleagues[68] reported long-term follow-up on cranial nerve preservation in 100 patients with lesions of the jugular foramen, including 59 patients with glomus jugulare tumors. In their report, patients with small tumors had excellent cranial nerve preservation, and excellent long-term functional recovery was reported in cases in which cranial nerve sacrifice was needed for tumor removal. On the basis of these data, Jackson and colleagues[68] concluded that the morbidity of cranial nerve loss associated with lateral skull base surgery does not support the use of radiation therapy as the primary treatment of lesions of the jugular fossa, particularly small tumors.

In 1996, Jackson and colleagues reported on the success of attempts to preserve hearing during surgery for glomus jugulare tumors.[69] In a series of 122 patients with glomus jugulare tumors treated for 24 years, hearing conservation was attempted in 41 patients. Hearing preservation was successful in 38 patients (93%). In six cases (14.6%), hearing actually improved.

Wound Healing and Cerebrospinal Fluid Leakage

Impaired wound healing after surgery for a glomus jugulare tumor may occur as the result of poor surgical technique, malnutrition, multiple medical problems, prolonged use of steroids, or previous radiation therapy. If a patient is malnourished preoperatively, surgery should be delayed until the nutritional status is normal. In all patients, nutrition should be resumed within several days of surgery. Patients with lower cranial nerve dysfunction and dysphagia often require tube feedings to maintain their nutritional status.

The prevention of CSF leakage depends on closure and healing of the surgical wound together with maintenance of normal intracranial CSF pressure. Small glomus jugulare tumors can often be removed with the dura intact. Adequate removal of large tumors often results in a large dural defect, which at the level of the jugular foramen can be difficult to close. Obliteration of the mastoid cavity with

adipose tissue or by rotating the temporalis muscle downward is essential. In addition, careful closure of the external auditory ear canal along with sealing off of the eustachian tube is mandatory. CSF leakage may occur directly through the incision, through the external auditory canal, or down the eustachian tube into the oropharynx. A postoperative CSF leak may be detected by the Dandy maneuver, in which the patient is examined in the sitting position with the head held forward below the waistline for several minutes; CSF should drip out the nostril if a leak is present.

The intracranial CSF dynamics are often altered in the postoperative period by contamination with blood, bone dust, and the ensuing inflammatory reaction. This impairment in reabsorption of CSF in the early postoperative period may result in elevated CSF pressures and a secondary CSF leak. The use of continuous lumbar CSF drainage for several days after surgery allows for the CSF to clear and maintains a normal CSF pressure during the early stages of wound healing.

Bleeding and Vascular Injury

The excessive bleeding encountered by earlier surgeons in their attempts to remove glomus jugulare tumors was one of the major factors that led to either limited surgery combined with radiation therapy or radiation therapy alone as the primary treatment of these lesions. The major blood supply of small to medium-sized glomus jugulare tumors is the tympanic branch of the ascending pharyngeal artery. Large tumors, however, may receive a large blood supply from other branches of the external carotid artery, the vertebrobasilar system, or the vasa vasorum of the ICA. Embolization has decreased the blood loss associated with operative excision, shortened operating time, and (we believe) decreased the incidence of cranial nerve deficits. Small tumors whose blood supply is derived solely from the external carotid artery can be almost completely devascularized by embolization. Large tumors with blood supply from the vasa vasorum of the petrous segment of the ICA or from the vertebrobasilar system cannot be fully devascularized, because these vessels are often too small to catheterize and embolization carries an unacceptable risk of stroke.

Injury to the ICA can be life threatening if not managed appropriately. Proximal and distal control of the ICA must be secured before the tumor is dissected off this artery. Patients with large tumors that encase the ICA should be evaluated with a preoperative ICA balloon occlusion test and either single photon emission CT scanning or xenon cerebral blood flow testing. If an adequate collateral cerebral circulation is present, there is some assurance (though not definitive) that carotid sacrifice will be tolerated. If the balloon occlusion test is not tolerated; however, the surgeon must be prepared to perform interposition saphenous vein grafting or an extracranial-intracranial bypass to the middle cerebral artery.

Infection and Meningitis

Infections occurring with glomus jugulare tumor surgery are rare despite the extensive dissection, long duration of surgery, and potential for CSF leak. The presence of CSF leak, fever, elevated white blood cell count, changes in mentation, or signs of meningeal irritation should alert the surgeon to the possibility of meningitis. If meningitis is suspected, CSF should be obtained for the appropriate studies, and broad-spectrum CSF-penetrating antibiotics should be started.

Miscellaneous Complications

A few glomus jugulare tumors may produce and secrete catecholamines. Surgical manipulation of these tumors may produce surges in blood pressure as catecholamines are released. This may be prevented by preoperatively screening for excess catecholamine production and by treating patients found to have catecholamine secretion with alpha and beta blockers preoperatively, as stated earlier in this chapter.

A history of previous bleeding problems should be thoroughly investigated because of the highly vascular nature of this neoplasm. In addition, medications with antiplatelet activity (e.g., aspirin) should be avoided during the week before surgery. The risk of lower extremity deep venous thrombosis can be minimized by the use of venous compression devices and early postoperative mobilization. Subcutaneous heparin is initiated on the first postoperative day. Catheterization of the veins of the neck or the contralateral subclavian vein is avoided because of the risk of thrombosis together with the plan to ligate one jugular vein during surgery.

Eustachian tube dysfunction may occur in patients with small tumors in whom the middle ear is preserved. This may result in serous otitis media, which can be managed with decongestants and antibiotics if needed. On occasion, a ventilation tube is required for definitive treatment if there is no evidence of CSF behind the tympanic membrane.

In patients with large glomus jugulare tumors encasing the ICA or extending up to the foramen lacerum, exposure of the infratemporal fossa is necessary. This can be accomplished by anteriorly dislocating the mandible. Early assessment by an oral surgeon to determine proper dental occlusion and an aggressive exercise program to increase range of motion is mandatory.

UNIVERSITY OF TENNESSEE EXPERIENCE

Table 70-1 summarizes the cases of glomus tumors treated at University of Tennessee, Memphis, from 1970 to 1998.

CASE REPORT 1
TYPICAL GLOMUS JUGULARE TUMOR IN A YOUNG PATIENT

A 24-year-old man developed right-sided pulsatile tinnitus and hearing loss. Physical findings were normal other than a red mass visible behind the right tympanic membrane. An MRI scan of the head with contrast showed a 3-cm enhancing mass enlarging the right jugular foramen and extending into the middle ear, consistent with a glomus jugulare tumor (Fig. 70-7). A cerebral arteriogram confirmed the typical vascular pattern of a glomus jugulare tumor and was followed by embolization. Two days after the embolization, the patient was taken to surgery for a combined lateral skull base approach and excision of the tumor. The mastoid segment of the facial nerve was found to be infiltrated by tumor over a 1-cm length. This segment of the facial nerve was resected, and through mobilization of the facial nerve from the geniculate ganglion to the soft tissue beyond the stylomastoid foramen, a primary facial nerve end-to-end anastomosis was performed. The tumor was found adjacent to, but not encasing, the petrous ICA and was carefully removed. Nonadherent, intraluminal tumor extension was found in the right transverse sinus as well as in the superior and inferior petrosal sinus. Resection of tumor after ligation of the upper sigmoid sinus and rostral jugular vein was accomplished with preservation of all lower cranial nerves.

The patient was neurologically intact after surgery, except for an immediate complete right facial palsy. A gold weight was placed in the right eyelid to assist in eye closure. The patient was discharged home on postoperative day 10. During the year after surgery, he returned to active employment in a lumber mill. Right facial nerve function returned but he had facial asymmetry and synkinesis when he smiled.

CASE REPORT 2
GLOMUS JUGULARE TUMOR IN A 64-YEAR-OLD PATIENT

A 64-year-old woman presented with several months of left hearing loss, a hoarse voice, tinnitus, mild swallowing difficulty, and posterior occipital neck pain. On physical examination, she had left sensorineural hearing loss and a left vocal cord paralysis. An MRI scan showed

TABLE 70-1 ▪ Treatment of Glomus Jugulare Tumors at University of Tennessee, Memphis (1970–1998)				
Treatment	Glomus Jugulare	Glomus Tympanicum	Glomus Vagale	Total
Surgery alone	31	30	4	65
Surgery + preoperative radiation therapy	7	0	0	7
Surgery + postoperative radiation therapy	4	0	0	4
Radiation therapy only	15	1	0	16
No treatment	5	5	1	11
Total	62	36	5	103

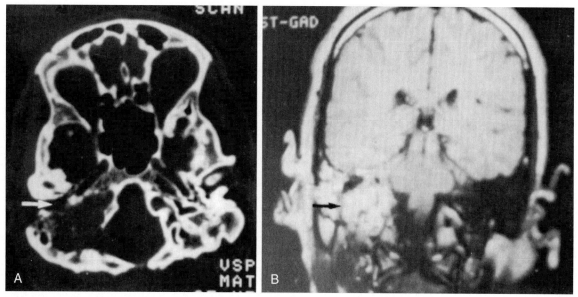

FIGURE 70-7 *A*, An axial CT scan showing extensive bone destruction in the bone surrounding the jugular foramen in Patient 1 (*arrow*). *B*, A coronal-enhanced T1-weighted MRI scan of the head in the same patient, demonstrating a glomus jugulare tumor extending out from the jugular foramen (*arrow*).

a 2.5- by 3-cm left jugular foramen mass (Fig. 70-8). An arteriogram showed a vascular tumor in the left jugular foramen with occlusion of the left jugular bulb consistent with a left glomus jugulare tumor. She was treated with gamma knife radiosurgery. A follow-up MRI scan 2 years after radiosurgery treatment showed that the tumor was stable in size. Her headache and neck pain resolved. She denied tinnitus, and her voice was slightly less hoarse.

CASE REPORT 3
PATIENT WITH A HORMONE-SECRETING GLOMUS JUGULARE TUMOR

A 35-year-old woman presented with a 3-month history of left-sided hearing loss and chronic hoarseness. She denied difficulty with swallowing. On physical examination, a red mass was visible behind the left tympanic membrane.

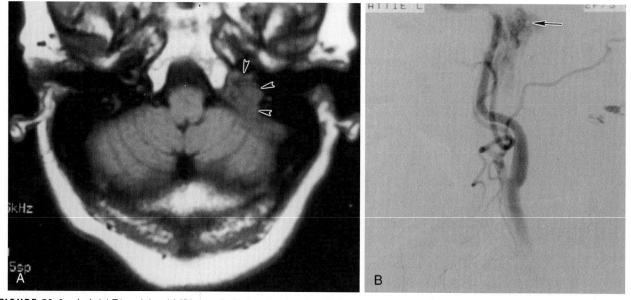

FIGURE 70-8 *A*, Axial T1-weighted MRI scan in Patient 2, showing a left glomus jugulare tumor (*arrowheads*). *B*, Lateral view of a left common carotid arteriogram showing the tumor blush in the jugular foramen (*arrow*).

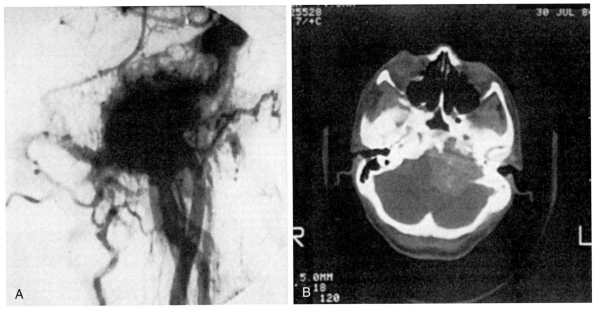

FIGURE 70-9 A carotid angiogram and an axial CT scan showing a large left glomus jugulare tumor with posterior fossa extension.

She had a complete left 10th, 11th, and 12th cranial nerve palsy. A CT scan of the head showed a large mass in the region of the left jugular foramen with extension into the posterior fossa (Fig. 70-9). A biopsy performed through the ear canal confirmed the diagnosis of a glomus jugulare tumor. Each manipulation of the tumor during the biopsy resulted in a brief but marked rise in the systolic blood pressure. Measurements of 24-hour urinary catecholamines were elevated both before and 1 week after the biopsy. The patient was treated with 4500 Gy of preoperative radiation therapy in an attempt to decrease the tumor's vascularity. (This patient was treated before the availability of embolization.)

Four months after the radiation treatment, the patient was admitted and received 3 days of phentolamine and a long-acting beta-blocker therapy. The large left glomus jugulare tumor was removed via the lateral skull base approach combined with a tracheostomy and a tarsorrhaphy. Tumor manipulation did not produce significant changes in blood pressure. Although surgery was well tolerated, a CSF leak developed 3 weeks postoperatively through an area of necrosis along the postauricular portion of the incision. This was treated successfully with débridement and primary closure.

Teflon was injected into the left vocal cord 1 month after tumor resection to help prevent aspiration and improve voice quality. The tracheostomy was removed. The patient returned to normal physical activities and has done well over the past 10 years, with mild facial asymmetry, left-sided hearing loss, and compensated left lower cranial nerve loss. Because of the complication associated with radiation therapy and the development of embolization techniques, preoperative radiation therapy was abandoned after this case.

CASE REPORT 4
PATIENT WITH SEVERAL GLOMUS TUMORS

A 26-year-old woman presented with complaints of left-sided hearing loss, tinnitus, headache, intermittent dizziness, and an enlarging left anterior cervical mass. Three of her six siblings have had glomus tumors. An MRI scan and cerebral angiography showed bilateral carotid body, glomus vagale, and glomus jugulare tumors (Fig. 70-10). The tumors involving the left neck and jugular fossa were larger than those on the right. General physical examination showed a mobile, nontender mass of 3 to 4 cm in the left midcervical region anterior to the sternocleidomastoid muscle. Neurologic examination was remarkable for mild left facial weakness and left-sided hearing loss. Embolization of the tumors on the left side was performed, followed by operative excision of all three of the left-sided glomus tumors. The mastoid segment of the facial nerve was encased by tumor, requiring excision of a 3-cm segment of the nerve; this was repaired by an interposition nerve graft using the greater occipital nerve. The lower cranial nerves were all anatomically preserved. Postoperatively, the patient had a complete left facial palsy and a partial left vagal palsy. A gold weight was implanted in the left eyelid to augment closure. The patient was able to tolerate oral feedings by postoperative day 7 without aspiration and was discharged home on postoperative day 10.

Ten months later, the patient had partial return of facial nerve function, but an incomplete left vagus nerve palsy and left hearing loss remained. Surgical excision of the remaining three glomus tumors was considered, and cerebral arteriography with embolization was performed.

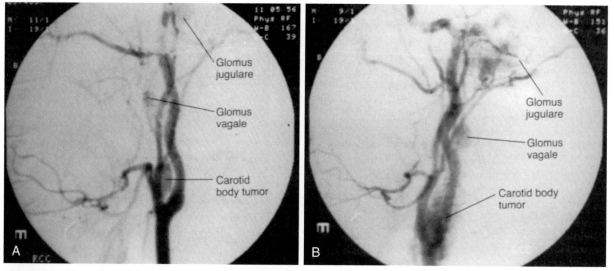

FIGURE 70-10 Right (*A*) and left (*B*) common carotid arteriograms in Patient 4 demonstrating bilateral carotid body tumors, glomus vagale tumors, and glomus jugulare tumors.

Arteriography showed patency of the right sigmoid–jugular vein system, which was providing the major venous outflow of the brain. Because of the risk of bilateral vagal nerve dysfunction and the fear of complications related to taking the dominant right sigmoid–jugular venous drainage, it was elected to resect only the right carotid body tumor and to treat the smaller right glomus vagale and right glomus jugulare tumors with radiation therapy. Two years after initiating treatment, the patient remains independent in all activities and is employed. Clinically, she has mild facial asymmetry, left hearing loss, and compensated vagal nerve function.

This patient may have benefited from a sigmoid sinus–jugular vein bypass on the left at the time of her first surgery. This technique has been reported by Sekhar.[70]

SUMMARY

Glomus jugulare tumors are uncommon, slow growing, and locally invasive. The tumor is thought to arise from glomus tissue in the region of the jugular bulb. The most common presenting symptom is hearing loss with pulsatile tinnitus. In a few patients, the disease may be familial or multiple. In rare cases, the tumor can metastasize. The relevant surgical anatomy is compact and complex. Preoperative embolization decreases the difficulty of surgical excision. In healthy patients, the primary treatment should be surgical excision, although patients who are elderly or have major medical problems may benefit from radiation therapy or a "wait and see" policy.

REFERENCES

1. Bickerstaff ER, Howell JS: The neurological importance of tumors of the glomus jugulare. Brain 76:576–592, 1953.
2. Krause W: Die Glandula tympanica des Menschen. Zentralbl Med Wiss 16:737–739, 1878.
3. Guild SR: A hitherto unrecognized structure: The glomus jugularis in man. Anat Rec 79(Suppl 2):28–107, 1941.
4. Rosenwasser H: Carotid body tumor of the middle ear and mastoid. Arch Otolaryngol 41:64–67, 1945.
5. Guild SR: Glomus jugulare in man. Ann Otol Rhinol Laryngol 62:1045–1071, 1953.
6. Rockley TJ, Hawke M: Glomus bodies in the temporal bone. J Otolaryngol 19:51–56, 1990.
7. Brown JS: Glomus jugulare tumors revisited: A ten year statistical follow-up of 231 cases. Laryngoscope 95:284–288, 1985.
8. Larner JM, Hahn SS, Spaulding CA, Constable WC: Glomus jugulare tumors: Long-term control by radiation therapy. Cancer 69:1813–1817, 1992.
9. Wang ML, Hussey DH, Doornbos JF, et al: A comparison of surgical and radiotherapeutic results. Int J Radiat Oncol Biol Phys 14:643–648, 1988.
10. McCabe BF, Fletcher M: Selection of therapy of glomus jugulare tumors. Arch Otolaryngol 89:182–185, 1969.
11. van der Mey AGL, Fruns JHM, Cornelisse CJ, et al: Does intervention improve the natural course of glomus tumors? A series of 108 patients seen in a 32-year period. Ann Otol Rhinol Laryngol 101:635–642, 1992.
12. Bhansali SA, Bojrab DI, Zarbo RJ: Malignant paragangliomas of the head and neck: Clinical and immunohistochemical characterization. Otolaryngol Head Neck Surg 104:132, 1991.
13. Bojrab DI, Bhansali SA, Glasscock ME: Metastatic glomus jugulare: Long-term followup. Otolaryngol Head Neck Surg 104:261–264, 1991.
14. Davis JM, Davis KR, Hesselink JR, et al: Malignant glomus jugulare tumor: A case with two unusual radiographic features. J Comput Assist Tomogr 4:415–417, 1980.
15. Dinges S, Budach V, Stuschke M, et al: Malignant paragangliomas: The results of radiotherapy in 6 patients. Strahlenther Onkol 169:114–120, 1993.
16. El Finky FM, Paparella MM: A metastatic glomus jugulare tumor: A temporal bone report. Am J Otol 5:197–200, 1984.
17. Johnston F, Symon L: Malignant paraganglioma of the glomus jugulare: A case report. Br J Neurosurg 6:255–259, 1992.
18. Taylor DM, Alford BR, Greenberg SD: Metastases of glomus jugulare tumors. Arch Otolaryngol 82:5–13, 1965.
19. Zak FG, Lawson W: Glomus jugulare tumors. The Paraganglionic Chemoreceptor System. New York: Springer-Verlag, 1982, pp 339–391.
20. Balatsouras DG, Eliopoulos PN, Economou CN: Multiple glomus tumors. J Laryngol Otol 106:538–543, 1992.
21. Tali ET, Sener RN, Ibis E, et al: Familial bilateral glomus jugulare tumors. Neuroradiology 33:171–172, 1991.
22. Thompson JW, Cohen SR: Management of bilateral carotid body tumors and a glomus jugulare tumor in a child. Int J Pediatr Otorhinolaryngol 17:75–87, 1989.
23. Azzarelli B, Felten S, Muller J, et al: Dopamine in paragangliomas of the glomus jugulare. Laryngoscope 98:573–578, 1988.
24. Blumenfeld JD, Cohen N, Laragh JH, Ruggiero DA: Hypertension and catecholamine biosynthesis associated with a glomus jugulare tumor [Letter]. N Engl J Med 327:894, 1992.

25. Farrior J: Surgical management of glomus tumors: Endocrine-active tumors of the skull base. South Med J 81:1121–1126, 1988.
26. Kremer R, Michel RP, Posner B, et al: Case report: Catecholamine-secreting paraganglioma of glomus jugulare region. Am J Med Sci 297:46–48, 1989.
27. Matishak MZ, Symon L, Cheeseman A, Pamphlett R: Catecholamine-secreting paragangliomas of the base of the skull. J Neurosurg 66:604–608, 1987.
28. Nelson MD, Kendall BE: Intracranial catecholamine-secreting paragangliomas. Neuroradiology 29:277–282, 1987.
29. Schwaber MK, Glasscock ME, Nissen AJ, et al: Diagnosis and management of catecholamine-secreting glomus tumors. Laryngoscope 94:1008–1015, 1984.
30. Makek M, Franklin DJ, Zhao JC, Fisch U: Neural infiltration of glomus temporale tumors. Am J Otol 11:1–5, 1990.
31. Jackson CG, Cueva RA, Thedinger BA, Glasscock ME: Conservation surgery for glomus jugulare tumors: The value of early diagnosis. Laryngoscope 100:1031–1036, 1990.
32. Troughton RW, Fry D, Allison RS, Nicholls MG: Depression, palpitations and unilateral pulsatile tinnitus due to a dopamine-secreting glomus jugulare tumor. Am J Med 104:310–311, 1998.
33. Di Chiro G, Fisher RL, Nelson KB: The jugular foramen. J Neurosurg 21:447–460, 1964.
34. Rhoton AL, Buza R: Microsurgical anatomy of the jugular foramen. J Neurosurg 42:541–550, 1975.
35. Hovelaque A: Osteologie, vol 2. Paris: G Doin, 1934, pp 155–156.
36. Graham MD: The jugular bulb: Its anatomic and clinical considerations in contemporary otology. Arch Otolaryngol 101:560–564, 1975.
37. Widick MH, Haynes DS, Jackson CG, et al: Slow-flow phenomena in magnetic resonance imaging of the jugular bulb masquerading as skull base neoplasms. Am J Otol 17:648–652, 1996.
38. Fisch U, Mattox D (eds): Microsurgery of the Skull Base. Stuttgart: Thieme, 1988.
39. Valavanis A: Preoperative embolization of the head and neck: Indications, patient selection, goals, and precautions. AJNR Am J Neuroradiol 7:943–952, 1986.
40. Wiet RJ, Harvey SA, O'Connor CA: Recent advances in surgery of the temporal bone and skull base. South Med J 86:5–12, 1993.
41. Hilal SK, Michelsen JW: Therapeutic percutaneous embolization for extra-axial vascular lesions of the head, neck, and spine. J Neurosurg 43:275–287, 1975.
42. Murphy TP, Brackmann DE: Effects of preoperative embolization on glomus jugulare tumors. Laryngoscope 99:1244–1247, 1989.
43. Simpson GT, Konrad HR, Takahashi M, et al: Immediate postembolization excision of glomus jugulare tumors. Arch Otolaryngol 105:639–643, 1979.
44. Young NM, Wiet RJ, Russell EJ, Monsell EM: Superselective embolization of glomus jugulare tumors. Ann Otol Rhinol Laryngol 97:613–620, 1988.
45. Hekster REM, Luyendijk W, Matricali B: Transfemoral catheter embolization: A method of treatment of glomus jugulare tumors. Neuroradiology 5:208–214, 1973.
46. Shapiro MJ, Neues DK: Technique for removal of glomus jugulare tumors. Arch Otolaryngol 79:219–224, 1964.
47. Gardner G, Cocke EW, Robertson JT, et al: Combined approach to surgery for removal of glomus jugulare tumors. Laryngoscope 87:665–688, 1977.
48. Glasscock ME, Harris PF: Glomus tumors: Diagnosis, classification, and management of large lesions. Arch Otolaryngol 108:401–410, 1982.
49. Fisch U: Infratemporal fossa approach for extensive tumors of the temporal bone and base of the skull. In Silverstein H, Norrell H (eds): Neurological Surgery of the Ear. Birmingham, AL: Aesculapius, 1977, pp 34–53.
50. Pensak ML, Jackler RK: Removal of jugular foramen tumors: The fallopian bridge technique. Otolaryngol Head Neck Surg 117:586–591, 1997.
51. Glasscock ME, Harris PF, Newsome G: Glomus tumors: Diagnosis and treatment. Laryngoscope 84:2006–2032, 1974.
52. Boyle JO, Shimm DS, Coulthard SW: Radiation therapy for paragangliomas of the temporal bone. Laryngoscope 100:896–901, 1990.
53. Cole JM, Beiler D: Long-term results of treatment of glomus jugulare and glomus vagale tumors with radiotherapy. Laryngoscope 104:1461–1465, 1994.
54. Ferrara P, Cimino A, Tortorici M: Role of radiation therapy in glomus tumor. Am J Otol 8:390–395, 1987.
55. Springate SC, Weichselbaum RR: Radiation or surgery for chemodectoma of the temporal bone: A review of local control and complications. Head Neck 12:303–307, 1990.
56. Gibbins KP, Henk JM: Glomus jugulare tumors in South Wales: A twenty year review. Clin Radiol 29:607–609, 1978.
57. Sharma PD, Johnson AP, Whitton AC: Radiotherapy of jugulotympanic paragangliomas. J Laryngol Otol 98:621–629, 1984.
58. Simko TG, Griffen TW, Gerdes AJ, et al: The role of radiation therapy in the treatment of glomus jugulare tumors. Cancer 42:104–106, 1978.
59. Spector GJ, Fierstein J, Ogura JH: A comparison of therapeutic modalities of glomus tumors in the temporal bone. Laryngoscope 86:690–696, 1976.
60. Pluta RM, Ram Z, Patronas NJ, Keiser H: Long-term effects of radiation therapy for a catecholamine-producing glomus jugulare tumor: Case report. J Neurosurg 80:1091–1094, 1994.
61. Foote RL, Coffey RJ, Gorman DA, et al: Stereotactic radiosurgery for glomus jugulare tumors: A preliminary report. Int J Radiat Oncol Biol Phys 38:491–495, 1997.
62. Liscak R, Vladyka V, Simonova G, et al: Leksell gamma knife radiosurgery of the tumor glomus jugulare and tympanicum. Stereotact Funct Neurosurg 70(Suppl 1):152–160, 1998.
63. Brackmann DE, House WF, Terry R, et al: Glomus jugulare tumors: Effect of radiation. Trans Am Acad Ophthalmol Otolaryngol 76:1423–1431, 1972.
64. Hawthorne MR, Makek MS, Harris JP, Fisch U: The histopathological and clinical features of irradiated and nonirradiated temporal paragangliomas. Laryngoscope 98:325–331, 1988.
65. Green JD, Brackman DE, Nguyen CD, et al: Surgical management of previously untreated glomus jugulare tumors. Laryngoscope 104:917–921, 1994.
66. Tucker HM: Rehabilitation of patients with postoperative deficits cranial nerves VIII through XII. Otolaryngol Head Neck Surg 88:576–580, 1980.
67. Netterville JL, Aly A, Ossoff RH: Evaluation and treatment of complications of thyroid and parathyroid surgery. Otolaryngol Clin North Am 23:529–552, 1990.
68. Jackson CG, Cueva RA, Thedinger BA, Glasscock ME: Cranial nerve preservation in lesions of the jugular fossa. Otolaryngol Head Neck Surg 105:687–693, 1991.
69. Jackson CG, Haynes DS, Walker PA, et al: Hearing conservation in surgery for glomus jugulare tumors. Am J Otol 17:425–437, 1996.
70. Sekhar LN, Tzortzidis FN, Bejjani GK, Schessel DA: Saphenous vein graft bypass of the sigmoid sinus and jugular bulb during the removal of glomus jugulare tumors: Report of two cases. J Neurosurg 86:1036–1041, 1997.

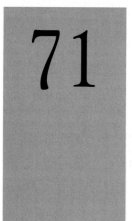

71 Surgical Management of Nonglomus Tumors of the Jugular Foramen

CHUNG-CHENG WANG, ALI LIU, and CHUN-JIANG YU

The occurrence of the nonglomus tumors within the jugular foramen is very rare; they account for only 0.3% of intracranial tumors. In the literature, chemodectoma is the most common tumor and schwannoma the second most common. Nonglomus tumors of the jugular foramen include schwannomas, meningiomas, chemodectomas, chordomas, myxomas, chondrosarcomas, and epidermoid cyst. Depending on the site and extent of the tumor, the jugular foramen tumor is classified into four groups: class A, tumor confined to the soft tissues of the neck; class B, tumor primary involvement of the neck with extension up to the jugular foramen; class C, tumor fills the jugular foramen with resultant bone expansion; and class D, comprising dumbbell-shaped tumors with both intracranial and extracranial extension. Because of their deep position and the complex surrounding neurovascular structures, surgical removal of jugular foramen tumors remains a difficult process. Over the past decade, a number of surgical procedures have been advocated for the removal of jugular foramen tumors. With advances in diagnostic methods, surgical approach, and microsurgical techniques, the prevailing goal for the management of extensive type C or D jugular foramen tumors is complete surgical excision with the preservation of cranial nerves. This chapter introduces some essential operative techniques.

Nonglomus tumors of the jugular foramen are rarely encountered and account for only 0.3% of intracranial tumors (84 of 28,462) operated on at the Beijing Neurosurgical Institute between 1975 and 2003. Our series included 60 schwannomas, 10 meningiomas, 9 chemodectomas, 4 chordomas, 3 myxomas, 3 chondrosarcomas, 2 epidermoid cysts, 1 choroid plexus papilloma, and 1 hemangiopericytoma. Other kinds of neoplasms, such as neurenteric cysts,[1] petrous bone carcinomas,[2,3] chondromyxoid fibromas,[4] plasmacytomas,[5] metastatic carcinomas,[6,7] peripheral primitive neuroectodermal tumors,[8] giant cell tumors,[9] lipomas,[10] myxoid chondrosarcomas,[11] and amyloidomas[12] have been reported in the literature. According to the literature, chemodectoma is the most common tumor, comprising 25% to 77% of jugular foramen tumors,[3,13-15] with schwannoma the second most common.

SCHWANNOMAS

The term *schwannoma* denotes a solitary nerve sheath tumor arising from perineural Schwann cells of the involved nerve.

It is also called neurinoma, neurilemmoma, and neurolemma. It is different from neurofibroma, which originates from the axon-encasing Schwann cell and therefore contains trapped axons. The neurofibroma usually surrounds nerve fibers, making resection of tumor without nerve sacrifice impossible, whereas most schwannomas can be resected without nerve injury.[16-18]

Incidence

Intracranial schwannomas constitute approximately 8% of all primary brain tumors.[19] Schwannomas arising from cranial nerves IX, X, and XI comprise 2.9% of all intracranial schwannomas.[20] Schwannomas involving the jugular foramen are rare, with approximately 169 cases reported in the world literature. The jugular foramen neurilemmoma is an unusual tumor,[2,20-27] and only a few centers have relatively large series. In 1984, Kaye and colleagues[28] reported 13 cases, Tan and colleagues[29] reported 14 cases, Sasaki and Takakara[30] reported 12 cases, Samii and colleagues[31] reported 16 cases, Mazzoni and colleagues[32] reported 19 cases, and Cokkeser and colleagues[33] reported 16 cases.

From 1975 to 2003, the Beijing Neurosurgical Institute accumulated 2797 operated cases of intracranial schwannomas. Of these cases, only 60 (2%) arose in the region of the jugular foramen. The group consists of 27 men and 33 women, ranging in age from 16 to 70 years, with a mean age of 43 years. The preadmission duration of disease ranges from 1 month to 16 years.

Anatomy

Cranial nerves IX, X, and XI emerge in a line from the medulla oblongata and then run laterally to the jugular foramen, leaving the posterior fossa. The jugular foramen is actually a canal. Tumors arising in the middle region tend to expand primarily into bone. The jugular foramen is bounded by the occipital bone medially and the temporal bone laterally and is divided by a fibrous or bony septum into an anteromedial (pars nervosa) compartment, containing the petrosal sinus and glossopharyngeal nerve, and a posterolateral (pars vasculara) compartment, containing the vagus and accessory nerves with the jugular vein.

Cranial nerves IX, X, and XI emerge from the anterior portion of the jugular foramen. Cranial nerve IX emerges between the internal carotid artery and the internal jugular vein, courses laterally to the internal jugular vein, and enters the sternocleidomastoid 1.5 to 2 inches (3.5 to 5 cm) below the mastoid tip. At the angle of the mandible, the cranial nerve XII parallels nerve X and is lateral to it. Nerves IX, X, and XI are anteroposterior, lateral to the internal carotid artery, and pass medially and then anterolaterally to the internal jugular vein, respectively. As the internal jugular vein comes to lie lateral to the internal carotid artery, the cranial nerve X lies behind and between the two vessels.

The parapharyngeal space is bounded medially by the vertebral column and the superior constrictor muscle and superiorly by the ramus of the mandible and the internal pterygoid muscle. It is a potential anatomic space and consists of the regions including the internal jugular vein, the carotid artery, four cranial nerves (IX, X, XI, and XII), and the cervical sympathetic chain. All the nerves are encased by Schwann cells, which may give rise to a schwannoma.

Disturbance of Cranial Nerves at Admission

The patient usually presents with a unilateral lesion of cranial nerves IX, X, or XI, or some combination of the three nerves. Occasionally, the patient presents with a retrocochlear lesion similar to a cerebellopontine angle tumor, such as an acoustic neuroma. In our series, 43 patients had initial symptoms involving cranial nerves IX to XI, and 17 had symptoms involving cranial nerves V to VIII (Table 71-1). All the initially involved nerves are summarized in Table 71-2. In addition, 30 (50%) patients had cerebellar signs: 6 contralateral hemiparalysis, 19 papilledema, 13 suboccipital pain without intracranial hypertension, and 1 pharyngeal mass.

Growth Patterns and Associated Symptomatology

The growth characteristics and associated symptomatology of these tumors are variable and can be grouped into three main categories. The first group is a jugular foramen syndrome with paralysis of the lower cranial nerves. The second common clinical picture is a cerebellopontine angle lesion with ipsilateral hearing loss, tinnitus, and vertigo, thus simulating acoustic neurinoma. Less frequently, patients present with pulsatile tinnitus and a hypotympanic mass.

At least two classification systems have been developed for jugular foramen schwannomas, depending on the site and extent of the tumor. Franklin and colleagues[34] classified the tumor into three groups: class A, tumor confined to the soft tissues of the neck; class B, tumor primary involvement of the neck with extension up to the jugular foramen; class C, tumor fills the jugular foramen with resultant bone expansion. Kaye and colleagues[28] classified the tumor as follows: type A tumors are primarily intracranial, with minimal extension into the bone foramen; type B tumors are primarily within the bone foramen, with or without an intracranial extension; and type C tumors are primarily extracranial, with only minor extension into the bone foramen or the posterior fossa. Samii and colleagues[31] and Pellet and colleagues[35] added another type, type D, comprising dumbbell-shaped tumors with both intracranial and extracranial extension.

Type A: Primarily Intracranial Tumors

Forty (66.7%) of the cases in our series are type A tumors. The tumors arise from the proximal nerve complex of cranial nerves IX, X, and XI, of which XI was the least involved. Patients had two types of symptoms: approximately half presented with a history of vertigo, tinnitus, or sensorineural hearing loss mimicking that of acoustic neuroma and half had disturbances of cranial nerves IX to XI, such as hoarseness, weakness, or atrophy of the trapezius and sternocleidomastoid muscles.

Twenty-six patients had jugular foramen enlargement, but none had an enlarged internal auditory meatus. All the tumors were confirmed by surgery. Seven patients had huge tumors, accompanied by hypoesthesia in the trigeminal distribution and hypodynamia of the facial nerve.

Type B: Intraosseous Tumors

There are eight (13.3%) cases of type B tumors in our series. Because the tumors grow in the jugular foramen, Vernet's syndrome provides the classic clinical signs. Motor and

TABLE 71-1 ▪ **Initial Symptoms of Jugular Foramen Schwannoma**

Initial Symptoms	No.	Percent
Swallowing difficulty	21	35
Glossal atrophy	11	18
Tinnitus	13	22
Hearing loss	20	33
Facial weakness	3	5
Headache	21	35
Vertigo	8	13
Cerebellar dysfunction	30	50
Facial paresthesias	1	2
Shoulder weakness	3	5

TABLE 71-2 ▪ **Cranial Nerve Disturbance at Admission**

Cranial Nerve Involved	No. of Cases
V	1
V, VII	1
XI, XII	2
IX–XI	2
VIII–X, XII	7
VIII–XII	3
V, VII–XII	3
VIII	11
IX–X	4
VIII–X	7
IX–XII	7
V, VII–X	6
VII–XII	2
V–XI	2
V, VIII–XII	1
V–X	1
Total	60

sensory disturbance of the soft palate, itching in the external auditory meatus, and tingling in the throat indicate a lesion of cranial nerve IX. Hoarseness results from vocal cord dysfunction due to a palsy of cranial nerve X, whereas weakness and atrophy of the sternocleidomastoid and trapezius indicate an accessory nerve lesion. The tumor tends to expand primarily into bone, with patients often exhibiting tinnitus, deafness, a middle ear mass, or involvement of the hypoglossal nerve.[28,34,36] The tumor in one case extended to the external auditory canal.

Type C: Primarily Extracranial Tumors

These tumors grow in the segments of cranial nerves IX to XI that lie in the lateral pharyngeal wall and can even reach the bifurcation of the carotid artery. They are primarily extracranial or have only a minor extension into the bone and usually manifest with single nerve palsy and a mass in the neck or lateral pharyngeal wall.[34] There are no cases of such tumors in our series.

Type D: Dumbbell-Shaped Tumors with Intracranial and Extracranial Extension

There are 12 cases (20%) of type D tumor in our series. This type includes two or three types mentioned earlier (Fig. 71-1). Clinically speaking, the three other types cannot be distinctly divided and are classified artificially according to their different growing periods and the main location of the tumor. If treatment is not administered in a timely fashion, the tumor grows into a dumbbell-like shape and extends upward and downward from the jugular foramen. In one case, a mass

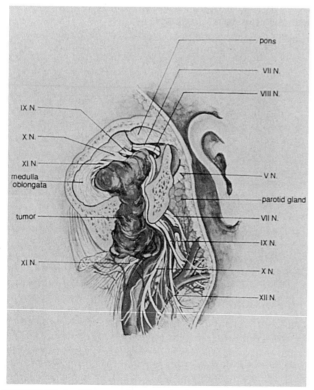

FIGURE 71-1   Diagram of a tumor in the jugular foramen (type D, dumbbell-shaped tumor).

was seen in the lateral pharyngeal wall. All the previously mentioned symptoms and signs can be noted on clinical examination.

Diagnosis

A jugular foramen tumor is highly likely to present in any adult who has initial symptoms of long duration originating from cranial nerves IX to XI and an enlarged jugular foramen. Most of them are glomus tumors, followed by schwannomas. The differential diagnosis of these tumors includes chemodectoma, acoustic neurinoma, and meningioma of the jugular fossa. Other tumors that involve the cerebellopontine angle, such as choroid plexus papillomas and exophytic pontine gliomas, should be considered.[5] The preoperative diagnosis of jugular foramen schwannoma, based only on neurologic signs, is difficult because the initial symptoms sometimes are hearing disturbances, indicating involvement of the acoustic nerve. Awareness of a mass in the throat or neck is the most common complaint for parapharyngeal neurinomas. Complete neurologic evaluation is imperative for a correct diagnosis. Patients with lesions involving the jugular foramen may present clinically with pain or lower cranial nerve palsies. This region is inaccessible to direct clinical examination and imaging studies are essential for evaluation. Both intracranial and extracranial lesions may affect the jugular foramen in addition to intrinsic abnormalities. As the anatomy of this region is complex, computed tomography (CT) and magnetic resonance imaging (MRI) in both the axial and coronal planes are desirable. MRI is the modality of choice for soft-tissue assessment, but lesions affecting small cortical bony structures may require CT for further evaluation.[37] CT and MRI outline the complete extent of these lesions. Angiography is helpful in determining the vascularity of the lesion and displacement of adjacent blood vessels as well as the status of blood flow in the jugular bulb and the internal carotid artery. Angiography shows characteristic rapid filling and intense tumor blush in glomus tumors, but such a finding usually is absent in schwannomas.

Computed Tomography

High-resolution CT has a decisive diagnostic value. CT was available for use with 53 of the patients in our series. It was of considerable help in showing the extent of the tumors, not only intracranially but throughout the bone and extracranially. Smooth widening of the jugular foramen with discrete margins and no signs of bone infiltration was the most characteristic manifestation of jugular foramen schwannoma, which differentiated it from an acoustic neuroma (Fig. 71-2). CT of the osseous skull base is extremely important. The simple enlargement or destruction of the foramen and adjoining area have a decisive differential diagnostic value. Contrast-enhanced CT scanning shows involvement of the base of the skull as well as extension into the posterior fossa. However, using only conventional CT, differentiation of an extra-axial tumor from an intra-axial one is difficult. CT cisternography is required for demonstrating small intracranial extra-axial masses and for differentiating an extra-axial mass from an intra-axial one.[38,39] The intracranial components of jugular foramen schwannomas showed as mixed low-density and isodense extra-axial masses, with ringlike enhancement in the cerebellopontine

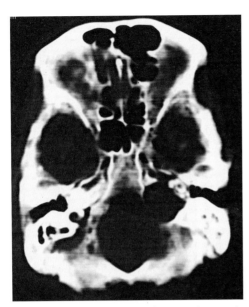

FIGURE 71-2   A computed tomography scan shows enlargement of the left jugular foramen.

angle; such lesions were easily misdiagnosed as acoustic neurinomas (Fig. 71-3).

Magnetic Resonance Imaging

MRI was performed in 54 patients, and all were correctly diagnosed. MRI gives better information than CT. On MRI, the T1 signal from tumor was low and T2 signal was high relative to white matter. Schwannoma of the jugular foramen is characteristically a sharply demarcated, contrast-enhancing tumor, typically centered on or based in an enlarged jugular foramen with sharply rounded bone borders and a sclerotic rim; intraosseous extension may be marked.[40] With the availability of different sequences, the absence of bone artifacts, and the ease of imaging in multiple planes, MRI showed jugular foramen schwannomas clearly as extra-axial posterior

fossa masses with or without extracranial extension and demonstrated the relationship of the tumor with the internal carotid artery. The coronal view clearly demonstrated the superior and inferior margins of the tumor, and the shape and nature of the tumor could be easily recognized (Fig. 71-4).

The intensities of jugular foramen schwannomas on T1- and T2-weighted images are similar to those of acoustic schwannomas, namely, long or isodense T1 and long T2 signals with or without cystic change, tumors are usually moderately enhanced after contrast enhancement. Because MRI can reveal the facial and acoustic nerves, it is helpful in differentiating jugular foramen schwannomas from acoustic schwannomas. In addition, jugular foramen schwannomas mainly press on the medulla oblongata, whereas acoustic schwannomas tend to press on the pons. MRI is useful not only for preoperative diagnosis but for planning the surgical approaches and postoperative follow-up.

Angiography

Carotid and vertebral angiography is helpful in determining the vascularity of the lesion and displacement of adjacent blood vessels, as well as the status of blood flow in the jugular bulb and the internal carotid artery. During the later phase of the angiography, when the dural sinuses are opacified, obstruction of the jugular bulb or sigmoid sinus by a tumor mass projecting into the vein may be seen. Retrograde jugular venography is valuable in determining the extent of obstruction of the internal jugular vein and the presence or absence of tumor in the lumen of the jugular vein. Schwannomas tend to occlude the vein by external compression, whereas glomus tumors often grow intraluminally.[20]

Angiographic studies were done in 19 patients in our series; 5 were normal, 6 had tumor blush (Fig. 71-5), and most had tumors noted only as displacements of adjacent blood vessels. Jugular foramen tumors are supplied by the ascending pharyngeal artery originating from the external carotid artery. In the patients with tumor blush, the diameter of the artery increased greatly. The tumor can also be supplied by the occipital artery.[21] Angiography may help

FIGURE 71-3   *A,* Unenhanced computed tomography (CT) scan shows a mixed low-density mass in the left cerebellopontine angle. *B,* An enhanced CT scan shows a ringlike enhancement.

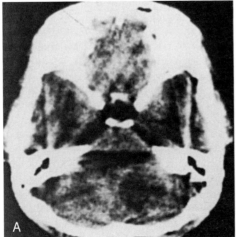
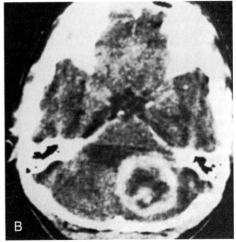

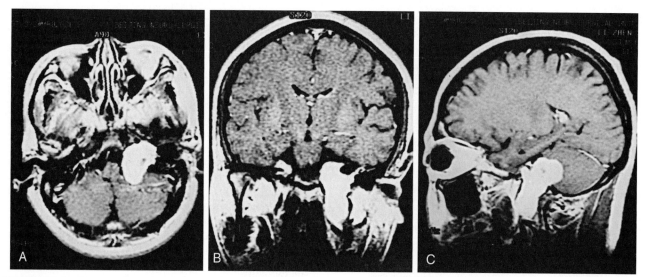

FIGURE 71-4   Preoperative enhanced magnetic resonance imaging shows a type D schwannoma at the left jugular foramen. *A,* Axial view; *B,* coronal view; *C,* sagittal view.

to differentiate a schwannoma from a glomus tumor because the glomus tumor is highly vascular, whereas the schwannoma has variable, often slight, vascularity. Preoperative arterial embolization during angiography may decrease operative blood loss and cause less injury to the four lower cranial nerves and other vital tissues during surgical manipulations.

Vessel displacements consist mainly of the anterior interior cerebellar artery being pushed upward and backward, and the posterior inferior cerebellar artery being pushed downward and backward. Large intracranial tumors can displace the proximal superior cerebellar artery superiorly and medially and can even affect the proximal end of the posterior cerebral artery. However, the latter effect is less significant than with proximal superior cerebellopontine angle tumors. Slight displacement of the basilar artery and vertebral artery

can be recorded. Large tumors in the jugular foramen can compress the internal carotid artery, leading to its stenosis or even complete occlusion.

Surgery

The jugular foramen, based on the studies of microsurgical anatomy, is divided into three compartments: two venous and one neural or intrajugular. The venous compartments consist of a larger posterolateral venous channel, the sigmoid part, which receives the flow of the sigmoid sinus, and a smaller anteromedial venous channel, the petrosal part, which receives the drainage of the inferior petrosal sinus. The petrosal part forms a characteristic venous confluens by also receiving tributaries from the hypoglossal canal, petroclival fissure, and vertebral venous plexus. The petrosal part empties into the sigmoid part through an opening in the medial wall of the jugular bulb between the glossopharyngeal nerve anteriorly and the vagus and accessory nerves posteriorly. The intrajugular or neural part, through which the glossopharyngeal, vagus, and accessory nerves course, is located between the sigmoid and petrosal parts at the site of the intrajugular processes of the temporal and occipital bones, which are joined by a fibrous or osseous bridge. The glossopharyngeal, vagus, and accessory nerves penetrate the dura on the medial margin of the intrajugular process of the temporal bone to reach the medial wall of the internal jugular vein. The operative approaches, which access the foramen and adjacent areas and are demonstrated in a stepwise manner, are the postauricular transtemporal, retrosigmoid, extreme lateral transcondylar, and preauricular subtemporal-infratemporal approaches.[41]

Because jugular foramen schwannomas are benign, the purpose of surgical treatment is to achieve complete resection in one procedure. Incomplete removal involves inevitable recurrence, and scarring from previous surgery adds greatly to the difficulties in preserving functional cranial nerves during a second procedure. Constantly evolving surgical approaches

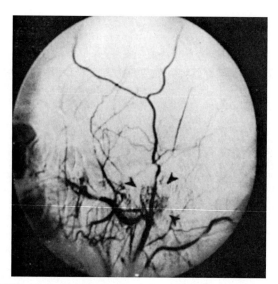

FIGURE 71-5   A right external carotid angiogram shows the tumor blush (*arrowheads*) supplied by ascending pharyngeal artery.

to the skull base, a better understanding of jugular foramen anatomy, improved electrophysiologic monitoring during operation, and improved microsurgical techniques have made the total removal of these tumors possible without causing major morbidity or mortality.

Accurate information about the size, location, and extent of the tumors and determination of involvement of the internal carotid artery and the internal jugular vein are very important in selecting an adequate surgical approach. Preoperative arterial embolization during angiography may decrease operative blood loss[42] and cause less damage to the lower cranial nerves. DasGupta and colleagues[43] indicated that benign schwannomas could be removed without resection of the involved nerves and the presumed nerve origin. In some of our cases, it seemed very easy to strip the tumor off its involved cranial nerves.

Operative Technique

Because of their deep position and the complex surrounding neurovascular structures, surgical removal of jugular foramen tumors remains a difficult process. With the aid of recent microsurgical techniques, a variety of approaches to the jugular foramen have been devised. Katsuta and colleagues[41] classified the approaches to the jugular foramen into three groups: (1) a lateral group directed through the mastoid bone, (2) a posterior group directed through the posterior cranial fossa, and (3) an anterior group directed through the tympanic bone. Arenberg and McCreary[20] and Neely[44] used the suboccipital approach on all their patients, but many authors have reported that for complete resection, removal of the petrous bone was needed. A transmastoid approach with subtotal removal was advocated by Gacek.[22] Crumley and Wilson[42] and Kinney and colleagues[45] advocated a two-stage combined otologic and neurosurgical approach. These authors used an infratemporal approach, followed by a suboccipital craniectomy for intracranial extension. Horn and colleagues[36] used a single-stage procedure, including transmastoid, translabyrinthine, and infratemporal approaches, and Kamitani and colleagues[46] used a combined extradural-posterior petrous and suboccipital approach. More recently, Mazzoni and colleagues[32] used the petro-occipital transsigmoid approach. Samii and colleagues[31] stated that any approach causing hearing loss is not recommended.

The jugular foramen is located under the middle ear, the labyrinth, and the internal auditory canal, behind the vertical part of the petrosal segment of the internal carotid artery, and lateral to the hypoglossal foramen. The infratemporal approach exposes the superior and anterior aspect of the jugular foramen by drilling part of the petrous bone. This approach requires a thorough knowledge of petrous bone anatomy and exposes the patient to postoperative complications such as auditory loss, facial nerve palsy, and cerebrospinal fluid leak.[47–50] George and colleagues[51] used the juxtacondylar approach to expose the posterior and inferior aspects of the jugular foramen. Exposing the inferior wall of the jugular foramen requires drilling a small part of the lateral aspect of the condyle and the bone above the condyle. This approach greatly reduces the risk of the complications.

The choice of surgical approach was determined by the type of tumor extension. Samii and colleagues[31] use a lateral suboccipital approach for type A tumors, and a cervical-transmastoid approach for type B, C, and D tumors, which

has the following advantages: (1) the facial nerve is left in its bone canal and (2) drilling of the petrous bone inferior to the labyrinth and cochlea allows preservation of hearing and vestibular function.[31] In type A tumors, standard lateral suboccipital craniectomy provides good exposure. But for exposure of these type B and D tumors, Pellet and colleagues[35] suggested that the widened transcochlear approach, which complements the transcochlear and infratemporal approaches, is best. This enlarges the route of access to the region, with disinsertion of the sternocleidomastoid, digastric, and stylohyoid muscles; removal of the petrous bone to displace the facial nerve, resection of the auditory canal, and subluxation of the temporomandibular joint and zygomatic process are involved.

Our jugular foramen schwannomas were mainly in the posterior fossa, with only 19 patients with tumors confined to the jugular foramen and bone. For these patients, we used a lateral suboccipital approach (Fig. 71-6). The tumors are usually large and occupy the space between the jugular bulb and cranial nerves VII and VIII, which splay over the tumor surface (Fig. 71-7). The petrosal vein is identified, coagulated, and cut near the dura, and the tumor is coagulated, gutted, and collapsed. Under a microscope, the tumor capsule is carefully dissected from its surrounding tissue, including the brain stem and cranial nerves IX to XI (Fig. 71-8). Generally we used the cervical-transmastoid approach in 10 patients with type D tumors. The incision extended into the neck along the anterior border of the sternocleidomastoid muscle to the level of the hyoid bone. The mastoid is exposed after mobilization of both the sternocleidomastoid muscle and the posterior belly of the digastric muscle (Fig. 71-9).

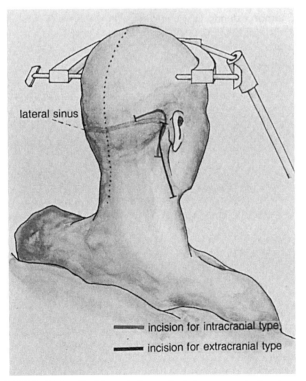

FIGURE 71-6 Position of the patient for removal of a tumor involving the jugular foramen.

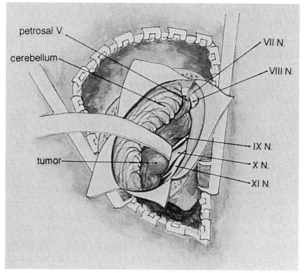

FIGURE 71-7   Exposure of a huge schwannoma and lower cranial nerves.

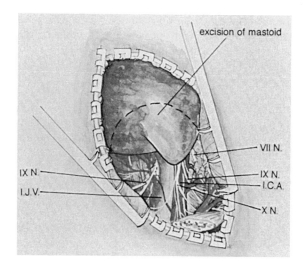

FIGURE 71-9   Excision of the mastoid.

The caudal cranial nerves are identified in the neck along with the internal jugular vein and followed cranially to the skull base. A part of the occipital squama is removed lateral to the occipitomastoid suture. The mastoid is removed, and to extend the exposure further, the posterior part of the occipital condyle may be removed, thus opening the jugular foramen dorsolaterally[31] (Fig. 71-10). Sometimes, successful total removal of skull base lesions requires complete control of the carotid artery and the internal jugular vein, so that the tumor may be removed from the vessels[48] (Fig. 71-11). In addition, in two type D tumors, we used the extreme lateral suboccipital transcondylar approach.

Most of the jugular foramen schwannomas were solid, but cystic degeneration of schwannomas is a well-known phenomenon, especially for acoustic schwannomas. Carvalho and

colleagues[52] reported that cystic tumors represented 20% of solid jugular foramen schwannomas. For cystic schwannomas, recognition of the plane between the tumor capsule and the arachnoid membrane, after opening of the cyst, may be more difficult.[52] Furthermore, despite the benign nature of these tumors, surgical findings after stripping of the tumor from the brain stem sometimes indicates a very fragile, friable brain stem surface. Fragile or very thin tumor capsules may not allow the surgeon to pull the tumor with a forceps and then peel it away, especially from the brain stem and cranial nerves. Punching the tumor capsule with a microdissector and then pulling it, in cases with thick tumor capsules, may help surgeons recognize the arachnoidal planes.[52]

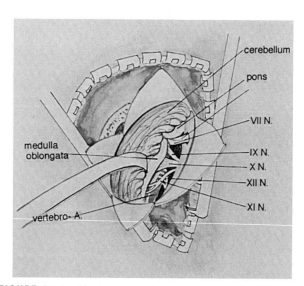

FIGURE 71-8   After removal of a schwannoma, the brain stem and cranial nerves VII to XII are exposed.

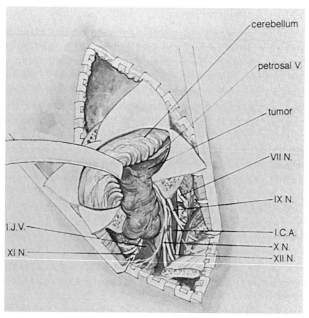

FIGURE 71-10   Exposure of the tumor involving the neck and related cranial nerves and vessels.

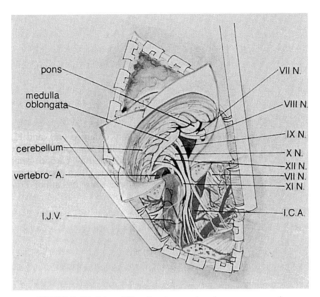

FIGURE 71-11   After the tumor has been removed.

Possible major complications include cerebrospinal fluid leak, the subsequent risk of meningitis, and lower cranial nerve deficits. Cerebrospinal fluid leak must be prevented when the tumor extends from the posterior fossa into the bone or outside it. A cerebrospinal fluid leak and subsequent risk of meningitis is much reduced by a watertight dural closure, sealing with fascia lata or lyophilized dura, the application of fibrin glue, postoperative lumbar drainage, no local drainage, and vigorous antisepsis.[53]

Preservation of adjacent cranial nerves in cases of schwannoma of the parapharyngeal space is usually possible at surgery, but those in the jugular foramen are extremely difficult to remove without damage to adjacent cranial nerves. If the vagus nerve is injured during tumor resection, microscopic reanastomosis or nerve grafting (greater auricular nerve) should be performed because nearly normal return of function has been reported with these techniques.[54] Often, lower cranial nerves are lost because of direct involvement by a pathologic state. However, morbidity of the facial nerve and acoustic nerve frequently result from the surgical procedure used to reach the tumor. When approaching jugular foramen lesions, the facial nerve presents the surgeon with the significant obstacle of how to adequately expose and remove the tumor while still preserving facial function.[55,56]

In our series, total excision of the tumor was achieved in 39 patients, subtotal in 16, and partial in five patients. There was no operative mortality. All patients presenting with lower cranial nerve dysfunction had the same or greater postoperative cranial nerve dysfunction. The long-term compensation for this deficit was good. Some patients had dramatic recovery from sensorineural hearing loss after total surgical removal of large intracranial jugular foramen schwannomas.[44]

MENINGIOMAS

There were 10 patients with a meningioma at the jugular foramen in our series. Such tumors arise from arachnoid granulations associated with the jugular bulb or venous sinuses, envelop the adjacent cranial nerves, and spread to the temporal bone, neck, and posterior fossa.[57] The clinical manifestation of meningiomas is similar to that of neurinomas and glomus tumors. Meningiomas grow slowly but have a greater tendency to recur than do glomus tumors, even after "complete" extirpation. Most of the tumors were meningothelial meningiomas (60%); malignant meningiomas are very rare.[58]

Imaging studies are helpful in the differential diagnosis. On CT, characteristic signs of sclerosis with little bone erosion at the edges of the tumor suggest a meningioma. Often, meningiomas show hyperostosis with loss of surrounding bony definition. Meningiomas are often hyperdense on noncontrast CT. MRI does not show a "salt-and-pepper" appearance or serpentine flow voids attributed to large vessels within the glomus tumor. Meningiomas strongly enhance with gadolinium, which indicates tumor size and involvement of adjacent soft tissue.[1] Angiography shows no tumor blush or less than that seen with glomus tumors. No early venous drainage can be seen, and differentiating a meningioma from a neurinoma in this area is not easy. If the lesion is rich with blood, embolization reduces blood loss during surgical procedures. For large dumbbell-type meningiomas extending to the infratemporal/parapharyngeal space, a two-stage operation is recommended. The intracranial tumor is removed in the first operation. The extracranial portion is resected in the second, and, if necessary, the involved cervical carotid artery is resected and simultaneous revascularization using a saphenous vein graft is performed with a vascularized free muscle graft.[59]

EPIDERMOID CYSTS

Epidermoid cysts of the central nervous system are described as rare, benign, slow-growing lesions with a high rate of recurrence even after surgical removal.[60] Surgeons at our institute operated on 394 patients with cerebellopontine angle epidermoids. Approximately half of these tumors involved the jugular foramen, but only two primary epidermoids were at the jugular foramen, and the patient had initial symptoms involving cranial nerves IX to XI, and the patient's jugular foramen was extremely enlarged with smooth margin.

CT usually shows a hypodense, irregular, or lobulated, nonenhancing mass, and MRI reveals an irregular, cauliflower-like surface. The most common signal pattern parallels that of cerebrospinal fluid but may occasionally be hyperintense on T1-weighted images if the solid cholesterin component is dominant.[61]

Surgical removal is the only treatment that provides a cure. Preoperative CT and MRI can indicate the size and extent of the tumor, and the approach should be planned accordingly. A combined supratentorial and infratentorial incision is sometimes required for huge tumors. If the tumor is closely adherent to vital neurovascular structures, this might complicate its removal. Removal of the whole capsule of a huge tumor is not usually necessary, lest it damage the cranial nerves, brain stem, and important vessels. However, the contents of tumor should be thoroughly cleared. Because a huge tumor of this kind cannot be completely exposed into the direct visual field, repeated physiologic saline irrigation should be applied after supposedly complete clearance of the contents, and the neurosurgeon should wait for new contents to flow out. This procedure must be performed several times until no new contents flow out. If clearance is not complete, tumor contents may flow into the subarachnoid space and cause arachnoid adhesion and intracranial hypertension.

The surgery achieves excellent results if the contents are completely cleared. The residue of the tumor capsule develops very slowly and takes a very long time to grow and give rise to recurrent symptoms. Some investigators advocate daubing the inner surface of the tumor capsule with formalin or alcohol to delay tumor development.

CHORDOMAS

Chordomas are rare tumors arising from remnants of the embryologic notochord. Because of their deep location, local infiltrative nature, and involvement of surrounding bone, treatment of chordomas is a challenge. Although chordomas are typically midline in site, we have encountered four cases of intracranial chordoma arising unilaterally in the petrous bone. All presented with Vernet's syndrome and bone erosion around the jugular foramen. The intraosseous portion of the internal carotid artery was displaced forward. CT demonstrated an extra-axial soft-tissue mass associated with foci of calcification accompanied by bone destruction. MRI showed heterogeneous hypodensity. Calcified or ossified portions of the chordomas showed as moderate hypodensity on MRI.

A chordoma is a locally invasive tumor with a high tendency for recurrence for which radical resection is generally recommended. Radical aggressive resection combined with radiotherapy seems to improve the prognoses of suboccipital and cervical chordomas when applied at the patient's first presentation with the disease.[62] In the four patients whom we encountered, the cranial nerve disturbance remained as it was before the operation. One patient died of other disease 2 years later; two patients were still alive and can take care of themselves 10 years after the operation; and the last patient is without recurrence at 4 years after surgery.

MYXOMAS

Intracranial primary myxomas are rare. Most of the reported cases were either embolic or metastatic cardiac myxomas.[63–65]

We had three female patients with primary myxomas, the first patient with a 3-year, the second with a 13-year, and the third with a 4-year history of illness. They all had Vernet's syndrome as the initial set of symptoms. The two patients with a shorter history had an intracranial tumor, and the third patient had a mixed tumor of the intracranium and extracranium. This patient's tumor extended upward, involving cranial nerve V and downward into the neck through the jugular foramen.

Differentiating the tumor from a neurinoma on neuroradiologic examination is difficult. CT shows a hypodense image that can be enhanced. MRI can show abnormal signals in long T1- and T2-weighted images of the clear margin of the jugular foramen. No tumor blush was seen on angiograms in either of these cases except for some displacement of adjacent blood vessels. One tumor in our series extended into the neck, pressing the internal carotid artery to occlusion at the C2 level (Fig. 71-12). Surgical removal is the best treatment for myxomas. Myxomas have a capsule with jelly-like contents that are easy to clear away.

Primary myxomas are benign tumors arising from mesenchymal tissues and composed of stellate and spindle-shaped cells set in a loose, mucoid stroma containing hyaluronic acid.[66] They may occur at any age, and no sex predominates.[67]

CHONDROSARCOMAS

Chondrosarcomas are malignant cartilage tumors arising from bone or preexisting exostosis. They usually occur in the long bone of the limbs with some calcification.[68] Intracranial chondrosarcomas are rare; intracranial chondrosarcomas have a predilection for the skull base, for which CT and MRI findings have been described.[69] Three patients in our series presented with unilateral disturbance of cranial nerves IX to XII. CT showed a mixed hypodense lesion in the posterior fossa with the tumor extended into the foramen. MRI indicated a sharply delineated ovoid mass at the jugular foramen, with mixed low density on T1-weighted images and low density with a high-signal rim on T2-weighted images. Its clinical manifestations and radiographic appearance were similar to those of chordoma. The tumor was tough in

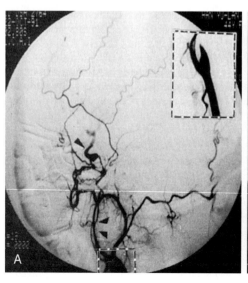
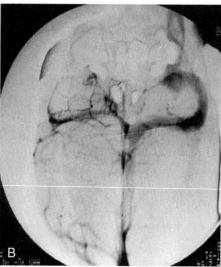

FIGURE 71-12 *A,* A left internal carotid artery (ICA) occluded at the C2 vertebra, appearing beaklike by external compression. The ascending pharyngeal artery is enlarged, and the ICA siphon is filled via the collateral circulation from the external carotid artery. *B,* The venous phase with occlusion of the left transverse sinus by tumor compression.

consistency, with a violet-red surface and yellowish substantial contents, and could not be easily suctioned to obtain total excision. Postoperative radiation therapy can improve the survival rate.[63] However, a better prognosis was observed in patients with a chondrosarcoms compared with those harboring a chordoma.[70]

REFERENCES

1. Harris CP, Dias MS, Brockmeyer DL, et al: Neurenteric cysts of the posterior fossa: Recognition, management and embryogenesis. Neurosurgery 29:893–897, 1991.
2. Maniglia AJ, Chandler JR, Goodwin WJ, et al: Schwannomas of the parapharyngeal space and jugular foramen. Laryngoscope 89:1405–1414, 1979.
3. Takahashi M, Kamito T, Hatayama N, et al: Clinical analysis of eight cases treated with lateral skull base surgery. Nippon Jibiinkoka Gakkai Kaiho 94:1683–1688, 1991.
4. Kitamura K, Niba K, Asai M, et al: Chondromyxoid fibroma of the mastoid invading the occipital bone. Arch Otolaryngol Head Neck Surg 115:384–386, 1989.
5. Comacchio F, Deredita R, Poletto E, et al: Hemangiopericytoma of skull base and Collet-Sicard syndrome: A case report. Ear Nose Throat J 74:845–847, 1995.
6. Schweinfurth JM, Johnson JT, Weissman J: Jugular foramen syndrome as a complication of metastatic melanoma. Am J Otolaryngol 14:168–174, 1993.
7. Chao CK, Sheen TS, Lien HC, et al: Metastatic carcinoma to the jugular foramen. Otolaryngol Head Neck Surg 122:922–923, 2000.
8. Yamazaki T, Kuroki T, Katsume M, et al: Peripheral primitive neuroectodermal tumor of the jugular foramen: Case report. Neurosurgery 51:1286–1289, 2002.
9. Rosenbloom JS, Storper IS, Aviv JE, et al: Giant cell tumors of the jugular foramen. Am J Otolaryngol 20:176–179, 1999.
10. Prasanna AV, Muzumdar DP, Goel A: Lipoma in the region of the jugular foramen. Neurol India 51:76–68, 2003.
11. Slaba S, Haddad A, Zafatayeff S, et al: Imaging of an exceptional tumor: myxoid chondrosarcoma of the jugular foramen. J Med Liban 49:231–233, 2001.
12. Matsumoto T, Tani E, Maeda Y, Natsume S: Amyloidomas in the cerebellopontine angle and jugular foramen: Case report. J Neurosurg 62:592–596, 1985.
13. Azm MEI, Samii M, Sepehrnia S, et al: Surgery of jugular foramen tumors. Paper presented at the First International Skull Base Congress, June 14–20, 1992, Hanover, Germany.
14. Jackson CG, Cueva RA, Thedinger BA, Glasscock ME 3rd: Cranial nerve preservation in lesions of the jugular fossa. Otolaryngol Head Neck Surg 105:687–793, 1991.
15. Ramina R, Manigha JJ, Barrionuevo CE, et al: Surgical treatment of jugular foramen lesions. Paper presented at the First International Skull Base Congress, June 14–20, 1992, Hanover, Germany.
16. Conley JJ: Neurogenous tumors in the neck. Arch Otolaryngol Head Neck Surg 61:167–180, 1955.
17. Harkin JC, Read RJ: Tumors of the Peripheral Nervous System. Washington, DC: Armed Forces Institute of Pathology, 1969.
18. Cokkeser Y, Brackmann DE, Fayad JN: Conservative facial nerve management in jugular foramen schwannomas. Am J Otol 21:270–274, 2000.
19. Russell DS, Rubinstein L: Pathology of Tumors of the Nervous System, 5th ed. Baltimore: Williams & Wilkins, 1989, p 537.
20. Arenberg IK, McCreary HS: Neurilemmoma of the jugular foramen. Laryngoscope 81:544–557, 1971.
21. Call WH, Pulec JL: Neurilemmoma of the jugular foramen, transmastoid removal. Ann Otol Rhinol Laryngol 87:313–317, 1978.
22. Gacek RR: Schwannoma of the jugular foramen. Ann Otol Rhinol Laryngol 85:215–224, 1976.
23. Maniglia AJ: Intra and extracranial meningiomas involving the temporal bone. Laryngoscope 88(Suppl 12):1–58, 1978.
24. Ito K, Suzuki M, Ottomo M, Suzuki S: Two cases of jugular foramen neurinoma—review of 48 cases in the literature. Rinsho Shinkeigaku 17:499–505, 1977.
25. Bordi L, Compton J, Symon L: Trigeminal neuroma. Surg Neurol 31:272–276, 1989.
26. Hiscott P, Symon L: An unusual presentation of neurofibroma of the oculomotor nerve: Case report. J Neurosurg 56:854–856, 1982.
27. Columella F, Delzanno GB, Nicola GC: Les neurinomes des quatre derniers neufs craniens. Neurochirurgie 5:280–295, 1959.
28. Kaye AH, Hahn JF, Kinney SE, et al: Jugular foramen schwannomas. J Neurosurg 60:1045–1053, 1984.
29. Tan LC, Bordi L, Symon L, et al: Jugular foramen neuromas: A review of 14 cases. Surg Neurol 34:205–211, 1990.
30. Sasaki T, Takakara K: Twelve cases of jugular foramen neurinoma. Skull Base Surg 1:152–160, 1991.
31. Samii M, Babu RP, Tatagiba M, et al: Surgical treatment of jugular foramen schwannomas. J Neurosurg 82:924–932, 1995.
32. Mazzoni A, Sanna M, Saleh E, Achilli V: Lower cranial nerve schwannomas involving the jugular foramen. Ann Otol Rhinol Laryngol 106:370–379, 1997.
33. Cokkeser Y, Brackmann DE, Fayad JN: Conservative facial nerve management in jugular foramen schwannomas. Am J Otol 21:270–274, 2000.
34. Franklin DJ, Moore GF, Fisch U: Jugular foramen peripheral nerve sheath tumors. Laryngoscope 99:1081–1087, 1989.
35. Pellet W, Cannoni M, Pech A: The widened transcochlear approach to jugular foramen tumors. J Neurosurg 69:887–894, 1988.
36. Horn KL, House WF, Hitselberger WE: Schwannomas of the jugular foramen. Laryngoscope 95:761–765, 1985.
37. Chong VF, Fan YF: Radiology of the jugular foramen. Clin Radiol 53:405–416, 1998.
38. Steele JR, Hoffman JC: Brainstem evaluation with CT cisternography. AJR Am J Roentgenol 136:287–292, 1981.
39. Uchino A, Hasuo K, Fukui M, et al: Computed tomography of jugular foramen neurinomas. Neurol Med Chir (Tokyo) 27:628–632, 1987.
40. Eldevik OP, Gabrielsen TO, Jacobsen EA: Imaging findings in schwannomas of the jugular foramen. AJNR Am J Neuroradiol 21:1139–1144, 2000.
41. Katsuta T, Rhoton AL, Jr, Matsushima T: The jugular foramen: Microsurgical anatomy and operative approaches. Neurosurgery 41:149–202, 1997 .
42. Crumley RL, Wilson C: Schwannomas of the jugular foramen. Laryngoscope 94:772–778, 1984.
43. DasGupta TK, Brasfield RD, Strong WE, et al: Benign solitary schwannomas (neurilemmomas). Cancer 23:355, 1969.
44. Neely JG: Reversible compression neuropathy of the eighth cranial nerve from a large jugular foramen schwannoma. Arch Otolaryngol Head Neck Surg 105:555–560, 1979.
45. Kinney SE, Dohn DF, Hahn JF, et al: Neuromas of the jugular foramen. In Brackmann DE (ed): Neurological Surgery of the Ear and Skull Base. New York: Raven Press, 1982, p 361.
46. Kamitani H, Masnzawa H, Kanazawa I, et al: A combined extradural-posterior petrous and suboccipital approach to the jugular foramen tumors. Acta Neurochir (Wien) 126:179–184, 1994.
47. Al-Mefty O, Fox JL, Rifar A, Smith RR: A combined infratemporal and posterior fossa approach for the removal of giant glomus tumors and chondrosarcomas. Surg Neurol 28:423–431, 1987.
48. Fisch U, Pillsburg HC: Infratemporal fossa approach to lesion in the temporal bone and base of the skull. Arch Otolargyngol 125:99–107, 1979.
49. Hakuba A, Hashi K, Fujitani K, et al: Jugular foramen neurinomas. Surg Neurol 11:83–94, 1979.
50. Patel SJ, Sekhar LN, Cass SP, Hirsch BE: Combined approaches for resection of extensive glomus jugular tumors. J Neurosurg 80:1026–1038, 1994.
51. George B, Lot G, Tran Ba Huy P: The juxtacondylar approach to the jugular foramen (without petrous bone drilling). Surg Neurol 44:279–284, 1995.
52. Carvalho GA, Tatagiba M, Samii M: Cystic schwannomas of the jugular foramen: Clinical and surgical remarks. Neurosurgery 46:560–566, 2000.
53. Yoo H, Jung HW, et al: Jugular foramen schwannomas: Surgical approaches and outcome of treatment. Skull Base Surg 9:243–252, 1999.
54. Reddick LP, Myers RT: Neurilemmoma of the cervical portion of the vagus nerve. Am J Surg 125:744–747, 1972.
55. Cokkeser Y, Brackmann DE, Fayad JN: Conservative facial nerve management in jugular foramen schwannomas. Am J Otol 21:270–274, 2000.
56. Kim CJ, Yoo SJ, Nam SY, et al: A hearing preservation technique for the resection of extensive jugular foramen tumors. Laryngoscope 111:2071–2076, 2001.

57. Molony TB, Brackmann DE, Lo WW: Meningiomas of the jugular foramen. Otolaryngol Head Neck Surg 106:128–136, 1992.

58. Tekkok IH, Ozcan OE, Turan E, et al: Jugular foramen meningioma. Report of a case and review of the literature. J Neurosurg Sci 41:283–292, 1997.

59. Kawahara N, Sasaki T, Nibu K, et al: Dumbbell type jugular foramen meningioma extending both into the posterior cranial fossa and into the parapharyngeal space: report of 2 cases with vascular reconstruction. Acta Neurochir (Wien) 140:323–331, 1998.

60. Zamzuri I, Abdullah J, Madhavan M, et al: A rare case of bleeding in a cerebellopontine angle epidermoid cyst. Med J Malaysia 57:114–117, 2002.

61. Osborn AG: Intracranial lesions: Cerebellopontine angle and internal auditory canals. In Osborn AG (ed): Handbook of Neuroradiology. St. Louis: Mosby-Year Book, 1991, p 347.

62. Carpentier A, Polivka M, Blanquet A, et al: Suboccipital and cervical chordomas: The value of aggressive treatment at first presentation of the disease. J Neurosurg 97:1070–1077, 2002.

63. Branch CL Jr, Laster DW, Kelly DL Jr: Left atrial myxoma with cerebral emboli. Neurosurgery 16:675–680, 1985.

64. Budzilovich G, Aleksic S, Greco A, et al: Malignant cardiac myxoma with cerebral metastasis. Surg Neurol 11:461–469, 1979.

65. Jungreis CA, Sekhar LM, Martinez AJ, Hirsch BE: Cardiac myxoma metastatic to the temporal bone. Radiology 170:244, 1989.

66. Stout AP: Myxoma, the tumor of primitive mesenchyme. Ann Surg 127:706–710, 1948.

67. Canalis RF, Smith GA, Konrad HR: Myxomas of the head and neck. Arch Otolaryngol 102:300–305, 1976.

68. Seidman MD, Nichols RD, Raju UB, et al: Extracranial skull base chondrosarcoma. Ear Nose Throat J 68:626–632, 1989.

69. Kothary N, Law M, Cha S, et al: Conventional and perfusion MR imaging of parafalcine chondrosarcoma. AJNR Am J Neuroradiol 24:245–248, 2003.

70. Colli B, Al-Mefty O: Chordomas of the craniocervical junction: Follow-up review and prognostic factors. J Neurosurg 95:933–943, 2001.

Section XII

Extracranial Vascular Disease

72 Surgical Management of Extracranial Carotid Artery Disease

BRIAN E. SNELL, JOHN H. HONEYCUTT, JR., and CHRISTOPHER M. LOFTUS

INTRODUCTION

Since the first description of a carotid endarterectomy (CEA) for the prevention of stroke,[1] the operation has been widely debated and often criticized; yet the numbers of endarterectomy procedures performed annually have steadily increased. Early studies suggested that medical management was superior to surgical intervention.[2,3] This is clearly no longer the case. Gratifying and unimpeachable results from recent multicenter trials have advocated surgical therapy over medical management in specific cases[4–6] of both asymptomatic and symptomatic carotid stenosis. The North American Symptomatic Carotid Endarterectomy Trial data indicate that CEA has benefit for all symptomatic patients with lesions of more than 70% linear stenosis and for specific subgroups of symptomatic patients with more than 50% stenosis. The Asymptomatic Carotid Atherosclerosis Study indicates that asymptomatic patients with more than 60% stenosis have a better outcome with CEA than with medical management.

In this chapter, we describe our standard technique for CEA and discuss the various surgical options and different variations of the procedure. Although there are numerous ways to perform CEA, one must adhere to several basic principles of carotid reconstruction. The surgeon must have complete preoperative knowledge of the patient's vascular anatomy, must maintain complete vascular control at all times, must have sufficient working anatomic knowledge to prevent harm to adjacent structures, and must assure the patient of having a widely patent repair free of technical errors.

SURGICAL TECHNIQUE

Surgical Magnification

We perform the operation with 3.5× loupe–magnified technique. Microscopic repair of the internal carotid artery (ICA), which we have also tried, allows a primary repair that is unquestionably finer and superior to a loupe-magnified technique,[2,7–9] but which in our experience did not alter the overall patient outcome or incidence of restenosis or acute occlusion. In the ongoing effort to reduce morbidity, we have instead adopted universal patch grafting with collagen-impregnated Dacron (Hemashield graft), which has essentially eliminated the problem of acute postoperative thrombosis or rapid restenosis. In our opinion, the graft procedure is more easily and expeditiously accomplished with 3.5× magnification rather than the microscope. There is no doubt that the suture lines are not as fine with this method, but the added lumen diameter with patch angioplasty renders the microscopic technique unnecessary in our routine practice.

Anesthetic Technique

General anesthesia and local anesthesia are both in common use for CEA. We routinely use general anesthesia with full-channel electroencephalographic monitoring. Proponents of local anesthesia cite the advantages of patient response to questioning as a superior method of assessing the need for intraoperative shunting while minimizing anesthetic risks, reducing postoperative morbidity, and shortening length of stay. The patient has local anesthesia with light sedation, which allows the patient to perform a simple task with the contralateral hand during cross-clamping. The disadvantages include risk of contamination and patient movement during the procedure, along with the increased psychological stress of remaining awake. A recent review comparing our technique with that of an institutional vascular surgeon using local anesthesia showed a decreased incidence of electroencephalographic changes and intraoperative shunting with local anesthesia. However, there was no difference in stroke rate, complications, length of stay, or overall outcome.[10]

We prefer general anesthesia for a number of reasons, not the least of which is the controlled environment. Additionally, all commonly used inhalational anesthetic agents and intravenous barbiturates significantly reduce the cerebral metabolic rate of oxygen,[11] giving a theoretical protective effect in the setting of cerebral ischemia. We keep our patients normocapnic. Although there has been much interest in arterial levels of carbon dioxide, in short, nonphysiologic hypercapnia and hypocapnia provide no cerebral protection.[12–15] Gross and colleagues[16] found that there was a 40% decrease in electroencephalographic changes with cross-clamping in those patients receiving either 1 or 2 units of 6% hetastarch (500 to 1000 mL). They had acceptable outcomes with a postoperative stroke and mortality rate of 1.3%. This finding warrants further research with a controlled, prospective study, although no study is planned at present. Finally, blood pressure is maintained at normotensive levels with a tolerance of as high as a 20% increase in systolic pressure.[11] Although some surgeons prefer to induce hypertension at cross-clamping if there are electroencephalographic changes and then shunting if no improvement is seen in the electroencephalographic recordings, we shunt immediately if electroencephalographic changes are evident.

Monitoring Techniques

Monitoring techniques can be divided into two categories: (1) tests of vascular integrity, such as stump pressure measurements, xenon regional cerebral blood flow studies, transcranial Doppler and, to a lesser extent, intraoperative oculoplethysmography (OPG), Doppler/duplex scanning, and angiography and (2) test of cerebral function, such as electroencephalography, electroencephalographic derivatives, and/or somatosensory evoked potential monitoring. The newly described near-infrared spectroscopy technique bridges both categories. We use a full-channel electroencephalography interpreted by a neurologist online. After completion of arteriotomy closure, an intraoperative Doppler examination is performed of the common carotid artery (CCA), the ICA, and the external carotid artery (ECA).

Intraoperative Shunting

Generally speaking, there are three schools of thought about intraoperative shunting.[17] Carotid surgeons shunt in every case, shunt when indicated by some form of intraoperative monitoring, or never place a shunt. In our institution, we perform monitor-dependent shunting based on electroencephalographic criteria. We use a custom commercial shunt of our own design (Loftus shunt, Heyer-Schulte Neurocare, Pleasant Prairie, WI). In our experience, we shunt approximately 15% of CEAs. This increases to approximately 25% if the contralateral carotid is occluded. After the shunt is placed, the monitoring should return to baseline. If this does not occur, the shunt must be inspected for possible kinking, thrombosis, or misplacement. We always auscultate the shunt with a Doppler probe that confirms patency and shunt flow.

Proponents of universal shunting tout the benefits of the maximal degree of cerebral protection in every case while eliminating dependence on specialized intraoperative monitoring techniques. They assert that shunt placement is benign and allows extra time to ensure meticulous intimal dissection and arteriotomy repair.[18–23]

Proponents of nonshunting believe that shunt placement is not benign. In one series, there was a higher stroke rate with shunting compared with nonshunting,[24] indicating that embolization from shunt placement, especially by surgeons inexperienced in the procedure, is a real risk. Another documented concern is distal intimal damage leading to embolization or carotid artery dissection.[25]

Many surgeons, in part because of the concerns previously discussed, choose not to shunt. There have been multiple series that have good surgical results with no shunts being used.[26–33] These authors do not deny the existence of postoperative stroke, but they strongly believe that neurologic deficits from carotid artery surgery are invariably embolic rather than hemodynamic in nature and that intraoperative monitoring and/or shunt placement will not further reduce the already low morbidity in their series.[32]

As discussed previously, we prefer to shunt when there are changes in the electroencephalogram with cross-clamping. This policy has been well supported by several reports of large series of patients.[34,35] Of note, there are also several authors who normally practice selective shunting but who advocate shunting all patients who have had recent strokes or reversible neurologic events (due to their belief that intraoperative monitoring is unreliable in the face of recent ischemic events).[36–38] Whereas we understand their concerns, this has not been our practice.

Patch Graft Angioplasty

Almost all carotid surgeons perform patch angioplasty for recurrent carotid stenosis. Many will also use selective patching in cases in which the internal carotid is small, where plaque, and, consequently, the arteriotomy have extended far up the ICA, or in any similar case in which compromise of the lumen and a high risk of thrombosis is anticipated. We have taken this policy one step further, and for 4 years have used a Hemashield patch graft primarily in all our patients. We have not encountered any restenosis or acute occlusions since using the patch universally. If patching is used, there are several synthetic grafts available along with using an autologous saphenous vein graft. There is the concern of central patch rupture in autologous vein grafts, especially in women and patients with diabetes, but the risk can be reduced with harvesting the graft from a high femoral site rather than at the ankle.

Heparinization

A single dose of intravenous heparin is given to the patient at some point before cross-clamping. This dose is between 2500 and 10,000 U of heparin, depending on the surgeon's preference. There are no published reports to support one dose versus another; however, Poisik and colleagues[31] recently reported their results using weight-based dosing of heparin at 85 U/kg. Although they did not see any statistically significant differences between fixed-dose heparinization (5000 U) and weight-based dosing, there were trends of decreased complications of hematoma formation and neuropsychometric testing differences. Some individuals reverse the heparinization with protamine after the operation.[32,33] We have not found any benefit in this practice. For those patients who come to the operating room on a continuous heparin drip, we continue the infusion until the arteriotomy closure is finished. With meticulous technique, bleeding in these cases has not been a problem.

Tacking Sutures

Tandem sutures to secure the distal intima in the ICA after plaque removal are considered a great advance by some[19] and are deemed unnecessary by others.[20,32,33] The concern with tacking sutures is that they may narrow the lumen, but to us this risk seems small compared with the concern of intimal dissection from an unsecured intimal flap. Several authors[21,32,33] state that, if the arteriotomy is carried far enough to see normal intima distal to the plaque, the tacking sutures are unnecessary. We strongly agree with an arteriotomy that extends past the plaque, but we are not always satisfied with how the intimal plaque tapers. In recent years, because of negative experiences with plaque that does not feather cleanly when pulled down from the distal ICA, we have adopted the use of fine scissors to "trim" the plaque cleanly in the ICA as it is removed. When this is done, tacking sutures are rarely necessary. We estimate that we selectively place tacking sutures in the distal ICA in approximately 5% of cases.

SURGERY

We think that the meticulous anatomic dissection and identification of vital cervical structures needed to minimize postoperative complications can be achieved only with a bloodless field. Accordingly, we do not consider elapsed time to be a factor in the performance of carotid artery surgery. In our institution, CEA requires from 2 to 2.5 hours of operating time and the average cross-clamp time is between 30 and 40 minutes. No untoward effects from the length of the procedure have been observed in any patient, and we are convinced that the risk of cervical nerve injury or postoperative complications related to hurried closure of the suture line is significantly reduced by meticulous attention to detail.[39]

Two surgeons trained in the procedure are always present during carotid surgery. Both surgeons may stand on the operative side, the primary surgeon facing cephalad and the assistant facing the patient's feet, or the surgeons may stand on each side of the table. The operative nurse may stand either behind or across the table from the primary surgeon. The patient is positioned supine on the operating room table with the head extended and turned away from the side of operation. Several folded pillowcases are placed between the shoulder blades to facilitate extension of the neck, and the degree of rotation of the head is determined by the relationship of the ECA and the ICA on preoperative angiography or magnetic resonance angiography. The carotid vessels are customarily superimposed in the anteroposterior plane, and moderate rotation of the head will swing the ICA laterally into a more surgically accessible position. In those patients in whom the ICA can be seen angiographically to be laterally placed, the head rotation need not be as great. Conversely, occasional patients will demonstrate an ICA that is rotated medially under the ECA, and in such cases, no degree of head rotation will yield a satisfactory exposure. When faced with such a case, the surgeon must be prepared to mobilize the ECA more extensively and swing it medially to expose the underlying internal carotid (even tacking it up to medial soft tissues if necessary).

The position of the carotid bifurcation has been likewise determined before surgery from the angiogram and the skin incision is planned accordingly. We always use a linear incision along the anterior portion of the sternocleidomastoid muscles (Fig. 72-1). This may go as low as the suprasternal notch and as high as the retroaural region depending on the level of the bifurcation. The skin and subcutaneous tissues are divided sharply to the level of the platysma, which is always identified and divided sharply as well. Hemostasis often requires the generous use of bipolar electrocautery.

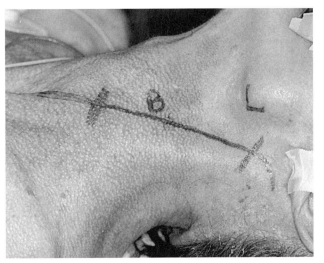

FIGURE 72-1 Positioning and surgical incision planning in a left carotid endarterectomy are shown. The incision parallels the anterior border of the sternomastoid muscle. B indicates the palpable position of the carotid bulb. The L-shaped mark indicates the angle of the mandible.

If careful attention is paid to all bleeding points during the opening, there will be little or no bleeding when heparin is administered and the closure will be much simpler.

Self-retaining retractors are next placed and the underlying fat is dissected to identify the anterior edge of the sternocleidomastoid muscle. Retractors are left superficial at all times on the medial side to prevent retraction injury to the laryngeal nerves but laterally may be more deeply placed. Dissection proceeds in the midportion of the wound down the sternomastoid muscle until the jugular vein is identified. Care must be taken under the sternomastoid muscle, however, to prevent injury to the spinal accessory nerve, which can be inadvertently transected or stretched.

It is to be emphasized that the jugular vein is the key landmark in this exposure and complete dissection of the medial jugular border should always be carried out before proceeding to the deeper structures. In some corpulent individuals, the vein is not readily apparent and a layer of fat between it and the sternomastoid must be entered to locate the jugular itself. If this is not done, it is possible to fall into an incorrect plane lateral and deep to the jugular vein. As soon as the jugular is identified, dissection is shifted to come along the medial jugular border and the vein is held back with blunt retractors. The importance of the blunt retractor in preventing vascular injury at this point cannot be overemphasized. In this process, several small veins and one large common facial vein are customarily crossing the field and need to be doubly ligated and divided (Fig. 72-2). The underlying carotid artery is soon identified once the jugular is retracted. Most often we come upon the CCA first, and at the point of first visualization, the anesthesiologist is instructed to give 5000 U of intravenous heparin, which, as discussed previously, is never reversed. Dissection of the carotid complex is then straightforward, and the CCA, ECA, and ICA are isolated with the gentlest possible dissection and encircled with 00 silk ties (or vessel loops, if preferred) passed with a right-angle clamp. We no longer routinely inject the carotid sinus; however, the anesthesiologist is notified when the bifurcation is being dissected, and if any

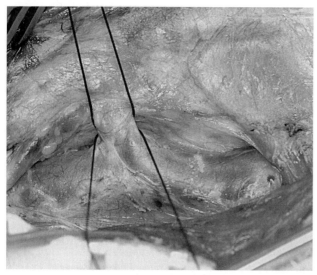

FIGURE 72-2 Intraoperative photograph shows the left jugular vein with 2-0 silk sutures around the left common facial vein. The carotid cannot be visualized yet.

changes in vital signs ensue, the sinus can be injected with 2 to 3 mL of 1% plain Xylocaine through a short 25-gauge needle (this has not been necessary for the past several years). Although the carotid complex is completely exposed, the CCA and ECA are not routinely dissected free from their underlying beds to prevent postoperative kinking and coiling of these vessels. These arteries are dissected circumferentially only in those areas where silk ties or clamps are placed around them. Posterior dissection is more extensive in the region of the ICA, where in an occasional case posterior tacking sutures may later be placed and tied.

The CCA 0 silk is passed through a wire loop that is then pulled through a rubber sleeve (Rummel tourniquet), thereby facilitating constriction of the vessel around an intraluminal shunt if this becomes necessary. The ECA and ICA ties or loops are merely secured with mosquito clamps. Particular attention is paid to the superior thyroid artery, which is dissected free and secured with a double loop 00 silk ligature (some prefer an aneurysm clip for this). A hanging mosquito clamp keeps tension on this occlusive Potts tie. Occasionally, multiple branches of this artery are identified on the preoperative angiogram and must be individually dealt with so that no troublesome backbleeding will ensue during the procedure through ignorance of these vessels. It is also essential that the ECA silk tie (and subsequent cross-clamp) be placed proximal to any major external branches, lest unacceptable back-bleeding occur during the arteriotomy and repair.

Proper placement of the retractors facilitates the control of the carotid system. The hanging mosquitoes and silk ties are draped over these retractor handles to keep the field uncluttered. Of particular note is a blunt, hinged retractor, which is invaluable in exposing the ICA when a far distal exposure is necessary. Dissection of the ICA must be complete and clearly beyond the distal extent of the plaque before cross-clamping is performed. A clear plane can be developed if the jugular vein is followed distally and dissection follows the plane between the lateral carotid wall and the medial jugular border. By following this plane, the hypoglossal

nerve is readily identified as it swings down medial to the jugular and crosses toward the midline over the ICA. The nerve is mobilized along its lateral wall adjacent to the jugular vein, after which it can be isolated with a vessel loop and gently retracted from the field. Hypoglossal paresis is rare and seems to result instead in cases in which the nerve is not visualized and is blindly retracted. On occasion, adequate mobilization of the hypoglossal nerve requires ligation of a small arterial branch of the ECA to the sternocleidomastoid muscle, which loops over the nerve. We have never seen inadvertent transection of the hypoglossal nerve.

There are several nerves that can be injured during carotid exposure and CEA. The spinal accessory and hypoglossal nerves have already been discussed. The vagus nerve lies deep to the carotid in the carotid sheath and can be inadvertently cross-clamped if not identified. The marginal mandibular branch of the facial nerve can be stretched by medial retraction in the high exposure of the ICA. The greater auricular nerve is at risk with a high incision, leaving the patient with a troublesome numb ear if it is transected. We have seen Horner's syndrome (always transient) from unrecognized injury to the pericarotid sympathetic chain. Cutaneous sensory nerves will always be transected with the skin incision, and we advise patients that the anterior triangle of their neck will be numb for approximately 6 months after endarterectomy, after which sensation customarily reverts to normal.

It is vital to have adequate exposure of the ICA and control distal to the plaque before opening the vessel. The extent of the plaque can be readily palpated with some experience by a moistened finger. There is also a visual cue when the vessel becomes pinker (instead of hard and yellow) and more normal appearing distal to the extent of the plaque. If high exposure is needed, the posterior belly of the digastric muscle can be cut with impunity, although this is necessary only in a small percentage of cases. When complete exposure is achieved, the final step in preparation for cross-clamping is to ensure that the shunt clamp can be fitted around the ICA to secure the shunt if one is used. We formerly used a Javid clamp for this purpose but have switched to a custom-designed commercial spring-loaded pinch clamp (Loftus carotid shunt clamp, Scanlan Instruments, St. Paul, MN), which is available in several angles and has a special head exactly sized to grasp the ICA and indwelling shunt without leakage. The Loftus shunt clamp is illustrated in Figure 72-3.

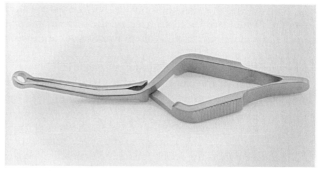

FIGURE 72-3 The Loftus shunt clamp. This customized spring-loaded clamp is slightly angled with an encircling atraumatic end. This clamp is used to secure the indwelling shunt in the internal carotid artery.

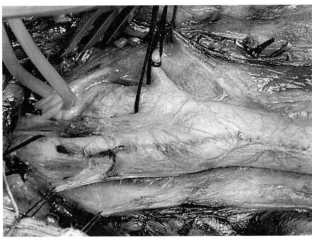

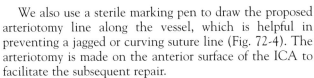

FIGURE 72-4 The carotid system has been cleanly dissected, and the arteriotomy site has been marked with a black marking pen. In the left upper quadrant, the hypoglossal nerve has been dissected and isolated with a vessel loop. The external carotid and superior thyroid arteries have silk ties around them. At the left edge, the internal carotid artery that is plaque free has a silk tie around it.

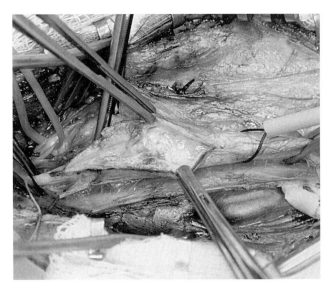

FIGURE 72-5 After the vessel has been opened, the plaque can be best seen by gently everting the edges of the artery with vascular forceps.

We also use a sterile marking pen to draw the proposed arteriotomy line along the vessel, which is helpful in preventing a jagged or curving suture line (Fig. 72-4). The arteriotomy is made on the anterior surface of the ICA to facilitate the subsequent repair.

The monitoring system is then rechecked, and the encephalographer is notified of impending cross-clamping. Once a suitable period of baseline electroencephalography has been recorded, the CCA is occluded with a large DeBakey vascular clamp and small, straight bulldog clamps or Yasargil aneurysm clips are used to occlude the ICA and ECA. We always occlude the ICA first in the belief that this approach has the lowest risk of embolization associated with clamping. A No. 11 blade is then used to begin the arteriotomy in the CCA and when the lumen is identified, a Potts scissors is used to cut straight up along the marked line into the region of the bifurcation and then up into the internal until normal ICA is entered (Fig. 72-5). In severely stenotic vessels with friable plaque, the lumen is not always easily discerned and false planes within the lesion are often encountered; great care must be taken to ensure that the back wall of the carotid is not lacerated and that the true lumen is identified before attempted shunt insertion.

Changes in the electroencephalogram mandate a rapid trial of induced hypertension. If there is no immediate reversal of these changes, an intraluminal shunt is used. The wisdom of shunt use is discussed elsewhere in the text. Numerous shunt types are available. We now use a customized indwelling shunt, the Loftus carotid endarterectomy shunt (Heyer-Schulte Neurocare) (Fig. 72-6). This is a 15-cm straight silicone tube, supplied in two diameters in the same kit, with tapered ends for easy insertion and a bulb

FIGURE 72-6 The Loftus shunt set. The set contains two shunts of differing diameters to allow for sizing preferences and a special scissors (disposable) to hook and cut the shunt cleanly for removal without damaging the back wall of the carotid. The shunt is a straight silicone tube beveled and rounded at both ends for safe insertion. A built-up bulb is present on the proximal (common carotid artery) end to anchor the shunt within the Rummel tourniquet.

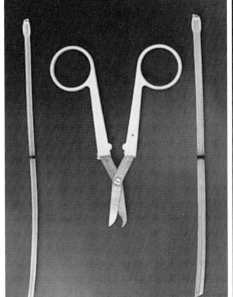

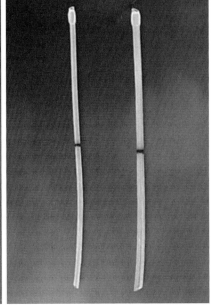

at the proximal end to facilitate anchoring by the Rummel tourniquet. This shunt has a black marker band directly in the center of the shunt, so that cephalad shunt migration can be readily discerned and corrected. The shunt is first inserted into the CCA and secured by pulling up on the silk ties; a mosquito clamp then holds the rubber sleeve in place to snug the silk around both the vessel and the intraluminal shunt. The shunt tubing is held closed at its midportion with a heavy vascular forceps and then briefly opened to confirm blood flow and evacuate any debris in the shunt tubing. Suction is then used by the assistant to elucidate the lumen of the ICA, and the distal end of the shunt tubing is placed therein. After the shunt is again bled, flushing any debris from the ICA, the bulldog clamp is removed and the shunt is advanced up the ICA until the black dot lies in the center of the arteriotomy. The shunt, if properly placed, should slide easily into the ICA, and no undue force should be employed to prevent intimal damage and possible dissection. The Loftus shunt clamp is then used to secure the shunt distally in the ICA. Visualization of the dot in the center of the arteriotomy confirms constant correct positioning of the shunt (Fig. 72-7). A hand-held Doppler probe can be applied to the shunt tubing to audibly confirm flow.

With or without the shunt, the plaque is next dissected from the arterial wall with a Freer elevator. A vascular pickup is used to hold the wall, and the Freer elevator is moved from side to side developing a plane first in the lateral wall of the arteriotomy (Fig. 72-8). The plaque is usually readily separated in a primary case, and we go approximately half way around the wall before proceeding to the other side. The plaque is then dissected on the medial side of the CCA and transected proximally with a Potts or Church scissors. A clean feathering away of the plaque is almost never possible in the CCA, and the goal here is to transect the plaque sharply, leaving a smooth

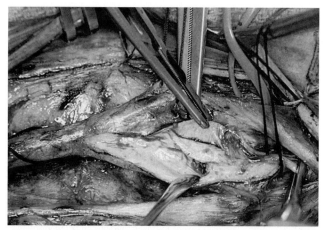

FIGURE 72-8 Plaque dissection is started by using a Freer elevator to develop a plane at the lateral edge of the arteriotomy. In this left carotid endarterectomy, the medial edge has already developed a plane, while the surgeon starts on the lateral edge.

transition zone. We like to pass a right-angle clamp between the plaque and the normal vessel and cut sharply along the clamp blade with the No. 15 knife (Fig. 72-9). It is important to note that, despite the direction of flow, the proximal end point can create a flap and the surgeon should ensure that the CCA end point is adherent. Attention is then directed to the ICA where likewise the plaque is dissected first laterally and then medially and then an attempt is made to feather the plaque down smoothly from the ICA (Fig. 72-10). However, we find that, in some cases no matter how far up the ICA we go, a shelf of normal intima remains and tacking sutures are required. Attention is finally directed to the final point of plaque attachment at the orifice of the ECA. The vascular pickup is used to grip across the entire plaque at the ECA opening, and, with some traction on the plaque, the ECA can be everted such that the plaque can be dissected quite far up into that vessel (Fig. 72-11). The eversion of the external and thus optimal plaque removal can be facilitated by "pushing" the distal external artery proximally with the clamp or forceps. The plaque is often tethered in the

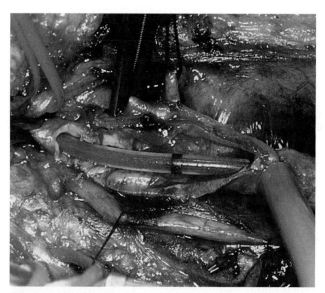

FIGURE 72-7 The Loftus shunt in place. The shunt is secured at the common carotid artery end by a Rummel tourniquet and in the internal carotid artery by the Loftus shunt clamp. The black band indicates the center of the shunt and helps prevent unrecognized shunt migration (which should also be prevented by the fat bulb on the common carotid artery end anchored by the Rummel tourniquet).

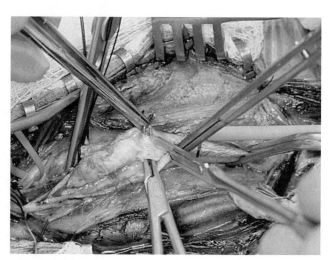

FIGURE 72-9 By using a right-angled clamp, the plaque can be incised in the common carotid artery by slipping the clamp under the plaque and then using a No. 15 knife to cut cleanly along the lower blade of the clamp.

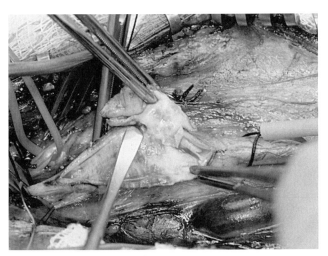

FIGURE 72-10 The dissection of the plaque is continued with the Freer elevator along the medial edge.

ECA by the clamp and as long as the lumen is held closed with the heavy forceps, this clamp can be removed without untoward bleeding, allowing avulsion of the distal plaque. The clamp must be quickly reapplied to stem back-bleeding that occurs when the plaque is removed from the ECA. It should be stressed that if plaque removal is inadequate in the ECA, thrombosis may ensue, which can occlude the entire carotid tree with disastrous results. If there is any question of incomplete removal of the external plaque, we do not hesitate to extend the arteriotomy up the ECA itself and close it via a separate suture line.

After gross plaque removal, a careful search is made for any remaining fragments adherent to the arterial wall (Fig. 72-12). Suspect areas are gently stroked with a peanut sponge, and every attempt is made to remove all loose fragments in a circumferential fashion, elevating them the complete width of the vessel until they break free at the arteriotomy edge. Although it is important to remove all

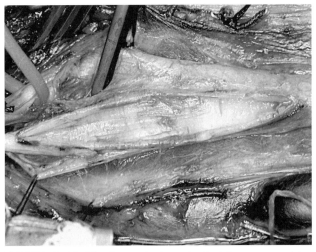

FIGURE 72-12 The lumen is then checked for any remaining fragments that are adherent to the wall.

loose fragments, no attempt is made to elevate firmly attached fragments, which pose no danger of elevating or breaking off.

Several special aspects of plaque removal need to be considered. The simplest plaque to remove is the soft, friable plaque with intraplaque hemorrhage and thrombus, which dissect quite readily and from which fragments are easily removed (Fig. 72-13). The more difficult is the severely stenotic, stony hard plaque in which a plane of dissection at the lateral border of the carotid may not be readily apparent. This situation is analogous to the gross appearance in a case of recurrent carotid stenosis. In these instances, even the most gentle plaque removal results in areas of thinning, where only an adventitial layer is left in the posterior wall of the carotid. These cases have been treated by primary plication with one or two double-armed interrupted stitches of 6-0 Prolene placed in the same fashion as the tacking sutures and no untoward consequences have ensued. Likewise, we have occasionally encountered an intraluminal thrombus emanating from a congenital web or shelf in the lumen of the vessel, and this has been successfully plicated with a posteriorly placed stitch of double-armed 6-0 Prolene.

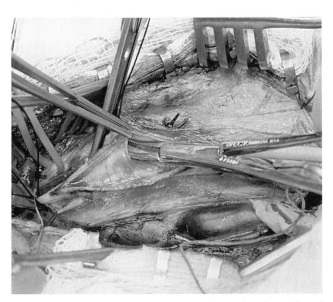

FIGURE 72-11 After plaque removal from the internal and common carotid arteries, attention is then turned to the external carotid artery. The plaque is gently removed from the external artery with a fine hemostat and gentle traction.

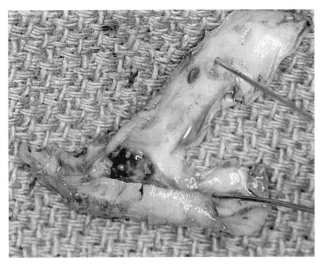

FIGURE 72-13 A soft, friable plaque with a small thrombus.

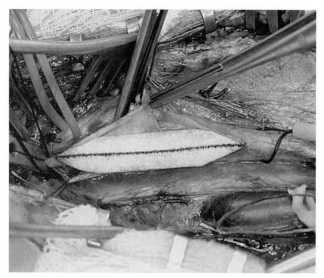

FIGURE 72-14 The Hemashield patch is attached to both ends of the arteriotomy with a double-armed 6-0 Prolene stitch. The needles are left attached to allow closure of the patch graft. Notice that both ends of the patch are tapered.

In all cases, the goal is to leave as smooth an arteriotomy bed as is possible with minimal areas of denudation or roughness available as sites of thrombus formation.

Attention is then directed to the arterial repair. If desired, the operating microscope can be brought into the field at this point or in some cases sooner to allow for removal of the small fragments under high magnification.[7-9,40] Our personal preference is to continue with 3.5× loupe magnification. If tacking sutures are required, double-armed sutures of 6-0 Prolene are placed vertically from the inside of the vessel out such that they traverse the intimal edge and are tied outside the adventitial layer. Most often two such sutures are used, placed at the 4- and 8-o'clock positions.

The patch, whatever material is employed, is then fashioned, if the surgeon has chosen this option. The patch material (Hemashield for the purposes of this description and illustrations) is placed over the arteriotomy and cut to the exact length of the opening. After removal from the field, the ends are trimmed and tapered to a point with fine Metzenbaum scissors. Each end of the patch is then anchored to the arteriotomy with double-armed 6-0 Prolene sutures, and the needles are left on and secured with rubber-shod clamps (Fig. 72-14). The medial wall suture line is closed first, and a running, nonlocking stitch is brought from the ICA anchor to the CCA anchor where it is tied to a free end of the CCA anchor Prolene (Fig. 72-15). The lateral wall is then closed (with the remaining limb of the ICA anchor stitch) from the ICA to just below the level of the carotid bulb. At this point, the second arm of the CCA anchor stitch is used to run up the CCA lateral wall to meet the ICA limb. Small bites are taken just at the arterial edge throughout (being certain, however, that all layers are included), and sutures are placed relatively close together to prevent leaks. Care is also taken so that no stray adventitial tags or suture ends are sewn into the lumen where they might induce thrombosis. Several millimeters of unsewn vessel are left on the lateral wall ensuring room to remove the shunt, if one has been used. After the electroencephalographer is again notified, the shunt is double-clamped with two parallel straight mosquitoes and then cut between them and removed in two sections, one from each end. A common error at this point is to mistakenly entangle the suture material in the shunt clamps and thereby hamper smooth shunt removal. With or without shunt, the arteriotomy is completely closed as follows: all three vessels are first opened and closed sequentially to ensure that back-bleeding is present from the ICA, ECA, and CCA. The ICA is back-bled last to ensure that it is free of debris. The two stitches are then held taut by the surgeon while the assistant introduces a heparinized saline syringe with a blunt needle into the arterial lumen. The vessel is filled with heparinized saline, and in this process, all air is evacuated from the intraluminal space. As the stitches are drawn up and a surgeons knot is thrown, the blunt needle is withdrawn, allowing no air to enter. Seven or eight more knots are then placed in this most crucial stitch (Fig. 72-16). The clamps are removed first from the ECA, then from the CCA, and, finally, some

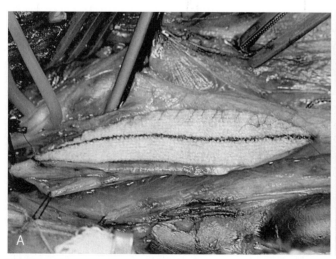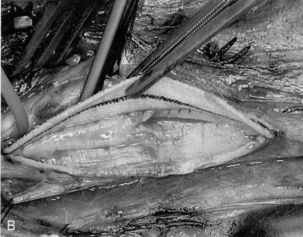

FIGURE 72-15 *A,* The medial wall is closed first from the internal to the common carotid arteries. *B,* The patch is lifted to show the sutures from the luminal side.

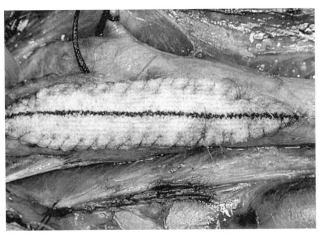

FIGURE 72-16 The lateral wall is then closed halfway down the internal carotid artery and then with the second stitch halfway up the common carotid artery.

10 seconds later, from the ICA. In this fashion, all loose debris and remaining microbubbles of air are flushed into the ECA circulation. Meticulous attention is paid to evacuation of all debris and air before opening the ICA in every case. However, in the rare case in which there is a known ECA occlusion (although most of these can be reopened at surgery with an ECA endarterectomy), this technique is extremely crucial as there is no ECA safety valve and all intraluminal contents will be shunted directly into the intracranial circulation.

An alternative method for completing the repair involves removal of the ligature or clip from the superior thyroid artery or ECA before final closure, allowing back-bleeding from that vessel to fill the lumen and eliminate the air and debris while the final stitches are placed and tied. We do not use this because we find the bleeding to be annoying.

When the clamps have been removed, the suture lines are inspected for leaks, which are customarily controlled with pressure, patience, and Surgicel gauze. In occasional cases, a single throw of 6-0 Prolene is necessary to close a persistent arterial hemorrhage. Suture repairs of bleeding points are more likely if a patch graft has been placed. It is almost never necessary to reapply clamps to the artery if the repair has been properly performed. The repair is then lined with Surgicel, and the three vessels are tested with a hand-held Doppler to ensure patency. Retractors are removed and hemostasis is confirmed both along the jugular vein and from the surrounding soft tissues. Persistent oozing is often encountered in these patients who have often received large doses of antiplatelet agents is addition to their intraoperative heparin. A final Doppler check is made, and the wound is closed in layers. The carotid sheath is first closed to provide a barrier against infection, and the platysma is then closed as a separate layer to ensure a good cosmetic result. Either running or interrupted subcuticular stitches may be used to close the skin edges. A Hemovac drain is left inside the carotid sheath. It is removed on the first postoperative day. Patients are continued on aspirin after surgery and are discharged in 1 to 2 days.

We manage any postoperative neurologic deficit, including a transient ischemic attack alone, with immediate assessment of the technical adequacy of repair. If high-quality color duplex ultrasonography is available, this may allow quick documentation of patency and identify any partially obstructing defects. Angiography is performed if ultrasonography is indeterminate or unavailable. Any occluded carotid artery postoperatively is re-explored and repatched immediately, although since adopting the primary Hemashield patch repair, the incidence of postoperative occlusion has been zero.

SPECIAL SITUATIONS

Complete Occlusion

Surgery is generally indicated for cases of acute carotid occlusion if the patient is not so debilitated as to make recovery untenable. Surgery is essentially always indicated for known acute postoperative occlusion, reflecting technical error in most cases. Surgery is sometimes indicated for cases of subacute carotid occlusion and in cases of chronic occlusion if the possibility of a "string sign" minimally patent vessel (which can usually be reopened) exists, justifying exploration. Our surgical technique for complete CCA/ICA occlusion involves opening (or reopening) of the CCA and ICA once the vessels have been controlled. The thrombus is usually seen at the carotid bulb and extending into the distal ICA; in our experience, the ECA is usually patent. Removal of thrombus and associated ICA plaque may establish back-bleeding; if not, the ICA can be explored with a No. 8 feeding tube cut to a 15-cm length and attached to a 10-mL syringe. The tube is advanced into the ICA, and the syringe is drawn back to establish suction, which often will pull down the distal thrombus as the tubing is withdrawn. If this fails, Fogarty catheters are passed into the ICA, but the risk of establishing a carotid-cavernous fistula with these must be considered. If back-bleeding cannot be established, we cleanly ligate the distal and proximal ICA stumps and perform a CCA/ECA endarterectomy and repair. If 6 hours or more have passed since occlusion, the likelihood of successful neurologic salvage is diminished, and the risk of intracerebral hemorrhage appears to increase.

Stump Syndrome

The term stump syndrome describes the continuation of ipsilateral ischemic symptoms after ICA occlusion due to emboli from the ICA intraluminal thrombus that enter the intracranial circulation via the ECA and its collateral blood flow. After strict criteria are met,[41] surgical correction is undertaken via a standard common to external carotid CEA. After removal of the thrombus from the ICA stump, we attempt to reopen the ICA and establish back-bleeding. If this is not possible (it usually is not), the stump is obliterated with inside-out sutures or with external application of large Weck clips. We stress that the ICA lumen must be obliterated. A standard external CEA is then performed (we place a CCA to ECA patch graft), and the arteriotomy is closed in the usual fashion.

Bilateral Carotid Endoarterectomy

Bilateral CEA runs the risk of extreme swings in blood pressure from concurrent denervation of both carotid sinuses[42] and from the risk of bilateral cranial nerve injury. For those patients who require bilateral endarterectomy, we recommend a staged procedure, with at least a 6-week window between the procedures. We customarily have the patient examined by an otolaryngologist to rule out an occult cranial nerve injury before the second procedure is undertaken. Unilateral nerve dysfunction in the cervical region is troublesome, but a bilateral one can be disabling. We have on occasion deferred the second surgery due to an occult vocal cord paralysis. When this happens, the patient is maintained on medical management until such time as cord function returns (as it usually does), after which the second side CEA is performed.

Plaque Morphology

The correlation of plaque ulceration with ischemic neurologic symptoms and the need for surgery is difficult for several reasons. First, studies have shown poor interobserver variability, either on ultrasound or arteriographic examinations, and poor correlation between pathologic specimens and radiographically demonstrated ulceration. Second, in symptomatic patients, deep ulceration is most commonly found in conjunction with significant degrees of carotid stenosis, and it becomes difficult to separate clinical symptomatology between these two findings.[43,44] The most recent data from the North American Symptomatic Carotid Endarterectomy Trial[6] show that in medically treated patients with 50% to 99% stenosis (now proven to be unequivocal surgical candidates), the presence of plaque ulceration in conjunction with stenosis significantly increases the risk of stroke.[45] Whether the presence of ulceration in plaques of less than 50% linear stenosis significantly increases the risk of stroke remains an unanswered question that has not been addressed by cooperative trial data.

The significance of intraplaque hemorrhage as a predictor of ischemic symptoms is also unclear. Heterogeneous plaque morphology on duplex scanning (consistent with intraplaque hemorrhage) was a significant risk factor for subsequent neurologic events in one study if the underlying stenosis was more than 50%.[46] Although one recent review also suggested that intraplaque hemorrhage was found more commonly in patients with symptomatic carotid artery disease,[43] other studies suggest that there is a low correlation between ischemic symptoms and plaque hematoma in patients who undergo CEA.[47]

CRITICAL STENOSIS/EMERGENCY SURGERY

Intraluminal Thrombi

The problem of surgical timing in patients with angiographically demonstrated propagating intraluminal thrombus remains an open question among cerebrovascular experts.[48–50] In patients who present with a transient ischemic attack (which, in our experience, has always resolved with anticoagulation) and an intraluminal thrombus, we have opted for delayed surgery (at 6 weeks after repeat angiography) in every case and have never seen a negative outcome from intercurrent embolization once heparin is instituted.

Likewise, there is a small subset of patients with postoperative neurologic events (most often transient ischemic attacks) after CEA who are found to have a fresh thrombus adherent to the suture line (by angiography), partially occluding the artery, and which is presumably the source of embolic phenomena. If there is no other angiographic evidence of technical inadequacy, we have chosen to manage these patients conservatively as well, with full anticoagulation and 6-week follow-up angiography. In every case, the thrombus has resolved, and there have been no negative neurologic outcomes in our series with this plan of management. Despite the surgeon's natural inclination to fix a problem with bold action, we have found that a measured conservative approach yields good results in cases of fresh or propagating thrombus and in our experience is superior to undertaking a high-risk surgical procedure.

Tandem Lesions of the Carotid Siphon

In the North American Symptomatic Carotid Endarterectomy Trial, symptomatic patients were excluded if the degree of siphon stenosis exceeded that at the carotid bifurcation.[6] The presence of stenotic disease at the carotid siphon has been proposed as a contraindication to CEA because of both the inability to pinpoint the symptomatic source and the reputed increased possibilities of postoperative occlusion from decreased carotid flow velocity. This has not been our experience, and we do not hesitate to operate on patients with tandem lesions if we are convinced that an active plaque at the carotid bifurcation is the source of their embolic phenomena.

Concurrent Coronary Artery Disease and Intracranial Aneurysm

There is always a concern that cervical carotid revascularization (for either symptomatic or asymptomatic carotid stenosis, especially high grade) will lead to rupture of a known intracranial aneurysm when both lesions are present. Although this is no doubt a small risk, several articles have shown that it is safe to proceed with a CEA with a silent intracranial aneurysm discovered on angiography.[51,52] Obviously, the symptomatic lesion should be treated first. We do not hesitate to operate in the light of an asymptomatic intracranial aneurysm, but we do customarily recommend subsequent craniotomy and aneurysm clipping as well.

Concurrent Coronary/Carotid Disease

It is well established that patients with extracranial carotid artery disease have a higher than normal incidence of coronary artery disease as well as other peripheral vascular problems.[53,54] Indeed, the risk of perioperative myocardial infarction exceeds the risk of perioperative stroke in many clinical series of CEA. Several major questions arise when planning treatment for concurrent coronary/carotid artery disease. These include first, what is the risk of coronary revascularization in a patient with a high-grade asymptomatic stenosis or bruit; second, in patients with symptomatic carotid artery disease, what is the appropriate workup of the coronary circulation; and third, if surgical degrees of both carotid artery and coronary artery disease are identified in the same patient, what is the appropriate surgical management (staged carotid and then coronary revascularization, combined procedure, or reverse-staged coronary revascularization and then delayed CEA).

The first question regarding asymptomatic bruit in patients symptomatic with coronary artery disease is straightforward. The Asymptomatic Carotid Atherosclerosis Study has now shown a surgical benefit for lesions of more than 60%, and we recommend that these be staged before coronary revascularization whenever possible.

The second question regarding the appropriate workup of coronary artery disease in patients with symptomatic carotid arteries is a more difficult one. In this situation, the workup is customarily guided by the history and symptomatology of the patient. It has been our practice to obtain cardiology consultation on any patient with a history of angina, known heart disease, or abnormal resting electrocardiogram. The workup proceeds with a thallium stress test with exercise or dipyridamole, and, if there is any evidence of myocardial ischemia, coronary angiography is performed.[55,56]

When the results of cardiac evaluation indicate the need for coronary revascularization, the question becomes one of timing of the surgical procedures. Our preference is to do staged procedures whenever possible. With careful hemodynamic monitoring and good anesthetic technique, we are able to routinely perform a safe unilateral CEA before coronary revascularization. An occasional patient with severe unstable angina may require a combined procedure, but this entails a significantly higher surgical risk, and we attempt staged procedures whenever possible.[55,57]

Most series dealing with reverse-staged coronary carotid procedures (coronary artery revascularization first with delayed CEA) discuss them in the context of asymptomatic carotid disease. Whereas we previously thought that reverse-staged procedures in asymptomatic patients were not indicated, we now believe that for unstable coronary disease with an unacceptable cardiac anesthetic risk, a reverse-staged procedure may be appropriate because the Asymptomatic Carotid Atherosclerosis Study data have validated surgery on silent carotid lesions.

In conclusion, then, it is our preference to aggressively work up any patient with cardiac symptoms before CEA. If procedures in both circulations are indicated, staged procedures are preferable unless the coronary circulation disease makes anesthesia for CEA an untenable proposition. In such cases, a combined procedure may be acceptable. We see no indication for reverse-staged procedures in symptomatic patients and prefer to reconstruct asymptomatic carotid stenosis of more than 60% first, whenever possible.

Recurrent Stenosis

There is a small but finite incidence of recurrent carotid stenosis after primary CEA. We have seen a decrease in our restenosis rate after adopting patching in all our cases. Piepgras and colleagues[58] show a symptomatic restenosis rate of 1% with an asymptomatic restenosis rate of 4% to 5% at a 2-year follow-up using a patch graft. Aside from technical inadequacies, it has been difficult to identify risk factors associated with recurrent carotid stenosis, although continuation of smoking habits after endarterectomy has proved to be a significant risk factor in several studies,[59,60] whereas hypertension, diabetes mellitus, family history, lipid

studies, aspirin use, and coronary disease may not be as important.

Reoperation for carotid stenosis is a technically difficult procedure. It is associated with significantly higher risks than primary endarterectomy. In our institution, the possibility of reoperation for carotid stenosis is entertained in patients who present with angiographically proven disease and classic neurologic symptoms referable to the appropriate artery or with documented progression to severe stenosis while being followed with annual serial duplex examinations.

CONCLUSIONS

Now that cooperative study data are available to support the clear superiority of surgery in the management of both asymptomatic (>60%) and symptomatic (>50%) carotid stenosis, carotid artery reconstruction will undergo continued technical refinements. Many of the basic neurovascular principles are standard, but conditions formerly thought to be unsuitable for CEA (such as contralateral occlusion, tandem stenosis, and fresh stroke) no longer prevent successful surgery in competent hands. In our opinion, this expanded acceptance of carotid surgery arises from more rigorous training and credentialing of surgeons, improved monitoring and anesthetic techniques, and the scientific application of cooperative trial methodology to the carotid problem.

The surgical methods presented here have been successful in producing acceptable postoperative results in patients who are candidates for CEA. Minor technical details, which may vary among surgeons, are probably of little significance. Conversely, subtleties of technique, which may add operative time to the routine CEA, assume greater importance when difficult lesions or high exposures are encountered or when the patient is unstable. The importance of a good outcome under these more difficult circumstances leads us to approach all carotid surgery, no matter how simple it may seem, with the same technical approach. Perhaps the most important factor in ensuring technically acceptable carotid surgery is the availability of a skilled cerebrovascular surgeon with demonstrable morbidity and mortality of less than 3% and a proper understanding of both vascular principles and cerebral physiology.

SUMMARY

Multicenter trials have advocated surgical therapy over medical management in the cases of symptomatic patients with more than 70% linear stenosis, for specific subgroups of symptomatic patients with more than 50% stenosis, and asymptomatic patients with more than 60% stenosis. We perform the operation using a 3.5× loupe–magnified technique. Universal patch grafting has essentially eliminated the problem of acute postoperative thrombosis or rapid restenosis. We prefer general anesthesia with full-channel electroencephalographic monitoring. We perform selective shunting based on electroencephalographic criteria. This has resulted in an approximately 15% shunt placement rate in our experience. We do not reverse heparinization with protamine after the operation. We only place tacking sutures in approximately 10% of cases due to the use of fine scissors to trim the plaque cleanly in the ICA as it is removed. We emphasize meticulous hemostasis in our technique.

We recommend a staged procedure in those requiring bilateral CEA, with at least a 6-week window between procedures. In the case of intraluminal thrombi, we recommend full anticoagulation and repeat angiography in 6 weeks. We do not hesitate to operate on patients with tandem lesions if we are convinced that an active plaque at the carotid bifurcation is the source of their embolic phenomena. We do not hesitate to perform CEA in the setting of an asymptomatic intracranial aneurysm, but we do customarily recommend subsequent craniotomy and aneurysm clipping as well. In the setting of concurrent coronary and carotid disease, we recommend staged procedures with endarterectomy first in symptomatic patients. We prefer to reconstruct asymptomatic carotid stenosis of more than 60% first, whenever possible. Reoperation for carotid stenosis is entertained in patients who present with angiographically proven disease and classic neurologic symptoms referable to the appropriate artery or with documented progression to severe stenosis while being followed with annual serial duplex examinations.

REFERENCES

1. Eastcott HHG, Pickering GW, Rob CG: Reconstruction of internal carotid artery in a patient with intermittent attacks of hemiplegia. Lancet 2:994–996, 1954.
2. Fields WS, Maslenikov V, Meyer JS, et al: Joint study of extracranial arterial occlusion. V: Progress report of prognosis following surgery or nonsurgical treatment for transient cerebral ischemic attacks and cervical carotid artery lesions. JAMA 211:1993–2003, 1970.
3. Shaw DA, Venables GS, Cartlidge NEF, et al: Carotid endarterectomy in patients with transient cerebral ischaemia. J Neurol Sci 64:45–53, 1984.
4. Executive Committee for the Asymptomatic Carotid Atherosclerosis Study: Endarterectomy for asymptomatic carotid stenosis. JAMA 273:1421–1428, 1995.
5. MRC European Carotid Surgery Trial: Interim results for symptomatic patients with severe (70–99%) or with mild (0–29%) carotid stenosis. Lancet 337:1235–1243, 1991.
6. North American Symptomatic Carotid Endarterectomy Trial Collaborators: Beneficial effect of carotid endarterectomy in symptomatic patients with high grade stenosis. N Engl J Med 325:445–453, 1991.
7. Bailes J, Spetzler RF: Microsurgical Carotid Endarterectomy. New York: Lippincott-Raven, 1996.
8. Spetzler RF, Martin N, Hadley MN, et al: Microsurgical endarterectomy under barbiturate protection: A prospective study. J Neurosurg 65:63–73, 1986.
9. Steiger HJ, Schaffler L, Liechti S: Results of microsurgical carotid endarterectomy. Acta Neurochir (Wien) 100:31–38, 1989.
10. Wellman BJ, Loftus CM, Kresowik T, et al: The differences in electroencephalographic changes in awake versus anesthetized carotid endarterectomy patients. Paper presented at the AANS/CNS Joint Section on Cerebrovascular Surgery, 2nd Annual Meeting. February 4–6, 1997, Anaheim, CA.
11. Gelb AW: Anesthetic considerations for carotid endarterectomy. Int Anesthesiol Clin 22:153–164, 1984.
12. Baker WH, Rodman JA, Barnes RW, et al: An evaluation of hypocarbia and hypercarbia during carotid endarterectomy. Stroke 7:451–454, 1976.
13. Boysen G, Ladegaard-Pedersen HG, Henriksen H, et al: The effect of $PaCO_2$ on regional cerebral blood flow and internal carotid arterial pressure during carotid clamping. Anesthesiology 35:286–300, 1971.
14. Fourcade HE, Larson CP, Ehrenfeld WK, et al: The effects of CO_2 and systemic hypertension on cerebral perfusion pressure during carotid endarterectomy. Anesthesiology 33:383–390, 1970.
15. Pistolese GR, Citone G, Faragilia V, et al: Effects of hypercapnia on cerebral blood flow during the clamping of the carotid arteries in surgical management of cerebrovascular insufficiency. Neurology 21:95–100, 1971.
16. Gross CE, Bednar MM, Lew SM, et al: Preoperative volume expansion improves tolerance to carotid artery cross-clamping during endarterectomy. Neurosurgery 43:222–228, 1998.
17. Loftus CM: Overview of shunt controversy. In Loftus CM, Kresowik TF (eds): Carotid Artery Surgery. New York: Thieme, 2000, pp 409–419.
18. Benoit BG, Navavi NL: The "routine" use of intraluminal shunting in carotid endarterectomy. Can J Neurol Sci 5:339, 1978.
19. Gianotta SL, Dicks RE, Kindt GW: Carotid endarterectomy: Technical improvements. Neurosurgery 7:309–312, 1980.
20. Javid H, Julian OC, Dye WS, et al: Seventeen year experience with routine shunting in carotid artery surgery. World J Surg 3:167–177, 1979.
21. Patterson RH: Technique of carotid endarterectomy. In Smith RR (ed): Stroke and the Extracranial Vessels. New York: Raven Press, 1984, pp 177–185.
22. Schiro J, Mertz GH, Cannon JA, et al: Routine use of a shunt for carotid endarterectomy. Am J Surg 142:735–738, 1981.
23. Thompson JE: Protection of the brain during carotid endarterectomy. Int Anesthesiol Clin 22:123–128, 1984.
24. Prioleau WH, Aiken AF, Hairston P: Carotid endarterectomy: Neurologic complications as related to surgical techniques. Ann Surg 185:678–683, 1977.
25. Loftus CM, Dyste GN, Reinarz SJ, et al: Cervical carotid dissection following carotid endarterectomy: A complication of indwelling shunt? Neurosurgery 19:441–445, 1986.
26. Allen GS, Preziosi TJ: Carotid endarterectomy: A prospective study of its efficacy and safety. Medicine (Baltimore) 60:298–309, 1981.
27. Baker WH, Dorner DB, Barnes RW: Carotid endarterectomy: Is an indwelling shunt necessary? Surgery 82:321–326, 1977.
28. Bland JE, Lazar ML: Carotid endarterectomy without shunt. Neurosurgery 8:153–157, 1981.
29. Ferguson GG: Carotid endarterectomy: Indications and surgical technique. Int Anesthesiol Clin 22:113–121, 1984.
30. Ferguson GG: Carotid endarterectomy: To shunt or not to shunt? Arch Neurol 43:615–617, 1986.
31. Poisik A, Heyer EJ, Solomon RA, et al: Safety and efficacy of fixed-dose heparin in carotid endarterectomy. Neurosurgery 45:434, 1999.
32. Ferguson GG: Extracranial carotid artery surgery. Clin Neurosurg 29:543–574, 1982.
33. Ferguson GG: Intra-operative monitoring and internal shunt: Are they necessary in carotid endarterectomy? Stroke 13:287–289, 1982.
34. Ferguson GG: Shunt almost never. Int Anesthesiol Clin 22:147–152, 1984.
35. Messick JM, Sharbrough F, Sundt T: Selective shunting on the basis of EEG and regional CBF monitoring during carotid endarterectomy. Int Anesthesiol Clin 22:137–145, 1984.
36. Sundt TM: The ischemic tolerance of neural tissue and the need for monitoring and selective shunting during carotid endarterectomy. Stroke 14:93–98, 1983.
37. Moore WS, Yee JM, Hall AD: Collateral cerebral blood pressure: An index to tolerance to temporary carotid occlusion. Arch Surg 106:520–523, 1973.
38. Rosenthal D, Stanton PE, Lamis PA: Carotid endarterectomy: The unreliability of intraoperative monitoring in patients having had a stroke or reversible ischemic neurological deficit. Arch Surg 116:1569–1575, 1981.
39. Honeycutt JH, Loftus CM: Carotid endarterectomy: General principles and surgical technique. Neurosurg Clin N Am 11:279–297, 2000.
40. Findlay JM: Carotid microendarterectomy. Neurosurgery 32:792–798, 1993.
41. Honeycutt JH, Loftus CM: Carotid stump syndromes and external revascularization. In Loftus CM, Kresowik TF (eds): Textbook of Carotid Artery Surgery. New York: Thieme, 2000, pp 315–320.
42. Wade JG, Larson CP, Hickey RF, et al: Effect of carotid endarterectomy on carotid chemoreceptor and baroreceptor function in man. N Engl J Med 282:F823–F829, 1970.
43. Gomez CR: Carotid plaque morphology and risk for stroke. Stroke 21:148–151, 1990.
44. Wechsler LR: Ulceration and carotid artery disease. Stroke 19:650–653, 1998.
45. Eliasziw M, Streifler JW, Fox AJ, et al: Significance of plaque ulceration in symptomatic patients with high-grade carotid stenosis. Stroke 25:304–308, 1994.
46. Sterpetti AV, Schultz RD, Feldhaus RJ, et al: Ultrasonographic features of carotid plaque and the risk of subsequent neurologic deficits. Surgery 104:652–660, 1988.

47. Lennihan L, Kupsky WJ, Mohr JP, et al: Lack of association between carotid plaque hematoma and ischemic cerebral symptoms. Stroke 18:879–881, 1987.
48. Biller J, Adams HP, Boarini D, et al: Intraluminal clot of the carotid artery. Surg Neurol 25:467–477, 1986.
49. Heros RC: Carotid endarterectomy in patients with intraluminal thrombus. Stroke 19:667–668, 1990.
50. Loftus CM: Propagating intraluminal carotid thrombus: surgery or anticoagulation? In Loftus CM, Kresowik TF (eds): Carotid Artery Surgery. New York: Thieme, 2000, pp 321–327.
51. Ladowski JS, Webster MW, Yonas HO, et al: Carotid endarterectomy in patients with asymptomatic intracranial aneurysms. Ann Surg 200:70–73, 1984.
52. Stern J, Whelan M, Brisman R, et al: Management of extracranial carotid stenosis and intracranial aneurysms. J Neurosurg 51:147–150, 1979.
53. Gerraty RP, Gates PC, Doyle JC: Carotid stenosis and perioperative stroke risk in symptomatic and asymptomatic patients undergoing vascular or coronary surgery. Stroke 24:1115–1118, 1993.
54. Newman DC, Hicks RG: Combined carotid and coronary artery surgery: A review of the literature. Ann Thorac Surg 45:574–581, 1988.
55. Graor RA, Hertzer NR: Management of coexistent carotid artery and coronary artery disease. Curr Concepts Cerebrovasc Dis Stroke 23:19–23, 1988.
56. Jones RH, Loftus CM, Sheldon WC, et al: Concomitant carotid and coronary disease. Patient Care 15:49–66, 1992.
57. Cosgrove DM, Hertzer RN, Loop FD: Surgical management of synchronous carotid and coronary artery disease. J Vasc Surg 3:690–692, 1986.
58. Piepgras DG, Sundt TM, Marsh WR, et al: Recurrent carotid stenosis: Results and complications of 57 operations. In Sundt TM (ed): Occlusive Cerebrovascular Disease: Diagnosis and Surgical Management. Philadelphia: WB Saunders, 1987, pp 286–297.
59. Clagett G, Rich N, McDonald P, et al: Etiologic factors for recurrent carotid artery stenosis. Surgery 2:313–318, 1983.
60. Dempsey RJ, Moore R, Cordero S: Factors leading to early reoccurrence of carotid plaque after carotid endarterectomy. Surg Neurol 43:278–283, 1995.

73

Management of Dissections of the Carotid and Vertebral Arteries

BRIAN L. HOH, ROBERT J. SINGER, BOB S. CARTER, and CHRISTOPHER S. OGILVY

INTRODUCTION: EXTRACRANIAL VERSUS INTRACRANIAL DISSECTION

The management of carotid and vertebral artery dissections has evolved immensely since the 1970s when Fisher and colleagues, and other groups, first described the modern diagnosis and treatment of extracranial[1] and intracranial dissections.[2] Certainly, in recent years, the advent of neuroendovascular therapies has altered the armamentarium of neurovascular physicians treating patients with such lesions.

Although this chapter reviews the management of both extracranial and intracranial dissections, in essence, these are two separate clinicopathologic entities with differing symptomatology, natural history, pathology, and management. Extracranial dissections are more likely to present with ischemic or thromboembolic complications, whereas intracranial dissections can present with subarachnoid hemorrhage. Extracranial dissections of the carotid and vertebral arteries account for 2% of all ischemic strokes.[3–8] Conversely, in a nationwide study in Japan of intracranial vertebral artery and carotid artery dissections, 58% presented with subarachnoid hemorrhage.[9] The dissimilarities are primarily due to the difference in the vascular histology and the surrounding milieu of the extracranial and intracranial segments. The management of such lesions reflects these differences.

Vascular Histology

Cervicocerebral artery dissections arise from a tear in the intima that allows hemodynamic flow to enter the wall of the artery within the layers of the tunica media, forming an intramural hematoma or false lumen. Subintimal dissections tend to cause stenosis of the parent artery, whereas subadventitial dissections may cause aneurysmal dilation of the artery, so-called pseudoaneurysms, which have been pointed out to differ from true pseudoaneurysms because their walls consist of vessel elements.[6,10]

The intradural arteries have a thinner media and adventitia with fewer elastic fibers than the extradural arteries, so intradural dissections are more likely to be subadventitial causing pseudoaneurysms and subarachnoid hemorrhage,[11] whereas the extradural arteries are more likely to have subintimal dissections presenting with arterial stenosis or thromboembolic complications.[1,6]

Surrounding Milieu

The difference in presentation, natural history, and management of extracranial versus intracranial dissection is also based on the surrounding milieu of the location of the pathology. Because the cervical bone and tissues surround an extracranial dissection of the carotid or vertebral artery, these lesions are associated with ischemic complications, mostly thromboembolic rather than hemorrhagic. Intracranial dissections of the carotid and vertebral arteries, however, are surrounded by cerebrospinal fluid in the subarachnoid space and can thus be associated with hemorrhagic as well as ischemic complications. Others have also proposed that the greater mobility of the extradural carotid and vertebral arteries and their proximity to bony structures such as the cervical vertebrae or styloid process put them at risk of subintimal dissections.[1,6,12]

EXTRACRANIAL CAROTID ARTERY DISSECTION

Presentation

The incidence of extracranial carotid artery dissection is thought to be 2.5 to 3.0 per 100,000,[4,6,8] and the extracranial carotid artery is the most common site of arterial dissection.[13–15] Patients with heritable connective tissue disorders, such as Ehlers-Danlos syndrome type IV, Marfan syndrome, autosomal dominant polycystic kidney disease, and osteogenesis imperfecta type I, have an increased risk of spontaneous dissections of either the carotid or vertebral artery,[16,17] and one fifth of patients with spontaneous carotid or vertebral artery dissection have an apparent but as yet unnamed connective tissue disorder.[18] In approximately 15% of patients with spontaneous carotid or vertebral artery dissection, fibromuscular dysplasia is seen angiographically.[7,12,16]

The classic triad for clinical presentation of extracranial carotid artery dissection is (1) pain on one side of the head, face, or neck, (2) partial Horner's syndrome, and (3) cerebral or retinal ischemia, although all three elements are found in fewer than one third of patients.[6]

The most common presenting complaint is ipsilateral neck or head pain.[19] The pain is usually described as throbbing and constant with varying intensity. The second most common presentation is focal neurologic symptoms. These may consist of transient ischemic attacks or overt stroke. These symptoms are often the result of either stenosis of the true lumen with hypoperfusion or thromboembolism and tend to occur in the subacute period after dissection. Oculosympathetic paresis is the third most commonly seen clinical manifestation of carotid dissection.[19] The paresis typically involves the oculomotor nerve while sparing those fibers traveling on the external carotid artery. Subsequently, patients have a classic third nerve lesion (involving the pupil) but have preserved facial sweating except for a small area in the frontosupraorbital region.[19] Pulsatile tinnitus has been noted in as many as one third of patients and has been suggested to signify the onset of the dissection.[20]

The risk of extracranial carotid dissection is stroke. Although dissections of the extracranial carotid and vertebral artery account for 2% of all ischemic strokes in the general population,[3–8] they account for as many as 20% of ischemic strokes in the young adult population. Most strokes are thought to be thromboembolic in nature. In one series of 78 patients with extracranial carotid artery dissection, 71% presented with cerebral infarction, 13% with transient ischemic attack, and 17% with local signs.[21] Most patients recover, however, there is a significant risk of morbidity and mortality. In that same series, on clinical follow-up, 69% had no sequelae or symptoms only, 15% had mild to moderate handicap, and 15% had severe handicap or death.[21]

Diagnosis

Cervicocerebral angiography has in the past been the gold standard in establishing diagnosis.[19] Cervical internal carotid artery dissection typically occurs approximately 2 cm distal to the artery's origin and usually terminates proximal to its entry into the petrous bone.[1,13,19,22] Extension into the petrous bone, however, has been reported. Stenosis is the most common angiographic finding, but a wide variety of dissection patterns have been noted.[1] Approximately 18% of cases are occluded at onset.[13] Aneurysms associated with dissection and stenosis are present in 35% to 40%. Aneurysms alone are seen in approximately 10%[19] (Figs. 73-1 and 73-2). They are not likely to rupture but manifest clinically because of thromboembolic phenomena or by compressive cranial neuropathy.[13]

Computed tomography (CT) and magnetic resonance (MR) angiography are rapidly replacing conventional cervicocerebral angiography as noninvasive, highly sensitive diagnostic techniques for aneurysms[23] and for dissection.[24–27] CT angiography has become the primary imaging modality of our neurovascular group at Massachusetts

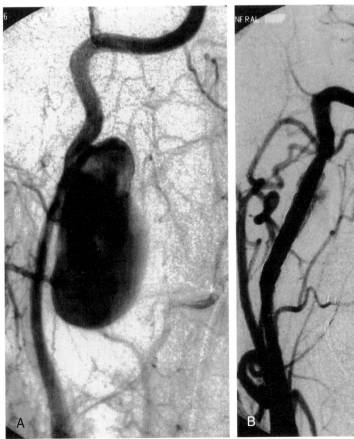

FIGURE 73-1 *A,* Digital subtraction angiogram demonstrates extracranial carotid artery dissection resulting in giant pseudoaneurysm. *B,* Treated with endovascular stent placement and angioplasty.

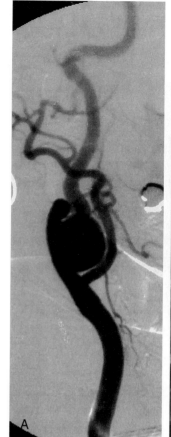
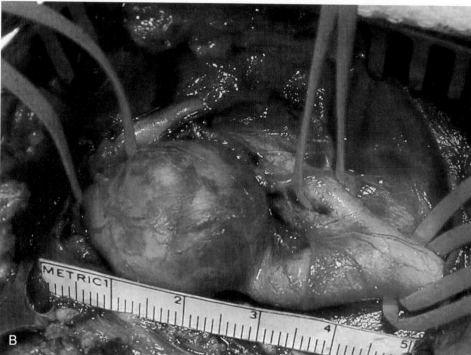

FIGURE 73-2 *A,* Digital subtraction angiogram demonstrates extracranial carotid artery dissection resulting in pseudoaneurysm. *B,* Intraoperative photograph demonstrates surgical view of an internal carotid artery pseudoaneurysm.

General Hospital.[23] Additionally, we have found MR angiography and fat suppression techniques for T1-weighted axial MR imaging to be extremely useful in demonstrating the intramural hematoma that appears as a crescent adjacent to the vessel lumen. Over a 12-month period at Massachusetts General Hospital, of 22 patients with clinical suspicion of cervical carotid or vertebral dissection, 19 underwent CT angiography and MR imaging/MR angiography, 2 underwent MR imaging/MR angiography, and 1 underwent conventional catheter angiography (Pomerantz and colleagues, unpublished data). CT angiography and MR imaging/MR angiography correctly detected dissection in all 21 patients in whom they were performed. In our practice, we find the two modalities of CT angiography and MR imaging/MR angiography complementary, although CT angiography is preferred in the acute setting (T1-hyperintense crescent on MR angiography is due to methemoglobin, which can take 1 to 3 days to become conspicuous) and especially with trauma (Pomerantz and colleagues, unpublished data).

Treatment

Anticoagulation with intravenous heparin followed by conversion to oral warfarin has been recommended as the first-line treatment of patients with extracranial carotid dissections to prevent the risk of thromboembolic complications.[6,28] However, no randomized trial has ever been performed to validate this treatment. After 3 to 6 months of warfarin anticoagulation with a goal of an international normalized ratio of 2.0 to 3.0, repeat imaging can be performed with a change to antiplatelet therapy if luminal irregularities are found to persist, a strategy based on the high rate of recanalization within 3 to 6 months and that most extracranial carotid dissections heal spontaneously.[6,28]

Intervention is performed for anticoagulation treatment failures or persistent luminal irregularities. Endovascular therapies have become the preferred treatment for these lesions. Carotid angioplasty and stent placement can achieve excellent results with long-term patency of the carotid artery[29] (Fig. 73-3).

Surgical treatment can consist of simple endarterectomy if the involved segment can be adequately exposed and the vessel integrity is sufficient. Unfortunately, these lesions often result in thin and friable vessel walls with the dissection extending to the skull base. If endovascular angioplasty and stent placement or surgical endarterectomy fail or are not possible, then surgical or endovascular ligation of the carotid artery may be required, with or without a surgical bypass procedure (external carotid artery to internal carotid

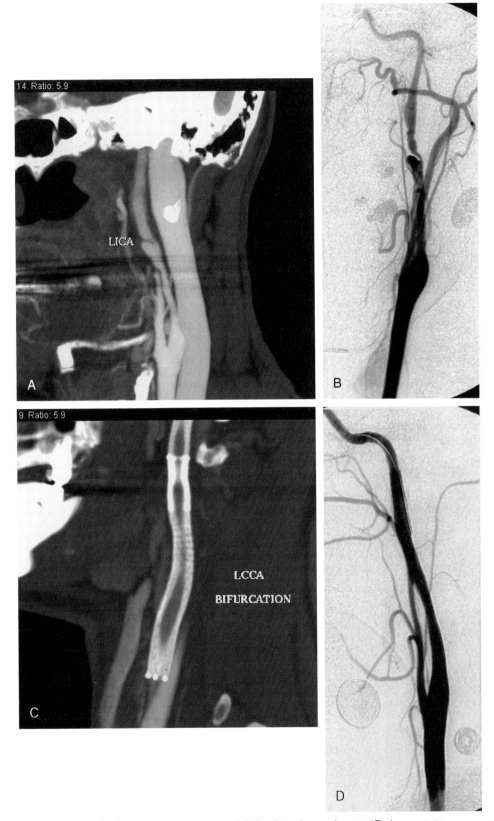

FIGURE 73-3 Computed tomography (CT) angiogram (*A*) and digital subtraction angiogram (*B*) demonstrate severe extracranial carotid artery dissection. CT angiogram (*C*), and digital subtraction angiogram (*D*) demonstrate results after endovascular stent placement and angioplasty. LICA, left internal carotid artery; LCCA, left common carotid artery.

artery bypass) depending on predicted tolerance to carotid occlusion.

EXTRACRANIAL VERTEBRAL ARTERY DISSECTION

Presentation

The incidence of extracranial vertebral artery dissection is estimated to be 1.0 to 1.5 per 100,000.[3,5-7] As mentioned previously, patients with heritable connective tissue disorders and patients with fibromuscular dysplasia are at increased risk of extracranial vertebral artery dissection. There is also a reported risk of vertebral artery dissection after chiropractic spinal manipulative therapy.[30] It has been estimated that as many as one in 20,000 spinal manipulations causes a stroke.[31]

Patients can present with posterior neck pain or occipital headache, but more than 90% present with ischemic symptoms of the brain stem, particularly the lateral medulla (Wallenberg syndrome), the thalamus, or the cerebral or cerebellar hemisphere.[15] In a series of 46 patients with extracranial vertebral artery dissection, 85% presented with cerebral infarction, 11% with transient ischemic attack, and 4% with local signs.[21]

The risk of extracranial vertebral artery dissection is stroke. Although the natural history risk of extracranial vertebral artery dissection is not well known, in one series, 70% had no sequelae or symptoms only, 22% had mild to moderate handicap, and 9% had severe handicap or death.[21]

Diagnosis

As mentioned above for extracranial carotid artery dissection, cervicocerebral angiography has in the past been the gold standard imaging modality for the diagnosis of extracranial vertebral artery dissection. However, CT angiography, MR angiography, and fat suppression techniques with T1-weighted axial MR imaging are rapidly becoming the diagnostic studies for vertebral artery dissection rather than conventional angiography.

Treatment

As with external carotid artery dissection, the first-line treatment for extracranial vertebral artery dissection is anticoagulation with intravenous heparin converted to oral warfarin for a target international normalized ratio 2.0 to 3.0 for 3 to 6 months.[6,28] With anticoagulation, angiographic improvement has been documented in 26% to 33% of cases, normalization was seen in 61% to 63%, and progression to occlusion occurred in 6% to 11%. Angiographic improvement has been described by as early as 7 days. Healing is expected by 3 months. Overall, with anticoagulation alone, a good outcome has been reported in 70% to 80% of patients.[19]

For cases in which anticoagulation has failed or there are persistent luminal irregularities, endovascular intervention can be performed typically as angioplasty and stent placement[32-34] (Fig. 73-4) or as vertebral artery sacrifice if it can be tolerated.

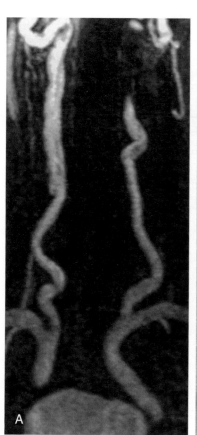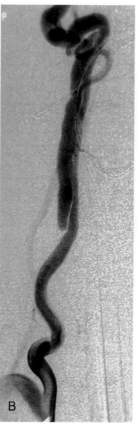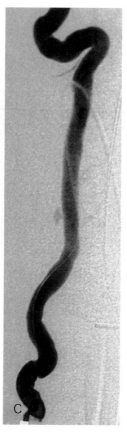

FIGURE 73-4 Magnetic resonance angiogram (*A*) and digital subtraction angiogram (*B*) demonstrate extracranial vertebral artery dissection. *C,* Treated with endovascular stent placement and angioplasty.

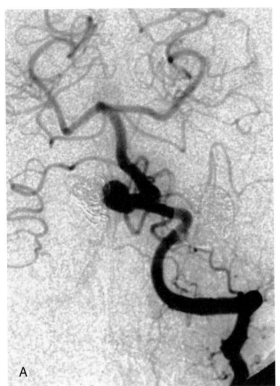
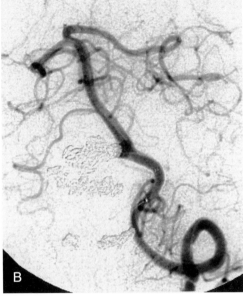

FIGURE 73-5 *A,* Digital subtraction angiogram demonstrates vertebrobasilar junction dissecting pseudoaneurysm recurrent after endosaccular coiling. *B,* Treated with endovascular intracranial stent placement and endosaccular coiling.

INTRACRANIAL ARTERIAL DISSECTION

Presentation

The incidence of intracranial arterial dissections is rare. The most common site of intracranial dissection is the intradural vertebral artery. In one series of 338 intracranial arterial dissections, the dissection occurred at the vertebral artery in 60% and 9% at the internal carotid artery.[35] Although the risk of extracranial cervicocerebral artery dissection is ischemic stroke, the risk of intracranial arterial dissections is subarachnoid hemorrhage. In Japan, 58% of patients with intracranial vertebral artery or carotid artery dissections presented with subarachnoid hemorrhage.[9] Subarachnoid hemorrhage was more common in intracranial vertebral artery dissections (67%) than in intracranial carotid artery dissections (22%).[9] Vertebral artery dissection accounted for 3% to 7% of all nontraumatic subarachnoid hemorrhage cases in one series.[11]

The intradural vertebral artery has a thin media and adventitia with fewer elastic fibers, so dissections result in pseudoaneurysms and subarachnoid hemorrhage.[36] The natural history of vertebral artery dissecting pseudoaneurysms is believed to be dangerous, with the rebleeding rate from these lesions reported to be 21% to 71%, with an associated 50% to 100% mortality rate, with the highest risk in the acute stage after initial bleeding.[37–41]

Diagnosis

Conventional catheter angiography has been the gold standard technique for intracranial arterial dissections; however, CT angiography and MR angiography are rapidly replacing it. At our center, we have adopted CT angiography as the primary diagnostic and pretreatment planning study for such lesions.[23]

Treatment

Unlike for extracranial disease, for intracranial dissection, anticoagulation is not recommended, particularly because of the high rate of rebleeding. Endovascular therapies, such as intracranial stenting or coiling or parent artery sacrifice, are the preferred treatment for these lesions. Various strategies of endovascular treatment have been reported.[38,42–45]

Our neurovascular group has managed 35 patients with intradural vertebral artery dissecting aneurysms between 1992 and 2002, 26 endovascularly and two surgically.[36,44] Twelve lesions were treated with trapping and 14 with proximal occlusion, of which 2 were eventually trapped. On angiographic long-term follow-up, complete cure was evident in 19 of 24 patients. There were two cases of recurrent hemorrhage after treatment, of which one patient died. The overall mortality rate was 20% in the treated group and 50% in the untreated group.[36,44]

Recently, we have treated intracranial vertebral dissecting pseudoaneurysms with endovascular intracranial stent placement and endosaccular coiling with excellent results (Fig. 73-5).

REFERENCES

1. Fisher CM, Ojemann RG, Roberson GH: Spontaneous dissection of cervico-cerebral arteries. Can J Neurol Sci 5:9–19, 1978.
2. Ojemann RG, Fisher CM, Rich JC: Spontaneous dissecting aneurysm of the internal carotid artery. Stroke 3:434–440, 1972.

3. Bassetti C, Carruzzo A, Sturzenegger M, Tuncdogan E: Recurrence of cervical artery dissection: a prospective study of 81 patients. Stroke 27:1804–1807, 1996.

4. Giroud M, Fayolle H, Andre N, et al: Incidence of internal carotid artery dissection in the community of Dijon. J Neurol Neurosurg Psychiatry 57:1443, 1994.

5. Leys D, Moulin TH, Stojkovic T, et al and DONALD Investigators: Follow-up of patients with history of cervical artery dissection. Cerebrovasc Dis 5:43–49, 1995.

6. Schievink WI: Spontaneous dissection of the carotid and vertebral arteries. N Engl J Med 344:898–906, 2001.

7. Schievink WI, Mokri B, O'Fallon WM: Recurrent spontaneous cervical-artery dissection. N Engl J Med 330:393–397, 1994.

8. Schievink WI, Mokri B, Whisnant JP: Internal carotid artery dissection in a community: Rochester, Minnesota, 1987–1992. Stroke 24:1678–1680, 1993.

9. Yamaura A, Ono J, Hirai S: Clinical picture of intracranial non-traumatic dissecting aneurysm. Neuropathology 20:85–90, 2000.

10. Bostrom K, Liliequist B: Primary dissecting aneurysm of the extracranial part of the internal carotid and vertebral arteries: A report of three cases. Neurology 17:179–186, 1967.

11. Sasaki O, Ogawa H, Koike T, et al: A clinicopathological study of dissecting aneurysms of the intracranial vertebral artery. J Neurosurg 75:874–882, 1991.

12. Hart RG, Easton JD: Dissections of the cervical and cerebral arteries. Neurol Clin N Am 1:155–182, 1983.

13. Anson J, Crowell RM: Cervicocranial arterial dissection. Neurosurgery 29:89–96, 1991.

14. Biller J, Hingtgen WL, Adams HP Jr, et al: Cervicocephalic arterial dissections: A ten-year experience. Arch Neurol 43:1234–1238, 1986.

15. Caplan LR, Zarins CK, Hemmati M: Spontaneous dissection of the extracranial vertebral arteries. Stroke 16:1030–1038, 1985.

16. Schievink WI, Bjornsson J, Piepgras DG: Coexistence of fibromuscular dysplasia and cystic medial necrosis in a patient with Marfan's syndrome and bilateral carotid artery dissections. Stroke 25:2492–2496, 1994.

17. Schievink WI, Michels VV, Piepgras DG: Neurovascular manifestations of heritable connective tissue disorders: A review. Stroke 25:889–903, 1994.

18. Schievink WI, Wijdicks EFM, Michels VV, et al: Heritable connective tissue disorders in cervical artery dissections: A prospective study. Neurology 50:1166–1169, 1998.

19. Sila CA, Awad IA: Arterial trauma and dissection. In Awad IA (ed): Cerebrovascular Occlusive Disease and Brain Ischemia. Parkridge, IL: American Association of Neurological Surgeons, 1992, pp 187–202.

20. Sila CA, Furlan AJ, Little JR: Pulsatile tinnitus. Stroke 18:252–256, 1987.

21. Dziewas R, Konrad C, Drager B, et al: Cervical artery dissection—Clinical features, risk factors, therapy and outcome in 126 patients. J Neurol 250:1179–1184, 2003.

22. O'Connell BK, Towfighi J, Brennan RW, et al: Dissecting aneurysms of head and neck. Neurology 35:993–997, 1985.

23. Hoh BL, Cheung AC, Rabinov JD, et al: Results of a prospective protocol of computed tomographic angiography in place of catheter angiography as the only diagnostic and pre-treatment planning study for cerebral aneurysms by a combined neurovascular team. Neurosurgery 54:1329–1342, 2004.

24. Djouhri H, Guillon B, Brunereau L, et al: MR angiography for the long-term follow-up of dissecting aneurysms of the extracranial internal carotid artery. AJR Am J Roentgenol 174:1137–1140, 2000.

25. Egelhof T, Jansen O, Winter R, Sartor K: CT angiography in dissections of the internal carotid artery: Value of a new examination technique in comparison with DSA and Doppler ultrasound. Radiologe 36:850–854, 1996.

26. Kasner SE, Hankins LL, Bratina P, Morgenstern LB: Magnetic resonance angiography demonstrates vascular healing of carotid and vertebral artery dissections. Stroke 28:1993–1997, 1997.

27. Kirsch E, Kaim A, Engelter S, et al: MR angiography in internal carotid artery dissection: Improvement of diagnosis by selective demonstration of the intramural haematoma. Neuroradiology 40:704–709, 1998.

28. Schievink WI: The treatment of spontaneous carotid and vertebral artery dissections. Curr Opin Cardiol 15:316–321, 2000.

29. Albuquerque FC, Han PP, Spetzler RF, et al: Carotid dissection: technical factors affecting endovascular therapy. Can J Neurol Sci 29:54–60, 2002.

30. Smith WS, Johnston SC, Skalabrin EJ, et al: Spinal manipulative therapy is an independent risk factor for vertebral artery dissection. Neurology 60:1424–1428, 2003.

31. Vickers A, Zollman C: The manipulative therapies: osteopathy and chiropractic. BMJ 319:1176–1179, 1999.

32. Malek AM, Higashida RT, Phatouros CC, et al: Treatment of posterior circulation ischemia with extracranial percutaneous balloon angioplasty and stent placement. Stroke 30:2073–2085, 1999.

33. Phatouros CC, Higashida RT, Malek AM, et al: Endovascular treatment of noncarotid extracranial cerebrovascular disease. Neurosurg Clin N Am 11:331–350, 2000.

34. Piotin M, Spelle L, Martin JB, et al: Percutaneous transluminal angioplasty and stenting of the proximal vertebral artery for symptomatic stenosis. AJNR Am J Neuroradiol 21:727–731, 2000.

35. Yamaura A: Nontraumatic intracranial arterial dissection: Natural history, diagnosis, and treatment. Contemp Neurosurg 16:1–6, 1994.

36. Rabinov JD, Hellinger FR, Morris PP, et al: Endovascular management of vertebrobasilar dissecting aneurysms. AJNR Am J Neuroradiol 24:1421–1428, 2003.

37. Aoki N, Sakai T: Rebleeding from intracranial dissecting aneurysms of the posterior circulation. Stroke 21:1623–1631, 1990.

38. Hoh BL, Ogilvy CS: Vertebral artery, posterior inferior cerebellar artery, and vertebrobasilar junction aneurysms. In Winn HR (ed): Youmans Neurological Surgery. Philadelphia: WB Saunders, 2004, pp 2007–2023.

39. Kawaguchi S, Sakaki T, Tsunoda S, et al: Management of dissecting aneurysms of the posterior circulation. Acta Neurochir (Wien) 131:26–31, 1994.

40. Mizutani T, Aruga T, Kirino T: Recurrent subarachnoid hemorrhage from untreated ruptured vertebrobasilar dissecting aneurysms. Neurosurgery 36:905–911, 1995.

41. Yamaura A, Watanabe Y, Saeki N: Dissecting aneurysms of the intracranial vertebral artery. J Neurosurg 72:183–188, 1990.

42. Anxionnat R, de Melo Neto JF, Bracard S, et al: Treatment of hemorrhagic intracranial dissections. Neurosurgery 53:289–300, 2003.

43. Hamada J, Kai Y, Morioka M, et al: Multimodal treatment of ruptured dissecting aneurysms of the vertebral artery during the acute stage. J Neurosurg 99:960–966, 2003.

44. Hoh BL, Putman CM, Budzik RF, et al: Combined surgical and endovascular techniques of flow alteration to treat fusiform and complex wide-necked intracranial aneurysms that are unsuitable for clipping or coil embolization. J Neurosurg 95:24–35, 2001.

45. Lylyk P, Cohen JE, Ceratto R, et al: Combined endovascular treatment of dissecting vertebral artery aneurysms by using stents and coils. J Neurosurg 94:427–432, 2001.

74 Surgical Management of Intracerebral Hemorrhage

MANISH AGHI, CHRISTOPHER S. OGILVY, and BOB S. CARTER

EPIDEMIOLOGY

Intracerebral hemorrhage (ICH), or hemorrhage within the brain parenchyma, occurs with an incidence estimated to range from 15 to 35 cases per 100,000 people per year. The incidence is up to twice that of subarachnoid hemorrhage by some estimates. Each year, approximately 37,000 to 52,000 people in the United States have an ICH. The rate is expected to double during the next 50 years as a result of the increasing age of the population and changes in racial demographics. Only 38% of patients affected with ICH survive the first year.[1]

Six risk factors for ICH have been identified: age, male sex, race, hypertension, high alcohol intake, and low serum cholesterol. Regarding other possible risks, current or past smoking and diabetes mellitus are weak risk factors, if at all.[2] The incidence of ICH increases significantly after age 55 and doubles with each decade of age until the age of 80, at which point the incidence increases 25-fold during each decade.[3] ICH is more common in men than women. ICH also affects blacks and Japanese more than whites. During the 20-year period covered by the National Health and Nutrition Examination Survey Epidemiologic Follow-up Study, the incidence of ICH among blacks was 50 per 100,000, a little more than twice the incidence among whites.[4] It has been hypothesized that hypertension and factors leading to limited access to health care result in the higher incidence of ICH within the African-American community. The higher incidence of ICH in Japan has been attributed to a higher incidence of hypertension in Japanese populations and diets leading to low serum cholesterol, another risk factor for ICH. The reversibility of the dietary factor may lead to the reductions in ICH seen when Japanese people emigrate to the United States, whereas their persistent hypertension may explain why their rates never drop to the same level as whites even after they emigrate to the United States.

There have been 11 case-controlled studies on hypertension and risk of ICH, with all showing a positive association between hypertension and ICH. Hypertension is classified as high normal (systolic 130 to 139 or diastolic 85 to 89), stage I hypertension (systolic 140 to 159 or diastolic 90 to 99), stage II hypertension (systolic 160 to 179 or diastolic 100 to 109), or stage III hypertension (systolic > 180 or diastolic > 110). Suh and colleagues[5] found a relative risk of 2.2 for high normal, 5.3 for stage I hypertension, 10.4 for stage II hypertension, and 33 for stage III hypertension. Iribarren and colleagues[6] found for each one standard deviation increase in systolic blood pressure (18 mm Hg in men and 19 mm Hg in women) a relative risk of 1.14 in men and 1.17 in women. Leppala and colleagues[7] found a relative risk of 2.20 for systolic blood pressure 140 to 159 mm Hg and 3.78 for systolic blood pressure more than 160 mm Hg compared with systolic blood pressure less than 139 mm Hg. The correlation between blood pressure and ICH also leads to diurnal and seasonal variations in the onset of ICH. In general, ICH onset is usually during activity and rarely during sleep, which may be related to elevated blood pressure or increased cerebral blood flow. One study covering a decade of ICH cases in a Japanese city found that men 69 years of age and younger had a bimodal distribution of time of ICH onset, with an initial peak between 8:00 and 10:00 AM and a second, lower peak between 6:00 and 8:00 PM. Men 70 years of age or older and women of all ages exhibited only a single evening peak, between 6:00 and 10:00 PM.[8] Men exhibited peak ICH in winter and a trough in summer, whereas women had no seasonal patterns.[8] The incidence of ICH correlates with the daily times of blood pressure peaks in the sexes, and the ability of the autonomic nervous system to increase blood pressure during the winter may particularly affect men because they tend to work outdoors more often.

Alcohol consumption is a risk factor in both the short term and long term. During the 24 hours preceding an ICH, moderate alcohol consumption (41 to 120 g of ethanol, where one standard drink averages 12 g of ethanol) causes a 4.6 relative risk of ICH, whereas heavy alcohol consumption (>120 g of ethanol) causes an 11.3 relative risk of ICH. During the week preceding ICH, low (1 to 150 g of ethanol), moderate (151 to 300 g of ethanol), and heavy (>300 g of ethanol) alcohol consumption carry relative risks of 2.0, 4.3, and 6.5, respectively.[9] ICH in patients with high ethanol consumption tends to be lobar.[10] Ethanol promotes ICH by impairing coagulation and directly affecting the integrity of cerebral vessels.[10]

A counterintuitive finding has been the identification of low serum cholesterol as a risk factor for ICH. Iribarren and colleagues[6] found that for each one standard deviation increase in serum cholesterol (1.45 mmol/L in men and 1.24 mmol/L in women), there was a relative risk reduction of 0.84 in men and 0.92 in women. One potential mechanism may be that patients with low serum cholesterol may exhibit reduced consumption of animal products, and such patients will have reduced concentrations of arachidonic acid in their cell membranes.[11] Arachidonic acid is a vital structural component of the cell membranes of vascular endothelium and its metabolites are involved in regulation of vascular tone and repair of injured vascular endothelium.[11] Defects in this pathway may increase the risk of ICH. However, hypercholesterolemia is a proven risk factor for morbidities such as myocardial infarction that are far more common than ICH and should therefore be avoided.

ETIOLOGY

Depending on the underlying cause of bleeding, ICH is classified as either primary or secondary. Primary ICH, accounting for nearly 80% of all ICH cases, originates from the spontaneous rupture of small vessels damaged by chronic hypertension or amyloid angiopathy, more commonly the former. Secondary ICH occurs in a minority of patients with ICH in association with vascular abnormalities, tumors, cerebral infarction, or impaired coagulation. Although primary ICH from vessels damaged by chronic hypertension remains the most common etiology of ICH, secondary ICH from vascular abnormalities should always be investigated as a possible source because of the high risk of recurrent hemorrhage and the necessity of surgical or endovascular treatment to prevent recurrent hemorrhage. Underlying vascular abnormalities can be searched for using computed tomographic angiography (CTA) or digital subtraction angiography (DSA) when the combined opinion of the medical team and radiologist interpreting the computed tomography (CT) scan deems it necessary.

In primary ICH, the hemorrhage arises from vessels damaged by chronic hypertension or amyloid angiopathy. Chronic hypertension causes degenerative changes in the walls of small penetrating arteries originating from the anterior, middle, or posterior cerebral arteries. These changes reduce vessel compliance and increase the likelihood of spontaneous rupture. Patients with chronic hypertension incur an annual risk of recurrent ICH of 2%, but this risk can be reduced by treatment of hypertension.[12] In 1868, Charcot and Bouchard attributed ICH to rupture at points of dilation in the walls of small arterioles that they called microaneurysms.[13] These microaneurysms were later found to be subadventitial hemorrhages or extravascular clots resulting from endothelial damage by the hematoma. Electron microscopy studies have since suggested that most ICH occurs at or near the bifurcation of affected arteries, where prominent degeneration of the media presumably caused by chronic hypertension can be seen.

In amyloid angiopathy, β-amyloid protein, an acellular eosinophilic material, is deposited within the media of small and medium-sized arteries in the cerebral cortex and leptomeninges, which causes primary ICH in the white matter of the cerebral lobes, particularly the parietal and occipital areas, in persons older than 70 years of age who exhibit no evidence of systemic amyloidosis. These patients face an annual risk of recurrent hemorrhage of 10.5%.[14] Cerebral amyloid angiopathy is present in the brains of 50% of people older than the age of 70; however, most do not experience ICH. Amyloid angiopathy may be associated with genetic factors including the apolipoprotein E allele and may be more prevalent in patients with Down syndrome. O'Donnell and colleagues[14] reported that the presence of the ε2 or ε4 alleles of the apolipoprotein E gene was associated with a tripling of the risk of recurrent ICH among survivors of primary lobar ICH attributable to amyloid angiopathy. Among patients with lobar ICH, those with the apoE ε4 allele typically have their first ICH more than 5 years earlier than noncarriers, an average age of 73 versus 79,[15] and experience a statistically independent decrease in survival.[16] Although they are distinct

diseases, there is some overlap between amyloid angiopathy and Alzheimer's disease, in that the amyloid in amyloid angiopathy is identical to that found in the senile plaques of Alzheimer's disease and apolipoprotein ε4 is associated with both the parenchymal plaque amyloid seen in Alzheimer's disease and the deposits of β-amyloid protein in cerebral vessel walls seen in amyloid angiopathy. Cerebral amyloid angiopathy may increase the risk of ICH by potentiating plasminogen, a finding that may be of some relevance to patients receiving tissue plasminogen activator to treat myocardial infarcts or cerebrovascular accidents. Amyloid angiopathy can be diagnosed suggestively based on radiologic findings such as hemosiderin deposits from small cortical and subcortical petechial hemorrhages on gradient echo magnetic resonance imaging (MRI). Histologic findings include deposits of acellular eosinophilic material in the media of vessels in the hematoma or in noninvolved brain (Fig. 74-1). Perivascular microglia, thickened vessel walls, vessel dilatation, and microaneurysms are also seen in the vessels of patients with cerebral amyloid angiopathy. After staining with Congo red, the amyloid in the media of vessel walls exhibits apple-green birefringence under polarized light. A definitive diagnosis can be made based on all three of the following findings: lobar, cortical, or corticosubcortical ICH; severe cerebral amyloid angiopathy on histopathologic examination; and the absence of another diagnostic lesion. A probable diagnosis with supporting pathologic evidence occurs with all three of the following findings: lobar, cortical, or corticosubcortical ICH; some degree of vascular amyloid deposition on histopathologic exam; and absence of another diagnostic lesion. Probable amyloid angiopathy without pathologic evidence occurs with all three of the following findings: age over 60; a history of multiple hemorrhages in the lobar, cortical, or subcortical

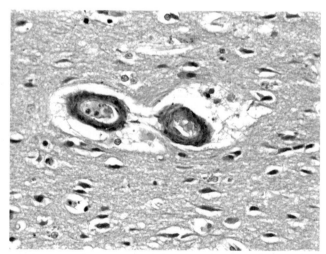

FIGURE 74-1 A pair of lobar intracerebral blood vessels from autopsy of a patient who experienced a lobar intracerebral hemorrhage with radiographic findings consistent with amyloid angiopathy. Shown here is peroxidase immunostaining using an antibody to the β-amyloid protein, an alternative to the Congo red staining that can also detect β-amyloid protein. Note that the β-amyloid protein localizes to the thickened media of both involved blood vessels, a typical finding in amyloid angiopathy. (Courtesy of Matthew P. Frosch, MD, PhD, Department of Neuropathology, Massachusetts General Hospital, Boston, MA.)

regions; and absence of another cause of hemorrhage. A diagnosis of possible amyloid angiopathy occurs with age over 60 combined with either a single lobar, cortical, or corticosubcortical hemorrhage without another cause or multiple hemorrhages with a possible but not a definitive cause.

Secondary ICH is far less common than primary ICH, but because the etiologies of secondary ICH include tumors and vascular malformations that will need surgical intervention or coagulopathies that need to be immediately corrected, attention must always be paid to secondary ICH as a possibility with any ICH. Tumors that produce ICH are usually malignant metastases. Hemorrhage is present in 3% to 14% of metastases and is most commonly seen in metastases from renal cell carcinoma, choriocarcinoma, melanoma, and thyroid cancer, with hemorrhage occurring in 70%, 50%, 40%, and 25% of the brain metastases from these respective primaries.[17] However, bronchogenic carcinoma represents the most common source of hemorrhagic cerebral metastases because, although only 9% of metastatic bronchogenic carcinomas undergo hemorrhage, it is a much more common metastasis than the other four tumor types. When ICH appears on an initial CT scan, the presence of nonhemorrhagic necrotic or hypodense tissue and pronounced surrounding vasogenic edema are radiologic clues to the underlying neoplasm and warrant an MRI with gadolinium to look for tumor. Vascular malformations that can give rise to secondary ICH are usually arteriovenous malformations (AVMs), with 81% of hemorrhages from AVMs having a significant intraparenchymal component. Cavernous malformations also tend to cause hemorrhage with a significant intraparenchymal component but only represent 10% of central nervous system vascular malformations. The diagnosis is strongly suggested by finding a mixed signal core indicative of old hemorrhage and a T2 dark rim on an MRI. ICH is unusual from aneurysmal rupture, which usually causes subarachnoid hemorrhage. Aneurysms that become adherent to the brain surface due to fibrosis from inflammation or previous hemorrhage can sometimes produce ICH rather than subarachnoid hemorrhage when they rupture. Oral anticoagulant therapy is a known source of secondary ICH. The relative risk of ICH during oral anticoagulant therapy increases more than 10-fold in patients over the age of 50.[18] Bleeding is more protracted and hematomas are larger in patients treated with anticoagulants than in those with spontaneous ICH.[19] The management of these patients requires rapid reversal of their coagulopathy. Vitamin K provides long-term reversal and stabilization of international normalized ratio, whereas fresh frozen plasma provides faster reversal. One study showed that 24 hours after administering 1000 mL of fresh frozen plasma, patients on Coumadin with ICH dropped their international normalized ratio (INR) from 3.35 to 1.40.[20] However, slightly less than one third of these patients experienced radiographic hematoma enlargement within 24 hours of their initial CT scan,[20] suggesting that the time that it takes fresh frozen plasma to reverse a coagulopathy may be too slow, particularly in elderly patients who cannot tolerate rapid administration of volume. A suggested alternative is prothrombin complex concentrate, which can counteract the effects of warfarin as early as 10 minutes in much smaller volumes than fresh frozen plasma.[20]

PATHOPHYSIOLOGY

Edematous parenchyma, often discolored by degradation products of hemoglobin, is visible adjacent to the clot and correlates with areas of CT and MRI T1 hypodensity and MRI T2 hyperdensity. Histologic sections are characterized by edema, neuronal damage, macrophages, and neutrophils in the region surrounding the hematoma. The hemorrhage spreads between planes of white matter, causing varying degrees of tissue destruction, leaving nests of intact neural tissue within and surrounding the hematoma. This pattern of spread accounts for the presence of viable and salvageable neural tissue in the immediate vicinity of the hematoma.

The presence of hematoma initiates edema and neuronal damage in the surrounding parenchyma. Animal models of ICH have identified three phases of perihematoma edema: immediate (within 24 hours), intermediate (24 hours to 5 days), and late onset (from 5 days to several weeks after ICH). Immediate edema occurs within the first 24 hours and can often be seen at a histologic but not radiographic level. This initial edema develops secondary to osmotically active plasma proteins accumulating in the extravascular space.[21] The blood-brain barrier is intact at this point, so the proteins most likely arise from the hematoma. After the initial hemorrhage, the clotting cascade activates thrombin, which disrupts the blood-brain barrier and activates the complement cascade, leading to lysis of red blood cells and other bystander cells. Vasogenic edema and cytotoxic edema subsequently follow owing to the disruption of the blood-brain barrier, the failure of the sodium pump, and the death of neurons.[22] This represents the intermediate edema seen at 24 hours to 5 days. This intermediate edema is noticeable radiographically and histologically. Red blood cell lysis releases hemoglobin and leads to formation of free radicals, which account for the late-onset edema. The role of the coagulation cascade in intermediate perihematoma edema may explain why ICH related to thrombolysis or coagulopathy causes less perihematoma edema than spontaneous ICH.

Studies in animals and humans have refuted the notion that cerebral ischemia in areas of ICH occurs due to mechanical compression by the hematoma and have suggested that secondary mediators may cause the delayed development of neuronal injury adjacent to a hematoma.[21] It is currently thought that blood products mediate most secondary processes initiated after ICH.[23] Recent evidence has suggested the presence of apoptosis or programmed cell death in neurons adjacent to ICH associated with nuclear factor-kB expression in neuronal nuclei.[24]

PRESENTATION BY LOCATION

ICH commonly occurs in the cerebral white matter (10% to 20%); basal ganglia, usually the putamen but also including the lenticular nucleus, internal capsule, and globus pallidus (50%); thalamus (15%); the pons (10% to 15%); other brain stem sites (1% to 6%); and the cerebellum (10%). Common arterial feeders of ICHs are the lenticulostriate branches of the anterior and middle cerebral arteries, which form Charcot-Bouchard microaneurysms and are the source of putaminal ICH; thalamoperforators branching off the anterior and middle cerebral arteries, which are the source of thalamic

ICH; and paramedian branches of the basilar artery, which are the source of pontine and cerebellar ICH.

ICH into the cerebral white matter includes ICH into the occipital, temporal, frontal, and parietal lobes, including ICH arising from the cortex and subcortical white matter, as opposed to ICH of deep structures such as the basal ganglia, thalamus, and infratentorial structures. Frontal lobe ICH causes frontal headache with contralateral hemiparesis, usually in the arm with mild leg and facial weakness. Parietal lobe ICH causes contralateral hemisensory deficit with mild hemiparesis. Occipital lobe ICH causes ipsilateral eye pain and contralateral homonymous hemianopsia, with some sparing of the superior quadrant. Temporal lobe ICH can be asymptomatic on the nondominant side, but, on the dominant side, produces fluent dysphasia with poor auditory comprehension but relatively good repetition. Lobar ICH is more likely to be associated with structural abnormalities such as AVMs or tumors than deep hemorrhages. Lobar ICH is also more common in patients who consume alcohol. In one study, significant independent risk factors for lobar ICH included the presence of an apoE ε2 or ε4 allele, frequent alcohol use, previous stroke, and first-degree relative with ICH, whereas significant independent risk factors for nonlobar ICH were hypertension, previous stroke, and first-degree relative with ICH,[25] suggesting different etiologies for lobar ICH than the other locations of ICH. Lobar ICH may also have a more benign outcome than basal ganglia and thalamic ICH.

In putaminal ICH, 62% of the patients experience smooth gradual deterioration with only 30% exhibiting their maximal deficit at the onset. In some studies, the 30-day mortality rate has been 50%.[26] The clinical presentation of putaminal hemorrhage may vary from relatively minor pure motor hemiparesis to profound weakness, sensory loss, eye deviation, hemianopsia, aphasia, and depressed level of consciousness. Headache is a presenting symptom in only 14% of putaminal ICHs. In putaminal ICH, intraventricular extension portends a poor prognosis because the hematoma must be quite large to track through the internal capsule and reach the ventricle.

Thalamic ICH usually causes contralateral hemisensory loss out of proportion to any weakness. Hemiparesis can ensue when the internal capsule becomes involved. Extension into the upper brain stem can cause vertical gaze palsy, retraction nystagmus, skew deviation, loss of convergence, ptosis, miosis, and anisocoria. Nearly 30% of patients with thalamic ICH present with headache. Hydrocephalus may result from obstruction of cerebrospinal fluid reabsorption pathways. In a series of 41 patients with thalamic ICH, all with a hemorrhage diameter greater than 3.3 cm on CT died, with smaller hematomas causing permanent disability.

Patients with supratentorial ICH involving the putamen, caudate, or thalamus have contralateral sensorimotor deficits of varying severity due to involvement of the internal capsule. Higher level cortical dysfunction, including neglect, gaze deviation, hemianopsia, and, for dominant hemisphere lesions, aphasia, can occur as a result of disruption of connecting fibers in the subcortical white matter and functional suppression of overlying cortex, known as diaschisis.[27]

Any deep, large hematoma can extend into the ventricles causing intraventricular hemorrhage. Common nonspecific initial symptoms include headache and vomiting due to increased intracranial pressure (ICP) and meningismus resulting from blood in the ventricles. As any hematoma becomes larger, patients will exhibit a decreased level of consciousness due to increased ICP and direct compression or distortion of the thalamic and brain stem reticular activating system. Small, deep lesions can occasionally impair consciousness due to decreased central benzodiazepine receptor binding on cortical neurons.[28]

Cerebellar ICH can cause a patients' level of consciousness to progress from impaired to comatose due to direct compression of the brain stem, without any associated hemiparesis, unlike supratentorial ICH. Cerebellar ICH can present with the abrupt onset of vertigo, headache, vomiting, and inability to walk without any associated hemiparesis. Cranial nerve palsies are common, particularly an abducens palsy or peripheral facial palsy. In one study, at least two of the three characteristic clinical signs, appendicular ataxia, ipsilateral gaze palsy, and peripheral facial palsy, were present in 73% of cases of cerebellar ICH.[29]

EVALUATION

Initial evaluation is typically through a CT scan, which is rapid and easily demonstrates ICH as high-density material within the brain parenchyma. Although mass effect on adjacent brain is common, the tendency for the hemorrhage to dissect through brain tissue often results in less mass effect than would be anticipated from the size of the clot. Clot volume can be estimated by computer programs that allow one to outline the hematoma on each slice and then model the hematoma in three dimensions and estimate a volume, or it can be approximated using the established practice of the modified ellipsoid volume = $A \times B \times C/2$ where A, B, and C are the diameters of the clot in each of three orthogonal dimensions, with one of the dimensions, C, being superoinferior such that C = number of slices with hematoma × slice thickness.[30] Clot volume carries significant prognostic significance. One study demonstrated a much steeper dependence of mortality on clot volume for deep ICH than lobar ICH, consistent with the fact that deep areas of the brain are less able to accommodate large volumes. Hematomas were divided into small (≤ 30 cm^3), medium (30 to 60 cm^3), and large (≥ 60 cm^3). The 30-day mortalities for small, medium, and large hematomas were 23%, 60%, and 71%, respectively, for lobar ICH, compared to 7%, 64%, and 93%, respectively, for deep ICH.[31] The overall 30-day mortality was 39% for lobar ICH and 48% for deep ICH. Hematoma volume also correlates with risk of rehemorrhage, with one retrospective study showing that 39% of patients with ICH who experienced rehemorrhage had initial clot volumes ≥ 25 cm,[3] compared to only 23% of patients with ICH who did not experience rehemorrhage.[32]

MRI is not the initial study of choice, as it is more time consuming, makes it difficult to access a patient who may acutely deteriorate, and does not show blood well within the first few hours. MRI may, however, be useful later once a patient stabilizes to identify cerebral amyloid angiopathy, cavernous malformations, or underlying tumors. Gradient-echo MRI is the most useful modality for identifying ICH of various ages. Gradient-echo MRI increases the amount of signal dropout from deposits of iron representing residual blood products as a result of past hemorrhage. This increases the potential for detecting two findings that are typical of patients with cerebral amyloid angiopathy: (1) small previous punctuate petechial hemorrhages; and (2) previous lobar ICH, as manifested by a dark hemosiderin ring around an area of lobar encephalomalacia (Fig. 74-2). MRI has improved to the point that gradient echo can now detect ICH as early as 2.5 hours with 99.5% sensitivity.[33] However, the specificity of MRI is limited in the hyperacute stage.[34] Overall, MRI remains a secondary study compared with CT and is most useful when a CT scan has findings listed above that suggest an underlying lesion such as a tumor or cavernous malformation. In these cases, MRI with gadolinium can be used to search for enhancing areas consistent with tumor; MR spectroscopy can be used to identify areas with high choline peaks, an inverted lactate peak, and absence of creatinine and N-acetyl-aspartate peaks; or T2 MRI can show a central mixed density core suggesting old hemorrhages surrounded by a hypodense rim.

Cerebral angiography is used to identify AVMs and aneurysms in patients with ICH. In a prospective study in which 206 ICH cases were investigated with CT and angiography, angiographic yield was significantly higher in patients (1) 45 years of age or younger and (2) without preexisting hypertension.[35] Analysis of angiographic yield of different sites of hemorrhage taken together with these two factors showed that (1) lobar ICH had a 10% angiographic yield in patients older than 45 years of age with preexisting hypertension; (2) putaminal, thalamic, and posterior fossa hemorrhages in patients of all ages with preexisting hypertension had a 0% angiographic yield; (3) lobar ICH had a 65% angiographic yield in normotensive patients younger than 45; (4) putaminal, thalamic, and posterior fossa hemorrhages in normotensive patients younger than 45 had a 48%

angiographic yield; and (5) putaminal, thalamic, and posterior fossa hemorrhages in normotensive patients older than 45 had a 7% angiographic yield. Patients with isolated intraventricular hemorrhage had 63% yield in the older and 67% yield in the younger groups. Taken together, these findings led the authors to recommend digital subtraction angiography in patients with ICH except those older than 45 who also have preexisting hypertension and thalamic, putaminal, or posterior fossa hemorrhages. In the future, the safer and more rapid technique of 3-dimensional computed tomographic angiography may replace digital subtraction angiography. Computed tomographic angiography involves a head CT scan with thin 2.5-mm axial cuts occurring 5 seconds after administering a 45-mL contrast bolus at 7 mL/second. Imaging software programs, which reformat the axial cuts and subtract out all but the contrast and adjacent brain tissue, are used to generate 3-dimensional images of the cerebral circulation. Preliminary studies have shown that CT angiography (CTA) is 95% as sensitive and just as specific as digital subtraction angiography in the detection of cerebral aneurysms,[36] a gap that is expected to close as CTA technology improves.

ACUTE REHEMORRHAGE

Although it was initially believed that ICH was largely a monophasic event that stopped quickly as a result of clotting and tamponade by the surrounding regions, a number of investigators have shown that rehemorrhage is common, with one study of 627 patients with ICH showing a 14.0% rehemorrhage rate within 24 hours of admission.[37] Brott and colleagues[38] found that the hematoma expanded in 26% of patients with ICH within 1 hour of the initial CT scan and in another 12% within 20 hours. Expansion has been attributed to continued bleeding from the primary source and to the mechanical disruption of surrounding vessels from compression by the hematoma. Acute hypertension after the initial ICH, a local coagulation deficit, or both may be associated with expansion of hematoma.[39]

Factors associated with rehemorrhage in the initial 24-hour period include: (1) a history of brain infarction; (2) liver disease; (3) uncontrolled diabetes; (4) systolic blood pressure on admission more than 195; (5) a history of alcohol abuse; (6) coagulation abnormalities; (7) a hematoma more than 25 cm³ on the initial CT scan; (8) irregular hematoma shape because irregularly shaped hematomas seem to indicate active bleeding from multiple sources; (9) a large peripheral white cell count; and (10) elevated body temperature on admission.[37] Computed tomographic angiography performed within 12 hours of the ICH revealing extravasation of contrast predicts rehemorrhage on a 24-hour post-ICH CT scan with 60% specificity and 100% sensitivity.[40]

Systolic blood pressure control using an arterial line and intravenous drips of antihypertensives like nitroprusside remains the primary medical intervention designed to prevent rehemorrhage. Recommendations written by a panel of experts commissioned by the American Heart Association in 1999 are to maintain the mean arterial blood pressure below 130 mm Hg (systolic < 180 and/or diastolic < 105) in patients with a history of chronic hypertension,[41] but therapeutic trials are needed. In patients with elevated ICP documented by an ICP monitor, cerebral perfusion pressure should be kept above 70 mm Hg.

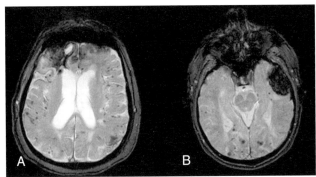

FIGURE 74-2 Axial magnetic resonance imaging (MRI) susceptibility pulse sequence images of the brain from patients shows findings consistent with amyloid angiopathy. *A,* This 74-year-old man presented with mental status changes. MRI susceptibility identified extensive areas of punctate darkness in both cerebral hemispheres, consistent with hemosiderin deposition from previous punctate petechial hemorrhages and cystic encephalomalacia with gliosis in right frontal lobe, consistent with a previous lobar intracerebral hemorrhage (ICH). The combination of these two findings is consistent with cerebral amyloid angiopathy. *B,* The susceptibility pulse sequences on this 82-year-old man with confusion, headache, and speech difficulty show a 3 × 2 × 3-cm anterior left temporal hypodensity, which was also hypointense on T1 and T2 (not shown), consistent with acute lobar ICH and numerous punctate foci of abnormal signal dropout throughout the right and left cerebral hemispheres, concentrated in the occipital, parietal, and temporal lobes. The findings are consistent with hemosiderin deposits from multiple foci of chronic hemorrhage, likely secondary to amyloid angiopathy. (Courtesy of Stuart R. Pomerantz, MD, Department of Neuroradiology, Massachusetts General Hospital, Boston, MA.)

MEDICAL MANAGEMENT

Whether ICH is best managed surgically or medically remains a subject of considerable debate. Regardless of which therapy is chosen, the goal is improvement in function, an objective that is based on the concept of a penumbra around ICH. There is now mounting evidence that there is a penumbra of functionally impaired, but potentially reversible, neuronal injury surrounding a hematoma. Adjacent brain tissue is displaced and compressed by extravasated blood. Animal models have shown that compression causes edema, ischemia, and hemorrhagic necrosis at the margin of the clot.[42] The volume of this penumbra may exceed the volume of the ICH severalfold. Single photon emission CT studies have confirmed that the penumbra tissue exhibits reversible ischemia.

We admit all patients with ICH to the neurologic intensive care unit. An arterial line is placed and systolic blood pressure is kept between 100 and 140 mm Hg using intravenous antihypertensives. Traditional medical measures used in the treatment of ICH include therapies that directly or indirectly treat intracranial pressure (ICP) such as mannitol, external ventricular drainage, and antiepileptics; therapies that protect the penumbra adjacent to the ICH such as maintaining normal blood sugars and body temperature; and administration of hemostatic agents to reduce the incidence or rehemorrhage.

Mannitol has been shown to improve mortality in patients with ICH, primarily by acting as an osmotic agent that lowers ICP caused by the hematoma.[43] Because of issues of mannitol failure and rebound increases in ICP, new osmolar agents have been investigated, including hypertonic saline, which can be given in 30-mL boluses of 23.4% saline as needed for refractory ICP documented via an ICP monitor. Such treatments can lower ICP, with the effect lasting 15 hours in our experience. Randomized studies are needed for these alternative osmolar agents.

External ventricular drains (EVDs) are placed for ICH cases with associated intraventricular hemorrhage that has led to an obstructive hydrocephalus. Unfortunately, in the presence of a large amount of intraventricular hemorrhage, the EVD will fill with blood, which will clot and occlude the EVD frequently. For these cases, we administer 5 mg of intraventricular tissue plasminogen activator twice daily for 5 days, in a fashion similar to that of previous reports.[44] After each administration, the EVD is clamped for 30 minutes if the ICP transduced by the EVD does not elevate to prevent the tissue plasminogen activator from leaking out of the ventricles. We have experienced no complications from the use of intraventricular tissue plasminogen activator in at least two dozen patients to treat EVDs occluded with blood products, although it is not our policy to use this therapy in the presence of an unsecured vascular lesion.

Convulsive seizures occur in 5% to 10% of patients with supratentorial ICH. Because seizures increase ICP, prophylactic antiepileptic medications are given to patients with lobar ICH, the group of patients with ICH at the greatest seizure risk. The 1999 American Heart Association guidelines acknowledge the lack of good data but recommend that prophylactic antiepileptic medication be given to patients with lobar ICH.[41] The antiepileptic may be tapered off after 1 month if no seizures are documented during that period.

Fever of 37.5°C or higher is seen in more than 90% of patients with supratentorial ICH.[45] The incidence, duration, and magnitude of fever are even greater in patients with ventricular hemorrhage.[45] The duration of fever is associated with poor long-term outcome.[45] Therefore, we aggressively treat fever with acetaminophen and cooling blankets, targeting a temperature of 37.5°C or less.

Hyperglycemia in patients without diabetes and worsening of baseline blood sugars in patients with diabetes both occur after ICH.[46] Regardless of whether there is preexisting diabetes, hyperglycemia is a predictor of poor outcome after supratentorial ICH.[46] We use intravenous insulin infusions titrated to maintain a blood glucose between 80 and 110 mg/dL rather than treating high blood glucose levels with subcutaneous insulin based on a sliding scale. Although this type of strict blood sugar control has been shown to reduce mortality, particularly due to septic end-organ failure in surgical intensive care units,[47] a study focusing on the outcomes associated with strict blood sugar control in neurosurgical patients is still needed.

Given the evidence that ongoing bleeding can occur for several hours after the onset of ICH, it is plausible that ultraearly hemostatic therapy may minimize hematoma volume and improve outcome by preventing early worsening related to hematoma growth and late deterioration related to perihematoma edema and mass effect. Replacement therapies such as fresh frozen plasma, prothrombin complex concentrate, and factor IX concentrate are used to treat bleeding in patients with coagulopathy with ICH, such as those who take Coumadin, but would not enhance hemostasis in patients with normal coagulation. Human and recombinant factors VIII and IX are used as replacement therapy for patients with hemophilia A or B, respectively, but, similarly, a strong procoagulant effect in patients with normal levels of these factors would not be expected. Cryoprecipitate enhances hemostasis in patients with hypofibrinogenemia, and desmopressin diacetate arginine vasopressin is used in patients with primary or acquired platelet disorders. In patients with normal coagulation, the most feasible hemostatic agents for ultraearly ICH therapy include the antifibrinolytic amino acids aminocaproic acid and tranexamic acid, aprotinin, and activated recombinant factor VII. The amino acids have a risk of cerebral ischemia, whereas aprotinin can cause hypersensitivity reactions and arterial or venous thrombosis, so attention in patients with ICH has focused on factor VII. Factor VIII, of which only 1% circulates in the active form, forms a complex with exposed tissue factor in the subendothelial layer of a damaged vessel wall, activating the hemostatic mechanism locally to form a hemostatic plug. Pharmacologic doses of recombinant factor VII have been shown to amplify this process.

Agents that have shown promise in the laboratory whose benefit remains to be proven clinically include neuroprotectants such as the γ-aminobutyric acid antagonist muscimol and the N-methyl-D-aspartate receptor antagonists MK801 and D-(E)-4-(3-phosphonoprop-2-enyl)-piperazine-2-carboxylic acid (D-CPP-ene), which have been shown to increase tolerance of larger hematomas, reduce edema 24 hours after ICH, and protect adjacent white matter in animal models.[48]

There are other medical agents that some have suggested for ICH but have not proven to be beneficial. A randomized study following 93 patients with ICH showed no statistical difference in neurologic outcome in patients who received Decadron, with the group receiving Decadron exhibiting 11 times more complications than the control group, including hyperglycemia, septicemia, and gastrointestinal bleeding.[49]

Hyperventilation is not recommended for patients with ICH because homeostatic mechanisms adjust to the lowered pH rapidly and the cerebral vasoconstriction causes increased ischemia and worse outcomes.

Parenchymal ICP monitors are infrequently used in our institution for ICP monitoring because we prefer to place ventricular catheters in those situations (particularly ICH associated with intraventricular hemorrhage) in which the combination of ICP monitoring and ventricular drainage to reduce ICP can be useful. In addition, a focal parenchymal ICP monitor can lend a false sense of security in that a hematoma typically causes a variety of focal pressure gradients, such that the pressure transduced in the right frontal lobe, where the monitor is typically placed, will not always reflect the pressure near the hematoma or in the brain stem.

MEDICAL VERSUS SURGICAL MANAGEMENT

There are relatively few randomized clinical trials on which the choice of medical versus surgical management of ICH can be based. The vast majority of studies comparing medical and surgical management of ICH have been retrospective, meaning that they are limited by biases inherent in the retrospective methodology. A total of seven prospective, randomized trials have compared surgical and medical treatment of ICH. The number of patients enrolled in these trials ranged from 20 to 180 in six smaller, earlier trials and culminated in 1033 patients enrolled in the largest trial, the International Surgical Trial in Intracerebral Hemorrhage (STICH), the results of which were released in January 2005. The results of all seven trials are summarized in Table 74-1. The two earliest trials, released in 1961 and 1989, showed better outcomes with medical treatment, while four subsequent trials, released in 1989, 1990, 1998, and 1999, all showed somewhat better outcomes with surgical treatment. This suggests that improvements in surgical technologies were rendering surgical treatment preferable in some cases. The STICH trial reported by Mendelow and colleagues[83] showed that surgical intervention within 24 hours of randomization offered no benefit in survival or prognosis-based indices for patients with lobar, basal ganglia, or thalamic ICH measuring greater than 2 cm in diameter and a Glasgow Coma

Score (GCS) of 5 or more. Analysis of subgroups defined by age, GCS, ICH laterality, ICH location, ICH volume, distance from cortical surface, method of evacuation, motor and speech deficits, anticoagulant treatment, and country found that the only subgroups to show heterogeneity of outcome were those defined by distance of the ICH from the cortical surface, with a favorable outcome from early surgery more likely if the hematoma was 1 cm or less from the cortical surface (absolute benefit 8%; p = 0.02). Of note is the fact that of patients randomized to initial conservative treatment, 26% went on to require surgery a few days after randomization due to clinical deterioration, and the outcome for this group was poorer than for patients who had early surgery or who were maintained on conservative management. Thus the STICH trial suggests that a significant benefit for early operative intervention existed only for patients with superficial hematomas. For deeper ICH, until factors are identified that predict which patients will go on to experience clinical deterioration, the results of the STICH trial suggest that operative intervention should be reserved for patients who experience clinical deterioration, at which time surgery will improve outcomes relative to not operating but will unfortunately not restore outcomes to what they would have been had the deterioration not occured.

Overall, there remains considerable variability in ICH management among physicians worldwide. Recently reported operation rates for spontaneous supratentorial ICH spanned a wide range, including 2% in Hungary, 20% in the United States, 50% in Germany and Japan, and 74% in Lithuania.[50]

The choice of intervention is influenced by the location of the ICH. We routinely operate on lobar ICH associated with a structural lesion such as an AVM or tumor that is surgically accessible in noneloquent cortex. In stable patients, we avoid operating on dominant hemisphere lobar ICH near Broca's or Wernicke's area. Operations are also performed on otherwise healthy patients with large lobar ICH who are clinically deteriorating.

The basal ganglia is the most common site of ICH, representing 60% of hypertensive ICHs, and basal ganglia ICH is associated with a 50% mortality rate.[26] The majority of these basal ganglia hemorrhages occur in the putamen. In an early study by Kanaya and Kuuoda,[51] patients who received medical treatment for basal ganglia hemorrhages less than 30 mL in

---

TABLE 74-1 ▪ Summary of Prospective, Randomized, Controlled Trials Comparing Surgery with Medical Treatment for Intracerebral Hemorrhage

| | | | | No. of Patients | | Outcome at 6 Months | | | | | |
| | | | | | | % of Patients Independent | | % of Patients Dependent | | % Dead | |
Ref.	Year	ICH Location	Surgery Method	M	S	M	S	M	S	M	S
McKissock et al.[79]	1961	All	Craniotomy	91	89	34	20	15	15	51	65
Juvela et al.[80]	1989	All	Craniotomy	26	26	19	4	42	50	39	46
Auer et al.[53]	1989	All	Endoscopic	50	50	26	44	4	14	70	42
Batjer et al.[81]	1990	Putamen	Craniotomy	9	8	22	25	0	25	78	50
Morgenstern et al.[60]	1998	Lobar and putamen	Craniotomy	17	17	41	35	35	47	24	18
Zucarrello et al.[82]	1999	All	Craniotomy	11	9	36	56	36	22	18	22
Mendelow et al.[83]	2005	All	All	530	503	N/S	N/S	N/S	N/S	37	36

ICH, intracerebral hemorrhage; M, medical treatment; S, surgery; N/S, not stated.

volume fared better than those treated surgically. A follow-up study by Tan and colleagues[52] randomized 34 patients with basal ganglia hematomas greater in volume than 30 mL into surgical and nonsurgical treatment groups. No difference in outcome was reported at 1-year follow-up. Although stereotactic and endoscopic techniques minimize surgical morbidity from basal ganglia hematoma evacuation, Auer and colleagues[53] failed to demonstrate any benefit from stereotactically guided endoscopic basal ganglia hematoma evacuation. While recent studies[54–56] have shown that stereotactic aspiration of basal ganglia hematomas can aspirate more than 80% of the hematoma, this volume reduction has not proven to be of benefit, perhaps due to the ability of residual blood products to trigger persistent and consequential perihematoma edema. In the end, complete surgical clot evacuation through open craniotomy may prove beneficial if the proper

patient group is selected, and the surgery is performed by a group experienced in the surgical approach to the basal ganglia. A study by Kaya and colleagues[56] 2 years after the study by Tan and colleagues compared conservative medical treatment with open craniotomy for putaminal hematomas of more than a 30-mL volume. The surgical group had 34% mortality at 6 months, compared with 63.1% in the medically treated group. When subdivided by initial neurologic grade, patients in stupor or semicoma without herniation signs fared better with nonsurgical treatment, whereas patients in semicoma with herniation signs fared better with surgical treatment. The more favorable results for surgery obtained by Kaya and colleagues compared with those of Tan and colleagues may reflect improved ability to evacuate basal ganglia hematomas safely through open craniotomies during the 2 years that transpired between the studies. Figure 74-3 illustrates results

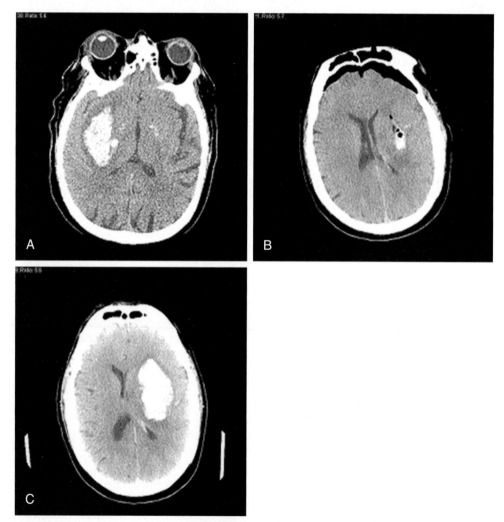

FIGURE 74-3   Management of hypertensive basal ganglia hemorrhages based on the size of the clot and other radiographic and clinical findings. Kaya and colleagues[56] suggest that patients with basal ganglia hematomas larger than 30 cm^3 who exhibit diminished mental status and radiographic signs of herniation fare better with surgical rather than medical treatment. *A* and *B*, A 62-year-old man with a history of hypertension presented with right hemiparesis and aphasia. Computed tomography (CT) scan (*A*) identified a left basal ganglia hemorrhage measuring 6 cm anteroposterior (AP) × 3 cm left to right (LR) × 8 cuts or 4 cm superoinferior (SI) = 144 cm^3, causing a 9-mm midline shift, and effacement of the cisterns. We went to the operating room and evacuated the hematoma, through a left frontal craniotomy, eliminating much of the midline shift and herniation (*B*), consistent with the recommendations of Kaya and colleagues.[56] Unfortunately, the patient succumbed to an aspiration pneumonia 45 days after his surgery. *C*, A 69-year-old man with a history of hypertension presented with left arm weakness but intact mental status. CT scan (*C*) identified a right basal ganglia hemorrhage measuring 5 cm (AP) × 2 cm (LR) × 7 cuts (3.5 cm SI) = 35 cm^3 causing a 2-mm midline shift with no cisternal effacement. He was managed conservatively, consistent with the recommendations of Kaya and colleagues,[56] and remains awake and conversant with stable left arm weakness.

when we used an algorithm similar to that followed by Kaya and colleagues in the management of two different basal ganglia hematomas.

Thalamic ICH is almost always managed medically with external ventricular drain placement when third ventricular outlet obstruction is present. Anatomically, the thalamus is difficult to access safely. There is a high risk of causing neurologic deficits from the parietal lobe, internal capsule, or transcallosal transventricular dissection when approaching thalamic hematomas. Regardless of whether the approach is open craniotomy, stereotactic, or endoscopic, the risk of damaging adjacent functional thalamic tissue often precludes a surgical approach. The only study comparing surgical versus medical treatment for thalamic ICH showed no benefit to endoscopic evacuation compared with medical treatment.[53]

Most patients with pontine hematoma are managed conservatively due to the difficulty achieving safe surgical access to the brain stem and the morbidity associated with the brain stem manipulation required for hematoma evacuation. The mortality from pontine ICH is estimated to be approximately 18% during hospitalization[57] and 69% at 1 year.[58] The majority of mortalities are associated with hypertensive pontine ICH and large paramedian pontine ICH, with pontine ICH from cavernous malformation and lateral tegmental pontine ICH having a better outcome.[57,58] Uncontrolled case series have documented successful stereotactic aspiration of pontine hematomas, but the effect on outcomes remains uncertain.

Cerebellar ICH is unique in that the posterior fossa is unable to tolerate large changes in volume without causing significant brain stem compression, which can lead to rapid, often fatal deterioration. A second source of morbidity and mortality in these patients is hydrocephalus when the hematoma compresses the fourth ventricle. Although the use of external ventricular drainage would seem a reasonable, less invasive means of addressing the hydrocephalus, there is concern of upward cerebellar herniation and rostral brain stem compression if surgical decompression of the posterior fossa is not performed simultaneously. Cohen and colleagues[59] studied 37 patients with cerebellar ICH and found that patients with hematomas less than 3 cm in maximal diameter had 100% good outcomes, compared with 57% of these patients who underwent surgery. On the other hand, patients with hematomas larger than 3 cm in maximal diameter who were not operated on immediately had a good outcome in only 33% of cases, compared with a good outcome in 50% of surgical patients with hematomas of this size.[59] Other studies have confirmed 3 cm in diameter as the recommended threshold for surgical intervention for cerebellar hematomas (Fig. 74-4), with an EVD placed if hydrocephalus is present.

Regarding the timing of surgery, Morgenstern and colleagues[60] demonstrated improved neurologic function regardless of hematoma location if patients with ICH were operated on within 12 hours of the onset of symptoms. In a follow-up study evaluating ultraearly surgery at less than 4 hours after the onset of symptoms, they found an increased rehemorrhage rate associated with increased mortality, with rebleeding occurring in 40% of the patients operated on within 4 hours compared with 12% of the patients operated on at 12 hours.[61] These results suggest that the optimal timing

for surgical clot evacuation may be within the 4- to 12-hour window after symptoms begin.

As a result of the paucity of data at the time, guidelines for ICH management written in 1999 by a panel of experts commissioned by the American Heart Association were largely limited to grade C recommendations based on case series and nonrandomized cohort studies.[41] The only grade A or B recommendations (based on randomized trials) were to use head CT for ICH diagnosis; to avoid corticosteroid therapy for ICH; to avoid surgical evacuation in patients with a Glasgow Coma Scale score of 4 or less, or ICH volume below 10 cm³; and to consider surgical evacuation in young patients with moderate or large lobar hemorrhages who are clinically deteriorating. Surgical evacuation was recommended for the following three categories of patients: (1) patients with cerebellar hemorrhages greater than 3 cm in diameter who have brain stem compression and hydrocephalus or who are neurologically deteriorating (grade C recommendation); (2) ICH associated with a structural lesion such as an AVM or tumor that is surgically accessible (grade C recommendation); and (3) young patients with moderate or large lobar ICH who are clinically deteriorating (grade B recommendation). The degree of neurologic deterioration must also be considered before recommending surgery, as one study of lobar ICH evacuated in patients with a mental status of stupor or worse or midline shift greater than 1 cm with cisternal obliteration showed that 22% of operated patients regained independence afterward, 22% remained severely disabled, and 56% died.[62] All patients who had absent papillary, corneal, or oculocephalic reflexes combined with extensor posturing died, indicating a level of severity beyond salvage surgically.

SPECIFIC SURGICAL TECHNIQUES

Craniotomy

Lobar hemorrhages are evacuated using craniotomies and corticectomies centered over the hematoma, with sparing of eloquent tissue. The head should be positioned so that the trajectory to the clot is as vertical as possible. Self-retaining brain retractors are attached to the Mayfield fixation device. After the corticectomy, superficial hematomas can be accessed by using a combination of bipolar cautery and small suction tips until the hematoma cavity is entered. Once in the hematoma, tumor forceps or a pituitary biter can be used to remove solid portions of the hematoma. Semisolid portions of the hematoma can be removed using suction tips. Hemostasis can then be achieved with a combination of Avitene, hydrogen peroxide–soaked cotton balls, thrombin-soaked Gelfoam, and Surgicel. The systolic blood pressure can be increased 10 to 20 points before closure to identify any potential bleeding sources. The mass effect is typically relieved after hematoma removal, and the bone flap can be replaced. For deeper lobar hematomas, intraoperative ultrasonography can be used for hematoma localization and to verify complete removal of the hematoma. Ultrasonography can also be used to guide placement of a ventriculostomy catheter into the hematoma cavity. Self-retaining retractors can then be placed alongside the ventriculostomy and a 1-cm corticectomy can be opened down to the clot by following the ventriculostomy catheter, thereby minimizing damage to nearby cortex.

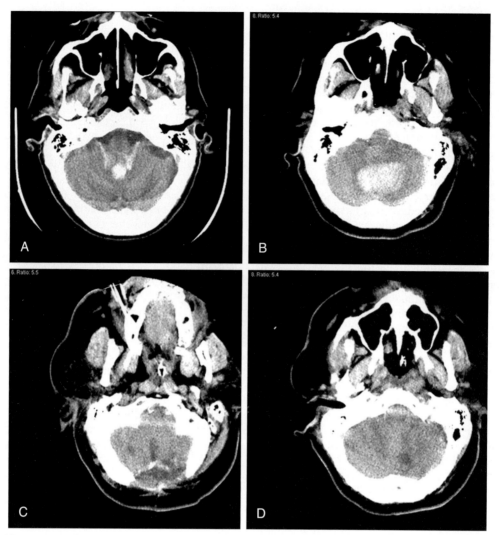

FIGURE 74-4 Management of cerebellar intracerebral hemorrhage (ICH) depends on the clinical status of the patient and the size of the blood clot. *A,* A 75-year-old man with a history of hypertension presented with headache, nausea, vomiting, and syncope. Head computed tomography (CT) identified a 1.7 cm (AP) × 1.5 cm (LR) × 2 cuts (1 cm SI) vermian cerebellar hemorrhage extending into the fourth ventricle, causing moderate hydrocephalus. Because of his intact mental status and the hematoma was less than 3 cm in maximal diameter, he was managed medically with an admission to the ICU and an external ventricular drain placed for the hydrocephalus. The hydrocephalus subsequently resolved, the drain was discontinued, and he was discharged from the hospital 10 days later. *B* to *D,* A 65-year-old woman with a history of hypertension collapsed. She was unresponsive to painful stimuli with intact brain stem reflexes in the emergency department. A head CT (*B*) identified a 4.6 cm (AP) × 3.1 cm (LR) × 6 cuts (3 cm SI) cerebellar hematoma centered in the dentate nucleus but favoring the left over the right cerebellar hemisphere, causing moderate hydrocephalus. Because of her clinical condition, she was brought emergently to the operating room, where a suboccipital craniectomy (*C*) and cerebellar hematoma evacuation (*D*) were performed. Unfortunately, she did not regain neurologic function, and care was withdrawn by her family 1 week later. These two cases illustrate the finding documented before that 3 cm in maximal diameter is the cutoff after which cerebellar hematomas are likely to impair mental status and will likely require immediate surgery to have any chance for clinical improvement.[59]

For putaminal hemorrhages, two approaches can be used: transtemporal or transsylvian. The transsylvian approach involves a pterional craniotomy, sylvian dissection under the microscope, and a 0.5- to 1-cm long corticectomy along the insular cortical surface in an area determined by the largest and closest point of hematoma on the CT scan. This is followed by clot evacuation and hemostasis. In the hands of an experienced surgeon who can dissect the middle cerebral branches in the insular cortex, the transsylvian approach puts the smallest amount of brain at risk because the insular cortical point of entry is closest to the putamen.

For putaminal hematomas that extend significantly into the temporal lobe, the transtemporal approach can be used.

Thalamic and pontine hemorrhages are not evacuated with open craniotomies, due to the amount of intact cerebral tissue put at risk during such a procedure. The stereotactic or endoscopic procedures described below have been somewhat successful in evacuating pontine hemorrhages, but a benefit has yet to be shown in a large randomized trial.

Cerebellar hemorrhages are evacuated using a suboccipital craniotomy for medial hemorrhages or a paramedian straight incision for unilateral cerebellar hemorrhage. Because the posterior fossa has less room to accommodate any postoperative bleeding than supratentorial sites after evacuating lobar ICH, we prefer doing a suboccipital craniectomy and not restoring the bone, which better accommodates posterior fossa bleeding and swelling than a bone flap craniotomy, an advantage that often outweighs the disadvantage of craniectomy headaches. A ventriculostomy is placed to relieve hydrocephalus.

Stereotactic Aspiration

Benes and colleagues[63] first reported the use of stereotactic hematoma drainage in 1965, with limited success. With improvement in techniques, including administration of fibrinolytics, the success rate has improved. Although no randomized, prospective, controlled studies have compared stereotactic aspiration with craniotomy and conservative therapy, studies show favorable outcomes, especially with deep-seated lesions such as those in the basal ganglia or pons. Use of a stereotactic frame or endoscopy and frameless stereotaxy approaches described below are less invasive procedures than open craniotomies but still require that the patient be intubated if not already because patients with ICH often have too tenuous a mental status to tolerate the sedation and lack of airway access associated with awake stereotactic procedures. Honda and colleagues[64] retrospectively compared stereotactic aspiration and medical therapy for thalamic hemorrhage. Patients with hematomas smaller than 2.5 cm in diameter had significantly higher activities of daily living scores with aspiration. In another study, 71 patients with ICH were randomized into a group that received stereotactic aspiration and administration of urokinase and another group that received systemic medical management only.[55] Although stereotactic aspiration reduced hematoma volume by 18 mL over 7 days, compared with 7 mL of reduction in the control group, no difference in morbidity or mortality was noted at 180 days.[55] The volume reduction achieved by stereotactic aspiration may be less beneficial than the more complete hematoma evacuation achieved by a craniotomy because residual hematoma can still cause considerable edema and mass effect. To make hematomas more amenable to stereotactic aspiration, various techniques have been incorporated into the stereotactic hematoma drainage, including (1) repeated injection of urokinase or recombinant tissue plasminogen activator into the hematoma to liquefy the clot and render it amenable to subsequent aspiration and (2) equipment aimed at physical fragmentation of the clot like systems based on the Archimedes screw,[65] devices using high-pressure fluid irrigation,[66] ultrasonic aspirators,[67] or the Nucleotome probe.[68] The lack of direct visualization and the risk of rebleeding may still limit this technique to patients whose neurologic condition warrants drainage rather than medical treatment alone but whose hemorrhages are deep and whose overall medical condition precludes open craniotomy, especially during the hyperacute phase of hemorrhage. In fact, the inability to control intraoperative bleeding has led some to recommend that stereotactic aspiration only be performed subacutely, as late as 3 days after the onset of symptoms,[54] which would limit this procedure to patients with deep hematomas who can tolerate a delayed operation.

Endoscopy

Endoscopy represents another minimally invasive means of draining ICH, which, unlike stereotaxy, is not limited to the chronic stage of ICH. In a recent technical note, four pontine hematomas were removed using a 1.7-mm fiberscope placed through a burr hole 3 cm from the midline at the bregma.[69] After entering the third ventricle through the foramen of Monro, patients with acute hydrocephalus were treated by forming a third ventriculostomy, followed by slight dilation of the aqueduct of Sylvius. The guide tube was advanced into pontine areas found to have yellow discoloration. Hematoma was evacuated by repeated rinsing with physiologic saline. Hemostasis was achieved using a KTP laser. An external ventricular drain was left in place and flushed with 6000 U urokinase 3 hours after surgery. The urokinase must be administered because only liquid blood products could be washed out of the pons using the endoscope, and areas of clot had to be treated with intraventricular urokinase. The procedure typically took 1 hour. The advantages of endoscopic treatment over stereotaxy and open craniotomy were rapidity of the procedure and ability to treat associated hydrocephalus. The ability to anticoagulate is an additional advantage over stereotaxy.

Frameless Stereotaxy and Intraoperative Magnetic Resonance Imaging

Tyler and Mandybur[70] reported on 10 patients harboring intracerebral hematomas who were treated by frameless stereotactic means without fiducial markers. Using an intraoperative MRI scanner, these patients underwent frameless stereotactic evacuation of 70% to 90% of each clot, with no complications or rehemorrhages. All patients showed some improvement. Similarly, Bernays and colleagues[71] reported complete evacuation in 62% of their 13 patients with ICH treated with a specially designed artifact-free aspiration cannula using intraoperative MRI. No rebleeding was demonstrated and neurologic function improved in 11 of 12 patients.

LONG-TERM OUTCOME

Recently, Becker and colleagues[72] pointed out that the most important variable predicting poor outcome in patients with ICH is the level of provided medical support. Perception of futility of aggressive therapy leads to early withdrawal of medical support, which is less likely in patients with ICH who are surgically treated. It may be worth studying whether patients with ICH have better outcomes in high-volume centers that frequently treat patients with ICH medically and surgically, a phenomenon demonstrated in the operative management of unruptured aneurysms.[73]

Reported 30-day mortalities for lobar, basal ganglia, thalamic, pontine, and cerebellar ICH have been 13%, 50%, 23%, 13%, and 16%, respectively.[74,75] Lobar ICH has consistently been shown to have the lowest mortality and best long-term outcomes and basal ganglia ICH the worst.

One of the sources of debate in long-term post-ICH management remains the issue of when it is safe to resume anticoagulation. In one study, epidemiologic data from the medical literature was used to generate a Markov state transition decision model, in which effectiveness of therapy was measured in quality-adjusted life-years.[76] The authors found that, for patients with previous lobar ICH, withholding anticoagulation therapy indefinitely led to the best outcome regardless of the indication for anticoagulation, leading to an improvement of life expectancy by 1.9 quality-adjusted life-years. On the other hand, patients with deep interhemispheric ICH because of a lower risk of recurrent ICH due to the lack of amyloid angiopathy in this group should never receive anticoagulation for nonvalvular atrial fibrillation but should resume anticoagulation with aspirin when the risk of a thromboembolic event is moderately higher and with Coumadin when the risk of a thromboembolic event is in the highest range.

The overall long-term recurrence rate of ICH has been estimated to be 2.4% per year and is 3.8-fold higher after lobar ICH caused by cerebral amyloid angiopathy (Fig. 74-5) than it is with hypertensive deep ICH.[77] Factors that are positive predictors of recurrent hemorrhage include age greater than 65 and male sex.[78] Use of anticoagulation after ICH triples the risk of recurrent hemorrhage.[78]

CONCLUSION

ICH remains an area where clinicians have far too little evidence on which to base clinical decision making. The randomized clinical trials showed a trend that gradually became favorable to surgical management over time as the ability of surgeons to safely perform clot evacuation improved, but recently-released results of the STICH trial have raised questions about the role of early operative intervention. It remains to be definitely determined what subset of patients with ICH is best served by surgical evacuation. In the meantime, clinicians caring for patients with ICH must continue to

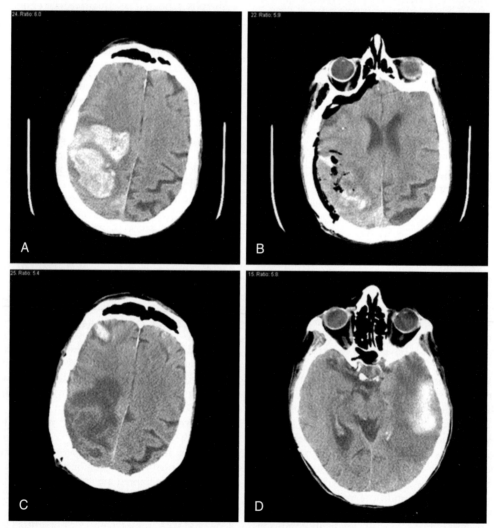

FIGURE 74-5 Amyloid angiopathy causes a high risk of recurrent intracerebral hemorrhage (ICH). A 77-year-old woman presented to our institution with left hemiparesis. A computed tomography (CT) scan (A) showed 7 cm (AP) × 6 cm (LR) × 11 cuts (5.5 cm SI) = 231 cm^3 right frontoparietal hematoma with surrounding edema, causing an 8-mm midline shift. She was brought to the operating room, where a right frontoparietal craniotomy enabled nearly complete hematoma evacuation and resolution of midline shift (B). Pathologic analysis of the clot confirmed the diagnosis of amyloid angiopathy. She was discharged from the hospital with some improvement in left-sided strength. Unfortunately, 1 month later, she was found unresponsive. A CT scan showed encephalomalacia in the area of the evacuated right frontoparietal hematoma and two new hematomas: a 1.8 cm (AP) × 0.7 cm (LR) × 3 cuts (1.5 cm SI) = 2 cm^3 right frontal hematoma (C) and a 4.9 cm (AP) × 1.9 cm (LR) × 7 cuts (3.5 cm SI) = 33 cm^3 left temporal hematoma (D). She was managed medically because her history of ICH and the bilateral nature of her most recent ICH meant that surgery would have a high morbidity. She remained unresponsive, and was eventually discharged to a nursing home after a tracheostomy.

make decisions regarding the treatment of this critically ill group of patients by combining clinical insights specific to the patient in question with the existing body of evidence.

REFERENCES

1. Dennis MS, Burn JP, Sanderock PA, et al: Long-term survival after first-ever stroke: The Oxfordshire Community Stroke Project. Stroke 24:796–800, 1993.
2. Ariesen MJ, Claus SP, Rinkel GJE, et al: Risk factors for intracerebral hemorrhage in the general population: A systematic review. Stroke 34:2060–2066, 2003.
3. Giroud M, Gras P, Chandan N, et al: Cerebral hemorrhage in a French prospective population study. J Neurol Neurosurg Psychiatry 54:595–598, 1991.
4. Qureshi AI, Giles WH, Croft JB: Racial differences in the incidence of intracerebral hemorrhage: Effects of blood pressure and education. Neurology 52:1617–1621, 1999.
5. Suh I, Jee SH, Kim HC, Appel LJ: Low serum cholesterol and hemorrhagic stroke in men: Korean Medical Insurance Corporation Study. Lancet 357:922–925, 2001.
6. Iribarren C, Jacobs DR, Sadler M, et al: Low total serum cholesterol and intracerebral hemorrhagic stroke: Is the association confined to elderly men? The Kaiser Permanente Medical Care Program. Stroke 27:1993–1998, 1996.
7. Leppala JM, Virtamo J, Fogelholm R, et al: Different risk factors for different stroke subtypes: Association of blood pressure, cholesterol, and antioxidants. Stroke 30:2535–2540, 1999.
8. Inagawa T: Diurnal and seasonal variations in the onset of primary intracerebral hemorrhage in individuals living in Izumo City, Japan. J Neurosurg 98:326–336. 2003.
9. Juvela S, Hillbom M, Palomaki H: Risk factors for spontaneous intracerebral hemorrhage. Stroke 26:1558–1564, 1995.
10. Monforte R, Estruch R, Graus F, et al: High ethanol consumption as risk factor for intracerebral hemorrhage in young and middle-aged people. Stroke 21:1529–1532, 1990.
11. Golfetto I, Min Y, Wang Y, et al: Serum cholesterol and hemorrhagic stroke. Lancet 358:508, 2001.
12. Furlan AJ, Whisnant JP, Elveback LR: The decreasing incidence of primary intracerebral hemorrhage: A population study. Ann Neurol 5:367–373, 1979.
13. Fisher CM: Pathological observations in hypertensive cerebral hemorrhage. J Neuropathol Exp Neurol 30:536–550, 1971.
14. O'Donnell HC, Rosand J, Knudsen KA, et al: Apolipoprotein E genotype and the risk of recurrent lobar intracerebral hemorrhage. N Engl J Med 342:240–245, 2000.
15. Greenberg SM, Rebeck GW, Vonsattel JPV, et al: Apolipoprotein E e4 and cerebral hemorrhage associated with amyloid angiopathy. Ann Neurol 38:254–259, 1995.
16. McCarron MO, Weir CJ, Muir KW, et al: Effect of apolipoprotein E genotype on in-hospital mortality following intracerebral haemorrhage. Acta Neurol Scand 107:106–109, 2003.
17. Weisberg, LA: Hemorrhagic metastatic intracranial neoplasms: Clinical-CT correlations. Comput Radiol 9:105–114, 1985.
18. Winzem AR, de Jonge H, Loelinger EA, et al: The risk of intracerebral hemorrhage during oral anticoagulant treatment: A population study. Ann Neurol 16:553–558, 1984.
19. Franke CL, deJonge J, van Swieten JC, et al: Intracerebral hemorrhage during anticoagulant treatment. Stroke 21:726–730, 1990.
20. Yasaka M, Minematsu K, Naritomi H, et al: Predisposing factors for enlargement of intracerebral hemorrhage in patients treated with warfarin. Thromb Haemost 89:278–283, 2003.
21. Zakulia AR, Diringer MN, Deredeyn CP, et al: Progression of mass effect after intracerebral hemorrhage. Stroke 30:1167–1173, 1999.
22. Wagner KR, Xi G, Hau Y, et al: Early metabolic alterations in edematous perihematomal brain regions following experimental intracerebral hemorrhage. J Neurosurg 88:1058–1065, 1998.
23. Lee KR, Kawai N, Kim S, et al: Mechanisms of edema formation after intracerebral hemorrhage: Effects of thrombin on cerebral blood flow, blood-brain barrier permeability, and cell survival in a rat model. J Neurosurg 86:272–278, 1997.
24. Hickenbottom SL, Grotta JC, Strong R, et al: Nuclear factor-kappaB and cell death after experimental intracerebral hemorrhage in rats. Stroke 30:2472–2477, 1999.
25. Woo D, Sauerbeck LR, Kissela BM, et al: Genetic and environmental risk factors for intracerebral hemorrhage: Preliminary results of a population-based study. Stroke 33:1190–1195, 2002.
26. Little KM, Alexander MJ: Medical versus surgical therapy for spontaneous intracranial hemorrhage. Neurosurg Clin N Am 13:339–347, 2002.
27. Tanaka A, Yoshinaga S, Nakayama Y, et al: Cerebral blood flow and clinical outcome in patients with thalamic hemorrhages: A comparison with putaminal hemorrhages. J Neurol Sci 144:191–197, 1996.
28. Hatazawa J, Shimosegawa E, Satoh T, et al: Central benzodiazepine receptor distribution after subcortical hemorrhage evaluated by mans of [123] iomazenil and SPECT. Stroke 26:2267–2271, 1995.
29. Ott KH, Kase CS, Ojemann RJ, et al: Cerebellar hemorrhage: Diagnosis and treatment: A review of 56 cases. Arch Neurol 31:160–167, 1974.
30. Kothari RU, Brott T, Broderick JP, et al: The ABCs of measuring intracerebral hemorrhage volumes. Stroke 27:1304–1305, 1996.
31. Broderick J, Brott T, Duldner J, et al: Volume of intracerebral hemorrhage: A powerful and easy-to-use predictor of 30-day mortality. Stroke 24:987–993, 1993.
32. Kazui S, Minematsu K, Yamamoto H, et al: Predisposing factors to enlargement of spontaneous intracerebral hematoma. Stroke 28:2370–2375, 1997.
33. Shellinger P, Jansen O, Fiebach JB, et al: A standardized MRI stroke protocol comparison with CT in hyperacute intracerebral hemorrhage. Stroke 30:765–768, 1999.
34. El-Koussy M, Guzman R, Bassetti C, et al: CT and MRI in acute hemorrhagic stroke. Cerebrovasc Dis 10:480–482, 2000.
35. Zhu XL, Chan MSY, Poon WS, et al: Spontaneous intracranial hemorrhage: Which patients need diagnostic cerebral angiography? A prospective study of 206 cases and review of the literature. Stroke 28:1406–1409, 1997.
36. Dehdashti AR, Rufenacht DA, Delavelle J, et al: Therapeutic decision and management of aneurysmal subarachnoid hemorrhage based on computed tomographic angiography. Br J Neurosurg 17:46–53, 2003.
37. Fujii Y, Takeuchi S, Sasaki O, et al: Multivariate analysis of predictors of hematoma enlargement in spontaneous intracerebral hemorrhage. Stroke 29:1160–1166, 1998.
38. Brott T, Broderick J, Kothari R, et al: Early hemorrhage growth in patients with intracerebral hemorrhage. Stroke 28:1–5, 1997.
39. Kazui S, Minematsu K, Yamamoto H, et al: Predisposing factors to enlargement of spontaneous intracerebral hematoma. Stroke 28:2370–2375, 1997.
40. Murai Y, Takagi R, Ikeda Y, et al: Three-dimensional computerized tomography angiography in patients with hyperacute intracerebral hemorrhage. J Neurosurg 91:424–431, 1999.
41. Broderick JP, Adams HP, Barsan W, et al: Guidelines for the management of spontaneous intracerebral hemorrhage: A statement for healthcare professionals from a special writing group of the Stroke Council, American Heart Association. Stroke 30:905–915, 1999.
42. Bullock R, Mendelow AD, Teasdale GM, et al: Intracranial hemorrhage induced at arterial pressure in the rat. Part 1: Description of technique, ICP changes, and neuropathological findings. Neurol Res 6:184–188, 1984.
43. Duff TA, Ayeni S, Levin AB, et al: Nonsurgical management of spontaneous intracerebral hematoma. Neurosurgery 9:387–393, 1981.
44. Goh KY, Poon WS: Recombinant tissue plasminogen activator for the treatment of spontaneous adult intraventricular hemorrhage. Surg Neurol 50:526–532, 1998.
45. Schwarz S, Hafner K, Aschoff A, et al: Incidence and prognostic significance of fever following intracerebral hemorrhage. Neurology 54:354–361, 2000.
46. Passero S, Ciacci G, Ulivelli M: The influence of diabetes and hyperglycemia on clinical course after intracerebral hemorrhage. Neurology 61:1351–1356, 2003.
47. van den Berghe G, Wouters P, Weekers F, et al: Intensive insulin therapy in critically ill patients. N Engl J Med 345:1359–1367, 2001.
48. Mendelow AD: Mechanisms of ischemic brain damage with intracerebral hemorrhage. Stroke 24(Suppl):115–117, 1993.
49. Poungvarin N, Bhoopat W, Viriyavekajul A: Effects of dexamethasone in primary supratentorial intracerebral hemorrhage. N Engl J Med 316:1229–1233, 1987.
50. Mendelow AD: International surgical trial in intracerebral hemorrhage: 668 patients randomized. J Neurosurg 96:186A–187A, 2002.
51. Kanaya H, Kuuroda K: Development in neurosurgical approaches to hypertensive intracerebral hemorrhage in Japan. In Kaufman HH (ed): Intracerebral Hematomas. New York: Raven Press Ltd., 1992.

52. Tan SH, Ng PY, Yeo TT, et al: Hypertensive basal ganglia hemorrhage: A prospective study comparing surgical and nonsurgical management. Surg Neurol 56:287–293, 2001.

53. Auer LM, Deinsberger W, Niederkorn K, et al: Endoscopic surgery versus medical treatment for spontaneous intracerebral hematoma: A randomized study. J Neurosurg 70:530–535, 1989.

54. Marquardt G, Wolff R, Siefert V: Multiple target aspiration technique for subacute stereotactic aspiration of hematomas within the basal ganglia. Surg Neurol 60:8–14, 2003.

55. Teernstra OPM, Evers SMAA, Lodder J, et al: Stereotactic treatment of intracerebral hematoma by means of a plasminogen activator—a multicenter randomized control trial (SICHPA). Stroke 34:968–974, 2003.

56. Kaya RA, Turkmenoglu O, Ziyal IM, et al: The effects on prognosis of surgical treatment of hypertensive putaminal hematomas through transsylvian transinsular approach. Surg Neurol 59:176–183, 2003.

57. Rabinstein AA, Tisch SH, McClelland RL, et al: Cause is the main predictor of outcome in patients with pontine hemorrhage. Cerebrovasc Dis 17:66–71, 2004.

58. Dziewas R, Kremer M, Ludemann P, et al: The prognostic impact of clinical and CT parameters in patients with pontine hemorrhage. Cerebrovasc Dis 16:224–229, 2003.

59. Cohen ZR, Ram Z, Knoller N, et al: Management and outcome of non-traumatic cerebellar hemorrhage. Cerebrovasc Dis 14:207–213, 2002.

60. Morgenstern LB, Frankowski RF, Shedden P, et al: Surgical treatment for intracerebral hemorrhage (STICH): A single-center, randomized clinical trial. Neurology 51:1359–1363, 1998.

61. Morgenstern LB, Demchuk AM, Kim DH, et al: Rebleeding leads to poor outcome in ultra-early craniotomy for intracerebral hemorrhage. Neurology 56:1294–1299, 2001.

62. Rabinstein AA, Atkinson JL, Wijdicks EF: Emergency craniotomy in patients worsening due to expanded cerebral hematoma: To what purpose? Neurology 58:1367–1372, 2002.

63. Benes V, Vladyka V, Zyverina E: Stereotaxic evacuation of typical brain hemorrhage. Acta Neurochir (Wien) 13:419–426, 1965.

64. Honda E, Hayashi T, Shimamoto H, et al: A comparison between stereotaxic operation and conservative therapy for thalamic hemorrhage. No Shinkei Geka 16(Suppl):665–670, 1988.

65. Nguyen JP, Decq P, Brugieres P, et al: A technique for stereotactic aspiration of deep intracerebral hematoma under computed tomographic control using a new device. Neurosurgery 24:814–819, 1992.

66. Mukai H, Yamashita J, Kitamura A, et al: Stereotactic aqua-stream and aspirator in the treatment of intracerebral hematoma. Stereotact Funct Neurosurg 57:221–227, 1991.

67. Hondo H, Uno M, Sasaki K, et al: Computed tomographic controlled aspiration surgery for hypertensive intracerebral hemorrhage: Experience of more than 400 cases. Stereotact Funct Neurosurg 54:432–437, 1990.

68. Kaufman HH: Treatment of deep spontaneous intracerebral hematomas. Stroke 24(Suppl 1):101–106, 1993.

69. Takimoto H, Iwaisako K, Kubo S, et al: Transaqueductal aspiration of pontine hemorrhage with the aid of a neuroendoscope. J Neurosurg 98:917–919, 2003.

70. Tyler D, Mandybur G: Interventional MRI-guided stereotactic aspiration of acute/subacute intracerebral hematomas. Stereotact Funct Neurosurg 72:129–135, 1999.

71. Bernays RL, Kollias SS, Romanowski B, et al: Near-real-time guidance using intraoperative magnetic resonance imaging for radical evacuation of hypertensive hematomas in the basal ganglia. Neurosurgery 47:1081–1090, 2000.

72. Becker KJ, Baxter AB, Cohen WA, et al: Withdrawal of support in intracerebral hemorrhage may lead to self-fulfilling prophecies. Neurology 56:766–772, 2001.

73. Barker FG, Amin-Hanjani S, Butler WE, et al: In-hospital mortality and morbidity after surgical treatment of unruptured intracranial aneurysms in the United States, 1996–2000: The effect of hospital and surgeon volume. Neurosurgery 52:995–1009, 2003.

74. Cheung RTF, Zou L-Y: Use of the original, modified, or new intracerebral hemorrhage score to predict mortality and morbidity after intracerebral hemorrhage. Stroke 34:1717–1722, 2003.

75. Salvati M, Cervoni L, Raco A, et al: Spontaneous cerebellar hemorrhage: Clinical remarks on 50 cases. Surg Neurol 55:156–161, 2001.

76. Eckman MH, Rosand J, Knudsen KA, et al: Can patients be anticoagulated after intracerebral hemorrhage? A decision analysis. Stroke 34:1710–1716, 2003.

77. Hill MD, Silver FL, Austin PC, et al: Rate of stroke recurrence in patients with primary intracerebral hemorrhage. Stroke 31:123–127, 2000.

78. Vermeer SE, Algra A, Franke CL, et al: Long-term prognosis after recovery from primary intracerebral hemorrhage. Neurology 59:205–209, 2002.

79. McKissock W, Richardson A, Taylor J: Primary intracerebral haemorrhage: A controlled trial of surgical and conservative treatment in 180 unselected cases. Lancet 2:221–226, 1961.

80. Juvela S, Heiskanen O, Poranen A, et al: The treatment of spontaneous intracerebral hemorrhage: A prospective randomized trial of surgical and conservative treatment. J Neurosurg 70:755–758, 1989.

81. Batjer HH, Reisch JS, Allen BC, et al: Failure of surgery to improve outcome in hypertensive putaminal hemorrhage: A prospective randomized trial. Arch Neurol 47:1103–1106, 1990.

82. Zuccarello M, Brott T, Derex L, et al: Early surgical treatment for supratentorial intracerebral hemorrhage: A randomized feasibility study. Stroke 30:1833–1839, 1999.

83. Mendelow AD, Gregson BA, Fernandes HM, et al: Early surgery versus initial conservative treatment in patients with spontaneous intracerebral hematomas in the International Surgical Trial in Intracerebral Hemorrhage (STICH): A randomised trial. Lancet 365:387–397, 2005.

75 Surgical Management of Moyamoya Disease in Adults

ALI H. MESIWALA, DAVID W. NEWELL, and GAVIN W. BRITZ

INTRODUCTION

Moyamoya disease is a rare cerebrovascular condition characterized by progressive, idiopathic occlusion of the bilateral supraclinoid internal cerebral arteries, proximal middle cerebral arteries (MCAs), and anterior cerebral arteries (Fig. 75-1). Since its first description by Takeuchi and Shimizu[1] in 1957, and subsequent angiographic characterization and naming by Suzuki and Takaku[2] in 1969, several thousand cases have been documented worldwide.

Depending on the country of origin, there appear to be differences in age distribution and clinical features in patients with moyamoya disease. In Japan, where the vast majority of cases have been documented, a bimodal age distribution exists, with the first peak in early childhood and a second peak in the fourth decade of life.[3] Ischemic symptoms are more common in children, whereas hemorrhagic events are more characteristic in adults.[3] Similar findings have been reported in Europe.[4] In contrast, studies from the United States suggest that moyamoya disease differs in its clinical expression in American populations.[5-7]

Nonetheless, surgical revascularization is considered beneficial in patients with moyamoya disease. This is true in the pediatric population, regardless of the country of origin.[8-11] There is less experience with adult patients, particularly in North America, and the majority of published results relate to indirect revascularization. Recently, however, direct revascularization techniques have shown benefits.[7,12,13]

CLINICAL PRESENTATION

Patients with moyamoya disease commonly present with ischemic or hemorrhagic symptoms. As the major intracranial vessels progressively narrow and occlude, cerebral blood flow (CBF), perfusion, and vascular reserve decrease. As a result, ischemic episodes may develop. Hemorrhagic events, generally thought to be more common than ischemic events in adults, may consist of intraventricular, parenchymal, or subarachnoid hemorrhages. The most common type of bleed is an intraventricular hemorrhage secondary to rupture of the fragile moyamoya vessels of the basal ganglia, thalamus, and ventricle. Alternatively, pseudoaneurysms, also peculiar to moyamoya disease, may rupture. They typically arise from the peripheral portions of the perforating and anterior and posterior choroidal arteries in a paraventricular location. In Japanese patients, the incidence of aneurysms is approximately 5.6%.[14] Other studies have shown a high incidence of major artery aneurysms in the posterior circulation[15]; this is thought to be due to increased flow in the posterior circulation due to compromised anterior circulation blood flow. The incidence of arteriovenous malformations associated with moyamoya disease has also been reported to be as high as 3%.[16] The pathophysiology of adult hemorrhage is thought to be related to long-term hemodynamic stress on the moyamoya vessels and pathologic changes of the vessel wall (thinning of the wall, mural fibrin deposits, fragmented elastic lamina, and arteriosclerotic disease).[17-19]

Recent studies suggest that the clinical presentation of moyamoya disease varies depending on the country evaluated. In Asia, hemorrhagic events are far more common than ischemic episodes in adults. Hemorrhagic presentations may account for as many as 65%, depending on the particular study.[20-22] This same pattern holds true in Europe.[4] In North America, however, ischemic presentations appear to be more common. In three series of patients from different regions of the United States and Canada, ischemic episodes were noted in 74% to 84% of cases.[5-7]

Other presenting symptoms may include seizures, movement disorders, and progressive cognitive decline.

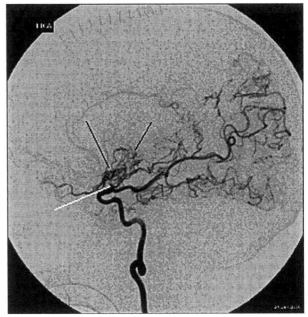

FIGURE 75-1 Lateral left carotid angiogram demonstrates occlusion of the supraclinoid internal cerebral arteries (*white line*), and no filling of the middle cerebral and anterior cerebral arteries. In addition, the classic moyamoya collateral vessels are seen (*black arrows*).

DIAGNOSTIC STUDIES AND PREOPERATIVE ASSESSMENT

Angiography

Cerebral angiography remains the gold standard for the diagnosis of moyamoya disease and is critical to obtain for surgical planning. As described by Suzuki and Takaku,[2] the natural history of the disease can be broken down into six angiographic stages (Table 75-1). The earlier stages relate to bilateral narrowing of the carotid arteries, the middle stages describe the development of moyamoya vessels, and the later stages note the appearance of extracranial to intracranial collateral pathways and regression of moyamoya vessels. Based on this, the Ministry of Health and Welfare in Japan developed the following four diagnostic criteria for moyamoya disease: (1) stenosis or occlusion of the intracranial internal cerebral arteries, adjacent anterior cerebral arteries, or MCAs; (2) abnormal vascular network adjacent to the stenosed artery identified during the arterial phase of angiography; (3) bilateral findings on angiography; and (4) no other identifiable cause.[23]

Computed Tomography and Magnetic Resonance Imaging

Despite advances in computed tomography (CT) and magnetic resonance imaging, these studies have not replaced angiography for the diagnosis of moyamoya disease. CT remains the imaging modality of choice for rapid detection of acute hemorrhage and stroke, whereas magnetic resonance imaging better detects ischemic changes and can be used for noninvasive assessment of the extent of moyamoya disease. When used for diagnostic purposes, however, magnetic resonance angiography overestimates the degree of disease.[24]

Cerebral Blood Flow Studies

The role of CBF studies in the treatment of adult moyamoya disease is not well defined. CBF dynamics and vasomotor reactivity can be evaluated using xenon-CT (Xe-CT) with acetazolamide challenge, single photon emission CT with acetazolamide challenge, positron emission tomography, and transcranial Doppler with CO_2 challenge. Many authors have demonstrated abnormal CBF in patients with moyamoya disease using these techniques and clearly showed improvements in CBF and vasomotor reserve after surgical revascularization.[7,13,25–30] The necessity of performing these studies preoperatively, however, is not established. In our experience, these studies may be useful in determining which cerebral hemisphere is at greater risk of ischemic

compromise; in this way, one can choose which cerebral hemisphere should be treated first.

SURGICAL INDICATIONS

The diagnosis of adult moyamoya disease is generally made during comprehensive workup for a new ischemic or hemorrhagic event. As such, virtually all adults with moyamoya disease are treated with surgical revascularization. Since moyamoya disease is bilateral in nature, both cerebral hemispheres will likely require surgical treatment. As a general rule, we prefer to treat the more impaired or symptomatic hemisphere first. For patients with ischemic symptoms, we perform CBF evaluations (as described previously) to determine which side has greater impairment. For those patients with hemorrhagic events, the ipsilateral hemisphere is initially addressed. Once the patient has recovered from their initial revascularization procedure, we wait approximately 6 to 8 weeks and then revascularize the contralateral hemisphere.

Although there is general agreement that revascularization procedures should be performed in adults with moyamoya disease, the appropriate surgical procedure remains controversial. Surgical revascularization for the treatment of moyamoya disease can be divided into two different techniques: direct bypass surgery and indirect revascularization. Direct bypass surgery usually consists of a direct anastomosis between the superficial temporal artery (STA) and MCA. In some cases, the anterior cerebral artery may be used instead of the MCA, and for posterior circulation procedures, the occipital artery and posterior cerebral arteries are used. Indirect revascularization is a simple surgical technique in which vascular-rich tissues such as the dura mater and temporalis muscle are placed on the surface of the brain to induce neovascularization to the ischemic part of the brain.

In pediatric patients, indirect revascularization using encephaloduroarteriomyosynangiosis (EDAMS) has been found to induce excellent neovascularization and prevent further ischemic episodes.[8–11] In adults, indirect revascularization procedures have been used with mixed success. Houkin et al[31] studied 22 hemispheres before and after surgery in adults. They found that direct STA-MCA anastomosis resulted in good revascularization of the MCA territory in 94% of cases. After indirect procedures, however, induction of neovascularization by the STA was observed in only 9% of cases, by the middle meningeal artery in 36% of cases, and by the deep temporal artery in 45% of cases. Mizoi et al[32] studied 16 adults who underwent direct and indirect bypass surgery and follow-up angiography an average of 6 months after surgery. In patients older than 30 years of age, direct bypass demonstrated excellent filling; in the same patients, however, the effectiveness of indirect bypass declined with advancing age, particularly after the age of 40 years. These patients all presented with ischemia, and during the follow-up period of 3.4 years, none of them had any further ischemic or hemorrhagic events.

Although these small studies have revealed some benefit of indirect revascularization on the clinical outcome of adults with moyamoya disease, the literature generally favors direct arterial bypass for ischemic disease.[13,27,29,31–34] The potential benefit of revascularization in hemorrhagic

---

TABLE 75-1 ▪ The Angiographic Stages of Moyamoya Disease

Stage 1	Narrowing of the carotid fork
Stage 2	Initiation of the moyamoya
Stage 3	Intensification of the moyamoya
Stage 4	Minimization of the moyamoya
Stage 5	Reduction of the moyamoya
Stage 6	Disappearance of the moyamoya

disease is thought to result from the reduction of hemodynamic stress on the basal moyamoya vessels. Published series of revascularization procedures, however, have not demonstrated a significant correlation between reduction in moyamoya vessels and prevention of hemorrhagic events. In fact, reduction in moyamoya vessels is observed in only 25% to 65% of patients.[21,27] Moreover, the ability of surgery to prevent or reduce the frequency of hemorrhagic events has been disappointing. Okada et al[27] reported that 20% of patients who presented with hemorrhagic events had additional hemorrhagic events after direct STA-MCA bypass. Yonekawa et al[35] reported that the rate of rebleeding after surgery was no different than the natural history of the disease. Houkin et al[21] reported on 35 adult patients with moyamoya disease. Twenty-four of these patients presented with hemorrhagic events and 11 with ischemic symptoms. All 35 underwent direct bypass surgery. Over a mean follow-up period of 6.4 years, 5 of the 35 patients (14.3%) had rehemorrhage. There were no postoperative ischemic events. These investigators concluded that surgery was effective in preventing ischemic attacks but remained uncertain about its effectiveness in preventing hemorrhagic events. Kawaguchi et al[33] described 22 patients with hemorrhagic moyamoya disease. Eleven patients were not surgically treated, six underwent direct bypass, and five EDAMS. During an average follow-up period of 7 years, 54% of the nonsurgically treated patients presented with rebleeding or ischemic events, and three of the five (60%) patients treated with EDAMS also presented with a bleed or ischemic event. Of the six patients who underwent direct bypass, no patients had any further events. In our cohort of 38 patients, 5 presented with hemorrhagic events, and 33 with ischemic episodes.[7] Thirty-five patients underwent direct bypass procedures, and 3 had EDAMS performed. During an average follow-up of 3.4 years, 6 of 35 (17%) patients who underwent direct STA-MCA bypass had an ischemic event, and 1 of 3 (33%) of the patients who underwent an indirect procedure experienced an ischemic attack. Interestingly, all patients demonstrated improved CBF and vasomotor reserve on CBF testing. Of the five patients who presented with hemorrhagic events, only one (20%) had another hemorrhage after a direct STA-MCA bypass; a follow-up cerebral angiogram performed at the time of his new bleed revealed a complete resolution of moyamoya vessels. This suggests that the presence of these abnormal collaterals, or the lack thereof, may be unrelated to the predisposition to hemorrhage.

In cases in which patients present with a subarachnoid hemorrhage secondary to a ruptured saccular aneurysm, the conventional treatment of obliteration of the aneurysm by surgical clipping or coiling is recommended.

PREOPERATIVE ASSESSMENT

All patients should undergo standard preoperative assessment, including evaluation of cardiovascular risk factors when presenting with ischemic disease. Imaging studies generally include noncontrast head CT and four-vessel cerebral angiography with selective external carotid runs for mapping the STA. In patients with ischemic disease, we believe that preoperative CBF evaluation is useful, as described previously, and can include transcranial Doppler, single photon emission CT, Xe-CT, and perfusion CT studies.

ANESTHESIA AND CEREBRAL PROTECTION

Patients are generally placed under general anesthesia with a combination of isoflurane and intravenous agents. Hyperventilation is not used, and the arterial P_{CO_2} is kept between 35 and 40 mm Hg. To maximize cerebral protection and minimize neurologic risks, mild hypothermia is induced (33°C to 34.5°C), barbiturate anesthesia is used, and mean arterial blood pressure is slightly elevated during arterial cross-clamping. Brain relaxation via osmotic or diuretic agents or cerebrospinal fluid drainage is not used so as to maintain proximity of the cerebral cortex to the dural surface and prevent any stretching or tension on the graft. Last, patients are given aspirin 325 mg the morning of surgery to reduce the risk of graft occlusion due to a platelet plug.

SURGICAL TECHNIQUE

Direct Bypass

The patient is placed in the supine position with the head turned to the contralateral side, parallel to the floor. A roll is tucked under the shoulder and side, thus relieving any tension on the ipsilateral neck. Based on the preoperative external carotid runs of the cerebral angiogram, one should decide whether the frontal or parietal branch of the STA will be used; the hair is then shaved so that an appropriate skin incision can be made to access the particular STA branch. Portable continuous-wave Doppler ultrasound is then used to surface map the course of the parietal branch of the STA, and this is clearly demarcated with a marking pen (Fig. 75-2). At this point, we find it helpful to use a fine needle to gently scratch the skin along the marked out

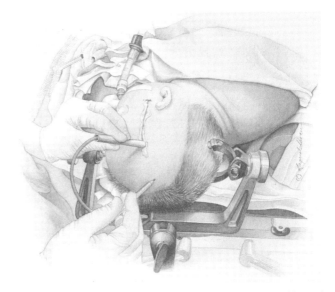

FIGURE 75-2 Drawing illustrates how Doppler ultrasound is used to map out the course of the STA. (From Newell DW, Vilela MD: Superficial temporal artery to middle cerebral artery bypass. Neurosurgery 54:1441–1449, 2004.)

course of the STA to ensure that the surface map is not lost during the skin prep. If only the parietal branch of the STA is to be used for the bypass, the incision will be made directly over the artery (retracing the scratch mapped out by Doppler) to its distal extent, approximately 4 cm from the sagittal midline. The incision must be of adequate length to allow enough retraction of the scalp so that an appropriate bone flap can be fashioned. If the frontal branch of the STA is to be used, the incision is extended anteriorly, as a second limb, toward the frontal region. The flap is then retracted forward so that the frontal branch can be dissected from the galea along the underside of the scalp flap. When making the incision immediately overlying the STA branch, extreme care must be taken not to damage the artery. As an alternative to a scalpel, we commonly use a needlepoint (Colorado tip) cautery unit (Colorado Biomedical, Inc., Evergreen, CO).

The STA branch is then dissected from the surrounding galeal tissue using the needlepoint cautery unit (Fig. 75-3). This is advantageous when compared with a purely sharp technique because the small branches off of the STA branch can be simultaneously cut and cauterized. For dealing with larger branches, a jeweler's bipolar forceps are particularly useful. After isolating the STA branch, the distal end of the artery is sharply transected and a temporary

clamp is placed proximally. Care must be taken when selecting the point of transection so that there is adequate length of the artery to perform the bypass. The lumen of the artery is then catheterized and irrigated with heparinized saline. It is then brought down toward the inferior aspect of the incision where it is gently wrapped in moist gauze and protected. Next, the temporalis muscle is divided down to bone beginning at the root of the zygomatic arch and extending superiorly, the full extent of the scalp incision. After the temporalis muscle is mobilized from the bone and retracted appropriately, a craniotomy flap is fashioned that maximizes the use of the exposed bone directly over the sylvian fissure; this is critical because it permits one to select the most appropriate cortical branch as a recipient artery (many M4 branches of the MCA emanate from the distal portion of the sylvian fissure). A temporal burr hole is placed at the root of the zygomatic arch and another at the superior aspect of the exposed bone. A high-speed drill is then used to perform the craniotomy (Fig. 75-4). The dura is then opened in a Y-shaped fashion, creating three triangular dural flaps (Fig. 75-5). Dural retraction stitches are placed, the cortex is exposed, and a suitable recipient artery is sought. Ideally, the recipient artery is on the surface, has an adequate straight portion without significant branching, and has a diameter of approximately 1.5 mm (Fig. 75-6).

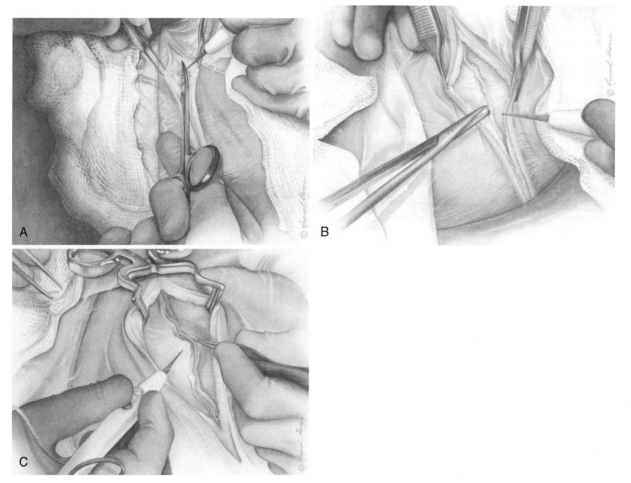

FIGURE 75-3 Drawings illustrate how, after identification of the artery, tenotomy scissors (*A*) are used to help isolate the artery and the needle point cautery is used to incise the galea adjacent to the artery on either side (*B* and *C*), which minimizes bleeding. (From Newell DW, Vilela MD: Superficial temporal artery to middle cerebral artery bypass. Neurosurgery 54:1441–1449, 2004.)

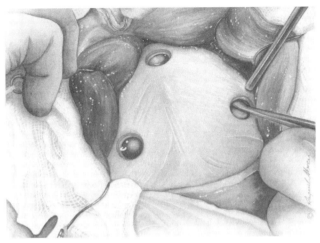

FIGURE 75-4 Drawing illustrates the craniotomy. (From Newell DW, Vilela MD: Superficial temporal artery to middle cerebral artery bypass. Neurosurgery 54:1441–1449, 2004.)

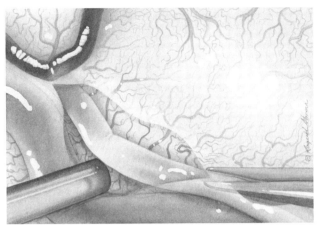

FIGURE 75-6 A surface artery is chosen for the recipient vessel, which is preferably the largest on the surface with a relatively long surface course and devoid of major branches. The drawing illustrates how the arachnoid membrane is divided along the surface of the artery, and small side branches are cauterized with a jeweler's forceps cautery. (From Newell DW, Vilela MD: Superficial temporal artery to middle cerebral artery bypass. Neurosurgery 54: 1441–1449, 2004.)

The microscope is then used to optimize dissection and isolation of the appropriate cortical artery. The arachnoid is then sharply opened directly over the recipient artery with an arachnoid knife and microscissors. A jeweler's microforceps are used to dissect the arachnoid away from the artery. It is equally important to separate the recipient artery from the surrounding veins. After isolating the artery, small side branches are cauterized with a fine jeweler's bipolar forceps and then divided with microscissors. A 1.5- to 2-cm segment of the artery is thus isolated, and a small rubber dam is placed under the artery, allowing the arteriotomy and the anastomosis to be performed.

Attention is now turned to the distal portion of the STA branch (Fig. 75-7). The distance between the donor artery and the recipient artery is carefully assessed, and approximately 3 cm of redundancy should be permitted to facilitate rotating the artery backward and forward to allow sutures to be easily placed on both sides of the arteriotomy. The periadventitial tissue is then dissected from the distal end of the STA branch, skeletonizing the artery for approximately

2 cm to allow an adequate working portion of the donor artery. The soft tissue is then trimmed back, and any small arterial branches are cauterized and divided. The STA branch is then dilated using topically applied dilute papaverine (Bedford Laboratories, Bedford, OH) solution (15 mg/100 mL of 0.9% saline). It is crucial that dilute papaverine solution be used; concentrated papaverine will cause permanent damage to the vessel wall. The distal end of the artery is cut with sharp scissors in an angled fashion and then spatulated using microscissors. The length of the spatulation should be approximately two times the diameter of the artery. After preparation of the donor artery, it is then brought down onto the rubber dam, where the recipient artery has been isolated.

At this time, the anesthesiologist should be notified that cross-clamping is about to take place, and cerebral protection should be initiated. Medhorn-Beamer clips, which occlude

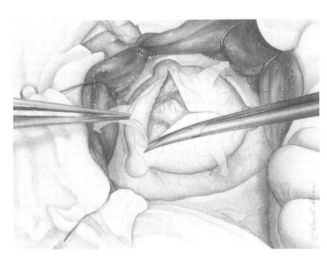

FIGURE 75-5 Drawing illustrates the dural opening. (From Newell DW, Vilela MD: Superficial temporal artery to middle cerebral artery bypass. Neurosurgery 54:1441–1449, 2004.)

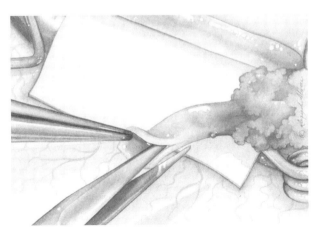

FIGURE 75-7 Drawing illustrates how the final preparation of the donor artery is performed by spatulating the end and irrigating the lumen with heparinized saline. (From Newell DW, Vilela MD: Superficial temporal artery to middle cerebral artery bypass. Neurosurgery 54:1441–1449, 2004.)

the artery with minimal trauma, are placed on both ends of the prepared anastomotic site on the recipient artery (Fig. 75-8). Van Ness scissors are used to make the arteriotomy, which is approximately twice the arterial diameter in length (Fig. 75-9). Next, the open lumen of the recipient vessel is irrigated with heparinized saline solution. With a tapered needle, a 10-0 nylon microsuture is then used to anchor the spatulated end (toe) of the donor artery to the end of the arteriotomy made on the recipient vessel. A second suture is then placed at the heel of the donor vessel, and it is anchored to the contralateral end of the arteriotomy site. Surgeon's knots are tied at both ends to prevent slippage. Interrupted sutures are then placed on each side of the arteriotomy to perform the anastomosis. Alternatively, a running suture technique can be used.

Next, the Medhorn-Beamer clips are removed and the anastomotic site is inspected. If significant bleeding is noted along the suture line, additional sutures are placed. Alternatively, if oozing occurs from the anastomosis, small Surgicel pledgets (Ethicon, Inc., Somerville, NJ) can be used on top of the suture line to tamponade and seal the leak. The temporary clip is then removed from the proximal STA, establishing flow through the anastomosis. A micro-Doppler ultrasound device (Mizuho America, Inc., Beverly, MA) is used to check the blood flow in the donor artery and in both limbs of the recipient artery. The flow velocity profile should be continuous, with no interruption of flow in diastole. Papaverine is then used to irrigate along the donor and recipient arteries to prevent vasospasm. From this point one, warm irrigation solution should be used for the remainder of the procedure to prevent spasm of the artery (Fig. 75-10). The dura is then closed, taking care to leave a generous durotomy through which the STA branch can pass. A dural graft, such as a piece of muscle or dural substitute, can be used to gently cover the durotomy, taking care not to occlude or kink the STA branch. The bone flap is then rongeured around the entry site of the donor artery through the craniotomy to ensure that there is no compression. In some cases, the inside of the bone flap must be drilled out to create a groove for the donor artery. After plating the

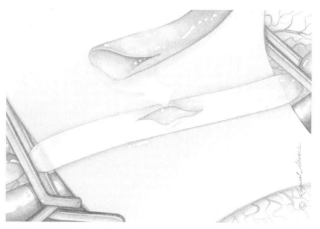

FIGURE 75-9   Drawing illustrates how the arteriotomy is made using small, curved Van Ness scissors. The length of the arteriotomy should be 2 to 2.5 times the diameter of the artery. (From Newell DW, Vilela MD: Superficial temporal artery to middle cerebral artery bypass. Neurosurgery 54:1441–1449, 2004.)

bone flap to the surrounding cranium, the temporalis muscle is reapproximated using sutures. A generous space for the artery to pass through the muscle is left.

The scalp is then closed over a subgaleal drain. This is done to reduce the chances that a hematoma or seroma will form within the operative site, causing compression and occlusion of the STA branch. Proper and meticulous closure of the scalp is critical because dissection of the STA branch from the galea creates a galeal defect. Thus care must be taken to ensure that the free edges of the galea are pulled together. We prefer to use 3-0 Vicryl sutures (Ethicon, Inc.) to close the remaining galeal layer, which can be 1 to 2 cm away from the skin edge. The skin is then closed with an absorbable suture, such as 4-0 Monocryl (Ethicon Inc.), taking care not to puncture the STA graft at the inferior portion of the incision. Although nonabsorbable suture can be used, we have found that patients prefer not having their

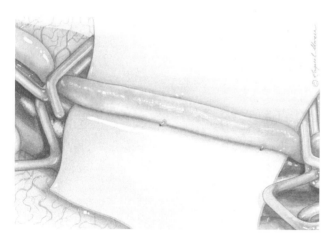

FIGURE 75-8   Drawing illustrates how the recipient artery is then cross-clamped. (From Newell DW, Vilela MD: Superficial temporal artery to middle cerebral artery bypass. Neurosurgery 54:1441–1449, 2004.)

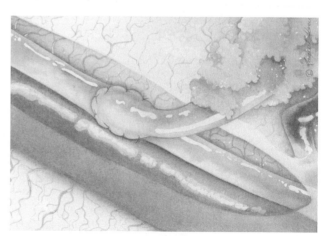

FIGURE 75-10   Drawing illustrates how the final anastomosis is visualized after all the clamps are removed. It is common to have some bleeding initially from the anastomotic site, which can be stopped by applying a small amount of a hemostatic agent. (From Newell DW, Vilela MD: Superficial temporal artery to middle cerebral artery bypass. Neurosurgery 54:1441–1449, 2004.)

stitches removed and the incision disturbed. After closure, dressings are placed.

Of note, the STA trunk and graft should be intermittently insonated with the Doppler probe throughout the closure process. If graft patency is in doubt and slow or poor flow is noted on Doppler ultrasound scan while closing, 500 mL dextran 40 can be administered at 50 mL/hr to inhibit platelet function.

Direct Bypass Using Vein Interposition Graft

In some cases, the STA branches may be absent, damaged, or too small so that a direct STA-MCA bypass is not possible. In these situations, a saphenous vein interposition graft may be useful. Harvesting of the saphenous vein is beyond the scope of this chapter; we describe, however, the interposition technique.

To identify the STA trunk, an incision is made in front of the tragus and carried down to the base of the ear. The dissection is carried along the tragus down to the tragal point; care must be taken to identify and avoid damaging the facial nerve. The posterosuperior portion of the parotid gland is encountered and is mobilized forward so that the trunk of the STA can be identified. Frequently, intraoperative Doppler ultrasound is very helpful in locating the artery. The artery is then dissected to allow a 1- to 2-cm working segment.

A craniotomy flap similar to that described previously, but centered over the anterior portion of the sylvian fissure, is created. This allows for more proximal exposure of the sylvian fissure. The sylvian fissure is opened widely, gently separating the temporal and frontal lobes. The M2 and M3 branches of the MCA are located, and a suitable recipient vessel is found. The distal anastomosis is performed first, allowing free manipulation of the saphenous vein graft and technically facilitating the end-to-side anastomosis. After completion of the distal anastomosis in a manner similar to that described previously, the vein graft is brought into apposition with the trunk of the STA. The vein is cut to the appropriate length in an angled fashion, and the end is spatulated. The STA trunk is prepared in a similar fashion, with an angled cut and spatulation. A 7-0 running vascular suture is then used to complete the end-to-end anastomosis.

Indirect Bypass

The technique for indirect revascularization is similar to that described for direct bypasses. Stepwise, the indirect bypass technique deviates from that described previously at the point at which the STA branches are dissected.

Using the needlepoint cautery device, the STA branches are carefully dissected and separated from the connective tissue of the scalp. Ideally, both the frontal and parietal branches are preserved in continuity with their distal ends. The arteries are isolated with a small amount of connective tissue on either side of the artery. The temporalis muscle and pericranium are then carefully mobilized off of the frontotemporal region so that the vascular and myofascial pedicles are preserved along the zygomatic arch. A frontotemporal craniotomy flap is then created using standard technique. Care is taken when elevating the bone off the underlying dura so that the middle meningeal artery is preserved. The dura is then opened in stellate fashion, preserving the middle meningeal artery and its large branches. The STA branches are then laid over the exposed surface of the brain. The dural flaps are then tucked into the subdural space, and the dural defect is covered by the temporalis muscle and pericranium. Meticulous hemostasis must be achieved or a subdural hematoma will result. The bone flap is then carefully plated to the surrounding cranium in a manner to prevent compression of the STA. In some cases the bone flap must be thinned out with a high-speed drill. A subgaleal drain is then placed. The soft-tissue flap is then closed in a manner analogous to that described previously.

POSTOPERATIVE CARE

Postoperatively, patients are monitored in an intensive care unit. Graft patency is assessed hourly at the bedside using a Doppler ultrasound device, and postoperative angiography is recommended (Figs. 75-11 and 75-12). Blood pressure parameters are provided to prevent hypotension and graft thrombosis or hypertension and possible hyperperfusion. Aspirin (325 mg), started on the morning of surgery, is continued daily thereafter. A cerebral angiogram with selective external carotid artery runs should be obtained on postoperative day 1 to confirm adequacy of the blood flow through the anastomosis. Last, tight head dressings should be avoided to reduce the risk of graft compression. We generally use simple dressings, such as tape and nonadherent gauze. Similarly, it is important to prevent patients from wearing eyeglasses during the first several postoperative days; the earpiece can cause compression and occlusion of the graft.

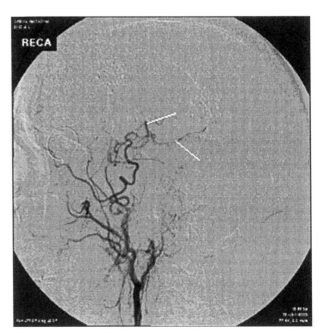

FIGURE 75-11 Lateral right external carotid angiogram demonstrates filling of the middle cerebral vessels (*white arrows*).

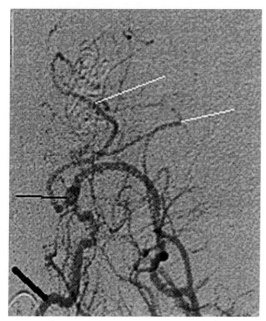

FIGURE 75-12 High-resolution anteroposterior right external carotid angiogram demonstrates the external carotid angiogram (*thick black line*), anastomosis (*thin black line*) and filling of middle cerebral vessels (*white arrows*).

COMPLICATIONS

The risks of surgical intervention in these relatively high-risk patients must be considered. Perioperative ischemic events are more common in moyamoya disease than in other cerebrovascular occlusive diseases. Attention must be paid to intraoperative fluid dynamics, blood loss, anesthetic cerebral protection, and blood pressure control. Similarly, fragility of abnormal moyamoya vessels may predispose them to hemorrhage; hypertensive spikes must be avoided, while ensuring that an adequate pressure head exists to maximize graft patency and cerebral perfusion. Graft occlusions may occur if there is prolonged hypotension, technical difficulties in creating an anastomosis between the graft and recipient vessel, relative intravascular hypovolemia, or increased blood viscosity. Last, systemic comorbidities, such as diabetes mellitus, hypertension, and cardiovascular disease, may lead to complications.

SUMMARY

Surgical revascularization for the treatment of moyamoya disease provides long-term reduction in ischemic and hemorrhagic events. Regardless of the differences that exist between the demographic characteristics of patients with moyamoya disease in the Western and Eastern hemispheres, improvement in cerebral perfusion and vasomotor reactivity can be expected, correlating to a reduction in ischemic events. While a similar reduction in hemorrhagic events has been observed, the mechanism by which this occurs is unclear.

Acknowledgments

The authors acknowledge Raquel Abreu, medical illustrator, for the surgical technique drawings. This project did not have any financial support or contribution, and neither of the authors has any financial agreement or relationship with any of the companies or pharmaceuticals mentioned in this chapter.

REFERENCES

1. Takeuchi K, Shimizu K: Hypogenesis of bilateral internal carotid arteries. No To Shinkei 9:37–43, 1957.
2. Suzuki J, Takaku A: Cerebrovascular "moyamoya" disease. Arch Neurol 20:288–299, 1969.
3. Fukui M: Current state of study on moyamoya disease in Japan. Surg Neurol 47:138–143, 1997.
4. Yonekawa Y, Ogata N, Kaku Y, et al: Moyamoya disease in Europe, past and present status. Clin Neurol Neurosurg 99(Suppl 2):S58–S60, 1997.
5. Chiu D, Shedden P, Bratina P, Grotta JC: Clinical features of moyamoya disease in the United States. Stroke 29:1347–1351, 1998.
6. Cloft HJ, Kallmes DF, Snider R, Jensen ME: Idiopathic supraclinoid and internal carotid bifurcation steno-occlusive disease in young American adults. Neuroradiology 41:772–776, 1999.
7. Mesiwala A, Sviri G, Newell D: Long-term outcome of STA-MCA bypass in moyamoya disease in North America. Presented at Joint Annual Meeting of the AANS/CNS Cerebrovascular Section and the ASITN, New Orleans, February 1–4, 2005.
8. Matsushima T, Fujiwara S, Nagata S, et al: Surgical treatment for paediatric patients with moyamoya disease by indirect revascularization procedures (EDAS, EMS, EMAS). Acta Neurochir (Wien) 98:135–140, 1989.
9. Matsushima T, Inoue T, Suzuki SO, et al: Surgical treatment of moyamoya disease in pediatric patients—comparison between the results of indirect and direct revascularization procedures. Neurosurgery 31:401–405, 1992.
10. Scott RM, Smith JL, Robertson RL, et al: Long-term outcome in children with moyamoya syndrome after cranial revascularization by pial synangiosis. J Neurosurg 100:142–149, 2004.
11. Suzuki Y, Negoro M, Shibuya M, et al: Surgical treatment for pediatric moyamoya disease: Use of the superficial temporal artery for both areas supplied by the anterior and middle cerebral arteries. Neurosurgery 40:324–330, 1997.
12. Iwama T, Hashimoto N, Miyake H, Yonekawa Y: Direct revascularization to the anterior cerebral artery territory in patients with moyamoya disease: Report of five cases. Neurosurgery 42:1157–1162, 1998.
13. Morimoto M, Iwama T, Hashimoto N, et al: Efficacy of direct revascularization in adult Moyamoya disease: Haemodynamic evaluation by positron emission tomography. Acta Neurochir (Wien) 141:377–384, 1999.
14. Yabumoto M, Funahashi K, Fujii T, et al: Moyamoya disease associated with intracranial aneurysms. Surg Neurol 20:20–24, 1983.
15. Nagamine Y, Takahashi S, Sonobe M: Multiple intracranial aneurysms associated with moyamoya disease: Case report. J Neurosurg 54:673–676, 1981.
16. Mawad ME, Hilal SK, Michelsen WJ, et al: Occlusive vascular disease associated with cerebral arteriovenous malformations. Radiology 153:401–408, 1984.
17. Suzuki J, Kodama N: Moyamoya disease—a review. Stroke 14:104–109, 1983.
18. Takeuchi K, Hara M, Yokota H, et al: Factors influencing the development of moyamoya phenomenon. Acta Neurochir (Wien) 59:79–86, 1981.
19. Yamashita M, Oka K, Tanaka K: Histopathology of the brain vascular network in moyamoya disease. Stroke 14:50–58, 1983.
20. Houkin K: [Cerebral revascularization surgery for moyamoya disease]. No Shinkei Geka 27:211–222, 1999.
21. Houkin K, Kamiyama H, Abe H, et al: Surgical therapy for adult moyamoya disease: Can surgical revascularization prevent the recurrence of intracerebral hemorrhage? Stroke 27:1342–1346, 1996.
22. Iwama T, Hashimoto N, Tsukahara T, Murai B: Peri-operative complications in adult moyamoya disease. Acta Neurochir (Wien) 132:26–31, 1995.
23. Nishimoto A: [Moyamoya disease] (author's transl). Neurol Med Chir (Tokyo) 19:221–228, 1979.
24. Houkin K, Aoki T, Takahashi A, Abe H: Diagnosis of moyamoya disease with magnetic resonance angiography. Stroke 25:2159–2164, 1994.
25. Inoue Y, Momose T, Machida K, et al: SPECT measurements of cerebral blood volume before and after acetazolamide in occlusive cerebrovascular diseases. Radiat Med 12:225–229, 1994.
26. Nariai T, Suzuki R, Hirakawa K, et al: Vascular reserve in chronic cerebral ischemia measured by the acetazolamide challenge test: Comparison with positron emission tomography. AJNR Am J Neuroradiol 16:563–570, 1995.

27. Okada Y, Shima T, Nishida M, et al: Effectiveness of superficial temporal artery-middle cerebral artery anastomosis in adult moyamoya disease: Cerebral hemodynamics and clinical course in ischemic and hemorrhagic varieties. Stroke 29:625–630, 1998.

28. Olsen AA, Ottenlips JR, Douville CM, et al: Use of cerebral vasoreactivity testing in the evaluation of moyamoya disease. J Vasc Tech 24:163–168, 2000.

29. Watanabe H, Ohta S, Oka Y, et al: Changes in cortical CBF and vascular response after vascular reconstruction in patients with adult onset moyamoya disease. Acta Neurochir (Wien) 138:1211–1217, 1996.

30. Yamashita T, Kashiwagi S, Nakano S, et al: The effect of EC-IC bypass surgery on resting cerebral blood flow and cerebrovascular reserve capacity studied with stable XE-CT and acetazolamide test. Neuroradiology 33:217–222, 1991.

31. Houkin K, Kuroda S, Ishikawa T, Abe H: Neovascularization (angiogenesis) after revascularization in moyamoya disease: Which technique is most useful for moyamoya disease? Acta Neurochir (Wien) 142:269–276, 2000.

32. Mizoi K, Kayama T, Yoshimoto T, Nagamine Y: Indirect revascularization for moyamoya disease: Is there a beneficial effect for adult patients? Surg Neurol 45:541–549, 1996.

33. Kawaguchi S, Okuno S, Sakaki T: Effect of direct arterial bypass on the prevention of future stroke in patients with the hemorrhagic variety of moyamoya disease. J Neurosurg 93:397–401, 2000.

34. Nussbaum ES, Erickson DL: Extracranial-intracranial bypass for ischemic cerebrovascular disease refractory to maximal medical therapy. Neurosurgery 46:37–43, 2000.

35. Yonekawa Y, Yamashita K, Taki W, et al: Clinical features of hemorrhagic type moyamoya disease: Special emphasis on cases with rebleeding. In Kikuchi H (ed): Annual Report 1988 of the Research Committee on the Spontaneous Occlusion of the Circle of Willis. Tokyo: Ministry of Health and Welfare, 1988, pp 81–88.

Management of Intracranial Aneurysms

76 Management of Unruptured Cerebral Aneurysms

P. ROC CHEN, DONG H. KIM, ARTHUR L. DAY, and
KAI FRERICHS

OVERVIEW

Subarachnoid hemorrhage (SAH), due to rupture of an intracranial aneurysm, carries a 30-day mortality rate of 45%, with approximately half the survivors sustaining irreversible brain damage.[1] As a result of the increasing use and the improving noninvasive brain imaging techniques such as computed tomography (CT), CT angiography, magnetic resonance imaging (MRI), and magnetic resonance angiography (MRA), a growing number of unruptured and often asymptomatic intracranial aneurysms are being diagnosed. The management of unruptured intracranial aneurysms (UIAs) remains controversial because of still incomplete and often conflicting data about the natural history of these lesions and the risks associated with their repair. Among the various types of aneurysms saccular (or berry) aneurysms, fusiform (or dissecting) aneurysms, and inflammatory (mycotic), this chapter focuses on the most common entity, unruptured intracranial saccular aneurysms.

NATURAL HISTORY

Intracranial aneurysms are common.[2-7] Autopsy studies have shown that the overall frequency in the general population ranges from 0.2% to 9.9% (mean frequency, approximately 5%).[6-10] The population-based incidence of aneurysmal SAH varies from 6 to 21.6 cases per 100,000 persons per year.[11-16] Management decisions of patients with UIAs, therefore, require an accurate assessment of the risks of various treatment options compared with the natural history of the condition.

To date, there has been no prospective study definitively noting the natural history of UIAs. Juvela[17] retrospectively examined the long-term natural history of UIAs and the risk factors for aneurysm rupture in 142 patients (131 with previous SAH). Before 1979, unruptured aneurysms were not treated in Helsinki. These patients were followed from 1956 to 1978, with a median follow-up duration of 19.7 years. During 2575 person-years, 33 of the 142 patients (23%) had SAH, resulting in an annual incidence of 1.3%. The cumulative rates of SAH were 10.5% at 10 years, 23% at 20 years, and 30.3% at 30 years.[17] Twenty-nine of 33 aneurysms that eventually ruptured were smaller than 10 mm in diameter at the time of the original diagnosis (18 were ≤6 mm).[8,17,18] One important observation of this study is that aneurysms that ruptured had increased in size (≥1 mm) more than aneurysms that did not rupture. Although this study was limited by the relatively small sample size, its annual rupture rate of 1.3% was similar to previously published reports

(1% to 2.3%).[19-21] In most of these reports, the unruptured aneurysm that was followed was in patients who had had a subarachnoid bleed from another aneurysm.

In another study, Tsutsumi and colleagues[28] observed 62 patients with saccular, nonthrombotic, noncalcified unruptured aneurysms at locations other than the cavernous sinus, which were detected on cerebral angiography studies performed for causes other than SAH between 1976 and 1997. The 5- and 10-year cumulative risks of CT confirmed SAH from small (<10 mm) aneurysms were 4.5% and 13.9%, respectively; the 5- and 10-year cumulative risks from large (>10 mm) aneurysms were 33.5% and 55.9%, respectively. This result is similar to that of Juvela's series.[8,17,18]

In 1998, the International Study of Unruptured Intracranial Aneurysm (ISUIA) Investigators published the retrospective part of their cohort of patients to assess the risk of aneurysm rupture and risks of surgical intervention for UIAs.[23] The natural history of 1937 UIAs in 1449 patients was evaluated. Results are summarized in Table 76-1. In group I, the cumulative rate of rupture of aneurysms that were less than 10 mm in diameter at diagnosis was less than 0.05% per year, and in group II, the rate was approximately 11 times higher (0.5% per year). The rupture rate of aneurysms that were 10 mm or more in diameter was less than 1% per year in both groups, but in group I, the rate was 6% in the first year for giant aneurysms (≥25 mm in diameter). The size and location of the aneurysm were independent predictors of rupture. Aneurysms 10 mm or more in diameter had a relative risk of rupture of 11.6. For posterior circulation aneurysms, the relative risk was 13.8 and 13.6 for basilar summit and vertebrobasilar locations, respectively.

Because of the exceedingly low rupture rate suggested by this study in the patients in group I with aneurysms less than 10 mm in diameter and relatively higher morbidity and mortality rates associated with surgical repair, as detailed later in this chapter, the ISUIA Investigators would seem to suggest that it is unlikely that surgery will reduce the rates of disability and death in patients with UIAs smaller than 10 mm in diameter and no history of SAH. These findings became the subject of significant controversy and had an impact on neurosurgical practice in the management of UIAs.

The ISUIA's results of rupture rates from unruptured aneurysms less than 10 mm of 0.05% to 0.5% annually are in disagreement with previously published data of 1% to 2.3% yearly.[8,17-21]

What are the possible sources of this discrepancy? There are several potential shortcomings of the ISUIA that may have affected the results.

TABLE 76-1 ▪ ISUIA Retrospective Cohort Results in 1998 (Follow-up for Mean 7.5 years) 1449 Patients with 1937 Unruptured Aneurysms

Size (mm)	Group I Yearly Rupture Rate (727 Cases without History of SAH [41% of ICA Aneurysms])	Group II Yearly Rupture Rate (722 Cases with History of SAH from a Different Aneurysm [27% of ICA Aneurysm])
<10	<0.05%	0.5%
10–24	<1%	<1%
≥25	6% first year	N/A

ICA, internal carotid artery; ISUIA, International Study of Intracranial Unruptured Aneurysms; N/A, not available; SAH, subarachnoid hemorrhage.

1. *Selection bias:* most of the patients in the ISUIA were identified retrospectively from hospital records, and only survivors with persistently asymptomatic aneurysms for whom a complete set of angiography studies could be traced were included.[23] Therefore, subjects who had had a fatal SAH, those in whom unruptured aneurysms had been treated since the study started, or those who had only incomplete angiography were not included in the ISUIA. The number of patients who may have harbored a UIA and underwent treatment is not known but may represent a selection bias as to which patients would be treated conservatively and which would be offered surgical repair.

2. *Internal carotid artery (ICA) aneurysms with a lower risk of SAH:* Some ICA aneurysms, particularly in the cavernous portion, carry a lower risk of SAH. Yet they represented 41% in group I and 27% in group II; of these, cavernous segment ICA aneurysms were represented by 16.9% in group I and 9.5% in group II.

3. *Short follow-up (7.5 years):* Juvela and colleagues[18] followed their patients for 19.5 years. These shortcomings may have contributed to the low annual rupture rate in small (≤10 mm) unruptured aneurysms reported in the ISUIA in comparison to the results of Juvela[18] and Tsutumis.[28]

Phase II of the ISUIA, a prospective study, was published in 2003. The aneurysms were categorized as less than 7 mm, 7 to 12 mm, 13 to 24 mm, and ≥25 mm in size. Their 5-year cumulative rupture rates of aneurysms located in anterior circulation were 0%, 2.6%, 14.5%, and 40%, respectively, for the patients who did not have a history of SAH. For aneurysms in posterior circulation, the cumulative rupture rates were 2.5%, 14%, 18.4%, and 50%.[24] The annual rupture rate for 7- to 12-mm aneurysms was found to be 0.5% of in the anterior circulation and 2.9% in the posterior circulation. This result reflects a much higher rate of small aneurysm rupture compared with the ISUIA phase I results. This is despite a possible selection bias in the prospective component as in the retrospective component, which may have contributed to a lower than expected rupture rate.

Winn and colleagues[10] reviewed 3684 cerebral angiography studies at the University of Virginia between April 1969 and January 1980 that yielded a prevalence rate of unruptured aneurysms of 0.65%. Nearly 80% of them were smaller than 10 mm in diameter. Authors normalized the prevalence rate from 0.65% to 1.3% because only 53% of the patients underwent a complete angiography study. A simple mathematical analysis based on the population of North America (250 million people during 1970 to 1980), and the prevalence rate yields 1.625 to 3.25 million people

who harbored an unruptured aneurysm during this period. There were 28,000 aneurysmal SAHs yearly during the same period.[25,26] The annual rupture rate would therefore have to range from 0.9% to 1.7%. Eighty percent of the 28,000 (or 22,500) aneurysmal SAHs were from aneurysms smaller than 10 mm, which suggested a 0.72% to 1.36% annual rupture rate for this group. In contrast, a 0.05% annual rupture rate, as defined in the ISUIA for aneurysms smaller than 10 mm, would yield a prevalence of unruptured small aneurysms of 45 million (22,500/0.0005), which would represent approximately 18% of the population of United States and Canada (1970 to 1980). In phase I of the ISUIA, 67% of aneurysms smaller than 10 mm were larger than 5 mm. This means that more than 12% (18% × 67%) of the population should have MRI-detectable cerebral aneurysms (>5 mm).[27] Certainly, the discovery of unruptured aneurysms of any size seems much less frequent than this number, even in busy MRI centers. However, a 1% to 2% risk of SAH would be in good agreement with the results from the data of Juvela and colleagues[18] and of Tsutsumi and colleagues.[28]

RISK FACTORS FOR ANEURYSM RUPTURE

The ISUIA pointed out that the size and location of aneurysms were independent predictors of rupture.

Size of Aneurysm

As mentioned previously, little controversy exists regarding a strong correlation between aneurysm size and the risk of rupture. For example, aneurysms larger than 25 mm in diameter have an annual rupture rate of approximately 6%.[23] This was confirmed not only in the retrospective but also prospective part of the ISUIA.

Locations of Aneurysms

In group I, the relative risk of rupture was 13.8 for aneurysms at the basilar summit and 13.6 for those in the vertebrobasilar or posterior cerebral distribution, as compared with other locations. For posterior communicating aneurysms, the relative risk of rupture was 8.0. In group II, the relative risk of rupture was 5.1 for aneurysm at the basilar summit. Asari and Ohmoto[29] found that aneurysms of the vertebrobasilar and middle cerebral arteries have a statistically higher probability of subsequent bleeding.

Shape of the Aneurysms

Few reports address the relationship between the risk of rupture and the shape (multilobed or with daughter domes) of unruptured aneurysms. Asari and Ohmoto[29] reported that SAH occurred in 7 of 22 multilobed aneurysms and 2 of 50 unilobed ones. Multilobed aneurysms have a significantly higher risk of hemorrhage than the unilobed unruptured aneurysms. Wiebers and colleagues[20] and Sampei and colleagues[30] both had similar findings in their small retrospective aneurysm series.

Age and Gender

Female gender seems to be a risk factor affecting both aneurysm formation and growth.[17] There are two peaks in the prevalence of aneurysms in women from the 1230 consecutive autopsy series of Iwamoto and colleagues[15]: 40- to 49-year and 60- to 69-year age groups. This corresponds with the finding of spontaneous SAH occurring most commonly in subjects between 40 and 60 years of age. There is approximately a 1.6-fold female predominance in the prevalence of aneurysms.[31] Interestingly, among men, the prevalence of aneurysms remained unchanged across the range of age groups.[15]

Cigarette Smoking (Active versus Cessation)

There is evidence that cigarette smoking may hasten growth of a preexisting aneurysm.[17] The mechanism of this remains unknown. Some observations, however, suggest that a change of the ratio of elastase/alpha$_1$-antitrypsin in plasma and arterial wall in cigarette smokers, that is, increased elastase activity and/or decreased alpha$_1$-antitrypsin, may contribute either to aneurysm formation or to SAH.[18,32] The faster the growth is, the more likely there may be a rupture.[17]

Genetic Conditions

Autosomal dominant polycystic kidney disease (ADPKD) is associated with a 15% prevalence[31] of cerebral aneurysms. Patients with type IV Ehlers-Danlos syndrome, hereditary hemorrhagic telangiectasia, neurofibromatosis type 1, alpha$_1$-antitrypsin deficiency, Klinefelter's syndrome, tuberous sclerosis, Noonan's syndrome, and alpha-1,4-glucosidase deficiency may have a higher incidence of intracranial aneurysms compared with the general population, but this is uncertain.

DETECTING ANEURYSMS

Intra-arterial Digital Subtraction Angiography

Digital subtraction angiography (DSA) with selective cerebral arterial injections and multiple projections, particularly with use of a 3-dimensional DSA technique, remains the gold standard to evaluate intracranial aneurysmal or other vascular conditions. Three-dimensional DSA offers a detailed 360-degree virtual view of the anatomic characteristics of the aneurysm, the neck shape and size, and the relationship to the parent and other blood vessels, which are crucial in planning potential interventions, especially endovascular interventions. High-quality angiography helps neurosurgeons and neurointerventionalists to optimally assess the anatomic risks of surgical clipping and endovascular coiling. Understanding the 3-dimensional relationships of the aneurysms, surgeons are able to preselect a suitable clip fit for the configuration, minimizing the risk of injuring adjacent vessels or leaving residual aneurysms behind; neurointerventionalists are able to avoid futile attempts to embolize aneurysms. Conventional or 3-dimensional DSA, however, only reveals the patent lumens of aneurysms. In aneurysms with heavy calcification or partial thrombosis, DSA can be misleading (Fig. 76-1). Cerebral CT and MRI provide useful complementary information in these patients.[33]

However, DSA is invasive and requires 2- to 6-hour hospital stays after the procedure. The permanent neurologic morbidity of the procedure has been reported to be in the range of 0.07% to 0.5%.[34,35] Therefore, DSA should not be used as a screening procedure.

Magnetic Resonance Imaging and Magnetic Resonance Angiography

Intra-arterial DSA should be considered the standard-of-reference investigative tool for intracranial aneurysmal disease, but it is invasive and carries a risk, even though this risk is very small in experienced hands. With the development of MRA, the absolute reliance on DSA for aneurysm detection and surgical planning is changing.[36] The spatial resolution of MRI/MRA is approaching that of formal angiography, and aneurysms with diameters smaller than 2 mm and vessels smaller than 1 mm can now be detected.[37] MRI/MRA is useful as a screening modality. Aneurysms of 6 mm or more in diameter have been detected with 100% sensitivity. The sensitivity decreased to 87.5%, 68.2%, 60%, and 55.6% for aneurysms with a diameter of 5, 4, 3, and 2 mm, respectively. Three-dimensional, contrast-enhanced MRA and 3-dimensional time-of-flight MRA can be useful adjuncts to conventional angiography in the assessment of intracranial aneurysms, and 3-dimensional, contrast-enhanced MRA is superior to 3-dimensional, time-of-flight MRA in detection of aneurysms.[33,38,39] In addition, MRI with MRA are useful in delineation of intra-aneurysmal thrombus; in such cases, DSA alone will misrepresent the size of an aneurysm.[33]

Multislice Computed Tomography Angiography

Multislice CT systems allow simultaneous acquisition of as many as four slices by using multirow detector systems. The concurrent acquisition of multiple slices results in a dramatic reduction of scan time. The major advantages of multislice CT are a longer scanning range, shorter scanning times, and a higher z-axis resolution.[40] The high scan speed of multislice helical CT permits helical scanning to be performed with a smaller slice thickness than is possible with conventional helical CT.[41] As a result, volumetric data with superior resolution in the z-axis can be obtained. This characteristic is useful in the visualization of vascular details in three dimensions. Acquired data can be reformatted to provide 3-dimensional angiographic images, called CT angiography (CTA). Many physicians routinely use

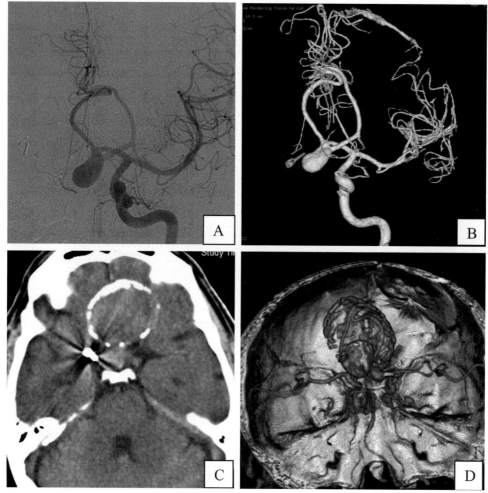

FIGURE 76-1   A 67-year-old man with history of anterior communicating artery aneurysm treated with clipping 30 years ago presented with worsening headache. Computed tomography (CT) revealed a giant interhemispheric mass with a rim of calcification (*C*). Digital subtraction angiography (DSA) confirmed a recurrent anterior communicating artery aneurysm (*A* and *B*); however, only a small part of the aneurysm was seen on angiography due to aneurysm thrombosis and calcification. CT angiography with 3-dimensional reconstruction (*D*) in this case provided a more complete view of the aneurysm, the thrombosed part, and the patent portion. Without combining CT images, DSA can be misleading in this case.

CTA in clinical practice. The sensitivity of the CTA ranged from 53% (95% confidence interval, 44% to 62%) for 2-mm aneurysms (Fig. 76-2) to 95% (95% confidence interval, 92% to 97%) for 7-mm aneurysms. The overall specificity was 98.9% (95% confidence interval, 91.5% to 99.99%), but there was between-study heterogeneity.[42] A recent meta-analysis comparing CTA with DSA (not 3-dimensional) in the diagnosis of cerebral aneurysms revealed a sensitivity of 93.3% and a specificity of 87.8% of CTA.[43]

The advantages of CTA are the following:

1. Data can be obtained more quickly and less expensively.
2. CTA provides additional anatomic information (information on bony and adjacent vessel relationships, neck-to-dome relationships, and the presence of calcium or atheromas).
3. CTA can be used for rapid planning, including planning of craniotomies for clip obliteration and preliminary determination of whether aneurysms are suitable for coil embolization.
4. CTA subjects patients to virtually no risk and negligible discomfort.

The disadvantages of CTA are as follows:

1. CTA is less sensitive and specific than the standard method, DSA, for the detection of cerebral aneurysms.
2. CTA has difficulty detecting aneurysms at the skull base, for example, aneurysms of clinoidal ICA and cavernous ICA due to the proximity to high-density structures such as bone.
3. CTA is sensitive to bolus timing, and opacified veins may be incorporated into the reconstructed image,[33] making interpretation of the arterial tree anatomy difficult.
4. CTA may be inadequate in those patients with left ventricular failure due to suboptimal opacification of the intracranial vasculature.[44]
5. CTA, like standard CT, is still subject to motion artifact.
6. CTA provides no information regarding flow in all phases of the bolus transit in the cerebral vessels.
7. CTA has not been validated to detect vasospasm or other flow-limiting lesions with the same reliability as DSA.

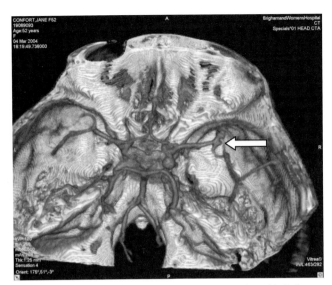

FIGURE 76-2 Computed tomography angiography with 3-dimensional volume rendering is able to detect a small intracranial aneurysm. The *arrow* points to a right middle cerebral artery bifurcation aneurysm that measured 2 mm in diameter. In addition, there is a readily identifiable right posterior communicating artery aneurysm (8 mm in diameter).

At present DSA is the standard method for the diagnosis and treatment planning of cerebral aneurysms. This approach will likely be diminished in the future as cross-sectional technology continues to improve. DSA will remain closely linked to any endovascular intervention, which still depends on fluoroscopic technology.

CLINICAL MANAGEMENT (CONSERVATIVE VERSUS TREATMENT)

Aneurysmal SAH carries a high fatality rate. In the retrospective part of the ISUIA, 66% of the patients (83% in group I and 55% in group II) who had an SAH from a previously unruptured aneurysm died.[23] Fifty-two percent of patients who sustained an aneurysm rupture during the follow-up period in the study of Juvela and colleagues[8] died. Tsutsumi and colleagues[28] reported a mortality rate of 86% as a result of aneurysm rupture. Ideally, the aneurysm should be secured before it ruptures. However, given the discrepancy of the data regarding the natural history of an unruptured aneurysm to subsequently rupture[8,17–21] and the morbidity and mortality associated with a prophylactic treatment,[24,45–49] decisions regarding the treatment of unruptured cerebral aneurysms are challenging and must be individualized for each patient.

Because only a proportion of aneurysms actually rupture, the key to the management of UIAs is (1) to identify those at greatest risk of harboring an aneurysm and (2) which of those aneurysms are at greatest risk of rupture. At present, however, both the natural course of unruptured cerebral aneurysms and outcome after treatment continue to be controversial subjects.

For example, Juvela[17] advocated that patients with unruptured aneurysms should be surgically treated, especially young and middle-aged adults regardless of the size of the aneurysm and of patients' smoking status. White and

Wardlaw[50] argues that in patients with no history of SAH, the risk/benefit analysis favors treatment in subjects younger than 50 years of age for all aneurysms except anterior circulation aneurysms smaller than 7 mm in size. For subjects older than 50 years of age, treatment is only favored for aneurysms larger than 12 mm and possibly posterior circulation aneurysms larger than 7 mm.

In 2000, before the publication of the prospective results from phase II of the ISUIA,[24] the Stroke Council of the American Heart Association issued a scientific statement to offer guidelines for the management of patients with UIAs.[51] These guidelines[51] remain appropriate at present.

The existing body of knowledge supports the following recommendations (options) regarding the treatment of UIAs:

1. *The treatment of small incidental intracavernous ICA aneurysms is not generally indicated. For large symptomatic intracavernous aneurysms, treatment decisions should be individualized on the basis of patient age, severity and progression of symptoms, and treatment alternatives. The higher risk of treatment and shorter life expectancy in older individuals must be considered in all patients and favors observation in older patients with asymptomatic aneurysms.*
2. *Symptomatic intradural aneurysms of all sizes should be considered for treatment, with relative urgency for the treatment of acutely symptomatic aneurysms. Symptomatic large or giant aneurysms carry higher surgical risks that require a careful analysis of individualized patient and aneurysmal risks and surgeon and center expertise.*
3. *Coexisting or remaining aneurysms of all sizes in patients with SAH due to another treated aneurysm carry a higher risk for future hemorrhage than do similar sized aneurysms without a prior SAH history and warrant consideration for treatment. Aneurysms located at the basilar apex carry a relatively high risk of rupture. Treatment decisions must take into account the patient's age, existing medical and neurological condition, and relative risks of repair. If a decision is made for observation, re-evaluation on a periodic basis with CT/MRA or selective contrast angiography should be considered, with changes in aneurysmal size sought, although careful attention to technical factors will be required to optimize the reliability of these measures.*
4. *In consideration of the apparent low risk of hemorrhage form incidental small (<10 mm) aneurysms in patients without previous SAH, treatment rather than observation cannot be generally advocated. However, special consideration for treatment should be given to young patients in this group. Likewise, small aneurysms approaching the 10-mm diameter size, those with daughter sac formation and other unique hemodynamic features, and patients with a positive family history for aneurysms or aneurysmal SAH deserve special consideration for treatment. In those managed conservatively, periodic follow-up imaging evaluation should be considered and is necessary if a specific symptom should arise. If changes in aneurysmal size or configuration are observed, this should lead to special consideration for treatment.*

5. *Asymptomatic aneurysms of ≥10 mm in diameter warrant strong consideration for treatment, taking into account patient age, existing medical and neurological conditions, and relative risks for treatment.*

INTERVENTIONS

Surgical Treatment

Should one decide to treat an unruptured intracranial aneurysm, the risks of the intervention must be thoroughly considered. Surgical aneurysm clipping has been the means of the treatment for approximately 40 years since the microscope was introduced to neurosurgery and is considered the time-tested treatment for aneurysms.[52–54] Like any other surgeries, high-volume centers and experienced surgeons offer better outcomes and fewer complications.[48]

Risks of Surgical Treatment

A systemic meta-analysis of surgical treatment for unruptured aneurysms identified 61 studies published between 1966 and June 1996 with a total of 2460 patients (57% female; mean age, 50 years) and at least 2568 unruptured aneurysms (27% > 25 mm, 30% located in the posterior circulation) with a mean follow-up at 24 weeks (range, 2 to 234).[45] Mortality was 2.6% (95% confidence interval, 2.0% to 3.3%). Permanent morbidity occurred in 10.9% (95% confidence interval, 9.6% to 12.2%) of patients. Postoperative mortality and morbidity were significantly lower in more recent years for nongiant aneurysms and aneurysms with an anterior location. The lowest morbidity and mortality were found with small anterior circulation aneurysms (0.8% mortality, 1.9% morbidity), and the worst with large posterior fossa aneurysms (9.6% mortality, 37.9% morbidity).

Phase II of the ISUIA, that is, the prospective arm of the ISUIA, found the surgery-related mortality at 1 year to be 2.7% in patients with no previous SAH and 0.6% in patients who had previously had an SAH. Morbidity rates were 9.9% and 9.8%, respectively.[24] Unlike most of previous studies, patient's cognitive impairment was included as a morbidity.

These data are similar to the in-hospital mortality rates of 2.5% and 3.0% in a statewide analysis of New York[55] and California[47] discharge data, respectively. A similar result was obtained through the Nationwide Inpatient Sample hospital discharge database (1996 to 2002).[48] Of 3498 patients who were treated at 463 hospitals with 585 identified surgeons in the database, 2.1% died and 16.1% were discharged to skilled-nursing facilities or other facilities other than home after UIA repair surgery. However, mortality was lower in high-volume hospitals (1.6% vs. 2.2%); discharge other than to home occurred in 15.6% of patients after surgery at high-volume hospitals (20 or more cases per year) compared with 23.8% in low-volume hospitals (fewer than four cases per year).

Factors Associated with Surgical Outcome

There are various risk factors that are potential predictors of surgical outcome besides hospital case volume and the experience of surgeons such as patient age and the size and location of an aneurysm.[24,56,57]

RELATIONSHIP OF AGE TO OUTCOME

In the ISUIA prospective arm, a 2.4 relative risk increase was observed in patients 50 years of age and older.[24] Takahashi[58] found the worst surgical outcome of patients at age 80 or older. Khanna and colleagues[59] report a sixfold higher risk of a poor outcome of a 70-year-old patient after surgery compared with a 30-year-old patient, keeping aneurysm size and location constant. This could be due to an increased incidence of atherosclerotic and/or calcified aneurysm necks and domes in addition to medical comorbidities in the older age group.

RELATIONSHIP OF ANEURYSM SIZE TO OUTCOME

Solomon and colleagues[57] found that aneurysm size had an important influence on surgical outcome. The morbidity and mortality of unruptured aneurysms were 0% for aneurysms 10 mm or smaller, 6% for aneurysms between 10 and 25 mm, and 20% for aneurysms greater than 25 mm. Drake[56] reported 15% morbidity and mortality in nongiant posterior circulation aneurysms compared with 39% for giant posterior circulation aneurysms, although ruptured aneurysms were also included in his series. The ISUIA[24] revealed a 2.6 relative risk of poor surgical outcome of an aneurysm greater than 12 mm in diameter.

RELATIONSHIP OF ANEURYSM LOCATION

Aneurysm location within the posterior circulation is associated with an increased incidence of poor outcome in the ISUIA.[24] Solomon and colleagues[57] observed 50% morbidity and mortality with surgery for unruptured giant basilar aneurysms compared with 13% for anterior circulation giant aneurysms. Drake[56] found a 14.3% morbidity rate with surgical treatment of unruptured asymptomatic aneurysms in the posterior circulation compared with 0% morbidity in the anterior circulation. Other aneurysm locations such as posterosuperior projecting anterior communicating aneurysms[60] and clinoidal segment and the cavernous portion ICA aneurysms are also associated with higher morbidity and mortality due to technical difficulties of safe intracranial exposure and acquisition of proximal control.[61,62]

Despite all the risks of surgical treatment for a UIA, decision of surgical treatment does require mathematical calculation. For instance, a group of patients with longest follow-up (23.4 years)[17] had a cumulative rate of bleeding in the whole patient population of 10.5% at 10 years after diagnosis of the unruptured aneurysm, 23.0% at 20 years, and 30.0% at 30 years. If the patient's age is 50 years or younger at the time of diagnosis and the projected life expectancy is 80 years, the risk of a devastating SAH in the next 30 years will outweigh the surgical risks. In many situations, however, a high-risk natural history is associated with a high surgical risk. For example, a 30-mm unruptured basilar apex aneurysm would have a 5-year rupture risk of approximately 50% to 60% and 40% to 50% risk of death or severe disability, and an operative risk of mortality may be approaching the same range if surgical clipping was the only option.[24] In such a situation, patient age, comorbidities, patient will, and availability of alternative treatment modalities will influence the decision-making process.

Endovascular Treatment

In 1991, Guglielmi and colleagues[63,64] introduced the detachable coil in treating intracranial aneurysms. The technique revolutionized endovascular treatment of intracranial aneurysms. In 1995, the Guglielmi detachable coil (GDC) system (Boston Scientific/Target, Inc., Fremont, CA) received U.S. Food and Drug Administration approval. Aneurysms considered not suitable for surgery formed the candidates for GDC coil embolization. In subsequent years, criteria for endovascular treatment broadened. In 1999, Guglielmi's group was the first to report a large series of 115 cases with 120 incidentally found intracranial aneurysms.[65] The efficacy of coil occlusion in preventing subsequent hemorrhage of intracranial aneurysms is based on GDC mechanical hemodynamic exclusion of intra-aneurysm flow.[66] Currently available data on endovascular treatment of intracranial aneurysms with GDC are derived mostly from relatively small series comprising several hundred patients. There are two meta-analysis reviews of outcomes of aneurysm coiling.[67,68] Brilstra and colleagues[67] reviewed 48 studies including 1383 patients. Permanent complications (death/disability) of embolization with GDC occurred in 3.7%; 54% (95% confidence interval, 50% to 57%) of aneurysms were completely occluded after one procedure. The other review focused on GDC embolization of posterior circulation aneurysms[68] and found procedural complication and morbidity rates of 12.5% and 5.1%, respectively. Procedural and 30-day mortality rates were 1.4% and 6.7%, respectively. The overall mortality rate was 9.8%. Complete aneurysm occlusion was achieved in 47.6%, nearly complete occlusion (90% to 99%) in 43.4%, and incomplete occlusion in 9.0%. The annual risk of SAH after embolization was 0.8%. These data indicate that embolization with a coil is a reasonably safe treatment for patients with a UIA. The effectiveness in terms of complete occlusion of the aneurysm at the first procedure is moderate. There are also concerns about aneurysm recurrences in 20.7% of treated aneurysms[49] and a higher rebleed rate of 0.9% for completely coiled aneurysm versus 0.4% for completely clipped aneurysms.[54]

However, it is important to understand that these case series are based on retrograde data analysis of a technology in flux, and patient selection bias may have skewed the results:

1. There was a learning curve for using GDC and related catheter-based techniques. For instance, in the endovascular series of 324 patients of Debrun and colleagues,[69,70] the initial series of 25 patients (May 1994 to February 1995) were treated without taking the geometry of the aneurysms as an important criterion for coiling into account, which led to high morbidity and mortality rate, and less than 50% of these aneurysms were angiographically occluded at 6-month follow-up.
2. Endovascular treatment has been offered as the alternative option for those patients "too sick" or simply "too old" to tolerate surgical clipping for aneurysms.
3. Unlike microsurgery, which is stable technologically after 40 years of development; endovascular techniques continue to evolve rapidly. For instance, in the not too distant past, broad-necked aneurysms were considered

unsuitable for GDC coiling; with new emerging technologies such as remodeling techniques using balloons or stents, these aneurysms have now become suitable targets for endovascular treatment.[71] Introduction of a specific microcatheter-deliverable, self-expandable stent designed exclusively for the intracranial circulation (Neuroform; BSCI, Natick, MA) has further broadened the endovascular armamentarium.

In 2002, the International Subarachnoid Aneurysm Trial (ISAT) Collaborative Group published the first prospective randomized trial in 2143 patients with ruptured intracranial aneurysms comparing outcomes after endovascular coiling versus surgical clipping.[72] In the endovascular group, 23.7% of patients either required assistance with their activities or were dead at 1 year compared with 30.6% after surgical clipping. Despite some shortcomings, including only 1 year of follow-up, the relative and absolute risk reductions in dependency or death after endovascular versus surgical treatment were 22.6% and 6.9%, respectively, and enrollment was halted as significance was reached before reaching the target enrollment number. The risk of rehemorrhage from the ruptured aneurysm after 1 year was 2 per 1276 and 0 per 1081 patient-years for patients allocated to endovascular or surgical treatment, respectively. The ISAT results suggest that if both treatments are suitable for a ruptured aneurysm, endovascular coil treatment is significantly more likely to result in survival free of disability 1 year after SAH, although long-term durability of coiling remains to be determined in the future.

For unruptured aneurysms, the ISUIA phase II data on treatment outcomes make direct comparisons of clipping versus coiling difficult because patient characteristics were different. There were disproportionately more elderly patients and posterior circulation and large aneurysms (predisposing to poorer outcome) in the endovascular cohort. Nevertheless, group I patients (without history of SAH from a different aneurysm) had a combined morbidity and mortality rate at 1 year of 12.6% for clipping and 9.8% for coiling and a 22.3% relative risk reduction for coiling. For group II patients (with a history of SAH from a different aneurysm that had been repaired), the rates were 10.1% for clipping and 7.1% for coiling, with a relative risk reduction for coiling at 1 year of 29.7%.[24]

Long-term follow-up data after coiling of an unruptured aneurysm will be needed to prove not just short-term efficacy but also durability of this new treatment. This is the subject of current and future trials[73] including the long-term follow-up from the ISAT.

Obstacles to Endovascular Treatments

Advances in endovascular technology have made possible the treatment of increasingly complex aneurysms over time. Prohibitive tortuosity in the access vessels may make an endovascular approach impossible. Combining an open surgical approach to provide access closer to the lesion may be suitable in some rare cases. Incorporation of a daughter dome in the neck may make it unlikely that an endovascular cure can be achieved. Incorporation of the parent artery into the aneurysm may be more amenable to surgical reconstruction of the artery unless readily amenable to stent or balloon remodeling techniques. Partial thrombosis of the aneurysm makes recurrence of the aneurysm due to shifting and compaction of the coil mass very likely. Controversial is the role of endovascular treatment in the management of mass effect–producing aneurysms. Intuitively, only an open surgical approach would have a reasonable chance to relieve the consequences of mass effect. On the other hand, some evidence exists that cranial neuropathies improve also after endovascular coiling.[74] The mechanism of recovery in cranial nerve function after endovascular aneurysm occlusion is unclear. It has been speculated that reduction in the aneurysm's size, the degree of pulsatility, and adjacent cerebral edema[74] may play a role in cranial nerve recovery after coiling.

Combining Surgical and Endovascular Modalities in Treating an Unruptured Aneurysm: The Multidisciplinary Approach

It has become clear that surgical clipping is no longer the only treatment option for obliteration of cerebral aneurysms, and surgical and endovascular modalities have become complementary technologies in the treatment of these patients. As part of a multidisciplinary approach, open cerebrovascular surgeons and endovascular surgeons evaluate every aneurysm case as a team to decide on the optimal treatment modality, that is, observation, surgical clipping, endovascular coiling, or combination approaches. This could include surgical reconstruction of parent arteries or bypass procedures followed by coiling and vice versa. The optimal treatment plan would strive to find the delicate balance between maximizing aneurysm obliteration and minimizing treatment-related morbidity to maximize the benefit to the patient (Fig. 76-3).

No formal or generally accepted guidelines exist to choose between the various treatment modalities. This choice would also be influenced by the available expertise of operators in each modality. The following factors, however, influence the selection of treatment modalities:

1. Location of the aneurysm
2. Relationship of the aneurysm with its parent vessels and other branches
3. Aneurysm dome-to-neck ratio
4. Surgical and endovascular accessibility
5. Age and general medical condition of the patient
6. Patient's preference

1. *Location:* For unruptured middle cerebral artery aneurysms, surgical clipping may still be the most efficient treatment option.[75,76] The two major anatomic features responsible for failure of the endovascular procedures are a dome/neck ratio of 1.5 or less and an arterial branch (proximal M2 segment) originating from the aneurysm neck. These features are frequently seen in middle cerebral artery aneurysms. In contrast, surgical clipping of middle cerebral artery aneurysms has a very low morbidity.[75,76] For anterior cerebral artery aneurysms, especially superoposterior projecting aneurysms, endovascular coiling avoids brain retraction and septal branch injury.[60] Aneurysms in the cavernous or paraclinoid ICA are associated with higher surgical risk, and an endovascular approach may be

the more appropriate treatment option.[77,78] For aneurysms in the posterior circulation, especial basilar apex aneurysms, endovascular treatment offers lower procedure-related morbidity and mortality.[79,80]

2. *Relationship to parent vessel:* Aneurysms with parent vessels incorporated into the neck or dome are generally not suitable for endovascular coiling, although remodeling techniques have created new opportunities for an endovascular option.[75,76] In this situation, however, strong consideration to an open surgical approach should be given unless contraindicated.

3. *Aneurysm dome and neck ratio:* An aneurysm neck size less than 4 mm or a dome/neck ratio of 2 are favorable parameters for coiling; otherwise, surgical clipping will be the better option.[69,70,81] However, the new endovascular remodeling techniques, that is, stent- or balloon-assisted coiling, have created new opportunities for endovascular treatment.[71,82,83]

4. *Surgical and endovascular accessibility:* Intracavernous ICA aneurysms are surgically difficult to access. Direct clipping, ipsilateral ICA occlusion, or external carotid artery to ICA bypass followed by ICA occlusion have been used as treatment options. The high morbidity and mortality of the procedures may not justify using them for this type of aneurysm. Endovascular coiling, on the other hand, may provide a safer alternative.[78] Conversely, the extreme vascular tortuosity of the aortic arch, carotid or vertebral arteries, and chronic carotid or vertebral artery occlusion can be the obstacles to catheter access to the aneurysm.

5. *Age and medical condition:* Elderly patients and patients with comorbidities tolerate endovascular approaches better than open surgery and craniotomy.[77]

In summary, it is likely that a combined microsurgical-endovascular team approach will provide the means to achieve the best outcomes for the entire population of patients with UIAs.

Conservative Management

If conservative management is chosen for a new-found unruptured aneurysm, it is crucial to reduce the risks of the rupture, which collectively can have a useful effect. Problems such as the following may arise: Should these patients be given anticoagulants or aspirin to treat other comorbidities?

Reduction of Risk Factors

CESSATION OF TOBACCO SMOKING

In the ISUIA retrospective data, 60.6% of patients with aneurysms were current smokers.[23] With longer follow-up data, Juvela and colleagues[17,32,84] revealed the prevalence of smoking in patients with SAH ranging from 45% to 75%, whereas in the general adult population in Finland, it is only 20% to 35%. It is likely that smoking is associated with an increased risk of SAH by formation of an aneurysm and increasing its rate of growth. Among smokers, the number of cigarettes smoked daily seems to be more significantly associated with aneurysm growth than the duration of or age at starting of smoking. Those who had quit smoking had no increased risk of aneurysm growth.[17,32,84] Therefore, cessation of cigarette smoking may help reduce both the risk of formation of aneurysms and the risk of rupture.

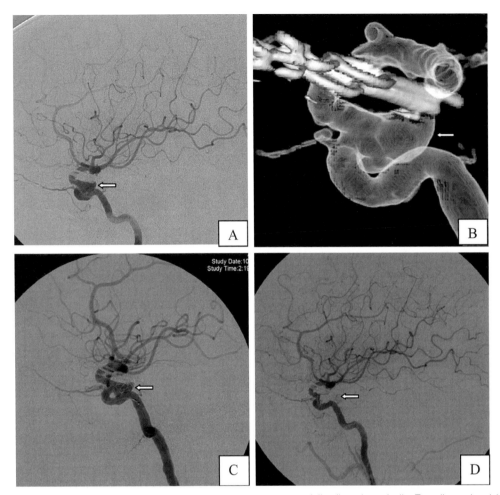

FIGURE 76-3   Left ophthalmic-clinoid internal carotid artery aneurysm was partially clipped surgically. Two-dimensional (*A*) and 3-dimensional (*B*) angiography. The patient then underwent Neuroform (Boston Scientific, Natick, MA) stent placement–assisted residual aneurysm coiling. *C*, After the first coil placement. *D*, There is complete obliteration of the aneurysm without compromising the internal carotid artery.

CONTROL HYPERTENSION AND RISK FACTORS FOR ATHEROSCLEROSIS

The risk factors for SAH and for growth of an aneurysm are very similar. Hypertension, alcohol consumption (particularly binge drinking),[8,18,32,85] cocaine and amphetamine abuse,[86] oral contraceptive use,[87] and cholesterol level more than 6.3 mmol/K[88] in addition to cigarette smoking may all be associated with an increased risk of aneurysm formation and SAH. Controlling hypertension and the risk factors for atherosclerosis may reduce the risks of aneurysm formation and its rupture.

Issues of Anticoagulation and Aspirin/Nonsteroidal Anti-inflammatory Drug Use in Patients with Unruptured Cerebral Aneurysms

There is no evidence of an increased risk of SAH using anticoagulation medications in patients with unruptured aneurysms. However, avoidance of anticoagulants in patients known to harbor an unruptured aneurysm may reduce the risk of a poor outcome should the aneurysm rupture. There is evidence of worse outcomes after aneurysmal SAH in patients on anticoagulants. The mortality of this group is at least twice as high.[31]

Use of aspirin or other nonsteroidal anti-inflammatory drugs, however, preceding aneurysmal SAH does not significantly affect outcome. Interestingly, nonsteroidal anti-inflammatory drugs given after SAH might actually reduce morbidity by reducing the risk of secondary ischemia events.[89]

FOLLOW-UP

Postsurgical and/or Endovascular Treatments

Risk of Aneurysm Regrowth and Subarachnoid Hemorrhage after Surgical Clipping

In a recent report,[90] the annual rate of postoperative SAH was 0.18% for all clipped aneurysms and 0% for completely clipped lesions during 7.4 ± 3.7 years of follow-up. With 12-year follow-up, another center reported that a rebleed incidence in 1170 subjects with completely clipped aneurysms was 0.4%.[54] A study of long-term (2.6 to 9.6 years) angiographic outcome of surgically treated aneurysms by David and colleagues[91] demonstrated 1.5% recurrent aneurysms of 135 aneurysms that were clipped without residual. Of 12 aneurysms with known residual, 25% enlarged.

Therefore, the long-term result of surgical clipping is very good, although periodic follow-up may also be necessary in surgically treated patients.

Risk of Aneurysm Regrowth and Subarachnoid Hemorrhage after Endovascular Coil Embolization

Although there are no long-term prospect data to demonstrate the risk of regrowth of an unruptured aneurysm after treatment, the ISAT revealed a higher risk of rebleeding from the endovascularly treated aneurysms in the first year after the treatment. The risk of rebleeding from the ruptured aneurysms 1 year after coil embolization was 2 per 1276 and 0 per 1081 patient-years for patients treated endovascularly and surgically, respectively, although the relative and absolute risk reductions in dependency or death after allocation to endovascular or surgical treatment were 22.6% and 6.9%, respectively.[72] The continued follow-up on those patients included in the ISAT will provide useful data on this issue in the future.

De Novo Aneurysms

The annual rate of new aneurysm formation in patients treated for aneurysmal SAH is reported to be as high as 1.8%, especially with history of multiple aneurysms.[91] Follow-up in this study was 4.4 ± 1.6 years. During 1789 patient-years of follow-up in 89 patients with unruptured aneurysms, Juvela[17] found 19 de novo aneurysms in 15 patients of which 2 caused SAH. The probability of de novo aneurysm formation cases was 0.84% per year. A similar annual rate of 0.89% was reported by Tsutsumi and colleagues.[22] The cumulative risk becomes significant after 9 to 10 years. These findings support the rationale for late (10 years) angiographic follow-up in patients with aneurysms that were treated surgically or endovascularly. In addition, female gender and current smoking were significant independent risk factors for new aneurysm formation.[17] Cessation of smoking is very important for patients with unruptured aneurysms and possibly also for those with a history of SAH.

SCREENING FOR OCCULT INTRACRANIAL ANEURYSMS

Familial or Patients with a Family History of Aneurysmal Subarachnoid Hemorrhage

In families with two or more first-degree family members, especially siblings and a mother-daughter pair, or two first- and second-degree family members with SAH, the risk of family members harboring UIAs is approximately 9% to 11%.[45,46,92] This is much higher than the prevalence in the general population. Therefore, it has been recommended that these family members be screened. MRI/MRA and CTA provide adequate noninvasive options for screening. The optimal age at which screening should be performed is not known. It has been reported that SAH occurs at a younger age in subsequent generations.[93] In siblings with SAH, aneurysmal rupture occurs within the same decade

of life significantly more often than it does in randomly selected pairs of patients with SAH.[94,95] It, therefore, seems reasonable to start screening first-degree relatives, especially siblings, in families with two or more affected patients at a younger age than the age at which their affected family members had their SAH. However, cost effectiveness has not been evaluated in clinical studies, and screening should be considered on an individual basis.[51]

Autosomal Dominant Polycystic Kidney Disease

Approximately 500,000 persons in the United States carry a mutant gene for ADPKD, making it one of the most common inherited disorders.[96] ADPKD is associated with an increased prevalence of cerebral aneurysms and increased risk of SAH. The clinical literature reports that the prevalence of asymptomatic aneurysms in patients with ADKDP is 14% to 16% by autopsy and conventional angiography studies.[97] There is a lack of population-based data on the rates of aneurysm rupture specifically in patients with ADPKD; however, the mean age at rupture in patients with ADPKD is between 35 and 40 years,[98–100] that is, 10 to 20 years earlier than in patients with sporadic SAH. This suggests that ADPKD per se is a risk factor for aneurysm rupture. Using decision analysis, a statistical technique for assisting in making decisions that involve competing risks and benefits, Butler and colleagues[97] demonstrated that an MRA screening strategy increased the life expectancy of young patients with ADPKD and reduced the financial impact of ADPKD on society.

REFERENCES

1. Graves EJ: Detailed diagnoses and procedures, national hospital discharge survey, 1990. Vital Health Stat 13:1–225, 1992.
2. Chason JL, Hindman WM: Berry aneurysms of the circle of Willis: Results of a planned autopsy study. Neurology 8:41–44, 1958.
3. Housepian EM, Pool JL: A systematic analysis of intracranial aneurysms from the autopsy file of the Presbyterian Hospital, 1914 to 1956. J Neuropathol Exp Neurol 17:409–423, 1958.
4. Stehbens WE: Aneurysms and anatomical variation of cerebral arteries. Arch Pathol 75:45–64, 1963.
5. McCormick WF, Acosta-Rua GJ: The size of intracranial saccular aneurysms: An autopsy study. J Neurosurg 33:422–427, 1970.
6. Jellinger K: Pathology of intracerebral hemorrhage. Zentralbl Neurochir 38:29–42, 1977.
7. Jakubowski J, Kendall B: Coincidental aneurysms with tumours of pituitary origin. J Neurol Neurosurg Psychiatry 41:972–979, 1978.
8. Juvela S, Porras M, Heiskanen O: Natural history of unruptured intracranial aneurysms: A long-term follow-up study. J Neurosurg 79:174–182, 1993.
9. Menghini VV, Brown RD Jr, Sicks JD, et al: Incidence and prevalence of intracranial aneurysms and hemorrhage in Olmsted County, Minnesota, 1965 to 1995. Neurology 51:405–411, 1998.
10. Winn HR, Jane JA Sr, Taylor J, et al: Prevalence of asymptomatic incidental aneurysms: Review of 4568 arteriograms. J Neurosurg 96:43–49, 2002.
11. Ingall TJ, Whisnant JP, Wiebers DO, O'Fallon WM: Has there been a decline in subarachnoid hemorrhage mortality? Stroke 20:718–724, 1989.
12. Sarti C, Tuomilehto J, Saloman V, et al: Epidemiology of subarachnoid hemorrhage in Finland from 1983 to 1985. Stroke 22:848–853, 1991.
13. Broderick JP, Brott T, Tomsick T, et al: The risk of subarachnoid and intracerebral hemorrhages in blacks as compared with whites. N Engl J Med 326:733–736, 1992.

14. Mayberg MR, Batjer HH, Dacey R, et al: Guidelines for the management of aneurysmal subarachnoid hemorrhage: A statement for healthcare professionals from a special writing group of the Stroke Council, American Heart Association. Stroke 25:2315–2328, 1994.

15. Iwamoto H, Kiyohara Y, Fujishima M, et al: Prevalence of intracranial saccular aneurysms in a Japanese community based on a consecutive autopsy series during a 30-year observation period: The Hisayama study. Stroke 30:1390–1395, 1999.

16. Hamada J, Morioka M, Yano S, et al: Incidence and early prognosis of aneurysmal subarachnoid hemorrhage in Kumamoto Prefecture, Japan. Neurosurgery 54:31–38, 2004.

17. Juvela S: Natural history of unruptured intracranial aneurysms: Risks for aneurysm formation, growth, and rupture. Acta Neurochir Suppl 82:27–30, 2002.

18. Juvela S, Porras M, Poussa K: Natural history of unruptured intracranial aneurysms: Probability of and risk factors for aneurysm rupture. J Neurosurg 93:379–387, 2000.

19. Winn HR, Almaani WS, Berga SL, et al: The long-term outcome in patients with multiple aneurysms: Incidence of late hemorrhage and implications for treatment of incidental aneurysms. J Neurosurg 59:642–651, 1983.

20. Wiebers DO, Whisnant JP, Sundt TM Jr, O'Fallon WM: The significance of unruptured intracranial saccular aneurysms. J Neurosurg 66:23–29, 1987.

21. Yasui N, Suzuki A, Nishimura H, et al: Long-term follow-up study of unruptured intracranial aneurysms. Neurosurgery 40:1155–1160, 1997.

22. Tsutsumi K, Ueki K, Morita A, et al: Risk of aneurysm recurrence in patients with clipped cerebral aneurysms: Results of long-term follow-up angiography. Stroke 32:1191–1194, 2001.

23. International Study of Unruptured Intracranial Aneurysms Investigators: Unruptured intracranial aneurysms—risk of rupture and risks of surgical intervention. N Engl J Med 339:1725–1733, 1998.

24. Wiebers DO, Whisnant JP, Huston J 3rd, et al: Unruptured intracranial aneurysms: Natural history, clinical outcome, and risks of surgical and endovascular treatment. Lancet 362:103–110, 2003.

25. Phillips LH 2nd, Whisnant JP, O'Fallon WM, Sundt TM Jr: The unchanging pattern of subarachnoid hemorrhage in a community. Neurology 30:1034–1040, 1980.

26. Kassell NF, Torner JC: Size of intracranial aneurysms. Neurosurgery 12:291–297, 1983.

27. Winn HR: Unruptured aneurysms. J Neurosurg 96:1–2, 1983.

28. Tsutsumi K, Ueki K, Morita A, Kirino T: Risk of rupture from incidental cerebral aneurysms. J Neurosurg 93:50–53, 2000.

29. Asari S, Ohmoto T: Natural history and risk factors of unruptured cerebral aneurysms. Clin Neurol Neurosurg 95:205–214, 1993.

30. Sampei T, Mizuno M, Nakajima S, et al: [Clinical study of growing up aneurysms: Report of 25 cases]. No Shinkei Geka 19:825–830, 1991.

31. Rinkel GJ, Djibuti M, Algra A, van Gijn J: Prevalence and risk of rupture of intracranial aneurysms: A systematic review. Stroke 29:251–256, 1998.

32. Juvela S, Poussa K, Porras M: Factors affecting formation and growth of intracranial aneurysms: A long-term follow-up study. Stroke 32:485–491, 2001.

33. Adams WM, Laitt RD, Jackson A: The role of MR angiography in the pretreatment assessment of intracranial aneurysms: A comparative study. AJNR Am J Neuroradiol 21:1618–1628, 2000.

34. Heiserman JE, Dean BL, Hodak JA, et al: Neurologic complications of cerebral angiography. AJNR Am J Neuroradiol 15:1401–1411, 1994.

35. Cloft HJ, Joseph GJ, Dion JE: Risk of cerebral angiography in patients with subarachnoid hemorrhage, cerebral aneurysm, and arteriovenous malformation: A meta-analysis. Stroke 30:317–320, 1999.

36. Graves MJ: Magnetic resonance angiography. Br J Radiol 70:6–28, 1997.

37. Huston J 3rd, Nichols DA, Luetmer PH, et al: Blinded prospective evaluation of sensitivity of MR angiography to known intracranial aneurysms: Importance of aneurysm size. AJNR Am J Neuroradiol 15:1607–1614, 1994.

38. Metens T, Rio F, Baleriaux D, et al: Intracranial aneurysms: detection with gadolinium-enhanced dynamic three-dimensional MR angiography—initial results. Radiology 216:39–46, 2000.

39. Suzuki IM, Matsui Ueda F, et al: Contrast-enhanced MR angiography (enhanced 3-D fast gradient echo) for diagnosis of cerebral aneurysms. Neuroradiology 44:17–20, 2002.

40. Fuchs T, Kachelriess M, Kalender WA: Technical advances in multi-slice spiral CT. Eur J Radiol 36:69–73, 2000.

41. Dillon EH, van Leeuwen MS, Fernandez MA, Mali WP: Spiral CT angiography. AJR Am J Roentgenol 160:1273–1278, 1993.

42. van Gelder JM: Computed tomographic angiography for detecting cerebral aneurysms: Implications of aneurysm size distribution for the sensitivity, specificity, and likelihood ratios. Neurosurgery 53:597–606, 2003.

43. Chappell ET, Moure FC, Good MC: Comparison of computed tomographic angiography with digital subtraction angiography in the diagnosis of cerebral aneurysms: A meta-analysis. Neurosurgery 52:624–631, 2003.

44. Vieco PT: CT angiography of the intracranial circulation. Neuroimaging Clin N Am 8:577–592, 1998.

45. Raaymakers TW, Rinkel GJ, Limburg M, Algra A: Mortality and morbidity of surgery for unruptured intracranial aneurysms: A meta-analysis. Stroke 29:1531–1538, 1998.

46. Raaymakers TW, Rinkel GJ, Ramos LM: Initial and follow-up screening for aneurysms in families with familial subarachnoid hemorrhage. Neurology 51:1125–1130, 1998.

47. Johnston SC, Zhao S, Dudley RA, et al: Treatment of unruptured cerebral aneurysms in California. Stroke 32:597–605, 2001.

48. Barker FG 2nd, Amin-Hanjani S, Butler WE, et al: In-hospital mortality and morbidity after surgical treatment of unruptured intracranial aneurysms in the United States, 1996–2000: The effect of hospital and surgeon volume. Neurosurgery 52:995–1009, 2003.

49. Raymond J, Guilbert F, Weill A, et al: Long-term angiographic recurrences after selective endovascular treatment of aneurysms with detachable coils. Stroke 34:1398–1403, 2003.

50. White PM, Wardlaw JM: Unruptured intracranial aneurysms. J Neuroradiol 30:336–350, 2003.

51. Bederson JB, Awad IA, Wiebers DO, et al: Recommendations for the management of patients with unruptured intracranial aneurysms: A Statement for healthcare professionals from the Stroke Council of the American Heart Association. Stroke 31:2742–2750, 2000.

52. Yasargil MG, Antic J, Laciga R, et al: Microsurgical pterional approach to aneurysms of the basilar bifurcation. Surg Neurol 6:83–91, 1976.

53. Jane JA, Winn HR, Richardson AE: The natural history of intracranial aneurysms: Rebleeding rates during the acute and long term period and implication for surgical management. Clin Neurosurg 24:176–184, 1977.

54. Asgari S, Wanke I, Schoch B, Stolke D: Recurrent hemorrhage after initially complete occlusion of intracranial aneurysms. Neurosurg Rev 26:269–274, 2003.

55. Berman MF, Solomon RA, Mayer SA, et al: Impact of hospital-related factors on outcome after treatment of cerebral aneurysms. Stroke 34:2200–2207, 2003.

56. Drake CG: Progress in cerebrovascular disease. Management of cerebral aneurysm. Stroke 12:273–283, 1981.

57. Solomon RA, Fink ME, Pile-Spellman J: Surgical management of unruptured intracranial aneurysms. J Neurosurg 80:440–446, 1994.

58. Takahashi T: The treatment of symptomatic unruptured aneurysms. Acta Neurochir Suppl 82:17–19, 2002.

59. Khanna RK, Malik GM, Qureshi N: Predicting outcome following surgical treatment of unruptured intracranial aneurysms: A proposed grading system. J Neurosurg 84:49–54, 1996.

60. Proust F, Debono B, Hannequin D, et al: Treatment of anterior communicating artery aneurysms: Complementary aspects of microsurgical and endovascular procedures. J Neurosurg 99:3–14, 2003.

61. Guidetti B, La Torre E: Carotid-ophthalmic aneurysms. A series of 16 cases treated by direct approach. Acta Neurochir (Wien) 22:289–304, 1970.

62. Guidetti B, La Torre E: Management of carotid-ophthalmic aneurysms. J Neurosurg 42:438–442, 1975.

63. Guglielmi G, Vinuela F, Dion J, Duckwiler G: Electrothrombosis of saccular aneurysms via endovascular approach. Part 2: Preliminary clinical experience. J Neurosurg 75:8–14, 1991.

64. Guglielmi G, Vinuela F, Sepetka I, Macellari V: Electrothrombosis of saccular aneurysms via endovascular approach. Part 1: Electrochemical basis, technique, and experimental results. J Neurosurg 75:1–7, 1991.

65. Murayama Y, Vinuela F, Duckwiler GR, et al: Embolization of incidental cerebral aneurysms by using the Guglielmi detachable coil system. J Neurosurg 90:207–214, 1999.

66. Sorteberg A, Sorteberg W, Rappe A, Strother CM: Effect of Guglielmi detachable coils on intraaneurysmal flow: Experimental study in canines. AJNR Am J Neuroradiol 23:288–294, 2002.

67. Brilstra EH, Rinkel GJ, van der Graaf Y, et al: Treatment of intracranial aneurysms by embolization with coils: A systematic review. Stroke 30:470–476, 1999.

68. Lozier AP, Connolly ES Jr, Lavine SD, Solomon RA: Guglielmi detachable coil embolization of posterior circulation aneurysms: A systematic review of the literature. Stroke 33:2509–2518, 2002.

69. Debrun GM, Aletich VA, Kehrli P, et al: Selection of cerebral aneurysms for treatment using Guglielmi detachable coils: The preliminary University of Illinois at Chicago experience. Neurosurgery 43:1281–1297, 1998.

70. Debrun GM, Aletich VA, et al: Aneurysm geometry: An important criterion in selecting patients for Guglielmi detachable coiling. Neurol Med Chir (Tokyo) 38(Suppl):1–20, 1998.

71. Han PP, Albuquerque FC, Ponce FA, et al: Percutaneous intracranial stent placement for aneurysms. J Neurosurg 99:23–30, 2003.

72. Molyneux A, Kerr R, Stratton I, et al: International Subarachnoid Aneurysm Trial (ISAT) of neurosurgical clipping versus endovascular coiling in 2143 patients with ruptured intracranial aneurysms: A randomised trial. Lancet 360:1267–1274, 2002.

73. Qureshi AI, Hutson AD, Harbaugh RE, et al: Methods and design considerations for randomized clinical trials evaluating surgical or endovascular treatments for cerebrovascular diseases. Neurosurgery 54:248–267, 2004.

74. Birchall D, Khangure MS, McAuliffe W: Resolution of third nerve paresis after endovascular management of aneurysms of the posterior communicating artery. AJNR Am J Neuroradiol 20:411–413, 1999.

75. Regli L, Uske A, de Tribolet N: Endovascular coil placement compared with surgical clipping for the treatment of unruptured middle cerebral artery aneurysms: A consecutive series. J Neurosurg 90:1025–1030, 1999.

76. Regli L, Dehdashti AR, Uske A, de Tribolet N: Endovascular coiling compared with surgical clipping for the treatment of unruptured middle cerebral artery aneurysms: An update. Acta Neurochir Suppl 82:41–46, 2002.

77. Martin NA: The combination of endovascular and surgical techniques for the treatment of intracranial aneurysms. Neurosurg Clin N Am 9:897, 1998.

78. Park HK, Horowitz M, Jungreis C, et al: Endovascular treatment of paraclinoid aneurysms: Experience with 73 patients. Neurosurgery 53:14–24, 2003.

79. Eskridge JM, Song JK: Endovascular embolization of 150 basilar tip aneurysms with Guglielmi detachable coils: Results of the Food and Drug Administration multicenter clinical trial. J Neurosurg 89:81–86, 1998.

80. Gruber DP, Zimmerman GA, Tomsick TA, et al: A comparison between endovascular and surgical management of basilar artery apex aneurysms. J Neurosurg 90:868–874, 1999.

81. Fernandez Zubillaga A, Guglielmi G, Vineula F, Duckwiler GR: Endovascular occlusion of intracranial aneurysms with electrically detachable coils: Correlation of aneurysm neck size and treatment results. AJNR Am J Neuroradiol 15:815–820, 1994.

82. Bendok BR, Hanel RA, Hopkins LN: Coil embolization of intracranial aneurysms. Neurosurgery 52:1125–1130, 2003.

83. Henkes H, Fischer S, Weber W, et al: Endovascular coil occlusion of 1811 intracranial aneurysms: Early angiographic and clinical results. Neurosurgery 54:268–285, 2004.

84. Juvela S: Risk of subarachnoid hemorrhage from a de novo aneurysm. Stroke 32:1933–1934, 2001.

85. Juvela S: [Alcohol and the prognosis of subarachnoid hemorrhage]. Duodecim 109:355–357, 1993.

86. Oyesiku NM, Colohan AR, Barrow DL, Reisner A: Cocaine-induced aneurysmal rupture: An emergent negative factor in the natural history of intracranial aneurysms? Neurosurgery 32:518–526, 1993.

87. Johnston SC, Colford JM Jr, Gress DR: Oral contraceptives and the risk of subarachnoid hemorrhage: A meta-analysis. Neurology 51:411–418, 1998.

88. Adamson J, Humphries SE, Ostergaard JR, et al: Are cerebral aneurysms atherosclerotic? Stroke 25:963–966, 1994.

89. Juvela S, Hillbom M, Numminen H, Koskinen P: Cigarette smoking and alcohol consumption as risk factors for aneurysmal subarachnoid hemorrhage. Stroke 24:639–646, 1993.

90. Lozier AP, Kim GH, Sciacca RR, et al: Microsurgical treatment of basilar apex aneurysms: Perioperative and long-term clinical outcome. Neurosurgery 54:286–299, 2004.

91. David CA, Vishteh AG, Spetzler RF, et al: Late angiographic follow-up review of surgically treated aneurysms. J Neurosurg 91:396–401, 1999.

92. Ronkainen A, Hernesniemi J, Puranen M, et al: Familial intracranial aneurysms. Lancet 349:380–384, 1997.

93. Bromberg JE, Rinkel GJ, Algra A, et al: Familial subarachnoid hemorrhage: Distinctive features and patterns of inheritance. Ann Neurol 38:929–934, 1995.

94. Leblanc R, Melanson D, Tampieri D, Guttmann RD: Familial cerebral aneurysms: A study of 13 families. Neurosurgery 37:633–639, 1995.

95. Ronkainen A, Hernesniemi J, Tromp G: Special features of familial intracranial aneurysms: Report of 215 familial aneurysms. Neurosurgery 37:43–47, 1995.

96. Parfrey PS, Bear JC, Morgan J, et al: The diagnosis and prognosis of autosomal dominant polycystic kidney disease. N Engl J Med 323:1085–1090, 1990.

97. Butler WE, Barker FG 2nd, Crowell RM: Patients with polycystic kidney disease would benefit from routine magnetic resonance angiographic screening for intracerebral aneurysms: A decision analysis. Neurosurgery 38:506–516, 1996.

98. Lozano AM, Leblanc R: Cerebral aneurysms and polycystic kidney disease: A critical review. Can J Neurol Sci 19:222–227, 1992.

99. Chauveau D, Pirson Y, Verellen-Dumoulin C, et al: Intracranial aneurysms in autosomal dominant polycystic kidney disease. Kidney Int 45:1140–1146, 1994.

100. Fick GM, Johnson AM, Hammond WS, Gabow PA: Causes of death in autosomal dominant polycystic kidney disease. J Am Soc Nephrol 5:2048–2056, 1995.

77

Surgical Management of Paraclinoid Aneurysms

KAZUHIKO KYOSHIMA, MASATO SHIBUYA, and SHIGEAKI KOBAYASHI

Paraclinoid aneurysms include aneurysms in the C2 and distal C3 portions (Fisher's classification) of the internal carotid artery (ICA).[1] Surgery for these aneurysms presents special difficulties because of their anatomic features and their proximity to complicated bony and dural structures. Some of these aneurysms were considered unclippable or associated with disastrous results when approached surgically, mainly because of the difficulty in securing the proximal parent artery. Furthermore, these aneurysms are often large and adhere tightly to the surrounding structures. Temporary carotid occlusion is often necessary during dissection and clip application, necessitating both preoperative complete circulation study including balloon occlusion test and protection of the brain from ischemic damage during occlusion. In addition to straight clips, special clips are often necessary; a combination of ring clips is essential for ventrally developed aneurysms.[2] With the recent refinement of microsurgical techniques and advancement of surgical anatomic study, their management has changed from conservative surgery to direct neck clipping. With the advent of intravascular surgery, the treatment strategy is gradually changing, but direct clipping is currently the treatment of choice whenever feasible.

ANATOMIC CONSIDERATIONS

Characteristic anatomic features of aneurysms in this area are their relationship to the anterior clinoid process, cavernous sinus, optic nerve, and ophthalmic artery.

The ICA enters into the intracranial space through the carotid canal, which is covered with periosteum. The ICA courses in the space between the dura propria and the periosteum (cavernous sinus) at the middle skull base, where it occasionally produces a mild bony impression called the carotid groove. The ICA then turns posteriorly to form a curve at the bony sulcus at the foundation of the anterior clinoid process; this definite bony sulcus is called the infraclinoid carotid groove.[3] The ICA finally courses into the intradural space and penetrates the dura propria. This penetrating portion is the carotid dural ring (distal ring). The venous space around the ICA in the infraclinoid carotid groove is called the infraclinoid carotid groove sinus (infraclinoid sinus), which is surrounded by the periosteum at the bony side of the carotid groove and the dura propria at the other side and is a peripheral venous space of the cavernous sinus similar to the intercavernous or basilar venous sinus.[3] The entrance of the infraclinoid sinus is the proximal ring, and it ends by the dural ring distally. The infraclinoid sinus, which is a peripheral venous space and not a venous lake like the cavernous sinus, could be differentiated from the

cavernous sinus. The ICA in this sinus is called the clinoid segment (infraclinoid carotid groove or infraclinoid segment).[3] On the medial side of the dural ring in most cases, a dural pouch called the carotid cave is present.[4] It is an intradural space seated in the infraclinoid carotid groove with its apex pointing proximally. The connection of the dural ring with the ICA in this area is relatively loose. A few superior hypophyseal arteries often arise from the ICA in the carotid cave. The carotid cave may not always exist.

This anatomic relationship is obtained by removing the anterior clinoid process and opening the optic canal. In the operating field via the pterional approach with the patient's head rotated to the opposite side approximately 45 degrees (Fig. 77-1); the carotid cave is located approximately in the ventral side of the ICA. After the anterior clinoid process is completely removed, the periosteal wall of the infraclinoid sinus is seen. By opening the periosteal wall, the infraclinoid segment of the ICA is exposed. The ICA penetrates the dural ring obliquely, and the lateral side of the ICA at this level of the carotid cave, therefore, belongs to extradural area. The curved portion of the ICA, before it penetrates the dural ring, is called the surgical genu of the ICA. The genu is usually observed horizontally in the operating field, and the concave portion of the genu is called the axilla of the ICA.[4]

The ophthalmic artery usually originates from the superior wall of the carotid artery (Table 77-1) immediately after the carotid artery penetrates the dura propria and enters the optic canal penetrating the dura propria.[5-7] The ophthalmic artery originates occasionally from the extradural portion of the ICA.[7-9] The segment of the ICA between the branching points of the ophthalmic and posterior communicating arteries is the ophthalmic segment; its length varies from 6 to 15 mm (mean, 9.6 mm) because of anatomic variation of the branching point of the posterior communicating artery along the ICA.[5]

TERMINOLOGY AND DEFINITION

With regard to surgical difficulty in clipping aneurysms arising from the C2 portion of the ICA, the anterior clinoid process has formerly been considered an important landmark to describe the limitation of "clippability" of these aneurysms. Aneurysms in the supraclinoid portion are clippable because they are in the subarachnoid space, whereas those in the infraclinoid portion cannot be clipped because they are in the cavernous sinus. With recent surgical and anatomic advancements, it has become feasible for aneurysms in the infraclinoid portion to be directly treated surgically with removal of the anterior clinoid process, and the surgical attention is now

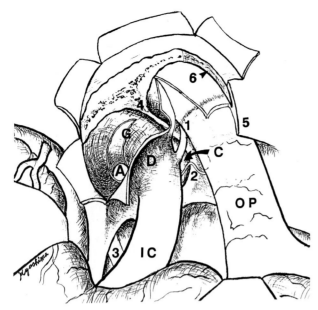

FIGURE 77-1 Schematic drawing of surgical anatomy in the operating field after removal of the anterior clinoid process and optic roof via the left pterional approach with the patient's head rotated to the opposite side approximately 45 degrees.[11] Note that the internal carotid artery (ICA) penetrates the dural ring obliquely in the field, and the carotid cave is located ventrally where the superior hypophyseal artery originates from the ICA. The infraclinoid portion of the ICA is partially exposed by dissecting the periosteum. The ICA in this area runs horizontally, and the dural ring adheres to the ICA tightly in the dorsal to lateral side. A, axilla of the ICA; C, carotid cave; D, dural ring; G, surgical genu of the ICA; OP, optic nerve; IC, internal carotid artery; 1, ophthalmic artery; 2, superior hypophyseal artery; 3, oculomotor nerve; 4, optic strut; 5, falciform fold; 6, optic roof. (From Kyoshima K, Koike G, Hokama M, et al: A classification of juxtadural ring aneurysms with reference to surgical anatomy. J Clin Neurosci 2:61–64, 1996.)

focused more appropriately on the aneurysm's relationship to the dural ring instead of the anterior clinoid process. Many aneurysms arising from the C2 and distal C3 portions, however, have no direct relationship to the branching arteries such as the ophthalmic or superior hypophyseal artery. As a result, these lesions are often described according to their relationship to adjacent anatomic landmarks or to the location of the aneurysm neck on the ICA, hence, the varying terms of para-, supra-, and infraophthalmic; para- and supraclinoid; sub-, para-, and suprachiasmal; and carotid cave aneurysms, or proximal ICA, global, ventral, and dorsal aneurysms.[10,11]

We consider that paraclinoid aneurysms in distal C3 and C2 portions can then be classified into two categories as intradural aneurysms near the carotid dural ring. In the first category, aneurysms arising from the ICA within the

TABLE 77-1 ▪ Origin of the Ophthalmic Artery from the Superior Wall of the Carotid Artery (%)

	Medial Third	Central Third	Lateral Third
Renn and Rhoton[8]	72	13	4
Gibo et al[6]	78	22	0
Lang[7]	55	25	20

ophthalmic segment, which is between the branching points of the ophthalmic and posterior communicating arteries and also includes the branching point of the ophthalmic artery, are defined as ophthalmic segment aneurysms abbreviated as ophthalmic aneurysms (Figs. 77-2 and 77-3; see also Figs. 77-7 and 77-8). In the ophthalmic aneurysms, those that have a clear relationship to the definite branching artery are described as carotid-ophthalmic artery aneurysms, abbreviated as carotid-ophthalmic aneurysms, if in relation to the ophthalmic artery (see Fig. 77-5) or carotid-superior hypophyseal (artery) aneurysms (see Fig. 77-6), if in relation to the superior hypophyseal artery.[10,12] Ophthalmic segment aneurysms have been classically called ophthalmic artery aneurysms, but the term ophthalmic artery aneurysm should be used only for an aneurysm arising from the ophthalmic artery itself.[13] Some ophthalmic aneurysms are located far distally from the anterior clinoid process because of anatomic variations of the arterial branching points. In these cases, the proximal parent artery and aneurysm neck are easily exposed, such as in the ordinary carotid–posterior communicating artery aneurysms. These cases may not be included in paraclinoid aneurysms. In the second category, intradural aneurysms arising from the ICA proximal to the branching level of the ophthalmic artery (usually in the carotid cave) are carotid cave aneurysms (Fig. 77-4).[3,4] Most of these aneurysms could not be recognized by removal of the anterior clinoid process alone; additional opening of the dural ring enabled their exposure. They were traditionally considered as infraclinoid or cavernous sinus aneurysms and therefore were considered unclippable.

Aneurysms may arise at any locations around the cross section of the ICA,[14,15] and the difficulties in clipping paraclinoid aneurysms depend not only on the existence of an arterial division or complicated anatomic features but also on their locations in the cross section of the ICA in the operating field. Therefore, from the surgical point of view, these aneurysms may be categorized. In the operating field, these aneurysms are seen via the pterional approach with the patient's head rotated to the opposite side approximately 45 degrees, according to their location in relation to the cross section of the ICA, as a lateral, medial, ventral, or dorsal type.[15]

Lateral-type ICA aneurysms are those that are directed laterally under the tentorium. Medial-type ICA aneurysms are directed medially toward or occasionally under the optic nerve. Ventral-type ICA aneurysms are located in the far side of the approaching route behind the ICA. Dorsal-type ICA aneurysms are located above the tentorium or the optic nerve projecting toward the approaching route in the operative field. A rare type of aneurysm also exists, called a global-type aneurysm,[16] which involves the whole circumference of the carotid artery and whose origins are not easy to identify.

Carotid-ophthalmic aneurysms are usually seen as a medial (Fig. 77-5) type protruding from the medial or dorsomedial wall of the ICA in the operating field. Ventral-type aneurysms may also arise from the medial side of the branching orifice on the ICA.

Carotid cave aneurysms are all the ventral type depending on the anatomic location of the carotid cave (see Fig. 77-4). They may grow out of the cave into the intradural subarachnoid space or the infraclinoid carotid groove sinus

FIGURE 77-2 A 66-year-old woman with a left ruptured giant ophthalmic aneurysm (ventral type). *A* and *B,* Preoperative angiograms, anteroposterior and lateral views. Note that the aneurysm is directed medially on the anteroposterior view and inferiorly on the lateral view. *C* and *D,* Postoperative angiograms show that the aneurysm was clipped with multiple clips preserving the natural curvature of the internal carotid artery (ICA). OPA, ophthalmic artery. *E,* Intraoperative view. A giant aneurysm was seen projecting ventrally. After exposure of the cervical ICA, removal of the anterior clinoid process, unroofing of the ophthalmic artery, sectioning of the dural ring, mobilization of the ophthalmic artery, and exposure of the infraclinoid segment, multiple clipping with ring clips was done in tandem fashion with direct puncture method under temporary occlusion of the cervical ICA, the ICA distal to the posterior communicating artery (PCoA), the OPA, and the PCoA. Postoperatively, the patient showed temporary right hemiparesis. In this earlier case, the dural ring was not dissected circumferentially. D, dural ring; G, surgical genu of the ICA; OP, optic nerve; 1, ophthalmic artery; 3, oculomotor nerve. (From Kyoshima K, Kobayashi K, Orz YI: Ophthalmic aneurysms. In Kaye AH, Black PM (eds): Operative Neurosurgery. London: Churchill Livingstone, 1999.)

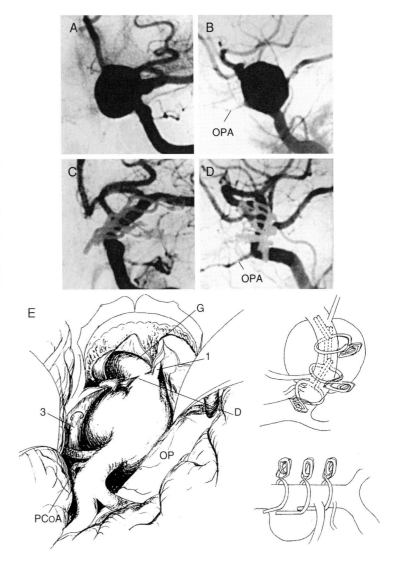

beyond the thin dura (propria). When a carotid cave aneurysm has grown distally, it may sometimes be difficult to differentiate from a carotid-ophthalmic aneurysm.

INCIDENCE

The reported incidence of ophthalmic aneurysms, which may include different types of aneurysms, varies from 0.5% to 5.4%.[14,17-19]

We have operated on 129 patients with paraclinoid aneurysms, including 44 patients with large to giant aneurysms (34%) at Nagoya University Hospital, Shinshu University Hospital, and their affiliated hospitals. At Nagoya University, there were 41 patients with paraclinoid aneurysms: 7 with carotid cave aneurysms and 34 with ophthalmic aneurysms, including 16 global aneurysms. At Shinshu University, there were 88 patients with 92 paraclinoid aneurysms: 42 carotid cave aneurysms and 50 ophthalmic aneurysms.

Paraclinoid aneurysms have a female preponderance, a high incidence of multiple aneurysms, symmetric aneurysms, large size (75% are >10 mm), and a high incidence of visual disturbance as the initial symptom as well as subarachnoid hemorrhage (Table 77-2).[14,17,19-21] In carotid cave aneurysms, no patients showed preoperative visual symptoms.

PREOPERATIVE EVALUATION

Cerebral Angiography

Transfemoral four-vessel cerebral angiography is preferable to delineate the anatomic relationships among the aneurysm; the carotid, ophthalmic, posterior communicating, and anterior choroidal arteries; the anterior clinoid process; and the optic canal. In addition to straight anteroposterior (AP) and lateral views, oblique and basal views are often helpful to identify the neck of an aneurysm. Cross circulation through the anterior communicating artery and the posterior communicating artery must also be fully examined. Vertebral angiography with ipsilateral carotid compression often helps to determine the collateral flow through the posterior communicating artery and to identify the distal neck of the aneurysm. A balloon occlusion test is mandatory for most patients with paraclinoid aneurysms.

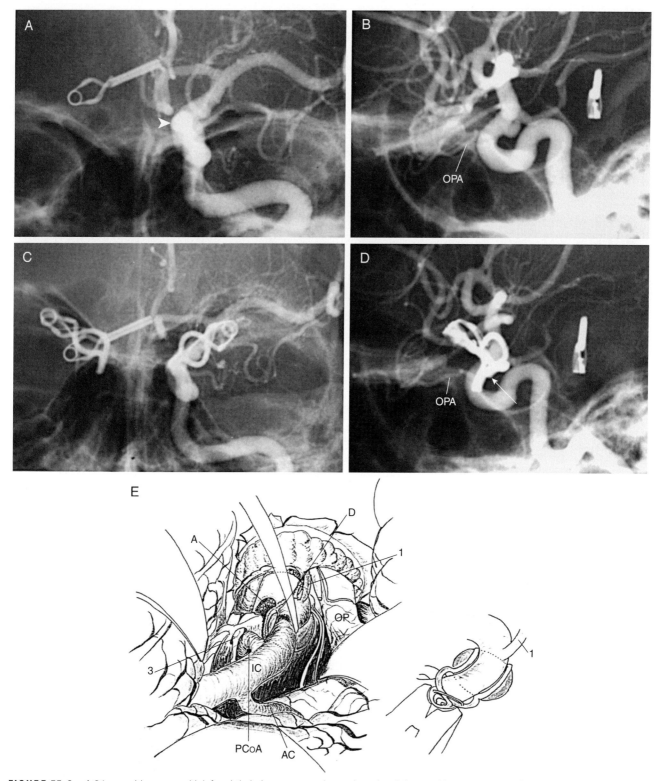

FIGURE 77-3 A 34-year-old woman with left ophthalmic aneurysms (ventral type), a right carotid cave aneurysm (ventral type), and a ruptured basilar aneurysm (which was clipped earlier). A and B, Preoperative left carotid angiograms with anteroposterior and lateral views. Note that the left ophthalmic aneurysm is located distally to the ophthalmic artery and directed just medially on the anteroposterior view and inferiorly on the lateral view. C and D, Postoperative angiograms are taken after clipping both internal carotid aneurysms. The *arrowhead* indicates the aneurysms. The *arrow* indicates a clip for the aneurysm. OPA, ophthalmic artery. E, This intraoperative view of the left ophthalmic aneurysm shows that the aneurysm is projecting ventrally. The aneurysm is located just distally to the branching level of the ophthalmic artery and was clipped with a curved-blade ring clip after the procedures of untethering exposure method. A, axilla of the internal carotid artery; D, dural ring; AC, anterior cerebral artery; OP, optic nerve; PCoA, posterior communicating artery; *Arrow*, left ophthalmic aneurysm; 1, ophthalmic artery; 3, oculomotor nerve. (From Kyoshima K, Kobayashi K, Orz YI: Ophthalmic aneurysms. In Kaye AH, Black PM (eds): Operative Neurosurgery. London: Churchill Livingstone, 1999.)

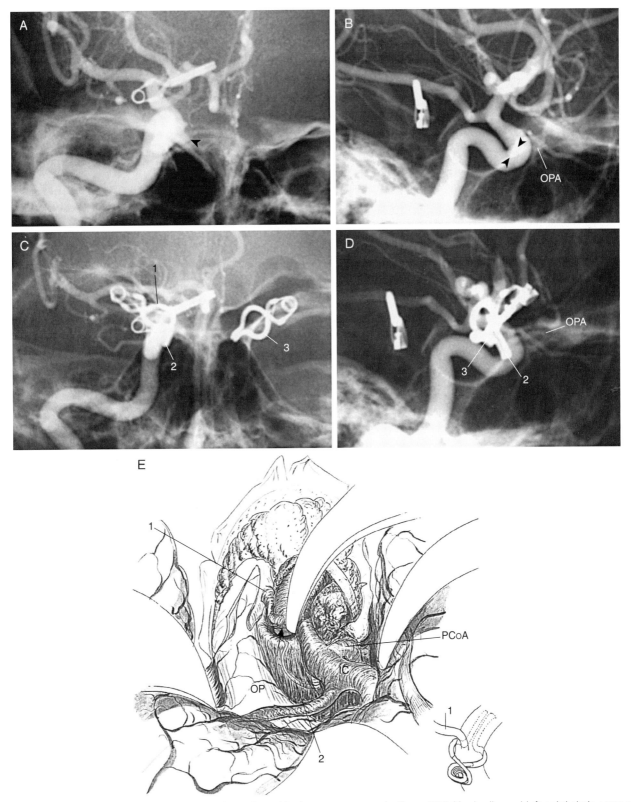

FIGURE 77-4   A right carotid cave aneurysm (ventral type) in the same case as in Figure 78-3 (the basilar and left ophthalmic segment aneurysms were previously clipped). *A* and *B,* Preoperative right carotid angiograms with anteroposterior and lateral views. Note that the carotid cave aneurysm is directed medially on the anteroposterior view and located proximally to the ophthalmic artery, superimposing at the hairpin curve of the angiographic genu on the lateral view. *C* and *D,* Postoperative angiograms, which were obtained after clipping both internal carotid aneurysms, show that the site of the aneurysm is precisely confirmed by the position of the clip blades. The *arrowhead* indicates a carotid cave aneurysm. *E,* This intraoperative view shows that the aneurysm is ventrally located in the carotid cave and was clipped with a curved-blade ring clip after the untethering exposure method (see text) with prior exposure of the cervical internal carotid artery (ICA). The ophthalmic artery originated from the ICA extradurally in this case. The *arrow* indicates the aneurysm. OPA, ophthalmic artery; PCoA, posterior communicating artery; 1, clip for the basilar aneurysm; 2, clip for the carotid cave aneurysm; 3, clip for the opposite ophthalmic segment aneurysm. (From Kyoshima K, Kobayashi K, Orz YI: Ophthalmic aneurysms. In Kaye AH, Black PM (eds): Operative Neurosurgery. London: Churchill Livingstone, 1999.)

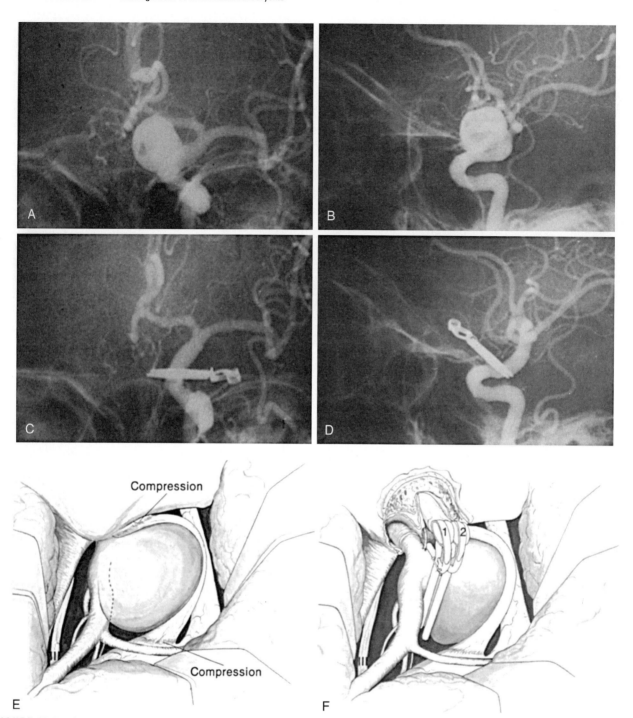

FIGURE 77-5   A carotid-ophthalmic aneurysm (medial type). *A* and *B,* Preoperative left carotid angiograms with anteroposterior and lateral views. *C* and *D,* Postoperative anteroposterior and lateral views. *E,* An intraoperative view before clipping shows that the left optic nerve was greatly displaced dorsomedially. The optic nerve was compressed anteriorly by the falciform process and posteriorly by the A1 segment of the anterior cerebral artery. *F,* Intraoperative view during clipping. Clip No. 1, which was applied perpendicularly, was not strong enough to close the aneurysm and opened with each pulsation. The larger clip No. 2 closed the aneurysm completely, and clip No. 1 was removed.

The anatomic relationship between large to giant paraclinoid aneurysms and the optic nerve is often difficult to predict from preoperative angiography alone. Results of comparative studies of angiographic and intraoperative findings suggest that paraclinoid aneurysms with a closed carotid siphon and aneurysms that grow inferiorly to the carotid artery stay beneath the optic nerve and compress the nerve from inferiorly (ventral type), although some ophthalmic

aneurysms grow above the optic nerve (medial type) and displace it medially.[22] Compression by these aneurysms is usually much less than that by ventral-type aneurysms.

On angiography, it is difficult to predict the location of the dural ring. However, the ophthalmic artery, when visible, and the angiographic genu of the ICA will give approximate landmarks of the ring, which is usually proximal to the ophthalmic artery and located at the

TABLE 77-2 ▪ Demographic Characteristics of Patients with Paraclinoid Aneurysms

	Yasargil[14]*	Weir[19]*	Current Series
Total no. of patients	272	207	129
Male/female (%)	25/75	19/81	23/77
Multiple aneurysms (%)	18	49	40
Symmetric aneurysms (%)	21	11	12
Initial symptoms: visual (%)	11	30	20
Subarachnoid hemorrhage (%)	76	56	23

*Patients with "classic" ophthalmic artery aneurysms.

level of the angiographic genu. The medial side of the hairpin curve portion of the angiographic genu corresponds to the level of the carotid cave, and its lateral side is the extradural portion. Because the ICA penetrates the dural ring obliquely (see Fig. 77-1), there is a discrepancy between the angiographic genu and the surgical genu as obtained by the pterional approach. The surgical genu is located more proximally than the angiographic genu.[3] The ophthalmic aneurysm is located at or distal to the branching point of the ophthalmic artery (see Figs. 77-2, 77-3, and 77-7), whereas the carotid cave aneurysm is located proximally (see Fig. 77-4).

In relation to the cross section of the ICA, the direction of aneurysm projection seen in the operating field can roughly be estimated from the preoperative angiogram. In lateral-type aneurysms, they are directed laterally on the AP view and inferiorly on the lateral view. In medial-type aneurysms, they are directed medially on the AP view and superiorly on the lateral view. In ventral-type aneurysms, they are directed medially on the AP view and inferiorly on the lateral view (see Fig. 77-3). In dorsal-type aneurysms, they are directed laterally on the AP view and superiorly on the lateral view. When dorsal-type aneurysms are superimposed with the ICA on the AP view, many of them are adherent to the basal surface of the frontal lobe in the operative field, and when they are superimposed with the ICA on the lateral view, many of them are adherent to the medial surface of the temporal lobe.[23]

Carotid cave aneurysms are located medially on the AP view and posteriorly or laterally on the lateral view and proximally to the origin of the ophthalmic artery. Then, they project ventrally in the operating field approached pterionally with the patient's head rotated approximately 45 degrees contralaterally. They are anatomically intradural aneurysms and located angiographically at the angiographic genu or the anterior siphon knee (see Fig. 77-4).

Computed Tomography and Magnetic Resonance Imaging

Computed tomography (CT) will reveal all giant aneurysms and most large aneurysms as an uniformly enhancing masses. Three-dimensional CT is useful for the planning surgical approach. Thin-slice CT scans are especially helpful in the surgical planning for large to giant paraclinoid aneurysms. Both plain and enhanced CT scans are needed. The former may reveal calcification of the carotid artery and aneurysmal

wall,[14] which often disturbs clipping. The shape and size of the anterior clinoid process must also be examined carefully. Air cells in the anterior clinoid process may lead to postoperative cerebrospinal fluid leakage. The anterior clinoid process may coalesce with the middle clinoid process to form a bony foramen around the carotid artery; drilling of the anterior clinoid process is extremely difficult in such cases.[24-26] Enhanced CT help to determine each relationship of the aneurysm, the carotid artery, and the anterior clinoid process, so that characteristics can be clearly kept in mind when the anterior clinoid process is drilled. Partial intramural thrombus may be revealed by CT as irregular enhancement, but magnetic resonance imaging is superior for such purposes as well as for 3-dimensional display of anatomic relationships between the aneurysm and optic nerve and surrounding structures. A 3-dimensional CT scan would give better operative view of the aneurysm in relation to the parent artery than that provided by magnetic resonance imaging; however, finer arteries such as the superior hypophyseal artery are not shown.

SURGICAL TREATMENT

All the information about the patient's condition, age, and the multiplicity and characteristics of the aneurysm as well as the collateral circulation must be carefully evaluated so that the most appropriate form of treatment is selected, that is, direct clipping, carotid occlusion with or without bypass surgery, or endovascular surgery. The results of a balloon occlusion test of the carotid artery provide important information for making such a decision.[27]

POSITIONING AND CRANIOTOMY

The ipsilateral pterional approach is usually taken for most paraclinoid aneurysms. Contralateral and interhemispheric approaches are limited to special cases of symmetric aneurysms or small, medially directed aneurysms.[28,29] The patient's head is elevated 25 to 45 degrees (depending on the estimation of intraoperative bleeding from the infraclinoid and cavernous sinus) and then rotated 45 degrees to the contralateral side and fixed to the headholder with four pins. In the direct approach to paraclinoid aneurysms, more contralateral rotation of the head than in other cases of ICA aneurysms is required because the optic nerve and ICA overlap at their proximal portions, and ophthalmic aneurysms have an intimate relationship with the optic nerve, which covers and tends to hide their origin. By more head rotation, the optic nerve and the ICA can be seen more or less in parallel, allowing less retraction of the ICA or optic nerve.

The ipsilateral neck must be cleaned and draped in the same operative field so that the carotid artery can be compressed manually in case of emergency. We usually expose the cervical carotid artery to allow temporary occlusion in difficult cases.

A semicoronal skin incision is made from just anterior to the tragus, crossing the midline behind the hairline to the contralateral side by approximately 4 cm. The frontal branch of the superficial temporal artery should always be preserved as a donor for anastomosis if needed.[30] A frontotemporal craniotomy is made with three burr holes. Medial enlargement of the craniotomy by 2 to 3 cm gives more freedom for clip application. After substantial removal of the sphenoid wing to the lateral corner of the superior orbital fissure, we usually open the dura and dissect the Sylvian fissure to inspect the aneurysm and to secure the carotid artery distal to the aneurysm.

Dissection of the Aneurysm

Wide splitting of the Sylvian fissure may allow easier retraction of the brain. In large to giant aneurysms that compress the optic nerve, sectioning the falciform ligament of the optic canal should be undertaken first before proceeding to the following procedures.

In acute-stage surgery performed when the brain is swollen, lumbar cerebrospinal fluid drainage or ventricular drainage may be helpful for easy and safe brain retraction. We use a soft suction tube made of a ventricular tube from a ventriculoperitoneal shunt to keep the operating field clean and dry by constantly removing blood, cerebrospinal fluid, and bone dust.

The important procedure in direct surgery of paraclinoid aneurysms is freeing the parent ICA by untethering it from the surrounding structures. Surgical procedures such as extensive removal of the anterior clinoid process, unroofing of the optic canal, mobilization of the ophthalmic artery, exposure of the infraclinoid segment by opening the infraclinoid sinus, and circumferential sectioning of the dural ring allow excellent exposure and mobilization of the parent ICA (untethering exposure method), thus providing enough proximal exposure for temporary carotid clipping, if required, to facilitate clip application.

On removal of the anterior clinoid process, we prefer to observe it both extradurally and intradurally by cutting the dura mater vertically toward the anterior clinoid process as needed[26] because premature rupture of the aneurysm during an exclusively epidural drilling can be catastrophic. Dural covering must be left to protect the aneurysm or parent ICA, and temporary cervical carotid occlusion may be helpful to decrease the tension and size of the aneurysm during critical drilling; however, this has to be done carefully and for a short time to avoid thromboembolism. Constant irrigation is mandatory to protect the optic nerve from heat injury. The optic canal should be completely opened anteriorly to the orbit and laterally to the floor by drilling the optic strut along with the anterior clinoid process with a high-speed diamond drill.[24,25] The medial wall of the optic canal must be carefully drilled, and the surgeon should try not to open the sphenoid air sinus. Once opened, it should be packed with muscle, fibrin glue, or Biobond. Exenteration of the sinus is not recommended; rather, it should be covered by the mucosa to keep the sinus clean.

The ophthalmic artery is mobilized from the dura in the optic canal. To find the origin of the ophthalmic artery, direct retraction of the ICA laterally is helpful as the optic sheath is opened.

The infraclinoid segment of the ICA is exposed by opening the periosteum over the infraclinoid sinus. Bleeding from the infraclinoid sinus is easily controlled by elevation of the patient's head and packing with Oxycel cotton, Gelfoam, or Surgicel proximally along the wall of the ICA. However, excessive packing may compress the cranial nerves and

disturb further dissection by forming a mass. The dural ring is finally cut circumferentially, and thus substantial untethering of the ICA is obtained. When sectioning the dural ring on the medial side, the surgeon should be mindful of rare cases in which the ophthalmic artery originates from the interdural portion of the ICA at the carotid dural ring and courses within the dura, if the ophthalmic artery detected by preoperative angiography is not seen intradurally or extradurally.[31]

Although the extent of bone removal of the optic canal and the anterior clinoid process depends on the characteristics of each aneurysm, the untethering exposure method is necessary in cases of a paraclinoid aneurysm in which the neck is located close to the dural ring or in cases of large to giant aneurysms to secure the proximal parent artery and aneurysm neck. Without sectioning the dural ring, it may disturb the advancement of the clip blades and result in incomplete clipping.

Gentle retraction of the tip of the temporal lobe preserving bridging veins is required. Cutting the dura at the medial side of the attachment of bridging veins and retraction of the temporal tip with the dura including the sphenoparietal sinus will facilitate further retraction of the temporal tip, if necessary.[32]

Dissection of the aneurysm from the carotid artery and optic nerve is carried out with silver dissectors. Those with various shapes and sharpness of blades or bends of the tips should be prepared. The most difficult part of surgery for large to giant aneurysms in this location is dissection of the thin aneurysmal wall from thick fibrous adhesion to the basal dura. Unless more than two thirds of the circumference of the aneurysmal wall is dissected free, clipping cannot be performed well without slipping. Sharp dissection with a knife or scissors and the use of a solid and less malleable dissector shorten the time to dissect tough and fibrous adhesions around the aneurysm.

Direct retraction of the ICA and optic nerve may facilitate the procedures. Careful retraction of the ICA laterally or the optic nerve medially brings the proximal portion of the ICA and the neck of the aneurysm into view. Retraction of the optic nerve should be undertaken as minimally as possible. However, if it is necessary, a normal optic nerve can be retracted as much as 5 mm intermittently, and during the procedure, protection of the optic nerve with a Silastic sheet is advisable.[33]

Carotid Occlusion

Temporary or permanent occlusion of the carotid artery may be needed for surgical treatment of the paraclinoid aneurysms. Temporary occlusion is performed when a critical region is drilled or dissected or when the aneurysm is trapped and punctured. Permanent occlusion may be performed as the final treatment with or without bypass surgery.[34] Before the carotid artery is occluded, the brain should be protected from ischemic injury. We usually administer the following drugs: heparin sodium (3000 to 4000 IU),[35] thiamylal sodium (150 to 250 mg), methylprednisolone (250 mg), mannitol (20%, 100 mL), or low-molecular-weight dextran (10%, 40 mL/hr), and diphenylhydantoin (125 to 250 mg). Although the brain is monitored continuously by electroencephalography or somatosensory evoked potentials, the duration of temporary occlusion should be kept as short as possible.

When longer trapping time is needed, it should be divided into several intermittent occlusions, and during periods of occlusion, the systemic blood pressure should be elevated above the preoperative level. Brain ischemia is usually more severe during surgery than at the time of the preoperative balloon occlusion test because of the additional factor of brain retraction. If the patient cannot tolerate a balloon occlusion test because of poor collateral circulation, an extracranial-intracranial bypass must be performed before the surgery to occlude the aneurysm.

Decompression of Aneurysm

In large to giant aneurysms, it is important to collapse the aneurysm to achieve satisfactory clipping and also to decompress the optic apparatus in cases with visual signs.

Aneurysms do not collapse by the temporary trapping of the carotid artery alone; however, to make them collapse, blood must be withdrawn by direct puncture of the aneurysmal dome,[36] the ICA,[37] or a branch of the external carotid artery in the neck.[38] We use a 21-gauge butterfly-type needle. Recently, we have used a specially designed puncture needle[39] to puncture the aneurysm after temporary trapping, with the needle held by a small hemostat that is fixed to a self-retaining retractor. Fifty to 200 mL of blood is withdrawn from the tube connected to the butterfly needle. When an aneurysm is punctured, the needle must be inserted at a point as distal from the neck as possible so that the puncture site will not be involved in the clipping site. When multiple clips are applied, a 1.5- to 2-mm width of aneurysmal wall is needed for each blade. Sometimes this method of withdrawing blood is unsatisfactory, and the aneurysm does not collapse because blood comes through the ophthalmic artery when temporary trapping is done between the infraclinoid segment and the ICA proximal to the posterior communicating artery or through anastomoses between the internal and external carotid arteries when proximal trapping is done at the cervical ICA. Under these circumstances, rapid suction is used; once the aneurysm is collapsed, its wall must be dissected from the surrounding tissues as quickly as possible to shorten the trapping time, and special care should be taken not to traumatize the optic nerve.

Clip Application

Clipping techniques vary depending on the anatomic situation and the size of the aneurysm. A large clip with a stronger closing force is often needed because of high intramural pressure and a thick aneurysmal wall. In these cases, a Sugita booster clip, with which 250 g can be added to the closing force, is useful.

For aneurysms free of the arterial division, perpendicular clipping (the clip blades are placed perpendicularly to the axis of the ICA) may be applied, but parallel clipping (clip blades are placed parallel to the axis) is generally recommended. When an aneurysm is obliterated perpendicularly, the neck becomes tensive and tearing at the neck or kinking of the parent artery may occur. Neck tearing is more likely to occur because the ICA is larger and often harder than other major cerebral arteries. For small aneurysms located free of the arterial division, however, the parallel clipping is occasionally difficult because clip blades may slip off the small dome of the aneurysm.

For aneurysms related to the arterial division, perpendicular clipping is possible (see Fig. 77-5). As the clip blades close the aneurysm neck, a branching artery approximates the side of the parent artery, and this will reduce the tension at the aneurysm neck by the decreased angle between the branching artery and the parent ICA. For aneurysms with a wide neck, however, parallel clipping or multiple clipping is required.

In lateral-type aneurysms, it is important to try to identify the posterior communicating artery during surgery, even though it is not seen on the preoperative angiogram. Medial-type aneurysms are often related to the ophthalmic artery, and most of them are carotid-ophthalmic aneurysms. Ventral-type aneurysms are located in the far side of the approaching route under the ICA and sometimes have a relationship to the ophthalmic artery. It is usually very difficult to occlude them with conventional clips; however, with the introduction of ring clips, especially an angled ring clip with or without curved blades, their obliteration has become relatively easy.[2,4,40] Using an angled ring clip, clip blades naturally become parallel to the axis of the ICA and the parent artery is reconstructed by the ring portion of the clip. All carotid cave aneurysms belong to this type. On clipping of carotid cave aneurysms, the untethering exposure method is essential. It is important to dissect the ICA from the dural ring completely and to place the tips of clip blades in the axilla to prevent parent artery stenosis or obstruction by clipping. Dorsal-type aneurysms include not only blister-like aneurysms but also usual saccular aneurysms.[23,41,42] They are frequently adherent to the frontal or temporal lobe. Large to giant aneurysms are rare in this type. Blister aneurysms are unlikely to grow large without rupture. They are usually small, fragile, and wide based, and at surgery, intraoperative rupture occurs very frequently, requiring special techniques.[23,42] Parallel clipping should be undertaken with an L-shaped or curved blade clip, and a clip should be placed in such a way that the clip blades partially include the wall of the parent artery causing some stenosis. Reversed parallel clipping (a clip is applied from the proximal side of the ICA) is advisable to avoid tearing of the aneurysm neck caused by pressure on the clip head when brain retraction is released. Temporary occlusion of the parent artery at the time of clipping is necessary. Perpendicular clipping is contraindicated because it may cause tearing of the fragile neck.

Large to Giant Aneurysms

A large to giant aneurysm with a very broad neck presents a much greater problem. A single long clip may not completely close the aneurysm neck, owing to high intraluminal pressure and a thick, broad aneurysm neck, and is likely to kink or occlude the ICA because the clip is pushed down by a bulbous sac. A multiple clipping technique in various combinations[40,41,43] is feasible to prevent straightening of the ICA to conform to its natural curvature at the C2–C3 portion and to obtain a sufficient closing force to occlude the neck completely.

Most of the large to giant aneurysms are of the ventral type and rarely of the dorsal type. Ventral-type aneurysms may grow very large because their wall is protected by the overlying ICA and underlying dura of the pituitary fossa.

In large to giant ventral-type aneurysms, it is easier to expose the aneurysm neck or to identify arteries around the neck than in smaller ones. In those aneurysms, the neck is spread almost in the same plane of the dorsal wall of the ICA, whereas in small aneurysms with a diameter less than that of the ICA, the aneurysm neck is likely hidden by the ICA. To clip large to giant ventral-type aneurysms, ring clips are usually the first choice. Clips must be applied along the course of the artery to keep the lumen of the artery adequately wide. For such purposes, using multiple ring clips[2] with short blades is better than using a single clip with long blades, and ring clips with curved blades that fit the C2–C3 curve are especially useful (see Figs. 77-3, 77-4, and 77-6). Clips are made specifically for such purposes for the right and left carotid arteries. A side-angled clip applier is also useful in this location, especially for medially directed aneurysms. Apertures of the Sugita ring clips are 3 or 5 mm in diameter, and the diameter of the carotid artery is usually a little less than 5 mm. To keep the lumen of the carotid artery as wide as possible, the clip must be inserted deep enough so that the near rim of the ring almost touches the dorsal wall of the carotid artery. When multiple ring clips are applied, the spring portion of the clips must be placed as parallel to each other as possible to keep good alignment and to avoid cross-biting of the blades. Narrowing of the carotid artery caught in the ring almost always results from a lack of dissection of adhesion of the aneurysm to the surrounding tissue, usually the dura mater. When the branching artery does not originate from the aneurysm, the aneurysm can be occluded with ring clips in tandem fashion (see Fig. 77-2). When the major branching artery originates from the neck or near the body of the aneurysm, the branching artery can be reconstructed with a straight ring clip (branching artery formation clipping).[2] It is often preferable to occlude the distal part of the aneurysm neck by a regular nonring clip from the lateral or medial side of the ICA to preserve fine perforating arteries.[2] After the clips are applied and the patency of the carotid artery is preserved, care must be taken not to constrict the posterior communicating and anterior choroidal arteries and their perforating branches when brain retraction is released because the angled clips tend to rotate when the brain returns to its original place. Such rotation can be avoided by breaking the pia mater of the frontal lobe where the spring portion of the clip is hitting.

In lateral- or medial-type large to giant aneurysms with a wide neck, clipping is often more difficult than for large to giant ventral aneurysms. Sometimes, in the case of a giant aneurysm, it is impossible because ring clips cannot be used as for ventral aneurysms, and the perpendicular clipping may cause tearing of the neck or kinking of the parent artery and placing clip blades parallel to the parent artery is technically difficult. In this situation, an attempt should be made to place the clip blades as parallel as possible with multiple clips. If the clip blades are placed perpendicularly, it is advisable to place them away from the aneurysm neck to the dome side.[2]

In some cases, kinking of the anterior or middle cerebral artery caused by elongation or displacement of the ICA by clipping a large aneurysm may occur and result in cerebral infarction. When the kinking is observed, alternative methods, which include relocation of the clip(s), replacement of the clip(s) to another clip(s) with shorter blades, or changing of the combination of clips may be tried.[43]

Partially thrombosed aneurysms are particularly difficult to clip. Clips applied to the neck of these aneurysms may not close completely but slide to or away from the parent artery unless the thrombus is removed. Intra-aneurysmal endarterectomy is often needed in such cases. Great care must be taken to prevent thrombi from migrating into the carotid stream; use of heparin and careful application of clips are important for this purpose. A Doppler ultrasound flow meter and intraoperative angiography help to check the clipping and to avoid kinking of the parent artery.

Closure

The defected portion of the dura and bone by opening the infraclinoid carotid groove is covered with a piece of temporalis muscle. If fibrin glue is applied, care should be taken to avoid direct contact of the glue with the optic or oculomotor nerve. Small titanium plates are useful to prevent a depression of the bone flap postoperatively.

Bypass Surgery

The carotid artery may be occluded without causing neurologic deficits in patients with sufficient collateral flow. Balloon occlusion of the carotid artery is often the treatment of choice in elderly patients with difficult extradural aneurysms, but the long-term results of such treatment in patients with paraclinoid aneurysm are not known. Furthermore, later development of hypertension or aneurysm in the remaining carotid artery[44] may have to be considered, especially in younger patients. Occlusion of the carotid artery in patients with poor collateral flow must be preceded by an intracranial-extracranial bypass, which can rescue patients with unclippable aneurysms, or those with hard calcification in the wall, fusiform aneurysm, or rupture of the aneurysm near the neck. Superficial temporal artery–to–middle cerebral artery anastomosis[30] may be performed if the superficial temporal artery is well developed, but flow through such a bypass is usually small and an insufficient substitute for that of the carotid artery. External carotid artery–to–middle cerebral artery bypass using either a saphenous vein or a radial artery graft are usually superior to superficial temporal artery–to–middle cerebral artery anastomosis. However, data on the long-term follow-up of patients who have had these bypass surgeries must be accumulated to evaluate the most appropriate methods. Such bypass surgery may have to be performed even temporarily for patients with very poor collateral flow yet who need temporary carotid occlusion. After successful clipping of the aneurysm, with patency of the carotid artery preserved, the bypass may close spontaneously.

Results

Of 129 patients with paraclinoid aneurysms, direct clipping was performed in 123 patients, wrapping in 4, and trapping in 2. Prophylactic superficial temporal artery–to–middle cerebral artery anastomosis was performed in one patient. External carotid artery to M2 bypass using a saphenous vein graft was performed in three sides of two patients whose aneurysms were trapped together with the ICA. Patency was obtained in all anastomoses.

In small aneurysms, 80 of 85 patients obtained excellent results (94%) and resumed their full daily activities; 12 patients showed some postoperative visual deficits due to surgical manipulation. Wrapping was performed in two carotid cave aneurysms in the early stage of this series. Results in three patients were poor; two patients did not improve from their poor preoperative condition due to rupture of the accompanying aneurysms, and another patient became disabled due to intraoperative thrombosis related to temporary occlusion of the ICA. Two patients died owing to worsening of the preoperative poor condition; one was due to ICA occlusion, and the other was due to subcortical hematoma.

In large to giant aneurysms, however, the results of these patients were not as good, with 33 of 44 patients obtaining excellent results (75%) and 4 of the 44 patients with unruptured large or giant aneurysms becoming moderately or severely disabled, probably because of complications of temporary carotid occlusion. Three patients had no improvement from their poor preoperative condition because of subarachnoid hemorrhage. Another patient (Hunt grade IV) who had bilateral ophthalmic aneurysms did not improve after surgery. One patient in whom a giant basilar tip aneurysm and a large ophthalmic aneurysm were clipped on the same day became severely disabled because of intraoperative midbrain ischemia complicating the clipping of the basilar aneurysm. Two patients died; one patient with a giant global aneurysm died of progressive thrombosis because of narrowing of the ICA caused by a dislocated clip, and another patient with a giant nonruptured aneurysm died of postoperative rupture owing to slipping out of the clip.

Representative cases are described in the following case reports.

CASE REPORT 1 (SEE FIGURE 77-5)

A carotid-ophthalmic aneurysm occurred in a 61-year-old woman with finger counting ability only in the left eye, a homonymous right lower quadrantanopia with a central scotoma in the left eye, and a mild left ptosis. A left carotid angiogram revealed a 16-mm aneurysm protruding superomedially from the C2 portion of the ICA. The angiogram also showed a defect due to an intramural thrombus (see Fig. 77-5A and B). The left carotid artery was secured in the neck. Intracranially, the left optic nerve was markedly pinched between the aneurysm and the falciform process anteriorly and between the aneurysm and the A1 posteriorly (see Fig. 77-5E). The optic canal was opened, and the anterior clinoid process was removed with a diamond burr. The aneurysm originated just distal to the ophthalmic artery and was protruding medially in the operating field (medial type). A No. 18 straight clip (1 in Fig. 77-5F) was applied perpendicularly to the neck of the aneurysm, but this clip opened with each pulsation, which required the addition of a stronger, No. 19a clip (2 in Fig. 77-5F) parallel to the first clip, which was then removed (see Fig. 77-5C and D). The oculomotor nerve was compressed by the carotid artery, which was displaced laterally by the aneurysm. The patient's visual acuity was unchanged after the surgery, but her ptosis disappeared.

Comment

Securing the carotid artery in the neck is safer for difficult ophthalmic aneurysms, or the neck should at least be draped along with the operative field so that the carotid artery can be compressed without delay in an emergency. Carotid-ophthalmic aneurysms usually grow underneath the optic nerve, as seen in this case. Straight clips can be applied perpendicularly for most carotid-ophthalmic aneurysms, which arise at the branching point of the ophthalmic artery medially to the carotid artery in the operating field. A booster clip (or a larger clip) should be used when the closing force of a clip is insufficient. The extent of opening of the optic canal and removal of the anterior clinoid process should be decided after inspection of the anatomic relationship of the aneurysm to the surrounding structures such as the optic nerve, the carotid artery, and the anterior clinoid process.

CASE REPORT 2 (FIGURE 77-6)

A superior hypophyseal aneurysm occurred in a 51-year-old woman. This patient had a subarachnoid hemorrhage 6 weeks before surgery. A ventriculoperitoneal shunt had been inserted for the treatment of hydrocephalus in another hospital. At admission, the patient had no neurologic deficits. A right carotid angiogram showed a small aneurysm protruding medially from the C2 portion (see Fig. 77-6A and B). Intraoperatively, the aneurysm was hidden underneath the optic nerve and the anterior clinoid process (medial type) (see Fig. 77-6E). The proximal neck of the aneurysm was found when the well-pneumatized roof of the optic canal and the anterior clinoid process were removed. The superior hypophyseal artery originated from the proximal part of the aneurysm (see Fig. 77-6F). A No. 73 ring clip with curved blades successfully obliterated the aneurysm, as confirmed by postoperative angiography (see Fig. 77-6C and D). It should be noted that the clip blades follow the natural curve of the carotid artery. The opened air cells in the roof of the optic canal and the anterior clinoid process were packed with muscle and fibrin glue. The patient was discharged without neurologic deficits.

Comment

Curved blades of the clip fit the natural curve of the carotid artery without causing kinking. Both bayonet and angled clips had been tried over the carotid artery, but their tips did not proceed deeply enough, and they hit a bone of the sella turcica. Consequently, they would have to be applied perpendicularly and not in parallel to the long axis of the carotid artery if such a clip as used in this patient was not available.

CASE REPORT 3 (FIGURE 77-7)

A giant ventral-type (or global-type) aneurysm occurred in a 60-year-old woman who came to the hospital complaining of poor vision in the right eye (20/600) but good vision in the left (20/25). Angiograms showed a 40-mm aneurysm projecting inferomedially from the C2 portion

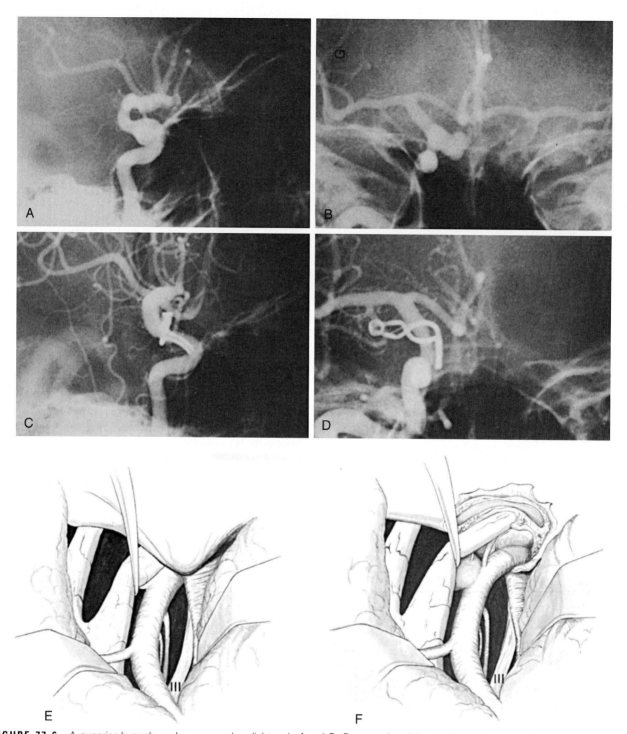

FIGURE 77-6   A superior hypophyseal aneurysm (medial type). *A* and B, Preoperative right carotid angiograms with lateral and antero-posterior views with manual compression of the left carotid artery. *C* and *D*, Postoperative angiograms show that the fenestrated clip with curved blades fits the curve without causing narrowing of the carotid artery. *E* and *F*, Intraoperative views show that the aneurysm was hidden behind the optic nerve and the anterior clinoid process and was well visualized after opening the optic canal and removing the anterior clinoid process.

of the left carotid artery that occupied the suprasellar space (see Fig. 77-7A and B). Collateral flow through both the anterior and posterior communicating arteries was good, and the patient tolerated the balloon occlusion test for 20 minutes. During surgery, the aneurysm markedly elevated the bilateral optic nerves and chiasm, especially in the right optic nerve, which was severely pinched between

the aneurysm and the right A1, and it was considered to be the cause of poor vision in the right eye (see Fig. 77-7E). After heparinization and brain protection, the aneurysm was trapped and collapsed by puncturing it with a butterfly needle held by a hemostat and a self-retaining retractor and connected to a syringe for suctioning blood. Severe adhesion of the aneurysmal wall to the basal dura was sharply dissected, and the aneurysm was occluded with three ring clips applied in tandem or vis-à-vis fashion (facing or crossing fashion[40]) (see Fig. 77-7F). Total trapping time of the carotid artery was 21 minutes. Postoperative angiograms showed obliteration of the aneurysm and patency of the carotid artery with its branches well preserved (see Fig. 77-7C and D). However, the patient had moderate right hemiparesis due to infarction in the territory of the lenticulostriate arteries, which

could not be detected by the intraoperative electroencephalographic monitoring.

Comment

Application of multiple ring clips is the treatment of choice for such a giant ventral carotid aneurysm. Multiple clips with shorter blades must be used rather than a single clip with longer blades so that the lumen of the carotid artery is kept open. Collapse of the aneurysm

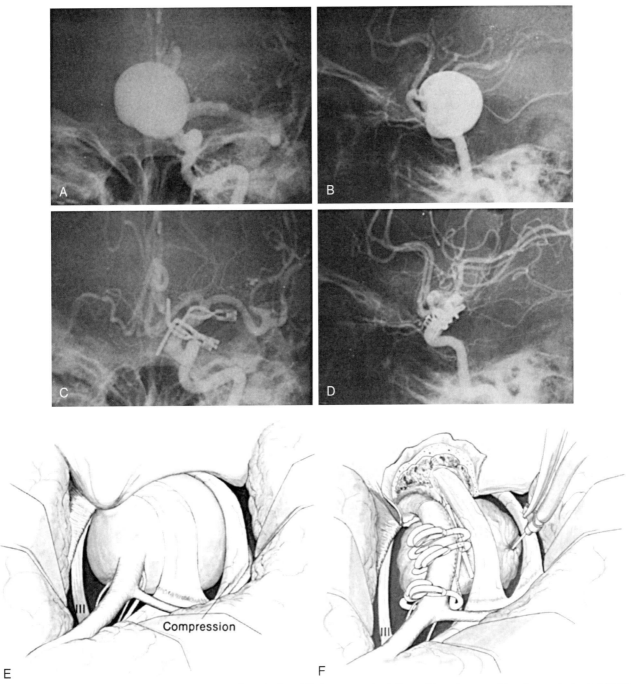

FIGURE 77-7   A giant ophthalmic aneurysm (ventral type). *A* and *B,* A preoperative left carotid angiogram with anteroposterior and lateral views. *C* and *D,* Postoperative angiograms show that the aneurysm has been excluded and the lumen of the internal carotid artery is well preserved. *E* and *F,* Intraoperative views show that the giant aneurysm developed ventral to the internal carotid artery, compressing both optic nerves from below. After the internal carotid artery was temporarily trapped, the aneurysm was punctured with a butterfly needle, which was held by a self-retaining retractor. The aneurysm was occluded with three fenestrated clips that were applied in tandem and vis-à-vis fashion.

is essential for clipping. We prefer a direct aneurysmal puncture to withdrawal of blood from the carotid artery in the neck. The aneurysm must be punctured at the dome, leaving enough distance from the parent artery (more than 6 mm when three clips are applied) so that the punctured hole is not involved under the clip blades.

CASE REPORT 4 (FIGURE 77-8)

Bilateral ophthalmic aneurysms occurred in a 67-year-old woman who suffered subarachnoid hemorrhage and was admitted in a semicomatose state. A CT scan revealed a severe subarachnoid hemorrhage in the basal cistern. Carotid angiograms showed a giant dorsal-type left and a large medial-type right ophthalmic aneurysm. The left A1 was hypoplastic, and bilateral anterior cerebral arteries were supplied by the right carotid artery (see Fig. 77-8A and B). Collateral flow through the posterior communicating artery was also not seen. Cerebral blood flow measured with Tc-hexamethylpropyleneamine oxime showed that the blood flow was severely decreased during compression of the carotid artery in the cervical region on the left side. Because of the lack of collateral circulation, bypass surgery was considered essential, even during temporary carotid occlusion. Although no preoperative evidence existed to determine which aneurysm had ruptured, the larger one on the left side was operated on first.

Two weeks after the hemorrhage, a left external carotid–to–M2 vein bypass with a saphenous vein graft was performed immediately before direct surgery via a frontotemporal craniotomy. The aneurysm was so large that dissection could not proceed without proximal occlusion of the ICA in the neck. The aneurysm displaced the optic nerve medially and grew above the left optic nerve (dorsal type) (see Fig. 77-8F). The optic canal was opened, and the anterior clinoid process was removed to dissect the C3 portion of the ICA. The anterior aneurysmal wall was calcified near the neck, as suggested by a preoperative CT scan, making neck clipping impossible. The posterior wall was so thin and tightly adhered to the dura that it prematurely ruptured near the neck during dissection, which made body clipping useless. Thus the left ICA was permanently trapped between the common carotid bifurcation and the C2, just proximal to the posterior communicating artery. Patency of the bypass was confirmed by the postoperative carotid angiogram (see Fig. 77-8D).

One week after this surgery, the right ophthalmic aneurysm was operated on via a right frontotemporal craniotomy. Because of absent collateral flow, a prophylactic external carotid artery–to–M2 vein bypass was performed in a similar fashion. The aneurysm on this side was beneath the optic nerve (medial type) (see Fig. 77-8E). After removal of the roof of the optic canal and anterior clinoid process, the dural ring was cut to free the C3 portion. During dissection of the aneurysm from the surrounding tissues, the right ICA was occluded intermittently for as long as 35 minutes. The aneurysm was successfully obliterated perpendicularly with a No. 18 straight clip. During both surgeries, the patient was heparinized, and brain protection was instituted before carotid occlusion (using the drug regimen as described earlier in the text). Postoperative angiography 1 week after surgery showed that the aneurysm had been obliterated and that patency of both the bypass and the ICA were well preserved (see Fig. 77-8C). Postoperative CT scans showed no evidence of ischemia; however, the patient's condition remained unchanged from the preoperative, severely disabled state 1 month after the last surgery.

Comment

External carotid artery–to–M2 vein bypass surgery is preferred in these patients because direct surgery can be performed without the concern about blood flow when trapping of the internal carotid ICA is needed because abundant collateral flow can be expected through the bypass. Temporary external carotid artery–to–M2 vein bypass using synthetic material would be ideal for such conditions as existed on the right side of this patient because of the high possibility of successful neck clipping and preservation of the carotid flow in patients in whom the bypass is needed only during surgery.

SUMMARY

Paraclinoid aneurysms are characterized by a female preponderance, multiple or symmetric aneurysms, frequent visual symptoms, and surgical difficulty. The most appropriate form of treatment is determined by considering the patients' age, specific characteristics of the aneurysm, the collateral circulation, and whether direct clipping or carotid occlusion with bypass surgery is indicated.

We propose classification of paraclinoid aneurysms according to the long axis and cross section of the ICA from surgical points.

Although the extent of opening of the optic canal and removal of the anterior clinoid process depends on the location and size of the aneurysms, the untethering exposure method is basically necessary in cases of a paraclinoid aneurysm whose neck is located close to the dural ring or large to giant aneurysms. It allows an excellent exposure of the ICA freed from the surrounding structures, providing enough space for temporary carotid occlusion and enabling necessary mobilization of the ICA at clipping.

For difficult or complicated cases involving large to giant aneurysms, the carotid artery should be isolated in the neck initially. The patient should be heparinized, and the brain should be protected from ischemic injury during carotid occlusion. Clips should be applied after most of the aneurysm wall is dissected free from the surrounding structures; clips are usually placed with the carotid artery trapped and the aneurysm punctured and collapsed. Surgeons should be prepared to perform bypass surgery on patients with poor collateral circulation.

In lateral or medial type aneurysms, straight clips can usually be applied; in the case of a large to giant aneurysm, the clip blades should be tried to be placed as parallel as possible with multiple clips. If the clip blades are placed perpendicularly, it is advisable to place the clip blades away from the aneurysm neck toward the dome side. In large to giant ventral-type aneurysms, multiple clipping with ring clips, especially in tandem fashion, would be the treatment of choice.

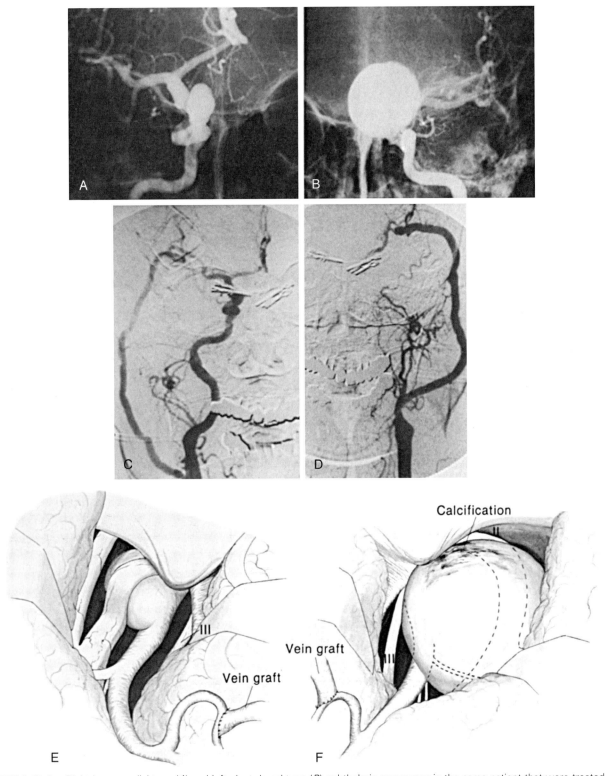

FIGURE 77-8 Right large medial-type (*A*) and left giant dorsal-type (*B*) ophthalmic aneurysms in the same patient that were treated with clipping after a bilateral saphenous vein external carotid–internal carotid artery bypass. Preoperative four-vessel angiography shows that blood flow through the A1 segment of the left anterior cerebral artery and both posterior communicating arteries was absent. The patient did not tolerate the balloon occlusion test. *C* and *D*, Postoperative carotid angiograms show exclusion of the aneurysms and patent external carotid–middle cerebral artery bypasses. *E* and *F,* Intraoperative views. The right large aneurysm required 35 minutes of intermittent carotid occlusion, but it was clipped successfully. The left giant aneurysm developed dorsally distal to the origin of the ophthalmic artery compressing the left optic nerve medially. Hard calcifications at the neck of the aneurysm made clipping impossible. The aneurysm was cut, and the carotid artery was trapped permanently.

In 129 patients, good results were obtained in almost all the patients with small aneurysms (94%); 12 patients had postoperative visual impairment caused by surgical manipulation. Good results were accomplished in only 75% of patients with large to giant aneurysms. To improve these results, further refinement and advancement in operative techniques and management of ischemia are needed.

Acknowledgement

The authors dedicate this chapter to the late Professor Kenichi Sugita.

REFERENCES

1. Knosp E, Muller G, Perneczky A: The paraclinoid carotid artery: Anatomical aspects of a microneurosurgical approach. Neurosurgery 22:896–901, 1988.
2. Sugita K, Kobayashi K, Kyoshima K, et al: Fenestrated clips for unusual aneurysms of the carotid artery. J Neurosurg 57:240–246, 1982.
3. Kyoshima K, Koike G, Hokama M, et al: A classification of juxta-dural ring aneurysms with reference to surgical anatomy. J Clin Neurosci 2:61–64, 1996.
4. Kobayashi S, Kyoshima K, Gibo H, et al: Carotid cave aneurysms of the internal carotid artery. J Neurosurg 70:216–221, 1989.
5. Gibo H, Lenkey C, Rhoton AL Jr: Microsurgical anatomy of the supraclinoid portion of the internal carotid artery. J Neurosurg 55: 560–574, 1981.
6. Lang J: Clinical Anatomy of the Head, Neurocranium-Orbit-Craniocervical Regions [translated by Wilson RR, Winstanley DP]. Berlin: Springer-Verlag, 1983.
7. Renn WH, Rhoton AL Jr: Microsurgical anatomy of the sellar region. J Neurosurg 43:288–298, 1975.
8. Engel A: Ursprungs- und Verlaufsvariationen der ersten Ophthalmica-Strecke. Wurzburg: Diss, 1975.
9. Hayreh SS: The ophthalmic artery. I: Normal gross anatomy. In Newton TH, Potts DG (eds): Radiology of the Skull and Brain; Angiography. St. Louis: CV Mosby, 1974, pp 1333–1410.
10. Day AL: Aneurysms of the ophthalmic segment: A clinical and anatomical analysis. J Neurosurg 72:677–691, 1990.
11. Kobayashi S, Koike G, Orz Y, et al: Juxta-dural ring aneurysms of the internal carotid artery. J Clin Neuroscience 2:345–349, 1995.
12. Gibo H, Kobayashi S, Kyoshima K, et al: Microsurgical anatomy of the arteries of the pituitary stalk and gland as viewed from above. Acta Neurochir (Wien) 90:60–66, 1988.
13. Kyoshima K, Kobayashi K, Orz YI: Ophthalmic aneurysms. In Kaye AH, Black PM (eds): Operative Neurosurgery. London: Churchill Livingstone, 1999, pp 973–984.
14. Yasargil MG: Internal carotid artery aneurysms. In Yasargil MG (ed): Microneurosurgery II. Stuttgart; Georg Thieme Verlag, 1984, pp 33–123.
15. Kyoshima K, Kobayashi S, Nitta J, et al: Clinical analysis of internal carotid artery aneurysms with reference to classification and clipping techniques. Acta Neurochir (Wien) 140:933–942, 1998.
16. Thurel C, Rey A, Thiebaut JB, et al: [Carotido-ophthalmic aneurysms]. Neurochirurgie 20:25–39, 1974.
17. Locksley HB: Report on the cooperative study of intracranial aneurysms and subarachnoid hemorrhage. Section V, Part I: Natural history of subarachnoid hemorrhage, intracranial aneurysms and arteriovenous malformations: Based on 368 cases in the cooperative study. J Neurosurg 25:219–239, 1966.
18. Kodama N, Mineura K, Fujiwara S, Suzuki J: Surgical treatment of the carotid-ophthalmic aneurysms. In Suzuki J (ed): Cerebral Aneurysms. Tokyo: Neuron Publishing Company, 1979, p 269.
19. Weir B: Carotid ophthalmic aneurysm. In Weir B (ed): Aneurysms Affecting the Nervous System. Baltimore: Williams & Wilkins, 1987, p 447.
20. Drake CG, Vanderlinden RG, Amacher AL: Carotid-ophthalmic aneurysms. J Neurosurg 29:24–31, 1968.
21. Ferguson GG, Drake CG: Carotid-ophthalmic aneurysms: Visual abnormalities in 32 patients and the results of treatment. Surg Neurol 16:1–8, 1981.
22. Kothandaram P, Dawson BH, Kruyt RC: Carotid ophthalmic aneurysms: A study of 19 patients. J Neurosurg 34:544–548, 1971.
23. Shigeta H, Kyoshima K, Nakagawa F, et al: Dorsal internal carotid artery aneurysms with special reference to angiographic presentation and surgical management. Acta Neurochir (Wien) 119:42–48, 1992.
24. Dolenc VV: A combined epi- and subdural direct approach to carotid-ophthalmic artery aneurysm. J Neurosurg 62:667–672, 1985.
25. Nutik SL: Removal of the anterior clinoid process for exposure of the proximal intracranial carotid artery. J Neurosurg 69:529–534, 1988.
26. Perneczky A, Knosp E, Czech TH: Para- and infraclinoidal aneurysms. Anatomy, surgical technique and report on 22 cases. In Dolenc VV (ed): The Cavernous Sinus. Vienna: Springer-Verlag, 1987, p 253.
27. Linskey ME, Sekhar LN, Horton JA, et al: Aneurysms of the intracavernous internal carotid artery: A multidisciplinary approach to treatment. J Neurosurg 75:525–534, 1991.
28. Kakizawa Y, Tanaka Y, Orz Y, et al: Parameters of contralateral approach to ophthalmic segment aneurysms of the internal carotid artery. Neurosurgery 47:1130–1137, 2000.
29. Nakao S, Kikuchi H, Takahashi N: Successful clipping of carotid-ophthalmic aneurysms through a contralateral pterional approach. J Neurosurg 54:532–536, 1981.
30. Gelber BR, Sundt TM Jr: Treatment of intracranial and giant carotid aneurysms by combined internal carotid ligation and extra- to intracranial bypass J Neurosurg 52:1–10, 1980.
31. Kyoshima K, Oikawa S, Kobayashi S: Interdural origin of the ophthalmic artery at the dural ring of the internal carotid artery. Report of two cases. J Neurosurg 92:488–489, 2000.
32. Kyoshima K, Oikawa S, Kobayashi S: Preservation of large bridging veins of the cranial base: Technical note. Neurosurgery 48:447–449, 2001.
33. Shibuya M, Sugita K, Kobayashi S: Intraoperative protection of cranial nerves and perforating arteries by silicone rubber sheet. J Neurosurg 74:677–679, 1991.
34. Nishioka JH: Report on the cooperative study of intracranial aneurysms and subarachnoid hemorrhage: Section VIII, Part 1. Results of the treatment on intracranial aneurysms by occlusion of the carotid artery in the neck. J Neurosurg 25:660–682, 1966.
35. Diaz FG, Ausman JI, Pearce JE: Ischemic complications after combined internal carotid occlusion and extracranial-intracranial anastomosis. Neurosurgery 10:563–570, 1982.
36. Flamm ES: Suction decompression of aneurysms: Technical note. J Neurosurg 54:275–276, 1981.
37. Samson DS, Batjer HH: Aneurysms of the anterior carotid wall (ophthalmic). In Samson DS, Batjer HH (eds): Intracranial Aneurysm Surgery Techniques. Mount Kisco, NY: Futura Publishing, 1990, p 41.
38. Tamaki N, Kim S, Ehara K, et al: Giant carotid-ophthalmic artery aneurysms: Direct clipping utilizing the "trapping-evacuation" technique. J Neurosurg 74:567–572, 1991.
39. Kyoshima K, Kobayashi S, Wakui K, et al: A newly designed puncture needle for suction decompression of giant aneurysms. J Neurosurg 76:880–882, 1992.
40. Kobayashi S, Tanaka Y: Aneurysm clip design, selection, and application. In Apuzo MLJ (ed): Brain Surgery. London: Churchill Livingstone, 1993, pp 825–846.
41. Diraz A, Kyoshima K, Kobayashi S: Dorsal internal carotid artery aneurysms: Classification, pathogenesis, and surgical considerations. Neurosurg Rev 16:197–204, 1993.
42. Nakagawa F, Kobayashi S, Takemae T, et al: Aneurysms protruding from the dorsal wall of the internal carotid artery. J Neurosurg 66:303–308, 1986.
43. Tanaka Y, Kobayashi S, Kyoshima K, et al: Multiple clipping technique for large to giant internal carotid artery aneurysms and complications: Angiographic analysis. J Neurosurg 80:635–642, 1994.
44. Keravel Y, Sindou M: Surgical occlusion of the carotid axis. In Keravel Y, Sindou M (eds): Giant Intracranial Aneurysms. Berlin: Springer-Verlag, 1984, pp 62–85.

Surgical Management of Posterior Communicating, Anterior Choroidal, and Carotid Bifurcation Aneurysms

JONATHAN A. FRIEDMAN

Aneurysms of the supraclinoid internal carotid artery (ICA) are typically named after the arterial branch from the ICA with which they are associated. This chapter discusses supraclinoid ICA aneurysms located distal to the ophthalmic segment, namely, posterior communicating (PCOM) artery aneurysms, anterior choroidal (ACHO) artery aneurysms, and ICA bifurcation (ICB) aneurysms. Ophthalmic and superior hypophyseal artery aneurysms are discussed elsewhere in this book.

HISTORY

The history of surgical repair of intracranial aneurysms began with early efforts to treat supraclinoid ICA aneurysms. Norman Dott successfully treated a PCOM aneurysm that had presented with third nerve paresis using cervical carotid ligation in 1933.[1] Later in that decade, Walter Dandy[2] described the first direct attack on an intracranial aneurysm. Dandy was the first to develop the use of a clip applied directly to the base of the aneurysm, occluding the lesion and preserving the parent vessel. His first description of this technique in 1938 was the treatment of a PCOM artery aneurysm causing third nerve paresis. The aneurysm was found adherent to the third nerve, and the patient regained oculomotor function postoperatively. The efforts of these and other pioneering neurosurgeons initiated an extensive, concerted effort by the neurosurgical community to understand and surgically treat intracranial aneurysms.

INCIDENCE AND PRESENTATION

Aneurysms of the PCOM artery are among the most common of the intracranial circulation, accounting for 20% to 25% of saccular intracranial aneurysms. ACHO artery aneurysms account for 2% to 5% of all intracranial aneurysms,[3] whereas ICB aneurysms represent approximately 5% of intracranial aneurysms.[1,3,4] Intracranial aneurysms are generally sporadic and occur in adults. However, patients with polycystic kidney disease, connective tissue disorders such as Ehler-Danlos syndrome, and aortic coarctation have a higher likelihood of aneurysm formation and tend to present at a younger age.

Supraclinoid ICA aneurysms most commonly present with subarachnoid hemorrhage (SAH). Patients with ruptured supraclinoid ICA aneurysms are more likely to present with good clinical grade than patients with ruptured posterior circulation aneurysms[5] and less likely to have focal neurologic deficits due to intracerebral hemorrhage extension than patients with middle cerebral artery aneurysms.[4,6,7] A recent prospective multicenter natural history study suggests that aneurysm location is related to risk of future rupture.[8] Unruptured aneurysms of the PCOM artery may be twice as likely as other ICA aneurysms to hemorrhage in the future, regardless of aneurysm size.[8] No increased or decreased risk of future rupture was found for unruptured ACHO artery or ICB aneurysms.[8]

Supraclinoid ICA aneurysms may cause symptoms other than rupture. The most common symptom is unilateral oculomotor nerve dysfunction due to mass effect from an unruptured PCOM or ACHO artery aneurysm. Considering both ruptured and unruptured aneurysms, approximately 40% of patients presenting with PCOM artery aneurysms will have third nerve dysfunction.[1] This is classically a complete third nerve palsy with pupillary dilation, as opposed to an ischemic oculomotor paresis, which may be pupil sparing. Symptoms other than rupture are much more common in larger lesions.[8,9] Large and giant lesions may cause visual field defects and neurologic deficit due to mass effect. However, even aneurysms less than 1 cm can cause such symptoms.[10] Rarely, supraclinoid ICA aneurysms can cause symptoms referable to cerebral ischemia, presumably as a result of artery-to-artery embolus from thrombus that had originated within the aneurysm. This is substantially more common in large and giant lesions but rarely occurs with smaller lesions.[10,11] Aneurysms presenting with symptoms other than rupture have an uncertain natural history.[10] Such aneurysms should be considered dynamic lesions and urgent treatment strongly considered.

IMAGING AND ANATOMY

Computed tomography (CT) scanning is the initial imaging modality in patients presenting acutely with SAH (Fig. 78-1). With current CT scanners, the sensitivity for SAH within 12 hours is greater than 95%. Supraclinoid ICA aneurysms are frequently difficult to localize based on the pattern of blood on admission CT alone.[12] Rarely, PCOM and ACHO artery

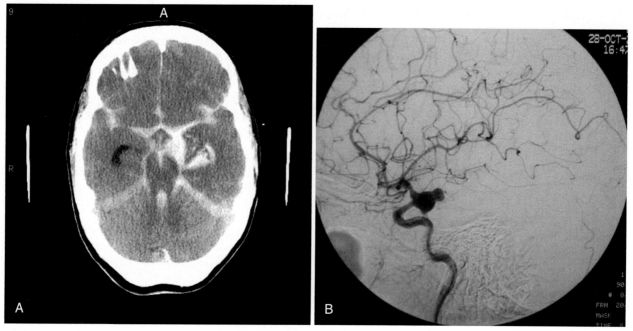

FIGURE 78-1 *A*, Noncontrast computed tomography scan shows extensive subarachnoid hemorrhage, more prominent in left-sided cisterns. *B*, Lateral view. Left internal carotid angiogram shows a large bilobed posterior communicating artery aneurysm.

aneurysms rupture with unusual hemorrhage patterns, including subdural hematoma.[13,14] ICB aneurysms, because of their projection superiorly into the basal frontal lobe, can cause predominantly frontal intracerebral and intraventricular hemorrhage from rupture cephalad into the ventricular system. Such a hemorrhage can mimic a hypertensive basal ganglia hemorrhage, and a high clinical suspicion must be maintained to pursue definitive imaging, particularly in young patients. The CT scan may provide valuable information regarding calcifications within the aneurysm,

particularly in large and giant lesions. In patients with symptoms other than rupture, magnetic resonance imaging is generally more useful provided that it can be obtained expeditiously.

Patients with SAH or clinical suspicion of intracranial aneurysm generally undergo conventional four-vessel cerebral angiography (Fig. 78-2). In addition to the obvious characteristics of size and morphology, additional information of value must be assessed including relationship of the aneurysm to the parent ICA and branching arteries, adult

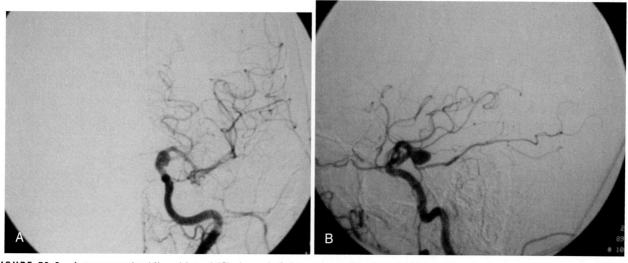

FIGURE 78-2 Anteroposterior (*A*) and lateral (*B*) views. Left internal carotid artery angiogram shows classic appearance of a recently ruptured 1.2-cm posterior communicating (PCOM) artery aneurysm. The PCOM artery supplies the posterior cerebral territory in a fetal-type pattern. Because the lesion projects directly posteriorly, it is difficult to visualize on anteroposterior views.

or fetal origin of the ipsilateral posterior cerebral artery (PCA), neck width, and determination of which aneurysm ruptured in the setting of multiple aneurysms.

More recently, improvements in the quality of CT angiography have made this a viable alternative or supplement to conventional cerebral angiography.[15–20] This is particularly the case with supraclinoid ICA aneurysms in which the skull base does not obscure the anatomy, and CT angiography seems likely to supplant conventional angiography for aneurysms at this location. An occasional limitation of CT angiography is that the supply of the ipsilateral PCA (adult or fetal origin) may be difficult to ascertain because a hypoplastic ipsilateral P1 segment may fill with contrast even if not providing relevant supply to a fetal type PCA. Additionally, the ACHO artery may not be adequately defined by CT angiography, necessitating conventional angiography.

The PCOM artery typically arises from the posteromedial ICA and courses posteriorly 5 to 10 mm to anastomose with the ipsilateral PCA. When the arterial supply to the PCA is mainly from the carotid via the PCOM artery, instead of from the basilar artery, it is considered a fetal-type circulation. The PCOM artery gives rise to several small perforating branches supplying the internal capsule and thalamus.

In understanding the anatomy of a PCOM artery aneurysm on the preoperative imaging, a key consideration is the relationship of the aneurysm to the PCOM artery itself. Although most PCOM artery aneurysms have a neck originating entirely from the ICA in the region of the PCOM artery origin (Fig. 78-3), occasional PCOM artery aneurysms will incorporate the origin of the PCOM artery itself at the neck (Fig. 78-4). Rarely, a PCOM artery aneurysm will originate entirely from the PCOM artery itself (Fig. 78-5); these are typically small and precarious lesions. Determination of the supply of the ipsilateral PCA is central in preoperative assessment of the imaging. Although every effort should be made to preserve the PCOM artery during aneurysm repair regardless of PCA

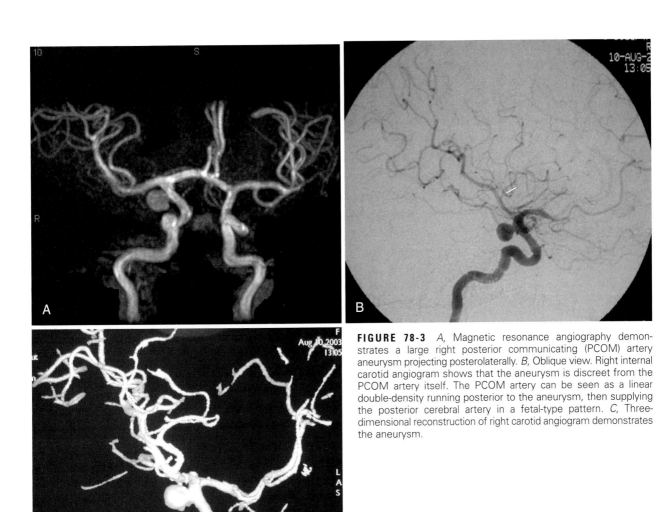

FIGURE 78-3 *A,* Magnetic resonance angiography demonstrates a large right posterior communicating (PCOM) artery aneurysm projecting posterolaterally. *B,* Oblique view. Right internal carotid angiogram shows that the aneurysm is discreet from the PCOM artery itself. The PCOM artery can be seen as a linear double-density running posterior to the aneurysm, then supplying the posterior cerebral artery in a fetal-type pattern. *C,* Three-dimensional reconstruction of right carotid angiogram demonstrates the aneurysm.

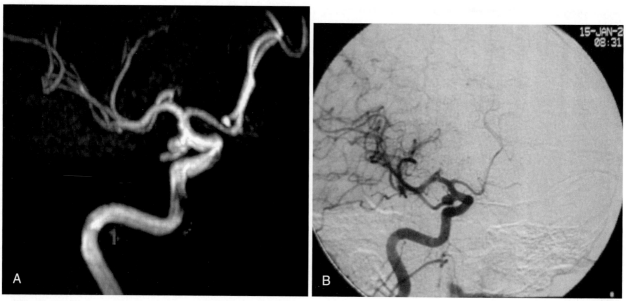

FIGURE 78-4 Magnetic resonance angiogram (*A*) and oblique view (*B*). Right internal carotid artery angiogram shows right posterior communicating (PCOM) artery aneurysm with the base of aneurysm involving origin of PCOM artery.

supply, this consideration is paramount with a fetal-type PCA origin and should also be considered when counseling the patient regarding surgical risk preoperatively. The relationship of the aneurysm to both the ACHO artery origin and the ACHO artery as it courses near the aneurysm in the carotid cistern must be considered to plan to avoid ACHO artery injury intraoperatively.

The projection of the PCOM artery aneurysm should be considered in visualizing the surgical approach. If the projection is lateral and suggests that the aneurysm is buried

into the temporal lobe or the third nerve, this may modify any retraction of the temporal lobe at surgery (Fig. 78-6). If the aneurysm projects predominantly posteriorly and/or medially, it is possible that direct visualization of the neck will be limited, and a fenestrated clip encompassing the ICA within the fenestration will be required for satisfactory repair. Finally, the relationship between the PCOM artery aneurysm and the anterior clinoid process should be assessed, as some proximal PCOM artery aneurysms may require clinoidal removal for adequate access to the entire

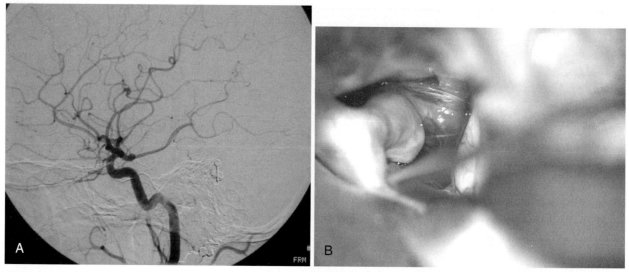

FIGURE 78-5 *A,* Lateral view. Right internal carotid angiogram shows posterior communicating (PCOM) artery aneurysm overlying a PCOM artery with fetal-type supply of the posterior cerebral circulation. The aneurysm origin is not obvious from the angiogram. *B,* Intraoperative photograph. A right pterional craniotomy has been performed. The right internal carotid artery is gently being deflected medially with a dissector, showing the PCOM artery and the aneurysm arising directly from the artery itself, remote from the internal carotid artery. The distal PCOM and several perforators arising from the PCOM artery, as well as the third nerve, are seen beyond the aneurysm.

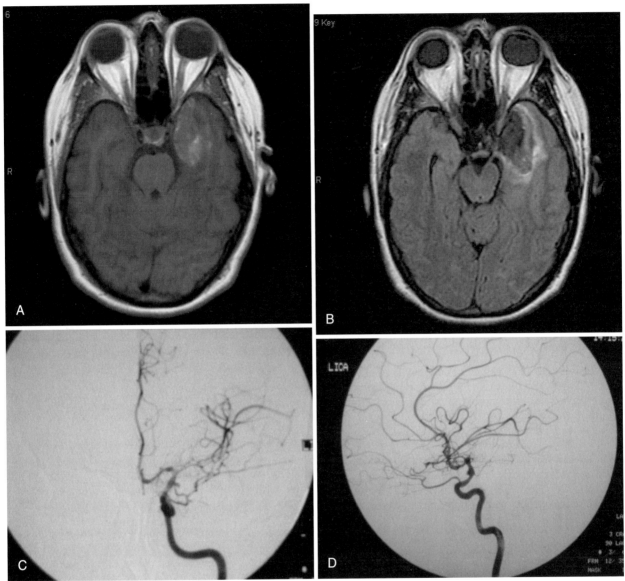

FIGURE 78-6   T1- (A) and T2- (B) weighted axial magnetic resonance imaging scans show a temporal lobe mass consistent with hematoma. Anteroposterior (C) and lateral (D) views. Left internal carotid artery angiogram shows irregular aneurysm of the supraclinoid internal carotid artery in the region of the posterior communicating artery.

aneurysm neck and for proximal control. In such unusual cases, the surgeon must consider the possible need for carotid exposure in the neck, endovascular balloon assist for proximal control, or extradural skull base removal. It is imperative to study the anatomic data on the imaging studies preoperatively and to use them to visualize the approach and repair of the aneurysm. This visualization will facilitate surgical success, particularly in situations in which the anatomy is partially obscured as in premature intraoperative aneurysm rupture.

Anatomic descriptions of the ACHO artery distinguish between the phylogenetically old (inferior cerebral artery) parenchymal ramification, named the cisternal segment, and its newly acquired choroidal ramification, named the plexal segment.[21–23] The cisternal segment supplies the optic tract, cerebral peduncle, uncus, lateral geniculate body, anterior perforated substance (globus pallidus and posterior

limb of the internal capsule), tip of the temporal lobe, hippocampus, dentate gyrus, fornix, and pulvinar. The plexal segment generally originates as a single branch, passing through the choroidal fissure to supply the choroid plexus. There are profuse anastomotic communications along the choroid plexus with the PCA and somewhat lesser communications with pial branches of the PCA in the region of the lateral geniculate body. Perforating arteries passing through the anterior perforating substance to the globus pallidus and posterior limb of the interior capsule have little collateral supply.[22,23]

The ACHO artery is most commonly the first branch of the ICA distal to the PCOM artery. However, it may be the second, third, or even fourth artery beyond the PCOM artery, and therefore its anatomic relationship with the posterior wall of the carotid and the posterior communicating artery may vary. Other perforating arteries may arise from the

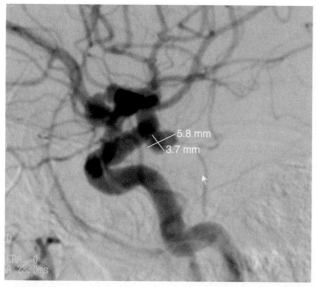

FIGURE 78-7   Lateral view. Left common carotid artery angiogram shows a bilobed anterior choroidal artery aneurysm. In this common carotid injection, the superficial temporal artery is also demonstrated (*arrow*).

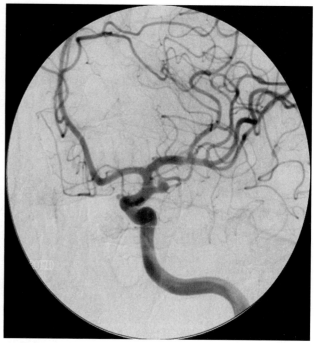

FIGURE 78-9   Oblique view. Left internal carotid artery angiogram shows an anterior choroidal artery aneurysm with indiscreet origin. At surgery, the aneurysm arose directly from the anterior choroidal artery itself and was fusiform.

posterior wall of the carotid artery and may also supply the posterior limb of the internal capsule and related structures through the anterior perforated substance but by definition do not provide arterial supply to the choroid plexus.[24]

The anatomy of ACHO artery aneurysms is varied and can be used to predict surgical risk (Figs. 78-7 to 78-10).[25] Like other supraclinoid ICA aneurysms, most ACHO artery aneurysms originate entirely from the ICA (see Figs. 78-7 and 78-8), but some lesions (particularly larger ones) may incorporate the ACHO artery origin in the aneurysm neck.

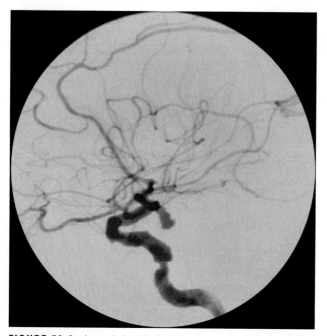

FIGURE 78-8   Lateral view. Left internal carotid artery angiogram shows an irregular, inferolaterally projecting anterior choroidal artery aneurysm causing third nerve dysfunction.

In 15% to 20% of cases, the aneurysm may arise partially or entirely from the ACHO artery itself (see Fig. 78-9).[25] When the aneurysm involves the ACHO artery itself, the risk of postoperative stroke is significantly elevated.[25] Unfortunately, this is very difficult to delineate on preoperative imaging studies and is frequently only discovered at surgical exploration. When the ACHO artery is large, CT angiography is superior to conventional angiography for displaying these subtleties and may contribute to treatment decision making and planning, particularly for small unruptured lesions.

Aneurysms of the ICB generally have straightforward angiographic anatomy (Fig. 78-11). With broad-necked lesions, the aneurysm neck will frequently extend along either A1 or M1 segments. ICB aneurysms are more likely to reach giant size as compared with PCOM or ACHO artery aneurysms.[26–29] Assessment of the aneurysm projection can help predict ease of surgical repair; anteriorly projecting aneurysms are generally easier to dissect at the neck and to separate from perforating arteries than are posteriorly projecting ICB aneurysms.

TREATMENT PLANNING

Ruptured intracranial aneurysms have a poor natural history with regard to rebleeding and should be treated when possible.[30] Unruptured lesions frequently require careful consideration and discussion with the patient to establish the most appropriate plan of action. Based on a recent prospective multicenter study, aneurysm size is a key predictor of the risk of rupture in patients with no history of SAH.[8] Over a 5-year interval, anterior circulation aneurysms less than

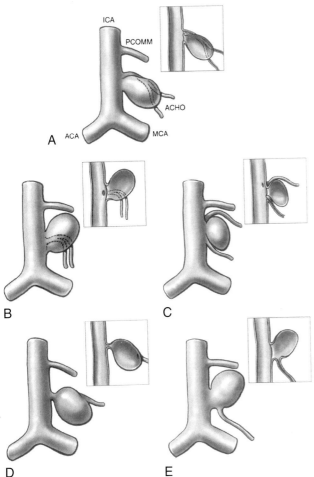

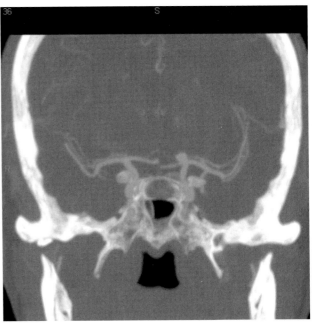

FIGURE 78-11 Computed tomography angiogram of classic superiorly projecting internal carotid artery bifurcation aneurysm.

FIGURE 78-10 Schematic representation of common anatomic variations of anterior choroidal artery aneurysms. *A,* Aneurysm arises from the internal carotid artery (ICA) distal to the origin of the anterior choroidal (ACHO) artery. ACA, anterior cerebral artery; MCA, middle cerebral artery; PCOM, posterior communicating (artery). *B,* Aneurysm arises lateral to the ACHO artery origin, obscuring the artery from view. *C,* Aneurysm arises from the ICA between perforating arteries in the ACHO artery region. Anatomic configurations at highest risk of postoperative stroke. *D,* Aneurysm originates from main ACHO artery trunk. *E,* ACHO artery arises from the base of a wide-necked aneurysm. (From Friedman JA, Pichelmann MA, Piepgras DG, et al: Ischemic complications of surgery for anterior choroidal artery aneurysms. J Neurosurg 94:565–572, 2001.)

7 mm in size had a very low risk of rupture, those 7 to 12 mm in size had a 2.6% risk of rupture, 13 to 24 mm had a 14.5% risk of rupture, and 25 mm or greater had a 40% risk of rupture.[8] The predictive value of aneurysm size for future rupture is apparently less relevant in patients with a history of SAH from a second aneurysm.[8,9] PCOM artery aneurysms may have a rupture rate of twice that of other supraclinoid aneurysms.[8] Other factors that must be considered in the decision to treat an unruptured aneurysm, despite the absence of definitive natural history data, are young age, aneurysm morphology, and family history.[31]

The emergence of endovascular coil occlusion as a viable treatment alternative to surgical repair has expanded the therapeutic armamentarium for intracranial aneurysms.

Endovascular tools and techniques continue to evolve rapidly, and the effectiveness and safety of the technique are gradually being established, despite large regional differences in availability, technology, facilities, and practitioner experience. To date, the only prospective, randomized trial suggests an absolute reduction of 6.9% in significant neurologic morbidity with endovascular coiling as compared with surgical clipping at 1 year.[32] However, the rate of complete angiographic aneurysm obliteration with endovascular coiling is suboptimal, and the need for serial angiography and repeat treatments is high.[33–40] The efficacy of coil occlusion with regard to long-term aneurysm occlusion and prevention of hemorrhage is not known, although the technique seems effective with regard to short-term prevention of rebleeding.[33,35,38,40–42]

In general, PCOM artery aneurysms can be surgically approached with ease and repaired with low risk; thus the endovascular alternative has a significant burden of proof in terms of therapeutic efficacy and safety to supplant surgical repair as the treatment of choice for most PCOM artery aneurysms. Anterior choroidal artery aneurysms may be associated with slightly higher surgical risks due to the highly eloquent territory supplied by this small artery.[25] Theoretically, endovascular treatment may carry increased therapeutic risks for the same reason, and the optimal treatment strategy for ACHO artery aneurysms awaits definition. With ICB aneurysms, the risk of cerebral infarction due to perforator injury is likely higher with surgical repair than with endovascular coiling. However, the rate of incomplete aneurysm occlusion with coils is also elevated at this location, perhaps due to the pattern of blood flow and pressure dynamics in terminus aneurysms, analogous to aneurysms of the basilar apex. New technologies, including recently developed stents for intracranial use, continue to improve clinical outcomes and angiographic occlusion rates.

OPERATIVE MANAGEMENT

The surgical approach for PCOM artery, ACHO artery, and ICB aneurysms is similar. In patients with ruptured aneurysms, placement of a lumbar drain before craniotomy may facilitate exposure, particularly for ICB aneurysms in which a significant amount of brain retraction is anticipated. A radiolucent pinion headholder and retractor system should be used in preparation for intraoperative angiography, along with placement of a sheath in the femoral artery sheath during positioning of the patient. In the rare cases of giant or unusually proximal lesions, the cervical carotid artery may be exposed for proximal control, although this control can be accomplished without cervical incision using endovascular balloon assistance. Antibiotics, steroids, and anticonvulsants may be administered intraoperatively, at the surgeon's discretion.

The patient is positioned supine on the operating table in modest reverse Trendelenburg, with the head turned 20 to 30 degrees opposite the side of the lesion. Modest extension is employed such that the malar eminence is the most superior facial or cranial prominence. A more pronounced extension of the head may be appropriate for some ICB lesions to facilitate the gravitational relaxation of the frontal lobe. A standard pterional craniotomy is performed. After a minimal hair shave, an incision is placed 1 cm behind the hairline in curvilinear fashion from the ipsilateral zygoma to the midline, and the scalp reflected anteriorly. A cuff of temporalis muscle is left along the superotemporal line to facilitate repair of the muscle at closure and reduce cosmetic deficits related to temporalis atrophy. A standard pterional craniotomy is performed with a high-speed drill. The sphenoid wing is removed with a high-speed drill to the level of the superior orbital fissure. Extradural removal of the clinoid process is considered for some proximal PCOM artery aneurysms. The dura is opened in curvilinear fashion and reflected anteriorly.

Either a transsylvian or subfrontal approach may be used for most PCOM or ACHO artery aneurysms. The subfrontal approach is faster and allows early establishment of proximal control. Care must be taken not to retract on the frontal lobe excessively, which may result in tearing the arachnoid of the Sylvian fissure or avulsion of temporopolar veins draining into the sphenoparietal sinus. When the supraclinoid ICA is long and the aneurysm is located distally on this segment, a transsylvian approach may be preferred for safer and more effective brain retraction.

Most ICB aneurysms are better approached via a transsylvian route, particularly since early retraction on the frontal lobe before the aneurysm has been dissected may cause premature rupture. However, for some ruptured and complex lesions, it is advisable to first gently place the retractor subfrontally, identify and prepare a site on the proximal ICA for temporary clipping if necessary for proximal control, then remove the retractor, and initiate a transsylvian approach.

In the surgical repair of PCOM artery aneurysms, the central element in the dissection is to identify the aneurysm neck and its relationship to the origins of the PCOM and ACHO arteries. These vessels must be preserved because, even if the PCA is not supplied via the PCOM artery, there are thalamoperforators originating from this vessel that are at risk if the artery is occluded. It is preferable to define the anatomy of the PCOM and ACHO artery origin and their relationship to the aneurysm before clipping. Occasionally, the origin of the PCOM artery is immediately behind the aneurysm, obscuring it completely from the surgeon. In such cases, identification of the distal PCOM artery and the preoperative imaging should allow the surgeon to predict the likely location of the origin of the PCOM artery. The aneurysm is clipped, and then the patency of the PCOM artery is expeditiously confirmed. The clip is readjusted if necessary.

For ACHO artery aneurysms, the ACHO artery must be identified early in the microdissection. Occasionally, there may be more than one small ACHO artery or a short stem arising off the ICA with an early leash of perforators originating from this stem. These small branches of the ACHO artery must be protected at all times. The origin of the ACHO is generally quite small compared with the neck of the aneurysm. This origin is unforgiving of overaggressive clip placement nearby and will occlude easily. When clipping the ACHO artery aneurysm, the surgeon should overcompensate to leave the ACHO artery origin unoccluded. The view from the external ICA surface will underestimate intraluminal compromise of the ACHO artery origin by the clip, and the surgeon must be deliberately overcautious; a small aneurysm remnant is preferable to occlusion of the ACHO artery. Despite reports from the mid- century from Cooper and others that the ACHO artery might be safely occluded, contemporary experience suggests that occlusion of the ACHO artery is frequently accompanied by cerebral infarction and permanent neurologic deficit.[4,25,43–46] Operative repair of ACHO artery aneurysms carries a risk of postoperative stroke as high as 16%, and the risk of stroke is associated with the anatomy of the aneurysm as discussed previously.[25] Many postoperative ACHO artery territory strokes occur in a delayed fashion 6 to 36 hours after surgery, suggesting a potential therapeutic window for aggressive hyperdynamic, hypervolemic therapy or endovascular therapy if new deficits are detected early.[25]

ICB aneurysms vary in their complexity. Behind all ICB aneurysms are lenticulostriate arteries from the A1 and M1 segments (and occasionally from the bifurcation itself) coursing superoposteriorly through the anterior perforating substance to supply the basal ganglia. The main surgical challenge is the dissection of the neck of the aneurysm from these small perforators and preventing perforator occlusion at the time of clip placement. Anterior choroidal artery branches and the recurrent artery of Huebner may also be at risk during dissection and repair of ICB aneurysms. Because these perforating arteries are found deep and posterior to the ICB aneurysm, anteriorly projecting lesions are generally easier to dissect from the underlying perforators than posteriorly projecting lesions. Surgical results of ICB aneurysm repair are generally quite good.[3,29,47,48]

Giant lesions can occur anywhere along the supraclinoid ICA but are more common at the ICB than PCOM or ACHO artery sites.[26–29] Surgical repair of large or giant lesions requires additional preoperative considerations, similar to considerations in the repair of giant aneurysms at other sites. Preoperative trial balloon occlusion may be valuable in the event that the aneurysm must be trapped with ICA sacrifice intraoperatively. In patients who do not tolerate trial balloon occlusion and in whom a high risk of ICA sacrifice is predicted, preparation must be made for vascular bypass preoperatively. Prediction of calcification and atheroma within the neck of the aneurysm and intra-aneurysmal thrombus on preoperative imaging studies is useful to the surgeon intraoperatively. Calcification or atheroma at the aneurysm base may require complex and multiple clip application to occlude the aneurysm while preserving the parent vessel. Intra-aneurysmal thrombus may require thrombectomy to achieve clip occlusion.

Achieving proximal control may be difficult in giant PCOM artery, ACHO artery, or ICB aneurysms because the lesion may fill the operative corridor. This needs to be predicted preoperatively and planned for, and cervical carotid exposure or proximal endovascular control must be achieved, if necessary. Most giant aneurysms will require temporary trapping to achieve clip placement, and many will need to be opened, thrombus removed, and the aneurysm partially resected to achieve satisfactory reconstruction.

Intraoperative angiography is expanding in its utility. Imaging equipment has improved such that even the ACHO artery can reliably be visualized on intraoperative studies. Although intraoperative angiography adds operative time, this tends to diminish as the technique is used more frequently. Several recent retrospective series suggest that intraoperative angiography should be used routinely.[49,50] The main value of intraoperative angiography is to identify incomplete aneurysm clipping and parent vessel compromise. Identifying such suboptimal findings intraoperatively allows the problem to be addressed with clip repositioning. This is preferable to identifying these problems on postoperative angiography and should improve clinical outcomes and lessen the likelihood of reoperation.

Surgical outcomes for the management of supraclinoid ICA aneurysms are largely determined by the presenting clinical grade in patients with SAH. For good-grade patients (Hunt-Hess score 1 to 3), excellent outcomes should be expected.[1,3,51] Poor-grade patients are less likely to return to independent function and more likely to suffer complications of SAH such as vasospasm and hydrocephalus. Giant lesions carry significantly higher surgical morbidity, but, given the dramatically worse natural history of giant aneurysms, treatment is usually warranted.[27]

Acknowledgment

The author is deeply indebted to Henry H. Schmidek, M.D., for his thoughtful contributions to this chapter.

REFERENCES

1. Schmidek HH: Surgical management of posterior communicating, anterior choroidal, and carotid bifurcation aneurysms. In Schmidek HH (ed): Operative Neurosurgical Techniques. Philadelphia: WB Saunders, 2000, pp 1129–1134.
2. Dandy WE: Intracranial aneurysm of the internal carotid artery cured by operation. Ann Surg 107:654, 1938.
3. Flamm E: Other aneurysms of the internal carotid artery. In Wilkins R, Rengachary SS (eds): Neurosurgery, vol 2. New York: McGraw-Hill, 1996, pp 2301–2310.
4. Yasargil M: Microneurosurgery II: Clinical Considerations, Surgery of the Intracranial Aneurysms and Results, vol. II. New York: Thieme, 1984.
5. Schievink WI, Wijdicks EFM, Piepgras DG, et al: The poor prognosis of ruptured intracranial aneurysms of the posterior circulation. J Neurosurg 82:791–795, 1995.
6. Friedman JA, Piepgras DG: Middle cerebral artery aneurysms. In Winn H (ed): Youman's Neurological Surgery. Philadelphia: WB Saunders, 2004, pp 1959–1970.
7. Rinne J, Hernesniemi J, Niskanen M, et al: Analysis of 561 patients with 690 middle cerebral artery aneurysms: Anatomical and clinical features as correlated to management outcome. Neurosurgery 38:2–11, 1996.
8. Wiebers DO, Whisnant JP, Huston J 3rd, et al, International Study of Unruptured Intracranial Aneurysms Investigators: Unruptured intracranial aneurysms: Natural history, clinical outcome, and risks of surgical and endovascular treatment. Lancet 362:103–110, 2003.
9. Unruptured intracranial aneurysms—risk of rupture and risks of surgical intervention. International Study of Unruptured Intracranial Aneurysms Investigators. N Engl J Med 339:1725–1733, 1998.
10. Friedman JA, Piepgras DG, Pichelmann MA, et al: Small cerebral aneurysms presenting with symptoms other than rupture. Neurology 57:1212–1216, 2001.
11. Qureshi AI, Mohammad Y, Yahia AM, et al: Ischemic events associated with unruptured intracranial aneurysms: Multicenter clinical study and review of the literature. Neurosurgery 46:282–290, 2000.
12. van der Jagt M, Hasan D, Bijvoet HWC, et al: Validity of prediction of the site of ruptured intracranial aneurysms with CT. Neurology 52:34–39, 1999.
13. Barton E, Tudor J: Subdural haematoma in association with intracranial aneurysm. Neuroradiology 23:157–160, 1982.
14. Strang RR, Tovi D, Hugosson R: Subdural hematomas resulting from the rupture of intracranial arterial aneurysms. Acta Chir Scand 121:345–350, 1961.
15. Chappell ET, Moure FC, Good MC: Comparison of computed tomographic angiography with digital subtraction angiography in the diagnosis of cerebral aneurysms: A meta-analysis. Neurosurgery 52:624–631, 2003.
16. Dehdashti AR, Rufenacht DA, Delavalle J, et al: Therapeutic decision and management of aneurysmal subarachnoid hemorrhage based on computed tomographic angiography. Br J Neurosurg 17:46–53, 2003.
17. Jayaraman MV, Mayo-Smith WW, Tung GA, et al: Detection of intracranial aneurysms: Multi-detector row CT angiography compared with DSA. Radiology 230:510–518, 2004.
18. van Gelder JM: Computed tomographic angiography for detecting cerebral aneurysms: Implications of aneurysm size distribution for the sensitivity, specificity, and likelihood ratios. Neurosurgery 53:597–605, 2003.
19. Villablanca JP, Hooshi P, Martin N, et al: Three-dimensional helical computerized tomography angiography in the diagnosis, characterization, and management of middle cerebral artery aneurysms: Comparison with conventional angiography and intraoperative findings. J Neurosurg 97:1322–1332, 2002.
20. Wintermark M, Uske A, Chalaron M, et al: Multislice computerized tomography angiography in the evaluation of intracranial aneurysms: A comparison with intraarterial digital subtraction angiography. J Neurosurg 98:828–836, 2003.
21. Goldberg H: The anterior choroidal artery. In Newton T, Potts DG (eds): Radiology of the Skull and Brain, vol 2. St. Louis: CV Mosby, 1974, pp 1628–1658.
22. Rhoton AJ, Fujii K, Fradd B: Microsurgical anatomy of the anterior choroidal artery. Surg Neurol 12:171–187, 1979.
23. Stephens R, Stillwell DL: Arteries and Veins of the Human Brain. Springfield, IL: Charles C Thomas, 1969.
24. Rosner S, Rhoton AL, Ono M, Barry M: Microsurgical anatomy of the anterior perforating arteries. J Neurosurg 61:468–185, 1984.
25. Friedman JA, Pichelmann MA, Piepgras DG, et al: Ischemic complications of surgery for anterior choroidal artery aneurysms. J Neurosurg 94:565–572, 2001.
26. Drake CG, Peerless SJ, Ferguson GG: Hunterian proximal arterial occlusion for giant aneurysms of the carotid circulation. J Neurosurg 81:656–665, 1994.
27. Lawton MT, Spetzler RF: Surgical strategies for giant intracranial aneurysms. Acta Neurochir Suppl 72:141–156, 1999.
28. Morley TP, Barr HWK: Giant intracranial aneurysms: Diagnosis, course, and management. Clin Neurosurg 16:73–94, 1969.
29. Yasargil MG, Boehm WB, Ho REM: Microsurgical treatment of cerebral aneurysms at the bifurcation of the internal carotid artery. Acta Neurochir (Wien) 41:61–72, 1978.
30. Locksley HB: Report on the cooperative study of intracranial aneurysms and subarachnoid hemorrhage. Section V, Part II.

Natural history of subarachnoid hemorrhage, intracranial aneurysms and arteriovenous malformations. J Neurosurg 25:321–368, 1966.

31. Bederson JB, Awad IA, Wiebers DO, et al: Recommendations for the management of patients with unruptured intracranial aneurysms: A statement for healthcare professionals from the Stroke Council of the American Heart Association. Stroke 31:2742–2750, 2000.

32. Molyneux A, Kerr R, Stratton I, et al, International Subarachnoid Aneurysm Trial (ISAT) Collaborative Group: International Subarachnoid Aneurysm Trial (ISAT) of neurosurgical clipping versus endovascular coiling in 2143 patients with ruptured intracranial aneurysms: A randomised trial. Lancet 360:1267–1274, 2002.

33. Brilstra EH, Rinkel GJE, van der Graaf Y, et al: Treatment of intracranial aneurysms by embolization with coils. Stroke 30:470–476, 1999.

34. Debrun GM, Aletich VA, Kehrli P, et al: Selection of cerebral aneurysms for treatment using Guglielmi detachable coils: The preliminary University of Illinois at Chicago experience. Neurosurgery 43:1281–1297, 1998.

35. Friedman JA, Nichols DA, Meyer FB, et al: Guglielmi detachable coil treatment of ruptured saccular cerebral aneurysms: Retrospective review of a 10-year single center experience. AJNR Am J Neuroradiol 24:526–533, 2003.

36. Kuether TA, Nesbit GM, Barnwell SL: Clinical and angiographic outcomes, with treatment data, for patients with cerebral aneurysms treated with Guglielmi detachable coils: A single-center experience. Neurosurgery 43:1016–1025, 1998.

37. Malisch TW, Guglielmi G, Vinuela F, et al: Intracranial aneurysms treated with the Guglielmi detachable coil: Midterm clinical results in a consecutive series of 100 patients. J Neurosurg 87:176–183, 1997.

38. Murayama Y, Nien YL, Duckwiler G, et al: Guglielmi detachable coil embolization of cerebral aneurysms: 11 years' experience. J Neurosurg 98:945–947, 2003.

39. Raymond J, Roy D: Safety and efficacy of endovascular treatment of acutely ruptured aneurysms. Neurosurgery 41:1235–1246, 1997.

40. Vinuela F, Duckwiler G, Mawad M: Guglielmi detachable coil embolization of acute intracranial aneurysm: Perioperative anatomical and clinical outcome in 403 patients. J Neurosurg 86:475–482, 1997.

41. Graves VB, Strother CM, Duff TA, Perl J: Early treatment of ruptured aneurysms with Guglielmi detachable coils: Effect on subsequent bleeding. Neurosurgery 37:640–648, 1995.

42. Hayakawa M, Murayama Y, Duckwiler GR, et al: Natural history of the neck remnant of a cerebral aneurysm treated with the Guglielmi detachable coil system. J Neurosurg 93:561–568, 2000.

43. Cooper I: Surgical alleviation of parkinsonism: Effect of occlusion of the anterior choroidal artery. J Am Geriatr Soc 11:691–718, 1954.

44. Rand R, Brown WJ, Stern WE: Surgical occlusion of the anterior choroidal artery in parkinsonism. Neurology 6:390–401, 1956.

45. Sundt TJ: Surgical Techniques for Saccular and Giant Intracranial Aneurysms. Baltimore: Williams & Wilkins, 1990.

46. Yasargil M, Yonas H, Gasser JC: Anterior choroidal artery aneurysms: Their anatomy and surgical significance. Surg Neurol 9:129–138, 1978.

47. Reynier Y, Lena G, Vincentelli F, Vigouroux RP: Aneurysms of the internal carotid artery bifurcation: Technical reflections apropos of a series of 10 cases. Neurochirurgie 35:242–245, 1989.

48. Sengupta RP, Lassman LP, de Moraes AA, Garvan N: Treatment of internal carotid bifurcation aneurysms by direct surgery. J Neurosurg 43:343–351, 1975.

49. Klopfenstein JD, Spetzler RF, Kim LJ, et al: Comparison of routine and selective use of intraoperative angiography during aneurysm surgery: A prospective assessment. J Neurosurg 100:230–235, 2004.

50. Tang G, Cawley CM, Dion JE, Barrow DL: Intraoperative angiography during aneurysm surgery: A prospective evaluation of efficiency. J Neurosurg 96:993–999, 2002.

51. Lee KC, Lee KS, Shin YS, et al: Surgery for posterior communicating artery aneurysms. Surg Neurol 59:107–113, 2003.

79 Distal Anterior Cerebral Artery Aneurysms

WILLIAM A. SHUCART and JAMES T. KRYZANSKI

SURGICAL MANAGEMENT

Aneurysms arising from the anterior cerebral artery (ACA) distal to the anterior communicating artery (ACoA) are uncommon: the reported incidence is 2% to 9% of all intracranial aneurysms.[1-9] Reviews emphasize that patients with distal anterior cerebral aneurysms have a high incidence of multiple aneurysms.[1,5,6,9] Although these aneurysms are relatively small, they are notoriously difficult to treat surgically.

Distal ACA aneurysms are similar to intracranial aneurysms found at other locations. They are saccular and are probably flow related, and they occur at arterial bifurcations. The most common location for aneurysms of the distal ACA is where it branches into the pericallosal and callosal marginal arteries (Fig. 79-1).[10] Aneurysms also arise just distal to the ACoA where the orbitofrontal branch arises, at the origin of the frontopolar branch, and much less commonly at the callosal marginal branches. Mycotic aneurysms can occur in the distal ACA as the result of septic emboli, and traumatic aneurysms from both penetrating and closed head injuries have also been described.[11] In closed head injury, the aneurysm is presumed to form as the result of arterial wall injury occurring as the brain and ACA impact against the falx. Finally, aneurysms can form on vessels that feed arteriovenous malformations, and malignant aneurysms may occur in the distal ACA territory as the result of tumor emboli.[12,13]

Most patients who have a distal ACA aneurysm come to medical attention because of subarachnoid hemorrhage. Imaging studies typically show a focal interhemispheric hemorrhage and sometimes a frontal lobe hematoma. Other patients may present with diffuse subarachnoid hemorrhage, intraventricular hemorrhage, corpus callosal hemorrhage, or interhemispheric subdural hematoma.[14,15] With wider use of magnetic resonance imaging (MRI), an increasing number of patients have aneurysms that are found incidentally.

Some authors have stated that distal ACA aneurysms tend to bleed when relatively small, an effect that leads to technical problems that differ from those associated with large aneurysms (e.g., clip placement may compromise the lumen of the parent vessel, and these aneurysms commonly have a sessile base, which makes perfect clip placement more difficult). Some authors report that these aneurysms rupture infrequently intraoperatively, whereas others (ourselves included) have been impressed with how easily they can rupture intraoperatively. They rupture easily because the dome of the aneurysm is often embedded in a frontal lobe and during retraction the dome can be torn from the aneurysm.

The surgical mortality rate for distal ACA aneurysms remains at 8% to 10%, despite advances in surgical and anesthetic techniques; however, most series remain small, thus variation in one or two cases greatly affects the percentages. Reported complications of surgical treatments of these aneurysms include recent memory problems, hemiparesis (generally with the leg more severely involved than the arm), and decreased verbal output, which is usually temporary but may last for months.

Surgical intervention is often more difficult than would be suspected from either the size or the angiographic appearance of the aneurysm, particularly for aneurysms occurring from the ACoA to the top of the genu of the corpus callosum. The reasons for the difficulty are numerous. The narrowness of the space between the hemispheres limits exposure. The subarachnoid space between the hemispheres (the callosal cistern) is small; therefore, the release of cerebrospinal fluid does not provide the excellent exposure that it gives in other locations. The neck of the aneurysm is often atherosclerotic and broad; moreover, dense adhesions often exist between the cingulated gyri. The approach is also difficult, partly because this area is not commonly dealt with.

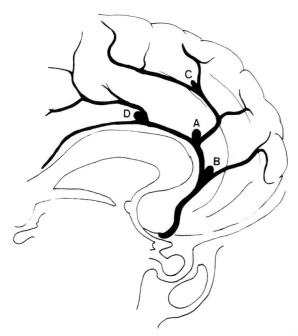

FIGURE 79-1 Anatomic location of pericallosal aneurysms. The junction of the pericallosal and callosal marginal arteries (A) is the most common location. The junction of the frontopolar and pericallosal arteries (B) is probably the second most common location. The callosal marginal artery bifurcation is also shown (C). The pericallosal artery bifurcation (D) is a typical location for aneurysms that develop after a closed head injury.

Endovascular approaches have emerged as an alternative to surgical clipping for selected patients. In general, distal ACA aneurysms are challenging to treat endovascularly because the ACA is often tortuous, making catheterization difficult, and because these aneurysms frequently have a poor neck-to-dome ratio.[16,17] For these reasons, we prefer surgery as the primary mode of treatment and reserve endovascular approaches for patients who are poor grade or have prohibitively high surgical risk factors. In the specific case of giant or ruptured fusiform distal ACA aneurysms, endovascular parent vessel occlusion and flow reversal is also a useful management tool.[18]

OPERATIVE PLANNING

We prefer to operate on patients early if they are in reasonably good condition. The usual preoperative routine of ensuring that the patient is in good cardiopulmonary status is followed. Anticonvulsants are started when the patient is admitted to the hospital, and corticosteroids are started just before surgery. Lumbar or ventricular drainage is used when necessary to facilitate brain retraction. Mannitol is given when the bone flap is being elevated; the usual adult dose is 12.5 to 25 g administered intravenously. Systemic hypotension is seldom used during surgery for distal ACA aneurysms. With these aneurysms, we prefer to begin with known anatomy and proceed toward the abnormal site. Without the aid of intraoperative image-guided navigation systems, attempts to descend directly on the dome of the aneurysm are often confusing; the surgeon can have difficulty deciding whether the parent artery first identified is proximal or distal to the aneurysm or whether it is on the right or left side.

The use of image-guided navigation systems can allow dissection directly to the aneurysm instead of localizing using a proximal-to-distal dissection. A magnetic resonance angiogram (MRA) or computed tomography angiogram (CTA) can be used depending on the specifics of the aneurysm; CTA allows better visualization of slow turbulent flow or thrombus in the aneurysm, features that are not as well seen on the MRA. Both MRA and CTA are limited to imaging aneurysms greater than 3 mm in size.[19,20] We generally use 2-dimensional time-of-flight (TR 35/TE 7.3) MRA source images at our institution (Fig. 79-2). Schwartz and associates[19] compared the use of helical CTA and MRA and concluded that they are comparable in demonstrating aneurysms. Harbaugh and colleagues[21] state that they prefer 3-dimensional CT over MRA for preoperative evaluation of cerebrovascular lesions, because it provides better detail.

The operative trajectory is mapped out using the navigational wand, and this becomes the center of the scalp incision and craniotomy for interhemispheric approach. If the planned entry is in front of the hairline, a bicoronal incision is used to avoid a forehead scar. A craniotomy is planned with the medial edge just to the right of the midline. Burr holes are placed as needed, and a craniotomy is done. The dura is opened in a horseshoe pattern with the flap hinged on the sagittal sinus. The falx adjacent to the aneurysm is located using the wand. The dissection is then directed toward the ACA approximately 1 cm proximal to the neck of the aneurysm. Once located, the aneurysm-artery complex is dissected free and secured as described in the section on Surgical Approach. It must be appreciated that the

frameless navigation system is most accurate in the beginning of the case before the drainage of cerebrospinal fluid, administration of mannitol, or retraction of intracranial structures. Brain relaxation often visibly shifts the frontal cortex more than 1 cm, with a corresponding decrease in the accuracy of frameless navigation.[22]

SURGICAL APPROACH

We use three different approaches to distal ACA aneurysms, depending on location. For those on the A2 segment just distal to the ACoA, a standard pterional craniotomy is used, and partial unilateral gyrus rectus resection is often needed. Aneurysms more than 1 cm beyond the ACoA to the top of the genu of the corpus callosum are approached differently than those located on the top of the body of the corpus callosum.

All distal ACA aneurysms are approached from the right unless specific reasons exist to do otherwise, such as when the dome of the aneurysm is large and embedded in the right hemisphere so that retraction would be hazardous. For aneurysms arising more than 1 cm distal to the ACoA up to the genu of the corpus callosum, a basal frontal interhemispheric approach is used (Fig. 79-3).[6,7] In this operation, the patient is placed in the supine position with the neck slightly extended. The head is kept straight or turned approximately 5 degrees to the left and is fixed in head pins. A bicoronal incision is made that extends slightly farther toward the zygomatic process on the right side than on the left, and the scalp flap is reflected to the supraorbital ridge. A unilateral right frontal bone flap is made that extends from the supraorbital ridge to a point approximately 8 cm above the ridge in the midline. The bone flap must be long enough in the sagittal plane to provide room to operate around the draining veins without the need to sacrifice a vein of significant size. If the frontal sinus is small, the anteromedial burr hole is placed just above it with the medial edge just to the right of the midline. If the frontal sinus is large, the surgeon should go through it to facilitate exposure. If the sinus is entered, it is repaired in the usual fashion of stripping the mucosa, packing it with fat, and swinging down a pericranial flap to the dura to exclude the frontal sinus. As the bone flap is being removed, the patient is given 12.5 to 25 g of mannitol intravenously. The floor of the frontal fossa must be reached, and the lateral aspect of the sagittal sinus must be exposed. The surgeon does not have to go across the midline. A dural flap about the same size as the bone flap is then raised and hinged along the sagittal sinus. As the dura is elevated, care is taken not to tear away any of the underlying corticodural veins. One or two small draining veins to the sagittal sinus usually have to be cauterized and divided to allow hemispheric retraction.

Without an image-guided navigation system, we find it least confusing to approach the aneurysm from normal proximal arteries, a method that also provided proximal vascular control. The closer the aneurysm is to the ACoA, the more imperative it is to begin as inferiorly and proximally as possible. The right cerebral hemisphere is gently retracted to expose the falx, which is then followed to the crista galli. Care is taken to avoid injury to the olfactory tracts. Once the crista has been identified, the right frontal lobe is gently retracted, and the adhesions between the

FIGURE 79-2 *A,* The monitor screen of the Radionics Optical Tracking System showing images of a patient with a ruptured right pericallosal ACA aneurysm. For intraoperative localization, 2-dimensional time-of-flight MRA source images were downloaded into the system. The *arrow* points to the pericallosal aneurysm. *B,* An oblique angiogram of the case shown in *A*. The *arrow* points to the pericallosal ACA aneurysm.

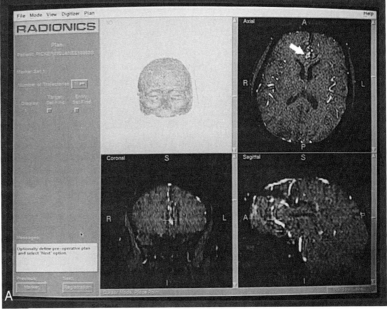

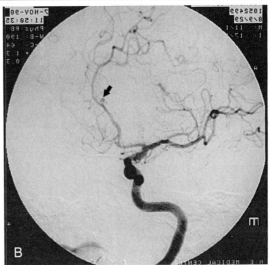

hemispheres are sharply divided. Retraction is carried back to expose the optic chiasm and the ACoA complex just above it. The two pericallosal arteries are then sharply dissected free in the subarachnoid space. The surgeon should know from the preoperative studies how far distally on the pericallosal artery dissection must be carried out, and, if MRI has been obtained, whether or not and where the dome is embedded in the brain.

The farther distally toward the genu the aneurysm is located, the greater the surgeon's temptation to come directly down on it and not to do the tedious dissection required when approaching from the ACoA. Unfortunately, without the aid of image-guided navigation systems, the surgeon often ends up exposing the pericallosal arteries distal to the aneurysm without realizing it, or the aneurysm may rupture secondary to retraction before the proximal or distal vascular anatomy has been identified.

As dissection proceeds distally on the pericallosal arteries above the ACoA complex, the pericallosal arteries run more anteriorly, closer to the surgeon. When the proximal portion of the neck of the aneurysm is reached, careful retraction and dissection are used to identify the distal pericallosal arteries before the aneurysm neck is approached. Determining the exact anatomy of the origin of the aneurysm before surgery is not always possible, but this finding must be made at the time of surgery. The magnification on the microscope is progressively increased as the aneurysm is approached. Because the aneurysm neck is often broad, the clip is best applied along the long axis of the parent artery (Fig. 79-4). If the aneurysm neck is very atherosclerotic, care is taken to avoid fracturing it during clip application. Occasionally, temporary clips proximal and distal to the aneurysm facilitate the dissection and the clipping by decreasing the turgor in the aneurysm. If temporary clipping is used, a cerebral protectant (either etomidate or thiopental) is given, and the blood pressure is elevated slightly. After the clip is applied, the dome of the aneurysm should be further shriveled, either by aspiration or with bipolar cautery, thus allowing complete inspection around the clip to ensure that the parent vessel is patent.

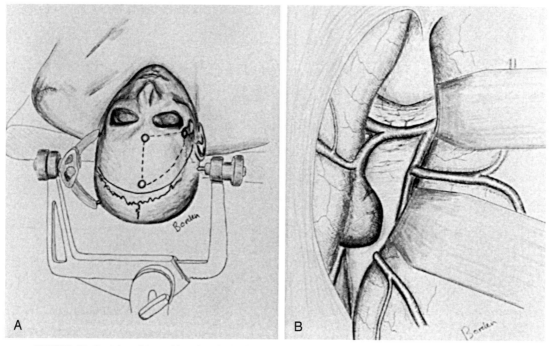

FIGURE 79-3 A basal frontal interhemispheric approach. *A,* Patient positioning. *B,* Operative exposure.

Aneurysms that are more distal on the corpus callosum are easier to deal with, but the surgeon should still obtain proximal control. We use a direct interhemispheric approach for these aneurysms (Fig. 79-5). A shorter coronal skin incision can be used that is guided by the location of the aneurysm. Even without image-guided navigational systems, MRI is helpful when planning the incision and bone flap. The coronal suture can often be identified on the sagittal MRI, and its location relative to the aneurysm dictates where the incision should be made relative to the coronal suture (Fig. 79-6). The same policy of careful, limited retraction of the hemisphere and preservation of the larger draining

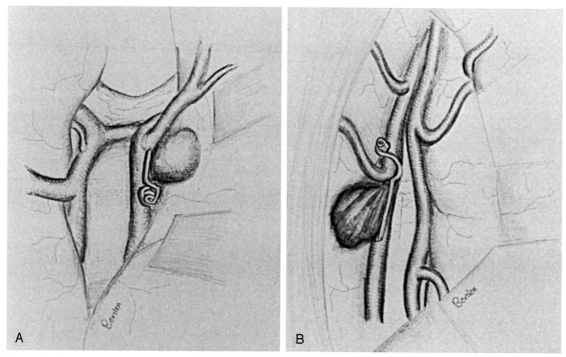

FIGURE 79-4 Optimal clip placement is often parallel to the pericallosal artery. *A,* A basal frontal interhemispheric approach. *B,* A direct interhemispheric approach.

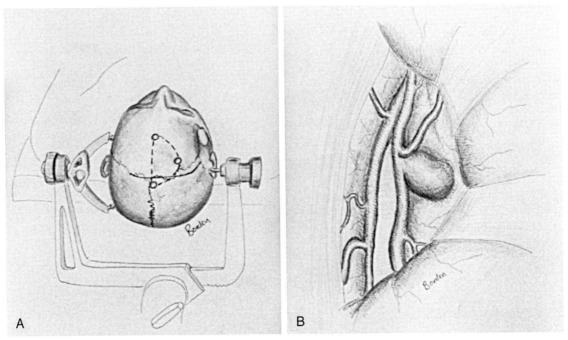

FIGURE 79-5 A direct interhemispheric approach. *A,* Patient positioning. *B,* Operative exposure.

veins is followed. The exposure to reach the proximal portion of the pericallosal artery as it comes around the curve of the genu of the corpus callosum is the same as the approach to the corpus callosum itself. A self-retaining retractor is used to gently hold the frontal lobe away from the falx. In some patients, fenestrations are present in the falx where dense arachnoid adhesions must be divided sharply. The vertical depth of the falx varies, but it rarely extends deep enough to separate the cingulated gyri, which are often adherent to one another. The corpus callosum is identified by its very white color, and in the absence of

hydrocephalus, the two pericallosal arteries are usually close together and must both be identified. If only one pericallosal artery is identified, it may not be the parent vessel. As before, both the proximal and distal portions of the ACA should be seen before the clip is applied. These aneurysms are rarely large enough to require aspiration of the aneurysm before the clip is placed. Because of the small size of the distal ACA, clip placement perpendicular to the parent vessel can compromise the vessel lumen; clip placement parallel to the pericallosal artery usually provides the best anatomic result.

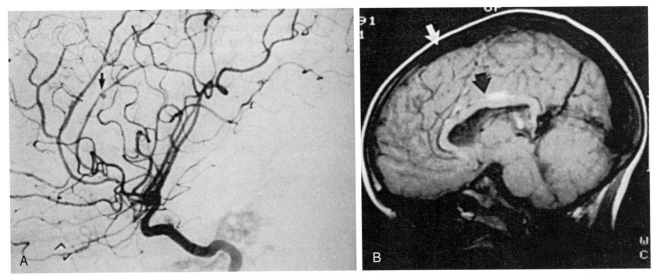

FIGURE 79-6 *A,* A lateral carotid arteriogram of a patient with a traumatic distal pericallosal artery aneurysm. *B,* A sagittal MRI scan of the same patient. The *small arrow* is on the coronal suture. The *large arrow* is on the aneurysm. Note that the relationship between the coronal suture on the surface of the skull and the location of the aneurysm can be determined from the MRI scan. In addition, the distance from the skull to the aneurysm can be measured. This information can help when planning the bone flap once the skin incision has been made and the coronal suture has been identified.

COMPLICATIONS

Complications that arise with these aneurysms are much the same as those occurring with other aneurysms. Delayed ischemic deficits remain a significant problem and are treated the same as ischemic deficits occurring with aneurysms in other locations, primarily with hypervolemia and moderate hypertension. The interhemispheric exposure creates some of its own problems, especially if retraction is too aggressive and prolonged against the cingulated gyri. Such prolonged retraction can give rise to a syndrome similar to akinetic mutism that is usually transient. A similar picture can be seen with rupture of the aneurysm if significant hemorrhage has occurred in or around the cingulated gyri. Intentional sacrifice or accidental damage to the medial frontal draining veins can result in venous hemorrhagic infarction. This risk can be minimized by meticulous technique, limited retraction, and avoidance of deliberate sacrifice of medially draining veins, if possible. The small size of the pericallosal arteries and the fact that the neck is often atherosclerotic make compromise of the lumen of the parent vessel a hazard. The status of this anatomy can be difficult to evaluate at the time of surgery, and complications are best avoided by the surgeon's awareness of the possibility and the use of meticulous technique. Topical papaverine can be helpful for increasing the size of the pericallosal arteries at least temporarily to evaluate the adequacy of the clipping and the lack of compromise of the parent vessel. The small hematomas often associated with these aneurysms are best left alone, unless they are more than a few cubic centimeters in volume or they interfere with the dissection, or both.

REFERENCES

1. Hernesneimi J, Tapaninaho A, Vapalahti M, et al: Saccular aneurysms of the distal anterior cerebral artery and its branches. Neurosurgery 31:994–999, 1992.
2. Laitenen L, Snellman A: Aneurysms of the pericallosal artery. J Neurosurg 17:447–458, 1960.
3. Mann KS, Yue CP, Wong G: Aneurysms of the pericallosal-callosal marginal junction. Surg Neurol 21:261–266, 1984.
4. McKissock W, Paine KWE, Walsh LS: An analysis of the results of treatment of ruptured intracranial aneurysms. J Neurosurg 17:726–776, 1960.
5. Ohno K, Monma S, Suzuki R, et al: Saccular aneurysms of the distal anterior cerebral artery. Neurosurgery 27:907–913, 1990.
6. Wisoff JH, Flamm ES: Aneurysms of the distal anterior cerebral artery and associated vascular anomalies. Neurosurgery 20:735–741, 1987.
7. Shucart WA: Distal anterior cerebral artery aneurysms. In Apuzzo MLJ (ed): Brain Surgery: Complication Avoidance and Management. New York: Churchill Livingstone, 1993, pp 1035–1040.
8. Yasargil MG, Carter LP: Saccular aneurysms of the distal anterior cerebral artery. J Neurosurg 40:218–223, 1974.
9. Yoshimoto T, Uchida K, Suzuki J: Surgical treatment of distal anterior cerebral artery aneurysms. J Neurosurg 50:40–44, 1979.
10. Sindou M, Pelissou-Guyotat I, Mertens P, et al: Pericallosal aneurysms. Surg Neurol 30:434–440, 1988.
11. Becker D, Newton T: Distal anterior cerebral artery aneurysm. Neurosurgery 4:495–503, 1979.
12. Montaut J, Hepner H, Tridon P, et al: Aspects pseudo-vasculaires des metastases intracraniennes des chorio-epitheliomes. Neurochirurgie 19:119–128, 1971.
13. New PFJ, Price DL, Carter B: Cerebral angiography in cardiac myxoma: Correlation of angiographic and histopathological findings. Radiology 96:335–345, 1970.
14. Batjer HH, Samson D: Distal anterior cerebral artery aneurysms. In Neurosurgical Operative Atlas, vol 2. Baltimore: Williams & Wilkins, 1992, pp 119–132.
15. Fein JM, Rovit RL: Interhemispheric subdural hematoma secondary to hemorrhage from a calloso-marginal artery aneurysm. Neuroradiology 1:183–186, 1970.
16. Debrun GM, Aletich VA, Kehrli P, et al: Selection of cerebral aneurysms for treatment using gugielmi detachable coils: The preliminary University of Illinois at Chicago experience. Neurosurgery 43:1281–1297, 1998.
17. Graves V: Advancing loop technique for endovascular access to the anterior cerebral artery. Am J Neuroradiol 19:778–780, 1998.
18. Proust F, Toussaint P, Hannequin D, et al: Outcome in 43 patients with distal anterior cerebral artery aneurysms. Stroke 28:2405–2409, 1997.
19. Schwartz RB, Tice HM, Hooten SM, et al: Evaluation of cerebral aneurysms with helical CT: Correlation with conventional angiography and MR angiography. Radiology 192:717–722, 1994.
20. Tampieri D, LeBlanc R, Oleszek J, et al: Three-dimensional computed tomographic angiography of cerebral aneurysms. Neurosurgery 36:749–755, 1995.
21. Harbaugh RE, Schlusselberg DS, Jeffery R, et al: Three-dimensional computed tomographic angiography in the preoperative evaluation of cerebrovascular lesions. Neurosurgery 36:320–327, 1995.
22. Roberts DW, Hartov A, Kennedy FE, et al: Intraoperative brain shift and deformation: A quantitative analysis of cortical displacement in 28 cases. Neurosurgery 43:749–760, 1998.

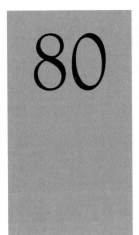

80 Microsurgical Management of Anterior Communicating Artery Aneurysms

RENE O. SANCHEZ-MEJIA, ALFREDO QUIÑONES-HINOJOSA,
PETER JUN, and MICHAEL T. LAWTON

The anterior communicating artery (ACoA) aneurysm is the one most commonly encountered in neurosurgical practice, accounting for one quarter to one third of all microsurgically treated aneurysms in published experience[1-3] and 21% of the senior author's experience with more than 1000 aneurysms. This aneurysm has a propensity to hemorrhage, often at or below size limits considered to be safe for conservative management, and often in younger patients for whom microsurgical clipping might be favored over endovascular coiling.[2,4] Consequently, neurosurgeons must be prepared to treat this lesion. This particular aneurysm, more than any other, has an unusually wide variety of complexity and technical difficulty that depends on variations in parent artery anatomy, aneurysm projection, and clinical presentation. In addition, the ACoA complex is adjacent to the hypothalamus, to optic apparatus, and to cognitive-emotional centers in the basal frontal lobes, while arteries emanating from the ACoA complex affect the basal ganglia, internal capsule, and motor-sensory cortex. Therefore, surgery for ACoA aneurysms is associated with elevated risks. This review will discuss the variables and techniques that facilitate surgical management of ACoA aneurysms and help to improve patient outcome.

ANATOMY

Nomenclature

The anterior cerebral artery (ACA) is divided into five segments. The A1 segment, also known as the precommunicating or horizontal segment of the ACA, originates with the ACA at the internal carotid artery bifurcation and extends to the junction with ACoA. The A2 segment, also known as the postcommunicating segment, originates at the ACoA and extends to the genu of the corpus callosum, following the contour of the rostrum. The A3 segment curves around the genu and extends to the body of the corpus callosum, where it assumes a posterior course. The A4 and A5 segments continue over the body of the corpus callosum, the division between them being located at the plane of the coronal suture. Contrary to popular opinion, this nomenclature is not defined by the bifurcation into pericallosal and callosomarginal arteries. This bifurcation is usually located along the A3 segment (approximately 60% of patients) but can be more proximal on the A2 segment

(10%) or more distal on the A4 segment (12%); or the pericallosal artery can be absent (18%).[5]

Normal Anatomy

The A1 segment courses medially and anteriorly over the optic tract and chiasm to the ACoA complex. There are numerous penetrating branches (average, 8; range, 2–15)[5] that originate from this segment and course superiorly to supply the anterior perforated substance, subfrontal area, dorsal surface of the optic apparatus, hypothalamus, anterior commissure, septum pellucidum, and paraolfactory structures. These perforators are known as the medial lenticulostriate arteries, as opposed to the lateral lenticulostriate arteries that originate from the M1 segment of the middle cerebral artery (MCA). The most important of these perforators is the recurrent artery of Heubner, which originates from the proximal A2 segment on its lateral wall, just distal to the ACoA. This artery can arise from the distal A1 segment, just proximal to ACoA, in 14% of patients, or at the level of ACoA in 8%, but is within 4 mm of ACoA in 95%.[5] The artery is almost always present (98%), and can be duplicated (2%).[5] The artery follows a course parallel to the A1 segment, either superior (60%) or anterior (40%) to it.[5] The recurrent artery is typically seen before the A1 segment when the frontal lobe is retracted, making it a useful landmark to identify the A1 segment and also the ACoA. The recurrent artery of Heubner supplies the head of the caudate nucleus, putamen, the outer segment of globus pallidus, and the anterior limb of the internal capsule. Therefore, arterial injury can produce weakness involving the contralateral face and arm, and an expressive aphasia in the dominant hemisphere.[6]

The anterior communicating artery joins the two ACAs as they arrive in the interhemispheric fissure, completing the anterior part of the circle of Willis. Normally, the ACoA diameter is about half that of the A1 segments, but there is a direct correlation between asymmetry in the A1 segments and ACoA diameter. In other words, ACoA diameter increases as the caliber of a hypoplastic A1 segment decreases, thereby compensating for the asymmetry in the A1 inflow.[7] The ACoA can be duplicated in one third of patients and triplicated in 10% of patients, but it is always present.[5] An inability to visualize an ACoA angiographically is usually explained by an absence of cross-filling rather than an absence of the ACoA itself, which can be visualized by a carotid cross-compression maneuver during angiography. The ACoA gives rise to important perforating arteries that originate from its superior (54%) and posterior (36%) surfaces.[5] These perforators course to the hypothalamus, median paraolfactory nuclei, genu, columns of the fornix, septum pellucidum, and anterior perforated substance. There can be perforators originating from the anterior and inferior aspects of the ACoA, supplying the dorsal optic chiasm, but these are few in number.

After making a right-angle turn from the horizontal A1 ACA, the A2 ACA runs superiorly in the interhemispheric fissure, coursing in front of the lamina terminalis and tracing the curvature of the genu. The branches arising from this segment are important more for correctly deciphering the anatomy of the ACoA complex than for their vascular supply. The orbitofrontal artery is the first cortical ACA branch, arising from the A2 segment approximately 5 mm distal to ACoA from the anterolateral surface and coursing perpendicularly over the gyrus rectus and olfactory tract.[6] This artery supplies the gyrus rectus, orbital gyri (anterior, posterior, medial, and lateral), and olfactory bulb and tract. It is important not to mistake the recurrent artery of Heubner for this orbitofrontal artery. Both can be seen on the medial aspect of the gyrus rectus, but their origins from the A2 segment are separated and their courses are different, with the recurrent artery of Heubner eventually rejoining the A1 segment, even if it meanders under the gyrus rectus along its more proximal course. Correctly identifying the recurrent artery is especially important when resecting the gyrus rectus. The recurrent artery is also typically small in caliber, with a diameter of approximately 1 mm.[5] Often encountered draped over or adherent to the dome of a superiorly projecting aneurysm, the orbitofrontal artery can tether the dome and make it more difficult to mobilize. The course of the orbitofrontal artery can also lead it across the neck of an ACoA aneurysm, requiring additional dissection before clipping.

The last relevant branch artery is the frontopolar artery, which originates from the A2 segment 14 mm, on average, from the ACoA near the genu.[5] This artery courses anteriorly in the interhemispheric fissure and supplies the ventromedial frontal lobes. Rarely, it can originate from a common trunk with the orbitofrontal artery. Like the orbitofrontal artery, the frontopolar artery can be draped over the dome of a superiorly projecting aneurysm and should be identified.

The terminal branches of the ACA are the pericallosal and callosomarginal arteries, bifurcating at a variable point along the genu of the corpus callosum. The callosomarginal artery, usually the smaller of the two, runs across the cingulate gyrus to the cingulate sulcus, where it continues posteriorly. It gives rise to the anterior, middle, and posterior internal frontal arteries, which supply the medial frontal lobes back to the precentral gyrus. The pericallosal artery courses over the corpus callosum, giving rise to the paracentral, superior internal parietal (precuneal), and inferior internal parietal arteries. These cortical branches extend over the convexity to supply the superomedial surfaces of the hemisphere, anastomosing laterally with the MCAs and posteriorly with posterior cerebral arteries in these watershed areas.

Variant Anatomy

Variations from the normal ACoA anatomy are common and probably contribute to the abnormal hemodynamics that forms aneurysms. While the effects of variant anatomy on aneurysm pathogenesis are poorly understood, the anatomy itself must be thoroughly understood if the neurosurgeon is to correctly interpret the anatomy intraoperatively and safely clip an aneurysm. Variations can be categorized as involving the afferent arteries (A1 segments), efferent arteries (A2 segments), or the ACoA itself.

Asymmetry in the caliber of the A1 segments is seen in approximately 10% of patients, with a hypoplastic segment defined arbitrarily as having a diameter of 1.5 mm or less.[5] Smaller diameters are observed less frequently, with approximately 2% of patients having an A1 segment diameter of 1 mm or less.[5] Aplastic A1 segments are rare, despite their suggestion on angiography with a contralateral A1 ACA that fills both distal ACAs. At surgery, a small A1 segment is typically found. The dominance of an A1 segment is relevant to the aneurysm formation, projection of the dome, site of hematoma, and choice of side. Dominant A1 segments are frequently seen in association with ACoA aneurysms, which typically project in the direction of blood flow in that segment.[7] As will be discussed later, it is usually advantageous to approach these aneurysms surgically from the side of the dominant A1 ACA, both for easier proximal control of the aneurysm and for a better clipping of the neck. One final variant, the duplicated A1 segment, is rare (2%) and almost always unilateral.[5]

Variations in ACoA anatomy include duplications, triplications, and fenestrations.[8,9] Accessory ACoAs are typically small and without significant perforators, making it important to recognize the primary ACoA and preserve both it and its perforators. Fenestrations can be the site of aneurysm formation and require special attention to differentiate the normal artery from the pathology. More important than these structural variations in the ACoA is its orientation. In only 18% of patients is the ACoA oriented in the transverse plane, as illustrated in anatomic textbooks.[5] Instead, the ACoA complex is usually rotated or tilted, causing the A2 ACAs to course obliquely to one another in the interhemispheric fissure. This variation in orientation can direct an A2 segment more posteriorly, making its visualization more difficult. Rotation of the ACoA can shift the location of perforators from posterior to lateral, again making visualization more difficult, particularly when the aneurysm lies between the neurosurgeon and the perforators. These subtle changes in angles can be misleading, particularly when visualization is compromised by other conditions like a swollen brain, a large aneurysm, and thick hematoma.

Variant anatomy in the efferent arteries can be the most difficult to treat and is best understood in terms of the classification by Baptista.[10] After analyzing 381 brain specimens, he defined three types of efferent artery anomaly. The type I anomaly, referred to as the azygos or "unpaired" ACA, is a single midline vessel arising from the confluence of the A1 segments (Fig. 80-1). Distally, the azygos ACA divides into pericallosal and callosomarginal arteries, with bifurcations, trifurcations, and quadrifurcations having been reported. This variant occurs in 0.3% to 2% of patients. The type II anomaly, referred to as the bihemispheric ACA, is an A2 ACA that transmits branches across the midline

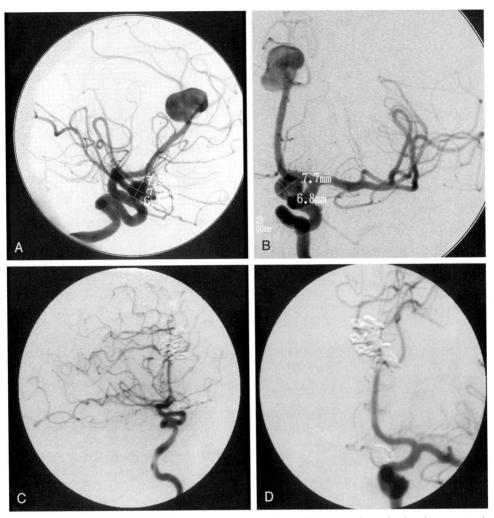

FIGURE 80-1 A 67-year-old woman with chronic headaches underwent left carotid artery angiography that demonstrated a 1.5-cm-diameter azygos ACA aneurysm and a 7-mm ophthalmic artery aneurysm in oblique (*A*) and anteroposterior (AP) (*B*) views. The ophthalmic artery aneurysm was coiled and the azygos ACA aneurysm was clipped through a bifrontal craniotomy and anterior interhemispheric approach. No residual aneurysms were seen on postoperative lateral (*C*) and AP (*D*) projection angiograms.

to supply both hemispheres, usually in the presence of a contralateral A2 segment that is either hypoplastic or terminates early in its course toward the genu. This anomaly can be seen in as many as 12% of patients. The type III anomaly, referred to as an accessory ACA, is defined as a third artery originating from the ACoA in addition to the paired A2 segments, usually between them (Fig. 80-2). This accessory ACA variant is the most difficult one surgically because it results in some of the most unusual anatomic puzzles, and if this variation is not appreciated, then a critical A2 ACA could be missed or, worse, sacrificed inadvertently during the aneurysm clipping. The accessory ACA varies in caliber from a small remnant of the median artery of the corpus callosum to a hyperplastic ACA that can resemble an azygos ACA when the two A2 segments are small in caliber and terminate early. A careful analysis of the angiogram preoperatively can alert the neurosurgeon to this challenging variant.

The median artery of the corpus callosum (MACC) mentioned earlier originates during embryogenesis when elongating ACAs coalesce in the midline to form plexiform

anastomoses at 44 days.[11] Normally, the MACC regresses and disappears as the A2 segments mature, but vestigial remnants can account for the accessory ACA.

Aneurysm Anatomy

Anterior communicating artery aneurysms, as a group, arise from the complex of arteries around the ACoA, but their precise location can be subdivided into true ACoA aneurysms, A1–A2 junction aneurysms, A1 ACA aneurysms, and variant aneurysms associated with the anatomic variants already described. In addition, the distal ACA aneurysms, notably the pericallosal artery aneurysms, are often included in this group.

The true ACoA aneurysm arises from the ACoA and is defined further by the projection of its dome in an anterior, posterior, superior, or inferior direction. In Yasargil's experience with ACoA aneurysms, the superiorly and anteriorly projecting aneurysms were most common (34% and 23%, respectively), while posteriorly and inferiorly projecting aneurysms were least common (14% and 13%, respectively).[12]

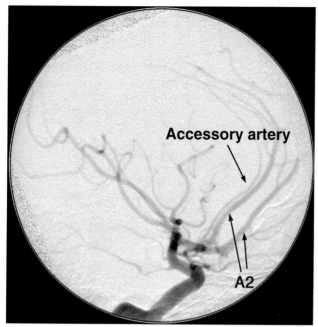

FIGURE 80-2 A 65-year-old man presented with severe headache and diffuse SAH. Two cerebral angiograms failed to reveal any aneurysms. His angiogram demonstrates a small accessory A2 ACA.

There are aneurysms (~16%) that have mixed projection or several lobes.

The anteriorly projecting aneurysm is a favorable one from the neurosurgeon's perspective because the parent arteries are separated from the aneurysm. The two A2 ACAs course at right angles to the aneurysm's axis, making their identification in the interhemipheric fissure straightforward. The neurosurgeon has a good view across the neck of the aneurysm, with the dome and its probable rupture site removed from where this crucial dissection takes place. Posteriorly projecting perforators are located well away from the aneurysm and are easily preserved. The anterior

projection of the dome typically leaves room under the neck to view across to the contralateral A1 segment to complete the exposure for proximal control of the aneurysm. This orientation often adheres the dome to the frontal lobes, which can limit the mobility of the aneurysm, but the dome can be freed as a final step in the dissection if greater mobility is needed to see the contralateral anatomy or to increase the aneurysm's maneuverability for clip application. In addition to their anterior projection, these aneurysms typically tilt to one side, most commonly away from the dominant A1 segment.

The superiorly projecting aneurysm is a less favorable prospect than the anterior projecting aneurysm, mainly because of the contralateral A2 ACA and the perforators (Fig. 80-3). Proximal control is straightforward, since the aneurysm is located away from the A1 segments and the view to the contralateral side is unobstructed. However, the aneurysm is interposed between the neurosurgeon and the contralateral A2 ACA, requiring some manipulation of the aneurysm to locate this artery. Furthermore, larger aneurysms can displace perforators laterally or posteriorly, and their adherence to the aneurysm necessitates some delicate dissection. In addition, the A2 segments can be adherent as well, requiring aggressive dissection along the plane between this efferent artery and the fundus to fully expose the neck. Whereas the view behind the anteriorly projecting aneurysm is panoramic, the view behind a superiorly projecting aneurysm requires more extensive dissection. The ipsilateral A2 ACA must be mobilized anteriorly and can require dissection of its branches (i.e., the orbitofrontal and frontopolar arteries). The clip application is often more complex with these aneurysms, sometimes requiring fenestrated clips that encircle the ipsilateral A2 ACA.

Posteriorly projecting ACoA aneurysms are arguably the most challenging to clip. With these lesions, the A1 and A2 segments can be identified readily, but the perforators are markedly more difficult to visualize and preserve. They are often displaced laterally, where they become obstacles to the clip blades during clip application, and/or they are

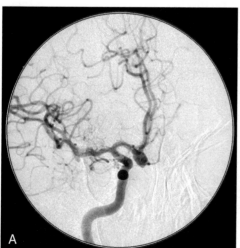
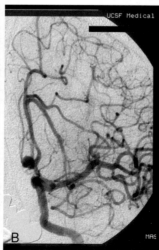
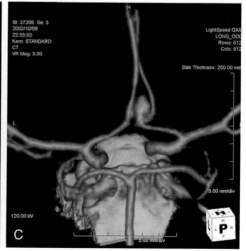

FIGURE 80-3 Cerebral angiograms demonstrate the different projections of ACoA aneurysms: inferiorly (A) and (B) anteriorly projecting. C, A CTA demonstrates a superiorly projecting right A1–A2 junction aneurysm at the ACoA complex.

displaced posteriorly, where they can easily elude detection. In addition, the parent arteries of the ACoA complex are interposed between the surgeon and the aneurysm neck, making it more difficult to dissect and apply the clips to the neck. Fortunately, these aneurysms are uncommon.[12]

The aneurysm that projects inferiorly is relatively favorable to treat, with the one caveat that its dome is often adherent to the optic apparatus, making it susceptible to avulsion and rupture early in the dissection with frontal lobe retraction. From that standpoint, approaching it can be treacherous because at that point in the dissection, proximal control is inadequate and the aneurysm anatomy has not been analyzed or even exposed. However, care in retracting the frontal lobe can avert this complication, and the advantages of an inferior projection make it a relatively straightforward aneurysm. As with the anteriorly projecting aneurysm, the ipsilateral A1 and bilateral A2 segments are easily visualized. The contralateral A1 segment can be obscured, which could compromise proximal control of the aneurysm, but the other crucial anatomy is accessible. Perforators are rarely a problem, and the necks of these aneurysms are easily closed. These aneurysms can be adherent to the optic nerves, the chiasm, or both, and it is often preferable either to leave the dome undissected or to amputate it after clipping the neck, rather than manipulating the optic nerves with unnecessary dissection.

A1–A2 junction aneurysms arise at the bifurcation of the A1 into the ACoA and A2 ACA, with a distinctly separate ACoA. These aneurysms have the same variability in their projection (anterior, posterior, superior, and inferior) but also tend to have a lateral projection leftward or rightward. This lateral deviation can result in rupture into frontal lobe parenchyma opposite from the dominant A1 ACA. The perforators tend to be more manageable with these aneurysms than with the ACoA aneurysms. A1 segment aneurysms are uncommon and tend to be located more proximally toward the carotid bifurcation than the ACoA complex. They are associated with the perforators from this segment, or with curves and bends in the artery as it courses to the ACoA complex.

Variant aneurysms include aneurysms that arise from a fenestration, duplicated or accessory ACoA, accessory A2 ACA, or azygos ACA. Accessory anatomy can pose additional risks because it can mislead the surgeon and result in inadvertent arterial occlusions if not carefully protected. For example, the neurosurgeon might erroneously clip and occlude an important accessory A2 segment if both ipsilateral and contralateral A2 segments have already been identified. Therefore, thorough preoperative review of the anatomy and intraoperative dissection is crucial before the final clipping is performed. Infundibula arising from the ACoA have been observed, particularly with other vascular lesions like arteriovenous malformations. These infundibula, like those at the posterior communicating artery and elsewhere, can appear similar to aneurysms on angiography but transmit normal arteries and must be preserved. Dissection along the course of these arteries will distinguish them from an aneurysm. ACoA aneurysms can be giant, atherosclerotic, calcified, or thrombotic. Aneurysms at this location can also be nonsaccular and due to other causes, including infection, trauma, and dissection.

CLINICAL PRESENTATION

Aneurysm rupture is the most common presentation of patients with ACoA aneurysms, with the classic headache characterized by its sudden onset and severity.[1] Patients can present in much worse neurologic condition, with obtundation or coma depending on the extent of hemorrhage and presence or absence of hydrocephalus. ACoA aneurysms are notoriously small in size, often rupturing at sizes below what would be considered a threshold for treatment. Therefore, advance symptoms are uncommon. When large or giant in size, ACoA aneurysms can produce symptoms from mass effect on the optic apparatus (visual field deficits), hypothalamus (endocrine dysfunction), hydrocephalus (obstruction of the foramen of Monro), or frontal lobes (cognitive dysfunction, memory impairment, and seizure).[13,14]

DIAGNOSTIC IMAGING

The diagnosis of subarachnoid hemorrhage (SAH) requires the confirmation of blood in the subarachnoid space, which can be accomplished best with computed tomography (CT) scan. Blood is easily seen on noncontrast CT scan, with a sensitivity of greater than 95%.[15] CT can also pinpoint aneurysm location based on SAH distribution, in addition to revealing the presence of intraparenchymal or intraventricular blood. Subarachnoid blood from a ruptured ACoA aneurysm tends to localize in the interhemispheric fissure.[16] The direction of aneurysm projection influences this pattern of blood distribution, with superior and posterior projecting aneurysms filling the interhemispheric fissure, while anterior and inferior projecting aneurysms can bleed more diffusely. While interhemispheric SAH is the most common finding with ruptured ACoA aneurysms, intracerebral hemorrhage can be observed in the gyrus rectus with laterally projecting aneurysms, and intraventricular hemorrhage can be observed with aneurysms that rupture through the lamina terminalis. Pericallosal artery aneurysms tend to have blood more distally located over the genu or body of the corpus callosum. CT scanning is quick, definitive, can diagnose associated conditions like hydrocephalus, and with an additional bolus of intravenous contrast, can generate a CT angiogram (CTA) (see Fig. 80-3).

Ultimately, the diagnosis of an aneurysm depends on its identification with catheter angiography. A complete angiogram includes injections of all four major intracranial arteries (both internal carotid arteries [ICAs] and both vertebral arteries [VAs]), filmed in two orthogonal views (anteroposterior and lateral). Additional views of the aneurysm (oblique, Townes, and Schuller views) are often needed to fully visualize its anatomy. Digital subtraction angiograms provide detailed information about the aneurysm location, anatomy, hemodynamics, other aneurysms, and collateral circulation. With ACoA aneurysms, balanced flow in symmetric A1 segments may prevent opacification of the aneurysm, and cross-compression angiograms may be needed to visualize these aneurysms. It should be remembered that angiographic images show the internal anatomy of an aneurysm, which may be much smaller than the external diameter of the aneurysm seen on axial imaging studies if it is filled with thrombus or coil material, or thickened with calcium or atherosclerotic changes.

While catheter angiography remains the "gold standard" for the diagnosis of aneurysms, it has disadvantages: it is invasive, time consuming, costly, and associated with some risk of dissection, embolization, and groin hematoma. Angiograms generated with CT or MR data (CTA and MRA, respectively) are superb and, with computerized 3-dimensional reconstruction, can generate images with startlingly high resolution that are adequate for preoperative and intraoperative planning.[17,18] CTA in particular is noninvasive, easy to obtain, and fast, offering an alternative to catheter angiography in unstable patients with ruptured aneurysms that require emergent surgery.

Lumbar puncture is considered in the evaluation of an aneurysm patient when the patient's history is strongly suggestive of SAH but the CT scan is normal.[19] There are two explanations for this inconsistency. The first explanation is a sentinel hemorrhage that has leaked so little blood that it is not radiographically apparent, in which case cerebrospinal fluid (CSF) may be tinged with blood and will not clear in successive tubes. The second explanation is a delayed CT scan performed days after the SAH. A delay in seeking medical attention or in ordering the CT scan allows subarachnoid blood to disperse, making it difficult to detect on the imaging study. CSF will be xanthochromic. CSF from a lumbar puncture that is positive for new or old blood indicates further evaluation with an angiogram.

Anterior communicating artery aneurysms have a rate of false-negative angiography that is higher than that observed with other aneurysms.[16,20] Patients with a characteristic aneurysmal SAH on CT scan and a negative angiogram should undergo repeat angiography within 1 week with careful attention focused on the ACoA region. This region is notorious for hiding small aneurysms that might elude detection as a result of intraluminal thrombus in the aneurysm, extraluminal thrombus compressing the aneurysm, or vasospasm in the afferent arteries.

PREOPERATIVE MANAGEMENT

After a ruptured aneurysm is diagnosed, the aneurysm is secured as quickly as possible, typically within 48 to 72 hours of the hemorrhage. In the meantime, efforts are made to stabilize the patient and minimize the risk of rerupture. There is a 4% risk of rehemorrhage in the first 24 hours after hemorrhage, with an associated mortality rate of 27% to 43%.[1] Most important is blood pressure control. Rehemorrhage is caused not only by absolute elevations in blood pressure but also by rapid variations. Blood pressure should be carefully monitored with invasive arterial lines in an intensive care setting where intravenous agents or drips can be administered to keep the systolic blood pressure under 140 mm Hg. Hydrocephalus is present in approximately one fourth of SAH patients[21] and resolves with the insertion of a ventriculostomy. External ventricular drainage can improve the clinical status of patients considerably and is recommended in all obtunded or comatose patients. In addition, ventriculostomy allows intracranial pressure to be transduced and can guide preoperative management of increased pressures. In poor-grade patients, intubation and mechanical ventilation is usually needed to protect the airway and sometimes to hyperventilate the patient for intracranial pressure management.

Other comfort measures, such as bed rest, sedation, and analgesics, help to minimize agitation that might precipitate rerupture. Seizures can precipitate rerupture, and anticonvulsants are given in the immediate post-SAH period when there is intraparenchymal hematoma.

MICROSURGICAL MANAGEMENT

The successful treatment of an ACoA aneurysm depends on three crucial elements: first, adequate exposure of the aneurysm and its associated anatomy; second, proper clipping technique; third, using alternative techniques for complex aneurysms that are not amenable to conventional clipping.

Exposure

The first decision in the surgical plan for an ACoA aneurysm is the choice of approach. For most aneurysms, a standard pterional craniotomy is sufficient. The alternative approach is the orbitozygomatic approach, which increases the exposure for large, giant, or complex ACoA aneurysms. The orbitozygomatic approach is, in essence, an application of skull base surgery principles, removing the orbital rim, roof, and inferior frontal skull to maximize the operating space under the brain and minimize retraction. The difference in exposure between the standard pterional and orbitozygomatic approaches is well documented in cadaveric and clinical studies,[22,23] but the decision to remove the orbitozygomatic unit should be made judiciously. In the senior author's experience with 214 ACoA aneurysms, the orbitozygomatic approach was used in only 16%. As with most maneuvers to expose ACoA aneurysms, the orbitozygomatic approach should be used only when absolutely necessary, since additional surgery adds to the patient's cumulative risk and impact from surgery.

The second decision in the surgical plan is the side of the craniotomy. In general, ACoA aneurysms are approached from the side of the dominant A1 segment, because this gives the neurosurgeon the best proximal control, avoids the dome of the aneurysm, and presents a more favorable vantage point for dissecting the aneurysm and applying the clips. When the A1 segments are symmetric, the aneurysm is approached from the side of the nondominant hemisphere. With as many as 85% of ACoA aneurysms having asymmetric or dominant A1 segments, this approach to choosing the craniotomy side results in a significant number of left-sided craniotomies. In the senior author's ACoA experience, exactly half of the craniotomies were left-sided. While there is some theoretical concern about operating on the dominant hemisphere, there has been no observable difference in neurologic or cognitive outcomes based solely on the side of the craniotomy in our experience. Therefore, the real anatomic advantages of a craniotomy ipsilateral to the dominant A1 segment outweigh the theoretical disadvantages of a craniotomy on the patient's dominant hemisphere. In cases involving an intraparenchymal hematoma in the frontal lobe contralateral to the dominant A1 segment, there may be some inclination to approach the aneurysm from the side of the hematoma. However, in our experience, the hematoma connects to the aneurysm dome and can be easily evacuated from the contralateral side. In cases involving several aneurysms, the choice of side may be influenced by the location of these other aneurysms so as to maximize the number of aneurysms that can be treated with a single craniotomy.

The technique of the pterional approach is well described and will not be discussed in detail, except for the crucial aspects. The patient is placed in the supine position and secured to the table with bolsters to permit extreme table tilting. The head is positioned in the Mayfield head-holder with the midline rotated 30 degrees away from the operative side and the head extended to allow gravity to retract the frontal lobes. In this position, the malar eminence becomes the highest point in the surgical field. The skin incision extends from the zygomatic arch to the hairline in the midline, coursing in a semicircular arc. The CT scan and angiogram are reviewed preoperatively to determine the likelihood of encountering the frontal sinuses at the anteroinferior edge of the craniotomy. In patients with large sinuses, the pericranium is harvested as a separate layer after just the scalp is reflected forward, since it is easiest at this point in the procedure to prepare a large and competent graft to cover the sinus during the closure. When the pericranium is dissected down from an elevated scalp flap at the end of the case, it is often more difficult, smaller in size, and susceptible to perforations. The temporalis muscle is mobilized anteriorly after fashioning a cuff along the temporal line, to be used to reattach the muscle during the closure. Fish hooks under tension retract and flatten this muscle to keep it from obscuring the operative field.

The pterional craniotomy is cut from a single burr hole in the temporal bone superior to the zygomatic arch. Extensive drilling of the greater and lesser wings of the sphenoid bone is essential to maximize the exposure. The inner table of the inferior frontal bone is drilled until flush with the anterior cranial fossa floor, and the ridges of the orbital roof are flattened. Temporal bone is drilled until flush with the middle fossa floor, and anterior temporal bone is drilled until the exposure is contiguous with the lateral orbital wall. All intervening pterional bone is drilled away until the superior orbital fissure is identified and opened. Drilling is continued down the medial sphenoidal ridge to the base of the anterior clinoid process, which can leave a prominence in the surgical corridor if it is not flattened. Blood from the base of the anterior clinoid process can well up and run into the surgical field during microdissection, making absolute hemostasis mandatory. The dura is opened in a semicircular flap based on this hinge point at the anterior clinoid process. When reflected and tacked with suture, this dura flap should form a flat surface and afford an unobstructed view to the carotid cistern.

The orbitozygomatic approach differs only in the dissection of the temporalis muscle and in the osteotomies of the orbit and zygoma.[24] We prefer the subfascial dissection to expose the zygoma and lateral orbit, but an interfascial dissection can also be used.[25] The osteotomies are performed after the craniotomy, yielding a separate bone flap and orbitozygomatic unit that can be reassembled with excellent cosmetic results postoperatively. The plates that replace the orbitozygomatic unit are applied and screw holes predrilled before the unit is detached to ensure proper realignment. In addition, we prefer a reciprocating saw over a high-speed

drill to make the osteotomies, and we prefer stepped cuts rather than linear cuts because they interlock the orbitozygomatic unit to the skull, enhancing the reconstruction.

A crucial decision in the microdissection is whether to dissect the sylvian fissure. There is no need to expose the MCA or its branches, but the sylvian dissection separates the frontal and temporal lobes to open the corridor to the ACoA complex. The important maneuver is the gentle elevation of the frontal lobe to expose the recurrent artery of Heubner and the A1 ACA; then, without splitting the sylvian fissure, the temporal lobe often is pulled into that corridor. Therefore, some degree of sylvian fissure dissection is required, sometimes just the proximal portion extending several centimeters from the carotid cistern, but other times a full fissure split down to the limen insulae. In older patients this extensive dissection can be straightforward, but in younger patients with edematous brains after SAH, this dissection can be difficult. The neurosurgeon must weigh the facility of opening the fissure with its necessity in determining the extent of dissection.

With the proximal sylvian fissure dissected and the carotid bifurcation exposed, a retractor can be placed with its tip on the posterior portion of the medial orbital gyrus. This retractor gently elevates the frontal lobe and exposes the A1 segment. A site should be prepared along this segment early in the procedure to place a temporary clip for proximal control. The A1 segment can then be followed to the ACoA complex. The recurrent artery of Heubner can also be used as a guide to the ACoA complex and is often seen before the A1 ACA. The exposure of an ACoA aneurysm requires progressively shifting the frontal retraction forward, from the posterior medial orbital gyrus to the gyrus rectus. In anticipation of greater retraction and to optimize brain relaxation, the lamina terminalis is opened early in the dissection to release CSF. The arachnoid around the optic nerves is incised, extending the dissection into the chiasmatic cistern and across the chiasm to the contralateral optic nerve. The lamina terminalis is then identified posterior to the chiasm and beneath the ipsilateral A1 ACA and ACoA. Inferiorly projecting aneurysms and some anteriorly projecting aneurysms may impede access to the lamina terminalis, in which case this maneuver is best deferred until after the aneurysm has been clipped.

The frontal retractor can then be advanced forward on the medial orbital gyrus, with the tip just lateral to the olfactory tract. The recurrent artery of Heubner is dissected away from the frontal lobe so that it lies with the A1 ACA. It is important to identify and mobilize this delicate artery to avoid inadvertent occlusion by the retractor blade, or inadvertent injury with gyrus rectus resection. When the retractor is lateral to the olfactory tract, the gyrus rectus overlies the ACoA complex and the neurosurgeon can evaluate whether it should be resected, or alternatively whether the interhemispheric fissure can be opened to elevate the gyrus rectus. Patients with unruptured aneurysms or atrophy often have interhemispheric fissures that can be opened widely to expose the ACoA complex without gyrus rectus resection. In others, gyrus rectus resection is the simplest, safest maneuver to expose the ipsilateral A2 ACA and proximal neck of the aneurysm.

The pia over the gyrus rectus is coagulated and incised, and brain is removed until the pia on the medial frontal lobe is reached. The orbitofrontal artery often courses across the gyrus rectus and should be avoided. When sufficient gyrus rectus has been removed, the retractor can be advanced again, with the tip of the blade within the resection cavity. The tip of the retractor should lie over the shoulder of the recurrent artery as it originates from the ipsilateral A2 ACA, to protect this artery. The medial arachnoid is then incised to enter the interhemispheric fissure where the A2 ACA and it distal branches can be visualized.

Clipping

Successful clipping depends on thorough dissection and interpretation of the anatomy, which at the ACoA complex can be challenging. There are 11 arteries that must be identified: bilateral A1 ACA, bilateral A2 ACA, bilateral recurrent arteries of Heubner, the ACoA, bilateral orbitofrontal arteries, and bilateral frontopolar arteries. The last two arteries are often outside the surgical field and are relevant only in rare cases where they course inferiorly into the surgical field. The first two arteries are the most important, because they provide the proximal control. Identification of the contralateral A1 ACA requires dissection across the region of the aneurysm, so its projection must be appreciated and the dissection should steer clear of the dome. Gyrus rectus resection or interhemispheric fissure dissection identifies the ipsilateral A2 ACA. The contralateral A2 ACA is the most difficult of the arteries to identify because it is the deepest artery in the surgical field and its visualization is usually obscured to some degree by the aneurysm. Therefore, the contralateral A2 ACA is typically the last of the five major arteries (two A1 ACAs, two A2 ACAs, and the ACoA) to be found, often requiring some manipulation of the aneurysm. Alternatively, it can sometimes be seen in the interhemispheric fissure distal to the aneurysm and traced back to the ACoA complex. The orbitofrontal arteries, which are identified at their origin just distal to the recurrent artery, not infrequently course over the aneurysm or region of the dissection. It should be remembered that the anatomic variations at the ACoA complex may add to or subtract from the projected number of 11 arteries.

After visualizing the parent arteries, attention is directed to the aneurysm neck and perforator dissection. ACoA aneurysms are notoriously adherent to surrounding structures. Aneurysms projecting superiorly typically adhere to the A2 ACAs, while those projecting inferiorly adhere to the optic apparatus. Posteriorly projecting aneurysms typically adhere to perforators, while anteriorly projecting aneurysms adhere to the frontal lobes. Therefore, the final steps in the dissection are often completed with the aneurysm softened with temporary clips on the A1 segments, mobilizing it from its surrounding adhesions and preparing it for the clip application. For this, cerebroprotection with barbiturates is used in conjunction with neurophysiologic monitoring.[26] Electroencephalography and somatosensory evoked potentials are monitored during administration of barbiturates, titrating the anesthetic dose to achieve electroencephalographic burst suppression. Mild hypothermia is also used routinely for cerebroprotection. Temporary clips can then be applied, with neurophysiologic monitoring indicating the patient's tolerance to parent artery occlusion during the dissection. If changes in neurophysiologic monitoring are

observed, temporary clips can be removed to reperfuse the ischemic territory, or the blood pressure can be elevated with vasopressor agents. Typically only several minutes are needed to complete the dissection and apply the clips. Minimizing temporary clip times requires maximizing the dissection that can be done beforehand, preselecting permanent clips, and having an experienced scrub nurse. Surgeon speed is of utmost importance during temporary clipping to reduce risk of ischemic injury. Temporary clipping relaxes the aneurysm to give the neurosurgeon the opportunity to perform the final, risky maneuvers, whether mobilizing the aneurysm to identify the remaining anatomy, clearing the perforators from the path of the clip blades, and/or establishing the cleavage planes between branch arteries and the aneurysm neck.

Permanent clipping depends on the aneurysm projection, size, and anatomy of the A1–A2 junction. Aneurysms that project anteriorly and inferiorly can usually be clipped with a straight clip, since the aneurysm and the afferent-efferent arteries are on opposite sides of the ACoA. With these aneurysms, the viewing angle is along the length of the neck, parallel to the ACoA, with good visualization of posterior perforators and parent arteries. Aneurysms that project superiorly can be difficult because of the intimate relationship between the neck and the A2 segments. A clip that parallels the ACoA must be positioned so that its tips do not compromise the contralateral A2 ACA, with the tips either stopping just short of this segment or passing anterior or posterior to it. On the ipsilateral side, a fenestrated clip is often needed to close the proximal neck without compromising the ipsilateral A2 ACA. These requirements demand a very precise clip application, but fortunately the perforators are not as difficult to dissect as with posteriorly projecting aneurysms. Alternatively, a more posteriorly directed clip can sometimes be applied perpendicular to the ACoA. This clip application can produce a dog-ear remnant below the clip, which might require additional clips below the original one. Aneurysms that project posteriorly can be difficult because not only are the A2 segments intimately associated with the neck on its anterior aspect, but so are the perforators on its posterior aspect. These aneurysms often require fenestrated clips like the superiorly projecting aneurysms, because the clip blades pass through or around the ACA vessels. Most importantly, the back blade must course safely through a complex array of treacherous perforators.

The large and giant ACoA aneurysms have challenges associated with their size, as they do at other locations. Wide necks, fusiform morphology, or an atherosclerotic artery contribute to the complexity for endovascular and microsurgical treatment. Often these aneurysms must be closed with multiple clips. Single straight clips on these aneurysms tend to fail, because tissue in the proximal blades prevents the distal tip from closing. Fenestrated clips address this problem, with the fenestration encircling only the proximal neck of the aneurysm rather than an A2 segment. Then, a second clip can close the proximal neck encircled by the first clip, thereby completing the repair and contouring the reconstruction. Some of the most challenging aneurysms are those with A2 ACAs originating from the base of the aneurysm (Fig. 80-4), with acute angles between the A1 and A2 segments or, even worse, with A2 segments that

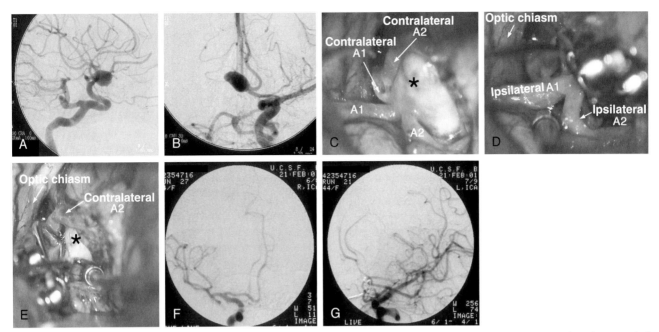

FIGURE 80-4 A 44-year-old woman with a family history of intracranial aneurysms underwent screening neuroimaging that revealed aneurysms. Lateral (A) and AP (B) views of a left carotid artery angiogram demonstrated a large ACoA aneurysm measuring approximately 14 mm by 7 mm with an ill-defined neck, as well as a small right superior hypophyseal artery (SHA) aneurysm (not shown). Note the incidental persistent left trigeminal artery. Endovascular coiling of the aneurysm was attempted, but the anatomy was not favorable for this modality. She then underwent a left orbitozygomatic-pterional craniotomy for clipping of the ACoA and right SHA aneurysms. The aneurysm anatomy is demonstrated before clipping (C) and after clipping, with views below the clips (D) and above them (E). The aneurysm is indicated by the asterisk. Postoperative cerebral angiography showed exclusion of both ACoA and SHA aneurysms, and flow in bilateral ACAs. F, Right carotid artery angiogram, AP view; G, left carotid artery angiogram, anterior oblique view.

leave the aneurysm parallel to the A1 segments. Clip reconstruction for this unusual anatomy is associated with a significant risk of efferent artery compromise and often requires intraoperative angiography.

Once the aneurysm has been clipped, it is essential to inspect the anatomy carefully to be certain that the aneurysm no longer fills, that there is no neck remnant, and that the parent arteries are patent. Gross inspection and palpation of the dome with a Rhoton No. 6 instrument (Codman) can often indicate whether an aneurysm still fills, with persistent pulsations observed in those that are incompletely occluded. Incompletely occluded aneurysms typically have some neck remaining distal to the tips that may not have been appreciated during clip application, or the neck may have elongated as the blades closed. This situation requires advancement of the clip across this remnant. If the clips are across the neck completely but the aneurysm still fills, it may require an additional stacked clip to reinforce the closure. When the aneurysm appears completely closed, it is punctured and deflated to be sure. At this point, the dome can be transected or aggressively mobilized to visualize anatomy that might have been poorly appreciated before clipping. Sometimes additional dissection after an aneurysm has been clipped can confirm the interpretation of anatomy or proper clip application, or can reveal technical errors. Therefore, it is essential to dissect beyond the point of aneurysm clipping. The neck beneath the clips along the ACoA is inspected next to ensure that no dog-ear remnants remain. These remants are easily closed with additional microclips. Finally, the 11 parent arteries are inspected for patency, often with a micro-Doppler probe and/or intraoperative angiography.

Alternative Techniques

The ACoA complex is home to complex aneurysms that cannot be treated with conventional clipping, including giant aneurysms, thrombotic aneurysms, calcified-atherosclerotic aneurysms, fusiform aneurysms, and mycotic-infectious aneurysms. For these aneurysms, other techniques may be required. Giant aneurysms require techniques not unlike the ones already discussed. The additional room provided by the orbitozygomatic approach makes it routine for these aneurysms.[23] Temporary clipping is particularly valuable, because a giant aneurysm that no longer has antegrade filling is deflated and mobile, thereby opening up the surgical field and facilitating the dissection and clipping.

With thrombotic aneurysms, the aneurysm does not respond to temporary clipping because thrombus transforms the aneurysm into a solid mass. Therefore, thrombectomy is needed to convert this mass into a deformable sac (Fig. 80-5). After trapping the aneurysm with temporary clips on both A1 and A2 ACAs bilaterally, it is entered by incising the wall. With some giant aneurysms, complete control is not possible at the outset because the bulk of the aneurysm prevents visualization of contralateral anatomy. In these cases, bleeding can be controlled from inside the aneurysm with a cottonoid over the orifice of the artery, until the involved artery is isolated and temporarily clipped. A Cavitron Ultrasonic Surgical Aspirator (CUSA) is typically

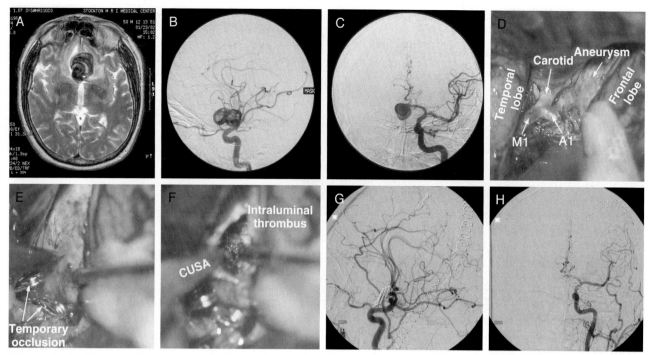

FIGURE 80-5 A 50-year-old man presented with a grand mal seizure and was diagnosed with an unruptured giant ACoA aneurysm. An axial T2-weighted MRI (*A*) revealed a giant, partially thrombosed aneurysm in the anterior interhemispheric fissure, with surrounding cerebral edema. Lateral (*B*) and AP (*C*) views of the left carotid artery angiogram demonstrated an inferiorly and anteriorly projecting, bilobed aneurysm. He underwent a left orbitozygomatic craniotomy to widely expose the aneurysm (*D*). Before the aneurysm neck could be clipped, the aneurysm was incised (*E*) and an intraluminal thrombus was removed with a CUSA (*F*). Postoperative left carotid artery angiography revealed good flow in the A1 and A2 branches bilaterally and no residual aneurysm filling (*G*, lateral view; *H*, AP view).

used to break up thrombi and clean out the aneurysm lumen, with attention focused at the neck where the clip needs to be placed. Transecting the aneurysm can expedite thrombectomy by freeing the essential tissue needed to reconstruct a neck, rather than gutting the entire lumen and mobilizing the sac. This transaction maneuver can be important, because it minimizes ischemia time and risk of neurologic complication.

Previously coiled aneurysms that have residual filling or that recur are often managed similarly to thrombotic aneurysms (Fig. 80-6). They too behave like a solid mass, and their intraluminal content is largely thrombotic. Ideally, coils that have compacted will create a neck beneath the coils that will accept a clip, thereby simplifying the management. In other cases, thrombectomy is required to mobilize the neck for clip reconstruction. The CUSA can be used as with purely thrombotic aneurysms, leaving the coil mass in place and clipping around the coils. Only rarely is it advisable to attempt to extract coils from the aneurysm.

Bypass techniques allow complex aneurysms to be proximally occluded or trapped with minimal risk of ischemic complications. However, revascularization of the distal ACA territory for ACoA aneurysms is more difficult than with other vascular territories and aneurysms. The superficial temporal artery and occipital artery, the two most commonly used donor arteries for other extracranial-to-intracranial bypasses, are not long enough for a distal ACA bypass. Interposition grafts, such as the radial artery or saphenous vein, bridge from the carotid artery or superficial temporal artery to the ACA. They are long, require an extensive exposure, and are prone to late occlusions. In situ

bypasses that connect the A3 or A4 ACA segments in the interhemispheric fissure with a side-to-side anastomosis can be used when blood flow in one of the efferent A2 arteries can be preserved during the aneurysm occlusion (Fig. 80-7). Most of these bypass procedures requires an interhemispheric approach, separate from the pterional approach used for the ACoA aneurysm. A multimodality approach that creates a surgical bypass first and then occludes the aneurysm endovascularly in a separate stage has appeal. It minimizes the extent of surgery, limiting the craniotomy to just an interhemispheric approach rather than a combined pterional-bifrontal approach. It also confirms bypass patency before arterial sacrifice and allows the patient's medical status and hemodynamics to be optimized for the second stage of the procedure. This multimodality strategy has proved effective with atherosclerotic, fusiform, mycotic-infectious, and traumatic aneurysms involving the ACoA complex.[27]

POSTOPERATIVE MANAGEMENT

Postoperatively, patients are assessed neurologically and radiographically with CT scan and digital subtraction angiogram. Angiography is essential in documenting complete aneurysm obliteration, patency of parent and branch arteries, and the presence of vasospasm. Patients at risk of developing vasospasm are monitored closely in intensive care. All patients are given nimodipine, starting within 4 days of SAH and continuing for 21 days, regardless of admission grade, at a dose of 60 mg every 4 hours.[28,29] Vasospasm is detected with angiography, transcranial

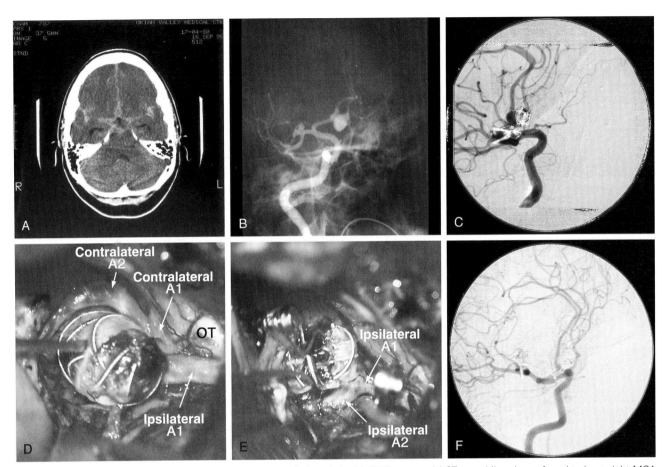

FIGURE 80-6 A 40-year-old woman presented to an outside hospital with SAH on an axial CT scan (*A*) and was found to have right MCA and ACoA aneurysms on a right carotid artery angiogram (*B*). After undergoing a right pterional craniotomy to clip the right MCA aneurysm, she was then referred to this institution for coiling of the ACoA aneurysm. Three years later, the ACoA aneurysm recurred (*C*), and the patient was referred for microsurgical clipping. She underwent a right orbitozygomatic craniotomy (*D*), and the coiled anterior portion of the aneurysm could be visualized. The recurrent posterior portion of the aneurysm was located behind this coil mass and was occluded with a fenestrated clip that encircled the coils (*E*). Postoperative angiography revealed no residual filling of the aneurysm (*F*).

Doppler (TCD) ultrasonography, or changes in neurologic signs. Angiography is the optimal diagnostic study, but it is limited by its invasiveness. TCD ultrasonography is non-invasive and can be done repeatedly to detect trends. Rising TCD velocities guide the timing of more aggressive measures, such as hypertensive therapy and angioplasty.

The mainstay of medical management is hypervolemia, hypertension, and hemodilution (HHH therapy).[30] Volume expansion is achieved with packed red blood cells, albumin solution, or hypertonic saline solution. Invasive monitoring with either a central venous pressure line or a pulmonary artery catheter is required to guide fluid management. Volume expansion to central venous pressure greater than 8 mm Hg or diastolic pulmonary artery pressure greater than 14 mm Hg is usually enough to dilute the hematocrit to less than 35%. In addition, volume expansion may increase systolic blood pressure to desired end points. As the patient's clinical condition demands, the blood pressure is elevated further with pressor agents to systolic values between 180 and 220 mm Hg.[31]

Endovascular therapies for vasospasm are used when aggressive medical management fails, when TCD velocities rise, or when there are several risk factors for severe vasospasm. Transluminal balloon angioplasty mechanically dilates segments of large cerebral arteries that are in spasm, restoring the normal caliber of the lumen, improving blood flow to ischemic brain, and resulting in clinical improvement.[32] Furthermore, the effects of angioplasty appear to last up to a week, which corresponds to the duration of vasospasm.[33] The success of this intervention is largely dependent on timing. Early angioplasty before or immediately after neurologic deterioration enhances its efficacy. Transluminal balloon angioplasty is limited to large cerebral arteries like the internal cerebral artery (ICA), MCA, and ACA. Smaller distal arteries, notably the A2 ACA segments, are not amenable to angioplasty and instead are treated with an intra-arterial papaverine or verapamil infusion. Superselective infusion of a vasodilator can improve the caliber of vasospastic arteries, but the effects are short-lived (<12 hours). The repeated treatments that may be needed for severe distal vasospasm limit its usefulness.

Hydrocephalus is a common complication of SAH, especially when there is significant intraventricular hemorrhage. Up to 65% of all patients requiring an external ventricular drain for hydrocephalus or intraventricular hemorrhage require permanent ventriculoperitoneal shunting.[34] Fenestration of the lamina terminalis during surgery appears to reduce the need for ventriculoperitoneal shunting.

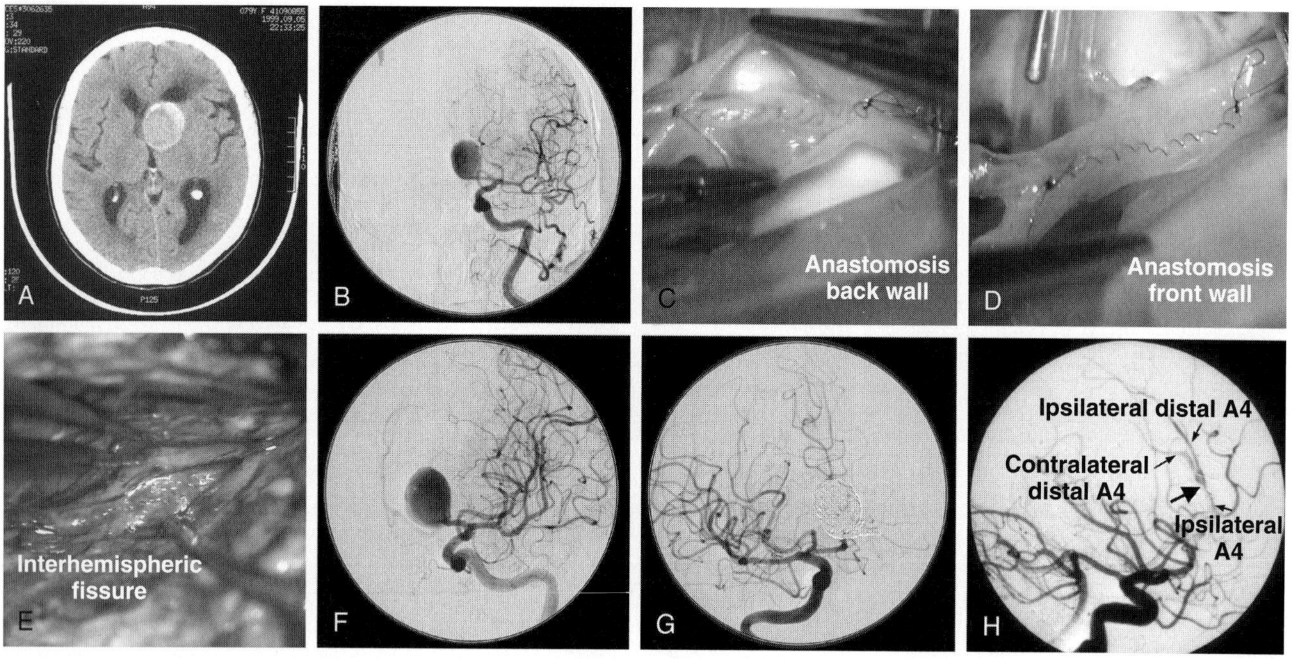

FIGURE 80-7 A 78-year-old woman presented with aphasia and headaches. Her head CT scan demonstrated obstructive hydrocephalus due to a giant, partially thrombosed ACoA aneurysm (A). Left carotid artery angiogram (AP view) revealed a superiorly projecting aneurysm without a discrete, clippable neck (B). The left A1 ACA and A2 ACA segments were separated by the base of the aneurysm, indicating a fusiform morphology. A multimodality treatment was planned, with a bypass to the distal ACA as a first stage and endovascular coil occlusion of the aneurysm as a second stage. She underwent bifrontal craniotomy, interhemispheric approach, and A3–A3 ACA side-to-side anastomosis to revascularize the ACA territory distal to the aneurysm. The back walls of the anastomosis are sutured from within the arterial lumen first (C), followed by the front walls (D). The depth of this surgical corridor is shown (E). Postoperative left carotid artery angiography demonstrated a patent bypass with good distal flow in bilateral ACA territories (F). The patient then underwent coil occlusion of the aneurysm and the proximal left A1 ACA segment, with right carotid artery angiography demonstrating obliteration of the aneurysm and blood flow in bilateral ACA territories that originates from the right A2 ACA and crosses to the left hemisphere through the bypass (G and H). The anastomosis site is indicated by the large black arrow (H).

Patients with ACoA aneurysms are susceptible to two postoperative entities, namely electrolyte abnormalities and the ACoA syndrome. Hyponatremia is frequently seen in patients with SAH, with an incidence around 18%, lasting from 1 to 5 days.[35] This electrolyte abnormality is the result of cerebral salt wasting, a natriuresis, and secondary water loss due to the kidneys' inability to retain sodium. Clinically, cerebral salt wasting can mimic the ischemic neurologic deterioration observed in patients with vasospasm. The laboratory picture of cerebral salt wasting is similar to that of the syndrome of inappropriate antidiuretic hormone secretion (SIADH), except that extracellular fluid volumes are low with cerebral salt wasting and elevated with SIADH. The routine treatment of SIADH, namely fluid restriction, can be dangerous in patients with cerebral salt wasting, since further dehydration can exacerbate the diminished cerebral blood flow and ischemia in patients with vasospasm. Instead, cerebral salt wasting is treated with normal saline infusion, supplemental salt intake, and sometimes hypertonic saline infusion. The ACoA syndrome after SAH is characterized by impaired memory, personality changes, and confabulation.[36]

REFERENCES

1. Kassell NF, Torner JC, Haley EC, et al: The International Cooperative Study on the Timing of Aneurysm Surgery. Part 1: Overall management results. J Neurosurg 73:18–36, 1990.
2. Molyneux A, Kerr R, Stratton I, et al: International Subarachnoid Aneurysm Trial (ISAT) of neurosurgical clipping versus endovascular coiling in 2143 patients with ruptured intracranial aneurysms: A randomised trial. Lancet 360:1267–1274, 2002.
3. Rhoton AL, Jr: Aneurysms. Neurosurgery 51(Suppl 4):S121–S158, 2002.
4. Barker FG, 2nd, Amin-Hanjani S, Butler WE, et al: Age-dependent differences in short-term outcome after surgical or endovascular treatment of unruptured intracranial aneurysms in the United States, 1996–2000. Neurosurgery 54:18–30, 2004.
5. Perlmutter D, Rhoton AL, Jr: Microsurgical anatomy of the anterior cerebral–anterior communicating–recurrent artery complex. J Neurosurg 45:259–272, 1976.
6. Avci E, Fossett D, Aslan M, et al: Branches of the anterior cerebral artery near the anterior communicating artery complex: An anatomic study and surgical perspective. Neurol Med Chir (Tokyo) 43:329–333, 2003.
7. Kerber CW, Imbesi SG, Knox K: Flow dynamics in a lethal anterior communicating artery aneurysm. AJNR Am J Neuroradiol 20:2000–2003, 1999.
8. Stefani MA, Schneider FL, Marrone AC, et al: Anatomic variations of anterior cerebral artery cortical branches. Clin Anat 13:231–236, 2000.
9. Namiki J, Doumoto Y: Microsurgically critical anomaly of the anterior communicating artery complex during the pterional approach to a ruptured aneurysm: Double fenestration of the proximal A2 segments. Neurol Med Chir (Tokyo) 43:304–307, 2003.
10. Baptista AG: Studies on the arteries of the brain. II: The anterior cerebral artery: Some anatomic features and their clinical implications. Neurology 13:825–835, 1963.
11. Serizawa T, Saeki N, Yamaura A: Microsurgical anatomy and clinical significance of the anterior communicating artery and its perforating branches. Neurosurgery 40:1211–1218, 1997.
12. Yasargil MG: Microneurosurgery. New York: Georg Thieme Verlag/Thieme Stratton, 1984.

13. Chan JW, Hoyt WF, Ellis WG, et al: Pathogenesis of acute monocular blindness from leaking anterior communicating artery aneurysms: Report of six cases. Neurology 48:680–683, 1997.

14. Lownie SP, Drake CG, Peerless SJ, et al: Clinical presentation and management of giant anterior communicating artery region aneurysms. J Neurosurg 92:267–277, 2000.

15. Sames TA, Storrow AB, Finkelstein JA, et al: Sensitivity of new-generation computed tomography in subarachnoid hemorrhage. Acad Emerg Med 3:16–20, 1996.

16. Iwanaga H, Wakai S, Ochiai C, et al: Ruptured cerebral aneurysms missed by initial angiographic study. Neurosurgery 27:45–51, 1990.

17. Villablanca JP, Jahan R, Hooshi P, et al: Detection and characterization of very small cerebral aneurysms by using 2D and 3D helical CT angiography. AJNR Am J Neuroradiol 23:1187–1198, 2002.

18. Dehdashti AR, Rufenacht DA, Delavelle J, et al: Therapeutic decision and management of aneurysmal subarachnoid haemorrhage based on computed tomographic angiography. Br J Neurosurg 17:46–53, 2003.

19. Vermeulen M: Subarachnoid haemorrhage: Diagnosis and treatment. J Neurol 243:496–501, 1996.

20. Bradac, GB, Bergui M, Ferrio MF, et al: False-negative angiograms in subarachnoid haemorrhage due to intracranial aneurysms. Neuroradiology 39:772–776, 1997.

21. Dorai Z, Hynan LS, Kopitnik TA, et al: Factors related to hydrocephalus after aneurysmal subarachnoid hemorrhage. Neurosurgery 52:763–771, 2003.

22. Schwartz MS, Anderson GJ, Horgan MA, et al: Quantification of increased exposure resulting from orbital rim and orbitozygomatic osteotomy via the frontotemporal transsylvian approach. J Neurosurg 91:1020–1026, 1999.

23. Gonzalez LF, Crawford NR, Horgan MA, et al: Working area and angle of attack in three cranial base approaches: Pterional, orbitozygomatic, and maxillary extension of the orbitozygomatic approach. Neurosurgery 50:550–557, 2002.

24. Lemole GM, Jr, Henn JS, Zabramski JM, et al: Modifications to the orbitozygomatic approach: Technical note. J Neurosurg 99:924–930, 2003.

25. Coscarella E, Vishteh AG, Spetzler RF, et al: Subfascial and submuscular methods of temporal muscle dissection and their relationship to the frontal branch of the facial nerve: Technical note. J Neurosurg 92:877–880, 2000.

26. Spetzler RF, Hadley MN, Rigamonti D, et al: Aneurysms of the basilar artery treated with circulatory arrest, hypothermia, and barbiturate cerebral protection. J Neurosurg 68:868–879, 1988.

27. Lawton MT, Quinones-Hinojosa A, Sanai N, et al: Combined microsurgical and endovascular management of complex intracranial aneurysms. Neurosurgery 52:263–275, 2003.

28. Allen GS, Ahn HS, Preziosi TJ, et al: Cerebral arterial spasm—a controlled trial of nimodipine in patients with subarachnoid hemorrhage. N Engl J Med 308:619–624, 1983.

29. Barker FG, 2nd, Ogilvy CS: Efficacy of prophylactic nimodipine for delayed ischemic deficit after subarachnoid hemorrhage: A metaanalysis. J Neurosurg 84:405–414, 1996.

30. Sen J, Belli A, Albon H, et al: Triple-H therapy in the management of aneurysmal subarachnoid haemorrhage. Lancet Neurol 2:614–621, 2003.

31. Kassell NF, Peerless SJ, Durward QJ, et al: Treatment of ischemic deficits from vasospasm with intravascular volume expansion and induced arterial hypertension. Neurosurgery 11:337–343, 1982.

32. Bejjani GK, Bank WO, Dolan WJ, et al: The efficacy and safety of angioplasty for cerebral vasospasm after subarachnoid hemorrhage. Neurosurgery 42:979–987, 1998.

33. Weir B, Grace M, Hansen J, et al: Time course of vasospasm in man. J Neurosurg 48:173–178, 1978.

34. Klopfenstein JD, Kim LJ, Feiz-Erfan I, et al: Comparison of rapid and gradual weaning from external ventricular drainage in patients with aneurysmal subarachnoid hemorrhage: A prospective randomized trial. J Neurosurg 100:225–229, 2004.

35. Landolt AM, Yasargil MG, Krayenbuhl H: Disturbances of the serum electrolytes after surgery of intracranial arterial aneurysms. J Neurosurg 37:210–218, 1972.

36. Alexander MP, Freedman M: Amnesia after anterior communicating artery aneurysm rupture. Neurology 34:752–757, 1984.

81 Surgical Management of Aneurysms of the Middle Cerebral Artery

JAAKKO RINNE, KEISUKE ISHII, HU SHEN, RIKU KIVISAARI, and JUHA HERNESNIEMI

Surprisingly few reports deal with such a common aneurysm site as the middle cerebral artery (MCA) and especially the overall management outcome of this specific group of patients.[1-12] MCA aneurysms (MCAAs) might be considered too common and routine, or maybe the results of the treatment are too unfavorable to be reported. Because of the lack of sufficient collateral circulation, inadvertent occlusion of the MCA, or even of its branches, in most cases leads to calamitous infarction and death, especially in acute (0–1 day after subarachnoid hemorrhage [SAH]) and early surgery (2–3 days after SAH). In his pioneering work on surgery for intracranial aneurysms (IAs), Dandy considered MCAAs hazardous for surgical management, even inoperable.[13] Although currently only a few MCAAs are inoperable, they certainly still present striking problems of their own as compared with other aneurysms in the anterior circulation. These MCAAs are less suitable for endovascular surgery,[14,15] because of both their anatomy and their frequent association with expanding hematomas; thus neurosurgeons should focus especially on the safe treatment of these lesions.[16-22]

Typically, Finnish patients (along with other Arctic peoples) have a higher frequency of MCAAs than reported in other series.[19,23-26] Consequently, we have had a unique opportunity to treat and scrutinize a large group of patients with these particular aneurysms (as of this writing, the combined experience of Kuopio University Hospital and Helsinki University Central Hospital exceeds 3000 patients with MCAAs). This chapter is based on our scrutiny of 561 patients with a total of 690 MCAAs treated in our institution at Kuopio University Hospital in 1977 to 1992,[19] and updated with the neuroradiologic and operative experience of the following 10 years. The baseline characteristics of these patients are shown in Table 81-1. Up to one third of our patients with IAs harbor multiple lesions; among them, MCAAs are the most frequently seen.[19,27,28]

DIAGNOSTIC WORKUP

Most MCAAs are diagnosed as an etiology for hemorrhagic stroke, that is, SAH and/or intracerebral hematoma (ICH). Large or giant MCAAs can cause hemiparesis, seizures, or rarely even ischemic symptoms due to embolic seeding. Unruptured, asymptomatic MCAAs are found in patients with several lesions, incidentally, or by screening for possible

familial aneurysms.[27,29] Recent studies have shown that up to 10% of IAs have familial occurrence. In our series, the most frequent site for familial aneurysms is the MCA.[29-31]

The foundation of the surgical management of MCAAs is proper imaging. A plain computerized tomography (CT) scan remains the cornerstone for the diagnosis of SAH, for bleeding aneurysms in the case of several lesions, and for demonstration of intracerebral or intraventricular bleeding. Recent advances in CT have led to the ability to detect any aneurysm greater than 2 mm in diameter on CT angiography (CTA), covering thus the majority of aneurysms.[32-38] This technique has now become an extremely rapid and safe substitute for digital subtraction angiography (DSA). The advantages of CTA include its 3-dimensionality, which provides a view of the aneurysm from all angles; it also can take

TABLE 81-1 ■ Baseline Characteristics of 561 Patients with Middle Cerebral Artery Aneurysms

Variable	Single MCAA	MIA with One MCAA	MIA with Multiple MCAAs
No. of patients	340	110	111
Mean age (yr)			
All	47.7	51.0	50.3
Females	50.0	55.5	51.9
Males	45.5	47.5	49.0
Females (%)	48.2	43.6	45.0
Size range of MCAAs (%)			
2–7 mm	27	63	51
8–14 mm	45	27	32
15–24 mm	19	6	13
≥25 mm	9	4	4
SAH (%)	91.7	90.0	91.8
MCAA rupture (% of patients)	91.7	31.8	81.8
Preoperative or admission grade in SAH, HH (mean)	2.9	2.8	2.7
ICH (%) in SAH	43	45*	33*
Familial (%)	11	11	14
Arterial hypertension (%)	28	32	36

HH, preoperative or admission grade by Hunt and Hess; ICH, intracerebral hematoma; MCAA, middle cerebral artery aneurysm; MIA, multiple intracranial aneurysms; SAH, subarachnoid hemorrhage.
*With symptomatic MCAA.

into account the bony background and show thrombosed aneurysms; perhaps most importantly, it can be used in emergency cases. CTA is a promising tool for planning microsurgical procedures especially in giant, thrombosed, or otherwise complicated aneurysms. In MCAAs it can sometimes be very difficult to visualize the anatomic relations of the base of the aneurysm and the efferent branches of the vessel. Good-quality CTAs require the use of a fast spiral multirow CT scanner that is capable of scanning very thin slices.

Also, the timing between contrast injection and scanning is crucial to obtain acceptable images. In addition, the venous enhancement in acute SAH can lead to a misdiagnosis; for example, crossing veins can mimic small aneurysms, or cavernous sinus enhancement can be diagnosed as paraclinoid aneurysm of the internal carotid.[34]

Conventional angiography, with or without digital subtraction or as 3-dimensional (3D) angiography, is still the "gold standard" in many institutions (Fig. 81-1). The modern

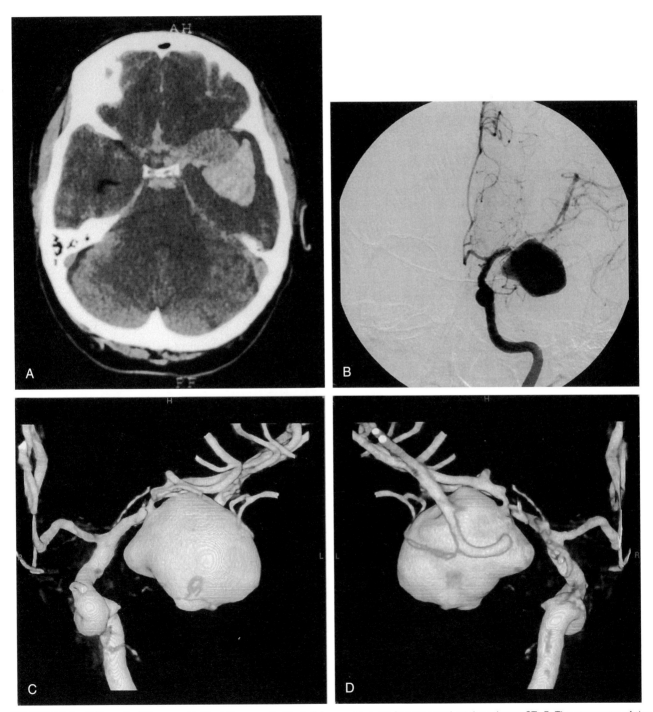

FIGURE 81-1 G.E., male, 66 years old, Hunt-Hess grade III. *A,* A large aneurysm is suspected on the primary CT. *B,* The aneurysm of the first bifurcation of the MCA diagnosed with DSA. Anterior (*C*) and posterior (*D*) 3D images clarify the anatomic details of the aneurysm and vasculature.

digital techniques and advances in catheters as well as in guiding wires have made this study safer with a 0.5% risk of permanent morbidity or mortality.[27,39] The technique, through femoral artery and selective internal carotid injection, allows the use of a considerably smaller amounts of contrast material. The complete angiographic study has at least three projections: lateral, anteroposterior (AP), and oblique. Sometimes more "tailor-made" views are mandatory to clarify the extent of the aneurysm or the neck, which is often broad and complex, especially in larger MCAAs. Because of the many vessel loops close to the MCA bi- or trifurcation, smaller aneurysms (recall that one fifth of

ruptured aneurysms are less than 5 mm in diameter) can remain undetected without special views. Except for the highly urgent cases with large hematomas, we try to study all four vessels at the first session, because associated aneurysms can be treated in the same operation. CTA has diminished the need for four-vessel angiography, and in most cases invasive angiography is not needed, since postoperative controls are also done by CTA (Fig. 81-2).

Magnetic resonance arteriography (MRA) allows the noninvasive imaging of intracranial vessels, even without contrast material. The major limitation of this technique is the (as yet) poorer resolution compared with DSA, leading

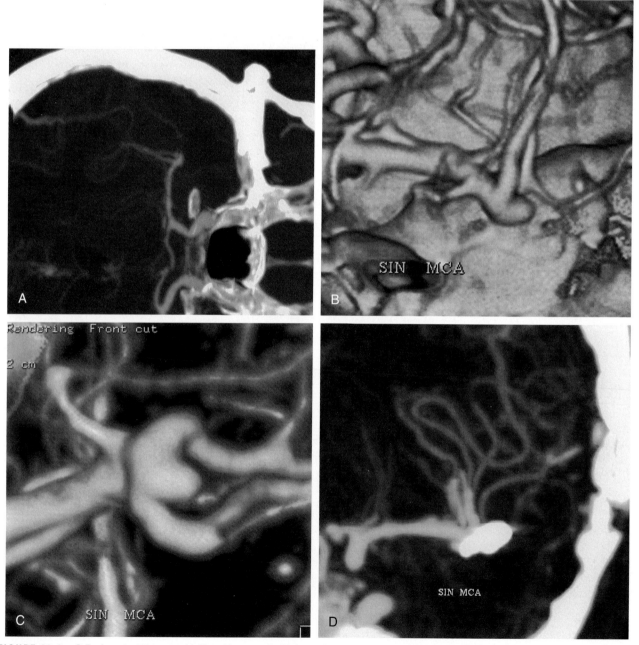

FIGURE 81-2 G.E., female, 59 years old, Hunt-Hess grade IV. A small aneurysm at the first bifurcation of the MCA diagnosed with CTA, 2D (*A*) and 3D (*B* and *C*) reconstruction images. The aneurysm was operated on day 1 after single bleeding. CTA control: complete closure of the aneurysm (*D*).

TABLE 81-2 ▪ **Number of Aneurysms at Various Sites in 1314 Patients with Intracranial Aneurysms**

Site of Aneurysm	All (1314 patients)	MIA (302 patients)	MIA with One MCAA (110 patients)	MIA with Multiple MCAAs (111 patients)
ICA	413	186	64	29
MCA	690	350	110	240
ACoA	433	115	60	16
Peric	96	53	25	9
VBA	119	34	9	2
Total	1751	738	268	296

ACoA, anterior communicating artery; ICA, internal carotid artery; MCA, middle cerebral artery; MCAA, middle cerebral artery aneurysm; MIA, multiple intracranial aneurysms; Peric, pericallosal artery; VBA, vertebrobasilar arteries.

to false-negative results in smaller lesions.[29,40,41] The longer study time and sensitivity to movement artifacts rule out this study from the basic workup toolbox for the often non-cooperative patients with acute SAH. However, MRA is the method of choice when screening for unruptured aneurysms.[29,30]

In the absence of CTA, in the extreme emergency situation with an unconscious patient harboring a large intraparenchymal hematoma, the diagnosis of MCAA can be based on a plain CT. The extent and more detailed anatomy of the ruptured aneurysm must be studied under the operating microscope.[42]

ANATOMIC FEATURES OF MIDDLE CEREBRAL ARTERY ANEURYSMS

Site and Directions

Among our patients with IAs, the MCAAs are the most frequently seen (Table 81-2). Of the frequently studied 1314 patients with IAs,[19,25,28,43] 43% had at least one MCAA (561 patients with 690 MCAAs), and of the patients with multiple IAs (MIAs), 73% had at least one MCAA. From the total number of 1751 IAs, 690 were MCAAs (39%). According to their site, MCAAs can be divided into three groups: proximal, bifurcation, and distal (Table 81-3).

Proximal MCAAs compose 16% of MCAAs, and their presence often indicates other associated aneurysms. Three fourths of the patients with proximal MCAAs have other aneurysm(s), complicating the planning of surgery. Typically, proximal MCAAs are located at the origin of the anterior temporal artery (first branch of the main trunk) and are pointing downward, or they are at the origin of lenticulostriate perforators and pointing upward (Fig. 81-3). A common feature among proximal MCAAs is that the neck is often wide and partially incorporated with the small efferent vessel, making them difficult to clip and coil. The same aneurysmal anatomy can be seen in basilar–superior cerebellar, vertebral–posteroinferior cerebellar, and some distal anterior cerebral artery aneurysms.

Most of the MCAAs (80%) are located at the bi- or trifurcation (see Table 81-3), usually pointing laterally and inferiorly (Figs. 81-4 to 81-6). In AP angiograms, 45% of MCAAs pointed laterally, 38% inferiorly, 15% superiorly, and 2% medially (Fig. 81-7), but the latter carries the highest risk for perforator injury during surgery. In lateral view, one third will projected inferiorly, the rest divided equally among other three directions.

Distal MCAAs are less frequently seen (Fig. 81-8); in our series 4% of MCAAs were located distally (see Table 81-3). Distal aneurysms may be fusiform or mycotic, but true saccular aneurysms are found in even the most distal parts of the MCA. All types of distal aneurysms are difficult to find during surgery, but today's neuronavigation systems have facilitated this task considerably.[8]

The frequency of MIAs in Finnish patients with cerebral aneurysms is at least 30%.[27] Because MCAAs are the most frequently seen, most of these patients harbor MIAs. The MCA is the most frequent site to present mirror aneurysms (i.e., IAs at the same site but on different sides). Two thirds of our patients with multiple MCAAs had mirror aneurysms. Most of the proximal MCAAs (72%) were in patients with MIAs, and a patient with a proximal MCAA has an almost three times higher risk for associated aneurysms than patients with bifurcation or distal MCAAs.

Size, Side, Shape, and Type

Middle cerebral artery aneurysms are larger than symptomatic aneurysms at other sites, although 77% of the symptomatic bifurcation and 92% of the symptomatic proximal MCAAs were 2 to 14 mm in size. More importantly, the broad necks often found on MCAAs make their open and especially endovascular treatment challenging. Among the single MCAAs, 9% were giant aneurysms, more than in any other aneurysmal site in our series.

Ruptured MCAAs were divided equally between both sides; two thirds of the proximal ones were left sided. Nearly all of the ruptured MCAAs are irregular in shape. The shape of the dome depends more on whether the aneurysm has ruptured than it does on its site, and is one of the most important signs to show the ruptured lesion in the absence

TABLE 81-3 ▪ **Frequencies (%) of Middle Cerebral Artery Aneurysms at Different Sites**

Site	Single MCAA (340 patients)	MIA with One MCAA (110 patients)	MIA with Multiple MCAAs (111 patients)
Proximal	9	24	22
Bifurcation	89	74	72
Distal	2	2	6

MCAA, middle cerebral artery aneurysm; MIA, multiple intracranial aneurysms.

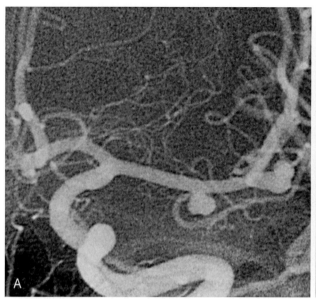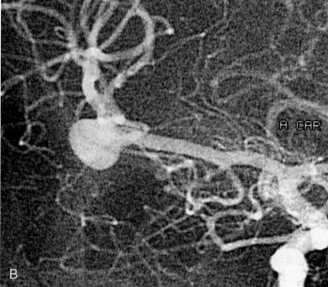

FIGURE 81-3 H.H., female, 64 years old, Hunt-Hess grade II. Multiple (three) aneurysms of the MCAs. The left bifurcation aneurysm had ruptured and was operated 3 days after single bleeding. *A,* Good recovery. *B,* Four months later a large unruptured aneurysm on the contralateral side was operated. Good recovery.

of CT scan or when a delay in admission has occurred. In our series the smaller MCAA often proves to be the one that has ruptured, even though statistically the larger ones are more commonly the ruptured aneurysms. Fusiform, atherosclerotic, or mycotic MCAAs are fortunately rare (0.6%), in that they remain one of the most difficult lesions to treat.[25,28,44-46]

SPECIAL CLINICAL FEATURES OF MIDDLE CRANIAL ARTERY ANEURYSMS

The MCAAs that rupture tend to do so more severely than do IAs at other sites. The mean preoperative or admission Hunt-Hess grade among our patients with ruptured MCAAs was 2.9, as compared with 2.4 at other anterior circulation sites. Also, severe bleeding causes death considerably more often among patients with MCAAs than among patients with other aneurysms. Partly explaining this outcome is the high frequency of ICHs (largest diameter ≥2.5 cm) associated with ruptured MCAAs (Fig. 81-9). The reported incidence of ICH in patients with aneurysmal SAH varies from 5% to 34%.[6,18,20,21,25,47,48] In our series the frequency of ICHs in patients with a single MCAA was very much higher than in patients with any other single aneurysm (43% vs. 11%), making the goals of surgery twofold: (1) securing the aneurysm and (2) evacuating the hematoma. The risk for ICH increased as the site of the ruptured aneurysm became more distal, because with a tighter cistern in that location, the aneurysm is more closely surrounded by the brain. The frequency of ICH was 12% with an aneurysm at the carotid bifurcation (i.e., the origin of the MCA), 29% with a proximal MCAA, 43% with a bifurcation MCAA, and 44% with a distal MCAA. With MCAAs at the bifurcation, the frequency of ICH was highest for aneurysms directed laterally in AP angiograms: 58%. The sacs and the bleeding sites of these aneurysms point toward the temporal lobe, and the fundi are more parallel to the main trunk and thus under a higher hemodynamic stress.

Moderate or severe intraventricular hemorrhage (IVH), one of the most important findings predicting poor outcome,[25,43,48] was observed in 24% of patients with ruptured bifurcation MCAAs, 19% for proximal MCAAs, and 11% for distal MCAAs. The frequencies for moderate or severe preoperative hydrocephalus were the same for each MCAA site as the frequencies for IVH. In a few cases with an acute hydrocephalus, an emergency ventricular drain can be life saving; in these instances we secure the aneurysm in the same session to prevent repeat hemorrhage.

SURGICAL MANAGEMENT

In the case of ruptured MCAA, the timing of the procedure has a crucial role. In SAH acute and early surgery (done in the first 72 hours) has a beneficial effect on outcome through two of the most important independent variables influencing outcome: it prevents repeat hemorrhage, and it allows active prevention and treatment of the vasospasm with intravenous nimodipine and HHH (hemodilution, hypervolemia, hypertension) therapy. However, in the extreme group of poor-grade (Hunt-Hess grade V) patients without a remarkable hematoma, the favorable effect of early surgery is less clear, and delay in the surgery might be justified.[49] With our recent clinical experience, we operate on even these patients if they improve or stabilize, since as long as the bleeding site is not secured, the aggressive treatment of vasospasm (HHH) may be equally hazardous to waiting. The incidence of surgical complications might be independent of the patient's grade.[50] In an unselected series of cases and in a series such as ours that lacks any referral bias, there are always patients arriving at the hospital with aneurysms that have bled so severely that the patients are beyond any treatment. Because these patients die within a few hours, they are not admitted to metropolitan tertiary centers, which consequently have better management or surgical results in their selected series. In our series the reasons for nonsurgical treatment were initial poor grade,[49]

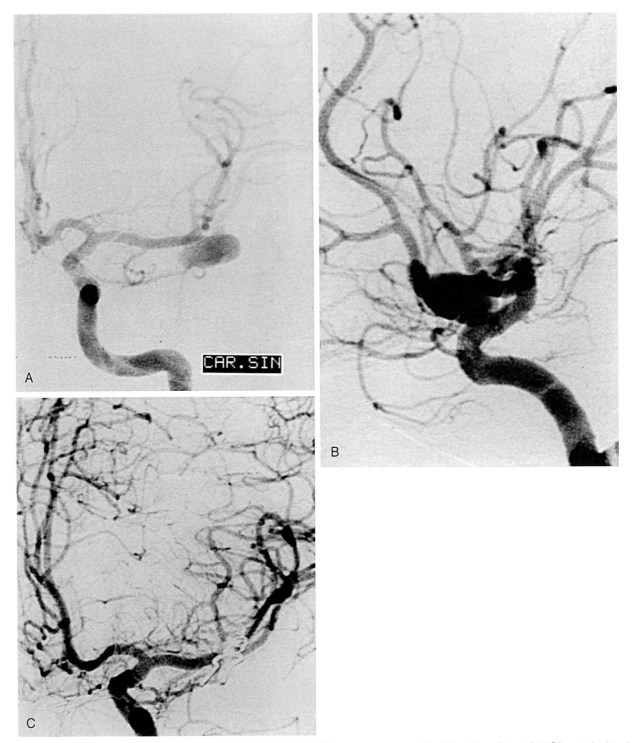

FIGURE 81-4   S.S., female, 31 years old, Hunt-Hess grade II. *A* to *C,* Large aneurysm at the bifurcation of the left MCA, attached to the sphenoidal wing. Clipping with two clips on day 1 after single bleed. Good recovery.

poor grade caused by repeat hemorrhage,[7] old age,[5] technical reasons,[3] or patients' refusal,[1] totaling 11% of all patients with MCAAs. Acute and early surgery (within 72 hours of SAH) was achieved in 60% of the ruptured MCAAs, but the number has clearly increased in more recent years.

Especially in aneurysm surgery, the results are reflected by the quality of the team, by the skills and experience of the surgeon, and surely by some of the aforementioned referral biases.[51] Unless the situation is an emergency, it

may be wise to delay an aneurysm operation from very late evening or night to the next morning, when a more experienced team and backup are available. However, in Helsinki, where an experienced team and backup are always available, aneurysms are usually operated on immediately on presentation. If the number of aneurysm operations in one institution is low, it is impossible to gather enough experience, and the overall results remain too unfavorable.[52,53] Very large and giant, or otherwise complex aneurysms should be treated by

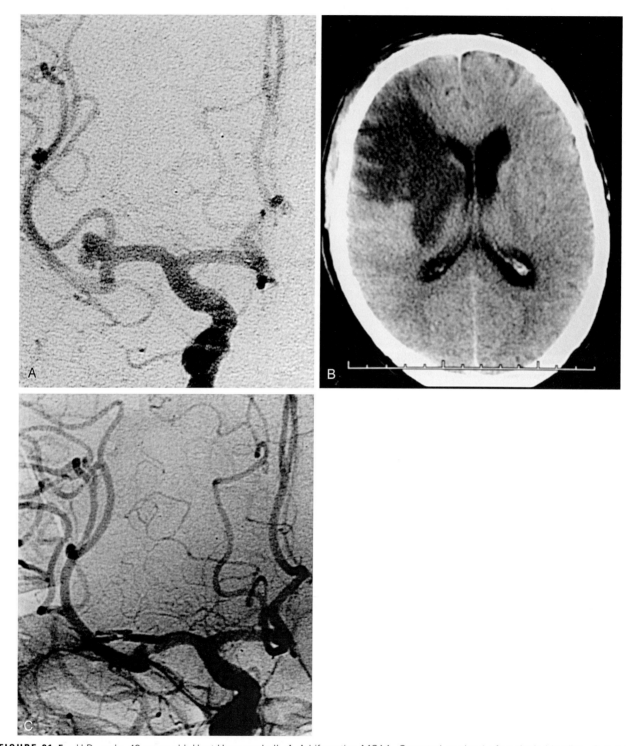

FIGURE 81-5   H.P., male, 49 years old, Hunt-Hess grade II. *A,* A bifurcation MCAA. Operated on day 1 after single bleeding. *B,* A large infarction due to closure of frontal bifurcation branch. *C,* No reoperation. Postoperative disability with left hemiparesis.

experienced vascular neurosurgeons, capable of reconstructing or bypassing the vessel(s).[54]

Positioning and Approach

All except those rare distal MCAAs can be reached through a standard pterional approach, which is used exclusively in our institutions. A more subfrontal approach, the lateral supraorbital approach, has been used by one of us (J.H.) in

hundreds of patients by creating only a small frontal flap with some removal of the sphenoid wing. For the surgery, the patient is positioned supine, the head elevated clearly above the cardiac level to reduce the cranial venous pressure and even the intra-aneurysmal arterial pressure. The head, fixed with three or four pins in the head frame (Mayfield or Sugita), is rotated some 15 to 20 degrees toward the opposite side, tilted slightly downward (Fig. 81-10). The most common error is overrotation, which causes the

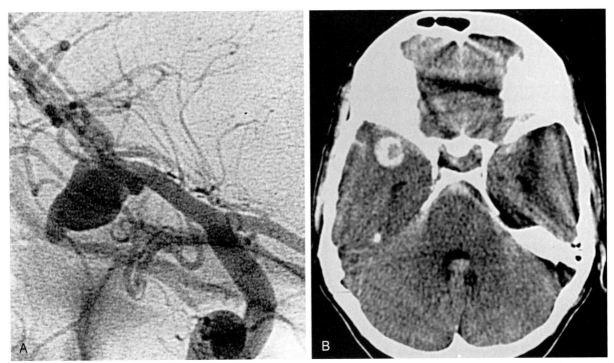

FIGURE 81-6   A.H., female, 39 years old, Hunt-Hess grade III. *A*, Large calcified aneurysm in the MCA bifurcation. *B*, Calcification seen in nonenhanced CT scan. Presence of calcification may predict difficult clipping. Operated on day 1. Good recovery.

temporal lobe to "cover" the sylvian fissure, leading the surgeon to retract the temporal lobe further and predisposing to a difficult dissection of the aneurysm. If the head is tilted downward too much, the basal orbital bony structures may obscure the operating field. The working channel parallel to the skull base is adequate, and removal of the superior orbital rim or the zygomatic arch to gain a more upward working direction is not necessary. The anesthesiologic staff must be prepared to adjust the position of the operating table frequently.

Shaving should be minimal but should allow for a sufficiently large oblique frontotemporal skin incision, behind the hairline if possible. In ordinary cases we prefer a short incision placed slightly over the estimated location of the

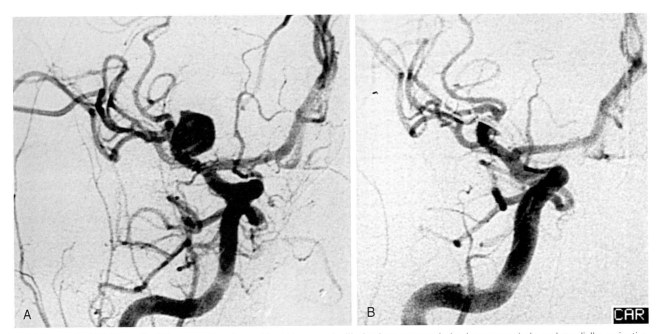

FIGURE 81-7   V-M.K., male, 34 years old, seizure, Hunt-Hess grade III. Angiogram revealed a large superiorly and medially projecting bifurcation MCAA. *A*, Postoperative angiogram shows closure of the aneurysm. *B*, Good recovery.

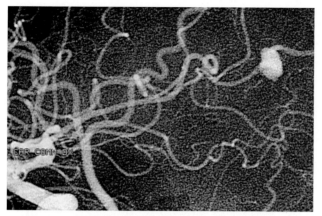

FIGURE 81-8   J.L., male, 39 years old, Hunt-Hess grade II. A distal fusiform MCA aneurysm. Operated on day 1 after second bleeding, a bypass from superficial temporal artery to the median cerebral artery was performed before the resection of the aneurysm. After operation there was a slight left hemiparesis, but it subsided rapidly; the anastomosis was patent. Good recovery.

sylvian fissure and more frontally as the approach to the sylvian fissure is made from the frontal side. A more fronto-basal approach can be used if necessary to achieve proximal control of the MCA. In the case of large hematomas and/or giant aneurysms, the skin flap is planned slightly more posteriorly to allow for better handling of the giant aneurysm or evacuation of hematomas that project posteriorly and many times deeply and centrally. The incision line is infiltrated abundantly with a mixture of lidocaine and epinephrine to prevent both unnecessary oozing of the wound and an increase in the patient's blood pressure during the incision. The area of the skin flap is covered with self-adhesive transparent plastic.

After stepwise detachment from the bone by diathermy in one layer, the skin-galea-muscle flap is elevated until the superior orbital rim and the anterior zygomatic arch are exposed, thus avoiding any injury of the facial nerve branches by spring hooks. The number of burr holes is determined by the size of the flap, thickness of the bone, and adherence of the dura. Usually one or two burr hole(s) are placed, one posteriorly just below the insertion line of the temporal muscle,

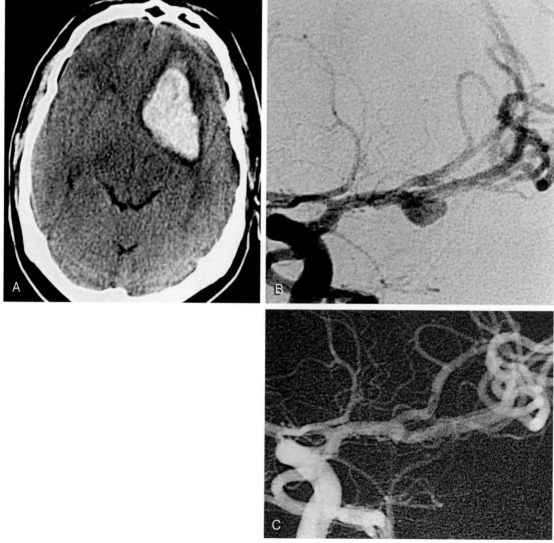

FIGURE 81-9   E.L., male, 38 years old, Hunt-Hess grade II. *A*, ICH without SAH. *B*, Bifurcation MCAA. *C*, Hematoma was evacuated and aneurysm clipped on day 3 after single bleeding. Good recovery.

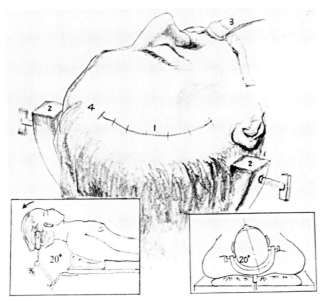

FIGURE 81-10 For operation, the head is elevated clearly above the level of the heart to reduce the cranial venous pressure and even the intra-aneurysmal pressure. The head, which is fixed with three or four pins in the head frame (Mayfield or Sugita), is rotated approximately 20 degrees toward the opposite side and is tilted slightly downward. The most common error is overrotation, which causes the temporal lobe to "cover" the sylvian fissure. If the head is tilted downward too much, the basal orbital bone structures may obscure the operating field. The working channel parallel to the skull base is adequate, and removal of the superior orbital rim or the zygomatic arch to gain a more upward-working direction is unnecessary. 1, Scalp incision; 2, head frame; 3, intubation tube; 4, hairline.

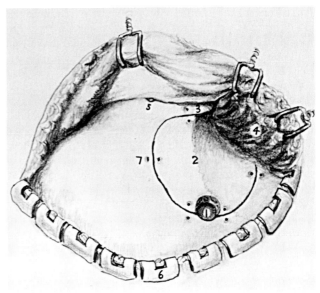

FIGURE 81-11 The skin-galea-muscle flap is elevated after stepwise detachment from the bone by diathermy in one layer, thus avoiding any injury to the branches of the facial nerve by spring hooks, until the superior orbital rim and the anterior zygomatic arch are exposed. The number of burr holes is determined by the size of the flap, the thickness of the bone, and adherence of the dura. Usually one or two burr holes are placed, one posteriorly just below the insertion line of the temporal muscle, and, if necessary, the other just over the pterion. The flap is detached mainly by a side-cutting craniotome, but the basal part is drilled off before lifting the flap. 1, Burr hole; 2, temporal line; 3, zygomatic process; 4, temporal muscle; 5, supraorbital foramen; 6, scalp clip; 7, burr holes for bone flap fixation.

and if necessary the other just over the pterion (Fig. 81-11). The flap is detached mostly by side-cutting craniotome, but the basal part is drilled off partially before lifting the flap. The operating microscope can be introduced at this point for high-speed drilling of the frontal and of the lateral sphenoid bone. The lateral sphenoid ridge and vertical bone on both sides are drilled off until the bony exposure is

along the skull base; oozing from the cut bony surfaces is best treated by "hot drilling" (i.e., drilling with a large diamond burr without irritation with water) or with bone wax. Oozing from the dura is controlled by bone wax and bipolar coagulation of the dural vessels (Fig. 81-12).

The dura is opened with a curvilinear incision pointing anterolaterally and elevated with stitches. The operating

FIGURE 81-12 An operating microscope can be introduced for high-speed drilling of the lateral sphenoid bone. The lateral sphenoid ridge and vertical bone on both of its sides are drilled off until the bony exposure is along the skull base; oozing of blood from the cut bone surfaces and the dura is controlled by bone wax and bipolar coagulation of the dural vessels. The dura is opened in a curvilinear incision pointing anterolaterally and is elevated with stitches. 1, Dura; 2, temporal muscle; 3, drill; 4, sphenoid; 5, sucker.

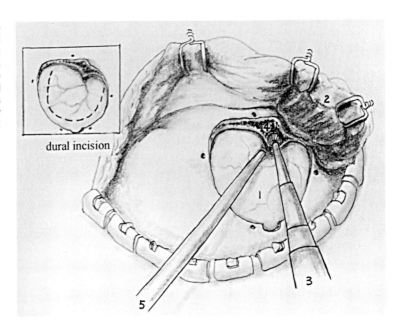

dural incision

microscope is brought into position. We try to minimize the use of spatulas for brain dislocation. The suction apparatus can be used in the left hand for intermittent brain retraction, while using the bipolar coagulating forceps or microscissors in the right hand. This technique necessitates frequent adjustment of the operating microscope to the proper position to keep the working channel minimum. Therefore, we prefer a mouth-controlled and balanced microscope with magnetic brakes as designed by Yasargil. In addition to the benefits of magnification, light view, and stereoscopic view, the modern microscope allows the surgeon to move freely— especially with the use of a mouthpiece—thus keeping the exposure as atraumatic as possible. The elbow and arm support is provided by a slim adjustable table that can be lifted frequently as needed to maintain the proper working direction and height (also designed by Yasargil). Successful microsurgery involves equipment, technique, knowledge of anatomy, and careful planning.

Strategy

The strategy for exposure depends for the most part on site, size, and especially direction of the aneurysm as well as the existence of hematomas or associated aneurysms. When positioning the head of the patient in the skull clamp, it is wise to imagine 3-dimensionally the exact location and projection of the aneurysm. With proximal MCAAs and with bifurcation MCAAs with a very short MCA main trunk, the sylvian fissure can be opened medially. The optico-carotid cisterns are approached frontobasally and opened. Cerebrospinal fluid (CSF) is drained slowly, providing more space. The frontal lobe is gently retracted, after taking into account the direction of the aneurysm, especially when dealing with recently ruptured aneurysms. The carotid bifurcation is exposed by opening the cisterns widely. The dissection is then carried along the main trunk of the MCA, opening the fissure mediolaterally, until the aneurysm is encountered. Any injury to the perforators at the bifurcation and at the medial wall of the MCA must be carefully avoided. Proximal MCAAs are usually small, but their necks are wide. When the aneurysm is located at the origin of the anterior temporal artery, the neck is always incorporated with that vessel; thus careless clip placement can lead to kinking and closure of the vessel. Those proximal MCAAs pointing upward and/or medially are involved with lenticulostriatal perforators. To properly secure these aneurysms and avoid calamitous infarcts, all small vessels must be meticulously separated from the neck before clipping. If the aneurysm is at the bifurcation, at this point in the dissection the part of main trunk free of perforators is observed for possible temporary clip placement.

We usually approach nearly all MCAAs directly by opening the fissure laterally. Even in acute SAH, in most cases enough space can be obtained by patiently removing CSF after the fissure has been initially opened. If the brain is very edematous and swollen and the fissure very tight, CSF can be first removed by opening the frontobasal cisterns or (more effectively) the lamina terminalis, or both. Gentle injection of fluid into the sylvian fissure aids considerably in its opening (water dissection introduced by Toth). Spinal CSF drainage has not been used in MCAAs. Once enough working space has been created, the lateral dissection is

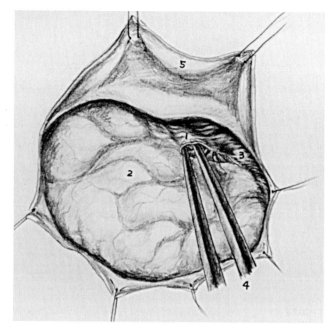

FIGURE 81-13 We usually approach almost all MCAAs directly by opening the fissure laterally. Even in an acute SAH, in most cases enough space can be obtained by patiently removing CSF after the fissure is first opened. If the brain is very edematous and swollen and the fissure is very tight, CSF can first be removed by opening the frontobasal cisterns or the lamina terminalis or both. Gentle injection of fluid inside the sylvian fissure helps to open it (via water dissection). CSF drainage from the spine has not been used in MCAAs. Once sufficient working space has been created, the lateral dissection is carried deeper into the fissure, and one of the distal MCA branches is followed to the aneurysm. Often, the sylvian fissure is opened straight over the aneurysm. 1, Arachnoid; 2, frontal lobe; 3, sylvian veins; 4, bipolar forceps; 5, dura.

carried deeper into the fissure, and one of the distal MCA branches is followed to the aneurysm. Often the sylvian fissure is opened directly over the aneurysm (Fig. 81-13). At this stage of dissection the need for lobe retraction is usually minimal and is achieved with small cotton patties. If additional retraction is needed, it should be directed away from the lobe toward which the aneurysm dome is pointing. When the bifurcation area is encountered, the main trunk of the MCA is identified to achieve proximal control or if temporary occlusion is to be applied. The main trunk can usually be found by dissecting under or beside the bifurcation away from the aneurysm. Thereafter the dissection is concentrated in the aneurysmal neck, and all manipulation of the dome and the bleeding site must be avoided as long as possible (Fig. 81-14). All main branches must be identified and carefully dissected free. After a clip has been applied, the dome is dissected free and the position of the blades is checked (Fig. 81-15).

If the clip is closing the neck, the sac is punctured or opened by scissors and coagulated (Fig. 81-16). It is essential to ascertain that there is no obstruction in the main trunk or branches and that none of the medial perforators has been trapped between the blades. Sometimes it is hard to visually assess whether sufficient flow remains in the M2 branches after clipping, especially under hypotension. The new mini-Doppler ultrasound is a practical tool for this purpose: it is simple and easy to use, it gives an unmistakable

FIGURE 81-14 Once the bifurcation area is encountered, the main trunk of the MCA can be identified to obtain proximal control. The main trunk can usually be found by dissecting under or beside the bifurcation away from the aneurysm; in this case M1 is below the bifurcation and its aneurysms. Thereafter, the dissection is concentrated in the neck, and all manipulation of the dome (and the bleeding site) must be avoided for as long as possible. All the main branches must be identified and carefully dissected free. 1, M2; 2, aneurysm; 3, sylvian veins; 4, frontal lobe; 5, arachnoid; 6, temporal lobe; 7, hook; 8, retractor; 9, sucker.

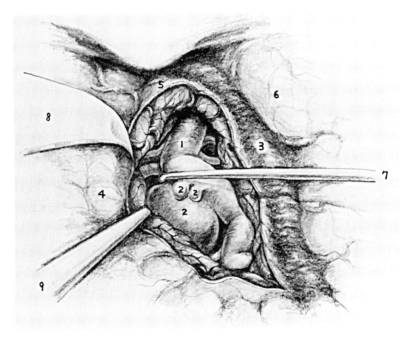

sound effect if there is flow, and it is relatively inexpensive. In the more complicated aneurysms, intraoperative angiography is more helpful.[55,56] This technique, however, not only is more costly but requires specialized equipment and personnel: it must be prepared preoperatively and requires adequate fluoroscopy, a special headrest and operating table, as well as a neuroradiologist. Despite these drawbacks, it has been proved to be cost effective in cases with higher risk for technical troubleshooting.[55,56] We use it routinely when treating large or giant aneurysms, because it is certainly capable of detecting unexpected arterial occlusions that otherwise would lead to clinically evident strokes if not immediately corrected.

In certain cases, one must consider leaving a small neck remnant ("dog ear") rather than risking possible closure of a branch (Fig. 81-17). If the remnant is thin, it must be pursued to catch with a miniclip; if it is strong walled, it should be left unclipped, because an overly tight clip could lead to occlusion of the branch(es) (see Fig. 81-5). With larger aneurysms, the force in the tips of the clipblades might be insufficient to close the neck completely. In those cases a booster clip must be applied above the first one, either parallel with it or crossing with the tips of the blades of the first one. The techniques of Drake and Peerless, involving tandem and piggyback clips, can also be used.[57] Local administration of papaverine has been used routinely to prevent vasospasm.

FIGURE 81-15 After a clip has been applied, the dome is dissected free and the position of the blades is checked. 1, Aneurysm; 2, M2; 3, aneurysm clip; 4, sylvian veins; 5, clip applier; 6, sucker; 7, retractor; 8, frontal lobe; 9, arachnoid; 10, temporal lobe.

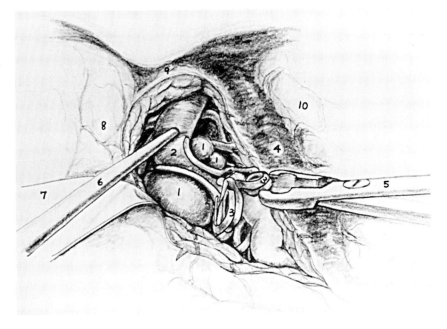

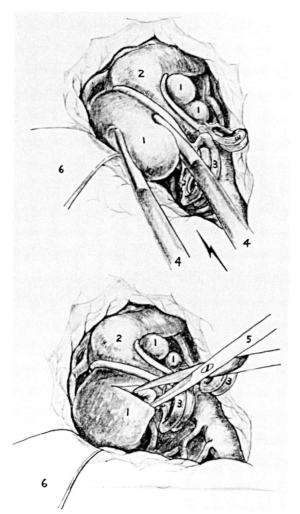

FIGURE 81-16 If the clip is closing the neck, the sac is punctured and coagulated. It must be secured so that there is not the slightest obstruction in the main trunk or branches and so that none of the medial perforators is trapped between the blades. It is sometimes difficult to assess visually whether there is enough flow in the M2 branches after clipping, especially under hypotension. Mini-Doppler ultrasound is a practical tool for this purpose. It is simple and easy to use; it gives an unmistakable sound effect if there is flow; and it is relatively inexpensive. 1, Aneurysm; 2, M2; 3, aneurysm clip; 4, bipolar forceps; 5, microscissors; 6, retractor.

In a few cases it has caused an alarming uni- or bilateral mydriasis lasting several hours.

Hematoma

A significant ICH (>2.5 cm) is often associated with a ruptured MCAA. This alters surgical strategy, not only by necessitating emergency surgery. The hematoma cavity can be used as a route to the aneurysm, but this route is unclear and dangerous. The aneurysm is pointing toward the cavity, and thus the first part of the aneurysm to be encountered is usually the bleeding site, increasing the risk of intraoperative rupture. It is preferable to remove only enough of the hematoma to create sufficient working space and then to continue with the clear anatomy of the transsylvian approach. Once the aneurysm has been secured, the rest of the hematoma can be sucked away. It is not uncommon for the

superiormost and posteriormost parts of the hematoma to remain unevacuated if the 3D anatomy of the hematoma is not carefully taken into account. In these cases edema increases postoperatively, and these hematoma remnants frequently require evacuation. In these second operations, we have additionally removed some parts of the temporal lobe and even done lifesaving large decompressive craniectomies.

Multiple Aneurysms

Our series consisted of 221 patients with multiple aneurysms and at least one MCAA. Surgical management of these patients should follow the guidelines for treatment of multiple aneurysms.[28,52] The symptomatic aneurysm must be treated first. In our experience, if the associated aneurysms could be secured during the same session, the overall outcome of these patients seemed to be slightly better. However, the decision whether to perform the operation in one or two stages is strongly biased and depends on the severity of SAH, extent of brain edema, sites of the aneurysms, and even the experience of the surgeon and the team. In troublesome perioperative conditions the pursuit of the intact sac(s) is abandoned. Our analysis also showed that in cases of multiple aneurysms, only two thirds of all the aneurysms could be secured.

Of our patients with multiple MCAAs, 100 had bilateral and 11 unilateral MCAAs. Two thirds[58] of the patients with bilateral MCAAs had mirror aneurysms, and in half of these cases they were the only aneurysms the patient had. Thirty-four percent of the associated bifurcation MCAAs were directed inferiorly in both angiogram projections, perhaps making them most suitable at this site for contralateral clipping. In 124 patients out of 221 with MIA and at least one MCAA, all aneurysms were secured—in 46 in a one-stage operation. In 18 patients ipsi- and contralateral aneurysms were clipped through the same craniotomy (Fig. 81-18), this experience is now tripled since initial scrutiny. Contralateral aneurysms should not be clipped in the presence of reddened edematous brain tissue associated with recent severe SAH. It is clear that contralateral surgery should be done only by highly experienced neurosurgeons.

Giant Aneurysms

About 5% of all aneurysms are giant (diameter ≥2.5 cm by definition). Of our MCAAs, 6% were giant aneurysms, and the MCA proved to be the most frequent site for these lesions (Fig. 81-19). Surgery for giant aneurysms requires exceptionally careful imaging and planning, including even preparation for bypass surgery and/or surgery with circulation arrest under hypothermia.[54,59–61] Direct clipping is reported to be possible in about two thirds of the cases (ranging from 38% to 71%), and reconstructive surgery is often needed, at least to some extent[61] (Figs. 81-20 to 81-23). To soften the aneurysm dome, temporary occlusion is almost mandatory. Occlusion times are frequently considerably longer than with smaller lesions. The risk of a permanent iatrogenic ischemic lesion might be lowered by perioperative electroencephalographic (EEG) monitoring, but we have not used EEG.[62] The lateral asymmetry in wave patterns indicates hypoxia, which can develop into ischemia if the circulation remains restricted.

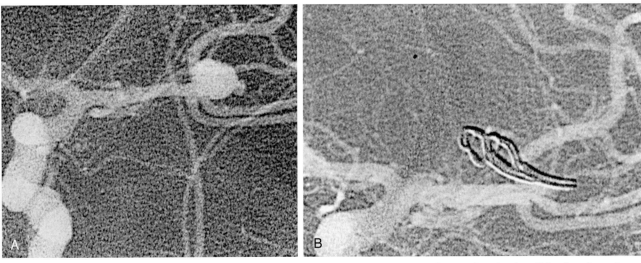

FIGURE 81-17 L.L., female, 48 years old, Hunt-Hess grade II. Left sided MCA aneurysm. *A,* Operated on the day of bleeding. A small remnant of the neck seen on the follow-up. *B,* Good recovery. An unruptured contralateral MCA aneurysm was operated uneventfully 6 weeks later.

The thrombosed mass inside the aneurysm can be removed by ultrasound aspirator. In some cases the securing of the aneurysm leads to occlusion of the parent artery. Sufficient circulation can be preserved by bypassing the MCA with the superficial temporal artery or the external carotid artery, using a venous graft with conventional occlusive technique (or with the ELANA [excimer laser-assisted nonocclusive anastomosis] technique, after training in Utrecht by Professor Cornelis Tulleken). Only in children can adequate oxygen content be provided by the collateral network. The majority of recent experience suggests that the only indications for aneurysm clipping under circulatory arrest with hypothermia and barbiturate brain protection are giant and/or complicated posterior fossa lesions.

Ruptured giant aneurysms seem to carry about the same risk for repeat hemorrhage as the smaller ones. In a series

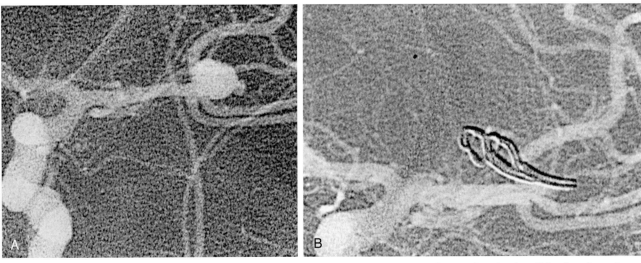

FIGURE 81-18 M.V., female, 53 years old, bleeding from a basilaris aneurysm that had been treated successfully with coils. Angiograms revealed bilateral unruptured MCA aneurysms. Both of them were treated in a single right-sided craniotomy. Good recovery.

from Mayo Clinic the risk for repeat hemorrhage was over 18% in the first 14 days after admission.[61,63] Although this experience seems to indicate the importance of early surgery, the actual pros and cons remain controversial. In the same series, of patients surviving for surgery, 72% had a favorable outcome. This is clearly higher than usually reported. The outcome figures are, however, affected more by the site of the aneurysm (anterior vs. posterior) and clinical grade (Hunt-Hess I–II vs. IV–V) than by early surgery alone. The clinical experience of the entire surgical team and the referral pattern also have an important impact on the overall outcome. Since Helsinki and Kuopio are the only neurosurgical units in their service area, no referral bias exists.

Temporary Arterial Occlusion

The indications for temporary arterial occlusion are: (1) premature aneurysm rupture during dissection and (2) the need to manipulate the sac for proper clip application as a result of the structure of the aneurysm (size, shape, location of the branches). Sometimes the backflow from the M2 branches is so strong that it is necessary to temporarily occlude not only the main trunk but also the branches to reduce the sac sufficiently. It is wise also to occlude M1 or at least the other M2—even both—to permit treatment of the aneurysms as soon as possible. It is common practice to protect the brain during temporary occlusion by raising blood pressure and by administering a bolus of mannitol and barbiturates before occlusion.[58,62,64] However, the actual independent influence of these actions in preventing iatrogenic infarction remains unproven. In Helsinki we have noted that increasing the blood pressure can result in excessive bleeding and an increase in the occlusion time. Consequently, we no longer raise the blood pressure, since under normotension the temporary occlusion time is considerably shorter. Moderate hypothermia (without cardiac arrest) may provide additional brain protection and can be used in complicated large or giant MCA aneurysms.

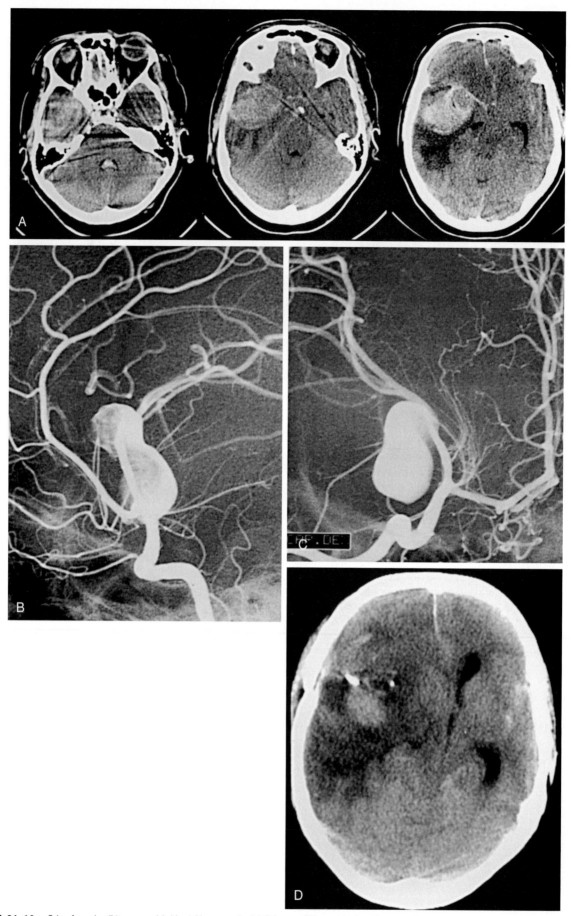

FIGURE 81-19 S.L., female, 51 years old, Hunt-Hess grade IV. Primary CT revealed an intracerebral hematoma and a large aneurysm in the right MCA, considerable edema, and expansion. *A,* Angiogram revealed a large aneurysm in the main bifurcation. *B* and *C,* At operation it was apparent that the whole expansion, which seemed like hematoma, was a giant aneurysm. *D,* On postoperative CT, strong edema and expansion led to the patient's death 2 days after the operation.

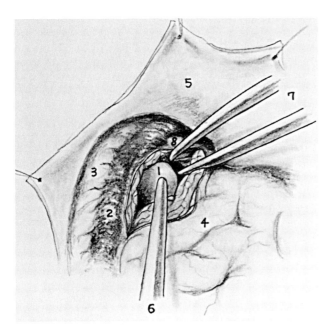

FIGURE 81-20 A small part of the fundus of a left-sided giant MCA aneurysm is seen after splitting of the sylvian fissure. Figures 81-21 to 81-23 illustrate the process of resecting this aneurysm. 1, Aneurysm; 2, sylvian veins; 3, temporal lobe; 4, frontal lobe; 5, dura; 6, sucker; 7, bipolar forceps.

The highest risk for an ischemic event during temporary occlusion is clearly related to duration of temporary occlusion (i.e., >30 minutes), placement of the clip (if perforators are being occluded as well), and operative conditions (emergency situation vs. elective occlusion).[64]

Temporary occlusion is safe when used for less than 5 minutes except for a few local technical complications. There is no safe upper limit, but caution is advisable with times more than 15 minutes. A single temporary occlusion is preferable. Considerable caution should be exercised when using temporary occlusion in aged patients and those in poor grades before surgery, and associated aneurysms should be left for a second craniotomy when using temporary occlusion. Temporary occlusion should be used with normo- or hypertensive levels of blood pressure and should be reserved mainly for those cases that absolutely cannot be managed without it.

The role of somatosensory evoked potential (SEPs) or EEG monitoring in helping to protect the brain from ischemic lesions during temporary occlusion is somewhat controversial.[58] There is evidence that SEPs will deteriorate in about 10 minutes after the closure of the MCA, but the brain tissue will recover completely without any new sequelae if recirculation is instituted in another 10 minutes. Asymmetric slowing of waves on EEG indicates hypoxia early enough to be reversible. These techniques have their limitations: there are false negatives, they require educated staff and special hardware, and they are most effective with elective surgery and not with cases treated very late at night.

Endovascular Treatment

Since the introduction of Guglielmi detachable coils (GDCs), the endovascular embolization of IAs with

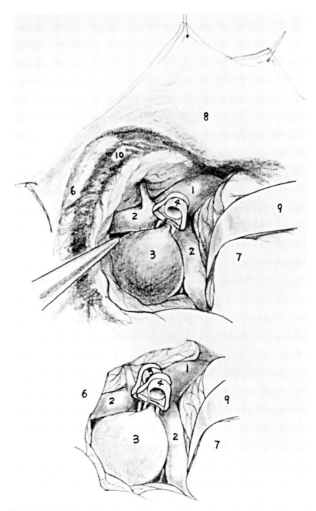

FIGURE 81-21 The first clip is applied on the sclerotic, thick neck of the aneurysm. Even with two clips, the aneurysm is still pulsating. 1, M1; 2, M2; 3, aneurysm; 4, aneurysm clip; 5, aneurysm clip; 6, temporal lobe; 7, frontal lobe; 8, dura; 9, retractor; 10, sylvian veins.

endosaccular coils (i.e., coiling) has provided an optional and increasingly used method of treatment.[14,15,17,65-68] With recent advances in microcatheters and guidewires, the site of the aneurysm is merely one issue in selecting patients for this treatment. Additional concerns are that the neck must be clearly visualized and free from efferent branches, and the width of the neck should preferably be less than the diameter of the dome.

Since follow-up studies of sufficient duration are lacking, the long-term effectiveness of this technique remains unclear. It has been increasingly used in the treatment of both unruptured and ruptured IAs, although many more studies are needed to aid in decision making and in selecting an optimal treatment modality for particular clinical situations. MCAAs are the aneurysms least suitable for coiling.[14,15,17,22,65,68] In giant aneurysms the experience of coiling is even more limited, but in a few cases the outcome has been dismal. The traditional endovascular parent vessel occlusion is not a real option in giant MCAAs.[67] Theoretically, coiling could be used as a first-stage treatment to secure the lesion from repeat hemorrhage and to allow delayed surgery and/or aggressive vasospasm management.

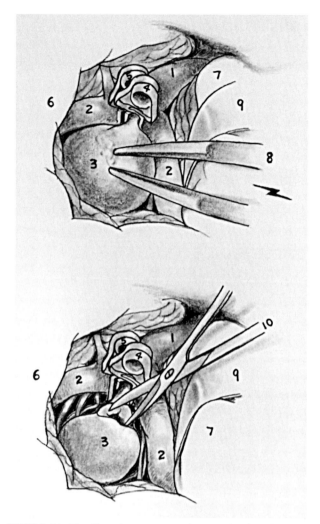

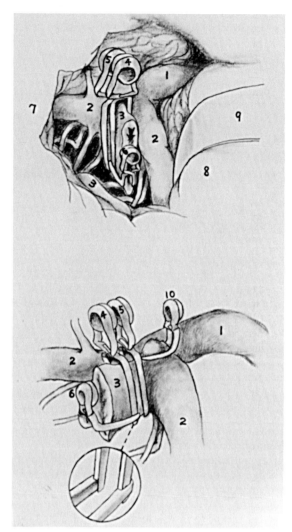

FIGURE 81-22   The giant aneurysm is coagulated and opened. 1, M1; 2, M2; 3, aneurysm; 4, aneurysm clip; 5, aneurysm clip; 6, temporal lobe; 7, frontal lobe; 8, bipolar forceps; 9, retractor; 10, scissors.

FIGURE 81-23   Finally, after the resection of the aneurysm, a booster clip is applied. A small additional aneurysm is ligated with a miniclip. 1, M1; 2, M2; 3, aneurysm remnant; 4, aneurysm clip; 5, aneurysm clip; 6, booster clip; 7, temporal lobe; 8, frontal lobe; 9, retractor; 10, miniclip.

According to our experience, delayed surgery for previously coiled aneurysms might be by far more complicated than had been thought as a result of the adhesions and lower mobility of the sac. Often the sac must be opened and the coils removed before clipping of the neck is possible. Also, the relief of other symptoms (e.g., in cases with epilepsy or mass symptoms) may be questionable with GDC treatment, even though the pulsatile effect might be diminished. Hypothetically, the risk for vasospasm might be higher in ruptured aneurysms with GDC treatment, since the thrombus in the subarachnoid space remains untouched.

A randomized study in our institution comparing the treatment of ruptured IAs with GDC or early surgery showed that in an unselected group, as many as one third of the symptomatic aneurysms are not suitable for GDC treatment.[22] At certain sites (e.g., MCA) the aneurysms are often structurally more suitable for surgery or present more complications with GDC. It is clearly evident that a modern neurovascular unit must be able to offer both of these treatment options at a high-standard level.

OUTCOME

Our patients with MCAAs fared surprisingly poorly overall, despite the good surgical results in good-grade patients: a good outcome occurred in more than 86% of grade 0 to II patients (Table 81-4). These were equal to our other patients with another symptomatic anterior circulation aneurysm. The immediate postoperative results were the same in all patients with symptomatic MCAAs as they were in patients with aneurysms at other sites, but 30% of the patients with a single MCAA had a poor outcome, being severely disabled or having died at the 12-month follow-up point, compared to a 23% frequency of unfavorable outcome in patients with a single IA at other sites in the anterior circulation. This significant difference is explained by the higher frequency of severe persistent deficits (i.e., dysphasia, severe hemiparesis, visual field deficits, and late epilepsy) associated with symptomatic MCAAs. In patients with MIA and one MCAA, the frequency for poor outcome was 38%, and in patients with multiple MCAAs 35%.

TABLE 81-4 ▪ Frequencies (%) of Outcome (GOS) at 12 Months in 457 Patients with Operated Middle Cerebral Artery Aneurysms*

Grade[†] (No. Patients)	Good Recovery	Moderate Disability	Severe Disability	Dead
0 (33)	88	12	–	–
I (46)	87	9	–	4
II (171)	85	6	4	5
III (124)	47	27	13	13
IV (59)	15	25	24	36
V (24)	8	17	29	46
Total	62	15	10	13

GOS, Glasgow Outcome Scale.
*No patient in a vegetative state at 12 months.
[†]Preoperative or admission grade according to Hunt and Hess.

These figures are worse than those generally seen in our patients with MIA. Table 81-5 shows the outcome of ruptured MCAAs in relation to their site and clinical grade.

In other published series of MCAAs, similar frequencies for surgical outcome can be seen.[7] In Suzuki's series (413 patients) 94% of the patients were in good or excellent condition 6 months after treatment.[10] Half of these patients had late surgery or their aneurysms were unruptured and/or had good grades (0–I). In a Hungarian series of 289 patients with MCAAs, only 18% had poor outcome after surgery in a long-term follow-up.[8] Yasargil reported unfavorable results only in 6% of his 231 patients with MCAAs.[12] Excellent results were published also by Sundt, with a 14% frequency for poor results after surgery for MCAAs.[46] All these are surgical series, and may reflect not only excellent surgical skills but also selection and referral bias.

The overall management outcome was almost equal for all MCAA sites: 34% poor outcome in patients with ruptured proximal, 32% with ruptured bifurcation, and 30% for ruptured distal MCAAs. The frequency for poor outcome in good-grade patients was highest among patients with a proximal MCAA. This is explained by a high frequency of anatomic variation in which the neck of the aneurysm is partly incorporated with the smaller efferent vessel, leading easily to its inadvertent occlusion by the clip. Poor results were most common in patients who had a bifurcation MCAA directed laterally in their AP angiogram, since

TABLE 81-5 ▪ Frequencies (%) of Poor Outcome (GOS 1–3) in Patients with Ruptured Middle Cerebral Artery Aneurysms at Different Sites

Grade[*]	Proximal MCAA (41 patients)	Bifurcation MCAA (376 patients)	Distal MCAA (9 patients)
I	12	3	–
II	18	11	20
III	40	25	100
IV	67	62	–
V	100	89	100

GOS, Glasgow Outcome Scale; MCAA, middle cerebral artery aneurysm.
*Preoperative or admission grade according to Hunt and Hess.

these patients had significantly more temporal ICHs. The best results were achieved in those patients with a bifurcation MCAA pointing inferiorly in both projections: a 9% frequency of poor outcome. This is reflected by the lower number of ICHs and the fewest technical problems in surgery with these aneurysms.

The larger the size of a ruptured MCAA, the poorer the long-term outcome: 29% of patients with very small MCAAs (2–7 mm), 33% with small (8–14 mm), 31 with large (15–24 mm), and 43% with giant ones had poor outcome (Figs. 81-24 and 81-25). Patients with large and giant MCAAs had significantly more ICHs (59%) than those with smaller MCAAs (34%). An irregular or multilobular shape of the MCAA correlated with a more unfavorable outcome, 33% compared with 7% in patients with a smooth-walled MCAA. This was not caused by more frequent intraoperative ruptures but chiefly by the significantly more severe (classified by CT according to Fisher) hemorrhages seen with these aneurysms, 60% and 23%, respectively. We also studied the influences on outcome by multivariate analysis in selected patients with SAH (MCAA ruptured) confirmed by early CT. The following four variables had the most significant independent contributions to outcome: grade, vasospasm, postoperative hematoma, and age. Temporal ICHs, together with vasospasm and inadvertent occlusion of main vessel(s) or thalamostriate perforators, explain those specific late disabilities (described in detail in the section, Specific Late Disabilities) seen in patients with MCAAs.

SPECIFIC LATE DISABILITIES

Epilepsy

The incidence of late epilepsy after SAH varies between 7% and 25% in different studies.[69–74] The risk factors have proved to be the site (MCA) of the symptomatic IA, temporal ICH, brain ischemia, and hypertension. Also, the existence of several IAs increases the risk for late epilepsy. In our series, late epilepsy occurred in 18% of the long-term survivors with a single MCAA. The frequencies were even higher in patients with MIA and one MCAA (20%) and with multiple MCAAs (27%). This is significantly higher than with any other symptomatic aneurysms. Whether the symptomatic MCAA was proximal, bifurcation, or distal, the frequencies for late epilepsy were not significantly different: 22%, 24%, and 30%, respectively. Of the patients with a bifurcation MCAA and late epilepsy, 52% had a temporal ICH, whereas only 23% of those who were seizure free had a temporal ICH. Half of the long-term survivors with symptomatic MCAAs and late epilepsy had had an ICH.

Hemiparesis

As a result of its feeding areas and the scarcity of the collateral circulation, as well as the high number of ICHs related to MCAAs, lesions (and spasm) of an MCA frequently cause hemiparesis and/or dysphasia. There were significantly more cases of severe hemiparesis among long-time survivors with symptomatic MCAAs than among those with symptomatic aneurysms at other sites. The frequency of severe hemiparesis was significantly higher in patients

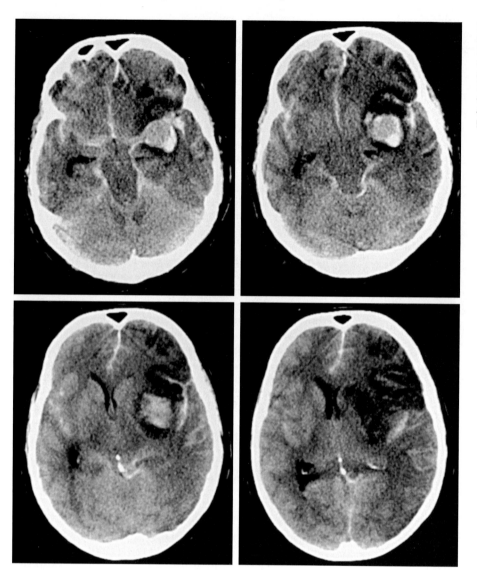

FIGURE 81-24 E.M., female, 58 years old, found unconscious at her home. Nonenhanced CT scan revealed an SAH and a large aneurysm in the left medial area surrounded with hematoma. Large infarction and edema were present. Patient died on the second day after hospitalization. No operation was performed.

with proximal MCAA than in those with bifurcation MCAA: 27% and 12%, respectively. This may be explained by technical difficulties associated with proper clipping of proximal MCAAs, leading to occlusion or kinking of the anterior temporal artery, or by occlusion of the thalamostriate perforator in superiorly directed aneurysms by the clip (Fig. 81-26). The frequencies for hemiparesis were equal whether the patient had a single MCAA, MIA with one MCAA, or multiple MCAAs.

Visual Field Deficits

Visual field deficits were significantly more common in patients with MCAAs than in patients with any other aneurysms: 20% and 11%, respectively. There were no differences in the frequencies among different MCAA sites. Also, visual impairment was equally common in patients with a single MCAA, with MIA and one MCAA, or with multiple MCAAs. In two thirds (69%) of the cases visual field deficits were at least partly caused by the close anatomic relationship between the course of the optic tract and temporal ICH.

CONCLUSIONS

Our conclusions from the eastern Finland and ISAT study[75–80] are that only competent aneurysm surgeons should continue open aneurysm surgery. Where such competence is unavailable, the aneurysms should be coiled. This is not possible in most case of MCAAs. Therefore, open microsurgery, with its slow learning curve as compared with endovascular surgery, must be continued.

Competence in aneurysm surgery means the ability to handle aneurysms at all sites and of all sizes, to manipulate the aneurysm and mold its base with bipolar coagulation, and to be knowledgeable in clip ligation and also about opening the aneurysm. Furthermore, the competent aneurysm surgeon should be skilled in aneurysm and vessel thrombectomy as well as in the use of temporary clipping, and should also be aware of cerebral protection during this procedure. He or she should be able to treat acute hydrocephalus by ventriculostomy and/or opening of the lamina terminalis. In cases of complex lesions, manual skill in reconstruction of arteries with clips or sutures is necessary, and the vessel bypassing techniques should be mastered.[12,81–85]

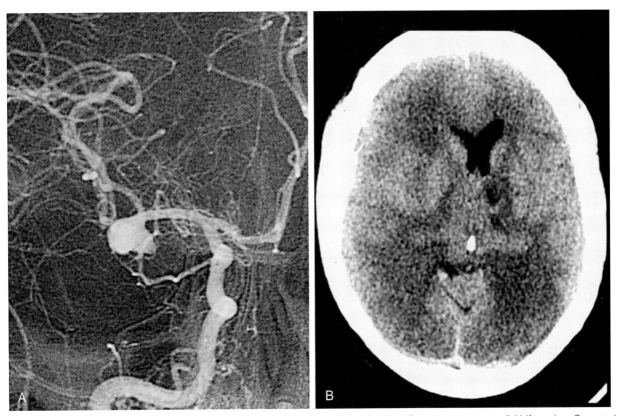

FIGURE 81-25   T.J., female, 37 years old, Hunt-Hess grade IV. *A,* After second bleeding of an aneurysm at medial bifurcation. Operated on day 1 after the second bleeding. *B,* Large, diffuse ischemic lesions were evident on CT scan 13 days postoperatively. The patient remained in poor condition.

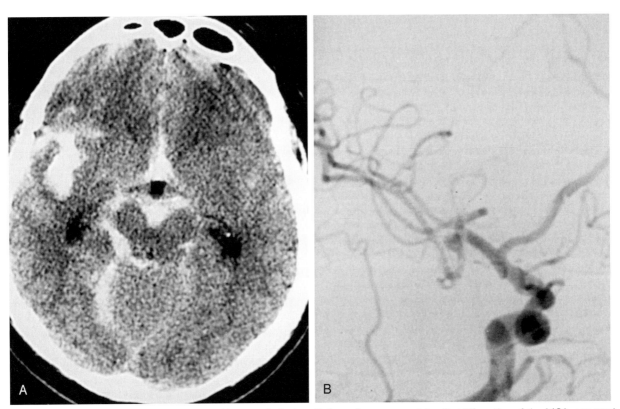

FIGURE 81-26   G. B., male, 59 years old, Hunt-Hess grade II. *A* to *C,* A small aneurysm at the first bifurcation of the MCA, operated on day 4 after bleeding. Left hemiparesis occurred postoperatively, and an infarction is seen on the CT scan. The ascending branch was narrowed at the operation due to kinking of the clip. Good recovery. Five months later a chronic subdural hematoma was evacuated.

(Continued)

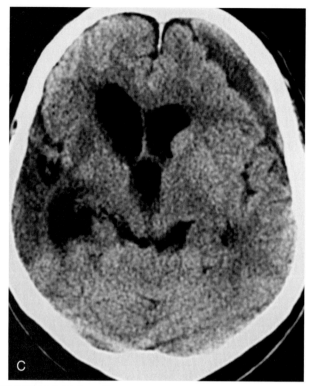

FIGURE 81-26 Cont'd

Finally, she or he should be also very well aware of the pitfalls and benefits of endovascular treatment. Competent exo- and endovascular aneurysm surgeons should form neurovascular teams to discuss and tailor together an individual treatment plan for each patient. Such teams are much more likely to achieve satisfactory results.

A competent aneurysm team should involve two or three cerebrovascular neurosurgeons, neuroanesthetists, good instrument nurses, good intensive care, good neuroradiologists (i.e., endovascular surgeons with preoperative angiography), and finally, sufficient facilities for rehabilitation after surgery.[80]

Competence in endovascular surgery means, in our opinion, aneurysm occlusion at all sites with knowledge of the limits of the method.[14,15] The competent neurosurgeon should be involved in clinics, discuss the options with patients and relatives, and be aware of cerebral protection. He or she should always be available, always remembering that acute and early aneurysm surgery is a heavy burden because of the high mortality and complication rate in acutely and severely ill patients.[84,85]

Furthermore, now and in the future, a large part of our research effort should concentrate on identification and treatment of aneurysms before they rupture, because this will surely improve management results far more than any technical or medical advance.[82]

REFERENCES

1. Aydin IH, Takci E, Kadioglu HH, et al: The variations of lenticulostriate arteries in the middle cerebral artery aneurysms. Acta Neurochir (Wien) 138:555–559, 1996.
2. Fox J: Technique of Aneurysm Surgery. IV: Middle Cerebral Artery Aneurysms. Intracranial Aneurysms, vol 2. New York: Springer-Verlag, 1983, pp 1012–1023.
3. Heros R: Middle cerebral artery aneurysms. In Wilkins RH, Rengachary SS (eds): Neurosurgery, vol. 2. New York: McGraw-Hill, 1985, pp 1376–1382.
4. Heros R: Aneurysms in the middle cerebral artery. In Symon L, Thomas DGT, Clarke K (eds): Rob & Smith's Operative Surgery: Neurosurgery. New York: Chapman & Hall, 1994, pp 171–179.
5. Hosoda K, Fujita S, Kawaguchi T, et al: Saccular aneurysms of the proximal (M1) segment of the middle cerebral artery. Neurosurgery 36:441–446, 1995.
6. Malik JM, Kamiryo T, Goble J, et al: Stereotactic laser-guided approach to distal middle cerebral artery aneurysms. Acta Neurochir (Wien) 1–3:138–144, 1995.
7. Ogilvy CS, Crowell RM, Heros RC: Surgical management of middle cerebral artery aneurysms: Experience with transsylvian and superior temporal gyrus approaches. Surg Neurol 43:15–24, 1995.
8. Pasztor E, Vajda J, Juhasz J, et al: The surgery of middle cerebral artery aneurysms. Acta Neurochirurcica (Wien) 82:92–101, 1986.
9. Peerless SJ: The surgical approach to middle cerebral and posterior communicating aneurysms. Clin Neurosurg 21:151–165, 1974.
10. Suzuki J, Yoshimoto T, Kayama T: Surgical treatment of middle cerebral artery aneurysms. J Neurosurg 61:17–23, 1984.
11. Weir BK, Findlay JM, Disney L: Middle cerebral artery aneurysms. In Apuzzo MLJ (ed): Brain Surgery, vol 1. New York: Churchill Livingstone, 1993, pp 983–1008.
12. Yasargil MG: Middle cerebral artery Aneurysms. Microneurosurgery, vol. 2. Stuttgart New York: Thieme Verlag, 1984, pp 124–164.
13. Dandy WE: Surgical Treatment of Aneurysms of the Middle Cerebral Artery: Intracranial Artery Aneurysms. Ithaca, NY: Comstock Publishing Company, Inc., 1945, p 129.
14. Regli L, Uske A, de Tribolet N: Endovascular coil placement compared with surgical clipping for the treatment of unruptured middle cerebral artery aneurysms: A consecutive series. J Neurosurg 90:1025–1030, 1999.
15. Henkes H, Fischer S, Weber W, et al: Endovascular coil occlusion of 1811 intracranial aneurysms: Early angiographic and clinical results. Neurosurgery 54:268–285, 2004.
16. Heiskanen O, Poranen A, Kuurne T, et al: Acute surgery for intracerebral haematomas caused by rupture of an intracranial aneurysm: A prospective randomized study. Acta Neurochir (Wien) 90:81–83, 1988.
17. Kuether TA, Nesbit GM, Barnwell SL: Clinical and angiographic outcomes, with treatment data, for patients with cerebral aneurysms treated with Guglielmi detachable coils: A single- center experience. Neurosurgery 43:1016–1025, 1998.
18. Papo I, Bodosi M, Doczi T: Intracerebral hematomas from aneurysm rupture: Their clinical significance. Acta Neurochir (Wien) 89:100–105, 1987.
19. Rinne J, Hernesniemi J, Niskanen M, et al: Analysis of 561 patients with middle cerebral artery aneurysms: Anatomic and clinical features as correlated to management outcome. Neurosurgery 38:2–11, 1996.
20. Tapaninaho A, Hernesniemi J, Vapalahti M: Emergency treatment of cerebral aneurysms with large haematomas. Acta Neurochir (Wien) 91:21–24, 1988.
21. Tokuda Y, Inagawa T, Katoh Y, et al: Intracerebral hematoma in patients with ruptured cerebral aneurysms. Surg Neurol 3:272–277, 1995.
22. Vanninen R, Koivisto T, Saari T, et al: Acute endovascular treatment of ruptured intracranial aneurysms with electrically detachable coils: A prospective randomized study. Radiology 211:325–336, 1999.
23. af Björkesten G, Halonen V: Incidence of intracranial vascular lesions in patients with subarachnoid hemorrhage investigated by four-vessel angiography. J Neurosurg 23:29–32, 1965.
24. Fogelholm R: Subarachnoid hemorrhage in middle-Finland: Incidence, early prognosis and indications for neurosurgical treatment. Stroke 3:296–301, 1981.
25. Hernesniemi J, Vapalahti M, Niskanen M, et al: One-year outcome in early aneurysm surgery: A 14-year experience. Acta Neurochir (Wien) 122:1–10, 1993.
26. Sarti C, Tuomilehto J, Narva E, et al: Epidemiology of subarachnoid hemorrhage in Finland during years 1982–85. Stroke:848–853, 1991.
27. Rinne J, Hernesniemi J, Puranen M, et al: Multiple intracranial aneurysms in a defined population: Prospective angiographic and clinical study. Neurosurgery 35:803–808, 1994.
28. Rinne J, Hernesniemi J, Niskanen M, et al: Management outcome for multiple intracranial aneurysms. Neurosurgery 36:31–38, 1995.

29. Ronkainen A, Puranen M, Hernesniemi JA, et al: Intracranial aneurysms: MR angiographic screening in 400 asymptomatic individuals with increased familial risk. Radiology 195:35–40, 1995.

30. Ronkainen A, Hernesniemi J, Puranen M, et al: Familial intracranial aneurysms. Lancet 349:380–384, 1997.

31. Ronkainen A, Miettinen H, Karkola K, et al: Risk of harboring an unruptured intracranial aneurysm. Stroke 29:359–362, 1998.

32. Dillon EH, van Leeuwen MS, Fernandez MA, et al: Spiral CT angiography. Am J Radiol 160:1273–1278, 1993.

33. Harbaugh RE, Schlusselberg DS, Jeffrey R, et al: Three-dimensional computerized tomography angiography in the diagnosis of cerebrovascular disease. J Neurosurg 32:408–414, 1992.

34. Nakajima Y, Yoshimine T, Yoshida H, et al: Computerized tomography angiography of ruptured cerebral aneurysms: Factors affecting time to maximum contrast concentration. J Neurosurg 88:663–669, 1998.

35. Ogawa T, Okudera T, Noguchi K, et al: Cerebral aneurysms: Evaluation with three-dimensional CT angiography. Am J Neuroradiol 3:447–454, 1996.

36. Tampieri D, Leblanc R, Oleszek J, et al: Three-dimensional computed tomography angiography of cerebral aneurysms. Neurosurgery 4:749–754, 1995.

37. Vieco PT, Shuman WP, Alsofrom GF, et al: Detection of circle of Willis aneurysms in patients with acute subarachnoid hemorrhage: A comparison of ct angiography and digital subtraction angiography. AJR Am J Roentgenol 165:425–430, 1995.

38. Young N, Dorsch NWC, Kingston RJ, et al: Spiral CT scanning in the detection and evaluation of aneurysms of the circle of Willis. Surg Neurol 50:50–61, 1998.

39. Kallmes DF, Kallmes MH, Lanzino G, et al: Routine angiography after surgery for ruptured intracranial aneurysms: A cost versus benefit analysis. Neurosurgery 41:629–641, 1997.

40. Horikoshi T, Fukamachi A, Nishi H: Detection of intracranial aneurysms by three-dimensional time-of-flight magnetic resonance angiography. Neuroradiology 36:203–207, 1994.

41. Nagasawa H, Ohta T, Tsuda E: Magnetic resonance angiographic source images for depicting topography and surgical planning for middle cerebral artery aneurysms: Technique application. Surg Neurol 50:62–64, 1998.

42. Le Roux PD, Dailey AT, Newell DW, et al: Emergent aneurysm clipping without angiography in the moribund patient with intracerebral hemorrhage: The use of infusion computed tomography scans. Neurosurgery 33:189–197, 1993.

43. Niskanen M, Hernesniemi J, Vapalahti M, et al: One-year outcome in early aneurysm surgery: Prediction of outcome. Acta Neurochir (Wien) 123:25–32, 1993.

44. Anson JA, Lawton MT, Spetzler RF: Characteristics and surgical treatment of dolichoectatic and fusiform aneurysms. J Neurosurg 84:185–193, 1996.

45. Hacein-Bey L, Connolly ES Jr, Mayer SA, et al: Complex intracranial aneurysms: Combined operative and endovascular approaches. Neurosurgery 43:1304–1313, 1998.

46. Sundt TM, Kobayashi S, Fode NC, et al: Results and complications of surgical management of 809 intracranial aneurysms in 722 cases: Related and unrelated to grade of patient, type of aneurysm, and timing of surgery. J Neurosurg 56:753–765, 1982.

47. Findlay JM: Current management of aneurysmal subarachnoid hemorrhage guidelines from the Canadian Neurosurgical Society. Can J Neurol Sci 24:161–170, 1997.

48. Säveland H, Hillman J, Brandt L, et al: Overall outcome in aneurysmal subarachnoid hemorrhage: A prospective study from neurosurgical units in Sweden during a 1-year period. J Neurosurg 76:729–734, 1992.

49. Fogelholm R, Hernesniemi J, Vapalahti M: Impact of early surgery on outcome after aneurysmal subarachnoid hemorrhage: A population-based study. Stroke 24:1649–1654, 1993.

50. Le Roux PD, Elliott JP, Newell DW, et al: The incidence of surgical complications is similar in good and poor grade patients undergoing repair of ruptured anterior circulation aneurysms: A retrospective review of 355 patients. Neurosurgery 38:887–894, 1996.

51. Whisnant JP, Sacco SE, O'Fallon WM, et al: Referral bias in aneurysmal subarachnoid hemorrhage. J Neurosurg 78:726–732, 1993.

52. Mayberg M, Batjer HH, Dacey R, et al: Guidelines for the management of aneurysmal subarachnoid hemorrhage: A statement for healthcare professionals from a special writing group of the Stroke Council, American Heart Association. Stroke 25:2315–2328, 1994.

53. Solomon RA, Mayer SA, Tarmey JJ: Relationship between the volume of craniotomies for cerebral aneurysm performed at New York state hospitals and in-hospital mortality. Stroke 27:13–17, 1996.

54. Lawton MT, Raudzens PA, Zabramski JM, et al: Hypothermic circulatory arrest in neurovascular surgery: Evolving indications and predictors of patient outcome. Neurosurgery 43:10–21, 1998.

55. Kallmes DF, Kallmess MH: Cost-effectiveness of angiography perfomed during surgery for ruptured intracranial aneurysms. Am J Neuroradiol 18:1453–1462, 1997.

56. Payner TD, Horner TG, Leipzig TJ, et al: Role of intraoperative angiography in the surgical treatment of cerebral aneurysms. J Neurosurg 3:441–448, 1998.

57. Drake CG: Giant intracranial aneurysms: Experience with surgical treatment in 174 patients. Clin Neurosurg 26:12–95, 1979.

58. Mizoi K, Yoshimoto T: Permissible temporary occlusion time in aneurysm surgery as evaluated by evoked potential monitoring. Neurosurgery 33:434–440, 1993.

59. Gewirtz RJ, Awad IA: Giant aneurysms of the anterior circle of Willis: Management outcome of open microsurgical treatment. Surg Neurol 5:409–420, 1996.

60. Lawton MT, Spetzler RF: Surgical management of giant intracranial aneurysms: Experience with 171 patients. Clin Neurosurg 42:245–266, 1995.

61. Piepgras DG, Khurana VG, Whisnant JP: Ruptured giant intracranial aneurysms. Part II: A retrospective analysis of timing and outcome of surgical treatment. J Neurosurg 3:430–435, 1998.

62. Samson DS, Batjer HH, Bowman G, et al: A clinical study of the parameters and effects of temporary arterial occlusion in the management of intracranial aneurysms. Neurosurgery 34:22–29, 1994.

63. Khurana VG, Piepgras DG, Whisnant JP: Ruptured giant intracranial aneurysms. Part I: A study of rebleeding. J Neurosurg 3:425–429, 1998.

64. Ogilvy CS, Carter BS, Kaplan S, et al: Temporary vessel occlusion for aneurysm surgery: Risk factors for stroke in patients protected by induced hypothermia and hypertension and intravenous mannitol administration. J Neurosurg 84:785–791, 1996.

65. Debrun GM, Aletich VA, Kehrli P, et al: Selection of cerebral aneurysms for treatment using Guglilemi detachable coils: The preliminary University of Illinois experience. Neurosurgery 43:1281–1297, 1998.

66. Eskridge JM, Song JK, and participants: Endovascular embolization of 150 basilar tip aneurysms with Guglielmi detachable coils: Results of the Food and Drug Administration multicenter clinical trial. J Neurosurg 89:81–86, 1998.

67. Standard SC, Guterman LR, Chavis TD, et al: Endovascular management of giant intracranial aneurysms. Clin Neurosurg 42:267–293, 1995.

68. Vinuela F, Duckwiler G, Mawad M: Guglielmi detachable coil embolization of acute intracranial aneurysm: Perioperative anatomical and clinical outcome in 403 patients. J Neurosurg 86:475–482, 1997.

69. Baker CJ, Prestigiacomo CJ, Solomon RA: Short-term perioperative anticonvulsant prophylaxis for the surgical treatment of low-risk patients with intracranial aneurysms. Neurosurgery 5:863–870, 1995.

70. Cabral RJ, King TT, Scott DF: Epilepsy after two different neurosurgical approaches to the treatment of ruptured intracranial aneurysm. J Neurol Neurosurg Psychiatry 39:1052–1056, 1976.

71. Fabinyi GCA, Artiola-Fortuny L: Epilepsy after craniotomy for intracranial aneurysms. Lancet 1:1299–1300, 1980.

72. Keränen T, Tapaninaho A, Hernesniemi J, et al: Late epilepsy after aneurysm operation. Neurosurgery 17:897–900, 1985.

73. Kotila M, Waltimo O: Epilepsy after stroke. Epilepsia 33:495–498, 1992.

74. Ukkola V, Heikkinen E: Epilepsy after operative treatment of ruptured cerebral aneurysms. Acta Neurochir (Wien) 106:115–118, 1990.

75. International Subarachnoid Aneurysm Trial (ISAT) Collaborative Group: International Subarachnoid Aneurysm Trial (ISAT) of neurosurgical clipping versus endovascular coiling in 2145 patients with ruptured intrcranial aneurysms: A randomized trial. Lancet 360:1267–1274, 2002.

76. Koivisto T, Vanninen R, Hurskainen H, et al: Outcomes of early endovascular versus surgical treatment of ruptured cerebral aneurysms: A prospective randomized study. Stroke 31:2369–2377, 2000.

77. Koivisto T, Vanninen E, Vanninen R, et al: Cerebral perfusion before and after endovascular or surgical treatment of acutely ruptured cerebral aneurysms: A 1-year prospective follow-up study. Neurosurgery 51:312–326, 2002.

78. Koivisto T: Prospective Outcome Study of Aneurysmal Subarachnoid Hemorrhage. Kuopio, Finland: Kuopio University Publications D. Medical Sciences, 2002.

79. Vanninen R, Koivisto T, Saari T, Hernesniemi J, Vapalahti M: Ruptured intracranial aneurysms: Acute endovascular treatment with electrolytically detachable coils—a prospective randomized study. Radiology 211:325–336, 1999.

80. Yasargil MG: Reflections on the thesis "Prospective Outcome Study of Aneurysmal Subarachnoid Hemorrhage" of Dr. Timo Koivisto. Kuopio, Finland: Kuopio University Publications D. Medical Sciences, 2002. (The original thesis of Dr. Timo Koivisto and the reflections on the thesis by Professor M.G. Yasargil are available at: www.uku.fi/tutkimus/vaitokset/2002/isbn951-781-884-X.pdf www.uku.fi/tutkimus/vaitokset/2002/isbn951-780-338-9.pdf)

81. Aboud E, Al-Mefty O, Yasargil MG: New laboratory model for neurosurgical training that simulates live surgery. J Neurosurg 97:1367–1372, 2002.

82. Drake CG, Peerless SJ, Hernesniemi JA: Surgery of Vertebrobasilar Aneurysms. London, Ontario Experience on 1767 patients. Vienna: Springer-Verlag, 1996.

83. Hernesniemi J, Vapalahti M, Niskanen M, Kari A, Luukkonen M: Saccular aneurysms of the distal anterior cerebral artery and its branches. Neurosurgery 31:994–999, 1992.

84. Hernesniemi J, Vapalahti M, Niskanen M, et al: One-year outcome in early aneurysm surgery: A 14 year experience. Acta Neurochir (Wien) 122:1–10, 1993.

85. Niskanen M, Hernesniemi J, Vapalahti M, Kari A: One-year outcome in early aneurysm surgery: Prediction of outcome. Acta Neurochir (Wien) 123:25–32, 1993.

Intraoperative Endovascular Techniques in the Management of Intracranial Aneurysms

KAZUO MIZOI and HIROYUKI KINOUCHI

With current advances in microsurgical techniques, the surgical treatment of cerebral aneurysms is approaching a satisfactory level. However, technical difficulties in aneurysm surgery are determined by two chief variables: the size and the location of the aneurysms. Many problems remain with surgery of large aneurysms of the proximal internal carotid artery (ICA) and the vertebrobasilar artery. In surgery of these aneurysms, there is considerable difficulty in gaining both proximal arterial control and a sufficient operative field. With the introduction of digital subtraction angiography (DSA) in our operating room, we have attempted to operate on surgically difficult aneurysms with the aid of intravascular catheter techniques. Such techniques include using (1) a balloon catheter placed into the parent artery of the aneurysm to obtain temporary proximal occlusion, (2) a double-lumen balloon catheter for large aneurysms to aspirate blood and collapse the aneurysm, and (3) intraoperative DSA to evaluate the result of aneurysm clipping. In this chapter, we review our experiences with the combined use of intravascular and neurosurgical approaches in surgically difficult aneurysms.

PATIENT SELECTION

Of 1276 patients with cerebral aneurysms who underwent surgery at our institution, 90 (7%) were treated with the aid of intravascular catheter techniques. All 90 patients had complex aneurysms with difficulty in gaining proximal arterial control or risk of arterial narrowing after clip placement. A total of 94 aneurysms were treated surgically in 90 patients: 69 aneurysms of the ICA in 65 cases and 25 posterior circulation aneurysms in 25 cases. The ICA aneurysms included 26 large paraclinoid carotid aneurysms, 18 carotid cave aneurysms, 18 broad-based posterior communicating artery (PCoA) aneurysms, 1 anterior choroidal artery (AChA) aneurysm, and 6 unusual dorsal ICA aneurysms. The paraclinoid aneurysms ranged from 15 to 30 mm in diameter, with an average size of 21 mm. Posterior circulation aneurysms included 10 basilar tip aneurysms, 12 basilar trunk aneurysms, 1 vertebral artery aneurysm, 1 distal anterior inferior cerebellar artery aneurysm, and 1 distal superior cerebellar artery aneurysm. The latter 2 distal aneurysms were associated with arteriovenous malformations (AVMs) located on their feeding arteries.

INTRODUCTION OF BALLOON CATHETER

The patient is placed on a radiolucent operating table. After induction of anesthesia, the head is fixed in the desired position with a radiolucent composite carbon headholder (Mizuho Medical Instrument Co., Tokyo, Japan; Fig. 82-1). A No. 7 or 5 French gauge heparinized angiographic catheter (Anthron; Toray Industries, Inc., Tokyo, Japan) is introduced coaxially through the femoral sheath to the vessels of interest under fluoroscopic control. For patients who undergo surgery in the prone or the lateral "park bench" position, transfemoral catheterization is done before fixation of the patient's position. Preoperative DSA is performed routinely to confirm that the aneurysm is not being obscured by the skull fixation pins. The silicone balloon (0.7–1.5 mm in uninflated diameter), attached to a No. 1.5 French gauge polyethylene catheter (DowCorning Corporation, Tokyo, Japan), is advanced through the angiographic catheter to the desired location for temporary vascular occlusion. The balloon is inflated temporarily to assess the appropriate inflation volume for occlusion of the parent artery, after which the balloon catheter is withdrawn back into the angiographic catheter to prevent

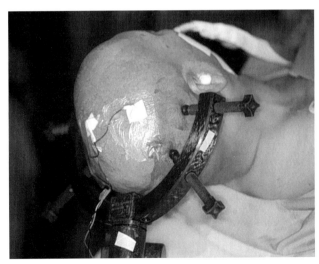

FIGURE 82-1 The patient's head is fixed with a radiolucent carbon composite headholder. The electrodes for evoked potential monitoring have also been placed.

thrombus formation. Both the femoral sheath and the angiographic catheter are flushed continually at 0.5 mL/minute with heparinized saline (10 U/mL). In some patients operated on in a prone position, the balloon catheter is left in place throughout the surgery because catheter manipulations are often difficult during surgery. The femoral sheath can also be used intraoperatively as the arterial line for systemic blood pressure monitoring. The groin is sterilely draped and covered for the subsequent intraoperative catheterization procedures, and the craniotomy is begun.

SURGICAL PROCEDURES

Internal carotid artery aneurysms are ordinarily exposed through a standard pterional craniotomy; however, when extensive removal of the anterior clinoid process is required for large paraclinoid ICA aneurysms or carotid cave aneurysms, we use Dolenc's combined epidural and intradural approach.[1] For posterior circulation aneurysms, various surgical approaches are used according to the location of the aneurysm: standard subtemporal approach, transzygomatic transsylvian approach, subtemporal transtentorial approach, transpetrosal approach, combined subtemporal and suboccipital approach, suboccipital retromastoid approach, and occipital transtentorial approach. In the case of aneurysms associated with AVMs, both lesions are treated in a single procedure.

The operation proceeds in a routine fashion until the stage of aneurysm dissection is reached, at which point the operation is temporarily interrupted. The operating microscope is moved, and the sterilely draped C-arm fluoroscope is positioned around the patient's head (Fig. 82-2). The balloon catheter is advanced again to the planned location under fluoroscopic guidance. After confirming that the tip of the balloon catheter is placed in a suitable position for proximal vascular control, the C arm is again moved and the operating microscope brought back for use. When these procedures have been completed, the balloon is inflated for temporary vascular occlusion. This maneuver can be performed without fluoroscopic control because the appropriate inflation volume has been verified beforehand. For cerebral protection during temporary occlusion, we administer a solution

of 500 mL of 20% mannitol with 500 mg of phenytoin and 500 mg of vitamin E.[2] In surgery for posterior circulation aneurysms, the occluding balloon is placed in the basilar or vertebral artery approximately 1 cm proximal to the aneurysm. For PCoA or carotid cave aneurysms, the balloon is inflated at the horizontal cavernous segment of the ICA.

A 40-year-old man had a moderate subarachnoid hemorrhage 2 weeks before surgery. Preoperative angiography demonstrated a small basilar trunk aneurysm arising from the basilar artery at the distal crotch of the anterior inferior cerebellar artery origin (Fig. 82-3A). After induction of anesthesia, a balloon catheter was introduced into the basilar artery to approximately 1 cm proximal to the aneurysm. The balloon was temporarily inflated under DSA control to determine its suitable inflation volume (see Fig. 82-3B). Craniotomy was then begun with the balloon catheter in place. Because the aneurysm was located relatively low (28 mm below the posterior clinoid process), it was approached through the right transpetrosal route. After the apex of the petrous bone had been drilled off extradurally, the tentorium was widely opened. The aneurysm was identified below the eighth cranial nerve without retraction of the brain stem and cranial nerves. At this point, the balloon within the basilar artery was inflated. The aneurysm was then dissected and successfully clipped. The duration of basilar artery occlusion was 30 minutes. The initial intraoperative DSA after clip placement demonstrated a false-positive finding of basilar artery occlusion, but the final DSA after removal of the balloon catheter from the basilar artery showed successful clipping and vessel patency (see Fig. 82-3C). The patient did not have any postoperative neurologic deficits and returned to his previous work.

RETROGRADE SUCTION DECOMPRESSION TECHNIQUE

For large or giant paraclinoid aneurysms, a retrograde suction decompression technique is used.[3,4] A No. 5 or 7 French gauge double-lumen occlusion balloon catheter (Medi-Tech, Hanako, Inc., Tokyo, Japan) is introduced into the cervical ICA and the balloon is inflated. After temporary trapping of the aneurysm by balloon occlusion of the cervical ICA and clipping of the intracranial ICA distal to the aneurysm, retrograde aspiration of blood is initiated manually using a 20-mL heparinized syringe (Fig. 82-4). With this procedure, the aneurysm is completely deflated and its dissection greatly facilitated. It is most important to preserve the patency of the AChA and clip the aneurysm while preserving sufficient lumen of the ICA.

In all of our cases, we confirm the results of clipping using intraoperative DSA, and if the results are unsatisfactory, the clip is readjusted. The catheter is removed after final examination of intraoperative DSA, but the femoral sheath is left in place until the end of the operation.

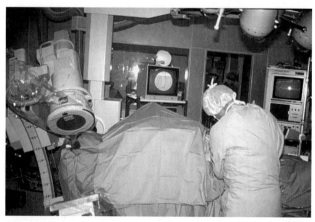

FIGURE 82-2 The operating room setup during intraoperative angiography. The operating microscope has been displaced and the sterilely draped C-arm fluoroscope positioned around the patient's head.

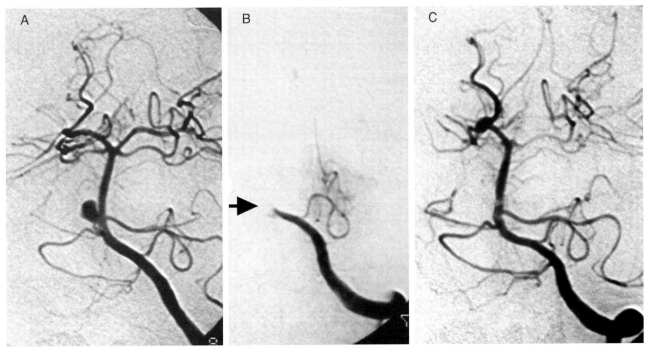

FIGURE 82-3 Case 1. *A,* Preoperative left vertebral angiogram, anteroposterior view, demonstrating a small basilar trunk aneurysm projecting laterally. This aneurysm was located 2.8 cm below the posterior clinoid process. *B,* Intraoperative DSA demonstrating temporary balloon occlusion *(arrow)* of the basilar artery just proximal to the aneurysm. *C,* Intraoperative angiogram following clip placement showing the successful obliteration of the aneurysm.

CASE REPORT 2

A 50-year-old woman presented with progressive loss of vision in the left eye. Computed tomography scan revealed a round mass lesion in the left suprasellar region, and angiography demonstrated a 26-mm left paraclinoid ICA aneurysm (Fig. 82-5). Surgery was performed using the retrograde balloon suction decompression method. Under general anesthesia, the double-lumen balloon catheter was introduced into the left ICA by the transfemoral route. After confirming sufficient balloon inflation volume, the catheter was temporarily withdrawn back into the introducing catheter. A left pterional craniotomy was then performed. The anterior clinoid process was removed extradurally and the optic canal was unroofed. Because this large aneurysm had projected inferiorly and expanded close to the carotid dural ring, the proximal dome of the aneurysm was tightly adherent to the surrounding dura mater (Fig. 82-6A). At this point, the balloon catheter was again advanced into the cervical ICA and inflated to occlude the cervical ICA. The intracranial ICA (C1 segment) was also occluded, and retrograde suctioning begun. The aneurysm collapsed completely and was easily dissected (see Fig. 82-6B). The AChA was recognized on the distal side of the aneurysm neck. Two Sugita fenestrated clips were applied in crosswise fashion to reconstruct the lumen of the ICA (see Fig. 82-6C). The duration of temporary trapping of the ICA was 20 minutes.

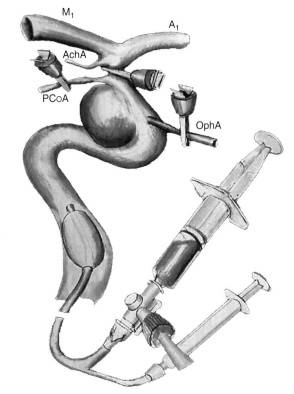

FIGURE 82-4 Schematic drawing showing the retrograde balloon suction decompression technique. A1, A1 segment of anterior cerebral artery; AChA, anterior choroidal artery; M1, M1 segment of middle cerebral artery; OphA, ophthalmic artery; PCoA, posterior communicating artery.

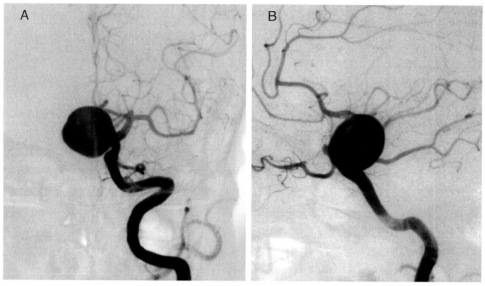

FIGURE 82-5   Case 2. Preoperative angiogram of the left ICA, demonstrating a giant paraclinoid aneurysm. *A,* Anteroposterior view. *B,* Lateral view.

Approximately 200 mL of blood was aspirated during this procedure and simultaneously returned to the patient. The operation was completed after confirming the results of clip placement by DSA (Fig. 82-7). The patient awoke from anesthesia with no new neurologic deficits. Three months later, she had full recovery of vision in the left eye.

CASE REPORT 3

A 57-year-old woman presented with the visual disturbance in the right eye. Angiography demonstrated a 28-mm right paraclinoid aneurysm and lateral inclination

of the ICA (Fig. 82-8). Surgery was performed using the same method as described in Case 2. Using retrograde suction decompression, the aneurysm was collapsed remarkably and dissected free from the surrounding structures. Several attempts were made to clip this aneurysm with parallel clipping method using the fenestrated clips. However, severe kinking of the ICA occurred on all such occasions. Finally, the aneurysmal neck was ligated to narrow the size of the neck, and perpendicular clipping was attempted using strong straight clips (Fig. 82-9). A booster clip was applied on the distal end of the first clip blades for reinforcement. The intraoperative angiogram showed a good result of clipping (Fig. 82-10). The postoperative course was uneventful.

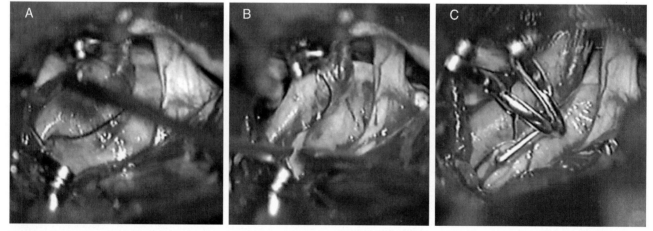

FIGURE 82-6   Case 2. *A,* Operative photographs of a giant paraclinoid aneurysm compressing the left optic nerve. *B,* The aneurysm was deflated and easily dissected with the aid of retrograde continuous blood aspiration. *C,* Two Sugita fenestrated clips were applied in crosswise fashion to reconstruct the sufficient lumen of the ICA.

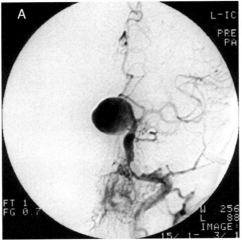
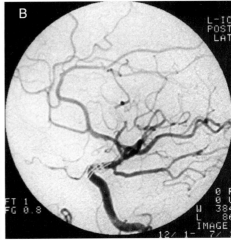

FIGURE 82-7 Case 2. *A*, Intraoperative angiogram before clip placement, demonstrating a large paraclinoid aneurysm. *B*, Intraoperative angiogram after aneurysmal clipping, showing a successful result.

RESULTS

Intraoperative Digital Subtraction Angiography

In 24 of 94 aneurysms (26%), a change in the surgical plan was required based on results obtained with intraoperative DSA. In 11 paraclinoid or carotid cave aneurysms, narrowing of the parent artery was demonstrated by DSA and corrected by clip replacement. In 13 aneurysms, residual neck of the aneurysm was identified and corrected by clip repositioning or additional clip placement. However, of these 13 aneurysms, 3 were cases of giant posterior circulation aneurysm. In those cases, complete neck occlusion was impossible and surgery resulted in clipping the body of the aneurysms. Most of the early series of patients underwent postoperative conventional angiography. The findings of postoperative angiography were essentially identical to those obtained with intraoperative DSA. There were no false-negative results in the intraoperative DSA studies.

Temporary Balloon Occlusion

In the operations for 48 aneurysms, the balloon catheter was placed in the vessels of interest, and temporary balloon occlusion was achieved in 37 aneurysms (77%). The remaining 11 aneurysms were treated without the use of temporary occlusion. The time required for the performance of preoperative vessel catheterization and intraoperative balloon technique was approximately 60 minutes. The duration of temporary occlusion among these 37 aneurysms ranged from 6 to 50 minutes, with a mean of 20.5 minutes. Intraoperative somatosensory evoked potential (SSEP) monitoring was performed in most cases. Significant changes in SSEPs were not observed during occlusion. There were no cases with postoperative sequelae attributable to ischemia caused by temporary balloon occlusion.

Balloon Suction Decompression

We have used balloon suction decompression in 26 aneurysms in 25 patients. Carotid stump pressure was monitored through the distal lumen of the double-lumen balloon catheter placed in the cervical ICA. On inflating the balloon, the stump pressure fell to approximately 50%; however, contrary to expectations, after occlusion of the intracranial ICA above the aneurysm, the pressure increased to above the preocclusion level (Fig. 82-11). Operative findings also indicated that the aneurysm became more tense.

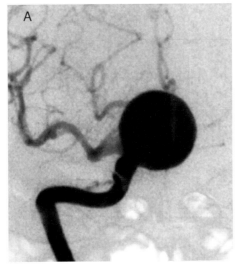
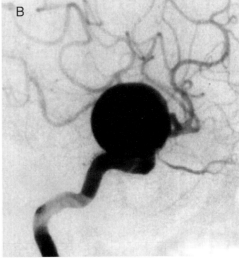

FIGURE 82-8 Case 3. Preoperative angiogram of the right ICA, demonstrating a giant paraclinoid aneurysm and lateral inclination of the ICA. *A*, Anteroposterior view. *B*, Lateral view.

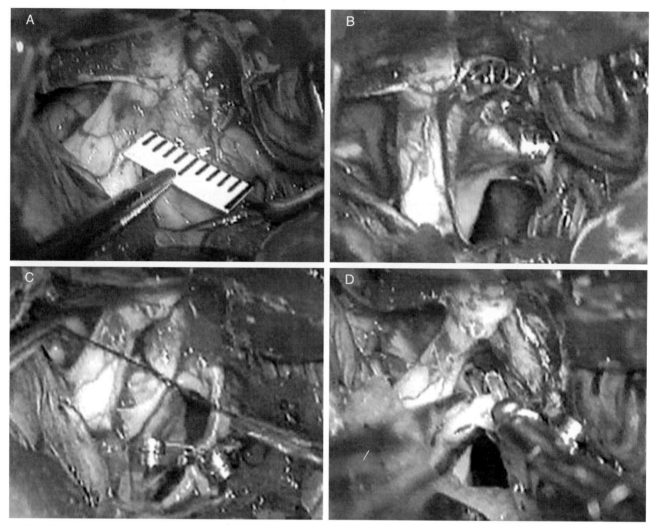

FIGURE 82-9 Case 3. *A,* Operative photographs of a giant paraclinoid aneurysm compressing the right optic nerve. *B,* The aneurysm sac was deflated completely with the aid of retrograde blood aspiration. *C,* At first, the angled fenestrated clip was used to clip the aneurysm. However, it was very difficult to apply the clip in parallel to the course of the ICA because of the limited working space. Then, the aneurysm neck was ligated to reduce its size. *D,* Finally, perpendicular clipping was performed using a strong straight clip.

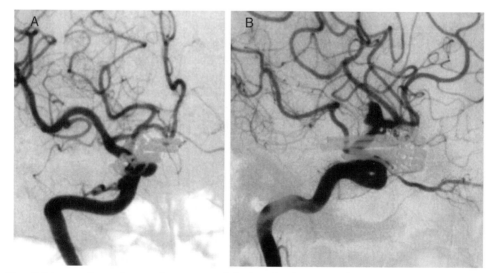

FIGURE 82-10 Case 3. Intraoperative angiogram after aneurysmal clipping, showing successful result. *A,* Anteroposterior view. *B,* Lateral view.

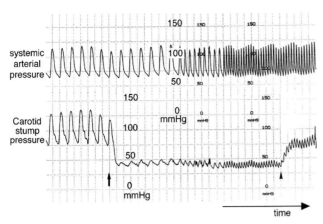

FIGURE 82-11 Continuous monitoring of the carotid stump pressure during the balloon suction decompression. On inflating the balloon within the cervical ICA (*arrow*), the stump pressure decreased to approximately 30% of the preocclusion level; however, subsequent occlusion of the ICA distal to the aneurysm (*arrowhead*) caused a paradoxic increase in stump pressure.

However, on beginning retrograde aspiration, the aneurysm collapsed completely. The rate of blood aspiration was between 10 and 20 mL/minute. When the syringe was exchanged and the aspiration temporarily interrupted, the aneurysm again inflated. The aspirated blood was returned to the patient intravenously. The total volume of aspirated blood differed among the patients but was between 200 and 500 mL.

The duration of temporary trapping of the ICA ranged from 5 to 60 minutes (mean, 25 minutes). Intraoperative SSEP monitoring was also done in all cases. Significant changes in the SSEPs were not observed during the occlusion in any case. However, only one case demonstrated postoperative sequelae attributable to the ischemia of the territory of the anterior cerebral artery, which could not be monitored by the median nerve SSEP.

Complications

Embolic complications attributable to the catheterization maneuver were seen in two cases. Both patients had large paraclinoid aneurysms treated using the retrograde suction decompression technique. In one patient, embolectomy was immediately carried out and no new neurologic deficits were observed after surgery. In another patient, the embolic complication was not detected during surgery and the patient had a postoperative persistent left hemiparesis.

DISCUSSION

Intraoperative Digital Subtraction Angiography

The need for intraoperative angiography in neurovascular surgery was recognized relatively early, and reports using such a technique in AVM surgery appeared by the late 1960s. More recently, the development of portable DSA equipment has led to its use in many institutions.[5–13] Although it has been used in cases of cerebral aneurysm, AVM, bypass surgery, carotid endarterectomy, and spinal AVM, DSA is not always essential in such cases. Because intraoperative

angiography is used primarily to detect inadequate surgical results before dural closure, its significance is not great in simple and uncomplicated operations. The experience and skill of the surgeon is the principal determinant of intraoperative angiography's usefulness.

Crucial for success in aneurysm surgery is complete closure of the aneurysm neck and preservation of patency of the parent artery and all adjacent arterial branches. Intraoperative DSA is used in complex aneurysms in which it may be difficult to accomplish these goals. From our experience, it is useful in surgery of large and broad-based aneurysms, as well as in surgery of aneurysms in deep locations where a wide operative field cannot be obtained, such as proximal ICA aneurysms and posterior circulation aneurysms. A wide operative field can usually be obtained for middle cerebral artery aneurysms. In complex anterior communicating artery aneurysms, a bifrontal interhemispheric approach allows for a sufficiently wide surgical field, and intraoperative DSA rarely is needed.

Clip repositioning was required in 24 of 94 aneurysms. As Barrow and associates[9] have argued, if intraoperative DSA is available, the initial attempt at clipping is apt to be relatively easy and the results immediately examined. In all cases, an effort should be made to complete aneurysm clipping at the first attempt.

Temporary Balloon Occlusion

Typically, proximal vascular control is difficult to obtain in large paraclinoid ICA and basilar trunk aneurysms. In such cases, temporary balloon occlusion can be used. Shucart and colleagues[14] and Bailes and co-workers[15] reported on a balloon occlusion method as an aid to clipping aneurysms of the basilar and paraclinoid ICAs. Some surgeons may argue that the traditional method for exposing the cervical ICA provides sufficient proximal control for ICA aneurysms, but for lower basilar trunk aneurysms there is no method for effective proximal control other than balloon occlusion.[16]

The most serious complication when using the intraoperative occlusion technique is embolism. To prevent this complication, in most cases we keep the balloon catheter within the heparinized angiographic catheter during the surgery, proceed with the operation until balloon occlusion is required, and then advance the balloon catheter. This method has the disadvantage that the surgical procedure must be temporarily interrupted, but the interruption usually lasts only 15 to 20 minutes. In all cases, a heparinized angiographic catheter is left in place throughout surgery. Systemic heparinization is not used, but embolic complications did not appear despite the catheter being kept in place for 4 to 8 hours. From our experiences with such cases, it seems that the heparinized catheter allows for prolonged intravascular placement without incurring embolic complications.

We usually initiate vascular occlusion before dissection of the aneurysm itself. In the current series, the duration of balloon occlusion was relatively long (average, 20.5 minutes), but there were no ischemic symptoms caused by temporary occlusion. The administration of brain-protective agents[2] might achieve such good results. However, because there were no changes in SSEP monitoring during occlusion, these findings indicate that there was sufficient collateral flow in most cases.[17]

Retrograde Balloon Suction Decompression

Flamm[18] was the first to report on a suction decompression method for giant aneurysms, in which the aneurysm was directly punctured using a No. 21 scalp vein needle. In puncturing the aneurysmal wall before treatment of the aneurysm, however, that technique may invite troublesome intraoperative bleeding. Subsequently, Batjer and Samson[19] and Tamaki and co-workers[20] reported retrograde suction methods in which the cervical ICA is exposed surgically and blood is aspirated from an angiocatheter inserted into the cervical ICA after clamping of both the cervical and intracranial ICA. Scott and colleagues[3] reported a less invasive modification of that method in which retrograde suction was done using a double-lumen balloon catheter. We had also developed the balloon suction decompression technique independently in 1993.[4]

The retrograde suction decompression technique is now the principal surgical adjunct to facilitate dissection and clipping of giant paraclinoid aneurysms.[21–26] However, even when the aneurysm is completely deflated, basic surgical procedures for the treatment of aneurysms in this location, such as extensive removal of the anterior clinoid process and sufficient exposure of the carotid dural ring, are still essential. Moreover, the duration of temporary occlusion of the ICA is an important issue. Even with the use of this technique, it is usually not possible to complete dissection and definitive clipping of aneurysms within a few minutes. In our series, the average occlusion time of the ICA was 25 minutes (ranging from 5 to 60 minutes). Accordingly, a balloon occlusion test should be performed routinely to select the best treatment. For patients at high risk from temporary arterial occlusion, the use of retrograde suction decompression technique should be considered more carefully. Although balloon test occlusion is not perfect in predicting the tolerable occlusion time in each case, this test can select patients who cannot withstand even a short period of temporary occlusion. Such patients usually develop motor disturbance, aphasia, or loss of consciousness within a minute after test occlusion. For patients who are intolerant of the test occlusion, we have used a combination of high-flow graft and proximal ICA occlusion, or direct clipping using the suction decompression technique after performing a high-flow bypass graft in the same operative session.

An interesting phenomenon has occurred routinely in our experience with this method.[4] While monitoring the carotid stump pressure by means of a double-lumen balloon catheter placed in the cervical ICA, inflation of the balloon (proximal occlusion) resulted in a sudden decrease in stump pressure to approximately 50% of the preocclusion level; subsequent occlusion of the intracranial ICA (distal occlusion), however, resulted in an increase in stump pressure to above the preocclusion level. This finding indicates that when an aneurysm is incompletely trapped, intra-aneurysmal pressure can be elevated by the retrograde flow through the remaining small branches. Even in cases in which the ophthalmic artery, PCoA, and AChA have been occluded, similar increases in stump pressure are observed, suggesting the notable participation of retrograde flow from the cavernous ICA branches involving the meningohypophyseal trunk.

To our knowledge, this paradoxic phenomenon has not been previously reported. However, as Batjer and Samson[19] pointed out, many neurosurgeons may empirically be aware of this phenomenon through their experience that simple trapping of a large aneurysm by cervical ICA clamping and intracranial distal clipping does not adequately soften the lesion because of a brisk retrograde flow through the ophthalmic artery and cavernous branches. This phenomenon also implies that risk of intraoperative aneurysmal rupture may increase after such a simple trapping as a result of the paradoxic rise in intra-aneurysmal pressure.

Clipping Technique for Paraclinoid Aneurysms

The basic clipping method of large/giant paraclinoid aneurysms is to apply the clip blades parallel to the direction of the ICA. This is relatively easily accomplished for anterior paraclinoid aneurysms (so-called ophthalmic aneurysms) but may prove difficult for posterior paraclinoid aneurysms (so-called ventral paraclinoid aneurysms). In all 21 cases with posterior paraclinoid aneurysms, we attempted to apply the angled fenestrated clips in tandem fashion to reconstruct the ICA. However, a parallel clip application method was possible in 18 cases. In the remaining 3 cases, the ICA had greatly shifted laterally, so that parallel clipping resulted in severe kinking of the ICA. In these cases, the aneurysm neck was narrowed with a ligature and then large straight clips were applied perpendicularly to the ICA.

From our experience, the direction of the ICA is the important variable influencing technical difficulty in reconstructing the parent artery (Fig. 82-12). Tanaka and colleagues reported a similar problem related to the clipping procedure in the cases of posterior (ventral) paraclinoid aneurysms with the ICA shifted far laterally.[27] They found that an excessive change of the longitudinal axis of the ICA occurred after tandem clipping using multiple angled fenestrated clips. They called such a change in the direction of the ICA "straightening of the parent carotid artery" and speculated that it could cause hemodynamic cerebral ischemia. It is important to trace the course of the ICA in the anteroposterior view angiogram, especially the degree of inclination of the ICA, for the preoperative planning of clipping method (Fig. 82-13). Although parallel clip

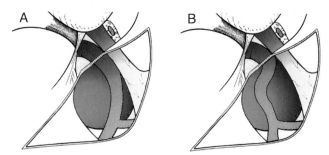

FIGURE 82-12   Schematic drawings demonstrating varying direction of the ICA. *A*, The ICA curves gently throughout its course; it is relatively easy to apply the angled ring clips parallel to the direction of the ICA. *B*, The ICA bends abruptly to the lateral direction at the clinoidal segment; in such a case, a parallel clip application can result in kinking and stenosis of the ICA.

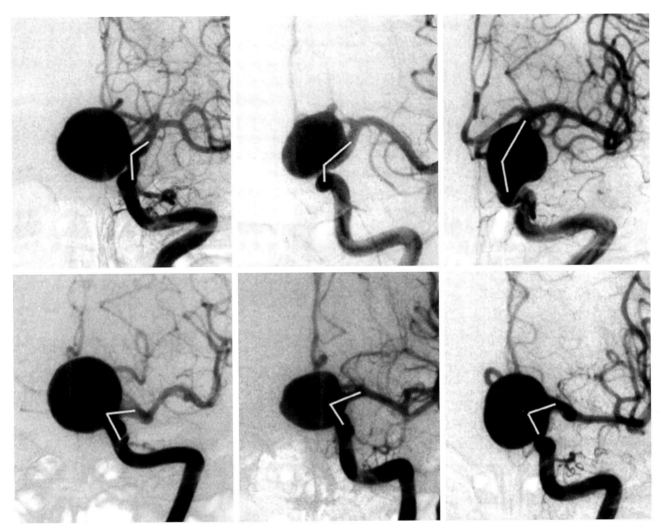

FIGURE 82-13 Angiograms (anteroposterior views) obtained in six patients with large paraclinoid aneurysms, demonstrating various angles of the longitudinal axis of the ICA.

application is more reasonable for reconstruction of the ICA, perpendicular clipping is the alternative option, especially when the ICA is displaced far laterally. Even if the aneurysm is giant size, with complete aneurysm deflation, the conventional technique of neck ligation and clipping does not result in significant stenosis of the parent artery.

REFERENCES

1. Dolenc VV: A combined epi- and subdural direct approach to carotid-ophthalmic artery aneurysms. J Neurosurg 62:667–672, 1985.
2. Suzuki J, Abiko H, Mizoi K, et al: Protective effect of phenytoin and its enhanced action by combined administration with mannitol and vitamin E in cerebral ischemia. Acta Neurochir (Wien) 88:56–64, 1987.
3. Scott JA, Horner TG, Leipzig TJ: Retrograde suction decompression of an ophthalmic artery aneurysm using balloon occlusion: Technical note. J Neurosurg 75:146–147, 1991.
4. Mizoi K, Takahashi A, Yoshimoto T, et al: Combined intravascular and neurosurgical approach for paraclinoid internal carotid artery aneurysms. Neurosurgery 33:986–992, 1993.
5. Foley KT, Cahan LD, Hieshima GB: Intraoperative angiography using a portable digital subtraction unit: Technical note. J Neurosurg 64:816–818, 1986.
6. Hieshima GB, Reicher MA, Higashida RT, et al: Intraoperative digital subtraction neuroangiography: A diagnostic and therapeutic tool. AJNR Am J Neuroradiol 8:759–767, 1987.
7. Batjer HH, Frankfurt AI, Purdy PD, et al: Use of etomidate, temporary arterial occlusion, and intraoperative angiography in surgical treatment of large and giant cerebral aneurysms. J Neurosurg 68:234–240, 1988.
8. Martin NA, Bentson J, Vinuela F, et al: Intraoperative digital subtraction angiography and the surgical treatment of intracranial aneurysms and vascular malformations. J Neurosurg 73:526–533, 1990.
9. Barrow DL, Boyer KL, Joseph GJ: Intraoperative angiography in the management of neurovascular disorders. Neurosurgery 30:153–159, 1992.
10. Alexander TD, Macdonald RL, Weir B, et al: Intraoperative angiography in cerebral aneurysm surgery: A prospective study of 100 craniotomies. Neurosurgery 39:10–18, 1996
11. Payner TD, Horner TG, Leipzig TJ, et al: Role of intraoperative angiography in the surgical treatment of cerebral aneurysms. J Neurosurg 88:441–448, 1998.
12. Chiang VL, Gailloud P, Murphy KJ, et al: Routine intraoperative angiography during aneurysm surgery. J Neurosurg 96:988–992, 2002.
13. Tang G, Cawley CM, Dion JE, et al: Intraoperative angiography during aneurysm surgery: A prospective evaluation of efficacy. J Neurosurg 96:993–999, 2002.
14. Shucart WA, Kwan ES, Heilman CB: Temporary balloon occlusion of a proximal vessel as an aid to clipping aneurysms of the basilar and paraclinoid internal carotid arteries: Technical note. Neurosurgery 27:116–119, 1990.
15. Bailes JE, Deeb ZL, Wilson JA, et al: Intraoperative angiography and temporary balloon occlusion of the basilar artery as an adjunct to surgical clipping: Technical note. Neurosurgery 30:949–953, 1992.

16. Mizoi K, Yoshimoto T, Takahashi A, et al: Direct clipping of basilar trunk aneurysms using balloon temporary occlusion. J Neurosurg 80:230–236, 1994.

17. Mizoi K, Yoshimoto T: Permissible temporary occlusion time in aneurysm surgery as evaluated by evoked potential monitoring. Neurosurgery 33:434–440, 1993.

18. Flamm ES: Suction decompression of aneurysms: Technical note. J Neurosurg 54:275–276, 1981.

19. Batjer HH, Samson DS: Retrograde suction decompression of giant paraclinoidal aneurysms: Technical note. J Neurosurg 73:305–306, 1990.

20. Tamaki N, Kim S, Ehara K, et al: Giant carotid–ophthalmic artery aneurysms: Direct clipping utilizing the "trapping-evacuation" technique. J Neurosurg 74:567–572, 1991.

21. Sinson G, Philips MF, Flamm ES: Intraoperative endovascular surgery for cerebral aneurysms. J Neurosurg 84:63–70, 1996.

22. Falbusch R, Nimsky C, Huk W: Open surgery of giant paraclinoid aneurysms improved by intraoperative angiography and endovascular retrograde suction decompression. Acta Neurochir (Wien) 139:1026–1032, 1997.

23. Arnautovic KI, Al-Mefty O, Angtuaco E: A combined microsurgical skull-base and endovascular approach to giant and large paraclinoid aneurysms. Surg Neurol 50:504–520, 1998.

24. Fan YW, Chan KH, Lui WM, et al: Retrograde suction decompression of paraclinoid aneurysm—a revised technique. Surg Neurol 51:129–131, 1999.

25. Jesus OD, Sekhar LN, Riedel CJ: Clinoid and paraclinoid aneurysms: Surgical anatomy, operative techniques, and outcome. Surg Neurol 51:477–488, 1999.

26. Ng PY, Huddle D, Gunel M, et al: Intraoperative endovascular treatment as an adjunct to microsurgical clipping of paraclinoid aneurysms. J Neurosurg 93:554–560, 2000.

27. Tanaka Y, Kobayashi S, Kyoshima K, et al: Multiple clipping technique for large and giant internal carotid artery aneurysms and complications: Angiographic analysis. J Neurosurg 80:635–642, 1994.

83 Surgical Techniques of Terminal Basilar and Posterior Cerebral Artery Aneurysms

JUHA HERNESNIEMI, AYSE KARATAS, MIKA NIEMELÄ,
KEISUKE ISHII, SYDNEY J. PEERLESS, and CHARLES G. DRAKE[†]

It is only recently that neurosurgeons have been able to attack aneurysms of the vertebral-basilar circulation with the same safety and assurance with which they attack aneurysms arising from the carotid circulation. The reasons for this late development are many. Aneurysms arising from the posterior circulation are relatively uncommon, amounting to less than 15% of all aneurysms of the brain, giving few surgeons the opportunity to gain the necessary experience and confidence to explore the confined space in front of the cerebellum and brain stem. The late refinement of routine vertebral angiography resulted in only a few of these lesions being diagnosed and then only when the aneurysms had grown to giant size and presented as tumors. Before 1950, a few large masses of unknown nature were explored, found to be thrombosed aneurysms, and shelled out and secured with proximal vessel ligation by Dandy,[1] Tönnis,[2] Falconer,[3] Poppen,[4] and Logue.[5] Schwartz[6] is credited with the first deliberate, direct attack on an aneurysm in the cerebellopontine angle. His dramatic description of controlling the bleeding and trapping the sac that was buried in the pons is memorable—the more so when one considers that the procedure was carried out without magnification and with the crude clips and instruments available at that time. The patient did well.

At the time of Drake's original report of his own experience with four patients with aneurysms of the basilar bifurcation, there was considerable skepticism about the value or safety of direct surgical attack on aneurysms of the posterior circulation. Of the 47 cases reported to that time, 14 had been treated indirectly with vertebral artery ligation, and almost half of the remainder were peripheral aneurysms arising distally on branches of the vertebral or basilar artery. The 10 aneurysms arising at the basilar bifurcation proved to be technically unapproachable; fewer than half were clipped, and the remainder were packed.[7] The first reported attempt to obliterate a basilar artery aneurysm was that made by Olivecrona. In 1954, using a subtemporal approach, he was able to clip a ruptured forward-projecting aneurysm at the basilar bifurcation. The patient improved remarkably

from postoperative hemiparesis and aphasia and was capable of part-time work. The same year another basilar tip aneurysm was successfully operated on by Bohm in the same clinic in Sweden.[8] Jamieson emphasized his discouragement in his index report on the direct surgical treatment of 19 aneurysms of the vertebrobasilar system. Ten of Jamieson's patients had died, and only four of the survivors were employable.[9] Although a note of optimism was evident in Drake's 1965 paper describing the treatment of aneurysms of the basilar trunk, the safe treatment of aneurysms of the basilar artery remained elusive.[10]

The first seven patients with aneurysms of the terminal basilar artery had not done well: four died, one was severely disabled, and only two returned to normal life. It was at this time that Drake realized the importance of identifying and sparing the tiny perforating vessels arising from the terminal basilar artery and proximal posterior cerebral arteries. It was evident that these small arteries, which were vital to the irrigation of the hypothalamus, midbrain, and pons, were often adhering to the posterior wall of the sac; moreover, they were surrounded by old blood and adhesions, and they were frequently difficult, if not impossible, to visualize in the confined space of the exposure.

At this time, there was a dramatic improvement in the technology of neurosurgery. The operating microscope, new fine instruments and clips, and the refinements of modern neuroanesthesia, including profound hypotension, all were combined to bring about a remarkable improvement in results.[11,12] In 1968, Drake[13] reported 12 additional cases with no direct operative deaths and 10 good results. In the following 25 years, the experience on all vertebrobasilar circulation aneurysms had grown to more than 1767 cases (1286 of them at the terminal basilar or posterior cerebral artery), and even now in the year 2005 still with the best microsurgical or endovascular series.[14] Poor results were almost entirely limited to patients harboring giant aneurysms or those who were in a poor clinical state before the operation. Recently, the introduction of endovascular techniques has reduced in many institutions direct operative microsurgery in the treatment of these difficult lesions.[15] Helsinki, with a high number of cerebral aneurysms treated yearly (350), has continued the legacy and techniques developed by Drake

[†]Deceased.

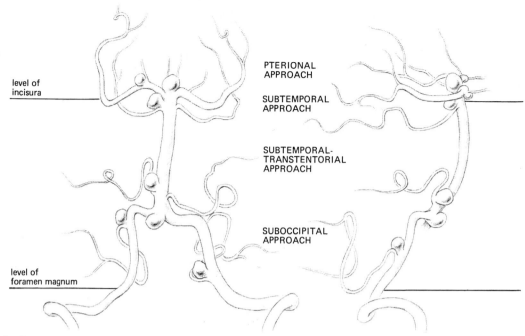

FIGURE 83-1 Common sites of posterior circulation aneurysms. The level of the tentorial incisura and foramen magnum is depicted at the usual site of the aneurysms relative to these fixed points. The surgical approaches to aneurysms of various regions is noted.

and Peerless, with the main principles remaining to perform fast, simple, clean surgery, and to preserve normal anatomy.[16–18] Many other neurosurgeons around the world continue to have good results with direct surgery but use more complicated skull base approaches.[19–24] In this chapter we describe the recent, slightly modified technique of subtemporal approach developed by Drake and Peerless, and we give, once again, the results of the London, Ontario series, by far the largest series of posterior circulation aneurysms (Fig. 83-1 and Tables 83-1 to 83-9).[14]

ANESTHESIA AND OPERATIVE ADJUNCTS

Much of the success of the actual technical procedure of approaching an aneurysm begins with the preparation of the patient and with careful, moment-to-moment assessment of the patient's condition during the procedure.[14] Patients are brought to the operating room lightly sedated and with

an accurate assessment of fluid balance. An arterial line is installed, usually with a flexible needle in the radial artery, where the arterial pressure can be continuously monitored. The patient is induced gently with pentothal, paralyzed, and then intubated with an armored tube. The anesthetic technique is basically an assisted controlled ventilation in most instances, using halothane, nitrous oxide, or a narcotic technique, depending on the preference of the anesthetist; the recent tendency is toward isoflurane. The anesthesia is kept generally light, with meticulous monitoring of blood gases to maintain the $PaCO_2$ in the range of 40 to 45 mm Hg, and the PaO_2 in excess of 100 mm Hg.

The success of the procedure largely depends on adequate intracranial relaxation. For this reason, we routinely give 1 g/kg of 20% mannitol, increasing this to 2 g/kg if we contemplate temporary occlusion of a major intracranial vessel. Furosemide (1 mg/kg) is given intravenously shortly after induction and the administration of mannitol only if intracranial relaxation is inadequate. While the patient is

TABLE 83-1 ▪ Preoperative Grade (Botterell) and Outcome in 361 Patients with Small and Upward-Projecting Basilar Bifurcation Aneurysms

Grade	Excellent	Good	Poor	Dead	Total
0	62	2	2	0	66
1	150	24	11	6	191
2	48	13	8	3	72
3	9	9	4	3	25
4	2	2	3	0	7
Total	271	50	28	12	361
	75.1%	13.9%	7.8%	3.3%	100%

TABLE 83-2 ▪ Preoperative Grade (Botterell) and Outcome in 61 Patients with Small and Posterior-Projecting Basilar Bifurcation Aneurysms

Grade	Excellent	Good	Poor	Dead	Total
0	7	0	1	0	8
1	29	6	0	0	35
2	9	3	0	3	15
3	2	0	1	0	3
Total	47	9	2	3	61
	77%	14.8%	3.3%	4.9%	100%

TABLE 83-3 ▪ Preoperative Grade (Botterell) and Outcome in 61 Patients with Small and Anterior-Projecting Basilar Bifurcation Aneurysms

Grade	Excellent	Good	Poor	Dead	Total
0	7	0	0	0	7
1	27	2	1	1	31
2	12	1	0	2	15
3	2	3	3	0	8
Total	48	6	4	3	61
	78.7%	9.8%	6.6%	4.9%	100%

TABLE 83-5 ▪ Preoperative Grade (Botterell) and Outcome in 137 Patients with Giant Basilar Bifurcation Aneurysms

Grade	Excellent	Good	Poor	Dead	Total
0	29	15	24	7	75
1	16	6	2	3	27
2	6	5	1	1	13
3	6	5	4	1	16
4	0	0	1	5	6
Total	57	31	32	17	137
	41.6%	22.6%	23.4%	12.4%	100%

being positioned, the neurosurgeon uses a Tuohy needle to insert a lumbar subarachnoid catheter (PE 100) into the lumbar subarachnoid space and attaches this tubing to a closed collection bag. The lumbar subarachnoid drain is kept clamped until the dura is opened, at which time cerebrospinal fluid (CSF) drainage is commenced to add to the intracranial relaxation.

We have frequently used intentional hypotension during the dissection and clipping of the aneurysm. The anesthetist prepares for this by connecting the transducer from the arterial line, at a level equal to the height of the brain, to an electronic monitor that gives systolic, diastolic, and mean pressures. Hypotension is induced by deepening the isoflurane anesthesia. Systemic arterial pressures of 50 to 60 mm Hg are routinely used during the initial dissection around the aneurysm, and when manipulation of the aneurysm itself or application of the clip begins, the pressure is lowered to 40 to 45 mm Hg. It has been our experience that these low pressures are routinely well tolerated for 30 to 40 minutes and have rarely been responsible for significant problems when prolonged for 60 to 90 minutes.

In more than 400 patients who have been operated on since 1981 (and since 1993 in Finland), we have frequently come to rely on temporary occlusion of the parent (basilar or vertebral) artery as a means to soften the aneurysmal sac while dissecting and preparing the neck for clipping. In fact, only one fifth of the patients were operated on under induced hypotension (<70 mm Hg) in the last 10 years in the Drake and Peerless series. The new small, temporary clips designed by Suzuki and Sugita are excellent for this purpose, not only for their reliably soft closing pressures, but

also for their relative ease of application and removal. The temporary clip must have a gentle closing pressure (<40 g) to prevent injury to the parent vessel, and it should not occlude any perforating vessels. Of course, before application of a temporary proximal clip, the patient should be normotensive and should receive an additional bolus of 1 g/kg 20% mannitol and pentothal. Under these circumstances, temporary occlusion of the basilar artery for up to 10 minutes is well tolerated. In longer single occlusion times, the mortality and morbidity rates seem to increase; admittedly these cases have been technically more difficult.

With the patient positioned, the anesthetist begins meticulous monitoring of fluid balance, electrocardiogram, systemic arterial blood pressure, and blood gases. Occasionally, we used brain retractor pressure monitoring but did not find it valuable. Electroencephalography, somatosensory evoked potentials, and intraoperative cerebral blood flow (CBF) monitoring have been used in unique situations of giant aneurysms or when we anticipate prolonged interruption of focal cerebral blood flow.[25]

POSITIONING

Almost all aneurysms of the basilar artery above the anterior inferior cerebellar arteries can be approached with the patient in the lateral decubitus, or "park bench," position. In that we normally aim to approach the aneurysm under the nondominant temporal lobe, the patient is placed on his or her left side, with a sandbag under the left axilla to elevate the shoulder from the table and provide free respiratory excursion of the chest. The back and chest of the

TABLE 83-4 ▪ Preoperative Grade (Botterell) and Outcome in 265 Patients with Large Basilar Bifurcation Aneurysms

Grade	Excellent	Good	Poor	Dead	Total
0	33	3	4	0	40
1	99	16	10	7	132
2	37	16	7	2	62
3	8	8	7	3	26
4	0	1	1	1	3
5	1	0	0	1	2
Total	178	44	29	14	265
	67.2%	16.6%	10.9%	5.3%	100%

TABLE 83-6 ▪ Preoperative Grade (Botterell) and Outcome in 210 Patients with Small and Large Superior Cerebellar Aneurysms

Grade	Excellent	Good	Poor	Dead	Total
0	40	2	1	1	44
1	96	3	4	3	106
2	24	11	4	2	41
3	6	8	4	0	18
4	0	0	1	0	1
Total	166	24	14	6	210
	79%	11.4%	6.7%	2.9%	100%

TABLE 83-7 ▪ Preoperative Grade (Botterell) and Outcome in 56 Patients with Giant Superior Cerebellar Artery Aneurysms

Grade	Excellent	Good	Poor	Dead	Total
0	11	8	5	7	31
1	4	6	1	1	12
2	4	1	1	1	7
3	1	1	0	2	4
4	0	0	2	0	2
Total	20	16	9	11	56
	35.7%	28.6%	16.1%	19.6%	100%

TABLE 83-9 ▪ Preoperative Grade (Botterell) and Outcome in 66 Patients with Giant Posterior Cerebellar Artery Aneurysms

Grade	Excellent	Good	Poor	Dead	Total
0	31	7	3	2	43
1	15	1	2	0	18
3	1	3	1	0	5
Total	47	11	6	2	66
	71.2%	16.7%	9.1%	3%	100%

patient are supported by rests attached to the table, and the head is fixed in a three- (or four-) point pin headrest. The alignment of the head is crucial for the subtemporal approach. The anteroposterior (AP) axis should be precisely parallel to the floor, and the sagittal plane of the head tipped 15 degrees toward the floor. The head does not move relative to the body following fixation in this position, but the whole table may be tipped head up or head down or rotated from one side to the other as necessary to gain further visual access to the upper basilar artery (Fig. 83-2). Only the operative area is shaved. Prophylactic antibiotics are not used; wound infection was seen in 7 out of 1767 patients with more than 2000 intracranial procedures.

In Drake's initial experience with aneurysms of the upper basilar artery, sizable temporal bone flaps were routinely turned. Later, in the last 1000 cases, this proved unnecessary. As is seen by the figures provided in this chapter, the aim of the exposure is to get as close to the base of the skull as possible at the junction of the anterior and middle thirds of the temporal lobe, where the temporal lobe has already begun to turn upward following the convex floor of the middle cranial fossa. Little is gained by fashioning a large bone flap up over the lateral surface of the temporal lobe or posteriorly, except in circumstances in which it is necessary to divide the tentorium to gain access to the middle portions of the basilar artery (Figs. 83-3 to 83-5).

We now routinely make a linear incision extending vertically upward, curving slightly backward at its upper extent, and originating at the zygomatic process of the temporal bone approximately one finger's width anterior to the ear. After the skin, subcutaneous tissue, and galea have been divided, the temporalis fascia and muscle are divided 5 mm

on either side of the vertical incision at the level of the zygomatic process. With the soft tissue held apart by a tic retractor, a single burr hole in the squamous portion of the temporal bone is enlarged with rongeurs, forming a somewhat pear-shaped opening that is widest at the base. It is important to remove the temporal squama with rongeurs— or recently with high-speed drill—down to the level of the zygomatic root so that the bony opening is as flush with the floor of the middle fossa as possible. The bony opening should be about 4 cm across at the base and 3 to 4 cm high. Recently we have returned to a small bone flap the same size as the craniectomy with less postoperative discomfort and deformity for better patient acceptance. The main stem and posterior branch of the superficial temporal artery are preserved in the posterior aspect of the scalp flap, but often the anterior branch of this vessel must be divided (Fig. 83-6).

The dura is opened in a triangle with the base inferior, and is sutured up to the overlying soft tissue so as not to obscure the view at the base. At this point, the lumbar subarachnoid drain is opened and CSF removal is begun. A slack brain is essential. The combination of the osmotic and loop diuretic and the removal of CSF is usually sufficient to produce excellent intracranial relaxation. If the brain remains full, however, and gentle retraction of the temporal lobe does not easily expose the middle intracranial fossa, it is imperative to wait, elevate the head, remove more CSF, check to ensure that the ventilation parameters are adequate, and wait again until adequate reduction of the intracranial contents has been achieved. Although cerebral edema is the most likely cause for a persistently swollen and tight brain, corticosteroids have not been used because they have little effect on cytotoxic edema and many potential complications. Most maneuvers on the operating table will not adequately relieve this, and further retraction and manipulation are very likely to aggravate the edema in the postoperative period. If the exposure is not easily accomplished, a ventriculostomy might be helpful, but it is also possible to abandon the procedure and return another day. With the brain relaxed, the surface of the temporal lobe should be covered with a compressed sheet of Gelfoam. With a hand-held retractor, the undersurface of the temporal lobe is inspected for the position of bridging veins. The vein of Labbé is usually seen just beyond the posterior limits of the craniectomy. It should, when visualized, be covered with several strips of Gelfoam and must be protected at all costs against rupture. Similarly, bridging veins at the tip of the temporal lobe seen just beyond the anterior limits of the bony removal also should be protected. Small bridging veins, from the undersurface of the temporal lobe to the tent,

TABLE 83-8 ▪ Preoperative Grade (Botterell) and Outcome in 59 Patients with Small or Large Posterior Cerebral Artery Aneurysms

Grade	Excellent	Good	Poor	Dead	Total
0	15	0	1	1	17
1	25	5	0	0	30
2	1	1	0	0	2
3	1	2	3	1	7
4	0	0	0	1	1
5	0	0	0	2	2
Total	42	8	4	5	59
	71.2%	13.6%	6.8%	8.5%	100%

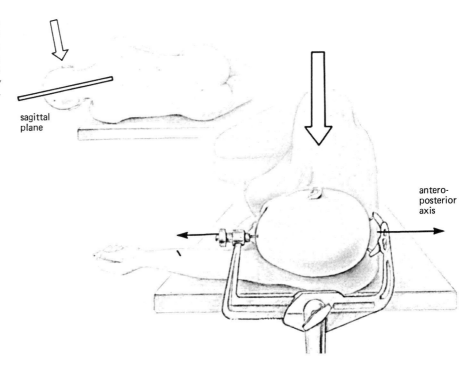

FIGURE 83-2 Patient position for the subtemporal approach. Note that the anteroposterior access of the head is fixed parallel to the floor and that the sagittal plane is tipped 15 degrees to the perpendicular. The *open arrow* shows the starting position of the operating microscope.

can be coagulated and divided with impunity; the larger veins on the surface, however, should never be sacrificed because of the danger of producing venous swelling or infarction.

With further retraction, the uncus of the temporal lobe is gently elevated, and the free edge of the tentorium comes into view. A Greenberg, Yasargil, or Sugita self-retaining retractor system should now be fixed without excessive retractor pressure to provide continuous support of the elevated temporal lobe. With this retractor in place and with a 2- to 3-mm gap visible between the uncus and the free surface of the tent, it is likely that the retractor will not need to

be moved again. The position of the tip of the retractor is important. It should just touch the uncus and its overlying arachnoid and be centered at about the midpoint of the concave curve of the free edge of the tent. Positioning the retractor anterior or posterior to this will lead the surgeon forward into the interpeduncular fossa and posterior clinoid or will lead backward onto the cerebral peduncle, instead of directly medially onto the terminal basilar artery (Fig. 83-7).

At this point, the operating microscope should be brought into position, and under 10–16× magnification the surgeon focuses on the layer of arachnoid covering the uncus

FIGURE 83-3 Subtemporal approach. Relationship of a scalp incision and a craniectomy to the skull and brain landmarks.

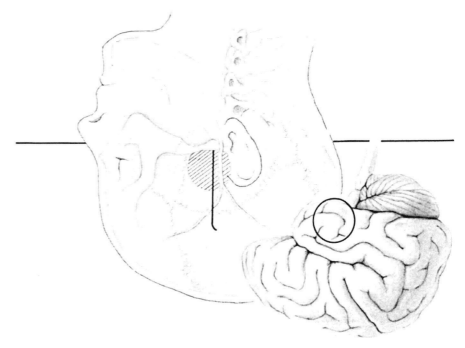

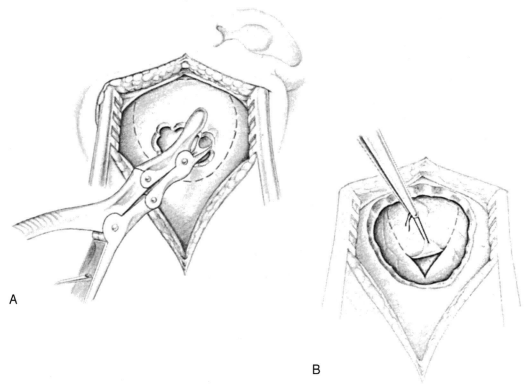

FIGURE 83-4 Subtemporal approach. Operative procedure. *A,* Exposure of the dura. *B,* Dural incision.

and cerebral peduncle, passing onto and under the free edge of the tentorium. It is usually possible to identify the oculomotor nerve at this point, coming up from the depths under the uncus and piercing the arachnoid in the anterior aspect of the exposure to enter its cavernous compartment. The trochlear nerve will also be seen posteriorly in the exposure, lying beneath the arachnoid and turning inferiorly underneath the tentorium. Popular textbooks of anatomy often depict the trochlear nerve passing between layers of the tentorium at this site, but it does not. It remains within its arachnoid layer, attached to the undersurface of the tentorium for about 2 cm, and swings in an arc laterally forward and then medially toward the cavernous sinus.

In most of the cases it is necessary at this point to pass a 4-0 silk suture through the free edge of the tentorium and to tie it back into the floor of the middle cranial fossa. This maneuver provides 3 to 5 mm more exposure by rolling back the free edge of the tentorium. We have developed a new surgical technique to retract the tentorial edge with the help of aneurysm clips during the subtemporal approach.[18] Only rarely (<10% of patients) will it be necessary to divide the tent in the exposure of aneurysms of the distal end of the basilar artery.

The initial arachnoid incision should then be made by picking up the arachnoid covering the side of the peduncle superior to the trochlear nerve and inferior to the uncus. This incision is extended forward below the course of the third nerve. This arachnoid is a rather thick and complex structure, dividing anteriorly to form a band running medially across the interpeduncular fossa known as the membrane of Liljequist. This band of arachnoid should also be sharply divided across the front of the pons to permit the

removal of clot in the interpeduncular fossa and to permit visualization of the opposite oculomotor nerve and posterior cerebral artery (Figs. 83-8 and 83-9).

At this stage, the inexperienced surgeon will often be surprised if he or she is unable to see the posterior cerebral artery. This vessel, of course, follows a compound curved course, bending upward laterally, forward, and then turning backward and is usually obscured by the third cranial nerve, the uncus, and the mesial portion of the temporal lobe as it winds its way back around the midbrain. Branches of the superior cerebellar artery are readily apparent at this stage as they wind around the peduncle, and these branches can be followed medially to the basilar artery. The surgeon must now have a clear mental picture of the anatomy gained from knowledge of the normal anatomy and by study of the angiograms (nowadays CT angiography in Helsinki), so that he or she can readily identify the structures in the depths of the exposure. It is usually best to begin removal of the blood clot in the region along the lateral aspects of the basilar artery between the superior cerebellar and the origin of Pl. Once the wall of the basilar artery is in view, dissection can be carried out in that plane anteriorly and posteriorly, removing clot with suction and forceps and working from the base of the presumed neck of the aneurysm and distally toward the fundus (Fig. 83-10). One should gain proximal control of the parent artery early.

BASILAR BIFURCATION ANEURYSMS

Basilar bifurcation aneurysms may be small (<1.25 cm in diameter), bulbous (1.25–2.5 cm in diameter), or giant (>2.5 cm in diameter). These aneurysms may point forward,

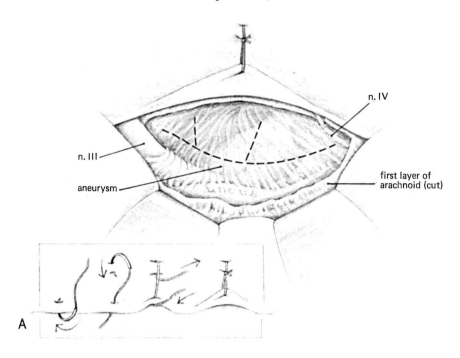

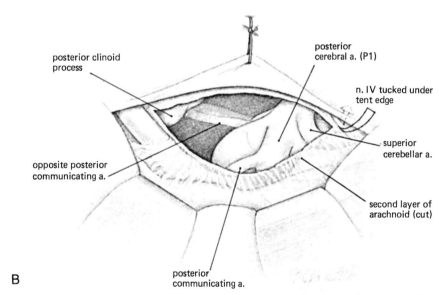

FIGURE 83-5 *A,* Subtemporal approach. The first layer of the arachnoid has been removed, showing the intact second layer. The tentorial edge has been sutured into the middle fossa. The *inset* depicts the technique of suturing the tentorium. *B,* Second layer of the arachnoid and the membrane of Lillequist has been divided to expose the terminal basilar artery and bifurcation aneurysm. Note that the fourth cranial nerve has been tucked back under the edge of the tentorium.

directly upward, or backward. For each size and orientation, there are special problems in dissection and clipping. The position of the basilar bifurcation relative to the posterior clinoid is also an important variable to be considered in one's approach to these aneurysms. In nearly half of the cases, the bifurcation lies precisely at the level of the posterior clinoid, but in nearly one third it lies several millimeters or up to 1 cm below the clinoid. In the remaining patients the basilar artery is elongated, with the bifurcation lying several millimeters or, rarely, as much as 1 cm above the clinoid. With aneurysms arising from the basilar

bifurcation located at the level of the posterior clinoid, the approach from this point will be quite straightforward. A very high bifurcation will require further retraction of the uncus and indeed may be preferentially approached from the frontotemporal exposure after splitting of the sylvian fissure. The low-lying basilar bifurcation is particularly hazardous because the interpeduncular space narrows to the apex of a cone, making manipulation and visualization difficult around the bulging belly of the pons, with the thin dome of the fundus obscuring the surgeon's path to the neck.

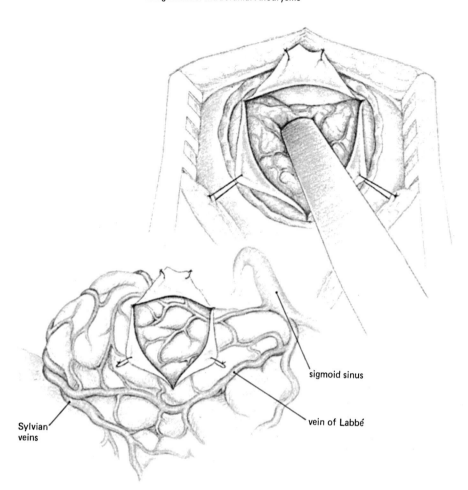

FIGURE 83-6 Subtemporal approach. Retraction of the temporal lobe and temporal lobe veins.

sigmoid sinus

vein of Labbé

Sylvian veins

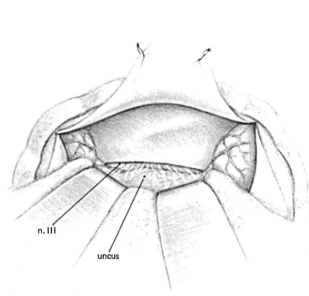

n. III

uncus

FIGURE 83-7 A subtemporal approach. Retraction of the temporal lobe to expose the edge of the tentorium and the first layer of the arachnoid.

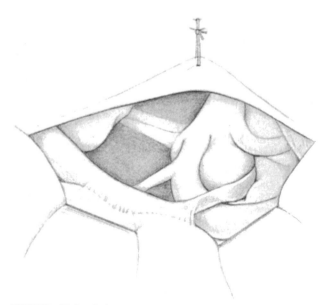

FIGURE 83-8 Subtemporal approach to show a superior cerebellar artery aneurysm in situ. Note that the third cranial nerve is displaced over the dome of the aneurysm.

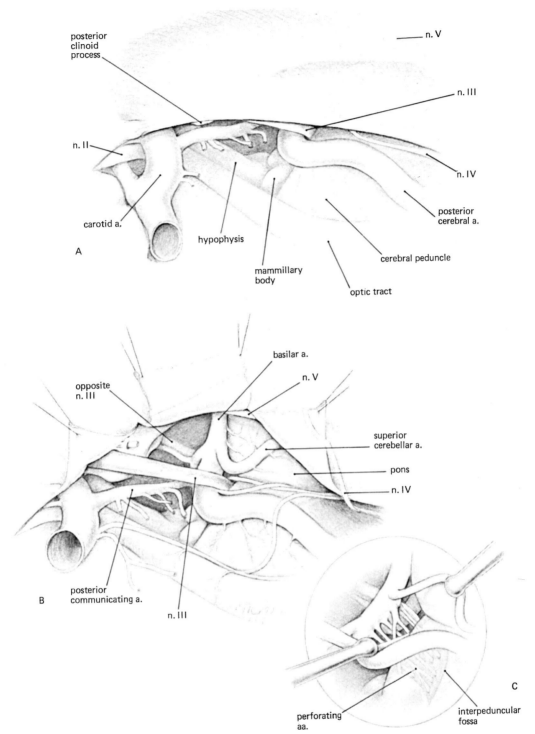

FIGURE 83-9 Microscopic anatomy of the interpeduncular fossa and its contents. *A*, Uncus and hippocampal gyrus of temporal removed and intact. *B*, Tentorium divided and retracted. *C*, Terminal basilar artery drawn out of the interpeduncular fossa to show perforating artery.

With an aneurysm of average size and in the usual position with the neck at the level of the clinoid, it is preferable at this stage to begin the dissection on the anterior surface of the aneurysm. By following the surface of the basilar artery anteriorly and superiorly, the origin of the Pl artery on the right side will be identified as well as the anterior aspect of the neck of the sac. The neck of the sac and the termination of the basilar artery are gently retracted backward into the interpeduncular fossa and, with further removal of clot, the opposite (left) Pl artery will be exposed and visualized through a layer of arachnoid, with the left oculomotor nerve passing forward. One must use this maneuver cautiously with aneurysms pointing forward for they are often fused to the clivus at the site of rupture; rough handling can tear away this point of junction and cause troublesome, even catastrophic, bleeding. It is important to

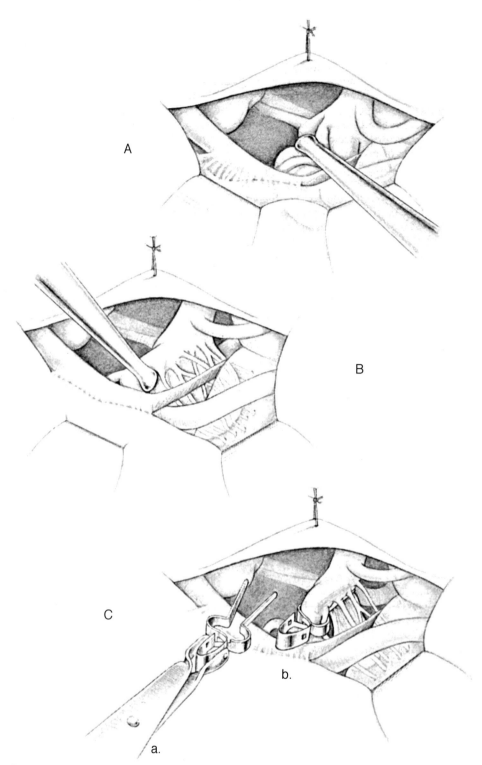

FIGURE 83-10 Subtemporal approach. Exposure and clipping of a basilar bifurcation aneurysm. *A,* Dissector compressing the anterior belly of the aneurysm in order to expose the opposite P1, the posterior communicating artery, and the oculomotor nerve. *B,* A microdissector displacing the right P1 anteriorly to display perforators on the side wall of the aneurysm. *C,* a, Drake aperture clip; b, an aperture clip in place, occluding the neck of the aneurysm and encircling the right P1 and one perforator in the aperture.

emphasize at this point that the termination of the basilar artery is usually widened and ectatic at the base of aneurysms arising from the bifurcation. One must have an appreciation of this variation in anatomy and identify the origin of the Pl artery precisely, lest one mistake the terminal basilar artery for a portion of the sac and position the clip dangerously low, resulting in occlusion of the terminal basilar artery. Furthermore, the distal basilar artery and the origin of both posterior cerebral arteries forms a V-shaped structure as viewed from the front, making the neck of these aneurysms quite narrow. This often comes as a surprise when the aneurysm is exposed in the operating room because the conventional angiographic projections of this area commonly superimpose the Pl artery and the neck of the aneurysm, giving the appearance of a spuriously wide base. Bearing this problem in mind, care must be taken to prevent placement of a clip with blades that are too long, because this would risk narrowing or occluding the opposite Pl artery. Moreover, the base of the aneurysm is narrower from front to back than from side to side, making application of the clip from the side somewhat safer because properly positioned clip blades are least likely to crimp the origins of the Pl artery.

After exposure of the front side of the aneurysm, dissection should be directed to the right lateral and posterior aspect of the aneurysm. Here the goal is to define the posterior aspect of the sac and, more importantly, to identify and separate the perforators that arise from the proximal, posterior portion of the Pl artery and that normally stream backward over the sac of the aneurysm to enter the posterior perforated substance and peduncle. These perforators are small vessels, often branching once or twice before penetrating the pia covering the brain. It is essential that each of these vital vessels be preserved, and any amount of time taken to separate these vessels from the sac can be justified. Often these perforators will have to be separated with a sharp hook or, after they have been stretched, by sharply dividing with a knife the fibrous bands fusing them to the sac. One must remember that the perforators are paired, with two to six vessels arising from each Pl artery, making it necessary to displace the terminal basilar artery and the sac away from the interpeduncular fossa and to dissect across the midline to visualize the perforators on the far side as well as those more readily seen on the near side. Displacement of the whole of the terminal basilar complex away from the interpeduncular fossa during periods of hypotension can be achieved by using a relatively wide blade dissector. It is important to re-emphasize that before any clip is placed, the origin of both of the Pl arteries must be identified on both the right and left sides. This is accomplished by looking across the front of the basilar artery and across the back and then all the perforators arising from both of the Pl arteries passing backward and upward must be seen and separated from the sac. Occasionally, with a low or highly placed basilar bifurcation, one may momentarily confuse the opposite superior cerebellar artery with the posterior cerebral artery. To inadvertently place the clip blades proximal to the origin of the opposite Pl artery is, of course, disastrous and can be avoided by identifying the opposite oculomotor nerve and recalling that this structure always runs between the superior cerebellar and posterior cerebral arteries. The absolute confirmation of this anatomy on both the near and far sides is fundamental to the success of the procedure.

In most instances, the dissection can be confined to the neck of the basilar bifurcation aneurysm and the adjacent proximal posterior cerebral arteries and their perforating branches. It is rarely necessary and indeed is hazardous to extend the dissection up onto the body or fundus for the wall is almost always thinner in this region and is the site of the original rupture; it will bleed again if not handled with care.

With the neck defined, the decision is now made regarding the type of clip to be used and its placement. For aneurysms that point forward or backward from the bifurcation, a simple straight clip may suffice after the sac is displaced away from the Pl arteries and, in the case of posterior projecting

aneurysms, working the blades under the perforators. The more common aneurysm, however, projects directly upward in the line of the basilar artery and the origins of the Pl artery and cannot be secured with a simple straight or angled clip. For this reason, we developed the aperture clip designed to enclose the Pl artery and, if necessary, adjacent perforators within the aperture, permitting the clip blades to compress only the neck of the aneurysm. Successful use of this clip depends on the precise choice of the correct blade length because blades that are too long will narrow or occlude the origin of the Pl segments of the posterior cerebral artery and blades that are too short will permit continued filling of the aneurysm.

There are three concerns when using the fenestrated clip. First, the fenestrating ring beyond the applier tips tends to obscure vision in the narrow confines, especially behind the aneurysm. Second, the clip blades must be no longer than the flattened, occluded neck or else the Pl origins and its perforators may be stenosed or occluded. A flattened neck is about 1.5 times the width of an open, circular neck. If the proper length blades are not available, longer blades may be trimmed with wire cutters and/or a diamond burr and polished with a whetstone. Two common errors are to use blades longer than necessary, which may occlude the opposite Pl or its perforators, or to place the clip too far out on the neck. It is remarkable how short the blades need to be when placed down at the very origin of the neck at the Pl roots. It must be certain, too, that the origin of the superior cerebellar artery (SCA) is not mistaken for Pl; otherwise inadvertent occlusion of the basilar bifurcation will occur. The third concern is that not uncommonly a bit of the neck is left open in the aperture just medial to the Pl root. This is usually the cause of an aneurysm that still pulsates or bleeds on needling, although it must be certain that the clip tips cross to the far side of the neck. Repositioning of the clip a little lower or with slightly longer blades may suffice to occlude the remaining neck. Otherwise a straight tandem clip can be added (see later). As the posterior blade is passed behind the neck, one must be certain that it is inside the perforators while using temporary basilar occlusion to soften a dangerously thin neck. As the blades are allowed to close and narrow the neck, the opposite Pl will come into view so that final alignment, flush with the neck at the upper origins of Pl on each side, can be made before final closure. The posterior blade must not be put too far across because the root of the opposite third nerve courses up just behind the opposite Pl and can be brushed or actually injured by this blade.

After placing the clip, one should not breathe a sigh of relief and step back. This is perhaps the most crucial part of the procedure, a time when the surgeon must quickly inspect both the anterior and posterior surfaces of the neck to ensure that the Pl segments are not kinked and to ensure that all perforators are entirely free. Rotating the clip handle forward usually exposes the posterior blade, and looking just above the blade will determine whether or not any perforators emerge from underneath it. If there is any suspicion that a perforator is trapped or kinked by the clip or that the origins of the Pl artery are narrowed, the clip should be removed immediately, further dissection accomplished, and the clip reapplied. Commonly the clip will have to be positioned and repositioned several times before a precise and accurate placement is achieved. Then the dome of the aneurysm should be punctured with a needle and its contents aspirated, and with the added room afforded by the collapsed sac, the whole anatomy can be reviewed and perfect positioning of the clip guaranteed.

One must recall that the height of the basilar bifurcation varies considerably. Most often, the bifurcation is at or just above the level of the dorsum sellae. Occasionally, it is higher, reaching the apex of the interpeduncular cistern and tucked in behind the mammillary bodies. Rarely, the bifurcation may be higher still, with the aneurysm indenting the floor of the third ventricle and posterior hypothalamus. The higher the placement of the bifurcation, the more temporal lobe retraction will be required, and retraction of the peduncle or mammillary body may even be necessary to expose the bifurcation and perforators. Retraction of these structures with a small spatula is normally well tolerated. As noted earlier, an aneurysm that is very high may be approached through the frontotemporal or so-called pterional exposure, using splitting and separation of the sylvian fissure.[12,13] With a moderately high bifurcation, it will occasionally be necessary to dissect above the oculomotor nerve in the space between the oculomotor nerve and the hippocampal gyrus. In this situation, it is sometimes necessary to enclose the oculomotor nerve along with the P1 segment in the aperture of the clip, a maneuver that is well tolerated by this hardy nerve. If the bifurcation is unusually low (at the base of the dorsum sellae or even lower), the exposure is considerably more difficult and hazardous. The interpeduncular fossa is cone shaped, with the apex pointing downward into the groove of the pons, forcing the surgeon to gain visual access around the belly of the pons in the depths of the wound. This line of sight can be enhanced by retracting the temporal lobe somewhat more posteriorly to view the anterior aspect of the pons and the pontomesencephalic junction. Although division of the tent may be used, it frequently does not improve the exposure at this site because both the trigeminal and trochlear nerves cross the sight line and obscure the view. Angled aperture clips are often essential for dealing with these low-placed aneurysms.

It should also be remembered that the sylvian approach to basilar bifurcation aneurysms is quite unsuitable for these low-lying lesions because it is impossible to see over the obstruction of the dorsum sellae. It should also be remembered that angiograms taken in the Townes projection usually show the P1 segments as entirely separate from the neck of the aneurysm and coming out almost straight laterally from the side of the basilar artery. The course of the posterior cerebral artery is complex, however, coursing forward and upward before it turns outward to cross above the oculomotor nerve and before swinging around the peduncle under the cover of the hippocampal gyrus. With this angiographic view in mind, the surgeon is often surprised, particularly when faced with a large or bulbous aneurysm, to see from the lateral exposure what appear to be the P1 segments and their perforators arising directly out of the sac. This is rarely, if ever, true but underscores the necessity of carefully dissecting between the P1 artery and the sac on both the near and far sides to clearly define the lowermost portion of the neck to be clipped. This anomalous appearance of vessels arising from the side wall of the aneurysm is particularly prominent when the terminal basilar artery is ectatic and shaped like the bell of a trumpet.

POSTERIORLY PROJECTING ANEURYSMS

Although the angiographic appearance of posteriorly projecting aneurysms would suggest that they would be the most difficult and dangerous to expose, as a group they have proved to be quite suitable for direct surgical treatment. With these aneurysms, it is usually necessary to work both above and below the third nerve to gain access to the neck. Often the perforators are fairly readily dissected from the neck but are densely adherent more distally on the dome, where they can and should be left untouched. With posteriorly projecting aneurysms, one can readily visualize the opposite P1 artery across the front of the aneurysm, and, with the position of the neck in view, it is then possible to work a fine sucker between the basilar artery and the crus with the left hand and gently draw the basilar artery forward, displacing the terminal basilar artery and the sac out of the interpeduncular fossa. By dissecting with a fine spatula in the right hand, it is then possible to see the perforators that have been stretched and to separate them from the neck on both the near and far sides. The fundus of this aneurysm is usually never seen because it is buried high up in the interpeduncular fossa, and because it is covered with brain stem, it is probably more secure and less likely to rupture. Because of the backward displacement of this aneurysm away from the curve of the posterior cerebral artery, one is frequently able to secure the neck with a simple straight clip, which, when placed across the neck and partially closed, allows excellent visualization across the back of the neck before final placement. A particular hazard with this aneurysm is the portion of the fundus bulging downward below the level of the neck posteriorly. This configuration makes blind application of the clip blades on the posterior aspect of the aneurysm hazardous because the inferior blade of the clip could pierce the sac. By beginning the dissection low on the back surface of the basilar artery at the origins of the superior cerebellar arteries and working distally, however, one will usually encounter this rolled-over portion of the fundus, allowing it to be separated from the parent vessel and tipped upward before the clip blades are applied.

ANTERIORLY PROJECTING ANEURYSMS: BILOBED ANEURYSMS

Anteriorly projecting aneurysms are the most straightforward to manage if they are located above or at the clinoid process. These aneurysms are, however, frequently fused to the dura of the dorsum and clivus, and care must be taken in the displacement of the aneurysm backward for fear of tearing away this attachment, which is usually at the site of rupture and therefore thin and friable. Low lying and attached to clivus, these aneurysms are the most dangerous. The anteriorly projecting aneurysm projects upward and forward from the line of the basilar artery, with the fundus usually placed above the dorsum sellae, free of the interpeduncular fossa and mammillary bodies. In the same way, the aneurysm is usually free of the posterior cerebral arteries and perforators, and only passing attention need be given to these structures in the definition of the terminal basilar anatomy. It is also important not to confuse these aneurysms with the bilobed, bulbous sac that typically has an upward-projecting or backward-projecting sac as well as the more obvious forward-projecting portion. These bilobed lesions are among the most complex and difficult aneurysms to deal with because of their bulk as well as the unusually wide and deformed terminal basilar artery. Eight small bilobed aneurysms were operated on with excellent results.

GIANT OR BULBOUS BASILAR BIFURCATION ANEURYSMS

Most giant or bulbous aneurysms of the basilar bifurcation project vertically and are always associated with a widened terminal basilar artery, giving the appearance that the posterior cerebral arteries are arising out of the neck and proximal fundus. As a group, these aneurysms are hazardous because they are difficult to expose and technically demanding to clip. The exceptional bulk of the aneurysm filling the interpeduncular cistern and deforming the parent and branch vessels makes definition of the anatomy difficult and at times impossible. It is usually necessary to firmly indent the waist of the sac anteriorly and posteriorly to visualize the neck, and often it must be held indented while the clip is being positioned. Again it is important to clearly identify the opposite Pl artery and its perforators before the clip is finally placed. It is frequently necessary to manipulate the clip into place with the left hand while holding perforators off with a small dissector in the right hand. Another major concern with this aneurysm is that, frequently, the neck of the aneurysm and the terminal ectatic basilar artery are firm and yellow with atherosclerosis. Instead of being soft and pliable, the neck and terminal basilar artery are solid and often calcified, and as the clip blades are closed, the clip tends to slide down and occlude the terminal basilar artery or the atherosclerotic plaque fractures, and fragments are driven into the Pl segments. If the clip does slip downward because of the firmness of the wall and the mass of the sac above, it may be necessary to place a clip high up across the body of the sac to occlude the fundus and permit its aspiration and then to seat a smaller clip more precisely across the neck. It is always safer, however, to clip these aneurysms somewhat more distally than at the actual neck because considerable narrowing several millimeters proximal to the clip is the rule as the blades approximate the firm wall, and this may impede flow through the Pl segments or the proximal perforators. If the dilatation and ectasia of the terminal basilar artery are extensive, the entire vessel and its major branches will be involved in the aneurysmal dilatation, making it impossible to secure the neck with a clip without occluding or seriously stenosing the orifice of one or both posterior cerebral arteries. In this situation, consideration must be given to proximal basilar artery occlusion as the only definitive form of treatment, particularly if generous posterior communicating arteries are known to be present.

SUPERIOR CEREBELLAR ARTERY ANEURYSMS

Superior cerebellar artery aneurysms arise at the distal carina of the origin of the superior cerebellar artery. The aneurysm almost always projects laterally forward or backward, with the fundus embedded in the peduncle. As the sac enlarges, it usually occupies the whole length of the basilar artery

between the distal carina of the superior cerebellar artery and the proximal origin of the posterior cerebral artery. The superior cerebellar artery usually arises separately from the necks of these large aneurysms rather than from the parent basilar arteries. Clip placement must not compromise this orifice, and it may be necessary to leave open a small wedge of neck just above to leave open the origin of the artery. The fundus frequently has an intimate association with the oculomotor nerve and often stretches this nerve above or below the sac as well as indenting the peduncle on that side.

Unless they are unusually large, these aneurysms can be dealt with in a relatively straightforward manner. The subtemporal exposure gives excellent visualization of the neck, and because there are no perforators arising off the segment of the basilar artery between the superior cerebellar and posterior cerebral arteries or off the superior surface of the superior cerebellar artery, the clip can be placed across the neck with concern only for preserving the integrity of the basilar artery and encompassing the whole of the neck between the blades. As noted earlier, these aneurysms normally project laterally and arise more frequently on the left side. As a consequence, one is faced with approaching the left-pointing aneurysm under the dominant temporal lobe. In our experience, this represents an additional and real hazard to the patient. When this aneurysm reaches large or giant proportions, the superior and anterior surface of the sac will be in direct contact with the perforators arising off the Pl artery. These should be identified and spared, as in the case of basilar bifurcation aneurysms. The larger aneurysms pointing toward the left side may be approached from the right, working across the midline and over the top of the basilar artery, because the basilar artery is usually deflected toward the right side as the sac enlarges (Fig. 83-11).

Superior cerebellar artery aneurysms are best dissected first on their anterior surface, again defining the plane of the basilar artery and the origins of the superior cerebellar and posterior cerebral arteries. It is then necessary to work on the distal and proximal surface of the sac to provide room for the clip blades. It is preferable to work a curved clip blade from the superior and anterior surface downward, following the curve of the inferior surface of the posterior cerebral artery and the lateral wall of the basilar artery as the clip blades are closed. In this way, one is able to locate the tips of the clip precisely to ensure that they are not impinging on the origin of the superior cerebellar artery. The fundus of the aneurysm can then be punctured and aspirated, and quick inspection of the posterior surface can be carried out to ensure that perforators from the Pl artery have not been picked up by the posterior blade. One must be cautious, particularly with larger aneurysms, that the clip does not slide medially and kink the basilar artery. Of course care should always be taken to avoid injuring the third nerve by these manipulations, and indeed it may be necessary to encircle the nerve in a curved aperture clip so that it is not deformed or compressed by the clip itself.

POSTERIOR CEREBRAL ARTERY ANEURYSMS

Aneurysms arise typically at four sites along the course of the posterior cerebral artery: (1) at the origin of the large perforating branches of the Pl artery, (2) at the junction of the

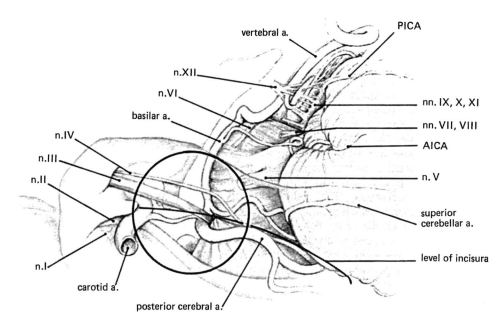

posterior communicating artery and the Pl artery, (3) at the origin of the anterior temporal and internal occipital arteries along the side of the brain stem, and (4) at the terminal branching of the vessel into its parietal and calcarine arteries. The most common sites are at the Pl and at the anterior temporal artery at the side of the brain stem.

The more proximal aneurysms are usually dealt with in exactly the same manner as are aneurysms of the terminal basilar artery. They may be easy aneurysms to dissect because they are relatively lateral and are generally situated a few millimeters away from the major perforators going to the peduncle. These perforators must be identified in the case of large or giant aneurysms, and separating these from the aneurysmal neck may provide a technical challenge. The most distal aneurysms are frequently hidden under the hippocampal gyrus and require retraction relatively posteriorly and, occasionally, require resection of a small portion of the gyrus. This is almost always necessary with those aneurysms lying in the mouth of the choroidal fissure. As with any aneurysm, the purpose is to secure the neck while maintaining normal flow through the parent and branching vessels in the region. Tiny posterior cerebral artery perforators are a lesser problem except for the segment that winds around the midbrain and normally gives rise to several circumferential vessels that must be seen and preserved. More distally (i.e., beyond the emergence of the anterior temporal artery), it is usually acceptable and quite safe to proximally occlude the parent vessel to a large posterior cerebral aneurysm.

In our experience, the posterior cerebral artery has perhaps the richest potential for collateralization of any of the major cerebral arteries. In 47 patients without visual field deficits in which we have deliberately or inadvertently occluded the posterior cerebral artery, we have noted only five cases of a persistent visual field defect, and one of these was only a superior quadrantic defect. One must be exceptionally cautious, however, not to occlude the vessel proximal to the posterior choroidal arteries because ischemia and infarction in the territory of these vessels can be devastating.

CONCLUSIONS AND RESULTS

The evolution of the surgical techniques for aneurysms of the vertebral basilar system has resulted in increasingly satisfactory results as our surgical expertise has grown and has been supported by refinements in neuroradiology and neuroanesthesia. It is now possible to attack aneurysms on the vertebral basilar system and to anticipate results as good as results obtained on aneurysms of the anterior circulation. In nearly 950 cases of smaller aneurysms in the posterior circulation, Drake and Peerless experienced a surgical mortality rate (all deaths within 90 days) of 3.6%, which included the earliest endeavors with these aneurysms as well as patients in poor condition. The risks and complications of surgical attack on large aneurysms increase proportionately with the size of the lesion, but, even so, in more than 1767 surgical cases they achieved excellent or good results in 83.9%, an overall surgical mortality rate of 6.6%, and an overall management morbidity rate of 9.6%. The basilar bifurcation remains the most hazardous site for large and small aneurysms of the posterior circulation, and it needs to be stressed again that it is the inadvertent rupture or occlusion of perforators of the Pl artery, or occlusion of the terminal basilar artery by the clip or atheroma, that accounts for most of the incidences of mortality and morbidity. It is essential for the surgeon to be completely familiar with the anatomy of the region and to accept only precise and accurate placement of the clip in every case. With technical experience and uniform excellence in neuroanesthesia, most, if not all, saccular aneurysms of the vertebral basilar system will be amenable to direct surgical treatment.

The rupture of an intracranial aneurysm continues to cause serious incidences of morbidity and mortality resulting from the direct effect of the hemorrhage and secondary cerebral ischemia.[26] The microsurgical repair of unruptured aneurysms of the vertebrobasilar system can, with the methods described above, be accomplished with a risk of less than 2.5%.[27] It is unlikely that further refinement of anesthesia, surgery, or medical management of subarachnoid hemorrhage will match the results obtained from recognition and treatment of these deadly sacs before their rupture.

REFERENCES

1. Dandy WE: Intracranial Arterial Aneurysms. Ithaca, NY: Comstock, 1944.
2. Tönnis W: Zur Behandlung intrakraniellar Aneurysmen. Arch Klin Chir 189:474, 1937.
3. Falconer MA: Surgical treatment of spontaneous intracranial hemorrhage. Br Med J 1:790, 1958.
4. Poppen JL: Vascular surgery of the posterior fossa. Proc Congr Neurol Surg 6:198, 1969.
5. Logue V: Posterior fossa aneurysms. In Shillito J, Mosberg WH (eds): Clinical Neurosurgery, vol 11. Baltimore: Williams & Wilkins, 1964, pp 183–207.
6. Schwartz HG: Arterial aneurysms of the posterior fossa. J Neurosurg 5:312, 1948.
7. Drake CG: Bleeding aneurysms of the basilar artery: Direct surgical management in four cases. J Neurosurg 23:230, 1961.
8. Hoeoek O, Norlen G, Guzman J: Saccular aneurysms of the vertebral-basilar arterial system: A report of 28 cases. Acta Neurol Scand 39:271–304, 1963.
9. Jamieson KG: Aneurysms of the vertebrobasilar system: Surgical intervention in 19 cases. J Neurosurg 21:781, 1964.
10. Drake CG: Surgical treatment of ruptured aneurysms of the basilar artery: Experience with 14 cases. J Neurosurg 23:457, 1965.
11. Yasargil MG, Antic J, Laciga R, et al: Microsurgical pterional approach to aneurysms of the basilar bifurcation. Surg Neurol 6:83, 1976.
12. Yasargil MG: Vertebrobasilar aneurysms. In Yasargil MG (ed): Microneurosurgery in 4 Volumes, vol II. Stuttgart: Georg Thieme Verlag, 1986, pp 232–295.
13. Drake CG: Further experience with surgical treatment of aneurysms of the basilar artery. J Neurosurg 29:372, 1968.
14. Drake CG, Peerless SJ, Hernesniemi JA: Surgery of Vertebrobasilar Aneurysms: London, Ontario Experience on 1767 Patients. Vienna: Springer-Verlag, 1996, pp 300–329.
15. Tateshima S, Murayama Y, Gobin YP, et al: Endovascular treatment of basilar tip aneurysms using Guglielmi detachable coils: Anatomic and clinical outcomes in 73 patients from a single institution. Neurosurgery 47:1332–1342, 2000.
16. Hernesniemi J, Ishii K, Niemelä M, et al: Subtemporal approach to basilar bifurcation aneurysms: Advanced technique and clinical experience. Acta Neurochir Suppl 94:1–38, 2005.
17. Niemelä M, Koivisto T, Kivipelto L, et al: Microsurgical clipping of cerebral aneurysms after the ISAT study. Acta Neurochir Suppl 94:3–6, 2005.
18. Hernesniemi J, Ishii K, Karatas A, et al: Surgical technique to retract the tentorial edge during subtemporal approach: Technical note. Neurosurgery (in press).
19. Samson D, Batjer HH, Kopitnik TA: Current results of the surgical management of aneurysms of the basilar apex. Neurosurgery 44:697–702, 1999.
20. Hsu FPK, Clatterbuck RE, Spetzler RF: Orbitozygomatic approach to basilar apex aneurysms. Neurosurgery 56(Suppl 1):172–177, 2005.
21. Lawton MT: Basilar apex aneurysms: Surgical results and perspectives from an initial experience. Neurosurgery 50:1–10, 2002.
22. Krisht AF, Kadri PA: Surgical clipping of complex basilar apex aneurysms: A strategy for successful outcome using the pretemporal transzygomatic transcavernous approach. Neurosurgery 56(Suppl 2):261–273, 2005.
23. Lozier AP, Kim GH, Sciacca RR, Connolly ES, Jr., Solomon R: Microsurgical treatment of basilar apex aneurysms: Perioperative and long-term clinical outcome. Neurosurgery 54:286–299, 2004.
24. Ogilvy CS, Hoh BL, Singer RJ, Putman CM: Clinical and radiographic outcome in the management of posterior circulation aneurysms by use of direct surgical or endovascular techniques. Neurosurgery 51:14–22, 2002.
25. Muizelaar JP: The use of electroencephalography and brain protection during operation for basilar aneurysms. Neurosurgery 25:899–903, 1989.
26. Hernesniemi JA, Vapalahti MP, Niskanen M, Kari A: Management outcome in vertebrobasilar artery aneurysms by early surgery. Neurosurgery 31:857–862, 1992.
27. Rice BJ, Peerless SJ, Drake CG: Surgical treatment of unruptured aneurysms of the posterior circulation. J Neurosurg 73:165–173, 1990.

84 Surgical Management of Midbasilar and Lower Basilar Aneurysms

MARK G. HAMILTON, IAN G. FLEETWOOD, and ROBERT F. SPETZLER

Aneurysms of the midbasilar and lower basilar artery are those that are located below the level of the superior cerebellar artery and involve the anteroinferior cerebellar artery (AICA), the inferior basilar trunk, and the vertebrobasilar junction.

Aneurysms of the midbasilar and lower basilar artery represent less than 1% of cerebral aneurysms in most neurosurgical series. Yamaura[1] reported a frequency of 10 midbasilar and lower basilar artery aneurysms in 202 posterior circulation aneurysms (5%), whereas Sano and colleagues[2] reported that they accounted for 7 of 1480 (0.5%) total cerebral aneurysms and for 7 of 116 (6%) posterior circulation aneurysms. In their earlier work, Peerless and Drake[3] reported that midbasilar and lower basilar artery aneurysms accounted for 193 of all 1266 (15.2%) of their cases of posterior circulation aneurysms. In their more recent publication describing 1767 patients, aneurysms of the basilar trunk and vertebrobasilar junction were seen in 14.7% of patients.[4] In the interval January 1988 to December 1992, 115 posterior circulation aneurysms were treated at the Barrow Neurological Institute, representing 11.2% of all aneurysms. Among these cases there were 17 patients with 18 midbasilar and lower basilar aneurysms, representing 15.7% of posterior circulation aneurysms and 1.8% of all aneurysms treated during this interval.

Recent large multicenter studies may overestimate the frequency of aneurysms in this anatomic location. In the original report from the International Study of Unruptured Intracranial Aneurysms (ISUIA), posterior circulation aneurysms (excluding basilar tip aneurysms) were seen in 6.2% of all patients.[5] In a subsequent report from this study, these compose 5.1% of all patients with unruptured aneurysms, 3.9% of those who had surgical clipping, and 8.9% of those who had their aneurysms coiled.[6] Alternatively, the International Subarachnoid Aneurysm Trial (ISAT) probably incorporates a preestablished treatment bias in Europe, since only 2.7% of randomized patients had posterior circulation aneurysms and only one of the 2143 patients (0.05%) analyzed had a basilar trunk aneurysm.[7]

The clinical features of subarachnoid hemorrhage (SAH) occurring in patients with aneurysms located in this region of the posterior circulation are the same as those associated with other cerebral aneurysms. Unruptured aneurysms that are of giant size may produce neurologic symptoms specific to their anatomic location (i.e., brain stem, cranial nerves). The natural history of hemorrhage in aneurysms located in the midbasilar or lower basilar artery is also identical to that in cerebral aneurysms located in other areas. The basic principles of management are, therefore, not markedly different.

MANAGEMENT PRINCIPLES

Patients presenting with SAH and aneurysms located on the midbasilar and lower basilar artery are managed utilizing the same protocols previously established for other patients with SAH[8]: cardiorespiratory and basic neurologic supportive care, early ventriculostomy with cerebrospinal fluid (CSF) drainage in patients with Hunt-Hess[9] grades IV and V SAH,[10] early surgery in suitable cases,[8,10] prophylaxis, and, when appropriate, aggressive management of post-SAH cerebral vasospasm with ischemic deficit[8,11,12] and aggressive management of raised intracranial pressure.[8,10] Patients presenting with neurologic symptoms related to the mass effect of the aneurysm are managed semiurgently. Typically, these patients present with signs of brain stem compression or cranial nerve deficits, and careful consideration of these deficits is required during planning of the treatment approach and the timing of intervention.

Endovascular management of aneurysms of the middle and lower basilar artery is increasingly reported.[13–17] However, evidence of treatment durability is currently lacking. Several recent reports also describe enhancements in surgical technique and outcomes associated with these improvements.[18–24]

The general rules for the anesthetic management of patients undergoing surgical clipping involve the use of preoperative corticosteroids and prophylactic intravenous antibiotics. Intraoperative hypotension is prevented, and the intraoperative blood pressure is allowed to run mildly hypertensive, especially during any temporary vessel clipping. In addition, during exposure and clipping of the aneurysm, all patients receive intravenous doses of a barbiturate (thiopental) titrated to achieve electroencephalographic (EEG) burst suppression.

GENERAL SURGICAL PRINCIPLES

The general principles for treatment of aneurysms located on this part of the basilar artery are the same as those for aneurysms anywhere in the cerebral circulation. The objective is complete isolation of the aneurysm from the cerebral circulation with preservation of the normal vasculature. Of particular importance in these aneurysms is preservation of the small perforating arteries from the basilar artery. This can be accomplished when maximum exposure of the basilar artery has been achieved with a minimum of brain retraction. With adequate visualization of the anatomic features and controlled application of an aneurysm clip of appropriate length and shape, the neck of the aneurysm can usually be obliterated and the parent vessels and perforators preserved.

Hypothermic Cardiac Standstill

In certain cases, the size of the aneurysm precludes adequate visualization of the parent vessel and of the perforators. This problem is often most difficult in basilar artery aneurysms. In these situations, additional exposure can be obtained through the use of hypothermic cardiac arrest with barbiturate cerebral protection.[25] During cardiac arrest, the aneurysm can be collapsed and the anatomic characteristics defined without the risk of hemorrhage. Since the original report from the Barrow Neurological Institute (BNI) in 1986[25] hypothermic cardiac arrest has been utilized in many patients with posterior circulation aneurysms.

The successful use of hypothermic cardiac standstill requires an experienced cardiovascular and cerebrovascular team. The success of hypothermic cardiac arrest in clipping of complex aneurysms is partially determined by four key variables: depth of hypothermia, duration of circulatory arrest, use of barbiturates, and hemostasis.[25] In the original BNI series, the mean brain temperature during standstill was 54°F, and the mean duration of standstill about 22 minutes (range, 3–72 minutes). The absolute maximum safe period of cerebral ischemia is not known. The duration of cerebral ischemia that can be safely tolerated is significantly increased, however, by the utilization of profound hypothermia and precooling intravenous barbiturates administered to achieve burst suppression of EEG activity.

The major complication of hypothermic cardiac standstill has been postoperative hemorrhage (11% in the BNI series). Meticulous, absolute hemostasis and close attention to the patient's clotting mechanisms must be used. Therefore, the inherent morbidity involved with circulatory arrest stipulates that it be used only in those patients for whom exposure and control of the parent vessels and aneurysm cannot be achieved with routine surgical techniques, including such measures as the application of multiple temporary aneurysm clips.

SURGICAL APPROACHES

Anatomic Issues in Surgical Exposure

Aneurysms of the midbasilar and inferior basilar artery are located in a small, restricted area encased within thick dense bone, situated within a subarachnoid space that is limited in size and filled with the densest collection of vital cranial nerve and vascular structures in the nervous system. The general goals of aneurysm surgery must, therefore, be accomplished with a minimum of brain retraction: (1) proximal and distal vascular control; (2) preservation of the

principal vessels, their branches, and the perforating vessels supplying the brain stem and cranial nerves; (3) complete obliteration of the aneurysm.

Previously, aneurysms at this location were treated through either a subtemporal-transtentorial approach or the suboccipital approach.[2,26–28] Although a transoral-transclival or transmaxillary-transclival approach has been utilized to expose the basilar artery by Peerless and Drake[3] and others,[2,29,30] it has notable technical limitations of exposure and a significant risk of postoperative CSF leak and meningitis.[3] These various techniques can provide access, but they do not meet the requirements of maximal exposure combined with minimal brain retraction. A number of techniques have been devised to maximize lateral bone removal and provide a relatively short and flat route of access to the front of the brain stem and the basilar artery: transpetrosal approach,[31,32] combined supratentorial-infratentorial approach,[33] far lateral approach,[34–36] and far lateral–combined supratentorial-infratentorial approach.[31] Each of these techniques, when appropriately matched to the location and size of the aneurysm, can provide excellent access to virtually any aneurysm located on the midbasilar and lower basilar artery (Table 84-1).

Transpetrosal Approaches

The anterior brain stem and clival regions can be reached through removal of portions of the petrosal bone with almost no brain or brain stem retraction. There are three variations of the temporal (petrous) bone dissection: the retrolabyrinthine technique, which involves petrous bone resection with preservation of hearing; the translabyrinthine technique, which utilizes greater petrous bone resection and

---

TABLE 84-1 ▪ Surgical Approaches in Treatment of Aneurysms of the Midbasilar and Lower Basilar Artery

Transpetrosal Approaches
Retrolabyrinthine
Translabyrinthine
Transcochlear

Combined Supra- and Infratentorial Approaches
Retrolabyrinthine
Translabyrinthine
Transcochlear

Far Lateral Approach

Extreme Lateral Craniocervical Approach

Far Lateral: Combined Supra- and Infratentorial ("Combined-Combined") Approaches
Retrolabyrinthine
Translabyrinthine
Transcochlear

Anterior Transclival Approaches
Transoral (transpalatal)
Transmaxillary
Transfacial

Other Approaches
Extended orbitozygomatic
Anterior petrosectomy
Subtemporal
Unilateral suboccipital

sacrifice of hearing; and the transcochlear technique, which involves maximal petrous bone resection with sacrifice of hearing and transposition of the facial nerve.[33] Moving through these three variations presents a gradual increase in the amount of petrous bone resected and in the exposure of the brain stem and of the clivus.

For these exposures, the patient is positioned supine on the operating table with the head positioned parallel to the floor, inclined slightly downward, and fixed to the operating table in the Mayfield headrest. A soft roll is placed under the ipsilateral shoulder to provide support.

The skin incision begins 3 cm posterior to the pinna and continues in a gentle curving fashion around the ear to the inferior border of the mastoid. The ear is retracted inferiorly with fishhooks attached to a Leyla bar. This maneuver exposes part of the temporal squama, external auditory meatus, and mastoid region. The neuro-otologist performs the approach through the temporal (petrous) bone and exposes the sigmoid sinus and dura 1 to 2 cm posterior to the sinus, after which the neurosurgeon performs the intradural part of the procedure. The mastoidectomy portion of the temporal bone procedure is completed with a high-speed drill (Medtronic Midas Rex, Midas Rex Institute, Inc., Fort Worth, TX), whereas the Osteon system (Linvatec Corporation, Largo, FL) is used with the operating microscope for the more detailed bone removal. Suction irrigation is used continuously during the temporal bone drilling.

Retrolabyrinthine Approach

The retrolabyrinthine approach provides excellent access into the cerebellopontine angle but does not allow significant anterior visualization of the brain stem; therefore, it has a limited, isolated role in management of aneurysms of the midbasilar and lower basilar artery. A retrolabyrinthine approach is used if hearing is to be preserved. The posterior and superior semicircular canals are skeletonized by drilling as far anteriorly as possible, both above and below the otic capsule, to expose as much dura as possible (Fig. 84-1A). The bone overlying the superior petrosal sinus and sigmoid sinus is removed with the drill. The endolymphatic sac and duct are preserved.

Recent studies describe a variation of the retrolabyrinthine approach designed to improve the surgical corridor to the midbasilar region but without necessarily jeopardizing hearing.[22,24] Noting that in some reports and series, incidental or accidental injuries to the semicircular canals are not universally associated with hearing loss, the transmastoid partial labyrinthectomy was described as a modification to the standard retrolabyrinthine approach. The posterior and superior semicircular canals are occluded and resected, but the vestibule and lateral semicircular canal are preserved. Serviceable hearing can be preserved in 80% of patients using this technique.[22]

Translabyrinthine Approach

If greater exposure is required, the standard translabyrinthine approach, which sacrifices hearing, can be used. The initial part of this approach is performed as described for the retrolabyrinthine approach but involves the additional complete removal of all three semicircular canals and skeletonization of the posterior half of the internal auditory canal (see Fig. 84-1B). More bone is removed from the face of the petrous pyramid than is possible with the retrolabyrinthine technique. Removal of all the bone overlying the sigmoid sinus and, if necessary, the jugular bulb provides greater exposure of the inferior aspect of the clivus. The posterior external auditory canal and the bone overlying the mastoid segment of the facial nerve should also be thinned to minimize the obstruction to visualization of the clivus. The distal end of the superior vestibular nerve in the vestibule is used as a reference for identification of the facial nerve as it exits the internal auditory canal. The bone overlying the labyrinthine segment of the facial nerve is also thinned with cautious drilling utilizing a diamond bit and continuous intraoperative monitoring of facial nerve function.

The translabyrinthine approach is a more direct, anterolateral approach to the cerebellopontine angle, allowing greater exposure of the anterolateral brain stem because of the removal of additional petrous bone. Although this exposure sacrifices ipsilateral hearing and is associated with an increased risk of CSF leakage, it is commonly required for these difficult aneurysms.

Transcochlear Technique

For the greatest exposure of the clivus, the transcochlear technique is used (see Fig. 84-1C). The external auditory canal is transected and oversewn in two layers. After the translabyrinthine exposure, the facial nerve is removed from its temporal bone canal,[37] the greater superficial petrosal nerve is sectioned, and the facial nerve is transposed posteriorly, utilizing the dura of the internal auditory canal to protect part of the nerve. The entire tympanic portion of the temporal bone is removed with exposure of the periosteum of the temporomandibular joint. The internal auditory canal and cochlea are then removed. Exposure of the jugular bulb is accomplished by removal of the bone that separates it from the internal carotid artery at the skull base. The bone surrounding the carotid artery is removed to the siphon.

If direct exposure of the internal carotid artery is unnecessary, a thin rim of bone can be left encasing the vessel. The option of extensive internal carotid artery exposure allows for a direct saphenous vein bypass graft from the petrous portion of the internal carotid artery to the subarachnoid internal carotid artery if necessary.[31,38] Bone is also removed from the floor of the plate of the middle fossa to the horizontal segment of the internal carotid artery. The difference in the amount of resection of the petrous ridge between the retrolabyrinthine and the transcochlear approaches can be appreciated on the postoperative computed tomographic (CT) reconstruction scans (Fig. 84-2).

The transcochlear technique gives a very flat angle of approach to the clivus and excellent exposure of both the anterior and anterolateral aspects of the brain stem. This exposure is gained, however, at the expense of sacrificing hearing and increasing the risk of facial nerve paralysis. In addition, the chance of CSF leakage is high.

Intradural Exposure and Closure

Whichever one of the aforementioned extradural bony exposures is used, the dura mater is incised just inferior and parallel to the superior petrosal sinus and just superior to the jugular bulb. These two dural incisions meet at the sinodural angle and the porus acusticus. The dura mater of the internal

FIGURE 84-1 The three variations in the combined supra- and infratentorial approach from the surgeon's viewpoint. *A*, Extended retrolabyrinthine approach with skeletonized posterior and superior semicircular canals and mastoidectomy. *B*, Translabyrinthine approach. Note that all three semicircular canals have been removed and a portion of the facial nerve has been skeletonized. *C*, The transcochlear approach, which involves extending the translabyrinthine technique by posteriorly transposing the facial nerve and aggressively drilling away the medial aspect of the petrous bone. (From Spetzler RF, Daspit CP, Pappas CT: The combined supra- and infratentorial approach for lesions of the petrous and clival regions: Experience with 46 cases. J Neurosurg 76:588–599, 1992.)

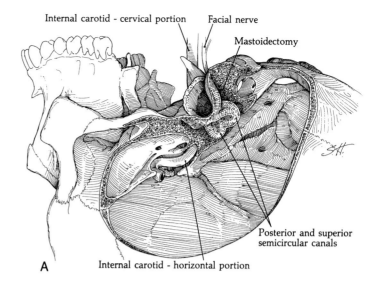

A

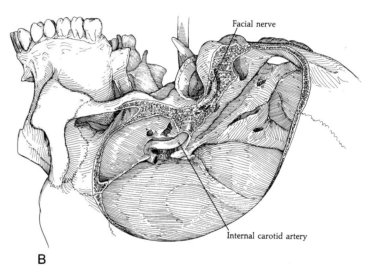

B

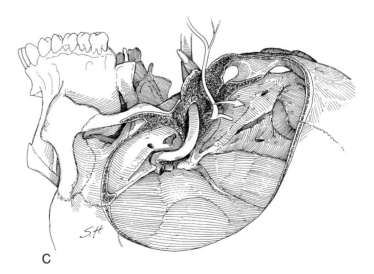

C

auditory canal is opened, and the cerebellopontine angle is entered. The surgical procedure is then carried out according to the specific principles of aneurysm surgery as elaborated on earlier. Following obliteration of the aneurysm, closure of the surgical field is accomplished in anatomic layers when possible. The temporal and occipital dura is reapproximated with 4-0 braided nylon suture. Abdominal adipose tissue, temporalis muscle, and fibrin glue are used to obliterate the eustachian tube in the translabyrinthine transcochlear approaches, as well as the void created by the

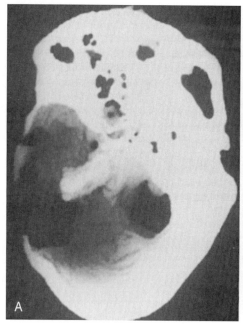 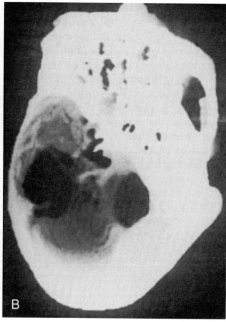

FIGURE 84-2 Postoperative 3-dimensional CT scans of bone window reconstruction comparing petrous bone resection by the retrolabyrinthine approach (*A*) with total petrous bone resection as performed with the transcochlear approach (*B*). (From Spetzler RF, Daspit CP, Pappas CT: The combined supra- and infratentorial approach for lesions of the petrous and clival regions: Experience with 46 cases. J Neurosurg 76:588–599, 1992.)

temporal bone resection. Temporary lumbar spinal drainage of CSF is used for 3 to 5 days to prevent CSF leakage through the wound.

Selection of Surgical Approach

The selection of the particular variation of the transpetrosal approaches for aneurysms of the midbasilar and lower basilar artery is based on: (1) the location of the aneurysm, (2) the size of the aneurysm, and (3) an estimation of the amount of temporal bone that must be removed to obtain an adequate exposure of the aneurysm and to obtain proximal and distal vascular control.

The salient features of the various approaches can be summarized as follows:

- The retrolabyrinthine approach provides excellent exposure of the cerebellopontine angle but not of the anterior brain stem and preserves function of both hearing and the facial nerves.
- The translabyrinthine approach offers greater exposure of the cerebellopontine angle and significantly improves exposure of the anterolateral and anterior brain stem, but at the expense of hearing and with an increased risk of CSF leakage.
- The transcochlear technique achieves the maximal exposure possible but accomplishes it with not only the disadvantages associated with the translabyrinthine technique but also an increased risk of facial nerve paralysis.

A generally problematic aspect of all the transpetrosal approaches, apart from the associated morbidity from the bone removal, is that the surgical corridor to the aneurysm is necessarily lateral to the lesion by the nature of the bony exposure. This can increase the difficulty with aneurysm clipping, because the surgeon may then need to explore around the dome of the aneurysm during dissection and preparation for clipping and may also need to manipulate the aneurysm during clipping to visualize the entire neck.

The senior author has explored the use of alternate approaches, specifically the extended orbitozygomatic approach for lesions of the distal two fifths of the basilar artery or the far lateral approach for lesions of the proximal two fifths of the basilar artery and vertebrobasilar junction.[20] These approaches leave only the truly midbasilar (i.e., middle one fifth of the basilar artery) for transpetrosal approaches. The advantage of these alternate strategies, with or without hypothermic cardiac arrest, is that they allow visualization along the axis of the basilar artery, with good exposure of the neck and perforating vessels, facilitating aneurysm obliteration with a straight clip.

Using this more selected approach led to good outcomes on the Glasgow Outcome Scale (GOS)[39] in 75% of patients (GOS 4 and 5).[20] Only 11% had permanent treatment-related neurologic deficits, and there were four deaths, but only one in the perioperative period.

Combined Supra- and Infratentorial Approaches

The exposure of the basilar artery provided by a transpetrosal approach can be considerably enhanced when it is combined with a supratentorial approach. Using a combined supra- and infratentorial surgical approach, in conjunction with the operating microscope, one gains an exposure extending from the sphenoid ridge and cavernous sinus to the foramen magnum and anterior cervical spinal cord with minimal brain retraction. The combined approach requires the skills of both a neurosurgeon and a neuro-otologist, in that it utilizes: (1) variable degrees of temporal bone removal, (2) a supra- and infratentorial craniotomy, and (3) division of the tentorium to connect the supra- and infratentorial compartments.

Although variations of the combined approach had been described since the first in 1905 by Borchardt, it had largely been abandoned, in part as a result of a high mortality rate and the improvements in the suboccipital approach offered by Cushing and Dandy. Hitselberger and House,[32] in 1966, described a combined suboccipital-petrosal approach for the removal of large cerebellopontine angle tumors and discussed how the wide exposure obtained with this technique overcame the individual limitations of the suboccipital and translabyrinthine approaches for dealing with extensive lesions. Their technique extended the translabyrinthine approach beyond the sigmoid sinus into the suboccipital areas, to achieve a wide view of the cerebellopontine angle with minimal brain retraction, and allowed the sigmoid sinus to be mobilized or divided to improve the surgical exposure.

Malis[40] popularized the idea of combining the subtemporal and posterior fossa (suboccipital) approaches to improve the surgical exposure when treating extensive lesions of the clivus or medial petrous region. In Malis' version, the petrosal bone is not extensively drilled, and the superior anastomotic vein (vein of Labbé) is preserved by ligation of the transverse sinus between the entrance of the superior anastomotic vein posteriorly and the sigmoid sinus and superior petrosal sinus anteriorly. After division of the transverse sinus, the tentorium is split along the petrosal apex with sparing of the superior petrosal sinus. Elevation of the tentorium, transverse sinus, temporal lobe, and superior anastomotic vein allows exposure of the clivus down to the foramen magnum.

Morrison and King[41] also described a translabyrinthine-transtemporal approach to provide extensive exposure, through drilling of the petrous bone, from the cerebellopontine angle upward into the middle fossa. Exposure is increased by division of the superior petrosal sinus and of the tentorium. In 1977, Fisch[42] described the infratemporal fossa approach for extensive tumors of the temporal bone and base of the skull. Fisch combined a partial posterior and inferior petrosectomy with a cervicofacial approach. This approach provided good exposure of the jugular foramen but frequently required permanent anterior displacement of the facial nerve, resection of the zygomatic arch and mandibular condyle, and complete obliteration of the pneumatic spaces of the temporal bone. House and Hitselberger[43] modified the translabyrinthine approach by adding the transcochlear technique. Pellet and colleagues[44] combined the infratemporal approach of Fisch[42] and the transcochlear approach of House and Hitselberger[43] to create the widened transcochlear approach. This approach utilizes a petrosectomy to connect the posterior fossa to the superior carotid region, allowing for the single-stage removal of lesions that extend from the infratemporal region to the posterior fossa. The basic principles for the combined approach had thus been defined: variable amounts of petrous bone dissection with a supratentorial-infratentorial craniotomy and division of the tentorium. An important variable in the combined approach concerns the significance and fate of both the dural sinuses (superior petrosal, sigmoid, or transverse sinus) and the superior anastomotic vein.

A number of authors have also presented their experiences using variations of the combined infratemporal and posterior fossa approach for removal of large lesions involving the clivus and medial petrous region.[33,45–48] Some advocate preservation of the major dural sinus,[47,48] and others, with appropriate consideration for patency of the opposite transverse sinus, commonly sacrifice the sigmoid[33,45] or transverse sinus.[40]

Surgical Technique

The patient is positioned supine on the operating table with the head positioned parallel to the floor, inclined slightly downward, and fixed to the operating table in a Mayfield headrest. A soft roll is placed under the ipsilateral shoulder to give appropriate support. The skin incision begins at the level of the zygoma, 1 cm anterior to the ear, and continues in a gentle curving fashion around the ear to just below the mastoid tip. To obtain greater exposure, the posterior part of the incision can be extended farther posteriorly. To obtain an exposure that includes the foramen magnum, this combined approach can be combined with the far lateral suboccipital approach (discussed later).[31,34–36] The scalp flap is retracted inferiorly with fishhooks attached to a Leyla bar. This maneuver exposes the lateral aspect of the skull: the zygoma, lateral temporal bone, external auditory meatus, and mastoid region. The neuro-otologist performs the approach through the temporal (petrous) bone, after which the neurosurgeon performs a craniotomy with exposure of the remaining sigmoid sinus and transverse sinus, followed by the intradural part of the procedure.

After the neuro-otologist has completed the petrous bone resection, the neurosurgeon proceeds with a subtemporal-suboccipital craniotomy that crosses the transverse sinus and exposes the remainder of the sigmoid sinus. This results in exposure of a large dural surface. Brain relaxation, if required, is achieved initially with hyperventilation, administration of mannitol or barbiturates, or spinal drainage of CSF. Comprehensive electrophysiologic monitoring is routinely used: compressed spectral EEG, somatosensory evoked potentials, brain stem auditory responses in both ears or just the contralateral ear if ipsilateral hearing is to be sacrificed, and functional evaluation of facial and other appropriate cranial nerves. The anterior part of the dural incision (Fig. 84-3) is made over the temporal lobe and extends posteriorly to at least 1 cm below the site where the superior petrosal sinus enters the sigmoid sinus. Uncommonly, a low-lying superior anastomotic vein is found attached to the temporal dura or tentorium, and care must be exercised to prevent damaging this important vascular structure. If the sigmoid sinus is to be preserved, the dural incision crosses the superior petrosal sinus to join with a dural incision in front of the sigmoid sinus. The superior petrosal sinus can usually be either cauterized or clipped and subsequently divided. Another incision can be made behind the sigmoid sinus (see Fig. 84-3, inset)[47] to allow access, if necessary, in front of and behind the sinus.

Sacrifice of Sigmoid Sinus

Sacrifice of the sigmoid sinus can be considered if the contralateral transverse sinus and sigmoid sinus are patent (Fig. 84-4) and if these sinuses communicate with the sagittal sinus and ipsilateral transverse sinus through a patent confluence of the sinuses (confluens sinuum). To allow for further assurance that the sigmoid sinus can be sacrificed, we assess intravascular pressures within the sigmoid sinus before and after temporary occlusion of the sinus. Once the superficial petrosal sinus has been divided, a No. 25 needle is inserted into the sigmoid sinus just proximal to the temporary clip location and pressure is recorded. It has been our experience that intravascular pressure has not increased by more than 7 mm Hg with sigmoid sinus occlusion when the sinuses are patent. Should pressure in the sigmoid sinus rise more than 10 mm Hg with temporary occlusion, the sinus should be kept intact. If the sigmoid sinus is sacrificed, the

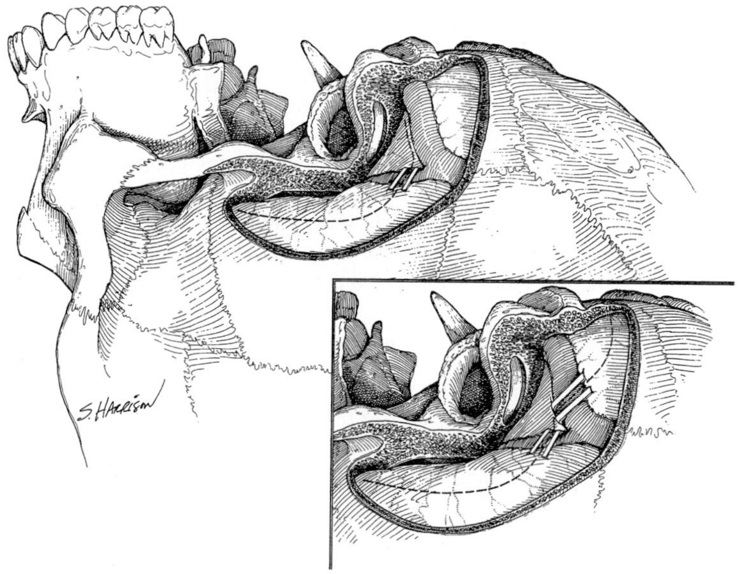

FIGURE 84-3 A right combined translabyrinthine approach. After the craniotomy and petrosal bone drilling have been completed, the dural opening is completed (*broken line*) along the floor of the middle fossa. The superior petrosal sinus is then divided between clips, and the dural opening is continued in the posterior fossa just anterior to the sigmoid sinus and the jugular bulb to the sinodural angle. An alternative dural incision (*inset*) crosses the sigmoid sinus. The sigmoid sinus can be sacrificed only if adequate collateral venous drainage can be demonstrated. (From Spetzler RF, Daspit CP, Pappas CT: The combined supra- and infratentorial approach for lesions of the petrous and clival regions: Experience with 46 cases. J Neurosurg 76:588–599, 1992.)

ipsilateral superior anastomotic vein drains contralaterally, because it consistently and reliably enters into the transverse sinus above the junction of the superior petrosal sinus and sigmoid sinus (see Fig. 84-4). We now keep the sigmoid sinus intact in the majority of patients.

Intradural Exposure

After the dural incisions have been completed, the superior petrosal sinus has been divided, and the fate of the sigmoid sinus has been determined, the dural incision is extended down through the tentorium (posterior to the fourth cranial nerve)

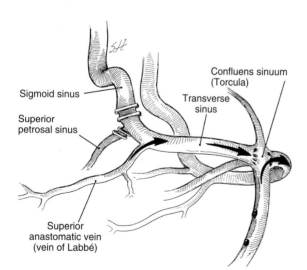

FIGURE 84-4 The major veins and dural venous sinuses that must be considered in the combined approaches. Orientation is as seen by the surgeon: the top of the figure is inferior anatomically, and the right side corresponds to the posterior anatomically. Before the sigmoid sinus can be ligated, a widely patent torcular and contralateral jugular venous system must be demonstrated angiographically. If the sigmoid sinus is sacrificed, the ipsilateral superior anastomotic vein (vein of Labbé) will drain contralaterally through the medial transverse sinus, across the confluens sinuum (Torcula) into the opposite jugular vein. (From Spetzler RF, Daspit CP, Pappas CTS: The combined supra- and infratentorial approach for lesions of the petrous and clival regions: Experience with 46 cases. J Neurosurg 76:588–599, 1992.)

to the tentorial hiatus, thus connecting the supra- and infratentorial compartments (Fig. 84-5). If the sigmoid sinus has been preserved, the posterior temporal lobe must be elevated, with care taken to protect the superior anastomotic vein, which is indirectly tethered to the skull base by the sigmoid sinus. The superior anastomotic vein can be mobilized by dissection from the cortical surface to minimize tension on the vessel.[48] These final maneuvers expose the ipsilateral petrous region, the entire clivus and brain stem, and the cranial nerves and major arterial vessels of the brain stem. With microscopic technique, tumors and vascular lesions can be resected or clipped between any pair of adjacent cranial nerves. These surgical approaches provide maximal angle of exposure along the base of the skull with minimal or no brain retraction (Fig. 84-6; see also Fig. 84-5).

Closure

Closure of the surgical field is accomplished in anatomic layers when possible. The temporal and occipital dura is reapproximated with 4-0 braided nylon suture. Abdominal adipose tissue, temporalis muscle, and fibrin glue are used to obliterate the eustachian tube (translabyrinthine) and the void created by temporal bone resection. Temporary lumbar spinal drainage of CSF is used for 3 to 5 days to prevent CSF leakage through the wound. A standard closure of the fascial and skin layers is then undertaken.

Selection of Surgical Approach

The selection of a particular variation of the combined approach for extensive lesions of the clivus and medial petrous region is based on the considerations outlined in the discussion concerning the transpetrosal approaches. Although sacrifice of the sigmoid sinus is optional, it provides further exposure, by permitting elevation of the temporal lobe, than is otherwise possible without stretching and potentially compromising the superior anastomotic vein. If the previously discussed procedure for verification of appropriate compensatory venous drainage is followed, no apparent risk appears to be associated with sacrifice of the sigmoid sinus.

FIGURE 84-5 A right transcochlear combined approach after the dura has been opened, the superior petrosal and sigmoid sinuses have been divided, and the tentorium has been divided down to the incisura. Division of the tentorium allows the superior anastomotic vein (vein of Labbé) to be retracted superiorly with the tentorial leaflets. The resultant approach to the brain stem and clivus is very flat and extends from the cavernous sinus down to the foramen magnum. (From Spetzler RF, Daspit CP, Pappas CT: The combined supra- and infratentorial approach for lesions of the petrous and clival regions: Experience with 46 cases. J Neurosurg 76:588–599, 1992.)

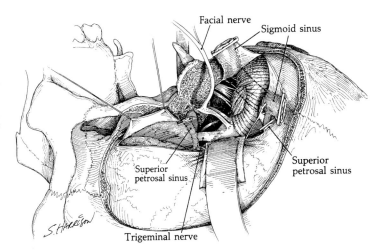

Treatment Complications

A detailed analysis of the first 46 patients reported in 1992[33] summarizes the operative risks associated with the combined approach. There was no operative mortality in this series, and the postoperative morbidity and mortality data compare favorably with those of previously published reports for this approach: the incidence of facial nerve paralysis in our patient series has remained about 30%, the incidence of CSF leak about 13%, and that of abducens paralysis about 7%. The incidence of other operative complications (numbness, aphasia, sepsis, hemiparesis, pneumonia, and hematoma) ranges between 2% and 4% for each.

The senior author has found that the combined supra- and infratentorial approach, with its appropriate variations, permits exquisite surgical exposure for treating most aneurysms involving the midbasilar and lower basilar artery. These approaches permit the surgeon to treat these lesions safely and adequately with a minimum of brain retraction.

Far Lateral Approach

The far lateral approach to the inferior clivus and upper cervical region is a technical modification that achieves lateral extension to the unilateral suboccipital approach

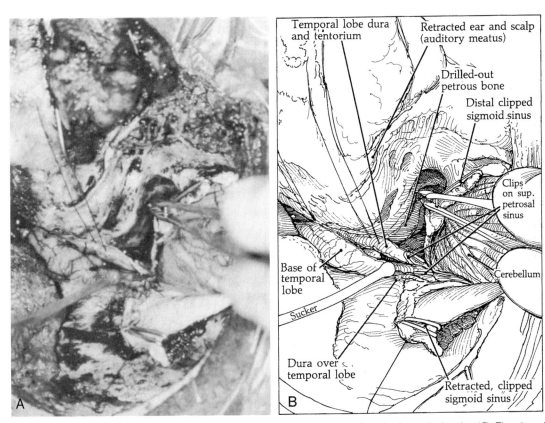

FIGURE 84-6 Translabyrinthine approach as illustrated by intraoperative photograph (*A*) and schematic drawing (*B*). The sigmoid sinus has been transected, and the dura of the temporal and posterior fossa has been opened. The tentorium will be divided along its entire length between the clips on the superior petrosal sinus. (From Spetzler RF, Daspit CP, Pappas CT: The combined supra- and infratentorial approach for lesions of the petrous and clival regions: Experience with 46 cases. J Neurosurg 76:588–599, 1992.)

and has been a neurosurgical "standard" for over a century.[34-36,49] This modification greatly enhances anterior exposure of this region (the inferior brain stem and clivus, upper cervical spine, and anterior spinal canal) and provides excellent access to the lower basilar artery and vertebrobasilar junction.

The main objective of the far lateral approach is to achieve a flat exposure to the anterior aspect of the inferior brain stem or upper cervical cord, and the associated neurovascular structures and cranial nerves, by removing the inferior rim of the foramen magnum as well as part of the occipital condyle and the posterolateral arch of C1 to the level of the sulcus arteriosus of the vertebral artery. The dural opening obtained after this bony removal provides maximal exposure and requires minimal retraction of neurovascular structures.

Patient Positioning

The patient is placed in a modified park-bench position that is different from the standard park-bench position in two features (Figs. 84-7 and 84-8): the position of the body and dependent arm, and the position of the head. Each of these features is critical to obtaining maximal exposure of the lesion with greatest ease for the surgeon and optimal safety for the patient.

The patient is placed in a Mayfield three-pin headrest (see Fig. 84-7) and positioned laterally on the operating table with the side to be treated facing upward. The operating table is extended by placing a 34-inch plastic board under the mattress and pulling the mattress and board 15 to 20 cm out past the table end. The patient's dependent arm is then allowed to drop off the extended end of the operating table and is carefully cradled in foam underneath the edge of the table, within the gap between the Mayfield headrest and the table attachment (see Figs. 84-7 and 84-8).

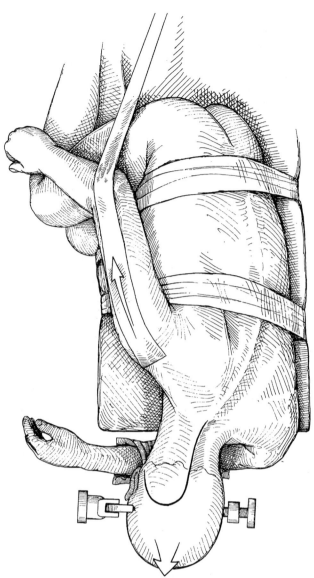

FIGURE 84-8 Schematic drawing of patient positioning for a right far lateral position viewed from above. The right arm is pulled downward with tape to open the craniocervical angle, and the patient is taped securely to the operating table to allow the angle to be changed during the procedure.

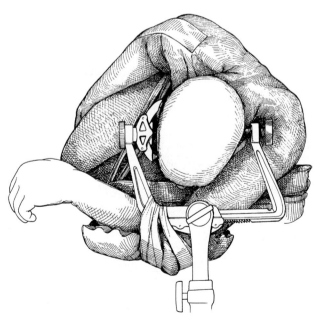

FIGURE 84-7 Schematic drawing of modified park-bench position for a right far lateral approach viewed from the cranial vertex. The three maneuvers outlined in the text have been performed. Note that the dependent arm has been padded and cradled beneath the Mayfield headrest. A foam roll is placed under the axilla for extra protection (not shown).

A foam roll is placed in the axilla. This placement of the arm improves venous return and decreases the risk of brachial plexus compression. In addition, the amount of cranial rotation and flexion that can be achieved is maximized by allowing the dependent arm to drop.

The head is not positioned in the standard straight lateral position. The position of the head is achieved with a sequence of three maneuvers that place the inferior clivus perpendicular to the floor and maximally open the posterior cervical-suboccipital angle, thereby allowing greater movement of the operating microscope around the operative field. The head is positioned with the midline parallel to the floor. Then, the head and neck are: (1) flexed in the anteroposterior plane until the chin is one fingerbreadth from the sternum, (2) rotated 45 degrees downward (to the contralateral side, away from the lesion), and (3) laterally flexed 30 degrees downward toward the opposite shoulder.

With the patient in this position, the ipsilateral mastoid process is at the highest point in the operative field. The upper shoulder is pulled down toward the feet and taped, thereby further enlarging the working space for the surgeon (see Fig. 84-8). The knees and upper arm are well padded, and the entire body is secured with tape to allow for full rotation of the operating table.

Surgical Technique

An inverted hockey-stick incision starts at the mastoid prominence and proceeds under the superior nuchal line to the midline, then follows the midline to the C3 or C4 spinous process (Fig. 84-9). A 1-cm edge of nuchal fascia and muscle is left at the upper incision to allow for anatomic closure of the wound. This nuchal cuff is obtained by dissecting under the muscle with a narrow periosteal elevator, starting from the midline and ending at the mastoid prominence. The fascia and muscle are then divided at the inferior edge of the instrument. At the time of closure, the Mayfield headrest is temporarily loosened from the table attachment, and the neck is extended to help reapproximate the cervical musculature to the nuchal fascia. The paraspinal muscles are split along the midline ligament until the spinous processes of C1 and C2 are identified. Subperiosteal dissection is used to expose the occipital bone as well as the spinous processes and ipsilateral laminae of C1 and C2. The myocutaneous flap is retracted inferiorly and laterally with fishhooks attached to a Leyla bar. The midline part of the incision can be retracted contralaterally with fishhooks from a second Leyla bar.

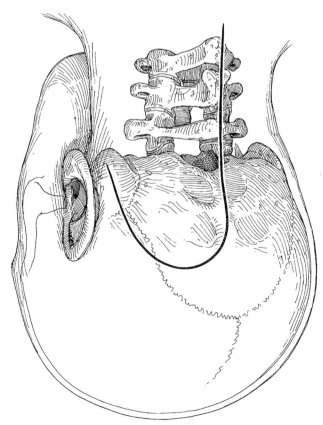

FIGURE 84-9 Close-up of the skin incision extending from the mastoid tip along the nuchal line to the midline, down to about C3 or C4 to allow for adequate muscle flap retraction.

The lateral mass of C1 and the vertebral artery from the sulcus of C1 to its point of posterior fossa dural entry are exposed. Bleeding from the venous plexus surrounding the vertebral artery is controlled with bipolar coagulation or small pieces of hemostatic material (e.g., Gelfoam, Surgicel). The Midas Rex drill with B1 bit and footplate is used to perform a C1 hemilaminectomy. The contralateral lamina is cut just across the midline, and the ipsilateral lamina is cut at the sulcus for the vertebral artery. The lamina can be replaced after the procedure is completed. A C2 hemilaminectomy can also be performed if additional caudal exposure is required.

A limited suboccipital, retrosigmoid craniotomy is performed with the same drill, extending from the contralateral margin of the foramen magnum (just past the midline) to as far lateral as possible and back down again to the foramen magnum, just medial to the level at which the vertebral artery enters the dura. The other dimension of the craniotomy—the height (the distance between the foramen magnum and the superior margin of the bone opening)—can extend to the level of the transverse sinus and is determined primarily by the location and size of the lesion (Fig. 84-10). Lesions confined to the foramen magnum do not require exposure to the transverse sinus. In addition, to provide access to clival lesions that extend beyond the reach of the far lateral approach, the craniotomy can be expanded with a transpetrosal procedure or past the level of the transverse sinus and tentorium when it is combined with the combined approach (see section on Far Lateral–Combined Supra- and Infratentorial Approach).

The next stage involves removal of bone from the remaining ipsilateral lateral rim of the foramen magnum and the occipital condyle. The rim of the foramen magnum is removed with a rongeur, and the posterior occipital condyle and the superior lateral mass and facet of C1 are removed with a high-speed drill. This is done by drilling away the inner portion of the condyle until only a thin shell of cortical bone remains. This "inside-out" approach, leaving a protective layer of cortical bone over the surrounding structures, facilitates safe removal in a restricted space. This shell is then carefully removed with microcurets. In addition, the extradural vertebral artery is protected with a small dissector while the condyle is drilled away. Entry into the condylar veins usually indicates that sufficient anterior bone has been removed, typically about 1 cm anterior (deep) to the point at which the vertebral artery enters the dura. Bleeding from these condylar vessels can readily be controlled with bone wax and bipolar coagulation. Because the hypoglossal canal is situated in the anterior medial third of the occipital condyle, it is not threatened by removal of the posterior lateral third of the condyle.[50] This extreme removal of lateral bone from the condyle and lateral mass of C1 is the crucial last step for approaching the anterior brain stem from an inferolateral angle with minimal brain retraction (see Fig. 84-10). Even more extensive exposure can be obtained by drilling away the mastoid process and the occipitoatlantal articular facet; however, bony fusion of the craniocervical junction is then needed to maintain postoperative stability.[51]

The dura is opened in a curvilinear fashion with its base hinged laterally and is pulled tight against the lateral aspect of the craniotomy with 4-0 braided nylon sutures. These tenting sutures are placed so that after passage of the needle

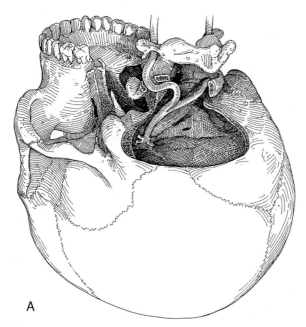

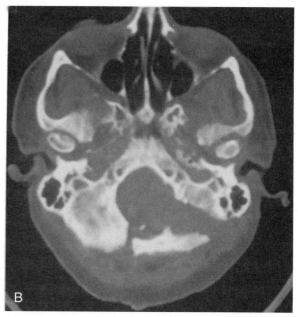

FIGURE 84-10 Illustration and postoperative CT scan illustrating the amount of bone resection. *A*, Schematic illustration demonstrating the perspective of the skull and vessels in relation to the amount of bone resection. It is important to resect the occipital and C1 condylar interface so that a gap of 1 cm is present between the extradural vertebral artery and the bone. *B*, Postoperative CT scan demonstrating the amount of bone removal that creates the lateral, extremely flat angle of approach to the clivus.

through the dura, both limbs of the suture are on the inside surface of the dura, thereby aiding in retracting the dura tightly against the underlying bone. The extensive extradural removal of the lateral bone eliminates the last obstruction to direct vision, without retraction, of the inferior clivus, anteroinferior brain stem, and upper anterior cervical spinal cord (Fig. 84-11). With arachnoidal microdissection and minimal elevation of the cerebellar tonsil, visualization is improved as far rostrally as the pontomedullary junction. In addition, this approach allows excellent proximal control of the vertebral artery and its branches.

Closure of the surgical field is accomplished in anatomic layers when possible. The cervical and occipital dura is reapproximated with 4-0 braided nylon suture. The C1 hemilamina and the craniotomy segment are returned to their normal positions and secured with small plates and screws or 2-0 braided nylon suture. A standard closure of the muscle, fascia, and skin layers is then accomplished.

Salas and colleagues have recently described a variation of the far lateral approach, which is designed to improve exposure and visualization of aneurysms at the vertebrobasilar junction.[21] The transtubercular approach initially involves extradural resection of the posteromedial one third of the occipital condyle and C1 lateral mass. Partial resection of jugular tubercle is also performed extradurally. The remainder of the tubercle is then craniectomized intradurally using a drill and working around the lower cranial nerves, with or without prior division of the sigmoid sinus (using similar principles for sinus division as described earlier).

Far Lateral–Combined Supra- and Infratentorial Approach

Occasionally, a more extensive lateral exposure of the clivus is required to deal with giant aneurysms involving the midbasilar and lower basilar artery. This can be accomplished by combining the far lateral approach with either a transpetrosal approach or the combined supra- and infratentorial approach.[31] This "combined-combined" approach offers a wide, flat route to the entire length of the clivus.

The combined-combined approach can be accomplished utilizing the principles previously outlined for the individual procedures. The skin incision for the far lateral approach is expanded to encompass the exposure needed for the transpetrosal or combined approach, thereby drawing

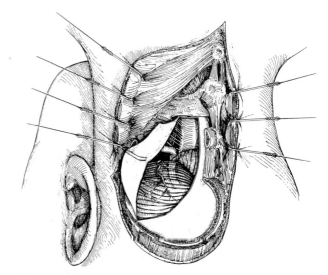

FIGURE 84-11 Schematic illustration demonstrating the dural opening and the amount of lateral exposure of the inferior clivus and associated neurovascular structures that can be obtained with the far lateral exposure. It is very important to have the superior and inferior limbs of the dural incision perpendicular to the wound edge to allow for maximum lateral retraction of the dural flap.

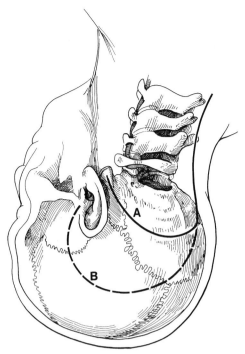

FIGURE 84-12 Schematic depiction of the skin incision used in the far lateral exposure (*A*) and the modification utilized in the combined-combined exposure (*B*). (From Baldwin HZ, Miller CG, Van Loveren HR, et al: The far lateral-combined supra- and infratentorial approach: A human cadaveric prosection model for routes of access to the petroclival region and ventral brain stem. J Neurosurg 81:60–68, 1994.)

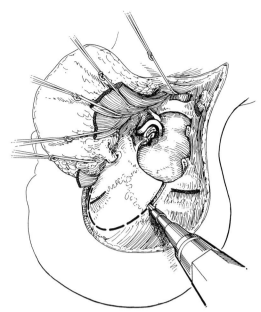

FIGURE 84-13 Schematic depiction of the craniotomy performed during the combined-combined procedure. In this illustration, the far lateral craniotomy has already been performed, and the craniotomy for the combined craniotomy is being performed. An alternative would be to perform the craniotomy as one segment that crosses the transverse sinus. Though not depicted, the neuro-otologist typically performs the petrosal drilling before the craniotomy flaps are turned. (From Baldwin HZ, Miller CG, Van Loveren HR, et al: The far lateral-combined supra- and infratentorial approach: A human cadaveric prosection model for routes of access to the petroclival region and ventral brain stem. J Neurosurg 81:60–68, 1994.)

the superior limb of the incision up over the ear, down to the level of the zygoma (Fig. 84-12). The transpetrosal drilling is completed by the neuro-otologist. The neurosurgeon then follows with the far lateral exposure. After the C1 hemilaminectomy has been completed, a craniotomy that starts at the foramen magnum and encompasses the suboccipital and temporal regions can be performed in two

sections (Fig. 84-13) or as a single unit. The dural opening for the far lateral and transpetrosal or combined techniques is completed, with joining of the two if the sigmoid sinus is ligated and divided (Fig. 84-14). The exposure of the anterior brain stem and basilar artery that can be obtained is exquisite. Closure of the dural opening and wound is performed as previously described.

FIGURE 84-14 Schematic illustration of the amount of intradural exposure provided in the retrolabyrinthine combined-combined approach. Note that the lateral view extends from about C2 up to the top of the basilar artery. The lateral angle can be greatly augmented by removal of the labyrinths (translabyrinthine approach). CN, cranial nerve; PCA, posterior cerebral artery; SCA, superior cerebral artery. (From Baldwin HZ, Miller CG, Van Loveren HR, et al: The far lateral-combined supra- and infratentorial approach: A human cadaveric prosection model for routes of access to the petroclival region and ventral brain stem. J Neurosurg 81:60–68, 1994.)

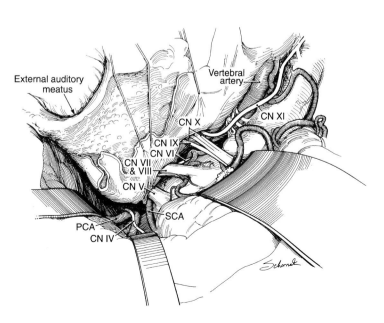

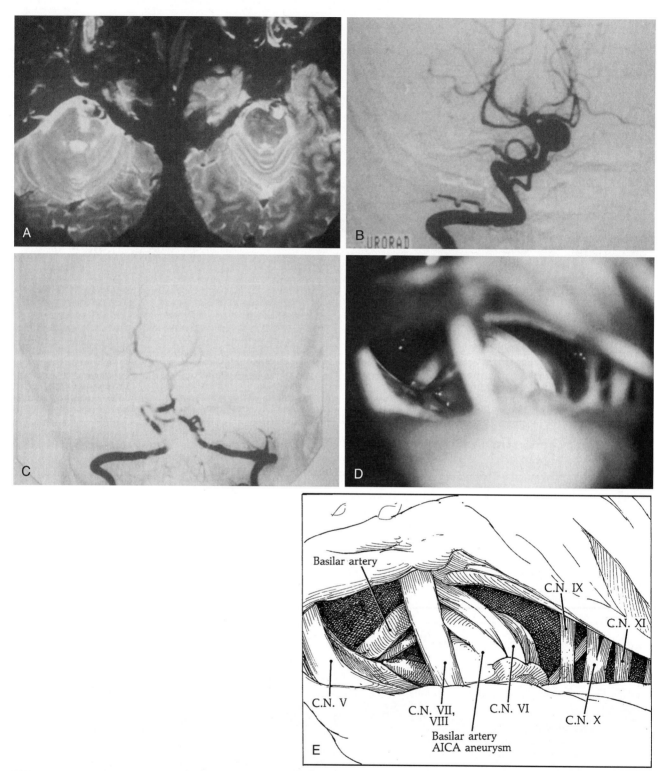

FIGURE 84-15 Case 1. A 20-year-old man presenting with a left hemiparesis. *A,* The preoperative magnetic resonance imaging (MRI) scan demonstrates the aneurysm and an area of increased T2 signal (representing an area of infarction) in the brain stem in the image on the left. *B,* Preoperative anteroposterior vertebral artery angiogram depicting the large left anteroinferior cerebellar artery (AICA) aneurysm. *C,* Postoperative anteroposterior vertebral artery angiogram demonstrates complete occlusion of the aneurysm. Intraoperative photograph (*D*) and schematic drawing (*E*) demonstrating the exposure of the basilar artery and neck of the aneurysm along with the associated cranial nerves. Roman numerals denote cranial nerves. (*D* and *E,* From Spetzler RF, Daspit CP, Pappas CT: The combined supra- and infratentorial approach for lesions of the petrous and clival regions: Experience with 46 cases. J Neurosurg 76:588–599, 1992.)

Anterior Transclival Approaches

The various transclival approaches are used infrequently to treat aneurysms of the midbasilar and lower basilar artery. They are generally the subject of case reports or small institutional series. In general, the risks of CSF leak and meningitis are higher than with the previously described approaches. There is also risk of palate dysfunction when the transpalatal route is used, and with a transmaxillary approach, Le Fort osteotomies are used. Ogilvy and colleagues developed the transfacial transclival approach through a lateral rhinotomy incision, an alternative to the other transclival approaches to optimize exposure without maxillotomy and minimize complications.[19] Using this approach, they treated five patients with excellent surgical exposure, good cosmetic results, and no palatal dysfunction. Although three developed CSF leaks, none had any long-term sequelae of meningitis.

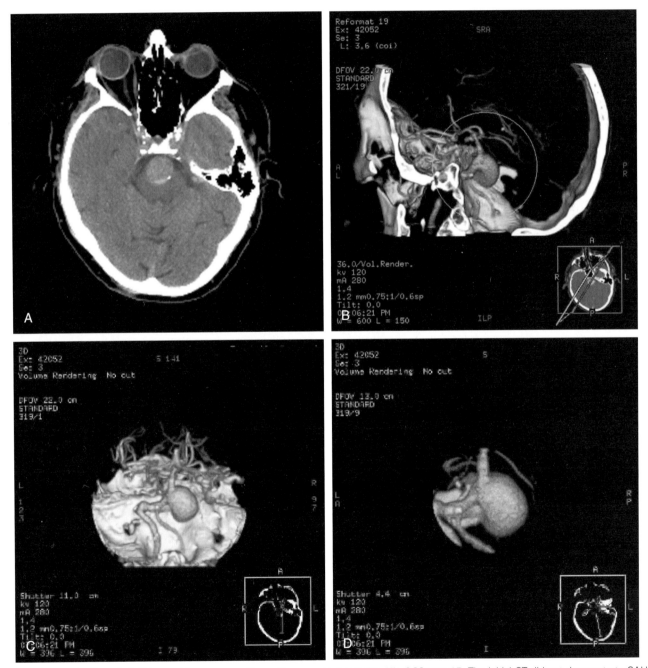

FIGURE 84-16   Case 2. A 77-year-old man presenting with an acute headache. His GCS was 15. The initial CT did not demonstrate SAH but did identify a 2.5-cm extra-axial mass (A) in the prepontine cistern consistent with a giant basilar aneurysm. The CTA superimposed on the skull (B) and CTA with progressive subtractions of bone (C and D) demonstrated a 2.5-cm left basilar artery aneurysm. On day 3 after presentation this patient developed sudden-onset tinnitus, vertigo, and nystagmus with right-sided incoordination.

(Continued)

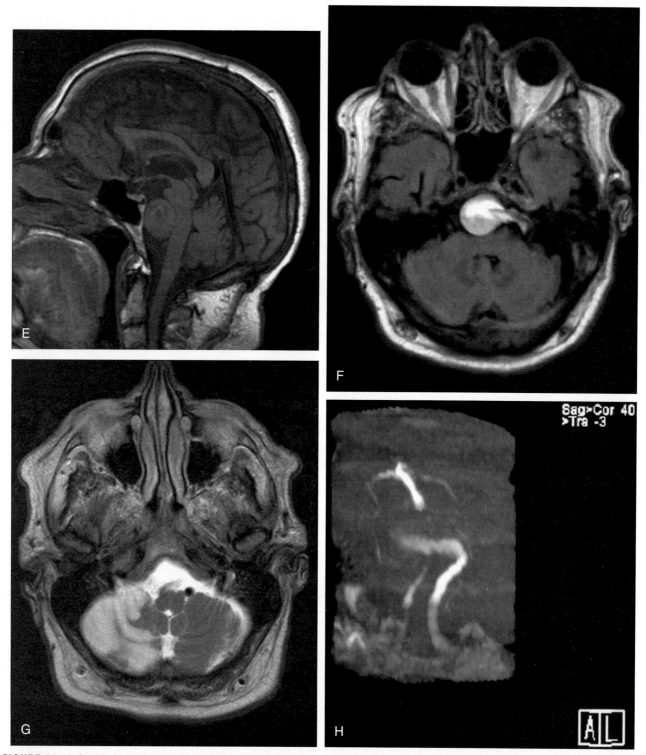

FIGURE 84-16 Cont'd His MRI (*E* to *G*) and MR angiogram (*H*) showed an acute to subacute posterior inferior cerebellar artery infarct (*G*), with some flow through the aneurysm and some thrombus present (*F* and *H*). This patient suffered a myocardial infarct and died on day 5 after presentation, before definitive therapy of the aneurysm could be considered.

Illustrative Cases

CASE REPORT 1

A 20-year-old man presented with an acute left hemiparesis. Investigations demonstrated a small pontine infarction related to a large (15–18 mm) left AICA aneurysm (Fig. 84-15). There was no evidence of SAH. Treatment of the aneurysm was initially attempted at another center with endovascular coils; however, the patient experienced a worsening of hemiparesis, and the coils were withdrawn. Over the next 24 hours, he experienced a return to baseline neurologic status. Subsequently, the senior author performed a left-sided combined (transcochlear) approach, utilizing 42 minutes of hypothermic cardiac arrest, to clip the AICA aneurysm. The patient did well and was discharged home from the hospital on postoperative day 14.

CASE REPORT 2

A 77-year-old man presented with an acute headache and normal Glasgow Coma Score (GCS). His initial CT demonstrated a 2.5-cm extra-axial prepontine mass consistent with a giant basilar aneurysm (Fig. 84-16). His subsequent CT angiogram (CTA) confirmed this. He was not medically suitable for surgical or endovascular management because of cardiovascular risk factors. He was admitted for observation and medical management. On day 3 he suffered a cerebellar infarct, and on day 5 died after a myocardial infarction. Definitive management of his aneurysm was not undertaken.

SUMMARY AND CONCLUSIONS

Aneurysms located on the midbasilar and lower basilar artery are uncommon, representing only a minority of cerebral aneurysms. They have the same natural history as aneurysms of other cerebral vessels. Because of their location, however, midbasilar and lower basilar artery aneurysms remain among the most difficult neurosurgical challenges. The principles of management of these lesions require maximal surgical exposure with minimal brain retraction, and proximal and distal vascular control with preservation of the parent vessel and perforators, to achieve complete obliteration of the aneurysm. A number of surgical exposures have been developed that fulfill these requirements, allowing aneurysms of the midbasilar and lower basilar artery to be managed effectively. Continuing advances in surgical technique lead to improved patient outcome. The mid- and lower basilar artery is a relatively uncommon location for cerebral aneurysms and there is an increasing use of endovascular methods to treat such lesions. Therefore, we feel that there is probably also an increasing role for subspecialized management of these complex aneurysms at experienced cerebrovascular centers.

REFERENCES

1. Yamaura A: Surgical management of posterior circulation aneurysms—part I. Contemp Neurosurg 7:1–6, 1985.
2. Sano K, Asano T, Tamura A: Surgical technique. In Sano K, Asano T, Tamura A (eds): Acute Aneurysm Surgery: Pathophysiology and Management. New York: Springer-Verlag, 1987, pp 194–246.
3. Peerless SJ, Drake CG: Surgical techniques of posterior circulation aneurysms. In Schmidek HHS, Sweet WH (eds): Operative Neurosurgical Techniques, vol 1, 2nd ed. Philadelphia: WB Saunders, 1988, pp 973–989.
4. Drake CG, Peerless SJ, Hernesniemi JA: Surgery of Vertebrobasilar Aneurysms: London, Ontario Experience on 1767 Patients. Vienna: Springer-Verlag, 1996.
5. ISUIA: Unruptured intracranial aneurysms—risk of rupture and risks of surgical intervention. International Study of Unruptured Intracranial Aneurysms Investigators. N Engl J Med 339:1725–1733, 1998.
6. Wiebers DO, Whisnant JP, Huston J, et al: Unruptured intracranial aneurysms: Natural history, clinical outcome, and risks of surgical and endovascular treatment. Lancet 362:103–110, 2003.
7. Molyneux A, Kerr R, Stratton I, et al: International Subarachnoid Aneurysm Trial (ISAT) of neurosurgical clipping versus endovascular coiling in 2143 patients with ruptured intracranial aneurysms: A randomised trial. Lancet 360:1267–1274, 2002.
8. Awad IA, Carter LP, Spetzler RF, et al: Clinical vasospasm after subarachnoid hemorrhage: Response to hypervolemic hemodilution and arterial hypertension. Stroke 18:365–372, 1987.
9. Hunt WE, Hess RM: Surgical risk as related to time of intervention in the repair of intracranial aneurysms. J Neurosurg 28:14–20, 1968.
10. Bailes JE, Spetzler RF, Hadley MN, Baldwin HZ: Management morbidity and mortality of poor-grade aneurysm patients. J Neurosurg 72:559–566, 1990.
11. Kassell NF, Peerless SJ, Durward QJ, et al: Treatment of ischemic deficits from vasospasm with intravascular volume expansion and induced arterial hypertension. Neurosurgery 11:337–343, 1982.
12. Findlay JM, Macdonald RL, Weir BKA: Current concepts of pathophysiology and management of cerebral vasospasm following aneurysmal subarachnoid hemorrhage. Cerebrovasc Brain Metab Rev 3:336–361, 1991.
13. Lanzino G, Wakhloo AK, Fessler RD, et al: Efficacy and current limitations of intravascular stents for intracranial internal carotid, vertebral, and basilar artery aneurysms. J Neurosurg 91:538–546, 1999.
14. Uda K, Murayama Y, Gobin YP, et al: Endovascular treatment of basilar artery trunk aneurysms with Guglielmi detachable coils: Clinical experience with 41 aneurysms in 39 patients. J Neurosurg 95:624–632, 2001.
15. Van Rooij WJ, Sluzewski M, Menovsky T, Wijnalda D: Coiling of saccular basilar trunk aneurysms. Neuroradiology 45:19–21, 2003.
16. Islak C, Kocer N, Kantarci F, et al: Endovascular management of basilar artery aneurysms associated with fenestrations. Am J Neuroradiol 23:958–964, 2002.
17. Yoon SM, Chun YI, Kwon Y, Kwun BD: Vertebrobasilar junction aneurysms associated with fenestration: Experience of five cases treated with Guglielmi detachable coils. Surg Neurol 61:248–254, 2004.
18. Seifert V, Stolke D: Posterior transpetrosal approach to aneurysms of the basilar trunk and vertebrobasilar junction. J Neurosurg 85:373–379, 1996.
19. Ogilvy CS, Barker FG, Joseph MP, et al: Transfacial transclival approach for midline posterior circulation aneurysms. Neurosurgery 39:736–741, 1996.
20. Lawton MT, Daspit CP, Spetzler RF: Technical aspects and recent trends in the management of large and giant midbasilar artery aneurysms. Neurosurgery 41:513–520, 1997.
21. Salas E, Sekhar LN, Ziyal IM, et al: Variations of the extreme-lateral craniocervical approach: Anatomical study and clinical analysis of 69 patients. J Neurosurg 90:206–219, 1999.
22. Sekhar LN, Schessel DA, Bucur SD, et al: Partial labyrinthectomy petrous apicectomy approach to neoplastic and vascular lesions of the petroclival area. Neurosurgery 44:537–550, 1999.
23. Seifert V, Raabe A, Stolke D: Management-related morbidity and mortality in unselected aneurysms of the basilar trunk and vertebrobasilar junction. Acta Neurochir (Wien) 143:343–348, 2001.
24. Shehab ZP, Walsh RM, Thorp MA, et al: Partial labyrinthectomy approach for brainstem vascular lesions. J Otolaryngol 30:224–230, 2001.
25. Spetzler RF, Hadley MN, Rigamonti D, et al: Aneurysms of the basilar artery treated with circulatory arrest, hypothermia and barbiturate cerebral protection. J Neurosurg 68:868–879, 1988.

26. Sugita K, Kobayashi S, Takemae T, et al: Aneurysms of the basilar trunk. J Neurosurg 66:500–505, 1987.

27. Sugita K, Kobayashi S, Shintani A, Mutsuga N: Microneurosurgery for aneurysms of the basilar artery. J Neurosurg 51:615–620, 1979.

28. Wascher TM, Spetzler RF: Surgical approaches to lesions involving the brain stem. Barrow Neurolog Inst Q 8:19–28, 1992.

29. Archer DJ, Young S, Uttley D: Basilar aneurysms: A new transclival approach via maxillotomy. J Neurosurg 67:54–58, 1987.

30. de los Reyes RA, Kantrowitz AB, Detwiler PW: Transoral-transclival clipping of giant lower basilar artery aneurysm. Surg Neurol 38:379–382, 1992.

31. Baldwin HZ, Miller CG, Van Loveren HR, et al: The far lateral–combined supra- and infratentorial approach: A human cadaveric prosection model for routes of access to the petroclival region and ventral brain stem. J Neurosurg 81:60–68, 1994.

32. Hitselberger WE, House WF: A combined approach to the cerebello-pontine angle: A suboccipital-petrosal approach. Arch Otolaryngol 84:49–67, 1966.

33. Spetzler RF, Daspit CP, Pappas CT: The combined supra- and infratentorial approach for lesions of the petrous and clival regions: Experience with 46 cases. J Neurosurg 76:588–599, 1992.

34. Spetzler RF, Graham TF: The far lateral approach to the inferior clivus and the upper cervical region: Technical note. Barrow Neurolog Inst Q 6:35–38, 1990.

35. Heros RC: Lateral suboccipital approach for vertebral and verte-brobasilar artery lesions. J Neurosurg 64:559–562, 1986.

36. Sen CN, Sekhar LN: An extreme lateral approach to intradural lesions of the cervical spine and foramen magnum. Neurosurgery 27:197–204, 1990.

37. House WF: Translabyrinthine approach. In House WF, Luetje CM (eds): Acoustic Tumors. II: Management. Baltimore: University Park Press, 1979, pp 43–87.

38. Spetzler RF, Fukushima T, Martin N, Zabramski JM: Petrous carotid-to-intradural carotid saphenous vein graft for intracavernous giant aneurysm, tumor, and occlusive cerebrovascular disease. J Neurosurg 73:496–501, 1990.

39. Jennett B, Bond M: Assessment of outcome after severe brain damage. Lancet 1:480–484, 1975.

40. Malis LI: Surgical resection of tumors of the skull base. In Wilkins RH, Rengachary SS (eds): Neurosurgery. New York: McGraw-Hill, 1985, pp 1011–1021.

41. Morrison AW, King TT: Experiences with a translabyrinthine-transtentorial approach to the cerebello-pontine angle. J Neurosurg 38:382–390, 1973.

42. Fisch U: Infratemporal fossa approach for extensive tumors of the temporal bone and base of the skull. In Silverstein H, Norell H (eds): Neurological Surgery of the Ear. Birmingham: Aesculapius, 1977, pp 34–53.

43. House WF, Hitselberger WE: The transcochlear approach to the skull base. Arch Otolaryngol 102:334–342, 1976.

44. Pellet W, Cannoni M, Pech A: The widened transcochlear approach to jugular foramen tumors. J Neurosurg 69:887–894, 1988.

45. Al-Mefty O, Fox JL, Rifai A, Smith RR: A combined infratemporal and posterior fossa approach for the removal of giant glomus tumors and chondrosarcomas. Surg Neurol 28:423–431, 1987.

46. Mayberg MR, Symon L: Meningiomas of the clivus and petrous bone: Report of 35 cases. J Neurosurg 65:160–167, 1986.

47. Samii M, Ammirati M, Mahran A, et al: Surgery of petroclival menin-giomas: Report of 24 cases. Neurosurgery 24:12–17, 1989.

48. Al-Mefty O, Fox JL, Smith RR: Petrosal approach for petroclival meningiomas. Neurosurgery 22:510–517, 1988.

49. Hammom WM, Kempe LG: The posterior fossa approach to aneurysms of the vertebral and basilar arteries. J Neurosurg 37:339–347, 1972.

50. De Oliveira E, Rhoton AL, Jr, Peace D: Microsurgical anatomy of the region of the foramen magnum. Surg Neurol 24:293–352, 1985.

51. Sen CN, Sekhar LN: Surgical management of anteriorly placed lesions at the craniocervical junction-an alternative approach. Acta Neurochir (Wien) 108:70–77, 1991.

85

Surgical Management of Aneurysms of the Vertebral and Posterior Inferior Cerebellar Artery Complex

HELMUT BERTALANFFY, LUDWIG BENES, STEFAN HEINZE, WUTTIPONG TIRAKOTAI, and ULRICH SURE

INTRODUCTION

Aneurysms of the vertebral artery–posterior inferior cerebellar artery (VA-PICA) complex comprise aneurysms that originate from any portion of the intradural VA up to the vertebrobasilar junction and from one of the five PICA segments. During the past decade, the treatment of these aneurysms became more sophisticated due to significant developments in diagnostic methods, improvements in microsurgical technique, further development of skull base surgery, better understanding of the microsurgical anatomy of the vertebrobasilar arterial territory, and dramatic advances in endovascular therapy. However, despite such continuous improvements, management of these complex lesions remains a challenging task. Several characteristic features distinguish VA and VA-PICA aneurysms from those of the anterior circulation: (1) they are relatively uncommon, occurring approximately one tenth as frequently as aneurysms in the anterior circulation[1]; (2) they show great variability in size, location, and morphology; the percentage of dissecting and fusiform aneurysms is much higher than in the other intracranial compartments; and (3) most of them are located deeply in the posterior fossa having a close relationship to the lower brain stem, the lower cranial nerves, and the cerebellum, making them difficult to access. The anatomic variability of the VA, the PICA, and the skull base around the jugular tubercle add further to the complexity of these lesions and increase the risk of their management. The infrequency of these lesions is the main reason why many neurosurgeons have only limited personal experience with the surgical treatment of VA-PICA aneurysms. With the advent of modern endovascular therapy, the number of lesions available for surgery, particularly the number of less complex VA and VA-PICA aneurysms, has further decreased, a situation that also raises problems in neurosurgical training. On the other hand, recent treatment strategies have gradually changed toward combined endovascular and surgical management, especially in the acute phase of severe subarachnoid hemorrhage (SAH) or in high-risk patients. It is obvious that only a limited number of specialized neurovascular centers can offer sufficient expertise for the safe management of this subgroup of vascular lesions.

EPIDEMIOLOGY

Aneurysms of the VA-PICA complex comprise 0.5% to 3% of all intracranial aneurysms.[2–6] Approximately two thirds of these aneurysms are located at the bifurcation of the VA-PICA junction, whereas distal PICA aneurysms account for approximately 0.3% to 1% of all aneurysms.[6–8] In a recently published series of 24 patients, distal PICA aneurysms accounted for only 0.3% of all intracranial aneurysms and for 3.7% of the vertebrobasilar lesions; 74% were saccular, 7% were fusiform, and 19% were dissecting.[7] Until 1992, only 140 patients harboring an aneurysm of the VA-PICA complex were reported in the literature[9]; of these, approximately 75% were VA or VA-PICA and 25% were distal PICA aneurysms. Multiple occurrence was occasionally reported.[4,10–13] Although the incidence of aneurysms arising in association with arteriovenous malformations may be as high as 46%, the combination of a VA-PICA aneurysm and an arteriovenous malformation is rarely reported in the literature.[14–16] With 85%, there is a clear predominance of female patients,[4,5,17,18] even more notable in saccular aneurysms.[19] Patients of virtually all ages may be affected, with an average age of 49.3 years.[20]

ANEURYSM CHARACTERISTICS

In contrast to intracranial aneurysms of other locations, only approximately 60% of VA-PICA aneurysms are saccular; approximately 30% are dissecting and 10% fusiform.[9,21,22] In Yamaura's[18] series, there were 60% saccular, 27% dissecting, and 13% arteriosclerotic fusiform aneurysms; moreover, he found three giant lesions with a diameter exceeding 25 mm and two partially thrombosed saccular aneurysms. Drs. Drake and Peerless and colleagues have treated the world's largest series of patients with vertebrobasilar aneurysms, comprising 1767 individual patients, of whom 217 (12.3%) harbored aneurysms of the VA-PICA complex.[19,20,23] One hundred sixty-six lesions were saccular (76.5%), 25 were dissecting (11%), 18 were fusiform (8%), 4 were atherosclerotic (1.8%), 3 were associated with an arteriovenous malformation (1.3%), and 1 was traumatic (0.4%). The majority (70%) were small (<12 mm); 27 aneurysms (12%) were large (13 to 24 mm) and 40 (18%) were giant (>25 mm).

Left-sided origin was more common (55%). Forty-three aneurysms (19%) were unruptured.[19,23]

Fusiform aneurysms appear as spindle-shaped dilatations, the vertebrobasilar trunk being the most frequent location for fusiform aneurysms.[24] Due to a clear difference in natural history and optimal therapy, they must be clearly distinguished from dissecting aneurysms. More than two decades ago, nontraumatic dissecting aneurysms were considered to be extremely rare. However, improved neuroradiologic imaging techniques have demonstrated such lesions with increasing frequency, and during the past years, this type of aneurysm has received great attention in the pertinent literature.[10,22,25] On arteriography, such aneurysms appear as a saccular or spindle-shaped vascular dilatation, occasionally combined with proximal stenosis. The classic arteriographic features of dissecting arteries include the double-lumen sign, retention of contrast medium, the pearl-and-string sign,[26] and focal outpouching.[22,27] Usually, they are not related to vascular branches of the VA. Such dissecting aneurysms of the VA may occur proximal as well as distal to the origin of the PICA, but occasionally they may involve the origin of the PICA as well.[28] Yasui and colleagues[29] believe that a fusiform VA aneurysm is one predisposing condition for a dissecting lesion. The sudden disruption of the internal elastic lamina is the primary mechanism underlying the development of dissecting aneurysms. The plane of dissection extends through the media, and most aneurysms have one entrance to this pseudolumen.[30] Dissecting aneurysms of the VA often cause SAH by rupture of the adventitia and present a high risk of rebleeding.[28,31,32] These lesions are not confined to the VA but may be observed on the distal PICA as well.[7,33,34] Occasionally, a dissecting distal PICA aneurysm can develop as a traumatic lesion.[35]

Extreme dilations of the VA, termed dolichoectasias, occur less frequently and are usually difficult to treat. The involved artery is elongated and tortuous. On histologic examination, large defects within the muscular and elastic lamina can be detected and sometimes also extensive arteriosclerotic changes.[30] Although dissecting aneurysms occur more frequently in male patients of younger age, dolichoectasias occur more frequently in the seventh decade.[9,22,36,37]

HISTORICAL BACKGROUND

According to Hudgins and colleagues,[4] the first case description of a saccular VA-PICA aneurysm was given by Cruveilhier in 1829. Rizzoli and Hayes[38] were the first to surgically treat such an aneurysm in 1947 by interrupting the parent artery with two silver clips. Interestingly, the aneurysm was detected by these authors on a ventriculogram that showed a displaced fourth ventricle. Lewis and colleagues[33] mentioned that the first case of an aneurysm arising from the distal segment of the PICA was reported in 1864 by Fernet and that the first surgical treatment of a peripheral PICA aneurysm is accredited to Olivecrona. In the 1950s and 1960s, vertebrobasilar aneurysms were associated with the highest mortality rate.[39] Rizzoli and Hayes[38] treated a peripheral PICA aneurysm with trapping in 1953. Uihlein and Hughes[40] described in 1955 the nonsurgical treatment of 14 patients harboring a posterior fossa aneurysm; eight of these patients died after the aneurysm ruptured. After the introduction of routine vertebral

angiography in patients with SAH, such aneurysms were detected with increasing frequency. In 1958, Desaussure and colleagues[41] reported the successful surgical obliteration of two PICA aneurysms found on vertebral angiograms. Further improvements of neuroradiologic techniques after the introduction of transfemoral catheter and subtraction angiography as well as the routine use of microsurgical techniques in neurosurgery have dramatically improved the outcome of surgical procedures for treatment of vertebrobasilar aneurysms.[42,43]

NEURORADIOLOGIC IMAGING

A meticulous preoperative neuroradiologic assessment is indispensable for successful treatment of VA and VA-PICA aneurysms. Neuroradiologic investigations should clarify the following features: (1) the exact location and origin of the aneurysm with respect to the VA and the various segments of the PICA (Fig. 85-1); (2) the size, shape, extent, and limits of the lesion to differentiate between saccular, fusiform, and dissecting aneurysms; (3) the orientation of the neck and the dome of the aneurysm; (4) the presence or absence of sufficient collateral circulation; (5) the patency of both VAs and the dominance of one of them, if present; (6) the presence or absence of multiple intracranial aneurysms or an associated arteriovenous malformation; (7) the precise relationship to the major surrounding anatomic structures as well as the degree of involvement of the brain stem and rootlets of the lower cranial nerves; and (8) the presence of hydrocephalus and/or intracerebellar/intraventricular hemorrhage.

Neuroradiologic studies include high-quality arterial digital angiography as well as various techniques of coronal, sagittal, and axial magnetic resonance imaging, and computed tomography (CT). Digital subtraction angiography may be complemented by rotational angiography with 3-dimensional rendering. Yonekawa and colleagues[44] described three distances that can be measured on preoperative angiograms that are important predictors of the difficulty of operative access to VA-PICA aneurysms: the distance of the aneurysm from the midline, the distance from the most lateral point of the

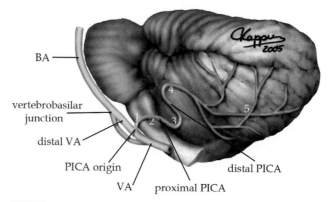

FIGURE 85-1 The segmental nomenclature of the posterior inferior cerebellar artery (PICA) and the vertebral artery complex (VA) for possible localizations of aneurysm formation. 1, Anterior medullary segment; 2, lateral medullary segment; 3, tonsillomedullary segment; 4, televelotonsillar segment; 5, cortical branch segments. (Courtesy of Christoph Kappus.)

foramen magnum, and the distance from the clivus. According to these authors, optimal results are obtained when these distances are more than 5 to 10 mm, less than 10 to 21 mm, and less than 13 mm, respectively.

In a previous communication, we emphasized that high-resolution CT using a bone tissue algorithm is most useful to demonstrate the configuration of the skull base around the jugular foramen, in particular showing the size and shape of the jugular tubercle, the size of the posterior condylar canal, and the distance between the dural entrance of the vertebral artery and the hypoglossal canal or jugular tubercle.[45] Special sections or 3-dimensional reconstructions may further add to the understanding of the individual skull base configuration or presence of bony anomalies. When performed with a bolus of contrast medium, this 3-dimensional CT image may demonstrate the relationship between the lesion, brain stem, and skull base, adding important information required for the planning of the procedure.[45] Huynh-Le and colleagues[46] have confirmed the utility of 3-dimensional CT angiography for the surgical management of VA-PICA aneurysms; this diagnostic technique was most valuable in demonstrating not only the exact site and shape of the aneurysm but also the relationships between parent vessel and malformation on the one side and the bony structures of the skull base on the other side. CT is important to demonstrate the SAH, the blood distribution within the basal cisterns, an associated hydrocephalus, and an intraventricular or intracerebellar hemorrhage. Intraventricular hemorrhage is present in as many as 82% of patients and associated hydrocephalus in approximately 75% of patients with ruptured aneurysms.[5,47,48] Magnetic resonance imaging is particularly valuable in fusiform, dissecting, or partially thrombosed aneurysms.[30,49] Magnetic resonance angiography can depict the aneurysm in relation to the brain stem, cerebellum, caudal cranial nerves, and skull base.

CLINICAL PRESENTATION

The most frequent presenting symptom of patients with aneurysms of the VA-PICA complex is SAH. Rupture of these aneurysms occurs similarly to the rupture of aneurysms of the anterior circulation. However, the clinical consequences are far more disastrous. Although only a few patients experience intracerebellar hemorrhage or deficits of caudal cranial nerves, in some instances, prolonged coma, hemiparesis, or pulmonary embolism can occur.[50,51] Aneurysm rupture occurs more frequently in lesions smaller than 12 mm. Large and giant aneurysms rarely rupture; they become symptomatic more frequently by their compressive effect on the lower brain stem or the caudal cranial nerves. Ischemic complications such as Wallenberg's syndrome may occur in dissecting aneurysms due to occlusion of perforating arteries that supply the lateral aspect of the medulla. Patients with dolichoectatic VA and/or basilar artery may have ischemic stroke, brain stem compression, and occasionally hemifacial spasm or trigeminal neuralgia.[52] In the series of Drake and Peerless[53] of 221 patients, 178 had SAH (80.5%). Sixth nerve palsy, not lower cranial nerve paresis, was the most frequent preoperative cranial nerve dysfunction, as one might have expected. It was nearly always associated with SAH and recovered in 75% completely.

MANAGEMENT

The decision as to whether an aneurysm of the VA-PICA complex should be treated, as well as the timing and choice of treatment modality in case treatment appears indicated, depends on criteria such as the patient's age, actual clinical condition, and neurologic status; progression or resolution of initial symptoms and signs; presence or absence of SAH; the interval between SAH and time of decision making; aneurysm characteristics; medical history; and the presence or absence of hydrocephalus and intraventricular or intracerebellar hemorrhage. Surgery, for instance, is preferable when a significant hematoma needs to be evacuated. For more than a decade, the concomitant availability of endovascular and microsurgical procedures has made possible a multimodal treatment of aneurysms of the VA-PICA complex.[54–57] Particularly, the technologic achievements in neurovascular instrumentation (i.e., coil technology, intracranial stent technique) of the recent years led to a continuing challenge for interventional neuroradiologists, enabling them to treat even previously "untreatable" aneurysms with a high success rate.[58–66] However, complications of the treatment such as brain stem infarction and hemorrhages are also reported for the interventional therapy of VA-PICA aneurysms.[61,67,68] For some rare complex cases, a combined interventional and microsurgical therapy may constitute a reasonable solution.[58]

In some aneurysms such as proximal PICA lesions, even in cases in which endovascular coil occlusion of the aneurysms seems possible, the direct microsurgical inspection of the affected segment of the PICA and of perforating brain stem–supplying arteries may offer significant advantages compared with endovascular therapy.[33] Considering the complexity and heterogeneity of VA and VA-PICA aneurysms, most lesions might require an individual case-by-case decision.

Surgical Approaches

To expose aneurysms of the VA-PICA complex surgically, a detailed analysis of aneurysm location, origin, extension, and orientation of the dome is necessary. Small saccular VA-PICA aneurysms may be exposed by a traditional sub-occipital medial or lateral approach when they are located proximal to the rootlets of the lower cranial nerves. Aneurysms located more distally or even at the vertebrobasilar junction, as well as large or giant saccular or complex dissecting aneurysms, may require more extensive skull base approaches. Aneurysms of the third, fourth, and fifth PICA segments are best visualized via a suboccipital medial craniotomy. The patient is placed in either the sitting or prone position with the head flexed. The craniotomy includes the posterior rim of the foramen magnum. A number of lateral approaches are available to expose various aneurysms of the VA or the first two PICA segments.[2,9,69–72] For exposure of some proximal VA aneurysms, a traditional retrosigmoid approach may be sufficient.[73] However, several authors have underscored the necessity of extending the exposure more laterally.[69] The retrolabyrinthine transsigmoidal approach was described by Giannotta and Maceri[74] in 1988 and used to expose distal VA-PICA aneurysms or those of the vertebrobasilar junction.

It is a complex and more time-consuming skull base approach because large portions of the petrous bone must be drilled away and the ipsilateral sigmoid sinus is ligated, provided the contralateral sinus is intact. This approach, however, is rarely described in the literature for treatment of aneurysms of the VA-PICA complex. The transcondylar approach and several variations have been widely used by several authors in this context.[33,75-79] A detailed description of the technique as we use it is given later in this chapter. Aneurysms that are not suitable for either surgical clipping or endovascular procedure may require other surgical techniques such as coating,[5,80] external (surgical) trapping,[4] or one of the various procedures of revascularization.

Saccular Aneurysms

Hernesniemi[81] mentioned that most saccular nongiant aneurysms of the VA-PICA complex can be clipped. Today, most authors prefer an early treatment of these aneurysms after rupture, including distal PICA aneurysms,[33] and also when they are associated with an arteriovenous malformation.[15,82] The decision as to whether surgical clipping or endovascular coil occlusion is preferable should be made by an experienced neurovascular team. In the series of Horiuchi and colleagues[7] comprising 27 PICA aneurysms in 24 patients, 22 lesions were clipped (81%), 2 (7%) were wrapped, 1 (4%) was proximally ligated with occipital artery–PICA bypass, and only 1 (4%) was occluded endovascularly with Guglielmi detachable (GD) coils.

Fusiform Aneurysms

For fusiform aneurysms of the VA and PICA, there is no safe surgical technique without major risk of severe morbidity. Moreover, the natural history of unruptured fusiform aneurysms is not well known. The rebleeding rate of such aneurysms is estimated at 10% per year, which is remarkably minor when compared with saccular or dissecting aneurysms. Observation and conservative treatment appear justified in view of the favorable history of many of these aneurysms.

Dissecting Aneurysms

With modern neuroimaging techniques, the diagnosis of dissecting aneurysms is now more precise than in the past.[49,83] Although a benign course has occasionally been documented,[84] the necessity of early treatment of dissecting aneurysms of the VA has been emphasized by many authors. An SAH from a dissecting aneurysm is considered a neurosurgical emergency because of a high incidence of rebleeding and a high mortality rate at the time of recurrent bleeding.[22,30,31,55] Conversely, the natural history of non-SAH cases is relatively benign and therefore the treatment remains controversial.[85-87] Despite early satisfactory results with a proximal occlusion of the VA,[88] it is now well recognized that proximal occlusion of the affected VA by clip placement or endovascular procedure may not be sufficient.[28] The primary goal of therapy is thus complete exclusion of the dissecting aneurysm from the circulation to avoid progression of the vascular dissection or a distal embolism with ischemic complications.[28] In most cases, clip occlusion is impossible and wrapping alone may not be efficient.[83] Test occlusion of

the vertebral artery is performed, and thereafter either surgical or endovascular occlusion (internal trapping) is recommended.[54] According to Hamada and colleagues,[28] when occlusion of the VA is chosen as treatment option, patients should undergo a 20-minute occlusion tolerance test using a nondetachable balloon. Yoshimoto and Wakai[87] have questioned the necessity of this balloon test because they doubt its reliability; these authors believe that definitive unilateral VA occlusion can be performed safely unless the contralateral VA is hypoplastic. Kitanaka and colleagues[89] have mentioned that the choice of surgical technique depends on the location of the dissecting aneurysm in relation to the origin of the PICA. The VA can usually be occluded distal to the PICA origin, whereas a proximal occlusion of the VA may cause a secondary thrombosis of the PICA. A number of revascularization techniques have therefore been applied to occlude the VA with a consecutive reanastomosis of the PICA: PICA-PICA bypass at the level of the caudal loop,[90-92] occipital artery–PICA,[93-98] VA-PICA anastomosis with the superficial temporal artery or radial artery,[99-101] and VA-PICA transposition.[102]

Giant Aneurysms

Despite the rare occurrence of giant aneurysms of the posterior circulation, these lesions have received much attention in the literature.[11,103-106]

The reasons for their frequent description are special characteristics of these lesions. The therapy of giant aneurysms is far more difficult that of those in the anterior circulation. Ausman and colleagues[93] have recommended surgical clip occlusion in cooperation with cardiosurgeons under hypothermia and circulatory arrest.[107] This method, however, has a specific morbidity and is associated with a certain mortality. The optimal therapy of giant aneurysms is the direct clip occlusion, which still bears a high risk for the patient. For this reason, the parent artery (VA) may be deliberately sacrificed or endovascularly occluded,[108] the same technique as that used for dissecting or fusiform aneurysms. According to Inamasu and colleagues[109] who treated six patients with giant VA and four patients with VA-PICA aneurysms surgically, more favorable results were obtained with surgical or endovascular rather than with conservative therapy.

THE AUTHORS' SERIES

A total of 69 patients with aneurysms of the VA-PICA complex were treated in the period 1992 to 2004. Thirty patients were treated surgically, 33 endovascularly and 6 conservatively. Patient data are summarized in Table 85-1.

AUTHORS' PREFERRED SURGICAL TECHNIQUE

Our preferred approach to VA and VA-PICA aneurysms, the suboccipital transcondylar approach, derives from the classic access route to the cerebellopontine angle and anterolateral aspect of the foramen magnum. The microsurgical exposure of these lesions usually requires extensive drilling of the bone around the jugular foramen. Among the pertinent anatomic structures of this area, the jugular tubercle plays a key role.

TABLE 85-1 ▪ Treatment Modalities for Patients with Vertebral Artery–Posterior Inferior Cerebellar Artery Aneurysms (Treated by the Authors)

Therapeutic Procedure	No. of Patients (n)	Average Age, Sex (M/F)	VA	VA-PICA Complex	Distal PICA	VA-Basilar Junction	Surgical Approach
Clipping	23	52, 0, 7/16	6	10	6	1	Transcondylar (n = 13), medial suboccipital (n = 7), lateral suboccipital (n = 3)
Coating	1	55, M	1	—	—	—	Transcondylar
Coagulation	1	61, F	—	1	—	—	Lateral suboccipital
PICA end-to-end anastomosis	2	39.5, 1/1	—	—	2	—	Lateral suboccipital (n = 1), transcondylar (n = 1)
VA-PICA anastomosis	2	55.5, 1/1	2	—	—	—	Transcondylar (n = 1), lateral suboccipital (n = 1)
Aneurysm excision	1	56, F	—	—	1	—	Medial suboccipital
Conservative treatment	6	46.7, 2/4	1	3	—	2	—
Endovascular treatment	33	47.4, 15/18	3	19	9	2	Coiling (n = 32), stenting and coiling (n = 1)
Total (n)	69	51.6, 27/42	13	33	18	5	—

PICA, posterior inferior cerebellar artery; VA, vertebral artery.

When drilling the jugular tubercle, we must control a number of vital anatomic structures around the jugular foramen, which are described in more detail later in this chapter. Considering the great variability of the aneurysms to be treated, we do not advocate a rigid surgical approach. Instead, with a precise knowledge of all individual morphologic, pathomorphologic, and functional details, we design and perform the procedure in an individually tailored fashion, according to the guiding principle of minimal invasiveness. In our understanding, this principle as applied to skull base surgery means obtaining maximal microsurgical exposure with the least possible amount of surgical trauma. Apart from aneurysms of the distal PICA that can be treated via the median suboccipital or the telovelar route, we usually start the procedure with a limited suboccipital transcondylar approach. This procedure is then gradually extended according to the specific requirements of each case. It is obvious that our policy of minimal invasiveness has important implications on the planning of the procedure, the positioning of the patient on the surgical table, the skin incision and muscle opening, the removal of bone at the base of the skull, and the intradural microsurgical technique.

Surgical Anatomy

The origin of the PICA at the VA varies from extradurally, below the foramen magnum, to the vertebrobasilar junction. The PICA arises from the posterior or lateral surfaces of the VA more often than from the anterior or medial surfaces.[110] The PICA is the artery with the most complex relationship to the cranial nerves of any artery.[111] By definition, the PICA originates from the VA. Although rarely encountered (5%), one must bear in mind the possibility of an extradural origin of the PICA and of an extracranial (intradural) site of distal PICA aneurysms.[110,112] In a few cases, the VA and the PICA are missing. If the PICA is present, it is the largest branch of the VA.[110] Lister and colleagues[113] have divided the artery into five segments based on its relationship to the medulla and the cerebellum. These five segments are the anterior

medullary, the lateral medullary, the tonsillomedullary (includes the caudal loop), the telovelotonsillar (includes the cranial loop), and the cortical.[113] Each segment sometimes includes more than one trunk. The PICA is closely related to the cerebellomedullary fissure, the inferior half of the ventricular roof, the inferior peduncle, and the suboccipital surface.[110] The PICA supplies perforating branches to the medullar, choroidal arteries and cortical arteries. Perforating arteries arise from the medullary segment terminating into the brain stem.[110] Recently, Marinkovic and colleagues[114] gave a detailed description of the perforating branches of the VA providing valuable information for those performing aneurysm surgery in this region.

From the microsurgical point of view, a number of muscular and osseous anatomic landmarks are essential for successful dissection in this region. The following is a brief description of these anatomic landmarks and their significance for the surgical procedure.

The upper portion of the sternocleidomastoid muscle and its posterior border indicate the region for the skin incision and further muscular opening. The most important muscles of the deep layer are the rectus capitis posterior major and minor muscles and the superior and inferior oblique muscles. The area between the medial rim of the superior oblique muscle, the upper rim of the inferior oblique muscle, and the lateral rim of the rectus capitis posterior major muscle, called the suboccipital triangle, contains the posterior rim of the atlantal arch, the horizontal portion of the vertebral artery, and the C1 root between these two structures. The posterior atlantal arch also serves as an important landmark for early localization of the VA during the stage of muscular dissection. Once this structure has been identified by palpation, the artery can readily be exposed in the sulcus dorsal and medial to the lateral atlantal mass. A C1 hemilaminectomy may not always be necessary but can be helpful when mobilization of the VA is required. The posterior edge of the occipital condyle is located just lateral to the dural entrance of the VA. To better expose the proximal intradural VA, this portion of the occipital condyle must be drilled away.

The diameter of the posterior condylar canal that contains the posterior condylar emissary vein varies widely. This canal is a very important landmark because it opens into the posteromedial margin of the jugular foramen and indicates the direction of bony drilling to expose the jugular tubercle. The jugular tubercle is a rounded prominence located at the junction between the basal part (clivus) and the condylar part of the occipital bone (jugular process). The jugular tubercle is one of the most important landmarks being surrounded by a number of vital neurovascular structures that must be exposed partially or totally.[45,77] Medially and superiorly, the jugular tubercle is overcrossed by the cranial nerves IX, X, and XI intradurally. Laterally, the jugular tubercle has a close relationship with the jugular bulb, reaching the medial wall of the jugular foramen. Inferiorly, there is the hypoglossal canal containing the hypoglossal nerve surrounded by its venous plexus. Seeger[115] was the first to document the necessity of resecting the jugular tubercle for an adequate visualization of near-midline aneurysms of the VA-PICA complex, later underscored by Perneczky.[116]

Positioning of the Patient

Proper positioning of the patient on the surgical table is essential for adequate access to the condylar fossa. Ideally, the patient's positioning should fulfill the following criteria: it should allow for an optimal view of the intradural VA without being hampered, for instance, by the patient's shoulder. It should also allow a wide range of movement with the operative microscope to be able to visualize the surgical field from different angles. This is important particularly for a narrow and deep exposure as in aneurysms of the distal VA. It should also allow the surgeon to adopt a neutral, relaxed position because this may influence the surgical result. Finally, it should reduce venous congestion and thus venous bleeding, particularly in this area with abundant venous channels within a narrow surgical field. On the other hand, one has to bear in mind that exaggerated negative venous pressure may favor the occurrence of air embolism during surgery. In our opinion, these criteria are best accomplished by the sitting position of the patient so that the legs are level with the heart. A disadvantage of the sitting position worth mentioning is the loss of cerebrospinal fluid from all basal cisterns and even from the ventricles during surgery. Especially in the elderly, this may delay postoperative awakening from anesthesia. In some instances, we therefore use the lateral park bench position for the patient. In either position, the head of the patient should be mobilized in three planes: flexion, axial rotation to the ipsilateral side, and slight tilting to the contralateral side. Flexion of the head is important because it exposes the posterior articular facet of the occipital condyle.

Anesthesia and Monitoring

The risk of air embolism in this position can be reduced to a minimum by an experienced neuroanesthetist who pays special attention to the blood volume and to normoventilation, particularly when carrying out the craniotomy and the bony drilling at the base of the skull. At present, all our procedures in the sitting position are performed with transesophageal Doppler monitoring, allowing for the early

detection of very small amounts of air bubbles within the atrium. The source of air embolism is identified after bilateral compression of the jugular vein, which is done when necessary by the anesthetist. With this management, we have not encountered serious problems or hemodynamic complications due to air embolism over many years of neurosurgical procedures using the sitting position. In the majority of skull base procedures, standard techniques of monitoring of somatosensory and brain stem auditory evoked potentials are routinely used at our institution. Monitoring the accessory and hypoglossal nerves may increase the safety in some procedures, provided the function of these nerves is intact preoperatively.

Skin Incision

Before skin incision, the scalp is infiltrated with local anesthetic and epinephrine (1:200,000). A proper selection of the skin incision is important for sufficient deep exposure but also for adequately reducing the surgical trauma. To expose the distal intradural VA, we prefer a longitudinal, slightly curved skin incision with the convexity oriented medially, approximately 3 cm medial to the mastoid process. If the aneurysm is located more laterally (proximal VA, first or second segment of PICA), a straight-line skin incision is placed more medially to allow an additional medial-to-lateral viewing trajectory. Some authors advocate an inverse U-shaped (horseshoe) 24, 61, 64; an S-shaped 112, 145; a C-shaped 22, 24, 72; or a so-called hockey stick 60, 96 incision, which, in our opinion, offer no obvious advantages over the straight-line or curved incision.

Exposure of the Deep Lateral Suboccipital Region

Basically, we have to deal with two muscular layers. The superficial muscle layer consists of the sternocleidomastoid and the splenius capitis muscles laterally, and the trapezius and the semispinalis capitis muscles medially. The occipital artery encountered either superficial or deep to the longissimus capitis and deep to the splenius capitis muscles is usually ligated and divided but may be preserved in case an occipital artery–PICA bypass is deemed necessary. From the deep muscle layer, the two oblique and the two rectus capitis posterior muscles deserve special attention. We start with freeing the attachment of the superficial and partially the deep muscles between the superior and inferior nuchal lines by using monopolar thermocautery. This instrument can be safely applied in this area when the tip of the instrument is permanently visualized and kept in contact with the occipital bone. The muscles are then divided in a craniocaudal direction layer by layer, as much as possible respecting the direction of the muscle fibers. Frequently, palpating the deep structures is helpful for avoiding injury to the VA, which sometimes may form a posterior loop that extends beyond the level of the atlantal arch. The surgeon should recognize this anatomic variation before surgery by carefully examining axial magnetic resonance imaging or CT slices taken at the C1 level. Instead of anatomically exposing the three suboccipital muscles that form the suboccipital triangle by extensive dissection, we prefer to identify the posterior arch of the atlas by palpation. The atlantal arch is then freed from its periosteal sheath using a sharp dissector, and the sulcus of the VA is thus exposed. The sulcus can easily be identified by observing the shape of the posterior rim of the atlantal arch. This structure is thick in its medial portion, changing into a thin and sharp osseous edge at the level of the sulcus more laterally. As the VA is surrounded by a venous plexus that may cause severe bleeding, it is advisable to identify the vessel at this stage by palpating its pulsations. Once the VA is identified, further detachment of the sub-occipital muscles is continued and the posterior condylar fossa containing abundant fatty tissue is exposed together with the posterior aspect of the atlantooccipital joint. It has proved favorable to perform this step under the operating microscope. The periarterial venous plexus may be coagulated or packed with collagen or Surgicel to control venous bleeding. Muscle and dural branches of the VA are coagulated and divided. Care is paid to the C1 root located beneath the horizontal portion of the VA. The fatty and connective tissue filling the condylar fossa is gradually removed and the posterior portion of the occipital condyle and lateral atlantal mass are exposed by subperiosteal dissection. When exposing the condylar fossa, the posterior condylar emissary vein is dissected free, coagulated, and then divided sharply. The remaining distal portion of the vein located within the posterior condylar canal is shrunk with bipolar forceps and serves as an important anatomic landmark, indicating the direction toward the posterior aspect of the jugular bulb (Fig. 85-2).

Suboccipital Craniectomy

Usually, we either perform a small bone flap or place several burr holes and preserve the bone dust for later wound closure. After placing the burr holes, the dura is gently detached from the bone. Craniectomy is continued step by step using a rongeur to preserve the bony fragments. The limits of the craniectomy are as follows: superiorly approximately 1 to 2 cm

below the transverse sinus; medially and superiorly approximately 1 to 2 cm from the midline; medially and inferiorly the dorsolateral rim of the foramen magnum is completely opened from the midline to the dural entrance of the VA, thus reaching the posterior condylar fossa and posterior medial aspect of the jugular process; and laterally to the medial rim of the sigmoid sinus. This stage of the procedure is carried out without the aid of the operating microscope (see Fig. 85-2).

Partial Drilling of the Occipital Condyle and Jugular Tubercle

The following surgical step is crucial for enabling direct access to the pathologic lesion at hand. It must be designed in great detail preoperatively because, on the one hand, it offers the working space necessary for microsurgical manipulation around the intradural VA. On the other hand, unnecessary drilling in this area should be avoided because of the potential of damage to vital neurovascular structures. The amount of bony resection depends on the location, site, and extent of the aneurysm and on the specific anatomic configuration of the skull base.

Because drilling around the jugular foramen is a highly demanding procedure, it is carried out extradurally with the aid of a high-speed drill and under magnification. Before drilling, however, we gently separate the bone from the adjacent dura mater and distal sigmoid sinus that may firmly adhere to the bone. In the early stage, a cutting burr is used that never touches the dura. Thereafter, we use diamond burrs of different sizes under continuous irrigation with saline solution. Drilling begins with removing the medial aspect of the posterior wall of the distal sigmoid sinus and continues to the medial aspect of the jugular process of the occipital bone. At this stage, the point where the VA pierces the dura serves as an important landmark. By measuring the distance from this point to the area of drilling in the depth, we can estimate the remaining distance to the hypoglossal canal and jugular tubercle as known from preoperative neuroradiologic studies. To expose the dura lateral to the point of entrance of the VA, the posteromedial aspect of the occipital condyle is gradually removed, leaving the vast majority of the articular surface intact. Venous bleeding from the marginal sinus at the level of the foramen magnum is controlled with bipolar coagulation and packing with Surgicel. While using the high speed drill in this region, the VA is protected from damage with the suction tube or a self-retaining brain retractor. Drilling is continued to expose the posterior aspect of the hypoglossal canal. Because the dural sheet of the hypoglossal nerve is surrounded by a venous plexus, the exposure may require packing with Surgicel to achieve hemostasis. Once the hypoglossal canal is exposed, the dura overlying the jugular tubercle is gently detached. In many instances, the jugular tubercle is a very high prominence. In such cases, this structure hampers visualization of the distal VA. To obtain a wide exposure, this bony structure is drilled partially or totally, depending on the specific anatomic situation and microsurgical requirements. Occasional bleeding from the jugular bulb or venous channels draining into the bulb is controlled by packing small amounts of Surgicel and, if necessary, fibrin glue is applied as well. It has proved advantageous to drill the cancellous bone until

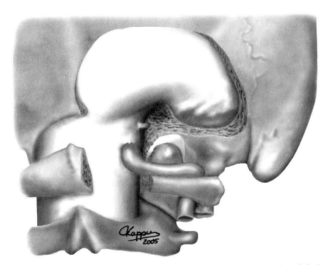

FIGURE 85-2 The bone resection of the approach. The suboccipital craniotomy exposes the inferior part of the cerebellum and edge of the jugular bulb. A resection of the medial part of the jugular tubercle and the occipital and C1 condylar interface has been done, producing a gap between the vertebral artery and the bone. Also a hemilaminectomy of C1 was performed for maximal lateral retraction of the dural flap. (Courtesy of Christoph Kappus.)

a thin shallow of cortical bone remains in place. This shallow is then removed piece by piece with a small rongeur. Such a technique is crucial to avoid injury to the jugular bulb or cranial nerves that traverse the jugular foramen. The skull base surgeon working in this area must bear in mind that the wall of the jugular bulb and also the dura overlying the jugular tubercle are thin and very vulnerable structures. Damaging the dura around the jugular tubercle may cause injury to the cranial nerves IX, X, and XI located immediately above this bony prominence or even premature aneurysm rupture. To avoid by all means such damage at this stage, we use very cautiously a conventional drill at low speed.

To enlarge the exposure, in most cases only small amounts of the occipital condyle must be drilled away in the posteromedial portion of this structure. We have always been able to preserve the function of the atlanto-occipital joint (see Fig. 85-2).

Dural Incision

The dura is opened in a longitudinal or Y-shaped fashion, usually medial to the dural entrance of the VA. The dural ring around the VA is left intact save for the cases with proximal artery involvement. Opening the dura exposes the lobulus biventer of the cerebellum rostrally and the medulla oblongata caudally. The dural edges are sutured to the muscles in the vicinity so that the dural entrance of the VA is gently reflected laterally together with the dura. This becomes possible only after sufficient resection of bone lateral to the dural entrance of the VA (Fig. 85-3).

Intradural Stage

The intradural procedure begins with opening the arachnoid membrane of the great cistern. Gentle elevation of the cerebellum gradually exposes the spinal root of the accessory nerve, the proximal intradural portion of the VA, the proximal PICA, the first dentate ligament, and the C1 root. To further retract the cerebellum, the arachnoid around cranial nerves IX through XI must be divided using microscissors. The rootlets of the caudal cranial nerves are then dissected free up to their origin from the antero-olivary and retro-olivary grooves. Anterior to these rootlets, the distal portion of the VA is visualized. The artery and aneurysm may be covered by the rootlets of the hypoglossal nerve, which may cross the PICA anteriorly as well as posteriorly. Close to the midline, the sixth nerve and the junction of both VAs become visible. Superior to the glossopharyngeal nerve, the exit zone of the statoacoustic and more anteriorly of the facial nerve can be seen. However, these anatomic structures may be covered, distorted, or displaced by the underlying aneurysm (Fig. 85-4).

Aneurysms located at the level of the jugular tubercle, such as proximal aneurysms of the VA at the origin of the PICA or true PICA aneurysms located at the anterior or posterior medullary portion of this artery, were readily visualized with this technique. Apart from sufficient exposure of the vascular malformation, it was of great importance to obtain enough control of the VA distal to the aneurysm. Sufficient drilling of the jugular tubercle from extradurally was essential in these particular cases. Before applying an aneurysm clip, the rootlets of the lower cranial nerves including the 12th nerve were dissected free from the vascular malformation. After complete arachnoidal dissection, clipping was performed through a corridor between these rootlets. Only rarely, temporary clipping of the proximal and distal VA and/or PICA was necessary, usually to minimize

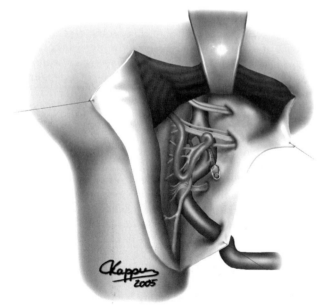

FIGURE 85-3   The dura opened by incision giving access to an aneurysm of the proximal posterior inferior cerebellar artery near its origin. A retractor is positioned to permit visualization of the caudal cranial nerves up to nerve VII. The lateral angle is augmented by partial removal of the jugular tubercle and the occipital and the C1 condylar interface. The remaining jugular tubercle appears as a bulge of the dura directly behind the aneurysm between the dural orifice of nerves XI and XII. (Courtesy of Christoph Kappus.)

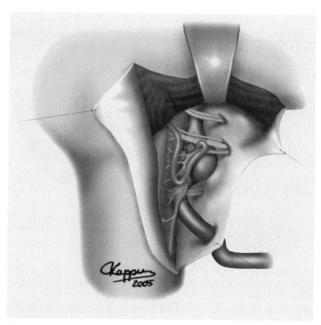

FIGURE 85-4   A clip positioned on the aneurysm. (Courtesy of Christoph Kappus.)

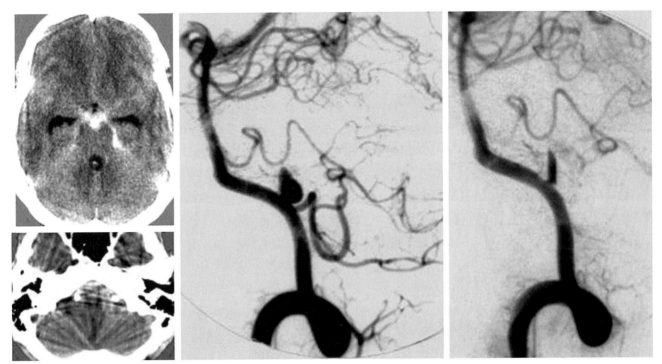

FIGURE 85-5 A 37-year-old woman with a subarachnoid hemorrhage (SAH) (Hunt & Hess grade III). *Upper and lower left:* Computed tomography scan demonstrates the SAH. *Middle:* Angiography reveals a left-sided vertebral artery–posterior inferior cerebellar artery (PICA) aneurysm. *Right:* During endovascular intervention before coiling, both the anterior medullary segment of the PICA and the aneurysm thrombosed.

the inner luminal pressure and shrink a larger aneurysm dome before definitive clipping. Dissecting aneurysms were wrapped or coated by either muscle or cottonoids. Before, during, and after aneurysm clipping, we routinely used a micro Doppler probe for the control of vascular patency (see Fig. 85-4).

Wound Closure

One of the main purposes of wound closure is to avoid postoperative cerebrospinal fluid leak. A watertight dural suture or reconstruction is also essential to prevent postoperative meningitis and to avoid local hemorrhage, wound infection, and compression to the caudal cranial nerves. The bony

FIGURE 85-6 Intraoperative view and postoperative angiography of the same patient as shown in Figure 85-5. *Upper left:* View of the thrombosed aneurysm and distal posterior inferior cerebellar artery (PICA) segment. *Lower left:* After thrombus removal from the aneurysm and the PICA, the aneurysm is clipped by two curved titanium clips. *Right:* Postoperative angiography reveals the patency of the PICA.

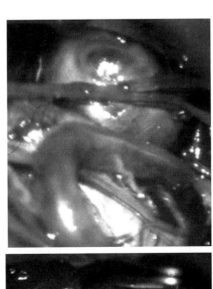

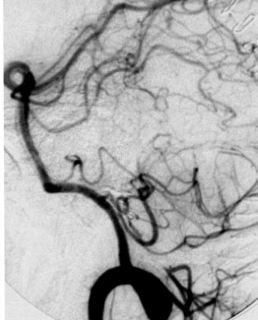

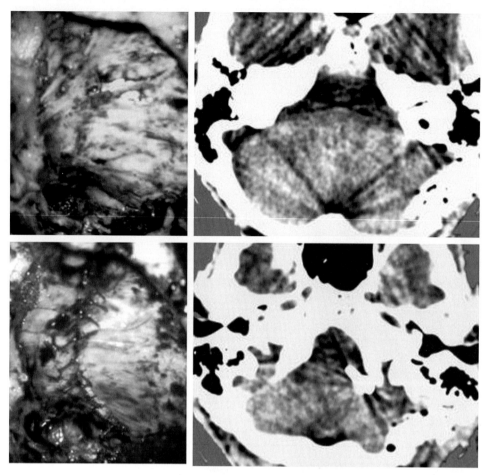

FIGURE 85-7 Intraoperative view and postoperative computed tomography (CT) of the same patient as shown in Figures 85-5 and 85-6. *Upper and lower left:* Microscopic view before (*upper*) dural opening and after (*lower*) watertight dura closure. *Upper and lower right:* Postoperative CT shows the approach and clip artifacts (*lower*).

FIGURE 85-8 A 37-year-old man with recent history of occipital headache. *Upper left:* Magnetic resonance angiography displays a mass suspected to be a right vertebral artery aneurysm (*arrows*). *Upper right:* Plain computed tomography scan with a suspected mass within the right medullary cistern (*arrow*). *Lower left and right:* T1-weighted magnetic resonance imaging demonstrates a berry-like lesion within the medullary cistern.

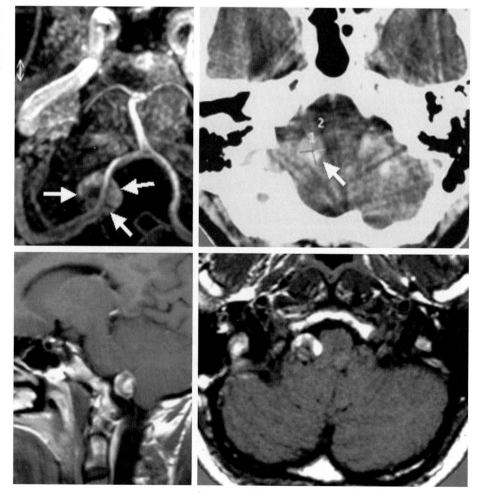

contour of the suboccipital region is restored for cosmetic reasons. In the majority of cases, a primary watertight dural closure is possible without the necessity of dural graft, except for small pieces of muscle. When the proximal portion of the intradural VA is involved, a small amount of dura mater may have to be resected. In such cases, we use a small graft of muscle fascia taken from the nuchal region. The bone flap and bone dust obtained from craniectomy are replaced, if necessary using osteosynthetic microplates.

CLINICAL OUTCOME AND PERIOPERATIVE MORBIDITY AND MORTALITY

Both intra- and perioperative conditions might influence the long-term outcome of patients. Intraoperatively, aneurysm rupture, perforating vessel injury, inadvertent arterial occlusion, or an inadequate arterial hypotension might cause postoperative new deficits. Perioperatively, a postoperative hematoma, postoperative significant vasospasm, rebleeding from a treated aneurysm, septicemia, meningitis, and bleeding

diathesis were observed as negative outcome predictors along with further intensive care–related complications such as respiratory insufficiency or pulmonary embolism. However, most patients can be managed without such problems and thus can expect a favorable outcome.[45,71,117,118] Even for complex VA-PICA aneurysms, good or excellent clinical results predominate in the larger surgical series.[33,34,45,71,78,117,118] One of the key issues for the management of these difficult lesions is the maintenance of cranial nerve function, which remains a challenging microsurgical problem during the treatment of VA-PICA aneurysms. In all major series, the most common postoperative neurologic deficit was a lower cranial nerve malfunction that can be observed in as many as 60% of the patients.[4,5,9,45,51,78,118–120] D'Ambrosio and colleagues[118] stated that the occurrence of lower cranial nerve dysfunction might be related to the extension of the approach. Our own data support this assumption.[45,78]

Severe morbidity or even mortality can be as high as 15% of the patients in the larger series but is mostly related to a poor preoperative state of the patients.[78,117]

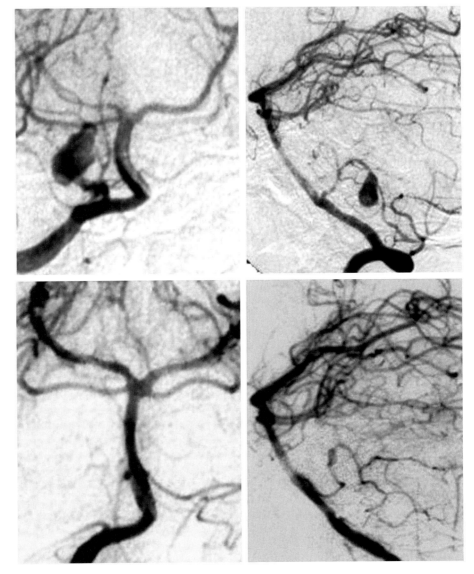

FIGURE 85-9 Pre- and postoperative angiography of the same patient as shown in Figure 85-5. Angiography before (*upper left and right*) surgery reveals an aneurysm of the tonsillomedullary segment of the right posterior inferior cerebellar artery that could not be treated by coiling due to the small caliber of the parent vessel. *Lower left and right:* Postoperative angiography displays the complete clip occlusion of the aneurysm.

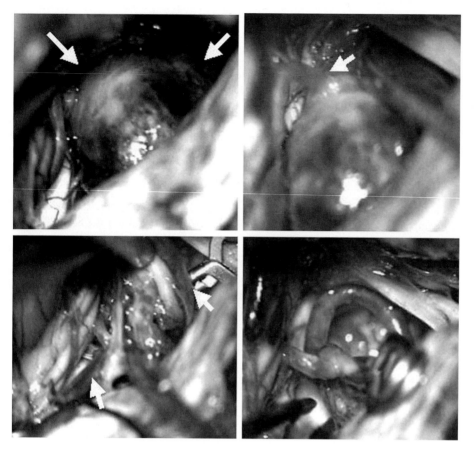

FIGURE 85-10 Intraoperative view of the same patient as shown in Figures 85-8 and 85-9. The aneurysm was approached by the transcondylar route. *Upper left:* Aneurysm (*arrows*) after arachnoidal dissection. *Upper right:* Vision of the aneurysm neck (*arrows*). Note that the distal posterior inferior cerebellar artery cannot be observed during this state of dissection because it originates at the back of the aneurysm neck. *Lower left:* Proximal and distal clipping after (*arrows*) and removal of a thrombus inside the aneurysm. *Lower right:* Final clipping with parent vessel reconstruction.

FIGURE 85-11 Postoperative computed tomography (CT) scans and photograph of the same patient as shown in Figures 85-8 to 85-10. *Upper and lower left:* CT scan shows the transcondylar approach and the clip. Note the partial condylar drilling in the small image. *Right:* Cosmetic result after 1 year.

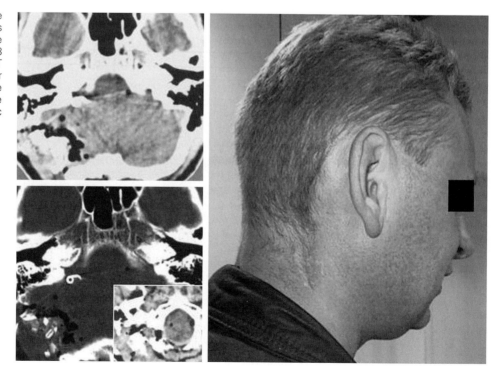

Generally, VA-PICA aneurysms can be treated with a fair degree of safety by an experienced neurovascular microsurgeon.

Illustrative Cases

CASE REPORT 1

A 37-year-old woman with a history of SAH Hunt & Hess grade III from a left-sided VA-PICA aneurysm was admitted to our department from an another hospital primarily for endovascular treatment. During the intervention with a GD coil, both the aneurysm and the anterior medullary segment of the PICA were spontaneously occluded by a thrombus. Local lysis was not attempted due to the risk of rebleeding from the recently ruptured aneurysm. Instead, emergency surgery was carried out, the thrombus was removed, and the aneurysm was successfully clipped with a restored patency of the PICA. Postoperatively, there was no additional morbidity (Figs. 85-5 to 85-7).

CASE REPORT 2

A 37-year-old man was admitted to our hospital with a recent history of occipital headache. Magnetic resonance imaging showed a right perimedullary hyperintense signal compatible with a partially thrombosed aneurysm of the PICA located slightly above the foramen magnum level. Angiography revealed a saccular aneurysm of the tonsillomedullary segment of the right PICA with the dome oriented downward. Endovascular treatment was judged inadequate by the endovascular interventionalist because of the reduced vessel diameter. The aneurysm was surgically exposed via the transcondylar approach and could be clipped successfully after endovascular thrombectomy. Temporary vocal cord paresis occurred postoperatively. No additional cranial nerve deficit was found. The patient returned to work (Figs. 85-8 to 85-11).

REFERENCES

1. Kassell NF, Torner JC: The International Cooperative Study on Timing of Aneurysm Surgery—an update. Stroke 15:566–570, 1984.
2. Drake CG: The treatment of aneurysms of the posterior circulation. Clin Neurosurg 26:96–144, 1979.
3. Friedman AH, Drake CG: Subarachnoid hemorrhage from intracranial dissecting aneurysm. J Neurosurg 60:325–334, 1984.
4. Hudgins RJ, Day AL, Quisling RG, et al: Aneurysms of the posterior inferior cerebellar artery: A clinical and anatomical analysis. J Neurosurg 58:381–387, 1983.
5. Lee KS, Gower DJ, Branch CL Jr, et al: Surgical repair of aneurysms of the posterior inferior cerebellar artery—a clinical series. Surg Neurol 31:85–91, 1989.
6. Peerless SJ, Drake CG: Posterior circulation aneurysms. In Wilkins RH, Rengachary SS (eds): Neurosurgery. New York: McGraw-Hill, 1985, pp 1422–1436.
7. Horiuchi T, Tanaka Y, Hongo K, et al: Characteristics of distal posteroinferior cerebellar artery aneurysms. Neurosurgery 53:589–595, 2003.
8. Yamamoto I, Tsugane R, Ohya M, et al: Peripheral aneurysms of the posterior inferior cerebellar artery. Neurosurgery 15:839–845, 1984.
9. Andoh T, Shirakami S, Nakashima T, et al: Clinical analysis of a series of vertebral aneurysm cases. Neurosurgery 31:987–993, 1992.
10. Beyerl BD, Heros RC: Multiple peripheral aneurysms of the posterior inferior cerebellar artery. Neurosurgery 19:285–289, 1986.
11. Dernbach PD, Sila CA, Little JR: Giant and multiple aneurysms of the distal posterior inferior cerebellar artery. Neurosurgery 22:309–312, 1988.
12. Gacs G, Vinuela F, Fox AJ, et al: Peripheral aneurysms of the cerebellar arteries: Review of 16 cases. J Neurosurg 58:63–68, 1983.
13. Hiscott P, Crockard A: Multiple aneurysms of the distal posterior inferior cerebellar artery. Neurosurgery 10:101–102, 1982.
14. Kaptain GJ, Lanzino G, Do HM, et al: Posterior inferior cerebellar artery aneurysms associated with posterior fossa arteriovenous malformation: Report of five cases and literature review. Surg Neurol 51:146–152, 1999.
15. Meisel HJ, Mansmann U, Alvarez H, et al: Cerebral arteriovenous malformations and associated aneurysms: Analysis of 305 cases from a series of 662 patients. Neurosurgery 46:793–800, 2000.
16. Westphal M, Grzyska U: Clinical significance of pedicle aneurysms on feeding vessels, especially those located in infratentorial arteriovenous malformations. J Neurosurg 92:995–1001, 2000.
17. Rothman SL, zar-Kia B, Kier EL, et al: The angiography of posterior inferior cerebellar artery aneurysms. Neuroradiology 6:1–7, 1973.
18. Yamaura A: Diagnosis and treatment of vertebral aneurysms. J Neurosurg 69:345–349, 1988.
19. Hernesniemi J: Distal PICA aneurysms. J Neurosurg 98:1144, 2003.
20. Drake CG, Peerless SJ, Hernesniemi JA: Surgery of Vertebrobasilar Aneurysms: London, Ontario, Experience on 1767 Patients. Vienna: Springer-Verlag, 1996.
21. Tiyaworabun S, Wanis A, Schirmer M, et al: Aneurysms of the vertebrobasilar system: Clinical analysis and follow-up results. Acta Neurochir (Wien) 63:221–229, 1982.
22. Yamaura A, Watanabe Y, Saeki N: Dissecting aneurysms of the intracranial vertebral artery. J Neurosurg 72:183–188, 1990.
23. Hernesniemi J: Clinical and radiographic outcome in the management of posterior circulation aneurysms by use of direct surgical or endovascular techniques. Neurosurgery 52:1505–1506, 2003.
24. Shokunbi MT, Vinters HV, Kaufmann JC: Fusiform intracranial aneurysms: Clinicopathologic features. Surg Neurol 29:263–270, 1988.
25. Kai Y, Hamada JI, Morioka M, et al: Endovascular coil trapping for ruptured vertebral artery dissecting aneurysms by using double microcatheters technique in the acute stage. Acta Neurochir (Wien) 145:447–451, 2003.
26. Yonas H, Agamanolis D, Takaoka Y, et al: Dissecting intracranial aneurysms. Surg Neurol 8:407–415, 1977.
27. Waga S, Fujimoto K, Morooka Y: Dissecting aneurysm of the vertebral artery. Surg Neurol 10:237–239, 1978.
28. Hamada J, Kai Y, Morioka M, et al: Multimodal treatment of ruptured dissecting aneurysms of the vertebral artery during the acute stage. J Neurosurg 99:960–966, 2003.
29. Yasui T, Komiyama M, Nishikawa M, et al: Fusiform vertebral artery aneurysms as a cause of dissecting aneurysms: Report of two autopsy cases and a review of the literature. J Neurosurg 91:139–144, 1999.
30. Mizutani T, Aruga T, Kirino T, et al: Recurrent subarachnoid hemorrhage from untreated ruptured vertebrobasilar dissecting aneurysms. Neurosurgery 36:905–911, 1995.
31. Aoki N, Sakai T: Rebleeding from intracranial dissecting aneurysm in the vertebral artery. Stroke 21:1628–1631, 1990.
32. Wakhloo AK, Lanzino G, Lieber BB, et al: Stents for intracranial aneurysms: The beginning of a new endovascular era? Neurosurgery 43:377–379, 1998.
33. Lewis SB, Chang DJ, Peace DA, et al: Distal posterior inferior cerebellar artery aneurysms: Clinical features and management. J Neurosurg 97:756–766, 2002.
34. Kanou Y, Arita K, Kurisu K, et al: Dissecting aneurysm of the peripheral posterior inferior cerebellar artery. Acta Neurochir (Wien) 142:1151–1156, 2000.
35. Schuster JM, Santiago P, Elliott JP, et al: Acute traumatic posteroinferior cerebellar artery aneurysms: Report of three cases. Neurosurgery 45:1465–1467, 1999.
36. Berger MS, Wilson CB: Intracranial dissecting aneurysms of the posterior circulation: Report of six cases and review of the literature. J Neurosurg 61:882–894, 1984.
37. Tanaka K, Waga S, Kojima T, et al: Non-traumatic dissecting aneurysms of the intracranial vertebral artery: Report of six cases. Acta Neurochir (Wien) 100:62–66, 1989.
38. Rizzoli HV, Hayes GJ: Congenital berry aneurysm of the posterior fossa: Case report with successful operative excision. J Neurosurg 10:550–551, 1953.

39. Richardson AE: The natural history of patients with intracranial aneurysm after rupture. Prog Brain Res 30:269–273, 1968.

40. Uihlein A, Hughes RA: The surgical treatment of intracranial vestigial aneurysms. Surg Clin North Am Mayo Clinic 1071–1083, 1955.

41. Desaussure RL, Hunter SE, Robertson JT: Saccular aneurysms of the posterior fossa. J Neurosurg 15:385–391, 1958.

42. Drake CG: The surgical treatment of vertebral-basilar aneurysms. Clin Neurosurg 16:114–169, 1969.

43. Rand RW, Jannetta PJ: Micro-neurosurgery for aneurysms of the vertebral-basilar artery system. J Neurosurg 27:330–335, 1967.

44. Yonekawa Y, Kaku Y, Imhof HG, et al: Posterior circulation aneurysms. Technical strategies based on angiographic anatomical findings and the results of 60 recent consecutive cases. Acta Neurochir Suppl 72:123–140, 1999.

45. Bertalanffy H, Gilsbach JM, Mayfrank L, et al: Planning and surgical strategies for early management of vertebral artery and vertebrobasilar junction aneurysms. Acta Neurochir (Wien) 134:60–65, 1995.

46. Huynh-Le P, Matsushima T, Miyazono M, et al: Three-dimensional CT angiography for the surgical management of the vertebral artery-posterior inferior cerebellar artery aneurysms. Acta Neurochir (Wien) 146:329–335, 2004.

47. Kayama T, Sugawara T, Sakurai Y, et al: Early CT features of ruptured cerebral aneurysms of the posterior cranial fossa. Acta Neurochir (Wien) 108:34–39, 1991.

48. Yeh HS, Tomsick TA, Tew JM Jr: Intraventricular hemorrhage due to aneurysms of the distal posterior inferior cerebellar artery: Report of three cases. J Neurosurg 62:772–775, 1985.

49. Iwama T, Andoh T, Sakai N, et al: Dissecting and fusiform aneurysms of vertebro-basilar systems: MR imaging. Neuroradiology 32:272–279, 1990.

50. Duvoisin RC, Yahr MD: Posterior fossa aneurysms. Neurology 15:231–241, 1965.

51. Salcman M, Rigamonti D, Numaguchi Y, et al: Aneurysms of the posterior inferior cerebellar artery-vertebral artery complex: Variations on a theme. Neurosurgery 27:12–20, 1990.

52. Day JD, Giannotta SL: Surgical Management of vertebro-PICA aneurysms. In Schmidek HH, Sweet WH, et al (eds): Operative Neurosurgical Techniques. Philadelphia: WB Saunders, 1994, pp 1103–1111.

53. Drake CG, Peerless SJ: Giant fusiform intracranial aneurysms: Review of 120 patients treated surgically from 1965 to 1992. J Neurosurg 87:141–162, 1997.

54. Halbach VV, Higashida RT, Dowd CF, et al: Endovascular treatment of vertebral artery dissections and pseudoaneurysms. J Neurosurg 79:183–191, 1993.

55. Iihara K, Sakai N, Murao K, et al: Dissecting aneurysms of the vertebral artery: A management strategy. J Neurosurg 97:259–267, 2002.

56. Kurata A, Ohmomo T, Miyasaka Y, et al: Coil embolization for the treatment of ruptured dissecting vertebral aneurysms. AJNR Am J Neuroradiol 22:11–18, 2001.

57. Lylyk P, Cohen JE, Ceratto R, et al: Combined endovascular treatment of dissecting vertebral artery aneurysms by using stents and coils. J Neurosurg 94:427–432, 2001.

58. Ponce FA, Albuquerque FC, McDougall CG, et al: Combined endovascular and microsurgical management of giant and complex unruptured aneurysms. Neurosurg Focus 17:E11, 2004.

59. Rabinov JD, Hellinger FR, Morris PP, et al: Endovascular management of vertebrobasilar dissecting aneurysms. AJNR Am J Neuroradiol 24:1421–1428, 2003.

60. Manabe H, Hatayama T, Hasegawa S, et al: Coil embolisation for ruptured vertebral artery dissection distal to the origin of the posterior inferior cerebellar artery. Neuroradiology 42:384–387, 2000.

61. Levy EI, Horowitz MB, Koebbe CJ, et al: Transluminal stent-assisted angioplasty of the intracranial vertebrobasilar system for medically refractory, posterior circulation ischemia: Early results. Neurosurgery 48:1215–1221, 2001.

62. Horowitz MB, Levy EI, Koebbe CJ, et al: Transluminal stent-assisted coil embolization of a vertebral confluence aneurysm: Technique report. Surg Neurol 55:291–296, 2001.

63. Barakate MS, Snook KL, Harrington TJ, et al: Angioplasty and stenting in the posterior cerebral circulation. J Endovasc Ther 8:558–565, 2001.

64. Rasmussen PA: Transluminal stent-assisted angioplasty of the intracranial vertebrobasilar system for medically refractory, posterior circulation ischemia: Early results. Neurosurgery 49:1489–1490, 2001.

65. Kremer C, Groden C, Hansen HC, et al: Outcome after endovascular treatment of Hunt and Hess grade IV or V aneurysms: Comparison of anterior versus posterior circulation. Stroke 30:2617–2622, 1999.

66. Lubicz B, Leclerc X, Gauvrit JY, et al: Giant vertebrobasilar aneurysms: Endovascular treatment and long-term follow-up. Neurosurgery 55:316–323, 2004.

67. Sugiu K, Takahashi K, Muneta K, et al: Rebleeding of a vertebral artery dissecting aneurysm during stent-assisted coil embolization: A pitfall of the "stent and coil" technique. Surg Neurol 61:365–370, 2004.

68. Nomura M, Kida S, Kita D, et al: Cerebellar hemorrhage after coil embolization for a ruptured vertebral dissecting aneurysm. Surg Neurol 53:239–242, 2000.

69. Heros RC: Lateral suboccipital approach for vertebral and vertebrobasilar artery lesions. J Neurosurg 64:559–562, 1986.

70. Pritz MB: Evaluation and treatment of aneurysms of the vertebral artery: Different strategies for different lesions. Neurosurgery 29:247–256, 1991.

71. Matsushima T, Matsukado K, Natori Y, et al: Surgery on a saccular vertebral artery-posterior inferior cerebellar artery aneurysm via the transcondylar fossa (supracondylar transjugular tubercle) approach or the transcondylar approach: Surgical results and indications for using two different lateral skull base approaches. J Neurosurg 95:268–274, 2001.

72. Matsushima T, Fukui M: [Lateral approaches to the foramen magnum: with special reference to the transcondylar fossa approach and the transcondylar approach]. No Shinkei Geka 24:119–124, 1996.

73. Pia HW: Classification and treatment of aneurysms of the vertebrobasilar system. Neurol Med Chir (Tokyo) 19:575–594, 1979.

74. Giannotta SL, Maceri DR: Retrolabyrinthine transsigmoid approach to basilar trunk and vertebrobasilar artery junction aneurysms: Technical note. J Neurosurg 69:461–466, 1988.

75. Day JD, Fukushima T, Giannotta SL: Cranial base approaches to posterior circulation aneurysms. J Neurosurg 87:544–554, 1997.

76. Todaka T, Hamada J, Yano S, et al: Successful clipping of a distal posterior inferior cerebellar artery aneurysm located on the anterior surface of the medulla oblongata—case report. Neurol Med Chir (Tokyo) 42:158–161, 2002.

77. Bertalanffy H, Seeger W: The dorsolateral, suboccipital, transcondylar approach to the lower clivus and anterior portion of the craniocervical junction. Neurosurgery 29:815–821, 1991.

78. Bertalanffy H, Sure U, Petermeyer M, et al: Management of aneurysms of the vertebral artery-posterior inferior cerebellar artery complex. Neurol Med Chir (Tokyo) 38(Suppl):93–103, 1998.

79. Kawase T, Bertalanffy H, Otani M, et al: Surgical approaches for vertebro-basilar trunk aneurysms located in the midline. Acta Neurochir (Wien) 138:402–410, 1996.

80. Chou SN, Ortiz-Suarez HJ: Surgical treatment of arterial aneurysms of the vertebrobasilar circulation. J Neurosurg 41:671–680, 1974.

81. Hernesniemi J: Comment on Matsushima T, et al.: Surgery on a saccular vertebral artery-posterior inferior cerebellar artery aneurysm via the transcondylar fossa (supracondylar transjugular tubercle) approach or the transcondylar approach: Surgical results and indications for using two different lateral skull base approaches. J Neurosurg 95:638–640, 2001.

82. Perata HJ, Tomsick TA, Tew JM Jr: Feeding artery pedicle aneurysms: Association with parenchymal hemorrhage and arteriovenous malformation in the brain. J Neurosurg 80:631–634, 1994.

83. Nagahiro S, Goto S, Yoshioka S, et al: Dissecting aneurysm of the posterior inferior cerebellar artery: Case report. Neurosurgery 33:739–741, 1993.

84. Pozzati E, Padovani R, Fabrizi A, et al: Benign arterial dissections of the posterior circulation. J Neurosurg 75:69–72, 1991.

85. Kitanaka C, Tanaka J, Kuwahara M, et al: Nonsurgical treatment of unruptured intracranial vertebral artery dissection with serial follow-up angiography. J Neurosurg 80:667–674, 1994.

86. Mokri B, Houser OW, Sandok BA, et al: Spontaneous dissections of the vertebral arteries. Neurology 38:880–885, 1988.

87. Yoshimoto Y, Wakai S: Unruptured intracranial vertebral artery dissection: Clinical course and serial radiographic imagings. Stroke 28:370–374, 1997.

88. Fujiwara S, Yokoyama N, Fujii K, et al: Repeat angiography and magnetic resonance imaging (MRI) of dissecting aneurysms of the intracranial vertebral artery: Report of four cases. Acta Neurochir (Wien) 121:123–129, 1993.

89. Kitanaka C, Sasaki T, Eguchi T, et al: Intracranial vertebral artery dissections: Clinical, radiological features, and surgical considerations. Neurosurgery 34:620–626, 1994.

90. Lemole GM Jr, Henn J, Javedan S, et al: Cerebral revascularization performed using posterior inferior cerebellar artery-posterior inferior cerebellar artery bypass: Report of four cases and literature review. J Neurosurg 97:219–223, 2002.

91. Kakino S, Ogasawara K, Kubo Y, et al: Treatment of vertebral artery aneurysms with posterior inferior cerebellar artery-posterior inferior cerebellar artery anastomosis combined with parent artery occlusion. Surg Neurol 61:185–189, 2004.

92. Nussbaum ES, Mendez A, Camarata P, et al: Surgical management of fusiform aneurysms of the peripheral posteroinferior cerebellar artery. Neurosurgery 53:831–834, 2003.

93. Ausman JI, Lee MC, Klassen AC, et al: Stroke: What's new? Cerebral revascularization. Minn Med 59:223–227, 1976.

94. Ausman JI, Pearce JE, Vacca DF, et al: Tandem bypass: occipital artery to posterior inferior cerebellar artery side-to-side anastomosis and occipital artery to anterior inferior cerebellar artery end-to-side anastomosis—a case report. Neurosurgery 22:919–922, 1988.

95. Ausman JI, Diaz FG, Mullan S, et al: Posterior inferior to posterior inferior cerebellar artery anastomosis combined with trapping for vertebral artery aneurysm: Case report. J Neurosurg 73:462–465, 1990.

96. Lawton MT, Hamilton MG, Morcos JJ, et al: Revascularization and aneurysm surgery: Current techniques, indications, and outcome. Neurosurgery 38:83–92, 1996.

97. Yasui T, Komiyama M, Nishikawa M, et al: Subarachnoid hemorrhage from vertebral artery dissecting aneurysms involving the origin of the posteroinferior cerebellar artery: Report of two cases and review of the literature. Neurosurgery 46:196–200, 2000.

98. Ali MJ, Bendok BR, Tawk RG, et al: Trapping and revascularization for a dissecting aneurysm of the proximal posteroinferior cerebellar artery: Technical case report and review of the literature. Neurosurgery 51:258–262, 2002.

99. Ausman JI, Nicoloff DM, Chou SN: Posterior fossa revascularization: Anastomosis of vertebral artery to PICA with interposed radial artery graft. Surg Neurol 9:281–286, 1978.

100. Hamada J, Nagahiro S, Mimata C, et al: Reconstruction of the posterior inferior cerebellar artery in the treatment of giant aneurysms: Report of two cases. J Neurosurg 85:496–499, 1996.

101. Hamada J, Todaka T, Yano S, et al: Vertebral artery-posterior inferior cerebellar artery bypass with a superficial temporal artery graft to treat aneurysms involving the posterior inferior cerebellar artery. J Neurosurg 96:867–871, 2002.

102. Durward QJ: Treatment of vertebral artery dissecting aneurysm by aneurysm trapping and posterior inferior cerebellar artery reimplantation: Case report. J Neurosurg 82:137–139, 1995.

103. Kurokawa Y, Okamura T, Watanabe K: Transcerebellar thrombectomy for the successful clipping of thrombosed giant vertebral

104. Drake CG: Giant intracranial aneurysms: experience with surgical treatment in 174 patients. Clin Neurosurg 26:12–95, 1979.

105. Sugita K: Microsurgical Atlas. New York: Springer-Verlag, 1985, pp 106–135.

106. Sugita K, Kobayashi S, Takemae T, et al: Giant aneurysms of the vertebral artery: Report of five cases. J Neurosurg 68:960–966, 1988.

107. Ausman JI, Malik GM, Tomecek FJ, et al: Hypothermic circulatory arrest and the management of giant and large cerebral aneurysms. Surg Neurol 40:289–298, 1993.

108. Steinberg GK, Drake CG, Peerless SJ: Deliberate basilar or vertebral artery occlusion in the treatment of intracranial aneurysms: Immediate results and long-term outcome in 201 patients. J Neurosurg 79:161–173, 1993.

109. Inamasu J, Suga S, Sato S, et al: Long-term outcome of 17 cases of large-giant posterior fossa aneurysm. Clin Neurol Neurosurg 102:65–71, 2000.

110. Rhoton AL Jr: The cerebellar arteries. Neurosurgery 47:S29–S68, 2000.

111. Katsuta T, Rhoton AL Jr, Matsushima T: The jugular foramen: Microsurgical anatomy and operative approaches. Neurosurgery 41:149–201, 1997.

112. Ito K, Tanaka Y, Kakizawa Y, et al: Aneurysm at the posterior inferior cerebellar artery of extradural origin for preoperative evaluation of safe clipping: Case report and review of the literature. Surg Neurol 60:329–333, 2003.

113. Lister JR, Rhoton AL Jr, Matsushima T, et al: Microsurgical anatomy of the posterior inferior cerebellar artery. Neurosurgery 10:170–199, 1982.

114. Marinkovic S, Milisavljevic M, Gibo H, et al: Microsurgical anatomy of the perforating branches of the vertebral artery. Surg Neurol 61:190–197, 2004.

115. Seeger W: Atlas of Topographical Anatomy of the Brain and Surrounding Structures. Wien: Springer-Verlag, 1978, pp 486–489.

116. Perneczky A: The posterolateral approach to the foramen magnum. In Samii M (ed): Surgery in and around the Brain Stem and the Third Ventricle. Berlin: Springer, 1986, pp 460–466.

117. Hernesniemi J: Posterior fossa aneurysms. J Neurosurg 96:638–640, 2002.

118. D'Ambrosio AL, Kreiter KT, Bush CA, et al: Far lateral suboccipital approach for the treatment of proximal posteroinferior cerebellar artery aneurysms: Surgical results and long-term outcome. Neurosurgery 55:39–50, 2004.

119. Horowitz M, Kopitnik T, Landreneau F, et al: Posteroinferior cerebellar artery aneurysms: Surgical results for 38 patients. Neurosurgery 43:1026–1032, 1998.

120. Peerless SJ, Hernesniemi JA, Gutman FB, et al: Early surgery for ruptured vertebrobasilar aneurysms. J Neurosurg 80:643–649, 1994.

artery-posterior inferior cerebellar artery aneurysm: Case report. Surg Neurol 33:217–220, 1990.

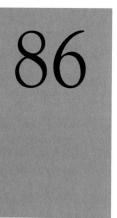

86 Diagnosis and Management of Traumatic Intracranial Aneurysms

DANIEL J. GUILLAUME, FUAD S. HADDAD,
GEORGES F. HADDAD, and PATRICK W. HITCHON

INTRODUCTION

Reports of aneurysm after head injury date back to the early 19th century. A post-traumatic middle meningeal artery aneurysm, proven by autopsy, was reported in 1829.[1] It was subsequently hypothesized that delayed apoplexy, after head injury, could occur because of the rupture of an aneurysm that was caused by trauma.[2] A few scarce reports of traumatic intracranial aneurysm (TICA) followed this[3,4] and in 1934, the first TICA was demonstrated by angiography.[5] Since then, a larger number of case reports and series have been published.[6-8] There are, at present, more than 500 reported cases.

CLASSIFICATION

TICAs are classified according to anatomy, etiology, or pathology as follows:

 I. Anatomic classification
    A. Cerebral
       i) Proximal to the circle of Willis (infraclinoid carotid, supraclinoid carotid, or vertebrobasilar)
       ii) Distal to the circle of Willis (subcortical or cortical)
    B. Extracerebral (middle meningeal artery)
 II. Etiological classification
    A. Blunt trauma
    B. Penetrating injury
       i) Missiles
       ii) Stab wounds
    C. Iatrogenic injury
 III. Pathologic classification
    A. True aneurysms occur after partial laceration of the vessel wall (i.e., disruption of intima, adventitia, or both) and subsequent ballooning of the remaining layers through the injured arterial wall.
    B. False or pseudoaneurysms occur after complete disruption of the arterial wall and subsequent hematoma formation that undergoes fibrous reorganization, enclosing the lumen and forming the wall of the aneurysm.
    C. Mixed aneurysms occur when a true aneurysm ruptures, forming a false aneurysm attached to it.

The majority of missile-induced aneurysms are false, caused by direct trauma from low-velocity, sharp-edged shrapnel, or by bone fragments grazing the artery.

EPIDEMIOLOGY

The overall incidence of reported cases of TICA is low. In adults, they represent less than 1% of all intracranial aneurysms.[9,10] In children, the proportion is approximately 30% according to Ventureyra and Higgins.[8] This apparent higher percentage in children may be caused by the lower incidence of saccular aneurysms in this age group[11] (Table 86-1).

Because the formation of TICAs is secondary to trauma, the population affected reflects those most at risk for blunt and penetrating head trauma, namely adults in their 20s and those in combat. Along these same lines, there appears to be a male predominance, with a male:female ratio reported as high as 12:1,[12] and 15:0[7] in missile-penetrating TICAs. In children, aneurysms can occur with a less severe trauma. Shaken baby syndrome, for instance, can lead to aneurysm formation.[13]

The relative incidence rates of TICA vary according to etiology. Blunt head trauma accounts for 60% to 70%, penetrating injuries for 16% to 26%, and iatrogenic accounts for approximately 10%.[8,9] The incidence of TICA in the group of penetrating brain injury is difficult to determine and may depend on the timing of angiography. Moreover, a negative angiogram does not exclude the possibility of delayed appearance of TICA. Haddad and colleagues reported the delayed appearance of a second TICA 2 weeks after an initial angiogram showed only a single one.[7]

The incidence of TICA following stab wounds is higher than that following gunshot wounds. Stab wounds to the head carry a very high risk of vascular injury in general (approximately 30%), and TICAs occur in 10% to 12% of stab wounds to the head.[14,15]

PATHOGENESIS

The mechanism of production of TICAs differs in each of the etiologic categories.

Blunt (Nonpenetrating) Trauma

In blunt trauma there are several possible mechanisms, as follows:

 1. The vessel can be directly injured by a contiguous skull fracture. Infraclinoid internal carotid artery (ICA) and basilar artery aneurysms are commonly

TABLE 86-1 ▪ **Differentiating Saccular from Traumatic Intracranial Aneurysms**

	Saccular Aneurysms	Traumatic Intracranial Aneurysms
Location in circulation	Large blood vessels at base of brain or major branch	Usually secondary branches
Location on vessel	Bifurcation of major arteries	Along course of artery, often near sharp edges
Pathology	Wall is well-defined (endothelial, fibrohyaline, and advential layers usually intact)	Wall is usually disrupted with organized clot forming part of wall
Patient age	Usually sixth decade	Any, but usually third decade

associated with basilar fractures because of the proximity of these arteries to the skull base.[16]

2. The second mechanism of injury is a shearing injury whereby the artery is partially torn because of the torque imparted on it by the moving brain. A relatively movable part or branch is stretched away from a fixed artery. In this process the ICA can be stretched or injured by traumatic movement along the anterior clinoid process.[17]

3. A tearing process may occur when a freely movable branch is rubbed against and traumatized by a relatively fixed hard edge such as the falx or the tentorial edges, as is seen in TICAs of the pericallosal artery and the posterior cerebral artery (PCA), respectively[18] (Fig. 86-1).

4. Another mechanism of etiology is entrapment of a cortical branch within a widened linear skull fracture. The pulsations of the brain squeeze a small part of the cortex within this aperture in the skull and rub the cortical vessel against the rugged edges of the fracture, thus injuring it.[19]

Case Reports

CASE REPORT 1

This 49-year-old man was involved in a motor vehicle collision, sustaining a closed head injury and a hangman's fracture. At that time, noncontrast head CT demonstrated cerebral contusion and subarachnoid hemorrhage. He recovered fully over the next 3 weeks and was discharged in halo immobilization. Eight months later, while standing in line at a bank, he lost consciousness and was transferred to the University of Iowa Hospital. On arrival, he had regained consciousness but was confused, displaying left hemiparesis. Noncontrast head CT (see Fig. 86-1A) revealed a right frontal paramedian hematoma with subdural and subarachnoid hemorrhage. Cerebral angiography (see Fig. 86-1B) demonstrated right callosomarginal post-traumatic saccular and fusiform aneurysms. On that same day, the patient underwent evacuation of the right frontoparietal subdural and parenchymal clot and aneurysm trapping. A clip was placed across the parent vessel (see Fig. 86-1C) and the aneurysm was found to harbor clot within it. Postoperative angiography (see Fig. 86-1D) revealed the aneurysm to have been removed from the circulation. The aneurysm was not submitted to histopathology.

Comments:
The callosomarginal artery is not a usual location for a saccular aneurysm.
The aneurysm is at the base of the falx and presumably formed as a result of injury by this structure.
The patient presented with sudden loss of consciousness.
The aneurysm is associated with an intracerebral and subdural hematoma.

Penetrating Trauma

In penetrating missile injuries the wall of the vessel is injured by a low-speed (at the time of vessel impact) fragment (metal or bone) with sharp edges (Fig. 86-2). Thus TICAs are more likely associated with ricochet bullets or with spent bullets that have irregular and sharp edges that develop after colliding with the skull. Traumatic aneurysms are seen in the distal path of the missile, after it has lost most of its energy and speed. Lacking the kinetic energy to exit the skull, these missiles are often retained within the skull. A high-speed fragment that has retained its smooth surface is less likely to be associated with aneurysmal formation.

CASE REPORT 2

This 25-year-old, left-handed male was admitted to the American University of Beirut (AUB) Medical Center with a shrapnel injury to the skull. A few hours previously, shrapnel had entered the right frontal pole and settled in the left parietal region (see Fig. 86-2A). On admission he was aphasic with a left hemiparesis. The next day he became restless, drowsy, and febrile. Débridement of the right frontal wound was carried out through a right frontal craniotomy. On day 12, a routine right carotid angiogram revealed aneurysmal dilatation of one of the left pericallosal branches (see Fig. 86-2B). Because of deterioration, a follow-up angiogram on day 16 revealed a 3 × 4 × 4 mm aneurysm at the apex of one of the middle cerebral candelabra vessels (see Fig. 86-2C and D), with delayed filling and emptying. The small aneurysmal dilatation of the proximal pericallosal artery was again observed. Follow-up angiography on day 59 revealed enlargement of the middle cerebral artery (MCA) warranting craniotomy. At surgery, a 12.5-mm aneurysm adherent to the frontal branch of the left middle cerebral artery was found. The aneurysm had no neck and was surrounded by a small blood clot; it was trapped and excised. The pathology revealed an organizing clot arising from the wall of a blood vessel. The hemiparesis gradually regressed, and the patient was discharged home on day 71. Two weeks after discharge (day 85) the motor aphasia disappeared and he recovered fully.

Comments:

This is a true penetrating missile traumatic aneurysm and not an iatrogenic one because it was in the hemisphere opposite to the one débrided.

The aneurysm lies in the distal portion of the trajectory of the shrapnel and is associated with a blood clot.

The offending shrapnel is still contained within the skull.

The aneurysm was on a branch of a major artery.

The aneurysm became apparent 16 days after injury and grew appreciably in size.

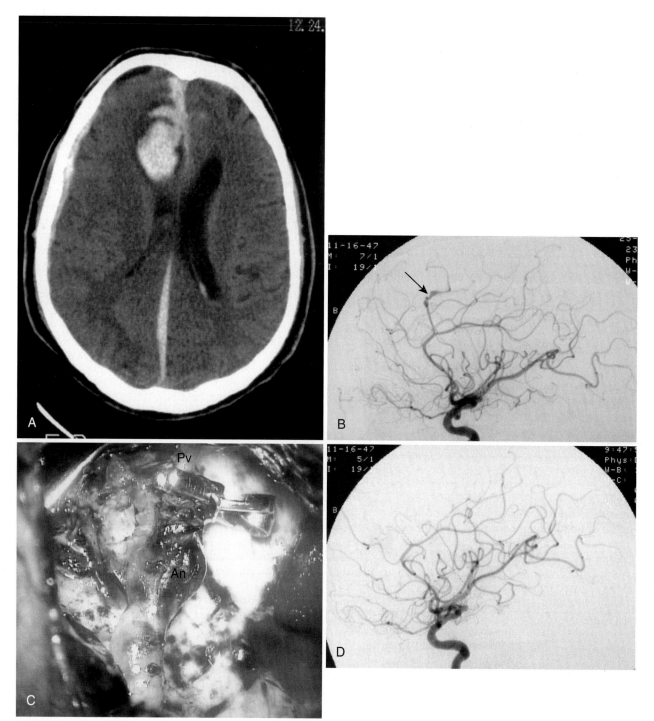

FIGURE 86-1 Noncontrast head CT reveals a right frontal paramedian hematoma with subdural and subarachnoid hemorrhage (*A*). Cerebral angiography shows right callosomarginal post-traumatic saccular and fusiform aneurysms (*arrow*) (*B*). Intra-operative photograph (*C*) demonstrates the aneurysm (An) excluded from circulation with aneurysm clip. Parent vessel (Pv) is seen proximal to aneurysm clip. Postoperative cerebral angiogram reveals that the aneurysm has been removed from the circulation (*D*).

Explosive bullets may act like shrapnels. Because most of these TICAs are false aneurysms, it is very common to find an associated blood clot in their vicinity. This could be an intracerebral (80%) or a subdural hematoma (26%).[7] Shearing forces, however, can also tear the wall or avulse the artery at a bifurcation, causing an aneurysm.[9] Peripheral branches of the MCA and anterior cerebral artery (ACA) are more vulnerable than are branches of the ICA or PCA.

This is because injuries to the skull base, below the external meatal line, are most commonly fatal.

Nonprojectile penetrating trauma with knives,[20] spurs, radio or TV antennae,[21] tent poles,[11] umbrella tips,[22] and other objects[23] have also been described to produce TICAs. These injuries may be accidental or provoked. They most commonly affect branches of the MCA and intracavernous ICA.[18]

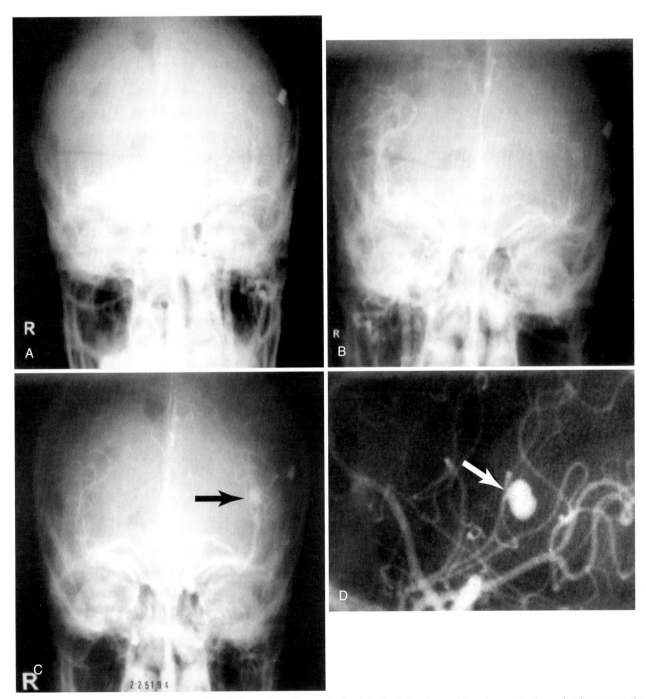

FIGURE 86-2   Plain skull x-ray shows the burr holes and craniotomy in the right frontal region and the shrapnel in the parietal cortex on the left side (*A*). A routine right carotid angiogram with cross compression performed on day 12 shows the mild dilatation of the pericallosal artery but no aneurysm on the left MCA (*B*). On day 16 a right carotid angiogram with cross compression reveals an aneurysm (*arrow*) on a left MCA branch (*C*). An enlarged view of the left MCA aneurysm in lateral projection is shown. The aneurysm (*arrow*) measures 3 × 4 × 4 mm (*D*).

Iatrogenic Injury

The first iatrogenic aneurysm was described by Finkemeyer in 1955 in a 55-year-old male operated on for an orbital roof meningioma.[24] Iatrogenic aneurysms may form because of traction on an arterial branch or be caused by direct injury that goes unnoticed because of the absence of bleeding. An iatrogenic aneurysm may occur anywhere in the brain subsequent to any of the following procedures: craniotomy, transsphenoidal, endoscopic, or endovascular.[24–26]

CASE REPORT 3

A 49-year-old female underwent endoscopic sphenoid sinus surgery for sinusitis that was complicated by perforation of the cribriform plate and laceration of both ACA A2 segments. She subsequently developed a left frontal hemorrhage and medial frontal lobe infarction (Fig. 86-3A). On examination she remained awake and alert, with mild weakness in both upper extremities (grading 4/5) and moderate to severe weakness in both lower extremities (grading 2/5 on the right and 3/5 on the left). Six days later, routine MRI and MRA were performed, revealing the above-mentioned hemorrhage and infarction, as well as a pseudoaneurysm between both A2 segments. She was transferred to the University of Iowa Hospital, where cerebral angiography demonstrated a 3-mm pseudoaneurysm arising from the right ACA A2 segment (see Fig. 86-3B and C). After clinically passing balloon test occlusion of the right ACA, she underwent successful coil embolization of aneurysm and parent right ACA A2 segment. Postprocedural angiogram (see Fig. 86-3D and E) demonstrates removal of parent vessel from circulation and good collateral flow to the ACAs distal to the site of injury. After the procedure, the patient initially developed depressed level of consciousness, diminished motivation for speech, and increased weakness of both lower extremities. She improved and, after a short stay in a rehabilitation facility, has fully recovered.

Comments:

This is a true iatrogenic aneurysm.
It is associated with a hemorrhage.
It was treated by endovascular technique.

CLINICAL PRESENTATION

The typical patient harboring a TICA suffers initial major blunt (in children the trauma may be minor) or penetrating head trauma that usually leads to intracranial hemorrhage. The location of the hemorrhage can be either intraparenchymal, intraventricular, subarachnoid, or subdural. Patients will have levels of consciousness varying from awake and complaining of headache to comatose. Initial management of these patients focuses on diagnosis and management of their presenting brain injuries.

Most TICAs occur 2 to 8 weeks following the instigating traumatic event, although they have been reported to occur within hours of the injury.[7] The presence of orbitofaciocranial trauma and intracerebral hemorrhage should lead to the suspicion of an underlying aneurysm. In projectile injuries, a retained fragment associated with a hematoma in the distal part of its trajectory should also alert the physician to the possibility of a TICA.[7]

The most common symptoms include delayed depressed level of consciousness, seizure, and new neurologic deficit.[27] TICAs occurring on different segments of the ICA can produce specific clinical findings. Supraclinoid ICA aneurysms can present with headache, memory changes, and visual loss (see Case Report 1). Neurologic signs suggesting aneurysm formation within the infraclinoid ICA include diabetes insipidus or compressive cranial nerve palsies caused by the enlarging aneurysm. A sixth nerve palsy may occur with increased intracranial pressure and is nonlocalizing. Massive epistaxis can occur when a petrous or intracavernous ICA aneurysm ruptures in association with a basilar skull fracture. TICAs located at the skull base can also cause visual deficits from compression of the optic nerve.[28,29] The triad of unilateral blindness, cranial base fractures, and recurrent severe epistaxis prompts the suspicion of ICA injuries originating in the cranial base.[28] An intracavernous TICA can also rupture into the cavernous sinus, leading to carotid-cavernous-fistula formation and its associated neurologic signs (i.e., proptosis, chemosis, retro-orbital pain, and fifth nerve deficit).

Aneurysms that occur on distal branches produce deficits that correspond to their locations. Pericallosal and distal cortical aneurysms can present with hydrocephalus.[11,30] In infants, a growing aneurysm may lead to a growing skull fracture.[30–32] In 10% to 20% of cases, the aneurysm may be asymptomatic and discovered incidentally during neuroimaging studies. (For a review of clinical presentations, see reference 29.)

DIAGNOSIS

There are certain radiologic and clinical indicators that should lead the clinician to suspect vascular injury with subsequent TICA formation. Development of aneurysm after trauma should be suspected in the following: when trauma to the orbitofaciocranial region is recent and is associated with delayed neurologic deterioration; with unusual location of intracerebral hemorrhage; with recurrent massive epistaxis; with enlarging skull fractures; and with progressive cranial nerve palsies caused by compression. When the injury is caused by a missile, an aneurysm should be suspected in the case of a low velocity fragment or ricochet bullet that is still retained in the skull; and where there is evidence of a hematoma toward the distal part of the fragment, especially if a previous CT scan failed to show it.

Neurologic deterioration after head trauma should always be initially worked up with high-resolution head CT. This will reveal the presence of intracranial hemorrhage, cerebral edema, hydrocephalus, missile tracts, bone, other fragments, and other lesions.

Four-vessel cerebral angiography should be performed in patients with intracranial hemorrhage; stab wounds to the

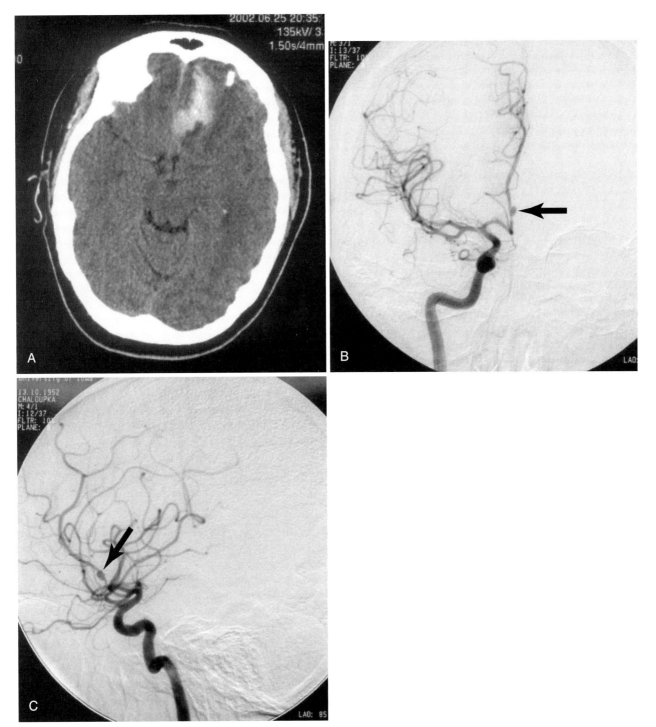

FIGURE 86-3   Noncontrast head CT demonstrates left frontal hemorrhage and medial frontal lobe infarction (*A*). Cerebral angiography AP (*B*) and lateral (*C*) views reveal a 3-mm pseudoaneurysm (*arrows*) arising from the right ACA A2 segment.

(Continued)

head with dural penetration; shrapnel wounds; spent or ricochet bullet; absent exit wound; a trajectory that enters through the pterion, crosses the midline, or passes through the basal cisterns, sylvian, or interhemispheric fissures; or when the inciting instrument remains embedded in the brain.[7,9] In general, angiography is recommended in workup for penetrating brain injury whenever a vascular injury is suspected.[33] Although aneurysms can occur within a few hours after injury, most develop over days and may be missed by early angiography. MRA or CT angiography (CTA) has also been used for evaluation, but these have not been utilized to the same degree as conventional cerebral angiography. Furthermore, artifact from metal can interfere with interpretation of these studies.

It is difficult to angiographically distinguish an aneurysm caused by trauma from one that was not. TICAs range in

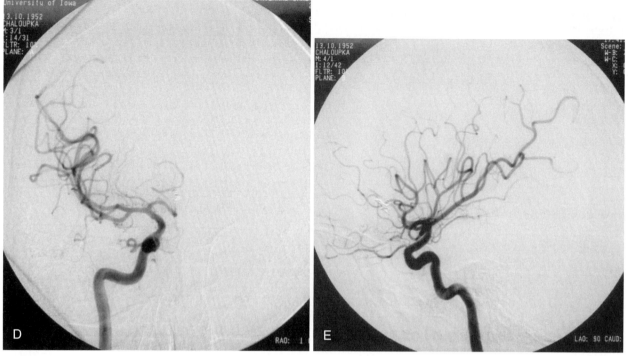

FIGURE 86-3 Cont'd Following intravascular occlusion, angiography shows occlusion of the parent vessel proximal to the aneurysm with good collateral flow to the ACAs distal to the site of injury (*D* and *E*).

size from 2 to 15 mm.[7,34] The angiographic features suggestive of traumatic etiology include delayed filling and/or excessive delayed emptying of the sac (Case Report 2), lack of relationship with bifurcations, irregular appearance, and absence of a neck.[35] These aneurysms usually have a well-defined border but may occasionally be irregular and lobulated in the early phase. Spasm is not a salient feature, and in the presence of multiple aneurysms does not provide a clue to the ruptured one.[7] Table 86-1 lists differentiating features of saccular and traumatic intracranial aneurysms.

MANAGEMENT OPTIONS

Although a small number of TICAs can thrombose spontaneously over time[36,37] (more commonly, those caused by closed head injury or that are iatrogenic, rather than penetrating ones), they typically enlarge and rupture.[7,38] Histologic classification does not influence management. For this reason, it is strongly recommended that, once diagnosed, a TICA should be excluded from the circulation regardless of its size or location, either by surgical or endovascular means. Surgical method depends on location and morphology of the aneurysm and the nature of the injury. It is preferable to clip the aneurysm, leaving the parent vessel patent; however, this is only possible in about 10% to 15% of cases because of the lack of a discrete aneurysm neck.[6,9] The morbidity and mortality of non-treated ruptured TICAs is 50% to 70%, whereas the morbidity and mortality of surgical treatment is 15% to 30%, or approximately one third.[9,18] The relative high surgical morbidity and mortality is generally caused by the preoperative

state of the patient (because of the original trauma) and reflects the propensity of these aneurysms to rupture during treatment because of the absence of a true wall. Additionally, they are adherent to brain tissue, which leads to difficulty with dissection.

A large portion of TICAs, particularly those located close to the skull base, result from rupture of the entire arterial wall.[39] These two obstacles (skull base location and rupture of entire wall thickness) cause difficulty in exploration and with obtaining proximal and distal control. The complex exposures needed to achieve proximal and distal vessel control can be complicated by significant cranial nerve damage,[40] cerebral ischemia, or thromboembolism.[41] In these situations, ICA trapping with or without external carotid–internal carotid (EC-IC) bypass (depending on tolerance of test occlusion) may be a better option.[42]

Endovascular aneurysm obliteration is another option that is gaining in attractiveness (see Case Report 3). This is partially in response to the obstacles associated with TICAs located near the skull base, discussed above. Moreover, the development of detachable balloon catheters has aided in more safely treating TICAs of the skull base.[43]

Endovascular procedures have their own associated morbidities. Placement of balloon or coil directly into pseudoaneurysms may lead to massive hemorrhage, because these aneurysms lack a formal wall. Endovascular treatment can also be difficult because of high neck:fundus ratio. Endovascular trapping or occlusion of the parent artery with a detachable balloon is the safest endovascular procedure.[43] More recently, endovascular stent placement with parent artery preservation has been described for traumatic skull base vascular lesions.[44]

Intraoperative cerebral protection (e.g., barbiturate use and moderate hypothermia) should be considered when vessel reconstruction would require temporary occlusion of the parent vessel. In awake patients, continuous neurologic examination can be performed during balloon test occlusion. In intubated or comatose patients, cerebral circulation can be assessed during test occlusion with electroencephalography or somatosensory evoked potentials. In those who do not tolerate parent artery occlusion, consideration can be given to EC-IC bypass or parent vessel stenting.[43,44]

CONCLUSIONS

Penetrating, nonpenetrating (blunt), and iatrogenic injuries can lead to aneurysm formation; however, aneurysms most commonly occur following nonpenetrating head injury. Missile-induced TICAs are usually false. Most TICAs occur 2 to 8 weeks following the traumatic event. Symptoms and signs include depressed level of consciousness, seizure, de novo neurologic deficit, diabetes insipidus, cranial nerve palsies, epistaxis, proptosis, chemosis, retro-orbital pain, headache, memory changes, visual loss, growing skull fracture, and hydrocephalus. Delayed neurologic deterioration after head trauma should always be worked up with head CT. Cerebral angiography should be performed whenever a vascular injury is suspected. The angiographic features suggestive of traumatic etiology include delayed filling or emptying of the sac, distal location of aneurysm away from a bifurcation, irregular appearance, and absence of a neck. Treatment should exclude the aneurysm from the circulation as soon as the patient is stable by either surgical or endovascular means.

REFERENCES

1. Smith S: On the difficulties attending the diagnosis of aneurism, being a contribution to surgical diagnosis and to medical jurisprudence. Am J Med Sci 4:237, 1829.
2. Bollinger O: Uber traumatische Spat-Apoplexie; Ein Beitrag zum Lahre von Hirnerschutterung. Festschr Rud Virshow 2:45; 7i–470, 1891.
3. Guibert: Aneurysme arteriel de la carotide interne au niveau du sinus caverneux gauche; comminication avec le sinus sphenoidal droit; hemorrhagies nasals; mort, autopsie. Ann d'Oculist 113:314–318, 1895.
4. Birly JL, Trotter W: Traumatic aneurysm of intracranial portion of internal carotid artery: Note on effects of effects of obstruction of carotid circulation on homolateral eye. Brain 51:184–208, 1928.
5. Tonnis W: Traumatisches aneurysma der linken art carotid int. mit embolie der linken art. Cerebri ant und retinae. Zentralbl Chir 61: 844–848, 1934.
6. Aarabi B: Traumatic aneurysms of brain due to high velocity missile head wounds. Neurosurgery 22:56–63, 1988.
7. Haddad FS, Faddad GF, Taha J: Traumatic intracranial aneurysms caused by missiles: Their presentation and management. Neurosurgery 28:1–7, 1991.
8. Ventureyra EC, Higgins MJ: Traumatic intracranial aneurysms in childhood and adolescence: Case report and review of the literature. Childs Nerv Syst 10:361–379, 1994.
9. Aarrabi B: Management of traumatic aneurysms caused by high-velocity missile head wounds. Neurosurg Clin N Am 6:775–797, 1995.
10. Kassell NF, Torner JC, Haley EC Jr, et al: The international cooperative study on the timing of aneurysm surgery: Part 1. Overall management results. J Neurosurg 73:18–36, 1990.
11. Thompson JR, Harwood-Nash DC, Fitz CR: Cerebral aneurysms in children. Am J Roentgenol Radium Ther Nucl Med 118:163–175, 1973.
12. Meyer FB, Sundt TM Jr, Fode NC, et al: Cerebral aneurysms in childhood and adolescence. J Neurosurg 70:420–425, 1989.
13. Lam CH, Montes J, Farmer JP, et al: Traumatic aneurysm from shaken baby syndrome: Case report. Neurosurgery 39:1252–1255, 1996.
14. Kieck CF, de Villiers JC: Vascular lesions due to transcranial stab wounds. J Neurosurg 60:42–46, 1984.
15. du Trevou MD, Takaku A, Aihara H, et al: Traumatic cerebral aneurysm associated with widening skull fracture: Report of two infancy cases. Childs Brain 6:131–139, 1980.
16. Shaw CM, Alvord EC Jr: Injury of the basilar artery associated with closed head trauma. J Neurol Neurosurg Psychiatry 35:247–257, 1972.
17. Pozzat E, Gaist G, Servadei F: Traumatic aneurysms of the supraclinoid internal carotid artery: Report of two cses. J Neurosurg 57:418–422, 1982.
18. Fleischer AS, Patton JM, Tindall GT: Cerebral aneurysms of traumatic origin. Surg Neurol 4:233–239, 1975.
19. Rumbaugh CL, Bergeron RT, Talalla A, et al: Traumatic aneurysms of the cortical cerebral arteries: Radiographic aspects. Radiology 96:49–54, 1970.
20. McDonald EJ, Winestock DP, Hoff JT: The value of repeat cerebral arteriography in the evaluation of trauma. AJR Am J Roentgenol 126: 792–797, 1976.
21. Cressman MR, Hayes GJ: Traumatic aneurysm of the anterior choroidal artery. Case report. J Neurosurg 24:102–104, 1966.
22. Carothers A: Orbitofacial wounds and cerebral artery injuries caused by umbrella tips. JAMA 239:1151–1152, 1978.
23. Chadduck WM: Traumatic aneurysm due to speargun injury: Case report. J Neurosurg 31:77–79, 1969.
24. Finkemeyer H: Eine säckenförmiges Aneurysma den Arteria Cerebralis media als postoperative Komplication. Zentrabl Neurochir 15:302–304, 1955;
25. McLaughlin MR, Wahlig JB, Kaufmann AM, et al: Traumatic basilar aneurysm after endoscopic third ventriculostomy: Case report. Neurosurg 41:1400–1404, 1997.
26. Raskind R: An intra-cranial aneurysm associated with a recurrent meningioma. J Neurosurg 23:622–625, 1965.
27. Larson PS, Reisner A, Morassutti DJ, et al: Traumatic intracranial aneurysms. Neurosurg Focus 8:1–4, 2000.
28. Maurer JJ, Mills M, German WJ: Triad of unilateral blindness, orbital fractures, and massive epistaxis after head injury. J Neurosurg 18:837–840, 1961.
29. Menezes AH, Graf CJ: True traumatic aneurysm of anterior cerebral artery. J Neurosurg 40:544–548, 1974.
30. Endo S, Takaku A, Aihara H, et al: Traumatic cerebral aneurysm associated with widening skull fracture: Report of two infancy cases. Childs Brain 6:131–139, 1980.
31. Almeida GM, Pindaro J, Plese P, et al: Intracranial arterial aneurysms in infancy and childhood. Childs Brain 3:193–199, 1977.
32. Yazbak PA, McComb JG, Raffel C: Pediatric traumatic intracranial aneurysms. Pediatr Neurosurg 22:15–19, 1995.
33. Aarabi B, Alden TD, Chesnut RM, et al: Neuroimaging in the management of penetrating brain injury. In Pruitt BA (ed): Guidelines for the management of penetrating brain injury. J Trauma 51(Suppl): S7-S11, 2001.
34. Achram M, Rizk G, Haddad FS: Angiographic aspects of traumatic intracranial aneurysms following war injuries. Br J Radiol 53: 1144–1149, 1980.
35. Takakura K, Saito I, Sasaki T: Special problems associated with subarachnoid hemorrhage. In Youmans JR (ed): Neurological Surgery: A Comprehensive Reference Guide to the Diagnosis and Management of Neurological Problems, 3rd ed. Philadelphia: Saunders, 1990, pp 1867–1868.
36. Brenner H: Frontale schädelspaltung mit traumatischen aneurysma der aeteria pericallosa. Acta Neurochir (Wien) 10:145–152, 1962.
37. Funakoshi T, Tsuchiya J, Sakai N, et al: Peripheral arterial aneurysm of the brain occurring after brain abscess extirpation and healing spontaneously: Report on a case and review of the literature. Neurol Surg (Tokyo) 4:405–410, 1976.
38. Umebayashi Y, Kuwayama M, Handa Y, et al: Traumatic aneurysm of a peripheral cerebral artery: Case report. Clin Radiol 21:36–38, 1970.

39. Benoit BG, Wortzman G: Traumatic cerebral aneurysms: Clinical features and natural history. J Neurol Neurosurg Psychiatry 36:127–138, 1973.

40. Fleischer AS, Patton JM, Tindall GT: Cerebral aneurysms of traumatic origin. Surg Neurol 4:233–239, 1975.

41. Mokri B, Piepgras DG, Houser OW: Traumatic dissections of the extracranial internal carotid artery. J Neurosurg 68:189–197, 1988.

42. du Trevou M, Bullock R, Teasdale E, et al: False aneurysms of the carotid tree due to unsuspected penetrating injury of the head and neck. Injury 22:237–239, 1991.

43. Uzan M, Cantasdemir M, Seckin MS, et al: Traumatic intracranial carotid tree aneurysms. Neurosurgery 43:1314–1320, 1998.

44. Redekip G, Marotta T, Weill A: Treatment of traumatic aneurysms and arteriovenous fistulas of the skull base by using endovascular stents. J Neurosurg 95:412–419, 2001.

87 Surgical Management of Intracranial Aneurysms Caused by Infection

ROBERT N. N. HOLTZMAN, JOHN M. D. PILE-SPELLMAN,
JOHN C. M. BRUST, JAMES E. O. HUGHES, and
P. C. TAYLOR DICKINSON

TERMINOLOGY

The term *mycotic aneurysm*, initially attributed to Osler and used to describe bacterial intracranial aneurysms, is a misnomer. Most investigators currently agree that its use should be strictly limited to descriptions of aneurysms of fungal origin. Yet efforts to establish an accurate nomenclature have been generally unsuccessful. Therefore, we are resigned to the fact that the term *mycotic aneurysm* will remain in general parlance. At the same time, we prefer the use of a more specific and accurate heading, namely, *infected intracranial aneurysm*, to include the categories of intracranial bacterial aneurysm,[1-3] fungal aneurysm,[4-6] spirochetal aneurysm,[7] infested or amebic aneurysm,[8] viral aneurysm,[9] and phytotic aneurysm,[10] according to the specific infecting organism or agent. The terms *infectious aneurysm*[2,11,12] and *infective aneurysm*[3,13] are flawed because they imply that the aneurysm itself is the infecting agent rather than being the end point of an infecting process. Until such a pathogenesis has been detected, it is the intention of the authors to avoid catachresis and the application of archaic language (Marcus S, The George Delacorte Professor of English and Comparative Literature, Columbia University, New York, personal communication, 1993: "The correct usage is 'infected.' The term 'infectious' died out as a usage in terms of infected in 1726." And Jost DA, Former Senior Lexicographer of *The American Heritage Dictionary*, Boston, personal communication, 1996: "[I]nfectious aneurysm will be interpreted by most users of English as an aneurysm that can communicate infection.").

The term *infected intracranial aneurysm* lacks the properties of complete definition because it refers to the initial process that affects the arterial wall and to aneurysms found to have bacteria in their walls at the time of excision (Table 87-1, Patient 3; see Case Report 9, Fig. 87-9), but not to the processes of focal dilatation or subsequent aneurysm formation and enlargement. It also accurately describes the congenital or berry aneurysm that has become secondarily infected.[1,14,15] The terms *septic aneurysm*,[16,17] *septic embolism*, and *septic arteritis* are also commonly used.[18] However, the word *septic* refers to infection involving the blood stream and is not really descriptive of the aneurysms themselves.

INTRODUCTION

Etiologies

Infected intracranial aneurysms have several possible origins:

1. Infected emboli, most often of cardiac valvular origin, lodge in cerebral vessels, usually at a bifurcation, obstruct the lumen, and cause damage to the tunica intima if rapid thrombolysis does not occur. Focal arteritis then disrupts the internal elastic lamina and the tunica media, weakening the vessel wall and causing focal enlargement in either a saccular or fusiform shape without a distinct "neck." Branches are incorporated in these focal dilatations as the hydrodynamic forces of pulsatile blood act on the weakened walls. Supportive experimental evidence for this mechanism has been provided by Foote and colleagues.[19] In most instances these aneurysms cannot be clipped or occluded endovascularly without sacrificing the parent artery or branching vessels.

2. Embolic infection of preexisting congenital aneurysms occurring by a similar mechanism appears angiographically as an enlarging aneurysm with a "neck" at sites characteristic for congenital aneurysms in the setting of endocarditis.[1,14,15] These aneurysms may have an accessible neck permitting endovascular occlusion or clipping in some instances with preservation of the parent artery.

3. Contiguous extravascular exposure to infective processes, such as cavernous sinus thrombophlebitis,[20-23] meningitis,[1,24-27] cerebral abscess (Stein BM, personal communication, 1993),[27a-30] and subdural empyema,[31] has resulted in focal infection of a vessel wall and subsequent aneurysm formation. Precisely how this phenomenon occurs is unknown. The manner by which infection is communicated to a blood vessel wall was explained as an initial infection spreading to the vasa vasorum with subsequent centripetal extension into the tunica media. This explanation was based on models in which bacteria were introduced systemically or locally into a vessel lumen.[32-35] Contiguous extravascular

TABLE 87-1 ■ Symptoms, Cerebrospinal Fluid, and Computed Tomography

Patient	Sex, Age (yr)	Systemic Symptoms and Signs	Neurologic Symptoms and Signs on Admission	Later Neurologic Symptoms and Signs	Cerebrospinal Fluid Findings*	Computed Tomographic Findings	Aneurysms at Angiography	Surgery	Outcome
1	F, 15	Abdominal and hip pain, fever × 4 wk	Sudden left hemiparesis, seizure	d 41: Right hemiparesis, aphasia	d 1: RBC 421, WBC 6, protein 120, not xanthochromic	ND	d 24: Right MCA, distal; d 46: Left MCA, distal	d 30: Excision and hematoma evacuation; d 51: Excision and hematoma evacuation	d 73: Died, sepsis
2	M, 66	Fever × 5 d, splinter hemorrhages	Normal	d 10: Seizure, right hemiparesis, aphasia	d 11: Bloody, xanthochromic	ND	d 11: Left MCA, distal	d 20: Excision and hematoma evacuation	Discharged aphasic
3	F, 11	Fever, headache × 1 wk	Sudden severe headache, stiff neck, confusion, left hemiparesis	—	d 1: Bloody, xanthochromic	ND	d 2: Right MCA, distal; d 11: Bigger	d 11: Excision	Discharged, cognitive impairment
4	M, 82	Urinary tract infections × 8 wk	Sudden left hemiparesis	—	ND	ND	d 2: 2 on right MCA, both distal	d 3: Excision of both, hematoma evacuation	d 19: Died; GI hemorrhage
5	F, 25	Fever, headache × 1 wk	Sudden left hemiparesis	—	ND	d 1: Normal	d 2: Left and right MCA, distal; d 63: Right gone, left still patent	d 69: Excised left	Discharged asymptomatic
6	F, 24	Fever, weight loss, "salpingitis"	Normal	d 12: Sudden headache, hemiparesis, aphasia	d 12: Bloody, xanthochromic	ND	d 20: Left MCA, distal; d 26: 2 on right MCA, distal; d 68: Left bigger; d 91: 1 on right gone, the other bigger	d 75: Excised left; d 104: Excised right	Discharged asymptomatic
7	M, 23	Migratory arthralgias × 4 d, splinter hemorrhages	Nuchal rigidity	d 5: Sudden right hemiparesis, seizure	d 1: RBC 450, WBC 264 (PMN 90%), protein 54, not xanthochromic	d 5: Normal; d 13: Enhancing parietal left lucency	d 5: Negative; d 27: Bilateral MCA, distal; d 38: Both gone	None	Discharged asymptomatic
8	M, 45	Headache, fever × 6 wk, microabscesses on fingers, splenomegaly	Mild right hemiparesis	—	d 1: RBC 72, WBC 12, normal protein, glucose, not xanthochromic	d 2: Left parietal hemorrhagic infarct	d 2: Left MCA, distal; d 41: Bigger	d 46: Excised	Discharged asymptomatic
9	M, 45	Cellulitis of foot × 10 d	Sudden left hemiparesis	d 66: Sudden right hemiparesis	d 3: RBC 4, WBC 8, normal protein, glucose, not xanthochromic	d 2: Normal; d 11: biparietal hemorrhagic infarcts	d 25: 3 on right distal MCA, 2 on left distal MCA, 1 on anterior communicating; d 52: 2 on left MCA smaller, 1 on right MCA smaller, 2 on right MCA unchanged, ACoA unchanged; d 69: 2 on left MCA smaller, 1 on right MCA gone, 1 on right MCA smaller, 1 on right MCA unchanged, ACoA unchanged	None	d 75: Died, rupture of hepatic aneurysm

10	F, 28	Fever × 5 d	Headache	d 5: Sudden left hemiparesis	ND	d 29: Right basal ganglia infarct	d 28: Right MCA, proximal, fusiform; d 48: Unchanged	d 35: Wrapped	Discharged, left hemiparesis
11	M, 37	Fever, lethargy × 6 d	Headache	d 3: Sudden left hemiparesis	d 1: RBC 15, WBC 0, protein 126, glucose normal, xanthochromic	d 18: Right frontoparietal infarct	d 35: Left MCA; d 72: bigger	d 75: Excised	Discharged asymptomatic after transient right hemiparesis
12	M, 24	Fever, headache, weight loss × 6 wk	Headache, stiff neck, mild weakness of right arm	d 15: Coma, transtentorial herniation	d 2: RBC 120 WBC 9, normal protein, glucose, not xanthochromic	d 7: Aneurysm, left middle cerebral artery; d 14: Aneurysm larger; d 15: Left intracerebral hemorrhage	ND (aneurysm seen on CT)	None	d 17: Died, intracerebral hemorrhage
13	M, 29	Shoulder abscess, fever	Normal	d 29: Coma, transtentorial herniation	ND	d 29: Left intracerebral hematoma	d 43: Right MCA, distal	d 29: Left hematoma evacuation; d 47: right excised	Discharged with mild aphasia
14	F, 41	Fever	Sudden severe headache, stiff neck, seizure, left homonymous hemianopia	—	d 1: RBC 700, WBC 450, protein 390, normal glucose, xanthochromic	d 1: Right parietotemporal hematoma	d 3: Right PCA, distal; d 16: smaller; d 36: Gone	None	Discharged asymptomatic
15	F, 36	Fever, Janeway's lesions, hepatomegaly	Delirium	d 20: Sudden left hemiparesis	d 1: WBC 2000 (PMN 90%), protein 86, glucose 43	d 14: Bihemispheric enhancing lucencies	d 20: Right MCA, distal; d 46: Smaller; d 81: Smaller; d 124: Smaller	None	Discharged, left hemiparesis
16	M, 54	—	Sudden headache, then coma with extensor posturing	—	ND	d 3: Third ventricular and subarachnoid hemorrhage	d 4: Right superior cerebellar	d 9: Excised	Discharged asymptomatic
17	M, 11	Fever	Lethargy	d 8: Stupor, right hemiparesis	d 2: RBC 48, WBC 39 (PMN 56%), normal protein, glucose, not xanthochromic	d 8: Right parietal hematoma	d 10: Right MCA distal	d 10: Excised, hematoma evacuation	Discharged asymptomatic

*Values are expressed as follows: RBC, per mm³; WBC, per mm³; protein, mg/dL; glucose, mg/dL.

ACoA, anterior communicating artery; CT, computed tomography; d, day; GI, gastrointestinal; MCA, middle cerebral artery; ND, not done; PCA, posterior cerebral artery; PMN, polymorphonuclear cells; RBC, red blood cell count; WBC, white blood cell count.

From Brust JC, Dickinson PCT, Hughes JEO, Holtzman RNN: The diagnosis and treatment of cerebral mycotic aneurysms. Ann Neurol 27:238–246, 1999.

infection of a vessel wall has been suggested[36] and should involve the vasa vasorum, but no experimental model exists. Infection of the vasa vasorum as a mechanism was considered less tenable for the cerebral than for the systemic circulation because a true vasa vasorum had rarely been found beyond the supraclinoid internal carotid[37-43] and the proximal intracranial vertebral arteries (Fukushima T, personal communication, 1993),[37a] although it had been seen in more distal locations in conjunction with certain pathologic processes.[39,40] Recent immunohistochemical[41] and routine hematoxylin and eosin[42] human autopsy studies detected vasa vasorum in the proximal internal carotid artery, in its A1 and M1 segments,[41] and in the basilar artery,[42] establishing this system as a potential pathway for cerebral arterial infection. The unique anatomic finding on electron microscopy of cerebral arterial stomata and the adventitial labyrinthine structure called the rete vasorum[43] could well be a component of the vasa vasorum and thereby also a portal of entry for infecting organisms.

4. Immune complexes in vessel walls have been theoretically implicated in the delayed appearance of infected intracranial aneurysms occurring after adequate treatment of endocarditis.[16] They may also be a mechanism of aneurysm formation occurring with bacteremia during antibiotic therapy, in which "bacterial debris encourages inflammation and its consequences"[44] and in aneurysms occurring in the nonbacterial settings of marantic[45,46] or myxomatous[47-50] embolization. The primary underlying factor may specifically relate to endothelial damage accompanied by "complement activation and release of lysosomal enzymes and prostaglandins," which disrupt and weaken the vessel wall.[51,52]

Natural History

The natural history of infected intracranial aneurysms is statistically uncertain and unpredictable because of the paucity of documented cases and an overall decreasing incidence.[3] There are, however, recognized patterns in their evolution:

1. Progressive enlargement, either rapid (see Table 87-1, Patient 12; Case Report 1, Fig. 87-1) or slow (see Table 87-1, Patient 6; Case Report 2, Fig. 87-2A and C) with or without rupture
2. Unchanging aneurysm size for long periods without rupture (see Table 87-1, Patient 6; Case Report 2, Fig. 87-2D)
3. Spontaneous thrombosis of small aneurysms with (see Table 87-1, Patient 15; Case Report 7, Fig. 87-7C) or without (see Table 87-1, Patient 14; Case Report 6, Fig. 87-6D) preservation of their parent vessel lumens
4. Delayed appearance of new aneurysms during and after appropriate antibiotic therapy[16,53]

Infected intracranial aneurysms complicate between 1% and 10% of all cases of infective endocarditis.[54,55]

Their formation probably occurs during acute flare-ups of endocarditis, when showers of emboli enter the cerebral circulation. The most dangerous lesions may be small aneurysms under 1 cm that rapidly enlarge. Aneurysms that remain patent and steadily diminish in size are likely to be less dangerous than those that remain patent and unchanged in size over many months, but some aneurysms enlarge again after becoming smaller.[56,57] Infected aneurysms that grow to a large size over weeks or months often appear threatening radiographically, yet may be less likely to rupture because of their thick walls (see Table 87-1, Patient 6; Case Report 2).[58] Reported mortality with aneurysm rupture ranges from 25% to 90%.[54,59] In settings of multiple coexisting infected aneurysms of different sizes, assessing the likelihood of individual aneurysm rupture is very difficult.[1,58,60-64] This lack of predictability does not detract from our fundamental concept that all of these infected intracranial aneurysms are potentially life threatening.

THE CLINICAL PROFILE

Transient ischemia or infarction occurring after embolic occlusion of a cerebral vessel (see Table 87-1, Patients 5 and 7 through 10) may precede aneurysm formation or rupture. Hemorrhage itself may present as acute subdural hematoma,[65,66] subarachnoid hemorrhage (SAH) (see Table 87-1, Patients 2, 3, and 6), parenchymal hemorrhage (see Table 87-1, Patients 2, 12, and 13), or ventricular hemorrhage (see Table 87-1, Patients 13 and 16). Small leaks, or sentinel hemorrhages, may occur soon after aneurysm formation, causing mild headache and perhaps meningismus[67]; they can be indistinguishable from similar hemorrhages that accompany widespread arteritis, which has been observed at autopsy without frank aneurysm formation.[13,68-70] More serious or even lethal rupture may accompany rapid enlargement when an aneurysm is still only millimeters in size or when it is larger (see Table 87-1, Patient 12; Case Report 1, Fig. 87-1), even during or after antibiotic therapy (see Table 87-1, Patient 6; Case Report 2, Fig. 87-2A and C). The absence of predictive angiographic features, the rarity of focal or diffuse vasospasm,[57,71-73] and the fact that chronically persisting aneurysms may develop very thick or leathery walls (see Table 87-1, Patient 6; Case Report 2) and may even calcify[20,58] add to the difficulty in foretelling rupture in individual cases.

Because of the variable course of these aneurysms and the risks of surgical intervention—especially with proximal aneurysms and inaccessible distal aneurysms—different strategies have been proposed. Some clinicians favor antibiotic therapy, serial angiography, and watchful waiting.[74] Others advocate early surgical intervention[1] with excision (see Table 87-1, Patients 4 through 6 and 16; Case Reports 2 and 5),[67,75] or open clipping, including stereotactic clipping,[15] of accessible secondary or tertiary branch and more distal aneurysms (see Table 87-1, Patient 13; Case Report 3). Wrapping with parent artery preservation (see Table 87-1, Patient 10; Case Report 4) is a feasible option for proximal aneurysms. Petrous aneurysms that are surgically inaccessible have been treated with extracranial carotid ligation,[76,77] trapping techniques,[78] and endovascular occlusion with preservation of the parent artery.[79] Cavernous sinus aneurysms have been managed using extracranial-to-intracranial arterial bypass procedures[80-83] or autologous saphenous vein grafts.[81,82] Endovascular balloon, platinum minicoils and *n*-butyl cyanoacrylate (NBCA) gluing (see Case Report 8, Fig. 87-8*H* to *L*) have been successfully used to occlude distal infected aneurysms.[84-86] Endovascular techniques that have been successfully applied to congenital or traumatic aneurysms will probably be used for infected aneurysms of the internal carotid artery at the base of the skull as well.[79,81,82,84,85,87-91]

Our experience has led us to conclude that single accessible infected aneurysms in medically stable patients should be promptly excised, with individualization of multiple or proximal aneurysms.[1] We would include the option of endovascular occlusion as more experience is gained with those procedures (see Case Report 8, Figs. 87-8A to O).[84-87]

PATIENT SELECTION AND DECISIONS IN MANAGEMENT

Identifying the Patient with Endocarditis Who May Have an Infected Intracranial Aneurysm

An aneurysm should be suspected in any patient with endocarditis who has neurologic symptoms or signs that are unexplained by systemic illness or toxicity,[1] including severe persistent headache or back pain, seizures,[59] altered mentation,[55] focal signs,[13,55,59,69,74,75,92] painful ophthalmoplegia with or without exophthalmos,[20-22,93,94] and evidence of central nervous system infection. Suspicion is also raised by computed tomographic (CT) (see Table 87-1, Patient 11; Case Report 4, Fig. 87-4B) or magnetic resonance imaging (MRI) (see Case Report 8, Figs. 8A to D, M to O) evidence of infarction or intracranial hemorrhage (see Table 87-1, Patient 14; Case Report 6, Fig. 87-6A and B) and by cerebrospinal fluid (CSF) pleocytosis, indicating purulent meningitis[20,24-27,95] or sterile meningitis (see Table 87-1, Patient 15; Case Report 7),[55] which in some cases may result from a parameningeal focus.

A significant number of infected aneurysms are silent or clinically deceptive until a fatal or near-fatal hemorrhage signals their presence (see Table 87-1, Patient 13; Case Report 3),[92] and although hemorrhagic transformation of ischemic infarction due to septic embolization[96] is the most common cause of cerebral hemorrhage, we remain sufficiently concerned to investigate and monitor the neurologically symptomatic patient with endocarditis.[1,97] A thorough history that screens for episodes that might be representative of ischemic events or "sentinel" hemorrhages should be taken for patients with endocarditis, and serial detailed neurologic examinations[1] searching for minute focal deficits and neuropsychiatric disturbances should be performed.[55] In addition, weekly CT scanning[1,12,67,75] or MRI (see Case Report 8, Fig. 87-8A to O)[98] should be performed to search for signs of infarction (e.g., hypodensities, luxury perfusion, hyperintensities) or aneurysm formation that might be seen with contrast enhancement (see Table 87-1, Patient 12; Case Report 1, Fig. 87-1) or partial thrombosis, as seen with flow void and flow phenomena (see Case Report 8, Fig. 87-8A to O). Magnetic resonance angiography (MRA) can identify congenital aneurysms at least

4 mm in diameter and, perhaps more importantly, those with partial thrombosis.[12,98-102] Contrast-enhanced MRA in conjunction with multislice surface anatomy scanning has been used for localization of a peripheral infected aneurysm.[103] Four-vessel angiography still remains the gold standard[84,85] and should promptly follow CT scanning or MRI if results of these studies are positive. Others have recommended that four-vessel angiography also be repeated at the end of adequate therapy[67,75,104] to check for new aneurysms and to ensure thrombosis of those less than 4 mm.[67,98-102]

These recommendations apply also to children suspected of harboring infected intracranial aneurysms. However, appropriate modifications, such as the use of transfontanelle ultrasonography, MRI, and CT scanning[17] for hematomas before angiography in neonates[105] and infants,[106] should be made. Recently, the entity of cerebral aneurysmal arteriopathy in children with long-standing acquired immunodeficiency syndrome (AIDS) has been suggested by CT, MRI, and MRA[107] findings of subacute infarction and fusiform dilation of the major vessels of the circle of Willis.[108] Once this diagnosis was established, death followed in less than 6 months and the findings were confirmed at autopsy. Both varicella zoster virus and human immunodeficiency virus (HIV) vasculitis were suspected.[107,108]

Treating the Patient with Endocarditis Who Has an Infected Intracranial Aneurysm

When the neurologically symptomatic patient with endocarditis is found to have signs of infarction by CT scanning or MRI, four-vessel cerebral angiography is mandatory for confirmation not only of the suspected aneurysm, but for

1. Determination of the coexistence of other aneurysms, which occurs in 25% in some series[13]
2. Analysis of aneurysms less than 4 mm
3. Establishment of the character of the vessels in the vicinity of the aneurysm for surgical or interventional endovascular purposes
4. Preparation for a bypass procedure if that is a consideration in management[80-83]

Nonsurgical versus Surgical Approaches

The decision at this juncture is whether to proceed with urgent surgical excision or to observe the evolution or resolution of the infected aneurysm or aneurysms with appropriate antibiotic coverage, serial CT scanning or MRI,[12] or serial angiography.[67,98] Based on our experience, we recommended that "single accessible mycotic aneurysms in medically stable patients be promptly excised." We now note that endovascular occlusion should also be considered as an option (see Case Report 8, Fig. 87-8A to O). "Recommendations for patients with multiple or proximal aneurysms must be individualized; however, the goal in such patients should also be definitive treatment as soon as possible."[1,109]

The dangers of not intervening promptly are demonstrated by

1. The patient who was being observed in a hospital setting while taking appropriate antibiotics for

Streptococcus viridans endocarditis (see Table 87-1, Patient 12; Case Report 1). Sequential CT scans showed an enlarging left middle cerebral artery (MCA) infected aneurysm and its rupture, with a fatal intracerebral hematoma 17 days after admission (see Fig. 87-1A to C).

2. The patient who was treated with appropriate antibiotics for *Streptococcus sanguis* endocarditis. There was MRI evidence of cerebral embolization and neurologic signs. The patient had subarachnoid and parenchymal hemorrhage from a left MCA aneurysm on day 12, lapsed into a coma, and died.[18]

Nonsurgical management was employed in two patients with single aneurysms (see Table 87-1, Patients 14 and 15; Case Reports 6 and 7) and in two patients with multiple aneurysms (see Patients 7 and 9) who were followed up with serial cerebral angiograms while they received appropriate antibiotic coverage. In one (Patient 7), 39 days elapsed to the spontaneous thrombosis of both aneurysms, seen on the third angiogram. Another (see Case Report 6, Patient 14) was followed up conservatively because the aneurysm, most likely located in the occipitotemporal sulcus, was not thought to be easily found at surgery (see Figs. 87-6A to D); 36 days elapsed until spontaneous thrombosis and disappearance of the parent vessel (see Fig. 87-6D). Another (see Case Report 7, Patient 15) was also followed up conservatively because the aneurysm was thought to be difficult to locate surgically. On the day after angiographic documentation of the infected aneurysm, the patient developed cardiac failure, which necessitated urgent valve replacement. At repeat angiography, the aneurysm was smaller (see Fig. 87-7A and B). The aneurysm resolved with preservation of the parent lumen 3.5 months later (see Fig. 87-7C). With the newer diagnostic technologies for localization and intraoperative guidance systems,[15,110–114] these single aneurysms would now be considered operable.

Patient 9, who had five distal aneurysms and one proximal aneurysm, presented a complex management problem. Such patients, in whom the site of bleeding is uncertain and the aneurysms are not enlarging, would have been treated nonsurgically by most clinicians.[1,55,57–61] However, some investigators report 100% mortality in patients with multiple intracranial infected aneurysms.[13] With current endovascular technological capabilities, that modality should be given therapeutic consideration (see Case Report 8, Fig. 87-8A to O).[109] In fact, this patient suffered a fatal rupture of a hepatic artery–infected aneurysm. With today's technology, that aneurysm could have been treated by superselective embolization,[115] but identification would have been difficult. A clue to identification might have been anicteric cholestasis.[116]

Surgical Management

We believe that the intraoperative risk—either surgically[1] or endovascularly (see Case Report 8, Fig. 87-8A to O)[84,85,86,109]—in superficial intracranial infected aneurysms is usually low. Superficial aneurysms in areas of gliosis or scar tissue appearing after craniotomy for cerebral abscess might be considered inaccessible, justifying conservative treatment (Stein BM, personal communication, 1993[27a]). Proximal aneurysms in the region of the circle of Willis and the primary bifurcations should be treated with caution; as their walls thicken, they may become more amenable to clipping,[15] excision with bypass,[117] reinforcement with wrapping (see Case Report 4, Patient 10), endovascular balloon, or Hilal minicoil occlusion.[85] Balloon occlusion with bypass[80–83] or a trapping procedure[78] may be used for common carotid occlusion.[76,77] Endovascular treatment may be considered for aneurysms of the petrous carotid[76,77,79,87,87] and intracavernous carotid.[80–83]

Emergency craniotomy without angiography is warranted for evacuation of hematoma when mass effect and worsening neurologic status are present. In such patients, the aneurysm may not be found (see Table 87-1, Patient 13; Case Report 3). Some patients with intracerebral hemorrhage may be sufficiently stable to undergo cerebral angiography in an attempt to define the source of bleeding. However, at least 10% of infected aneurysms are missed by angiography[55]; some are detected only with repeated studies[118] or after recovery from endocarditis.[74]

Cardiovascular Considerations

Affecting the decision to proceed with craniotomy is the underlying medical condition of the patient, especially the cardiovascular status. Patients in acute heart failure may require cardiac surgery, as in the case of our patient (see Case Report 7, Patient 15), who received a bioprosthetic porcine valve replacement and systemic heparin during the procedure while the aneurysm was patent, although clearly decreasing in size.

With present technologic advances and intracardiac support systems, a patient with acute cardiac failure may be successfully assisted through an emergency craniotomy. Certainly, endovascular balloon, NBCA gluing (see Case Report 8, Fig. 87-8A to O), or Hilal minicoil occlusions seem more feasible under these circumstances.[84–87]

Cardiac valve surgery may be indicated for

1. Impending congestive heart failure due to persisting valve or chordae tendineae infection with disruption either before[119,120] or after management of the aneurysm[120,121]
2. Persisting evidence of embolization during antibiotic therapy
3. Persisting infection manifested by recurrent bacteremia (see Table 87-1, Patient 13; Case Report 3)

Anticoagulation

Although "there has been no increased morbidity with the cardiopulmonary bypass and associated heparinization,"[2] valve replacement with a bioprosthesis is sometimes performed without the postoperative administration of anticoagulation (see Table 87-1, Patient 15; Case Report 7).[119] Valve replacement after aneurysm excision (see Table 87-1, Patient 13; Case Report 3)[121] negates the risk for aneurysmal rupture during intraoperative and postoperative systemic heparinization.

Anticoagulation in the management of embolization during attacks of endocarditis carries significant risk. A pregnant woman suffered a fatal SAH while receiving anticoagulants.[122] Of seven patients with endocarditis and cerebral emboli who were being treated with anticoagulant therapy, 43% developed massive intracerebral hematomas, whereas in a comparable group of 211 patients not treated with anticoagulation, only 5% developed intracranial hemorrhages.[13] In this regard, heparinization might also aggravate SAH or parenchymal hemorrhage secondary to aneurysm rupture.[120] Nevertheless, anticoagulation in selected patients with infective endocarditis has its advocates.[120] Anticoagulation may be useful in the post-NBCA aneurysmal occlusion period when there have been parent artery and branch occlusions (see Case Report 8, Fig. 87-8A to O).

REGIONAL SURGICAL ANATOMY AND CHOICE OF SURGICAL APPROACH

The surgical anatomy of the infected intracranial aneurysm is affected by three factors: the shape and form of the aneurysm itself, the adjacent blood vessels, and the aneurysm location in relation to brain parenchyma and meninges.

Infected aneurysms in distal locations represent focal dilatations of the arterial wall that incorporate branching vessels in the process. They often lie within a sulcus and may not be visible until the sulcus is opened (see Fig. 87-2E and F). Whether they are saccular or fusiform, excision entails the resection of a portion of each vessel entering or emerging from the aneurysm. Favorable environmental signs include immediate retrograde bleeding from the distal artery signifying good collateral supply and surrounding infarction or encephalomalacia rendering the area less vulnerable to surgical manipulation, as was noted in the excision of the Broca's area aneurysm (see Table 87-1, Patient 6; Case Report 2), which had no postoperative deficit. Within vascular territories, no specific cortical sulci are more likely to be affected than others. Combined data from two studies involving 219 cases show that the MCA distribution is most commonly involved (in 39%), followed by the anterior cerebral artery (in 5%), the basilar artery (in 5%), the intradural internal carotid (in 4%), and the posterior cerebral artery (in 4%).[3,7,36]

Proximal locations, such as the MCA bifurcation or the anterior communicating artery–anterior cerebral artery complex (see Table 87-1, Patient 9)[15] may be the sites of infected congenital aneurysms. Standard approaches to these are well known and have been described in great detail.[39,40] These approaches involve routes through the subarachnoid spaces and cisterns. These aneurysms may be in the subarachnoid space, or they may be embedded in the adjacent brain parenchyma. The early friable nature of their walls makes them extremely dangerous from a surgical standpoint. Clipping is possible, however, with meticulous microscopic dissection at the neck.[15] Alternatively, an endovascular approach with NBCA (see Case Report 8, Fig. 87-8A to O), balloon occlusion, or Hilal minicoils may carry less risk.[84–87]

Infected aneurysms may be located within the walls of the cavernous sinus[21,22,80] and may present with massive epistaxis and shock.[123] That anatomy has been extensively described by Dolenc.[124] Infected aneurysms in the cavernous sinus have been treated with trapping and bypass[80–83] procedures.

Infected aneurysms of the petrous carotid have also been suspected and described,[76,77,79,87,88] and the anatomy of that region has been presented in detail.[125] Congenital aneurysms in the carotid canal have been approached directly and with present technology could be amenable to direct resection with saphenous graft interposition,[81,89–91] trapping,[78] or bypass.[81,91] Common carotid artery occlusion has also been valuable in managing severe otorrhagia from aneurysms in this region.[76,77] Alternatively, endovascular occlusion and trapping procedures of the carotid artery have been successfully performed with[79] and without preservation of the parent artery with a small risk for thrombotic complications.[87] Since experience with platinum coil endovascular occlusion of petrous infected aneurysms with preservation of the parent artery[79] now exists, this technology certainly represents a treatment option. In view of the frequent circumferential involvement of the vessel wall, preservation of the parent artery lumen may not be possible in all instances.

ANESTHETIC CONSIDERATIONS AND AIDS TO SURGICAL MANAGEMENT

The requirement of general anesthesia for surgical management of infected intracranial aneurysms is widely accepted. Although craniotomy with the patient under local anesthesia has been recommended for those with cardiovascular instability,[75,126] it no longer need be considered except in the most unusual circumstances and is of course limited to the management of only the distally located infected aneurysms.

In our patients, induction and intubation were followed by standard inhalation techniques without any apparent complications. At no time was induced hypotension employed, and postoperative hypertension was unnecessary because vasospasm was not observed preoperatively.[1]

Neuroanesthetic techniques[127,128] depend on the age and clinical condition of the patient, particularly if increased intracranial pressure or altered cardiovascular function are present. Differing clinical situations requiring the use of adjunctive techniques in addition to the administration of anesthetic agents include the following.

General Considerations in Elective Surgical Excision or Endovascular Occlusion

1. Preoperative analyses may include balloon test occlusion to assess the patient's tolerance for occlusion or excision. In addition, a Wada test may be similarly employed.
2. Preparation for intraoperative monitoring of the patient's neurologic function may include somatosensory evoked potentials and electroencephalography.[129] Where facilities are available, xenon 133 cerebral blood flow measurements (^{133}Xe washout) can be a useful adjunct[130] in the endovascular occlusion of proximal aneurysms. A central venous line monitoring for venous air embolus may be necessary for patients in the sitting or couch position with posterior fossa aneurysms,

particularly those on the dorsal surface of the cerebellum, where gravity facilitates exposure (see Table 87-1, Patient 16; Case Report 5). Similarly, a Swan-Ganz catheter may be useful in instances of cardiovascular instability where the central venous pressure might not reflect left heart function along with transesophageal echocardiography in circumstances where there is severe cardiac valvular damage due to endocarditis.

3. Smooth induction with minimal hemodynamic changes usually begins with small amounts of curare, followed by nondepolarizing muscle relaxants such as vecuronium bromide. Three minutes of oxygen by facemask are followed by the administration of rapid-acting agents such as thiopental, propofol, or etomidate followed by fentanyl and mild or modest hyperventilation. Intubation then follows.

4. Maintenance anesthesia can be continued with potent agents such as isoflurane, desflurane, or sevoflurane or infusion of narcotics.

5. Staff must ensure that the intraoperative hemodynamic status is closely monitored and that changes are kept to a minimum; at the termination of the procedure the patient must be sufficiently awake before being extubated.

EMERGENCY CRANIOTOMY FOR EVACUATION OF HEMATOMA

The same outline used for anesthesia can be used for hematoma evacuation, with several modifications. In somnolent patients, intubation should be performed as soon as possible. High concentrations of potent agents such as isoflurane and desflurane should be avoided if mass effect or increased intracranial pressure exists. Dexamethasone in large doses can be administered in a loading dose of up to 100 mg in adult patients. Mannitol, 0.5 g/kg, can be given in one or more boluses, as required. Judicious management of blood pressure is required; systemic hypertension may reflect increased intracranial pressure, and hypotensive agents, such as sodium nitroprusside, should be used with caution.

Elective or Urgent Craniotomy in the Face of Incipient or Frank Cardiovascular Collapse

Most surgeons prefer to perform craniotomy first in patients with incipient congestive failure, which can often be managed by a cardiotonic medical regimen (see Table 87-1, Patient 13; Case Report 3). High-dose fentanyl-oxygen anesthesia has been used in patients with incipient cardiac failure.[131]

In extreme cases of frank cardiovascular collapse, an intra-aortic balloon pump or a left ventricular assist devices (LVAD) may be implanted, and a combined effort of craniotomy for aneurysm excision or wrapping or encasement may be followed by cardiac valvular repair. Permanent pacemaker implantation may be required (see Table 87-1, Patient 13). The general principles of anesthesia

administration during the phases of induction, maintenance, and reversal remain otherwise unchanged. Of course, in emergency situations, monitoring facilities may not be as readily available.

SURGICAL TECHNIQUES AND CASE REPORTS

Calvarial craniotomies, posterior fossa craniectomies, and dural flaps are well described in this volume and elsewhere.[39,40] Once the cortex is exposed, the immediate problem facing the surgeon is the precise localization of the infected aneurysm. If it is superficially protruding from a sulcus, it may be easily seen (see Fig. 87-2E). After the arachnoid surrounding the parent cortical artery is opened, the lips of the adjacent gyri are easily parted, creating a sulcal plane and exposing the aneurysm, its parent artery, and branches that may be cauterized or clipped. The aneurysm is then excised (see Fig. 87-2F).

When the aneurysm is not seen, the surgeon faces considerable difficulty and frustration. To avoid such circumstances, we suggest preoperative and intraoperative preparations that provide coordinates for the target aneurysm such that accurate localization by guidance systems is assured for both cortical and subcortical aneurysms. The list includes the older Brown-Roberts-Wells or Cosman-Roberts-Wells (CRW) CT- or MRI-guided localization systems[111] and the newer StealthStation (Sofamor Danek, Minneapolis, MN, U.S.A.), BrainLab AG or Viewing Wand (ISG Technologies, Salina, KS, U.S.A.) frameless stereotactic guidance systems among others.

1. These systems are well understood and may guide the surgeon to cortical or subcortical lesions. The use of CT scanning has been reported in conjunction with the Leksell Steiner-Lindquist microsurgical guide for excision of a distal infected aneurysm.[114]

2. CRW stereotactic angiography–guided localization using the Suetens-Gybels Vandermeulen angiographic localizer has permitted the clipping of a saccular aneurysm at the MCA bifurcation through a 4-cm craniotomy after hematoma evacuation[15] and at the distal anterior cerebral artery.[132]

3. Sonic stereometry, a frameless, computerized navigating system that permits localization in space by measuring the traveling time of sonic waves, has been used with CT scanning and is being optimized for use with MRI and digital subtraction angiography.[102,103]

4. The future use of MRA for digital image-based localization.[110]

Once the system is in place and guidance to the aneurysm has been performed, clot removal and aneurysm excision or clipping[15,114,132] may be undertaken with greater assurance.

In endovascular treatment of infected cerebral aneurysms, selective catheterization of a distal middle cerebral and posterior cerebral branch was performed in two patients with a microcatheter followed by superselective amobarbital testing of the parent vessel before the occlusion of that vessel with autologous clot or glue. A third patient was treated by selective occlusion of the aneurysm by intra-aneurysmal placement of platinum minicoils. All three infected aneurysms, two of which had bled and one of which was found at angiography, were excluded from the circulation. One balloon deflation required retreatment with coils. The authors of this report concluded that endovascular embolization is indicated in patients who are at special risk for hemorrhage and that the procedure is safe and effective for distal infected aneurysms.[84,85] Case Report 8, Figure 87-8A to O (courtesy of John M. D. Pile-Spellman) fully documents the clinical course and the successful endovascular occlusion of an MCA infected aneurysm with NBCA. Clearly this technology now represents a major development in the future management of these aneurysms.

The following case reports from our series illustrate the various problems associated with the surgical and medical management of infected intracranial aneurysms.

Case of Mortality

CASE REPORT 1 (TABLE 87-1, PATIENT 12)
SPONTANEOUS HEMORRHAGE WITH A FATAL OUTCOME IN A DOCUMENTED RAPIDLY ENLARGING INFECTED ANEURYSM

The patient was a 24-year-old man whose history included juvenile rheumatoid arthritis since the age of 5 and recurrent arthralgias and vascular migraine.

3/14/83: Patient admitted with bilateral calf tenderness and swelling, fever, sweating, and 20-pound weight loss.

3/15/83: Echocardiogram showed aortic insufficiency with valvular vegetations.

3/16/83: Blood cultures were positive for *S. viridans*. Treatment was begun with ampicillin, oxacillin, and gentamicin, and the following day, aqueous penicillin, 20 million U/day replaced the initial regimen.

3/21/83: CT scan with contrast showed a small left MCA infected aneurysm (Fig. 87-1A).

3/28/83: CT scan with contrast showed that the infected aneurysm was three times larger than before (Fig. 87-1B).

4/1/83: The decision was made to proceed with cardiac valve surgery and to treat the infected aneurysm medically. On that day, the patient suddenly lapsed into a coma and developed fixed, dilated pupils. A CT scan obtained before death showed a large left intracerebral hematoma with a massive left-to-right shift (Fig. 87-1C). Respiratory failure ensued, and the patient died.

Comment

This case clearly demonstrates the lethal nature of patent infected intracranial aneurysms, which appear to rupture especially during rapid enlargement and supports our contention that single, accessible, infected aneurysms in medically stable patients should be promptly excised[1] or managed with endovascular occlusion techniques (see Case Report 8, Fig. 87-8A to O).[79,84–87]

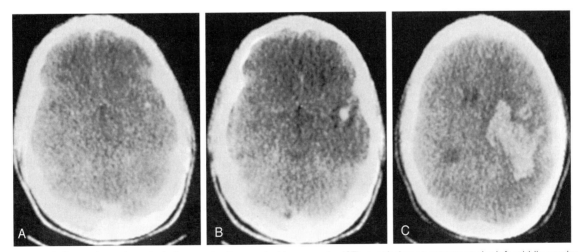

FIGURE 87-1 *A,* Seven days after admission, contrast computed tomography (CT) revealed an aneurysm on the left middle cerebral artery in the sylvian fissure. *B,* One week later, the same aneurysm was larger. *C,* The next day, an intracerebral hemorrhage was adjacent to the site of the aneurysm. Between the CT scan shown in *B* and *C,* the patient, who was receiving appropriate antibiotics, became abruptly comatose with left pupillary dilatation and died a few hours later.

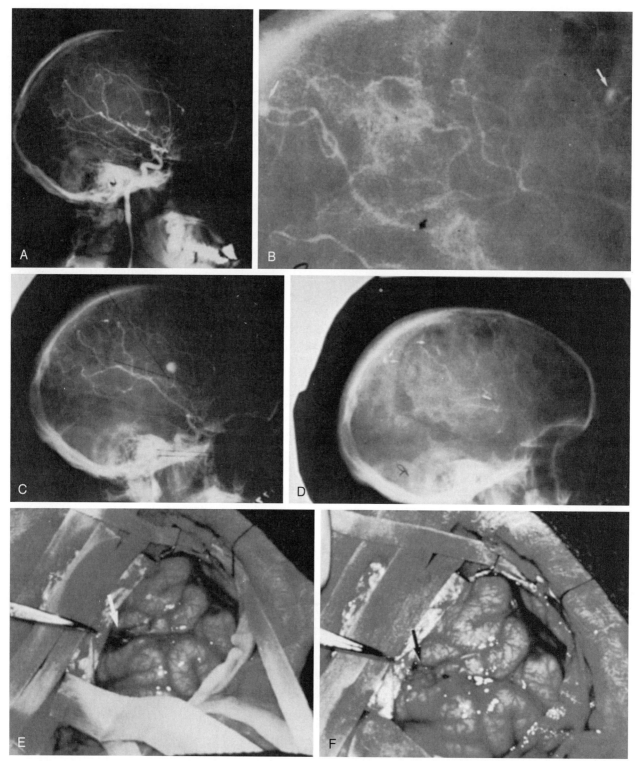

FIGURE 87-2   *A,* Twenty days after admission (and 8 days after subarachnoid hemorrhage), a left frontal aneurysm distal to the middle cerebral artery bifurcation was evident. *B,* Twenty-six days after admission, angiography disclosed additional right frontal and parietal aneurysms (*large white arrows*). *C,* Sixty-nine days after admission (and following antibiotic treatment), the left frontal aneurysm was bigger. *D,* Ninety-one days after admission and after craniotomy and excision of the left frontal aneurysm, the right frontal aneurysm disappeared and the right parietal aneurysm persisted (*two small white arrows*). *E,* The right parietal aneurysm exposed in its sulcus (*large white arrow*). *F,* The sulcal bed after excision of the aneurysm with its parent artery (*large black arrow*).

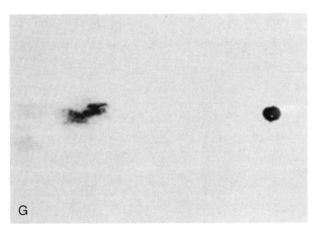

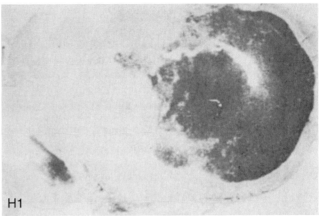

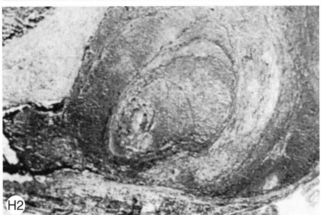

FIGURE 87-2 Cont'd *G,* Gross specimen: a small symmetric saccular aneurysm, 0.4 cm in diameter, with a moderately thickened wall attached to a feeding vessel. *H,* Microscopic examination: Masson's trichrome (*1*) and Verhoff's elastic (*2*) stains show a small cerebral artery with the internal elastic lamina intact leading into the saccular structure. At the point of dilatation, there is a mild thickening of the intima and fragmentation and then disappearance of the internal elastic lamina. The tunica media shows marked stretching around the circumference of the dilatation but was otherwise intact and did not show evidence of inflammatory changes. Within the deeper layer of the thickened intima, there are aggregates of chronic inflammatory cells, predominantly mononuclear.

Cases of Survival and Recovery with Surgical and Endovascular Management

CASE REPORT 2 (TABLE 87-1, PATIENT 6)
THREE INFECTED ANEURYSMS IN A SINGLE PATIENT WITH INDIVIDUAL PATTERNS OF EVOLUTION

This 24-year-old woman presented at one hospital with vomiting, headaches, fever of 101°F, systolic murmur, an erythrocyte sedimentation rate of 96, a white blood cell count of 14,500, and pyuria. The patient signed out against medical advice.

6/24/77: The patient returned 21 days later with lower abdominal pain and headaches, and pelvic inflammatory disease was diagnosed. She was treated with intramuscular penicillin and referred to the clinic for follow-up. Blood cultures obtained from the patient grew *Streptococcus viridans.* Attempts to contact the patient failed.

8/2/77: Patient was admitted to Harlem Hospital Center with fatigue, weight loss, and headaches. Her medical history included rheumatic fever and a cardiac murmur. Examination showed a grade III/VI heart murmur and splenomegaly. CSF: two red blood cells; protein, 30 mg/dL; glucose, 51 mg/dL. Positive results on blood cultures for *S. viridans* and *Micrococcus.* Treatment was begun with aqueous penicillin, 4 million U every 4 hours.

12th day: Sudden severe headaches, right hemiparesis, and Broca's aphasia. CSF was bloody and xanthochromic; OP, 410; glucose, 54 mg/dL; protein, 74 mg/dL.

20th day: Cerebral angiogram showed aneurysm in the left suprasylvian location (Fig. 87-2A).

26th day: Cerebral angiogram showed two additional aneurysms in the right frontal and parietal lobes (Fig. 87-2B).

33rd day: Streptomycin, 1 g/day added to treatment regimen.

68th day: Cerebral angiogram showed marked enlargement of the left suprasylvian aneurysm (Fig. 87-2C).

75th day: Craniotomy and excision of the left suprasylvian aneurysm performed.

91st day: Cerebral angiogram showed spontaneous thrombosis of the right posterior frontal aneurysm (Fig. 87-2D).

104th day: Craniotomy and excision of the right superior parietal lobule infected aneurysm (Fig. 87-2E and F). Pathology (see Fig. 87-2G and H).

During 4-year follow-up, patient had no symptoms or neurologic deficits.

Comment

This patient demonstrates the different evolutionary patterns seen with infected aneurysms. The ruptured left suprasylvian aneurysm was addressed initially. Its wall was firm and almost leathery, and it was embedded in Broca's area in the brain that was encephalomalacic. Brisk retrograde bleeding from the distal cortical artery was seen at the time of excision highlighting several of the mechanisms of cerebrocortical collateral blood supply, namely, pial-pial collaterals through the anterior cerebral artery to the MCA and collaterals from MCA branches to MCA branches through short and long gyral anastomoses.

CASE REPORT 3 (TABLE 87-1, PATIENT 13)
EMERGENCY CRANIOTOMY FOR PARIETO-OCCIPITAL HEMATOMA WITH LEFT UNCAL HERNIATION AND DECEREBRATION

This 29-year-old male intravenous drug user was admitted for his third episode of endocarditis with fever, chills, shortness of breath, and weakness.

7/8/84: Examination disclosed multiple skin ulcers at the sites of heroin injection. Blood culture results were initially negative. A shoulder abscess due to a central venous line was drained. Positive results on blood cultures for *Pseudomonas aeruginosa* and *Providencia*. Treatment was begun with gentamicin and carbenicillin.

8/6/84: Emergency craniotomy was performed for evacuation of a left parieto-occipital intracerebral hematoma (Fig. 87-3A), which presented clinically with a left uncal herniation syndrome and decerebration. No aneurysm was found.

8/17/84: Piperacillin was added to the regimen.

8/20/84: Cerebral angiography revealed right distal MCA infected aneurysm (Fig. 87-3B). No aneurysms were seen on the left.

8/24/84: Craniotomy performed for excision of the right parieto-occipital aneurysm with clipping of the feeding vessels (Fig. 87-3C).

9/10/84: Cardiac catheterization performed for aortic regurgitation. Blood culture results continued to be positive for *Pseudomonas*. Clinical appearance: patient in fetal position in bed, used monosyllabic speech, had spastic quadriparesis.

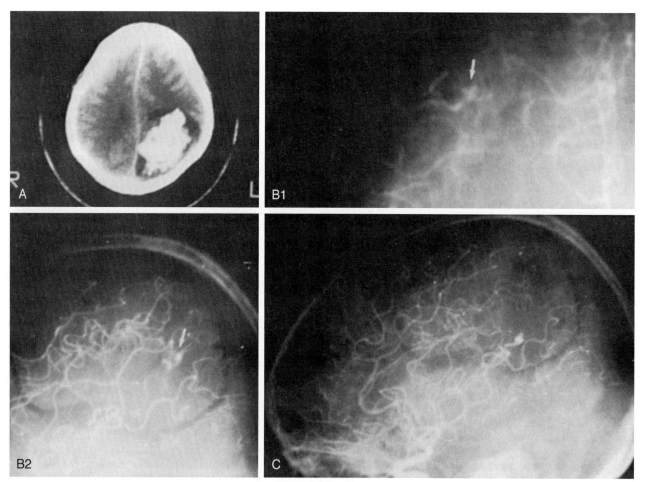

FIGURE 87-3   *A,* Computed tomography scan shows a left parieto-occipital hematoma with mass effect. The patient was comatose and decerebrate. *B,* Fourteen days later, an infected right distal middle cerebral artery aneurysm was seen on angiography (*anteroposterior and lateral views with large white arrows*). *C,* Four days later, the aneurysm was successfully clipped.

9/20/84: Cardiac surgery: Aortic valve replacement was performed, and an aortic ring abscess was found. Resection involved disruption of the bundle of His, and a permanent pacemaker was required.

7/1/85: The patient made a remarkable recovery. He was fully independent and ambulatory, with only a mild residual encephalopathy and incomplete left dominant parietal and occipital lobe syndromes.

Comment

Despite the desperately poor clinical state of this patient, aggressive management resulted in a good outcome. We managed the right parieto-occipital infected aneurysm before proceeding with cardiac valve surgery, which was mandated by aortographic documentation of the abscess cavity and persisting septicemia.

CASE REPORT 4 (TABLE 87-1, PATIENT 10)

ELECTIVE CRANIOTOMY WITH WRAPPING OF A PROXIMAL RIGHT M1 SEGMENT FUSIFORM INFECTED ANEURYSM PRESENTING WITH A RIGHT BASAL GANGLIA INFARCT

This 28-year-old female intravenous heroin and cocaine user was treated 1 year previously for *Staphylococcus aureus* endocarditis with 6 weeks of intravenous oxacillin. Cardiac catheterization at that time showed mitral regurgitation.

4/5/81: 5 days of headaches and temperature elevation of 102°F.

4/10/81: Acute left hemiparesis and dysarthria. Grade III/VI murmur.

4/15/81: *S. viridans* endocarditis documented. Patient treated with aqueous penicillin, 3 million U every 4 hours. CSF was normal.

5/8/81: Cerebral angiogram showed a right M1 segment fusiform infected aneurysm with an MCA branch occlusion (Fig. 87-4A). CT scan revealed right basal ganglia infarction (Fig. 87-4B).

6/4/81: Right pterional craniotomy performed with wrapping of a multilobar fusiform aneurysm. Antibiotic regimen: 4/15 to 5/21, aqueous penicillin; 5/21 to 6/22, oral penicillin V-K; 6/22, oxacillin.

6/22/81: Patient discharged. Left hemiparesis improving.

Comment

This patient with endocarditis presented with a left hemiparesis. Angiography disclosed a proximal M1 segment fusiform aneurysm. Subsequent CT scan showed a right basal ganglia infarction without evidence of hemorrhage. The aneurysm could not be clipped or excised, and therefore wrapping was undertaken. The infarction was related to lenticulostriate occlusion by embolus or arteritis in the M1 segment.

CASE REPORT 5 (SEE TABLE 87-1, PATIENT 16; CASE COURTESY OF DR. GEORGE V. DIGIACINTO)

SUPERIOR CEREBELLAR ARTERY INFECTED ANEURYSM WITH VENTRICULAR HEMORRHAGE AND RECOVERY

This 54-year-old man was admitted with a sudden severe headache, which he described as "the worst headache of my life"; transient blindness; and a temperature of 102°F.

10/28/85: Patient's clinical condition rapidly deteriorated. He became comatose and decerebrate, and intubation was required on an emergency basis.

10/29/85: Recovery of consciousness was noted.

10/31/85: Blood cultures grew *S. aureus*. Echocardiogram showed aortic valve sclerosis and mitral valve fibrosis.

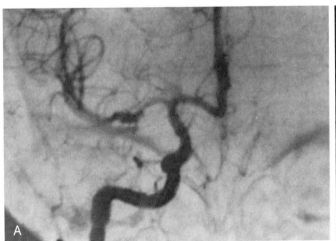
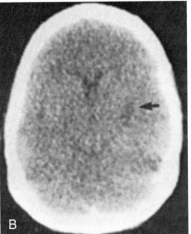

FIGURE 87-4 *A,* Anteroposterior view cerebral angiogram shows an irregular fusiform aneurysm of the right M1 segment. *B,* Computed tomography scan shows a right basal ganglia infarction (*large black arrow*).

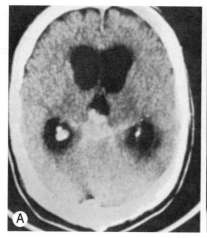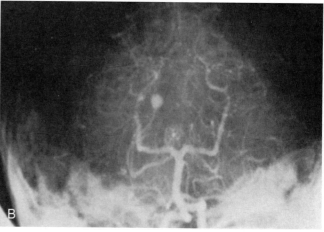

FIGURE 87-5 *A,* Computed tomography scan shows posterior third ventricular hemorrhage, subarachnoid hemorrhage, and acute hydrocephalus. *B,* Anteroposterior view of posterior circulation angiography demonstrates a right distal superior cerebellar artery aneurysm.

11/1/85: CT scan showed subarachnoid and third ventricular hemorrhage with acute hydrocephalus (Fig. 87-5A). Cerebral angiography revealed superior cerebellar artery infected aneurysm (Fig. 87-5B and C).

11/7/85: Suboccipital craniectomy was performed with excision of the aneurysm. Postoperative recovery was excellent.

Comment

An example of a posterior circulation distal infected aneurysm with ventricular hemorrhage in a patient who presented in coma with decerebrate rigidity and made a complete recovery.

Cases of Survival and Recovery with Medical Management

CASE REPORT 6 (TABLE 87-1, PATIENT 14)
RUPTURED INFECTED ANEURYSM WITH SPONTANEOUS THROMBOSIS

This 41-year-old female intravenous drug user had presented 1 year previously (7/84) at another hospital with anemia and fever. Left upper extremity cellulitis was noted, and she was treated with antibiotics. Electrocardiographic results were negative. Subsequently, she medicated herself with antibiotics intermittently for recurrent fever.

4/9/85: Patient admitted to the hospital with recent history of intravenous drug use (inflamed leg), then the onset of sudden severe headache, stiff neck, vertigo, vomiting, and a focal seizure. Examination disclosed multiple cutaneous scars, grade II/VI murmur, Brudzinski's sign, and left homonymous hemianopia.

Echocardiography revealed no valvular abnormalities or left ventricular hypertrophy.

CSF showed OP, 350; xanthochromic; 700 red blood cells, 450 white blood cells (100% polymorphonuclear cells); protein, 390 mg/dL, glucose, 63 mg/dL. Blood and CSF culture results were negative.

CT scan revealed right posterior temporoparietal intracerebral hematoma (Fig. 87-6A).

Treatment was initiated with cefotaxime, 2 g every 6 hours; vancomycin, 500 mg every 6 hours; and oxacillin, 2 g every 6 hours. All antibiotics were discontinued on 4/20/85, when cultures conclusively demonstrated no growth.

4/11/85: First cerebral angiogram revealed right posterior temporal artery branch infected aneurysm (Fig. 87-6B).

4/24/85: Second cerebral angiogram showed aneurysm decreased in size (Fig. 87-6C).

5/14/85: Third cerebral angiogram showed that aneurysm disappeared with apparent thrombosis of a portion of the parent vessel (Fig. 87-6D).

5/15/85: Patient discharged completely well.

Comment

This patient with a history of intravenous heroin use and associated subarachnoid and parenchymal hemorrhage had an angiographically documented infected aneurysm in the absence of positive culture results and cardiac valve abnormalities. She was treated for 11 days with antibiotics, and spontaneous thrombosis of the aneurysm was documented 36 days after initial symptoms appeared. This aneurysm may have formed in the presence of a transient bacteremia associated with the liberation of immune complexes.[16,36,44] Surgery was not undertaken initially because it was felt that the aneurysm would be difficult to localize in a sulcus under the temporal lobe, and guidance systems were not available. On repeat angiography, the aneurysm was smaller and then disappeared.

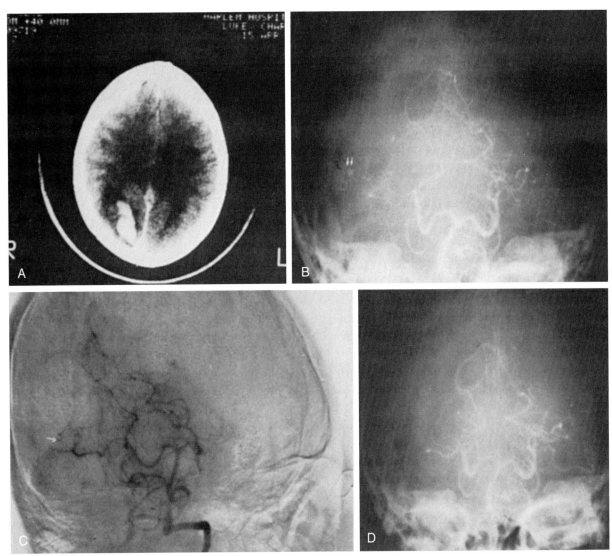

FIGURE 87-6   *A,* Computed tomography scan demonstrates a right posterior temporoparietal intracerebral hematoma. *B,* Cerebral angiography shows a right posterior temporal artery branch aneurysm (*two small white arrows*). *C,* Second cerebral angiogram: Thirteen days later, the aneurysm has decreased in size (*small white arrows*). *D,* Third cerebral angiogram: Twenty days later, the aneurysm has disappeared with apparent thrombosis of a portion of the parent vessel.

CASE REPORT 7 (TABLE 87-1, PATIENT 15)
INFECTED ANEURYSM ASSOCIATED WITH STAPHYLOCOCCUS AUREUS SEPTICEMIA AND MENINGITIS

This 36-year-old female intravenous drug user on maintenance methadone treatment was admitted to the hospital.

2/8/85: Patient was found delirious without focal neurologic signs. Temperature was 104°F; positive meningeal signs were present; and patient had grade III/VI murmur, Janeway's spots, and hepatomegaly. Ethyl alcohol level, 404 mg/dL. Blood culture results were positive for *S. aureus.* CSF had 2000 white blood cells; 90% polymorphonuclear cells; glucose, 43 mg/dL; and protein, 86 mg/dL. Echocardiogram showed mitral valve

vegetations. Treatment was begun with oxacillin, 2 g intravenously every 4 hours.

2/22/85: CT scan showed multiple enhancing lesions compatible with embolization and luxury perfusion (Fig. 87-7A).

2/27/85: Cerebral angiogram showed right MCA branch aneurysm (Fig. 87-7B).

2/28/85: Acute congestive heart failure with pulmonary edema required intubation. Left hemiparesis was noted.

3/7/85: Mitral valve replacement with a porcine prosthesis was performed under systemic heparinization. Left anterior leaflet vegetations involving the papillary muscle with chorda tendineae rupture were seen. Cultures of the valvular vegetations revealed no growth. Postoperatively, the patient was given vancomycin for 6 weeks.

3/25/85: Second cerebral angiogram showed that aneurysm was smaller.

4/29/85: Third cerebral angiogram showed that aneurysm continued to decrease in size.

6/11/85: Fourth cerebral angiogram showed aneurysm had virtually resolved, but a focal area of dilatation persisted. Patency of the parent vessel was preserved (Fig. 87-7C).

7/12/85: The patient made a full recovery. One year later, she was readmitted with cardiac arrhythmia and died.

Comment

This case illustrates the probable formation of an infected aneurysm in close temporal proximity to a flare-up of endocarditis with clinical and CT evidence of multifocal embolization. Moreover, meningitis may have produced focal arteritis and aneurysm formation through the rete vasorum[43] or vasa vasorum[41,42] of the cerebral arteries. Surgical excision of the infected aneurysm would have been considered had the patient not developed

acute heart failure and required valve replacement. She tolerated systemic heparinization during the cardiac procedure, probably because her aneurysm was undergoing involution. After surgery, the aneurysm was clearly decreasing in size angiographically, and it was then decided to follow its course without attempts at excision.

CASE REPORT 8 (COURTESY OF DR. JOHN M. D. PILE-SPELLMAN)
RUPTURED RIGHT MIDDLE CEREBRAL ARTERY BRANCH INFECTED ANEURYSM SUCCESSFULLY MANAGED WITH ENDOVASCULAR NBCA ANEURYSM AND ANTICOAGULATION WITH PARENT ARTERY OCCLUSION

This 29-year-old man noted an 18-pound weight loss since June 1997 following the extraction of four wisdom teeth. In the last week of September 1997 and on two subsequent occasions he experienced episodes of

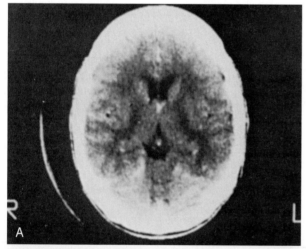

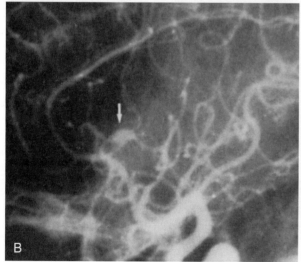

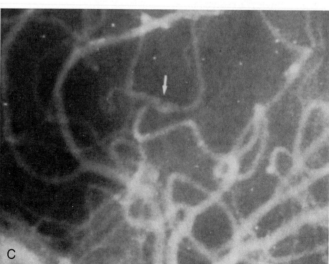

FIGURE 87-7 *A,* Computed tomography scan shows multiple enhancing lesions compatible with embolization and "luxury perfusion." *B,* Cerebral angiogram shows a right middle cerebral artery branch aneurysm (*large white arrow*). *C,* Fourth cerebral angiogram: Three and a half months later, the aneurysm has virtually resolved, but a focal area of dilatation persists. Patency of the parent vessel is preserved (*large white arrow*).

numbness and tingling of the left side of his tongue, lips, and face lasting several hours. An evaluation for multiple sclerosis and HIV testing was negative. Thereafter, he complained of malaise, night sweats, chills, and fever. Evaluation revealed microscopic hematuria, and he was treated with antibiotics for a urinary tract infection. An IVP demonstrated left ureteral obstruction.

10/22/97: He was admitted to the hospital for placement of a ureteral stent. Examination disclosed a cardiac systolic III/VI murmur, anemia, and hepatosplenomegaly. Blood cultures were positive for *Streptococcus bovis*.

11/03/97: MRI of the brain was performed to evaluate his episodes of facial numbness, which disclosed small punctate hyperintensities in the frontal and parietal regions. He had no focal neurologic deficits.

11/11/97: He was transferred to another hospital for cardiac valve surgery. He complained of pounding temporal headaches. Examination showed splinter hemorrhages, Roth spots, conjunctival hemorrhages, and grade III/VI systolic murmur hepatosplenomegaly. Left facial weakness and left hemiparesis of one day's duration were noted along with lethargy. Abdominal CT scan showed evidence of splenic infarction. He was treated with ceftriaxone sodium 2 g intravenously every 24 hours, digoxin, and Capoten, and was begun on anticoagulation. His diagnoses were aortic and mitral valve endocarditis.

11/14/97: He underwent aortic and mitral valve replacement with prosthetic St. Jude's valves.

11/19/97: MRI of the brain demonstrated a 1.5-cm area of subacute ischemic change involving the right insular cortex and subacute ischemic changes in the right centrum semiovale which could not be completely distinguished from cerebritis (Fig. 87-8A and B). Enhancement with gadolinium suggested inflammatory change consistent with cerebritis in the insula at the sites of subacute ischemic change (Fig. 87-8C and D).

11/25/97: Cerebral angiography disclosed a right MCA opercular branch 6-mm saccular infected aneurysm without evidence of vasospasm (Fig. 87-8E).

12/05/97: Repeat angiography demonstrated dramatic enlargement of the aneurysm over a 10-day period with loss of fine branching candelabra vessels in the region of the sylvian triangle (Fig. 87-8F). Emergency superselective aneurysmography (Fig. 87-8H) followed by superselective angiography (see Fig. 87-8I) with opacified NBCA injection resulted in occlusion of the aneurysm and a segment of the proximal and distal right MCA parent artery (Fig. 87-8J and K). Following the procedure he was maintained on anticoagulation.

03/26/98: He remained generally well, having recovered from his hemiparesis with a mild residual left facial weakness and complaints of dizziness. Repeat angiography demonstrated no recurrent or new aneurysms. MRI demonstrated resolving chronic ischemic change in the right insular cortex and persisting chronic ischemic change in the right centrum semiovale and resolving cerebritis (Fig. 87-8M to O). He then returned to his prior gainful employment.

MAJOR INTRAOPERATIVE AND POSTOPERATIVE COMPLICATIONS AND THEIR MANAGEMENT

In our series, no major intraoperative complications occurred in 15 craniotomies.[1] The surgical risks with distal infected aneurysm excision are related to uncontrolled rupture, cerebral ischemia, and infection. If the aneurysm with its feeding and draining parent vessels are well visualized and fully exposed in its sulcal bed, complete hemostatic control should be anticipated. The potential risk for cerebral ischemic damage could be assessed by a preoperative Wada test or test balloon occlusion.

The problems with proximal aneurysms are more profound. In our case of wrapping an M1 segment fusiform aneurysm, no complication occurred. However, anecdotal reports of fatal rupture during manipulation of proximal aneurysms have discouraged attempts to manage them surgically. The techniques of bypass[80–83,117] and reanastomosis[87–90] have been employed. Endovascular occlusions with balloons, Hilal minicoils, and NBCA have been successful for distal aneurysms (see Case Report 8; Fig. 87-8A to O),[84–86] and now are beginning to be used for more proximal lesions.[79,87] One approach is to allow thickening of the wall to occur over time, making the aneurysm more amenable to direct handling. Endovascular occlusion with preservation of the parent vessel[79] or combined with a bypass procedure if the parent vessel must be sacrificed are now tenable options.

Balloon occlusion for high cervical carotid[89] infected aneurysm was associated with distal embolization, subsequently controlled by ligation of the supraclinoid carotid 8 days later. Superficial temporal to MCA bypass was established before balloon occlusion of a petrous artery aneurysm in another case that successfully averted an ischemic event.[88] Carotid ligation without bypass has similarly been used successfully.[76,77,123] Closure of a major vessel is always fraught with hazard, and the neurosurgeon should perform Wada testing and test balloon occlusion preoperatively. If an ischemic event occurs, hypertensive techniques and volume expansion may reverse the symptoms.[80,133] It may be necessary to perform angiography to ensure patency of a bypass or cross filling.

If an intraoperative rupture occurs, efforts to control the bleeding should include the use of temporary clips, induced hypotension, and, for more proximal lesions, direct common carotid compression or even open ligation.

The outcome for patients with intracranial fungal aneurysms is discouraging. Despite adequate intraoperative aneurysm management and appropriate antibiotic therapy, there had been no recorded cases of survival.[2–6] The recent successful surgical management of an infected posterior communicating artery aneurysm found to have hyphae of *Aspergillus* in the granulation tissue of its wall treated with superficial temporal artery to MCA bypass followed by

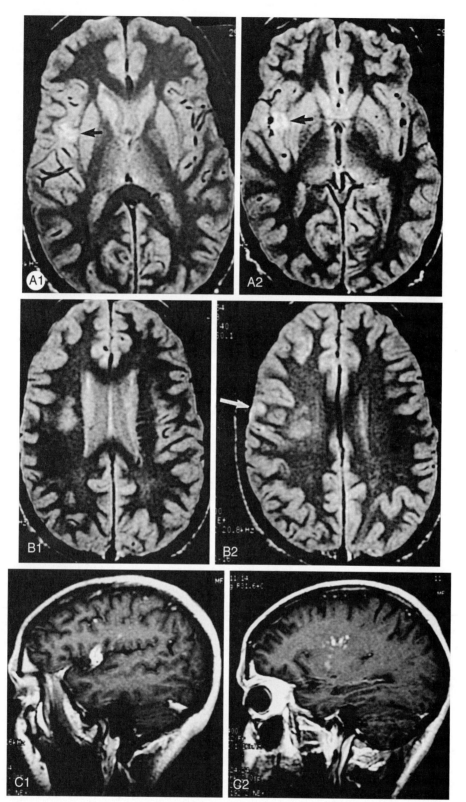

FIGURE 87-8   *A,* 11/19/97: Proton density axial magnetic resonance images (MRIs) (A1 and A2) showing a focal area of hyperintensity in the right insular cortex (*black arrows*) compatible with subacute ischemic change or cerebritis. *B,* 11/19/97: Proton density axial MRIs showing an area of hyperintense signal compatible with subacute ischemic change in the region of the right centrum semiovale (*B1*) and one cortical gyrus (*B2, white arrow*). *C,* 11/19/97: Postcontrast sagittal T1-weighted MRIs showing a focal area of discrete enhancing cortex or extravasation in the right insular cortex surrounding a middle cerebral artery (MCA) branch and the infected aneurysm denoted by the flow voids (*C1*) and patchy enhancement in the centrum semiovale suggestive of inflammation (*C2*).

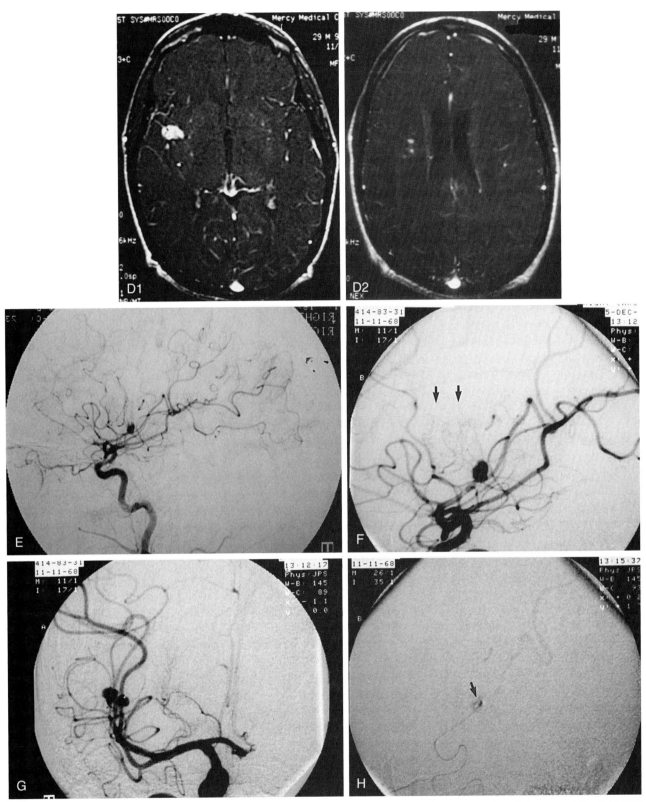

FIGURE 87-8 Cont'd *D,* 11/19/97: Postcontrast axial T1-weighted images demonstrating the extravasation of dye around the right MCA branch and the infected aneurysm (*D1*) and enhancement medially in the centrum semiovale suggestive of inflammation and comparable to the sagittal images seen in *C2* (*D2*). *E,* 11/25/97: Lateral angiogram demonstrating the infected aneurysm on an M2–M3 branch of the right MCA. *F,* 12/05/97: Lateral angiographic view showing dramatic aneurysmal enlargement with loss of at least two of the MCA candelabra branching vessels in the sylvian triangle (*black arrows*). *G,* 12/05/97: Anteroposterior (AP) angiographic view demonstrating the enlarged bilobed aneurysm. *H,* 12/05/97: Lateral superselective aneurysmography demonstrating the Magic 1.8 French catheter tip (Balt, Paris, France) in the fundus of the infected aneurysm (*black arrow*).

(Continued)

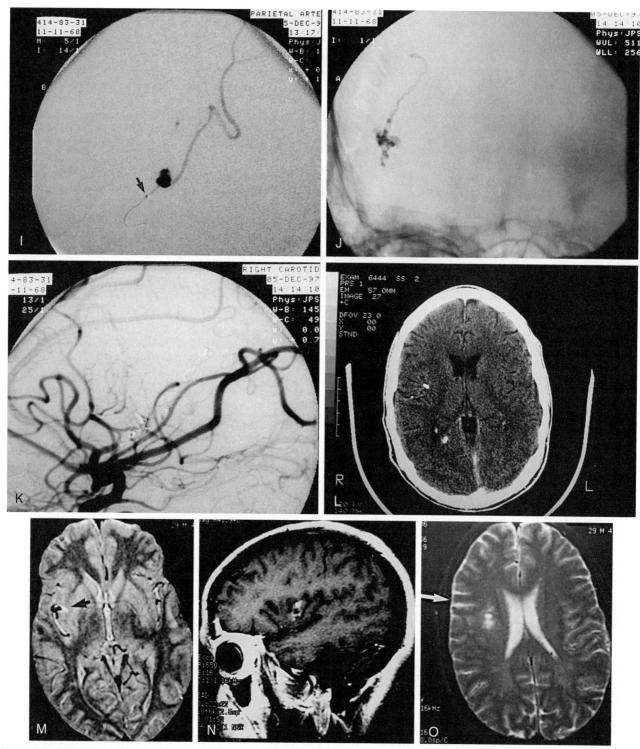

FIGURE 87-8 Cont'd *I,* 12/05/97: Superselective angiogram with the catheter tip extracted from the aneurysm into the proximal parent artery (*black arrow*). This view shows the aneurysm and its parent artery just prior to instillation of 0.2 mL of the quick-polymerizing *n*-butyl cyanoacrylate (NBCA) mixture composed of 3 mL of NBCA opacified with 0.5 mL of pantopaque and 10 g of Tantalum powder. *J,* 12/05/97: AP film showing the NBCA cast of the bilobed infected aneurysm and a segment of its parent artery. *K,* 12/05/97: Postembolization lateral angiogram showing occlusion of the aneurysm, loss of the parent artery, and the absent small candelabra branches in the sylvian triangle. *L,* 12/08/97: Axial computed tomography scan showing NBCA within the infected aneurysm. *M,* 03/26/98 (3 months later): Proton density axial MRI view showing a smaller area of chronic insular cortex ischemic change in the right insular region (compare with *A1* and *A2*) and probable associated resolving cerebritis along with an area of signal void compatible with NBCA casting of the infected aneurysm (*black arrow*). *N,* 03/26/98: Postcontrast T1-weighted sagittal MRI of the right sylvian fissure showing the NBCA signal void indicative of the aneurysmal occlusion with NBCA, the surrounding resolving chronic ischemic change, and resolving inflammation. *O,* T2-weighted axial MRI demonstrating the hyperintense signal in the right centrum semiovale compatible with the MCA territory chronic ischemic change and widened sulci (*white arrow*) in an area of resolving cortical ischemic change seen initially on 11/19/97 as subacute ischemic change (*B2*).

trapping and excision of the aneurysm[134] along with the report of recovery from *Candida albicans* meningitis in which miconazole was used[135] may offer some hope.

POSTOPERATIVE MANAGEMENT

Postoperative management includes continuation of appropriate antibiotics, anticonvulsants, dexamethasone when indicated (see Table 87-1, Patient 13), and post-NBCA embolization anticoagulation when small branch and parent artery occlusions have occurred (see Case Report 8; Fig. 87-8A to O). Extubation should be performed as soon as possible, and occupational and physical therapy and drug counseling are provided as needed. Testing for AIDS is advised in selected patients.[107,108] Strict attention must be directed to the potential development of additional aneurysms,[16] to close monitoring of coexisting aneurysms,[12,98-102] and to cardiovascular status (see Table 87-1, Patients 13 and 15; Case Reports 3 and 7).

THE AUTHORS' SERIES

Our series consisted of 17 patients 11 to 82 years of age (see Table 87-1; Table 87-2) who harbored a total of 28 infected aneurysms.[1] In 16 patients, the aneurysms were detected angiographically, and in one patient (Patient 12; see Case Report 1), the aneurysm was demonstrated by CT scan (see Fig. 87-1A and B). Four patients had two aneurysms, one had three, and one had six. In five of these six patients, infected aneurysms were seen bilaterally. Twenty-five aneurysms were on distal branches of the MCA, three were more proximally located on the middle cerebral and anterior communicating arteries, and one was on the superior cerebellar artery.

Eight patients had known valvular heart disease. Seven were parenteral drug users. All except one had "infective" endocarditis (see Table 87-1; Table 87-3); one patient (Patient 4), despite an aortic systolic murmur and positive blood culture result for *Staphylococcus epidermidis*, had no evidence of endocarditis at autopsy; he had had a urinary tract infection several weeks before the intracerebral hemorrhage from a pathologically documented infected aneurysm. Another patient (Patient 14; see Case Report 6),

a parenteral drug user, had negative findings on blood culture but had had endocarditis with bacteremia 9 months earlier and had subsequently self-administered illicitly obtained antibiotics. Except for these two patients (Patients 4 and 14), blood culture results were positive more than once in all patients in the group.

The behavior of the aneurysms during antimicrobial therapy was varied and unpredictable (see Tables 87-1 and 87-4). Five patients experienced aneurysm rupture during or at the conclusion of antimicrobial treatment. Intracerebral hematoma developed in one patient (Patient 2) after 5 days of treatment with ampicillin and then 3 days of penicillin and streptomycin for *S. viridans*; in another (Patient 6; see Case Report 2) after 12 days of penicillin treatment for *S. viridans* and *Micrococcus* species; in one patient (Patient 12; see Case Report 1) after 3 days of treatment with ampicillin, gentamicin, and oxacillin and then 15 days of penicillin for *S. viridans* (see Fig. 87-1A to C); and in a fourth patient (Patient 17), after 7 days of vancomycin treatment for *S. aureus*. In one patient (Patient 1) who had had only right cerebral angiography, a left cerebral

TABLE 87-3 ▪ Results of Blood Cultures

Result	No. of Patients
Streptococcus viridans	5
Staphylococcus aureus	5
Diphtheroids	1
Staphylococcus epidermidis	1
S. viridans plus *Micrococcus* spp	1
Corynebacterium pseudodiphtheroid hoffmannis	1
Serratia marcessens	1
Pseudomonas sp plus *Providencia* sp	1
No growth	1

From Brust JC, Dickinson PCT, Hughes JEO, Holtzman RNN: The diagnosis and treatment of cerebral mycotic aneurysms. Ann Neurol 27:238–246, 1990.

TABLE 87-4 ▪ Aneurysm Behavior in Relation to Antibiotic Therapy

Behavior During Therapy	No. of Aneurysms
Bled before treatment, early excision	4
Bled before treatment, then enlarged during treatment	1
Bled during treatment, then continued to enlarge	1
Bled during treatment after enlarging	1
Bled during treatment, then early excision	2
Bled following treatment, then early excision	1
Never bled, early excision	1
Never bled, but enlarged or unchanged during or after treatment	7
Never bled, became smaller or disappeared during or after treatment	10
Total	28

From Brust JC, Dickinson PCT, Hughes JEO, Holtzman RNN: The diagnosis and treatment of cerebral mycotic aneurysms. Ann Neurol 27:238–246, 1990.

TABLE 87-2 ▪ Patient Backgrounds

Age (yr)	
Range	11–82
Mean	35
Median	29
Sex	
Male	10
Female	7
Risk Factor (No. of Patients)	
Rheumatic heart disease	6
Congenital heart disease	2
Parenteral drug abuse	7
Uncertain	2

From Brust JC, Dickinson PCT, Hughes JEO, Holtzman RNN: The diagnosis and treatment of cerebral mycotic aneurysms. Ann Neurol 27:238–246, 1990.

aneurysm ruptured on the last day of a 6-week course of ampicillin and streptomycin for diphtheroid bacilli; blood culture results had been negative for at least 16 days. Of these five patients with aneurysm rupture during antibiotic treatment, two died; one of these had rapid transtentorial herniation (Patient 12), and the other lapsed into a coma after emergency craniotomy and died 73 days later. In one patient (Patient 3), the aneurysm ruptured on the day of admission and then continued to enlarge angiographically; it was excised after 11 days of antibiotic therapy and showed histologically persistent inflammation, with clumps of gram-positive cocci in the wall, intraluminal thrombus, and destruction of the internal elastic lamina. Cultures of the aneurysm confirmed the presence of S. aureus (Fig. 87-9).

Eleven intracranial hemorrhages occurred either before or during hospitalization in 10 patients (twice in Patient 1, once in Patients 2, 3, 4, 6, 12, 13, 14, 16, and 17). Two hemorrhages were preceded by focal neurologic signs: one patient's (Patient 1) second hemorrhage occurred 41 days after the first, and another's (Patient 12) hemorrhage occurred after 15 days of mild weakness of the right arm. The other nine hemorrhages (eight of which were caused by documented ruptured aneurysms) occurred without neurologic prodrome.

Ten aneurysms became smaller or disappeared with medical treatment (including four of the six in Patient 9), but 10 (including one that had already bled before treatment) became larger or remained the same size (see Fig. 87-2).

Fifteen craniotomies were performed in 12 patients (see Table 87-1; Table 87-5). Eight aneurysms in seven patients (Patients 1, 2, 3, 4, 6, 16, and 17) were excised after rupture. Two of these patients died, one patient (Patient 1) with sepsis and one (Patient 4) with gastrointestinal bleeding; two others (Patients 2 and 3) had residual aphasia or cognitive impairment. Six unruptured aneurysms in six patients were excised. In one (Patient 6), the unruptured aneurysm was excised a month after surgery for a contralateral ruptured aneurysm. Another (Patient 13, see Case Report 3) had evacuation of a left cerebral hematoma, but an aneurysm was not found; the patient later underwent excision of a right-sided unruptured aneurysm. An unruptured fusiform

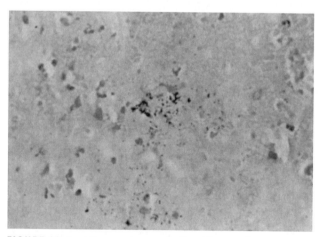

FIGURE 87-9 Microscopic examination: Clumps of gram-positive cocci are seen in the wall and thrombus of the excised aneurysm 11 days after the institution of appropriate antibiotic therapy. Cultures of the aneurysm confirmed the presence of *Staphylococcus aureus*

TABLE 87-5 ▪ Surgical Procedures

Procedure	No. of Aneurysms
Aneurysms excised after rupture*	8
Unruptured aneurysms excised†	6
Aneurysm wrapped‡	1
Hematoma evacuated, aneurysm not found	1

*Seven patients.
†One within a hematoma secondary to an adjacent ruptured aneurysm.
‡Fusiform, proximal middle cerebral artery.
From Brust JC, Dickinson PCT, Hughes JEO, Holtzman RNN: The diagnosis and treatment of cerebral mycotic aneurysms. Ann Neurol 27:238–246, 1990.

aneurysm in the proximal MCA M1 segment was surgically wrapped in one patient (Patient 10, see Case Report 4). All four patients whose only surgery was for an unruptured aneurysm made uneventful recoveries. One patient (Patient 9) had angiographic shrinkage or disappearance of five distal aneurysms and persistence of a proximal aneurysm on the anterior cerebral artery; while surgery for the latter was being considered, the patient had fatal rupture of a hepatic artery–infected aneurysm.

DISCUSSION

Consistent with previous literature, our patients demonstrated that infected intracranial aneurysms should be suspected in any patient, adult or child, with endocarditis who has neurologic symptoms not explained by systemic illness or toxicity. Infected aneurysms occur proportionately more frequently in children than in adults; studies suggest that between 27% and 55% of patients with infected aneurysms are children.[136] Approximately 10% of all pediatric intracranial aneurysms are infected aneurysms,[137] with risk factors resembling those for adults (see Table 87-2).[139] Serious attention must be given to the recently described entity of cerebral aneurysmal arteriopathy in children with immunodeficiency syndrome and AIDS characterized by findings of subacute infarction and fusiform dilatation of the major vessels of the circle of Willis[107,108] because fatal outcomes occurred within 6 months after the diagnosis was established.

As noted, the mechanism of formation and evolution of infected intracranial aneurysms remains uncertain. Results of experimental studies of systemic arteries[32–35] may not apply to cerebral arteries. Although it now appears that cerebral vessels have true vasa vasorum,[41,42] their detailed anatomy and physiologic roles, as in the case of the rete vasorum,[43] still remain unclear. Theories of embolic infection of the tunica intima[19] imply initial endothelial injury, either mechanical or rheological. Possibly important in pathogenesis are adherence of the embolus itself; vessel wall penetration by infectious organisms; liberation of immune complexes[16] alone or in conjunction with antibiotics[44]; and endothelial injury related to focal anoxia, impaired nutrition, interference with DNA synthesis, complement activation, or release of lysosomal enzymes and prostaglandins, including prostacyclin.[51,52]

Destruction of the internal elastic lamina and the tunica media produces focal weakness. Reparative processes, however, produce thickening of the aneurysm wall. In some cases, the parent artery is spontaneously occluded (see Table 87-1, Patient 14; Case Report 6, Fig. 87-6A to D) or operatively occluded (see Case Report 8; Fig. 87-8I to O), whereas in others it is preserved with resolution of the aneurysm (see Table 87-1, Patient 15; Case Report 7, Fig. 87-7A to C).[79] Antibiotics suppress the infecting organisms sufficiently to facilitate these reparative processes, but in some instances bacteria may remain in the arterial wall despite antibiotic therapy (see Fig. 87-9, Patient 3).

The serious nature of infected intracranial aneurysms is not diminished by the fact that they occur infrequently,[98] because frank rupture carries a mortality statistic of 25% to 90%. There is an absolute need to document their presence in patients with endocarditis and unexplained neurologic symptoms or signs, including pleocytosis in the CSF or apparent infarction on CT scan or MRI.[1] Infected intracranial aneurysms may also occur in patients with meningitis,[1,24–26] cavernous sinus thrombophlebitis,[20–23] cerebral abscess (Stein BM, personal communication, 1993),[27a–30] and subdural empyema.[31]

Recognizing that infected aneurysms could become larger or smaller during antibiotic treatment,[13,55,56,60–62,71,118,137–142] Bingham[74] suggested "early four-vessel angiography" in selected patients with endocarditis and then "effective antibiotic therapy" with monitoring by "serial cerebral angiography every 2 to 3 weeks." He advised prompt surgery for enlarging lesions and after a course of antibiotics for lesions that were unchanged in size. (As an option, he suggested "definitive surgery for smaller lesions," presumably with or without enlargement.)

A more aggressive approach was advocated by Frazee and colleagues,[67] who noted that intracranial infected aneurysms could rupture "at any point in the course of appropriate antibiotic therapy." They recommended serial cerebral angiography every 7 to 10 days in patients with bacterial endocarditis and "sudden severe headache, focal neurological signs or symptoms or seizures," as well as prompt excision of aneurysms "whenever possible." Such a policy, they noted, would lead to angiography in 19% of patients with bacterial endocarditis; 25% to 33% of them (and 4% to 6% of all patients with bacterial endocarditis) would have an intracranial mycotic aneurysm.

Sharing this sense of urgency, Roach and Drake[143] advised that mycotic aneurysms "should be suspected" in any patient with bacterial endocarditis and that "peripheral aneurysms should be excised or ligated immediately." Similarly, Bohmfalk and associates[75] recommended "complete cerebral angiography" on all patients with bacterial endocarditis, whether or not they had neurologic symptoms, as well as surgical excision of "aneurysms with mass lesions" or "single superficial aneurysm." They proposed serial angiography for multiple peripheral aneurysms and surgery for those that enlarged; for proximal aneurysms, their recommendations were more tentative but included serial angiography and consideration of various surgical procedures.

In other anecdotal reports, investigators described infected intracranial aneurysms that ruptured, sometimes fatally, during or after presumed appropriate antimicrobial therapy.[9,13,53,75,138,144–159] New aneurysms have also formed during or after therapy.[16,55,63] In one patient, an infected aneurysm ruptured after 4 weeks of appropriate antimicrobial therapy and 2 weeks after normal findings on cerebral angiography.[147] Aneurysms have also persisted[160] or enlarged,[140] sometimes after getting smaller.[56,57] Ojemann[161] reviewed the cases of 81 patients with documented infected aneurysms and "definite or probable endocarditis." Of 30 patients "treated with antibiotics where the outcome was known," 13 died. Of 29 who had elective surgery, 2 died, but both had recovered from surgery "only to die from rupture of a second unrecognized aneurysm."

Our experience with 17 patients leads us to agree with advocates of early detection and surgical management. Nonsurgical treatment with serial angiography presupposes that in every patient, aneurysm appearance or enlargement will be identified in time for prophylactic surgery to be carried out. However, neurologic symptoms may be absent in patients with infected aneurysms, and when symptoms are present, they are hardly specific. Moreover, animal experiments have demonstrated that aneurysm formation and rupture can occur with greater rapidity than any reasonable serial angiographic schedule could safely predict.[19,34,35]

Salgado and colleagues[104] recommended that 48 hours elapse between symptoms of embolic infarction and cerebral angiography because in experimental animals, aneurysms tended to form during such an interval after embolization. Among our patients, intracranial hemorrhage frequently occurred without prior neurologic symptoms; in two patients without hemorrhage, aneurysms were detected angiographically within 24 hours after the appearance of hemiparesis.

Our experience and that of numerous previous authors does not enable us to identify in advance those aneurysms that will become smaller or disappear with appropriate antimicrobial therapy, those that will slowly enlarge before rupturing, and those that will rupture without angiographic enlargement. We therefore recommend MRI/MRA followed by four-vessel angiography without delay when an infected aneurysm is suspected in patients with endocarditis who have neurologic abnormalities that are not attributable to systemic toxicity (including CSF pleocytosis or apparent infarction on CT). We also recommend that single accessible infected aneurysms in medically stable patients be promptly excised.[1] We further suggest that patients with cavernous sinus thrombophlebitis, meningitis, cerebral abscess, and subdural empyema also be considered as potentially harboring an infected aneurysm. Recommendations for patients with multiple or proximal aneurysms must be individualized; however, the goal in such patients should also be definitive treatment as soon as possible.[1,109]

Salgado and colleagues[104] advised repeat angiography on completion of antibiotic therapy when long-term anticoagulation treatment is planned in patients with initially negative results. Recognizing that aneurysms can form during treatment, we agree. Long-term follow-up is mandatory to assess delayed appearance of aneurysms[16,53] and to manage the problems of cardiac failure and valve disruption.

The recent advances in cerebral endovascular technology have permitted superselective catheterization[162] of both proximal[79] and distal (see Case Report 8, Fig. 87-8E to K)[86] vessels and selective occlusion of infected aneurysms with[79] and without (see Case Report 8, Fig. 87-8E to K) preservation of the parent arteries. Patients have tolerated these procedures well, and with the accumulation of further experience, perhaps in combination with bypass procedures in certain instances, it is likely that the role of interventional endovascular neuroradiology in the management of infected cerebral aneurysms will steadily increase.[162]

SUMMARY

Recognizing the retrospective and anecdotal nature of our data and the differing views of previous investigators, we recommend that

1. Careful neurologic examination, CT, and, unless contraindicated, lumbar puncture is performed on any patient with endocarditis.
2. Those with neurologic abnormalities not attributable to systemic toxicity, including pleocytosis in the CSF or apparent infarction on CT scans, undergo four-vessel cerebral angiography.
3. Single accessible infected aneurysms in medically stable patients are promptly excised, with individualization of multiple or proximal aneurysms. Endovascular management may be an option in certain cases.
4. Repeat angiography is performed at the conclusion of antibiotic therapy in patients requiring long-term anticoagulation.

Our data do not allow us to predict whether performing repeat angiography on all neurologically abnormal patients or initial angiography on all endocarditis patients would do more harm than good.

Acknowledgments

We thank Dr. Robert L. DeLa Paz, Director of Neuroradiology, New York Presbyterian Hospital for his interpretations of the MRI scans; Dr. George V. DiGiacinto, Director, Division of Neurosurgery, St. Luke's-Roosevelt Hospital Center, for the contribution of his case (Table 87-1, Patient 16) to our series; Dr. Harold "Russ" Gaetz, Assistant Chief of Anatomic Pathology, St. Luke's-Roosevelt Hospital Center, for his analysis and identification of the bacteria in the aneurysm excised from Table 87-1, Patient 3; Dr. Edward B. Healton, Senior Associate Dean and Assistant Vice-President, Columbia University College of Physicians & Surgeons, for his clinical insight and contributions to the management of our cases at the Harlem Hospital Center; Dr. Mark D. Krieger, Resident, Department of Neurosurgery, University of Southern California, for his contribution to the discussion in the section on terminology; Richard A. Rand, Ph.D., Professor of English, University of Alabama for contributing the concept of catachresis to the section on terminology; Dr. Henry Spotnitz, the George H. Humphreys II Professor of Surgery, Columbia University College of Physicians & Surgeons, for his care and successful cardiac surgical management of Table 87-1, Patients 13 and 15; Dr. William L. Young, Professor of Anesthesiology (in Neurosurgery and in Radiology), Columbia University College of Physicians & Surgeons, for his contributions to the section on anesthetic considerations; Mr. Ronald H. Winston, Chairman, Harry Winston Medical Foundation, for his insight, critiquing, and support of the manuscript; and Little, Brown & Company for permission to reproduce portions of our article from *Annals of Neurology* 27:238–246, 1990 (reference 1).

REFERENCES

1. Brust JCM, Dickinson PCT, Hughes JEO, Holtzman RNN: The diagnosis and treatment of cerebral mycotic aneurysms. Ann Neurol 27:238–246, 1990.
2. Ojemann RG, Heros RC, Crowell RM: Infectious aneurysms. In Surgical Management of Cerebrovascular Diseases, 2nd ed. Baltimore: Williams & Wilkins, 1988, pp 337–346.
3. Weir B: Special aneurysms (nonsaccular and saccular)— "Infective." In Aneurysms Affecting the Nervous System. Baltimore: Williams & Wilkins, 1987, pp 159–171.
4. Horton BC, Abbott GF, Porro RS: Fungal aneurysms of intracranial vessels. Arch Neurol 33:570–576, 1976.
5. Mielke B, Weir B, Oldring D, Von Westrap C: Fungal aneurysms: Case report and review of the literature. Neurosurgery 9:578–582, 1981.
6. Komatsu Y, Narushima K, Kobayashi E, et al: *Aspergillus* mycotic aneurysm—Case report. Neurol Med Chir (Tokyo) 31:346–350, 1991.
7. Stehbens WE: Subarachnoid hemorrhage. In Pathology of the Cerebral Blood Vessels. St. Louis: CV Mosby, 1972, pp 252–283.
8. Martinez AJ, Sotelo-Avila C, Alcala H, Willaert E: Granulomatous encephalitis, intracranial arteritis and mycotic aneurysm due to a free-living ameba. Acta Neuropathol (Berl) 49:7–12, 1980.
9. O'Donohue JM, Enzmann DR: Mycotic aneurysm in angiitis associated with herpes zoster ophthalmicus. AJNR Am J Neuroradiol 8:615–619, 1987.
10. Steele JJ, Kilburn KL, Leech RW: Phytotic (mycotic) intracranial aneurysm with an unusual pathogenesis: A case report. Pediatrics 50:936–939, 1972.
11. Clare CE, Barrow DL: Infectious intracranial aneurysms. Neurosurg Clin N Am 3:551–566, 1992.
12. Ahmadi J, Tung H, Giannotta SL, Destian S: Monitoring of infectious intracranial aneurysms by sequential computed tomographic/magnetic resonance imaging studies. Neurosurgery 32:45–50, 1993.
13. Pruitt AA, Rubin RH, Kachmer AW, Gold GW: Neurological complications of bacterial endocarditis. Medicine 57:329–343, 1978.
14. Ray H, Wahal KM: Subarachnoid hemorrhage in subacute bacterial endocarditis. Neurology 7:265–269, 1957.
15. Steinberg GK, Guppy KH, Adler JR, Silverberg GD: Stereotactic, angiography-guided clipping of a distal, mycotic intracranial aneurysm using the Cosman-Roberts-Wells System: Technical note. Neurosurgery 30:408–411, 1992.
16. Venger BH, Aldama AE: Mycotic vasculitis with repeated intracranial aneurysmal hemorrhage: Case report. J Neurosurg 69:775–779, 1988.
17. Daltroff G, Lamit J, Bichet J, et al: Intracranial septic aneurysm in an infant: Apropos of a case and review of the literature. Pediatrie 39:125–132, 1984.
18. Scully RE, Mark EJ, McNeely WF, McNeely BU: Case records of the Massachusetts General Hospital-weekly clinicopathological exercises. Case 10-1993. N Engl J Med 328:717–725, 1993.
19. Foote RA, Reagen TJ, Sandok BA: Cerebral arterial lesions resulting from inflammatory emboli. Stroke 9:498–503, 1978.
20. Suwanwela C, Suwanwela N, Charuchinda S, Hongsoprabhas C: Intracranial mycotic aneurysms of extravascular origin. J Neurosurg 36:552–559, 1972.
21. Tomita T, McClone D, Naidich TP: Mycotic aneurysm of the intracavernous portion of the carotid artery in childhood: Case report. J Neurosurg 54:681–684, 1981.
22. Rout D, Sharma A, Mohan PK, Rao VRK: Bacterial aneurysms of the intracavernous carotid artery. J Neurosurg 60:1236–1242, 1984.
23. Shibuya S, Igarashi S, Amo T, et al: Mycotic aneurysms of the internal carotid artery: Case report. J Neurosurg 44:105–108, 1976.
24. Heidelberger KP, Layton WM, Jr, Fisher RG: Multiple cerebral mycotic aneurysms complicating posttraumatic *Pseudomonas* meningitis: Case report. J Neurosurg 26:631–635, 1968.
25. Hannesson B, Sachs E, Jr: Mycotic aneurysms following purulent meningitis: Report of a case with recovery and review of the literature. Acta Neurochir (Wien) 24:305–313, 1971.
26. Sypert GW, Young HF: Ruptured mycotic pericallosal aneurysm with meningitis due to *Neisseria meningitidis* infection: Case report. J Neurosurg 37:467–469, 1972.
27. Shimosaka S, Waga S: Cerebral chromoblastomycosis complicated by meningitis and multiple fungal aneurysms after resection of a granuloma: Case report. J Neurosurg 59:158–161, 1983.

27a. Stein BM: Byron Stookey Professor of Neurological Surgery, Emeritus, New York Neurological Institute. Personal communication, 1993. Regarding the successful conservative management of an infected aneurysm at the site of prior brain abscess excision.

28. Sato T, Sakuta Y, Suzuki J, Takaku Y: Successful surgical treatment of intracranial mycotic aneurysm with brain abscess: Report of a case. Acta Neurochir (Wien) 47:53–61, 1979.

29. Funakoshi T, Tsuchiya J, Sakai N, et al: Peripheral arterial aneurysm of the brain occurring after brain abscess extirpation and healing spontaneously—Report of a case and review of the literature. No Shinkei Geka Apr 4:405–410, 1976.

30. Pozzati E, Tognetti F, Padovani R, Gaist G: Association of cerebral mycotic aneurysm and brain abscess. Neurochirurgia (Stuttg) 26:18–20, 1983.

31. Fujita Y, Kohira R, Yanagida K, et al: A case of multiple subdural empyema complicated by intracranial mycotic aneurysm. No To Hattatsu 19:507–511, 1987.

32. Eppinger H: Pathogenesis (Histogenesis unde Aetiologie) der aneurysmen einschliesslich des Aneurysma equi verminosum. IV: Parasitöre aneurysmen Arch Klin Chir 35:126–440, 1887.

33. Nakata Y, Shionoya S, Kamiya: Pathogenesis of mycotic aneurysm. Angiology 19:593–610, 1968.

34. Molinari GF: Septic cerebral embolism. Stroke 3:117–122, 1972.

35. Molinari GF, Smith L, Goldstein MN, Satran R: Pathogenesis of cerebral mycotic aneurysms. Neurology 23:325–332, 1973.

36. Stengel A, Wolferth CC: Mycotic (bacterial) aneurysms of intravascular origin. Arch Intern Med 31:505–508, 1923.

37. Clower BR, Sullivan DM, Smith RR: Intracranial vessels lack vasa vasorum. J Neurosurg 61:44–48, 1984.

37a. Fukushima T: Professor of Neurological Surgery, Allegheny General Hospital. Personal communication, Winter Neurosurgical Conference, Alberta, Canada, March, 1993.

38. Atkinson JLD, Okazaki H, Sundt TM, Jr, Nichols DA, Rufenacht DA: Intracranial cerebrovascular vasa vasorum associated with atherosclerosis and large thick-walled aneurysms. Surg Neurol 36:365–369, 1991.

39. Yasargil MG: Microneurosurgery, vol 1. New York: Thieme Medical, 1984, p 57.

40. Yasargil MG: Microneurosurgery, vol 4. New York: Thieme Medical, 1988, pp 333, 342, 389.

41. Connolly ES, Huang J, Goldman JE, Holtzman RNN: Immunohistochemical detection of intracranial vasa vasorum: A human autopsy study. Neurosurgery 38:789–793, 1996.

42. Takaba M, Endo S, Kurimoto M, et al: Vasa vasorum of the intracranial artery. Acta Neurochir (Wien) 140:411–416, 1998.

43. Zervas NT, Liszczak TM, Mayberg MR, Black PMCL: Cerebrospinal fluid may nourish cerebral vessels through pathways in the adventitia that may be analogous to systemic vasa vasorum. J Neurosurg 56:475–481, 1982.

44. Tuomanen E: Breaching the blood brain barrier. Sci Am 268:80–85, 1993.

45. Garvey GJ, Neu HC: Infective endocarditis—An evolving disease: A review of endocarditis at the Columbia-Presbyterian Medical Center, 1968–73. Medicine (Baltimore) 57:105–127, 1978.

46. Biller J, Challa VR, Toole JF, Howard VJ: Nonbacterial thrombotic endocarditis: A neurologic perspective of clinicopathologic correlations of 99 patients. Arch Neurol 39:95–98, 1982.

47. Castaigne P, Laplane D, Ricou P, Mallacourt J: Multiple intracranial arterial aneurysms of mycotic appearance: Repeated vascular embolic accidents. Myxoma of the left atrium. Rev Neurol (Paris) 131:339–345, 1975.

48. Hofmann E, Becker T, Romberg-Hahnloser R, et al: Cranial MRI and CT in patients with left atrial myxoma. Neuroradiology 34:57–61, 1992.

49. Branch CL, Laster DW, Kelly DL, Jr: Left atrial myxoma with cerebral emboli. Neurosurgery 16:675–680, 1985.

50. Michael AS, Mikhael MA, Christ M: Myxoma of the heart presenting with recurrent episodes of hemorrhagic cerebral infarction: MR findings. J Comput Assist Tomogr 13:123–135, 1989.

51. Oyesiku NM, Barrow DL, Eckman JR, et al: Intracranial aneurysms in sickle-cell anemia: Clinical features and pathogenesis. J Neurosurg 75:356–363, 1991.

52. Engelberg H: Endothelium in health and disease. Semin Thromb Hemost 15:178–181, 1989.

53. Bamford J, Hodges J, Warlow C: Late rupture of a mycotic aneurysm after "cure" of bacterial endocarditis. J Neurol 233:51–53, 1986.

54. Monsuez JJ, Vittecoq D, Rosenbaum A, et al: Prognosis of ruptured intracranial mycotic aneurysms: A review of 12 cases. Eur Heart J 10:821–825, 1989.

55. Ziment I, Johnson BL, Jr: Angiography in the management of intracranial mycotic aneurysms. Arch Intern Med 122:349–352, 1968.

56. Pootrakul A, Carter LP: Bacterial intracranial aneurysm: Importance of sequential angiography. Surg Neurol 17:429–431, 1982.

57. Kamiya K, Inagawa Y, Ogasawara H: A case of ruptured mycotic cerebral aneurysm associated with repeated arterial narrowing and remission. No Shinkei Geka 16:275–280, 1988.

58. Iwabuchi T, Kurashima Y, Fukawa O, Suzuki J: Multiple mycotic cerebral aneurysms—A case report. In Suzuki J (ed): Cerebral Aneurysms. Tokyo: Neuron, 1979, pp 690–696.

59. Greenlee JE, Mandell GE: Neurological manifestations of infective endocarditis: A review. Stroke 4:958–963, 1973.

60. Valadarez JB, de Souza MT, Hankinson J, et al: Multiple intracranial mycotic aneurysms: Case report. Arq Neuropsiquiatr 37:311–318, 1979.

61. Morawetz RB, Karp RB: Evolution and resolution of intracranial bacterial (mycotic) aneurysms. Neurosurgery 15:43–49, 1984.

62. Morawetz RB, Acker JD, Harsh GR: Management of mycotic (bacterial) intracranial aneurysms. Contemp Neurosurg 3:1–6, 1981.

63. Kowada M, Watanabe K, Takahashi M, Nishimura H: Multiple intracranial mycotic aneurysms: Report of a case. No Shinkei Geka 3:255–260, 1975.

64. Hadley MN, Martin NA, Spetzler RF, Johnson PC: Multiple intracranial aneurysms due to *Coccidioides immitis* infection: Case report. J Neurosurg 66:453–456, 1987.

65. Bandoh K, Sugimura J, Hosaka K, Takagi S: Ruptured intracranial mycotic aneurysm associated with acute subdural hematoma—Case report. Neurol Med Chir (Tokyo) 27:56–59, 1987.

66. Ho KL: Acute subdural hematoma and intracerebral hemorrhage: Rare complications of rhinocerebral mucuromycosis. Arch Otolaryngol Head Neck Surg 105:279–281, 1979.

67. Frazee JG, Cahan LD, Winter J: Bacterial intracranial aneurysms. J Neurosurg 53:633–641, 1980.

68. Jones HR, Jr, Siekert RG: Neurological manifestations of infective endocarditis: Review of clinical and therapeutic challenges. Brain 112:1295–1315, 1989.

69. Kanter MC, Hart RG: Neurologic complications of infective endocarditis. Neurology 41:1015–1020, 1991.

70. Hart RG, Kagan-Hallet K, Joerns SE: Mechanisms of intracranial hemorrhage in infective endocarditis. Stroke 18:1048–1056, 1987.

71. McNeel D, Evans RA, Ory EM: Angiography of cerebral mycotic aneurysms. Acta Radiol 9:407–412, 1969.

72. Mohr JP, Kase CS: Cerebral vasospasm. Part I. In cerebral vascular malformations. Rev Neurol (Paris) 139:99–113, 1983.

73. Yasargil MG: Microneurosurgery, vol. 1. New York: Thieme Medical, 1984, p 282.

74. Bingham WF: Treatment of mycotic intracranial aneurysms. J Neurosurg 46:428–437, 1977.

75. Bohmfalk GL, Story JL, Wissinger JP, Brown WE, Jr: Bacterial intracranial aneurysms. J Neurosurg 48:369–382, 1979.

76. Chiapetta F, Vangelista S, Pirrone R: Recurrent massive otorrhagia caused by a petrous carotid aneurysm. J Neurosurg Sci 26:205–207, 1982.

77. Holtzman RNN, Parisier SC: Acute spontaneous otorrhagia resulting from a ruptured petrous carotid aneurysm. J Neurosurg 51:258–261, 1979.

78. Anderson RD, Liebeskind A, Schechter M, et al: Aneurysms of the internal carotid artery in the carotid canal of the petrous temporal bone. Radiology 102:639–642, 1972.

79. Kawakami K, Kayama T, Kondo R, et al: A case of mycotic ICA petrous portion aneurysm treated with endovascular surgery. No Shinkei Geka 24(3):253–257, 1996.

80. Eguchi T, Nakagomi T, Teraoka A: Treatment of bilateral carotid cavernous aneurysms: Case report. J Neurosurg 56:443–447, 1982.

81. Al-Mefty O, Yamamoto Y: Neurovascular reconstruction during and after skull base surgery. Contemp Neurosurg 15:4–6, 1993.

82. Linskey ME, Sekhar LN, Horton JA, et al: Aneurysms of the intracavernous carotid artery: A multidisciplinary approach to treatment. J Neurosurg 75:525–534, 1991.

83. Wascher TM, Spetzler RF, Zabramski JM: Improved transdural exposure and temporary occlusion of the petrous internal carotid artery for cavernous sinus surgery: Technical note. J Neurosurg 78:834–837, 1993.

84. Aymard A, Herbreteau D, Khayata M, et al: Endovascular treatment of mycotic cerebral aneurysms [Abstract]. Neuroradiology 33 (Suppl):146, 1991.

85. Khayata MH, Aymard A, Casasco A, et al: Selective endovascular techniques in the treatment of cerebral mycotic aneurysms. J Neurosurg 78:661–665, 1993.

86. Bishop RC, Fisher WS, Morawetz RB: Infectious intracranial aneurysm. In Batjer HH, Caplan LR, Greenlee RG, Jr, et al (eds): Cerebrovascular Disease. Philadelphia: Lippincott-Raven, 1997, pp 1183–1188.

87. Halbach VV, Higashida RT, Hieshima GB, et al: Aneurysms of the petrous portion of the internal carotid artery: Results of treatment with endovascular or surgical occlusion. AJNR Am J Neuroradiol 11:253–257, 1990.

88. McGrail KM, Heros RC, Debrun G, Beyerl BD: Aneurysm of the ICA petrous segment treated by balloon entrapment after EC-IC bypass: Case report. J Neurosurg 65:249–252, 1986.

89. Bolender NF, Bassett MR, Loeser JD, Patterson HC: Mycotic aneurysm of the internal carotid artery: A surgical emergency. Ann Otol Rhinol Laryngol 93(3 Part 1):273–276, 1984.

90. Sandmann W, Hennerici M, Aulich A, et al: Progress in carotid artery surgery at the base of the skull. J Vasc Surg 1:734–743, 1984.

91. Monson RC II, Alexander RH: Vein reconstruction of a mycotic internal carotid aneurysm. Ann Surg 191:47–50, 1980.

92. Katz RI, Goldberg HI, Selzer ME: Mycotic aneurysm: Case report with novel sequential angiographic findings. Arch Intern Med 134:939–942, 1974.

93. Saff G, Frau M, Murtagh FR, Silbiger ML: Mucormycosis associated with carotid cavernous fistula and cavernous carotid mycotic aneurysm. J Fla Med Assoc 76:863–865, 1989.

94. Van Dellen JR, Haffejee IE: Mycotic intracavernous carotid artery aneurysm in childhood. Ann Trop Paediatr 4:51–54, 1984.

95. Harwood-Nash DC: The angiography of intracranial infections in children. In Salamon G (ed): Advances in Cerebral Angiography. Berlin, Springer-Verlag, 1975, pp 282–290.

96. Masuda J, Yutani C, Waki R, et al: Histopathological analysis of the mechanisms of intracranial hemorrhage complicating infective endocarditis. Stroke 23:843–850, 1992.

97. Kantor MC, Hart RG: Cerebral mycotic aneurysms are rare in infective endocarditis [Letter and reply]. Ann Neurol 28:590–591, 1990.

98. Lanfermann H, Gross-Fengels W, Steinbrich W: Intracranial aneurysms: A comparison between magnetic resonance tomography and arteriography. Rofo Fortschr Geb Rontgenstr Neuen Bildgeb Verfahr 157:118–123, 1992.

99. Louail C, Raynaud M, Gense de Beaufort D, Gréselle JF, Caillé JM: MRI-angiography in the evaluation of intracranial aneurysms [Abstract]. Neuroradiology 33(Suppl):128, 1991.

100. Gotsis ED, Kapsalaki E, Stylopoulos L, et al: Magnetic resonance angiography (MRA) of the brain and neck: Evaluation of state of the art methods on 200 patients [Abstract]. Neuroradiology 33 (Suppl):128, 1991.

101. Rovira A, Romero FJ, Ibarra B, et al: Evaluation of intracranial aneurysms using three-dimensional time of flight MR angiography [Abstract]. Neuroradiology 33(Suppl):128, 1991.

102. Volle E, Gustorf-Aeckerle R, Kraft R, et al: 3-D-MR angiography for acute subarachnoid hemorrhage. Neuroradiology 33(Suppl):129, 1991.

103. Kato Y, Yamaguchi S, Sano H, et al: Stereoscopic synthesized brain-surface imaging with MR angiography for localization of a peripheral mycotic aneurysm: Case report. Minim Invasive Neurosurg 39(4):113–115, 1996.

104. Salgado AV, Furlan AJ, Keys TF: Mycotic aneurysm, subarachnoid hemorrhage and indications for cerebral angiography in infective endocarditis. Stroke 18:1057–1067, 1987.

105. Lee KS, Liu SS, Spetzler RF, Rekate HL: Intracranial mycotic aneurysm in an infant: Report of a case. Neurosurgery 26:129–133, 1990.

106. Zee CS, Segall HD, McComb JG, et al: Intracranial arterial aneurysms in childhood: More recent considerations. J Child Neurol 1:99–114, 1986.

107. Dubrovsky T, Curless R, Scott G, et al: Cerebral aneurysmal arteriopathy in childhood AIDS. Neurology 51(2):560–656, 1998.

108. Shah SS, Zimmerman RA, Rorke LB: Cerebrovascular complication of HIV in children. AJNR Am J Neuroradiol 17(10):1913–1917, 1996.

109. Katakura K, Kayama T, Kondo R, et al: A case of multiple cerebral mycotic aneurysms treated with endovascular surgery. No Shinkei Geka 23(12):1127–1132, 1995.

110. Guthrie BL: Comment on stereotactic, angiography-guided clipping of a distal, mycotic intracranial aneurysm using the Cosman-Roberts-Wells system: Technical note. Neurosurgery 30:411, 1992.

111. Sisti MB, Solomon RA, Stein BM: Stereotactic craniotomy in the resection of small arteriovenous malformations. J Neurosurg 75:40–44, 1991.

112. Reinhardt HF, Horstmann GA, Gratzl O: Sonic stereometry in microsurgical procedures for deep-seated brain tumors and vascular malformations. Neurosurgery 32:51–57, 1993.

113. Barnett GH, Kormos DW, Steiner CP, Weisenberger J: Intraoperative localization using an armless, frameless stereotactic wand: Technical note. J Neurosurg 78:510–514, 1993.

114. Elowitz EH, Johnson WD, Milhorat TH: Computerized tomography (CT) localized stereotactic craniotomy for excision of a bacterial intracranial aneurysm. Surg Neurol 44(3):265–269, 1995.

115. Charlier P, Cohen A, Eiferman C, et al: Selective embolization of mycotic aneurysm of the branches of the abdominal aorta. Arch Mal Coeur Vaiss 81:1269–1274, 1988.

116. Kaufman SL, White RI, Jr, Harrington DP, et al: Protean manifestations of mycotic aneurysms. AJR Am J Roentgenol 131:1019–1025, 1978.

117. Day AL: Extracranial intracranial bypass grafting in the surgical treatment of bacterial aneurysms: Report of 2 cases. Neurosurgery 9:583–588, 1981.

118. Cantu RC, LeMay M, Wilkinson HA: The importance of repeated angiography in the treatment of mycotic-embolic intracranial aneurysms. J Neurosurg 25:189–193, 1966.

119. Shiraishi Y, Awazu A, Harada T, et al: Valve replacement in a patient with infective endocarditis and ruptured mycotic cerebral aneurysm. Nippon Kyobu Geka Gakkai Zasshi 40:118–123, 1992.

120. Jara FM, Lewis JF, Jr, Magilligan DJ, Jr: Operative experience with infective endocarditis and intracerebral mycotic aneurysm. J Thorac Cardiovasc Surg 80:28–30, 1980.

121. Yoshida K, Wanibuchi Y, Kanda T, et al: Valve replacement in infective endocarditis with mycotic aneurysm. Nippon Kyobu Geka Gakkai Zasshi 38:2162–2165, 1990.

122. Weigle EH: Pregnancy complicated by subarachnoid hemorrhage following anticoagulant therapy of subacute bacterial endocarditis. Am J Obstet Gynecol 69:888–891, 1955.

123. Shike T, Hoshino H, Takagi M, et al: Bacterial intracavernous carotid aneurysm presented as massive epistaxis. Rinshi Shinkeigaku 35(5):531–536, 1995.

124. Dolenc VV: Anatomy and Surgery of the Cavernous Sinus. New York: Springer-Verlag, 1989.

125. Paullus WS, Pait TG, Rhoton AL, Sr: Microsurgical exposure of the petrous portion of the carotid artery. J Neurosurg 47:713–726, 1977.

126. Amine AR: Neurosurgical complications of heroin addiction: Brain abscess and mycotic aneurysm. Surg Neurol 7:385–386, 1977.

127. Ornstein E, Shenkman Z, Young WL: Subarachnoid hemorrhage: Concerns of the neuroanesthesiologist. In Batjer HH, Caplan LR, Greenlee RG, Jr, et al (eds): Cerebrovascular Disease. Philadelphia: Lippincott-Raven, 1997, pp 843–855.

128. Young WL, Ornstein E, Baker KZ, Pile-Spellman J: Neuroanesthetic considerations for surgical and endovascular therapy of arteriovenous malformations. In Batjer HH, Caplan LR, Greenlee RG, Jr, et al. (eds): Cerebrovascular Disease. Philadelphia: Lippincott-Raven, 1997, pp 843–855.

129. Young WL, Solomon RA, Pedley TA, et al: Direct cortical EEG monitoring during temporary vascular occlusion for cerebral aneurysm surgery. Anesthesiology 71:794–799, 1989.

130. Young WL, Prohovnik I, Schroeder T, et al: Intraoperative ^{133}Xe cerebral blood flow measurements by intravenous versus intracarotid methods. Anesthesiology 73:637–643, 1990.

131. Shupak RC, Rosenwasser RH, Harp JR: High dose fentanyl-oxygen anaesthesia for intracranial mycotic aneurysm surgery: A clinical report. Neurosurgery 13:160–162, 1983.

132. Cunha e Sa M, Sisti M, Solomon R: Stereotactic angiographic localization as an adjunct to surgery of cerebral mycotic aneurysms: Case report and review of the literature. Acta Neurochir (Wien) 139(7):625–628, 1997.

133. Solomon RA: Management of symptomatic cerebral vasospasm. Contemp Neurosurg 13(1), 1991.

134. Ishikawa T, Kazumata K, Yoshimasa N, et al: Subarachnoid hemorrhage as a result of fungal aneurysm at the posterior communicating artery associated with occlusion of the internal carotid artery. Surg Neurol 58:261–265, 2002.

135. Fukui S, Tahata H, Hayashi H, Matsushima Y: Successful treatment of *Candida* meningitis with miconazole. No To Shinkei 42:863–866, 1990.

136. Meyer FB, Reeves AL: Pediatric and adolescent aneurysms. Contemp Neurosurg 12:1–5, 1990.

137. Bell WE, Butler C: Cerebral mycotic aneurysms in children: Two case reports. Neurology 18:81–86, 1968.

138. Blum L: Development of current concepts of mycotic aneurysm. NY State J Med 64:1317–1320, 1964.

139. Moskowitz MA, Rosenbaum AE, Tyler HR: Angiographically monitored resolution of cerebral mycotic aneurysms. Neurology 24:1103–1108, 1974.

140. Leipzig TJ, Brown FD: Treatment of mycotic aneurysm. Surg Neurol 23:403–407, 1985.

141. Stilhart B, Aboulker J, Khouadja F, et al: Faut-il rechercher et opérer les anevrismes de la maladie d'Osler avant l'hemorrhagie? Neurochirurgie 32:410–417, 1986.

142. Almazen V, Pulpon A, de Teresa L, et al: Aneurisma micotico secundario a endocarditis bacteriana: Revision a propositio de un caso. Arch Inst Cardiol Mex 48:1224–1232, 1978.

143. Roach MR, Drake CG: Ruptured cerebral aneurysms caused by microaneurysms. N Engl J Med 273:240–244, 1965.

144. Gilroy J, Andaya L, Thomas VJ: Intracranial mycotic aneurysms and subacute bacterial endocarditis in heroin addiction. Neurology 23:1193–1198, 1973.

145. Cates JE, Christie RV: Subacute bacterial endocarditis—A review of 442 patients treated in 14 centers appointed by the Penicillin Trials Committee of the Medical Research Council. Q J Med 20:93–130, 1971.

146. Lerner PI, Weinstein L: Infective endocarditis in the antibiotic era. N Engl J Med 274:259–266, 1966.

147. Schold C, Earnest MP: Cerebral hemorrhage from a mycotic aneurysm developing during appropriate antibiotic therapy. Stroke 9:267–268, 1978.

148. Dean RH, Waterhouse G, Meacham PW, et al: Mycotic embolism and embolomycotic aneurysms: Neglected lessons of the past. Ann Surg 204:300–307, 1986.

149. Morin MA, Talalla A: Angiography for mycotic aneurysm. N Engl J Med 281:1249–1250, 1969.

150. O'Connor TW, Lord RSA, Tracy GD: Treatment of mycotic aneurysms. Med J Aust 2:1161–1164, 1972.

151. Nelson RJ, Harley DP, Frency WJ, Bayer AJ: Favorable ten-year experience with valve procedures for active infective endocarditis. J Thorac Cardiovasc Surg 87:493–502, 1984.

152. Languna J, Derby BM, Chase R: *Cardiobacterium hominis* endocarditis with cerebral mycotic aneurysm. Arch Neurol 324:438–439, 1975.

153. North-Coombes D, Schonland MM: Cerebral mycotic aneurysms: A case report. S Afr Med J 48:1808–1810, 1974.

154. Bullock R, Van Dellen JR, Van den Heever CM: Intracranial mycotic aneurysms: A review of 9 cases. S Afr Med J 60:970–973, 1981.

155. Mendelsohn DB, Hertzanu Y: Ruptured mycotic aneurysm during computed tomogram brain scan. J Neurol Neurosurg Psychiatry 46:285–286, 1983.

156. Hourihane JB: Ruptured mycotic intracranial aneurysm: A report of three cases. Vasc Surg 4:21–29, 1970.

157. Ng KK, Wong WK, Skene-Smith H: Ruptured mycotic intracranial aneurysm. Aust Radiol 19:255–257, 1975.

158. Simmons KC, Sage MR, Reilly PL: CT of intracerebral hemorrhage due to mycotic aneurysms—Case report. Neuroradiology 19:215–217, 1980.

159. Love JW, Medina D, Anderson S, Braniff B: Infective endocarditis due to *Corynebacterium diphtheriae*: Report of a case and review of the literature. Johns Hopkins Med J 148:41–42, 1981.

160. Isaacs BA, van Dellen JR: Persistence of a mycotic aneurysm of the intracavernous carotid artery. Surg Neurol 26:577–580, 1986.

161. Ojemann RF: Surgical management of bacterial intracranial aneurysms. In Schmidek HH, Sweet WH (eds): Operative Neurosurgical Techniques. Orlando: Grune & Stratton, 1988, pp 997–1001.

162. Holtzman RNN, Stein BM (eds): Endovascular interventional neuroradiology. New York: Springer-Verlag, 1995, pp 1–434.

INDEX

Note: Page numbers followed by f indicate figures; those followed by t indicate tables; those followed by b indicate boxed material.